Lippincott®
Q&A Review for
NCLEX-RN®

FOURTEENTH EDITION

Lippincott®
Q&A Review for
NCLEX-RN®

FOURTEENTH EDITION

Diane M. Billings, EdD, RN, ANEF, FAAN
Chancellor's Professor Emeritus
Indiana University School of Nursing
Indianapolis, Indiana

Desiree Hensel, PhD, RN, PCNS-BC, CNE
Chief Executive Officer
Hensel Nursing Education Consulting
Dorset, Vermont

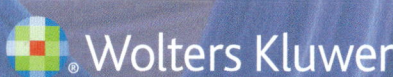

Philadelphia • Baltimore • New York • London
Buenos Aires • Hong Kong • Sydney • Tokyo

Vice President and Publisher: Julie K. Stegman
Senior Acquisitions Editor: Joyce Berendes
Director of Product Development: Jennifer K. Forestieri
Content Strategist: Bernadette Enneg
Editorial Coordinator: Erin E. Hernandez
Editorial Assistant: Devika Kishore
Marketing Manager: Amy Whitaker
Senior Production Project Manager: Alicia Jackson
Manager, Graphic Arts & Design: Stephen Druding
Art Director, Illustration: Jennifer Clements
Senior Manufacturing Coordinator: Margie Orzech
Prepress Vendor: Straive

14th Edition

Copyright © 2024 Wolters Kluwer

13th edition © 2020 Wolters Kluwer. All rights reserved. This book is protected by copyright. No part of this book may be reproduced or transmitted in any form or by any means, including as photocopies or scanned-in or other electronic copies, or utilized by any information storage and retrieval system without written permission from the copyright owner, except for brief quotations embodied in critical articles and reviews. Materials appearing in this book prepared by individuals as part of their official duties as U.S. government employees are not covered by the above-mentioned copyright. To request permission, please contact Wolters Kluwer at Two Commerce Square, 2001 Market Street, Philadelphia, PA 19103, via email at permissions@lww.com, or via our website at shop.lww.com (products and services). 1/2023

9 8 7 6 5 4 3 2 1

Printed in Mexico

Cataloging-in-Publication Data available on request from the Publisher
ISBN: 978-1-9751-8038-6

This work is provided "as is," and the publisher disclaims any and all warranties, express or implied, including any warranties as to accuracy, comprehensiveness, or currency of the content of this work.

This work is no substitute for individual patient assessment based upon healthcare professionals' examination of each patient and consideration of, among other things, age, weight, gender, current or prior medical conditions, medication history, laboratory data and other factors unique to the patient. The publisher does not provide medical advice or guidance and this work is merely a reference tool. Healthcare professionals, and not the publisher, are solely responsible for the use of this work including all medical judgments and for any resulting diagnosis and treatments.

Given continuous, rapid advances in medical science and health information, independent professional verification of medical diagnoses, indications, appropriate pharmaceutical selections and dosages, and treatment options should be made and healthcare professionals should consult a variety of sources. When prescribing medication, healthcare professionals are advised to consult the product information sheet (the manufacturer's package insert) accompanying each drug to verify, among other things, conditions of use, warnings and side effects and identify any changes in dosage schedule or contraindications, particularly if the medication to be administered is new, infrequently used or has a narrow therapeutic range. To the maximum extent permitted under applicable law, no responsibility is assumed by the publisher for any injury and/or damage to persons or property, as a matter of products liability, negligence law or otherwise, or from any reference to or use by any person of this work.

shop.lww.com

Contributor List

Editors and Contributors

Editors

Diane Billings, EdD, RN, ANEF, FAAN
Chancellor's Professor Emeritus
Indiana University School of Nursing
Indianapolis, Indiana

Desiree Hensel, PhD, RN, PCNS-BC, CNE
Chief Executive Officer
Hensel Nursing Education Consulting
Dorset, Vermont

Contributors

Jana Ambrogne, PhD, PMHNP-BC
Professor
School of Nursing
Curry College
Milton, Massachusetts

Diane Billings, EdD, RN, ANEF, FAAN
Chancellor's Professor Emeritus
Indiana University School of Nursing
Indianapolis, Indiana

Emily Davis, DNP, RN, CNE
Clinical Assistant Professor
Indiana University School of Nursing
Indianapolis, Indiana

Deborah DeMeester, PhD, RN, CNE
Clinical Associate Professor
Indiana University School of Nursing
Indianapolis, Indiana

Desiree Hensel, PhD, RN, PCNS-BC, CNE
Chief Executive Officer
Hensel Nursing Education Consulting
Dorset, Vermont

Maureen M. Hillier, DNP, RN, CCRN, CHSE
Senior Lecturer, Nursing
Curry College
School of Nursing
Milton, Massachusetts

Bertha Lee, PhD, RN
Assistant Professor
School of Nursing
Curry College
Milton, Massachusetts

Meg Moorman, PhD, RN, CNE, ANEF
Director of Faculty Innovation in Nursing Education Center
Coordinator of MSN in Nursing Education
Associate Clinical Professor
Indiana University School of Nursing
Indianapolis, Indiana

Tonja Marie Padgett, RN, DNP, ACNS-BC, CNE
Clinical Assistant Professor
Indiana University School of Nursing
Indianapolis, Indiana

Contributors to the Previous Edition

Don Anderson, RN, EdD
Diane Billings, EdD, RN, FAAN, ANEF
Ann Butt, MSN, RN
Desiree Hensel, PhD, RNC-NIC, CNE
Kathy Jorgensen, RN, MA, MSN
Cindy Kohtz, RN, EdD, CNE
Julie Poore, DNP, RN, CHSE
Evelyn Stephenson, DNP, RNC-NIC, NNP-BC, CHSE
Jean Yockey, RN, PhD, FNP, CNE
Judith Young, DNP, RN, CNE
Wendy Zeiher, MSN, RN

Reviewers

Andrea Barron, BN, RN, MN, CCNE
Nurse Educator
Centre for Nursing Studies
St. John's, Newfoundland and Labrador, Canada

Susan Boland-Shepherd, PhD, MPH, BSN, RN
Professor
Quinsigamond Community College
Worcester, Massachusetts

Ruth A. Chaplen, RN, MSN, DNP, ACNS BC
Director, Nursing Program
Alma College
Alma, Michigan

Rachel Coats, MS, RN, CNE
Assistant Professor of Nursing
Lander University
Greenwood, South Carolina

Linda Copel, PhD, RN, PMHCNS, BC, CNE, ANEF, NCC, FAPA
Professor
Villanova University
Malvern, Pennsylvania

Louis Davis, DNP, APRN, FNP-C
Assistant Professor
McAuley School of Nursing
University of Detroit Mercy
Detroit, Michigan

Vicky DeWick, RN, MSN
Professor of Nursing
Valencia College
Orlando, Florida

Brenda Dafoe Enns, BA, MN, RN
Nursing Instructor
Red River College
Winnipeg, Manitoba

Amy Ertwine, EdD, MSN, RN, CM/DN
Associate Professor
Community College of Baltimore County
Dundalk, Maryland

Tracey Fallak, RN, BScN, MN
Curriculum Coordinator
Theory Instructor Mentor
Nursing Department
Red River College
Winnipeg, Manitoba, Canada

Nancy J. Frank, PhD(c), RN, CNE
Assistant Professor of Nursing
Clinical Track
Messiah University
Mechanicsburg, Pennsylvania

Susan Gallagher, MSN, ACNP-BC, ANP-BC, CNE
Clinical Instructor
Northeastern University
Boston, Massachusetts

Cheryl Green, PhD, DNP, RN, LCSW, CNL, CNE, ACUE, MAC, FAPA
Associate Professor of Nursing
Southern Connecticut State University
New Haven, Connecticut

Millie Hepburn, PhD, RN, ACNS-BC, SCRN
Assistant Professor
Lienhard School of Nursing
Pleasantville, New York

Kynthia James, MSN, APRN, FNP-C, CNL, CMSRN
Instructor
Valdosta State University
Valdosta, Georgia

Paul Jeffrey, DNP, NP-Adult
Professor, Nursing
Humber College
Toronto, Ontario, Canada

Joanne Jones, RN, MSN, CCNE
Senior Lecturer
Thompson Rivers University
Kamloops, British Columbia, Canada

Debra Kantor, PhD, RN, CNE
Associate Professor
Molloy University
Rockville Centre, New York

Paula Lynne Littlejohn, ID, GNC(C), RN, BSN, MA
Nursing Instructor
Victoria BSN Program
Camosun College
Victoria, British Columbia, Canada

Keisha Lovence, DNP, MSN, ACNP-BC, RN
Associate Professor
Eastern Michigan University
Ypsilanti, Michigan

Janice Lowden-Stokley, PhD, RN
Professor, Coordinator of Nursing Research and Student Success
Advent Health University
Sorrento, Florida

Jeanette H. (Bjurback) Lupinacci, EdD, CRRN
Associate Professor
Department of Nursing Chair
Western Connecticut State University
Danbury, Connecticut

Janice MacIntosh, RN, BScN, MScN
Clinical Nursing Teacher–Fanshawe–Western Collaborative BScN Program
Western University
London, Ontario, Canada

Bernadette Mandrick, RN, BN, MEd
Instructor/Clinical Mentor
Red River College
Winnipeg, Manitoba, Canada

Jaime Mantesso, RN, MN, PhD(c)
Instructor
Faculty of Nursing
University of Regina
Regina, Saskatchewan, Canada

Jaimee A. McGuire, DNP, NP-C, CHC, CHPSE
Nursing Faculty
Oklahoma Panhandle State University
Goodwell, Oklahoma

Marg Olfert, RN, MN, EdD
Assistant Professor
Mount Royal University
Calgary, Alberta, Canada

Jennifer Ort, DNS, RNC MN-N
Associate Professor
Western Connecticut State University
Danbury, Connecticut

Dr. Barbara Jeanne Pinchera, DNP, ANP-BC
Professor
Curry College
Milton, Massachusetts

Monica Pozowicz, MSN, CCRN, CEN, CFRN, CAPA, CNE-cl
Assistant Professor of Nursing
Mary Inez Grindle School of Nursing
Brenau University
Gainesville, Georgia

Debbie Rickeard, DNP, MSN, BScN, BA, RN, CNE, CCRN
Experiential Learning Specialist
University of Windsor
Windsor, Ontario, Canada

Jeffrey Ross, EdD, RN, CNE
Dean and Professor of Nursing
Abraham Baldwin Agricultural College
Tifton, Georgia

Shelley Sadler, RN, MSN, APRN, WHNP-BC
Instructor of Nursing
Morehead State University
Morehead, Kentucky

Lynette Scianna-DeBellis, MA, RN, CMSRN
Instructor of Nursing
Mount Saint Mary College
Newburgh, New York

Katherine Scott, DNP, CPNP
Assistant Professor
Mercy College of Health Sciences
Des Moines, Iowa

Elizabeth B. Simon, PhD, RN, ANP-BC
Professor and Assistant Dean of Clinical Affairs
Department of Nursing
School of Health Professions
New York Institute of Technology
Old Westbury, New York

Diane F. Smith, DNP, MSN, FNP, RN
Assistant Professor
Bon Secours Memorial College of Nursing
Richmond, Virginia

Pam Smyth, MSN, RN, CHSE
Assistant Professor
School of Nursing
Ferris State University
Big Rapids, Michigan

Elizabeth Stuesse, MSN, RNC-OB, RNC-MNN
Clinical Assistant Professor of Nursing
Maryville University
Pevely, Missouri

Kathryn J. Vanderzwan, DNP, APRN-BC
Clinical Assistant Professor
University of Illinois at Chicago
Chicago, Illinois

Laura A. Vasel, PhD, RN, CPNP, CNE
Assistant Director of Nursing and Assistant Professor
Randolph-Macon College
Ashland, Virginia

Lisa Wallace, DNP, RNC-OB, NE-BC
Assistant Professor of Nursing
Morehead State University
Morehead, Kentucky

Jason Woodsome, MS, RN-BC
Faculty
St. Joseph's College of Nursing
Syracuse, New York

Preface

INTRODUCTION TO THE Q&A REVIEW FOR NCLEX-RN®

Endorsed by the National Student Nurses' Association (NSNA), the *Lippincott Q&A Review for NCLEX-RN®* has been developed to help you prepare for—and pass!—the National Council Licensing Examination for Registered Nurses (NCLEX-RN®). It will also help you prepare for course exams, final exams, NCLEX-RN® assessment exams, or other standardized or competency exams.

This 14th edition has been prepared for students preparing to take the NCLEX-RN® in the United States and its territories and provinces and in Canada. It was guided by an editorial board composed of faculty from schools of nursing in both countries, and every question item has been written and reviewed by clinical experts in each. Item revision was data-driven, with each item evaluated based on analysis derived from *Lippincott® NCLEX-RN PassPoint* data.

About the Questions and Practice Exams

- All questions are written to test components of the nursing clinical judgment model used by the National Council of State Boards of Nursing to guide your preparation for the NCLEX-RN® exam.
- There are more than 5700 test questions of every question type found on the actual NCLEX®—multiple-choice, multiple-response (including extended multiple response, Select N, and multiple response grouping), matrix, cloze (drop-down and drag-and-drop), highlight text, highlight table, drag-and-drop rationale, drop-down, bow-tie, trend, hot-spot, fill-in-the-blank, drag-and-drop/ordered response, chart/exhibit, as well as graphic option and audio questions.
- Examples of all "Next Gen NCLEX" types of questions are also included to help you prepare for the inclusion of NGN questions on the exam.
- Questions cover all clinical areas of nursing—childbearing family and newborn; nursing care of infants, children, and adolescents; nursing care of adults with medical and surgical health problems; and nursing care of clients with psychiatric disorders and mental health problems.
- All questions are edited for readability and cultural appropriateness.
- The material is organized by major health problems in the United States and Canada to help you review for course-specific exams.
- Questions are coded by client needs to ensure practice in *all* areas of the NCLEX-RN® test plan. They are also coded by cognitive level to guide study and test-taking at higher levels of the cognitive domain.
- Questions highlight integrative processes (nursing process, caring, communication and documentation, teaching/learning, culture and spirituality, and clinical judgment) and are designed to emphasize nursing clinical judgment, prioritization, delegation, and management of care.
- Items are developed to provide practice in calculating drug dosages, intravenous drip rates, and intake and output, and there are a variety of questions that require calculation and reporting of a numerical response to the question.
- Questions emphasize pharmacology, medication safety, complementary and alternative modalities, and the nurse's role in administering pharmacotherapeutic agents.
- All items point out current nursing practice in the areas of client safety, managing care quality, home care, health promotion, care of the older adult, cancer nursing, end-of-life care, perioperative care, community health nursing, and emergency and disaster nursing.
- Every question provides detailed rationales for correct and incorrect answers.
- Six comprehensive postreview tests, each of which has been designed to resemble the testing format and content of the NCLEX-RN® test plan, are offered. The tests are of varying lengths and include those that have the minimum (85) and maximum (150) possible questions on the licensing exam.
- One practice test is devoted entirely to pharmacology test questions.

Look for These Features

- NEW! A new section explains the NCSBN Nursing Clinical Judgment Model and practice questions for new test item types that will be used to test nursing clinical judgment.
- NEW! A table of definitions lists terms commonly used by health providers; it also includes health care terminology for which the meaning may vary in the United States and Canada.
- NEW! A tear-out sheet of common laboratory values. Laboratory values are presented in U.S.

Standard Units and in the International System of Units.
- NEW! Measurements in test items are presented in both U.S. Standard Units and in metric measurements.
- NEW! An entire chapter explains the various test question formats and strategies for answering each type of test item and at each level of the cognitive domain.
- NEW! A detailed description of the NCLEX-RN® test plan in effect from April 1, 2023, through March 31, 2026, is provided.
- Risk factors for *not* passing the NCLEX-RN® exam—as well as related study strategies—are listed in a table.
- A *Content Mastery and Test-Taking Skill Self-Analysis* worksheet helps you assess your exam readiness. The tear-out worksheet can be copied and used with each test in this book; reviewing all worksheets will help you analyze the reasons for not answering test questions correctly and allow you to revise your study plan accordingly.
- A study plan and checklist to help you study for and pass the exam.
- Information about developing study skills, taking tests, and managing test anxiety.
- Tips for studying from students who have successfully passed the NCLEX-RN® exam.
- Addresses, telephone numbers, and websites for the National Council of State Boards of Nursing, Inc., and each state board of nursing.

More Ways to Prepare

thePoint®

http://thepoint.lww.com/Billings14e

With the purchase of this book, you receive access to thePoint®, where you will find more than 1600 EXTRA practice questions! On thePoint®, questions can be used in several ways. For example, you may take a test composed of the four content areas, arrange a test to present questions in random order, or select questions for a particular review and practice. thePoint® simulates the actual NCLEX-RN® exam by formatting questions on a computer screen and requiring you to use the keyboard and mouse to enter answers to the questions. It also features a pop-up calculator for questions that require you to calculate drug doses and drip rates for intravenous infusions.

PassPoint

By purchasing this text, you are also offered a free 7-day trial of *Lippincott PassPoint NCLEX-RN | Powered by prepU! PassPoint NCLEX-RN* is a separate, personalized, and comprehensive learning system designed to help you fully prepare for the NCLEX-RN® exam. *PassPoint* gives you multiple options for individualized review, quizzing, and practice, helping you pinpoint areas that require additional study. As you take Practice Quizzes, *PassPoint* quickly determines current knowledge and delivers questions with just the right difficulty. Learn more about how PassPoint works, request a demo, and sign up for your free trial! Visit https://www.wolterskluwer.com/en/solutions/lippincott-nursing-faculty/passing-nclex-rn-with-passpoint#request-a-demo.

Organization of the Book

The book is organized into three sections. Each section is designed to build on the previous section.

The book's first section provides information about the licensing exam and how to prepare for, take, and pass high-stakes examinations. A full chapter is devoted to explaining the various types of test question formats and cognitive levels of questions used on the licensing exam. The chapter also gives you examples of all types and levels of questions and strategies for answering them.

In the second section of the book, there are five major units:

1. Nursing care of the childbearing family and their neonate
2. Nursing care of infants, children, and adolescents
3. Nursing care of adults with medical and surgical health problems
4. Nursing care of clients with psychiatric disorders and mental health problems
5. Nursing care of clients receiving pharmacological and parenteral therapies

Within each unit, chapter tests are grouped according to health problems and include questions that are matched to the NCLEX-RN® test plan. At the end of each chapter, there is a section of questions about managing client safety and quality care. These questions will help you understand the important concepts of client safety and quality. Because the test questions in this section are organized around health problems, use this section when preparing for tests that focus on specific content in your curriculum.

The third section of the book contains six comprehensive exams written to simulate the NCLEX-RN® by placing test items in random order of content area. Tests present a variety of situations commonly encountered in nursing practice and include test questions from all components of the NCLEX-RN® test plan and all types of questions used on the licensing exam (except audio questions, which are found only on thePoint®).

HOW TO USE THIS BOOK TO PREPARE FOR EXAMS

Before using the practice questions and taking the postreview tests in this book, read Chapter 2: *NCLEX-RN® Test Questions and Strategies for Answering Them*. This chapter includes a description of the nursing clinical judgment model used by the NCSBN to guide test item development and examples of item types that will be included on the licensing exam.

Next, use the practice exams to identify areas of strength and areas in which you need further study. The answers include rationales for both correct and incorrect answer options to help reinforce your learning, and by scoring the results of each practice test, you can identify areas in which you need further review. After completing each exam, divide the number of your correct responses by the total number of questions in the test and multiply by 100. This will give you the percentage of correct responses. For example, if you answered 72 of 90 items correctly, you would divide 72 by 90 and multiply by 100, for a result of 80%. If you answered more than 75% of the items in an area correctly, you are most likely prepared to answer questions in that area on the NCLEX-RN®. If you answered fewer than 75% of the questions correctly, you need to determine why. Did you answer incorrectly because of a lack of content knowledge or because you did not read carefully?

As you take each test, use the *Content Mastery and Test-Taking Skill Self-Analysis* worksheet to tally your reasons for not answering the test questions correctly. Understanding why you are not answering the questions correctly or which content area is most difficult for you is the **most** important aspect of preparing for any exam. Use this information to guide your study.

After reviewing the specific content areas in the practice exams, take the comprehensive tests. These tests reflect the NCLEX-RN® because each test presents a variety of situations commonly encountered in nursing practice and across all clinical disciplines. Underlying knowledge, skills, and abilities related to the basic sciences, fundamentals of nursing, pharmacology and other therapeutic measures, communicable diseases, legal and ethical considerations, and nutrition are included in the items as applicable to plan nursing care for individual clients or groups of clients. The comprehensive tests also include test items related to client safety and care quality. These tests are designed with varying numbers of questions, so you can time yourself and determine how long it will take you to complete the minimum and the maximum number of possible questions on the licensing exam.

Finally, as you take each test, use the *Content Mastery and Test-Taking Skill Self-Analysis* tear-out worksheet at the back of the book to tally your reasons for not answering the test questions correctly. Understanding why you are not answering the questions correctly or which content area is most difficult for you is the **most** important aspect of preparing for any exam. Use this information to guide your study.

And don't forget to check the online resources available at http://thepoint.lww.com/Billings14e and log into your free 7-day trial of *Lippincott NCLEX-RN PassPoint*! The study tips, study plan, additional questions, and testing will provide you with a solid foundation to begin to prepare for and pass your exam!

DIVERSITY, EQUITY, AND INCLUSION

A note about the language used in this book: Wolters Kluwer Health recognizes that people have a diverse range of identities, and we are committed to using the most inclusive, nonbiased language possible in our products. In line with the principles of nursing, we strive not to define people by their diagnoses, but to recognize their personhood first and foremost, using as much as possible the language diverse groups use to define themselves, and including only information that is relevant to nursing care. We strive to better address the unique perspectives, complex challenges, and lived experiences of diverse populations traditionally underrepresented in health literature. When describing or referencing populations discussed in research studies, we will adhere to the identities presented in those studies to maintain fidelity to the evidence presented by the study investigators. We follow best practices of language set forth by the Publication Manual of the American Psychological Association, 7th edition, but acknowledge that language evolves rapidly, and we anticipate continuing to modify our language in future editions of our products.

Acknowledgments

This book has been developed with the expertise of an Advisory Board of faculty from schools of nursing in the United States and Canada along with a team of internationally recognized test item writers and reviewers. We appreciate the clinical expertise of these faculty and their willingness to develop and review the test questions in this book. We have been most fortunate to have excellent support from Joyce Berendes, Senior Acquisitions Editor; Bernadette Enneg, Content Strategist; and Erin Hernandez, Editorial Coordinator whose wisdom, managerial skills, and editorial eyes have helped us prepare this book. Many future nurses in both the United States and Canada who are preparing for the licensing exam will reap the benefits of their dedication to making this the highest quality review book possible. The authors would like to thank their loved ones who have provided support over the years to make this book possible. They also thank the faculty and students who use this book to help build nursing's future.

Diane M. Billings, EdD, RN, ANEF, FAAN
Chancellor's Professor Emeritus
Indiana University School of Nursing
Indianapolis, Indiana

Desiree Hensel, PhD, RN, PCNS-BC, CNE
Chief Executive Officer
Hensel Nursing Education Consulting
Dorset, Vermont

About the Authors

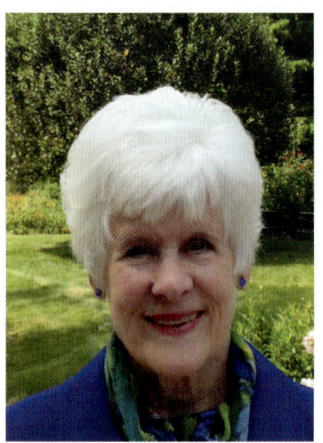

Diane M. Billings, EdD, RN, ANEF, FAAN, is an award-winning author and nursing educator who has taught students in associate degree through doctoral programs, with a special focus on preparing students to pass the NCLEX-RN® examination. Dr. Billings has taught NCLEX-RN® review courses and workshops to prepare faculty for writing NCLEX-RN® test questions. A nationally recognized test-item writer, her NCLEX-RN® preparation books have helped thousands of students pass the NCLEX-RN® exam. Dr. Billings is the recipient of the National League for Nursing's Award for Outstanding Leadership in Nursing Education, the President's Award for Distinguished Teaching at Indiana University, and the Founders Award for Excellence in Teaching from Sigma Theta Tau, International. She is a fellow and Living Legend in the American Academy of Nursing.

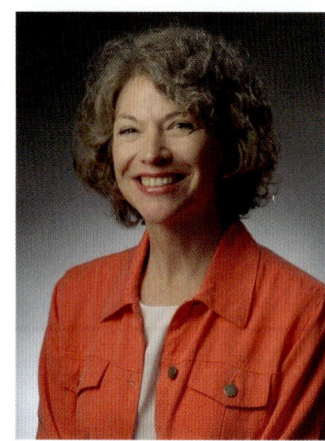

Desiree Hensel, PhD, RN, PCNS-BC, CNE, is the Chief Executive Officer of Hensel Nursing Education Consulting and is the the former Dean of of Curry College School of Nursing. Her education includes a PhD in Health Services from Walden University, an MSN from Ball State University, and a BS in Nursing from Indiana University. She is certified as a Pediatric Clinical Nurse Specialist and a Certified Nurse Educator. Dr. Hensel's scholarship centers on curriculum design, evaluation, and the use of high-impact teaching strategies while more closely examining how nurses define themselves in the 21st century. Dr. Hensel has unique expertise using Q methodology for research, quality improvement, and program evaluation. She has published over 40 peer-reviewed manuscripts, many of these in collaboration with BSN students. She has been recognized for her leadership and innovation in undergraduate research, teaching, and service. As coeditor of *Lippincott's Q&A Review for NCLEX-RN*, Dr. Hensel lectures to faculty and students nationally and internationally about NCLEX preparation, including conducting mini NCLEX reviews for the National Student Nurses Association.

Contents

PART 1
Introduction to the NCLEX-RN® Licensing Examination and Preparation for Test Taking 1

CHAPTER 1
The NCLEX-RN® Licensing Examination........2

CHAPTER 2
NCLEX-RN® Test Questions and Strategies for Answering Them........12

CHAPTER 3
Study Skills for Taking the NCLEX-RN® and Other Nursing Exams........34

PART 2
Practice Tests 53

CHAPTER 1
The Nursing Care of the Childbearing Family........54
- Test 1: Antepartum Care........54
- Test 2: Complications of Pregnancy........87
- Test 3: The Birth Experience........114
- Test 4: Postpartum Care........141
- Test 5: The Neonatal Client........170

CHAPTER 2
The Nursing Care of Children........205
- Test 1: Health Promotion........205
- Test 2: The Child with Respiratory Health Problems........228
- Test 3: The Child with Cardiovascular and Hematologic Health Problems........248
- Test 4: The Child with Health Problems of the Gastrointestinal Tract........264
- Test 5: The Child with Health Problems Involving Ingestion, Nutrition, or Diet........290
- Test 6: The Child with Health Problems of the Urinary System........301
- Test 7: The Child with Neurologic Health Problems........315
- Test 8: The Child with Musculoskeletal Health Problems........339
- Test 9: The Child with Dermatologic and Endocrine Health Problems........359

CHAPTER 3
The Nursing Care of Adults with Medical and Surgical Health Problems........374
- Test 1: The Adult with Cardiac Health Problems........374
- Test 2: The Adult with Vascular Disease........404
- Test 3: The Adult with Hematologic Health Problems........428
- Test 4: The Adult with Respiratory Health Problems........452
- Test 5: The Adult with Upper Gastrointestinal Tract Health Problems........490
- Test 6: The Adult with Lower Gastrointestinal Tract Health Problems........503
- Test 7: The Adult with Pancreatic and Biliary Tract Disorders........521
- Test 8: The Adult with Endocrine Health Problems........535
- Test 9: The Adult with Urinary Tract Health Problems........562
- Test 10: The Adult with Reproductive Health Problems........588
- Test 11: The Adult with Neurologic Health Problems........627
- Test 12: The Adult with Musculoskeletal Health Problems........660
- Test 13: The Adult with Cancer........692
- Test 14: The Adult Having Surgery........728
- Test 15: The Adult with Health Problems of the Eyes, Ears, Nose, and Throat........762
- Test 16: The Adult with Health Problems of the Integumentary System........776
- Test 17: Responding to Emergencies, Mass Casualties, and Disasters........794

CHAPTER 4
The Nursing Care of Clients with Psychiatric Disorders and Mental Health Problems........804
- Test 1: Mood Disorders........804
- Test 2: Schizophrenia, Other Psychoses, and Cognitive Disorders........832
- Test 3: Personality Disorders, Substance-Related Disorders, Anxiety Disorders, and Anxiety-Related Disorders........857
- Test 4: Stress, Crisis, Anger, and Violence........893
- Test 5: Abuse and Mental Health Problems of Children, Adolescents, and Families........917

CHAPTER 5
The Nursing Care of Clients Receiving Pharmacological and Parenteral Therapies........945
- Test 1: Managing Care, Quality, and Safety of Clients Receiving Pharmacological and Parenteral Therapies........945

PART 3
Postreview Tests — 965

Comprehensive Test 1 966
Comprehensive Test 2 1002
Comprehensive Test 3 1044
Comprehensive Test 4 1093
Comprehensive Test 5 1125
Comprehensive Test 6 1166

Appendices 1217

PART 1

INTRODUCTION TO THE NCLEX-RN® LICENSING EXAMINATION AND PREPARATION FOR TEST TAKING

The NCLEX-RN® Licensing Examination

OVERVIEW

The National Council Licensure Examination for Registered Nurses (NCLEX-RN®) is administered to graduates of nursing schools in the United States and Canada to test the knowledge, abilities, and skills necessary for entry-level safe and effective nursing practice. The examination is developed by the National Council of State Boards of Nursing, Inc. (NCSBN; www.ncsbn.org), an organization with representation from all state boards of nursing in the United States and provincial/territorial regulatory bodies in Canada. The same examination is used in all 50 states, the District of Columbia, United States possessions, Canada, and Australia. The exam is also administered at international test centers worldwide. Students who have graduated from prelicensure programs must pass this examination to meet licensing requirements in the United States and Canada.

THE TEST PLAN

The NCSBN prepares the test plan used to develop the licensing examination. The test plan is based on an analysis of current nursing practice and the skills, abilities, and processes nurses use to provide nursing care. The plan also describes the structure of the test, general information about the content, and the distribution of the content.

Practice Analysis: The Foundation of the Test Plan

The NCLEX-RN test plan is based on the results of a practice analysis conducted every 3 years of the entry-level performance of newly licensed registered nurses and on expert judgment provided by members of the National Council's Examination Committee as well as a job analysis panel of experts. The job analysis panel asks newly graduated nurses to rank the nursing activities that they perform on a regular basis. The questions used on the test plan, therefore, include those activities that nurses commonly perform. For example, the practice analysis, conducted in 2019 and published in 2022, revealed that nursing practice commonly involves activities such as maintaining client confidentiality and privacy, using approved terminology when documenting care, reviewing pertinent data prior to medication administration, protecting the client from injury, performing procedures necessary to safely admit, transfer, or discharge a client; providing and receiving reports on assigned clients; advocating for client rights and needs; applying principles of infection control; and prioritizing the delivery of care (National Council of State Boards of Nursing, Inc., 2022).

Test Plan Details

Test plans, or test blueprints, are developed to indicate the components and the relative weights of the components that will be tested on an exam. The test plan structure for the NCLEX-RN addresses two components of nursing care: (1) client needs categories and (2) integrated processes, such as the nursing process, caring, communication and documentation, teaching/learning, and culture and spirituality, and clinical judgment (Table 1.1). Representative items test knowledge of these components as they relate to specific health care situations in all of the four major areas of client needs. The questions developed for the test plan are written to test entry-level nursing knowledge and the ability to apply nursing knowledge to client situations.

Client Needs

The health needs of clients are grouped under four broad categories: (1) safe, effective care environment, (2) health promotion and maintenance, (3) psychosocial integrity, and (4) physiologic integrity.

The NCLEX-RN® Licensing Examination

TABLE 1.1
Test Plan Structure

The framework of client needs was selected for the examination because it provides a universal structure for defining nursing actions and competencies and focuses on clients in all settings.

Client Needs

The content of the NCLEX-RN test plan is organized into four major client needs categories. Two of the four categories are divided into subcategories:

A. Safe and Effective Care Environment
1. Management of care: 15% to 21%
2. Safety and infection control: 10% to 16%

B. Health Promotion and Maintenance: 6% to 12%

C. Psychosocial Integrity: 6% to 12%

D. Physiological Integrity
1. Basic care and comfort: 6% to 12%
2. Pharmacological and parenteral therapies: 13% to 19%
3. Reduction of risk potential: 9% to 15%
4. Physiological adaptation: 11% to 17%

Integrated Processes

The following processes are fundamental to the practice of nursing and are integrated throughout the client needs categories and subcategories:

- Nursing Process
- Caring
- Communication and Documentation
- Teaching/Learning
- Culture and Spirituality
- Clinical Judgment

Copyright by the National Council of State Boards of Nursing, Inc. All rights reserved.

Two of these categories include subcategories of related and specified needs (Table 1.2). The percentage of test items in each subcategory on the NCLEX-RN examination is shown in Figure 1.1. Because candidates receive individualized tests, the percentage of questions any candidate receives from each category varies within a range of ±3%. Understanding the category of client needs is essential to recognize the types of questions that are found on the licensing exam and the relative emphasis given to the category based on the percentage of questions from that category on the exam.

Integrated Processes

The NCLEX-RN test plan also is organized according to six integrated processes. These include the nursing process, caring, communication and documentation, teaching/learning, clinical judgment, and culture and spirituality (see Table 1.1 and Fig. 1.1).

The Nursing Process

The nursing process is a scientific approach to client care. The NCLEX-RN test plan includes questions from all steps of the nursing process. The five phases of the nursing process are (1) assessment, (2) analysis, (3) planning, (4) implementation, and (5) evaluation.

Assessment. Assessment involves recognizing cues and establishing a database. The nurse gathers objective and subjective information about the client and then verifies the data and communicates information gained from the assessment.

TABLE 1.2
Overview of Content

All content categories and subcategories reflect client needs across the life span in a variety of settings.

A. Safe, Effective Care Environment
The nurse promotes the achievement of client outcomes by providing and directing nursing care that enhances the care delivery setting to protect clients and health care personnel.

1. *Management of care*—Providing and directing nursing care that enhances the care delivery setting to protect clients and health care personnel. Related content includes but is **not limited** to:
    - Advance Directives/Self-Determination/Life Planning
    - Advocacy
    - Case Management
    - Client Rights
    - Collaboration with Interdisciplinary Team
    - Concepts of Management
    - Confidentiality/Information Security
    - Continuity of Care
    - Assignment, Delegation, and Supervision
    - Establishing Priorities
    - Ethical Practice
    - Informed Consent
    - Information Technology
    - Legal Rights and Responsibilities
    - Organ Donation
    - Performance Improvement (quality improvement)
    - Referrals

(Continued)

TABLE 1.2
Overview of Content (*Continued*)

   2. *Safety and infection control*—Protecting clients and health care personnel from health and environmental hazards. Related content includes but is **not limited** to:
- Accident/Error/Injury Prevention
- Emergency Response Plan
- Ergonomic Principles
- Handling Hazardous and Infectious Materials
- Home Safety
- Reporting of Incident/Event/Irregular Occurrence/Variance
- Safe Use of Equipment
- Security Plan
- Standard Precautions/Transmission-Based Precautions/Surgical Asepsis
- Use of Restraints/Safety Devices

B. Health Promotion and Maintenance

The nurse provides and directs nursing care of the client that incorporates the knowledge of expected growth and development principles, prevention and/or early detection of health problems, and strategies to achieve optimal health. Related content includes but is **not limited** to:
- Aging Process
- Ante/Intra/Postpartum and Newborn Care
- Developmental Stages and Transitions
- Health Promotion/Disease Prevention
- Health Screening
- High-Risk Behaviors
- Lifestyle Choices
- Self-Care
- Techniques of Physical Assessment

C. Psychosocial Integrity

The nurse provides and directs nursing care that promotes and supports the emotional, mental, and social well-being of the client experiencing stressful events, as well as clients with acute or chronic mental illness. Related content includes but is **not limited** to:
- Abuse/Neglect
- Behavioral Interventions
- Chemical and Other Dependencies/Substance Use Disorder
- Coping Mechanisms
- Crisis Intervention
- Cultural Awareness/Cultural Influences on Health
- End-of-Life Care
- Family Dynamics
- Grief and Loss
- Mental Health Concepts
- Religious and Spiritual Influences on Health
- Sensory/Perceptual Alterations
- Stress Management
- Support Systems
- Therapeutic Communication
- Therapeutic Environment

D. Physiological Integrity

The nurse promotes physical health and wellness by providing care and comfort, reducing client risk potential, and managing health alterations.

   1. *Basic care and comfort*—Providing comfort and assistance in the performance of activities of daily living. Related content includes but is **not limited** to:
- Assistive Devices
- Elimination
- Mobility/Immobility
- Nonpharmacological Comfort Interventions
- Nutrition and Oral Hydration
- Personal Hygiene
- Rest and Sleep

TABLE 1.2
Overview of Content (Continued)

2. *Pharmacological and parenteral therapies*—Providing care related to the administration of medications and parenteral therapies. Related content includes but is **not limited** to:
   - Adverse Effects/Contraindications/Side Effects/Interactions
   - Blood and Blood Products
   - Central Venous Access Devices
   - Dosage Calculation
   - Expected Actions/Outcomes
   - Medication Administration
   - Parenteral/Intravenous Therapies
   - Pharmacological Pain Management
   - Total Parenteral Nutrition
3. *Reduction of risk potential*—Reducing the likelihood that clients will develop complications or health problems related to existing conditions, treatments, or procedures. Related content includes but is **not limited** to:
   - Changes/Abnormalities in Vital Signs
   - Diagnostic Tests
   - Laboratory Values
   - Potential for Alterations in Body Systems
   - Potential for Complications of Diagnostic Tests/Treatments/Procedures
   - Potential for Complications from Surgical Procedures and Health Alterations
   - System Specific Assessments
   - Therapeutic Procedures
4. *Physiological adaptation*—Managing and providing care for clients with acute, chronic, or life-threatening physical health conditions. Related content includes but is **not limited** to:
   - Alterations in Body Systems
   - Fluid and Electrolyte Imbalances
   - Hemodynamics
   - Illness Management
   - Medical Emergencies
   - Pathophysiology
   - Unexpected Response to Therapies

Copyright by the National Council of State Boards of Nursing, Inc. All rights reserved.

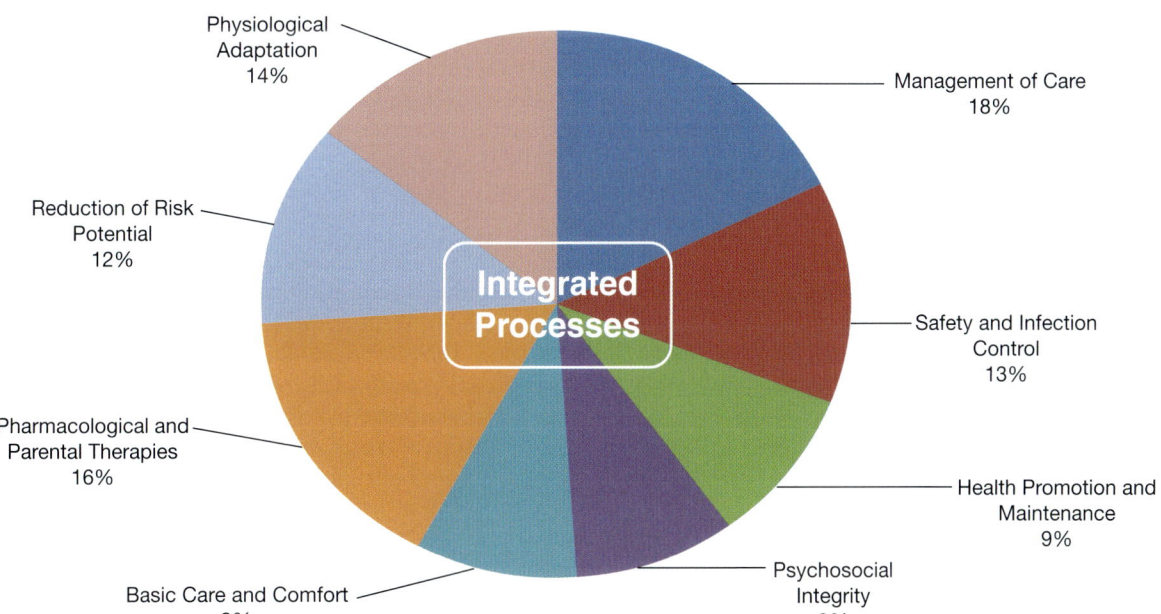

FIGURE 1.1 Distribution of Content for the NCLEX-RN Test Plan

Distribution of Content Copyright by the National Council of State Boards of Nursing, Inc. All rights reserved.

Analysis. Analysis involves making a hypothesis and identifying actual or potential health care needs or problems based on assessment data. The nurse interprets the data, collects additional data as indicated, and identifies and communicates the client's nursing problem. The nurse also determines the congruency between the client's needs and the ability of the health care team members to meet those needs.

Planning. Planning involves setting outcomes and goals for meeting the client's needs and designing strategies to attain them. Prioritization is an important aspect of planning. The nurse determines the goals of care, develops and modifies the plan, collaborates with other health team members for delivery of the client's care, and formulates expected outcomes of nursing interventions.

Implementation. Implementation involves initiating and completing actions necessary to accomplish the defined goals. The nurse organizes and manages the client's care; performs or assists the client in performing activities of daily living; counsels and teaches the client, significant others, and health care team members; and provides care to attain the established client goals. The nurse also provides care to optimize the achievement of the client's health care goals; supervises, coordinates, and evaluates delivery of the client's care as provided by nursing staff; and records and exchanges information.

Evaluation. Evaluation determines goal achievement. The nurse compares actual with expected outcomes of therapy, evaluates compliance with prescribed or proscribed therapy, and records and describes the client's response to therapy or care. The nurse also modifies the plan, as indicated, and reorders priorities.

The NCSBN has identified that newly licensed nurses must make increasingly complex decisions to safely care for clients. Therefore, it is important to understand all steps of the nursing process and how they relate to clinical judgment. All phases are integrated throughout the exam. In this book, you will have opportunities to respond to questions involving all five steps of the nursing process.

Caring

The caring process refers to interaction between the nurse, client, and family in a way that conveys mutual respect and trust. The nurse offers encouragement and hope to clients and their families while providing nursing care. Questions about the caring process are threaded throughout the licensing exam to test the candidate's attitudes and values for caring for and about clients. In this book, you will have the opportunity to respond to questions that test your ability to apply the caring process in a variety of situations.

Communication and Documentation

Another element of the licensing exam test plan evaluates the nurse's ability to communicate with clients, families, and health team members. The test also includes questions about documenting nursing care according to standards of nursing practice. In this book, you will be presented with questions that ask you to determine the most effective way to communicate with clients, families, and other health professionals. You will also have the opportunity to respond to questions that require you to select the appropriate information to document or chart.

Teaching/Learning

An important aspect of nursing care is to teach clients and their families about managing their own health status. Nurses also teach other members of the health care team. Questions in this book are designed to assist you in answering questions about the teaching and learning process for a variety of clients and health care team members.

Culture and Spirituality

Culture and spirituality are integral to person-centered health care and involve the interaction of the nurse and the client (individual, family, or group, including significant others and population) in a way that conveys respect for the client's culture and spiritual beliefs. The nurse assesses the client's self-reported and unique individual preferences and incorporates them into the plan of care.

Clinical Judgment

Clinical judgment is an observed outcome of critical thinking and decision-making. It is considered to be a iterative process that uses nursing knowledge to observe and assess presenting situations, identify a prioritized client concern, and generate the best possible evidence-based solutions to deliver safe client care. The steps of the NCSBN Clinical Judgment Measurement Model are described in more detail in Chapter 2. On the NCLEX, each test-taker will receive three scored case studies; however, some candidates may receive more as pretest items. Depending on how many total questions a candidate takes, they may receive up to 10 standalone clinical judgment questions. In this book, you will be able to practice taking case studies with six linked questions and standalone item types to test clinical judgment.

Test Item Writers

Nurse clinicians and nurse educators volunteer to become item writers. All item writers are approved by the Council of State Boards of Nursing or the provincial/territorial regulatory bodies. Because the item writers come from a variety of geographical areas and practice settings, the test items reflect nursing practice in all parts of the United States and provinces/territories that are using the NCLEX-RN.

EXAM ADMINISTRATION

Computer Adaptive Testing

The NCLEX-RN is administered using a combination of computer adaptive testing (CAT) and static procedures. CAT uses the memory and speed of the computer to administer a test individualized for each candidate. When the examination begins, the computer randomly selects a relatively easy question. The next question is based on the candidate's response to the previous question. If the question is answered correctly, an item of similar or greater difficulty is generated; if it is answered incorrectly, a less difficult item is selected. The computer selects items that the candidate has a 50/50 chance of answering correctly, so test-takers should not be concerned that they are not answering every question correctly. Approximately 50% of the test items every candidate will receive may be too difficult (and will be answered incorrectly), and 50% of the test items will be easily answered based on the candidate's ability. Thus, the test is adapted for each candidate. Once competence has been determined, the exam is completed at a passing level. Since the NCLEX-RN is designed to address specific test plan categories, not content areas, candidates should also not be concerned if it seems they are receiving a large proportion of questions about a specific health problem or client age group. For the six-item case study questions, the computer adaptive testing will be suspended, and each item will be scored according to the published scoring procedures for those individual items (see Chapter 2).

Each NCLEX-RN test is generated from a large pool of questions (a test item bank) based on the NCLEX-RN test plan and is reviewed each quarter to ensure questions reflect current practice. The test item bank includes all item types, but an individual candidate may or may not receive each type of question, depending on the questions generated from the item bank for each candidate. The exams for all candidates are derived from the same large pool of test items. They contain comparable questions for each component of the test plan. Although the questions are not exactly the same, they test the same knowledge, skills, and abilities from the test plan. All candidates receive comparable percentages of questions from each client need category that aligns with the test plan and must attain the passing standard from this balanced test plan. Each candidate, therefore, has the same opportunity to demonstrate competence. Although one candidate may answer fewer questions, all candidates have the opportunity to answer a sufficient number of questions to demonstrate competence until the stability of passing or failing is established or the time limit expires.

Each exam includes both "operational" questions (the actual questions used to determine competency) and 15 "pretest" questions (those questions that are being tested for use on subsequent exams). The pretest questions are not included in your final score on the exam. The pretest questions are administered during the early part of the exam, but you will not be able to differentiate pretest items from operational items on the exam. All candidates must answer at least 70 operational test questions. Thus, the minimum number of questions you might receive is 85 (70 operational test questions and 15 pretest questions); the maximum number of possible questions a candidate might receive is 150 (135 operational questions and 15 pretest questions). Historically, the average candidate received about 110 test questions.

Five hours are available to each candidate for completing the test. This time includes rest breaks. Students are expected to complete an online tutorial before arriving for the exam. Although some candidates may finish in a shorter time, others will use the entire 5 hours. The amount of time used during testing is not an indication of passing or failing the examination but rather reflects the time required to establish competence for each candidate.

Scheduling the Examination

Information about scheduling the exam will be included in the *Candidate Bulletin*. Refer to the most current information when you are ready to register for the exam. The first step to scheduling your NCLEX-RN exam is to apply to the board of nursing/regulatory body (BON/RB) where you wish to be licensed and meet all of their requirements. Submit any requests for testing accommodations with your application. Next, register with Pearson VUE by phone or web. Have a credit card, name on the identification (ID) you will use the day of the test, and an email ready. You will receive an NCLEX-RN registration acknowledgment via email from Pearson VUE, so it is important that you provide an email address that you will continue to have access to after graduation. The BON/RB makes you eligible in the Pearson VUE system. You will then receive an Authorization to Test (ATT) email from Pearson VUE. The ATT contains the authorization number, the candidate identification number, and an expiration date. You are then ready to schedule your exam with Pearson VUE. You may select a preferred testing center and preferred dates via the Pearson VUE website or telephone. You must schedule your exam before the expiration of the ATT. Confirmation of appointments comes by email. Check for current information in the *Candidate Bulletin* at the NCSBN website (www.ncsbn.org) and the website of your board of nursing/regulatory body. (See the appendix for state, provincial, and territorial boards of nursing.) Scheduling to take the examination at an international test center requires additional steps and fees; consult the NCSBN website for current information.

Test Center Locations

The Council of State Boards of Nursing contracts with vendors in each state, province, and territory to serve as exam sites. Your school of nursing can inform you of the nearest location, but you may take the exam at any location. You can also contact your board of nursing/

regulatory body for information. (See the appendix for state, provincial, and territorial boards of nursing for the address.) You can also find updated information from the NCSBN on its website (www.ncsbn.org).

Computer Use and Screen Design

Test questions are presented on the computer screen (monitor); you select your answer and use the keyboard or a mouse to enter your answer. To practice using computer-generated questions, use the questions on thePoint. To log into thePoint, go to http://thepoint.lww.com. (The code for accessing the site is printed on the inside front cover of this book along with specific instructions for accessing the questions.) To practice with item types that are computer generated and adaptable, a 7-day free trial to *Lippincott® NLCEX-RN PassPoint* is included with this book.

Before you take the licensing exam, you should also take the tutorial about the design of computer-generated questions at the Pearson VUE website (www.pearsonvue.com/nclex) and available from the NCSBN (https://nclex.com/next-generation-nclex.page). At every testing site, written directions are provided at each computer exam station.

The computer used at the testing site has a drop-down clock that indicates elapsed time for taking the exam. This clock can be turned "off" or "on" depending on your preference. Some test takers wish to watch the time as they take the test; others wish to monitor their time periodically. When the exam ends, there will be a message on the screen that indicates, "Examination is ended."

The computer used at the testing site also has a drop-down calculator. The calculator can be used to answer test items requiring calculation. You can use the mouse to drag the calculator to a position on the screen where it is most helpful to you.

Exam Security

Each testing site maintains a high level of security for the exam and for the candidate. The exam is administered on a secured file server and uses password security and host site authentication. All exam sites use test administrators (TAs) and video/audio monitoring. Candidates are required to undergo identification verification, which includes showing a valid and recent photo ID (for example, driver's license or passport—a passport is required at international test centers—provincial/territorial or state identification card, permanent residence card, or military identification card) with signature (the name must match *exactly* the name on the ATT), and a biometric test such as a palm vein scan. You will also have your photograph taken. The photo will be used to confirm your identity and will be included with your exam score report. Check with your board of nursing/regulatory body, the NCSBN, and the *Candidate Bulletin* for details about exam security

in the jurisdiction in which you are taking the exam, and review information on the testing service website (www.pearsonvue.com/nclex). Additionally testing sites will have infection-control practices in place based on local and national trends.

Exam Confidentiality

The NCSBN takes significant steps to protect exam confidentiality. You will not be allowed to bring anything into the exam area. Lockers will be available at the testing site to store items such as cellular telephones, wallets, watches (smartwatches must be placed in a plastic bag), hats/coats/scarves/gloves, medical aids/devices, lip balm, food or drink, or gum/candy.

During the break you will not be allowed to access study notes (any educational or test preparation materials); mobile phones, MP3 players, fitness bands, jump drives, cameras, or any other electronic device or weapons of any kind.

While taking the exam, you are not allowed to give or receive test-taking assistance, and you cannot review study materials during a break from the exam; a test administrator will be monitoring these areas. Additionally, you will be asked to sign a confidentiality agreement that you will not share information about the test or the test items with others. Social media sites are also monitored to determine if information is shared by way of electronic communication. Students who have posted information through social media about the test will be reported to their state board of nursing or provincial/territorial nursing regulators with a possible consequence of having their license denied. For additional information see the *Candidate Bulletin*.

Special Accommodations

Special accommodations for Americans or Canadians with disabilities can be made with authorization from the individual boards of nursing/regulatory bodies and the NCSBN.

Accommodations that are frequently requested are extended time, readers, large font or adaptations for use of color, and quiet/distraction-reduced environments. Only your board of nursing/regulatory body (BON/RB) can approve testing accommodations. Typically, the BON/RB will require proof of a condition requiring accommodations and proof that you were provided the requested accommodations while in your prelicensure program. It is important to know that there is no option to take a paper-pencil test and readers may not be approved by some BON/RBs. If approved, the accommodations will be noted on the ATT. Check with your BON/RB for additional information. Accommodation requests are not needed for approved comfort aids, including certain medical devices, hearing aids, and cough drops. These aids must be disclosed at the testing site to the test administrator. Find a complete list of approved comfort aids on the Pearson VUE website.

The Test Center

Although each test center is configured differently, each center will have a small waiting area, a registration area, and a proctored testing area; lockers are provided for valuables. Since the waiting area is small, you should advise your friends or family to return to the test center when you have completed the exam.

You should arrive at the test center 30 minutes before you are scheduled to take the test. You should bring your ATT and two forms of identification with you, one of which has photo identification. It is important that the name on the ID matches the name provided when registering with Pearson VUE. See the Pearson VUE website for a list of approved IDs. Leave all unnecessary items in your car or with friends or family. Personal items such as coats, medical devices, and snacks must be placed in provided, lockable storage. If test takers access their phone, or any electronic device, during a break, an incident report will be generated that could result in an exam failure. When you register at the test center, the test center staff will obtain your biometric identification and digital signature. No watches, pencils, or cell phones will be allowed in the test-taking area.

Taking the Exam

Once you have entered the testing area and have settled comfortably at the desk, the test administrator (TA) will turn the computer on. You may request earplugs from the TA if the noise of other test takers using the computers in the area is distracting. You may also request an erasable note board with a marking pen, which may be used to make notes or perform math calculations as the test progresses. Previous computer experience is not necessary to take the NCLEX-RN exam.

You are expected to complete the tutorial on item types before arriving for the examination. The test questions are presented on the computer screen. You should answer each question; the next question will not appear until you have submitted an answer to the question on the screen. you should make a reasonable attempt to answer the question correctly. Rapid guessing to answer as many questions as possible is not recommended and can drastically reduce your score.

As you progress through the test, pace yourself. You should answer the questions at a comfortable speed, not spending too much time on any one question. There is a clock on the computer that can be turned off or on. Some students prefer to turn the clock on periodically rather than watching the time on the clock and feeling rushed. The clock will appear during the last 5 minutes of the test.

You will be given an opportunity to take a break during a "scheduled" break time at 2 hours and again at 3.5 hours after you have begun the exam. Break time counts as test-taking time. Raise your hand, and the TA will escort you to the restroom. You will be given a lanyard to wear indicating you are on break. Biometric identification (palm vein scan) will be obtained on your return to the computer desk.

Once you have answered a sufficient number of questions to determine if you have passed or failed the test, or if the allotted time (5 hours) has ended, the exam will end. You may be asked to take a survey about the test experience following the exam or invited to answer 15 questions that are being tested for future use on the NCLEX-RN exam. When you are finished, you can raise your hand to indicate to the proctor that you are done. The TA then will collect all items at the desk and escort you to the exit.

Results Reporting

Computerized testing allows timely reporting of examination results. The results of the examination are first scored at the testing site and then are verified by Pearson VUE before being forwarded to the board of nursing/regulatory body. The candidate will not receive any results on the day of the exam. Results are reported to the candidate up to 6 weeks after taking the exam. Some candidates in the United States can obtain "unofficial" results after 48 business hours through the Quick Results Service available on the NCLEX candidate website at www.pearsonvue.com/nclex. The Quick Results Service is not available in all states, and there is a minimal fee for this service. The Quick Results Service is not available for candidates in Canada. For current information, read the *Candidate Bulletin*.

Exam Failure

If you have failed the exam, you will receive a Candidate Performance Report (CPR), which provides the number of items that you completed and a summary of your relative strengths and weaknesses based on the test plan. You can use this report to guide your study for taking the exam again.

The exam can be retaken as soon as 45 days after the previous test date. Failing the licensing exam can be devastating, but it does not mean that you will never pass the exam or be a good nurse. While you are waiting to retake the exam, you should make a study plan that includes studying for a few hours most days of the week and prepare to take the exam as soon as possible. As a first step, try to determine why you did not pass. Possible reasons include fatigue, stress, illness on the day of the exam, or inadequate preparation. Many students say that the main reason that they do not succeed is test anxiety. Taking practice exams, such as those in Part 3 of this book, can help you feel more prepared and help reduce your anxiety. Review the information in Chapter 3 about test preparation, and review or complete the Content Mastery and Test-Taking Skill Self-Analysis (Table 3.3) to identify your particular problems with test taking or your knowledge of the content. You can find a blank version of this document that you are able to pull out and use at the back of this textbook. Students also find it helpful to form study groups or enroll in an NCLEX-RN test review course.

When to Take the NCLEX-RN

You should plan to take the exam as soon as possible after graduating. Suggestions for developing a study plan are discussed in Chapter 3 of this book.

TERMINOLOGY, MEASUREMENTS, AND LABORATORY VALUES USED IN THIS BOOK

Specific terminology is used on the licensing exam to be inclusive of the variety of health care providers, registered, licensed, and unlicensed assistive personnel (Table 1.3). Measurements are presented in both U.S. Standard Units and in metric measurements; laboratory

TABLE 1.3
Definitions of Terms, Measurements, and Laboratory Values Used in This Book

Definition of Terms

Client
- Individual, family, or group that includes significant others and population.

NCLEX Integrated Processes
- Themes such as the nursing process, caring, communication, documentation, teaching, learning, culture and spirituality, and clinical judgment are fundamental to the practice of nursing and are integrated throughout the Client Needs categories and subcategories.

Prescription
- Orders, interventions, remedies, or treatments ordered or directed by an authorized health care provider.

Exhibit
- Denotes a client chart or medical record type of item. Additional information is available behind tabs listed on the screen. Click on a tab to review the additional information.

Primary Health Care Provider
- Member of the health care team (usually a medical physician [or other specialty, e.g., surgeon, nephrologist, etc.], nurse practitioner, etc.), licensed and authorized to formulate prescriptions on behalf of the client.

Unlicensed Assistive Personnel (UAP)
- Any unlicensed personnel, regardless of title, to whom nursing tasks are delegated.

Other Terms

Informed Consent
- Informed consent is a mechanism for communication between a client and a health care provider in which the client makes an informed decision about the type of health care, tests, procedures, or treatments they are about to receive. There are legal and ethical aspects of informed consent. While each state and province has its own definition of informed consent, in general, the client must be legally able to sign the consent, not be pressured to do so, and must understand the implications of giving the consent. Typically, it is the responsibility of the physician, surgeon, or other health care provider who is performing the procedure or treatment to obtain the consent. The nurse's role is to verify that the consent form is signed by the client or designated representative, serve as a witness to the client's signature, document in the nurse's notes that the signature was obtained, and advocate for the client in ensuring the client fully understands the consent.

Handoff of Care
- Handoff of care, or handoff communication, is a process of communicating information about a client from one health care professional, or a team to another person or team in order to ensure high-quality care and client safety.

Medical Record
- The term medical record is used to refer to a "chart," a "health record," "electronic medical record," or an "electronic health record." A medical record is the documentation of health care provided to a client and includes prescriptions, history and physical, laboratory results, miscellaneous reports, imaging results, flow sheets, intake and output records, medication administration records, progress notes, and vital signs.

Rapid Response Team
- A rapid response team is composed of physicians, nurses, hospitalists, and other health care providers who are prepared to respond to a situation when a client demonstrates signs of imminent clinical deterioration. The team is called to assess and treat a client with the goal of preventing the need to transfer the client to an intensive care unit or preventing a cardiac arrest. Nurses and health care providers may initiate a call to the rapid response team.

Time Out
- A "time out" refers to a protocol for preventing wrong site, wrong procedure, and wrong person surgery. The purpose of a "time out" is to address any discrepancies before the surgery begins or to clarify concerns of any of the surgical team prior to making the incision. This protocol provides an opportunity for nurses and other members of the health care team, including the client, to verify the presurgery checklist prior to beginning the surgery or invasive procedure.

TABLE 1.3
Definitions of Terms, Measurements, and Laboratory Values Used in This Book (*Continued*)
Measurements
Measurements such as weight, temperature, height, distance, and volume are presented in U.S. Standard Units and metric representation. Examples include the following: ■ A client weighs 125 lb (56.7 kg). ■ Measurements are rounded to the nearest tenth. ■ Blood pressure is presented as mm Hg. Temperature is reported first as Fahrenheit with Centigrade in parentheses.
Laboratory Values
Lab values are presented in U.S. Standard Units and in the International System of Units (SI units). Examples include the following: ■ 140 mEq/L (140 mmol/L) ■ A BUN of 26 mg/dL (26 mmol/L) ■ Creatinine of 1.2 mg/dL (1.2 μmol/L) ■ Reference ranges will be provided in questions that require you to interpret lab results. Common lab values will include ABGs (pH, PO2, PCO2, SaO2, HCO3), BUN, cholesterol (total) glucose, hematocrit, hemoglobin, glycosylated hemoglobin (HgbA1C), platelets, potassium, sodium, WBC, creatinine, PT, PTT and APTT, INR.

Copyright by the National Council of State Boards of Nursing, Inc. All rights reserved.

values are presented in U.S. Standard Units and in International System of Units (SI units) (see Table 1.3). Reference values will be provided for all laboratory reports with numeric data. A reference sheet of normal laboratory values is found in the tear-out section in the back of this book. We encourage you to use this resource as you answer questions in the book.

ADDITIONAL INFORMATION

For further and up-to-date information about the NCLEX-RN, the test plan, test questions, exam format, or testing procedures, visit the NCSBN website at www.ncsbn.org. For information about the dates, requirements, and specifics of writing the examination in your state, contact your board of nursing/regulatory body. The addresses and telephone numbers of the NCSBN and board of nursing/regulatory body are provided in the appendix. Information can also be obtained from the vendor who has contracted to provide the testing center for the NCLEX-RN exam. The current vendor is Pearson VUE, and information can be found on their website (www.pearsonvue.com/nclex).

REFERENCES

National Council of State Boards of Nursing, Inc. (2022). Research Brief: Volume 81, April 2022. 2021 RN Practice Analysis: Linking the NCLEX-RN examination to practice—U.S. and Canada. Retrieved from https://www.ncsbn.org

National Council of State Boards of Nursing, Inc. (2022). Virtual NCLEX Conference.

2

NCLEX-RN® Test Questions and Strategies for Answering Them

INTRODUCTION

The test questions used on the NCLEX-RN exam are written to test the knowledge, skills, and abilities essential to provide safe client care. Understanding the types of questions, the cognitive level of the questions, as well as the thinking and nursing clinical judgment processes used to answer the questions is essential for test success. This chapter provides information about the traditional and new test items used on the NCLEX-RN exam and offers strategies for answering questions for various types of test items, levels of the cognitive domain, and clinical judgment steps.

TYPES OF TEST ITEMS

Beginning in April of 2023, the National Council of State Boards of Nursing (NCSBN) will use a combination of single, standalone questions and six-question case studies (NGN News, Winter 2022). Case studies will test the six steps of the NCSBN Clinical Judgment Measurement Model. The standalone items can test either client needs or clinical judgment.

The updated NCLEX-RN, referred to as *Next Generation NCLEX*, will include item formats used on previous versions of the NCLEX-RN and introduce new technology-enhanced item types. Item formats used on previous versions of NCLEX-RN include multiple-choice, multiple-response, fill-in-the-blank (calculation), chart/exhibit, ordered-response, and graphic options. The five new item types are extended multiple-response, drag-and-drop, matrix/grid, highlight, and drop-down (NGN News Winter, 2022). Each of these new item types has variations summarized in Table 2.1. The two types of standalone clinical judgment item formats are bowtie, a drag-and-drop variation, and trends that show changes over time and can be any new item type.

Although each type of item tests your understanding of nursing content and is developed using the same test development process, each type of test item requires you to respond in a different way. Because alternate item formats test knowledge, skills, and abilities in a variety of ways, there are increased opportunities for you to demonstrate your competence. This book contains case studies and standalone item types that will be used on Next Generation NCLEX-RN. To practice with additional items and computerized formats, log into thePoint at http://thepoint.lww.com. (The code for accessing the site is printed on the inside front cover of the book along with specific instructions for accessing the questions.)

TABLE 2.1
Summary of Item Types

Traditional Items	Extended multiple-response	Drag & Drop	Drop-Down	Matrix/Grid	Highlight	Standalone
- Multiple-choice - Multiple-response - Fill-in-the-blank - Exhibit/chart - Graphic - Ordered response	- Select all that apply - Select N - Multiple-response grouping	- Cloze - Rationale	- Cloze - Rationale - Table	- Multiple-choice - Multiple-response	- In text - In table	- Bowtie - Trend (can be any new item type except bowtie)

SCORING

Beginning in April 2023, the NCSBN will introduce multiple scoring methods (NGN News Summer, 2021). Items will be worth different point values based on how many correct options each question contains. Unlike previous versions of NCLEX-RN where questions were scored as correct or incorrect, you will be able to earn partial credit on items worth more than one point. The question key in this book will indicate which of the three scoring models applies. If no key is shown, the item is scored as correct or incorrect with no partial credit. The three models are summarized below.

0/1 Scoring

Scoring is used when there are limits set on how many options you may select. You earn one point for each correct option selected in a multipoint item. You earn zero points for selecting incorrect options. Points earned on the question equals the sum of correct responses (Fig. 2.1). Questions that have only one correct response, such as multiple-choice questions, fall under the 0/1 scoring rule. You earn one point for selecting the correct response, but no credit if you do not.

FIGURE 2.1 Sample 0/1 Scoring

The nurse reassesses the client 1 hour after implementing the treatment protocol and giving a second uterotonic agent.

Which four findings suggest that the client's status is declining?
- ☒ 1. Fundus [correct] ✓
- ☒ 2. Peripads ✗
- ☒ 3. Skin [correct] ✓
- ☐ 4. Pulse [correct]
- ☐ 5. Respirations
- ☒ 6. Blood pressure [correct] ✓
- ☐ 7. Nausea
- ☐ 8. Hemoglobin

This item is worth a possible 4 points. Three correct items are selected. Score = 3 points.

–/+ Scoring

Scoring applies when you are able to select an unlimited number of options, such as in a select all that apply question. Total points possible equals the number of options identified as being correct. You will earn one point for each correct option selected, but you will lose one point for every incorrect option selected. The total score for the item is the sum of correct responses minus the sum of incorrect options. However, there is no negative scoring (Fig. 2.2). The lowest score you can receive on a question is zero. When items are scored using the +/– rule, guessing incorrectly is penalized. Therefore, you should only select options that you are reasonably confident are correct.

FIGURE 2.2 Sample +/– Scoring

The nurse reassesses the client 1 hour after implementing the treatment protocol and giving a second uterotonic agent.

Which finding(s) would suggest that the patient's status is declining? Select all that apply.
- ☒ 1. Fundus [correct] ✓
- ☒ 2. Peripads ✗
- ☒ 3. Skin [correct] ✓
- ☐ 4. Pulse [correct]
- ☐ 5. Respirations
- ☒ 6. Blood pressure [correct] ✓
- ☐ 7. Nausea
- ☐ 8. Hemoglobin

Item is worth a possible 4 points. Three correct items were selected; one incorrect item was selected. Score = 2 points.

Rationale scoring

R Rationale scoring applies to items that appear as a single sentence and show a relationship between selectable options. You must understand the relationships and select the correct pairings to earn full credit. Questions may be worth one point if it has one concept and one justification. Both answers must be correct to earn credit. The item is worth two points if it contains one concept and two justifications. Partial credit of one point may be earned if the correct concept and only one correct justification are selected (Fig. 2.3).

FIGURE 2.3 Sample Rationale Scoring

The nurse assesses the adolescent on postoperative day 2 after a tibial fasciotomy.

▸ Complete the sentences from the list of drop-down options.

The nurse is concerned that the client is developing the complication of [infection / muscle necrosis / **nerve damage** ✗] as evidenced by the client's [swelling / **urine** / pain ✓].

Item is worth 1 point. The correct options are muscle necrosis and urine. Only one of two parts is correct. Score = 0 points.

To give you the opportunity to learn how to answer different types of questions, this review book contains the item formats you can expect to see on the NCLEX-RN beginning in April 2023. Additional materials are available on thePoint. You can also find examples of these types of questions in the *Detailed Test Plan* and the *Candidate Bulletin* found on the NCSBN website (www.ncsbn.org). The candidate tutorial, available from the NCSBN at https://nclex.com/next-generation-nclex.page, gives you an opportunity to practice with the different item types exactly as they will appear on NCLEX-RN.

Multiple-Choice Items

Multiple-choice items include a scenario/situation, a question, and four answers—only *one* of which is correct (Fig. 2.4). The scenario provides information about the client or care management situation. The question (stem) poses the problem to solve. The question is written as a direct question, such as "What should the nurse do **first**?" The answers (options) are possible responses to the question (stem). Each question has one correct option and three incorrect options. Multiple-choice items are the most common type of test item used on the licensing exam.

FIGURE 2.4 Sample Multiple-Choice Item

The nurse is instructing a client with a new colostomy about protecting the skin around the colostomy. Which skin barrier is **best** to apply around the ostomy?
  ☐ 1. adhesive barrier
  ☐ 2. petroleum jelly
  ☐ 3. cornstarch
  ☐ 4. antiseptic cream

Strategies for Answering Multiple-Choice Items

- Read the scenario, and relate the question and answers to the data provided in the scenario. Pay particular attention to information, if included, about the client's age, family status, health status, ethnicity, place of care, changes in assessment data, or point in the care plan (e.g., early admission vs. preparation for discharge).
- Note particular key words such as **first, except, not, most,** or **last**.
- Answer the question before looking at the possible answers.
- Eliminate answers you know are wrong.
- Choose the answer that best matches the answer you first thought was correct.
- Double-check your answer to be sure you have fully responded to the question.
- Base your answer on best nursing practice, not experience with one client or in a particular clinical agency.

Multiple-Response Select All that Apply Items

Multiple-response select all that apply items are similar to multiple-choice items, except that they include more than four options, and one or all may be correct. In previous versions of the NCLEX-RN, multiple-response questions had five or six answers. With the introduction of extended multiple-response items, candidates will see questions with a minimum of five and a maximum of ten answer options (Fig. 2.5). These questions will ask you to identify all of the answers that are correct ("Select all that apply"). This item type will be scored using the +/− rule. Points earned on a question equals the sum of correct responses minus the sum of incorrect responses. The lowest possible score on an item is zero.

FIGURE 2.5 Sample Multiple-Response Select All That Apply Item

➤ A client is scheduled for insertion of a coronary stent with right groin access. Which teaching point(s) should the nurse include in this client's preoperative teaching plan? Select all that apply.

  ☐ 1. "If you have a hearing aid, you'll need to remove it before leaving for the procedure."
  ☐ 2. "If you have chest pain during this procedure, please tell the staff when this occurs."
  ☐ 3. "The stitches at your right groin will be able to be removed in 7 to 10 days after the procedure."
  ☐ 4. "You'll be given general anesthesia and will be asleep throughout this procedure."
  ☐ 5. "You'll need to remain flat during the procedure and for 3 to 6 hours after the procedure."
  ☐ 6. "You'll need to keep your right leg in a flexed position for 1 to 2 hours after the procedure."

When using the text pages in this book to answer the multiple-response questions, you can make check marks or circle the answers. When taking the actual NCLEX-RN exam, you will place your cursor on the box in front of the answer you wish to select and click on the box; a checkmark will appear, indicating that you wish to select that answer. To change an answer, you can use the mouse to remove the checkmark from that box.

Strategies for Answering Multiple-Response Items

- If a case study or scenario is used in the question, read all pages of the medical record.
- Read the question carefully, and determine what it is you are to select, for example, all client findings that need follow-up, all intended outcomes of a particular nursing intervention, or all of the elements of a teaching plan for a client with a particular health problem.
- Read each answer, and determine if it is true or false as it pertains to the question.
- Consider how the answers are "clustered" and how the correct answers are related.
- Select options you are reasonably sure are correct. Avoid guessing because incorrect responses will lower your score.

- Be sure you have selected ALL of the possible correct answers.
- Double-check your answer by reviewing the answers you did NOT check, and be sure they are incorrect and should not be included in the answer.

Multiple-Response Select N Items

Select N items have a minimum of five and a maximum of ten answer options. What differentiates them from select all that apply items is that they tell you how many options to select. The "N" is equal to the number of correct options (Fig. 2.6). When taking the NCLEX-RN, it is possible to select less than the number stated, but you cannot select more. When answering questions in this book, pay close attention to "N," and select only that number of answer options. These items are scored using the 0/1 rule. The total possible points equals the number of options you are directed to select. You earn one point for every correctly selected option in these items. There is no guessing penalty.

FIGURE 2.6 Sample Multiple-Response Select N

A child receives a diagnosis of varicella.
➤ Which two complications is the child most at risk for developing?

- ☐ 1. dehydration
- ☐ 2. meningitis
- ☐ 3. pneumonia
- ☐ 4. skin infection
- ☐ 5. seizures

Strategies for Answering Multiple-Response Select N Items

- If a case study or scenario is used in the question, read all pages of the medical record.
- Read the question carefully, and determine what it is you are to select, for example, all client findings that are urgent, possible side effects of a particular drug, or all instructions a nurse should give to a client who is being discharged.
- Read each answer, and determine if it is true or false as it pertains to the question.
- Consider how the answers are "clustered" and how the correct answers are related.
- Always select the number of options asked for in the question. It does not count against you if you guess incorrectly.
- Be sure you have selected ALL of the possible correct answers. Do not submit the item with less than the number of answers required.
- Double-check your answer by reviewing the answers you did NOT check, and be sure they are incorrect.

Multiple-Response Grouping Items

This form of a multiple-response item appears as a table with a minimum of two and a maximum of five groupings (Fig. 2.7). Each grouping has a minimum of two and a maximum of four options. All groups will have the same number of options. You must select at least one option from each group. One to all of the options in a group may be correct. The number of points possible equals the number of correctly keyed options. Scoring is done per group using the +/– rule with a guessing penalty. The number of incorrect options is subtracted from the number of correct options in each group. The minimum score per group is zero. The total points earned for a question equals the sum of points earned per group.

FIGURE 2.7 Sample Multiple-Response Grouping

The health care provider diagnoses a client with anorexia nervosa (restricting type) and orders inpatient psychiatric hospitalization for safety.

➤ Select the anticipated provider orders from each of the following categories. Each category must have at least one option selected.

Category	Possible Order
Nursing	☐ Activity ad lib ☐ Intake and output ☐ Daily weights
Consults	☐ Dietary ☐ Psychiatry ☐ Cardiology
Medications	☐ IV 5% dextrose in 0.45% normal saline ☐ Total parenteral therapy ☐ Potassium supplements

Strategies for Answering Multiple-Response Grouping Items

- If a case study or scenario is used in the question, read all pages of the medical record.
- Read the question carefully, and determine what it is you are to select. These will often be groups of related orders or interventions.
- Read each answer, and determine if it is true or false as it pertains to the question.
- Select at least one option per group. Do not leave a group with no response selected.
- Select more options, up to all, if you are reasonably sure they are correct. Avoid guessing.
- Be sure you have selected ALL of the possible correct answers.
- Double-check your answer by reviewing the answers you did NOT check, and be sure they are incorrect and should not be included in the answer.

Fill-in-the-Blank (Calculation) Items

Fill-in-the-blank items involve calculations, such as determining a drug dose, calculating an IV drip rate, or totaling intake-output records (Fig. 2.8). These items can be answered with a number. On the NCLEX-RN exam, if you do not enter a number, you will receive an error message that will prompt you to "enter a numeric answer." When an answer includes a measurement amount such as milliliters (mL), grams (g), or centimeters (cm), the measurement unit will be stated in the stem of the question and supplied in the answer box; thus, you will not include the unit of measure as part of your answer. The question will indicate how many decimal places to include in the answer. These items will be scored as correct or incorrect with no partial credit.

FIGURE 2.8   Sample Fill-in-the-Blank Item

The nurse administers 10 mg of morphine sulfate to a client with three fractured ribs. The available concentration for this drug is 15 mg/mL. How many milliliters should the nurse administer? Round to one decimal place.

_____0.7_____ mL.

When answering fill-in-the-blank questions on the text pages of this book, you can use paper and pencil, a handheld device with a calculator, or a calculator to determine your answers. However, on the actual NCLEX-RN exam, you will be given a whiteboard to write on, and a drop-down calculator will be available for you to use to calculate your answers. The division sign used is similar to the one used on the Microsoft Calculator (/); be sure to familiarize yourself with the mathematical function keys. To practice calculations required for fill-in-the-blank questions, use the calculator on your computer.

Strategies for Answering Fill-in-the-Blank Items

- Determine what calculation the question is asking you to perform (e.g., add, subtract, or use a formula).
- Write the calculation on the whiteboard provided at the testing center.
- Access the drop-down calculator from the computer to perform the appropriate mathematical function.
- To avoid calculation errors, be sure that you do not enter numbers rapidly when you are using the calculator.
- Round the numbers, as directed, to one or two decimal points after completing the calculation.
- Place your answer on the appropriate line.
- Double-check your answer using a logic test—is this answer plausible? Did I perform the correct mathematical function? Is the answer appropriate for the unit of measure required in the question?

Chart/Exhibit Items

Chart/exhibit items present data from a chart, medical record, graph, or table. Data from a client's chart will be presented from one or more chart "tabs" such as nurse's notes, orders, history and physical, laboratory results, diagnostic reports, flow sheets, intake and output, medication administration records, progress notes, and vital signs (Fig. 2.9). On the actual NCLEX-RN exam, you will be prompted to "click on the exhibit button below for additional client information." You will then use the data presented in the scenario and on the chart or exhibit to make a nursing judgment. You will need to locate and interpret data, validate if the data are correct or sufficient, and then be asked to respond to a question based on the data.

FIGURE 2.9   Sample Chart/Exhibit Item

The nurse is reviewing the history and physical and health care provider prescriptions on the chart of a newly admitted client.

History and Physical

Subjective:	A 19-year-old reports a constant cough for the past "few weeks" with dark sputum for the past few days. The client has night sweats, 10-lb (4.5-kg) weight loss in the past month, and is "always" feeling tired. The client took one acetaminophen about an hour before arrival.
Objective:	
Blood pressure	120/64 mm Hg
Heart rate	84/regular
Respiration rate	26/unlabored/slight wheezing in right lower lobe posteriorly
Oxygen saturation	92%
Temperature	99.9°F (37.7°C) oral
Skin	Warm, slight diaphoretic
Nonproductive cough at this time	
Assessment:	Possible respiratory infection
Physician prescription tab	
	Chest x-ray
	Sputum specimen
	Oxygen at 2 L per nasal cannula

What action should the nurse take **first**?
- ☐ 1. Initiate airborne precautions.
- ☐ 2. Apply oxygen at 2 L per nasal cannula.
- ☐ 3. Collect a sputum sample.
- ☐ 4. Reassess vital signs.

In this book, chart/exhibit questions show data on one or more "tabs" and then ask you to use the data to respond to the question. When these types of questions are administered by the computer (as in the NCLEX-RN exam), you may be asked to determine which tab to use to locate the information that is required to answer the question. You will click on the tab to open the tab(s), and a "pop-up" window will appear on the computer screen. Only one page may be open at a time. Different scoring rules may apply depending on if you are asked to select one or more answers.

Strategies for Answering Chart/Exhibit Items

- Read the scenario and question carefully to understand the context for the data to be provided in the chart or exhibit. For example, are you looking for vital signs? Would an elevated pulse or drop in blood pressure be consistent with the context of the question and provide data for making a nursing decision?
- Read the information provided on the chart or exhibit, and identify the information that is essential to answer the question. Make sure you have reviewed all tabs available.
- Review the chart or exhibit pop-up box as many times as needed.
- If necessary, take notes on the whiteboard provided at the testing center.
- Answer the question only from data provided in the chart or exhibit and from the data presented in the scenario.
- Double-check your answer by being sure you have obtained all of the data necessary to answer the question and that the answer is complete and plausible.

Ordered-Response Items

Ordered-response items are drag and drop–type items that require you to place information in a specified order (Fig. 2.10). For example, the question might ask you to put steps of a procedure in order or provide information about several clients and ask you to determine the order of priority in which each client should receive nursing care. All options must be used in ordered-response questions.

When answering ordered-response items in the text of *this book*, you will write the appropriate step number next to the answer choice. For example, write #1 next to the first step in the process, #2 for the second step in the process, and so on until all answer choices have been used. Or you may write the answers in the correct order in the additional spaces provided. On the actual licensing exam, you will use the computer mouse to drag each response from the left-hand column and drop it into the correct order on the right-hand column. You can move the items around until you have them in the correct order and then click "Next" to enter your answer. If you need to change your answer, you can drag the response to another position and reorder the responses. The questions on thePoint function in much the same way.

FIGURE 2.10 Sample Ordered-Response Item

The nurse's assignment consists of the following four clients. From highest to lowest priority, in which order should the nurse assess the clients after receiving the morning report? All options must be used.

1. the client with cirrhosis who became confused and disoriented during the night

2. the client who is 1 day postoperative following a cholecystectomy and has a T tube inserted

3. the client with acute pancreatitis who is requesting pain medication

4. the client with hepatitis B who has questions about discharge instructions

Strategies for Answering Ordered-Response Items

- Read the key words in the stem of the question that indicate the order in which you are to place the answers. This sequence will often be from first to last.
- Test the logic of your answer. Apply a decision-making framework if applicable.
- Be sure all items have been placed.
- Double-check your answer by reviewing the correct order for the answers and that you have placed your answers in the order in which you intend to answer the question. One answer out of order will cause the question to be counted as incorrect.

Graphic Option Items

While graphics can be used as a part of the *question*, graphic option items use graphics (figures, illustrations, photos) as the answer(s) to the question (Fig. 2.11). You will select the correct answer(s) from the graphic options offered as possible answer(s) to the question. Scoring will depend on whether you are asked to select one or multiple answers.

In the text of this book, you can use your pencil to mark the correct answer to a graphic option question. On thePoint and on the actual NCLEX-RN exam, you will click on the circle or box in front of the graphic that represents your answer. To change your answer, click on another circle or box.

FIGURE 2.11 Sample Graphic Option Item

Which is the correct knot used to secure a restraint to the bed frame?

1.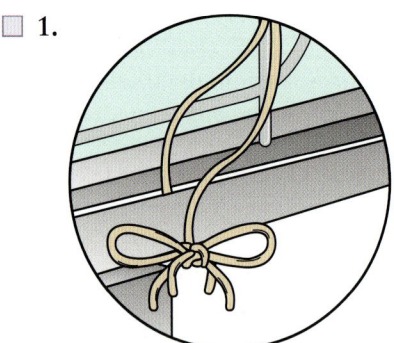

2.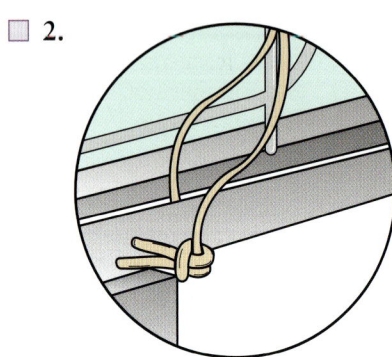

3.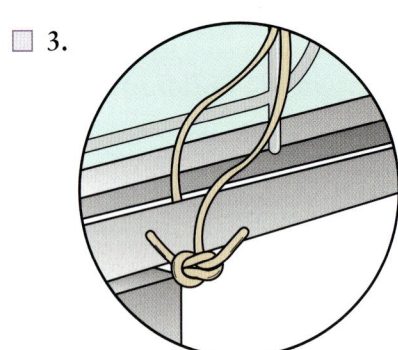

4.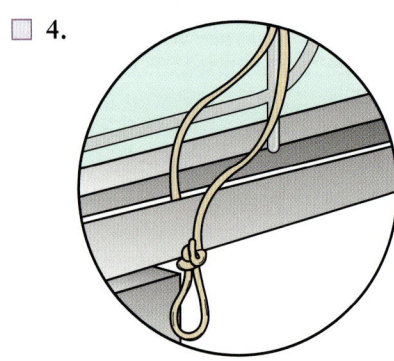

Strategies for Answering Graphic Option Items

- Read the question carefully, and visualize the answer before looking at the options presented with the test item.
- Look carefully at each graphic option, and be certain you understand the visual differences among the options.
- Select the option that best answers the question.
- Double-check your answer by reviewing the question, answering the question based on best nursing practice, and matching the answer to the graphic option.

Multiple-Choice Matrix Items

A multiple-choice matrix is used to categorize information into two or three groups. On the NCLEX-RN, you will be prompted to complete the matrix with the term "click to specify" followed by specific instructions for answering the question (Fig. 2.12). In this book, you will just be asked to "specify" or "indicate." The first column lists client findings, orders, interventions, or nursing actions. You must select which category the item belongs to. Possible questions might ask if the finding is a risk factor or not a risk factor for a condition; if teaching was understood or not understood; if an order was essential, not essential, or contraindicated; or if the finding shows the client's status has improved, declined, or has not changed. You may select only one option per row. On the licensure exam, you will click a radio dial. In this book, you may put an X or a checkmark in the cell of the desired options. The 0/1 scoring rule applies to multiple-choice matrix items. Each row is worth one point. You earn one point for each row that is correct and zero points for rows that are incorrect. There is no penalty for guessing.

FIGURE 2.12 Sample Multiple-Choice Matrix Item

The nurse receives orders from the health care provider.

➤ When the nurse is screening for postpartum depression, indicate whether each action is essential or not essential.

Action	Essential	Not Essential
Screen for postpartum depression with a standardized screening tool	○	○
Have a second provider repeat the screen	○	○
Compare screening results with screenings done before hospital discharge	○	○
Refer clients with positive screens for a confirmatory diagnosis	○	○
Seek immediate care for clients who answer positively to self-harm questions	○	○

Strategies for Answering Multiple-Choice Matrix Items

- Read the scenario carefully. If the item is a case study, note if any new information has been added to update the case. Also be mindful of how you may have answered previous questions in the case.

- Make sure you understand what the client findings are. Findings may list parameters like "blood pressure," but you may have to read the case to learn what the actual value is to answer the question.
- Treat each row as an independent multiple-choice question as you look to see which category the finding, order, intervention, or action best fits.
- Each row must have one response option selected. The radio dial will only let you select one option per row, but you may change your answer up until you submit your response. You cannot continue to the next item until you respond to all rows.
- Double-check that you have not clicked the wrong answer before selecting "Next."

Multiple-Response Matrix Items

Multiple-choice matrix items are used to categorize findings into at least two groups that have overlapping features (Fig. 2.13). On the licensure exam, you will be prompted to complete the matrix with the term "click to specify" followed by specific instructions for answering the question. In this book, you will just see instructions to "specify." The first column lists client findings, factors, orders, interventions, or nursing actions. You must determine if the finding belongs to one or more of the listed categories. This item type is frequently used to analyze if client findings are consistent with certain conditions. Unlike a multiple-choice matrix question, you may select multiple options in a row, and it is possible that there may be no correct options in some rows. Instructions for this item include factors or findings may reflect more than one condition, and each column must have at least one response. In this book, you may place an X in the cell of each desired option.

FIGURE 2.13 Sample Multiple-Response Matrix Item

> For each client finding below, specify if the finding is consistent with the complication of compartment syndrome, deep vein thrombosis (DVT), or hypovolemic shock. Each finding may support more than one complication. Each column must have at least one finding.

	Compartment Syndrome	Deep Vein Thrombosis	Hypovolemic Shock
Delayed capillary refill	☐	☐	☐
Throbbing pain	☐	☐	☐
Swelling	☐	☐	☐
Impaired movement	☐	☐	☐

Total points possible equals the number of correct options for the item. A multiple-response matrix is scored using the +/– rule, but the item is first scored by columns. The column total equals one point for each correct response minus one point for each incorrect response, but there is no negative scoring. The minimum score per column is zero. The points awarded for the item equals the sum of column scores.

Strategies for Answering Multiple-Response Matrix Items

- Read the scenario carefully. If the item is a case study, note if any new information has been added to update the case. Also, be mindful of how you may have answered previous questions in the case.
- Read the case, and make sure you understand what the client findings are. Findings may list parameters like "respiratory status," but you must read the case to know what the status is to answer the question.
- Read the question carefully to determine what relationship is being assessed.
- Treat each row as an independent multiple-response select all that apply question. Ask if each category is true or false.
- Each column must have at least one response option selected. If a column does not have an option selected, review your answers.
- Select as many options per row as you are reasonably certain are correct. All categories may apply to some factors or findings. Remember that some rows may have no correct options.
- The penalty that reduces scores will be applied for wrong answers, so avoid guessing.
- Double-check that you have not clicked the wrong answer before selecting "Next."

Drop-down Items

In a drop-down, you supply information that has systematically been deleted in a sentence, paragraph, or table (Fig. 2.14). Using a cloze format, this type of item uses one or more drop-down items containing a list of single words or short phrases to fill in the missing information. On the NCLEX, the missing information will appear as the word "select." Clicking "select" opens the options available for completing the item. In this text, all options are visible. Circle or underline the best option for each drop-down item. When drop-downs appear in paragraphs or tables, the total points possible for the item equals the number of drop-downs. This item type is scored using the 0/1 rule. There is no guessing penalty.

FIGURE 2.14 Sample Drop-Down Cloze Item

The nurse receives laboratory results.
> Complete the following sentences by choosing from the list of drop-down options.

The nurse should recognize that the client has a [microcytic / macrocytic / normocytic] anemia most likely caused by a(n) [iron / vitamin B12 / folate] nutritional deficit. Untreated, the client is at most risk for developing more [cardiac / neurological / digestive] symptoms as pregnancy progresses.

A drop-down may also use a rationale format, in which you select paired information to complete a single sentence. The question includes a concept that is justified by one or two rationales. The question might state that "the nurse must do (drop-down) because of (drop-down)," or "the client has (drop-down) as evidenced by the (drop-down) and (drop-down)." The same process used for answering drop-down cloze items is used for answering drop-down rationale items, but the scoring is different. Using the rationale scoring rule, the item is worth one point if there is one justification and two points if there are two justifications. Full credit is only awarded if *all* parts are correct.

Strategies for Answering Drop-down Cloze and Table Items

- Review the scenario. For case studies, consider where you are in a case and how you have made decisions up to this point. Note if any new information has been added to update the scenario.
- Read the table, sentence, or sentences carefully, inserting each available drop-down option.
- Determine if the sentence/table is true or false when the option is selected.
- If more than one option is true, select the best option.
- If there are multiple sentences or table rows, review the question after making all selections to determine if your answers make sense as a group.
- There is no guessing penalty, so do not submit questions with unanswered drop-downs.

Strategies for Answering Rationale Drop-down Items

- Follow the steps for answering a cloze or table question, but answer the first part of the sentence by carefully inserting each available drop-down option.

- Determine which option you think is most correct, and then look for the best rationale in the second drop-down.
- If the justifications do not seem to match the first option you selected, recheck your first answer.
- There is no guessing penalty, so do not submit questions with unanswered drop-downs.

Drag-and-Drop Items

In a drag-and-drop question, you drag tokens (words or phrases), to targets (blanks) or answer spaces to complete information that has systematically been deleted in a sentence or paragraph (Fig. 2.15). This type of item uses a list of choices to fill in the answer spaces. Choices are a list of 4 to 10 words or short phrases. Not all choices in the list need to be used. On the licensure exam, you will use your mouse to drag the token to the target. You may send the token back to the choices or just remove it to select another option to change your answer. In this text, write the selected word or phrase in the blank.

Items may use a cloze or rationale format. Using the cloze format, there is one box of word choices to complete one or more sentences. The total points possible for the item equals the number of targets. Cloze items are scored using the 0/1 rule. There is no guessing penalty. In the rationale variation, you select paired information to complete a single sentence. The question includes a concept that is justified by one or two rationales just like a drop-down rationale item. There will be two boxes of word choices instead of one. One box is used for the first target. The justifications are selected from a second box of choices. The rationale scoring rule applies. The item is worth one point if there is one justification and two points if there are two justifications. Full credit is only awarded if all parts are correct.

FIGURE 2.15 Sample Extended Drag-and-Drop

The nurse is caring for a newborn on the mother-baby unit with suspected exposure to maternal substance use disorder.

Nurse's Notes

Day 2

0700:
S: Two-day-old term newborn who is breastfeeding.
B: Neonate born by spontaneous vaginal birth to a primigravid parent who used opioids during pregnancy. Apgar scores were 9 and 10. Birthweight was 3100 g.
A: Vital signs: temperature 99.5°F (37.5°C); heart rate 140 bpm; respiration rate 62 breaths/min. Irritable with moderate tremors when disturbed and regurgitates two to three times with feedings. Today's weight is 2950 g.
R: The baby has routine orders and needs to be reassessed.

➤ Drag words from the choices below to fill in each blank found in the following sentences.

The nurse is most concerned that the client has
[_____].

The nurse should take immediate actions to prevent the complications of
[_____] and
[_____].

Word Choices
dehydration
hyperbilirubinemia
neonatal abstinence syndrome
neonatal sepsis
respiratory arrest
seizure

Strategies for Answering Drag-and-Drop Cloze Items

- Review the scenario. For case studies, consider where you are in a case and how you have made decisions up to this point. Note if any new information has been added to update the scenario.
- Read each sentence carefully to determine what type of information is missing. Is it an assessment, condition, outcome, intervention, or action?
- Look at the choices to find options that align with the missing information in the sentence.
- Select the best option to complete the sentence.
- If there are multiple sentences, answer each one first, and then go back to determine if your answers make sense as a group.
- There is no guessing penalty, so do not submit questions with unanswered blanks.

Strategies for Answering Drag-and-Drop Rationale Items

- Use the same rules for answering drag-and-drop cloze questions, but read the first part of the sentence carefully, inserting each available option from the corresponding box of choices.
- Determine which option you think is most correct.
- Next, look for the best options for answering the second and/or third blanks from the second box of choices.
- If the justifications do not seem to match the first option you selected, recheck your first answer.
- Make sure you have correctly placed your answers.
- There is no guessing penalty, so do not submit the question with unanswered blanks.

Highlighting Text or Table Items

Highlighting items are a variation of hotspots where you must select parts of the text or a table to answer the question (Fig. 2.16). The item might ask you to identify what information needs immediate follow-up, what actions to take first, or what findings suggest a client's condition is deteriorating. It is quite common for a highlighting item to be the first question in a case study. Selectable options in the text or table have been tokenized or broken into units. These may be single words or short phrases. Each question may have up to 10 selectable options. On the licensure exam, hovering over areas of the text or table will show if the area is selectable. Clicking anywhere in the selectable text will automatically highlight the word or entire phrase. In this book, options for selecting have been underlined. You may use a highlighter or circle your choices. The number of points possible equals the number of identified correct options. Highlighting questions will be scored like a multiple-response select all that apply question. Here the +/− rule applies with a guessing penalty.

FIGURE 2.16 Sample Highlighting Item

Progress Notes

Day 2: 1100
The client slept 5 hours last night and has eaten a total of two spoons of scrambled eggs and drank 250 mL of coffee. Vital signs are T 98.0°F (36.7°C); pulse 52 bpm and regular; respiration rate 16 breaths/min; and blood pressure 82/50 mm Hg. The client's morning weight is 89 lb (40.1 kg), which is up 0.5 kg. Repeat potassium this morning is 3.3 mEq/L (3.3 mmol/L). The client insists that they are fine and need to be discharged because they need to practice for a track meet. The client has spent most of the day in their room, refusing to participate in group.

The nurse evaluates the client's progress on day 2.

➤ Highlight the findings that indicate the client's status is improving.

Progress Notes

Day 2: 1100
The client <u>slept 5 hours last night</u> and has <u>eaten a total of two spoons of scrambled eggs and drank 250 mL of coffee</u>. Vital signs are temperature 98.0°F (36.7°C); <u>pulse 52 bpm and regular; respiration rate 16 breaths/min; and blood pressure 82/50 mm Hg</u>. The client's <u>morning weight is up 0.5 kg from admission to 89 lb (40.1 kg)</u>. Repeat potassium this morning is 3.3 mEq/L (3.3 mmol/L). The client <u>insists that they are fine and need to be discharged because they need to practice for a track meet</u>. The client has spent most of the day in their room, refusing to participate in group.

Strategies for Answering Highlighting Items

- The most important factor in a highlighting question is to carefully read the scenario and look for what is being asked.
- Pay attention to all cues, including the environment, client observation, medical records, and time pressures.
- Treat all selectable options as a multiple-response item.
- Select the options you are reasonably sure are correct. Avoid guessing unless the item specifies how many options to select. In that case, make sure you have selected the correct number of options.
- Make sure that you have clicked to highlight the options you want and that they have remained highlighted.

Bowtie Items

A bowtie is a standalone item used to test all 6-steps of the NCSBN Clinical Judgment Measurement Model in one item (NGN News, Spring 2021). The item is formatted as a three-column, drag-and-drop variation with options of five actions in the left well, four potential conditions in the center, and five parameters in the right well (Fig. 2.17). After reviewing a scenario, you select the condition the client is most likely experiencing, two actions to take to address the condition, and two parameters to monitor to assess a client's progress. Targets are arranged in a configuration that resembles a bowtie. On the NCLEX, the tokens and targets are color coded to help ensure you place information in the correct space. In the book, complete the diagram by writing in the selected options or circling your answers. These items are always worth 5 points and are scored using the 0/1 rule.

Strategies for Answering Bowtie Items

- Review the scenario. Make sure you have read all available electronic medical record (EMR) pages.
- Treat the bowtie like a care plan with a problem, interventions, and outcomes.
- Answer the middle column with what condition the client is most likely experiencing first.
- Based on the condition you selected, determine which two actions you would take to address that condition. Order does not matter.
- Finally, select two parameters, or assessments, to monitor to evaluate outcomes. These should be specific to the identified condition. Order does not matter.
- Review the completed diagram before submitting.
- All targets must be filled before you can move to the next question.

Trend Items

Trends are a standalone item type designed to test one or more steps of the NCSBN Clinical Judgment Measurement Model in a single item (NGN News, Spring 2021). The primary characteristic of these items is that they present a clinical scenario with a series of

FIGURE 2.17 Sample Bowtie Item

The nurse is caring for an older adult who had a right hip replacement 2 days ago.

Nurse's Notes

Today: 0705
The client has incisional pain and requires 4 mg of morphine every 3 to 4 hours since surgery. Morphine 4 mg IV push was administered as per health care provider order of 4 mg every 3 to 4 hours for pain. The client voided 300 mL of urine. Vital signs are temperature (T) 99°F (37.2°C); heart rate (HR) 86 bpm; respiration rate (RR) 20 breaths/min; blood pressure (BP) 126/82 mm Hg; oxygen saturation on room air 93%.

1000:
Vital signs T 99°F (37.2°C); HR 86 bpm; RR 16 breaths/min; BP 126/82 mm Hg; and oxygen saturation on room air 93%. The client reports pain of 9 on a scale of 0 to 10 at the incision site on the right hip.

> Complete the diagram by circling the choices below to specify what condition the client is most likely experiencing at 1000, two actions the nurse should take to address that condition, and two parameters the nurse should monitor to assess the client's progress.

Actions to Take	Potential Conditions	Parameters to Monitor
Administer 3 mg morphine	Narcotic dependence	Activity level
Ask the client to wait 30 minutes before the next dose	Narcotic tolerance	Respirations
Administer 4 mg of morphine	Postoperative pain	Pain level
Notify physical therapy to ambulate the client in 20 minutes	Depression of respirations	Urinary output
Ambulate the client before administering morphine		Oxygen saturation

FIGURE 2.18 Sample Trend Item

The nurse cares for a client in labor who received an epidural anesthetic.

Flow Sheet			
	1030	1100	1115
Vital Signs	Temperature 98.6°F (37.0°C) Pulse (P) 90 bpm Respiration rate (RR) 18 breaths/min Blood pressure (BP) 130/80 mm Hg Pulse oximeter 98%	P 88 bpm RR 18 breaths/min BP 124/76 mm Hg Pulse oximeter 98%	P 80 bpm RR 18 breaths/min BP 98/56 mm Hg Pulse oximeter 96%
Nurse's Notes 10:30	Primigravid client with contractions lasting 60 seconds every 3 minutes. Cervical exam 5 cm, 0 station, 75% effaced. Category I tracing; fetal heart rate (FHR) 140 bpm. Requesting an epidural. 1000-mL fluid bolus started.		
11:30	Fluid bolus complete. Epidural placed by anesthesiology. Category I tracing FHR 145		
11:15	The client is vomiting.		

The nurse reviews the client trends.

➤ Complete the following sentences by using the list of options.

The nurse determines that the client is most likely experiencing [anaphylaxis / hypotension / spinal headache]

The first action the nurse should take is to [activate the emergency response team. / turn the client on their side. / dim the room lights.]

---

time-stamped data requiring you to make judgments about client care. Trends can be any of the new item formats listed in table 2.0 except bowtie. Figure 2.18 shows one example of a trend item.

Strategies for Answering Trend Items

- Review the scenario, paying special attention to changes in the client's status.
- Answer the question based on the item type and previously listed strategies.

Cognitive Levels of Test Items

The cognitive level of questions refers to the type of mental activity, such as critical thinking or making a nursing clinical judgment, required to answer the question. The cognitive levels used to write test items for the NCLEX-RN are derived from the original Bloom's taxonomy and Bloom's revised taxonomy of the cognitive domain (Anderson & Krathwohl, 2001); (Su, Osiek, & Starnes, 2005) (Table 2.2). The lowest level of the taxonomy is the *knowledge* (or *remember*) level and involves the ability to remember or recall facts. The next level of the cognitive domain, *comprehension* (or *understand*), requires you to interpret, explain, or understand the knowledge. The *application* (or *apply*) level involves using information that you remember and understand and can apply in new situations. *Analysis* (or *analyze*) requires recognizing and differentiating relationships between parts and using clinical reasoning and critical thinking skills. The next level of the cognitive domain is *evaluation* (or *evaluate*). Here, you must check data, critique information, or judge the outcome of nursing care. The final level of the cognitive domain in Bloom's revised taxonomy is *creation* (or *create*), formerly referred to as "synthesize" in the original taxonomy. At this level, you must be able to generate new approaches to nursing care or order nursing care based on available information.

Test items can be written to test all levels of the cognitive domain, but questions that are written for the NCLEX-RN exam are generally written at application levels and above because nursing requires the ability to apply knowledge to clinical situations, analyze data, think critically, prioritize information, make clinical decisions for client care, evaluate outcomes of nursing interventions or health care treatments, and create care plans based on specific client needs. This book and the questions on thePoint present questions at the application level and higher.

TABLE 2.2
Levels of the Cognitive Domain

- **Knowledge/Remember:** Recognizing, recalling
- **Comprehension/Understand:** Interpreting, exemplifying, classifying, summarizing, inferring, comparing, explaining
- **Application/Apply:** Executing, implementing, using knowledge appropriately in new or different situations
- **Analysis/Analyze:** Differentiating, organizing, attributing
- **Evaluation/Evaluate:** Checking, critiquing, judging against standards or protocols
- **Creation/Create:** Generating, planning, producing

TABLE 2.3
Keys to Answering Test Questions from Various Levels of the Cognitive Domain

Cognitive Level	Descriptions	Examples of Question Stems	Strategies for Answering Questions
Apply	Transfer knowledge from classroom to clinical practice.	To assess the breath sounds of a client with heart failure, where should the nurse place the stethoscope?	Use knowledge and understanding of how to auscultate breath sounds to assess a particular client.
	Use a formula or guidelines to perform calculations.	The client is to receive 1000 mL of fluids in 8 hours. The intravenous administration set delivers 15 drops per minute. The nurse should regulate the infusion to provide how many milliliters per minute?	Apply the appropriate formula to calculate an intravenous fluid drip rate.
	Apply knowledge and understanding to new situations.	Which nursing intervention is appropriate for this client?	Use knowledge and understanding about nursing interventions, and apply them to the client's particular situation.
		The nurse should instruct the client about which side effects that may occur when the client takes this drug? Select all that apply.	Apply knowledge and understanding about drug side effects to instruct a particular client.
		The nurse is teaching a client to use a metered-dose inhaler. Specify which information is indicated or not indicated to include in the teaching plan.	Use knowledge and understanding of the skill or procedure to teach a particular client.
		The nurse is communicating with an agitated client. Which communication technique is most appropriate?	Use knowledge and understanding of communication techniques to apply to this particular client.
Analyze	Organize clinical data into relevant parts in order to identify a client need, form a conclusion, or make a clinical decision.	Based on the clinical assessment, the nurse determines the client has which need?	Review the client's signs and symptoms to determine an appropriate nursing problem.
	Review all data to determine if sufficient data are available to make a decision.	Which finding indicates the need for nursing action?	Analyze data to determine which nursing action to take next.
	Analyze data to determine priorities.	Which client should the nurse care for first?	Organize information about a group of clients, and determine which client requires nursing care first.
	Distinguish relevant from irrelevant data.	Which findings require immediate follow-up?	Analyze data, and determine if additional data are needed.
	Determine what data are needed to plan or implement care.	Based on these findings, the nurse determines the client is in xxx stage of development.	Analyze data/findings, and determine the appropriate stage (of development).
		Which client is at risk for falls?	Analyze data about a group of clients with risk factors, and determine the client's risk.
		The client is expressing concerns about safety and the nurse observes restless behaviors. What is the nurse's best response?	Analyze clients' verbal and behavioral responses to determine what to say to the client.

TABLE 2.3
Keys to Answering Test Questions from Various Levels of the Cognitive Domain (*Continued*)

Cognitive Level	Descriptions	Examples of Question Stems	Strategies for Answering Questions
Evaluate	Make judgments about the effectiveness of nursing care.	Which statement indicates the client has understood the nurse's teaching?	Determine if the client understands the instructions based on the criteria established in the teaching plan.
	Use standards of care to determine the extent to which the client has met them.	Which finding indicates the intended therapeutic effect has occurred?	Evaluate the effectiveness of a nursing intervention, drug, or treatment based on the intended or expected outcome.
	Critique care given by others.	The nurse is observing an unlicensed assistive personnel (UAP) turn a client. Which observation indicates the nurse should intervene?	Evaluate the appropriateness of care given by others according to standards of care and knowledge of scope of practice.
		The nurse has administered nitroglycerin to a client with chest pain. In 30 seconds, the client's chest pain should be?	Judge effectiveness of outcome of a nursing action (administering a drug) based on expected therapeutic effect.
Create	Create or organize a unique or individualized plan, report, or protocol based on client needs.	Complete the diagram by circling the choices below to specify the condition the client is most likely experiencing, two actions to take immediately, and two parameters the nurse should monitor to assess the client's progress.	Develop a care plan with multiple components.

Clinical judgment refers to the higher-order information processing skills used to provide safe client care. Understanding the types of test items written at various levels of the cognitive domain and strategies to answer them is key (🔑) to success on the licensing exam. Examples of questions at higher levels of the cognitive domain are provided here to assist you in further understanding the types of questions used on the licensing exam and the strategies you can use to answer them. A summary of the cognitive levels, with examples of question stems and strategies for answering them, is given in Table 2.3.

Apply-Level Items

Apply-level items test your ability to apply knowledge to a specific scenario. These questions draw on your ability to know and understand nursing content and then apply this information to a specific scenario or situation (Fig. 2.19).

Strategies for Answering Apply-Level Items

- Read the question, and consider what information you already know and how that information should be used to answer this particular question.
- Consider how information you can recall should be applied to nursing care for the client described in the scenario for the question.
- Apply known formulas (divided dose/drip rate calculation), frameworks (e.g., Maslow's hierarchy, developmental stages, stages of moral development), and procedural steps (how to administer a particular medication) to answer the question posed in the new clinical situation (scenario). Pay close attention to client characteristics or care settings that may require different approaches to care.
- Double-check your answer by recognizing what information you are applying to answer the question.

FIGURE 2.19 Sample Apply-Level Item

The health care provider prescribes a serum lithium level tomorrow for a client with bipolar disorder, manic phase, who has been receiving lithium 300 mg orally three times daily for the past 5 days. At what time should the nurse plan to have the blood specimen obtained?
- ☐ 1. before bedtime
- ☐ 2. after lunch
- ☐ 3. before breakfast
- ☐ 4. during the afternoon

Analyze-Level Items

Questions at this level ask you to analyze data, examine clusters of symptoms, or scrutinize implementation plans and then make an interpretation or clinical decision. These questions can also ask about what additional information should be obtained to make a clinical decision or plan care (Fig. 2.20).

FIGURE 2.20 Sample Analyze-Level Item

Which statement(s) by the parent of a toddler should lead the nurse to suspect that the child is at risk for iron deficiency anemia? Select all that apply.

- ☐ 1. "He drinks over four glasses of milk per day."
- ☐ 2. "I can't keep enough apple juice in the house; he must drink over 10 oz (300 mL) per day."
- ☐ 3. "He refuses to eat more than two different kinds of vegetables."
- ☐ 4. "He doesn't like meat, but he'll eat small amounts of it."
- ☐ 5. "He sleeps 12 hours every night and takes a 2-hour nap."

Strategies for Answering Analyze-Level Items

- Identify the data presented in the scenario that lead you to draw a conclusion.
- Identify how the parts are related and how the nurse should assemble them to make a complete care plan.
- Determine if you have sufficient information to make a decision or interpretation.
- Review data from all sources possible (client's vital signs, client's responses to medication and treatments, chart information, client assignment list, etc.).
- Double-check your answer by determining that you have understood all of the components of care and have made the correct nursing decision based on those components.

Evaluate-Level Items

Evaluate-level items ask you to make judgments about care, determine the effectiveness of nursing care, or evaluate the extent to which an intended outcome has been achieved. Evaluation-level test items can also ask you to determine if the care given by others (client/family, health care team, health care provider) is appropriate (Fig. 2.21).

FIGURE 2.21 Sample Evaluate-Level Item

A nurse is reviewing the chart of a male client with cancer. The health care provider has prescribed filgrastim 400 mcg, subcutaneously once daily. What laboratory result indicates the medication has been effective?

Laboratory Results

Test	Result	Reference range
Hemoglobin	12.0 g/dL (120 g/L)	Males: 13–18 g/dL (130–180 g/L)
Platelet count	108,000/mm³ (108 × 10⁹/L)	4.5–10.5 × 10³ cells/mm³ (4.5–10.5 × 10⁹/L)
White blood cell (WBC) count	1600/mm³ (1.6 × 10⁹/L)	140,000–450,000/mm³ (140–450 × 10⁹/L)
Absolute neutrophil count (ANC)	Less than 1000/mm³ (1 × 10⁹/L)	2500–8000 per mm³ (2.5–8 × 10⁹/L)

- ☐ 1. Hemoglobin is 16 g/dL (160 g/L).
- ☐ 2. WBC count is 3500/mm³ (3.5 × 10⁹/L).
- ☐ 3. Platelet count is 200,000/mm³ (200 × 10⁹/L).
- ☐ 4. Red blood cell count is 4.3 million/mm³ (4.3 × 10¹²/L).

Strategies for Answering Evaluate-Level Items

- Review the question to determine what is to be evaluated. Consider if the question is asking you to verify a client's understanding or if the question is asking if a particular outcome has been attained.
- Before looking at possible answers, consider the accepted standard of care, the ideal level of care, or the intended outcome.
- Match the answers with your understanding of the standard of care.
- Double-check your answer with the scenario and expected standard of care in that scenario.

Create-Level Items

Create-level test items require you to synthesize information obtained from a client, family, or clinical situation and develop a new, client-centered, or unique or complete approach to solving the clinical problem. For example, bowtie items may be considered create-level items because they require you to organize a condition, actions, and parameters into a coherent pattern (Fig. 2.22).

FIGURE 2.22 Sample Create-Level Item

The nurse cares for a 72-year-old female client with a history of alcohol use disorder on the medical-surgical unit the day after a left knee placement.

Nurse's Notes

Postoperative Day 2

0700:
The client was agitated, reported sleeping little last night, and refused breakfast. The client was given oral (PO) pain medication for left knee pain that was rated as a 6 on a scale of 0 to 10.

0800:
The nurse entered the room because the client was heard from the hall to be shouting "get the spiders out of here!" The client was found highly agitated, confused, and oriented to person only and had moderate hand and tongue tremors. Beads of sweat were visible on the client's forehead. A pool of vomit was found by the bed. The left knee dressing was also found on the floor. The incision remains intact. The client's spouse, returning from the cafeteria, verifies that the client's typical alcohol consumption included drinking a bottle of vodka a day. Vital signs are temperature 100°F (37.8°C); pulse 116 bpm; respiration rate 24 breaths/min; blood pressure 168/94 mm Hg; and pulse oximetry reading 96% in room air. The health care provider and the rapid response team were paged.

The nurse reviews the client's changes and updates the plan of care.

➤ Complete the diagram by circling the choices below to specify the condition the client is most likely experiencing, two actions to take immediately, and two parameters the nurse should monitor to assess the client's progress.

Action to Take	Potential Conditions	Parameters to Monitor
Administer intramuscular (IM) haloperidol	Korsakoff psychosis	Blood alcohol levels
Perform gastric lavage	Delirium tremens	Alcohol withdrawal assessment scores
Administer intravenous (IV) diazepam	Wernicke encephalopathy	Vital signs
Initiate seizure precautions	Alcohol overdose	Memory changes
Administer PO thiamine		Glasgow Coma Scale score

Strategies for Answering Create-Level Test Items

- Read the question to determine what is to be developed or organized.
- Consider all of the elements necessary to have a complete plan of care, discharge plan, etc.
- Understand what is and is not appropriate to include in the plan being created, and rule out inappropriate aspects of care for the client or situation presented in the scenario.
- Double-check your answer by reviewing the appropriateness of each of the elements in the plan you have developed.

Nursing Clinical Judgment and Case Studies

The NCSBN defines clinical judgment as "the observed outcome of critical thinking and decision making. It is an iterative process that uses nursing knowledge to observe and assess presenting situations, identify a prioritized client concern, and generate the best possible evidence-based solutions in order to deliver safe client care (NGN News, Winter 2019)." Studies of newly employed nurses indicate that a lack of clinical judgment skills is contributing to a significant number of client errors (Muntean, 2012). Because content knowledge by itself is not sufficient to ensure critical thinking and accurate decision-making, the NCSBN has updated testing procedures to better test new graduates' clinical judgment skills.

Nursing Clinical Judgment Measurement Model

The Next Generation NCLEX-RN uses the NCSBN's Clinical Judgment Measurement Model as a framework to guide the development of items to test clinical judgment in this large-scale, high-stakes examination (NGN News, Spring 2019). Figure 2.23 depicts the most current version of the model. As with other thinking process models, such as the nursing process or Tanner's (2006) model of clinical judgment in nursing, the steps in the NCSBN Clinical Judgment Measurement Model information-processing framework are sequential and iterative. Layer 3 shows the 6-steps of the clinical judgment process. Layer 4 of the model shows environmental and individual factors that add context to a clinical encounter. These factors influence the clinical judgment process meaning nurses make different decisions based on the combination of multiple factors. You can expect to find environmental factors included in clinical judgment questions. Case studies may unfold over a short time period or over weeks, and care settings may change.

Case studies on the NCLEX-RN will test the 6-steps of the NCSBN Clinical Judgment Measurement Model in order (NGN News, Spring 2020). Beginning with step 1, candidates will review a clinical scenario and the client's electronic medical record (EMR). The scenario will include an overview sentence that includes

FIGURE 2.23 NCSBN Clinical Judgment Measurement Model

The NCSBN Clinical Judgment Measurement Model

Layer 0: Client Needs → Clinical Judgment → Clinical Decisions (Satisfied)

Layer 1: Clinical Judgment

Layer 2: Form Hypotheses → Refine Hypotheses → Evaluation (Not Satisfied loops back)

Layer 3: Recognize Cues | Analyze Cues | Prioritize Hypotheses | Generate Solutions | Take Actions | Evaluate Outcomes

Layer 4:
- Environmental Factor Examples: Environment, Client Observation, Resources, Medical Records, Consequences & Risks, Time Pressure, Task Complexity, Cultural Consideration
- Individual Factor Examples: Knowledge, Skills, Specialty, Candidate Characteristics, Prior Experience, Level of Experience

Nursing Process: Assessment → Analysis → Planning → Implementation → Evaluation

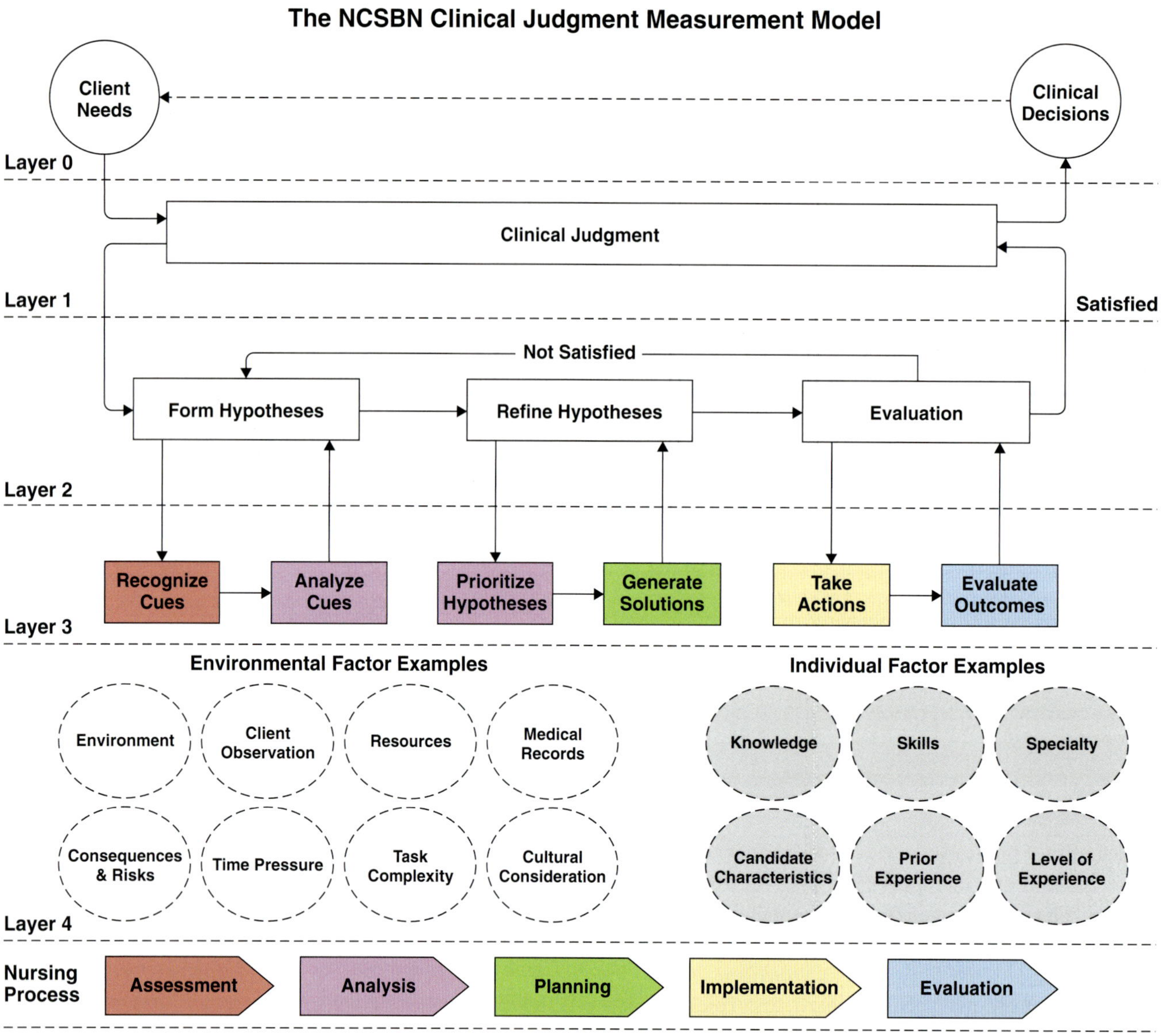

Copyright by the National Council of State Boards of Nursing, Inc. All rights reserved.

a brief description of the client, setting, and reason for the encounter before the medical record. Candidates will then be asked a question that tests their ability to recognize cues. After the candidate submits the answer, the next question in the case study appears. Each question in the case study is numbered to let candidates know which of the six steps they are on. The medical record will appear again with each question. New information may be added to the record at any point. Candidates must answer the questions in the order they are presented and may not go back and change answers. Figures 2.24 through 2.29 show an example of a case study. Keep in mind that item types to test the different steps will vary.

Recognize Cues

The first step of a case study involves observing and assessing the client and determining what matters most (Fig. 2.24). The nurse obtains information from the client's health record (history, labs, tests, orders), notes vital sign trends, and identifies signs and symptoms. In this step, the nurse differentiates relevant from irrelevant data, differentiates normal from abnormal findings, and recognizes what is most important and urgent. These questions typically ask the candidate to identify what the most important findings are, or which findings are most urgent to follow up on.

Strategies for Answering Recognize Cues Questions

- Review all pages of the medical record. Pay close attention to the environmental factors. If there are entries for more than one time point, notice any changes in the client's status.
- Determine which values are normal for this client and which are abnormal or unexpected.
- From the abnormal findings, determine if the issues you are seeing represent an acute or chronic

NCLEX-RN® Test Questions and Strategies for Answering Them   29

FIGURE 2.24 Sample Recognize Cues

Nurse's Notes

Today: 0900
A 75-year-old client was brought to the emergency department by their spouse who reports the client is experiencing sudden-onset drowsiness. The client has had a urinary tract infection treated with oral cephalexin for the past 5 days. The client's pupils are equal, round, and respond to light, and the client is oriented to time and place.
Admission vital signs are temperature (T) 101.8°F (38.8°C); pulse (P) 92 bpm; respiration rate (RR) 28 breaths/min; and blood pressure (BP) 88/40 mm Hg. Oxygen saturation per pulse oximeter is 95%.

➤ Highlight the findings that require the nurse to follow up. Answer choices have been underlined.

Nurse's Notes

Today: 0900
A <u>75-year-old</u> client was brought to the emergency department by their spouse who reports the client is experiencing sudden-onset <u>drowsiness</u>. The client has had a <u>urinary tract infection</u> treated with oral cephalexin for the past 5 days. The client's pupils are equal, round, and respond to light, and the client is oriented to time and place.
Admission vital signs are <u>temperature (T) 101.8°F (38.8°C)</u>; <u>pulse (P) 92 bpm</u>; <u>respiration rate (RR) 28 breaths/min</u>; and <u>blood pressure (BP) 88/40 mm Hg</u>. <u>Oxygen saturation per pulse oximeter is 95%.</u>

---

problem. If it is a chronic problem, is it stable or has it been exacerbated?
- Of the findings, determine which are most serious and have the greatest potential to lead to a bad outcome.
- Read the question, and select the answers that best match your assessment. Reread the scenario as needed.

Analyze Cues

In step 2, the nurse analyzes data by clustering it into patterns and thinking through what could be happening (Fig. 2.25). They look for consistencies and inconsistencies in the client's presentation and history. The nurse must identify relevant pathophysiology, determine why findings are concerning, and consider possible causes. This step might ask questions like which client findings are consistent with a specific condition or what risk factors does the client have for a specific problem?

Strategies for Answering Analyzing Cues Questions

- Review the case, and determine if any new information has been added.
- Read the question, and consider how you answered the first question in the case study. Does the question match your original assessment? For instance, if you thought the respiratory assessment findings were most urgent, does this question build on your initial thoughts and ask about a respiratory problem? If not, reread the scenario.
- Pay close attention to the item types. If the question is a multiple-response select all that apply or multiple-response matrix, avoid guessing, and only select options you are reasonably sure about.

FIGURE 2.25 Sample Analyze Cues

The nurse is caring for a 75-year-old male client who has been brought to the emergency department by the client's spouse.

Nurse's Notes

Today: 0900
A 75-year-old client was brought to the emergency department by their spouse who reports the client is experiencing sudden-onset drowsiness. The client has had a urinary tract infection treated with oral cephalexin for the past 5 days. The client's pupils are equal, round, and respond to light, and the client is oriented to time and place.
Admission vital signs are temperature (T) 101.8°F (38.8°C); pulse (P) 92 bpm; respiration rate (RR) 28 breaths/min; and blood pressure (BP) 88/40 mm Hg. Oxygen saturation per pulse oximeter is 95%.

➤ For each assessment finding below, specify if the finding is consistent with urinary tract infection or septic shock. Each finding may support more than one disease process.

Client Findings	Urinary Tract Infection	Septic Shock
T 101.8°F (38.8°C)	☐	☐
RR 28 breaths/min	☐	☐
BP 98/40 mm Hg	☐	☐
P 94 bpm	☐	☐
Oxygen saturation 91%	☐	☐

Note: Each column must have at least one response option selected.

FIGURE 2.26 Sample Prioritize Hypotheses

The nurse is caring for a 75-year-old male client who has been brought to the emergency department by the client's spouse.

Nurse's Notes

Today: 0900
A 75-year-old client was brought to the emergency department by their spouse who reports the client is experiencing sudden-onset drowsiness. The client has had a urinary tract infection treated with oral cephalexin for the past 5 days. The client's pupils are equal, round, and respond to light, and the client is oriented to time and place.
Admission vital signs are temperature (T) 101.8°F (38.8°C); pulse (P) 92 bpm; respiration rate (RR) 28 breaths/min; and blood pressure (BP) 88/40 mm Hg. Oxygen saturation per pulse oximeter is 95%.

0930:
Vital signs are T 101.8°F (38.8°C); P 96 bpm; RR 28 breaths/min; BP 84/38 mm Hg; and oxygen saturation 91%.
The client is becoming confused and unable to follow commands. The client voided 150 mL of cloudy urine.

➤ Complete the following sentence by choosing from the list of options.

The client is at risk for developing [stroke / hypoxia / renal failure / septic shock]

as evidenced by the client's [vital signs. / oxygen level. / neurologic assessment. / urinary output.]

Prioritize Hypotheses

Step 3 asks about where the nurse should start when planning care for the client. The nurse must narrow down the possibilities from step 2 to the one or two things the client is most likely experiencing, the client's greatest risk, or the most urgent priority (Fig. 2.26). This step of the case study might ask what condition is most likely causing the client's symptoms, what is the client's greatest risk, or which problem should the nurse address first. This question may also ask for a rationale for why you selected a condition or priority, or it may ask you what might happen if the nurse does not act.

Strategies for Answering Prioritize Hypotheses Questions

- Review the case, and determine if any new information has been added.
- Read the question, and consider how you answered question 2 in the case study. Does this question build on patterns you identified in the last question? If not, reread the question.
- Apply decision-making frameworks you may have learned, remembering to prioritize physiological and safety needs.
- Pay close attention to the item types. If the question is a multiple-response select all that apply, avoid guessing, and only select options you are reasonably sure about.

Generate Solutions

In step 4, nurses generate solutions by beginning to create a plan of care. They determine outcomes and select multiple appropriate interventions while avoiding interventions that are not helpful or are potentially harmful. They also gather more information if needed. It is very common for more information to be added to the medical record at this stage of the case. The client might receive a medical diagnosis or test results might return. This question will typically require a response type with multiple answer options because most problems require more than one intervention.

Strategies for Answering Generate Solutions Questions

- Review the case, and determine if any new information has been added.
- Read the question stem, and consider how you answered question 3 in the case study. Does this question reflect the priority you identified in the last question? If not, reread the question.
- Consider what interventions you want to include in the plan of care before reading the options provided. Also consider if you know that there are things you have learned that would be harmful and should be avoided.
- Review the answer options, and select the ones that best match the interventions you thought were needed.
- Pay close attention to the item types. If the question is a multiple-response select all that apply, grouping, or multiple-response matrix, avoid guessing, and only select options you are reasonably sure about.

FIGURE 2.27 Sample Generate Solutions

The nurse is caring for a 75-year-old male client who has been brought to the emergency department by the client's spouse.

Nurse's Notes

Today: 0900
A 75-year-old client was brought to the emergency department by their spouse who reports the client is experiencing sudden-onset drowsiness. The client has had a urinary tract infection treated with oral cephalexin for the past 5 days. The client's pupils are equal, round, and respond to light, and the client is oriented to time and place.
Admission vital signs are temperature (T) 101.8°F (38.8°C); pulse (P) 92 bpm; respiration rate (RR) 28 breaths/min; and blood pressure (BP) 88/40 mm Hg. Oxygen saturation per pulse oximeter is 95%.

0930:
Vital signs are T 101.8°F (38.8°C); P 96 bpm; RR 28 breaths/min; BP 84/38 mm Hg; and oxygen saturation 91%.
The client is becoming confused and unable to follow commands. The client voided 150 mL of cloudy urine.

Orders

- Start oxygen at 2 L per minute per nasal cannula
- 5% dextrose in normal saline (D5NS) 1000 mL every 8 hours
- Vancomycin 500 mg intravenously (IV) every 6 hours
- Norepinephrine 0.01 to 3.3 mcg/kg per minute IV infusion
- Insert an indwelling urinary catheter
- Urine culture and sensitivity stat
- Arterial blood gas (ABG) stat
- Blood urea nitrogen (BUN) and creatinine

The nurse reviews the health care provider's orders and develops a care plan.

➤ Which nursing action(s) should the nurse include when developing a care plan and preparing to implement the health care provider's orders? Select all that apply.

☐	1. Start a peripheral IV.
☐	2. Start an arterial line.
☐	3. Question the order for oxygen at 2 L per minute.
☐	4. Place leads for continuous cardiac monitoring.
☐	5. Question the order for the indwelling catheter.
☐	6. Maintain accurate intake/output records.
☐	7. Explain the plan of care to the client and spouse.

Take Action

In step 5, the nurse takes action and implements the plan of care (Fig. 2.28). This step may take one aspect of step 4 and break it down into how specifically the nurse requests a prescription, performs a skill or procedure, administers a medication, communicates with team members, teaches clients, or documents care. Like step 4, it is very common for more information to be added to the medical record at this point, such as a new order. A step 5 question might ask which action(s) the nurse should take immediately, or what step(s) to take when performing a procedure or administering a medication. These steps will focus on using clinical judgment rather than listing the order to perform steps that may have been found in nursing textbooks.

Strategies for Answering Take Action Questions

- Review the case, and determine if any new information has been added.
- Read the question, and consider how you answered question 4 in the case study.
- Pay close attention to client characteristics. Does the client have an allergy, a learning barrier, or a physical characteristic that will influence how the plan of care must be implemented?
- If the question involves team members, consider the client's needs in relation to the expertise and training of those team members. Remember that the nurse cannot delegate assessment, teaching, or evaluation.
- Pay close attention to the item types. If the question is a multiple-response, select all that apply, grouping, multiple-response matrix, or highlighting item, avoid guessing, and only select options you are reasonably sure of.

FIGURE 2.28 Sample Take Action

The nurse is caring for a 75-year-old male client who has been brought to the emergency department by the client's spouse.

Nurse's Notes

Today: 0900
A 75-year-old client was brought to the emergency department by their spouse who reports the client is experiencing sudden-onset drowsiness. The client has had a urinary tract infection treated with oral cephalexin for the past 5 days. The client's pupils are equal, round, and respond to light, and the client is oriented to time and place.
Admission vital signs are temperature (T) 101.8°F (38.8°C); pulse (P) 92 bpm; respiration rate (RR) 28 breaths/min; and blood pressure (BP) 88/40 mm Hg. Oxygen saturation per pulse oximeter is 95%.

0930:
Vital signs are T 101.8°F (38.8°C); P 96 bpm; RR 28 breaths/min; BP 84/38 mm Hg; and oxygen saturation 91%.
The client is becoming confused and unable to follow commands. The client voided 150 mL of cloudy urine.

Orders

- Start oxygen at 2 L per minute per nasal cannula
- 5% dextrose in normal saline (D5NS) 1000 mL every 8 hours
- Vancomycin 500 mg intravenously (IV) every 6 hours
- Norepinephrine 0.01 to 3.3 mcg/kg per minute IV infusion
- Insert an indwelling urinary catheter
- Urine culture and sensitivity stat
- Arterial blood gas (ABG) stat
- Blood urea nitrogen (BUN) and creatinine

The nurse has established IV access and inserted the indwelling urinary catheter.

➢ Highlight the three orders the nurse should implement right away. Answer choices have been underlined.

Orders

- <u>Start oxygen at 2 L per minute per nasal cannula</u>
- <u>5% dextrose in normal saline (D5NS) 1000 mL every 8 hours</u>
- <u>Vancomycin 500 mg intravenously (IV) every 6 hours</u>
- <u>Norepinephrine 0.01 to 3.3 mcg/kg per minute IV infusion</u>
- Insert an indwelling urinary catheter
- Urine culture and sensitivity
- Arterial blood gas (ABG) stat
- Blood urea nitrogen (BUN) and creatinine

Evaluate Outcomes

In step 6, the nurse compares observed and desired outcomes, recognizes changes in the client's status, and determines the effectiveness of actions (Fig. 2.29). It is very common for reassessment data to be added at this point to the case study. If no new data is provided, the question will most likely ask what data would the nurse gather to determine the effectiveness of the plan of care. Other questions might ask what conclusions does the nurse make after implementing the treatment plan, which findings suggest the teaching is understood, which assessments indicate that the client's condition has improved, stayed the same, or declined, or what additional intervention should the nurse implement based on the findings.

Strategies for Answering Evaluate Outcomes Questions

- Review the case, and determine if any new information has been added.
- Read the question, and consider how you answered questions 4 and 5 in the case study. Does the case unfold the way you anticipated based on the solutions and actions you selected? If not, reread the scenario.
- Pay close attention to the item types. If the question is a multiple-response, select all that apply, highlighting item, or multiple-response matrix, avoid guessing, and only select options you are reasonably sure of.

FIGURE 2.29 Sample Evaluate Outcomes

The nurse is caring for a 75-year-old male client who has been brought to the emergency department by the client's spouse.

Nurse's Notes

Today: 0900
A 75-year-old client was brought to the emergency department by their spouse who reports the client is experiencing sudden-onset drowsiness. The client has had a urinary tract infection treated with oral cephalexin for the past 5 days. The client's pupils are equal, round, and respond to light, and the client is oriented to time and place.
Admission vital signs are temperature (T) 101.8°F (38.8°C); pulse (P) 92 bpm; respiration rate (RR) 28 breaths/min; and blood pressure (BP) 88/40 mm Hg. Oxygen saturation per pulse oximeter is 95%.

0930:
Vital signs are T 101.8°F (38.8°C); P 96 bpm; RR 28 breaths/min; BP 84/38 mm Hg; and oxygen saturation 91%.
The client is becoming confused and unable to follow commands. The client voided 150 mL of cloudy urine.

Orders

- Start oxygen at 2 L per minute per nasal cannula
- 5% dextrose in normal saline (D5NS) 1000 mL every 8 hours
- Vancomycin 500 mg intravenously (IV) every 6 hours
- Norepinephrine 0.01 to 3.3 mcg/kg per minute IV infusion
- Insert an indwelling urinary catheter
- Urine culture and sensitivity
- Arterial blood gas (ABG) stat
- Blood urea nitrogen (BUN) and creatinine

Vital Signs

Vital Signs	0900	0930	1000
HR	92 bpm	96 bpm	94 bpm
BP systolic	88 mm Hg	84 mm Hg	92 mm Hg
BP diastolic	40 mm Hg	38 mm Hg	50 mm Hg
RR	28 breaths/min	28 breaths/min	28 breaths/min
Oxygen saturation	95%	91%	94%
Temp	101.8°F (38.8°C)		101.8°F (38.8°C)
Urinary output	Voided 150 mL		Per catheter 40 mL

➤ The nurse administered norepinephrine at 0930 and reassesses the client's condition at 1000. Which vital sign(s) indicate the order for norepinephrine has been effective? Select all that apply.

- ☐ 1. HR
- ☐ 2. Systolic BP
- ☐ 3. Diastolic BP
- ☐ 4. RR
- ☐ 5. Oxygen saturation
- ☐ 6. Temp
- ☐ 7. Urinary output

REFERENCES

Anderson, L. W., & Krathwohl, D., eds. (2001). *A taxonomy for learning, teaching, and assessing: A revision of Bloom's taxonomy of educational objectives.* New York: Longman.

Muntean, W. J. (2012). Nursing clinical decision-making: A literature review. Available at: https://www.ncsbn.org/11507.htm

NGN News. (Winter, 2022). https://www.ncsbn.org/16640.htm

NGN News. (Summer, 2021). https://www.ncsbn.org/15991.htm

NGN News. (Spring, 2021). https://www.ncsbn.org/15800.htm

NGN News. (Spring, 2020). https://www.ncsbn.org/14425.htm

NGN News. (Winter, 2019). https://www.ncsbn.org/13342.htm

NGN News. (Spring, 2019). https://www.ncsbn.org/13444.htm

Su, W. M., Osiek, P. J., & Starnes, B. (2005). Using the revised Bloom's Taxonomy in the clinical laboratory. *Nurse Educator,* 30(3), 117–122. https://www.ncbi.nlm.nih.gov/pubmed/15900205

Tanner, C. A. (2006). Thinking like a nurse: A research-based model of clinical judgment in nursing. *Journal of Nursing Education,* 45(6), 204–211. https://www.ncbi.nlm.nih.gov/pubmed/16780008

Study Skills for Taking the NCLEX-RN® and Other Nursing Exams

INTRODUCTION

Studying for the NCLEX-RN or exams offered at your school requires careful planning and preparation. Evidence from research studies indicates that the students who do best on exams have done three things: (1) learned the content in a way that they can apply it to nursing practice (deep learning), (2) learned how to control their anxiety, and (3) fine-tuned their test-taking skills (Thomas & Baker, 2011). This chapter provides information about each of these factors associated with exam success.

You can begin developing your study skills by following these five steps:

- Assess your study skills.
- Make a study plan.
- Develop effective test-taking strategies.
- Practice managing test anxiety.
- Evaluate your progress.

Use these five steps as you take your first test in nursing school. Refine your test-taking strategies as you evaluate your progress at each step of the way so that when you are ready to take the licensing exam, you will be an experienced and successful test taker. Use the Personal Study Plan in Table 3.1 to help develop your own study plan.

ASSESS YOUR STUDY SKILLS

The first step toward test success is to determine your strengths and limitations. Even students who have been successful throughout their academic life, and nurses who are excellent caregivers, have areas in which they need improvement. Be honest with yourself as you assess your own study needs. These steps can help you in your assessment:

- *Review your success in your nursing program.* Review your grades in science courses and the courses in the nursing curriculum. Success on the NCLEX-RN and other nursing exams tends to correlate with grades (grade point average) achieved in science and nursing courses. Subjects in which you received high grades, that you found easy to learn, or in which you have had additional clinical practice or work experience are likely to be areas of strength. On the other hand, subjects you found difficult to learn (or in which you did not achieve high grades) should be areas for concentrated review. Also, consider content areas that you have not studied for a while. Recent coursework will be the most familiar and, therefore, may require the least amount of study. Candidates should have a strong mastery of materials learned in fundamental skills or assessment courses, which are typically offered early in a program. All students, even students who have achieved success in nursing courses, benefit from identifying areas requiring study and spending time practicing test-taking skills. You also can use the practice exams in this book to identify areas needing further study. Begin with the subjects you find most difficult or in which you have the least confidence.

- *Read the NCLEX-RN test plan.* The test plan includes the common activities new nurses perform. Assess your knowledge level of these activities, and create a study plan for the areas that you feel you did not master in your nursing program. Test plans are updated every 3 years and can be found on the National Council of State Board of Nursing website (www.ncsbn.org/testplans.htm).

- *Assess your test-taking skills.* Using effective test-taking skills contributes to exam success. What have you done in the past to make you confident about taking a test? How do you feel when you are in an exam situation? What has worked in the past to help you be successful? Review these strategies to build on past successes and work on problem areas. Consider additional strategies suggested in the section "Develop Effective Test-Taking Strategies," page XX. You can practice these skills

TABLE 3.1
Personal Study Plan

Assess Study Needs

1. **Review your success in nursing school.**
   - I did best in these courses:
     _____
     _____
   - I needed to study harder in these courses:
     _____
     _____
   - I took these courses near the beginning of the curriculum:
     _____
     _____
   - I scored best on these practice exams in this book:
     _____
     _____
   - I am not satisfied with my scores on these practice exams in this book:
     _____
     _____
   - I need further study in these content areas:
     _____
     _____
   - I need further study in these areas of the nursing process:
     _____
     _____
   - I need further study to understand the steps of making a clinical judgment using the National Council of State Boards of Nursing's Clinical Judgment Measurement Model:
     _____
     _____
   - I need further study in these areas of client needs:
     _____
     _____

2. **Review your test-taking skills.**
   - I can identify the components of a test question.
   - I read questions carefully before answering.
   - I can make reasonable guesses if I am not certain of the correct answer.
   - I understand the National Council State Boards of Nursing Clinical Judgment Measurement Model (CJMM), and I can answer the three types of Next Generation (NextGen) questions: case studies, bow-ties, and trends.

3. **I can recognize patterns of why I miss questions.**

4. **I can pace myself to complete questions in the allotted time.**

5. **Review your test-anxiety management skills.**
   - I can do relaxation and deep-breathing exercises.
   - I can visualize success.
   - I can give myself positive feedback.
   - I can concentrate for extended periods of time.

6. **Review your computer skills.**
   - I am able to use a computer to read and answer test questions.

Develop a Study Plan
- I will study in this location:
  _____
  _____
- I will study at these times and dates:
  _____
  _____
- I have assembled all of the materials I need to study:
  _____
  _____
- I will study with a study group:
  _____
  _____

Evaluate Progress
- I have completed the practice tests in this book.
- I have completed the comprehensive tests in this book.
- I need to improve my scores in these areas:
  _____
  _____
- I am prepared to take the NCLEX-RN examination.

by simulating the testing situation using the practice tests and comprehensive exams in this review book and on the National Council of State Boards of Nursing's website: https://www.nclex.com/nclex-practice-exam.htm.

- *Assess your ability to take tests that require application, analysis, and evaluation.* Test questions used on the licensing exam are written at higher levels of the cognitive domain. Many candidates' experience with taking tests has come from taking "teacher-made" tests—tests developed by the faculty at your school of nursing. These tests are commonly written to test students' knowledge and understanding of course content and may not include questions that require you to apply and analyze nursing actions or make clinical judgments. Additionally, there may be types of questions on the computer-administered licensing exam that faculty cannot replicate in their exams. Finally, some students are able to "second-guess" the teacher and use this ability to their advantage when taking teacher-made classroom tests. However, it is not as easy to anticipate test questions on standardized and licensing exams, and you will need to develop skills that will help you think critically when presented with an unfamiliar situation. As you prepare to take the licensing exam, spend time on questions where you need to "figure out" the best approach to answering the question. You can use the questions in this book and on thePoint, as well as tests offered by the NCSBN, to be sure you understand the difference between questions that require only recall and understanding and those that require you to apply information to provide client care, make clinical judgments, and initiate nursing actions. Use the *Content Mastery and Test-Taking Skill Self-Analysis* table at the end of this chapter and in the back of this book to identify your ability to answer questions in the higher levels of the cognitive domain.

- *Assess your ability to answer questions that require you to think critically and make clinical judgments.* The licensing exam tests more than just your knowledge of nursing content, it also tests your ability to *use* that knowledge to make decisions about safe nursing care. Can you answer questions that require you to use your knowledge and apply it to a specific client situation? Can you use the six steps of the NCSBN Clinical Judgment Measurement Model to answer questions that require you to make clinical judgments?

- *Assess your language skills.* If English or French is not your primary language, or if you do not have well-developed reading and comprehension skills, you may require additional practice in reading and answering NCLEX-RN–style test questions. If you are one of these persons, plan additional time to practice reading and answering questions, time yourself when answering questions, and validate that you understand the question correctly. If necessary, seek assistance. As you study, keep a list of words you do not understand, and practice using them.

- *Assess your ability to take timed tests.* Are you always the last one to finish a test? Do you request additional time to complete a test? If so, you will want to practice taking timed tests and doing your best, while completing as many questions as possible. The licensing exam is designed to be completed in 5 hours; only questions completed within that time frame will be scored. As you use the practice questions and tests in this book, time yourself and, if needed, determine ways that you can increase your speed without sacrificing accuracy. The comprehensive tests in this book have been intentionally designed with the minimum (70 questions) and maximum (135) number of operational (scored) questions on the licensing exam; time yourself as you take these tests. A typical response time on the exam is under 2 minutes per question.

- *Assess your skills for taking computer-administered exams.* Although previous computer experience is not necessary to take the NCLEX-RN, you should familiarize yourself with the differences between taking a paper-and-pencil exam and taking exams administered by the computer. If you have not used a computer before, find a learning resource center at your college, university, library, or hospital where you can become familiar with basic computer keyboard skills. *Lippincott NCLEX-RN® PassPoint*, which simulates the computerized NCLEX-RN, offers you the opportunity to practice taking computer-administered test questions. See the inside cover of this textbook for a code to activate a free 7-day trial for *Lippincott NCLEX-RN® PassPoint*. Use these questions to practice reading questions from the computer screen and become acquainted with answering questions in a computerized format. If you are accustomed to underlining key words or making notes in the margins of paper-and-pencil tests, adapt these strategies to reading and answering the questions on the computer screen. Also, be sure that you can use a drop-down calculator to answer questions requiring the use of math skills. Use the tutorial offered by the testing company, Pearson VUE, at http://www.pearsonvue.com/nclex/, to learn how the test questions will be computer-administered. You can also purchase access to two tests offered by the NCSBN at https://www.nclex.com/nclex-practice-exam.htm. These tests are comprised of questions used on previous exams and simulate the types of questions and the amount of time of the actual exam.

- *Assess your reason(s) for not answering the test question correctly.* There are many reasons why students select an incorrect answer. These could include not reading the question carefully (not reading all of the words in the sentence; missing key words), not reading the options carefully, not knowing the answer (lack of knowledge or deep learning), not recognizing the rationale for the correct answer, guessing, not being rested, or dealing with health problems when taking the exam.

- Another reason for not answering the questions correctly is that you may be experiencing anxiety. Students who do not manage their anxiety during the exam are likely to change their answers (George, Muller, & Bartz, 2016). If you find yourself changing your answer during tests you are taking now or when taking the practice tests in this book, review the questions for which you changed the answer, and determine the underlying reason for the change.

- The most important thing you can do is assess the *reason* why you are not answering questions correctly. Evidence about test taking indicates that understanding the *pattern* of missed questions is essential to changing how you study. Using *Exam Wrappers* is one way to develop an awareness of the pattern of why you have not answered a question correctly. Schuler and Chung (2019) recommend using a questionnaire such as the one in Table 3.3 after each test you take. For the tests you take during your academic program, request a meeting with your faculty, and use the questionnaire in Table 3.3 or the tear-out copy of the *Content Mastery and Test-Taking Skill Self-Analysis* table at the back of the book. You can make as many copies of this self-analysis questionnaire as you need. You should also use this questionnaire for *each* test in this book to determine the reason for each incorrect answer. As you reflect on the results of using the exam wrapper questionnaire, consider how much you studied, your attendance and participation in the class, and if you studied alone or in a group. The final step is to use what you have learned from the exam wrapper to revise your study habits. When using exam wrappers, students tend to improve their study skills and achieve higher test scores (Sethares & Asselin, 2021).

- *Assess your risk for not passing the licensing exam.* Factors associated with not passing the licensing exam are listed in Table 3.2; having more factors is associated with a higher risk for exam failure. Note that the three top risk factors are poverty, low science grade point average prior to the nursing major, and repeating college science courses. It is important that you identify your risk for not passing the licensing exam and take advantage of all resources available to assist you to lower your risk. Interventions include forming study groups, attending review sessions, establishing effective study habits, practicing test taking on a regular basis, determining reasons for not answering questions correctly, and taking action steps to improve knowledge of nursing content and test-taking strategies. The earlier in the academic program that you can identify your risk, use interventions, and monitor your progress, the more likely you are to minimize your risk and improve your chance of passing!

TABLE 3.2 Factors Associated with Risk for Failure on NCLEX-RN

- Income at or below the poverty level
- Science grade point average (GPA) (low grades in science courses—biology, chemistry, microbiology)
- Repeating college science courses
- English is a second language
- Low score on standardized admission tests (SAT, ACT)
- Low score on standardized progression tests (ATI, HESI)
- Failure of one or more nursing prerequisite courses (more courses, higher risk)
- Failure of one or more nursing courses (more courses, higher risk)
- GPA (<3.0)
- Working (more hours worked, higher risk)
- Lack of sufficient support to care for children while in school or studying
- First in family to attend college

MAKE A STUDY PLAN

Once you have identified areas of strength and areas needing further study, develop a specific plan and begin to study regularly. Students who study a small amount of content over a longer period of time tend to have higher success rates than students who wait until the last few weeks before the exam and then "cram." Additionally, if you are at risk for not passing the exam (see Table 3.3), participate in study groups, tutoring sessions, or other resources offered at your school of nursing. Remember, the longer you wait to take the licensing exam after becoming eligible, the less likely you are to be successful on the exam (Eich & O'Neill, 2007). So, plan to start studying while you are still in your nursing program.

Here are some study suggestions to consider:

- *Identify a place for study.* The area should be quiet and have room for your books and papers or electronic study materials. Do not study while playing music, responding to text messages, or listening to the television; background noise is distracting and will not be allowed at the actual NCLEX-RN testing site. Your area for study might be in your home, at your nursing school, at your

(text continues on page 13)

TABLE 3.3
Content Mastery and Test-Taking Skill Self-Analysis

Use the chart below to identify the subject matter and the reason you missed the question. Place a checkmark in the columns for questions you did not answer correctly and why, and then total each column. The key (🔑) to effective review is to understand your knowledge deficits and focus additional review on those subjects and reasons for not answering the question.

Review Strategies

Test Number	Subject (care of childbearing family, care of children, care of adults, care of clients with psychiatric disorders and mental health problems)	Score

Total number of questions missed: _____

Use the chart below to identify the subject matter and the reason you missed the question. Use the following codes to note the client need area of the question you missed:
MC, management of care; SI, safety and infection control; HM, health promotion and maintenance; PA, physiological adaptation; PI, psychosocial integrity; PP, pharmacological and parenteral therapies; RR, reduction of risk potential; BC, basic care and comfort.

Question #	Client need	Misread/ Misunderstood the question	Missed key word(s)	Did not read all options	Changed answer	Missed certain types of questions (often multiple-response questions)	Missed Next Generation (NGN) types of questions (Case studies; Bow Ties; Trends)	Did not understand the subject matter	Did not recognize rationale for the correct answer	Made an incorrect guess	Did not understand the meaning of the term in question	Other
1												
2												
3												
4												
5												
5												

Question #	Client need	Misread/ Misunderstood the question	Missed key word(s)	Did not read all options	Changed answer	Missed certain types of questions (often multiple-response questions)	Missed Next Generation (NGN) types of questions (Case studies; Bow Ties; Trends)	Did not understand the subject matter	Did not recognize rationale for the correct answer	Made an incorrect guess	Did not understand the meaning of the term in question	Other
6												
7												
8												
9												
10												
11												
12												
13												
14												
15												
16												
17												
18												
19												
20												
21												
22												
23												
24												
25												
26												
27												
28												

(Continued)

Question #	Client need	Misread/ Misunderstood the question	Missed key word(s)	Did not read all options	Changed answer	Missed certain types of questions (often multiple-response questions)	Missed Next Generation (NGN) types of questions (Case studies; Bow Ties; Trends)	Did not understand the subject matter	Did not recognize rationale for the correct answer	Made an incorrect guess	Did not understand the meaning of the term in question	Other
29												
30												
31												
32												
33												
34												
35												
36												
37												
38												
39												
40												
41												
42												
43												
44												
45												
46												
47												
48												
49												
50												
51												
52												

Question #	Client need	Misread/ Misunderstood the question	Missed key word(s)	Did not read all options	Changed answer	Missed certain types of questions (often multiple-response questions)	Missed Next Generation (NGN) types of questions (Case studies; Bow Ties; Trends)	Did not understand the subject matter	Did not recognize rationale for the correct answer	Made an incorrect guess	Did not understand the meaning of the term in question	Other
53												
54												
55												
56												
57												
58												
59												
60												
61												
62												
63												
64												
65												
66												
67												
68												
69												
70												
71												
72												
73												
74												

(Continued)

Question #	Client need	Misread/ Misunderstood the question	Missed key word(s)	Did not read all options	Changed answer	Missed certain types of questions (often multiple-response questions)	Missed Next Generation (NGN) types of questions (Case studies; Bow Ties; Trends)	Did not understand the subject matter	Did not recognize rationale for the correct answer	Made an incorrect guess	Did not understand the meaning of the term in question	Other
75												
76												
77												
78												
79												
80												
81												
82												
83												
84												
85												
86												
87												
88												
89												
90												
91												
92												
93												
94												
95												
96												
97												
98												

Question #	Client need	Misread/ Misunderstood the question	Missed key word(s)	Did not read all options	Changed answer	Missed certain types of questions (often multiple-response questions)	Missed Next Generation (NGN) types of questions (Case studies; Bow Ties; Trends)	Did not understand the subject matter	Did not recognize rationale for the correct answer	Made an incorrect guess	Did not understand the meaning of the term in question	Other
99												
100												
101												
102												
103												
104												
105												
106												
107												
108												
109												
110												
111												
112												
113												
114												
115												
116												
117												
118												
119												
120												

(Continued)

Question #	Client need	Misread/ Misunderstood the question	Missed key word(s)	Did not read all options	Changed answer	Missed certain types of questions (often multiple-response questions)	Missed Next Generation (NGN) types of questions (Case studies; Bow Ties; Trends)	Did not understand the subject matter	Did not recognize rationale for the correct answer	Made an incorrect guess	Did not understand the meaning of the term in question	Other
121												
122												
123												
124												
125												
126												
127												
128												
129												
130												
131												
132												
133												
134												
135												
136												
137												
138												
139												
140												
141												
142												
143												
144												

Question #	Client need	Misread/ Misunderstood the question	Missed key word(s)	Did not read all options	Changed answer	Missed certain types of questions (often multiple-response questions)	Missed Next Generation (NGN) types of questions (Case studies; Bow Ties; Trends)	Did not understand the subject matter	Did not recognize rationale for the correct answer	Made an incorrect guess	Did not understand the meaning of the term in question	Other
145												
146												
147												
148												
149												
150												

- How many questions in each area of client needs did you miss?
- How does this compare with other exam results from this review?

Lower _____ Same _____ Higher _____ NA _____

If you missed questions because you misread questions, missed key words, or changed answers, review *Lippincott Q&A Review for NCLEX-RN* Part I.

If you missed questions because you did not remember or understand the content, review that content in *Lippincott Q&A Review for NCLEX-RN* Part II and your other nursing references.

If you missed questions because you guessed, were you missing because of "rapid guessing" to complete the test on time, or because of "random guessing," making a reasoned attempt to answer the question? Consider how you will approach "guessing" when you do not know the answer.

If you missed questions because you did not pace yourself, practice taking timed test questions and pacing yourself to allow sufficient time for all questions.

What is the pattern of the types of questions you are missing?

What is your action plan for further study?

_____

_____

workplace, or in a library. Be sure your friends and family understand the importance of not interrupting you when you are studying.

- *Establish regular study times.* Make appointments with yourself to ensure a commitment to study. Frequent, short study periods (1 or 2 hours) are preferable to sporadic, extended study periods. Test yourself often by taking test questions or generating test questions yourself; using practice test questions is more effective than rereading your textbooks or notes (Shellenbarger, 2011). Plan to finish your studying 1 week before the NCLEX-RN; last-minute cramming tends to increase anxiety.

- *Obtain all necessary resources.* As you begin to study, it is helpful to have easy access to textbooks, electronic resources, notes, and study guides.

- *Make the best use of your time.* Make review cards that you can carry with you to study during free moments throughout the day. Some students review notes and listen to tapes or podcasts while driving or exercising. Use electronic devices and smartphones to add test review "apps" to practice test questions on a regular basis.

- *Reduce or eliminate stressful situations.* Students who are juggling multiple responsibilities (such as working, managing a family, taking courses, planning a wedding, or caring for older adult parents) may find it difficult to find time to study or to concentrate when studying. Managing a variety of stressful situations puts students at risk for failing exams. If possible, reduce the number of stressful situations you are involved in during the time you are preparing to take the NCLEX-RN exam.

- *Develop effective study skills.* Study skills enable you to acquire, organize, remember, and use the information you need to take the NCLEX-RN. These skills include outlining, summarizing, applying, synthesizing, reviewing, and practicing test-taking strategies. Some students make concept maps or use reflective journaling to help them learn and remember important content. Use these study skills each time you prepare for an exam.

- *Use study skills with which you are familiar and that have worked well for you in the past.* Recall effective study behaviors that you used in nursing school, such as reviewing highlighted text, outlines, or content/concept maps.

- *Study to learn, not to memorize.* The NCLEX-RN tests application and analysis of knowledge. When reviewing content, continually ask yourself, "How is this information used in client care?" "What clinical decision-making will be required of this information?" and "What is the role of the nurse in using this information?" Being able to apply information, rather than just being able to list or recognize information, is one of the most important study skills to master. Study for "deep learning," not surface learning, which emphasizes only comprehension and short-term recall.

- *Study through the repetitive use of questions.* Using practice questions helps you know if you can retrieve and understand the information that you have studied (Pence & Wood, 2018). Known as "retrieval practice," this study technique uses questions to recall what you have just learned to strengthen your memory (Froehlich & Rogers, 2022). You can do this by using practice questions in this book, participating in study groups, or making up your own questions that will require you to recall information that you just learned and how to use it to plan nursing care and make clinical judgments. Repeated practice with test questions over time helps imbed knowledge in your long-term memory and makes it easier to recall than just reading or rereading the material. In addition to using the questions in this book, Computer Adaptive Quizzing, available on *Lippincott NCLEX-RN® PassPoint*, offers a way to study using retrieval practices.

- *Use deliberate practice study strategies.* Deliberate practice involves the repetitive performance of cognitive (and motor) skills followed by immediate feedback and practice until the correct answer is obtained consistently. In this book, all practice questions offer the opportunity for immediate feedback and provide instruction about both the correct and incorrect answers. After answering each question on these tests, turn to the rationale at the end of the test to determine if you answered correctly. If you did not, use the feedback that is offered for both the correct and incorrect answers, and do additional learning about the concept being tested, followed by using similar questions to test your understanding of the concept to solidify your learning.

- *Identify your learning and study style preferences.* Each student has a preferred way of learning. For example, some students prefer learning material by listening; they are considered *auditory* learners. If this describes your preference, you will benefit from reviewing recorded notes or class lectures. Some students learn best in a visual mode. They learn by reading, reviewing slide presentations, or looking at illustrations. For these *visual* learners, reading and looking at images is helpful. *Kinesthetic* learners, those who like to touch and manipulate to learn, benefit from working with models and manikins to reinforce their learning. While you likely have one learning style and study preference, using a variety of styles will enhance the study experience.

- *Affirm your language skills.* If English or French is not your first or only language, focus on developing your language skills (Hansen & Beaver, 2012).

Make note cards of words that are unfamiliar, or keep a list of words from practice tests that you do not know, and review these words. Study with a friend for whom English is the native language, and discuss practice questions to understand the meaning of the words and the nursing context. Using concept maps is another useful strategy when studying particular health problems.

- *Consider forming a study group.* Some students prefer to study alone, whereas others benefit from study groups; know which approach works best for you, and develop your study plan accordingly. If you participate in a study group, limit the group size to about seven people. The group should develop norms for working together that focus on understanding and applying nursing content, rather than memorizing facts. Talking out loud about the thought processes that go into answering a question is a helpful approach, particularly when students or faculty can provide corrective feedback. In a study group, students can pose questions to each other and discuss rationale or divide the topics for review and practice, but every member must come prepared to contribute. If your school has software that allows you to form online groups of students, set up a study forum. Some students study with a "study buddy." With just a few people, it is easy to use video meeting technology that permits seeing the person with whom you are studying.

- *Attend faculty-led test review sessions.* Most faculty provide opportunities for group or individual review after each test. Attend these sessions or ask to discuss your exam scores with your faculty. Interaction with faculty and advisors about your test-taking skills is an important element to success on nursing exams and has been shown to improve course grades. Determine the reasons for and patterns of missing particular questions, and plan to use this information in your study plan.

- *Study the most difficult material before bedtime.* Research indicates that sleeping consolidates information in your memory (Shellenbarger, 2011).

- *Anticipate questions.* As you study, formulate questions around the content. Practice giving a rationale for your answer to these questions. If you work in a study group, have each member contribute questions that the entire group answers. Frequent testing solidifies learning.

- *Study common, not unique, nursing care situations.* The NCLEX-RN tests minimum competence for nursing practice; therefore, focus on common health problems and client needs. Review the *RN Practice Analysis*, published by the National Council of State Boards of Nursing, and the current licensing exam test plan to determine common nursing care activities. Both can be found on the NCSBN website at www.ncsbn.org.

- *Study broad concepts, rather than insignificant details.* Be sure you understand the underlying pathophysiology and nursing implications across the life span for broad concepts such as oxygenation, perfusion, comfort, delegation, and so on. Answers to test questions can be derived from understanding the basic concept and then determining how to implement nursing care for specific client needs.

- *Simulate test taking.* The comprehensive tests in Part Three of this book are designed to simulate the random order in which questions appear in the NCLEX-RN and the possible number of questions you might receive. Make additional copies of answer sheets and retake the exams on which you had low scores. Use the *Content Mastery and Test-Taking Skill Self-Analysis* table (see Table 3.3 and the worksheet at the back of the book) to review the *reason* you have missed a question and note *patterns* that may become evident, and use these to guide further study.

DEVELOP EFFECTIVE TEST-TAKING STRATEGIES

Knowing how to take a test is as important as knowing the content being tested. Strategies for taking tests can be learned and used to improve test scores. Here are some suggestions for building a repertoire of effective test-taking strategies:

- *Understand the type of test item, the cognitive level, and related thinking processes.* (See Chapter 2 for more information on question types and cognitive levels found on the NCLEX-RN exam.)

- *Understand which integrated process* (step of the nursing process, caring, communication, documentation, teaching/learning, culture, spirituality, and clinical judgment) is being tested. For example, as you read the question, determine whether the question is asking you to set priorities (planning) or judge outcomes (evaluation).

- *Understand client needs.* As you read the question, consider the question in the context of client needs. Be sure to understand if the question is asking you to determine what to do "**first**" or to select the nursing action that is "**best**."

- *Understand the age of the client, if noted in the test question.* If relevant to answering the question, the age of the client will be specified; consider what information about that age group will be important to answering the question.

- *Understand the "process" and "step of the process" being tested.* Nursing care involves the use of many processes that involve a sequence of interrelated steps such as the nursing process, nursing clinical judgment process, management of care, and communication processes. Read the question to be sure you understand which part of the process the question is asking about or how the component parts of the process are interrelated.

- *Read the question carefully.* This is one of the most important aspects of effective test-taking. Read the stem carefully; do not rush. Ask yourself, "What is this question asking?" and "What is the expected response?" If necessary, rephrase the question in your own words, but do not change the meaning of the question when putting the question in your own words, as this is one of the reasons for obtaining an incorrect response.

- *Do not read meaning into a question that is not intended, and do not make a question more difficult than it is.* If you do not understand the question, try to figure it out. If, for example, the question is asking about the fluid balance needs of a client with pheochromocytoma and you do not remember what pheochromocytoma is, try to answer the question based on your knowledge of the concept of fluid balance.

- *Base your answer to a question on evidence for best nursing practice.* The exam questions reflect national nursing practice standards and are not written to test knowledge of procedures or practices at specific health care agencies. Thus, it is important to answer the question from the framework of best nursing practice, not unique practices or procedures that are specific to one clinical agency. For example, "code blue" may be a specific term for a cardiac arrest in one agency but not in another, or there may be specific steps in the procedure for intravenous line care at each agency. When answering the question, refer to evidence-based practices more than your personal clinical experiences.

- *Determine if the question is asking you to set priorities or place steps of a procedure in a particular order.* Read the stem of the question carefully, and be clear about the priority (first, last) or order (first, last) in which you are to answer the question. Base your answer on commonly used nursing frameworks for setting priorities, such as the nursing process: assess, plan, implement, and evaluate; Maslow's hierarchy of needs: physiological, safety and security; love and belonging, self-esteem; and self-actualization; principles of emergency care: breathing, bleeding, and circulation; principles of triage: resuscitation, emergency, urgent, less urgent, and nonurgent; fire response priorities: rescue, alarm, confine, and extinguish; the role of the nurse versus the role of the primary care provider versus role of the licensed practical/vocational nurse (LPN/VN) and unlicensed assistive personnel (UAP); or procedures for delegation: scope of practice, workload, ability, and follow-up.

- *Look for key words that provide clues to the correct answer.* For instance, words such as "except," "not," and "but" can change the meaning of a question; words such as "first," "next," and "most" ask you to establish a priority or use an order or sequence of steps; key words such as "most likely" or "least likely" are asking you to determine a probability of a successful outcome. When the question asks you to "select all that apply," be sure you are considering each option as having the possibility of being correct and have ruled out the ones you have not selected as being incorrect.

- *Be certain you understand the meaning of all words in the question.* If you see a word you do not know, try to figure out its meaning from a familiar base of the word or from the context of the question.

- *Attempt to answer the question before you see the answers, and then look for the answer(s) that is/are similar to the one(s) you generated.* If you do not see the answer you thought was correct, stop and reread the question, be sure you understand what the question is asking, and determine what will help you choose the correct answer.

- *Eliminate answers that you know are not correct.* This will improve your chances of selecting the correct answer. Treat each option in multiple-response questions as "true" or "false"; this will help eliminate incorrect answers.

- *Base answers on nursing knowledge.* Remember that the NCLEX-RN is used to test for safe practice and that you have learned the information needed to answer the question.

- *If you do not know an answer, make a reasonable guess.* Hunches and intuition are often correct. Do not waste time and energy; give yourself permission to not know every question and move on to the next one. In the computerized adaptive testing format of the NCLEX-RN test, you must answer each question before the next item is administered, and because the level of difficulty will be adjusted as you answer each question, it is likely that you will know the answer to one of the next questions.

- *Be cautious about changing an answer.* If you know that you have made a mistake, definitely change your first choice to the correct answer, but if you are changing an answer for other reasons, do not make the change. Current evidence indicates students change incorrect answers to correct answers about 50% of the time (George, Muller, & Bartz, 2016). Well-prepared and confident students rarely change answers, while students who are anxious tend to change answers more often. Changing answers results in only a slight increase in scores.

- *Learn to pace yourself.* Pacing has been noted to be an important test-taking skill (Thomas & Baker, 2011). Pacing involves spending an appropriate time on each question as well as monitoring the overall amount of time during the test so that you are not rushing at the end. Some students, when they realize they are running out of time, tend to do "rapid guessing," that is, making quick decisions in order to answer more questions. This approach leads to answering with an incorrect response. "Random guessing" on the other hand is a more strategic approach in which you think carefully and make a reasonable guess based on the information you can recall to help you answer the question. Pacing also involves recognizing when you need a break. Attention span and concentration levels can start to decline in about 45 minutes, and you should request a break when needed. *Use the comprehensive tests in this book to time yourself and develop an appropriate pace for taking the test.*

Practice Managing Test Anxiety

All test takers experience some anxiety. A certain amount of anxiety is motivating; extreme anxiety contributes significantly to poor test performance by causing test takers to change answers, lose concentration, misread or misunderstand questions, or become unable to control the pace of their response to the questions. Be prepared to control unwanted anxiety using the suggestions that follow.

Anxiety can be managed by both physical and mental activities. Practice anxiety management strategies while you are taking the comprehensive examinations in this book, and use them with *each* exam you take in school or elsewhere. Practicing managing test anxiety when taking "low-stakes" tests, such as practice tests and classroom tests, will make managing test anxiety much easier when you are taking the "high-stakes" tests, such as course or program final exams and, of course, the licensing exam. Changing thought processes that contribute to anxiety is an effective way to reduce test anxiety (Quinn & Peters, 2017). Commonly used anxiety management strategies include:

- *Mental rehearsal.* Mental rehearsal involves reviewing the events and environment during the examination. Anticipate how you will feel, what the setting will be like, how you will take the exam, what the computer screen will look like, and how you will talk to yourself during the exam. To see an example of a testing center, go to the Pearson VUE website, and use the video to take a tour of a typical test center (http://home.pearsonvue.com/test-taker/Pearson-Professional-Center-Tour.aspx). Rehearse what you will do if you have test anxiety.

- *Relaxation exercises.* Relaxation exercises involve tensing and relaxing various muscle groups to relieve the physical effects of anxiety. Practice systematically contracting and relaxing muscle groups from your toes to your neck to release energy for concentration. You can do these exercises during the exam to promote relaxation. Smile! Smiling relaxes tense facial muscles and reminds you to maintain a positive attitude.

- *Deep breathing.* Taking deep breaths by inhaling slowly while counting to 5 and then exhaling slowly while counting to 10 increases oxygen flow to the lungs and brain. Deep breathing also decreases tension and helps manage anxiety by focusing your thoughts on the breathing and away from worries.

- *Positive self-talk.* Talking to yourself in a positive way serves to correct negative thoughts (e.g., "I can't pass this test" and "I don't know the answers to any of these questions") and reinforces a positive self-concept. Replace negative thoughts with positive ones, for example, tell yourself, "I can do this," "I studied well and am prepared," or "I can figure this out." Visualize yourself as a nurse—you have passed the test!

- *Imagery.* Visualizing a calm environment or visualizing success on the exam is another strategy to manage your anxiety. You can practice this strategy every time you are taking a test.

- *Distraction.* Thinking about something else can clear your mind of negative or unwanted thoughts. Think of something fun, something you enjoy. Plan now what you will think about to distract yourself during the exam.

- *Concentration.* During the exam, be prepared to concentrate. Have tunnel vision. Do not worry if others finish the test before you. Remember that everyone has their own speed for taking tests and that each test is individualized. Do not rush; you will have plenty of time. Focus; do not let noises from the keyboard next to you divert your attention. Do not become overwhelmed by the testing environment. Use positive self-talk as you begin the exam. Some students become bored during the exam and then become careless as they answer questions toward the end of the exam. Practice taking tests of at least 150 questions and discover how long you can focus your attention on the test questions. Practice taking breaks if you begin to lose your concentration. During the actual test, be sure to take breaks when you need them.

- *Seek help.* If you find that you are not able to manage your test anxiety, consult your faculty or resources on your campus. Consider obtaining professional help if needed.

Evaluate Your Progress

The last step of your study plan is to check your progress. Review all of your responses using the tear-out *Content Mastery and Test-Taking Skill Self-Analysis* table (at the back of the book) to identify the number of incorrect responses, the reasons for not answering the question correctly, and how many questions in any one clinical area or categories of client needs you have missed. Note if your scores on the practice and comprehensive tests improve. Do not spend time on content you have mastered, on areas in which you obtained high scores on the practice exam, or on areas with which you feel confident. Use the results of your evaluation to set priorities for study on areas needing additional review. As noted previously, evaluate your study skills, your test-taking abilities, and the use of test anxiety management strategies as you take *each* test throughout your academic program. Doing so now will prepare you to test for success.

Tips from Students Who Have Passed the NCLEX-RN

Students who have successfully passed the NCLEX-RN offer these tips for preparing for, and taking, this exam:

- Study regularly for several months before taking the exam. Be sure you are well prepared. Accept responsibility for your study plan—being prepared is up to you!
- Practice taking randomly generated test questions. Most students are accustomed to taking teacher-made exams that cover several topics in the same content area. When taking the NCLEX-RN examination, however, each question will come from a different topic or content area, and you will need to be prepared to shift your focus to a different practice area for each question.
- Use practice questions until you can score at least 75% on the exam. Practice with at least 2000 questions so you test yourself with a wide range of content and types of questions.
- Create a study plan that includes how many questions you will answer each day.
- Use an app on your phone to practice taking questions when you have short breaks.
- Use a timer to determine how many questions you can answer in a specified amount of time. Use the timer to be sure you are keeping a steady pace, but not rushing through the test.
- Schedule to take the exam when YOU are ready, but as soon after graduation as is feasible. Candidates who take the exam before they are prepared are not as successful. You are in control of when you take the exam!
- Make sure you know the date, time, and place the exam will be given; how to get to the exam site; how long it takes to drive there; and where you can park. Locate the exam site, drive to it, and see the room where the exam will be given. Exam sites may be located in small offices in shopping centers and could be difficult to find.
- Visualize yourself in the room taking the test. Use mental rehearsal to practice anxiety-managing strategies.
- Organize the information you will need to bring to the testing center the night before the exam. You will need to present your Authorization to Test. You will also need to provide the required identification.
- Make sure you are physically prepared. Get enough rest before the examination; fatigue can impair concentration. If you work, it may be advisable not to work the day before the exam; if you work on a shift that is different from the time of the exam, adjust your work schedule several days ahead of time.
- Avoid planning time-consuming activities (e.g., weddings, vacation trips) immediately before the exam.
- Do not use any drugs you usually do not use (including caffeine and nicotine), and do not use alcohol for 2 days before the exam.
- Eat regular meals before the exam. Remember that high-carbohydrate foods provide energy, but excessive sugar and caffeine can cause hyperactivity. Experts recommend that before taking a test, test takers eat high-fiber, high-carbohydrate foods that are slow to digest, such as oatmeal. Eating well-balanced meals the week before the test is also helpful; the diet should include fruits and vegetables; avoid meals high in meat, eggs, and cheese (Shellenbarger, 2011).
- Learn your stress cues so you implement strategies early to keep your anxiety from rising.
- Dress comfortably, in layers that can be added or removed according to your comfort level.
- Include planned rewards for sticking to your study goals, such as a dinner with friends.

The authors of this review book offer you our best wishes for success on all of the exams you will be taking throughout your academic career. We are confident that your review and preparation have given you a good foundation for a positive testing experience!

REFERENCES

Eich, M., & O'Neill, T. (2007). NCLEX® delay pass rate study. *NCLEX® Psychometric Research Brief*, January 2007. Available at: https://www.ncsbn.org/delaystudy2006.pdf

Froehlich, A., & Rogers, E. B. (2022). Four keys to unlocking equitable learning: Retrieval, spacing, interleaving, and elaborative encoding. In *Teaching and learning for social justice and equity in higher education* (pp. 249–275). Cham: Palgrave Macmillan.

George, T. M., Muller, A., & Bartz, J. (2016). A mixed-methods study of prelicensure nursing students changing answers on multiple choice examinations. *Journal of Nursing Education, 55*(4), 220–223. doi: 10.3928/01484834-20160316-07

Hansen, E., & Beaver, S. (2012). Faculty support for ESL nursing students: Action plan for success. *Nursing Education Perspectives, 33*(4), 246–250. Available at: https://www.ncbi.nlm.nih.gov/pubmed/22916628

Pence, J., & Wood, F. (2018). Using computer-adaptive quizzing as a tool for National Council Licensure Examination success. *Nursing Education Perspectives, 39*(3), 164–166. doi: 10.1097/01.NEP.0000000000000289

Quinn, B. L., & Peters, A. (2017). Strategies to reduce nursing student test anxiety: A literature review. *Journal of Nursing Education, 56*(3), 145–151. doi: 10.3928/01484834-20170222-05

Quinn, B. L., Smolinski, M., & Peters, A. B. (2018). Strategies to improve NCLEX-RN success: A review. *Teaching and Learning in Nursing, 13*(1), 18–26. https://doi.org/10.1016/j.teln.2017.09.002

Schuler, M., & Chung, J. (2019). Exam wrapper use and metacognition in a fundamentals course: Perceptions and reality. *Journal of Nursing Education, 58*(7), 417–421.

Sethares, K., & Asselin, M. (2021). Use of exam wrapper metacognitive strategy to promote student self-assessment of learning. *Nurse Educator, 47*(1), 37–41.

Shellenbarger, S. (2011, October 26). Toughest exam question: What is the best way to study? *Wall Street Journal*, D1.

Thomas, M. H., & Baker, S. S. (2011). NCLEX-RN success: Evidence-based strategies. *Nurse Educator, 36*(6), 246–249. doi: 10.1097/NNE.0b013e3182333f70

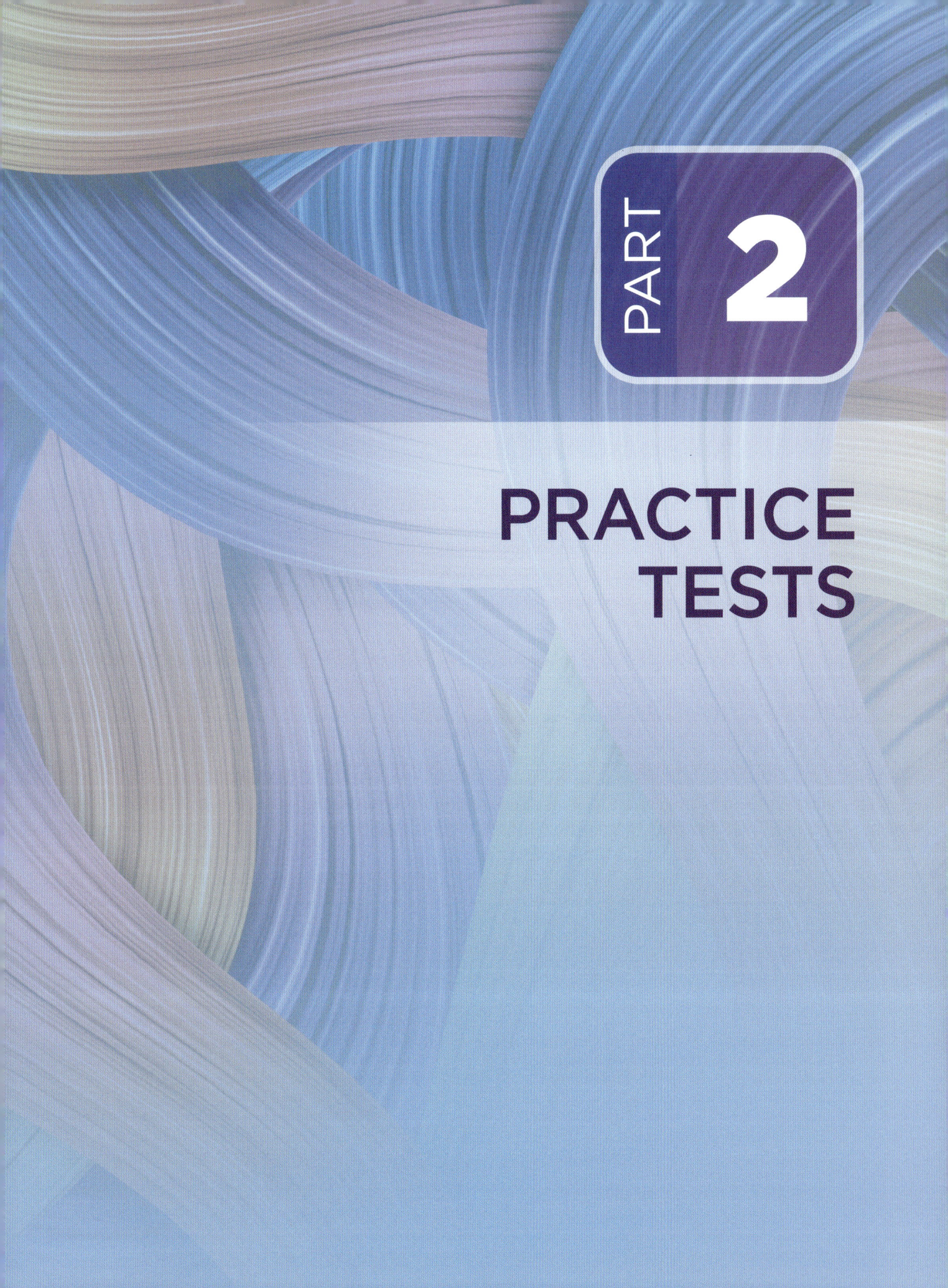
PART 2

PRACTICE TESTS

1

The Nursing Care of the Childbearing Family

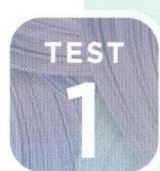

Antepartum Care

- The Preconception Client
- The Pregnant Client Receiving Prenatal Care
- The Pregnant Client in Birth Preparation Classes
- The Pregnant Client with Risk Factors
- Managing Care, Quality, and Safety for Childbearing Clients

The Preconception Client

1. A client has obtained levonorgestrel as emergency contraception. After unprotected intercourse, the client calls the clinic to ask questions about taking the contraceptives. The nurse realizes the client needs further explanation when they make which statement?
   - ☐ 1. "I can wait up to 4 days after intercourse to start taking these to prevent pregnancy."
   - ☐ 2. "My partner can buy levonorgestrel from the pharmacy if they are over 18 years old."
   - ☐ 3. "The birth control works by preventing ovulation or fertilization of the egg."
   - ☐ 4. "I may feel nauseated and have breast tenderness or a headache after using the contraceptive."

2. An antenatal G2, T1, P0, A0, L1 client is discussing postpartum plans for birth control with their health care provider (HCP). In analyzing the available choices, which factor has the **greatest** impact on their birth control options?
   - ☐ 1. satisfaction with prior methods
   - ☐ 2. preference of their sexual partner
   - ☐ 3. breast- or bottle-feeding plan
   - ☐ 4. desire for another child in 2 years

3. Which information would be important to include in the teaching plan for the client who wants more information on ovulation and fertility management?
   - ☐ 1. The ovum survives for 96 hours after ovulation, making conception possible during this time.
   - ☐ 2. The basal body temperature falls at least 0.2°F (0.17°C) after ovulation has occurred.
   - ☐ 3. Ovulation usually occurs on day 14, plus or minus 2 days, before the onset of the next menstrual cycle.
   - ☐ 4. Most women can tell they have ovulated because of severe pain and thick, scant cervical mucus.

4. Which instructions about activities during menstruation would the nurse include when counseling an adolescent who has just begun to menstruate?
   - ☐ 1. Take a mild analgesic if needed for menstrual pain.
   - ☐ 2. Avoid cold foods if menstrual pain persists.
   - ☐ 3. Stop exercising while menstruating.
   - ☐ 4. Avoid tampons until 1 year after periods begin.

5. After conducting a class for female adolescents about human reproduction, the nurse concludes teaching has been effective when a student makes which statement?
☐ 1. "Under ideal conditions, sperm can reach the ovum in 15 to 30 minutes, resulting in pregnancy."
☐ 2. "I will not become pregnant if I abstain from intercourse during the last 14 days of my menstrual cycle."
☐ 3. "Sperms from a healthy male usually remain viable in the female reproductive tract for 96 hours."
☐ 4. "After an ovum is fertilized by a sperm, the ovum contains 21 pairs of chromosomes."

6. A 20-year-old nulligravid client expresses a desire to learn more about the symptothermal method of family planning. Which information would the nurse include in the teaching plan?
☐ 1. This method has a 50% failure rate during the first year of use.
☐ 2. Couples must abstain from coitus for 5 days after the menses.
☐ 3. Cervical mucus is carefully monitored for changes.
☐ 4. The male partner uses condoms for significant effectiveness.

7. Before advising a 24-year-old client desiring oral contraceptives for family planning, the nurse would assess the client for which signs and symptoms?
☐ 1. anemia
☐ 2. hypertension
☐ 3. dysmenorrhea
☐ 4. acne vulgaris

8. After instructing a 20-year-old nulligravid client about the adverse effects of oral contraceptives, the nurse determines that further instruction is needed when the client states which factor as an adverse effect?
☐ 1. weight gain
☐ 2. nausea
☐ 3. headache
☐ 4. ovarian cancer

9. Which information would the nurse include in the teaching plan for a 32-year-old female client requesting information about using a diaphragm for family planning?
☐ 1. Douching with an acidic solution after intercourse is recommended.
☐ 2. Diaphragms should not be used if the client develops acute cervicitis.
☐ 3. The diaphragm should be washed in a weak solution of bleach and water.
☐ 4. The diaphragm should be left in place for 2 hours after intercourse.

10. After being examined and fitted for a diaphragm, a 24-year-old client receives instructions about its use. Which client statement indicates a need for further teaching?
☐ 1. "I can continue to use the diaphragm for about 2 to 3 years if I keep it protected in the case."
☐ 2. "If I get pregnant, I will have to be refitted for another diaphragm after birth."
☐ 3. "Before inserting the diaphragm, I should coat the rim with contraceptive jelly."
☐ 4. "If I gain or lose 20 lb (9 kg), I can still use the same diaphragm."

11. A couple is inquiring about vasectomy as a permanent method of contraception. Which teaching statement would the nurse include in the teaching plan?
☐ 1. "Another method of contraception is needed until the sperm count is 0."
☐ 2. "Vasectomy is easily reversed if children are desired in the future."
☐ 3. "Vasectomy is contraindicated in males with prior history of cardiac disease."
☐ 4. "Vasectomy requires only a yearly follow-up once the procedure is completed."

12. A 39-year-old multigravida client asks the nurse for information about female sterilization with a tubal ligation. Which client statement indicates effective teaching?
☐ 1. "My fallopian tubes will be tied off through a small abdominal incision."
☐ 2. "Reversal of a tubal ligation is easily done, with a pregnancy success rate of 80%."
☐ 3. "After this procedure, I must abstain from intercourse for at least 3 weeks."
☐ 4. "Both of my ovaries will be removed during the tubal ligation procedure."

13. A 23-year-old nulliparous client visiting the clinic for a routine examination tells the nurse that they desire to use the basal body temperature method for family planning. What instructions should the nurse give the client?
☐ 1. Check the cervical mucus to see if it is thick and sparse.
☐ 2. Take the client's temperature at the same time every morning before getting out of bed.
☐ 3. Document ovulation when their temperature decreases at least 1°F (0.56°C).
☐ 4. Avoid coitus for 10 days after a slight rise in temperature.

14. A couple visiting the infertility clinic for the first time states that they have been trying to conceive for the past 2 years without success. After a history and physical examination of both partners, what would be the **most** appropriate outcome for the couple to accomplish by the end of this visit?
☐ 1. Choose an appropriate infertility treatment method.
☐ 2. Acknowledge that only 50% of infertile couples achieve a pregnancy.
☐ 3. Discuss alternative methods of having a family, such as adoption.
☐ 4. Describe each of the potential causes and possible treatment modalities.

15. A 20-year-old primigravid client tells the nurse that their mother had a friend who died from hemorrhage about 10 years ago during a vaginal birth. Which response would be **most** helpful?
☐ 1. "Today's modern technology has resulted in a low maternal mortality rate."
☐ 2. "Do not concern yourself with things that happened in the past."
☐ 3. "In North America, birth parents seldom die in birth."
☐ 4. "What is it that concerns you about pregnancy, labor, or birth?"

16. A 19-year-old nulligravid client visiting the clinic for a routine examination asks the nurse about cervical mucus changes that occur during the menstrual cycle. Which information would the nurse expect to include in the client's teaching plan?
☐ 1. About midway through the menstrual cycle, cervical mucus is thick and sticky.
☐ 2. During ovulation, cervical mucous is decreased and cloudy.
☐ 3. As ovulation approaches, cervical mucus becomes clear and stretchy.
☐ 4. Cervical mucus disappears immediately after ovulation, resuming with menses.

17. When instructing a client about the proper use of condoms for pregnancy prevention, the nurse should include which instruction to ensure maximum effectiveness?
☐ 1. Place the condom over the erect penis before coitus.
☐ 2. Withdraw the condom after coitus when the penis is flaccid.
☐ 3. Ensure that the condom is pulled tightly over the tip of the penis before coitus.
☐ 4. Obtain a prescription for a condom with nonoxynol 9.

18. The nurse teaches a client about using medroxyprogesterone as a birth control method. Which client statement indicates effective teaching?
☐ 1. "This method of family planning requires monthly injections."
☐ 2. "I should have my first injection during my menstrual cycle."
☐ 3. "One possible adverse effect is the absence of a menstrual period."
☐ 4. "This drug will be given by subcutaneous injections."

19. Which instruction should the nurse include in the teaching plan for a 30-year-old multiparous client who will be using an intrauterine device (IUD) for family planning?
☐ 1. Amenorrhea is a common adverse effect of IUDs.
☐ 2. Additional conception protection will be needed.
☐ 3. IUDs are more costly than other forms of contraception.
☐ 4. Severe cramping may occur when the IUD is inserted.

20. Which information would the nurse include in a teaching plan about treatments for sexually transmitted infections?
☐ 1. Acyclovir can be used to cure herpes genitalis.
☐ 2. *Chlamydia trachomatis* infections are usually treated with penicillin.
☐ 3. Ceftriaxone may be used to treat *Neisseria gonorrhoeae* infections.
☐ 4. Metronidazole is used to treat condylomata acuminata.

21. A couple is visiting the clinic because they have been unable to conceive a baby after 3 years of frequent coitus. The nurse determines that the couple needs further instruction when they identify which factor as a cause of male infertility?
☐ 1. seminal fluid with an alkaline pH
☐ 2. frequent exposure to heat sources
☐ 3. abnormal hormonal stimulation
☐ 4. immunologic factors

The Pregnant Client Receiving Prenatal Care

22. A primigravid client at 15 weeks' gestation has received teaching about concerning signs and symptoms to report following an amniocentesis. Which statement indicates that the client needs further teaching?
☐ 1. "I need to call if I start to leak fluid from my vagina."
☐ 2. "If I start bleeding, I will need to call back."
☐ 3. "If my baby does not move, I need to call my health care provider."
☐ 4. "If I start running a fever, I should let the office know."

23. The nurse is caring for a client who is 12 weeks pregnant and speaks Spanish only. Which intervention(s) should the nurse include in the plan of care at the client's initial visit? Select all that apply.
☐ 1. Provide brochures in the client's native language.
☐ 2. Discuss differences with the dominant culture.
☐ 3. Arrange for an interpreter for their appointments.
☐ 4. Discuss contraception and options.
☐ 5. Review nutritional preferences.

24. During a visit to the prenatal clinic, a pregnant client at 32 weeks' gestation has heartburn. The client needs further instruction when they say they must do what to manage heartburn?
☐ 1. Avoid highly seasoned foods.
☐ 2. Avoid lying down right after eating.
☐ 3. Eat small, frequent meals.
☐ 4. Consume liquids only between meals.

25. The nurse is teaching a new prenatal client about their iron deficiency anemia during pregnancy. Which statement indicates that the client needs further instruction about their anemia?
☐ 1. "I will need to take iron supplements now."
☐ 2. "I may have anemia because my family is of Asian descent."
☐ 3. "I am considered anemic if my hemoglobin is below 11 g/dL (110 g/L)."
☐ 4. "The anemia increases the workload on my heart."

26. Following a positive pregnancy test, a client begins discussing the changes that will occur in the next several months with the nurse. The nurse should include which information about a change the client can anticipate in the first trimester?
☐ 1. differentiating the self from the fetus
☐ 2. enjoying the role of nurturer
☐ 3. preparing for the reality of parenthood
☐ 4. experiencing ambivalence about pregnancy

27. An antenatal primigravid client has just been informed that they are carrying twins. The plan of care includes educating the client concerning factors that put them at risk for problems during the pregnancy. The nurse realizes the client needs further instruction when they indicate carrying twins puts them at risk for which complication?
☐ 1. preterm labor
☐ 2. twin-to-twin transfusion
☐ 3. anemia
☐ 4. group B streptococcus

28. A 30-year-old multigravida client has missed three periods and now visits the prenatal clinic because they assume they are pregnant. The client is experiencing enlargement of their abdomen, a positive pregnancy test, and changes in the pigmentation on their face and abdomen. These assessment findings reflect this client is experiencing a cluster of which signs of pregnancy?
☐ 1. positive
☐ 2. probable
☐ 3. presumptive
☐ 4. diagnostic

29. When preparing a 20-year-old client for a serum pregnancy test, the nurse should include what information?
☐ 1. The test has a high degree of accuracy within 1 week after ovulation.
☐ 2. The test is identical in nature to an over-the-counter home pregnancy test.
☐ 3. A positive result is considered a presumptive sign of pregnancy.
☐ 4. A urine sample is needed to obtain quicker results.

30. After instructing a female client about the radioimmunoassay pregnancy test, the nurse determines that the client understands the instructions when the client states that which hormone is evaluated by this test?
☐ 1. prolactin
☐ 2. follicle-stimulating hormone
☐ 3. luteinizing hormone
☐ 4. human chorionic gonadotropin (hCG)

31. Using Nägele's rule for a client whose last normal menstrual period began on May 10, the nurse determines that the client's estimated date of birth is what date?
☐ 1. January 13
☐ 2. January 17
☐ 3. February 13
☐ 4. February 17

32. After instructing a primigravid client about the functions of the placenta, the nurse determines that the client needs additional teaching when they say that which hormone is produced by the placenta?
☐ 1. estrogen
☐ 2. progesterone
☐ 3. human chorionic gonadotropin (hCG)
☐ 4. testosterone

33. The nurse assesses a client at 24 weeks' gestation and is unable to find the fetal heartbeat. The fetal heartbeat was heard at the client's last visit 4 weeks ago. According to **priority**, the nurse should do the tasks in which order? All options must be used.

1. Call the health care provider (HCP).
2. Explain that the fetal heartbeat could not be found at this time.
3. Obtain different equipment and recheck.
4. Ask the client if the baby is or has been moving.

34. A primigravid client at 10 weeks' gestation questions the nurse about the need for an ultrasound. The client states, "I feel fine, so why should I have the test?" The nurse should incorporate which statement(s) as the underlying reason for performing the ultrasound now? Select all that apply.
☐ 1. "The test helps us view the gross anatomy of the fetus."
☐ 2. "Early ultrasound helps verify gestational age."
☐ 3. "The test will determine if the fetus is viable."
☐ 4. "It is important to determine the fetal position."
☐ 5. "The test helps verify that there is a sufficient nutrient supply for the fetus."

35. A 20-year-old married client with a positive pregnancy test states, "Is it really true? I cannot believe I am going to have a baby!" Which response by the nurse would be **most** appropriate at this time?
☐ 1. "Would you like some booklets on the pregnancy experience?"
☐ 2. "Yes, it is true. How does that make you feel?"
☐ 3. "You should be delighted that you are pregnant."
☐ 4. "What concerns you about this pregnancy?"

36. A newly diagnosed pregnant client tells the nurse, "If I am going to have all of these discomforts, I am not sure I want to be pregnant!" The nurse interprets the client's statement as an indication of which perception?
☐ 1. fear of pregnancy outcome
☐ 2. rejection of the pregnancy
☐ 3. normal ambivalence
☐ 4. limited self-care abilities

37. A client, approximately 11 weeks pregnant, and their spouse are seen in the antepartal clinic. The client's spouse tells the nurse that they have also been experiencing nausea and vomiting and fatigue along with the client. The nurse interprets these findings as suggesting that the client's husband is experiencing which complication?
☐ 1. ptyalism
☐ 2. mittelschmerz
☐ 3. couvade syndrome
☐ 4. pica

38. A primigravid client asks the nurse if they can continue to have a glass of wine with dinner during their pregnancy. Which statement would be the nurse's **best** response?
☐ 1. "The effects of alcohol on a fetus during pregnancy are unknown."
☐ 2. "You should limit your consumption to beer and wine."
☐ 3. "You should abstain from drinking alcoholic beverages."
☐ 4. "You may have one drink of 2 oz of alcohol per day."

39. Examination of a primigravid client having increased vaginal secretions since becoming pregnant reveals clear, highly acidic vaginal secretions. The client denies any perineal itching or burning. The nurse interprets these findings as a response related to which factor?
☐ 1. a decrease in vaginal glycogen stores
☐ 2. development of a sexually transmitted infection
☐ 3. prevention of expulsion of the cervical mucus plug
☐ 4. control of the growth of pathologic bacteria

40. When measuring the fundal height of a primigravid client at 20 weeks' gestation, the nurse will locate the fundal height at which point?
☐ 1. halfway between the client's symphysis pubis and umbilicus
☐ 2. at about the level of the client's umbilicus
☐ 3. between the client's umbilicus and xiphoid process
☐ 4. near the client's xiphoid process and compressing the diaphragm

41. A primigravida at 8 weeks' gestation tells the nurse that they want an amniocentesis because there is a history of hemophilia A in their family. The nurse informs the client that they will need to wait until they are at 15 weeks' gestation for the amniocentesis. Which is the **most** appropriate rationale for the nurse's statement regarding amniocentesis at 15 weeks' gestation?
☐ 1. Fetal development needs to be complete before testing.
☐ 2. The volume of amniotic fluid needed for testing will be available by 15 weeks.
☐ 3. Cells indicating hemophilia A are not produced until 15 weeks' gestation.
☐ 4. Performing an amniocentesis prior to 15 weeks' gestation carries a greater infection rate.

42. After instructing a primigravid client about desired weight gain during pregnancy, the nurse determines that the teaching has been successful when the client makes which statement?
- ☐ 1. "A total weight gain of approximately 20 lb (9 kg) is recommended."
- ☐ 2. "A weight gain of 6.6 lb (3 kg) in the second and third trimesters is considered normal."
- ☐ 3. "A weight gain of about 12 lb (5.5 kg) every trimester is recommended."
- ☐ 4. "Although it varies, a gain of 25 to 35 lb (11.4 to 14.5 kg) is about average."

43. When developing a teaching plan for a client who is 8 weeks pregnant, the nurse would suggest what food(s) to meet the client's need for increased folic acid? Select all that apply.
- ☐ 1. spinach
- ☐ 2. bananas
- ☐ 3. seafood
- ☐ 4. yogurt
- ☐ 5. beans

44. The nurse instructs a primigravid client about the importance of sufficient vitamin A in their diet. The nurse knows that the instructions have been effective when the client indicates that they should include which foods in their diet?
- ☐ 1. buttermilk and cheese
- ☐ 2. strawberries and broccoli
- ☐ 3. egg yolks and squash
- ☐ 4. oranges and tomatoes

45. The nurse is discussing dietary concerns with pregnant teens. Which choice(s) would be convenient for teens yet nutritious for both the birth parent and the fetus? Select all that apply.
- ☐ 1. milkshake or yogurt with fresh fruit or granola bar
- ☐ 2. chicken nuggets with tater tots
- ☐ 3. cheese pizza with spinach and mushroom topping
- ☐ 4. peanut butter with crackers and orange juice
- ☐ 5. buttery light popcorn with diet cola
- ☐ 6. cheeseburger, pickle, and ketchup

46. An antenatal client is discussing their anemia with the nurse in the prenatal clinic. After a discussion about sources of iron to be incorporated into their daily meals, the nurse knows the client needs further instruction when they respond with which statement?
- ☐ 1. "I can meet two goals when I drink milk: lots of iron and meeting my calcium needs at the same time."
- ☐ 2. "Drinking coffee, tea, and sodas decreases the absorption of iron."
- ☐ 3. "I can increase the absorption of iron by drinking orange juice when I eat."
- ☐ 4. "Cream of wheat and molasses are excellent sources of iron."

47. The nurse instructs a primigravid client to increase their intake of foods high in magnesium because of its role in which process?
- ☐ 1. prevention of demineralization of the birth parent's bones
- ☐ 2. synthesis of proteins, nucleic acids, and fats
- ☐ 3. amino acid metabolism
- ☐ 4. synthesis of neural pathways in the fetus

48. A client is at 24 weeks' gestation. The nurse is reviewing the report of laboratory tests as noted below.

Laboratory Results

Test	Result
Blood type	A-positive
Blood glucose	90 mg/dL (5 mmol/L)
VDRL	Positive
Rubella titer	Immune

The nurse should report which results to the health care provider (HCP)?
- ☐ 1. blood type
- ☐ 2. venereal disease research laboratory (VDRL) test
- ☐ 3. blood glucose
- ☐ 4. rubella titer

49. A prenatal client wants to know why the nurse is asking about their use of herbal supplements. What is the nurse's **best** response?
- ☐ 1. "I need to assess your risk because most dietary supplements have not been tested in pregnant parents, nursing parents, or children."
- ☐ 2. "You may need additional screening because herbal supplements often contain other ingredients that may affect your care."
- ☐ 3. "Understanding the full picture of what herbal supplements you use to manage your health will help us better provide coordinated and safe care."
- ☐ 4. "Many herbal supplements change the way your body processes many medications and make them less ineffective."

50. A 34-year-old multiparous client at 16 weeks' gestation who received regular prenatal care for all of their previous pregnancies tells the nurse that they have already felt the baby move. How does the nurse interpret this finding?
- ☐ 1. the possibility that the client is carrying twins
- ☐ 2. unusual because most multiparous clients do not experience quickening until 30 weeks' gestation
- ☐ 3. evidence that the client's estimated date of birth is probably off by a few weeks
- ☐ 4. normal because multiparous clients can experience quickening between 14 and 20 weeks' gestation

51. A 17-year-old gravid client presents for their regularly scheduled 26-week prenatal visit. The client appears disheveled, is wearing ill-fitting clothes, and does not make eye contact with the nurse. Which item(s) should the nurse discuss with the client? Select all that apply.
☐ 1. intimate partner violence
☐ 2. substance abuse
☐ 3. depression
☐ 4. blood glucose screening
☐ 5. hCG (human chorionic gonadotropin) levels

52. When performing Leopold maneuvers, the nurse would ask the client to perform which action to ensure optimal comfort and accuracy?
☐ 1. breathing deeply for 1 minute
☐ 2. emptying their bladder
☐ 3. drinking a full glass of water
☐ 4. lying on their left side

53. The nurse performed Leopold maneuvers and determined that the fetal position is right occiput anterior (ROA). Identify the area where the nurse would place the Doppler to hear fetal heart sounds **most** easily.

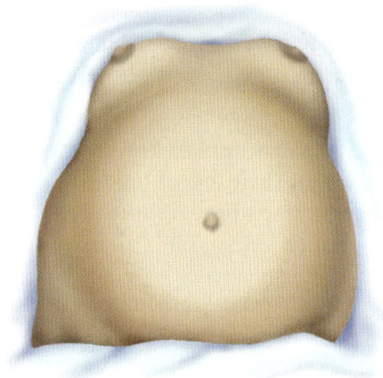

54. The nurse is assessing the fetal position for a 32-year-old client in their eighth month of pregnancy. As shown below, the fetus is in which position?

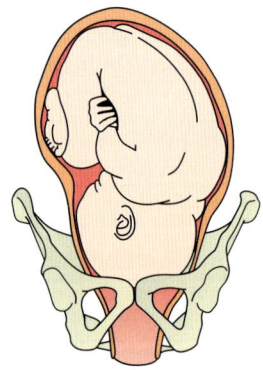

LOA

☐ 1. left occipitus transverse
☐ 2. left occipitus anterior
☐ 3. right occipitus transverse
☐ 4. right occipitus anterior

55. Which statement by the nurse would be **most** appropriate when responding to a primigravid client who asks, "What should I do about this brown discoloration across my nose and cheeks?"
☐ 1. "This usually disappears after birth."
☐ 2. "It is a sign of skin melanoma."
☐ 3. "The discoloration is due to dilated capillaries."
☐ 4. "It will fade if you use a prescribed cream."

56. A 36-year-old primigravid client at 22 weeks' gestation without any complications to date is being seen in the clinic for a routine visit. Why does the nurse need to assess the client's fundal height?
☐ 1. to determine the level of uterine activity
☐ 2. to identify the need for increased weight gain
☐ 3. to assess the fetal position
☐ 4. to estimate the fetal growth

57. After the nurse reviews the primary health care provider's (HCP's) explanation of amniocentesis with a multigravida client, which complication if stated by the client indicates that they need more teaching about the procedure?
☐ 1. risk for infection
☐ 2. possible miscarriage
☐ 3. risk for club foot
☐ 4. fetal organ malformations

58. A prenatal client wants to begin a yoga-based exercise class to keep healthy during pregnancy. What information should the nurse include in the plan of care? Select all that apply.
☐ 1. Drink plenty of water before, during, and after a workout.
☐ 2. Take precautions to prevent overheating.
☐ 3. Avoid jerky, high-impact motions.
☐ 4. Modify any positions that put a strain on the abdomen.
☐ 5. Participate only in classes specifically designed for pregnant clients.

59. A primigravid client at 28 weeks' gestation tells the nurse that they and their spouse wish to drive to visit relatives who live several hours away. Which recommendation by the nurse would be **best**?
☐ 1. "Try to avoid traveling anywhere in the car during your third trimester."
☐ 2. "Limit the time you spend in the car to a maximum of 4 to 5 hours."
☐ 3. "Taking the trip is okay if you stop every 1 to 2 hours and walk."
☐ 4. "Avoid wearing your seat belt in the car to prevent injury to the fetus."

60. The nurse teaches a client who is 18 weeks pregnant about seat belt safety. Identify the area that indicates that the client understands where the lap portion of the seat belt should be placed.

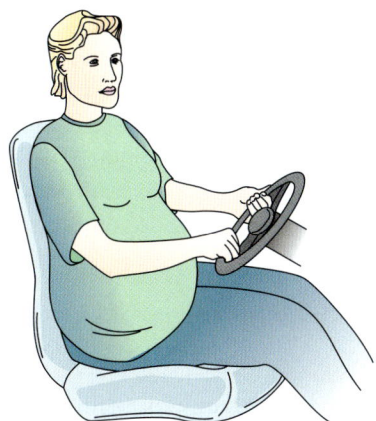

61. Which recommendation would be **most** helpful to suggest to a primigravid client at 37 weeks' gestation who has leg cramps?
- ☐ 1. Change positions frequently throughout the day.
- ☐ 2. Alternately flex and extend the legs.
- ☐ 3. Straighten the knees, and flex the toes toward the chin.
- ☐ 4. Lie prone in bed with the legs elevated.

62. A nurse sees a pregnant client showing signs of airway obstruction. When the nurse asks the client if they need help, the client nods their head yes. Indicate the area where the nurse's fist should be placed to effectively administer thrusts to clear the foreign body from the airway.

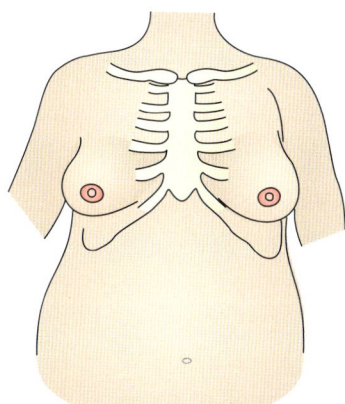

63. When performing Leopold maneuvers on a primigravid client at 22 weeks' gestation, the nurse performs the first maneuver to accomplish which action?
- ☐ 1. Locate the fetal back and spine.
- ☐ 2. Determine what is in the fundus.
- ☐ 3. Determine whether the fetal head is at the pelvic inlet.
- ☐ 4. Identify the degree of fetal descent and flexion.

64. A primigravid adolescent client at approximately 15 weeks' gestation is visiting the prenatal clinic to undergo maternal quad screening. What information should the nurse include in the teaching plan for this client?
- ☐ 1. Ultrasonography usually accompanies maternal quad screen testing.
- ☐ 2. Results are usually very accurate until 20 weeks' gestation.
- ☐ 3. A clean-catch midstream urine specimen is needed.
- ☐ 4. Increased levels of alpha-fetoprotein (AFP) are associated with neural tube defects.

65. Which statement **best** identifies the rationale for why the nurse reinforces the need for continued prenatal care throughout the pregnancy with an adolescent primigravid client?
- ☐ 1. Pregnant adolescents are at high risk for pregnancy-induced hypertension.
- ☐ 2. Gestational diabetes during pregnancy commonly develops in adolescents.
- ☐ 3. Adolescents need additional instruction related to common discomforts.
- ☐ 4. The client's spouse is rarely involved in the pregnancy.

66. Which information would be included in the teaching plan about pregnancy-related breast changes for a primigravid client?
- ☐ 1. Growth of the milk ducts is greatest during the first 8 weeks of gestation.
- ☐ 2. Enlargement of the breasts indicates adequate levels of progesterone.
- ☐ 3. Colostrum is usually secreted by about the 16th week of gestation.
- ☐ 4. Darkening of the areola occurs during the last month of pregnancy.

67. A primigravid client at 32 weeks' gestation is enrolled in a breastfeeding class. Which statement(s) would indicate that the client understands the breastfeeding education? Select all that apply.
- ☐ 1. "My milk supply will be adequate since I have increased a whole bra size during pregnancy."
- ☐ 2. "I can hold my baby several different ways during feedings."
- ☐ 3. "If my infant latches on properly, I will not develop mastitis."
- ☐ 4. "If I breastfeed, my uterus will return to prepregnancy size more quickly."
- ☐ 5. "I need to feed my baby when I see feeding cues and not wait until they are crying."

68. When planning a class for primigravid clients about the common physiologic changes of pregnancy, the nurse should include which information in the teaching plan?
    ☐ 1. The temperature decreases slightly early in pregnancy.
    ☐ 2. Cardiac output increases by 25% to 50% during pregnancy.
    ☐ 3. The circulating fibrinogen level decreases as much as 50% during pregnancy.
    ☐ 4. The anterior pituitary gland secretes oxytocin late in pregnancy.

69. When teaching a primigravid client about the diagnostic tests used in pregnancy, the nurse should include which information?
    ☐ 1. A fetal biophysical profile involves assessments of breathing movements, body movements, tone, amniotic fluid volume, and fetal heart rate reactivity.
    ☐ 2. Fetal heart rate increases during a nonstress test is an ominous sign and requires further evaluation with fetal echocardiography.
    ☐ 3. Contraction stress testing, performed on most pregnant women, can be initiated as early as 16 weeks' gestation.
    ☐ 4. Percutaneous umbilical blood sampling uses a needle inserted through the vagina to obtain a sample.

70. A client asks why they feel so much variability in fetal activity each day. The nurse explains that fetal movement is affected by which factor(s)? Select all that apply.
    ☐ 1. fetal sleep
    ☐ 2. barometric pressure
    ☐ 3. blood glucose
    ☐ 4. time of day
    ☐ 5. cigarette smoking

71. During a routine clinic visit, a 25-year-old multigravida client who initiated prenatal care at 10 weeks' gestation and is now in their third trimester states, "I've been having strange dreams about the baby. Last week I dreamed he was covered with hair." What should the nurse tell the client?
    ☐ 1. "Dreams like the ones that you describe are very unusual. Please tell me more about them."
    ☐ 2. "Commonly when a client has these dreams, they are trying to cope with becoming a parent."
    ☐ 3. "Dreams about the baby late in pregnancy usually mean that labor is about to begin soon."
    ☐ 4. "It is not uncommon to have dreams about the baby, particularly in the third trimester."

72. Which client statement indicates a need for additional teaching about self-care during pregnancy?
    ☐ 1. "I should use nonskid pads when I take a shower or bath."
    ☐ 2. "I should avoid using soap on my nipples to prevent drying."
    ☐ 3. "I should sit in a hot tub for 20 minutes to relax after working."
    ☐ 4. "I should avoid douching even if my vaginal secretions increase."

The Pregnant Client in Birth Preparation Classes

73. A new antenatal G6, T4, P0, A1, L4 client attends their first prenatal visit with their partner. The nurse is assessing this couple's psychological response to the pregnancy. Which finding requires the **most** immediate follow-up?
    ☐ 1. The couple is concerned with the financial changes this pregnancy causes.
    ☐ 2. The couple expresses ambivalence about the current pregnancy.
    ☐ 3. The client's spouse states that the pregnancy has changed the client's focus.
    ☐ 4. The client's spouse is irritated that the client is not like they were before pregnancy.

74. When preparing a prenatal class about endocrine changes that normally occur during pregnancy, the nurse should include information about which subject?
    ☐ 1. Human placental lactogen maintains the corpus luteum.
    ☐ 2. Progesterone is responsible for hyperpigmentation and vascular skin changes.
    ☐ 3. Estrogen relaxes smooth muscle in the respiratory tract.
    ☐ 4. The thyroid enlarges with an increase in basal metabolic rate.

75. When developing a series of parent classes on fetal development, the nurse should include which feature as being developed by the end of the third month (9 to 12 weeks)?
    ☐ 1. external genitalia
    ☐ 2. myelinization of nerves
    ☐ 3. brown fat stores
    ☐ 4. air ducts and alveoli

76. During a 2-hour birth preparation class focusing on the labor and birth process for primigravid clients, the nurse is describing the maneuvers that the fetus goes through during the labor process when the head is the presenting part. In which order do these maneuvers occur? All options must be used.

| 1. engagement |
| 2. flexion |
| 3. descent |
| 4. internal rotation |

| |
| |
| |
| |

77. A primigravid client in a preparation for parenting class asks how much blood is lost during an uncomplicated vaginal birth. What should the nurse tell the client?
☐ 1. "The maximum blood loss considered within normal limits is 500 mL."
☐ 2. "The minimum blood loss considered within normal limits is 1000 mL."
☐ 3. "Blood loss during birth is rarely estimated unless there is a hemorrhage."
☐ 4. "It would be very unusual if you lost more than 100 mL of blood during birth."

78. Which statement by a primigravid client about the amniotic fluid and sac indicates the need for further teaching?
☐ 1. "The amniotic fluid helps the fetus grow symmetrically."
☐ 2. "Fetal nutrients are provided by the amniotic fluid."
☐ 3. "Amniotic fluid provides a cushion against the impact of the maternal abdomen."
☐ 4. "The fetus is kept at a stable temperature by the amniotic fluid and sac."

79. During a birth preparation class, a primigravid client at 36 weeks' gestation tells the nurse, "My lower back has really been bothering me lately." Which exercise would be **most** helpful?
☐ 1. pelvic rocking
☐ 2. deep breathing
☐ 3. tailor sitting
☐ 4. squatting

80. A client is experiencing pain during the first stage of labor. What should the nurse instruct the client to do to manage their pain? Select all that apply.
☐ 1. Walk in the hospital room.
☐ 2. Use slow chest breathing.
☐ 3. Request pain medication on a regular basis.
☐ 4. Lightly massage the abdomen.
☐ 5. Sip ice water.

81. During a preparation for parenting class, one of the participants asks the nurse, "How will I know if I am really in labor?" What should the nurse tell the participant about true labor contractions?
☐ 1. "Walking around helps decrease true contractions."
☐ 2. "True labor contractions are irregular and intense."
☐ 3. "The duration and frequency of true labor contractions remain the same."
☐ 4. "True labor contractions are felt first in the lower back, then the abdomen."

82. After instructing participants in a birth education class about methods for coping with discomforts in the first stage of labor, the nurse determines that one of the pregnant clients needs further instruction when they say that they have been practicing which technique?
☐ 1. biofeedback
☐ 2. effleurage
☐ 3. guided imagery
☐ 4. pelvic tilt exercises

83. The topic of physiologic changes that occur during pregnancy is to be included in a parenting class for primigravid clients who are in their first half of pregnancy. Which topic would be important for the nurse to include in the teaching plan?
☐ 1. decreased plasma volume
☐ 2. increased risk for urinary tract infections
☐ 3. increased peripheral vascular resistance
☐ 4. increased hemoglobin levels

The Pregnant Client with Risk Factors

84. A multigravida client at 32 weeks' gestation has experienced hemolytic disease of the newborn in a previous pregnancy. The nurse should prepare the client for frequent antibody titer evaluations obtained from which source?
☐ 1. placental blood
☐ 2. amniotic fluid
☐ 3. fetal blood
☐ 4. maternal blood

85. Which diagnostic test would be the **most** important for a 40-year-old primigravid client to have in the second trimester of pregnancy?
☐ 1. beta strep screening
☐ 2. chorionic villus sampling
☐ 3. ultrasound testing
☐ 4. quad screen

86. The nurse is caring for a client who has a history of gastric bypass surgery and is now being seen for their first prenatal visit. Which intervention(s) should be included in the plan of care? Select all that apply.
☐ 1. Take a prenatal vitamin with 400 mcg of folic acid.
☐ 2. Refer the client to a registered dietician.
☐ 3. Draw glucose levels at each prenatal visit.
☐ 4. Counsel the client that they will most likely gain all of their weight back.
☐ 5. Check urine at each visit for protein and glucose.
☐ 6. Monitor with nonstress tests beginning at 20 weeks.

87. A client with a medical history of ventricular septal defect repaired in infancy is seen at the prenatal clinic. The client has dyspnea with exertion and is very tired. Their vital signs are oxygen saturation 98%; pulse 80 bpm; respiration rate 20 breaths/min; and blood pressure 116/72 mm Hg. The client has +2 pedal edema and clear breath sounds. The nurse determines the client's symptoms indicate which cardiac functional classification?
☐ 1. class I
☐ 2. class II
☐ 3. class III
☐ 4. class IV

88. A primigravid client has completed their first prenatal visit and blood work. Their laboratory test for the hepatitis B surface antigen (HBsAg) is positive. The nurse can advise the client that the plan of care for this newborn will include which intervention(s)? Select all that apply.
☐ 1. administering hepatitis B immune globulin within 12 hours of birth
☐ 2. beginning the hepatitis B vaccine series within 24 hours of birth
☐ 3. testing the newborn for hepatitis B before discharge.
☐ 4. isolating the infant during hospitalization
☐ 5. maintaining universal precautions for the client and the infant
☐ 6. permitting breastfeeding if the nipples are not cracked

89. A client with asthma controlled through the consistent use of medication is now pregnant for the first time. Which client statement concerning asthma during pregnancy indicates the need for further instruction?
☐ 1. "I need to continue taking my asthma medication as prescribed."
☐ 2. "It is my goal to prevent or limit asthma attacks."
☐ 3. "During an asthma attack, oxygen needs to continue to be high for the birth parent and fetus."
☐ 4. "Bronchodilators should be used only when necessary because of the risk they present to the fetus."

90. A client at 22 weeks' gestation has right upper quadrant pain radiating to their back. The client rates the pain as 9 on a scale of 0 to 10 and says that it has occurred two times in the last week for about 4 hours at a time. The client does not associate the pain with food. Which nursing measure is the **highest priority** for this client?
☐ 1. Educate the client concerning changes occurring in the gallbladder as a result of pregnancy.
☐ 2. Refer the client to their health care provider (HCP) for evaluation and treatment of the pain.
☐ 3. Discuss nutritional strategies to decrease the possibility of heartburn.
☐ 4. Support the client's use of acetaminophen to relieve pain.

91. A client in the triage area who is at 19 weeks' gestation states that they have not felt their baby move in the past week, and no fetal heart tones are found. While evaluating this client, the nurse identifies the client as being at the **highest** risk for developing which problem?
☐ 1. abruptio placentae
☐ 2. HELLP syndrome
☐ 3. disseminated intravascular coagulation (DIC)
☐ 4. threatened abortion

92. The nurse performs a routine prenatal assessment on a client at 35 weeks' gestation and finds these vital signs: blood pressure 138/88 mm Hg; pulse 82 bpm; respirations 18 breaths/min; and temperature 99.1°F (37.3°C). Which statement is **most** appropriate for the nurse to make at this time?
☐ 1. "Your pulse is low. Do you exercise a lot?"
☐ 2. "Your blood pressure is slightly high. I will check it again before you leave."
☐ 3. "You have a slight temperature. Do you feel hot?"
☐ 4. "Your vital signs are all normal. I will document them on your medical record."

93. A 40-year-old client at 8 weeks' gestation has a 3-year-old child with Down syndrome. The nurse is discussing amniocentesis and chorionic villus sampling (CVS) as genetic screening methods for the expected baby. The nurse is confident that the teaching has been understood when the client makes which statement?
☐ 1. "Each test identifies a different part of the infant's genetic makeup."
☐ 2. "CVS can be performed earlier in pregnancy."
☐ 3. "The test results take the same length of time to be completed."
☐ 4. "Amniocentesis is a more dangerous procedure for the fetus."

94. After conducting a presentation to a group of adolescent parents on the topic of adolescent pregnancy, the nurse determines that one of the parents needs further instruction when the parent says that adolescents are at greater risk for which complication?
☐ 1. denial of the pregnancy
☐ 2. low-birth-weight infant
☐ 3. cephalopelvic disproportion
☐ 4. congenital anomalies

95. A dilatation and curettage (D&C) is scheduled for a primigravid client admitted to the hospital at 10 weeks' gestation with abdominal cramping, bright red vaginal spotting, and passage of some of the products of conception. The nurse should assess the client further for the expression of which feeling?
☐ 1. ambivalence
☐ 2. anxiety
☐ 3. fear
☐ 4. guilt

96. When providing care to the client who has undergone a dilatation and curettage (D&C) after a spontaneous abortion, the nurse administers hydroxyzine as prescribed. What is an expected outcome?
☐ 1. absence of nausea
☐ 2. minimized pain
☐ 3. decreased uterine cramping
☐ 4. improved uterine contractility

97. On entering the room of a client who has undergone a dilatation and curettage (D&C) for a spontaneous abortion, the nurse finds the client crying. Which comment by the nurse would be **most** appropriate?
☐ 1. "Are you having a great deal of uterine pain?"
☐ 2. "Commonly spontaneous abortion means a defective embryo."
☐ 3. "I am truly sorry you lost your baby."
☐ 4. "You can try to get pregnant again after a normal period."

98. A multigravida client who stands for long periods while working in a factory visits the prenatal clinic at 35 weeks' gestation, stating, "The varicose veins in my legs have really been bothering me lately." Which instruction would be **most** helpful?
☐ 1. Perform slow contraction and relaxation of the feet and ankles twice daily.
☐ 2. Take frequent rest periods with the legs elevated above the hips.
☐ 3. Avoid support hose that reach above the leg varicosities.
☐ 4. Take a leave of absence from work to avoid prolonged standing.

99. A primigravid client at 8 weeks' gestation tells the nurse that since having had sexual relations with a new partner 2 weeks ago, the client has noticed flulike symptoms, enlarged lymph nodes, and clusters of vesicles on their vagina. The nurse refers the client to a primary health care provider (HCP) because the nurse suspects which sexually transmitted infection?
☐ 1. gonorrhea
☐ 2. *Chlamydia trachomatis* infection
☐ 3. syphilis
☐ 4. herpes genitalis

100. The nurse is caring for a 24-year-old primigravid client scheduled for emergency surgery because of a probable ectopic pregnancy. What is the **most** important thing for the nurse to do?
☐ 1. Prepare to witness an informed consent for surgery.
☐ 2. Assess the client for massive external bleeding.
☐ 3. Explain that the fallopian tube can be salvaged.
☐ 4. Monitor the client for uterine contractions.

101. **STEP 1**

The nurse is caring for a 22-year-old female client in the prenatal clinic with a history of Crohn's disease.

Nurse's Notes

0900:
The 22-year-old primigravid client with a history of Crohn's disease is seen for a routine prenatal visit at 24 weeks' gestation. The client reports that their feet are cold and sometimes swell at the end. The client reports that lately they are more tired than usual and sometimes feel short of breath. The client says that their appetite has been good and they especially like chewing ice but that they do not take prenatal vitamins because of stomach irritation. The client's prepregnant weight was 114 lb (51.7 kg) with a body mass index (BMI) of 18.4 kg/m². Today, the client weighs 122 lb (55.3 kg), for a total weight gain of 8 lb (3.6 kg). Vital signs are temperature 97.9°F (36.6°C); pulse 80 bpm; respiration rate 16 breaths/min; blood pressure 102/68 mm Hg; and oxygen saturation by pulse oximetry 97% on room air. A urine dipstick test is negative for protein, glucose, ketones, and nitrites. Other lab test results are pending. The fetal heart rate is 140 bpm. The fundal height increased 4 cm from the last visit at 20 weeks. The client appears pale.

➤ Which assessment finding(s) would require follow-up? Select all that apply.

☐ 1. Activity
☐ 2. Circulation
☐ 3. Diet
☐ 4. Fetal heart rate
☐ 5. Fundal height
☐ 6. Urine dipstick
☐ 7. Vital signs
☐ 8. Weight

102. STEP 2

The nurse is caring for a 22-year-old female client in the prenatal clinic with a history of Crohn's disease.

Nurse's Notes

0900:
The 22-year-old primigravid client with a history of Crohn's disease is seen for a routine prenatal visit at 24 weeks' gestation. The client reports that their feet are cold and sometimes swell at the end. The client reports that lately they are more tired than usual and sometimes feel short of breath. The client says that their appetite has been good and they especially like chewing ice but that they do not take prenatal vitamins because of stomach irritation. The client's prepregnant weight was 114 lb (51.7 kg) with a body mass index (BMI) of 18.4 kg/m². Today, the client weighs 122 lb (55.3 kg), for a total weight gain of 8 lb (3.6 kg). Vital signs are temperature 97.9°F (36.6°C); pulse 80 bpm; respiration rate 16 breaths/min; blood pressure 102/68 mm Hg; and oxygen saturation by pulse oximetry 97% on room air. A urine dipstick test is negative for protein, glucose, ketones, and nitrites. Other lab test results are pending. The fetal heart rate is 140 bpm. The fundal height increased 4 cm from the last visit at 20 weeks. The client appears pale.

➤ For each possible finding, indicate if the finding is consistent with iron deficiency anemia, vitamin B_{12} anemia, or folate deficiency anemia. Each finding may support more than one disease process.

Possible Finding	Iron Deficiency Anemia	Vitamin B_{12} Deficiency Anemia	Folate Deficiency Anemia
Chewing ice	☐	☐	☐
Fatigue	☐	☐	☐
Crohn's disease history	☐	☐	☐
Pallor	☐	☐	☐

Note: Each column must have at least one response selected.

103. STEP 3

The nurse is caring for a 22-year-old female client in the prenatal clinic with a history of Crohn's disease.

Nurse's Notes

0900:
The 22-year-old primigravid client with a history of Crohn's disease is seen for a routine prenatal visit at 24 weeks' gestation. The client reports that their feet are cold and sometimes swell at the end. The client reports that lately they are more tired than usual and sometimes feel short of breath. The client says that their appetite has been good and they especially like chewing ice but that they do not take prenatal vitamins because of stomach irritation. The client's prepregnant weight was 114 lb (51.7 kg) with a body mass index (BMI) of 18.4 kg/m². Today, the client weighs 122 lb (55.3 kg), for a total weight gain of 8 lb (3.6 kg). Vital signs are temperature 97.9°F (36.6°C); pulse 80 bpm; respiration rate 16 breaths/min; blood pressure 102/68 mm Hg; and oxygen saturation by pulse oximetry 97% on room air. A urine dipstick test is negative for protein, glucose, ketones, and nitrites. Other lab test results are pending. The fetal heart rate is 140 bpm. The fundal height increased 4 cm from the last visit at 20 weeks. The client appears pale.

Laboratory Results

Test	Result	Reference
Red blood cells	$3.38 \times 10^6/\mu L$ ($3.38 \times 10^{12}/L$)	Women: 3.6–5 million/μL ($3.6–5 \times 10^{12}/L$)
Hemoglobin	9.0 g/dL (90 g/L)	Women: 12–16 g/dL (120–160 g/L)
Hematocrit	27.2% (0.27 proportion of 1.0)	Women: 36%–48% (0.36–0.48)
Mean corpuscular volume (MCV)	75 μm^3 (75 fL)	Women: 80–100 μm^3 (80–100 fL)

The nurse receives the laboratory test results.

➤ Complete the following sentences by choosing from the list of drop-down options.

The nurse should recognize that the client has a [microcytic / macrocytic / normocytic]

anemia most likely caused by a(n) [iron / vitamin B_{12} / folate]

nutritional deficit. Untreated, the client is at **most** risk for developing more [cardiac / neurologic / digestive]

symptoms as the pregnancy progresses.

104. STEP 4

The nurse is caring for a 22-year-old female client in the prenatal clinic with a history of Crohn's disease.

Nurse's Notes

0900:
The 22-year-old primigravid client with a history of Crohn's disease is seen for a routine prenatal visit at 24 weeks' gestation. The client reports that their feet are cold and sometimes swell at the end. The client reports that lately they are more tired than usual and sometimes feel short of breath. The client says that their appetite has been good and they especially like chewing ice but that they do not take prenatal vitamins because of stomach irritation. The client's prepregnant weight was 114 lb (51.7 kg) with a body mass index (BMI) of 18.4 kg/m². Today, the client weighs 122 lb (55.3 kg), for a total weight gain of 8 lb (3.6 kg). Vital signs are temperature 97.9°F (36.6°C); pulse 80 bpm; respiration rate 16 breaths/min; blood pressure 102/68 mm Hg; and oxygen saturation by pulse oximetry 97% on room air. A urine dipstick test is negative for protein, glucose, ketones, and nitrites. Other lab test results are pending. The fetal heart rate is 140 bpm. The fundal height increased 4 cm from the last visit at 20 weeks. The client appears pale.

Laboratory Results

Test	Result	Reference
Red blood cells	$3.38 \times 10^6/\mu L$ ($3.38 \times 10^{12}/L$)	Women: 3.6–5 million/μL (3.6–5 $\times 10^{12}/L$)
Hemoglobin	9.0 g/dL (90 g/L)	Women: 12–16 g/dL (120–160 g/L)
Hematocrit	27.2% (0.27 proportion of 1.0)	Women: 36%–48% (0.36–0.48)
Mean corpuscular volume (MCV)	75 μm^3 (75 fL)	Women: 80–100 μm^3 (80–100 fL)

The client receives the diagnosis of iron deficiency anemia.

➢ Which intervention(s) should the nurse include in the plan of care? Select all that apply.

☐	1. Administer oxygen.
☐	2. Monitor lab values.
☐	3. Perform a stat 12-lead echocardiogram (ECG).
☐	4. Replace fluid volume.
☐	5. Request a prescription for iron.
☐	6. Provide nutritional education.
☐	7. Obtain a referral to a dietician.
☐	8. Teach strategies to reduce fatigue.

105. STEP 5

The nurse is caring for a 22-year-old female client in the prenatal clinic with a history of Crohn's disease.

Nurse's Notes

0900:
The 22-year-old primigravid client with a history of Crohn's disease is seen for a routine prenatal visit at 24 weeks' gestation. The client reports that their feet are cold and sometimes swell at the end. The client reports that lately they are more tired than usual and sometimes feel short of breath. The client says that their appetite has been good and they especially like chewing ice but that they do not take prenatal vitamins because of stomach irritation. The client's prepregnant weight was 114 lb (51.7 kg) with a body mass index (BMI) of 18.4 kg/m². Today, the client weighs 122 lb (55.3 kg), for a total weight gain of 8 lb (3.6 kg). Vital signs are temperature 97.9°F (36.6°C); pulse 80 bpm; respiration rate 16 breaths/min; blood pressure 102/68 mm Hg; and oxygen saturation by pulse oximetry 97% on room air. A urine dipstick test is negative for protein, glucose, ketones, and nitrites. Other lab test results are pending. The fetal heart rate is 140 bpm. The fundal height increased 4 cm from the last visit at 20 weeks. The client appears pale.

Laboratory Results

Test	Result	Reference
Red blood cells	$3.38 \times 10^6/\mu L$ ($3.38 \times 10^{12}/L$)	Women: 3.6–5 million/µL ($3.6–5 \times 10^{12}/L$)
Hemoglobin	9.0 g/dL (90 g/L)	Women: 12–16 g/dL (120–160 g/L)
Hematocrit	27.2% (0.27 proportion of 1.0)	Women: 36%–48% (0.36–0.48)
Mean corpuscular volume (MCV)	75 µm³ (75 fL)	Women: 80–100 µm³ (80–100 fL)

Orders

- Refer to the outpatient infusion clinic
- Intravenous (IV) iron dextran per protocol

The client returns the next day to the outpatient infusion clinic to receive IV iron dextran.

➤ For each possible step, indicate if the step is essential or nonessential when administering dextran.

Possible Steps	Essential	Nonessential
Instruct the client to remain nothing by mouth (NPO)	○	○
Assess for allergies	○	○
Have resuscitation equipment available	○	○
Administer a sedative	○	○
Monitor for anaphylaxis	○	○
Obtain a complete blood count (CBC) immediately after the infusion	○	○

106. STEP 6

The nurse is caring for a 22-year-old female client in the prenatal clinic with a history of Crohn's disease.

Nurse's Notes

0900:
The 22-year-old primigravid client with a history of Crohn's disease is seen for a routine prenatal visit at 24 weeks' gestation. The client reports that their feet are cold and sometimes swell at the end. The client reports that lately they are more tired than usual and sometimes feel short of breath. The client says that their appetite has been good and they especially like chewing ice but that they do not take prenatal vitamins because of stomach irritation. The client's prepregnant weight was 114 lb (51.7 kg) with a body mass index (BMI) of 18.4 kg/m^2. Today, the client weighs 122 lb (55.3 kg), for a total weight gain of 8 lb (3.6 kg). Vital signs are temperature 97.9°F (36.6°C); pulse 80 bpm; respiration rate 16 breaths/min; blood pressure 102/68 mm Hg; and oxygen saturation by pulse oximetry 97% on room air. A urine dipstick test is negative for protein, glucose, ketones, and nitrites. Other lab test results are pending. The fetal heart rate is 140 bpm. The fundal height increased 4 cm from the last visit at 20 weeks. The client appears pale.

Laboratory Results

Test	Result	Reference
Red blood cells	3.38 × 10^6/μL (3.38 × 10^{12}/L)	Women: 3.6–5 million/μL (3.6–5 × 10^{12}/L)
Hemoglobin	9.0 g/dL (90 g/L)	Women: 12–16 g/dL (120–160 g/L)
Hematocrit	27.2% (0.27 proportion of 1.0)	Women: 36%–48% (0.36–0.48)
Mean corpuscular volume (MCV)	75 μm^3 (75 fL)	Women: 80–100 μm^3 (80–100 fL)

Orders

- Refer to the outpatient infusion clinic
- Intravenous (IV) iron dextran per protocol

Discharge orders

- Ferrous sulfate 325 mg orally once a day to begin 5 days after the infusion
- Recheck the CBC in 3 weeks
- Call the office with any concerns

The iron infusion is complete. The nurse reviews the discharge orders with the client and performs home medication teaching.

➤ For each possible client statement, specify if the statement indicates teaching was understood or not understood.

Possible Client Statement	Understood	Not Understood
"I can take my iron with some food since it upsets my stomach."	○	○
"Taking my iron with orange juice will help the medication absorb."	○	○
"I can't take antacids at the same time I take my iron."	○	○
"I should drink more to help prevent constipation."	○	○
"I might have tarry or bloody stools."	○	○
"If I miss a pill, I can take two pills next time."	○	○
"I should call the office if I develop a rash while taking the medication."	○	○

Managing Care, Quality, and Safety for Childbearing Clients

107. The nurse is reviewing results for clients who are having antenatal testing. The assessment data from which client warrant prompt notification of the health care provider (HCP) and a further plan of care?
- ☐ 1. primigravida who reports fetal movement six times in 2 hours
- ☐ 2. multigravida who had a positive oxytocin challenge test
- ☐ 3. primigravida whose infant has a biophysical profile of 9
- ☐ 4. multigravida whose infant has a moderate variability on a nonstress test

108. A nurse is assigned to the obstetrical triage area. When beginning the assignment, the nurse is given a report about four clients waiting to be seen. Place the clients in the order in which the nurse should see them. All options must be used.

1. a primigravid client at 10 weeks' gestation stating they are not feeling well with nausea and vomiting, urinary frequency, and fatigue

2. a multiparous client at 32 weeks' gestation asking for assistance with finding a new primary health care provider (HCP)

3. a single parent at 4 months postpartum fearful of shaking their baby when it cries

4. an antenatal client at 16 weeks' gestation who has occasional sharp pain on their left side radiating from the client's symphysis to their fundus

109. The nurse is working in an ambulatory obstetrics setting. Which client safety procedure(s) would be emphasized for this setting? Select all that apply.

☐ 1. employing handwashing or antiseptic use when entering and leaving a room
☐ 2. using two client identifiers when initiating contact with a client
☐ 3. using the same abbreviations as in the hospital setting
☐ 4. conducting a preprocedure verification asking for the client's name and the procedure to be performed
☐ 5. preventing infection by isolating anyone with nausea and vomiting

Answers, Rationales, and Test-Taking Strategies

*The answers and rationales for each question follow below, along with keys (🔑) to the client need (CN) and cognitive level (CL) for each question. In addition, questions that measure clinical judgment will be coded (CJ). As you check your answers, use the **Content Mastery and Test-Taking Skill Self-Analysis** worksheet (tear-out worksheet in the back of the book) to identify the reason(s) for not answering the questions correctly. For additional information about test-taking skills and strategies for answering questions, refer to pages 12–51 in Part 1 of this book.*

The Preconception Client

1. 1. Levonorgestrel can reduce the chance of pregnancy if taken within 72 hours of unprotected intercourse, and then again 12 hours later. Waiting 4 days to take levonorgestrel reduces effectiveness. Males can purchase this contraceptive as long as they are over 18 years of age. Levonorgestrel works by preventing ovulation or fertilization depending on where a client is in the menstrual cycle. Common side effects include nausea, breast tenderness, vertigo, and stomach pain.

🔑 CN: Physiological adaptation; CL: Evaluate

2. 3. Birth control plans are influenced primarily by whether the birth parent is breast- or bottle-feeding their infant. The maternal milk supply must be well established prior to the initiation of most hormonal birth control methods. Low-dose oral contraceptives would be the exception. Use of estrogen/progesterone-based pills and progesterone-only pills are commonly initiated from 4 to 6 weeks postpartum because the milk supply is well established by this time. Prior experiences with birth control methods have an impact on the method chosen, as do the preferences of the client's partner; however, they are not the most influential factors. A desire to have another child in 2 years would make some methods, such as an intrauterine device (IUD), less attractive, but it would still be secondary to the choice to breastfeed.

🔑 CN: Pharmacological and parenteral therapies; CL: Analyze

3. 3. For a client with a typical menstrual cycle of 28 days, ovulation usually occurs on day 14, plus or minus 2 days, before the onset of the next menstrual cycle. Stated another way, the menstrual period begins about 2 weeks after ovulation has occurred. Ovulation does not usually occur during the menses component of the cycle when the uterine lining is being shed. In most women, the ovum survives for about 12 to 24 hours after ovulation, during which time conception is possible. The basal body temperature rises 0.5°F to 1°F (0.28°C to 0.56°C) when ovulation occurs. Although some women experience some pelvic discomfort during ovulation (mittelschmerz), severe or unusual pain is rare. After ovulation, the cervical mucus is thin and copious.

CN: Health promotion and maintenance; CL: Create

4. 1. The nurse should instruct the client to take a mild analgesic, such as ibuprofen, if menstrual pain or "cramps" are present. The client should also eat foods rich in iron and should continue moderate exercise during menstruation, which increases abdominal tone. Avoiding cold foods will not decrease dysmenorrhea. The use of pads or tampons is a personal choice. There is no evidence that it is necessary to wait to use tampons.

CN: Health promotion and maintenance; CL: Apply

5. 1. Under ideal conditions, sperm can reach the ovum in 15 to 30 minutes. This is an important point to make with adolescents who may be sexually active. Many people believe that the time interval is much longer and that they can wait until after intercourse to take steps to prevent conception. Without protection, pregnancy and sexually transmitted diseases can occur. When using the abstinence or calendar method, the couple should abstain from intercourse on the days of the menstrual cycle when the client is most likely to conceive. Using a 28-day cycle as an example, a couple should abstain from coitus 3 to 4 days before ovulation (days 10 through 14) and 3 to 4 days after ovulation (days 15 through 18). Sperm from a healthy male can remain viable for 24 to 72 hours in the female reproductive tract. If the female client ovulates after coitus, there is a possibility that fertilization can occur. Before fertilization, the ovum and sperm each contain 23 chromosomes. After fertilization, the conceptus contains 46 chromosomes unless there is a chromosomal abnormality.

CN: Health promotion and maintenance; CL: Evaluate

6. 3. The symptothermal method is a natural method of fertility management that depends on knowing when ovulation has occurred. Because regular menstrual cycles can vary by 1 to 2 days in either direction, the symptothermal method requires daily basal body temperature assessments plus close monitoring of cervical mucus changes. The method relies on abstinence during the period of ovulation, which occurs approximately 14 days before the beginning of the next cycle. Abstinence from coitus for 5 days after menses is unnecessary because it is unlikely that ovulation will occur during this time period (days 1 through 10). Typically, the failure rate for this method is between 10% and 20%. Although a condom may increase the effectiveness of this method, most clients who choose natural methods are not interested in chemical or barrier types of family planning.

CN: Health promotion and maintenance; CL: Create

7. 2. Before advising a client about oral contraceptives, the nurse needs to assess the client for signs and symptoms of hypertension. Clients who have hypertension, thrombophlebitis, obesity, or a family history of cerebral or cardiovascular accident are poor candidates for oral contraceptives. In addition, women who smoke, are older than 40 years of age, or have a history of pulmonary disease should be advised to use a different method. Iron deficiency anemia, dysmenorrhea, and acne are not contraindications for the use of oral contraceptives. Iron deficiency anemia is a common disorder in young women. Oral contraceptives decrease the amount of menstrual flow and thus decrease the amount of iron lost through menses, thereby providing a beneficial effect when used by clients with anemia. Low-dose oral contraceptives to prevent ovulation may be effective in decreasing the severity of dysmenorrhea (painful menstruation). Dysmenorrhea is thought to be caused by the release of prostaglandins in response to tissue destruction during the ischemic phase of the menstrual cycle. The use of oral contraceptives commonly improves facial acne.

CN: Reduction of risk potential; CL: Analyze

8. 4. The nurse determines that the client needs further instruction when the client says that one of the adverse effects of oral contraceptive use is ovarian cancer. Some studies suggest that ovarian and endometrial cancers are reduced in women using oral contraceptives. Other adverse effects of oral contraceptives include weight gain, nausea, headache, breakthrough bleeding, and monilial infections. The most serious adverse effect is thrombophlebitis.

CN: Pharmacological and parenteral therapies; CL: Evaluate

9. **2.** The teaching plan should include a caution that a diaphragm should not be used if the client develops acute cervicitis, possibly aggravated by contact with the rubber of the diaphragm. Some studies have also associated diaphragm use with an increased incidence of urinary tract infections. Douching after the use of a diaphragm and intercourse is not recommended because pregnancy could occur. The diaphragm should be inspected and washed with mild soap and water after each use. A diaphragm should be left in place for at least 6 hours but no longer than 24 hours after intercourse. More spermicidal jelly or cream should be used if intercourse is repeated during this period.

    🔑 CN: Reduction of risk potential;
    CL: Create

10. **4.** The client would need additional instructions when they say that they can still use the same diaphragm if they gain or lose 20 lb (9 kg). Gaining or losing more than 15 lb (6.8 kg) can change the pelvic and vaginal contours to such a degree that the diaphragm will no longer protect the client against pregnancy. The diaphragm can be used for 2 to 3 years if it is cared for and well protected in its case. The client should be refitted for another diaphragm after pregnancy and birth because the weight changes and physiologic changes of pregnancy can alter the pelvic and vaginal contours, thus affecting the effectiveness of the diaphragm. The client should use a spermicidal jelly or cream before inserting the diaphragm.

    🔑 CN: Reduction of risk potential;
    CL: Evaluate

11. **1.** Another method of contraception is needed until all sperm has been cleared from the body. The number of ejaculates for this to occur varies with the individual, and laboratory analysis is required to determine when that has been accomplished. Vasectomy is considered a permanent sterilization procedure and requires microsurgery for anastomosis of the vas deferens to be completed. Studies have shown that there is no connection between cardiac disease in males and vasectomy. There is no need for follow-up after verification that there is no sperm in the system.

    🔑 CN: Physiological adaptation; CL: Create

12. **1.** Tubal ligation, a female sterilization procedure, involves ligation (tying off) or cauterization of the fallopian tubes through a small abdominal incision (laparotomy). Reversal of a tubal ligation is not easily done, and the pregnancy success rate after reversal is about 30%. After a tubal ligation, the client may engage in intercourse 2 to 3 days after the procedure. The ovaries are not generally removed during a tubal ligation. An oophorectomy involves the removal of one or both ovaries.

    🔑 CN: Health promotion and maintenance;
    CL: Evaluate

13. **2.** The basal body temperature method requires that the client take their temperature each morning before getting out of bed, preferably at the same time each day before eating or any other activity. Just before the day of ovulation, the temperature falls by 0.5°F (0.28°C). At the time of ovulation, the temperature rises 0.4°F to 0.8°F (0.22°C to 0.44°C) because of increased progesterone secretion in response to the luteinizing hormone. The temperature remains higher for the rest of the menstrual cycle. The client should keep a diary of about 6 months of menstrual cycles to calculate "safe" days. There is no mucus for the first 3 or 4 days after menses, and then thick, sticky mucus begins to appear. As estrogen increases, the mucus changes to clear, slippery, and stretchy. This condition, termed *spinnbarkeit,* is present during ovulation. After ovulation, the mucus decreases in amount and becomes thick and sticky again until menses. Because the ovum typically survives about 24 hours and sperm can survive up to 72 hours, couples must avoid coitus when the cervical mucus is copious and for about 3 to 4 days before and after ovulation to avoid a pregnancy.

    🔑 CN: Health promotion and maintenance;
    CL: Apply

14. **4.** By the end of the first visit, the couple should be able to identify potential causes and treatment modalities for infertility. If their evaluation shows that a treatment or procedure may help them to conceive, the couple must then decide how to proceed, considering all of the various treatments before selecting one. Treatments can be difficult, painful, or risky. The first visit is not the appropriate time to decide on a treatment plan because the couple needs time to adjust to the diagnosis of infertility, a crisis for most couples. Although the couple may be in a hurry for definitive therapy, a thorough assessment of both partners is necessary before a treatment plan can be initiated. The success rate for achieving a pregnancy depends on both the cause and the effectiveness of the treatment, and in some cases, it may be only as high as 30%. The couple may desire information about alternatives to treatment, but insufficient data are available to suggest that a specific treatment modality may not be successful. Suggesting that the couple consider adoption at this time may inappropriately imply that the couple has no other choice. If a specific therapy may result in a pregnancy, the couple should have time to consider their options. After a thorough

evaluation, adoption may be considered by the couple as an alternative to the costly, time-consuming, and sometimes painful treatments for infertility.

🗝️ CN: Health promotion and maintenance; CL: Analyze

15. 4. The client is verbalizing concerns about death during birth, thus providing the nurse with an opportunity to gather additional data. Asking the client about these concerns would be most helpful to determine the client's knowledge base and to provide the nurse with the opportunity to answer any questions and clarify any misconceptions. Although the maternal mortality rate is low in the United States and Canada, maternal deaths do occur, even with modern technology. Leading causes of maternal mortality in the United States and Canada include embolism, pregnancy-induced hypertension, hemorrhage, ectopic pregnancy, and infection. Telling the client not to concern themselves about what has happened in the past is not useful. It only serves to discount the client's concerns and block further therapeutic communication. Also, postponing or ignoring the client's need for a discussion about complications of pregnancy may further increase the client's anxiety.

🗝️ CN: Health promotion and maintenance; CL: Apply

16. 3. As ovulation approaches, cervical mucus is abundant, clear, and stretchy, resembling raw egg white. Ovulation generally occurs 14 days (±2 days) before the beginning of menses. During the luteal phase of the cycle, which occurs after ovulation, the cervical mucus is thick and sticky, making it difficult for sperm to pass. Changes in the cervical mucus are related to the influences of estrogen and progesterone. Cervical mucus is always present.

🗝️ CN: Health promotion and maintenance; CL: Create

17. 1. To ensure maximum effectiveness, the condom should always be placed over the erect penis before coitus. Some couples find condom use objectionable because foreplay may have to be interrupted to apply the condom. The penis, covered by the condom, should be withdrawn before the penis becomes flaccid. Otherwise, semen may escape from the condom, providing an opportunity for possible fertilization. Rather than having the condom pulled tightly over the penis before coitus, space should be left at the tip of the penis to allow the condom to hold the sperm. The client does not need a prescription for a condom with nonoxynol 9 because these are sold over the counter.

🗝️ CN: Reduction of risk potential; CL: Apply

18. 3. With medroxyprogesterone acetate, irregular menstrual cycles and amenorrhea are common adverse effects. Other adverse effects include weight gain, breakthrough bleeding, headaches, and depression. This method requires deep intramuscular injections every 3 months. The first injection should occur within 5 days after menses.

🗝️ CN: Reduction of risk potential; CL: Evaluate

19. 4. Severe cramping and pain may occur as the device is passed through the internal cervical os. The insertion of the device is generally done when the client is having their menses because it is unlikely that they are pregnant at that time. Common adverse effects of IUDs are heavy menstrual bleeding and subsequent anemia, not amenorrhea. Uterine infection or ectopic pregnancy may occur. The IUD has an effectiveness rate of 98%. Therefore, additional protection is not necessary to prevent pregnancy. IUDs generally are less costly than other forms of contraception because they do not require additional expense. Only one insertion is necessary, in comparison to daily doses of oral contraceptives or the need for spermicides in conjunction with diaphragm use.

🗝️ CN: Reduction of risk potential; CL: Apply

20. 3. Ceftriaxone may be used to treat *N. gonorrhoeae* infections and is commonly combined with doxycycline. Both the client and their partner should be treated if gonorrhea is present. Acyclovir can be used to treat herpes genitalis; however, the drug does not cure the disease. *C. trachomatis* infections are usually treated with antibiotics such as doxycycline or azithromycin. Metronidazole is used to treat trichomoniasis vaginitis, not condylomata acuminata (genital warts).

🗝️ CN: Pharmacological and parenteral therapies; CL: Create

21. 1. The couple needs further instruction when they identify that one cause of male infertility is decreased sperm count due to seminal fluid that has an alkaline pH. A slightly alkaline pH is necessary to protect the sperm from the acidic secretions of the vagina and is a normal finding. An alkaline pH is not associated with decreased sperm count. However, seminal fluid that is abnormal in amount, consistency, or chemical composition suggests obstruction, inflammation, or infection, which can decrease sperm production. The typical number of sperm produced during ejaculation is

400 million. Frequent exposure to heat sources, such as saunas and hot tubs, can decrease sperm production, as can abnormal hormonal stimulation. Immunologic factors produced by the man against his own sperm (autoantibodies) or by the woman can cause the sperm to clump or be unable to penetrate the ovum, thus contributing to infertility.

CN: Health promotion and maintenance; CL: Evaluate

The Pregnant Client Receiving Prenatal Care

22. 3. At 15 weeks' gestation, a primipara will not feel the baby moving. Quickening typically occurs between 18 and 20 weeks' gestation for a primipara and between 16 and 18 weeks' gestation for a multipara. Leaking fluid from the vagina should not occur until labor begins and may indicate a rupture of the membranes. Bleeding and fever are complications that warrant further evaluation and should be reported at any time during the pregnancy.

CN: Health promotion and maintenance; CL: Evaluate

23. 1, 3, 5. Providing culturally sensitive care includes providing printed material in the client's native language. Discussing cultural differences is not a priority or important at the first visit. Clients need to have an interpreter for each prenatal visit to translate and interpret questions. Contraceptive options are not a priority for the first prenatal visit. Reviewing dietary intake and discussing nutrition are important components of early prenatal care.

CN: Health promotion and maintenance; CL: Create

24. 4. Consuming most liquids between meals rather than at the same time as eating is an excellent strategy to deter nausea and vomiting in pregnancy but does not relieve heartburn. During the third trimester, progesterone causes relaxation of the sphincter, and the pressure of the fetus against the stomach increases the potential of heartburn. Avoiding highly seasoned foods, remaining in an upright position after eating, and eating small, frequent meals are strategies to prevent heartburn.

CN: Physiological adaptation; CL: Evaluate

25. 2. Iron deficiency anemia is caused by insufficient iron stores in the body, poor iron content in the diet of the pregnant client, or both. Other thalassemias and sickle cell anemia, rather than iron deficiency anemia, can be associated with ethnicity but occur primarily in clients of African or Mediterranean origin. Because red blood cells increase by about 50% during pregnancy, many clients will need to take supplemental iron to avoid iron deficiency anemia. A pregnant client is considered anemic when the hemoglobin is below 11 mg/dL (110 g/dL). In most types of anemia, the heart must pump more often and harder to deliver oxygen to cells.

CN: Reduction of risk potential; CL: Evaluate

26. 4. Many clients in their first trimester feel ambivalent about being pregnant because of the significant life changes that occur for most people who have a child. Ambivalence can be expressed as a list of positive and negative consequences of having a child, consideration of financial and social implications, and possible career changes. During the second trimester, the infant becomes a separate individual from the birth parent. The birth parent will begin to enjoy the role of nurturer postpartum. During the third trimester, the birth parent begins to prepare for parenthood and all of the tasks that parenthood includes.

CN: Health promotion and maintenance; CL: Apply

27. 4. Group B streptococcus is a risk factor for all pregnant women and is not limited to those carrying twins. The multiple gestation client is at risk for preterm labor because uterine distention, a major factor initiating preterm labor, is more likely with a twin gestation. The normal uterus is only able to distend to a certain point, and when that point is reached, labor may be initiated. Twin-to-twin transfusion drains blood from one twin to the second and is a problem that may occur with multiple gestations. The donor twin may become growth restricted and can have oligohydramnios, while the recipient twin may become polycythemic with polyhydramnios and develop heart failure. Anemia is a common problem with multiple gestation clients. The birth parent is commonly unable to consume enough protein, calcium, and iron to supply their needs and those of the fetuses. A maternal hemoglobin level below 11 mg/dL (110 g/L) is considered anemic.

CN: Physiological adaptation; CL: Evaluate

28. 2. The plan of care should reflect that this client is experiencing probable signs of pregnancy. The client may be pregnant, but the signs and symptoms may have another etiology. An enlarging abdomen and a positive pregnancy test may also be caused by tumors, hydatidiform mole, or other disease processes as well as pregnancy. Changes in the pigmentation of the face may also be caused by oral contraceptive use. Positive signs of pregnancy are considered diagnostic and include evident fetal heartbeat, fetal movement felt by a trained examiner, and visualization of the fetus with ultrasound confirmation. Presumptive signs are subjective and can have another etiology. These signs and symptoms include lack of menses, nausea, vomiting, fatigue, urinary frequency, and breast changes. The word "diagnostic" is not used to describe the condition of pregnancy.

CN: Physiological adaptation; CL: Analyze

29. **1.** The serum pregnancy test measures human chorionic gonadotropin (hCG) in blood plasma and is highly accurate within 1 week after ovulation. The test is performed in a laboratory. Over-the-counter or home pregnancy tests are performed on urine and typically require higher levels of hCG to obtain a positive result. A positive pregnancy test is considered a probable sign of pregnancy. Certain conditions other than pregnancy, such as choriocarcinoma, can cause increased hCG levels.

CN: Reduction of risk potential; CL: Apply

30. **4.** The hormone analyzed in most pregnancy tests is hCG. In the pregnant client, trace amounts of hCG appear in the serum as early as 24 to 48 hours after implantation owing to the trophoblast production of this hormone. Prolactin, follicle-stimulating hormone, and luteinizing hormone are not used to detect pregnancy. Prolactin is the hormone secreted by the pituitary gland to prepare the breasts for lactation. Follicle-stimulating hormone is involved in follicle maturation during the menstrual cycle. Luteinizing hormone is responsible for stimulating ovulation.

CN: Reduction of risk potential; CL: Evaluate

31. **4.** When using Nägele's rule to determine the estimated date of birth, the nurse would count back 3 calendar months from the first day of the last menstrual period and add 7 days. This means the client's estimated date is February 17.

CN: Health promotion and maintenance; CL: Apply

32. **4.** The placenta does not produce testosterone. Human placental lactogen, hCG, estrogen, and progesterone are hormones produced by the placenta during pregnancy. The hormone hCG stimulates the synthesis of estrogen and progesterone early in the pregnancy until the placenta can assume this role. Estrogen results in uterine and breast enlargement. Progesterone aids in maintaining the endometrium, inhibiting uterine contractility, and developing the breasts for lactation. The placenta also produces some nutrients for the embryo and exchanges oxygen, nutrients, and waste products through the chorionic villi.

CN: Health promotion and maintenance; CL: Evaluate

33. **4, 3, 2, 1.** While initially continuing to attempt to find the fetal heartbeat, the nurse can ask the client if the baby has been moving. This will give a quick idea of the status. The next step would be to obtain different equipment and attempt to find the fetal heartbeat again. A simple statement of fact that the nurse cannot find the heartbeat and is taking steps to rule out equipment error is appropriate. Calling the HCP would be the last step after it is determined that the baby does not have a heartbeat.

CN: Reduction of risk potential; CL: Create

34. **1, 2.** Although ultrasounds are not considered part of routine care, the ultrasound is able to confirm the pregnancy, identify the major anatomic features of the fetus and possible abnormalities, and determine the gestational age by measuring the crown-to-rump length of the embryo during the first trimester. At this time, the ultrasound cannot confirm that the fetus is viable. The ultrasound will provide information about fetal position; however, this information would be more important later in the pregnancy, not during the first trimester. The ultrasound would provide no information about the nutrient supply for the fetus.

CN: Health promotion and maintenance; CL: Analyze

35. **2.** This client is expressing a feeling of surprise about having a baby. Therefore, the nurse's best response would be to confirm the pregnancy, which is something that the client already suspects, and then ascertain how the client is feeling now that the suspicion is confirmed. Studies have shown that a common reaction to pregnancy is summarized as ambivalence or "someday, but not now." Such feelings are normal and are experienced by many women early in pregnancy. Offering a pamphlet on pregnancy does not respond to the client's feelings. Telling the client that they should be delighted ignores, rather than addresses, the client's feelings. Also, doing so imposes the nurse's opinion on the client. Ambivalence is a common reaction to pregnancy. Telling the client that they should be delighted may lead to feelings of guilt. Asking about the client's concerns is premature until the nurse determines the client's overall feelings about the pregnancy.

CN: Psychosocial integrity; **CL:** Apply

36. 3. Clients normally experience ambivalence when pregnancy is confirmed, even if the pregnancy was planned. Although the client's culture may play a role in openly accepting the pregnancy, most new birth parents who have been ambivalent initially accept the reality by the end of the first trimester. Ambivalence also may be expressed throughout the pregnancy; this is believed to be related to the amount of physical discomfort. The nurse should become concerned and perhaps contact a social worker if the client expresses ambivalence in the third trimester. The client's statement reflects ambivalence, not fear. There is no evidence to suggest or imply that the client is rejecting the fetus. The client's statement reflects ambivalence about the pregnancy and is not in and of itself an indication that the client lacks support resources.

CN: Psychosocial integrity; **CL:** Analyze

37. 3. *Couvade syndrome* refers to the situation in which the expectant spouse or partner experiences some of the discomforts of pregnancy along with the pregnant client as a means of identifying with the pregnancy. *Ptyalism* is the term for excessive salivation. *Mittelschmerz* is the lower abdominal discomfort felt by some clients during ovulation. *Pica* refers to an oral craving for substances such as clay or starch that some pregnant clients experience.

CN: Psychosocial integrity; **CL:** Analyze

38. 3. Maternal alcohol use may result in fetal alcohol syndrome, marked by mild-to-moderate mental retardation, physical growth retardation, central nervous system disorders, and feeding difficulties. Because there is no definitive answer as to how much alcohol can be safely consumed by a pregnant client, it is recommended that they be taught to abstain from drinking alcohol during pregnancy. Smoking and other medications also may affect the fetus.

CN: Reduction of risk potential; **CL:** Apply

39. 4. An increase in clear, highly acidic vaginal secretions is a normal finding during pregnancy that aids in controlling the growth of pathologic bacteria. Vaginal secretions increase because of the influence of estrogen secretion and increased vaginal and cervical vascularity. The highly acidic nature of the vaginal secretions is caused by the action of *Lactobacillus acidophilus*, which increases the lactic acid content of the secretions. The increased acidity helps make the vagina resistant to bacterial growth. During pregnancy, estrogen secretion fosters a glycogen-rich environment. Unfortunately, this glycogen-rich, acidic environment fosters the development of yeast (*Candida albicans*) infections, manifested by itching, burning, and a cheese-like vaginal discharge. If the client had a sexually transmitted infection, most likely they would have additional symptoms, such as lesions in the genital area or changes in color, consistency, or odor of the vaginal secretions. An increase in vaginal secretions does not help prevent expulsion of the mucus plug. The mucus plug is held in place by the cervix until the cervix becomes ripe.

CN: Health promotion and maintenance; **CL:** Analyze

40. 2. Measurement of the client's fundal height is a gross estimate of fetal gestational age. At 20 weeks' gestation, the fundal height should be at about the level of the client's umbilicus. The fundus typically is over the symphysis pubis at 12 weeks. A fundal height measurement between these two areas would suggest a fetus with a gestational age between 12 and 20 weeks. The fundal height increases approximately 1 cm per week after 20 weeks' gestation. The fundus typically reaches the xiphoid process at approximately 36 weeks' gestation. A fundal height between the umbilicus and the xiphoid process would suggest a fetus with a gestational age between 20 and 36 weeks. The fundus then commonly returns to about 4 cm below the xiphoid process owing to lightening at 40 weeks. Additionally, pressure on the diaphragm occurs late in pregnancy. Therefore, a fundal height measurement near the xiphoid process with diaphragmatic compression suggests a fetus near the gestational age of 36 weeks or older.

CN: Health promotion and maintenance; **CL:** Apply

41. 2. The volume of fluid needed for amniocentesis is 15 mL, and this is usually available at 15 weeks' gestation. Fetal development continues throughout the prenatal period. Cells necessary for testing for hemophilia A are available during the entire pregnancy but are not accessible by amniocentesis until 12 weeks' gestation. Amniocentesis carries a slight risk for infection regardless of when the procedure is performed.

CN: Reduction of risk potential; **CL:** Apply

42. 4. The National Academy of Sciences Institute of Medicine and Health Canada recommends that women gain 25 to 35 lb (11.5 to 14.5 kg) during pregnancy. The pattern of weight gain is as important as the total amount of weight gained. Underweight women and women carrying twins should have a greater weight gain. Typically, women should gain 3.5 lb (1.6 kg) during the first trimester and then 1 lb (0.45 kg)/week during the remainder of the pregnancy (24 weeks) for a total of about 27 to 28 lb (12.2 to 12.7 kg). A weight gain of only 6.6 lb (3 kg) in the second and third trimesters is not normal because the client should be gaining about 1 lb (0.45 kg)/week, or 12 lb (5.4 kg) during the second and third trimesters. Gaining 12 lb (5.4 kg) during each trimester would total 36 lb (16.2 kg), which is slightly more than the recommended weight gain. In addition, nausea and vomiting during the first trimester can contribute to a lack of appetite and smaller weight gain during this trimester.

CN: Health promotion and maintenance; CL: Evaluate

43. 1, 5. Green, leafy vegetables, such as asparagus, spinach, brussels sprouts, and broccoli, are rich sources of folic acid. Beans, peas, and lentils are also good sources. The pregnant client needs to eat foods high in folic acid to prevent folic acid deficits, which may result in neural tube defects in the newborn. A well-balanced diet must include whole grains, dairy products, and fresh fruits; however, bananas are rich in potassium, seafood is rich in iodine, and yogurt is rich in calcium, not folic acid.

CN: Reduction of risk potential; CL: Apply

44. 3. Egg yolks and squash and other yellow vegetables are rich sources of vitamin A. Buttermilk and cheese are good sources of calcium. Strawberries, broccoli, citrus fruits (such as oranges), and tomatoes are good sources of vitamin C, not vitamin A.

CN: Basic care and comfort; CL: Evaluate

45. 1, 3, 4. Dairy products, fresh fruit, vegetables, and foods high in protein (like cheese and peanut butter) are excellent choices. Fried foods, such as chicken nuggets and tater tots, and foods such as cheeseburgers and buttered popcorn are high in fat; carbonated drinks such as diet colas and foods such as pickles and ketchup contain large amounts of sodium. These foods can lead to an increase in ankle edema and promote weight gain from empty calories.

CN: Health promotion and maintenance; CL: Apply

46. 1. Milk contains a large amount of calcium but contains no iron. Coffee, tea, and caffeinated soft drinks inhibit the absorption of iron. The vitamin C found in orange juice enhances the absorption of iron. Cream of wheat (1 cup/10 mg iron) and molasses (1 tbsp/3 mg iron) are considered excellent sources of iron as they contain the indicated amounts of iron.

CN: Physiological adaptation; CL: Evaluate

47. 2. Magnesium aids in the synthesis of protein, nucleic acids, proteins, and fats. It is important for cell growth and neuromuscular function. Magnesium also activates the enzymes for the metabolism of protein and energy. Calcium prevents demineralization of the birth parent's bones. Vitamin B_6 is important for amino acid metabolism. Folic acid assists in the development of neural pathways in the fetus.

CN: Basic care and comfort; CL: Apply

48. 2. The nurse reports the results of the VDRL test to the HCP. The pregnant client must be treated for syphilis to prevent perinatal transmission of the disease. The rubella titer and blood sugar values are within normal range. The blood type is not a significant factor in this situation.

CN: Reduction of risk potential; CL: Analyze

49. 3. Clients often do not tell providers about the use of complementary and alternative approaches because they fear they will be judged. By approaching care as a partnership, the nurse sets the stage for open communication. All other statements are true but begin the conversation in a way that suggests the client has done something wrong.

CN: Basic care and comfort; CL: Apply

50. 4. Although most multiparous women experience quickening at about 17½ weeks' gestation, some women may perceive it between 14 and 20 weeks' gestation because they have been pregnant before and know what to expect. Detecting movement early does not suggest a twin pregnancy. If the multiparous client does not experience quickening by 20 weeks' gestation, further investigation is warranted because the fetus may have died, the client has a hydatidiform mole, or the pregnancy dating is incorrect. There is no evidence that the client's expected date of birth is erroneous.

CN: Health promotion and maintenance; CL: Analyze

51. 1, 2, 3, 4. Anyone could be a victim of intimate partner violence. Health care workers should routinely assess women for intimate partner violence. Pregnant teens have an increased risk for not finishing school, smoking, and substance abuse. It is possible that the client is depressed and their appearance and lack of eye contact are symptoms of depression. The nurse expects the blood glucose screening test to be prescribed between 24 and 28 weeks' gestation to screen for gestational diabetes. hCG levels can identify the presence of a pregnancy or give information about an abnormal pregnancy. It would not be done at this time in a normal pregnancy.

🗝 CN: Health promotion and maintenance; CL: Apply

52. 2. Leopold's maneuvers involve abdominal palpation. The client should empty their bladder before the nurse palpates the abdomen. Doing so increases the client's comfort and makes palpation more accurate. Although breathing deeply may help relax the client, it has no effect on the accuracy of the results of Leopold maneuvers. The client does not need to drink a full glass of water before the examination. The client should be lying in a supine position with the head slightly elevated for greater comfort and with the knees drawn up slightly.

🗝 CN: Health promotion and maintenance; CL: Apply

53. Because the fetus is determined to be in an ROA, a vertex position, the convex portion of the fetus lying closest to the uterine wall would be located in the lower right quadrant of the abdomen. Placing the Doppler ultrasound over that area would produce the loudest fetal heart sounds.

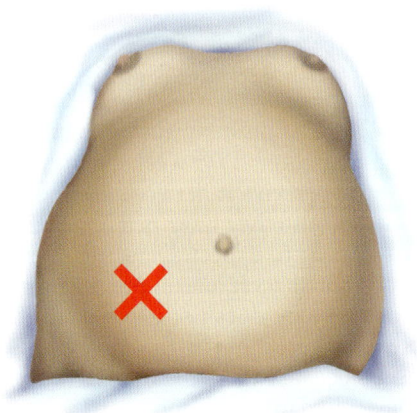

🗝 CN: Management of care; CL: Apply

54. 2. In left occipitus anterior lie, the occiput faces the left anterior segment of the client's pelvis. In left occipital transverse lie, the occiput faces the client's left hip. In right occipital transverse lie, the occiput faces the client's right hip. In right occipital anterior lie, the occiput faces the right anterior segment of the client's pelvis.

🗝 CN: Physiological adaptation; CL: Apply

55. 1. Discoloration on the face that commonly appears during pregnancy, called *chloasma* (mask of pregnancy), usually fades postpartum and is of no clinical significance. The client who is bothered by their appearance may be able to decrease the prominence of chloasma with ordinary makeup. Chloasma is not a sign of skin melanoma. It is not caused by dilated capillaries. Rather, it results from increased secretion of melanocyte-stimulating hormones caused by estrogen and progesterone secretion. No treatment is necessary for this condition.

🗝 CN: Health promotion and maintenance; CL: Apply

56. 4. Assessment of fundal height is a gross estimate of fetal growth. By 20 weeks' gestation, the height of the fundus should be at the level of the umbilicus, after which it should increase 1 cm for each week of gestation until approximately 36 weeks' gestation. A fundal height that is significantly different from that implied by the estimated gestational age warrants further evaluation (e.g., ultrasound examination) because it possibly indicates multiple pregnancy or fetal growth retardation. Fundal height estimation will not determine uterine activity or a need for increased weight gain. Leopold maneuvers will determine fetal position but are not typically done in the second trimester when the fetus is still freely moving.

🗝 CN: Health promotion and maintenance; CL: Apply

57. 4. There is little risk for fetal organ malformations from amniocentesis. One of the primary risks of amniocentesis is stimulation of the uterus and possible miscarriage. Other risks include hemorrhage from penetration of the placenta, infection of the amniotic fluid, and puncture of the fetus. Club foot has been associated with amniocentesis, especially when it is performed before 15 weeks.

🗝 CN: Reduction of risk potential; CL: Evaluate

58. -/+ 1, 2, 3, 4. Clients should keep well hydrated with any form of exercise. Dehydration can lead to dizziness and put the client at risk for falls. Later in pregnancy, dehydration can contribute to preterm labor. Becoming overheated can lead to dehydration. In the first trimester, heat can act as a teratogen. Ligaments become more relaxed during pregnancy, making joints more mobile. High impact, quick movements can lead to injury. Many yoga poses put pressure on the abdomen and would need to be modified as a pregnancy progresses. It is unnecessary to restrict participation to a prenatal yoga class only; however, the client should be advised to notify the instructor that they are pregnant and discuss if participating in that particular class is appropriate.

   CN: Basic care and comfort; CL: Create

59. 3. The client traveling by automobile should be advised to take intermittent breaks of 10 to 15 minutes, including walking, every 1 to 2 hours to stimulate the circulation, which becomes sluggish during long periods of sitting. Automobile travel is not contraindicated during pregnancy unless the client develops complications. There is no set maximum number of hours allowed. The pregnant client should always wear a seat belt when traveling by automobile. The client should be aware of the nearest health care facility in the city to which they are traveling.

   CN: Reduction of risk potential; CL: Apply

60. Seat belt safety is important for pregnant clients because proper use reduces maternal mortality in car crashes. Both lap and shoulder belts are to be used. The lap portion of the belt is placed snugly but comfortably to fit under the abdominal bulge. Wearing the lap belt over the abdomen could increase the risk for uterine rupture and fetal complications due to belt tightening as the client is propelled forward during an automobile collision. The shoulder belt is placed snugly across the shoulder, chest, and upper abdomen.

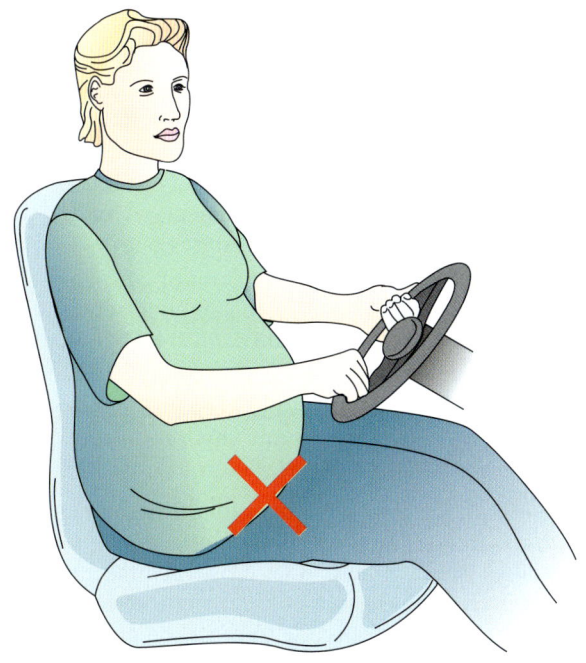

   CN: Safety and infection control; CL: Apply

61. 3. Leg cramps are thought to result from excessive amounts of phosphorus absorbed from milk products. Straightening the knee and flexing the toes toward the chin is an effective measure to relieve leg cramps. Also, decreasing milk intake and supplementing with calcium lactate may help reduce cramping. Keeping the legs warm and elevating them are good preventive measures. Changing positions frequently aids venous return but is not helpful in relieving leg cramps. Alternately flexing and extending the legs will not help relieve the leg cramp. Lying prone in the bed is a difficult position for a client at 37 weeks' gestation to achieve and maintain because of the increase in abdominal size and therefore is not considered helpful.

   CN: Basic care and comfort; CL: Apply

62. The fist is placed against the middle of the client's sternum, with backward thrusts until the foreign body is expelled. The pressure from the backward thrusts causes compression of the ribs, further adding to the chest and lung pressure, thereby forcing the foreign body to move upward.

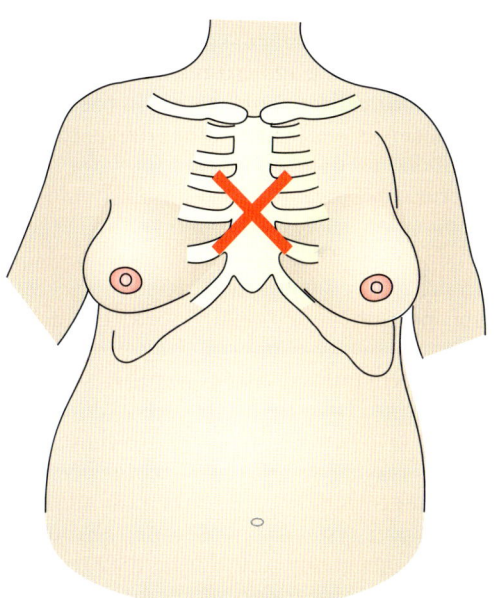

   CN: Safety and infection control; CL: Apply

63. 2. In the first maneuver, which is done with the nurse facing the client's head, both hands are used to palpate and determine which fetal body part (e.g., the head or buttocks) is in the fundus. This first maneuver helps determine the presenting part of the fetus. In the second maneuver, also done with the nurse facing the client's head, the palms of both hands are used to palpate the sides of the uterus and determine the location of the fetal back and spine. In the third maneuver, one hand gently grasps the lower portion of the abdomen just above the symphysis pubis to determine whether the fetal head is at the pelvic inlet. The fourth maneuver, done with the nurse facing the client's feet, determines the degree of fetal descent and flexion into the pelvis.

🔑 CN: Health promotion and maintenance; CL: Apply

64. 4. Increased AFP is one of the four laboratory values in a maternal quad screen. The labs are *human chorionic gonadotropin*, *estriol*, and *inhibin-A*. Increased AFP levels are associated with neural tube defects, such as spina bifida, anencephaly, and encephalocele. Ultrasonography is used to confirm a neural tube defect only when AFP levels are increased. Because AFP levels are usually highest at 15 to 18 weeks' gestation, this is the optimum time for testing. Performing the test after this time leads to inaccurate results. The client's blood, not urine, is used for the sample.

🔑 CN: Reduction of risk potential; CL: Create

65. 1. Prenatal care is commonly the most critical factor influencing pregnancy outcomes. This is especially true for adolescents because the most significant medical complication in pregnant adolescents is pregnancy-induced hypertension. Continued prenatal care helps allow for early detection and prompt intervention should the complication arise. Other risks for adolescents include low-birth-weight infant, preterm labor, iron deficiency anemia, and cephalopelvic disproportion. Gestational diabetes can occur with any pregnancy regardless of the age of the birth parent. Generally, all first-time birth parents need instruction related to discomforts. Adolescent birth parents have better nutrition when they attend group classes and are subject to peer pressure. No evidence demonstrates that most adolescents lack support systems. Spouses may abandon birth parents at any time during the pregnancy; other spouses, regardless of age, are supportive throughout the pregnancy.

🔑 CN: Health promotion and maintenance; CL: Apply

66. 3. Colostrum is usually secreted by about the 16th week of gestation in preparation for breastfeeding. Growth of the milk ducts is greatest in the last trimester, not in the first 8 weeks of gestation. Enlargement of the breasts is usually caused by estrogen, not progesterone. Darkening of the areola can occur as early as the sixth week of gestation.

🔑 CN: Health promotion and maintenance; CL: Create

67. -/+ 2, 4, 5. Understanding of breastfeeding education is demonstrated by statements involving knowledge of the several positions available for comfortable breastfeeding, oxytocin release from the pituitary gland leading to a let-down reflex and uterine contractions for involution, and feeding cues helpful in successful breastfeeding (because waiting until the infant is hungry and crying is stressful). Breast size does not ensure successful breastfeeding. Mastitis is an infectious process and is not influenced by latching on.

🔑 CN: Basic care and comfort; CL: Evaluate

68. 2. During pregnancy, the circulatory system undergoes tremendous changes. Cardiac output increases by 25% to 50%, and circulatory blood volume increases by about 30%. The client may experience transient hypotension and dizziness with sudden position changes. Early in pregnancy, there is a slight increase in the temperature, and clients may attribute this to a sinus infection or a cold. The client may feel warm, but this sensation is transient. The level of circulating fibrinogen increases as much as 50% during pregnancy, probably because of increased estrogen. Any calf tenderness should be reported because it may indicate a clot. Late in pregnancy, the posterior pituitary gland secretes oxytocin. The client may experience painful Braxton Hicks contractions or early labor symptoms.

🔑 CN: Health promotion and maintenance; CL: Create

69. 1. The fetal biophysical profile includes fetal breathing movements, fetal body movements, tone, amniotic fluid volume, and fetal heart rate reactivity. Normal nonstress test findings include at least two qualifying accelerations in the fetal heart rate from baseline in 20 minutes. A contraction stress test or oxytocin challenge test should be performed only on women who are at risk for fetal distress during labor. The contraction stress test is rarely performed before 28 weeks' gestation because of the possibility of initiating labor. Percutaneous umbilical cord sampling requires the insertion of a needle through the abdomen to obtain a fetal blood sample.

🔑 CN: Reduction of risk potential; CL: Apply

70. -/+ 1, 3, 4, 5. The fetus does go through sleep cycles, rendering it less likely to move while it is asleep. Blood glucose does cross the placenta and can affect fetal movement. Cigarette smoking causes carbon monoxide to cross the placenta, which reduces fetal oxygen. Pregnant women are more likely to notice fetal movement while they are sitting or lying down, and the time of day often determines this. Most pregnant women notice fetal movement in the evening. Barometric pressure does not affect fetal activity in utero.

🔑 CN: Health promotion and maintenance; CL: Analyze.

71. 4. During the third trimester, it is not uncommon for clients to have dreams or fantasies about the baby. Sometimes the dreams are about infants who are malformed or, in this example, covered with hair. There is no evidence to suggest that the client is trying to cope with becoming a parent. Having dreams about the baby does not mean that labor will begin soon.

🔑 CN: Psychosocial integrity; CL: Apply

72. 3. The client needs further instruction when they say it is permissible to sit in a hot tub for 20 minutes to relax after work. Hot tubs and saunas should be avoided, particularly in the first trimester, because their use can lead to maternal hyperthermia, which is associated with fetal anomalies such as central nervous system defects. The client should use nonskid pads in the shower or bath to avoid slipping because the client's center of gravity has shifted and they may fall. The client should avoid using soap on the nipples to prevent the removal of natural protective oils. Douching is not recommended for pregnant women because it can destroy the normal flora and increase the client's risk for infection.

🔑 CN: Health promotion and maintenance; CL: Evaluate

The Pregnant Client in Birth Preparation Classes

73. 4. Pregnancy creates changes in the parents. Being considerate, accepting changes, and being supportive of the current situation are considered acceptable responses by the client's spouse, rather than feeling irritation about these changes. Expressing concern over the financial changes of pregnancy and an expanded family is normal. The first trimester involves the client and family feeling ambivalent about pregnancy and moving toward acceptance of the changes associated with pregnancy. Maternal acceptance of the pregnancy and a subsequent change in the birth parent's focus are normal occurrences.

🔑 CN: Health promotion and maintenance; CL: Analyze

74. 4. Thyroid enlargement and increased basal body metabolism are common occurrences during pregnancy. Human placental lactogen enhances milk production. Estrogen is responsible for hyperpigmentation and vascular skin changes. Progesterone relaxes smooth muscle in the respiratory tract.

🔑 CN: Health promotion and maintenance; CL: Create

75. 1. Although sex is not easily discerned at 9 to 12 weeks, external genitalia are developed at this period of fetal development. Myelinization of the nerves begins at about 20 weeks' gestation. Brown fat stores develop at approximately 21 to 24 weeks. Air ducts and alveoli develop later in the gestational period, at approximately 25 to 28 weeks.

🔑 CN: Health promotion and maintenance; CL: Apply

76. 1, 3, 2, 4. Engagement refers to the fetus' entering the true pelvis and occurs before descent in primiparas and concurrently in multiparous clients. If the head is the presenting part, the normal maneuvers during labor and birth are (in order) descent, flexion, internal rotation, extension, external rotation, and expulsion. These maneuvers are called the *cardinal movements*. They occur as the fetal head passes through the maternal pelvis during the normal labor process.

🔑 CN: Health promotion and maintenance; CL: Create

77. 1. In a normal birth and for the first 24 hours postpartum, a total blood loss not exceeding 500 mL is considered normal. Blood loss during birth is almost always estimated because it provides a valuable indicator for possible hemorrhage. A blood loss of 1000 mL is considered hemorrhage.

🔑 CN: Health promotion and maintenance; CL: Apply

78. 2. Although the amniotic fluid promotes normal prenatal development by allowing symmetric development, it does not provide the fetus with nutrients. Rather, nutrients are provided by the placenta. The amniotic fluid helps protect the fetus from injury by cushioning against the impact of the maternal abdomen and allows room and buoyancy for fetal movement. The amniotic fluid and sac keep the fetus at a stable temperature by maintaining a neutral thermal environment.

🔑 CN: Health promotion and maintenance; CL: Evaluate

79. 1. Pelvic rocking helps relieve backache during pregnancy and early labor by making the spine more flexible. Deep-breathing exercises assist with relaxation and pain relief during labor. Tailor sitting and squatting help stretch the perineal muscles in preparation for labor.

🗝️ CN: Health promotion and maintenance; CL: Analyze

80. 🔢 **1, 2, 4.** Pain during the first stage of labor is primarily caused by hypoxia of the uterine and cervical muscle cells during contraction, stretching of the lower uterine segment, dilatation of the cervix and perineum, and pressure on adjacent structures. Ambulating will assist in increasing the circulation of blood to the area and relaxing the muscles. Slow chest breathing is appropriate during the first stage of labor to promote increased oxygenation as well as relaxation. The client or their coach can lightly massage the abdomen (effleurage) while using slow chest breathing. Chest breathing and massaging increase oxygenation and relaxation of uterine muscles. Pain medication is not used during the first stage of labor because most medications will slow labor; anesthesia may be considered during the second stage of labor. Sipping ice water, while helpful for maintaining hydration, will not be useful as a pain management strategy.

🗝️ CN: Health promotion and maintenance; CL: Apply

81. 4. With true labor, the contractions are felt first in the lower back and then the abdomen. They become more regular, gradually increase in frequency and duration, and do not disappear with ambulation, rest, or sleep. In true labor, the cervix dilates and effaces. Walking tends to increase true contractions. False labor contractions disappear with ambulation, rest, or sleep. False labor contractions commonly remain the same in duration and frequency. Clients who are experiencing false labor may have pain, even though the contractions are not very effective.

🗝️ CN: Health promotion and maintenance; CL: Apply

82. 4. Pelvic tilt exercises are useful to alleviate backache during pregnancy and labor but are not useful for the pain from contractions. Biofeedback (a conscious effort to control the response to pain), effleurage (light uterine massage), and guided imagery (focusing on a pleasant scene) are appropriate pain relief techniques to practice before labor begins. Various breathing exercises also can help alleviate the discomfort from contraction pain.

🗝️ CN: Health promotion and maintenance; CL: Evaluate

83. 2. During pregnancy, urinary tract infections are more common because of urinary stasis. Clients need instructions about increasing fluid volume intake. Plasma volume increases during pregnancy. The increase in plasma volume is more pronounced and occurs earlier than does the increase in red blood cell mass, possibly resulting in physiologic anemia. Peripheral vascular resistance decreases during pregnancy, providing a relatively stable blood pressure. Hemoglobin levels decrease during pregnancy even though there is an increase in blood volume.

🗝️ CN: Health promotion and maintenance; CL: Apply

The Pregnant Client with Risk Factors

84. 4. For the Rh-negative client who may be pregnant with an Rh-positive fetus, an indirect Coombs test measures antibodies in the maternal blood. Titers should be performed monthly during the first and second trimesters and biweekly during the third trimester and the week before the due date. A direct Coombs test can be done after birth to measure antibodies in baby's blood. An indirect Coombs is not done on placental blood or amniotic fluids.

🗝️ CN: Health promotion and maintenance; CL: Apply

85. 4. A maternal quad screen testing is done to screen for genetic and neural tube abnormalities between the 15th and 18th weeks of gestation. The four tests included are alpha-fetoprotein (AFP), *human chorionic gonadotropin*, estriol, and inhibin-A. Abnormally high levels of AFP found in maternal serum may be indicative of neural tube defects such as anencephaly and spina bifida. Low levels may indicate trisomy 21 (Down syndrome). Beta strep testing is done in the third trimester. Chorionic villus sampling is done as early as 10 weeks' gestation to detect anomalies. Ultrasound testing may be done in the first trimester to determine fetal viability and in the third trimester to determine pelvic adequacy and fetal or placental position.

🗝️ CN: Reduction of risk potential; CL: Apply

86. 🔢 **1, 2, 5.** Prenatal care includes a general supplementation of 400 mcg of folic acid, and clients with a history of gastric bypass should be referred to a dietician to determine adequate nutrient intake. All pregnant clients have their urine routinely checked for protein and sugar. There is no indication for checking glucose levels at each prenatal visit in clients who have undergone gastric bypass. Clients who have undergone gastric bypass are not at risk for gaining all of their weight back. No evidence supports implementing nonstress tests at 20 weeks.

CN: Health promotion and maintenance; CL: Create

87. **2.** According to both the New York Heart Association and the Canadian Cardiovascular Society, this client would fit under class II because they are symptomatic with increased activity (dyspnea with exertion). Class II clients have cardiac disease and a slight limitation in physical activity. When physical activity occurs, the client may experience angina, difficulty breathing, palpations, and fatigue. All of the client's other symptoms are within normal limits.

CN: Management of care; CL: Analyze

88. **1, 2, 5, 6.** The test result indicates that the client has an active hepatitis infection and is a carrier. The administration of hepatitis B immune globulin within 12 hours of birth provides the infant with passive immunity against hepatitis B and serves as a prophylactic treatment. Additionally, the infant will be started on the vaccine series of three injections within 24 hours of birth. The infant should not be isolated. Testing the infant before 9 months of age would detect antibodies from passive immunity versus true disease. As with all clients, universal precautions should be used and are sufficient to prevent transmission of the virus. Women who are positive for hepatitis B surface antigen are able to breastfeed as long as they do not have cracked nipples that may bleed.

CN: Management of care; CL: Create

89. **4.** Asthma medications and bronchodilators should be continued during pregnancy as prescribed before the pregnancy began. The medications do not cause harm to the birth parent or fetus. Regular use of asthma medication will usually prevent asthma attacks. Prevention and limitation of an asthma attack is the goal of care for a client who is or is not pregnant and is the appropriate care strategy. During an asthma attack, oxygen needs continue as with any pregnant client, but the airways are edematous, decreasing perfusion. Asthma exacerbations during pregnancy may occur as a result of infrequent use of medication rather than as a result of the pregnancy.

CN: Pharmacological and parenteral therapies; CL: Evaluate

90. **2.** The nurse seeing this client should refer the client to an HCP for further evaluation of the pain. This referral would allow a more definitive diagnosis and medical interventions that may include surgery. A referral would occur because of the client's high pain rating as well as the other symptoms, which suggest gallbladder disease. During pregnancy, the gallbladder is under the influence of progesterone, which is a smooth-muscle relaxant. Because bile does not move through the system as quickly during pregnancy, bile stasis and gallstone formation can occur. Although education should be a continuous strategy, with pain at this level, a brief explanation is most appropriate. Major emphasis should be placed on determining the cause and treating the pain. It is not appropriate for the nurse to diagnose pain at this level as heartburn. Discussing nutritional strategies to prevent heartburn is appropriate during pregnancy, but not in this situation. Acetaminophen is an acceptable medication to take during pregnancy, but it should not be used on a regular basis as it can mask other problems.

CN: Management of care; CL: Analyze

91. **3.** A fetus that has died and is retained in utero places the birth parent at risk for DIC because the clotting factors within the maternal system are consumed when the nonviable fetus is retained. The longer the fetus is retained in utero, the greater the risk for DIC. This client has no risk factors, history, or signs and symptoms that put them at risk for abruptio placentae such as sharp pain and a "woody," firm consistency of the abdomen. HELLP syndrome is a complication of preeclampsia that does not occur before 20 weeks' gestation unless a molar pregnancy is present. There is no evidence that the client is threatening to abort as they have no cramping or vaginal bleeding.

CN: Management of care; CL: Analyze

92. **2.** A blood pressure reading of 138/88 mm Hg is nearing the hypertension range and could be a sign of developing gestational hypertension. Conversely, the client may be experiencing "white coat" syndrome or could be anxious during the prenatal visit. To obtain an accurate blood pressure reading, the nurse should allow the client to rest for a period of time and recheck the blood pressure in the same arm while the client is in the same position. This blood pressure is considered approaching high. All other vitals are within normal range.

CN: Physiological adaptation; CL: Analyze

93. **2.** CVS can be performed from approximately 8 to 12 weeks' gestation, while amniocentesis cannot be performed until between 11 weeks' gestation and the end of the pregnancy. Eleven weeks' gestation is the earliest possible time within the pregnancy to obtain a sufficient amount of amniotic fluid to sample. Because CVS takes a piece of the membrane surrounding the infant, this procedure can be completed earlier in the pregnancy. Amniocentesis and chorionic villus sampling identify the genetic makeup of the fetus in its entirety, rather than a portion of it. Laboratory analysis of CVS takes less time to complete. Both procedures place the fetus at risk, and postprocedure teaching asks the client to report the same complicating events (bleeding, cramping, fever, and fluid leakage from the vagina).

🔑 CN: Management of care; CL: Evaluate

94. 4. Additional teaching is needed when the parent says that adolescents are at greater risk for congenital anomalies. Although adolescents are at greater risk for denial of the pregnancy, lack of prenatal care, low-birth-weight infant, cephalopelvic disproportion, anemia, and nutritional deficits and have a higher maternal mortality rate, studies reveal that congenital anomalies are not more common in adolescent pregnancies.

🔑 CN: Health promotion and maintenance; CL: Evaluate

95. 4. With a spontaneous abortion, many clients and their partners feel an acute sense of loss. Their grieving commonly includes feelings of guilt, which may be expressed as wondering whether the client could have done something to prevent the loss. Anger, sadness, and disappointment are also common emotions after a pregnancy loss. Ambivalence, anxiety, and fear are not common emotions after a spontaneous abortion.

🔑 CN: Psychosocial integrity; CL: Analyze

96. 1. Hydroxyzine has a tranquilizing effect and also decreases nausea and vomiting. It does not decrease fluid retention, reduce pain, decrease uterine cramping, or promote uterine contractility. One of the adverse effects of the medication is sleepiness. Ibuprofen may decrease pain from uterine cramping. Oxytocin may be used to increase uterine contractility.

🔑 CN: Pharmacological and parenteral therapies; CL: Evaluate

97. 3. The death of a fetus at any time during pregnancy is a tragedy for most parents. After a spontaneous abortion, the client and family members can be expected to suffer from grief for several months or longer. When offering support, a simple statement such as "I am truly sorry you lost your baby" is most appropriate. Therapeutic communication techniques help the client and family understand the meaning of the loss, move less stressfully through the grief process, and share feelings. Asking the client whether they are experiencing a great deal of uterine pain is inappropriate because this is a "yes-no" question and does not allow the client to express their feelings. Saying that the embryo was defective is inappropriate because this may lead the client to think that they contributed to the fetus's demise. This is not the appropriate time to discuss embryonic or fetal malformations. However, the nurse should explain to the client that this situation was not their fault. Telling the client that they can get pregnant again after a normal period may be factual, but it does not address the feelings of the expectant client who had already begun to bond with the fetus.

🔑 CN: Psychosocial integrity; CL: Apply

98. 2. The client with leg varicosities should take frequent rest periods with the legs elevated above the hips to promote venous circulation. The client should avoid constrictive clothing, but support hose that reach above the varicosities may help alleviate the pain. Contracting and relaxing the feet and ankles twice daily is not helpful because it does not promote circulation. Taking a leave of absence from work may not be possible because of economic reasons. The client should try to rest with their legs elevated or walk around for a few minutes every 2 hours while on the job.

🔑 CN: Reduction of risk potential; CL: Analyze

99. 4. The client is reporting symptoms typically associated with herpes genitalis. Some women have no symptoms of gonorrhea. Others may experience vaginal itching and a thick, purulent vaginal discharge. Women infected with *C. trachomatis* commonly do not have symptoms, but symptoms may include a yellowish discharge and painful urination. The first symptom of syphilis is a painless chancre.

🔑 CN: Physiological adaptation; CL: Apply

100. 1. The client may need surgery to remove a ruptured fallopian tube where the pregnancy has occurred, and the nurse is usually responsible for witnessing the signature on the informed consent. Typically, if bleeding is occurring, it is internal, and there is only scant vaginal bleeding with no discoloration. The nurse cannot determine whether the fallopian tube can be salvaged; this can be accomplished only during surgery. If the tube has ruptured, it must be removed. If the tube has not ruptured, a linear salpingostomy may be done to salvage the tube for future pregnancies. With an ectopic pregnancy, although the client is experiencing abdominal pain, they are not having uterine contractions.

🔑 CN: Physiological adaptation; CL: Analyze

101.
STEP 1

–/+ 1, 2, 3, 8. Being more tired than usual and short of breath are changes in activity that need investigation. Swelling in the feet at the end of the day is expected, but cold feet and being pale suggest the client may not have adequate perfusion. The history of Crohn's disease and not taking a prenatal vitamin increases the client's risk for nutritional deficits as the fetus grows. Craving ice, a nonfood item, may be an indication the client is anemic. The client had a BMI of 18.4 before pregnancy. The recommended weight gain for underweight clients is 28 to 40 lb (13 to 18 kg). More than midway through pregnancy, the client has not gained enough weight. All vital signs are within normal limits. Negative urine dipstick findings are desirable. A typical fetal heart rate is 110 to 160 bpm. Fundal height approximates gestational age. Increasing 4 cm over 4 weeks would reflect a typical growth pattern.

CJ: Case study; Step 1: Recognize cues; CL: Analyze

102.
STEP 2

Possible Finding	Iron Deficiency Anemia	Vitamin B_{12} Deficiency Anemia	Folate Deficiency Anemia
Chewing ice	X		
Fatigue	X	X	X
Crohn's disease history	X	X	X
Pallor	X	X	X

Iron deficiency anemia is the most common anemia affecting one in four pregnancies in the United States. Eating nonfood substances like eating ice is referred to as *pica* and is a symptom of iron deficiency anemia. All anemias cause fatigue, weakness, and circulatory changes associated with pallor. Gastrointestinal tract disorders, like Crohn's disease, affect the absorption of nutrients and can play a factor in all three types of anemia.

CJ: Case study; Step 2: Analyze cues; CL: Analyze

103.
STEP 3

0/1 *The nurse should recognize that the client has a* **microcytic** *anemia most likely caused by a(n)* **iron** *nutritional deficit. Untreated, the client is at most risk for developing more* **cardiac** *symptoms as pregnancy progresses.*

The low MCV indicates red blood cells are smaller than normal, indicating the presence of a microcytic anemia. The complete blood count and the symptoms of pallor, cold feet, pica, and poor weight gain indicate the client has symptomatic iron deficiency anemia. As the fetus grows and begins to store iron, the client can expect the untreated anemia to worsen. With less hemoglobin to carry oxygen, the client would likely see more cardiac symptoms such as tachycardia and increased fatigue. An elevated MCV would indicate macrocytic anemia, which can be caused by a vitamin B_{12} or folate deficiency. Clients with B_{12} or folate deficiencies experience neurologic changes along with cardiovascular changes.

CJ: Case study; Step 3: Prioritize hypothesis; CL: Create

104.
STEP 4

–/+ 2, 5, 6, 7, 8. The nurse will continue to monitor the hemoglobin and hematocrit to ensure anemia has not reached levels requiring transfusions. Iron therapy is key to treating anemia. Resuming prenatal vitamins will not be sufficient to treat this client's iron deficit. Dietary education is needed to help improve anemia and weight gain. The complexity of the client's history with Crohn's disease and the poor weight gain indicates that a consultation with a dietician is warranted. Teaching self-care strategies to help reduce fatigue will increase quality of life and may help with weight gain. The client's vital signs are normal, so there is no immediate need for oxygen, an ECG, or a fluid bolus.

CJ: Case study; Step 4: Generate solutions; CL: Analyze

105.
STEP 5

Possible Steps	Essential	Nonessential
Instruct the client to remain nothing by mouth (NPO)		X
Assess for allergies	X	
Have resuscitation equipment available	X	
Administer a sedative		X
Monitor for anaphylaxis	X	
Obtain a complete blood count (CBC) immediately after the infusion		X

IV iron carries a high risk for anaphylaxis. It is critical that the nurse assess the client for known allergies and have resuscitation equipment available before administering IV iron. Although anaphylaxis is most common with the test dose in the first few minutes, it can occur at any point during or after the infusion. Thus, clients should be observed carefully for hypersensitivity reactions throughout the infusion and at least another 30 minutes before sending them home. Keeping pregnant clients NPO for procedures is seldom recommended, and there is no need to be NPO for an IV iron infusion. Premedication with a sedative is not recommended. If a client has multiple drug allergies or known asthma, premedication with a steroid may be indicated. The body needs time to make red blood cells with the infused iron. A CBC is not needed because changes in hemoglobin would not be expected at the end of the infusion.

CJ: Case study; Step 5: Take action; CL: Apply

106.

STEP 6

	Possible Client Statement	Understood	Not Understood
0/1	"I can take my iron with some food since it upsets my stomach."	X	
	"Taking my iron with orange juice will help the medication absorb."	X	
	"I can't take antacids at the same time I take my iron."	X	
	"I should drink more to help prevent constipation."	X	
	"I might have tarry or bloody stools."		X
	"If I miss a pill, I can take two pills next time."		X
	"I should call the office if I develop a rash while taking the medication."	X	

Iron is best absorbed on an empty stomach. However, if it causes nausea, clients should take the medication with food. Taking iron with orange juice helps absorption, but taking iron with an alkalotic substance like an antacid or milk will decrease absorption. Clients frequently report that iron is constipating; therefore, increasing fluid and fiber intake along with increasing activity can help decrease constipation. If a client develops a rash while on iron, they should consult their health care provider to further assess for hypersensitivity to the medication. Although stools may turn hard and dark green, iron supplementation should not cause tarry or bloody stools. If a dose is missed, clients can take the medication as soon as remembered, but clients should not double up on doses to make up for missed doses because of the risk for toxicity.

CJ: Case study; Step 6: Evaluate outcomes; CL: Evaluate

Managing Care, Quality, and Safety for Childbearing Clients

107. **2.** Late decelerations during an oxytocin challenge test indicate that the infant is not receiving enough oxygen during contractions and is exhibiting signs of uteroplacental insufficiency. This client would need further medical intervention. Fetal movement 6 times in 2 hours is adequate in a healthy fetus, and a biophysical profile of 9 indicates that the risk for fetal asphyxia is rare. A normal nonstress test report shows that the fetal heart rate is between 110 and 160 bpm with moderate variability, with two fetal heart rate accelerations of 15 bpm above baseline and lasting for 15 seconds within a 20-minute period and no decelerations.

CN: Management of care; CL: Evaluate

108. **3, 4, 1, 2.** The first client to be seen should be the postpartum client who is fearful of shaking their infant. Postpartum depression is a disorder that may occur during the first year postpartum but peaks at 4 weeks postpartum, prior to menses, or upon weaning. As a single parent, this client may not have support, a large factor putting women at risk. Other factors accentuating risk include prior depressive or bipolar illness and self-dissatisfaction. Second, the nurse should see the 16-week antenatal client, who is likely experiencing round ligament syndrome. At this point in the pregnancy, the uterus is stretching into the abdomen, causing this type of pain. The pain is on the wrong side to be attributed to appendicitis or gallbladder disease. Nursing interventions to ease the pain include a heating pad or bringing the legs toward the abdomen. The nurse should next see the primigravid client who states they are not feeling well because they are exhibiting signs and symptoms of discomfort experienced by most clients in the first trimester. The multiparous client at 32 weeks' gestation is the lowest priority as they are physically well, while the other clients have physical and psychological problems. In most emergency department situations, the client may not be seen by medical or nursing staff but would be given the names of HCPs in the reception area.

CN: Management of care; CL: Create

109. **1, 2, 3, 4.** The same safety policies apply to both inpatient and ambulatory settings and are adapted to the individual specialty. Handwashing and the use of two client identifiers are standard procedures. Abbreviations that are used in the inpatient setting are also used in the ambulatory care setting because the same mistakes can occur in either setting, such as confusion in spelling or interpretation of letters and numbers. A preprocedure verification that asks for the client's name and the procedure to be performed is conducted in the operating room and in inpatient and ambulatory settings, regardless of the procedure. It is logical to place clients with obvious communicable diseases by themselves, but nausea and vomiting are a "normal" situation in early pregnancy and not contagious.

CN: Risk reduction; CL: Evaluate

TEST 2

Complications of Pregnancy

- The Pregnant Client with Preeclampsia or Eclampsia
- The Pregnant Client with a Chronic Hypertensive Disorder
- The Pregnant Client with Third-Trimester Bleeding
- The Pregnant Client with Preterm Labor
- The Pregnant Client with Premature Rupture of the Membranes
- The Pregnant Client with Diabetes Mellitus
- The Pregnant Client with Heart Disease
- The Client with an Ectopic Pregnancy
- The Pregnant Client with Hyperemesis Gravidarum
- The Client with a Gestational Trophoblastic Disease
- The Pregnant Client with Miscellaneous Complications
- Managing Care, Quality, and Safety for Pregnant Clients

The Pregnant Client with Preeclampsia or Eclampsia

1. A laboring client with preeclampsia is prescribed magnesium sulfate 2 g per hour intravenous (IV) piggyback. The pharmacy sends the IV to the unit labeled *magnesium sulfate 20 g/500 mL normal saline*. To deliver the correct dose, the nurse should set the pump to deliver how many milliliters per hour? Record your answer using one decimal place. _____ mL.

2. A 32-year-old multigravida client returns to the clinic for a routine prenatal visit at 36 weeks' gestation. The assessments during this visit include blood pressure, 140/90 mm Hg; pulse, 80 beats/min; and respiratory rate, 16 breaths/min. What further information should the nurse obtain to determine if this client is becoming preeclamptic?
   ☐ 1. headaches
   ☐ 2. blood glucose level
   ☐ 3. proteinuria
   ☐ 4. peripheral edema

3. The nurse instructs a preeclamptic client about monitoring the movements of their fetus to determine fetal well-being. Which statement by the client indicates that they need further instruction about when to call the health care provider (HCP) concerning fetal movement?
   ☐ 1. "if the fetus is becoming less active than before"
   ☐ 2. "if it takes longer each day for the fetus to move 10 times"
   ☐ 3. "if the fetus stops moving for 12 hours"
   ☐ 4. "if the fetus moves more often than three times an hour"

4. A 29-year-old multigravida at 37 weeks' gestation is being treated for severe preeclampsia and has magnesium sulfate infusing at 3 g per hour. What is the **priority** intervention to maintain safety for this client?
   ☐ 1. Maintain continuous fetal monitoring.
   ☐ 2. Encourage family members to remain at the bedside.
   ☐ 3. Assess reflexes, clonus, visual disturbances, and headache.
   ☐ 4. Monitor maternal liver studies every 4 hours.

5. At 32 weeks' gestation, a 15-year-old primigravid client who is 5 feet, 2 inches (151.7 cm) has gained a total of 20 lb (9.1 kg), with a 1-lb (0.45-kg) gain in the last 2 weeks. Urinalysis reveals negative glucose and a trace of protein. The nurse should advise the client that which factor increases the risk for preeclampsia?
   ☐ 1. total weight gain
   ☐ 2. short stature
   ☐ 3. adolescent age group
   ☐ 4. trace proteinuria

6. After instructing a primigravid client at 38 weeks' gestation about how preeclampsia can affect the client and the growing fetus, the nurse realizes that the client needs additional instruction when they say that preeclampsia can lead to which problem?
   ☐ 1. hydrocephalic infant
   ☐ 2. abruptio placentae
   ☐ 3. intrauterine growth restriction
   ☐ 4. poor placental perfusion

7. A nurse is completing a prenatal assessment on a client who is 28 weeks pregnant with gestational hypertension. Which finding(s) should be reported to the primary health care provider? Select all that apply.
   ☐ 1. dull headache
   ☐ 2. weight gain of 1 lb (500 g) per week
   ☐ 3. blurred vision
   ☐ 4. 1+ urine protein
   ☐ 5. fundal height of 28 cm

8. When teaching a multigravida client diagnosed with mild preeclampsia about nutritional needs, the nurse should discuss which type of diet?
   ☐ 1. low carbohydrate
   ☐ 2. restricted sodium
   ☐ 3. typical pregnancy
   ☐ 4. high protein

9. A client with preeclampsia is receiving magnesium sulfate via infusion pump at 1 g per hour. The nurse's assessment includes temperature 98.1°F (36.7°C); pulse 78 bpm; respirations 12 breaths/min; blood pressure 128/82 mm Hg; urinary output 90 mL in last 4 hours via urinary catheter; patellar-tendon reflex absent; ankle clonus absent; fetal heart rate 120 bpm; and cervix 4 cm dilated, 80% effaced, station −1. Which is the **most** appropriate action for the nurse to take?
   ☐ 1. Assess the urinary catheter for kinks in the drainage tubing, and obtain a urine sample.
   ☐ 2. Document findings, and continue to monitor the client's progress in labor.
   ☐ 3. Discontinue the magnesium sulfate infusion, and notify the health care provider (HCP).
   ☐ 4. Increase fluid intake intravenously, and measure intake and output.

10. A primigravid client at 38 weeks' gestation diagnosed with mild preeclampsia calls the clinic nurse to say they have had a continuous headache for the past 2 days accompanied by nausea. The client does not want to take aspirin. What should the nurse tell the client?
    ☐ 1. "Take two acetaminophen tablets. They are not as likely to upset your stomach."
    ☐ 2. "I think the health care provider (HCP) should see you today. Can you come to the clinic this morning?"
    ☐ 3. "You need to lie down and rest. Have you tried placing a cool compress over your head?"
    ☐ 4. "I will ask the HCP to call in a prescription for nausea medications. What is your pharmacy's number?"

11. When the nurse is preparing the room for admission of a multigravida client at 36 weeks' gestation diagnosed with severe preeclampsia, which item is **most** important for the nurse to obtain?
    ☐ 1. oxytocin infusion solution
    ☐ 2. disposable tongue blades
    ☐ 3. portable ultrasound machine
    ☐ 4. padding for the side rails

12. A client who is 34 weeks pregnant is admitted to the labor and birth room with the diagnosis of preeclampsia. The client has a blood pressure of 149/92 mm Hg; a pulse of 62 bpm; a respiratory rate of 18 breaths/min; and a temperature of 98.4°F (36.8°C). What is the **priority** intervention?
    ☐ 1. Encourage the client to lie in a lateral position.
    ☐ 2. Administer an antihypertensive agent.
    ☐ 3. Notify the health care provider (HCP) of the client's blood pressure.
    ☐ 4. Check the cervix.

13. For the client who is receiving intravenous magnesium sulfate for severe preeclampsia, which assessment finding would alert the nurse to suspect hypermagnesemia?
    ☐ 1. decreased deep tendon reflexes
    ☐ 2. cool skin temperature
    ☐ 3. rapid pulse rate
    ☐ 4. tingling in the toes

14. A client at 28 weeks' gestation presents to the emergency department with a "splitting headache." What action(s) would be indicated by the nurse at this time? Select all that apply.
    ☐ 1. Assess for the presence of urine ketones.
    ☐ 2. Assess the client for vision changes or epigastric pain.
    ☐ 3. Obtain a nonstress test.
    ☐ 4. Assess the client's reflexes and presence of clonus.
    ☐ 5. Determine if the client has a documented ultrasound for this pregnancy.

15. Which outcome would the nurse identify as the **priority** to achieve when developing the plan of care for a primigravid client at 38 weeks' gestation who is hospitalized with severe preeclampsia and receiving intravenous magnesium sulfate?
    ☐ 1. decreased generalized edema within 8 hours
    ☐ 2. decreased urinary output during the first 24 hours
    ☐ 3. sedation and decreased reflex excitability within 48 hours
    ☐ 4. absence of any seizure activity during the first 48 hours

16. The nurse is administering intravenous magnesium sulfate as prescribed for a client at 34 weeks' gestation with severe preeclampsia. Which outcome(s) of this therapy would be desired? Select all that apply.
    ☐ 1. temperature, 98°F (36.7°C); pulse, 72 bpm; respiratory rate, 14 breaths/min
    ☐ 2. urinary output less than 30 mL per hour
    ☐ 3. fetal heart rate with late decelerations
    ☐ 4. blood pressure of less than 140/90 mm Hg
    ☐ 5. deep tendon reflexes 2+
    ☐ 6. absence of seizures

17. Soon after admission of a primigravid client at 38 weeks' gestation with severe preeclampsia, the primary health care provider (HCP) prescribes a continuous intravenous infusion of 5% dextrose in Ringer's lactate solution and 4 g of magnesium sulfate. While the medication is being administered, which assessment finding should the nurse report **immediately**?
☐ 1. respiratory rate of 12 breaths/min
☐ 2. patellar reflex of +2
☐ 3. blood pressure of 160/88 mm Hg
☐ 4. urinary output exceeding intake

18. As the nurse enters the room of a newly admitted primigravid client diagnosed with severe preeclampsia, the client begins to experience a seizure. Which action should the nurse take **first**?
☐ 1. Insert an airway.
☐ 2. Note the time when the seizure begins and ends.
☐ 3. Call for immediate assistance.
☐ 4. Turn the client to the left side.

19. After administering hydralazine 5 mg intravenously as prescribed for a primigravid client with severe preeclampsia at 39 weeks' gestation, the nurse should assess the client for which complication?
☐ 1. tachycardia
☐ 2. bradypnea
☐ 3. polyuria
☐ 4. dysphagia

20. A primigravid client with severe preeclampsia exhibits hyperactive, very brisk patellar reflexes with two beats of ankle clonus present. How does the nurse document the patellar reflexes?
☐ 1. 1+
☐ 2. 2+
☐ 3. 3+
☐ 4. 4+

21. A 16-year-old primigravid client at 37 weeks' gestation with severe preeclampsia is in early active labor. The client's blood pressure is 164/110 mm Hg. Which finding would alert the nurse that the client may be about to experience a seizure?
☐ 1. decreased contraction intensity
☐ 2. decreased temperature
☐ 3. epigastric pain
☐ 4. hyporeflexia

22. Following an eclamptic seizure, the nurse should assess the client for which complication?
☐ 1. polyuria
☐ 2. facial flushing
☐ 3. hypotension
☐ 4. uterine contractions

The Pregnant Client with a Chronic Hypertensive Disorder

23. An obese 36-year-old multigravid client at 12 weeks' gestation has a history of chronic hypertension. The client was treated with methyldopa before becoming pregnant. When counseling the client about diet during pregnancy, the nurse realizes that the client needs additional instruction when they make which statement?
☐ 1. "I need to reduce my caloric intake to 1200 calories a day."
☐ 2. "A regular diet is recommended during pregnancy."
☐ 3. "I should eat more frequent meals if I get heartburn."
☐ 4. "I need to consume more fluids and fiber each day."

24. After instructing a multigravid client at 10 weeks' gestation diagnosed with chronic hypertension about the need for frequent prenatal visits, the nurse determines that the instructions have been successful when the client makes which statement?
☐ 1. "I may develop hyperthyroidism because of my high blood pressure."
☐ 2. "I need close monitoring because I may have a small-for-gestational-age infant."
☐ 3. "It is possible that I will have excess amniotic fluid and may need a cesarean birth."
☐ 4. "I may develop placenta accreta, so I need to keep my clinic appointments."

25. After the nurse reinforces the danger signs to report with a gravida 2 client at 32 weeks' gestation with an elevated blood pressure, which client statement(s) would demonstrate understanding of when to call the primary health care provider's (HCP's) office? Select all that apply.
☐ 1. "if I feel dizzy when I get up quickly"
☐ 2. "if I see any bleeding, even if I have no pain"
☐ 3. "if I have a pounding headache that will not go away"
☐ 4. "if I notice the veins in my legs getting bigger"
☐ 5. "if the leg cramps at night are waking me up"
☐ 6. "if the baby seems to be more active than usual"

The Pregnant Client with Third-Trimester Bleeding

26. A client presents to the obstetric triage unit with no prenatal care and painless, bright red vaginal bleeding. Which interventions are **most** indicated?
☐ 1. applying an external fetal monitor and completing a physical assessment
☐ 2. applying an external fetal monitor and performing a sterile vaginal examination
☐ 3. obtaining a fundal height physical assessment on the client
☐ 4. obtaining fundal height and a sterile vaginal examination

27. The nurse is caring for a 22-year-old gravida 2, para 2 client who has disseminated intravascular coagulation after the birth of a dead fetus. Which finding is the **highest priority** to report to the health care provider (HCP)?
    ☐ 1. activated partial thromboplastin time (APTT) of 30 seconds
    ☐ 2. hemoglobin of 11.5 g/dL (115 g/L)
    ☐ 3. urinary output of 25 mL in the past hour
    ☐ 4. platelets at 149,000/mm³ (149 × 10⁹/L)

28. A 24-year-old client, G3, T1, P1, A1, L1 at 32 weeks' gestation, is admitted to the hospital because of vaginal bleeding. After reviewing the client's history, the nurse might suspect abruptio placentae based on which factor?
    ☐ 1. several hypotensive episodes
    ☐ 2. previous low transverse cesarean birth
    ☐ 3. one induced abortion
    ☐ 4. history of cocaine use

29. When caring for a multigravid client admitted to the hospital with vaginal bleeding at 38 weeks' gestation, the nurse would anticipate administering intravenously which therapeutic agent if the client develops disseminated intravascular coagulation (DIC)?
    ☐ 1. Ringer's lactate solution
    ☐ 2. fresh frozen platelets
    ☐ 3. 5% dextrose solution
    ☐ 4. warfarin

30. When the nurse is assessing a 34-year-old multigravid client at 34 weeks' gestation experiencing moderate vaginal bleeding, which symptom would **most** likely alert the nurse that placenta previa is present?
    ☐ 1. painless vaginal bleeding
    ☐ 2. uterine tetany
    ☐ 3. intermittent pain with spotting
    ☐ 4. dull lower back pain

31. Following a cesarean birth for abruptio placentae, a multigravid client tells the nurse, "I feel like such a failure. None of my other births were like this." Which factor is **most** important for the nurse to consider when responding to the client?
    ☐ 1. The client will most likely have postpartum blues.
    ☐ 2. Maternal-infant bonding is likely to be difficult.
    ☐ 3. The client's feeling of grief is a normal reaction.
    ☐ 4. This type of birth was necessary to save the client's life.

32. A client has received epidural anesthesia to control pain during a vaginal birth. Place an X over the **highest** point on the body locating the level of anesthesia expected for a vaginal birth.

33. Which action should the nurse take **first** when admitting a multigravid client at 36 weeks' gestation with a probable diagnosis of abruptio placentae?
    ☐ 1. Prepare the client for a vaginal examination.
    ☐ 2. Obtain a brief history from the client.
    ☐ 3. Insert a large-gauge intravenous catheter.
    ☐ 4. Prepare the client for an ultrasound scan.

The Pregnant Client with Preterm Labor

34. The health care provider (HCP) has determined that a preterm labor client at 34 weeks' gestation has no fetal fibronectin present. Based on this finding, the nurse would anticipate which other client finding within the next week?
    ☐ 1. The client will develop preeclampsia.
    ☐ 2. The fetus will develop mature lungs.
    ☐ 3. The client will not develop preterm labor.
    ☐ 4. The fetus will not develop gestational diabetes.

35. Which statement by the client indicates an understanding of the teaching regarding the use of corticosteroids during preterm labor?
    ☐ 1. "I will be taking corticosteroids until my baby's due date so that they will have the best chance of doing well."
    ☐ 2. "The corticosteroids may help my baby's lungs mature."
    ☐ 3. "The goal of the corticosteroids is to stop contractions and help me get to my due date."
    ☐ 4. "If I take corticosteroids, my baby will not have to spend any time in the neonatal intensive care unit when they are born."

36. In which maternal locations would the nurse place the ultrasound transducer of the external electronic fetal heart rate monitor if a fetus at 34 weeks' gestation is in the left occiput anterior (LOA) position?
    ☐ 1. near the symphysis pubis
    ☐ 2. 2 inches (5.1 cm) above the umbilicus
    ☐ 3. below the umbilicus on the left side
    ☐ 4. at the level of the umbilicus

The Pregnant Client with Premature Rupture of the Membranes

37. The nurse is planning care for a multigravid client hospitalized at 36 weeks' gestation with confirmed rupture of membranes and no evidence of labor. What prescription would the nurse anticipate from the primary health care provider (HCP)?
    ☐ 1. frequent assessments of cervical dilation
    ☐ 2. intravenous oxytocin administration
    ☐ 3. cultures for chorioamnionitis
    ☐ 4. internal fetal monitoring

38. A primigravid client at 30 weeks' gestation has been admitted to the hospital with premature rupture of the membranes without contractions. The client's cervix is 2 cm dilated and 50% effaced. Which factor is **most** important for the nurse to assess **next**?
☐ 1. red blood cell count
☐ 2. degree of discomfort
☐ 3. urinary output
☐ 4. temperature

39. A multigravid client at 34 weeks' gestation with premature rupture of the membranes tests positive for group B streptococcus. The client is having contractions every 4 to 6 minutes. The client's vital signs are: blood pressure, 120/80 mm Hg; temperature, 100°F (37.8°C); pulse, 100 bpm; and respirations, 18 breaths/min. Which medication would the nurse expect the primary health care provider (HCP) to prescribe?
☐ 1. intravenous penicillin
☐ 2. intravenous gentamicin sulfate
☐ 3. intramuscular betamethasone
☐ 4. intramuscular cefaclor

40. A primigravid client at 34 weeks' gestation is experiencing contractions every 3 to 4 minutes lasting for 35 seconds. The client's cervix is 2 cm dilated and 50% effaced. While the nurse is assessing the client's vital signs, the client says, "I think my bag of water just broke." Which intervention would the nurse do **first**?
☐ 1. Check the status of the fetal heart rate.
☐ 2. Reassess the client's vital signs.
☐ 3. Test the leaking fluid for fetal fibronectin.
☐ 4. Perform a sterile vaginal examination.

The Pregnant Client with Diabetes Mellitus

41. The antenatal clinic nurse is educating a client with gestational diabetes soon after diagnosis. Evaluation for this client session will include which outcome(s)? Select all that apply.
☐ 1. The client states the need to maintain blood glucose levels between 70 and 110 mg/dL (3.9 and 6.2 mmol/L).
☐ 2. The client describes a planned walking program while pregnant.
☐ 3. The client will strive to maintain a hemoglobin A1C of less than 6%.
☐ 4. The client verbalizes the need to maintain a dietary intake of fewer than 1500 calories a day to prevent hyperglycemia.
☐ 5. The client will continue taking prenatal vitamins, iron, and folic acid.

42. A 27-year-old primigravid client with insulin-dependent diabetes at 34 weeks' gestation undergoes a nonstress test, the results of which are documented as reactive. What should the nurse tell the client that the test results indicate?
☐ 1. A contraction stress test is necessary.
☐ 2. The nonstress test should be repeated.
☐ 3. Chorionic villus sampling is necessary.
☐ 4. There is evidence of fetal well-being.

43. A primigravid client with insulin-dependent diabetes tells the nurse that the contraction stress test performed earlier in the day was suspicious. The nurse interprets this test result as showing which fetal heart rate pattern?
☐ 1. frequent late decelerations
☐ 2. decreased fetal movement
☐ 3. inconsistent late decelerations
☐ 4. lack of fetal movement

44. Which statement about a fetal biophysical profile would be incorporated into the teaching plan for a primigravid client with insulin-dependent diabetes?
☐ 1. It determines fetal lung maturity.
☐ 2. It is noninvasive using real-time ultrasound.
☐ 3. It will correlate with the newborn's Apgar score.
☐ 4. It requires the client to have an empty bladder.

45. A 30-year-old multigravid client at 8 weeks' gestation has a history of insulin-dependent diabetes since age 20. When explaining the importance of blood glucose control during pregnancy, the nurse should tell the client that what will occur regarding the client's insulin needs during the first trimester?
☐ 1. They typically increase slightly.
☐ 2. They may decrease.
☐ 3. They will remain constant.
☐ 4. They often double.

46. The nurse explains the possible complications of pregnancy to a primigravid client at 10 weeks' gestation who has a 5-year history of insulin-dependent diabetes. Which complication, if stated by the client, indicates the need for additional teaching?
☐ 1. *Candida albicans* infection
☐ 2. twin-to-twin transfusion
☐ 3. polyhydramnios
☐ 4. preeclampsia

47. When developing a teaching plan for a primigravid client with insulin-dependent diabetes about monitoring blood glucose control and insulin dosages at home, the nurse would expect to include which desired target range for blood glucose levels?
  ☐ 1. 40 to 60 mg/dL (2.2 to 3.3 mmol/L) between 14:00 and 16:00 hours
  ☐ 2. 70 to 100 mg/dL (3.3 to 5.6 mmol/L) before meals and bedtime snacks
  ☐ 3. 110 to 140 mg/dL (6.2 to 7.8 mmol/L) before meals and bedtime snacks
  ☐ 4. 140 to 160 mg/dL (7.8 to 8.9 mmol/L) 1 hour after meals

48. When teaching a primigravid client with diabetes about common causes of hyperglycemia during pregnancy, the nurse would include which information?
  ☐ 1. fetal macrosomia
  ☐ 2. decreased fetal insulin
  ☐ 3. maternal infection
  ☐ 4. gestational hypertension

49. After teaching a primigravid client with diabetes about the symptoms of hyperglycemia and hypoglycemia, the nurse determines that the client understands the instruction when they say that hyperglycemia may be manifested by which symptom?
  ☐ 1. dehydration
  ☐ 2. pallor
  ☐ 3. sweating
  ☐ 4. nervousness

50. At 38 weeks' gestation, a primigravid client with poorly controlled diabetes and severe preeclampsia is admitted for a cesarean birth. The nurse explains to the client that birth helps prevent which complication?
  ☐ 1. neonatal hyperbilirubinemia
  ☐ 2. congenital anomalies
  ☐ 3. perinatal asphyxia
  ☐ 4. stillbirth

51. With plans to breastfeed their neonate, a pregnant client with insulin-dependent diabetes asks the nurse about insulin needs during the postpartum period. Which statement about postpartum insulin requirements for the breastfeeding parent should the nurse include in the explanation?
  ☐ 1. They fall significantly in the immediate postpartum period.
  ☐ 2. They remain the same as during the labor process.
  ☐ 3. They usually increase in the immediate postpartum period.
  ☐ 4. They need constant adjustment during the first 24 hours.

The Pregnant Client with Heart Disease

52. After the nurse instructs a primigravid client at 8 weeks' gestation diagnosed with class I heart disease about self-care during pregnancy, which client statement would indicate the need for additional teaching?
  ☐ 1. "I should avoid being near people who have a cold."
  ☐ 2. "I may be given antibiotics during my pregnancy."
  ☐ 3. "I should reduce my intake of protein in my diet."
  ☐ 4. "I should limit my salt intake at meals."

53. While caring for a primigravid client with class II heart disease at 28 weeks' gestation, the nurse would instruct the client to contact their primary health care provider (HCP) immediately if the client experiences which symptom?
  ☐ 1. mild ankle edema
  ☐ 2. emotional stress on the job
  ☐ 3. weight gain of 1 lb (0.45 kg) in 1 week
  ☐ 4. dyspnea at rest

54. The nurse develops the collaborative plan of care with the health care provider (HCP) for a multigravid client at 10 weeks' gestation being treated with digitalis for a history of cardiac disease. Based on the understanding of renal function in pregnancy, the nurse anticipates which modification will be needed to the client's drug therapy regimen?
  ☐ 1. possible need for an increased dosage
  ☐ 2. need for weekly drug level monitoring
  ☐ 3. switching to a different medication
  ☐ 4. addition of a diuretic to the regimen

55. Which anticoagulants would the nurse expect to administer when caring for a primigravid client at 12 weeks' gestation who has class II cardiac disease due to mitral valve stenosis?
  ☐ 1. heparin
  ☐ 2. warfarin
  ☐ 3. enoxaparin
  ☐ 4. ardeparin

56. A primigravid client with class II heart disease who is visiting the clinic at 8 weeks' gestation tells the nurse that they have been maintaining a low-sodium, 1800-calorie diet. Which instruction should the nurse give the client?
  ☐ 1. void folic acid supplements to prevent megaloblastic anemia.
  ☐ 2. Severely restrict sodium intake throughout the pregnancy.
  ☐ 3. Take iron supplements with milk to enhance absorption.
  ☐ 4. Increase caloric intake to 2200 calories daily to promote fetal growth.

Complications of Pregnancy

The Client with an Ectopic Pregnancy

57. On arrival at the emergency department, a client tells the nurse that they suspect that they may be pregnant and they have been having a small amount of bleeding and severe pain in the lower abdomen. The client's blood pressure is 70/50 mm Hg, and the pulse rate is 120 bpm. The nurse notifies the primary health care provider (HCP) immediately because of the possibility of which complication?
☐ 1. ectopic pregnancy
☐ 2. abruptio placentae
☐ 3. gestational trophoblastic disease
☐ 4. complete abortion

58. The nurse is assessing a multigravid client at 12 weeks' gestation who has been admitted to the emergency department with sharp right-sided abdominal pain and vaginal spotting. Which information should the nurse obtain about the client's history? Select all that apply.
☐ 1. history of sexually transmitted infections
☐ 2. number of sexual partners
☐ 3. last menstrual period
☐ 4. cesarean birth
☐ 5. contraceptive use

59. Before surgery to remove an ectopic pregnancy and the fallopian tube, which sign or symptom would alert the nurse to the possibility of tubal rupture?
☐ 1. light vaginal bleeding and discharge
☐ 2. profuse sweating
☐ 3. slow, bounding pulse rate of 80 bpm
☐ 4. marked abdominal edema

60. A multigravid client diagnosed with a probable ruptured ectopic pregnancy is scheduled for emergency surgery. In addition to monitoring the client's blood pressure before surgery, which factor is **most** important for the nurse to assess?
☐ 1. uterine cramping
☐ 2. abdominal distention
☐ 3. hemoglobin and hematocrit
☐ 4. pulse rate

61. A 36-year-old multigravid client is admitted to the hospital with a possible ruptured ectopic pregnancy. When the nurse is obtaining the client's history, which finding would be **most** important to identify as a predisposing factor?
☐ 1. urinary tract infection
☐ 2. marijuana use during pregnancy
☐ 3. episodes of pelvic inflammatory disease
☐ 4. use of estrogen-progestin contraceptives

62. A multigravid client is admitted to the hospital with a diagnosis of ectopic pregnancy. Because the client's fallopian tube has not yet ruptured, the nurse anticipates that which medication may be prescribed?
☐ 1. progestin contraceptives
☐ 2. medroxyprogesterone
☐ 3. methotrexate
☐ 4. dyphylline

The Pregnant Client with Hyperemesis Gravidarum

63. A pregnant client is prescribed doxylamine succinate and pyridoxine hydrochloride to treat morning sickness that has not responded to lifestyle changes. Which information is appropriate for the nurse to include in this client's education?
☐ 1. Diarrhea may occur with antacid medication.
☐ 2. Corticosteroids may increase thirst.
☐ 3. Drowsiness is a common side effect of antihistamines
☐ 4. Dopamine antagonists may cause restlessness.

64. After the nurse instructs a primigravid client at 8 weeks' gestation about measures to overcome early morning nausea and vomiting, which client statement indicates the need for additional teaching?
☐ 1. "I will eat dry crackers or toast before arising in the morning."
☐ 2. "I will drink adequate fluids separate from my meals or snacks."
☐ 3. "I will eat two large meals daily with frequent protein snacks."
☐ 4. "I will snack on a small amount of carbohydrates throughout the day."

65. A prenatal client tells the nurse that they have been eating ginger cookies to treat nausea and vomiting. Which response by the nurse is **best**?
☐ 1. "When consumed as a spice in foods, ginger is generally considered safe in pregnancy."
☐ 2. "It is safer to use a prescription medication than eating ginger while you are pregnant."
☐ 3. "Wait at least 2 hours to take your prenatal vitamin after eating ginger cookies."
☐ 4. "You should immediately stop eating ginger-containing foods."

66. A multigravid client thought to be at 14 weeks' gestation reports that they are experiencing such severe morning sickness that they "have not been able to keep anything down for a week." The nurse should assess for signs and symptoms of which condition?
☐ 1. hypercalcemia
☐ 2. hypobilirubinemia
☐ 3. hypokalemia
☐ 4. hyperglycemia

67. A multigravid client is admitted at 16 weeks' gestation with a diagnosis of hyperemesis gravidarum. The nurse should explain to the client that hyperemesis gravidarum is thought to be related to high levels of which hormone?
☐ 1. progesterone
☐ 2. estrogen
☐ 3. somatotropin
☐ 4. aldosterone

68. The primary health care provider (HCP) prescribes 1000 mL of Ringer's lactate solution intravenously over an 8-hour period for a 29-year-old primigravid client at 16 weeks' gestation with hyperemesis. The drip factor is 12 gtts/mL. The nurse should administer the IV infusion at how many drops per minute? Record your answer using one decimal place.
_____ gtts/min.

69. In caring for a pregnant client with hyperemesis gravidarum, which is the **priority** nursing intervention?
☐ 1. providing adequate sleep for the client
☐ 2. correcting the fluid-electrolyte imbalance
☐ 3. reviewing dietary choices and food intake
☐ 4. administering acetaminophen suppositories

70. STEP 1

The nurse cares for a 28-year-old female client at 16 weeks' gestation in the prenatal clinic.

Nurse's Notes

1030:
The 28-year-old gravida 2, para 1 client with a singleton pregnancy has a history of mild intermittent asthma that the client treats approximately once a week with albuterol. The client reports that they continue to have morning sickness, which first presented at 6 weeks' gestation, and they are vomiting more than three times a day. The client stopped taking prenatal vitamins because they increased nausea. The client reports fatigue and has not gone to work for the last 3 days. The client's prepregnant weight was 120 lb (54.4 kg) with a body mass index (BMI) of 20.1 kg/m². Today's weight is 121 lb (54.8 kg) with a BMI of 20.3 kg/m². Vital signs are 98.2°F (36.7°C); pulse (P) 86 bpm; respiration rate (RR) 16 breaths/min; and blood pressure (BP) 96/60 mm Hg. Mucous membranes are dry. The results of a urine dipstick test show no protein, glucose, or nitrates and trace amounts of ketones. The fetal heart rate (HR) is 150 bpm. The fundal height is 15 cm.

➤ Which five client findings require follow-up?

☐ 1. vital signs
☐ 2. albuterol use
☐ 3. nausea and vomiting
☐ 4. urine dipstick test
☐ 5. weight changes
☐ 6. mucous membranes
☐ 7. fetal HR
☐ 8. fundal height
☐ 9. fatigue

71. STEP 2

The nurse cares for a 28-year-old female client at 16 weeks' gestation in the prenatal clinic.

Nurse's Notes

1030:
The 28-year-old gravida 2, para 1 client with a singleton pregnancy has a history of mild intermittent asthma that the client treats approximately once a week with albuterol. The client reports that they continue to have morning sickness, which first presented at 6 weeks' gestation, and they are vomiting more than three times a day. The client stopped taking prenatal vitamins because they increased nausea. The client reports fatigue and has not gone to work for the last 3 days. The client's prepregnant weight was 120 lb (54.4 kg) with a body mass index (BMI) of 20.1 kg/m². Today's weight is 121 lb (54.8 kg) with a BMI of 20.3 kg/m². Vital signs are 98.2°F (36.7°C); pulse (P) 86 bpm; respiration rate (RR) 16 breaths/min; and blood pressure (BP) 96/60 mm Hg. Mucous membranes are dry. The results of a urine dipstick test show no protein, glucose, or nitrates and trace amounts of ketones. The fetal heart rate (HR) is 150 bpm. The fundal height is 15 cm.

➤ For each client finding below, specify if the finding is most consistent with morning sickness or hyperemesis gravidarum.

Client Findings	Morning Sickness	Hyperemesis Gravidarum
Second-trimester nausea	○	○
Vomiting frequency	○	○
Weight gain pattern	○	○
Dry mucous membranes	○	○
Trace ketonuria	○	○
Missing work related to fatigue	○	○

72. STEP 3

The nurse cares for a 28-year-old female client at 16 weeks' gestation in the prenatal clinic.

Nurse's Notes

1030:
The 28-year-old gravida 2, para 1 client with a singleton pregnancy has a history of mild intermittent asthma that the client treats approximately once a week with albuterol. The client reports that they continue to have morning sickness, which first presented at 6 weeks' gestation, and they are vomiting more than three times a day. The client stopped taking prenatal vitamins because they increased nausea. The client reports fatigue and has not gone to work for the last 3 days. The client's prepregnant weight was 120 lb (54.4 kg) with a body mass index (BMI) of 20.1 kg/m². Today's weight is 121 lb (54.8 kg) with a BMI of 20.3 kg/m². Vital signs are 98.2°F (36.7°C); pulse (P) 86 bpm; respiration rate (RR) 16 breaths/min; and blood pressure (BP) 96/60 mm Hg. Mucous membranes are dry. The results of a urine dipstick test show no protein, glucose, or nitrates and trace amounts of ketones. The fetal heart rate (HR) is 150 bpm. The fundal height is 15 cm.

➤ Select words from the choices below to fill in each blank found in the following sentences.

The nurse should recognize that the nausea and vomiting are causing _____ and _____.

Untreated, these complications **most** likely will lead to the adverse pregnancy outcomes of _____ and _____.

Word Choices
- birth defects
- dehydration
- hypotension
- infection
- low birth weight
- malnutrition
- preeclampsia
- preterm labor

73. STEP 4

The nurse cares for a 28-year-old female client at 16 weeks' gestation in the prenatal clinic.

Nurse's Notes

1030:
The 28-year-old gravida 2, para 1 client with a singleton pregnancy has a history of mild intermittent asthma that the client treats approximately once a week with albuterol. The client reports that they continue to have morning sickness, which first presented at 6 weeks' gestation, and they are vomiting more than three times a day. The client stopped taking prenatal vitamins because they increased nausea. The client reports fatigue and has not gone to work for the last 3 days. The client's prepregnant weight was 120 lb (54.4 kg) with a body mass index (BMI) of 20.1 kg/m². Today's weight is 121 lb (54.8 kg) with a BMI of 20.3 kg/m². Vital signs are 98.2°F (36.7°C); pulse (P) 86 bpm; respiration rate (RR) 16 breaths/min; and blood pressure (BP) 96/60 mm Hg. Mucous membranes are dry. The results of a urine dipstick test show no protein, glucose, or nitrates and trace amounts of ketones. The fetal heart rate (HR) is 150 bpm. The fundal height is 15 cm.

Orders

- Intravenous (IV) fluids: 1000 mL 5% dextrose in lactated Ringer's solution over 60 minutes
- Medication: ondansetron 4 mg IV now
- Dietary: hold oral (PO) intake until nausea subsides
- Diagnostics: metabolic panel, complete blood count, urinalysis, and ultrasound
- Education: provide home management teaching
- Reassess in 2 hours

The client receives the diagnosis of hyperemesis gravidarum. The nurse receives these orders to try to manage the client as an outpatient.

➤ What outcome(s) does the nurse establish as needed to be met for discharge to home therapy? Select all that apply.

- ☐ 1. relief of nausea
- ☐ 2. able to retain PO fluids
- ☐ 3. return to baseline weight
- ☐ 4. correction of hypovolemia
- ☐ 5. normal sodium and potassium levels
- ☐ 6. normal hemoglobin and hematocrit levels
- ☐ 7. understands the home management plan

74. STEP 5

The nurse cares for a 28-year-old female client at 16 weeks' gestation in the prenatal clinic.

Nurse's Notes

1030:
The 28-year-old gravida 2, para 1 client with a singleton pregnancy has a history of mild intermittent asthma that the client treats approximately once a week with albuterol. The client reports that they continue to have morning sickness, which first presented at 6 weeks' gestation, and they are vomiting more than three times a day. The client stopped taking prenatal vitamins because they increased nausea. The client reports fatigue and has not gone to work for the last 3 days. The client's prepregnant weight was 120 lb (54.4 kg) with a body mass index (BMI) of 20.1 kg/m². Today's weight is 121 lb (54.8 kg) with a BMI of 20.3 kg/m². Vital signs are 98.2°F (36.7°C); pulse (P) 86 bpm; respiration rate (RR) 16 breaths/min; and blood pressure (BP) 96/60 mm Hg. Mucous membranes are dry. The results of a urine dipstick test show no protein, glucose, or nitrates and trace amounts of ketones. The fetal heart rate (HR) is 150 bpm. The fundal height is 15 cm.

Orders

- Intravenous (IV) fluids: 1000 mL 5% dextrose in lactated Ringer's solution over 60 minutes
- Medication: ondansetron 4 mg IV now
- Dietary: hold oral (PO) intake until nausea subsides
- Diagnostics: metabolic panel, complete blood count, urinalysis, and ultrasound
- Education: provide home management teaching
- Reassess in 2 hours

The client is ready to try some PO intake after the fluid bolus and antiemetic medications.

➢ For each possible action, specify if the action is indicated or not indicated to help the client tolerate PO fluids.

Possible Action	Indicated	Not Indicated
Position the client on their side	○	○
Offer fluids with a straw	○	○
Select a carbonated beverage	○	○
Ensure noxious stimuli have been removed	○	○
Loosen any tight waistbands	○	○
Offer crackers with the fluids	○	○

75. STEP 6

The nurse cares for a 28-year-old female client at 16 weeks' gestation in the prenatal clinic.

Nurse's Notes

1030:
The 28-year-old gravida 2, para 1 client with a singleton pregnancy has a history of mild intermittent asthma that the client treats approximately once a week with albuterol. The client reports that they continue to have morning sickness, which first presented at 6 weeks' gestation, and they are vomiting more than three times a day. The client stopped taking prenatal vitamins because they increased nausea. The client reports fatigue and has not gone to work for the last 3 days. The client's prepregnant weight was 120 lb (54.4 kg) with a body mass index (BMI) of 20.1 kg/m². Today's weight is 121 lb (54.8 kg) with a BMI of 20.3 kg/m². Vital signs are 98.2°F (36.7°C); pulse (P) 86 bpm; respiration rate (RR) 16 breaths/min; and blood pressure (BP) 96/60 mm Hg. Mucous membranes are dry. The results of a urine dipstick test show no protein, glucose, or nitrates and trace amounts of ketones. The fetal heart rate (HR) is 150 bpm. The fundal height is 15 cm.

1230:
The client states nausea is improved after the fluid bolus and ondansetron. The client retained 240 mL of clear liquids and voided 100 mL of straw-colored urine. Vital signs are T 98°F (36°C); P 84 bpm; RR 16 breaths/min; and BP 96/56 mm Hg. Fetal HR is 140 bpm. Electrolytes are within normal limits. The client understands ways to decrease nausea and understands when to call the health care provider.

Orders

- Intravenous (IV) fluids: 1000 mL 5% dextrose in lactated Ringer's solution over 60 minutes
- Medication: ondansetron 4 mg IV now
- Dietary: hold oral (PO) intake until nausea subsides
- Diagnostics: metabolic panel, complete blood count, urinalysis, and ultrasound
- Education: provide home management teaching
- Reassess in 2 hours

➢ The nurse implements the ordered interventions and reassesses the client's status. Which four assessments show the client has improved and meets discharge criteria?

- ☐ 1. improved nausea
- ☐ 2. retained PO intake
- ☐ 3. ability to urinate
- ☐ 4. normal electrolytes
- ☐ 5. improved vital signs
- ☐ 6. understanding of management plan
- ☐ 7. reassuring fetal HR

The Client with a Gestational Trophoblastic Disease

76. A client at 15 weeks' gestation presents to the obstetrical triage unit with dark brown vaginal bleeding and continuous nausea and vomiting. The client's blood pressure is 142/98 mm Hg, and the fundal height is 19 cm. Which prescription is **most** important for the nurse to request from the primary health care provider?
☐ 1. a transfer to the antenatal unit
☐ 2. nothing-by-mouth (NPO) status for 24 hours
☐ 3. intravenous magnesium sulfate
☐ 4. a stat ultrasound

77. A 38-year-old client at about 14 weeks' gestation is admitted to the hospital with a diagnosis of complete hydatidiform mole. Soon after admission, the nurse would assess the client for which signs and symptoms?
☐ 1. gestational hypertension
☐ 2. gestational diabetes
☐ 3. hypothyroidism
☐ 4. polycythemia

78. After a client undergoes a dilatation and curettage (D&C) to evacuate a molar pregnancy, it would be **most** important for the nurse to assess the client for which signs and symptoms?
☐ 1. urinary tract infection
☐ 2. hemorrhage
☐ 3. abdominal distention
☐ 4. chorioamnionitis

79. When preparing a multigravid client who has undergone evacuation of a hydatidiform mole for discharge, the nurse explains the need for follow-up care. The nurse determines that the client understands the instruction when they say that they are at risk for developing which problem?
☐ 1. ectopic pregnancy
☐ 2. choriocarcinoma
☐ 3. multifetal pregnancies
☐ 4. infertility

80. After suction and evacuation of a complete hydatidiform mole, a 28-year-old multigravid client asks the nurse when they can become pregnant again. The nurse would advise the client not to become pregnant again for at least how long?
☐ 1. 6 months
☐ 2. 12 months
☐ 3. 18 months
☐ 4. 24 months

81. A client is diagnosed with a complete molar pregnancy. The nurse understands that the client requires more teaching when they make which statement?
☐ 1. "I need to make follow-up appointments to have my hormone levels checked."
☐ 2. "I know the placenta caused problems, and my baby died in my uterus."
☐ 3. "I plan to get pregnant again next year."
☐ 4. "I understand I may develop a serious type of cancer."

The Pregnant Client with Miscellaneous Complications

82. The nurse is working with four clients on the obstetrical unit. Which client will be the **highest priority** for a cesarean birth?
☐ 1. client at 40 weeks' gestation whose fetus weighs 8 lb (3630 g) by ultrasound estimate
☐ 2. client at 37 weeks' gestation with the fetus in the right occiput posterior (ROP) position
☐ 3. client at 32 weeks' gestation with the fetus in the breech position
☐ 4. client at 38 weeks' gestation with active herpes lesions

83. The nurse notices that a client who has just given birth is short of breath and ashen in color and begins to cough. The client becomes limp on the birthing table. At last assessment 30 minutes ago, the client's temperature was 98°F (36.7°C), pulse was 78 bpm, and respirations were 16 breaths/min. Determine the nursing actions in the order they should occur. All options must be used.

| 1. Open the airway using the head tilt-chin lift. |
| 2. Ask staff to activate the emergency response system. |
| 3. Establish unresponsiveness. |
| 4. Give two breaths. |
| 5. Begin compressions. |

| |
| |
| |
| |
| |

84. A client in sickle cell crisis has been hospitalized during pregnancy. After giving discharge instructions, the nurse determines the client needs further teaching when they make which statement?
☐ 1. "I will need more frequent appointments during the remainder of the pregnancy."
☐ 2. "Signs of any type of infection must be reported immediately."
☐ 3. "At the earliest signs of a crisis, I need to seek treatment."
☐ 4. "I will need to take an iron supplement even if my laboratory values are normal."

85. A laboring client at −2 station has a spontaneous rupture of the membranes, and a cord immediately protrudes from the vagina. What should the nurse do **first**?
☐ 1. Place gentle pressure upward on the fetal head.
☐ 2. Place the cord back into the vagina to keep it moist.
☐ 3. Begin oxygen by face mask at 8 to 10 L per minute.
☐ 4. Turn the client on the left side.

86. A client has just had a cesarean birth for a prolapsed cord. In reviewing the client's history, which factor(s) place a client at risk for cord prolapse? Select all that apply.
☐ 1. −2 station
☐ 2. low-birth-weight infant
☐ 3. rupture of membranes
☐ 4. breech presentation
☐ 5. prior abortion
☐ 6. low-lying placenta

87. A client who has given birth to a healthy neonate is being discharged. As part of discharge teaching, the nurse should instruct the client to observe vaginal discharge for postpartum hemorrhage and notify the health care provider (HCP) of which finding?
☐ 1. bleeding that increases with breastfeeding
☐ 2. clots the size of grapes
☐ 3. saturating a pad in less than an hour
☐ 4. lochia that lasts longer than 1 week

88. A client who is Rh negative has given birth to an Rh-positive infant. The nurse explains to the client that they will receive Rho(D) immune globulin. The nurse determines that the client understands the purpose of the treatment when they report that Rho(D) immune globulin has which action?
☐ 1. protecting their next baby if it is Rh negative
☐ 2. preventing antibody formation in their blood
☐ 3. preventing antigen formation in the baby's blood
☐ 4. preventing jaundice in their baby

89. A client at 4 weeks postpartum tells the nurse that they cannot cope any longer and are overwhelmed by their newborn. The baby has old formula on the clothes and under the neck. The client does not remember when they last bathed the baby and states they do not want to care for the infant. The nurse should encourage the client and spouse to call their health care provider (HCP) because the client should be evaluated further for which complication?
☐ 1. postpartum blues
☐ 2. postpartum depression
☐ 3. poor bonding
☐ 4. infant abuse

90. The nurse and an unlicensed assistive personnel (UAP) are caring for clients in a birthing center. Which task(s) should the nurse delegate to the UAP? Select all that apply.
☐ 1. emptying a urinary catheter from a postpartum client
☐ 2. assisting an active labor client with breathing and relaxation
☐ 3. ambulating a postcesarean client to the bathroom
☐ 4. calculating hourly intravenous (IV) totals for a preterm labor client
☐ 5. intake and output catheterization for culture and sensitivity
☐ 6. teaching the birth parent how to take a newborn's temperature

Managing Care, Quality, and Safety for Pregnant Clients

91. Several pregnant clients are waiting to be seen in the triage area of the obstetrical unit. Which client should the nurse see **first**?
☐ 1. a client at 13 weeks' gestation who is experiencing nausea and vomiting three times a day with +1 ketones in their urine
☐ 2. a client at 37 weeks' gestation who has insulin-dependent diabetes and is experiencing three to four fetal movements per day
☐ 3. a client at 32 weeks' gestation who has preeclampsia and +3 proteinuria and who is returning for evaluation of epigastric pain
☐ 4. a client at 17 weeks' gestation who is not feeling fetal movement at this point in the pregnancy

92. The nurse is planning care for a group of pregnant clients. Which client should be referred to a health care provider (HCP) **immediately**?
- ☐ 1. a client at 10 weeks' gestation who reports vomiting three times a day and has +1 ketones in their urine
- ☐ 2. a client at 36 weeks' gestation with insulin-dependent diabetes who reports having two to three hyperglycemic episodes per week
- ☐ 3. a client at 32 weeks' gestation who is preeclamptic with +3 proteinuria
- ☐ 4. a client at 15 weeks' gestation who reports they have not felt fetal movement

93. A client with gestational hypertension is to receive magnesium sulfate to run at 3 g per hour with normal saline to maintain the total intravenous (IV) rate at 125 mL per hour. The nurse giving the end-of-shift report stated that the client's blood pressures have been elevated during the night. The oncoming nurse checked the client and found magnesium sulfate running at 2 g per hour. Identify the nursing actions to be taken from first to last. All options must be used.

1. Notify the primary health care provider (HCP) of the incident.
2. Assess the client's current status.
3. Correct the IV rates.
4. Initiate an incident report.

94. As the nurse enters the room of a newly admitted primigravid client diagnosed with severe preeclampsia, the client begins to experience a seizure. The nurse should do which in order of **priority** from first to last? All options must be used.

1. Call for immediate assistance.
2. Turn the client to their side.
3. Assess for ruptured membranes.
4. Clear airway secretions.
5. Apply oxygen.

95. The nurse is receiving the shift report on four clients on an antenatal unit. The four clients are (1) a client at 35 weeks' gestation with severe preeclampsia started on a maintenance dose of magnesium sulfate 1 hour ago; (2) a client at 30 weeks' gestation with preterm labor on an oral tocolytic and having no contractions in 6 hours; (3) a client with hyperemesis who has experienced emesis four times in the past 12 hours, and (4) a client at 33 weeks' gestation with placenta previa who began to feel pelvic pressure during the change of shift report. Which action should the nurse take **first**?
- ☐ 1. Evaluate the client with preeclampsia for maternal and fetal tolerance of magnesium sulfate and the labor pattern.
- ☐ 2. Assess the client with preterm labor for tolerance of tocolytics and the labor pattern.
- ☐ 3. Assess the client with hyperemesis for nausea, further emesis, or dehydration.
- ☐ 4. Evaluate the client with placenta previa without an examination.

96. Which client findings require the nurse's attention **first?**
☐ 1. a gravida 2, para 1 at 39 weeks' gestation with spontaneous rupture of membranes 1 hour ago but no contractions
☐ 2. a gravida 3, para 2 at 30 weeks' gestation with nausea, vomiting, and epigastric pain
☐ 3. a gravida 5, para 1 at 37 weeks' gestation with pink vaginal discharge and abdominal cramping
☐ 4. a gravida 1, para 0 at 39 weeks' gestation with bruises on the arms and abdomen at various stages of healing

Answers, Rationales, and Test-Taking Strategies

The answers and rationales for each question follow below, along with keys (🔑) to the client need (CN) and cognitive level (CL) for each question. In addition, questions that measure clinical judgment will be coded (CJ). As you check your answers, use the Content Mastery and Test-Taking Skill Self-Analysis worksheet (tear-out worksheet in the back of the book) to identify the reason(s) for not answering the questions correctly. For additional information about test-taking skills and strategies for answering questions, refer to pages 12–51 in Part 1 of this book.

The Pregnant Client with Preeclampsia or Eclampsia

1. 50 mL

$$\frac{500 \text{ mL}}{20 \text{ g}} \times \frac{2 \text{ g}}{\text{h}} = \frac{\cancel{1{,}000}^{\,50} \text{ g/mL}}{\cancel{20}_{1} \text{ g/h}} = \frac{50 \text{ mL}}{1 \text{ h}}$$

🔑 CN: Pharmacological and parenteral therapies; CL: Apply

2. 3. The two major defining characteristics of preeclampsia are blood pressure elevation of 140/90 mm Hg or greater and proteinuria. Because the client's blood pressure meets the gestational hypertension criteria, the next nursing responsibility is to determine if the client has protein in their urine. If the client does not, they may be having transient hypertension. The peripheral edema is within normal limits for someone at this gestational age, particularly because it is in the lower extremities. While the preeclamptic client may have significant edema in the face and hands, edema can be caused by other factors and is not part of the diagnostic criteria. Headaches are significant in pregnancy-induced hypertension but may have other etiologies. The client's blood glucose level has no bearing on a preeclampsia diagnosis.

🔑 CN: Physiological adaptation; CL: Analyze

3. 4. The fetus is considered well if it moves more often than three times in 1 hour. Daily fetal movement counting is part of all high-risk assessments and is a noninvasive, inexpensive method of monitoring fetal well-being. The HCP should be notified if there is a gradual slowing over time of fetal activity, if each day it takes longer for the fetus to move a minimum of 10 times, or if the fetus stops moving for 12 hours or longer.

🔑 CN: Reduction of risk potential; CL: Evaluate

4. 3. The central nervous system (CNS) functioning and freedom from injury is a priority in maintaining the well-being of the maternal-fetal unit. If the birth parent has CNS damage related to hypertension or stroke, oxygenation status is compromised, and the well-being of both the client and the infant is at risk. Continuous fetal monitoring is an assessment strategy for the infant only and would be of secondary importance to maternal CNS assessment because maternal oxygenation will dictate fetal oxygenation and well-being. In preeclampsia, frequent assessment of maternal reflexes, clonus, visual disturbances, and headache give clear evidence of the condition of the maternal CNS system. Monitoring liver studies gives an indication of the status of the maternal system, but the less invasive and highly correlated condition of the maternal CNS system in assessing reflexes, maternal headache, visual disturbances, and clonus is the highest priority. Psychosocial care is a priority and can be accomplished in ways other than having the family remain at the bedside.

🔑 CN: Safety and infection control; CL: Analyze

5. 3. Clients with increased risk for preeclampsia include primigravid clients younger than 20 years or older than 40 years, clients with five or more pregnancies, clients of color, clients with multifetal pregnancies, clients with diabetes or heart disease, and clients with hydramnios. A total weight gain of 20 lb (9.1 kg) at 32 weeks' gestation with a 1-lb (0.45-kg) weight gain in the last 2 weeks is within normal limits. Short stature is not associated with the development of preeclampsia. A trace amount of protein in the urine is common during pregnancy. However, protein amounts of 1+ or more may be a symptom of pregnancy-induced hypertension.

🔑 CN: Reduction of risk potential; CL: Apply

Complications of Pregnancy   101

6. **1.** Congenital anomalies such as hydrocephalus are not associated with preeclampsia. Conditions such as stillbirth, prematurity, abruptio placentae, intrauterine growth restriction, and poor placental perfusion are associated with preeclampsia. Abruptio placentae occurs because of severe vasoconstriction. Intrauterine growth restriction is possible owing to poor placental perfusion. Poor placental perfusion results from increased vasoconstriction.

   🔑 CN: Physiological adaptation; CL: Evaluate

7. **1, 3, 4.** The nurse must be alert for any signs and symptoms of superimposed preeclampsia in clients with gestational hypertension. Dull headache, blurred vision, and protein in urine are all classic signs of preeclampsia in pregnancy and must be reported to the primary care provider immediately. Weight gain of 1 lb (500 g) per week is an expected finding. A fundal height of 28 cm is an expected finding.

   🔑 CN: Management of care; CL: Analyze

8. **3.** For clients with mild preeclampsia, a regular diet with ample protein and calories is recommended. If the client experiences constipation, they should increase the fiber in their diet, such as by eating raw fruits and vegetables, and increase their fluid intake. A high-residue diet is not a nutritional need in clients with preeclampsia. Sodium and fluid intake should not be restricted or increased. A high-protein diet is unnecessary.

   🔑 CN: Basic care and comfort; CL: Apply

9. **3.** The nurse must be alert to signs of magnesium sulfate toxicity that include loss of deep tendon reflexes, which is often the first sign (patellar-tendon response is the most common reflex tested); urinary output decreases (should have at least 30 mL per hour); and respirations decrease (12 breaths/min is low and could be developing respiratory distress). The first action would be to stop magnesium sulfate infusion and notify the HCP. The urinary catheter tubing may be kinked; however, looking at all findings would indicate to the nurse that the client is experiencing magnesium sulfate toxicity. It is not a priority to obtain a urine sample. Documentation is extremely important to complete; however, the nurse must intervene by stopping the magnesium sulfate and notifying the primary HCP. Increasing fluid intake at this point is not appropriate for a client who has magnesium sulfate toxicity. Intake and output should be ongoing for a client on intravenous fluids and magnesium sulfate and a diagnosis of preeclampsia.

   🔑 CN: Pharmacological and parenteral therapies; CL: Apply

10. **2.** A client with preeclampsia and a continuous headache for 2 days should be seen by an HCP immediately. Continuous headache, drowsiness, and mental confusion indicate poor cerebral perfusion and are symptoms of severe preeclampsia. Immediate care is recommended because these symptoms may lead to eclampsia or seizures if left untreated. Advising the client to take two acetaminophen tablets would be inappropriate and may lead to further complications if the client is not evaluated and treated. Although the application of cool compresses may ease the pain temporarily, this would delay treatment. Treatment for nausea may be indicated, but only after the primary HCP has seen the client and determined if the preeclampsia requires further treatment.

    🔑 CN: Reduction of risk potential; CL: Apply

11. **4.** A client with severe preeclampsia may develop eclampsia, which is characterized by seizures. The client needs a darkened, quiet room and side rails with thick padding. This helps decrease the potential for injury should a seizure occur. Airways, a suction machine, and oxygen also should be available. If the client is to undergo induction of labor, an oxytocin infusion solution can be obtained at a later time. Tongue blades are not necessary. However, the emergency cart should be placed nearby in case the client experiences a seizure. The ultrasound machine may be used at a later point to provide information about the fetus. In many hospitals, the client with severe preeclampsia is admitted to the labor area, where the client and the fetus can be closely monitored. The safety of the client and fetus is the priority.

    🔑 CN: Physiological adaptation; CL: Apply

12. **1.** Although the client is being admitted, the first response would be to attempt to lower blood pressure by putting the client in the left lateral position. The other interventions may be appropriate later, but the left lateral position would be the priority.

    🔑 CN: Management of care; CL: Analyze

13. **1.** Typical signs of hypermagnesemia include decreased deep tendon reflexes, sweating or flushing of the skin, oliguria, decreased respirations, and lethargy progressing to coma as the toxicity increases. The nurse should check the client's patellar, biceps, and radial reflexes regularly during magnesium sulfate therapy. Cool skin temperature may result from peripheral vasodilation, but the opposite—flushing and sweating—are usually seen. A rapid pulse rate commonly occurs in hypomagnesemia. Tingling in the toes may suggest hypocalcemia, not hypermagnesemia.

    🔑 CN: Physiological adaptation; CL: Analyze

14. ⊟ **2, 3, 4.** Headaches could be a sign of preeclampsia/eclampsia in pregnancy. The client should be assessed for headache, vision changes, epigastric pain, hyper reflexes, and the presence of clonus. The fetus should be assessed using a nonstress test. Urine should be tested for proteinuria, not ketones. An ultrasound done in this pregnancy does not give information to assess the presence of preeclampsia or eclampsia.

🗝️ CN: Management of care; CL: Analyze

15. 4. The highest priority for a client with severe preeclampsia is to prevent seizures, thereby minimizing the possibility of adverse effects on the birth parent and fetus, and then to facilitate a safe birth. Efforts to decrease edema, reduce blood pressure, increase urine output, limit kidney damage, and maintain sedation are desirable but are not as important as preventing seizures. It would take several days or weeks for the edema to be decreased. Sedation and decreased reflex excitability can occur with the administration of intravenous magnesium sulfate, which peaks in 30 minutes, much sooner than 48 hours.

🗝️ CN: Physiological adaptation; CL: Create

16. ⊟ **1, 5, 6.** The use of magnesium sulfate as an anticonvulsant medication acts to depress the central nervous system by blocking peripheral neuromuscular transmissions and decreasing the amount of acetylcholine liberated. The primary goal of magnesium sulfate therapy is to prevent seizures. While this therapy is being used, the temperature and pulse of the client should remain within normal limits. The respiratory rate needs to be greater than 12 breaths/min. Rates at 12 breaths/min or lower are associated with respiratory depression and are seen with magnesium toxicity. Renal compromise is identified with a urinary output of less than 30 mL per hour. A fetal heart rate that is maintained within the range of 112 to 160 bpm is desired without later or variable decelerations. Although extreme elevations of blood pressure must be treated, achieving a normal pressure carries a risk for decreasing perfusion to the fetus. Deep tendon reflexes should not be diminished or exaggerated.

🗝️ CN: Pharmacological and parenteral therapies; CL: Evaluate

17. 1. A respiratory rate of 12 breaths/min suggests potential respiratory depression, an adverse effect of magnesium sulfate therapy. The medication must be stopped, and the HCP should be notified immediately. A patellar reflex of +2 is normal. The absence of a patellar reflex suggests magnesium toxicity. A blood pressure reading of 160/88 mm Hg would be a common finding in a client with severe preeclampsia. Urinary output exceeding intake is not likely in a client receiving intravenous magnesium sulfate. Oliguria is more common.

🗝️ CN: Pharmacological and parenteral therapies; CL: Analyze

18. 3. Principles of emergency management begin with calling for assistance. If a client begins to have a seizure, the first action by the nurse is to remain with the client and call for immediate assistance. The nurse needs to have some assistance in managing this client. After the seizure, the client needs intensive monitoring. An airway can be inserted, if appropriate, after the seizure ends. Noting the time the seizure begins and ends and turning the client to their left side should be done after assistance is obtained.

🗝️ CN: Reduction of risk potential; CL: Analyze

19. 1. One of the most common adverse effects of the drug hydralazine is tachycardia. Therefore, the nurse should assess the client's heart rate and pulse. Hydralazine acts to lower blood pressure by peripheral dilation without interfering with placental circulation. Bradypnea and polyuria are usually not associated with hydralazine use. Dysphagia is not a typical adverse effect of hydralazine.

🗝️ CN: Pharmacological and parenteral therapies; CL: Analyze

20. 4. These findings would be documented as 4+. 1+ indicates a diminished response; 2+ indicates a normal response; and 3+ indicates a response that is brisker than average but not abnormal. Mild clonus is said to be present when there are two movements.

🗝️ CN: Physiological adaptation; CL: Apply

21. 3. Epigastric pain or acute right upper quadrant pain is associated with the development of eclampsia and an impending seizure; this is thought to be related to liver ischemia. Decreased contraction intensity is unrelated to the severity of preeclampsia. Typically, the client's temperature increases because of increased cerebral pressure. A decrease in temperature is unrelated to an impending seizure. Hyporeflexia is not associated with an impending seizure. Typically, the client would exhibit hyperreflexia.

🗝️ CN: Physiological adaptation; CL: Analyze

22. 4. After an eclamptic seizure, the client commonly falls into a deep sleep or coma. The nurse must continually monitor the client for signs of impending labor because the client will not be able to verbalize that contractions are occurring.

Oliguria is more common than polyuria after an eclamptic seizure. Facial flushing is not common unless it is caused by a reaction to a medication. Typically, the client remains hypertensive unless medications such as magnesium sulfate are administered.

 CN: Physiological adaptation; CL: Analyze

The Pregnant Client with a Chronic Hypertensive Disorder

23. 1. Pregnancy is not the time for clients to begin a diet. Clients with chronic hypertension need to consume adequate calories to support fetal growth and development. They also need an adequate protein intake. Meat and beans are good sources of protein. Most pregnant clients report that eating more frequent, smaller meals decreases heartburn caused by the reflux of acidic secretions into the lower esophagus. Pregnant clients need adequate hydration (fluids) and fiber to prevent constipation.

 CN: Basic care and comfort; CL: Evaluate

24. 2. Clients with chronic hypertension during pregnancy are at risk for complications such as preeclampsia (about 25%), abruptio placentae, and intrauterine growth retardation, resulting in a small-for-gestational-age infant. There is no association between chronic hypertension and hyperthyroidism. Pregnant clients with chronic hypertension are not at an increased risk for hydramnios (polyhydramnios), an abnormally large amount of amniotic fluid. Clients with diabetes and multiple gestations are at risk for this condition. Placenta accreta, a rare placental abnormality, refers to a condition in which the placenta abnormally adheres to the uterine lining. It is not associated with chronic hypertension.

 CN: Reduction of risk potential; CL: Evaluate

25. 2, 3, 6. Vaginal bleeding with or without pain could signify placenta previa or abruptio placentae. A continuous or pounding headache could indicate an elevated blood pressure, and a change in the strength or frequency of fetal movements could indicate that the fetus is in distress. Orthostatic hypotension can occur during pregnancy and can be alleviated by rising slowly. Leg veins may increase in size as a result of additional pressure from the increasing uterine size; leg cramps may also occur and can commonly be decreased with calcium supplements.

 CN: Reduction of risk potential; CL: Evaluate

The Pregnant Client with Third-Trimester Bleeding

26. 1. Bright red vaginal bleeding without contractions could indicate placenta previa. A sterile vaginal examination should never be done on a client with known or suspected placenta previa. Applying the external fetal monitor will allow the nurse to assess fetal status. A complete physical assessment of the client is indicated. A fundal height is used to monitor fetal growth during pregnancy, but it does not provide information related to vaginal bleeding.

 CN: Reduction of risk potential; CL: Analyze

27. 3. Urinary output of less than 30 mL per hour indicates renal compromise and would be the most important assessment finding to report to the HCP. The APTT is within normal limits, and the hemoglobin is lower than values for an adult female but within normal limits for a pregnant female. Although the platelet level is slightly low and may impact blood clotting, when compared to renal failure, it is less important.

 CN: Management of care; CL: Analyze

28. 4. Although the exact cause of abruptio placentae is unknown, possible contributing factors include excessive intrauterine pressure caused by hydramnios or multiple pregnancy, cocaine use, cigarette smoking, alcohol ingestion, trauma, increased maternal age and parity, and amniotomy. A history of hypertension is associated with an increased risk for abruptio placentae. A previous low transverse cesarean birth and a history of one induced abortion are associated with increased risk for placenta previa, not abruptio placentae.

 CN: Physiological adaptation; CL: Analyze

29. 2. Treatment of DIC includes treating the causative factor, replacing maternal coagulation factors, and supporting physiologic functions. Intravenous infusions of whole blood, fresh frozen plasma, or platelets are used to replace depleted maternal coagulation factors. Although Ringer's lactate solution and 5% dextrose solution may be used as intravenous fluid replacement, the client needs blood component therapy. Therefore, normal saline must be used. Intravenous heparin, not warfarin, may be administered to halt the clotting cascade.

 CN: Physiological adaptation; CL: Analyze

30. 1. The most common assessment finding associated with placenta previa is painless vaginal bleeding. With placenta previa, the placenta is abnormally implanted, covering a portion or all of the cervical os. Uterine tetany, intermittent pain with spotting, and dull lower back pain are not associated with placenta previa. Uterine tetany is associated with oxytocin administration. Intermittent pain with spotting commonly is associated with a spontaneous abortion. Dull lower back pain is commonly associated with poor maternal posture or a urinary tract infection with renal involvement.

CN: Physiological adaptation; CL: Analyze

31. 3. Feelings of loss, grief, and guilt are normal after a cesarean birth, particularly if it was not planned. The nurse should support the client, listen with empathy, and allow the client time to grieve. The likelihood of the client experiencing postpartum blues is not known, and no evidence is presented. Although maternal-infant bonding may be delayed owing to neonatal complications or maternal pain and subsequent medications, it should not be difficult. Although the nurse is aware that this type of birth was necessary to save the client's life, using this as the basis for the response does not acknowledge the client's feelings.

CN: Psychosocial integrity; CL: Apply

32. The level of anesthesia achieved via epidural anesthesia for a vaginal birth is T10 (approximately the level of the umbilicus). Epidural anesthesia for a cesarean birth would be at the level of T4 to T6, approximately at the nipple line.

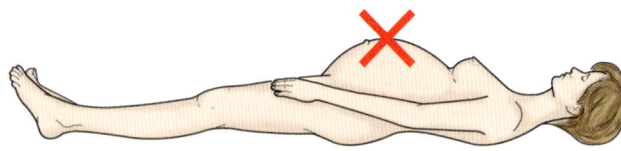

CN: Pharmacological and parenteral therapies; CL: Apply

33. 3. Abruptio placentae is a medical emergency because the degree of hypovolemic shock may be out of proportion to visible blood loss. On admission, the nurse should plan to first insert a large-gauge intravenous catheter for fluid replacement and oxygen by mask to decrease fetal anoxia. Vaginal examination usually is not performed on pregnant clients who are experiencing third-trimester bleeding due to abruptio placentae because it can result in damage to the placenta and further fetal anoxia. The client's history can be obtained once the client has been admitted and the intravenous line has been started. The goal is the birth of the fetus, usually by emergency cesarean birth. The nurse should also plan to monitor the client's vital signs and the fetal heart rate. Ultrasound is of limited use in the diagnosis of abruptio placentae.

CN: Reduction of risk potential; CL: Analyze

The Pregnant Client with Preterm Labor

34. 3. The absence of fetal fibronectin in a vaginal swab between 22 and 37 weeks' gestation indicates there is a less than 1% risk for developing preterm labor in the next week. Fetal fibronectin is an extracellular protein normally found in fetal membranes and deciduas and has no correlation with preeclampsia, fetal lung maturation, or gestational diabetes.

CN: Reduction of risk potential; CL: Evaluate

35. 2. Corticosteroids given intramuscularly have been shown to increase fetal lung maturity by increasing surfactant and reducing the risk for respiratory distress syndrome in premature infants. It is not a guarantee that a premature newborn would not have problems at birth that would require time in the neonatal intensive care unit. The administration of the corticosteroids is normally completed within 24 to 48 hours.

CN: Pharmacological and parenteral therapies; CL: Evaluate

36. 3. As the uterus contracts, the abdominal wall rises and, when external monitoring is used, presses against the transducer. This movement is transmitted into an electrical current, which is then recorded. With the fetus in the LOA position, the cardiotransducer should be placed below the umbilicus on the side where the fetal back is located and uterine displacement during contractions is greatest. If the fetal back is near the symphysis pubis, the fetus is presenting as a transverse lie. If the fetus is in a breech position, the fetal back may be at or above the umbilicus.

CN: Reduction of risk potential; CL: Apply

The Pregnant Client with Premature Rupture of the Membranes

37. 3. Because chorioamnionitis may occur when membranes have ruptured, vaginal cultures for *Neisseria gonorrhoeae*, group B streptococcus, and chlamydia are usually taken. Prophylactic antibiotics may be prescribed to reduce the risk for infection in the newborn. Frequent vaginal examinations should be avoided because they can further increase the client's risk for infection. Intravenous oxytocin to initiate labor may be used if an infection occurs. Bed rest can sometimes prolong the pregnancy and prevent a preterm birth. Internal fetal monitoring is not indicated if external monitoring is working sufficiently.

CN: Reduction of risk potential; CL: Apply

38. 4. Premature rupture of the membranes is commonly associated with chorioamnionitis, or an infection. A priority assessment for the nurse to make is to document the client's temperature every 2 to 4 hours. Temperature elevation may indicate an infection. Lethargy and an elevated white blood cell count also indicate an infection. The red blood cell count would provide information related to anemia, not infection. The client is not in labor. Therefore, assessing the degree of discomfort is not a priority at this time. Urinary output is not a reliable indicator of an infection such as chorioamnionitis.

🔑 CN: Reduction of risk potential; CL: Analyze

39. 1. Because group B streptococcus is a gram-positive bacterium, the HCP probably will prescribe intravenous penicillin to treat the client's infection and prevent fetal infection. Gentamicin sulfate, which acts on gram-negative bacteria, would be inappropriate. Administering a corticosteroid, such as betamethasone, is inappropriate because the premature rupture of the membranes enhances fetal lung maturity. The lack of amniotic fluid causes the early maturation of lung tissue. Cefaclor, which is available only in oral form, is used for upper and lower respiratory tract infections and urinary tract infections by gram-negative staphylococci.

🔑 CN: Pharmacological and parenteral therapies; CL: Analyze

40. 1. The priority is to determine whether a prolapsed cord has occurred as a result of the spontaneous rupture of membranes. The nurse's first action should be to check the status of the fetal heart rate. Complications of premature rupture of the membranes include a prolapsed cord or increased pressure on the fetal umbilical cord that inhibits fetal nutrient supply. Variable decelerations or fetal bradycardia may be seen on the external fetal monitor. The cord also may be visible. Turning the client to their right side is not necessary. If the cord does prolapse, the client should be placed in a knee-to-chest or Trendelenburg position. A vaginal examination may be appropriate once the status of the fetus has been evaluated. The nurse can continue to measure the client's vital signs at routine intervals.

🔑 CN: Reduction of risk potential; CL: Analyze

The Pregnant Client with Diabetes Mellitus

41. ➗ **1, 2, 3, 5.** A client with gestational diabetes needs to maintain blood glucose levels as close to "normal" as a pregnant client who does not have diabetes. Walking is an excellent form of exercise for anyone and works well for pregnant clients with diabetes as it burns calories, accelerates the heart rate, and, as a result, maintains the blood sugar at a lower level. During pregnancy, continuously high blood glucose levels measured by a hemoglobin A1C of greater than 6 mg/dL (60 g/L) carry risks for the dyad. The suggested diet for a pregnant client with diabetes is 1800 to 2400 calories a day to avoid the body breaking down maternal fat to maintain blood glucose levels. Continuing prenatal vitamins, iron, and folic acid (800 mcg per day) are general nutritional recommendations for pregnancy.

🔑 CN: Reduction of risk; CL: Evaluate

42. 4. The nonstress test is considered reactive when two or more fetal heart rate accelerations of at least 15 bpm occur (from a baseline fetal heart rate of 120 to 160 bpm), along with fetal movement, during a 10- to 20-minute period. A reactive nonstress test indicates fetal heart rate accelerations and well-being. There is no indication for further evaluation (such as a contraction stress test). However, contraction stress tests are commonly scheduled for pregnant clients with insulin-dependent diabetes in the latter part of pregnancy and are repeated periodically until birth. Chorionic villus sampling is usually performed early in the pregnancy to detect fetal abnormalities.

🔑 CN: Reduction of risk potential; CL: Apply

43. 3. A contraction stress test is used to evaluate fetal well-being during simulated labor. A suspicious contraction stress test indicates inconsistent late deceleration patterns requiring further evaluation. A negative contraction stress test indicates no late decelerations and is the desired outcome. A positive contraction stress test indicates fetal compromise with frequent late decelerations. Fetal movements are one of the parameters of a biophysical profile and are detected with nonstress testing. Decreased or absent fetal movements may indicate central nervous system dysfunction or prematurity. Lack of fetal movement or decreased fetal movement is not associated with contraction stress testing.

🔑 CN: Reduction of risk potential; CL: Analyze

44. 2. The fetal biophysical profile, a noninvasive test using real-time ultrasound, assesses five parameters: fetal heart rate reactivity, fetal breathing movements, gross fetal body movements, fetal tone, and amniotic fluid volume. Fetal heart rate reactivity is determined by a nonstress test; the other four parameters are determined by ultrasound scanning. The results are available as soon as the test is completed and interpreted. The lecithin-sphingomyelin ratio is used to determine fetal lung maturity. Although the fetal biophysical profile is useful in predicting which fetuses may be at greater risk for compromise, there is no correlation with the newborn's Apgar score. The biophysical score is sometimes referred to as the *fetal Apgar score*. A score of 8 to 10 indicates fetal well-being. The use of an ultrasound requires the client to have a full bladder.

🗝 CN: Pharmacological and parenteral therapies; CL: Apply

45. 2. During the first trimester, it is not unusual for insulin needs to decrease, commonly as a result of nausea and vomiting. Progressive insulin resistance is characteristic of pregnancy, particularly in the second half of pregnancy. It is not unusual for insulin needs to increase by as much as four times the nonpregnant dose after about the 24th week of gestation. This resistance is caused by the production of human placental lactogen, also called *human chorionic somatotropin,* by the placenta and by other hormones, such as estrogen and progesterone, which are insulin antagonists.

🗝 CN: Pharmacological and parenteral therapies; CL: Apply

46. 2. Clients who are pregnant and have diabetes are not at greater risk for multifetal pregnancy and subsequent twin-to-twin transfusion unless they have undergone fertility treatments. A pregnant client with diabetes is at higher risk for complications such as infection, polyhydramnios, ketoacidosis, and preeclampsia, compared with a pregnant client who does not have diabetes.

🗝 CN: Reduction of risk potential; CL: Evaluate

47. 2. The goal is to maintain blood plasma glucose levels at 70 to 100 mg/dL (3.5 to 5.6 mmol/L) before meals and bedtime snacks. Below 60 mg/dL (5.6 mmol/L) indicates hypoglycemia. A range of 110 to 140 mg/dL (6.2 to 7.8 mmol/L) suggests hyperglycemia. The target range 1 hour after meals is 100 to 120 mg/dL (5.6 to 6.7 mmol/L).

🗝 CN: Pharmacological and parenteral therapies; CL: Apply

48. 3. Maternal infection is the most common cause of maternal hyperglycemia and can lead to ketoacidosis, coma, and death. The client should notify the health care provider immediately if they experience symptoms of an infection. Fetal macrosomia results from maternal hyperglycemia but does not cause it. Fetal insulin production increases as maternal glucose crosses the placenta. This helps control glucose in the fetus, but it has no bearing on maternal glucose levels. Gestational hypertension does not cause maternal hyperglycemia during pregnancy.

🗝 CN: Physiological adaptation; CL: Create

49. 1. Dehydration, polyuria, fatigue, flushed hot skin, dry mouth, and drowsiness are manifestations of hyperglycemia. Hyperglycemia is a medical emergency and requires immediate action to prevent maternal and fetal mortality. Pallor, sweating, and nervousness are early signs of hypoglycemia, not hyperglycemia.

🗝 CN: Reduction of risk potential; CL: Evaluate

50. 4. Stillbirths caused by placental insufficiency occur with increased frequency in clients with diabetes and severe preeclampsia. Clients with poorly controlled diabetes may experience unanticipated stillbirth as a result of premature aging of the placenta. Therefore, labor is commonly induced in these clients before term. If induction of labor fails, a cesarean birth is necessary. Induction and cesarean birth do not prevent neonatal hyperbilirubinemia, congenital anomalies, or perinatal asphyxia.

🗝 CN: Reduction of risk potential; CL: Apply

51. 1. Insulin needs fall significantly during the first 24 hours postpartum because the client has usually been on nothing-by-mouth status for a period of time during labor and the labor process has used maternal glycogen stores. If the client breastfeeds, lower blood glucose levels decrease the insulin requirements. With insulin resistance gone, the client commonly needs little or no insulin during the immediate postpartum period. Although the need for insulin decreases during the intrapartum period, the insulin requirements fall further during the first 24 hours postpartum. After the first 24 hours postpartum, insulin requirements may fluctuate markedly, needing adjustment during the next few days as the birth parent's body returns to a nonpregnant state.

🗝 CN: Pharmacological and parenteral therapies; CL: Create

The Pregnant Client with Heart Disease

52. 3. The client needs a diet that is adequate in protein and calories to prevent anemia, which can place additional strain on the cardiac system, further compromising the client's cardiac status. The client should avoid contact with people who have infections because of the increased risk for developing endocarditis. The client may need antibiotics during the pregnancy to prevent endocarditis. Limiting sodium intake can help prevent excessive expansion of blood volume and decrease cardiac workload.

👉 CN: Reduction of risk potential; CL: Evaluate

53. 4. Clients with class II heart disease have dyspnea upon exertion but not at rest. Dyspnea at rest would indicate a change in condition that must be reported immediately because it may be indicative of increasing congestive heart failure. Mild ankle edema in the third trimester is a common finding. However, generalized or pitting edema, suggesting increasing congestive heart failure, must be reported immediately. Emotional stress on the job increases cardiac demand. However, it needs to be reported only if the client experiences symptoms, such as palpitations or irregular heart rate, indicating heart failure related to the increased stress. A weight gain of 1 lb (0.45 kg) per week is a normal finding during the third trimester.

👉 CN: Reduction of risk potential; CL: Apply

54. 1. Clients on cardiac medications may need dosage increases. As their blood volume and glomerular filtration rates increase, they may experience higher rates of drug excretion. Drug level monitoring may be needed after dose changes or if the client presents with toxicity, but weekly monitoring is unnecessary. The medication would be switched only if digitalis toxicity occurs. A diuretic is added only if congestive heart failure is not controlled by sodium and activity restrictions.

👉 CN: Management of care; CL: Apply

55. 1. Although there is no completely safe anticoagulant therapy during pregnancy, heparin is typically the drug of choice. Warfarin, a pregnancy category D drug, can cause fetal malformations. Enoxaparin is sometimes used, but clients are typically switched to heparin near labor because enoxaparin used along with spinal or epidural anesthesia presents an increased risk for bleeding in the epidural or spinal space. Ardeparin also can cause fetal malformations.

👉 CN: Pharmacological and parenteral therapies; CL: Apply

56. 4. The client can continue a low-sodium diet but should increase the caloric intake to 2200 calories daily to provide adequate nutrients to support fetal growth and development. Folic acid supplements, a standard component of care, are used to prevent folic acid deficiency, which is associated with megaloblastic anemia during pregnancy. Severe restriction of sodium intake is not recommended because sodium is necessary to maintain fluid volume. Iron supplements should be taken with acidic foods and fluids (e.g., citrus juices) for maximum absorption. Milk decreases the absorption of iron.

👉 CN: Reduction of risk potential; CL: Apply

The Client with an Ectopic Pregnancy

57. 1. The client's signs and symptoms indicate a probable ectopic pregnancy, which can be confirmed by ultrasound examination or by culdocentesis. The HCP is notified immediately because hypovolemic shock may develop without external bleeding. Once the fallopian tube ruptures, blood will enter the pelvic cavity, resulting in shock. Abruptio placentae would be manifested by a boardlike uterus in the third trimester. Gestational trophoblastic disease would be suspected if the client exhibited no fetal heart rate and symptoms of pregnancy-induced hypertension before 20 weeks' gestation. A client with a complete abortion would exhibit a normal pulse and blood pressure with scant vaginal bleeding.

👉 CN: Physiological adaptation; CL: Analyze

58. 1, 2, 3, 5. The client may be experiencing an ectopic pregnancy. Contributing factors to an ectopic pregnancy include a prior history of sexually transmitted infection that can scar the fallopian tubes. Multiple sex partners increase the risk for sexually transmitted infections. Knowledge of the client's last menstrual period and contraceptive use may support or rule out the possibility of an ectopic pregnancy. The client's history of cesarean births would not contribute information valuable to the client's current situation or a potential diagnosis of ectopic pregnancy.

👉 CN: Reduction of risk potential; CL: Analyze

59. 2. Diaphoresis, or profuse sweating, indicates shock, which occurs if the tube ruptures. Other common symptoms of tubal rupture include severe, knifelike lower quadrant abdominal pain, referred shoulder pain, and falling blood pressure. Slight vaginal bleeding, commonly described as *spotting* occurs for many reasons not related to tubal rupture. A rapid, thready pulse, a symptom of shock, is more common with tubal rupture than a slow, bounding pulse. Abdominal edema is a late sign of a tubal rupture in ectopic pregnancy.

🗝 CN: Reduction of risk potential; CL: Analyze

60. 4. Fallopian tube rupture is an emergency situation because of extensive bleeding into the peritoneal cavity. Shock soon develops if precautionary measures are not taken. The nurse readying a client for surgery should be especially careful to monitor blood pressure and pulse rate for signs of impending shock. The nurse should be prepared to administer fluids, blood, or plasma expanders as necessary through an intravenous line that should already be in place. Because the fertilized ovum has implanted outside the uterus, uterine cramping is unlikely. However, abdominal tenderness or knifelike pain may occur. Abdominal fullness may be present, but abdominal distention is rare unless peritonitis has developed. Although the hemoglobin and hematocrit values may be checked routinely before surgery, the laboratory results may not truly reflect the presence or degree of acute hemorrhage.

🗝 CN: Reduction of risk potential; CL: Analyze

61. 3. Anything that causes a narrowing or constriction in the fallopian tubes so that a fertilized ovum cannot be properly transported to the uterus for implantation predisposes an ectopic pregnancy. Pelvic inflammatory disease is the most common cause of constricted or narrow tubes. Developmental defects are other possible causes. Ectopic pregnancy is not related to urinary tract infections. The use of marijuana during pregnancy is not associated with ectopic pregnancy, but its use can result in cognitive reduction if the client's use during pregnancy is extensive. Progestin-only contraceptives and intrauterine devices have been associated with ectopic pregnancy.

🗝 CN: Physiological adaptation; CL: Analyze

62. 3. Because the fallopian tube has not yet ruptured, methotrexate may be given, followed by leucovorin. This chemotherapeutic agent attacks the fast-growing zygote and trophoblast cells. RU-486 is also effective. A hysterosalpingogram is usually performed after chemotherapy to determine whether the tube is still patent. Progestin-only contraceptives and medroxyprogesterone are ineffective in clearing the fallopian tube. Dyphylline is a bronchodilator and is not used.

🗝 CN: Pharmacological and parenteral therapies; CL: Analyze

The Pregnant Client with Hyperemesis Gravidarum

63. 3. Doxylamine succinate and pyridoxine hydrochloride is a combination drug of an antihistamine and vitamin B used to treat morning sickness. Drowsiness is the most common side effect of antihistamines. Antacid medications may cause diarrhea but are used to treat gastrointestinal reflux. Corticosteroids, like dexamethasone, do cause thirst but are more typically used to treat nausea associated with chemotherapy or surgery. Promethazine is an example of a dopamine antagonist sometimes used to treat nausea in pregnancy. These medications may cause restlessness, muscle spasms, constipation, and dry mouth.

🗝 CN: Pharmacological and parental therapies; CL: Apply

64. 3. The client needs further instructions when saying they should eat two meals a day with frequent protein snacks to decrease nausea and vomiting. The client should eat more frequent, smaller meals, with frequent carbohydrate snacks to decrease nausea and vomiting. Eating dry crackers or toast before arising, consuming fluids separately from meals, and avoiding greasy or spicy foods may also help decrease nausea and vomiting.

🗝 CN: Basic care and comfort; CL: Evaluate

65. 1. The herbal supplement ginger is taken to reduce nausea and vomiting. When consumed as a spice in foods, such as ginger cookies, there is a general consensus that ginger is safe. Prescription medications may be necessary to treat severe nausea and vomiting in pregnancy, but they can carry risks, such as sedation. Prenatal vitamins should be taken when clients are experiencing the least amount of nausea rather than waiting for a specific time period after eating food. There is no known pregnancy risk from eating ginger as a spice in foods.

🗝 CN: Basic care and comfort; CL: Apply

66. 3. Gastrointestinal secretion losses from excessive vomiting, diarrhea, and excessive perspiration can result in hypokalemia, hyponatremia, decreased chloride levels, metabolic alkalosis, and eventual acidosis if precautionary measures are not taken. Ketones may be present in the urine. Dehydration can lead to poor maternal and fetal outcomes. Persistent vomiting can lead to hypocalcemia, not hypercalcemia. Hyperbilirubinemia, not hypobilirubinemia, is typical in clients with hyperemesis. Persistent vomiting may affect liver function and subsequently the excretion of bilirubin from the body. Hypoglycemia, not hyperglycemia, may occur as a result of decreased intake of food and fluids, decreased metabolism of nutrients, and excessive vomiting.

🗝 CN: Reduction of risk potential; CL: Analyze

67. 2. Although the cause of hyperemesis is still unclear, it is thought to be related to high estrogen and human chorionic gonadotropin levels or to trophoblastic activity or gonadotropin production. Hyperemesis is also associated with infectious conditions, such as hepatitis or encephalitis, intestinal obstruction, peptic ulcer, and hydatidiform mole. Progesterone is a relaxant used during pregnancy and would not stimulate vomiting. Somatotropin is a growth hormone used in children. Aldosterone is a male hormone.

🗝 CN: Physiological adaptation; CL: Apply

68. 25 gtts/min

$$\frac{\text{gtts}}{\text{min}} = \frac{12 \text{ gtts}}{1 \text{ mL}} \times \frac{1000 \text{ mL}}{8 \text{ h}} \times \frac{1 \text{ h}}{60 \text{ min}} = 25 \text{ gtts/min}$$

🗝 CN: Pharmacological and parenteral therapies; CL: Apply

69. 2. Clients with hyperemesis gravidarum can experience severe vomiting. Some clients will require hospital care to treat dehydration, including intravenous fluids, antiemetics, and enteral nutrition. Sleep and dietary choices are important, but they are not the priority intervention. Acetaminophen suppositories are not indicated for the care of a client with hyperemesis gravidarum.

🗝 CN: Management of care; CL: Analyze

70.

STEP 1

0/1 **3, 4, 5, 6, 9.** Pregnancy-associated nausea and vomiting typically improve by the second trimester, but the client still reports vomiting more than three times a day. A client with a normal body weight would typically gain 4.4 lb (2 kg) in the first trimester. This client has gained only 1.1 lb (0.5 kg) by 16 weeks. Trace ketones in the urine indicate the client is having to burn stored fat for energy. While some fatigue is normal, fatigue so severe that it causes a client to miss work for several days is not. The vital signs all fall within a normal range, but the nurse should compare the pulse and blood pressure with baseline values. Albuterol use once week is consistent with the diagnosis of mild intermittent asthma. Albuterol can cause nausea, but once-a-week use does not explain the symptoms. Dry mucous membranes indicate dehydration. A normal fetal HR is 110 to 160 bpm. Fundal height is best interpreted on a fundal height chart and watched over time. A height of 15 cm at 16 weeks' gestation would fall within expected limits and not be concerning.

🗝 CJ: Case study; Step 1: Recognize cues; CL: Analyze

71.

STEP 2

Client Findings	Morning Sickness	Hyperemesis Gravidarum
Second-trimester nausea		X
Vomiting frequency		X
Weight gain pattern	X	
Dry mucous membranes		X
Trace ketonuria		X
Missing work related to fatigue		X

Morning sickness typically begins early in pregnancy but improves through the first trimester. Vomiting is infrequent. Weight loss is minimal, or clients may be able to continue to gain weight. Ketonuria would not be expected because nutritional deficits, if any, are minimal. Clients with morning sickness typically can continue to work and care for their families on most days. Hyperemesis gravidarum is more severe and can persist to mid pregnancy or longer. Vomiting is frequent, leading to poor oral intake, dehydration, fluid and electrolyte imbalances, and ketonuria. A weight loss of 5% or more of prepregnant weight with signs of dehydration is diagnostic of hyperemesis gravidarum. Dry mucous membranes indicate dehydration. Clients with hyperemesis gravidarum may be off work for long periods of time and may have difficulty caring for themselves.

🗝 CJ: Case study; Step 2: Analyze cues; CL: Analyze

72.

STEP 3

0/1 *The nurse should recognize that the nausea and vomiting are causing* **dehydration** *and* **malnutrition**. *Untreated, these complications most likely will lead to the adverse pregnancy outcomes of* **low birth weight** *and* **preterm labor**.

The client's nausea and vomiting are causing dehydration as evidenced by dry mucous membranes and fatigue, and malnutrition is evidenced by poor weight gain and ketonuria. The cause is most likely hyperemesis gravidarum; however, a diagnostic workup is indicated to rule out other causes, such as a molar pregnancy. Untreated, malnutrition may affect fetal growth, leading to low birth weight and dehydration, which contributes to preterm labor. The client's blood pressure is still within normal limits. There is no elevation of temperature or nitrites in the urine to suggest infection at this point. Birth defects, or congenital anomalies, are most associated with exposure to teratogens during the embryonic period, which ends after the eighth week of pregnancy. Hyperemesis gravidarum is not associated with hypertensive disorders of pregnancy.

🗝️ CJ: Case study; Step 3: Prioritize hypothesis; CL: Analyze

73.

STEP 4

−/+ 1, 2, 4, 5, 7. The ability to treat hyperemesis gravidarum on an outpatient basis depends on the severity of the symptoms. Relief of nausea is needed so the client can take PO fluids. Correcting the hypovolemia is essential to ensure adequate placental perfusion and prevent client injury. Untreated, electrolyte imbalances contribute to fatigue and neurologic and cardiac problems, including increased fatigue, dizziness, muscle spasms, and arrhythmias. Prior to discharge, the client needs to understand how to manage their nausea and vomiting and when to call their health care provider. The client would not be reweighed on the same day. Dehydration may increase the client's hematocrit level, but nutritional deficits may cause anemia. Unless the client's anemia is extreme enough to require a transfusion, it is managed on an outpatient basis.

🗝️ CJ: Case study; Step 4: Generate solutions; CL: Analyze

74.

STEP 5

0/1

Possible Action	Indicated	Not Indicated
Position the client on their side		X
Offer fluids with a straw		X
Select a carbonated beverage	X	
Ensure noxious stimuli have been removed	X	
Loosen any tight waistbands	X	
Offer crackers with the fluids		X

Carbonated beverages are often more soothing to the stomach than plain water. The nurse should remove triggers from the environment that cause nausea, including strong smells. Restrictive clothing can place pressure on the stomach that impedes digestion. Clients should be placed as upright as possible to facilitate gastric emptying. Drinking fluids with a straw increases air intake, which can increase distention that leads to vomiting. Crackers can help decrease nausea, but solids should be offered separately from fluids to help ensure fluids are rapidly absorbed.

🗝️ CJ: Case study; Step 5: Take action; CL: Apply

75.

STEP 6

0/1 1, 2, 4, 6. The nausea has improved, enabling the client to retain PO fluids. The electrolytes are within normal limits, suggesting the dehydration is not severe at this point. The client understands the plan of care. If the client had not been able to take PO fluids after treatment or if the electrolytes showed significant imbalances, the client would need hospitalization. Such treatment would include a gastrointestinal tract rest and parenteral fluids to restore hydration, electrolytes, vitamins, and other nutrients until foods could be reintroduced. The client was voiding when admitted to the clinic, so the urine output does not necessarily show improvement. The vital signs and fetal HR were stable and have not changed significantly.

🗝️ CJ: Case study; Step 6: Evaluate outcomes; CL: Evaluate

The Client with a Gestational Trophoblastic Disease

76. 4. The nurse should prepare the client for an ultrasound to determine the cause of the symptoms. Elevated blood pressure at this point in the pregnancy could indicate chronic hypertension as well as hydatidiform mole. The fundal height of 19 cm is higher than is typically found at 15 weeks' gestation and is indicative of a molar pregnancy (hydatidiform mole). The dark brown vaginal bleeding in isolation could indicate an abortion, but when placed in context with the other symptoms, it is likely related to a hydatidiform mole. The continuous nausea and vomiting is abnormal at this point in the pregnancy and can be a result of the high levels of progesterone from a molar pregnancy. There is no fetus involved; the blood pressure elevation and the continuous nausea and vomiting will resolve with evacuation of the mole, negating the need for magnesium sulfate therapy and placing the client on NPO status. Transferring the client to the antenatal unit is premature before a diagnosis has been made.

🗝️ CN: Reduction of risk potential; CL: Analyze

77. 1. Hydatidiform mole is suspected when the following findings are present: gestational hypertension before the 24th week of gestation, brownish or prune-colored vaginal bleeding, anemia, absence of fetal heart tones, passage of hydropic vessels, uterine enlargement greater than expected for gestational age, and increased human chorionic gonadotropin levels. Gestational diabetes is related to an increased risk for preeclampsia and urinary tract infections, but it is not associated with hydatidiform mole. Hyperthyroidism, not hypothyroidism, occurs occasionally with hydatidiform mole. If it does occur, it can be a serious complication that is possibly life-threatening to the client and the fetus as a result of cardiac problems. Polycythemia is not associated with hydatidiform mole. Rather, anemia from blood loss is associated with molar pregnancies.

CN: Reduction of risk potential; CL: Analyze

78. 2. After D&C to evacuate a molar pregnancy, the nurse should assess the client's vital signs and monitor for signs of hemorrhage because the surgical procedure may have traumatized the uterine lining, leading to hemorrhage. Urinary tract infections are not common after the evacuation of a molar pregnancy; they are most commonly related to urinary catheterization. Typically, urinary catheters are not used during the evacuation of a molar pregnancy. The client should not experience abdominal distention because the contents of the uterus have been removed. Chorioamnionitis is an inflammation of the amniotic fluid membranes. With complete mole, no embryonic or fetal tissue or membranes are present.

CN: Reduction of risk potential; CL: Analyze

79. 2. A client who has had a hydatidiform mole removed should have regular checkups to rule out the presence of choriocarcinoma, which may complicate the client's clinical picture. The client's human chorionic gonadotropin (hCG) levels are monitored for 1 year. During this time, the client should be advised not to become pregnant because this would be reflected in rising hCG levels. Ectopic or multifetal pregnancy is not associated with hydatidiform mole. Clients who have molar pregnancies have fertility rates similar to the general population.

CN: Reduction of risk potential; CL: Evaluate

80. 2. A client who has experienced a molar pregnancy is at risk for the development of choriocarcinoma and requires close monitoring of human chorionic gonadotropin (hCG) levels. Pregnancy would interfere with monitoring these levels. High hCG titers are common for up to 7 weeks after the evacuation of the mole, but then these levels gradually begin to decline. Clients should have a pelvic examination and a blood test for hCG titers every month for 6 months and then every 2 months for 1 year. Gradually declining hCG levels suggest no complications. Increasing levels are indicative of a malignancy and should be treated with methotrexate. If after 1 year the hCG levels are negative, the client is theoretically free of the risk for a malignancy developing and could plan another pregnancy.

CN: Reduction of risk potential; CL: Apply

81. 2. Although the client shows signs and symptoms typical of early pregnancy, in gestational trophoblastic disease, or molar pregnancy, gestational tissue exists, but the pregnancy is not viable. The client must have their human chorionic gonadotropin (hCG) levels assessed for the remaining 12 months to ensure the remaining tissue does not turn malignant. Because of the risk of developing a malignancy, the client must avoid pregnancy for at least 1 year following gestational trophoblastic disease. In a complete molar pregnancy, the villi swell and form cysts, and the client is at risk for choriocarcinoma, which is a rapidly spreading malignancy.

CN: Health promotion and maintenance; CL: Evaluation

The Pregnant Client with Miscellaneous Complications

82. 4. Herpes simplex virus can be transmitted to the infant during a vaginal birth. The neonatal effects of herpes are severe enough that a cesarean birth is warranted if active lesions—primary or secondary—are present. A client with a primary infection during pregnancy sheds the virus for up to 3 months after the lesion has healed. The client carrying an infant weighing 8 lb (3629 g) will be given a trial of labor before a cesarean. The client with a fetus in the ROP position will have a slow labor with increased back pain but can give birth vaginally. The fetus in a breech position still has many weeks to change positions before being at term. At 7 months' gestation, the breech position is not a concern.

CN: Physiological adaptation; CL: Evaluate

83. 3, 2, 5, 1, 4. The client's actions indicate distress, and the nurse should initiate emergency procedures. The nurse should first establish unresponsiveness and then ask staff to activate the emergency response system. Next, the nurse should follow the CABs (chest compressions first, then airway and breathing) of cardiopulmonary resuscitation (CPR). The nurse should check the pulse and begin CPR. After 30 compressions, the nurse should assure the open airway and give two breaths.

CN: Management of care; CL: Create

84. 4. Sickle cell disease is an autosomal recessive disorder requiring both parents to have a sickle cell trait to pass the disease to a child. Deoxygenated hemoglobin cells assume a sickle shape and obstruct tissues. Tissue obstruction causes hypoxia to the area (vasoocclusion) and results in pain, called *sickle cell crisis*. This type of anemia is an inherited disorder; it is not caused by a lack of iron in the diet. Iron supplementation is needed only if there is laboratory evidence of iron deficiency anemia. Self-monitoring for any type of infection or sickle cell crisis and increased frequency of antenatal care visits are part of the teaching plan of care.

🗝️ CN: Physiological adaptation; CL: Evaluate

85. 1. The nurse should place a hand on the fetal head and provide gentle upward pressure to relieve the compression on the cord. Doing so allows oxygen to continue flowing to the fetus. The cord should never be placed back into the vagina because doing so may further compress it. Administering oxygen is an appropriate measure but will not serve a useful purpose until the pressure is relieved on the cord, enabling perfusion to the infant. Turning the client to their left side facilitates better perfusion to the birth parent, but until the compression on the cord is relieved, the increased oxygen will not serve its purpose. Placing the client in a Trendelenburg or knee-chest position would be position changes to increase perfusion to the infant by relieving cord compression.

🗝️ CN: Management of care; CL: Analyze

86. -/+ 1, 2, 3, 4. Having the fetus at a negative station places the client at risk for a cord prolapse. With a negative station, there is room between the fetal head and the maternal pelvis for the cord to slip through. A small infant is more mobile within the uterus, and the cord can rest between the fetus and the inside of the uterus or below the fetal head. With a large infant, the head is usually in a vertex presentation and occludes the lower portion of the uterus, preventing the cord from slipping by. When membranes rupture, the cord can be swept through with the amniotic fluid. In a breech presentation, the fetal head is in the fundus, and smaller portions of the fetus settle into the lower portion of the uterus, allowing the cord to lie beside the fetus. Prior abortion and a low-lying placenta have no correlation with cord prolapse.

🗝️ CN: Physiological adaptation; CL: Analyze

87. 3. A postpartum client who saturates a pad in an hour or less at any time in the postpartum period is considered to be hemorrhaging. As the normal postpartum client heals, bleeding changes from red to pink to off-white. It also decreases in amount each day. It is also normal to have some increases in lochia early on with breastfeeding, which causes uterine contractions. Passing blood clots the size of a fist or larger is a reportable problem. Lochia varies in how long it lasts and is considered normal up to 6 weeks postpartum.

🗝️ CN: Health promotion and maintenance; CL: Create

88. 2. Rho(D) immune globulin is given to new birth parents who are Rh negative and not previously sensitized and who have given birth to an Rh-positive infant. Rho(D) immune globulin must be given within 72 hours of the birth of the infant because antibody formation begins at that time. The vaccine is used only when the client has borne an Rh-positive infant—not an Rh-negative infant. Rho(D) immune globulin is not given to a newborn and does not affect antigen formation. Administering Rho(D) immune globulin after birth reduces the risk for hyperbilirubinemia in newborns from future pregnancies, but it will not reduce the risk to the current newborn.

🗝️ CN: Pharmacological and parenteral therapies; CL: Evaluate

89. 2. The client is experiencing and verbalizing signs of postpartum depression, which usually appears at about 4 weeks postpartum but can occur at any time within the first year after birth. It is more severe and lasts longer than postpartum blues, also called "baby blues." Baby blues are the mildest form of depression and are seen in the latter part of the first week after birth. Symptoms usually disappear shortly. Depression may last several years and is disabling to the client. Poor bonding may be seen at any time but commonly becomes evident as the client begins interacting with the infant shortly after birth. Infant abuse may take the form of neglect or injuries to the infant. A depressed birth parent is at risk for injuring or abusing their infant.

🗝️ CN: Reduction of risk potential; CL: Analyze

90. -/+ 1, 2, 3. The UAP could assist the client with breathing and relaxation and ambulate the postcesarean client to the bathroom. UAP can empty catheters. Calculating the hourly IV totals for a preterm labor client would involve assessments that require nursing expertise. In-and-out catheterization, a sterile procedure, and client teaching are responsibilities of the nurse.

🗝️ CN: Management of care; CL: Evaluate

Managing Care, Quality, and Safety for Pregnant Clients

91. **3.** A client with preeclampsia who has +3 proteinuria and epigastric pain is at risk for seizing, which would jeopardize the client and the fetus. Thus, this client would be the highest priority. The client at 13 weeks' gestation with nausea and vomiting is a concern because the presence of ketones indicates that the client's body does not have glucose to break down. However, this situation is a lower priority than a client with preeclampsia or a client who is insulin dependent. The client with insulin-dependent diabetes is a high priority; however, the fetal movement indicates that the fetus is alive but may be ill. As few as four fetal movements in 12 hours can be considered normal. (The client may need additional testing to further evaluate fetal well-being.) The client who is at 17 weeks' gestation may be too early in their pregnancy to experience fetal movement and would be the last person to be seen.

CN: Management of care; CL: Evaluate

92. **3.** The nurse should refer the preeclamptic client with 3+ proteinuria to an HCP. The 3+ urine is significant, indicating there is much protein circulating. The client who is 37 weeks' gestation with insulin-dependent diabetes and who has experienced hypoglycemic episodes in the past week can be managed with food and glucose tablets until they can obtain an appointment with the care provider. The client at 10 weeks' gestation with nausea and vomiting and +1 ketones should also be seen by an HCP, but at this point, although this client is uncomfortable, their life is not in danger. The 15-week client would not be expected to feel their baby move this soon in the pregnancy, and this would not be considered a problem that requires immediate referral to an HCP.

CN: Management of care; CL: Evaluate

93. **3, 2, 1, 4.** The nurse should first change the IV magnesium sulfate and normal saline infusion to the ordered rates and then assess the current status of the client. The nurse should then notify the HCP to explain the error, provide the client assessment data, and report the action taken. A medication error has occurred, and the nurse will need to initiate an incident report.

CN: Management of care; CL: Create

94. **1, 4, 5, 2, 3.** If a client begins to have a seizure, the first action by the nurse is to remain with the client and call for immediate assistance. Next, the nurse should clear the airway if needed, and apply oxygen to help maintain oxygenation to the fetus. When help arrives, the team should turn the client to their side to decrease the risk for aspiration. When the seizure is over, the nurse should assess the client for ruptured membranes and assess the fetal status.

CN: Management of care; CL: Create

95. **4.** The first action taken should be to evaluate the client with placenta previa who has pelvic pressure. The pelvic pressure may be caused by a fetal head creating pressure in the pelvis indicating a potential birth. This client should be evaluated without a pelvic examination and then consult with the health care provider. A vaginal examination is contraindicated as it may stimulate bleeding of the placenta. The second action would be to complete an assessment of the client with preeclampsia and the client's fetus to evaluate the client's tolerance for and the effectiveness of the magnesium sulfate. The hyperemesis client needs to be evaluated for hydration status and for medication. The preterm labor client is stable on the oral medication and should be seen last.

CN: Management of care; CL: Apply

96. **2.** A client presenting at 30 weeks' gestation with nausea and vomiting and epigastric pain has signs and symptoms of preeclampsia and requires the nurse's attention first. Gravida 2, para 1 with spontaneous rupture of membranes, but no contractions, is not a priority. Gravida 5, para 1 at 37 weeks with pink discharge and abdominal cramping could be in early labor and is not a priority at this time. A gravida 1, para 0 at 39 weeks with bruises at various stages of healing could indicate they are in an abusive relationship, but this is not a priority at this time.

CN: Management of care; CL: Analyze

TEST 3

The Birth Experience

- The Primigravid Client in Labor
- The Multigravid Client in Labor
- The Labor Experience
- The Intrapartal Client with Risk Factors
- Managing Care, Quality, and Safety for Clients Giving Birth

The Primigravid Client in Labor

1. The nurse is managing the care of a primigravida at full term who is in active labor. What should be included in the plan of care for this client?
   - ☐ 1. oxygen saturation monitoring every half hour
   - ☐ 2. supine positioning on the back, if it is comfortable
   - ☐ 3. anesthesia and pain level assessment every 30 minutes
   - ☐ 4. vaginal bleeding, rupture of membrane assessment every shift

2. The health care provider (HCP) prescribes intermittent fetal heart rate monitoring for a 20-year-old primigravid client with obesity who is at 40 weeks' gestation and in the first stage of labor. The nurse should monitor the client's fetal heart rate pattern at which interval?
   - ☐ 1. every 15 minutes during the latent phase
   - ☐ 2. every 30 minutes during the active phase
   - ☐ 3. every 60 minutes during the pushing phase
   - ☐ 4. every 2 hours during the transition phase

3. The primigravid client is at +1 station and 9 cm dilated. Based on these data, what should the nurse do **first**?
   - ☐ 1. Ask the anesthesiologist to increase the epidural infusion rate.
   - ☐ 2. Assist the client to push if the client feels the need to do so.
   - ☐ 3. Encourage the client to breathe through the urge to push.
   - ☐ 4. Support family members in providing comfort measures.

4. An assessment of a primigravid client in active labor who has had no analgesia or anesthesia reveals complete cervical effacement, dilation of 8 cm, and the fetus at 0 station. The nurse should expect the client to exhibit which behavior during this phase of labor?
   - ☐ 1. excitement
   - ☐ 2. loss of control
   - ☐ 3. numbness of the legs
   - ☐ 4. feelings of relief

5. The nurse is explaining to a primigravida in labor that their baby is in a breech presentation, with the baby's presenting part in a left, sacrum, posterior (LSP) position. Which illustration should the nurse use to help the client understand how the baby is positioned?
   - ☐ 1.
   - ☐ 2.
   - ☐ 3.
   - ☐ 4.

6. The nurse is discussing pain relief methods for a pregnant first-time parent. The discussion should include which labor support method(s)? Select all that apply.
   ☐ 1. effleurage
   ☐ 2. positive reinforcement
   ☐ 3. guided imagery
   ☐ 4. pattern-paced breathing
   ☐ 5. progressive relaxation

7. A primigravid client is admitted as an outpatient for an external cephalic version. Which factor would be a contraindication for the procedure?
   ☐ 1. multiple gestation
   ☐ 2. breech presentation
   ☐ 3. maternal Rh-negative blood type
   ☐ 4. history of gestational diabetes

8. A primigravida is admitted to the labor area with ruptured membranes and contractions occurring every 2 to 3 minutes, lasting 45 seconds. After 3 hours of labor, the client's contractions are now every 7 to 10 minutes, lasting 30 seconds. The nurse administers oxytocin as prescribed. What is the expected outcome of this drug?
   ☐ 1. The cervix will begin to dilate 2 cm per hour.
   ☐ 2. Contractions will occur every 2 to 3 minutes, lasting 40 to 60 seconds, with moderate intensity resting tone between contractions.
   ☐ 3. The cervix will change from firm to soft, efface to 40% to 50%, and move from a posterior to anterior position.
   ☐ 4. Contractions will be every 2 minutes, lasting 60 to 90 seconds, with intrauterine pressure of 70 mm Hg.

9. A primigravid client in the second stage of labor feels the urge to push. The client has had no analgesia or anesthesia. Anatomically, what would be the **best** position for the client to assume?
   ☐ 1. dorsal recumbent
   ☐ 2. lithotomy
   ☐ 3. hands and knees
   ☐ 4. squatting

10. A 21-year-old primigravid client at 40 weeks' gestation is admitted to the hospital in active labor. The client's cervix is 8 cm and completely effaced at 0 station. During the transition phase of labor, which is a **priority** nursing problem?
    ☐ 1. urinary retention
    ☐ 2. hyperventilation
    ☐ 3. ineffective coping
    ☐ 4. pain

11. A 24-year-old primigravid client who gives birth to a viable term neonate is prescribed oxytocin intravenously after delivery of the placenta. Which sign would indicate to the nurse that the placenta is about to be delivered?
    ☐ 1. The cord lengthens outside the vagina.
    ☐ 2. There is decreased vaginal bleeding.
    ☐ 3. The uterus cannot be palpated.
    ☐ 4. The uterus changes to a discoid shape.

12. A primiparous client, who has just given birth to a healthy term neonate after 12 hours of labor, holds and looks at their neonate and begins to cry. The nurse interprets this behavior as a sign of which response?
    ☐ 1. disappointment in the baby's gender
    ☐ 2. grief over the ending of the pregnancy
    ☐ 3. a normal response to the birth
    ☐ 4. indication of postpartum "blues"

13. The cervix of a 15-year-old primigravid client who has been admitted to the labor area is 2 cm dilated and 50% effaced. Membranes are intact, and contractions are occurring every 5 to 6 minutes. Which intervention should the nurse recommend at this time?
    ☐ 1. resting in the right lateral recumbent position
    ☐ 2. lying in the left lateral recumbent position
    ☐ 3. walking around in the hallway
    ☐ 4. sitting in a comfortable chair for a period of time

14. Which technique to promote active relaxation would the nurse include in the teaching plan for a 16-year-old primigravid client in early labor?
    ☐ 1. relaxing uninvolved body muscles during uterine contractions
    ☐ 2. practicing being in a deep, meditative, sleeplike state
    ☐ 3. focusing on an object in the room during the contractions
    ☐ 4. breathing rapidly and deeply between contractions

15. The nurse is performing effleurage for a primigravid client in early labor. Which technique should the nurse use?
    ☐ 1. deep kneading of superficial muscles
    ☐ 2. secure grasping of muscular tissues
    ☐ 3. light stroking of the skin surface
    ☐ 4. prolonged pressure on specific sites

16. A 24-year-old primigravid client in active labor asks to use the jet hydrotherapy tub to aid in pain relief. Which condition would the nurse consider to be a contraindication for hydrotherapy?
    ☐ 1. ruptured membranes
    ☐ 2. multifetal gestation
    ☐ 3. diabetes mellitus
    ☐ 4. hypotonic labor patterns

17. The health care provider (HCP) prescribes an amniocentesis for a primigravid client at 37 weeks' gestation to determine fetal lung maturity. Which is an indicator of fetal lung maturity?
    ☐ 1. amount of bilirubin present
    ☐ 2. presence of red blood cells
    ☐ 3. Barr body determination
    ☐ 4. lecithin-sphingomyelin (L/S ratio)

18. A 19-year-old primigravid client at 38 weeks' gestation is 7 cm dilated, and the presenting part is at +1 station. The client tells the nurse, "I need to push!" What should the nurse do **next**?
    ☐ 1. Use the McDonald procedure to widen the pelvic opening.
    ☐ 2. Increase the rate of oxygen and intravenous fluids.
    ☐ 3. Instruct the client to use a pant-blow pattern of breathing.
    ☐ 4. Tell the client to push only when absolutely necessary.

19. To determine whether a primigravid client in labor with a fetus in the left occiput anterior (LOA) position is completely dilated, the nurse performs a vaginal examination. During the examination, the nurse should palpate which cranial sutures?
    ☐ 1. sagittal
    ☐ 2. lambdoidal
    ☐ 3. coronal
    ☐ 4. frontal

20. After a long labor process, a primigravid client gives birth to a healthy newborn with a moderate amount of skull molding. What information would the nurse include when explaining to the client about this condition?
    ☐ 1. It is typically seen with breech births.
    ☐ 2. It usually lasts a day or two before resolving.
    ☐ 3. It is typical when the brow is the presenting part.
    ☐ 4. Surgical intervention may be necessary to alleviate pressure.

21. The health care provider (HCP) has informed the labor nurse that they believe the uterus has inverted in a primiparous client who has just given birth. Which finding(s) would help confirm this diagnosis? Select all that apply.
    ☐ 1. hypotension
    ☐ 2. gush of blood from the vagina
    ☐ 3. intense, severe, tearing type of abdominal pain
    ☐ 4. uterus is hard and in a constant state of contraction
    ☐ 5. inability to palpate the uterus
    ☐ 6. diaphoresis

22. The nurse explains to a newly admitted primigravid client in active labor that, according to the gate-control theory of pain, a closed gate means that the client should experience what type of pain?
    ☐ 1. no pain
    ☐ 2. sharp pain
    ☐ 3. light pain
    ☐ 4. moderate pain

23. The cervix of a primigravid client in active labor who received epidural anesthesia 4 hours ago is now completely dilated, and the client is ready to begin pushing. What is **most** important for the nurse to assess before the client begins to push?
    ☐ 1. fetal heart rate variability
    ☐ 2. cervical dilation again
    ☐ 3. status of membranes
    ☐ 4. bladder status

24. For the past 8 hours, a 20-year-old primigravid client in active labor with intact membranes has been experiencing regular contractions. The fetal heart rate is 136 bpm with moderate variability. After determining that the client is still in the latent phase of labor, the nurse should observe the client for which problem?
    ☐ 1. exhaustion
    ☐ 2. chills and fever
    ☐ 3. fluid overload
    ☐ 4. meconium-stained fluid

25. A primigravid client whose cervix is 7 cm dilated with the fetus at 0 station and in a left occiput posterior (LOP) position has severe back pain. What intervention is **most** indicated?
    ☐ 1. Provide firm pressure to the client's sacral area.
    ☐ 2. Prepare the client for a cesarean birth.
    ☐ 3. Prepare the client for a precipitate birth.
    ☐ 4. Maintain the client in a left side-lying position.

26. A primigravid client in active labor, who has had no anesthesia, has managed contractions using slow chest breathing. The client's cervix is 7 cm dilated, and the client is starting to feel considerable discomfort during contractions. Which breathing technique should the nurse instruct the client to try next?
    ☐ 1. rapid, shallow chest breathing
    ☐ 2. deep chest breathing
    ☐ 3. rapid pant-blow breathing
    ☐ 4. slow abdominal breathing

27. Assessment of a primigravid client reveals cervical dilation at 8 cm and complete effacement. The client has severe back pain during this phase of labor. The nurse explains that the client's severe back pain is **most** likely caused by the fetal occiput being in which position?
    ☐ 1. breech
    ☐ 2. transverse
    ☐ 3. posterior
    ☐ 4. anterior

28. The nurse assesses a primiparous client with ruptured membranes who has been in labor for 20 hours. The nurse identifies late decelerations on the monitor and initiates standard procedures for the client with this wave pattern. Which intervention(s) should the nurse perform? Select all that apply.
    ☐ 1. administering oxygen via mask to the client
    ☐ 2. questioning the client about the effectiveness of pain relief
    ☐ 3. placing the client on their side
    ☐ 4. readjusting the monitor to a more comfortable position
    ☐ 5. applying an internal fetal monitor

29. When performing Leopold's maneuvers on a primigravid client, the nurse is palpating the uterus as shown below. Which maneuver is the nurse performing?

    ☐ 1. first maneuver
    ☐ 2. second maneuver
    ☐ 3. third maneuver
    ☐ 4. fourth maneuver

30. Before placing the fetal monitoring device on a primigravid client's fundus, the nurse performs Leopold's maneuvers. The nurse explains that the third maneuver is done for which reason?
    ☐ 1. to determine whether the fetal presenting part is engaged
    ☐ 2. to locate the fetal cephalic prominence
    ☐ 3. to distinguish between a breech and a cephalic presentation
    ☐ 4. to locate the position of the fetal arms and legs

The Multigravid Client in Labor

31. The nurse is caring for a client who is G2, T1, P0, A0, and L1 at term. The client is completely effaced and dilated to 2 cm and has contractions every 3 minutes that last for 45 seconds. The client is asking for an epidural to make them more comfortable. What is the **most** appropriate response by the nurse?
    ☐ 1. "We cannot give epidurals until you are 5 to 6 cm dilated. There is intravenous (IV) medication available if you would like it now."
    ☐ 2. "You cannot have an epidural until your membranes have ruptured."
    ☐ 3. "Your contraction pattern is slow at this point and will need to accelerate before you can have your epidural."
    ☐ 4. "It is too early in labor for the epidural, but you can have IV medication to keep you comfortable until you have dilated 1 to 2 cm more."

32. The nurse has just received a report on a G3, T1, P0, Ab1, L1 labor client, which states that they are 80% effaced, 3-cm dilated, and at 0 station. The nurse anticipates the plan of care for the shift will address what factor(s)? Select all that apply.
    ☐ 1. Birth should occur before the change of shift in 12 hours.
    ☐ 2. Stage 2 should take 30 minutes or less.
    ☐ 3. Contractions will remain irregular until transition.
    ☐ 4. Transition will be shorter for this multiparous client.
    ☐ 5. This client will withdraw into herself during transition.

33. A multigravida in active labor is 7 cm dilated. The fetal heart rate baseline is 130 bpm with moderate variability. The client begins to have variable decelerations from 100 to 110 bpm. What should the nurse do **next**?
    ☐ 1. Perform a vaginal examination.
    ☐ 2. Notify the health care provider (HCP) of the decelerations.
    ☐ 3. Reposition the client and continue to evaluate the fetal heart rate.
    ☐ 4. Administer oxygen via mask at 2 L per minute.

34. A nurse is preparing a change-of-shift report and has been caring for a multigravid client with a normally progressing labor. Which information should be part of this report? Select all that apply.
    ☐ 1. interpretation of the fetal monitor strip
    ☐ 2. analgesia or anesthesia being used
    ☐ 3. previous methods of birth control
    ☐ 4. support persons with the client
    ☐ 5. prior birth history

35. A multigravid client is admitted at 4-cm dilation and is requesting pain medication. The nurse gives the client an opioid agonist-antagonist. Within 5 minutes, the client tells the nurse they feel the need to have a bowel movement. What should the nurse do **first**?
☐ 1. Have naloxone available in the birthing room.
☐ 2. Complete a vaginal examination.
☐ 3. Prepare for birth.
☐ 4. Document the client's relief due to pain medication.

36. A 31-year-old multigravid client at 39 weeks' gestation admitted to the hospital in active labor is receiving intravenous lactated Ringer's solution and a continuous epidural anesthetic. During the first hour after administration of the anesthetic, the nurse should monitor the client for which adverse reaction?
☐ 1. hypotension
☐ 2. diaphoresis
☐ 3. headache
☐ 4. tremors

37. A 30-year-old G3, T2, P0, A0, L2 client is being monitored internally. The client is being induced with intravenous (IV) oxytocin because they are postterm. The nurse notes the pattern below. The client is wedged to their side while lying in bed and is approximately 6 cm dilated and 100% effaced. What should the nurse do **first**?

☐ 1. Continue to observe the fetal monitor.
☐ 2. Anticipate rupture of the membranes.
☐ 3. Prepare for fetal oximetry.
☐ 4. Discontinue the oxytocin infusion.

38. The nurse assists with a precipitous birth in an outpatient setting. While waiting for more advanced care, the nurse places the infant skin to skin with the parent and encourages breastfeeding. What would be the desired outcome(s) of skin-to-skin care with early breastfeeding? Select all that apply.
☐ 1. beginning the parental-infant bonding process
☐ 2. preventing neonatal hypothermia
☐ 3. providing glucose to the neonate
☐ 4. contracting the client's uterus
☐ 5. preventing maternal infection

39. Approximately 15 minutes after the birth of a viable term neonate, a multiparous client has chills. What should the nurse do **next**?
☐ 1. Assess the client's pulse rate.
☐ 2. Decrease the rate of intravenous (IV) fluids.
☐ 3. Provide the client with a warm blanket.
☐ 4. Assess the amount of blood loss.

40. The health care provider (HCP) plans to perform an amniotomy on a multiparous client admitted to the labor area at 41 weeks' gestation for labor induction. After the amniotomy, what should the nurse do **first**?
☐ 1. Monitor the client's contraction pattern.
☐ 2. Assess the fetal heart rate (FHR) for 1 full minute.
☐ 3. Assess the client's temperature and pulse.
☐ 4. Document the color of the amniotic fluid.

41. A multigravid client who is 10 cm dilated is admitted to the labor and birth unit. In addition to supporting the client, what is the **priority** nursing action?
☐ 1. preparing the room for birth
☐ 2. increasing intravenous (IV) fluids
☐ 3. determining the client's preferences for pain control
☐ 4. providing client education regarding care of the newborn

42. The nurse is assessing fetal presentation in a multiparous client. The illustration below indicates which type of presentation?

☐ 1. frank breech
☐ 2. complete breech
☐ 3. footling breech
☐ 4. vertex

43. Two hours ago, a multigravid client was admitted in active labor with their cervix dilated at 5 cm and completely effaced and the fetus at 0 station. Currently, the client is experiencing nausea and vomiting, a slight chill with perspiration beads on their lip, and extreme irritability. What should the nurse do **first**?
    ☐ 1. Warm the temperature of the room by a few degrees.
    ☐ 2. Increase the rate of intravenous fluid administration.
    ☐ 3. Obtain a prescription for an intramuscular antiemetic medication.
    ☐ 4. Assess the client's cervical dilation and station.

44. What interval should the nurse use when assessing the frequency of contractions of a multiparous client in active labor admitted to the birthing area?
    ☐ 1. acme of one contraction to the beginning of the next contraction
    ☐ 2. beginning of one contraction to the end of the next contraction
    ☐ 3. end of one contraction to the end of the next contraction
    ☐ 4. beginning of one contraction to the beginning of the next contraction

45. While a client is being admitted to the birthing unit they state, "My water broke last night, but my labor started 2 hours ago." Which finding(s) would be a concern? Select all that apply.
    ☐ 1. maternal vital signs: temperature 99.5°F (37.5°C); heart rate 80 bpm; respiration rate 24 breaths/min; blood pressure 130/80 mm Hg
    ☐ 2. blood and mucus on the perineal pad
    ☐ 3. baseline fetal heart rate of 140 bpm with a range between 110 and 160 bpm with contractions
    ☐ 4. peripad stained with green fluid
    ☐ 5. client stating, "This baby wants out—he keeps kicking me"

46. While the nurse is caring for a multiparous client in active labor at 36 weeks' gestation, the client tells the nurse, "I think my water just broke." What should the nurse do **first**?
    ☐ 1. Take the client's vital signs.
    ☐ 2. Assess the color, amount, and odor of the fluid.
    ☐ 3. Assess the fetal heart rate pattern.
    ☐ 4. Check the client's cervical dilation.

47. The nurse has obtained a urine specimen from a multiparous client admitted to the labor unit. The client asks to go to the bathroom and reports that they feel the need to move their bowels. Which action(s) would be appropriate? Select all that apply.
    ☐ 1. assisting the client to the bathroom
    ☐ 2. applying an external fetal monitor to obtain the fetal heart rate
    ☐ 3. assessing the client's stage of labor
    ☐ 4. asking if the client had back labor pains like this with any of their other birth experiences
    ☐ 5. allowing the client a support person to take them to the bathroom to maintain privacy
    ☐ 6. checking the degree of fetal descent

48. A multigravid client admitted to the labor area is scheduled for a cesarean birth under spinal anesthesia. Which client statement indicates that teaching about spinal anesthesia has been understood?
    ☐ 1. "The medication will be administered while I am in the prone position."
    ☐ 2. "The anesthetic may cause a severe headache, which is treatable."
    ☐ 3. "My blood pressure may increase if I lie down too soon after the injection."
    ☐ 4. "I can expect immediate anesthesia that can be reversed very easily."

49. The nurse is conducting preoperative teaching for a client with gestational diabetes scheduled for a repeat cesarean birth. The client tells the nurse that they have been taking ginkgo biloba to help manage their blood sugar. The nurse notifies the health care provider because this herbal supplement puts the client at risk for which complication?
    ☐ 1. medication interactions
    ☐ 2. hypertensive crisis
    ☐ 3. oversedation
    ☐ 4. prolonged bleeding

The Labor Experience

50. The nurse is performing a vaginal examination on a client in labor. The nurse finds the fetal presenting part 1 cm above the ischial spines. How should the nurse document the fetal station?
    ☐ 1. −1 station
    ☐ 2. +1 station
    ☐ 3. engaged
    ☐ 4. floating

51. The nurse is managing a pregnant client's second stage of labor. The nurse should intervene when observing which action?
    ☐ 1. closed glottis pushing
    ☐ 2. open glottis pushing
    ☐ 3. "rest and descent"
    ☐ 4. squatting while pushing

52. A client in the second stage of labor who planned an unmedicated birth is in severe pain because the fetus is in the right occiput posterior (ROP) position. The nurse should place the client in which position for pain relief?
☐ 1. lithotomy
☐ 2. right lateral position
☐ 3. hands and knees
☐ 4. squatting

53. A client who gave birth to their last infant by cesarean birth is admitted to the hospital at term with contractions every 5 minutes. The health care provider (HCP) intends to have the client undergo "a trial labor." What does the nurse explain to the client that trial of labor means?
☐ 1. Labor will be stimulated with exogenous oxytocin until birth.
☐ 2. The HCP needs more information to determine the presence of true labor.
☐ 3. Labor progress will be evaluated continually to determine appropriate progress for a vaginal birth.
☐ 4. Labor will be arrested with tocolytic agents after 2 hours even if no fetal distress is noted.

54. The nurse prepares a client for lumbar epidural anesthesia. Before anesthesia administration, the nurse instructs the client to assume which position?
☐ 1. lithotomy
☐ 2. side-lying
☐ 3. hands and knees
☐ 4. prone

55. A client in labor received an epidural for pain management. Before receiving the epidural, the client's blood pressure was 124/76 mm Hg. Ten minutes after receiving the epidural, the client's blood pressure is 98/56 mm Hg, and the client is vomiting. Before calling the health care provider (HCP), the nurse should perform which action?
☐ 1. Decrease the intravenous (IV) fluid rate.
☐ 2. Turn the client to their side.
☐ 3. Catheterize the client.
☐ 4. Perform a vaginal examination.

56. A nurse is caring for a gravida 1, para 0 client at 40 weeks' gestation who is in active labor. The client's cervix is 5 cm dilated and 90% effaced; the fetal station is 0, and the fetus is in cephalic presentation. The baseline fetal heart rate is 135 bpm; it decreases to 125 bpm shortly after the onset of five uterine contractions and returns to baseline before the uterine contraction ends. Based on this assessment, what action should the nurse take **first**?
☐ 1. Position the client on their left side and administer oxygen via a face mask.
☐ 2. Document findings on the client's chart, and continue to monitor labor progress.
☐ 3. Perform a vaginal examination to rule out umbilical cord prolapse.
☐ 4. Notify the health care provider (HCP) immediately, and prepare for an emergency cesarean birth.

57. The nurse is caring for a full-term, nonmedicated, primiparous client who is in the transition stage of labor. The client is writhing in pain and saying, "Help me, help me!" The client's last vaginal examination was 1 hour ago and showed that they were 8 cm dilated, +1 station, and in what appeared to be a comfortable position. What does the nurse anticipate as the **highest priority** intervention in caring for this client?
☐ 1. Help the client through contractions until a narcotic can be given.
☐ 2. Palpate the bladder to see if it has become distended.
☐ 3. Ask the client for suggestions to make them more comfortable.
☐ 4. Perform a vaginal examination to determine if the client is fully dilated.

58. A client at 33 weeks' gestation is admitted in preterm labor. The client is given betamethasone 12 mg intramuscularly now. Repeat in 24 hours. What is the expected outcome of this drug therapy?
☐ 1. The contractions will end within 24 hours.
☐ 2. The client will give birth to a neonate without infection.
☐ 3. The client will give birth to a full-term neonate.
☐ 4. The neonate will be born with mature lungs.

59. A full-term client is admitted for an induction of labor. The health care provider (HCP) has assigned a Bishop score of 10. Which drug would the nurse anticipate administering to this client?
☐ 1. oxytocin 30 units in 500 mL dextrose 5% in water (D_5W)
☐ 2. prostaglandin gel 0.5 mg
☐ 3. misoprostol 50 mcg
☐ 4. dinoprostone 10 mg

60. The health care provider (HCP) has performed an amniotomy on a laboring client. Which detail(s) must be included in the documentation of this procedure? Select all that apply.
☐ 1. time of the rupture
☐ 2. color and clarity of the fluid
☐ 3. fetal heart rate (FHR) and the pattern before and after the procedure
☐ 4. size of amnio hook used during the procedure
☐ 5. odor and amount of fluid

61. Following an epidural and placement of internal monitors, a client's labor is augmented with oxytocin. Contractions are lasting longer than 90 seconds and occurring every 1½ minutes. The uterine resting tone is greater than 20 mm Hg with an abnormal fetal heart rate and pattern. Which action should the nurse take **first**?
☐ 1. Notify the health care provider (HCP).
☐ 2. Turn off the oxytocin infusion.
☐ 3. Turn the client to their left side.
☐ 4. Increase the maintenance intravenous (IV) fluids.

62. A nurse notices repetitive late decelerations on the fetal heart monitor. What are the **best** initial actions by the nurse?
- ☐ 1. Prepare for birth, reposition the client, and tell the client to begin pushing.
- ☐ 2. Perform a sterile vaginal examination, increase intravenous (IV) fluids, and apply oxygen.
- ☐ 3. Notify the provider, explain the findings to the client, and tell the client to begin pushing.
- ☐ 4. Reposition the client, apply oxygen, and increase IV fluids.

63. What action(s) does the nurse anticipate completing at the end of the second stage of labor before the delivery of the placenta in a spontaneous vaginal birth of a term newborn? Select all that apply.
- ☐ 1. assigning the Apgar scores
- ☐ 2. administering oxytocin
- ☐ 3. assisting with perineal repairs
- ☐ 4. drying the newborn
- ☐ 5. initiating skin-to-skin care
- ☐ 6. taking newborn vital signs

64. As a nurse begins the shift on the obstetrical unit, there are several new admissions. The client with which condition would be a candidate for induction?
- ☐ 1. preeclampsia
- ☐ 2. active herpes
- ☐ 3. face presentation
- ☐ 4. fetus with late decelerations

65. A laboring client smiles pleasantly at the nurse when asked simple questions. The client speaks only Mandarin, and the interpreter is busy with an emergency situation. At the client's last vaginal examination, the client was 5 cm dilated, 100% effaced, and at 0 station. While working with this client, the nurse understands that which response indicates the client may be approaching birth?
- ☐ 1. The fetal monitor strip shows late decelerations.
- ☐ 2. The client begins to speak to family in their native language.
- ☐ 3. The fetal monitor strip shows early decelerations.
- ☐ 4. The client's facial expressions become animated.

66.

The nurse cares for a client in labor who received an epidural anesthetic.

Flow Sheet

Vital Signs

	1030	1100	1115
Temperature 98.6°F (37.0°C)		P 88 bpm	P 80 bpm
Pulse (P) 90 bpm		RR 18 breaths/min	RR 18 breaths/min
Respiration rate (RR) 18 breaths/min		BP 124/76 mm Hg	BP 98/56 mm Hg
Blood pressure (BP) 130/80 mm Hg		Pulse oximeter 98%	Pulse oximeter 96%
Pulse oximeter 98%			

Nurse's Notes

1030: The primigravid client is having contractions lasting 60 seconds every 3 minutes. A cervical examination shows the client is 5 cm dilated, at 0 station, and 75% effaced. Category I tracing shows the fetal heart rate (FHR) is 140 bpm. The client is requesting an epidural. A 1000-mL fluid bolus was started.

1130: The fluid bolus is complete. An epidural was placed by the anesthesiology team. Category I tracing shows the FHR is 145 bpm.

1115: The client is vomiting.

The nurse reviews the client trends.

➤ Complete the following sentences by using the list of options.

The nurse determines that the client is most likely experiencing [anaphylaxis / hypotension / spinal headache].

The first action the nurse should take is to [activate the emergency response team; turn the client on their side; dim the room lights].

The Intrapartal Client with Risk Factors

67. A client is admitted with a suspected abruptio placentae. The nurse should assess the client for which sign(s) or symptom(s)? Select all that apply.
- ☐ 1. bleeding that is concealed or apparent
- ☐ 2. abdominal rigidity
- ☐ 3. painful abdomen
- ☐ 4. painless bleeding
- ☐ 5. large placenta
- ☐ 6. bleeding that stops spontaneously

68. A 39-year-old multigravid client at 39 weeks' gestation admitted to the hospital in active labor has been diagnosed with class II heart disease. Which measure will the nurse encourage to ensure cardiac emptying and adequate oxygenation during labor?
- ☐ 1. Breathe slowly after each contraction.
- ☐ 2. Avoid the use of analgesics for labor pain.
- ☐ 3. Remain in a side-lying position with the head elevated.
- ☐ 4. Request local anesthesia for vaginal birth.

69. When developing the plan of care for a multigravid client with class III heart disease, the nurse should expect to assess the client frequently for which problem?
- ☐ 1. dehydration
- ☐ 2. nausea and vomiting
- ☐ 3. iron deficiency anemia
- ☐ 4. tachycardia

70. A primigravid client at 39 weeks' gestation is admitted to the hospital for induction of labor. The health care provider (HCP) has prescribed prostaglandin E2 gel for the client. Before administering prostaglandin E2 gel to the client, the nurse should perform which action **first**?
- ☐ 1. Assess the frequency of uterine contractions.
- ☐ 2. Place the client in a side-lying position.
- ☐ 3. Determine whether the membranes have ruptured.
- ☐ 4. Prepare the client for an amniotomy.

71. A primigravida near birth is experiencing a prolonged second stage of labor with a fetus suspected of weighing over 4000 g (4 kg). Which intervention is **most** important?
- ☐ 1. preparing for a vacuum-assisted birth
- ☐ 2. administering an intravenous (IV) fluid bolus
- ☐ 3. preparing for an emergency cesarean birth
- ☐ 4. performing the McRoberts maneuver

72. A multigravid client is receiving oxytocin augmentation. When the client's cervix is dilated to 6 cm, the client's membranes rupture spontaneously with meconium-stained amniotic fluid. Which action should the nurse perform **first**?
- ☐ 1. Increase the rate of the oxytocin infusion.
- ☐ 2. Turn the client to a knee-to-chest position.
- ☐ 3. Assess cervical dilation and effacement.
- ☐ 4. Assess the fetal heart rate.

73. A primigravid client who has had a prolonged labor but now is completely dilated has received epidural anesthesia. Which statement should the nurse include in the teaching plan about pushing?
- ☐ 1. The client needs to push for at least 1 to 3 minutes.
- ☐ 2. Pushing is most effective when the client holds their breath.
- ☐ 3. The client should be urged to push with an open glottis.
- ☐ 4. Pushing is limited to times when they feel the urge.

74. The health care provider (HCP) determines that outlet forceps are needed to assist in the birth of a primigravid client in active labor with a large-for-gestational-size fetus. The nurse understands that the fetus's skull must be at what point before this procedure can take place?
- ☐ 1. engaged past the inlet
- ☐ 2. at +1 station
- ☐ 3. visible at the perineal floor
- ☐ 4. reached the level of the ischial spines

75. The health care provider (HCP) prescribes an amnioinfusion for a primigravid client at term who is diagnosed with oligohydramnios. What does the nurse explain is the primary purpose of the procedure to the client?
- ☐ 1. decreases the frequency and severity of variable decelerations
- ☐ 2. minimizes the possibility of fetal metabolic alkalosis
- ☐ 3. increases the fetal heart rate accelerations during a contraction
- ☐ 4. raises the amniotic fluid index to more than 15 cm

76. The nurse is admitting a primigravid client at 37 weeks' gestation who has been diagnosed with preeclampsia to the labor and birth area. Which client care room is **most** appropriate for this client?
- ☐ 1. a brightly lit private room at the end of the hall from the nurses' station
- ☐ 2. a semiprivate room midway down the hall from the nurses' station
- ☐ 3. a private room with many windows that is near the operating room
- ☐ 4. a darkened private room as close to the nurses' station as possible

77. A multigravid client is admitted to the labor area from the emergency department. At the time of admission, the fetal head is crowning, and the client yells, "The baby is coming!" To help the client remain calm and cooperative during the imminent birth, which response by the nurse is **most** appropriate?
☐ 1. "You're right; the baby is coming, so just relax."
☐ 2. "Please do not push because you will tear your cervix."
☐ 3. "Your health care provider will be here as soon as possible."
☐ 4. "I'll explain what is happening to guide you as we go along."

78. The nurse is caring for a multigravid client and observes the client squatting on the bed and the fetal head crowning. After calling for assistance and helping the client lie down, the nurse should perform which action **next**?
☐ 1. Tell the client to push between contractions.
☐ 2. Provide gentle support to the fetal head.
☐ 3. Apply gentle upward traction on the neonate's anterior shoulder.
☐ 4. Massage the perineum to stretch the perineal tissues.

79. During the first hour after a precipitous birth, the nurse should monitor a multiparous client for signs and symptoms of which complication?
☐ 1. postpartum "blues"
☐ 2. uterine atony
☐ 3. intrauterine infection
☐ 4. urinary tract infection

80. A multigravid client in labor at 38 weeks' gestation has been diagnosed with Rh sensitization and probable fetal hydrops and anemia. Which fetal heart rate pattern would the nurse find is **most** concerning?
☐ 1. early deceleration pattern
☐ 2. sinusoidal pattern
☐ 3. variable deceleration pattern
☐ 4. late deceleration pattern

81. The nurse in the labor and birth area receives a telephone call from the emergency department announcing that a multigravid client in active labor is being transferred to the labor area. The client has had no prenatal care. When the client arrives by stretcher, they say, "I think the baby is coming … Help!" The fetal skull is crowning. The nurse should obtain which information **first**?
☐ 1. estimated date of birth
☐ 2. amniotic fluid status
☐ 3. gravida and parity
☐ 4. prenatal history

82. A primigravid client at 41 weeks' gestation is admitted to the hospital's labor and birth unit in active labor. After 25 hours of labor with membranes ruptured for 24 hours, the client gives birth to a healthy neonate vaginally with a midline episiotomy. Which problem should the nurse identify as the **priority** for the client?
☐ 1. activity intolerance
☐ 2. sleep deprivation
☐ 3. situational low self-esteem
☐ 4. risk for infection

83. The nurse is caring for a primiparous client and their neonate immediately after birth. The neonate was born at 41 weeks' gestation and weighs 4082 g (4.1 kg). Assessing for signs and symptoms of which condition should be a **priority** in this neonate?
☐ 1. anemia
☐ 2. hypoglycemia
☐ 3. delayed meconium
☐ 4. elevated bilirubin

84. A multigravid client in active labor at term is diagnosed with polyhydramnios. The health care provider (HCP) has instructed the client about possible neonatal complications related to polyhydramnios. The nurse determines that the client has understood the instructions when the client states that polyhydramnios is associated with which problem in the fetus or neonate?
☐ 1. renal dysfunction
☐ 2. intrauterine growth restriction
☐ 3. pulmonary hypoplasia
☐ 4. gastrointestinal disorders

85. The health care provider (HCP) who elects to perform a cesarean birth on a primigravid client for fetal distress has informed the client of possible risks during the procedure. When the nurse asks the client to sign the consent form, the client's spouse says, "I will sign it for them. The client is too upset by what is happening to make this decision." What should the nurse do?
☐ 1. Ask the client if this is acceptable to them.
☐ 2. Have the client and their spouse both sign the consent form.
☐ 3. Ask the client to sign the consent form.
☐ 4. Ask the HCP to witness the consent form.

86. A multigravid client at term is admitted to the hospital for a trial labor and possible vaginal birth. The client has a history of previous cesarean birth because of fetal distress. When the client is 4 cm dilated, they receive nalbuphine intravenously. While monitoring the fetal heart rate, the nurse observes minimal variability and a rate of 120 bpm. The nurse should explain to the client that the decreased variability is **most** likely caused by which factor?
☐ 1. maternal fatigue
☐ 2. fetal malposition
☐ 3. small-for-gestational-age fetus
☐ 4. effects of analgesic medication

87. During a scheduled cesarean birth of a primigravid client with a fetus at 39 weeks' gestation in a breech presentation, a neonatologist is present in the operating room. The nurse explains to the client that the neonatologist is present because neonates born by cesarean birth tend to have an increased incidence of which problem?
☐ 1. congenital anomalies
☐ 2. pulmonary hypertension
☐ 3. meconium aspiration syndrome
☐ 4. respiratory distress syndrome

88. A 28-year-old multigravid client at 28 weeks' gestation diagnosed with acute pyelonephritis is receiving intravenous fluids and antibiotics. After teaching the client about the rationale for the aggressive therapy, the nurse determines that the client needs further instruction when they say that acute pyelonephritis can lead to which complication?
☐ 1. preterm labor
☐ 2. maternal sepsis
☐ 3. intrauterine growth restriction
☐ 4. congenital fetal anomalies

89. A primigravid client at 38 weeks' gestation is admitted to the labor suite in active labor. The client's physical assessment reveals a chlamydial infection. The nurse explains that if the infection is left untreated, the neonate may develop which problem?
☐ 1. conjunctivitis
☐ 2. heart disease
☐ 3. harlequin sign
☐ 4. brain damage

90. A 34-year-old primigravid client at 39 weeks' gestation admitted to the hospital in active labor has type B Rh-negative blood. The nurse should instruct the client that if the neonate is Rh positive, the client will receive an Rh immune globulin injection for which reason?
☐ 1. to prevent Rh-positive sensitization with the next pregnancy
☐ 2. to provide active antibody protection for this pregnancy
☐ 3. to decrease the amount of Rh-negative sensitization for the next pregnancy
☐ 4. to destroy fetal Rh-positive cells during the next pregnancy

91. A 16-year-old primigravid client admitted at 38 weeks' gestation with severe preeclampsia is given intravenous magnesium sulfate and lactated Ringer's solution. The nurse should obtain which information?
☐ 1. urinary output every 8 hours
☐ 2. deep tendon reflexes every 12 hours
☐ 3. respiratory rate every hour
☐ 4. blood pressure every 6 hours

92. The nurse has received a telephone call from the emergency department indicating that a multigravid client in early labor and diagnosed with probable placenta previa will be arriving soon. What is the **priority** invention when the client arrives at the unit?
☐ 1. whole blood replacement
☐ 2. continuous blood pressure monitoring
☐ 3. internal fetal heart rate monitoring
☐ 4. an immediate cesarean birth

93. During admission, a multigravida in early active labor acts somewhat euphoric and tells the nurse that they smoked some crack cocaine before coming to the hospital. In addition to fetal heart rate assessment, the nurse should monitor the client for symptoms of which complication?
☐ 1. placenta previa
☐ 2. ruptured uterus
☐ 3. maternal hypotension
☐ 4. abruptio placentae

94. A primigravid client in early labor with abruptio placentae develops disseminated intravascular coagulation (DIC). Which agent should the nurse expect the health care provider (HCP) to prescribe?
☐ 1. magnesium sulfate
☐ 2. warfarin sodium
☐ 3. fresh frozen platelets
☐ 4. meperidine hydrochloride

95. A multigravid client diagnosed with chronic hypertension is now in preterm labor at 32 weeks' gestation. The health care provider (HCP) has prescribed magnesium sulfate at 3 g per hour. Which assessment finding indicates that the intended therapeutic effect has occurred?
☐ 1. decrease in fetal heart rate accelerations
☐ 2. decrease in the frequency and number of contractions
☐ 3. decrease in maternal blood pressure rate
☐ 4. decrease in maternal respiratory rate

96. A primigravid client at 37 weeks' gestation has been hospitalized for several days with severe preeclampsia. While caring for the client, the nurse observes that the client is beginning to have a seizure. What should the nurse do **first**?
☐ 1. Pad the side rails of the client's bed.
☐ 2. Turn the client to the right side.
☐ 3. Insert a padded tongue blade into the client's mouth.
☐ 4. Call for immediate assistance in the client's room.

97. While assessing a primigravid client admitted at 36 weeks' gestation, the nurse observes multiple bruises on the client's face, neck, and abdomen. When asked about the bruises, the client admits that their partner beats them now and then and says, "I want to leave because I am afraid they will hurt the baby." Which action is the nurse's **most** appropriate response?
   ☐ 1. Tell the client to leave the partner immediately.
   ☐ 2. Ask the client when they last felt the baby move.
   ☐ 3. Refer the client to a social worker for possible options.
   ☐ 4. Report the incident to the unit nursing supervisor.

Managing Care, Quality, and Safety for Clients Giving Birth

98. A newly postpartum client is asking to go to the bathroom 45 minutes after birth. The client had an epidural for labor and birth and has an intravenous (IV) line infusing, and every 15 minutes assessments are in progress. What should the nurse do to provide the safest care for this client?
   ☐ 1. Ask the client to remain in bed until the 15-minute assessments are complete.
   ☐ 2. Assess the client's ability to stand and bear weight before going to the bathroom.
   ☐ 3. Encourage the client to sit at the side of the bed before ambulating to the bathroom.
   ☐ 4. Ask the client to ambulate the first time with a staff member at their side.

99. The charge nurse is preparing for the day shift on the labor and birth unit. What would be included in the responsibilities for this position? Select all that apply.
   ☐ 1. Review the current status of each labor client with the primary nurse.
   ☐ 2. Admit the new labor client sent from the triage area.
   ☐ 3. Complete the work of the nurse who had to leave 30 minutes early.
   ☐ 4. Follow up with the primary nurse after a birth.
   ☐ 5. Complete the unit report with the oncoming charge nurse.

100. The labor and birth nurse is assigned to triage for the day. There are four clients already in rooms, and reports have been received about each of these clients. To provide the safest care and best manage time, the nurse should plan to see which client **first**?
   ☐ 1. a primipara in active labor who is 5 cm dilated and asking for admission and an epidural
   ☐ 2. a primipara who is 100% effaced, 8 cm dilated, and at +2 station with nausea
   ☐ 3. a client with no prenatal care, occasional contractions, a blood pressure of 148/90 mm Hg, and swollen feet
   ☐ 4. a client at 42 weeks' gestation with bloody show, no contractions, rupture of membranes 1 hour ago, and leaking green amniotic fluid

101. The triage nurse is giving a telephone report to the receiving nurse in the labor and birth unit. The multigravida client is 8 cm dilated and is being transferred to the labor and birth unit. How should the labor and birth nurse manage the next 10 minutes with the client? Select all that apply.
   ☐ 1. Begin fetal monitoring.
   ☐ 2. Call other staff to set up the birthing table.
   ☐ 3. Assess the comfort needs of the client.
   ☐ 4. Determine support systems for the client.
   ☐ 5. Prepare to give an early report to the nurse arriving on the next shift.

102. The health care provider (HCP) verbally prescribed carboprost tromethamine 0.25 mg intramuscularly stat for a client experiencing a postpartum hemorrhage. The nurse administers the medication but later finds that the HCP has written a prescription for 0.25 mg carboprost tromethamine intravenously stat. How should the nurse respond?
   ☐ 1. Ask the charge nurse to discuss the prescription with the HCP.
   ☐ 2. Initiate an incident report.
   ☐ 3. Call the HCP, discuss the prescription, and request a revision if heard correctly.
   ☐ 4. Wait until the HCP returns to the unit, and discuss the situation in person.

103. The nurse is asked to develop in-service training to explain documents guiding professional nursing practice on the obstetrical unit. One of the documents included is the Code of Ethics. The nurse correctly explains that the Code of Ethics asks nurses to demonstrate which behavior(s)? Select all that apply.
   ☐ 1. Maintain the integrity of practice and shape social policy.
   ☐ 2. Develop, maintain, and improve health care environments.
   ☐ 3. Ask the hospital systems for fair compensation for work.
   ☐ 4. Be responsible and accountable for individual practice.
   ☐ 5. Increase professional competence and personal growth.

104. The nurse is preparing to assist the health care provider (HCP) with a cervical check for a client whose membranes have ruptured. What equipment should the nurse have ready for the HCP? Select all that apply.
☐ 1. sterile speculum
☐ 2. sterile gloves
☐ 3. sterile lubricant
☐ 4. intrauterine pressure catheter
☐ 5. cervical dilators

105. Which client is the **best** candidate for a vaginal birth after a cesarean (VBAC)?
☐ 1. a client who had an emergency cesarean birth because of fetal distress during their last birth and who has a classic incision
☐ 2. a client who had a breech presentation in their last pregnancy, and this pregnancy is a vertex pregnancy
☐ 3. a client who dilated 6 cm in their last birth and failed to progress beyond this point despite 5 more hours of labor
☐ 4. a client with diabetes whose last infant was over 4536 g (4.5 kg) and whose fetus is larger according to ultrasound

Answers, Rationales, and Test-Taking Strategies

The answers and rationales for each question follow below, along with keys () to the client need (CN) and cognitive level (CL) for each question. In addition, questions that measure clinical judgment will be coded (CJ). As you check your answers, use the **Content Mastery and Test-Taking Skill Self-Analysis** *worksheet (tear-out worksheet in the back of the book) to identify the reason(s) for not answering the questions correctly. For additional information about test-taking skills and strategies for answering questions, refer to pages 12–51 in Part 1 of this book.*

The Primigravid Client in Labor

1. 3. The nurse should monitor anesthesia and pain levels every 30 minutes during active labor to ascertain that this client is comfortable during the labor process and particularly during active labor when pain often accelerates for the client. When in active labor, oxygen saturation is not monitored unless there is a specific need, such as heart disease. The client should not be on their back but wedged to the right or left side to take the pressure off the vena cava. When lying on the back, the fetus compresses the major blood vessels. Vaginal bleeding in active labor should be monitored every 30 minutes to 1 hour.

CN: Reduction of risk potential; CL: Create

2. 2. The first stage of labor is categorized into three phases: latent, active, and transition. During the active stage of labor, intermittent fetal monitoring is performed every 30 minutes to detect changes in fetal heart rate such as bradycardia, tachycardia, or decelerations in a low-risk labor. If complications develop, more frequent or continuous electronic fetal monitoring may be needed. During the latent phase, intermittent monitoring is usually performed every 1 hour because contractions during this time are usually less frequent. During the transition phase, intermittent monitoring is performed every 5 minutes because the client is getting closer to the birth of the baby. Pushing occurs in the second stage of labor, and monitoring continues to occur every 5 to 15 minutes.

CN: Reduction of risk potential; CL: Analyze

3. 3. The urge to push is often present when the fetus reaches + stations. This client does not have a cervix that is completely dilated, and pushing in this situation may tear the cervix. Encouraging the client to breathe through the urge to push is the most appropriate strategy and allows the cervix to dilate before pushing. Increasing the level of the epidural is inappropriate as nursing would like to have the client be able to push when they are fully dilated. Comfort measures are important for the client at this time, but they are not the highest priority for the nurse.

CN: Management of care; CL: analyze

4. 2. Assessment findings indicate that the client is in the transition phase of labor. During this phase, it is not unusual for clients to exhibit a loss of control or irritability. Leg tremors, nausea, vomiting, and an urge to bear down also are common. Excitement is associated with the latent phase of labor. Numbness of the legs may occur when epidural anesthesia has been given; however, it is rare when no anesthesia is given. Feelings of relief generally occur during the second stage, when the client begins bearing-down efforts.

CN: Health promotion and maintenance; CL: Analyze

5. 1. This figure shows the client's baby in a breech presentation with the baby facing the pelvis on the left, the sacrum as the presenting part, and the presenting part (sacrum) posterior in the pelvis. Figure 2 shows a vertex presentation with the baby in a left occiput anterior (LOA) position. Figure 3 shows a vertex presentation, left occiput posterior (LOP). Figure 4 shows a face position with the baby in a left mentotransverse (LMT) position.

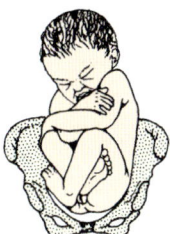

  CN: Physiological adaptation; CL: Apply

6. **1, 3, 4, 5.** Effleurage is a method of light massage that can provide pain relief. Guided imagery is a relaxation technique used in birth preparation, as is pattern-paced breathing. Positive reinforcement is not a labor support method.

  CN: Basic care and comfort; CL: Apply

7. **1.** External cephalic version is the turning of the fetus from a breech position to the vertex position to prevent the need for a cesarean birth. Gentle pressure is used to rotate the fetus in a forward direction to a cephalic lie. Contraindications to the procedure include multiple gestation because of the potential for fetal or uterine injury, severe oligohydramnios (decreased amniotic fluid), contraindications to a vaginal birth (e.g., cephalopelvic disproportion), and unexplained third-trimester bleeding. If the client has Rh-negative blood type, the procedure can be performed, and Rh immunoglobulin should be administered in case minimal bleeding occurs. A history of gestational diabetes is not a contraindication unless the fetus is large for gestational age and the client has cephalopelvic disproportion.

  CN: Reduction of risk potential; CL: Analyze

8. **2.** The goal of oxytocin administration in labor augmentation is to establish an adequate contraction pattern to enhance the forces of labor. The expected outcome is a pattern of contractions that occur every 2 to 3 minutes, last 40 to 60 seconds, and are of moderate intensity with a palpable resting tone between them. Other contraction patterns will cause the cervix to dilate too quickly or too slowly. Cervical changes in softening, effacement, and moving to an anterior position are associated with the use of cervical ripening agents, such as prostaglandin gel. Cervical dilation of 2 cm per hour is too rapid for the induction/augmentation process.

  CN: Pharmacological and parenteral therapies; CL: Evaluate

9. **4.** Anatomically, the best position for the client to assume is the squatting position because this enhances pelvic diameters and allows gravity to assist in the expulsion stage of labor. This position also provides for natural pressure anesthesia as the fetal presenting part presses on the stretched perineum. If the client is extremely fatigued from a long labor process, they may prefer the dorsal recumbent position. However, this position is not considered the best position anatomically. The lithotomy position may be ineffective and uncomfortable for a client who is ready to push. The hands and knees position may help alleviate some back pain. However, this position can cause discomfort to the arms and wrists and is tiring over a long period of time.

  CN: Health promotion and maintenance; CL: Apply

10. **4.** During the transition phase, contractions are increasing in frequency, duration, and intensity. The most appropriate nursing problem is pain related to the strength and duration of the contractions. Insufficient information is provided in the scenario to support the other listed nursing diagnoses. Urinary retention would be appropriate if the client had a full bladder and was unable to void. Hyperventilation might apply if the client was breathing too rapidly, but there is no evidence this is occurring. Ineffective coping might apply if the client said, "I can't do this" or something similar.

  CN: Health promotion and maintenance; CL: Analyze

11. **1.** The most reliable sign that the placenta has detached from the uterine wall is lengthening of the cord outside the vagina. Other signs include a sudden gush of (rather than a decrease in) vaginal blood. Usually, when placenta detachment occurs, the uterus becomes firmer and changes in shape from discoid to globular. This process takes about 5 minutes. If the placenta does not separate, manual removal may be necessary to prevent postpartum hemorrhage.

  CN: Health promotion and maintenance; CL: Analyze

12. **3.** Birth is a very emotional experience. An expression of happiness with tears is a normal reaction. Cultural factors, exhaustion, and anxieties over the new role can all affect maternal responses, so the nurse must be sensitive to the client's emotional expressions. There is no evidence to suggest that the client is disappointed in the baby's gender, grieving over the end of the pregnancy, or a candidate for postpartum "blues." However, approximately 80% of postpartum clients experience transient postpartum blues several days after birth.

🔑 CN: Health promotion and maintenance; CL: Analyze

13. 3. Most authorities suggest that a client in an early stage of labor should be allowed to walk if they wish as long as no complications are present. Birthing centers and single-room maternity units allow women considerable latitude without much supervision at this stage of labor. Gravity and walking can assist the process of labor in some clients. If the client becomes tired, they can rest in bed in the left lateral recumbent position or sit in a comfortable chair. Resting in the left lateral recumbent position improves circulation to the fetus.

🔑 CN: Health promotion and maintenance; CL: Apply

14. 1. Birth educators use various techniques and methods to prepare parents for labor and birth. Active relaxation involves relaxing uninvolved muscle groups while contracting a specific group and using chest breathing techniques to lift the diaphragm off the contracting uterus. A deep, meditative, sleeplike state is a form of passive relaxation. Focusing on an object in the room is part of the Lamaze technique for distraction. Breathing rapidly and deeply can lead to hyperventilation and is not recommended.

🔑 CN: Health promotion and maintenance; CL: Apply

15. 3. Light stroking of the skin, or *effleurage*, is commonly used with the Lamaze method of birth preparation. Light abdominal massage with just enough pressure to avoid tickling is thought to displace the pain sensation during a contraction. Deep kneading and secure grasping are typically associated with relaxation massages to relieve stress. Prolonged pressure on specific sites is associated with acupressure.

🔑 CN: Health promotion and maintenance; CL: Apply

16. 1. Some health care providers (HCPs) do not allow clients with ruptured membranes to use a hot tub or jet hydrotherapy tub during labor for fear of infections. The temperature of the water should be between 98°F and 100°F (36.7°C and 37.8°C) to prevent hyperthermia. Jet hydrotherapy is not contraindicated for clients with multifetal gestation, diabetes mellitus, or hypotonic labor patterns.

🔑 CN: Reduction of risk potential; CL: Analyze

17. 4. To determine fetal lung maturity, the sample of amniotic fluid will be tested for the L/S ratio. When fetal lungs are mature, the ratio should be 2:1. Bilirubin indicates hemolysis and, if present in the fluid, suggests Rh disease. Red blood cells should not appear in the amniotic fluid because their presence suggests fetal bleeding. Barr body determination is a chromosome analysis of the sex chromosomes that is sometimes used when a child is born with ambiguous genitalia.

🔑 CN: Health promotion and maintenance; CL: Analyze

18. 3. Pushing during the first stage of labor, when the urge is felt but the cervix is not completely dilated, may produce cervical swelling, making labor more difficult. The client should be encouraged to use a pant-blow (or blow-blow) pattern of breathing to help overcome the urge to push. The McDonald procedure is used for cervical cerclage for an incompetent cervix and is inappropriate here. Increasing the rate of oxygen and intravenous fluids will not alleviate the pressure that the client is feeling. The client should not push even if they feel the urge to do so because this may result in cervical edema at 7-cm dilation.

🔑 CN: Health promotion and maintenance; CL: Analyze

19. 1. The sagittal suture is the most readily felt during a vaginal examination. When the fetus is in the LOA position, the occiput faces the client's left. The lambdoid suture is on the side of the skull. The coronal suture is a horizontal suture across the front portion of the fetal skull that forms the anterior fontanelle. It may be felt with a brow presentation. The frontal suture may be felt with a brow or face presentation.

🔑 CN: Health promotion and maintenance; CL: Apply

20. 2. Molding occurs with vaginal births and is commonly seen in newborns. This is especially true with primigravid clients experiencing a long labor process. Parents need to be reassured that it is not permanent and that it typically lasts a day or two before resolving. Molding rarely is present if the fetus is in a breech or brow presentation. Surgical intervention is not necessary.

🔑 CN: Health promotion and maintenance; CL: Analyze

21. -/+ 1, 2, 5, 6. Uterine inversion is indicated by a sudden gush of blood from the vagina leading to decreased blood pressure and an inability to palpate the uterus since it may be in or protruding from the vagina; any signs of blood loss such as diaphoresis, paleness, or dizziness could be observed at this time. Intense pain and a hard, contracting uterus are not associated with uterine inversion.

🔑 CN: Reduction of risk potential; CL: Analyze

22. 1. According to the gate-control theory of pain, a closed gate means that the client should feel no pain. The gate-control theory of pain refers to the gate-control mechanisms in the substantia gelatinosa that are capable of halting an impulse at the level of the spinal cord so the impulse is never perceived at the brain level as pain (i.e., a process similar to keeping a gate closed).

🔑 CN: Health promotion and maintenance; CL: Evaluate

23. 4. The bladder status should be monitored throughout the labor process, but especially before the client begins pushing. A full bladder can impede the progress of labor and slow fetal descent. Because the client has had an epidural anesthetic, it is most likely that the client is receiving intravenous fluids, contributing to a full bladder. The client also does not feel the urge to void because of the anesthetic. Although it is important to monitor membrane status and fetal heart rate variability throughout labor, this does not affect the client's ability to push. There is no need to recheck cervical dilation because increasing the frequency of examinations can increase the client's risk for infection.

🔑 CN: Reduction of risk potential; CL: Analyze

24. 1. The normal length of the latent stage of labor in a primigravid client is 6 hours. If the client is having prolonged labor, the nurse should monitor the client for signs of exhaustion as well as dehydration. Hypotonic contractions, which are painful but ineffective, may be occurring. Oxytocin augmentation may be necessary. Chills and fever are manifestations of an infection and are not associated with a prolonged latent phase of labor. Fluid overload can occur from the rapid infusion of intravenous fluids administered if the client is experiencing hemorrhage or shock. It is not associated with a prolonged latent phase. The client's membranes are intact, so it would be difficult to assess meconium staining of the fluid. Meconium-stained fluid is associated with fetal distress, and this fetus appears to be in a healthy state, as evidenced by a fetal heart rate within normal range and good variability.

🔑 CN: Reduction of risk potential; CL: Analyze

25. 1. The client who has back pain during labor experiences marked discomfort because the fetus is in an LOP position. This pain is much greater than when the fetus is in the anterior position because the fetal head impinges on the sacrum in the course of rotating to the anterior position. Application of firm pressure to the sacral area can help alleviate the pain. Problems of severe back pain during labor do not typically require a cesarean birth. The health care provider (HCP) may elect to do an episiotomy, but it is not necessarily required. It is unlikely that a primigravid client with a fetus in an LOP position will have a precipitous birth; rather, labor is usually more prolonged. A hands-and-knees position or a right side-lying position may help rotate the fetal head and thus alleviate some of the back pain.

🔑 CN: Health promotion and maintenance; CL: Analyze

26. 1. The psychoprophylaxis method of birth suggests using slow chest breathing until it becomes ineffective during labor contractions, then switching to shallow chest breathing (mostly at the sternum) during the peak of a contraction. The rate is 50 to 70 breaths/min. Deep chest breathing is appropriate for the early phase of labor, in which the client exhibits less frequent contractions. When transition nears, a rapid pant-blow pattern of breathing is used. Slow abdominal breathing is very difficult for clients in labor.

🔑 CN: Health promotion and maintenance; CL: Apply

27. 3. When a client has severe back pain during labor, the fetus is most likely in an occiput posterior position. This means that the fetal head presses against the client's sacrum, causing marked discomfort during contractions. These sensations may be so intense that the client requests medication for relief of the back pain rather than the contractions. Breech presentation and transverse lie are usually known before 8-cm dilation, and a cesarean birth is performed. A fetal occiput anterior position does not increase the pain felt during labor.

🔑 CN: Health promotion and maintenance; CL: Apply

28. 🗂️ **1, 3, 5.** Decelerations alert the nurse that the fetus is experiencing decreased blood flow from the placenta. Administering oxygen will increase tissue perfusion. Placing the client on their side will increase placental perfusion and decrease cord compression. Using an internal fetal monitor would help in identifying the possible underlying cause of the decelerations, such as metabolic acidosis. Assessing for pain relief and readjusting the monitor would have no effect on correcting the late decelerations.

🗝 CN: Reduction of risk potential; CL: Apply

29. 3. The third maneuver involves grasping the lower portion of the abdomen just above the symphysis pubis between the thumb and index finger. This maneuver determines whether the fetal presenting part is engaged. The first maneuver involves facing the client's head and using the tips of the fingers to palpate the uterine fundus. This maneuver is used to identify the part of the fetus that lies over the inlet to the pelvis. The second maneuver involves placing the palms of each hand on either side of the abdomen to locate the back of the fetus. The fourth maneuver involves placing the fingers on both sides of the uterus and pressing downward and inward in the direction of the birth canal. This maneuver is done to determine fetal attitude and degree of extension and should only be done if the fetus is in the cephalic presentation.

🗝 CN: Physiological adaptation; CL: Apply

30. 1. Leopold's maneuvers are performed to determine the presentation and position of the fetus. The third maneuver determines whether the fetal presenting part is engaged in the maternal pelvis. The first maneuver distinguishes between a breech and a cephalic presentation through palpation of the top of the fundus. The second maneuver locates the fetal back, arms, and legs. The fetal heart rate monitoring device should be placed near the fetal skull and back for optimal fetal heart rate monitoring. The fourth maneuver is done to locate the fetal cephalic prominence if the fetus is in a cephalic position.

🗝 CN: Health promotion and maintenance; CL: Apply

The Multigravid Client in Labor

31. 4. Epidurals are given when labor is established, usually at 3- to 4-cm dilation. The effect of the epidural should be that labor will continue and not be slowed down by the administration of the epidural. The use of an epidural is not correlated with rupture of membranes. The contraction pattern for this client is adequate, not slow, and considered normal for 2-cm dilation. Epidurals are given at 3- to 4-cm dilation, and if there is medication available, it can be given to make the client comfortable until an epidural can be given.

🗝 CN: Management of care; CL: Apply

32. −/+ 1, 2, 4, 5. A multiparous client usually gives birth within 12 hours of the time labor began. The pushing phase statistically takes 30 minutes or less and many multiparous clients go immediately from 10-cm dilation to birth. Contractions become regular and increase in frequency, intensity, and duration as labor progresses for both primiparous and multiparous clients. Transition will be shorter for a multiparous client than it will for a primiparous client as the entire labor process takes less time for someone who has had a baby before. This client will withdraw into themselves during transition, and this is a common characteristic for those in the transition phase.

🗝 CN: Management of care; CL: Create

33. 3. The cause of variable decelerations is cord compression, which may be relieved by moving the client to one side or another. If the client is already on the left side, changing the client to the right side is appropriate. Performing a vaginal examination will let the nurse know how far dilated the client is but will not relieve the cord compression. If the decelerations are not relieved by position changes, oxygen should be initiated, but the rate should be 8 to 10 L per minute. Notifying the HCP should occur if turning the client and administering oxygen does not relieve the decelerations.

🗝 CN: Management of care; CL: Analyze

34. −/+ 1, 2, 4, 5. Knowledge of how the fetus is tolerating contractions as well as the frequency, intensity, and duration of contractions, as indicated on the fetal monitor strip, are extremely important. The type of analgesia or anesthesia being used, the client's response, and their pain rating should be included as well. The amount of vaginal bleeding indicates whether this labor is in the normal range. The support persons with the client are an integral part of the labor process and greatly influence how the client manages labor emotionally and, commonly, physically. A complete change-of-shift report would include the client's name, age, gravida and parity, current and prior illnesses that may influence this hospitalization, prior labor and birth history if applicable, last vaginal examination time and findings, vaginal bleeding, support persons with the client, current intravenous lines and other medications being used, and pertinent laboratory test results. Previous use of birth control is not important at this time.

🗝 CN: Physiological adaptation; CL: Create

35. 2. The feeling of needing to have a bowel movement is commonly caused by pressure on the receptors low in the perineum when the fetal head is creating pressure on them. This feeling usually indicates advances in fetal station and that the client may be close to birth. The nurse should respond initially to the client's signs and symptoms by completing a vaginal examination to validate current effacement, dilation, and station. If the fetus is ready to be born, having the room ready for the birth and having naloxone available are important. Naloxone completely or partially reverses the effects of natural and synthetic opioids, including respiratory depression. Documenting pain relief takes time away from the vaginal examination, preparing for birth, and obtaining naloxone. The birth may be occurring rapidly. Being prepared for the birth is a higher priority than documentation for this client.

CN: Safety and infection control; CL: Analyze

36. **1.** When a client receives an epidural anesthetic, sympathetic nerves are blocked along with the pain nerves, possibly resulting in vasodilation and hypotension. Other adverse effects include bladder distention, a prolonged second stage of labor, nausea and vomiting, pruritus, and delayed respiratory depression for up to 24 hours after administration. Diaphoresis and tremors are not usually associated with the administration of epidural anesthesia. Headache, a common adverse effect of many drugs, also is not associated with the administration of epidural anesthesia.

CN: Pharmacological and parenteral therapies; CL: Analyze

37. **4.** The fetal monitor strip shows late decelerations. The first intervention would be to turn off the oxytocin because the medication is causing the contractions. The stress caused by the contractions demonstrates that the fetus is not being perfused during the entire contraction (as shown by the late decelerations). There is no time to continue to observe in this situation; intervention is a priority. The client is attached to an internal fetal monitor, which would be possible only if their membranes had already ruptured. If the fetus continues to experience stress, fetal oximetry may be initiated.

CN: Physiological adaptation; CL: Analyze

38. **1, 2, 3, 4.** The nurse places the newborn skin to skin with the birth parent immediately following birth for many reasons. The practice facilitates transition to the extrauterine environment. Skin-to-skin contact helps begin the parental-infant bonding process and helps prevent neonatal hypothermia. Early breastfeeding provides the neonate with nutrients to prevent hypoglycemia. Breastfeeding stimulates the natural production of oxytocin, which helps reduce the potential for uterine atony. Skin-to-skin care with early breastfeeding does not reduce the risk for maternal infections.

CN: Reduction of risk potential; CL: Apply

39. **3.** A chill shortly after birth is a common, normal occurrence. Warm blankets can help provide comfort for the client. It has been suggested that the shivering response is caused by a difference between internal and external body temperatures. A different theory proposes that the client is reacting to fetal cells that have entered the maternal bloodstream through the placental site. Assessing the client's pulse rate will provide no further information about the chill. Decreasing the IV rate will not influence the length of time the client trembles. Assessing blood loss is a standard of care at this point postpartum but has no correlation with the chill.

CN: Health promotion and maintenance; CL: Analyze

40. **2.** After an amniotomy, the nurse should plan to first assess the FHR for 1 full minute. One of the complications of amniotomy is cord compression or a prolapsed cord, and an FHR of 100 bpm or less should be promptly reported to the HCP. A cord prolapse requires prompt birth by cesarean birth. The client's contraction pattern should be monitored once labor has been established. The client's temperature, pulse, and respirations should be assessed every 2 to 4 hours after rupture of the membranes to detect an infection. The nurse should document the color, quantity, and odor of the amniotic fluid, but this can be done after the FHR is assessed and a normal pattern is present.

CN: Health promotion and maintenance; CL: Analyze

41. **1.** When a client arrives at the labor and birth unit fully dilated, the nurse must prepare for a precipitous birth. Supplies should be gathered, personnel should be gathered, and the infant warmer should be turned on. Oxygen and IV fluids may be indicated if variable or late decelerations are noted on the fetal heart monitor, but decelerations are not indicated in the question. It is likely too late for pharmacologic pain relief for a multigravid client. Education regarding care of the newborn is not appropriate at this time.

CN: Management of care; CL: Apply

42. **1.** Breech presentations account for 5% of all births, and the most common is frank breech. In frank breech, there is flexion of the fetal thighs and extension of the knees. The feet rest at the side of the fetal head. In complete breech, there is flexion of the fetal thighs and knees; the fetus appears to be squatting. Footling breech occurs when there is an extension of the fetal knees and one or both feet protrude through the cervix. Vertex presentation occurs in 95% of births with the head engaged in the pelvis.

🗝 CN: Physiological adaptation; CL: Apply

43. 4. The nurse should assess the client's cervical dilation and station because the client's symptoms are indicative of the transition phase of labor. Multiparous clients can proceed 5 to 9 cm per hour during the active phase of labor. Warming the temperature of the room is not helpful because the client will soon be ready to begin expulsive pushing. Increasing the intravenous fluid rate is not warranted unless the client is experiencing dehydration. Administration of an antiemetic at this point in labor is not warranted and may result in neonatal depression should a rapid birth occur.

🗝 CN: Health promotion and maintenance; CL: Analyze

44. 4. To assess the frequency of the client's contractions, the nurse should assess the interval from the beginning of one contraction to the beginning of the next contraction. The duration of a contraction is the interval between the beginning and the end of a contraction. The acme identifies the peak of a contraction.

🗝 CN: Health promotion and maintenance; CL: Analyze

45. -/+ **3, 4, 5.** The range of fetal heart rate fluctuating more than 25 bpm could indicate fetal distress. The green fluid on the peripad indicates meconium, which could be associated with fetal distress. Increased fetal activity during labor may also indicate distress. The maternal vital signs noted and a perineal pad with blood and mucus are normal findings.

🗝 CN: Reduction of risk potential; CL: Analyze

46. 3. After spontaneous rupture of the amniotic fluid, the gushing fluid may carry the umbilical cord out of the birth canal. Sudden deceleration of the fetal heart rate commonly signifies cord compression and/or prolapse of the cord, which would require immediate birth. This client is particularly at risk because the fetus is preterm and the fetal head may not be engaged. Taking the client's vital signs is not a priority action. t. The nurse should assess the color, amount, and odor of the fluid, but this can be done once the fetal heart rate is assessed and no problems are detected. Cervical dilation should be checked but only after the fetal heart rate pattern is assessed.

🗝 CN: Reduction of risk potential; CL: Analyze

47. -/+ **3, 6.** The pressure from the fetus descending into the birth canal can cause the client to feel the need to move their bowels and could be near birth. Failure to assess the stage of labor and degree of fetal descent before allowing the client to go to the bathroom may lead to progression of labor and could result in a birth in the bathroom. Applying a fetal monitor may reassure the nurse that the fetus is doing well; however, it does not help determine if the fetus is ready to be born, which is the higher priority in this situation. Regardless of the client's prior experience with back labor pain, the fetal head moving lower into the birth canal causes pressure in the lower back area similar to the feeling of pressure with a bowel movement.

🗝 CN: Safety and infection control; CL: Apply

48. 2. Spinal anesthesia is used less commonly today because of the preference for epidural block anesthesia. One of the adverse effects of spinal anesthesia is a "spinal headache" caused by leakage of spinal fluid from the needle insertion. This can be treated by applying a cool cloth to the forehead, keeping the client in a flat position, and using a blood patch that can clot and seal off any further leakage of fluid. Spinal anesthesia is administered with the client in a sitting or side-lying position. Another adverse effect of spinal anesthesia is hypotension caused by vasodilation. General anesthesia provides immediate anesthesia, whereas the full effects of spinal anesthesia may not be felt for 20 to 30 minutes. General anesthesia can be discontinued quickly when the anesthesiologist administers oxygen instead of nitrous oxide. Epidural anesthesia may take 1 to 2 hours to wear off.

🗝 CN: Pharmacological and parenteral therapies; CL: Evaluate

49. 4. Ginkgo biloba is an herbal supplement commonly taken to improve memory or improve glycemic control. It has known antiplatelet effects and can put surgical clients at risk for bleeding. It is not known to cause hypertension or sedation. Ginkgo biloba's primary medication interaction relates to its potential to enhance the effects of other anticoagulants and lead to prolonged bleeding.

🗝 CN: Basic care and comfort; CL: Analyze

The Labor Experience

50. 1. If the presenting part is 1 cm above the ischial spines, the station is −1. If the presenting part is 1 cm below the ischial spines, the station is +1.

The terms *engaged* and *floating* are not used to describe station.

 CN: Reduction of risk potential; CL: Apply

51. 1. Closed glottis pushing, or when a client is told to hold their breath when they push (typically while the nurse counts to 10), creates the Valsalva maneuver and is associated with decreased perfusion. Open glottis pushing, on the other hand, encourages the client to listen to their body cues for when to breathe and when to bear down. "Rest and descent" and squatting have positive influences on the second stage of labor and birth.

 CN: Reduction of risk potential; CL: Analyze

52. 3. Placing the client in the hands and knees position pulls the fetal head away from the sacral promontory (relieving pain) and facilitates rotation of the fetus to the anterior position. Lithotomy is the position preferred by some health care providers for birth but does not facilitate rotation. The right lateral position will perpetuate the ROP position. Squatting facilitates descent in occiput anterior positions.

 CN: Basic care and comfort; CL: Apply

53. 3. A trial labor in this context means that the client is allowed to go into labor and their progress is assessed by cervical dilation and effacement as well as fetal descent evaluated to determine whether to allow the labor to progress to birth. If there are indications that labor is not progressing, other means of birth are considered. Labor stimulation is used cautiously and may not be safe. The presence of contractions every 5 minutes indicates true labor. If fetal distress is noted and an emergency cesarean birth cannot be done immediately, tocolytic agents may be considered to stop contractions.

 CN: Management of care; CL: Analyze

54. 2. Lumbar epidural anesthesia is usually administered with the client in a sitting or a left side-lying position with the shoulders parallel and the legs slightly flexed. These positions expose the vertebrae to the anesthesiologist. Paracervical and local anesthetics are usually administered with the client in the lithotomy position. The hands and knees and prone positions are not used for anesthesia administration.

 CN: Pharmacological and parenteral therapies; CL: Apply

55. 2. The nurse should turn the client to the side to reduce pressure on the abdominal aorta. The IV fluid rate would be increased, not decreased. There is no information indicating the client has a full bladder or requires a vaginal examination.

 CN: Management of care; CL Analyze

56. 2. The nurse would document these findings as "early" decelerations. Early decelerations are thought to be the result of vagal nerve stimulation caused by compression of the fetal head during labor. They are considered a normal physiologic response to labor and do not require any intervention. Early decelerations do not require a position change or the administration of oxygen as they are not a sign of fetal distress. Variable decelerations are thought to be due to umbilical cord compression. Early decelerations are considered to be an emergency and do not require immediate reporting to the HCP or preparing for a cesarean birth.

 CN: Management of care; CL: Analyze

57. 4. Transition is the most difficult period of the labor process, and often when clients are tired, pain becomes more intensified. Clients during this stage verbalize anger and are outspoken and difficult to comfort. The most logical next step would be to determine if the client has completed transition and is ready to begin pushing. Performing a vaginal examination would provide this answer. The use of narcotic medications is discouraged at this stage as they can lead to respiratory depression in the neonate. Palpating the bladder is an important intervention, but it is not the highest priority as it was done less than an hour ago. Since the nurse has correctly completed the most logical steps, asking for the client's input would certainly be in order but not the highest priority intervention.

 CN: Basic care and comfort; CL: Apply

58. 4. Betamethasone is a corticosteroid that induces the production of surfactant. The pulmonary maturation that results causes the fetal lungs to mature more rapidly than normal. Because the lungs are mature, the risk for respiratory distress in the neonate is lowered but not eliminated. Betamethasone also decreases the surface tension within the alveoli. Betamethasone has no influence on contractions or carrying the fetus to full term. It also does not prevent infection.

 CN: Pharmacological and parenteral therapies; CL: Evaluate

59. 1. A Bishop score evaluates cervical readiness for labor based on five factors: cervical softness, cervical effacement, dilation, fetal position, and station. A Bishop score of 5 or greater in a multipara or a score of 8 or greater in a primipara indicates that a vaginal birth is likely to result from the induction process. The nurse should expect that labor will be induced using oxytocin because the Bishop score indicates that the client is 60% to 70% effaced, 3 to 4 cm dilated, and in an anterior position. The cervix is soft, and the presenting part is at a −1 to 0 position. Prostaglandin gel, misoprostol, and dinoprostone are all cervical ripening agents, and the doses are accurate; however, cervical ripening has already taken place.

🗝 CN: Pharmacological and parenteral therapies; CL: Analyze

60. -/+ **1, 2, 3, 5.** The time of rupture; the color, odor, amount, and clarity of the amniotic fluid; and the FHR and pattern before and after the procedure are all information that must be documented on the client's record. There is only one size for an amnio hook.

🗝 CN: Management of care; CL: Create

61. 2. The client is experiencing uterine hyperstimulation from the oxytocin. The first intervention should be to stop the oxytocin infusion, which may be the cause of the long, frequent contractions, elevated resting tone, and abnormal fetal heart patterns. Only after turning off the oxytocin should the nurse turn the client to their left side to better perfuse the birth parent and fetus. Then, the nurse should increase the maintenance IV fluids to allow available oxygen to be carried to the client and fetus. When all other interventions are initiated, the nurse should notify the HCP.

🗝 CN: Management of care; CL: Analyze

62. 4. Late decelerations on a fetal heart monitor indicate uteroplacental insufficiency. Interventions to improve perfusion include repositioning the client and administering oxygen and IV fluids. A sterile vaginal examination is not indicated at this time. Late decelerations are not expected findings and do not indicate an imminent birth.

🗝 CN: Management of Care; CL: Analyze

63. -/+ **1, 4, 5, 6.** The second stage of labor ends with birth. Delivery of the placenta normally happens 5 to 30 minutes after birth. It is the nurse's responsibility to note the time of birth and complete or assist with the 1- and 5-minute Apgar scores. The infant should be dried immediately after birth to prevent heat loss from evaporation. Ideally, the infant is then placed skin to skin with the birth parent. Vital signs on the infant should be taken soon after birth. Oxytocin administration is done to actively manage the fourth stage of labor after the delivery of the placenta. Perineal repairs also happen after the delivery of the placenta.

🗝 CN: Health promotion and maintenance; CL: Apply

64. 1. The client with preeclampsia would be a candidate for the induction process because ending the pregnancy is the only way to cure preeclampsia. A client with active herpes would be a candidate for a cesarean birth to prevent the fetus from contracting the virus while passing through the birth canal. The client with a face presentation will not be able to give birth vaginally due to the extended position of the neck. The client whose fetus exhibits late decelerations without oxytocin would be at greater risk for fetal distress with use of this drug. Late decelerations indicate the fetus does not have enough placental reserves to remain oxygenated during the entire contraction. This client may require a cesarean birth.

🗝 CN: Management of care; CL: Evaluate

65. 3. When the fetal head is compressed, early decelerations are seen as a vagal response, during which the fetal heart rate decelerates and inversely mirrors the contraction. This response commonly occurs when the client is 9 to 10 cm dilated or pushing. If communication cannot be facilitated, early decelerations are one indicator that birth may be approaching. Late decelerations may occur at this time but indicate uteroplacental insufficiency rather than imminent birth. At any time during the labor process, the client may communicate with family in their native language. The client's facial expressions may change at any point during labor and cannot be used as an indicator of imminent birth.

🗝 CN: Physiological adaptation; CL: Analyze

66. 0/1 The nurse determines that the client is most likely experiencing **hypotension**. The first action the nurse should take is to **turn the client on their side**.

Nausea and vomiting after an epidural can be a reaction to the medication used or caused by a drop in blood pressure. The nurse should turn the client to the side to reduce pressure on the abdominal aorta, increase placental perfusion, and decrease the risk for aspiration. Although low blood pressure and nausea can be seen with allergic responses, the nurse would expect to see other symptoms, such as respiratory distress or hives, if the client had anaphylaxis. A spinal headache that causes nausea can occur after the administration of an epidural anesthetic, but the nurse would not expect this complication to occur immediately after the anesthetic was placed. The nurse would also expect the client to report having a headache. There is no need to activate the emergency response team. Dimming the room lights may be desirable to improve comfort, but it is not a priority for treating hypotension.

🗝 CJ: Standalone trend; CL: Analyze

The Intrapartal Client with Risk Factors

67. -/+ **1, 2, 3.** With abruptio placentae, bleeding may occur vaginally, be obstructed by the fetal head, or be hidden behind a portion of the placenta. Abdominal rigidity occurs, particularly with a concealed hemorrhage, because the girth and fundal height increase. Abdominal pain is one of the classic symptoms of abruption. The pain may be intermittent, as in labor contractions, or continuous. The placenta with abruption is not larger than a normal placenta, and the bleeding does not end spontaneously.

 CN: Physiological adaptation; CL: Analyze

68. 3. The multigravid client with class II heart disease has a slight limitation of physical activity and may become fatigued with ordinary physical activity. A side-lying or semi-Fowler position with the head elevated helps ensure cardiac emptying and adequate oxygenation. In addition, oxygen by mask, analgesics and sedatives, diuretics, prophylactic antibiotics, and digitalis may be warranted. Although breathing slowly during a contraction may assist with oxygenation, it would not affect cardiac emptying. It is essential that the laboring client with cardiac disease be relieved of discomfort and anxiety. Effective intrapartum pain relief with analgesia and epidural anesthesia may reduce cardiac workload by as much as 20%. Local anesthetics are effective only during the second stage of labor.

 CN: Reduction of risk potential; CL: Analyze

69. 4. Assessing for signs and symptoms associated with cardiac decompensation is the priority. Class III heart disease during pregnancy has a 25% to 50% mortality. These clients are markedly compromised, with marked limitation of physical activity. They frequently experience fatigue, palpitations, dyspnea, or anginal pain. A pulse rate greater than 100 bpm or a respiratory rate greater than 25 breaths/min may indicate cardiac decompensation that could result in cardiac arrest. Additional symptoms include dyspnea, peripheral edema, orthopnea, tachypnea, rales, and hemoptysis.

 CN: Reduction of risk potential; CL: Analyze

70. 1. Before administering prostaglandin E2 gel, the nurse would assess the frequency and duration of any uterine contractions first because prostaglandin E2 gel is contraindicated if the client is having contractions. If there are no contractions, the client should be placed in a semi-Fowler position to allow for vaginal insertion of the gel. Although determining whether the client's membranes have ruptured is part of the assessment of any client in labor, it is not specifically related to the administration of prostaglandin E2 gel. If the membranes remain intact, an amniotomy may be performed once the client begins to dilate and the fetal head is engaged. However, the nurse does not need to prepare the client for this procedure at this time.

 CN: Pharmacological and parenteral therapies; CL: Analyze

71. 4. A prolonged second stage of labor with a large fetus could indicate shoulder dystocia at birth. Immediate nursing actions for shoulder dystocia include suprapubic pressure and the McRoberts maneuver. If interventions for a vaginal birth with a shoulder dystocia fail, an emergency cesarean birth may be needed, but this is not indicated at this time. A vacuum-assisted birth would be contraindicated because of the increased risk for shoulder dystocia with an infant with macrosomia. An IV fluid bolus may be indicated for fetal distress, but there is not enough information to establish that it is needed at this time.

 CN: Physiologic adaptation; CL: Apply

72. 4. Assessing the fetal heart rate is always a priority after spontaneous rupture of membranes has occurred. Meconium-stained fluid is also a common sign of fetal distress related to an inadequate transfer of oxygen to the fetus. Because the fetus has suffered hypoxia, close fetal heart rate monitoring is necessary. In addition, all clients are monitored continuously after rupture of membranes for fetal distress caused by cord prolapse. If there are increasing signs of fetal distress (e.g., late decelerations), the health care provider (HCP) should be notified immediately. A cesarean birth may be performed for fetal distress. Increasing the rate of the oxytocin infusion could lead to further fetal distress. Turning the client to the left side, rather than a knee-chest position, improves placental perfusion. The HCP may wish to determine the extent of cervical dilation to decide whether a cesarean birth is warranted, but continuous fetal heart rate monitoring is essential to determine fetal status.

 CN: Reduction of risk potential; CL: Analyze

73. 3. The client should be urged to push with an open glottis to prevent the Valsalva maneuver. Pushing with a closed glottis increases intrathoracic pressure, preventing venous return. Blood pressure also falls, and cardiac output decreases. Pushing for at least 1 to 3 minutes is too long; prolonged pushing can lead to reduced blood flow and fatigue. Pushing for the duration of the contraction is sufficient. Pushing while holding the breath results in the Valsalva maneuver. Because the client has had an epidural anesthetic, they may not feel the urge to push and may need coaching during the pushing phase.

🔑 CN: Pharmacological and parenteral therapies; CL: Apply

74. 3. When the fetal skull is on the perineum with the scalp visible at the perineal floor or vaginal opening, this is considered outlet forceps application. When the head is higher in the pelvis but engaged and its greatest diameter has passed the inlet, the operation is termed *midforceps*. Midforceps births are not recommended because they are extremely dangerous for the birth parent and fetus because of the possibility of uterine rupture. If the head is not engaged, at −1 station, this is termed high forceps. High-forceps births also are exceedingly dangerous for both the birth parent and fetus because of the possibility of uterine rupture and are not recommended. Cesarean birth is preferred in these situations. The fetal head at station +2 or lower is termed low forceps.

🔑 CN: Reduction of risk potential; CL: Apply

75. 1. Oligohydramnios, or a decrease in the volume of amniotic fluid, is associated with variable fetal heart rate decelerations due to cord compression. Maintenance of an adequate amniotic fluid volume during labor provides protective cushioning of the umbilical cord and minimizes cord compression. Cord compression can result in fetal metabolic acidosis, not alkalosis. Amnioinfusion is used to minimize cord compression, not increase the fetal heart rate accelerations during a contraction. The goal is to maintain the amniotic fluid index at 8 cm. This can be determined by ultrasound.

🔑 CN: Reduction of risk potential; CL: Apply

76. 4. A primigravid client diagnosed with preeclampsia has the potential for developing seizures (eclampsia). This client should be in a room with the least amount of stimulation possible to reduce the risk for seizures and as close to the nurses' station as possible in case the client requires immediate assistance. Bright lighting and sunshine can be a stimulant, possibly increasing the risk for seizures, as can being in a semiprivate room with a roommate, visitors, conversation, and noise.

🔑 CN: Management of care; CL: Analyze

77. 4. The client is experiencing a precipitous birth. The nurse should remain calm during a precipitous birth. Explaining to the client what is happening as the birth progresses and how they can assist is likely to help the client remain calm and cooperative. Maintaining eye contact is also beneficial. Telling the client that they are right and to just relax is inappropriate because the client may not be able to relax because of the strong urge to push the fetus out of the birth canal. Telling the client not to push because they may tear the cervix can instill fear, not cooperation. Saying that the health care provider will be there soon may not be an accurate statement and is not reassuring if the client is concerned about the birth.

🔑 CN: Psychosocial integrity; CL: Apply

78. 2. During a precipitous birth, after calling for assistance and helping the client lie down, the nurse should provide support to the fetal head to prevent too rapid of emergence, which could lead to injury. It is not appropriate to tell the client to push between contractions because this may lead to lacerations. The shoulder should be delivered by applying downward traction until the anterior shoulder appears fully at the introitus, then upward pressure to lift out the other shoulder. Priority should be given to the safe birth of the infant rather than protecting the perineum by massage.

🔑 CN: Reduction of risk potential; CL: Analyze

79. 2. Because birth occurs so rapidly and the fetus is propelled quickly through the birth canal, the major complication of a precipitous birth is a boggy fundus caused by uterine atony. The neonate should be put to the breast, if the birth parent permits, to allow for the release of natural oxytocin. In a hospital setting, the health care provider will probably prescribe the administration of oxytocin. The nurse should gently massage the fundus to ensure that it is firm. There is no relationship between a precipitous birth and postpartum "blues" or intrauterine infection. Postpartum "blues" usually do not occur until about 3 days after birth, and symptoms of postpartum infection usually occur after the first 24 hours. There is no relationship between a precipitous birth and urinary tract infection even though the birth has been accomplished under clean rather than sterile technique. Symptoms of urinary tract infection typically begin on the first or second postpartum day.

🔑 CN: Reduction of risk potential; CL: Analyze

80. 2. A sinusoidal pattern is an ominous sign that reflects an absence of autonomic nervous control over the fetal heart rate resulting from severe hypoxia. Sinusoidal patterns, while rare, are associated with Rh sensitization, fetal hydrops, and anemia. This client will most likely require a cesarean birth to improve the fetal outcome.

Variable decelerations, associated with cord compression, and late decelerations, associated with poor placental perfusion, are concerning but may correct with appropriate interventions. Early decelerations are associated with head compression and are considered a normal variation.

🗝 CN: Reduction of risk potential; CL: Analyze

81. 1. A priority assessment for the nurse to make is to determine the estimated date of birth or probable gestational age of the fetus. If the gestation is less than 37 weeks, the neonatal team should be called to begin resuscitative efforts if needed. Amniotic fluid status is not important at this point because if the fetal skull is crowning, birth is imminent. Determination of gravida and parity is part of the normal nursing history, but the priority is the status of the fetus and a safe birth. Prenatal history is part of the nursing assessment, but this information is not especially relevant until the fetus is safely born and has been given immediate care.

🗝 CN: Health promotion and maintenance; CL: Analyze

82. 4. Birth trauma and prolonged ruptured membranes make the risk for infection the priority problem for this client. Infection can be a serious postpartum complication. Although the client may be fatigued, they should not be experiencing activity intolerance. Clients with heart disease may experience activity intolerance due to excessive cardiac workload. Although the client may be experiencing sleep deprivation, most clients are alert and awake after the birth of a neonate. Situational low self-esteem is not a priority. Clients who undergo a cesarean birth commonly feel a sense of failure because of not having a vaginal birth experience, but this is not the case for this client.

🗝 CN: Reduction of risk potential; CL: Analyze

83. 2. Postmature neonates commonly have difficulty maintaining adequate glucose reserves and usually develop hypoglycemia soon after birth. Other common problems include meconium aspiration syndrome, polycythemia, congenital anomalies, seizure activity, and cold stress. These complications result primarily from a combination of advanced gestational age, placental insufficiency, and continued exposure to amniotic fluid. Delayed meconium is not associated with postterm gestation. Hyperbilirubinemia occurs in term neonates as well as postterm neonates, but unless there is an Rh incompatibility, it does not develop until after the first 24 hours of life.

🗝 CN: Reduction of risk potential; CL: Analyze

84. 4. Polyhydramnios is an abnormally large amount of amniotic fluid in the uterus. The client has understood the instructions when the client states that polyhydramnios is associated with gastrointestinal disorders (e.g., tracheoesophageal fistula). Polyhydramnios is also associated with maternal illnesses such as diabetes and anemia. Other fetal/neonatal disorders associated with this condition include congenital anomalies of the central nervous system (e.g., anencephaly), upper gastrointestinal obstruction, and macrosomia. Polyhydramnios can lead to preterm labor, premature rupture of the membranes, and cord prolapse. Renal dysfunction and intrauterine growth restriction are associated with oligohydramnios, not polyhydramnios. Pulmonary hypoplasia (poorly developed lungs) is associated with prolonged oligohydramnios.

🗝 CN: Reduction of risk potential; CL: Evaluate

85. 3. Preparation for a cesarean birth is similar to preparation for any abdominal surgery. The client must give informed consent. Another person may not sign for the client unless the client is unable to sign the form. If this is the case, only certain designated people can do so legally. The spouse does not need to sign the form unless the client is unable to do so. In a life-threatening emergency, surgery may be performed without a written consent. The HCP does not need to witness the consent.

🗝 CN: Management of care; CL: Analyze

86. 4. Decreased variability may be seen in various conditions. However, it is most commonly caused by analgesic administration. Other factors that can cause decreased variability include anesthesia, deep fetal sleep, anencephaly, prematurity, hypoxia, tachycardia, brain damage, and arrhythmias. Maternal fatigue, fetal malposition, and a small-for-gestational-age fetus are not commonly associated with decreased variability.

🗝 CN: Health promotion and maintenance; CL: Apply

87. 4. Respiratory distress syndrome is more common in neonates born by cesarean birth than in those born vaginally. During a vaginal birth, pressure is exerted on the fetal chest, which aids in the fetal inhalation and exhalation of air and lung expansion. This pressure is not exerted on the fetus with a cesarean birth. Congenital anomalies are not more common with cesarean birth. Pulmonary hypertension occurs more commonly in infants with meconium aspiration syndrome, congenital diaphragmatic hernia, respiratory distress syndrome, or neonatal sepsis, not with cesarean birth. Meconium aspiration syndrome occurs more commonly with vaginal birth, postterm neonate, and prolonged labor, not with cesarean birth.

🗝 CN: Health promotion and maintenance; CL: Apply

88. 4. Congenital anomalies are not related to maternal urinary tract infections. A multigravid client with acute pyelonephritis is susceptible to preterm labor, premature rupture of the membranes, maternal sepsis, intrauterine growth restriction, and fetal loss. The most common organism responsible for urinary tract infection is *Escherichia coli*.

🗝 CN: Reduction of risk potential; CL: Evaluate

89. 1. Conjunctivitis is a common complication of neonates who are born to clients with untreated chlamydial infection. Neonatal pneumonia is another condition associated with chlamydial infection of the client. Untreated chlamydial infection is not associated with heart disease or brain damage. Exposure to rubella may lead to neonatal heart defects, and brain damage may occur as a result of prolonged shoulder dystocia or difficulty delivering the fetal head during a vaginal breech birth. Occasionally, because of immature circulation, a neonate who has been lying on their side appears red on one side of the body. This "harlequin sign" is transient and is of no clinical significance. The presence of a harlequin sign is unrelated to untreated chlamydial infection.

🗝 CN: Reduction of risk potential; CL: Apply

90. 1. The purpose of Rh immune globulin is to provide passive antibody immunity and prevent Rh-positive sensitization with the next pregnancy. It should be given within 72 hours after the birth of an Rh-positive neonate. Clients who are Rh negative and conceive an Rh-negative fetus do not need antibody protection. Rh-positive cells contribute to sensitization, not Rh-negative cells. Rh immune globulin does not cross the placenta and destroy fetal Rh-positive cells.

🗝 CN: Reduction of risk potential; CL: Apply

91. 3. Because magnesium sulfate is a central nervous system depressant, the nurse should plan to assess the client's respiratory rate and blood pressure every hour. If the respiratory rate is less than 12 breaths/min, the client may be experiencing magnesium sulfate overdose. Urinary output via an indwelling catheter should be assessed hourly and should be at least 30 mL per hour. Deep tendon reflexes should be assessed at least every 4 hours. At some institutions, continuous electronic blood pressure monitoring will be performed.

🗝 CN: Pharmacological and parenteral therapies; CL: Analyze

92. 2. For a client diagnosed with probable placenta previa, hypovolemic shock is a complication. Continuous blood pressure monitoring with an electronic cuff is the priority assessment after the client's admission. Once the client is admitted, an ultrasound examination will be performed to determine the placement of the placenta. Whole blood replacement is not warranted at this time. However, it may be necessary if the client demonstrates signs and symptoms of hemorrhage or shock. Internal fetal heart rate monitoring is contraindicated because the monitoring device may puncture the placenta and place both the birth parent and fetus in jeopardy. An immediate cesarean birth is not necessary until there has been an assessment of the amount of bleeding and the location of the placenta previa.

🗝 CN: Reduction of risk potential; CL: Apply

93. 4. Dramatic vasoconstriction occurs as a result of smoking crack cocaine. This can lead to increased respiratory and cardiac rates and hypertension. It can severely compromise placental circulation, resulting in abruptio placentae and preterm labor and birth. Infants of these women can experience intracranial hemorrhage and withdrawal symptoms of tremulousness, irritability, and rigidity. Placenta previa, a ruptured uterus, and maternal hypotension are not associated with cocaine use. Placenta previa may be associated with grand multiparity. A ruptured uterus may be associated with a large-for-gestational-age fetus.

🗝 CN: Reduction of risk potential; CL: Analyze

94. 3. To stop the process of DIC, the underlying insult that began the phenomenon must be halted. Treatment includes fresh frozen platelets or blood administration. The HCP also may prescribe heparin before the administration of blood products to restore the normal clotting mechanism. Immediate birth of the fetus is essential. Magnesium sulfate is given for pregnancy-induced hypertension or preterm labor. Heparin, not warfarin sodium, is used to treat DIC. Meperidine hydrochloride is used for pain relief.

🗝 CN: Pharmacological and parenteral therapies; CL: Apply

95. **2.** Magnesium sulfate may be used as an anticonvulsive or a tocolytic agent. The intended effect for this client is to decrease the number and frequency of contractions. Even though this client has chronic hypertension, the first goal is to delay birth in a client at 34 weeks' gestation so steroids can be given to accelerate lung maturity. If the blood pressure moves into the therapeutic range, that is a benefit for the client, but it is not the major goal. Magnesium sulfate may decrease the accelerations found in this fetus as it decreases the ability of the infant to respond, acting on the infant in the same way it does on the birth parent. Maternal respiratory rate may also decrease, and a lower respiratory rate of 12 breaths/min indicates that this level of magnesium sulfate is becoming toxic to this client.

CN: Pharmacological and parenteral therapies; CL: Evaluate

96. **4.** The nurse should respond using emergency response principles. The first action by the nurse should be to call for immediate assistance in the client's room. Throughout the seizure, the nurse should note the time and length of the seizure and continue to monitor the status of both the client and the fetus. The side rails should have been padded at the time of the client's admission to the hospital as part of seizure precautions. The client should be turned to their left side to improve placental perfusion. Inserting a tongue blade is not recommended because it can further obstruct the airway or cause injury to the client's teeth.

CN: Safety and infection control; CL: Analyze

97. **3.** In an abusive situation, the client's safety is the priority. The nurse should refer the client to a social worker who can provide the client with options such as a safe shelter. Clients who are battered often feel powerless and fear that the batterer will kill them. As a result, they remain in the abusive situation. Telling the client to leave the boyfriend immediately is not helpful and reflects the values of the nurse. Although asking about fetal movement is important and is part of a routine assessment, a sonogram can be performed to confirm fetal well-being. The referral is more important at this time. Although it may be part of the unit's policies and procedures to report any incidents such as this one to the unit supervisor, the client's immediate need for safety must be addressed first.

CN: Management of care; CL: Apply

Managing Care, Quality, and Safety for Clients Giving Birth

98. **2.** The nurse will need to assess the client's ability to bear weight before taking them to the bathroom. If the client cannot bear weight, they will be unable to ambulate. Asking the client to remain in bed until the assessments are complete sets the client up for increased postpartum bleeding because the bladder will displace the uterus. Encouraging the client to sit at the bedside is an excellent strategy to prevent orthostatic hypotension, but it will not give the nurse an idea if the client can ambulate. Having a staff member with the client is also correct for the first ambulation of this client, but the ability to bear weight and walk will need to be assessed first.

CN: Reduction of risk potential; CL: Analyze

99. **1, 4, 5.** In most settings, the charge nurse coordinates and directs the activities of the unit. Before the change of shift, the nurse will review and update the status of each of the laboring clients on the unit to include any difficulties or unusual situations that may be occurring with each of them, including following up with a primary nurse after a birth. A change-of-shift report with the oncoming charge nurse is among the last activities completed before ending the shift. Activities such as admitting a client in labor and completing the nursing responsibilities of the nurse who had to leave 30 minutes early can be delegated to staff members. In an emergency, the charge nurse could assume responsibility for client care.

CN: Management of care; CL: Create

100. **4.** The client at 42 weeks' gestation is the greatest concern, and the nurse should make rounds on this client first based on the length of the pregnancy and the green color of the amniotic fluid. Bloody show is a normal sign of impending labor as the cervix may be beginning to dilate. Not having contractions after rupture of membranes is not unusual within a 1-hour time frame. The green amniotic fluid indicates that fetal distress has recently occurred to the point that the fetus had a bowel movement in utero. This occurrence, along with the 42-week gestation, places this fetus at greatest risk. The nurse can see the primipara in active labor at 5-cm dilation last; this client is in pain, but nothing about the situation indicates anything but a normal labor process, and because the client is a primipara, the labor process will be slow. The client who is completely effaced, 8 cm dilated, and at +2 station is also a primipara and thus will move through labor at a slower pace than a multiparous client. Experiencing nausea is an expected situation as a laboring client enters transition. The client with no prenatal care is a cause for concern because the nurse knows nothing about their background. The client's blood pressure is elevated, which is an indicator of mild preeclampsia, but there are no other indications of worsening preeclampsia, such as headache, visual disturbances, or epigastric pain, so this client would not be the priority.

CN: Management of care; CL: Analyze

101. 1, 2, 3, 4. Assuring the safety of this client is the top priority. The nurse should begin either intermittent or continuous fetal and contraction monitoring, depending on the client's risk status. Since the client is 8 cm dilated and a multigravid client, asking other staff members to set up the birthing table would be in order. This client is not a candidate for medication as this may cause respiratory suppression in the baby. This client is past the point of getting an epidural as they may have given birth by the time the medication takes effect, but comfort measures such as warm or cool cloths and back rubs may be helpful. The support system is an important aspect of the birthing process and is an easily settled situation. Preparing to give an early report to the oncoming nurse does not apply in this situation.

CN: Management of care; CL: Create

102. 3. In emergency situations, verbal prescriptions should be entered into the medical record or chart and signed immediately after the emergency. The nurse taking this prescription and giving the medication needs to call the HCP, explain the prescription and that the medication was administered per the verbal prescription, and request that the HCP write the correct prescription. If the nurse misunderstood the prescription and gave the medication by the wrong route, an incident report will need to be initiated. The charge nurse would become involved if an error has occurred, an incident report is needed, or there is difficulty between the nurse and HCP that cannot be remediated. Rectifying this prescription is the responsibility of the implementing nurse. Waiting until the HCP comes back to the hospital unit may not occur quickly enough to safely care for the client.

CN: Management of care; CL: Synthesize

103. 1, 2, 4, 5. The Code of Ethics describes those actions by the nurse that guide their practice. It is the responsibility of each nurse to be active in determining policy for health care for all citizens and assuring that the way nursing is practiced is of the highest caliber. Nurses need to participate in the development of health care of the future while caring for all members of society. To be productive in shaping policy, nurses need to be politically astute while growing personally and professionally to meet the needs of clients. The Code of Ethics does not address compensation for work.

CN: Management of care; CL: Apply

104. 2, 3. Intact membranes act as a barrier to prevent infections. Once a client's membranes have ruptured, it is important to take precautions to limit the introduction of bacteria into the genital tract. Using sterile gloves and sterile lubricant for cervical checks helps reduce the risk for infection. A sterile speculum is only needed to diagnose if the membranes have ruptured. An intrauterine pressure catheter would only be indicated if the plan was to begin internal contraction monitoring. Cervical dilators are not used for cervical checks in labor.

CN: Management of care; CL: Apply

105. 2. The best candidate for a VBAC is a client who had a cesarean birth in their last birth because of a problem related to the infant that is not repeated in this pregnancy. The client with the breech presentation in their last birth and a vertex pregnancy in this pregnancy would be the best candidate, especially if they had other vaginal births. The client who was unable to dilate beyond 6 cm (failure to progress) may try a VBAC but is likely to experience the same problem with this birth. The client with the very large infant is likely to experience cephalopelvic disproportion with this birth if they experienced cephalopelvic disproportion with their last infant who was large. A classic cesarean birth scar is a contraindication for a VBAC because that type of scar may not be strong enough to withstand the stress of hours of uterine contractions and may result in uterine disruption.

CN: Management of care; CL: Analyze

TEST 4

Postpartum Care

- The Postpartum Client with a Vaginal Birth
- The Postpartum Client Who Breastfeeds
- The Postpartum Client Who Bottle-feeds
- The Postpartum Client with a Cesarean Birth
- The Postpartum Client with Complications
- Managing Care, Quality, and Safety of Postpartum Clients

The Postpartum Client with a Vaginal Birth

1. The nurse from the nursery is bringing a newborn to a client's room. The nurse took care of the client yesterday and knows the client and baby well. The nurse should implement which action **next** to ensure the safest transition of the infant to the birth parent?
   - ☐ 1. Assess whether the birth parent is able to ambulate to care for the infant.
   - ☐ 2. Ask the birth parent if there is anything else they need for the care of the baby.
   - ☐ 3. Check the crib to determine if there are enough diapers and formula.
   - ☐ 4. Complete the hospital identification procedure with the birth parent and infant.

2. A client is in the first hour of recovery after a vaginal birth. During an assessment, the lochia is moderate, bright red, and trickling from the vagina. The nurse locates the fundus at the umbilicus; it is firm and midline with no palpable bladder. The client's vital signs remain at their baseline. Based on this information, the nurse would implement which action?
   - ☐ 1. Massage the fundus and expel clots.
   - ☐ 2. Recheck the admission hematocrit and hemoglobin levels.
   - ☐ 3. Request that the health care provider (HCP) assess the client.
   - ☐ 4. Document the findings as normal.

3. The nurse is caring for a multigravida client who is 1 day postpartum following a vaginal birth. Which finding indicates a need for further assessment?
   - ☐ 1. hemoglobin 12.1 g/dL (121 g/L)
   - ☐ 2. white blood cell (WBC) count of 15,000/μL (15 × 10⁹/L)
   - ☐ 3. pulse of 60 bpm
   - ☐ 4. temperature of 100.8°F (38.2°C)

4. The nurse is providing follow-up care to a client 10 days after the birth. The nurse would anticipate what outcomes from the new parent? Select all that apply.
   - ☐ 1. The client feels tired but is able to care for themselves and the new infant.
   - ☐ 2. The family has adequate support from one another and others.
   - ☐ 3. Lochia is changing from red to pink and is smaller in amount.
   - ☐ 4. The client feeds the baby every 6 to 8 hours without difficulty.
   - ☐ 5. The client has positive comments about their new infant.

5. A client gave birth vaginally 2 hours ago and has a third-degree laceration. There is ice in place on the perineum. However, the perineum is slightly edematous, and the client is having pain rated 6 on a scale of 1 to 10. Which nursing intervention would be the **most** appropriate at this time?
   - ☐ 1. Begin sitz baths.
   - ☐ 2. Administer pain medication per prescription.
   - ☐ 3. Replace ice packs on the perineum.
   - ☐ 4. Initiate prescription anesthetic sprays to the perineum.

6. A primigravid client gave birth vaginally 2 hours ago with no complications. As the nurse plans care for this postpartum client, which postpartum goal would have the **highest priority**?
   - ☐ 1. By discharge, the family will bond with the neonate.
   - ☐ 2. The nurse will demonstrate self-care and infant care by the end of the shift.
   - ☐ 3. The nurse will state instructions for discharge during the first postpartum day.
   - ☐ 4. By the end of the shift, the nurse will describe a safe home environment.

7. In response to the nurse's question about how they are feeling, a postpartum client states that they are fine. The client then begins talking to the baby, checking the diaper, and asking infant care questions. The nurse determines that the client is in which postpartum phase of psychological adaptation?
   ☐ 1. taking in
   ☐ 2. taking on
   ☐ 3. taking hold
   ☐ 4. letting go

8. At which location would the nurse expect to palpate the fundus of a primiparous client immediately after the birth of a neonate?
   ☐ 1. halfway between the umbilicus and the symphysis pubis
   ☐ 2. at the level of the umbilicus
   ☐ 3. just below the level of the umbilicus
   ☐ 4. above the level of the umbilicus

9. The nurse assesses a swollen ecchymosed area to the right of a laceration on a primiparous client 6 hours after a vaginal birth. What should the nurse do **next**?
   ☐ 1. Apply an ice pack to the perineal area.
   ☐ 2. Assess the client's temperature.
   ☐ 3. Have the client take a warm sitz bath.
   ☐ 4. Contact the health care provider (HCP) for prescriptions for an antibiotic.

10. Two hours after a vaginal birth under epidural anesthesia, a client with a midline episiotomy ambulates to the bathroom to void. After voiding, the nurse assesses the client's bladder, finding it distended. The nurse interprets this finding based on the understanding that the client's bladder distention is **most** likely caused by which factor?
   ☐ 1. prolonged first stage of labor
   ☐ 2. urinary tract infection
   ☐ 3. pressure of the uterus on the bladder
   ☐ 4. edema in the lower urinary tract area

11. A primiparous client who is bottle-feeding their neonate at 12 hours after birth asks the nurse, "When will my menstrual cycle return?" Which response by the nurse would be **most** appropriate?
   ☐ 1. "Your menstrual cycle will return in 3 to 4 weeks."
   ☐ 2. "It will probably be 6 to 10 weeks before it starts again."
   ☐ 3. "You can expect your menses to start in 12 to 14 weeks."
   ☐ 4. "Your menses will return in 16 to 18 weeks."

12. While the nurse is preparing to assist the primiparous client to the bathroom to void 6 hours after a vaginal birth under epidural anesthesia, the client says that they feel dizzy when sitting up on the side of the bed. The nurse explains that this is **most** likely caused by which factor?
   ☐ 1. effects of the anesthetic during labor
   ☐ 2. hemorrhage during the birth process
   ☐ 3. effects of analgesic agents used during labor
   ☐ 4. decreased blood volume in the vascular system

13. Three hours postpartum, a primiparous client's fundus is firm and midline. On perineal inspection, the nurse observes a small, constant trickle of blood. Which condition should the nurse assess further?
   ☐ 1. retained placental tissue
   ☐ 2. uterine inversion
   ☐ 3. bladder distention
   ☐ 4. perineal lacerations

14. At a postpartum checkup 11 days after birth, the nurse asks the client about the color of their lochia. Which color is expected?
   ☐ 1. dark red
   ☐ 2. pink
   ☐ 3. brown
   ☐ 4. white

15. After instructing a primiparous client about suture care after a third-degree laceration repair, the nurse understands that which client statement indicates successful teaching?
   ☐ 1. "I will use hot, sudsy water to clean my stitches."
   ☐ 2. "I wipe the area from front to back using a blotting motion."
   ☐ 3. "Before bedtime, I will use a cold water sitz bath."
   ☐ 4. "I can use ice packs for 3 to 4 days after birth."

16. A primiparous client, 20 hours after birth, asks the nurse about starting postpartum exercises. Which instruction would be **most** appropriate to include in the plan of care?
   ☐ 1. Start in a sitting position, lie back, and then return to a sitting position, repeating this five times.
   ☐ 2. Assume a prone position, and then do push-ups by using the arms to lift the upper body.
   ☐ 3. Flex the knees while supine, and then inhale deeply and exhale while contracting the abdominal muscles.
   ☐ 4. Flex the knees while supine, bring the chin to the chest while exhaling, and then reach for the knees by lifting the head and shoulders while inhaling.

17. A multiparous client whose fundus is firm and midline at the umbilicus 8 hours after a vaginal birth tells the nurse that when they ambulated to the bathroom after sleeping for 4 hours, their dark red lochia seemed heavier. Which information would the nurse include when explaining to the client about the increased lochia on ambulation?
☐ 1. The increased lochia needs to be reported to the health care provider (HCP) immediately.
☐ 2. The increased lochia occurs from lochia pooling in the vaginal vault.
☐ 3. The increase in lochia may be an early sign of postpartum hemorrhage.
☐ 4. This increase in lochia usually indicates retained placental fragments.

18. A primiparous client who gave birth vaginally 8 hours ago desires to take a shower. The nurse anticipates remaining near the client to assess for which problem?
☐ 1. fatigue
☐ 2. fainting
☐ 3. bleeding
☐ 4. hygiene needs

19. A primiparous client who gave birth 12 hours ago under epidural anesthesia with a second-degree laceration tells the nurse that they are experiencing a great deal of discomfort when sitting in a chair with the baby. Which instruction would be **most** appropriate?
☐ 1. "Ask for some pain medication before you sit down."
☐ 2. "Squeeze your buttock muscles together before sitting down."
☐ 3. "Keep a relaxed posture before sitting down with your full weight."
☐ 4. "Ask the health care provider for some analgesic cream or spray."

20. Which information would the nurse include in the primiparous client's discharge teaching plan about measures to provide visual stimulation for the neonate?
☐ 1. Maintain eye contact while talking to the baby.
☐ 2. Paint the baby's room in bright colors accented with teddy bears.
☐ 3. Use brightly colored animals and cartoon figures on the wall.
☐ 4. Move a brightly colored rattle in front of the baby's eyes.

21. An adolescent primiparous client 24 hours postpartum asks the nurse how often they can hold their baby without "spoiling" them. Which response would be **most** appropriate?
☐ 1. "Hold them when they are fussy or crying."
☐ 2. "Hold them as much as you want to hold them."
☐ 3. "Try to hold them infrequently to avoid overstimulation."
☐ 4. "You can hold them periodically throughout the day."

22. On the first postpartum day, the primiparous client reports perineal pain of 5 on a scale of 1 to 10 that was unrelieved by ibuprofen 800 mg given 2 hours ago. The nurse should further assess the client for which complication?
☐ 1. puerperal infection
☐ 2. vaginal lacerations
☐ 3. history of drug abuse
☐ 4. perineal hematoma

23. The nurse working on the postpartum unit is in charge of a team that includes an unlicensed assistive personnel (UAP). Which task would the nurse question if completed by the UAP caring for a client who gave birth 1 day ago?
☐ 1. changing the perineal pad and reporting the drainage
☐ 2. teaching the client to latch the infant onto the breast
☐ 3. reinforcing good hygiene while assisting the client with washing the perineum
☐ 4. assisting the client with ambulation shortly after birth

24. While the nurse is caring for a primiparous client on the first postpartum day, the client asks, "How is that person doing who lost their baby from prematurity? We were in labor together." Which response by the nurse would be **most** appropriate?
☐ 1. Ignore the client's question and continue with morning care.
☐ 2. Tell the client, "I'm not sure how the other person is doing today."
☐ 3. Tell the client, "I need to ask the client's permission before discussing their well-being."
☐ 4. Explain to the client that "nurses are not allowed to discuss other clients on the unit."

25. A newly postpartum primiparous client asks the nurse, "Can my baby see?" Which statement about neonatal vision should the nurse include in the explanation?
☐ 1. Neonates primarily focus on moving objects.
☐ 2. They can see objects up to 12 inches (30.5 cm) away.
☐ 3. Usually they see clearly about 2 days after birth.
☐ 4. Neonates primarily distinguish light from dark.

26. While assessing the fundus of a multiparous client 36 hours after the birth of a term neonate, the nurse notes a separation of the abdominal muscles. What should the nurse tell the client?
☐ 1. that they will have a surgical repair at 6 weeks postpartum
☐ 2. to remain on bed rest until resolution occurs
☐ 3. that the separation will resolve on its own with the right posture and diet
☐ 4. to perform exercises involving head and shoulder raising in a lying position

27. A postpartum client gave birth 6 hours ago without anesthesia and just voided 100 mL. The nurse palpates the fundus 2 fingerbreadths above the umbilicus and off to the right side. What should the nurse do **first**?
☐ 1. Assess the lochia.
☐ 2. Reassess in 1 hour.
☐ 3. Catheterize the client.
☐ 4. Obtain a prescription for a fluid bolus.

28. A primiparous client who gave vaginal birth to a viable term neonate 48 hours ago has a repair of a third-degree laceration. When preparing the client for discharge, the nurse understands that which assessment would be **most** important?
☐ 1. constipation
☐ 2. diarrhea
☐ 3. excessive bleeding
☐ 4. rectal fistulas

29. While caring for a multiparous client 4 hours after the vaginal birth of a term neonate, the nurse notes that the client's temperature is 99.8°F (37.2°C), the pulse is 66 bpm, and the respirations are 18 breaths/min. The fundus is firm, midline, and at the level of the umbilicus. What should the nurse do?
☐ 1. Continue to monitor the client's vital signs.
☐ 2. Assess the client's lochia for large clots.
☐ 3. Notify the client's health care provider (HCP) about the findings.
☐ 4. Offer the client an ice pack for their forehead.

30. While assessing the episiotomy site of a primiparous client on the first postpartum day, the nurse observes a fairly large hemorrhoid at the client's rectum. After instructing the client about measures to relieve hemorrhoid discomfort, which client statement indicates the need for additional teaching?
☐ 1. "I should ask my health care provider about using a stool softener."
☐ 2. "Analgesic sprays and witch hazel pads can relieve the pain."
☐ 3. "I should lie on my back as much as possible to relieve the pain."
☐ 4. "I should drink lots of water and eat foods that have a lot of roughage."

31. A primiparous client is on a regular diet 24 hours postpartum. The client's parent asks the nurse if they can bring some "special foods from home." The nurse responds based on the understanding of which principle?
☐ 1. Foods from home are generally discouraged on the postpartum unit.
☐ 2. The parent can bring the client any foods that they desire.
☐ 3. This is permissible as long as the foods are nutritious and high in iron.
☐ 4. The client's health care provider (HCP) needs to give permission for the foods.

32. A primiparous client, 48 hours after a vaginal birth, is to be discharged with a prescription for vitamins with iron because they are anemic. To maximize absorption of the iron, the nurse instructs the client to take the medication with which liquid?
☐ 1. orange juice
☐ 2. herbal tea
☐ 3. milk
☐ 4. grape juice

33. Twelve hours after a vaginal birth with epidural anesthesia, the nurse palpates the fundus of a primiparous client and finds it to be firm, above the umbilicus, and deviated to the right. What should the nurse do **next**?
☐ 1. Document this as a normal finding in the client's record.
☐ 2. Contact the health care provider (HCP) for a prescription for oxytocin.
☐ 3. Encourage the client to ambulate to the bathroom and void.
☐ 4. Gently massage the fundus to expel the clots.

34. A nurse is discussing discharge instructions with a client. Which statement(s) would indicate that the client understands the discharge instructions? Select all that apply.
☐ 1. "My fertility can return as early as 21 days after my baby's birth."
☐ 2. "I have the hospital phone number if I have any questions."
☐ 3. "If I have any breathing problems, chest pain, or pounding fast heart rate, I will seek medical assistance."
☐ 4. "My parent is coming to help for a month, so I will be fine."
☐ 5. "I know if I get fever or chills or change in lochia to call the health care provider."
☐ 6. "I will continue my prenatal vitamins until my postpartum checkup or longer."

The Postpartum Client Who Breastfeeds

35. The nurse is reviewing discharge instructions with a postpartum breastfeeding client who is going home. They have chosen depot medroxyprogesterone acetate (DMPA) injections as birth control. Which statement by the client identifies that they need further instruction concerning birth control?
☐ 1. "I will wait for my 6-week checkup to get my first birth control injection."
☐ 2. "Depot injections last for 90 days."
☐ 3. "My milk supply should be well established before receiving a birth control injection."
☐ 4. "You will give me my first depot injection before I leave today."

36. A postpartum primiparous client is having difficulty breastfeeding their infant. The infant latches on to the breast, but the client's nipples are extremely sore during and after each feeding. The client needs further instruction about breastfeeding when they make which statement?
☐ 1. "The baby needs to have as much of the nipple and areola in the mouth as possible to prevent sore and cracked nipples."
☐ 2. "I can put breast milk on my nipples to heal the sore areas."
☐ 3. "As long as some of my nipple is in the baby's mouth, the baby will receive enough milk."
☐ 4. "Feeding the baby for a half-hour on each side will not make my breasts sore."

37. The nurse is caring for a primipara who gave birth yesterday and has chosen to breastfeed their neonate. Which assessment finding is considered unusual for the client at this point postpartum?
☐ 1. milk production
☐ 2. diaphoresis
☐ 3. constipation
☐ 4. diuresis

38. The nurse is caring for several birth mother and baby couplets. In planning the care for each of the couplets, the nurse would expect which birth mother to have the **most** severe afterbirth pains?
☐ 1. G4, P1 client who is breastfeeding their infant
☐ 2. G3, P3 client who is breastfeeding their infant
☐ 3. G2, P2 client who had a cesarean birth and who is bottle-feeding their infant
☐ 4. G3, P3 client who is bottle-feeding their infant

39. A breastfeeding client is seen at home by the visiting nurse 10 days after a vaginal birth. The client has a warm, red, painful breast, a temperature of 100°F (37.7°C), and flulike symptoms. What should the nurse do?
☐ 1. Encourage the client to breastfeed their infant using the unaffected breast.
☐ 2. Refer the client to their health care provider (HCP).
☐ 3. Inform the client that they need to discontinue breastfeeding.
☐ 4. Instruct the client to apply warm compresses to the affected breast.

40. A client with diabetes who just gave birth plans to breastfeed. The nurse determines that the client's understanding of breastfeeding instructions is sufficient when the client makes which statement?
☐ 1. "Insulin will be transferred to the baby through breast milk."
☐ 2. "Breastfeeding is not recommended for birth mothers with diabetes."
☐ 3. "Breast milk from birth mothers with diabetes contains few antibodies."
☐ 4. "Breastfeeding will assist in lowering maternal blood glucose."

41. A 1-day-old breastfed infant has a bilirubin level that is an intermediate risk for jaundice. Which statement by the infant's parent indicates an understanding of the teaching regarding jaundice?
☐ 1. "I should breastfeed my baby as often as possible."
☐ 2. "I should supplement with formula after every feeding."
☐ 3. "I should discontinue breastfeeding and change to formula feeding."
☐ 4. "I should place my baby in direct sunlight several times a day."

42. During a home visit, a breastfeeding client asks the nurse what contraception method they should use until their 6-week postpartum examination. Which method would be **most** appropriate for the nurse to suggest?
☐ 1. condom with spermicide
☐ 2. oral contraceptives
☐ 3. rhythm method
☐ 4. abstinence

43. A primiparous client who is beginning to breastfeed their neonate asks the nurse, "Is it important for my baby to get colostrum?" When instructing the client, the nurse would explain that colostrum provides the neonate with which factor?
☐ 1. more fat than breast milk
☐ 2. vitamin K, which the neonate lacks
☐ 3. delayed meconium passage
☐ 4. passive immunity from maternal antibodies

44. Which principle forms the basis for the teaching plan about avoiding nonprescription medication for a primiparous client who is breastfeeding?
☐ 1. Breast milk quality and richness are decreased.
☐ 2. The parent's motivation to breastfeed is diminished.
☐ 3. Medications may be excreted in breast milk to the nursing neonate.
☐ 4. Medications interfere with the parent's letdown reflex.

45. A multiparous client, 28 hours after cesarean birth, who is breastfeeding has severe cramps or afterpains. The nurse explains that these are caused by which factor?
☐ 1. flatulence accumulation after a cesarean birth
☐ 2. healing of the abdominal incision after cesarean birth
☐ 3. adverse effects of the medications administered after birth
☐ 4. release of oxytocin during the breastfeeding session

46. After the nurse counsels a primiparous, breastfeeding client about diet and nutritional needs during the lactation period, which client statement indicates a need for additional teaching?
☐ 1. "I need to increase my intake of vitamin D."
☐ 2. "I should drink at least five glasses of fluid daily."
☐ 3. "I need to get an extra 500 calories a day."
☐ 4. "I need to make sure I have enough calcium in my diet."

47. While assisting a primiparous client with their first breastfeeding session, the nurse should instruct the client to perform which action to stimulate the neonate to open the mouth and grasp the nipple?
☐ 1. Pull down gently on the neonate's chin and insert the nipple.
☐ 2. Squeeze both of the neonate's cheeks simultaneously.
☐ 3. Place the nipple into the neonate's mouth on top of the tongue.
☐ 4. Brush the neonate's lips lightly with the nipple.

48. A 25-year-old primiparous client who gave birth 2 hours ago has decided to breastfeed their neonate. Which instructions should the nurse address as the **highest priority** in the teaching plan about preventing nipple soreness?
☐ 1. keeping plastic liners in the brassiere to keep the nipple drier
☐ 2. placing as much of the areola as possible into the baby's mouth
☐ 3. smoothly pulling the nipple out of the mouth after 10 minutes
☐ 4. removing any remaining milk left on the nipple with a soft washcloth

49. After the nurse teaches a primiparous client planning to return to work about storing breast milk, which client statement indicates the need for further teaching?
☐ 1. "I can safely store freshly expressed breast milk at room temperature for 8 hours."
☐ 2. "I will be sure to label the breast milk with the date, time, and amount."
☐ 3. "I must discard any breast milk stored for more than 3 days in the refrigerator."
☐ 4. "I can keep the breast milk in a deep freeze in clean glass bottles for up to 1 year."

50. During a home visit on the fourth postpartum day, a primiparous client tells the nurse that they are aware of a "letdown sensation" in their breasts and asks what causes it. The nurse explains that the letdown sensation is stimulated by which hormone?
☐ 1. progesterone
☐ 2. estrogen
☐ 3. prolactin
☐ 4. oxytocin

51. A telehealth nurse receives a call from a breastfeeding 25-year-old female client who gave birth 4 weeks ago.

> **Nurse's Notes**
>
> **1000:**
> The client reports the infant has been breastfeeding well every 2 ½ to 3 hours, but this morning the client found a movable lump on the left breast. The client reports that the lump is painful but not red. The pain was worst during letdown but got better after feeding. The client also reports having symptoms of an upper respiratory infection and nasal congestion. The client denies any fever.

The nurse begins planning the client's care.

➤ Complete the diagram by circling the choices below to specify the condition the client is **most** likely experiencing, two actions to take, and two parameters the nurse should monitor for complications.

Action to Take — Condition Most Likely Experiencing — Parameter to Monitor
Action to Take — Parameter to Monitor

Action to Take	Potential Conditions	Parameters to Monitor
Request prescription for antibiotics	Mastitis	Temperature
Arrange a same-day office appointment	Breast abscess	Milk production
Encourage the use of moist heat	Plugged milk duct	Flulike symptoms
Schedule a mammogram	Breast cancer	Bruising or bleeding
Teach feeding techniques		Right breast changes

52. During a home visit on the fourth postpartum day, a primiparous client tells the nurse that they have been experiencing breast engorgement. To relieve engorgement, the nurse teaches the client to use which intervention before nursing their baby?
☐ 1. Apply an ice cube to the nipples.
☐ 2. Rub the nipples gently with lanolin cream.
☐ 3. Express a small amount of breast milk.
☐ 4. Offer the neonate a small amount of formula.

53. A breastfeeding primiparous client who gave birth 8 hours ago asks the nurse, "How will I know that my baby is getting enough to eat?" Which guideline should the nurse include in the teaching plan as evidence of adequate intake?
☐ 1. six to eight wet diapers by the fifth day
☐ 2. three to four transitional stools on the fourth day
☐ 3. ability to fall asleep easily after feeding on the first day
☐ 4. regain of lost birth weight by the third day

54. Which information should the nurse include in the teaching plan for a primiparous client who asks about weaning their neonate?
☐ 1. "Wait until you have breastfed for at least 4 months."
☐ 2. "Eliminate the baby's favorite feeding times first."
☐ 3. "Plan to omit the daytime feedings last."
☐ 4. "Gradually eliminate one feeding at a time."

55. A nurse is caring for a client who is 3 days postpartum and breastfeeding their baby. The nurse assesses that the episiotomy area is red and edematous; the breasts are firm and tender on palpation; and the fundus is firm and 2 fingerbreadths below the umbilicus. Which nursing action(s) would be indicated? Select all that apply.
☐ 1. Suggest that the client apply cool compresses to the breasts.
☐ 2. Encourage the client to sit on a supportive device.
☐ 3. Ask the client how often the baby feeds.
☐ 4. Suggest the client take cool sitz baths twice a day.
☐ 5. Obtain a specimen for culture and sensitivity from the episiotomy site.

56. Two weeks after a breastfeeding primiparous client is discharged, they call the birthing center and say that they are afraid they are "losing my breast milk. The baby had been nursing every 3 hours, but now the baby is crying to be fed every 2 hours." The nurse interprets the neonate's behavior as **most** likely caused by which factor?
☐ 1. lack of adequate intake to meet maternal nutritional needs
☐ 2. the client's fears about the baby's weight gain
☐ 3. preventing the neonate from sucking long enough with each feeding
☐ 4. the neonate's temporary growth spurt, which requires more feedings

57. During a home visit to a breastfeeding primiparous client 1 week after birth, the client tells the nurse that their nipples have become sore and cracked from the feedings. Which instruction should the nurse give the client?
☐ 1. Wipe off any lanolin creams from the nipple before each feeding.
☐ 2. Position the baby with as much of the areola as possible in the baby's mouth.
☐ 3. Feed the baby less often for the next several days.
☐ 4. Use a mild soap while in the shower to prevent an infection.

58. A new parent feels left out of the new family relationship because they are not bonding with the infant in the same way as the breastfeeding birth mother. What is the **most** appropriate response by the nurse?
☐ 1. "This is normal, and these feelings will go away within a few days."
☐ 2. "Holding, talking to, and playing with the infant will facilitate bonding."
☐ 3. "Bonding occurs later in the first year of life, and you become involved when the infant is better able to recognize you."
☐ 4. "Maternal infant bonding takes priority over other infant bonding."

59. The triage nurse in the pediatrician's office returns a call to a birth parent who is breastfeeding their 4-day-old infant. The parent is concerned about the yellow seedy stool that has developed since discharge home. What is the **best** reply by the nurse?
☐ 1. "This type of stool indicates the infant may have diarrhea and should be seen in the office today."
☐ 2. "The stool will transition into a soft, brown, formed stool within a few days and is appropriate for breastfeeding."
☐ 3. "The stool results from the gassy food eaten by the birth parent. Refrain from eating these foods while breastfeeding."
☐ 4. "Soft, seedy, unformed stools with each feeding are normal for this age infant and will continue through breastfeeding."

The Postpartum Client Who Bottle-feeds

60. The nurse is assessing a client at a postpartum checkup 6 weeks after a vaginal birth. The client is bottle-feeding their baby. Which client finding indicates a problem at this time?
☐ 1. firm fundus at the symphysis
☐ 2. menstrual discharge
☐ 3. striae that are silver in color
☐ 4. soft breasts without milk

61. A client gave birth 2 days ago and has been given instructions on breast care for bottle-feeding birth parents. Which statement indicates that the nurse should reinforce the instructions to the client?
☐ 1. "I will wear a sports bra or a well-fitting bra for several days."
☐ 2. "When showering, I will direct water onto my shoulders."
☐ 3. "I will use only water to clean my nipples."
☐ 4. "I will use a breast pump to remove any milk that may appear."

62. A 24-year-old primipara who has given birth to a healthy neonate plans to bottle-feed their neonate. What information regarding normal weight gain should the nurse include in the teaching plan?
☐ 1. A baby normally loses 15% of weight before beginning to gain weight.
☐ 2. Adding rice cereal to the bottle is a good way to increase calories if weight gain is slow.
☐ 3. Gaining 30 g a day is a normal weight gain pattern.
☐ 4. Babies typically double their birth weight by 3 months.

63. A primiparous client with a neonate who is 36 hours old asks the nurse, "Why does my baby spit up a small amount of formula after feeding?" The nurse explains that the regurgitation is thought to result from which factor?
☐ 1. an immature cardiac sphincter
☐ 2. a defect in the gastrointestinal system
☐ 3. burping the infant too frequently
☐ 4. moving the infant during the feeding

64. A primiparous client who will be bottle-feeding their neonate asks, "What is the **best** position for the baby to nap after feeding?" What should the nurse recommend?
☐ 1. Place the baby in a supine position after feedings.
☐ 2. Keep the baby wedged on their left side 20 minutes after feedings.
☐ 3. Place the baby prone after feedings if they spit up frequently.
☐ 4. Hold the baby upright for 15 to 20 minutes before placing them down for a nap.

65. A primiparous client who is bottle-feeding their neonate asks, "When should I start giving the baby solid foods?" The nurse instructs the client to introduce solid foods no sooner than at which age?
☐ 1. 2 months
☐ 2. 6 months
☐ 3. 8 months
☐ 4. 10 months

66. After instructing a primiparous client who is bottle-feeding about burping, which client statement indicates that the client needs further teaching?
☐ 1. "I will burp them after 15 minutes of feeding them formula."
☐ 2. "After they take a half-ounce of formula, I will burp them."
☐ 3. "I will burp them while they are in an upright position."
☐ 4. "I will gently pat their back to get them to burp."

67. The nurse reviews the contraception choices of a bottle-feeding postpartum client prior to discharge. The client wants to know why they need to wait to resume the use of oral contraceptives. What is the nurse's **best** response?
☐ 1. "The estrogen in combined hormonal contraceptives interferes with the involution process."
☐ 2. "Clients cannot resume intercourse for 6 weeks after birth, so contraception is not needed."
☐ 3. "Combined oral contraceptives potentiate the risk for blood clots immediately after birth."
☐ 4. "The risk for bleeding is increased from the progestin in combined hormonal contraceptives."

The Postpartum Client with a Cesarean Birth

68. The nurse places inflatable compression sleeves on the legs of a client undergoing a cesarean birth under a regional anesthetic. When does the nurse tell the client that the sleeves will be removed?
☐ 1. after sensation returns to the lower extremities
☐ 2. when the platelet levels return to normal
☐ 3. when the client resumes ambulating
☐ 4. just prior to the client's discharge

69. The nurse is assessing a client who had a cesarean birth 12 hours ago. Findings include a distended abdomen with faint bowel sounds, a firm fundus at the umbilicus, scant lochia rubra, and pain rated as a 2 on a scale of 0 to 10. The intravenous line and Foley catheter have been discontinued, and the client received medication 3 hours ago for pain. The client can have pain medication every 3 to 4 hours. What should the nurse do **first**?
☐ 1. Give the client pain medication.
☐ 2. Have the client use incentive spirometry.
☐ 3. Ambulate the client from the bed to the hallway and back.
☐ 4. Encourage the client to begin caring for their baby.

70. Carboprost was injected into the uterus of a client to treat uterine atony during a cesarean birth. In preparing to care for this client after birth, the nurse should assess the client for which common adverse effects of the medication?
☐ 1. vertigo and confusion
☐ 2. nausea and diarrhea
☐ 3. restlessness and increased vaginal bleeding
☐ 4. headache and hypertension

71. A multigravida 30-year-old client has given cesarean birth to a healthy term neonate due to an abnormal fetal heart rate tracing. At 2 hours after birth, the nurse assesses the client's urinary catheter and observes that the client's urine is slightly red-tinged. What should the nurse do **next**?
☐ 1. Continue to monitor the client's input and output.
☐ 2. Palpate the client's fundus gently every 15 minutes.
☐ 3. Assess the placement of the Foley catheter.
☐ 4. Contact the client's health care provider (HCP) for further instructions.

72. Four hours after the cesarean birth of a neonate weighing 4000 g (8 lb, 13 oz), the primiparous client asks, "If I get pregnant again, will I need to have a cesarean?" When responding to the client, the nurse should base the response to the client about vaginal birth after cesarean (VBAC) on which standard of practice?
☐ 1. VBAC may be possible if the client has not had a classic uterine incision.
☐ 2. A history of rapid labor is a necessary criterion for VBAC.
☐ 3. A low transverse incision contraindicates the possibility for VBAC.
☐ 4. VBAC is not possible because the neonate was large for gestational age.

73. A primiparous client who underwent a cesarean birth 30 minutes ago is to receive Rho(D) immune globulin. The nurse should administer the medication within which time frame after birth?
☐ 1. 12 hours
☐ 2. 24 hours
☐ 3. 48 hours
☐ 4. 72 hours

74. While the nurse is caring for a primiparous client with cephalopelvic disproportion 4 hours after a cesarean birth, the client requests assistance in breastfeeding. To promote maximum maternal comfort, which position would be **most** appropriate for the nurse to suggest?
☐ 1. football hold
☐ 2. scissors hold
☐ 3. cross-cradle hold
☐ 4. cradle hold

The Postpartum Client with Complications

75. A multigravida client gave birth vaginally 2 hours ago. A family member notifies the nurse that the client is pale and shaky. Which are the **priority** assessments for the nurse to make?
☐ 1. blood glucose and vital signs
☐ 2. temperature and level of consciousness
☐ 3. uterine infection and pain
☐ 4. fundus and lochia

76. A postpartum client has unrelenting pain in their rectum after vaginal birth despite the administration of pain medications. Which action is **most** indicated?
☐ 1. administering additional pain medications
☐ 2. assessing the perineum
☐ 3. reassuring the client that pain is normal after vaginal birth
☐ 4. preparing a warm sitz bath for the client

77. A multiparous client at 24 hours postpartum is found to have swelling and pain in their right leg. What should the nurse do **next**?
☐ 1. Place a cold pack on the client's perineal area.
☐ 2. Place the client in a semi-Fowler position.
☐ 3. Notify the client's health care provider (HCP) immediately.
☐ 4. Ask the client to ambulate around the room.

78. Prophylactic heparin therapy is prescribed to treat thrombophlebitis in a multiparous client who gave birth 24 hours ago. After instructing the client about the medication, the nurse determines that the client understands the instructions when they state which effect is the purpose of the drug?
☐ 1. to thin the blood clots
☐ 2. to increase the flow of lochia
☐ 3. to increase the perspiration for diuresis
☐ 4. to prevent further blood clot formation

79. While caring for a postpartum client who is receiving treatment with bed rest and intravenous heparin therapy for deep vein thrombosis, the nurse should contact the client's health care provider (HCP) immediately if the client exhibits which symptom?
☐ 1. pain in their calf
☐ 2. dyspnea
☐ 3. hypertension
☐ 4. bradycardia

80. A primiparous client who gave birth 3 days ago is to be discharged on heparin therapy. After teaching the client about the possible adverse effects of heparin therapy, the nurse determines that the client needs further instruction when they state that the adverse effects include which symptom?
☐ 1. epistaxis
☐ 2. bleeding gums
☐ 3. slow pulse
☐ 4. petechiae

81. After being treated with heparin therapy for thrombophlebitis, a multiparous client who gave birth 4 days ago is to be discharged on oral warfarin. After the nurse teaches the client about the medication and its possible effects, which client statement indicates successful teaching?
☐ 1. "I can take ibuprofen if I get uterine cramps."
☐ 2. "I will need my international normalized ratio (INR) drawn every week."
☐ 3. "I should use only waxed dental floss when caring for my teeth."
☐ 4. "I need to refrain from eating green leafy vegetables."

82. A nurse is explaining basic principles of asepsis and infection control to a client who has a respiratory tract infection after birth. The nurse determines that the client understands the principles of infection control to follow when the client makes which statement?
☐ 1. "I must ask visitors to wear a mask."
☐ 2. "I must wear gloves when I handle my baby."
☐ 3. "I must use individual client care equipment."
☐ 4. "I must practice frequent handwashing."

83. The nurse is caring for a client who gave birth vaginally 4 hours ago. Which factors would likely contribute to the development of endometritis in this client? Select all that apply.
☐ 1. manual removal of the placenta
☐ 2. in-and-out catheterization during labor
☐ 3. epidural use
☐ 4. prolonged labor
☐ 5. placement of a fetal scalp electrode

84. Which intervention would be **most** important for the nurse to encourage in a primiparous client diagnosed with endometritis who is receiving intravenous antibiotic therapy?
☐ 1. Ambulate to the bathroom frequently.
☐ 2. Discontinue breastfeeding temporarily.
☐ 3. Facilitate drainage in an upright position.
☐ 4. Restrict visitors to prevent contamination.

85. Which measure would the nurse expect to include in the teaching plan for a multiparous client who gave birth 24 hours ago and is receiving intravenous antibiotic therapy for cystitis?
☐ 1. limiting fluid intake to 1 L daily to prevent overload
☐ 2. emptying the bladder every 2 to 4 hours while awake
☐ 3. washing the perineum with povidone-iodine after voiding
☐ 4. avoiding the intake of acidic fruit juices until the treatment is discontinued

86. A primiparous client diagnosed with cystitis at 48 hours postpartum who is receiving intravenous ampicillin asks the nurse, "Can I still continue to breastfeed my baby?" What should the nurse tell the client?
☐ 1. "You can continue to breastfeed as long as you want to do so."
☐ 2. "Alternate your breastfeeding with formula feeding to help you rest."
☐ 3. "You will need to discontinue breastfeeding until the antibiotic therapy is stopped."
☐ 4. "You will need to modify your technique by manually pumping your breasts."

87. Four days after a vaginal birth, a client has excessive lochia rubra with clots. The health care provider (HCP) prescribes carboprost 0.25 mg intramuscularly. Which statement by the client reflects the need for more teaching about carboprost?
☐ 1. "This medication may cause nausea and vomiting."
☐ 2. "This medication sometimes causes hypotension that leads to dizziness."
☐ 3. "I will also receive medication to help prevent severe diarrhea."
☐ 4. "I may run a fever after being treated with carboprost."

88. During the first hour after birth, the assessment of a multiparous client who gave cesarean birth to a neonate weighing 4593 g (10 lb, 2 oz) reveals a soft fundus with excessive lochia rubra. The nurse should include which intervention in the client's plan of care?
☐ 1. administration of intravenous oxytocin
☐ 2. placement of the client in a side-lying position
☐ 3. rigorous fundal massage every 5 minutes
☐ 4. preparation for an emergency hysterectomy

89. A primiparous client who was diagnosed with hydramnios and breech presentation while in early labor is diagnosed with early postpartum hemorrhage 1 hour after a cesarean birth. The client asks, "Why am I bleeding so much?" The nurse responds based on the understanding that the **most** likely cause of uterine atony in this client is which factor?
☐ 1. trauma during labor and birth
☐ 2. moderate fundal massage after birth
☐ 3. lengthy and prolonged second stage of labor
☐ 4. overdistention of the uterus from hydramnios

90. Thirty-six hours after a vaginal birth, a multiparous client is diagnosed with endometritis. When assessing the client, the nurse would expect to find which symptom?
☐ 1. profuse amounts of lochia
☐ 2. abdominal distention
☐ 3. nausea and vomiting
☐ 4. fever higher than 100.4°F (38.0°C)

91. A multiparous client visits the urgent care center 5 days after a vaginal birth and reports experiencing moderate to heavy and persistent lochia rubra. The client asks the nurse, "Why am I continuing to bleed like this?" The nurse should instruct the client that this type of postpartum bleeding is **most** likely caused by which problem?
☐ 1. uterine atony
☐ 2. cervical lacerations
☐ 3. vaginal lacerations
☐ 4. retained placental fragments

92. A 26-year-old primiparous client is seen in the urgent care clinic 2 weeks after giving birth. The client, who is breastfeeding, is diagnosed with mastitis of the right breast. The client asks the nurse, "Can I continue breastfeeding?" What should the nurse tell the client?
☐ 1. "You can continue to breastfeed, feeding your baby more frequently."
☐ 2. "You can continue once your symptoms begin to decrease."
☐ 3. "You must discontinue breastfeeding until antibiotic therapy is completed."
☐ 4. "You must stop breastfeeding because the breast is contaminated."

93. A primiparous client who had a vaginal birth 1 hour ago voices anxiety because they have a nephew with Down syndrome. After teaching the client about Down syndrome, the nurse understands that which client statement indicates the need for additional teaching?
☐ 1. "Down syndrome is an abnormality that can result from a missing chromosome."
☐ 2. "Down syndrome usually results in some degree of intellectual disability."
☐ 3. "There are several methods available to determine whether my baby has Down syndrome."
☐ 4. "Older birth parents are more likely to have a baby with chromosomal abnormalities."

94. A 15-year-old primiparous client is being cared for in the hospital's birthing center after the vaginal birth of a viable neonate. The neonate is being placed for adoption through a social service agency. Four hours after birth, the client asks if they can feed their baby. Which response would be **most** appropriate?
☐ 1. "I'll bring the baby to you for feeding."
☐ 2. "I think we should ask your health care provider (HCP) if this is a good idea."
☐ 3. "It's not a good idea for you to have any contact with the baby."
☐ 4. "I'll check with the social worker to see if the adopting parents will permit this."

95. After teaching a primiparous client about treatment and self-care of mastitis of the right breast, the nurse determines that the client needs further instruction when they make which statement?
☐ 1. "I can apply localized heat to the infected area."
☐ 2. "I should increase my fluid intake to 2000 mL a day."
☐ 3. "I will need to take antibiotics for 7 to 10 days before I am cured."
☐ 4. "I should begin breastfeeding on the right side to decrease the pain."

96. A breastfeeding postpartum client experiencing breast engorgement tells the nurse that they have applied cabbage leaves to decrease their breast discomfort. What is the nurse's **best** response?
☐ 1. "Using cabbage leaves to relieve engorgement is considered a folk remedy."
☐ 2. "I'm concerned that the cabbage leaves may harm your nursing baby."
☐ 3. "I need to notify your health care provider immediately that you're using cabbage leaves."
☐ 4. "Let me know if you get relief using the cabbage leaves."

97. During a home visit to a primiparous client who gave birth vaginally 14 days ago, the client says, "I've been crying a lot the last few days. I just feel so awful. I'm a rotten parent. I just don't have any energy. Plus, my spouse just got laid off from their job." The nurse observes that the client's appearance is disheveled. What would be the nurse's **best** response?
☐ 1. "These feelings commonly indicate symptoms of postpartum blues and are normal. They will go away in a few days."
☐ 2. "You're doing the best you can as a parent. You should accept help from friends and family while you recover from birth."
☐ 3. "It's not unusual for some parents to feel depressed after the birth of a baby. I'm going to contact your health care provider (HCP)."
☐ 4. "This may be a symptom of a serious mental illness. I think you should probably go to the hospital."

98. A teen client, who gave birth 1 week ago, is concerned about the possibility of postpartum depression because they have a history of depression. Which comment by the client would indicate that they understood the nurse's teaching about the postpartum period and their risks for postpartum depression?
☐ 1. "Sleep should not be too much of a problem because the baby will soon start to sleep through the night."
☐ 2. "Since I am breastfeeding, I can eat all the food I want and not feel fat. The baby will use all the calories."
☐ 3. "If I'm feeling guilty or not capable of caring for the baby and am not sleeping or eating well, I need to contact the office."
☐ 4. "I'm going to give the baby the best care possible without asking anyone for help to show all those people who think I can't do it."

99. A multigravida prenatal client with a history of postpartum depression tells the nurse that they are taking measures to make sure they do not suffer that complication, including taking St. John's wort. What is the **most** important assessment for the nurse to make?
☐ 1. current medications
☐ 2. fetal growth
☐ 3. liver functions
☐ 4. mood status

Managing Care, Quality, and Safety of Postpartum Clients

100. The nurse is catheterizing a client who cannot void after a normal birth 8 hours ago. The nurse begins the catheterization process, and the client states, "I forgot to tell the nurse I get hives to povidone-iodine." The nurse should take which steps in order of priority from first to last? All options must be used.

1. Document the incident.

2. Clean the povidone-iodine from the client's vaginal area.

3. Notify the health care provider (HCP) prescribing catheterization.

4. File an incident report.

101. A nurse is walking down the hall in the main corridor of a hospital when the infant security alert system sounds and a code for an infant abduction is announced. The **first** responsibility of the nurse when this situation occurs is to take which action?
☐ 1. Move to the entrance of the hospital, and check each person leaving.
☐ 2. Go to the obstetrics unit to determine if they need help with the situation.
☐ 3. Call the nursery to ask which baby is missing.
☐ 4. Observe individuals in the area for large bags or oversized coats.

102. The nurse on a birth mother and baby unit who is working on the night shift is revising the planning worksheet for the remaining 2 hours of the shift. The nurse has tasks and prescriptions to complete prior to the change of shift at 0700. Using the work plan below, how should the nurse organize the tasks from first to last so that everything is completed by 0700? All options must be used.

1. Draw blood for the prescribed laboratory tests (complete blood counts [CBCs]) on three postpartum clients with a report on medical records by shift change.

2. Start an intravenous (IV) line of dextrose 5% in 0.45% saline at keep vein open (KVO) rate on a postpartum client just prior to the change of shift.

3. Complete the admission assessment of a newborn turned over to the nurse at 0500.

4. Draw a newborn's bilirubin level at 0600.

103. A nurse is caring for a client who gave birth to their baby boy 2 hours ago. The nurse notes that the client's perineal pad contains some small clots and a moderate amount of lochia has accumulated under the buttocks. What is the **first** action the nurse should take at this time?
☐ 1. Request a prescription to administer oxytocin.
☐ 2. Perform an in-and-out catheter immediately.
☐ 3. Measure blood loss by measuring the perineal pad.
☐ 4. Check the fundus for position and consistency.

104. The nurse is reviewing the laboratory values on the medical record of a client who gave birth 2 days ago.

Laboratory Results

Value	Units	Normal Range
White Blood Cell (WBC)	18,000 (18 x/L)	4.5 – 10.5 x 10^3 cells/mm³ (4.5 – 10.5 x 10^9/L)
Hematocrit	40% (0.40%)	36% to 48% (0.36 to 0.48)
Hemoglobin (Hgb)	9 g/dL (90 g/L)	12 to 16 g/dL (120 to 160 g/L)
Platelets	400,000 (40 x/L)	40,000 to 400,000/μL (140 to 400 × 10^9/L).

Based on this information, what should the nurse do?
☐ 1. Contact the health care provider (HCP).
☐ 2. Obtain a prescription for intravenous antibiotics.
☐ 3. Assess the client's vital signs.
☐ 4. Prepare to administer pain medication.

105. The nurse assesses a client, who delivered vaginally 6 days ago, during a home visit. Which finding(s) should the nurse report **immediately** to the health care provider (HCP)? Select all that apply.
☐ 1. foul-smelling lochia
☐ 2. engorged breasts bilaterally
☐ 3. client who cries easily
☐ 4. soaking one peripad every 3 to 4 hours
☐ 5. temperature of 100.8°F (38.2°C)

106. The night nurse has completed the change of shift report. As the day nurse makes rounds on a postpartum client receiving magnesium sulfate for preeclampsia, the magnesium sulfate rate is found to be infusing well below the prescribed rate. After the nurse adjusts the infusion rate and notifies the health care provider (HCP), what is the **most** important action by the nurse?
☐ 1. Complete an incident report.
☐ 2. Discuss the matter with the nurse the next time they work.
☐ 3. Ask the charge nurse if an incident report is necessary.
☐ 4. Evaluate the client's vital signs for 4 hours before making a decision.

107. The nurse is serving on the Quality Improvement Committee for the maternity unit. Quality improvement projects for this unit impacting safety and quality of care include which project(s)? Select all that apply.
☐ 1. use of recycling bins on the unit
☐ 2. infant identification system
☐ 3. sibling and family visitation policies
☐ 4. postpartum discharge instructions
☐ 5. rooming-in guidelines

108. A nurse working on the postpartum unit is asked to participate in the unit Client Safety Committee. What type of project(s) would the committee conduct for the unit? Select all that apply.
☐ 1. prevention of infant abduction
☐ 2. safe medication administration
☐ 3. adequate nourishment on unit
☐ 4. proper restraints during procedures
☐ 5. maternal/infant identification system

109. A nurse who works on an obstetric inpatient unit has been assigned to the client safety committee. What client safety goal(s) would be **most** applicable to this setting? Select all that apply.
☐ 1. completing effective and timely "hand-off reports" between labor and birth staff and birth mother and baby staff
☐ 2. ensuring that preprocedural verifications are completed by health care providers (HCPs) for any invasive procedure
☐ 3. involving clients in education about cord infections
☐ 4. identifying safety risks specific to the unit, such as infant abduction
☐ 5. performing car seat instruction that allows infants to ride facing backward in the front seat

110. The nurse is making a postpartum visit to the home of a client who gave birth 14 days earlier. After assessing the vital signs (temperature, 99°F [37.2°C]; pulse, 88 bpm; respiration rate, 20 breaths/min; and blood pressure, 112/60 mm Hg), the nurse records the other assessments. (See exhibit.)

Physical Assessment	
Breasts	Soft + Firm − Nipples intact + Cracks − Blisters −
Heart	Regular rate, 88
Lungs	Clear +
Abdomen	Soft + Distended − Bowel sounds + Fundus firm + Midline + 4 CM↓U Nontender + Bladder empty +
Perineum	Midline episiotomy redness − Ecchymosis − Edema − Discharge − Approximated + Hemorrhoids −
Lochia	Serosa scant
Extremities	Legs: 1+ ankles edema Redness − Tenderness − Homans −

Which finding indicates delayed involution?
☐ 1. vital signs
☐ 2. fundus
☐ 3. lochia
☐ 4. edema of the ankles

Answers, Rationales, and Test-Taking Strategies

*The answers and rationales for each question follow below, along with keys (🔑) to the client need (CN) and cognitive level (CL) for each question. In addition, questions that measure clinical judgment will be coded (CJ). As you check your answers, use the **Content Mastery and Test-Taking Skill Self-Analysis worksheet** (tear-out worksheet in the back of the book) to identify the reason(s) for not answering the questions correctly. For additional information about test-taking skills and strategies for answering questions, refer to pages 12–51 in Part 1 of this book.*

The Postpartum Client with a Vaginal Birth

1. **4.** The hospital identification procedures for clients and infants need to be completed each time a newborn is returned to a family's room. It does not matter how well the nurse knows the client and infant; this validation is a standard of care in an obstetric setting. Assessing the client's ability to ambulate, asking if there is anything else the client needs to care for the infant, and checking the crib to determine if there are enough supplies are important steps that are part of the process of transferring a baby to the client, but identification verification is a safety measure that must occur first.

   🔑 CN: Safety and infection control; CL: Create

2. **3.** At any point in the postpartum period, the lochia should be dark in color rather than bright red. The volume should not be great enough to trickle or run from the vagina. The information provided states the fundus is firm, midline, and at the umbilicus, which are the expected outcomes at this point after birth. These findings would indicate to the nurse that the bleeding is not coming from the uterus or from uterine atony. The bladder is not palpable, which indicates that the bleeding is not related to a full bladder, which is further validated by the fundus being at the umbilicus. The most likely etiology is cervical or vaginal lacerations or tears. The nurse is unable to do anything to stop this type of bleeding and request that the HCP assess the client. massaging the fundus does not decrease the amount or type of vaginal bleeding from a laceration or tear. Rechecking the hematocrit and hemoglobin will only provide background information for the nurse and identify the beginning levels for this client, rather than where they are now. It will do nothing

to stop the bleeding. The bleeding level and color are not normal, and documenting such findings as normal is incorrect.

🔑 CN: Management of care; CL: Analyze

3. 4. Within the first 24 hours postpartum, maternal temperature may increase to 100.4°F (38°C), a normal postpartum finding attributed to dehydration. A temperature above 100.4°F (38°C) after the first 24 hours indicates a potential for infection. The hemoglobin is in the normal range. The WBC count is normally elevated as a response to the inflammation, pain, and stress of the birthing process. A pulse rate of 60 bpm is normal at this period and results from an increased cardiac output (mobilization of excess extracellular fluid into the vascular bed, decreased pressure from the uterus on vessels, blood flow back to the heart from the uterus returning to the central circulation) and alteration in stroke volume.

🔑 CN: Physiological adaptation; CL: Analyze

4. –/+ **1, 2, 3, 5.** Outcome evaluation for a family about 7 days after birth would include a client who is tired but is able to care for themselves and the baby. Having adequate support systems enables the client to care better for themselves and family members, as they can provide the backup for situations that may arise and are a resource for new families. The normal progression for lochia is to change from red to pink to off-white while decreasing in amount. This is within the usual time periods for a postpartum client. The baby should be feeding more frequently than every 6 to 8 hours. It is expected that a 7-day-old infant feeds every 3 to 4 hours if bottle-feeding and every 1½ to 3 hours if breastfeeding. Follow-up questions the nurse would ask to further evaluate this situation include "How many wet diapers does the infant have daily? How alert is the infant? Did the infant gain any weight at the first checkup?" It is expected that the client has positive comments about the infant, but the nurse will evaluate to determine if there is at least one positive comment.

🔑 CN: Management of care; CL: Evaluate

5. 2. Pain medication is the first strategy to initiate at this pain level. When trauma has occurred in any area, the usual intervention is ice for the first 24 hours and heat after the first 24 hours. Sitz baths are initiated at the conclusion of ice therapy. Ice has already been initiated and will prevent further edema to the rectal sphincter and perineum and continue to reduce some of the pain. Anesthetic sprays can also be utilized for the perineal area when pain is involved but would not lower the pain to a level that the client considers tolerable.

🔑 CN: Physiological adaptation; CL: Analyze

6. 2. Educating the client about caring for themselves and the infant are the two highest priority goals. Following birth, all birth parents, especially the primigravida, require instructions regarding self-care and infant care. Learning needs should be assessed to meet the specific needs of each client. Bonding is significant, but it is only one aspect of the needs of this client, and the bonding process would have been implemented immediately postpartum, rather than waiting 2 hours. Planning the discharge occurs after the initial education has taken place for the client and infant and the nurse is aware of any need for referrals. Safety is an aspect of education taught continuously by the nurse and should include maternal as well as newborn safety.

🔑 CN: Management of care; CL: Create

7. 3. The client is in the taking-hold phase with a demonstrated focus on the neonate and learning about and fulfilling infant care and needs. The taking-in phase is the first period after birth where there is an emphasis on reviewing and reliving the labor and birth process, concern with self, and needing to be cared for. Eating and sleep are high priorities during this phase. Taking on is not a phase of postpartum psychological adaptation. Letting go is the process beginning about 6 weeks postpartum when the client may be preparing to go back to work. During this time, they can have other individuals assume care of the infant and begin the separation process.

🔑 CN: Psychosocial integrity; CL: Analyze

8. 1. Immediately after delivery of the placenta, the nurse would expect to palpate the fundus halfway between the umbilicus and the symphysis pubis. Within 2 hours postpartum, the fundus should be palpated at the level of the umbilicus. The fundus remains at this level or may rise slightly above the umbilicus for approximately 12 hours. After the first 12 hours, the fundus should decrease 1 fingerbreadth (1 cm) per day in size. By the ninth or tenth day, the fundus usually is no longer palpable.

🔑 CN: Health promotion and maintenance; CL: Apply

9. 1. The client has a hematoma. During the first 24 hours postpartum, ice packs can be applied to the perineal area to reduce swelling and discomfort. Ice packs usually are not effective after the first 24 hours. Although vital signs, including temperature, are important assessments, taking the client's temperature is unrelated to the hematoma and would provide no additional information about swelling. After 24 hours, the client may obtain more relief by taking a warm sitz bath. This moist heat is an effective way to increase circulation to the perineum and provide comfort. Usually, hematomas resolve without further treatment within 6 weeks. Additionally, the nurse should measure the hematoma to provide a baseline for subsequent measurements and should notify the HCP of its presence. An antibiotic is not warranted at this point because the client is not exhibiting any signs or symptoms of infection.

🗝 CN: Health promotion and maintenance; CL: Analyze

10. 4. Urinary retention soon after birth is usually caused by edema and trauma of the lower urinary tract; this commonly results in difficulty with initiating voiding. Hyperemia of the bladder mucosa also commonly occurs. The combination of hyperemia and edema predisposes to decreased sensation to void, overdistention of the bladder, and incomplete bladder emptying. A prolonged first stage of labor can contribute to exhaustion and uterine atony, not urinary retention. If the client had a urinary tract infection, they would exhibit symptoms such as dysuria and a burning sensation. After birth, the uterus is contracting, which leads to less pressure on the bladder. Pressure of the uterus on the bladder occurs during labor.

🗝 CN: Health promotion and maintenance; CL: Analyze

11. 2. For clients who are bottle-feeding, the menstrual flow should return in 6 to 10 weeks, after a rise in the production of follicle-stimulating hormone by the pituitary gland. Nonlactating parents rarely ovulate before 4 to 6 weeks postpartum. Therefore, 3 to 4 weeks is too early for the menstrual cycle to resume. For women who are breastfeeding, the menstrual flow may not return for 3 to 4 months (12 to 16 weeks) or, in some women, for the entire period of lactation, because ovulation is suppressed.

🗝 CN: Health promotion and maintenance; CL: Apply

12. 4. The client's dizziness is most likely caused by orthostatic hypotension secondary to the decreased volume of blood in the vascular system resulting from the physiologic changes occurring in the client after birth. The client is experiencing dizziness because not enough blood volume is available to perfuse the brain. The nurse should first allow the client to "dangle" on the side of the bed for a few minutes before attempting to ambulate. By 6 hours postpartum, the effects of the anesthesia should be worn off completely. Typically, the effects of epidural anesthesia wear off by 1 to 2 hours postpartum, and the effects of local anesthesia usually disappear by 1 hour. The client scenario provides no information to indicate that the client experienced any postpartum hemorrhage. Normal blood loss during birth should not exceed 500 mL.

🗝 CN: Health promotion and maintenance; CL: Apply

13. 4. A small, constant trickle of blood and a firm fundus are usually indicative of a vaginal tear or cervical laceration. If the client had retained placental tissue, the fundus would fail to contract fully (uterine atony), exhibiting as a soft or boggy fundus. Also, vaginal bleeding would be evident. Uterine inversion occurs when the uterus is displaced outside of the vagina and is obvious on inspection. Bladder distention may result in uterine atony because the pressure of the bladder displaces the fundus, preventing it from fully contracting. In this case, the fundus would be soft, possibly boggy, and displaced from the midline.

🗝 CN: Reduction of risk potential; CL: Analyze

14. 4. On about the eleventh postpartum day, the lochia should be lochia alba, clear or white in color. Lochia rubra, which is dark red to red, may persist for the first 2 to 3 days postpartum. From day 3 to about day 10, lochia serosa, which is pink or brown, is normal.

🗝 CN: Health promotion and maintenance; CL: Evaluate

15. 2. The nurse should instruct the client to cleanse the perineal area with warm water and to wipe from front to back with a blotting motion. Warm water is soothing to the tender tissue, and wiping from front to back reduces the risk for contamination. Hot, sudsy water may increase the client's discomfort and may even burn the client in a very tender area. After the first 24 hours, warm water sitz baths taken three or four times a day for 20 minutes can help increase circulation to the area. Ice packs are helpful for the first 24 hours.

🗝 CN: Health promotion and maintenance; CL: Evaluate

16. 3. After an uncomplicated birth, postpartum exercises may begin on the first postpartum day with exercises to strengthen the abdominal muscles. These are done in the supine position with the knees flexed, inhaling deeply while allowing the abdomen to expand and then exhaling while contracting the abdominal muscles. Exercises such as sit-ups (sitting, then lying back, and returning to a sitting position) and push-ups or exercises involving reaching for the knees are ordinarily too strenuous for the first postpartum day. Sit-ups may be done later in the postpartum period, after approximately 3 to 6 weeks.

🗝 CN: Health promotion and maintenance; CL: Apply

17. 2. Lochia can be expected to increase when the client first ambulates. Lochia tends to pool in the uterus and vagina when the client is recumbent and flows out when the client arises. If the client had reported that their lochia was bright red, the nurse would suspect bleeding. In this situation, the client would be put back in bed, and the HCP would be notified. Early postpartum hemorrhage occurs during the first 24 hours, but typically the fundus is soft or "boggy." The client's fundus here is firm and midline. Late postpartum hemorrhage, occurring after the first 24 hours, is usually caused by retained placental fragments or abnormal involution of the placental site.

CN: Health promotion and maintenance; CL: Analyze

18. 2. Clients sometimes feel faint or dizzy when taking a shower for the first time after birth because of the sudden change in blood volume in the body. Primarily for this reason, the nurse remains nearby while the client takes their first shower after birth. If the client becomes dizzy or expresses symptoms of feeling faint, the nurse should get the client back to bed as soon as possible. If the client faints while in the shower, the nurse should cover the client to protect privacy, stay with the client, and call for assistance. Fatigue postpartum is common and will precede taking a shower. Diuresis is a normal physiologic response during the postpartum period and is not associated with showering. The nurse determines a client's risk for bleeding before allowing them to shower. If the client was at high risk for bleeding, the shower should be delayed. Once in the shower, bleeding status would be difficult to determine.

CN: Safety and infection control; CL: Analyze

19. 2. The nurse should instruct the client to squeeze or contract the muscles of the buttocks together before sitting down in the chair; this contracts the pelvic floor muscles, which reduces the tension on the tender perineal area. Then the client should put their full weight slowly down on the chair. Pain medication may only be prescribed every 3 to 4 hours, so the client may not be able to receive pain medication every time they desire to sit in the chair. The perineal laceration pain usually fades by the fifth or sixth postpartum day. Maintaining a relaxed posture before sitting does not contract the pelvic floor muscles. Most health care providers prescribe an analgesic cream or spray when a client has an episiotomy, but these provide only temporary relief.

CN: Health promotion and maintenance; CL: Analyze

20. 1. Neonates like to look at eyes, and eye-to-eye contact is a highly effective way to provide visual stimulation. The parent's eyes are circular, move from side to side, and become larger and smaller. Neonates have been observed to fix on them. In general, neonates prefer circular objects of darkness against a white background. Sharp black and white images of geometric figures are appropriate. The use of bright colors on the walls and moving a colorful rattle do not provide as much visual stimulation as eye-to-eye contact with talking. Brightly colored animals and cartoon figures are more appropriate at approximately 1 year of age.

CN: Health promotion and maintenance; CL: Create

21. 2. According to Erikson, infants are in the trust versus mistrust stage. Holding, talking to, singing to, and patting neonates helps them develop trust in caregivers. Tactile stimulation is important and should be encouraged. Holding neonates often is unlikely to spoil them because they are totally dependent on other human beings to meet their needs. Being held makes infants feel loved and cared for and should be encouraged. The birth parent can hold the neonate as often as they want, not just when the baby is crying or fussy. Overstimulation typically does not result from holding an infant.

CN: Health promotion and maintenance; CL: Analyze

22. 4. If the client continues to have perineal pain after an analgesic medication has been given, the nurse should inspect the client's perineum for a hematoma because this is the usual cause of such discomfort. Ibuprofen is a nonsteroidal antiinflammatory medication used to relieve mild pain. Pain from a perineal hematoma can be moderate to severe, possibly requiring a stronger analgesic agent, such as acetaminophen with codeine. Ice applied to the perineum during the first 24 hours postpartum may decrease the severity of hematoma formation. Application of warm heat, such as a sitz bath three times daily for 20 minutes, also can help relieve the discomfort when implemented after the first 24 hours. Typically, hematomas resolve themselves within 6 weeks. A puerperal infection would be indicated if the client's temperature were 100.4°F (41°C) or higher. Also, lochia most likely would be foul smelling. A continuous trickle of lochia rubra would suggest a possible vaginal laceration. No evidence is presented to suggest a history of drug abuse.

CN: Reduction of risk potential; CL: Analyze

23. 2. Delegating care to UAP requires that the nurse knows which tasks are within that individual's capability. Changing the perineal pad and reporting drainage, reinforcing hygiene with perineal care, and assisting with ambulation are within the individual's capacity. It would be beyond the scope of the job of UAP to conduct client teaching.

CN: Management of care; CL: Analyze

24. 4. Legal regulations and ethical decision-making require that the nurse maintain confidentiality at all times. The nurse's best response is to explain to the client that nurses are not allowed to discuss other clients on the unit. Ignoring the client's question is inappropriate because doing so would interfere with the development of a trusting nurse-client relationship. Confidentiality must be maintained at all times. Telling the client that the nurse is not sure may imply that the nurse will find out and then tell the client about the other woman. Asking the other client's permission to discuss them with another client is inappropriate because confidentiality must be maintained at all times.

CN: Management of care; CL: Apply

25. 2. The neonate has immature oculomotor coordination, an inability to accommodate for distance, and poorly developed eyes, visual nerves, and brain. However, the normal neonate can see objects clearly within a range of 9 to 12 inches (22.9 to 30.5 cm), whether or not the neonate is moving. Visual acuity at birth is 20/100 to 20/150, but it improves rapidly during infancy and toddlerhood. Newborns can distinguish colors as well as light from dark.

CN: Health promotion and maintenance; CL: Apply

26. 4. The client is experiencing diastasis recti, a separation of the longitudinal muscles (recti) of the abdomen that is usually palpable on the third postpartum day. An exercise involving raising the head and shoulders about 8 inches (20.3 cm) with the client lying on their back with knees bent and hands crossed over the abdomen is preferred. This exercise helps pull the abdominal muscles together, and the client gradually works up to performing this exercise 50 times per day. However, until the diastasis has closed, the client should avoid exercises that rotate the trunk, twist the hips, or bend the trunk to one side because further separation may occur. The condition does not need a surgical repair, and limited activity and bed rest are not necessary. Correct posture and adequate diet assist the body to return to its prepregnancy state more quickly but do not resolve the separation of abdominal muscles.

CN: Reduction of risk potential; CL: Apply

27. 3. A uterine fundus located off to one side and above the level of the umbilicus is commonly the result of a full bladder. Although the client had voided, the client may be experiencing urinary retention with overflow. If anesthesia has been used for birth, the inability to void may be related to the lingering effects of anesthesia; however, that is not the case here. Health care providers commonly write a one-time prescription for catheterization, after which, typically, enough edema has subsided to make it easier and less painful for the client to void and completely empty their bladder. Administering ibuprofen would have no effect on the uterine fundus. Waiting to reassess in 1 hour could be detrimental since the client's distended bladder is interfering with uterine involution, predisposing them to possible hemorrhage. Administering a bolus of fluid would be inappropriate because it would only add to the client's full bladder.

CN: Reduction of risk potential; CL: Analyze

28. 1. The client with a third-degree laceration should be assessed for constipation because a third-degree laceration extends into a portion of the anal sphincter. Constipation, not diarrhea, is more likely because this condition is extremely painful, possibly causing the client to be reluctant to have a bowel movement. The laceration has been sutured and should not be bleeding at 48 hours postpartum. Rectal fistulas may develop at a later time, but not at 48 hours postpartum.

CN: Reduction of risk potential; CL: Analyze

29. 1. The nurse needs to continue to monitor the client's vital signs. During the first 24 hours postpartum, it is normal for the client to have a slight temperature elevation because of dehydration. A temperature of 100.4°F (38°C) that persists after the first 24 hours may indicate an infection. Bradycardia during the first week postpartum is normal because of decreased blood volume, diuresis, and diaphoresis. The client's respiratory rate is within normal limits. Large clots are indicative of hemorrhage. However, the client's vital signs are within normal limits and the fundus is firm and midline. Therefore, large clots and possible hemorrhage can be ruled out. The HCP does not need to be notified at this time. An ice pack is not necessary because the client's temperature is within normal limits.

CN: Health promotion and maintenance; CL: Apply

30. 3. The client needs more teaching when stating, "I should lie on my back as much as possible to relieve the pain." Instead, the client should lie in the lateral recumbent position as much as possible to aid venous return to the rectal area and to reduce discomfort. Stool softeners can decrease pain with defecation, but clients should discuss their use with their provider before taking them. Analgesic sprays and witch hazel pads are helpful in reducing the discomfort of hemorrhoids. Drinking lots of water and eating roughage aid in bowel elimination, minimizing the risk for straining and subsequent hemorrhoidal development or enlargement.

🔑 CN: Basic care and comfort; CL: Evaluate

31. 2. On most postpartum units, clients on regular diets are allowed to eat whatever kinds of food they desire. Generally, foods from home are not discouraged. The nurse does not need to obtain the HCP's permission. Although it is preferred, the foods do not necessarily have to be high in iron. In some cultures, there is a belief in the "hot-cold" theory of disease; certain foods (hot) are preferred during the postpartum period, and other foods (cold) are avoided. Therefore, the nurse should allow the parent to bring the client "special foods from home." Doing so demonstrates cultural sensitivity and aids in developing a trusting relationship.

🔑 CN: Basic care and comfort; CL: Analyze

32. 1. Iron is best absorbed in an acid environment or with vitamin C. For maximum iron absorption, the client should take the medication with orange juice or a vitamin C supplement. Herbal tea has no effect on iron absorption. Milk decreases iron absorption. Grape juice is not acidic and therefore would have no effect on iron absorption.

🔑 CN: Pharmacological and parenteral therapies; CL: Analyze

33. 3. At 12 hours postpartum, the fundus normally should be in the midline and at the level of the umbilicus. When the fundus is firm yet above the umbilicus and deviated to the right rather than in the midline, the client's bladder is most likely distended. The client should be encouraged to ambulate to the bathroom and attempt to void because a full bladder can prevent normal involution. A firm but deviated fundus above the level of the umbilicus is not a normal finding, and if voiding does not return it to midline, it should be reported to the HCP. Oxytocin is used to treat uterine atony. This client's fundus is firm, not boggy or soft, which would suggest atony. Gentle massage is not necessary because there is no evidence of atony or clots.

🔑 CN: Reduction of risk potential; CL: Analyze

34. -/+ **1, 2, 3, 5, 6.** The nurse is responsible for providing discharge instructions that include signs and symptoms that need to be reported to the health care provider as well as resources and follow-up for home care if needed. Phone numbers and health practices to promote healing, such as the use of prenatal vitamins, are also essential pieces of information. Fertility can return in as little as 21 days, especially among women who are not breastfeeding, so it is important to discuss the client's contraception plan. Although the client's parent may be helpful, the client's statement that they will be fine because their parent is coming indicates that they are unaware or ignoring information about valuable information and resources.

🔑 CN: Reduction of risk potential; CL: Evaluate

The Postpartum Client Who Breastfeeds

35. 4. DMPA is an injectable progestin contraceptive that can reduce the initial production of breast milk. It is given to breastfeeding clients when they return for the 6-week postpartum checkup. By this time, the milk supply is well established and will remain at that level. DMPA is effective as a contraceptive for 90 days. DMPA can be given within 5 days of birth only if a birth parent is not breastfeeding.

🔑 CN: Pharmacological and parenteral therapies; CL: Evaluate

36. 3. As much of the client's nipple and areola as possible need to be in the infant's mouth to establish a latch that does not cause nipple cracks or fissures. Having the nipple and the areola deep in the infant's mouth decreases the stress on the end of the nipple, therefore decreasing pain, cracking, and fissures. Breast milk has been found to heal nipples when placed on the nipple at the completion of a feeding. The length of time the baby feeds on each nipple is not a factor as long as the nipple is correctly placed in the infant's mouth.

🔑 CN: Health promotion and maintenance; CL: Evaluate

37. 1. New clients usually begin to produce milk at about the third day postpartum, and colostrum is produced until that time. For clients who have breastfed another infant during pregnancy, having milk shortly after birth is not unusual. Diaphoresis and diuresis are considered normal during this time as the body excretes the additional fluids that are no longer needed after the pregnancy. Constipation may continue for several days as a result of progesterone remaining in the system, the consummation of iron, and trauma to the perineum.

🔑 CN: Physiological adaptation; CL: Analyze

38. 2. The major reasons for afterbirth pains are breastfeeding, high parity, overdistended uterus during pregnancy, and a uterus filled with blood clots. Physiologically, afterbirth pains are caused by intermittent contraction and relaxation of the uterus. These contractions are stronger in multigravidas so they maintain a contracted uterus. The release of oxytocin when breastfeeding also stimulates uterine contractions. There are no data to suggest any of these clients has had an overdistended uterus or currently has clots within the uterus. The G3, P3 client who is breastfeeding has the highest parity of the clients listed, which—in addition to breastfeeding—places them most at risk for afterbirth pains. The G2, P2 client who had a cesarean birth may have cramping, but it should be less than the G3, P3 client. The G3, P3 client who is bottle-feeding would be at risk for afterbirth pains because they have given birth to several children, but their choice to bottle-feed reduces the risk for pain.

 CN: Physiological adaptation; CL: Evaluate

39. 2. The client is exhibiting signs and symptoms of a breast infection (mastitis). The nurse should instruct them to contact their HCP, who will likely prescribe a prescription for antibiotics. They should continue to breastfeed the infant from both breasts. Frequent breastfeeding is encouraged rather than discontinuing the process for anyone having a breast infection. Applying warm compresses may relieve pain. However, the underlying infection indicated by the elevated temperature indicates that additional treatment with antibiotics will be needed.

 CN: Management of care; CL: Analyze

40. 4. Breastfeeding consumes maternal calories and requires energy that increases the maternal basal metabolic rate and assists in lowering the maternal blood glucose level. Insulin is not transferred to the infant through breast milk. Breastfeeding is recommended for clients with diabetes because it lowers blood glucose levels. The number of antibodies in breast milk is not altered by maternal diabetes.

 CN: Physiological adaptation; CL: Evaluate

41. 1. Jaundice in a breastfeeding infant is common and is not pathological. Clients should be taught to breastfeed as often as possible, at least every 2 to 3 hours and until the infant is satiated. Breastfed babies rarely need to be supplemented with formula. Clients should be encouraged to continue breastfeeding their infants due to the numerous benefits it provides. Infants should never be placed in direct sunlight.

 CN: Health promotion and maintenance; CL: Evaluate

42. 1. If not contraindicated for moral, cultural, or religious reasons, a condom with spermicide is commonly recommended for contraception after birth until the client's 6-week postpartum examination. This method has no effect on the neonate who is breastfeeding. Oral contraceptives containing estrogen are not advised for women who are breastfeeding because the hormones decrease the production of breast milk. Women who are not breastfeeding may use oral contraceptive agents. The rhythm method is not effective because the client is unlikely to be able to determine when ovulation has occurred until their menstrual cycle returns. Although breastfeeding is not considered an effective form of contraception, breastfeeding usually delays the return of both ovulation and menstruation. The length of the delay varies with the duration of lactation and the frequency of breastfeeding. While abstinence is one form of birth control and safe while breastfeeding, it may not be acceptable to this couple who is asking about a method that will allow them to resume sexual relations.

 CN: Health promotion and maintenance; CL: Analyze

43. 4. Colostrum is a thin, watery, yellow fluid composed of protein, sugar, fat, water, minerals, vitamins, and maternal antibodies (e.g., immunoglobulin A). It is important for the neonate to receive colostrum for passive immunity. Colostrum is lower in fat and lactose than mature breast milk. Colostrum does not contain vitamin K. The neonate will produce vitamin K once a feeding pattern is established. Colostrum may speed, rather than delay, the passage of meconium.

 CN: Health promotion and maintenance; CL: Apply

44. 3. Various medications can be excreted in breast milk and affect the nursing neonate. The client should avoid all nonprescribed medications (such as acetaminophen) unless approved by the health care provider. Medications typically do not affect the quality of the client's breast milk. Medications usually do not interfere with or diminish the client's motivation to breastfeed, nor do they interfere with the client's letdown reflex.

 CN: Health promotion and maintenance; CL: Apply

45. 4. Breastfeeding stimulates oxytocin secretion, which causes the uterine muscles to contract. These contractions account for the discomfort associated with afterpains. Flatulence may occur after a cesarean birth. However, the client typically would have abdominal distention and a bloating feeling, not a "cramp-like" feeling. Stretching of the tissues or healing may cause slight tenderness or itching, not cramping feelings of discomfort. Medications such as mild analgesic agents or stool softeners, which are commonly administered after birth, typically do not cause cramping.

CN: Health promotion and maintenance; CL: Apply

46. 2. For the breastfeeding client, drinking at least 8 to 10 glasses of fluid a day is recommended. Breastfeeding women need an increased intake of vitamin D for calcium absorption. A breastfeeding client requires an extra 500 calories a day above the recommended nonpregnancy intake to produce quality breast milk. Breastfeeding women need adequate calcium for blood clotting and strong bones and teeth.

CN: Basic care and comfort; CL: Evaluate

47. 4. Lightly brushing the neonate's lips with the nipple causes the neonate to open the mouth and begin sucking. The neonate should be taught to open the mouth and grasp the nipple on their own. The neonate should not be forced to nurse.

CN: Health promotion and maintenance; CL: Apply

48. 2. Several methods can be used to prevent nipple soreness. Placing as much of the areola as possible into the neonate's mouth is one method. This action prevents compression of the nipple between the neonate's gums, which can cause nipple soreness. Other methods include changing position with each feeding, avoiding breast engorgement, nursing more frequently, and feeding on demand. Plastic liners are not helpful because they prevent air circulation, thus promoting nipple soreness. Instead, air drying is recommended. Pulling the baby's mouth out smoothly after only 10 minutes may prevent the baby from getting the entire feeding and increases nipple soreness. Any breast milk remaining on the nipples should not be wiped off because the milk has healing properties.

CN: Health promotion and maintenance; CL: Analyze

49. 3. Although there is some variation in recommendations, fresh breast milk can be safely kept in the refrigerator for 5 to 7 days. Storage recommendations for frozen breast milk vary per type of freezer. In a chest or upright deep freezer at −4°F (−20°C) breast milk can be stored for 12 months. Breast milk should be stored in glass containers because immunoglobulin tends to stick to plastic bottles. Freshly expressed breast milk can remain without refrigeration or loss of nutrients for up to 6 to 8 hours. The containers should be labeled with the date, time, and amount to prevent the inadvertent administration of spoiled milk. Frozen breast milk should be thawed in the refrigerator for a few hours, placed under warm tap water, and then shaken.

CN: Health promotion and maintenance; CL: Evaluate

50. 4. Oxytocin stimulates the letdown reflex when milk is carried to the nipples. A lactating client can experience the letdown reflex suddenly when they hear their baby cry or when they anticipate a feeding. Some birth parents have reported feeling the letdown reflex just by thinking about the baby. Progesterone plays an important role in pregnancy, but levels drop after giving birth. This hormone if taken for contraception too soon after birth may decrease milk supply. Estrogen influences the development of female secondary sex characteristics and controls menstruation. Prolactin stimulates milk production.

CN: Health promotion and maintenance; CL: Apply

51. 0/1

Action to Take	Potential Conditions	Parameters to Monitor
Encourage the use of moist heat	Plugged milk duct	Temperature
Teach feeding techniques		Flulike symptoms

A small painful knot that is not reddened most suggests a plugged milk duct. Systematic flulike symptoms of more than rhinitis such as fever, chills, body aches, or headaches are seen with mastitis. A breast abscess typically appears after mastitis. A firm painless lump that persists and does not change with milk flow would be more suggestive of a breast tumor. The nurse should encourage the client to use warm moist heat on the affected breast. Teaching the client about altering the infant's position and massaging the lump while feeding can assist with removing the plug. A mammogram and antibiotics are not needed at this point. The client should be told to call the office if they develop a fever or any flulike symptoms. Since breastfeeding has been going well, milk production should be considered adequate. There is reason to suggest monitoring for bruising or bleeding. It is not necessary to monitor for problems in the right breast because plugged milk ducts commonly develop in one only breast.

CJ: Standalone bowtie; CL: Create

52. 3. Expressing a little milk before nursing, massaging the breasts gently, or taking a warm shower before feeding also may help improve milk flow. Although various measures such as ice, heat, and massage may be tried to relieve breast engorgement, prevention of breast engorgement by frequent feedings is the method of choice. Applying ice to the nipples does not relieve breast engorgement. However, it may temporarily relieve the discomfort associated with breast engorgement. Using lanolin on the nipples does not relieve breast engorgement and is unnecessary. The use of lanolin may cause sensitivity and irritation. Having frequent breastfeeding sessions, rather than offering the neonate a small amount of formula, is the method of choice for preventing and relieving breast engorgement. In addition, offering the neonate small amounts of formula may result in nipple confusion.

CN: Health promotion and maintenance; CL: Apply

53. 1. The nurse should instruct the client that the baby is getting enough to eat when there are six to eight wet diapers by the fifth day of age. Other signs include good suckling sounds during feeding, dripping breast milk at the mouth, and quiet rest or sleep after the feeding. By the fourth day of age, the infant should have soft yellow stools, not transitional (greenish) stools. Falling asleep easily after feeding on the first day is not a good indicator because most infants are sleepy during the first 24 hours. Most infants regain their lost birth weight in 7 to 10 days after birth. An infant who has gained weight during the first well-baby checkup (usually at 2 weeks) is getting sufficient breast milk at feedings.

CN: Health promotion and maintenance; CL: Apply

54. 4. The client should wean the infant gradually, eliminating one feeding at a time. The baby can be weaned to a bottle (formula) anytime the birth parent desires; they do not have to breastfeed for 4 months. Most infants (and birth parents) develop a "favorite feeding time," so this feeding session should be eliminated last. The client may wish to begin weaning with daytime feedings when the infant is busy.

CN: Health promotion and maintenance; CL: Create

55. 1, 3. The client is experiencing symptoms of engorgement. Cool compresses between feedings can help decrease swelling. Determining when the baby last fed is critical because frequent feedings can help relieve symptoms. The nurse must also assess how long the baby feeds, if the baby has a correct latch, and if the baby empties the breast during feeds. Sitting on supportive devices is not necessary as the episiotomy is healing. Cool sitz baths do not promote circulation to the area; instead, they cause vasoconstriction and decrease blood flow to the area, therefore prolonging healing and increasing discomfort. Obtaining a specimen for culture and sensitivity from the episiotomy site is not warranted at this time. If edema and redness continue for more than 2 days, further assessment is required to rule out infection.

CN: Basic care and comfort; CL: Analyze

56. 4. Neonates normally increase breastfeeding during periods of rapid growth (growth spurts). These can be expected at age 10 to 14 days, 5 to 6 weeks, 2½ to 3 months, and 4½ to 6 months. Each growth spurt is usually followed by a regular feeding pattern. Lack of adequate intake to meet maternal nutritional needs is not associated with the neonate's desire for more frequent breastfeeding sessions. However, an intake of adequate calories is necessary to produce quality breast milk. The client's fears about weight gain and preventing the neonate from sucking long enough are not associated with the desire for more frequent breastfeeding sessions.

CN: Health promotion and maintenance; CL: Analyze

57. 2. Even if the nipples are sore and cracked, the client should position the baby with the entire areola in the baby's mouth so that the nipple is not compressed between the baby's gums during feeding. The best method is to prevent cracked nipples before they occur. This can be done by feeding frequently and using proper positioning. Warm, moist tea bags can soothe cracked nipples because of the tannic acid in the tea. Creams on the nipples should be avoided; wiping off any lanolin creams from the nipple before each feeding can cause further soreness. Feeding the baby less often for the next few days will cause engorgement (and possible neonatal weight loss), leading to additional problems. Soap use while in the shower should be avoided to prevent drying and removal of protective oils.

CN: Reduction of risk potential; CL: Analyze

58. 2. Time for bonding with their newborns is a frequent concern for partners of birth mothers who are breastfeeding. It is common for partners to express concern about having less intimate contact time. These feelings are normal, but they do not go away in a few days. The partner of the breastfeeding birth mother has to dedicate time to spend with the infant where they can talk to, hold, cuddle, or play with the infant. These strategies provide the infant with the contact and stimulation to establish a close bond between them. Bonding occurs from the moment of birth and continues in various ways between the client, the client's partner, and the infant. Infants recognize and respond to touch, light, and voice immediately after birth. Bonding between both parents is equally important, and one does not take priority over the other.

CN: Psychosocial integrity; CL: Analyze

59. 4. A soft seedy unformed stool is the norm for a 4-day-old infant. It may surprise the client as it is a change from the meconium the infant had since birth. This stool is not diarrhea even though it has no form. There is no need for the infant to be seen for this. As long as the infant is breastfeeding, the stools will remain of this color and consistency. Brown and formed stool is common for an infant who is bottle-fed or after the breastfeeding infant has begun eating food.

🔑 CN: Physiologic adaptation; CL: Analyze

The Postpartum Client Who Bottle-feeds

60. 1. By 4 to 6 weeks postpartum, the fundus should be deep in the pelvis and the size of a nonpregnant uterus. Subinvolution, caused by infection or retained placental fragments, is a problem associated with a uterus that is larger than expected at this time. Menstruation can normally return after 6 to 8 weeks in nonbreastfeeding clients. Other normal expectations include striae that are beginning to fade to silver and breasts that are soft without evidence of milk production (in a bottle-feeding client).

🔑 CN: Physiological adaptation; CL: Analyze

61. 4. The use of a breast pump to remove milk is contraindicated in bottle-feeding clients. Nipple and breast stimulation and emptying of the breasts produce milk, rather than eliminate milk production. The bottle-feeding client is discouraged from stimulating the breasts in any way. A sports bra that is well fitting provides support and decreases stimulation. (Binders are not suggested.) Having the water in a shower land on the shoulders of the client rather than the breasts also decreases stimulation. Only water is necessary to clean nipples when breast or bottle-feeding.

🔑 CN: Basic care and comfort; CL: Evaluate

62. 3. Gaining 1 oz (30 g) a day is normal for a neonate. Initial weight loss that exceeds 10% of birth weight is abnormal. Adding rice cereal to a bottle without a medical indication increases the risk for aspiration and may promote obesity. Doubling the birth weight is typical at 5 months.

🔑 CN: Basic care and comfort; CL: Apply

63. 1. Initial regurgitation in the neonate during the first 12 to 24 hours may be caused by excessive mucus and gastric irritation from foreign substances in the stomach. After the first 24 hours, regurgitation is thought to be caused by the neonate's immature cardiac sphincter. It represents an overflow of stomach contents and is probably a result of feeding the neonate too fast or too much. A defect in the gastrointestinal system usually results in more severe symptoms. A small amount of regurgitation is normal, but vomiting or forceful fluid expulsion is not. Burping the infant often during a feeding can decrease the amount of air in the stomach from swallowing. However, burping too often can lead the neonate to become tired or fussy. Moving the infant usually does not result in regurgitation.

🔑 CN: Health promotion and maintenance; CL: Apply

64. 4. The best recommendation is to keep the baby upright do 15 to 20 minutes before placing the baby down for a nap. This helps the stomach empty and decreases the risk for regurgitation. After the short waiting period, the baby should be placed in a supine position. Placing infants on their side or prone in a crib after a feeding is no longer recommended due to the increased risk for sudden infant death syndrome (SIDS).

🔑 CN: Health promotion and maintenance; CL: Apply

65. 2. Pediatricians recommend that infants be given either breast milk or formula until at least 6 months of age because of the neonate's difficulty digesting solid foods. Giving solid foods too early can lead to food allergies. Because chewing movements do not begin until 7 to 9 months of age, foods requiring chewing should be delayed until this time.

🔑 CN: Health promotion and maintenance; CL: Apply

66. 1. The client needs further instruction when they say burping should be done after 15 minutes of formula feeding. The entire feeding should take only 15 to 20 minutes, and the neonate should be burped before the feeding is complete. During initial feedings, the burping should be done after each half-ounce of formula with the neonate in an upright position, patting the neonate gently on the back.

🔑 CN: Health promotion and maintenance; CL: Evaluate

67. 3. Pregnancy and the immediate postpartum period is a hypercoagulable state that puts clients at risk for blood clots. Taking a combined hormonal contraceptive would expose the client to estrogen and further increase the risk for blood clots. Clients are advised to wait a minimum of 3 weeks after birth before taking estrogen-containing contraceptives. Oral contraceptives do not significantly affect the involution process in nonbreastfeeding women. For oral contraceptives to be effective, they must be started before intercourse resumes. Although some practitioners may advise clients to wait 6 weeks before resuming intercourse, other providers advise clients that they may resume after they no longer have lochia. Progestin does not significantly increase the risk for bleeding after birth, and there are no restrictions for beginning progestin-based contraceptives in nonbreastfeeding women.

CN: Pharmacological and parental therapies; CL: Apply

The Postpartum Client with a Cesarean Birth

68. 3. A cesarean birth is an independent risk factor for a thromboembolic event in pregnant women. Inflatable compression sleeves should be placed on the lower extremities of a client until the risk for venous stasis is reduced through ambulation. Although a return of sensation must happen before the client can safely ambulate, this finding alone does not significantly decrease the risk for venous stasis. Platelets continue to be significantly elevated for at least 3 weeks after birth, which is well after a client would be discharged. It is unnecessary to continue wearing the compression sleeves after ambulation has returned.

CN: Basic care and comfort; CL: Apply

69. 3. The client should have more active bowel sounds by this time after birth. Ambulation will encourage passing flatus and begin peristaltic action in the gastrointestinal tract. Medicating the client should be evaluated prior to ambulating, but it is probably too soon because the last dose was 3 hours ago and the pain assessment rating is fairly low. Pain medications should not have codeine as a component as it decreases peristaltic activity. Incentive spirometry or asking the client to turn, cough, and deep breathe is appropriate to encourage good oxygen exchange in the lungs prior to ambulation, and walking can be used concurrently with these interventions. Participating in infant care is another way to encourage the client to move about, but the primary goal would be to have them walk on the unit, a more purposeful activity.

CN: Physiological adaptation; CL: Analyze

70. 2. Carboprost is an oxytocic prostaglandin that causes uterine contraction in women who are bleeding heavily. Nausea, vomiting, diarrhea, and fever are common adverse effects of prostaglandin administration. Vertigo and confusion are not associated with this drug. Carboprost may not control all cases of hemorrhage, but it does not cause bleeding. Restlessness typically is a sign of shock, not a reaction to carboprost. If too large a dose is given, the client may experience headache and hypertension because carboprost contracts smooth muscles.

CN: Pharmacological and parenteral therapies; CL: Evaluate

71. 4. Slightly red-tinged urine may indicate that the bladder was accidentally cut during the cesarean birth. The nurse should notify the HCP as soon as possible about the urine color. Continuing to monitor the client's input and output should be done after the HCP is contacted. Palpating the fundus every 15 minutes is not necessary unless the client's fundus becomes soft or "boggy." Assessment of the urinary catheter is a normal part of the elimination assessment by the nurse, but displacement is not the cause of the red-tinged urine.

CN: Reduction of risk potential; CL: Analyze

72. 1. VBAC can be attempted if the client has not had a classic uterine incision. This type of incision carries a danger of uterine rupture. A health care provider (HCP) must be available, and a cesarean birth must be possible within 30 minutes. A history of rapid labor is not a criterion for VBAC. A low transverse incision is not a contraindication for VBAC. A classic (vertical) incision is a contraindication because the client has a greater possibility for uterine rupture. An estimated fetal weight of more than 4000 g (8 lb, 13 oz) by itself is not a contraindication if the client does not have diabetes.

CN: Health promotion and maintenance; CL: Apply

73. 4. For maximum effectiveness, Rho(D) immune globulin should be administered within 72 hours postpartum. Most Rh-negative clients also receive Rho(D) immune globulin during the prenatal period at 28 weeks' gestation and then again after birth. The drug is given to Rh-negative clients who have a negative Coombs test and give birth to Rh-positive neonates. If there is doubt about the fetus's blood type after the pregnancy is terminated, the client should receive the medication.

CN: Pharmacological and parenteral therapies; CL: Apply

74. 1. After a cesarean birth, most clients have the greatest comfort when the neonate is positioned in the football hold with the client in a semi-Fowler position, supporting the neonate's head in their hand and resting the neonate's body on pillows alongside their hip. This position prevents pressure on the uterine incision yet allows the neonate easy access to the breast. The scissors hold, where the birth parent places their hand well back on the breast to prevent touching the areola and interfering with the neonate's mouth placement, is used by the client to hold the breast and support it during breastfeeding. The cross-cradle hold is done when the parent holds the neonate's head in the hand opposite from the breast on which the neonate will feed and the parent's arm supports the neonate's body across their lap. This position can be uncomfortable because of the pressure placed on the client's incision line. For the cradle hold, the parent cradles the infant alongside the arm at the breast on which the neonate will feed. This position also can be uncomfortable because of the pressure placed on the incision line.

CN: Basic care and comfort; CL: Analyze

The Postpartum Client with Complications

75. 4. A client who is pale and shaking could be experiencing hypovolemic shock likely caused by blood loss. A primary cause of blood loss after the birth of an infant is uterine atony. Therefore, the priority assessments should be the fundus of the uterus for firmness and location. In addition, the amount of vaginal bleeding (lochia) should also be assessed. An immediate intervention for uterine atony is fundal massage that will help the uterus to contract and therefore stop additional bleeding. Assessing the client's level of consciousness does not require additional time and can be done by the nurse while the fundus and lochia are assessed. Obtaining vital signs, blood glucose, and temperature are important, but either should be done after the fundus has been assessed and massaged or should be obtained by a second responder. Assessing for uterine infection and pain should be done after treatment for hypovolemic shock has been initiated.

CN: Reduction of risk potential; CL: Analyze

76. 2. Pain after birth is generally well managed with pain-control medications; since they did not help this client, further assessment is necessary. The first nursing action would be to assess the source of the pain; the client may have sustained a laceration or a hematoma as a result of birth. Assessing the perineum may help the nurse to determine the source of the pain and may require follow-up by the health care provider. Subsequent nursing interventions may include pain medication, sitz bath, or education regarding the healing process.

CN: Basic care and comfort; CL: Analyze

77. 3. Pain and swelling may be indicative of thrombophlebitis. Redness at the site may be more reliable as an indicator of thrombophlebitis. The nurse should notify the HCP immediately and ask the client to remain in bed to minimize the risk for pulmonary embolus, a serious consequence of thrombophlebitis should a clot dislodge. Placing an ice pack on the perineal area is inappropriate. However, ice to the perineum would be useful for episiotomy pain and swelling. The client does not need to be positioned in a semi-Fowler position but should remain on bed rest to prevent dislodgement of a potential clot.

CN: Reduction of risk potential; CL: Analyze

78. 4. Heparin therapy is prescribed to prevent further clot formation by inhibiting further thrombus and clot formation. Heparin, an anticoagulant, does not make blood clots thinner. An adverse effect of heparin therapy during the puerperium is increased lochia flow, so the nurse must be observant for symptoms of hemorrhage, such as heavy lochia flow. Heparin does not increase diaphoresis, which is normal for the postpartum client.

CN: Pharmacological and parenteral therapies; CL: Evaluate

79. 2. A major complication of deep vein thrombosis is pulmonary embolism. Signs and symptoms, which may occur suddenly and require immediate treatment, include dyspnea, severe chest pain, apprehension, cough (possibly accompanied by hemoptysis), tachycardia, fever, hypotension, diaphoresis, pallor, shortness of breath, and friction rub. Pain in the calf is common with a diagnosis of deep vein thrombosis. Hypotension, not hypertension, would suggest a possible pulmonary embolism. It also could suggest possible hemorrhage secondary to intravenous heparin therapy. Bradycardia for the first 7 days in the postpartum period is normal.

CN: Reduction of risk potential; CL: Analyze

80. 3. A slow pulse (bradycardia) is normal for the first 7 days after birth as the body begins to adjust to the decrease in blood volume and return to the prepregnant state. Adverse effects of heparin therapy suggesting prolonged bleeding include hematuria, epistaxis, increased lochia flow, and bleeding gums. Typically, tachycardia, not bradycardia, would be associated with hemorrhage. Petechiae indicate bleeding under the skin or in subcutaneous tissue.

CN: Reduction of risk potential; CL: Evaluate

81. 3. Anticoagulant therapy can cause the gums to bleed, so a soft toothbrush and waxed dental floss should be used to minimize this adverse effect. Nonsteroidal antiinflammatory medications should be avoided because of the increased risk for possible hemorrhage. At the beginning of treatment, clients will need to have their INR levels assessed frequently, which could be more often than weekly. Once INR levels have stabilized, clients may need them checked only monthly. Clients should be advised to keep the consumption of foods high in vitamin K consistent from day to day rather than eliminate them totally from their diets.

 CN: Pharmacological and parenteral therapies; CL: Evaluate

82. 4. Frequent handwashing is the most important aspect of infection control. The nurse can emphasize, monitor, and ensure this strategy for all who come in contact with this client. The use of gloves is not needed for clients caring for their own infants. The best practice is to restrict visitation if the client has a respiratory illness. If visitation is necessary, it is better if the client with the known infection wears a mask. Individual client care equipment is not needed in this situation.

 CN: Reduction of risk potential; CL: Evaluate

83. 1, 4, 5. Endometritis is an ascending infection where organisms from the lower reproductive tract contaminate the normally sterile uterine lining. When the amniotic membranes rupture, bacteria from the cervix, vagina, perineum, and bowel can ascend into the uterus and infect the lining. Manual removal of the placenta, prolonged labor, and the use of fetal scalp electrodes all increase the risk for developing endometritis postpartum. The use of in-and-out catheters during labor is not a risk factor for developing endometritis. Epidural use for pain relief in labor is not a risk factor for developing endometritis after birth.

 CN: Reduction of risk potential; CL: Analyze

84. 3. The nurse should encourage the client to maintain a semi-Fowler position, which promotes comfort and facilitates drainage. Endometritis can make the client feel extremely uncomfortable and fatigued, so ambulation during intravenous therapy is not as important at this time. The client does not need to discontinue breastfeeding, though they may become quite fatigued and need assistance in caring for the neonate. Typically, breastfeeding would be discontinued only if the birth parent lacks the necessary energy. The institution's policy regarding visitors is to be followed. However, visitors do not need to be restricted to prevent contamination because the client is not considered to be contagious. The nurse should maintain the client's need for privacy and rest and should respect the client's wishes related to visitors.

 CN: Reduction of risk potential; CL: Analyze

85. 2. The client diagnosed with cystitis needs to void every 2 to 4 hours while awake to keep their bladder empty. In addition, they should maintain adequate fluid intake; 3000 mL a day is recommended. Intake of acidic fruit juices (e.g., cranberry, apricot) is recommended because of their association with reducing the risk for infection. The client should wear cotton underwear and avoid tight-fitting slacks. The client does not need to wash with povidone-iodine after voiding. Plain warm water is sufficient to keep the perineal area clean.

 CN: Basic care and comfort; CL: Create

86. 1. The client can continue to breastfeed as often as desired. Continuation of breastfeeding is limited only by the client's discomfort or malaise. Antibiotics for treatment are chosen carefully so that they avoid affecting the neonate through breast milk. Drugs such as sulfonamides, nitrofurantoin, and cephalosporins usually are not prescribed for breastfeeding parents. Manual pumping of the breasts is not necessary.

 CN: Health promotion and maintenance; CL: Apply

87. 2. Carboprost tromethamine may cause hypertension, not hypotension. More commonly carboprost tromethamine, a synthetic prostaglandin, causes nausea, vomiting, diarrhea, and fever. Gastrointestinal symptoms are so common that antiemetic and antidiarrheal medications are often given as a pretreatment or immediately following carboprost.

 CN: Pharmacological and parenteral therapies; CL: Analyze

88. 1. The client is exhibiting signs of early postpartum hemorrhage, defined as blood loss greater than 500 mL in the first 24 hours after birth. A rapid intravenous oxytocin infusion of 30 units in 500 mL of normal saline, oxygen therapy, and gentle fundal massage to contract the uterus are usually effective. If bleeding persists, the nurse should inspect the cervix and vagina for lacerations. Other pharmacologic interventions may be needed. Severe uncontrolled hemorrhage may require bimanual uterine compression, dilation and curettage to remove any retained placental tissue, or a hysterectomy to prevent maternal death from hemorrhage. The client should be placed in the supine position to allow evaluation of the fundus. The side-lying position is not helpful in controlling postpartum hemorrhage. Vigorous fundal massage every 5 minutes is unnecessary. In addition, it can be very painful for the birth parent. Rather, gentle massage along with oxytocin administration is used to stimulate the uterus to contract. A hysterectomy is used to remove fibroid tumors. With massive

Postpartum Care 167

hemorrhage, a hysterectomy (removal of the uterus) may be necessary to control the bleeding.

CN: Health promotion and maintenance; CL: Create

89. 4. The most likely cause of this client's uterine atony is overdistention of the uterus caused by the hydramnios. As a result, the stretched uterine musculature contracts less vigorously. Besides hydramnios, a large infant, bleeding from abruptio placentae or placenta previa, and rapid labor and birth can also contribute to uterine atony during the postpartum period. Trauma during labor and birth is not a likely cause, and no evidence of excessive trauma was described in the scenario. Moderate fundal massage helps contract the uterus; it does not contribute to uterine atony. Although a lengthy or prolonged labor can contribute to uterine atony, this client had a cesarean birth for breech presentation. Therefore, it is unlikely that they had a long labor.

CN: Physiological adaptation; CL: Apply

90. 4. The classic symptoms of endometritis are fever and foul-smelling lochia. Odorless heavy bleeding is associated with retained placental fragments. Abdominal distention is associated with parametritis as the pelvic cellulitis advances and spreads, causing severe pain and distention. Nausea and vomiting are associated with parametritis, resulting from an abscess and advancing pelvic cellulitis.

CN: Reduction of risk potential; CL: Analyze

91. 4. The most likely cause of delayed postpartum hemorrhage is retained placental fragments. The client may be scheduled for dilatation and curettage to remove remaining placental fragments. Uterine atony, cervical lacerations, and vaginal lacerations are commonly associated with early, not late, postpartum hemorrhage.

CN: Health promotion and maintenance; CL: Apply

92. 1. The client being treated for mastitis should continue to breastfeed often, or at least every 2 to 3 hours. Treatment also includes bed rest, increased fluid intake, local heat application, analgesic agents, and antibiotic therapy. Continually emptying the breasts decreases the risk for engorgement or breast abscess. The client should not discontinue breastfeeding unless they choose to do so. The client may continue breastfeeding while receiving antibiotic therapy. Generally, the breast milk is not contaminated by the offending organism and is safe for the neonate.

CN: Physiological adaptation; CL: Analyze

93. 1. Down syndrome is a genetic abnormality that is caused by an extra chromosome that results in intellectual disability. The degree of intellectual disability is difficult to predict in a neonate, though most children born with Down syndrome have some degree of intellectual disability. Various methods can be used to determine whether a neonate has Down syndrome, which is commonly manifested by hypotonia, poor Moro reflex, flat facial profile, up-slanting palpebral fissures, epicanthal folds, and hyperflexible joints. Genetic studies can be indicative of this disorder. Clients older than 35 years of age are at a higher risk for having a child with Down syndrome. However, chromosomal abnormalities can occur regardless of the client's age.

CN: Reduction of risk potential; CL: Evaluate

94. 1. After birth, the client should make the decision about how much they would like to participate in the neonate's care. Seeing and caring for the neonate commonly facilitates the grief process. The nurse should be nonjudgmental and allow the client any opportunity to see, hold, and care for the neonate. The HCP does not need to be contacted about the client's desire to see the baby, which is a normal reaction. The social worker and the adoptive parents do not need to give the client permission to feed the baby.

CN: Health promotion and maintenance; CL: Analyze

95. 4. The client needs further instruction when they say that they should begin feeding on the right (painful) breast to decrease the pain. Starting the feeding on the unaffected (left) breast can stimulate the milk ejection reflex in the right breast and thereby decrease the pain. Frequent nursing or pumping is recommended to empty the breast. For some birth parents, mastitis is so painful that they choose to discontinue breastfeeding, so these parents need a great deal of support. Applying heat to the infected area before starting to feed is appropriate because heat stimulates circulation and promotes comfort. Increasing fluid intake is advised to ensure adequate hydration. Antibiotics need to be taken until all medication has been used, usually 7 to 10 days to ensure eradication of the infection.

CN: Reduction of risk potential; CL: Evaluate

96. 4. Holistic nursing honors the client's preference for safe, alternative, and complementary practices. Cabbage leaves tucked into the bra is an alternative practice that may relieve pain and swelling caused by engorgement in some clients. Saying that using cabbage is a folk remedy does not address the safety or efficacy of the practice. There are no known safety risks to using cabbage as a treatment for engorgement. The nurse should document the client's use of cabbage leaves to treat the engorgement in the medical record, but there is no risk that warrants immediate notification of the health care provider.

🗝️ CN: Health promotion and maintenance; CL: Apply

97. 3. The client is probably experiencing postpartum depression, and the HCP should be contacted. Postpartum depression is usually treated with psychotherapy, social support groups, and antidepressant medications. Contributing factors include hormonal fluctuations, a history of depression, and environmental factors (e.g., job loss). An estimated 50% to 70% of women experience some degree of postpartum "blues," but these feelings of sadness disappear within 1 to 2 weeks after birth. However, the client is voicing more than just sadness. Telling the client that they are overreacting is not helpful and may make them feel even less worthy. They are not exhibiting symptoms of a serious mental illness (loss of contact with reality), and they do not need hospitalization.

🗝️ CN: Health promotion and maintenance; CL: Analyze

98. 3. Feelings of guilt combined with a lack of self-care (not eating or sleeping enough) can predispose a new parent to postpartum depression, especially one who has had previous episodes of depression. Sleep is essential to both the birth parent and baby, but sleeping through the night does not usually occur in the first few weeks after birth. Although breastfeeding parents need good nutrition, unlimited eating after birth may inhibit the return to a normal weight and could create depression in a new parent, especially a vulnerable one. Attempting to care for an infant with no help from others is likely to cause stress that could lead to depression, especially in an adolescent.

🗝️ CN: Psychosocial integrity; CL: Evaluate

99. 1. St. John's wort, an herbal supplement commonly used to treat mild depression, interacts with many medications, making them less effective. If the client is already taking a prescription antidepressant, they can be at risk for serotonin syndrome. St. John's wort is not known to cause fetal growth or liver problems. It would be important to assess the client's mood after determining if the client is at risk for medication interactions.

🗝️ CN: Basic care and comfort; CL: Analyze

Managing Care, Quality, and Safety of Postpartum Clients

100. 2, 3, 1, 4. The nurse should then clean the solution from the client, notify the HCP of the incident, and ask for a prescription for medication if needed to counteract the povidone-iodine. The nurse will need to document the incident on the client's medical record as soon as the client has physically been taken care of. The nurse also will need to file an incident report.

🗝️ CN: Management of care; CL: Create

101. 4. The process for infant abduction in a hospital system focuses on utilizing all health care workers to observe for anyone who may possibly be concealing an infant in a large bag or under an oversized coat and is attempting to leave the building. Moving to the entrances and exits and checking each individual would be the responsibility of the doorman or security staff within the hospital system. Going to the obstetrics unit to determine if they need help would not be advised as the doors to the unit will be locked and access will not be available. Calling the nursery to ask about a missing baby wastes time, and the nursery staff should not reveal such information.

🗝️ CN: Safety and infection control; CL: Analyze

102.

0500	3
0530	1
0600	4
0630	2

Drawing the bilirubin levels at 0600 must occur at a specific time. The admission assessment should be completed as soon after admission as possible; 0500 is available to complete this task. The IV should be started at 0630 and completed as close to the change of shift as possible. The nurse should then draw the blood at 0530, right after the newborn assessment.

🗝️ CN: Management of care; CL: Create

103. 4. Although the greatest risk for postpartum hemorrhage is within the first hour following birth, a client can develop an early postpartum hemorrhage anytime within the first 24 hours after birth. As soon as the nurse notices an increased amount of lochia and clots, the fundus must be assessed for firmness and position. Normally, it should be firm, midline, and either just above or below the umbilicus. Massaging the fundus if it is not firm will assist with a uterine contraction to help decrease blood loss postpartum.

Administering oxytocin would not be the first action for the nurse to take. Performing an in-and-out catheterization at this time is not appropriate. The nurse should assist the client to the washroom to void on their own first. The nurse can measure the blood loss by measuring the perineal pad; however, this would be done after the nurse has first assessed the fundus.

 CN: Management of care; CL: Analyze

104. 1. Hemoglobin (Hgb) values following birth remain close to those during pregnancy. This value would indicate a low Hgb value and requires further follow-up by notifying the HCP and documenting the finding. A white blood cell (WBC) count of 18,000 μL (18 ×10⁹/L) is considered normal during the postpartum period. This is a normal value for hematocrit. A value of 50.28 μg/dL (9 mmol/L) for serum iron is within the normal range. The WBC count is within normal range for the postpartum period and will not require parenteral antibiotics. Vital signs can be assessed after contacting the HCP. Pain medication is not indicated at this time based on these laboratory values.

 CN: Management of care; CL: Analyze

105. 1, 5. Foul-smelling lochia and a temperature of 100.8°F (38.2°C) or higher are signs of a postpartum infection and should be reported to the HCP. Bilateral engorgement is not an unusual finding and typically responds to nursing interventions such as the use of ice packs. Postpartum blues can cause the client to cry easily for up to 2 weeks after birth. Soaking a peripad every 3 to 4 hours is a normal amount of lochia for a postpartum client within a week of birth.

 CN: Management of care; CL: Analyze

106. 1. Safety is the highest priority, and a nursing error has occurred. If the day nurse decides to tell the night nurse, the timing of the notification will be up to the nurse initiating the incident report. The nurse should confer with the charge nurse concerning the incident, but completion of the report is required. Waiting for several hours to initiate the report based on changes in client data and assessment is not an ethical or professional decision and should not be considered; again, safety is the highest priority.

 CN: Reduction of risk; CL: Analyze

107. 2, 3, 4, 5. The use of recycling bins on the unit does not impact safety or contribute to the quality of care. The infant identification system is a safety practice. Nursing influences the type of system used and how monitoring and identification occur, which improves the quality of care. The sibling and family visitation policy can be an excellent project. Sibling policies regarding visitation can influence safety (safety of the birth parent and infant by keeping children with colds, cases of flu, and infections away from the obstetrics unit). Nursing influences the development of a policy that is used and implemented on a daily basis. Postpartum instructions represent an area where the skill level, quality, and quantity of instruction represent nursing contributions to care. The ability of a family to remain together during a hospital stay is important to families. The quality of the obstetric experience can be enhanced or determined to be negative by this particular policy, one that is often looked at by these committees.

 CN: Management of care; CL: Apply

108. 1, 2, 4, 5. The safety of clients on an obstetric unit includes the prevention of infant abduction. Safe medication administration guidelines apply in obstetrics as well as all units in the hospital system. Adequate nourishment on the unit is essential for the promotion of breastfeeding and for those clients who want to eat shortly after birth, but it is not a safety concern. Adequate restraints as used during procedures, such as circumcisions, are a safety concern. An infant always needs proper identification when admitted, discharged, and taken to or away from parents, and this is also a great safety issue.

 CN: Reduction of risk; CL: Apply

109. 1, 2, 3, 4. Specific safety concerns on an obstetric unit include a very specific "hand-off report" after birth and recovery has been completed and the couplet is transitioned to birth mother and baby care. In any invasive procedure including tubal ligations and circumcisions, preprocedural verification is a standard procedure. Client education concerning the potential for infection in obstetrics is essential for any incision areas. Infant abduction is an ever-present concern for those working in a birth mother and baby unit. Car seat instructions for new parents involve the infant being in the back seat of a car facing backward—**not** in the front seat. Education for the family includes this important area.

 CN: Reduction of risk potential; CL: Evaluate

110. 2. The fundus descends at the rate of 1 to 2 cm a day and by 2 weeks is no longer a pelvic organ. The vital signs, breasts, heart, lungs, abdomen (with exception of fundus), lochia, perineum, and extremities are within normal limits.

 CN: Reduction of risk potential; CL: Analyze

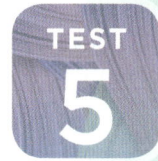

The Neonatal Client

- Neonatal Care
- Physical Assessment of the Neonatal Client
- The Preterm Neonate
- The Post-term Neonate
- The Neonate Who Needs Phototherapy
- The Neonate with Risk Factors
- Managing Care, Quality, and Safety of Neonatal Clients

Neonatal Care

1. A primiparous woman has just given birth to a term infant. What topic should the nurse teach the client about **first**?
   ☐ 1. sudden infant death syndrome (SIDS)
   ☐ 2. breastfeeding
   ☐ 3. newborn medications
   ☐ 4. infant sleep-wake cycles

2. A newborn who is 20 hours old has a respiratory rate of 66 breaths/min, is grunting when exhaling, and has occasional nasal flaring. The newborn's temperature is 98°F (36.6°C); the baby is breathing room air and is pink with acrocyanosis. The birth parent had membranes that were ruptured 26 hours before birth. What nursing action is **most** indicated?
   ☐ 1. Continue recording vital signs, voiding, stooling, and eating patterns every 4 hours.
   ☐ 2. Place a pulse oximeter, and request a prescription to draw blood cultures.
   ☐ 3. Arrange a transfer to the neonatal intensive care unit with a diagnosis of possible sepsis.
   ☐ 4. Draw a complete blood count (CBC) with differential, and feed the infant.

3. A neonate is born by cesarean birth at 36 weeks' gestation. The temperature in the birthing room is 70°F (21.1°C). To prevent heat loss from convection, the nurse should take which action?
   ☐ 1. Dry the neonate quickly after birth.
   ☐ 2. Keep the neonate away from air-conditioning vents.
   ☐ 3. Place the neonate away from outside windows.
   ☐ 4. Prewarm the bed.

4. The nurse cares for a term newborn on the third day of life.

   Progress Notes

Day	Pounds	Grams
Day 1 (birth)	7 lb 8 oz	3,401 g
Day 2	7 lb 4 oz	3,288 g
Day 3	7 lb	3,175 g

   The nurse reviews the daily weights of a breastfeeding term newborn.

   ➤ Complete the sentence from the list of options.

   The nurse's best action is to | reweigh the newborn.
   provide supplementation.
   continue routine monitoring.
   notify the health care provider.

5. The nurse makes a home visit to a 3-day-old full-term neonate who weighed 3912 g (3.91 kg) at birth. Today the neonate, who is being bottle-fed, weighs 3572 g (3.57 kg). Which instruction should the nurse give the parent?
☐ 1. Continue feeding every 3 to 4 hours since the weight loss is normal.
☐ 2. Contact the health care provider (HCP).
☐ 3. Switch to a soy-based formula because the current one seems inadequate.
☐ 4. Change to a higher-calorie formula to prevent further weight loss.

6. Commercial formulas contain 20 calories per 30 mL. A 1-day-old infant was fed 45 mL at 0200, 0530, 0800, 1100, 1400, 1630, 2000, and 2230. What is the total amount of calories the infant received today? Record your answer using one decimal place.
_____ calories.

7. A healthy neonate was just born in stable condition. In addition to drying the infant, what is the preferred method to prevent heat loss?
☐ 1. placing the infant under a radiant warmer
☐ 2. wrapping the infant in warm blankets
☐ 3. applying a knit hat
☐ 4. placing the infant skin to skin on the birth parent

8. The nurse is preparing to administer a vitamin K injection to a neonate shortly after birth. What statement by the birth parent indicates that they understand the purpose of the injection?
☐ 1. "My baby does not have the normal bacteria in their intestines to produce this vitamin."
☐ 2. "My baby is at a high risk for a problem involving their blood's ability to clot."
☐ 3. "The red blood cells my baby formed during pregnancy are destroying the vitamin K."
☐ 4. "My baby's liver is not able to produce enough of this vitamin so soon after birth."

9. The nurse is teaching the parent of a newborn to develop their baby's sensory system. To further improve the infant's most developed sense, the nurse should instruct the parent to perform which action?
☐ 1. Speak in a high-pitched voice to get the newborn's attention.
☐ 2. Place the newborn about 12 inches (30.5 cm) from the maternal face for best sight.
☐ 3. Stroke the newborn's cheek with the nipple to direct the baby's mouth to the nipple.
☐ 4. Give the infant formula with a sweetened taste to stimulate feeding.

10. The nurse has completed discharge teaching with new parents who will be bottle-feeding their term newborn. Which statement by the parents reflects the need for more teaching?
☐ 1. "Our baby will require feedings through the night for several weeks or months after birth."
☐ 2. "The baby should burp during and after each feeding with no projective vomiting."
☐ 3. "Our baby should have one to three soft, formed stools a day."
☐ 4. "We should weigh our baby daily to make sure they are gaining weight."

11. While making a home visit to a primiparous client and the client's 3-day-old infant, the nurse observes the parent changing the baby's disposable diaper. Before putting the clean diaper on the neonate, the parent begins to apply baby powder to the neonate's buttocks. Which information about baby powder should the nurse relate to the parent?
☐ 1. It may cause pneumonia to develop.
☐ 2. It helps prevent diaper rash.
☐ 3. It keeps the diaper from adhering to the skin.
☐ 4. It can result in allergies later in life.

12. After teaching a new parent about the care of their neonate after circumcision with a Gomco clamp, which statement by the parent indicates to the nurse that the parent needs additional instructions?
☐ 1. "The petroleum gauze may fall off into the diaper."
☐ 2. "A few drops of blood oozing from the site is normal."
☐ 3. "I will leave the gauze in place for 24 hours."
☐ 4. "I will remove any yellowish crusting gently with water."

13. After completing discharge instructions for a primiparous client who is bottle-feeding their term neonate, the nurse determines that the parent understands the instructions when the parent says that they should contact the health care provider (HCP) if the neonate exhibits which sign or symptom?
☐ 1. ability to fall asleep easily after each feeding
☐ 2. spitting up a tablespoon of formula after feeding
☐ 3. passage of a liquid stool with a watery ring
☐ 4. production of one to two light brown stools daily

14. The nurse is to draw a blood sample for glucose testing from a term neonate during the first hour after birth. The nurse should obtain the blood sample from the neonate's foot near which area?

☐ 1.

☐ 2.

☐ 3.

☐ 4.

15. After circumcision with a Plastibell, the nurse should instruct the neonate's parent to cleanse the circumcision site using which agent?
☐ 1. antibacterial soap
☐ 2. warm water
☐ 3. povidone-iodine solution
☐ 4. diluted hydrogen peroxide

16. Based on the understanding of periods of reactivity, what should the nurse encourage the parent of a term neonate to do approximately 90 minutes after birth?
☐ 1. Feed the neonate.
☐ 2. Allow the neonate to sleep.
☐ 3. Get to know the neonate.
☐ 4. Change the neonate's diaper.

Physical Assessment of the Neonatal Client

17. The nurse is to assess a newborn for incurving of the trunk. Which illustration indicates the position in which the nurse should place the newborn?

☐ 1.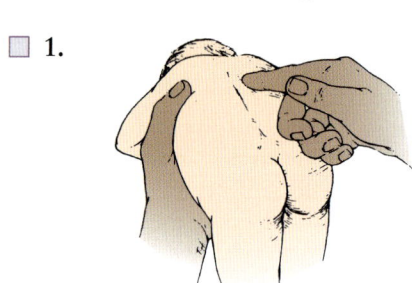

☐ 2.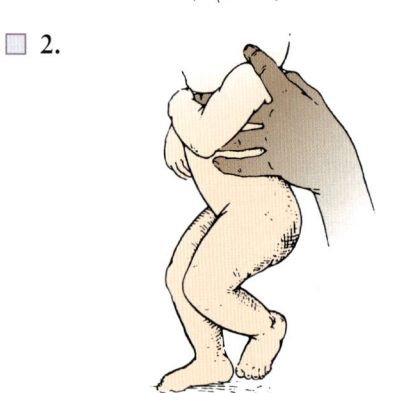

☐ 3.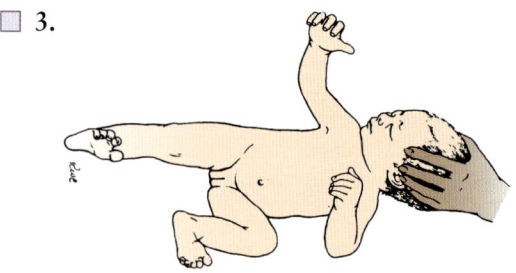

☐ 4.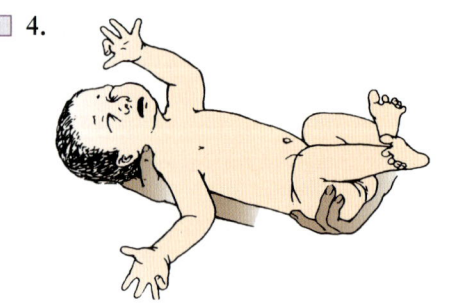

18. A full-term neonate is admitted to the newborn nursery. When lifting the baby out of the crib, the nurse notes the baby's arms move sideways with the palms up and the thumbs flexed. What should the nurse do **next**?
☐ 1. Activate rapid response teams.
☐ 2. Identify this reflex as a normal finding.
☐ 3. Place the neonate on seizure precautions.
☐ 4. Start supplemental oxygen.

19. After the birth of a neonate, a quick assessment is completed. The neonate is found to be apneic. After quickly drying and positioning the neonate, the nurse should do which action **next**?
☐ 1. Assign the first Apgar score.
☐ 2. Start positive pressure ventilation.
☐ 3. Administer oxygen.
☐ 4. Start cardiac compressions.

20. A 2948-g (2.94-kg) neonate was born vaginally at 38 weeks' gestation. At 5 minutes of life, the neonate has the following signs: heart rate of 110 bpm, intermittent grunting with a respiratory rate of 70 breaths/min, flaccid tone, no response to stimulus, and overall pale white in color. What is the Apgar score?
☐ 1. 2
☐ 2. 3
☐ 3. 4
☐ 4. 6

21. A neonate has a large amount of secretions. After vigorously suctioning the neonate, the nurse should assess for what possible result?
☐ 1. bradycardia
☐ 2. rapid eye movement
☐ 3. seizures
☐ 4. tachypnea

22. After the vaginal birth of a term neonate, the nurse observes that the neonate has one artery and one vein in the umbilical cord. The nurse notifies the health care provider (HCP) based on the analysis that this may be indicative of which anomalies?
☐ 1. respiratory anomalies
☐ 2. musculoskeletal anomalies
☐ 3. cardiovascular anomalies
☐ 4. intestinal anomalies

23. While changing the neonate's diaper, the client asks the nurse about some red-tinged drainage from the neonate's vagina. Which response would be **most** appropriate?
☐ 1. "It's of no concern because it's such a small amount."
☐ 2. "The cause is usually related to swallowing blood during the birth."
☐ 3. "Sometimes baby girls have this from hormones received from the birth parent."
☐ 4. "This vaginal spotting is caused by hemorrhagic disease of the newborn."

24. Which finding would the nurse expect as common when caring for a neonate born with the aid of a vacuum extractor at 41 weeks' gestation?
☐ 1. caput succedaneum
☐ 2. cephalohematoma
☐ 3. facial bruising
☐ 4. neonatal intracranial hemorrhage

25. After the nurse explains to a primiparous client the causes of their neonate's cranial molding, which statement by the client indicates the need for further instruction?
☐ 1. "The molding was caused by an overlapping of the baby's cranial bones during my labor."
☐ 2. "The amount of molding is related to the amount and length of pressure on the head."
☐ 3. "The molding will usually disappear in a couple of days."
☐ 4. "Brain damage may occur if the molding does not resolve quickly."

26. Which observation is expected when the nurse is assessing the gestational age of a neonate born at term?
☐ 1. ear lying flat against the head
☐ 2. absence of rugae in the scrotum
☐ 3. sole creases covering the entire foot
☐ 4. square window sign angle of 90 degrees

27. While the nurse is performing a complete assessment of a term neonate, which finding would alert the nurse to notify the health care provider (HCP)?
☐ 1. red reflex in the eyes
☐ 2. expiratory grunt
☐ 3. respiratory rate of 45 breaths/min
☐ 4. prominent xiphoid process

28. After instructing a parent about normal reflexes of term neonates, the nurse determines that the parent understands the instructions when they describe the tonic neck reflex as occurring when the neonate displays which behavior?
☐ 1. steps briskly when held upright near a firm, hard surface
☐ 2. pulls both arms and does not move the chin beyond the point of the elbows
☐ 3. turns the head to the left, extends the left extremities, and flexes the right extremities
☐ 4. extends and abducts the arms and legs with the toes fanning open

29. A primiparous client expresses concern to the nurse about why their neonate's eyes are crossed. Which information would the nurse include when teaching the parent about neonatal strabismus?
☐ 1. The neonate's eyes are unable to focus on light at this time.
☐ 2. Neonates commonly lack eye muscle coordination.
☐ 3. Congenital cataracts may be present.
☐ 4. The neonate is able to fixate on distant objects immediately.

30. While performing a physical assessment on a term neonate shortly after birth, the nurse would notify the health care provider (HCP) if which finding is noted?
☐ 1. deep creases across the soles of the feet
☐ 2. frequent sneezing during the assessment
☐ 3. single crease on each of the palms
☐ 4. absence of lanugo on the skin

31. Metabolic screening of an infant revealed a high phenylketonuria (PKU) level. Which statement(s) by the infant's parent indicates an understanding of the disease and its management? Select all that apply.
☐ 1. "My baby cannot have milk-based formulas."
☐ 2. "My baby will grow out of this by the age of 2 years."
☐ 3. "This is a hereditary disease, so any future children will have it, too."
☐ 4. "My baby will eventually become intellectually disabled because of this disease."
☐ 5. "We have to follow a strict low-phenylalanine diet."
☐ 6. "A dietitian can help me plan a diet that keeps a safe phenylalanine level but lets my baby grow."

32. Assessment of a term neonate at 2 hours after birth reveals a heart rate of less than 100 bpm, periods of apnea approximately 25 to 30 seconds in length, and mild cyanosis around the mouth. The nurse notifies the health care provider (HCP) based on the interpretation that these findings may lead to which condition?
☐ 1. respiratory arrest
☐ 2. bronchial pneumonia
☐ 3. intraventricular hemorrhage
☐ 4. epiglottitis

33. A new parent asks, "When will the soft spot near the front of my baby's head close?" When should the nurse tell the parent the soft spot will close?
☐ 1. 2 to 3 months
☐ 2. 6 to 8 months
☐ 3. 9 to 10 months
☐ 4. 12 to 18 months

34. Which assessment finding in a term neonate would cause the nurse to notify the health care provider (HCP)?
☐ 1. absence of tears
☐ 2. unequally sized corneas
☐ 3. pupillary constriction to bright light
☐ 4. red circle on pupils seen with a penlight

35. At 24 hours of age, assessment of the neonate reveals the following: eyes closed, skin pink, no sign of eye movements, heart rate of 120 bpm, and respiratory rate of 35 breaths/min. What is this neonate **most** likely experiencing?
☐ 1. drug withdrawal
☐ 2. first period of reactivity
☐ 3. a state of deep sleep
☐ 4. respiratory distress

36. While assessing a male neonate whose parent desires them to be circumcised, the nurse observes that the neonate's urinary meatus appears to be located on the ventral surface of the penis. The health care provider (HCP) is notified because the nurse suspects which complication?
☐ 1. phimosis
☐ 2. hydrocele
☐ 3. epispadias
☐ 4. hypospadias

The Preterm Neonate

37. The nurse is discussing kangaroo care with the parents of a premature neonate. The nurse should tell the parents that the advantages of skin-to-skin care include which benefit(s)? Select all that apply.
☐ 1. enhanced bonding
☐ 2. increased IQ
☐ 3. improved physiologic stability
☐ 4. decreased length of stay in the neonatal intensive care unit
☐ 5. improved breastfeeding

38. After a vaginal birth, a preterm neonate is to receive oxygen via mask. While administering the oxygen, the nurse would place the neonate in which position?
☐ 1. left side, with the neck slightly flexed
☐ 2. back, with the head turned to the left side
☐ 3. abdomen, with the head down
☐ 4. back, with the neck slightly extended

39. Which action should the nurse take when performing external chest compressions on a neonate born at 28 weeks' gestation?
☐ 1. Maintain a compression-to-ventilation ratio of 3:1.
☐ 2. Compress the sternum with the palm of the hand.
☐ 3. Compress the chest 70 to 80 times per minute.
☐ 4. Displace the chest wall at half the depth of the anterior-posterior diameter of the chest.

40. A preterm neonate who has been stabilized is placed in a radiant warmer and is receiving oxygen via an oxygen hood. Which action should the nurse take while administering oxygen in this manner?
☐ 1. Humidify the air being delivered.
☐ 2. Cover the neonate's scalp with a warm cap.
☐ 3. Record the neonate's temperature every 3 to 4 minutes.
☐ 4. Assess the neonate's blood glucose level.

41. Two hours ago, a neonate at 38 weeks' gestation and weighing 3175 g (3.18 kg) was born to a primiparous client who tested positive for beta-hemolytic *Streptococcus*. Which finding would alert the nurse to notify the health care provider (HCP)?
☐ 1. alkalosis
☐ 2. increased muscle tone
☐ 3. temperature instability
☐ 4. positive Babinski reflex

42. Assessment of a 2-day-old neonate born at 34 weeks' gestation reveals absent apical pulse left of the midclavicular line, cyanosis, grunting, and diminished breath sounds. After beginning oxygen, what is the **priority** intervention?
☐ 1. Obtain a prescription for a stat chest x-ray.
☐ 2. Reposition the neonate, and then assess if the grunting and cyanosis resolve.
☐ 3. Obtain a prescription for an echocardiogram.
☐ 4. Prepare for endotracheal intubation.

43. Twenty-four hours after cesarean birth, a neonate at 30 weeks' gestation is diagnosed with respiratory distress syndrome (RDS). When explaining to the parents about the cause of this syndrome, the nurse should include a discussion about an alteration in the body's secretion of which substance?
☐ 1. somatotropin
☐ 2. surfactant
☐ 3. testosterone
☐ 4. progesterone

44. A viable neonate born to a 28-year-old multiparous client by cesarean birth because of placenta previa is diagnosed with respiratory distress syndrome (RDS). Which factor would the nurse explain as the factor placing the neonate at the **greatest** risk for this syndrome?
☐ 1. birth parent's development of placenta previa
☐ 2. neonate born preterm
☐ 3. birth parent receiving analgesia 4 hours before birth
☐ 4. neonate with sluggish respiratory efforts after birth

45. While the nurse is caring for a neonate at 32 weeks' gestation in an isolette with continuous oxygen administration, the neonate's parent asks why the neonate's oxygen is humidified. What should the nurse tell the parent?
☐ 1. "The humidity promotes the expansion of the neonate's immature lungs."
☐ 2. "The humidity helps prevent viral or bacterial pneumonia."
☐ 3. "Oxygen is drying to the mucous membranes unless it is humidified."
☐ 4. "Circulation to the baby's heart is improved with humidified oxygen."

46. A preterm neonate admitted to the neonatal intensive care unit at about 30 weeks' gestation is placed in an oxygenated isolette. The neonate's birth parent tells the nurse that they were planning to breastfeed the neonate. Which instructions about breastfeeding would be **most** appropriate?
☐ 1. Breastfeeding is not recommended because the neonate needs increased fat in the diet.
☐ 2. Once the neonate no longer needs oxygen and continuous monitoring, breastfeeding can be done.
☐ 3. Breastfeeding is contraindicated because the neonate needs a high-calorie formula every 2 hours.
☐ 4. Gavage feedings using breast milk can be given until the neonate can coordinate sucking and swallowing.

47. What is the best reason for assessing a neonate weighing 1500 g (1.5 kg) at 32 weeks' gestation for retinopathy of prematurity (ROP)?
☐ 1. The neonate is at risk because of multiple factors.
☐ 2. Oxygen is being administered at a level of 21%.
☐ 3. The neonate was alkalotic immediately after birth.
☐ 4. Phototherapy is likely to be prescribed by the health care provider (HCP).

48. Which subject should the nurse include when teaching the parent of a neonate diagnosed with retinopathy of prematurity (ROP) about possible treatment for complications?
☐ 1. laser therapy
☐ 2. anti-inflammatory eye drops
☐ 3. frequent testing for glaucoma
☐ 4. corneal transplants

49. Three days after admission of a neonate born at 30 weeks' gestation, the neonatologist plans to assess the neonate for intraventricular hemorrhage (IVH). The nurse should plan to assist the neonatologist by preparing the neonate for which test?
☐ 1. cranial ultrasonography
☐ 2. arterial blood specimen collection
☐ 3. radiographs of the skull
☐ 4. complete blood count specimen collection

50. Which finding would the nurse **most** expect to find in a neonate born at 28 weeks' gestation who is diagnosed with intraventricular hemorrhage (IVH)?
☐ 1. increased muscle tone
☐ 2. hyperbilirubinemia
☐ 3. bulging fontanelles
☐ 4. hyperactivity

51. An infant born prematurely at 34 weeks is receiving gavage feedings. The client is holding their infant and asks why the nurse places a pacifier in the infant's mouth during these feedings. The nurse replies that the pacifier helps in what way(s)? Select all that apply.
    ☐ 1. coordinates the swallowing of feedings
    ☐ 2. encourages sucking behaviors
    ☐ 3. improves weight gain
    ☐ 4. instills a calming effect
    ☐ 5. improves digestion

52. While the nurse is caring for a neonate born at 32 weeks' gestation, which finding would **most** suggest the infant is developing necrotizing enterocolitis (NEC)?
    ☐ 1. the presence of 1 mL of gastric residual before a gavage feeding
    ☐ 2. jaundice appearing on the face and chest
    ☐ 3. an increase in bowel peristalsis
    ☐ 4. abdominal distention

53. Which statement by the parent of a neonate diagnosed with bronchopulmonary dysplasia (BPD) indicates effective teaching?
    ☐ 1. "BPD is an acute disease that can be treated with antibiotics."
    ☐ 2. "My baby may require long-term respiratory support."
    ☐ 3. "Bronchodilators can cure my baby's condition."
    ☐ 4. "My baby may have seizures later on in life because of this condition."

54. A preterm infant born 2 hours ago at 34 weeks' gestation is experiencing rapid respirations, grunting, no breath sounds on one side, and a shift in location of heart sounds. The nurse should prepare to assist with which procedure?
    ☐ 1. placement of the neonate on a ventilator
    ☐ 2. administration of bronchodilators through the nares
    ☐ 3. suctioning of the neonate's nares with wall suction
    ☐ 4. insertion of a chest tube into the neonate

55. Which finding would lead the nurse to suspect that a neonate born at 34 weeks' gestation receiving intravenous fluids has developed overhydration?
    ☐ 1. hypernatremia
    ☐ 2. polycythemia
    ☐ 3. hypoproteinemia
    ☐ 4. increased urine specific gravity

56. A newborn with an estimated weight of 3000 g (3 kg) requires full resuscitation. The provider prescribes 0.2 mL/kg of epinephrine in a standard concentration of 1 mg/10 mL concentration to be given in via the umbilical vein. How many milliliters would the newborn receive? Record your answer using two decimal places.
    _____ mg.

The Post-term Neonate

57. A neonate born by cesarean birth at 42 weeks' gestation, weighing 4100 g (4.1 kg), with Apgar scores of 8 at 1 minute after birth and 9 at 5 minutes after birth, develops an increased respiratory rate and tremors of the hands and feet 2 hours after birth. What is the **priority** problem for this neonate?
    ☐ 1. ineffective airway clearance
    ☐ 2. hyperthermia
    ☐ 3. decreased cardiac output
    ☐ 4. hypoglycemia

58. At a home visit, the nurse assesses a neonate born vaginally at 41 weeks' gestation 5 days ago. Which of these findings warrants further assessment?
    ☐ 1. frequent hiccups
    ☐ 2. loose, watery stool in the diaper
    ☐ 3. pink papular vesicles on the face
    ☐ 4. dry, peeling skin

59. The nurse assists the health care provider (HCP) with a lumbar puncture on a post-term neonate with signs of sepsis. What should the nurse do to assist in this procedure? Select all that apply.
    ☐ 1. Administer the intravenous (IV) antibiotic.
    ☐ 2. Hold the neonate steady in the correct position.
    ☐ 3. Ensure a patent airway.
    ☐ 4. Maintain a sterile field.
    ☐ 5. Obtain a serum glucose level.

60. A neonate is admitted to the neonatal intensive care unit for observation with a diagnosis of probable meconium aspiration syndrome (MAS). The neonate weighs 4650 g (4.65 kg) and is at 41 weeks' gestation. What would be the **priority** problem for this neonate?
    ☐ 1. impaired skin integrity
    ☐ 2. hyperglycemia
    ☐ 3. risk for impaired parent-infant-child attachment
    ☐ 4. impaired gas exchange

61. The neonate in the nurse's care has a pneumothorax. The nurse knows the signs of early decompensation and observes carefully for changes in which assessment(s)? Select all that apply.
    ☐ 1. blood pressure
    ☐ 2. temperature
    ☐ 3. urinary output
    ☐ 4. color
    ☐ 5. heart rate

The Neonate Who Needs Phototherapy

62. The nurse assesses the term newborn with facial bruising. The nurse knows to further assess for an elevation of which lab value?
    ☐ 1. bilirubin
    ☐ 2. blood urea nitrogen (BUN)
    ☐ 3. hematocrit
    ☐ 4. potassium

63. The nurse cares for a 2 day-old newborn born at 37 weeks' gestation on the birth parent and baby unit.

> **Nurse's Notes**
>
> **Day 2 0800:**
> The neonate is rooming in with the parent. Breastfeeding occurs every 3.5 hours, with an audible swallow. The neonate has had two wet diapers and one meconium stool since birth. The infant is quiet and alert, and the fontanelle is flat. Acrocyanosis and slight jaundice are noted at the clavicles. Cephalhematoma has been present since 2 hours after birth. Vital signs are temperature 97.8°F (36.5°C); heart rate 120 bpm; and respiration rate 52 breaths/min, which is irregular with pauses of 10 seconds. Today's weight of 3410 g (3.41 kg) is down 100 g (0.1 kg) from birth.

After reviewing the admission lab test results, the nurse updates the client's care.

➤ Complete the diagram by dragging from the choices below to specify the condition the client is most likely experiencing, two actions to take, and two parameters the nurse should monitor to assess the client's progress.

[Action to Take] — [Condition Most Likely Experiencing] — [Parameter to Monitor]
[Action to Take] — — [Parameter to Monitor]

Actions to Take	Possible Conditions	Parameters to Monitor
Obtain a bilirubin level	Dehydration	Intake and output
Offer supplemental feedings	Neonatal jaundice	Respiratory status
Provide lactation support	Infection	Color
Obtain a complete blood count	Respiratory distress	Temperature instability
Obtain a pulse oximetry reading		Heart rate

64. When developing a nursing care plan for an infant receiving phototherapy, the nurse should include what information in the plan of care? Select all that apply.
  ☐ 1. adequate skin exposure to phototherapy
  ☐ 2. allowing the birth parent to hold the infant as much as they wish
  ☐ 3. eye protection
  ☐ 4. supplemental water between feedings
  ☐ 5. thermoregulation

65. The nurse assesses a 15-hour-old infant and finds jaundice. What is the **priority** action the nurse needs to take?
  ☐ 1. Continue with normal newborn care.
  ☐ 2. Notify the health care provider of the finding.
  ☐ 3. Provide an extra feeding for the infant.
  ☐ 4. Wait and assess the skin color when the infant is over 24 hours old.

66. The nurse is providing teaching to the parent of a newborn with early jaundice about the condition's progression. The nurse knows that the teaching regarding hyperbilirubinemia was successful when the parent makes which response?
  ☐ 1. "Kernicterus is a consequence of elevated bilirubin levels and has possible lifelong effects."
  ☐ 2. "My baby should not get hyperbilirubinemia if I place them near a window in the sunlight."
  ☐ 3. "My baby will be 3 days old at discharge, and I will not need to worry about hyperbilirubinemia."
  ☐ 4. "Since I'm exclusively breastfeeding, the risk for my baby having hyperbilirubinemia is very low."

67. While performing an assessment, the nurse notes the infant's jaundice has moved from the nipple line to the umbilicus in the past 24 hours. How does the nurse interpret this physical finding?
  ☐ 1. A decrease in bilirubin level is probable.
  ☐ 2. An increase in bilirubin level is probable.
  ☐ 3. No further assessment is necessary.
  ☐ 4. Where jaundice is located on the baby is not indicative of bilirubin level.

68. Which instructions should the nurse give to the parents of a neonate diagnosed with hyperbilirubinemia who is receiving phototherapy?
☐ 1. Keep the neonate's eyes completely covered.
☐ 2. Use a regular diaper on the neonate.
☐ 3. Offer feedings every 4 hours.
☐ 4. Check the rectal temperature every 8 hours.

69. While caring for a term neonate who has been receiving phototherapy for 8 hours, the nurse should notify the health care provider (HCP) if which finding is noted?
☐ 1. bronze-colored skin
☐ 2. maculopapular chest rash
☐ 3. urine specific gravity of 1.018
☐ 4. absent Moro reflex

The Neonate with Risk Factors

70. A nurse is attempting to resuscitate a neonate. Thirty seconds of chest compressions have been completed. The neonate's heart rate remains less than 60 bpm. Epinephrine is given. What is the expected outcome for a neonate who has received epinephrine during resuscitation?
☐ 1. increased urine output
☐ 2. a normal heart rate
☐ 3. pain relief
☐ 4. sedation

71. A parent is visiting their neonate in the neonatal intensive care unit. The baby is fussy, and the parent wants to know what to do. To quiet a sick neonate, what can the nurse teach the parent to do?
☐ 1. Bring in toys for distraction.
☐ 2. Place a musical mobile over the crib.
☐ 3. Stroke the neonate's back.
☐ 4. Use a constant, gentle touch.

72. A neonate born at 40 weeks' gestation admitted to the nursery is found to be hypoglycemic. At 4 hours of age, the neonate appears pale, and the pulse oximeter is reading 75% on room air. What should the nurse do?
☐ 1. Increase the IV rate.
☐ 2. Provide supplemental oxygen.
☐ 3. Record the finding on the medical record and repeat the reading in 30 minutes.
☐ 4. Wrap the neonate to increase body temperature.

73. A neonate with heart failure is being discharged home. When the nurse is teaching the parents about the neonate's nutritional needs, what should the nurse explain?
☐ 1. Fluids must be restricted.
☐ 2. A decreased activity level should reduce the need for additional calories.
☐ 3. The formula should be low in sodium.
☐ 4. The neonate may need a more calorie-dense formula.

74. During an assessment of a neonate born at 33 weeks' gestation, a nurse finds and reports a heart murmur. An echocardiogram reveals patent ductus arteriosus, for which the neonate received indomethacin. What is the expected outcome after the administration of indomethacin to a neonate with patent ductus arteriosus?
☐ 1. closure of a patent ductus arteriosus
☐ 2. decreased bleeding time
☐ 3. increased gastrointestinal function
☐ 4. increased renal output

75. The nurse is receiving over the telephone a laboratory results report of a neonate's blood glucose level. What should the nurse do?
☐ 1. Write down the results, read back the results to the caller from the laboratory, and receive confirmation from the caller that the nurse understands the results.
☐ 2. Repeat the results to the caller from the laboratory, write the results on scrap paper first, and then transfer the results to the medical record.
☐ 3. Indicate to the caller that the nurse cannot receive verbal results from laboratory tests for neonates, and ask the laboratory to bring the written results to the nursery.
☐ 4. Request that the laboratory send the results by email to transfer to the client's medical record.

76. A multiparous client who has a neonate diagnosed with hemolytic disease of the newborn asks the nurse why the neonate has developed this problem. Which response(s) by the nurse would be appropriate? Select all that apply.
☐ 1. "Mixing of maternal and newborn blood that is incompatible has caused sensitization."
☐ 2. "You are Rh positive, and the baby is Rh negative."
☐ 3. "Your immune system saw the newborn's blood cells as foreign bodies."
☐ 4. "You are Rh negative, and the baby is Rh positive."
☐ 5. "The baby made antibodies against your red blood cells."

77. After teaching the multiparous parent about hemolytic disease of the newborn and Rh sensitization, the nurse determines that the client understands why they were not sensitized during their other pregnancy when they make which statement?
☐ 1. "My other baby had a different father."
☐ 2. "Like most women, I have immunity against the Rh factor."
☐ 3. "Antibodies are not usually formed until after exposure to an antigen."
☐ 4. "My blood could not neutralize antibodies formed from my first pregnancy."

78. After teaching a multiparous client about the effects of hemolysis due to Rh sensitization on the neonate at birth, the nurse determines that the client needs further instruction when the parent reports that the neonate may have which complication?
☐ 1. cardiac decompensation
☐ 2. polycythemia
☐ 3. anemia
☐ 4. splenic enlargement

79. After birth, a direct Coombs test is performed on the umbilical cord blood of a neonate with Rh-positive blood born to a parent with Rh-negative blood. The nurse explains to the client that this test is done to detect which information?
☐ 1. appropriate dose of Rho(D) immune globulin
☐ 2. degree of anemia in the neonate
☐ 3. initial bilirubin level
☐ 4. presence of maternal antibodies

80. The nurse recognizes that teaching about the need for an exchange transfusion in a neonate with erythroblastosis fetalis has been effective if the parents describe the purpose of the transfusion is to do what?
☐ 1. to replenish the neonate's leukocytes
☐ 2. to restore the fluid and electrolyte balance
☐ 3. to correct the neonate's anemia
☐ 4. to replace Rh-negative blood with Rh-positive blood

81. The nurse explains to the parent of a neonate diagnosed with erythroblastosis fetalis that the exchange transfusion is necessary to prevent damage primarily to which organ in the neonate?
☐ 1. kidneys
☐ 2. brain
☐ 3. lungs
☐ 4. liver

82. The nurse is caring for a newborn of a primiparous woman with insulin-dependent diabetes. When the parent visits the neonate 1 hour after birth, the nurse explains to the parent that the neonate is being closely monitored for symptoms of hypoglycemia because of which reason?
☐ 1. increased use of glucose stores during a difficult labor and birth process
☐ 2. interrupted supply of maternal glucose and continued high neonatal insulin production
☐ 3. a normal response that occurs during the transition from intrauterine to extrauterine life
☐ 4. increased pancreatic enzyme production caused by decreased glucose stores

83. While caring for a neonate of a birth parent with diabetes soon after birth, the nurse has fed the newborn formula to prevent hypoglycemia. The nurse checks the neonate's blood glucose level, and it is 60 mg/dL (3.3 mmol/L), but the neonate continues to exhibit jitteriness and tremors. What should the nurse do **first**?
☐ 1. Request a prescription for a blood calcium level.
☐ 2. Administer intravenous (IV) glucose.
☐ 3. Assess the neonate's temperature.
☐ 4. Refeed the infant.

84. The nurse is caring for a neonate weighing 4536 g (4.5 kg) who was born via cesarean birth 1 hour ago to a client with insulin-dependent diabetes. The client asks the nurse, "Why is my baby in the neonatal intensive care unit?" The nurse bases a response on the understanding that neonates of clients with diabetes commonly develop which condition?
☐ 1. anemia
☐ 2. persistent pulmonary hypertension
☐ 3. hemolytic disease
☐ 4. hypoglycemia

85. While assessing a neonate weighing 3175 g (3.2 kg) who was born at 39 weeks' gestation to a primiparous client who reports opiate use during pregnancy, the nurse understands that which finding would indicate possible opiate withdrawal?
☐ 1. bradycardia
☐ 2. high-pitched cry
☐ 3. sluggishness
☐ 4. hypothermia

86. The nurse recognizes that a parent needs more teaching about the complications of neonatal opioid exposure when the parent states that the baby may exhibit which gastrointestinal problem?
☐ 1. constipation
☐ 2. increased sucking
☐ 3. poor feeding
☐ 4. vomiting

87. When teaching a primiparous client who used cocaine during pregnancy how to comfort their fussy neonate, the nurse can advise the birth parent to use which intervention?
☐ 1. Tightly swaddle the neonate.
☐ 2. Feed the neonate extra, high-calorie formula.
☐ 3. Keep the neonate in a brightly lit environment.
☐ 4. Touch the baby only when they are crying.

88. A neonate born at 38 weeks' gestation is admitted to the neonatal nursery for observation. The neonate's birth parent, who is positive for human immunodeficiency virus (HIV) infection, has received no prenatal care. The parent asks the nurse if their neonate is positive for HIV. The nurse can tell the parent which information?
    ☐ 1. "More than 50% of neonates born to birth parents who are positive for HIV will be positive at 18 months of age."
    ☐ 2. "An enlarged liver at birth generally means the neonate is HIV positive."
    ☐ 3. "A complete blood count analysis is the primary method for determining whether the neonate is HIV positive."
    ☐ 4. "We will test your baby now, but testing will need to be repeated for an accurate diagnosis."

89. When caring for a multiparous client who is human immunodeficiency virus (HIV) positive and asking to breastfeed their neonate as soon as possible, the nurse should include which instructions about breast milk in the teaching plan?
    ☐ 1. It may help prevent the spread of the HIV virus.
    ☐ 2. It contains antibodies that can protect the neonate from HIV.
    ☐ 3. It can be beneficial for the bonding process.
    ☐ 4. It has been found to contain the retrovirus HIV.

90. While caring for the neonate of a human immunodeficiency virus (HIV)-positive birth parent, the nurse prepares to administer a prescribed vitamin K intramuscular injection 1 hour after birth. Which action should the nurse do **first**?
    ☐ 1. Bathe the neonate.
    ☐ 2. Place the neonate under a radiant warmer.
    ☐ 3. Wash the injection site with povidone-iodine solution.
    ☐ 4. Wait until the first dose of antiretroviral medication is given.

91. A 6-hour-old neonate born at 38 weeks' gestation by cesarean birth after prolonged rupture of the membranes and a maternal oral temperature of 102°F (38.8°C) is being observed for signs and symptoms of infection. Which sign would alert the nurse to notify the health care provider (HCP)?
    ☐ 1. white blood cell (WBC) count of 15,000 cells/mm³ (15 × 10⁹/L)
    ☐ 2. apical heart rate of 132 bpm
    ☐ 3. behavioral changes
    ☐ 4. warm, moist skin

92. The nurse is caring for a neonate diagnosed with early-onset sepsis who is being treated with intravenous antibiotics. Which instruction will the nurse include in the parents' teaching plan?
    ☐ 1. Wear protective gear near the isolation incubator.
    ☐ 2. Visit but do not touch the neonate.
    ☐ 3. Wash hands thoroughly before touching the neonate.
    ☐ 4. Wear a mask when holding the neonate.

93. A neonate born vaginally at term with a cleft lip and cleft palate is admitted to the regular nursery. Which action should the nurse take the **first** time the parents visit the neonate in the nursery?
    ☐ 1. Explain the surgical interventions that will be performed.
    ☐ 2. Stress that this defect is not life-threatening.
    ☐ 3. Emphasize the neonate's normal characteristics.
    ☐ 4. Reassure the parents about the success rate of the surgery.

94. After teaching the parents of a neonate born with a cleft lip and cleft palate about appropriate feeding techniques, the nurse determines that the parent needs further instruction when the parent makes which statement?
    ☐ 1. "I should clean my baby's mouth after each feeding."
    ☐ 2. "I should feed my baby in an upright position."
    ☐ 3. "I need to remember to burp my baby often."
    ☐ 4. "I may need to use a special nipple for feeding."

95. A neonate born at 36 weeks' gestation is admitted to the neonatal intensive care nursery with a diagnosis of probable fetal alcohol syndrome (FAS). The parent visits the nursery soon after the neonate is admitted. Which instructions should the nurse expect to include when developing the teaching plan for the parent about FAS?
    ☐ 1. Withdrawal symptoms usually do not occur until 7 days after birth.
    ☐ 2. Large-for-gestational-age size is common with this condition.
    ☐ 3. Facial deformities associated with FAS can be corrected by plastic surgery.
    ☐ 4. Symptoms of withdrawal include tremors, sleeplessness, and seizures.

96. Which characteristic should the nurse teach the birth parent about their neonate diagnosed with fetal alcohol syndrome (FAS)?
    ☐ 1. Neonates are commonly lethargic.
    ☐ 2. The IQ scores are usually average.
    ☐ 3. Neurologic disorders are common.
    ☐ 4. The mortality rate is 70% unless treated.

97. A newborn is diagnosed with fetal alcohol syndrome. The nurse is teaching the parent what to expect when they go home with the baby. The nurse determines the parent needs further instruction when they make which statement?
☐ 1. "The way my baby's face looks now will stay that way."
☐ 2. "My baby may be irritable as a newborn."
☐ 3. "I may need some help coping with my newborn."
☐ 4. "My baby will be fine soon after we are home."

98. The parent of a neonate diagnosed with gastroschisis tells the nurse that their spouse had planned on breastfeeding the neonate. Which information should the nurse include in the preoperative teaching plan about feeding the neonate?
☐ 1. The neonate will remain on nothing-by-mouth (NPO) status until after surgery.
☐ 2. An iron-fortified formula will be given before surgery.
☐ 3. The neonate will need total parenteral nutrition for nourishment.
☐ 4. The birth parent may breastfeed the neonate before surgery.

99. The nurse is developing a plan of care for a neonate who is to undergo gastroschisis surgery. What information should be included? Select all that apply.
☐ 1. prevention of hypothermia
☐ 2. maintenance of fluid and electrolyte balance
☐ 3. controlling preoperative pain
☐ 4. prevention of infection
☐ 5. providing developmental care

100. While caring for a male neonate diagnosed with gastroschisis, the nurse observes that the parents seem hesitant to touch the neonate because of his appearance. The nurse determines that the parents are **most** likely experiencing which stage of grief?
☐ 1. denial
☐ 2. shock
☐ 3. depression
☐ 4. anger

101. The nurse is caring for a neonate at 38 weeks' gestation when the nurse observes marked peristaltic waves on the neonate's abdomen. After this observation, the neonate exhibits projectile vomiting. The nurse notifies the health care provider (HCP) because these signs are indicative of which problem?
☐ 1. esophageal atresia
☐ 2. pyloric stenosis
☐ 3. diaphragmatic hernia
☐ 4. hiatal hernia

102. The nurse is caring for a term neonate who is diagnosed with patent ductus arteriosus. While performing a physical assessment of the neonate, the nurse anticipates that the neonate will exhibit which signs?
☐ 1. decreased cardiac output with faint peripheral pulses
☐ 2. profound cyanosis over most of the body
☐ 3. loud cardiac murmur through systole and diastole
☐ 4. harsh systolic murmur with a palpable thrill

103. Assessment of a term neonate at 8 hours after birth reveals tachypnea, diminished femoral pulses, and poor lower body perfusion. The nurse notifies the health care provider (HCP) based on the interpretation that these symptoms are associated with which complication?
☐ 1. coarctation of the aorta
☐ 2. atrioventricular septal defect
☐ 3. pulmonary atresia
☐ 4. transposition of the great arteries

104. The nurse assesses a neonate on the first day of life.

Vital Signs

Time	1100	1130
Color	Acrocyanosis	Central cyanosis
Respirations	92 breaths/min, no nasal flaring, retractions, or grunting	102 breaths/min, breath sounds clear, no nasal flaring, retractions, or grunting
Heart rate	128 bpm, no murmur	138 bpm, no murmur
Temperature	98.9°F (37.2°C)	98.6°F (37°C)

What action should the nurse take?
☐ 1. Change the position.
☐ 2. Encourage the baby to cry.
☐ 3. Notify the health care provider (HCP).
☐ 4. Suction the nose and mouth.

105. The nurse is performing an admission assessment on a neonate and finds the femoral pulses to be weaker than the brachial and radial pulses. What nursing action should the nurse take **next**?
☐ 1. Call for a cardiac consult.
☐ 2. Note and tell the health care provider (HCP) when rounds are made.
☐ 3. Place the neonate in reverse Trendelenburg position.
☐ 4. Take the neonate's blood pressure in all four extremities.

106. A neonate is 4 hours of age. The nursing assessment reveals a heart murmur. What should the nurse do?
☐ 1. Call the health care provider (HCP) immediately.
☐ 2. Continue routine care.
☐ 3. Apply oxygen
☐ 4. Further assess for signs of distress.

107. During the change-of-shift report, it was reported that a neonate was experiencing subcostal retractions. Identify where the nurse would expect to see the retractions.

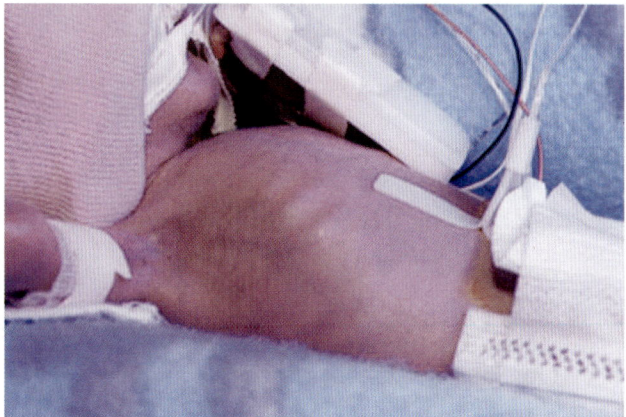

Managing Care, Quality, and Safety of Neonatal Clients

108.

STEP 1

The nurse is caring for a newborn on the birth parent and baby unit with suspected exposure to maternal substance use disorder.

Nurse's Notes

Day 2 0700:
S: A 2-day-old term newborn is breastfeeding.
B: The neonate was born by spontaneous vaginal birth to a primigravid parent who used opioids during pregnancy. The neonate's Apgar scores were 9 and 10. The birth weight was 3100 g (3.1 kg).
A: The neonate's vital signs are temperature (T) 99.5°F (37.5°C); heart rate (HR) 140 bpm; and respiration rate (RR) 62 breaths/min. The neonate is irritable with moderate tremors when disturbed and regurgitates two to three times with feedings. Today's weight is 2950 g (2.9 kg).
R: The baby has routine orders and needs to be reassessed.

The nurse reviews the end-of-shift handoff.

➢ Highlight the assessment findings that require follow-up. Answer choices have been underlined.

Nurse's Notes

Day 2 0700:
S: A 2-day-old term newborn is breastfeeding.
B: The neonate was born by spontaneous vaginal birth to a primigravid parent who used opioids during pregnancy. The neonate's Apgar scores were 9 and 10. The birth weight was 3100 g (3.1 kg).
A: The neonate's vital signs are <u>temperature (T) 99.5°F (37.5°C); heart rate (HR) 140 bpm</u>; and <u>respiration rate (RR) 62 breaths/min</u>. <u>The neonate is irritable with moderate tremors when disturbed</u> and <u>regurgitates two to three times with feedings. Today's weight is 2950 g (2.9 kg).</u>
R: The baby has routine orders and needs to be reassessed.

109. STEP 2

The nurse is caring for a newborn on the birth parent and baby unit with suspected exposure to maternal substance use disorder.

Nurse's Notes

Day 2 0700:
S: A 2-day-old term newborn is breastfeeding.
B: The neonate was born by spontaneous vaginal birth to a primigravid parent who used opioids during pregnancy. The neonate's Apgar scores were 9 and 10. The birth weight was 3100 g (3.1 kg).
A: The neonate's vital signs are temperature (T) 99.5°F (37.5°C); heart rate (HR) 140 bpm; and respiration rate (RR) 62 breaths/min. The neonate is irritable with moderate tremors when disturbed and regurgitates two to three times with feedings. Today's weight is 2950 g (2.9 kg).
R: The baby has routine orders and needs to be reassessed.

➤ For each of the findings, indicate if the symptoms are consistent with central nervous system (CNS) dysfunction; metabolic, vasomotor, and respiratory disturbances; or gastrointestinal dysfunction. Each finding may support more than one disease process.

Findings	CNS Dysfunction	Metabolic, Vasomotor, and Respiratory Disturbances	Gastrointestinal Dysfunction
Fever	○	○	○
Respiratory rate	○	○	○
Irritability	○	○	○
Moderate tremors	○	○	○
Frequent regurgitation	○	○	○

Note: Each column must have at least one response selected.

110. STEP 3

The nurse is caring for a newborn on the birth parent and baby unit with suspected exposure to maternal substance use disorder.

Nurse's Notes

Day 2 0700:
S: A 2-day-old term newborn is breastfeeding.
B: The neonate was born by spontaneous vaginal birth to a primigravid parent who used opioids during pregnancy. The neonate's Apgar scores were 9 and 10. The birth weight was 3100 g (3.1 kg).
A: The neonate's vital signs are temperature (T) 99.5°F (37.5°C); heart rate (HR) 140 bpm; and respiration rate (RR) 62 breaths/min. The neonate is irritable with moderate tremors when disturbed and regurgitates two to three times with feedings. Today's weight is 2950 g (2.9 kg).
R: The baby has routine orders and needs to be reassessed.

➤ Identify words from the choices below to fill in each blank found in the following sentences.

The nurse is most concerned that the client has

[_____].

The nurse should take immediate actions to prevent the complications of

[_____] and

[_____].

Word Choices

dehydration

hyperbilirubinemia

neonatal abstinence syndrome

neonatal sepsis

respiratory arrest

seizure

111. STEP 4

The nurse is caring for a newborn on the birth parent and baby unit with suspected exposure to maternal substance use disorder.

Nurse's Notes

Day 2 0700:
S: A 2-day-old term newborn is breastfeeding.
B: The neonate was born by spontaneous vaginal birth to a primigravid parent who used opioids during pregnancy. The neonate's Apgar scores were 9 and 10. The birth weight was 3100 g (3.1 kg).
A: The neonate's vital signs are temperature (T) 99.5°F (37.5°C); heart rate (HR) 140 bpm; and respiration rate (RR) 62 breaths/min. The neonate is irritable with moderate tremors when disturbed and regurgitates two to three times with feedings. Today's weight is 2950 g (2.9 kg).
R: The baby has routine orders and needs to be reassessed.

Orders

1. Begin nonpharmacological comfort measures.
2. Notify the health care provider and increase nonpharmacological therapy if the neonate is unable to:
   - eat at least 1 oz per feed or breastfeed well.
   - sleep for at least 1 hour undisturbed.
   - be consoled within 10 minutes.
3. If the neonate does not respond to increased nonpharmacological therapy,
   - begin morphine 0.03 mg/kg PO every 4 hours as needed (PRN).

The newborn receives the diagnosis of neonatal abstinence syndrome, and the health care provider writes new orders.

➤ What nonpharmacological comfort measure(s) should the nurse include in the plan of care? Select all that apply.

☐	1. Avoiding overstimulation
☐	2. Breastfeeding on demand
☐	3. Direct sunlight
☐	4. Gentle rocking
☐	5. Pacifier use
☐	6. Rooming-in
☐	7. Safe swaddling
☐	8. Side positioning

112. STEP 5

The nurse is caring for a newborn on the birth parent and baby unit with suspected exposure to maternal substance use disorder.

Nurse's Notes

Day 2 0700:
S: A 2-day-old term newborn is breastfeeding.
B: The neonate was born by spontaneous vaginal birth to a primigravid parent who used opioids during pregnancy. The neonate's Apgar scores were 9 and 10. The birth weight was 3100 g (3.1 kg).
A: The neonate's vital signs are temperature (T) 99.5°F (37.5°C); heart rate (HR) 140 bpm; and respiration rate (RR) 62 breaths/min. The neonate is irritable with moderate tremors when disturbed and regurgitates two to three times with feedings. Today's weight is 2950 g (2.9 kg).
R: The baby has routine orders and needs to be reassessed.

Orders

1. Begin nonpharmacological comfort measures.
2. Notify the health care provider and increase nonpharmacological therapy if the neonate is unable to:
   - eat at least 1 oz per feed or breastfeed well.
   - sleep for at least 1 hour undisturbed.
   - be consoled within 10 minutes.
3. If the neonate does not respond to increased nonpharmacological therapy,
   - begin morphine 0.03 mg/kg PO every 4 hours as needed (PRN).

The nurse implements the treatment plan and gathers more information while providing breastfeeding education.

➢ For each possible finding, specify if the finding would suggest breastfeeding is indicated or contraindicated.

Possible Findings	Indicated	Contraindicated
Negative maternal urine toxicology at birth	○	○
Positive maternal human immunodeficiency virus (HIV) diagnosis	○	○
Maternal referral to an addiction counselor	○	○
Previous maternal history of hepatitis A	○	○
Need to give the newborn a PRN dose of morphine	○	○
Positive meconium drug screen for opioids	○	○
Maternal use of an illicit street drug	○	○

113. STEP 6

The nurse is caring for a newborn on the birth parent and baby unit with suspected exposure to maternal substance use disorder.

Nurse's Notes

Day 2 0700:
S: A 2-day-old term newborn is breastfeeding.
B: The neonate was born by spontaneous vaginal birth to a primigravid parent who used opioids during pregnancy. The neonate's Apgar scores were 9 and 10. The birth weight was 3100 g (3.1 kg).
A: The neonate's vital signs are temperature (T) 99.5°F (37.5°C); heart rate (HR) 140 bpm; and respiration rate (RR) 62 breaths/min. The neonate is irritable with moderate tremors when disturbed and regurgitates two to three times with feedings. Today's weight is 2950 g (2.9 kg).
R: The baby has routine orders and needs to be reassessed.

Orders

1. Begin nonpharmacological comfort measures.
2. Notify the health care provider and increase nonpharmacological therapy if the neonate is unable to:
   - eat at least 1 oz per feed or breastfeed well.
   - sleep for at least 1 hour undisturbed.
   - be consoled within 10 minutes.
3. If the neonate does not respond to increased nonpharmacological therapy,
   - begin morphine 0.03 mg/kg PO every 4 hours as needed (PRN).

Progress Notes

Day 5:
The 5-day-old term breastfeeding newborn was diagnosed on day 2 of life with neonatal abstinence syndrome. PRN morphine was initiated on day 3 of life when nonpharmacological comfort measures alone did not control symptoms. Vital signs are T 98.6°F (37°C); HR 140 bpm; and RR 40 breaths/min. The newborn breastfeeds every 2 to 3 hours, sleeping 2 hours at a time. Mild tremors are noted when the infant is disturbed. The parent can console the neonate. The baby has been stable on 0.09 mg/kg morphine every 4 hours for 24 hours. The neonate's weight has increased by 30 g (0.03 kg). The parent has requested a meeting to discuss the plan for discharge.

The nurse implements the plan of care for a newborn with neonatal abstinence syndrome and evaluates the progress 3 days later.

➢ Which finding(s) would suggest the neonate is ready for discharge? Select all that apply.

- ☐ 1. gaining 30 to 60 mg of weight daily
- ☐ 2. stable on 0.09 mg/kg of morphine
- ☐ 3. breastfeeding every 2 to 3 hours
- ☐ 4. sleeping 2 hours at a time
- ☐ 5. can be consoled by the parent
- ☐ 6. parent agreeable with the plan of care

114. During a shift handoff, the nurse receives the following information: "The infant was born at 38 weeks' gestation to a gravida 1, para 1, 26-year-old birth parent by spontaneous vaginal birth. The birth parent is breastfeeding the infant." What additional information does the nurse need to make an accurate assessment? Select all that apply.
- ☐ 1. age of the infant in hours
- ☐ 2. length of labor
- ☐ 3. infant's output
- ☐ 4. birth parent's nutritional status
- ☐ 5. infant's weight

115. The nurse has received a shift report on a group of newborns. The nurse should make rounds on which client **first**?
- ☐ 1. a newborn who is large for gestational age (LGA) and who needs a repeat blood glucose prior to the next feeding in 15 minutes
- ☐ 2. a neonate born at 36 weeks' gestation weighing 2270 g (2.27 kg) who is due to breastfeed for the first time in 15 minutes
- ☐ 3. a neonate who was born 24 hours ago by cesarean birth and had a respiratory rate of 62 breaths/min 30 minutes ago
- ☐ 4. a newborn who had a borderline low temperature and was double-wrapped with a hat 30 minutes ago to bring up the temperature

116. The nurse is caring for a 2-hour-old, full-term, breastfeeding newborn. The nurse notes the following assessments: apical pulse, 122 bpm; axilla temperature, 96.6°F (35.9°C); and jitteriness. Based on this assessment, what should the nurse do **first**?
☐ 1. Assist the newborn to breastfeed.
☐ 2. Notify the health care provider (HCP).
☐ 3. Obtain a blood glucose sample.
☐ 4. Place the newborn under a radiant heater.

117. The nurse is assigned to care for four birth parents and their term newborns. Which parent and newborn couplet requires the nurse's attention **first**?
☐ 1. Birth parent: fundus is firm 2 cm below the umbilicus; minimal lochia rubra. Infant: color is pink on room air; respirations 67 breaths/min; bilateral crackles on auscultation.
☐ 2. Birth parent: fundus is firm 3 cm above the umbilicus and to the right; moderate rubra lochia. Infant: color is pink when active, currently dusky while quiet; respirations 70 breaths/min.
☐ 3. Birth parent: fundus is firm 1 cm above the umbilicus; small amount of lochia rubra. Infant: color is pink with acrocyanosis; respirations 68 breaths/min and intermittent expiratory grunting.
☐ 4. Birth parent: fundus is firm at the umbilicus; small amount of lochia rubra. Infant: pale pink, quiet, alert; respirations 65 breaths/min; periodic breathing noted.

118. The nurse in a postpartum couplet room is making rounds before ending the shift. Which finding(s) would indicate that the safety needs of the clients have been met? Select all that apply.
☐ 1. infant lying on the abdomen
☐ 2. security tags in place
☐ 3. identification system on the birth parent and infant
☐ 4. bulb syringe within sight
☐ 5. someone in the room able to care for the infant
☐ 6. infant in the parent's arms, both asleep

119. After receiving the change-of-shift report in the normal newborn nursery, the nurse should see which neonate **first**?
☐ 1. 3-hour-old neonate with increased respiratory secretions
☐ 2. 6-hour-old neonate with a blood glucose of 25 mg/dL (1.38 mmol/L)
☐ 3. 12-hour-old neonate with a temperature of 97.4°F (36.4°C)
☐ 4. 24-hour-old neonate with no urine output for the past 12 hours

120. The newborn nurse has just received the shift report about a group of newborns and is to receive another admission in 30 minutes. To provide the safest care and plan for the new admission, the nurse should do which tasks in order of first to last? All options must be used.

1. Move quickly from room to room, and assess all clients.
2. Check the room to which the new client will be admitted to ensure all supplies and equipment are available.
3. Log on to the clinical information system, and determine if there are new prescriptions.
4. Review notes from the shift report, and prioritize all clients; make rounds on the most critical first.

121. The charge nurse in the newborn nursery and an unlicensed assistive personnel (UAP) are working together on a shift. Under their care are eight babies rooming in with their birth parents, and one infant is in the nursery for the night on tube feedings. There is a new client whose infant will be brought to the nursery in 15 minutes. Which task(s) would the nurse assign to the UAP? Select all that apply.
☐ 1. newborn admission
☐ 2. vital signs of all stable infants
☐ 3. tube feeding
☐ 4. document feedings of infants
☐ 5. record voids/stools
☐ 6. bath and initial feeding for new admission

Answers, Rationales, and Test-Taking Strategies

*The answers and rationales for each question follow below, along with keys (🗝️) to the client need (CN) and cognitive level (CL) for each question. In addition, questions that measure clinical judgment will be coded (CJ). As you check your answers, use the **Content Mastery and Test-Taking Skill Self-Analysis** worksheet (tear-out worksheet in the back of the book) to identify the reason(s) for not answering the questions correctly. For additional information about test-taking skills and strategies for answering questions, refer to pages 12–51 in Part 1 of this book.*

Neonatal Care

1. **2.** Ideally, breastfeeding should begin immediately after birth while infants are still very awake. Successful breastfeeding will likely require sustained support, encouragement, and instruction from the nurse. Information on SIDS and sleep-wake cycles are also important topics for the new parent, but this information can be given at any time prior to discharge. Newborn medications, including vitamin K and eye ointments, are given soon after birth and can be given after the first breastfeeding session.

    🗝️ CN: Health promotion and maintenance; CL: Analyze

2. **2.** The concern with this infant is sepsis based on prolonged rupture of membranes before birth. Blood cultures would provide an accurate diagnosis of sepsis but will take 48 hours from the time drawn. Frequent monitoring of infant vital signs, looking for changes, and maintaining contact with the parents is also part of care management while awaiting culture results. Continuing with vital signs, voiding, stooling, and eating every 4 hours is the standard of care for a normal newborn, but a respiratory rate higher than 60 breaths/min, grunting, and occasional flaring are not normal. Although these findings are not normal, the need for the intensive care unit is not warranted as newborns with sepsis can be treated with antibiotics at the maternal bedside. The CBC does not establish the diagnosis of sepsis, but the changes in the white blood cell levels can identify an infant at risk. Many experts suggest that waiting until an infant is 6 to 12 hours old to draw a CBC will give the most accurate results.

    🗝️ CN: Reduction of risk potential; CL: Analyze

3. **2.** The neonate should be kept away from drafts, such as from air conditioning vents, which may cause heat loss by convection. Evaporation is one of the most common mechanisms by which the neonate will lose heat, such as when the moisture on the newly born neonate's body is converted to vapor. Drying the infant prevents heat loss by evaporation. Keeping infants away from outside windows helps prevent heat loss by radiation, which is defined as heat loss between solid objects that are not in contact with one another such as walls and windows. Conduction is when heat is transferred between solid objects in contact with one another, such as when a neonate comes in contact with a cold mattress or scale. Placing the infant in a radiant warmer or skin to skin with the birth parent reduces heat loss from conduction.

    🗝️ CN: Reduction of risk potential; CL: Analyze

4. **0/1** *The nurse's best action is to* **continue routine monitoring.**

    Up to a 10% weight loss in the first few days of life is normal in a breastfeeding newborn. This newborn's weight loss is under 10%, so the nurse can assume that breastfeeding is going as expected and just needs routine monitoring. There is no need to reweigh the newborn or notify the health care provider. Best breastfeeding practices do not include supplementation unless there is a medical reason.

    🗝️ CJ: Standalone trend; CL: Apply

5. **1.** This 3-day-old neonate's weight loss falls within a normal range, and therefore no action is needed at this time. Full-term neonates tend to lose 5% to 10% of their birth weight during the first few days after birth, most likely because of minimal nutritional intake. With bottle-feeding, the neonate's intake varies from one feeding to another. Typically, neonates regain any weight loss by 7 to 10 days of life. If the weight loss continues after that time, the HCP should be called.

    🗝️ CN: Health promotion and maintenance; CL: Analyze

6. **240 calories**

    Eight feedings × 45 mL per feeding equals 360 mL. 360 mL × 20 cal/30 mL = 240 calories.

    🗝️ CN: Basic care and comfort; CL: Apply

7. **4.** Placing an infant on the birth parent's bare chest or abdomen facilitates the transition to extrauterine life and is the preferred method of thermoregulation for stable infants. A radiant warmer should be used if an infant is unstable and needs medical intervention. Blankets may be placed over a

newborn and birth parent's chest. A hat may be added to prevent heat loss from the head, but these methods are supplemental to skin-to-skin care.

🔑 CN: Health promotion and maintenance; CL: Apply

8. 1. For vitamin K synthesis in the intestines to begin, food and normal intestinal flora are needed. However, at birth, the neonate's intestines are sterile. Therefore, vitamin K is administered via injection to prevent a vitamin K deficiency that may result in a bleeding tendency. When administered, vitamin K promotes the formation of clotting factors II, VII, IX, and X in the liver. Neonates are not normally susceptible to clotting disorders unless they are diagnosed with hemophilia or demonstrate a deficiency of or a problem with clotting factors. Hemolysis of fetal red blood cells does not destroy vitamin K. Hemolysis may be caused by Rh or ABO incompatibility, which leads to anemia and necessitates an exchange transfusion. Vitamin K synthesis occurs in the intestines, not the liver.

🔑 CN: Pharmacological and parenteral therapies; CL: Evaluate

9. 3. Currently, touch is believed to be the most highly developed sense at birth. It is probably why neonates respond well to touch. Auditory sense typically is relatively immature in the neonate, as evidenced by the neonate's selective response to the human voice. By 4 months, the neonate should turn the eyes and head toward a sound coming from behind. Visual sense tends to be relatively immature. At birth, visual acuity is estimated at 20/100 to 20/150, but it improves rapidly during infancy and toddlerhood. Taste is well developed, with a preference toward glucose; however, touch is more developed at birth.

🔑 CN: Health promotion and maintenance; CL: Analyze

10. 4. Healthy infants are weighed during their visits to their health care provider, so it is not necessary to monitor weights at home. Infants may require one to three feedings during the night initially. By 3 months, 90% of babies sleep through the night. Projective vomiting may indicate pyloric stenosis and should not be seen in a normal newborn. Bottle-fed infants may stool one to three times daily.

🔑 CN: Health promotion and maintenance; CL: Evaluate

11. 1. The nurse should inform the parent that baby powder can enter the neonate's lungs and result in pneumonia secondary to aspiration of the particles. The best prevention for diaper rash is frequent diaper changing and keeping the neonate's skin dry. The disposable diapers have moisture-collecting materials and generally do not adhere to the skin unless the diaper becomes saturated. Typically, allergies are not associated with the use of baby powder in neonates.

🔑 CN: Reduction of risk potential; CL: Analyze

12. 4. The parent needs further instruction when they say that a yellowish crust should be removed with water. The yellowish crust is normal and indicates scar formation at the site. It should not be removed because to do so might cause increased bleeding. The petroleum gauze prevents the diaper from sticking to the circumcision site, and it may fall off in the diaper. If this occurs, the parent should not attempt to replace it but should simply apply plain petroleum jelly to the site. The gauze should be left in place for 24 hours, and the parent should continue to apply petroleum jelly with each diaper change for 48 hours after the procedure. A few drops of oozing blood is normal, but if the amount is greater than a few drops, the parent should apply pressure and contact the health care provider. Any bleeding after the first day should be reported.

🔑 CN: Reduction of risk potential; CL: Evaluate

13. 3. The parent demonstrates an understanding of the discharge instructions when they say that they should contact the HCP if the baby has a liquid stool with a watery ring because this indicates diarrhea. Infants can become dehydrated very quickly, and frequent diarrhea can result in dehydration. Normally, babies fall asleep easily after a feeding because they are satisfied and content. Spitting up a tablespoon of formula is normal; however, projectile or forceful vomiting in larger amounts should be reported. Bottle-fed infants typically pass one to two light brown stools each day.

🔑 CN: Reduction of risk potential; CL: Evaluate

14. 1. In a neonate, the lateral aspect of the heel is the most appropriate site for obtaining a blood specimen. Using this area prevents damage to the calcaneus bone, which is located in the middle of the heel. The middle of the heel is to be avoided because of the increased risk for damaging the calcaneus bone located there. The middle of the foot contains the medial plantar nerve and the medial plantar artery, which could be injured if this site is selected. Using the base of the big toe as the site for specimen collection would cause a great deal of discomfort for the neonate; therefore, it is not the preferred site.

🔑 CN: Reduction of risk potential; CL: Apply

15. 2. After circumcision with a Plastibell, the most commonly recommended procedure is to clean the circumcision site with warm water with each diaper change. Other treatments are necessary only if complications, such as an infection, develop. Antibacterial soap or diluted hydrogen peroxide may cause pain and is not recommended. Povidone-iodine solution may cause stinging and burning, and therefore its use is not recommended.

🔑 CN: Health promotion and maintenance; CL: Apply

16. 2. As part of the neonate's physiologic adaptation to birth at 90 minutes after birth, the neonate typically is in the rest or sleep phase. During this time, the heart and respiratory rates slow, and the neonate sleeps, unresponsive to stimuli. At this time, the birth parent should rest and allow the neonate to sleep. Feedings should be given during the first period of reactivity, considered the first 30 minutes after birth. During this period, the neonate's respirations and heart rate are elevated. Getting to know the neonate typically occurs within the first hour after birth and then when the neonate is awake and during feedings. Changing the neonate's diaper can occur at any time, but at 90 minutes after birth, the neonate is usually in a deep sleep, unresponsive, and probably has not passed any meconium.

🔑 CN: Health promotion and maintenance; CL: Apply

Physical Assessment of the Neonatal Client

17. 1. When assessing the incurving of the trunk tests for automatic reflexes in the newborn, the nurse places the infant horizontally and in a prone position with one hand and strokes the side of the newborn's trunk from the shoulder to the buttocks using the other hand. If the reflex is present, the newborn's trunk curves toward the stimulated side. Option 2 shows a figure for testing for a stepping response. Option 3 shows a figure for testing for a tonic neck reflex. Option 4 shows a figure for testing for the Moro (startle) reflex.

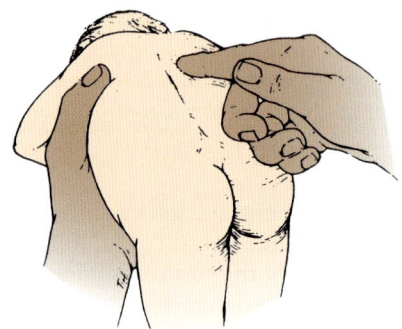

🔑 CN: Physiological adaptation; CL: Apply

18. 2. The baby is displaying a normal Moro reflex that occurs with a sudden loss of support and requires no intervention. Activating rapid response teams, placing the neonate on seizure precautions, and starting supplemental oxygen are not necessary for a normally occurring reflex.

🔑 CN: Basic care and comfort; CL: Analyze

19. 2. If an infant is not breathing after the initial steps of resuscitation, the next thing the nurse must do is begin positive pressure ventilation. Apgar scores are an evaluation of the neonate's status at 1 and 5 minutes of life. Waiting to restore respirations until after assigning an Apgar score would be a waste of valuable time. Oxygen alone does little good if the infant is not breathing. Chest compressions must be accompanied by adequate oxygenation.

🔑 CN: Physiological adaptation; CL: Analyze

20. 3. The neonate has a heart rate higher than 100 bpm, which earns them 2 points. The respiratory rate of 70 breaths/min is equivalent to a 2 on the scale. The flaccid muscle tone is equal to 0 on the scale. The lack of response to stimulus also equals 0, as does the neonate's overall pale white color. Thus, the total score equals 4.

🔑 CN: Basic care and comfort; CL: Apply

21. 1. After performing vigorous suctioning, the nurse must watch for bradycardia due to potential vagus nerve stimulation. Rapid eye movement is not associated with vagus nerve stimulation. Vagal stimulation will not cause seizures or tachypnea.

🔑 CN: Reduction of risk potential; CL: Analyze

22. 3. Normally, the umbilical cord has two umbilical arteries and one vein. When a neonate is born with only one artery and one vein, the nurse should notify the HCP for further evaluation of cardiac anomalies. Other common congenital problems associated with a missing artery include renal anomalies, central nervous system lesions, tracheoesophageal fistulas, trisomy 13, and trisomy 18. Respiratory anomalies are associated with dyspnea and respiratory distress; musculoskeletal anomalies include fractures or a dislocated hip; and intestinal anomalies are associated with increased amniotic fluid and failure to pass meconium.

🔑 CN: Reduction of risk potential; CL: Analyze

23. **3.** The most appropriate response would be to explain that vaginal spotting in female neonates is associated with hormones received from the birth parent. Estrogen is believed to cause slight vaginal bleeding or spotting in the female neonate. The condition disappears spontaneously, so there is no need for concern. Telling the parent that it is of no concern does not allay the parent's worry. The vaginal spotting is related to hormones received from the parent, not to swallowing blood during the birth or hemorrhagic disease of the neonate. Anemia is associated with hemorrhagic disease.

🔑 CN: Health promotion and maintenance; CL: Analyze

24. **1.** Caput succedaneum is common after the use of a vacuum extractor to assist the client's expulsion efforts. This edema may persist for up to 7 days. Vacuum extraction is not associated with cephalohematoma. Facial bruising may occur, but it is more common when forceps are used. Neonatal intracranial hemorrhage is a risk with both vacuum extraction and forceps births, but it is not a common finding.

🔑 CN: Health promotion and maintenance; CL: Analyze

25. **4.** The parent needs further instruction if they say the molding can result in brain damage. Brain damage is highly unlikely. Molding occurs during vaginal birth when the cranial bones tend to override or overlap as the head accommodates to the size of the birth parent's birth canal. The amount and duration of pressure on the head influence the degree of molding. Molding usually disappears in a few days without any special attention.

🔑 CN: Health promotion and maintenance; CL: Evaluate

26. **3.** Sole creases covering the entire foot are indicative of a term neonate. If the neonate's ear is lying flat against the head, the neonate is most likely preterm. An absence of rugae in the scrotum typically suggests a preterm neonate. A square window sign angle of 0 degrees occurs in neonates of 40 to 42 weeks' gestation. A 90-degree square window angle suggests an immature neonate of approximately 28 to 30 weeks' gestation.

🔑 CN: Health promotion and maintenance; CL: Apply

27. **2.** An expiratory grunt is significant and should be reported promptly because it may indicate respiratory distress and the need for further intervention such as oxygen or resuscitation efforts. The presence of a red reflex in the eyes is normal. An absent red reflex may indicate congenital cataracts. A respiratory rate of 45 breaths/min and a prominent xiphoid process are normal findings in a term neonate.

🔑 CN: Reduction of risk potential; CL: Analyze

28. **3.** The tonic neck reflex, also called the *fencing position*, is present when the neonate turns the head to the left side, extends the left extremities, and flexes the right extremities. This reflex disappears in a matter of months as the neonatal nervous system matures. The stepping reflex is demonstrated when the infant is held upright near a hard, firm surface. The prone crawl reflex is demonstrated when the infant pulls both arms but does not move the chin beyond the elbows. When the infant extends and abducts the arms and legs with the toes fanning open, this is a normal Babinski reflex.

🔑 CN: Health promotion and maintenance; CL: Apply

29. **2.** Convergent strabismus is common during infancy until about age 6 months because of poor oculomotor coordination. The neonate has peripheral vision and can fixate on close objects for short periods. The neonate can also perceive colors, shapes, and faces. Neonates can focus on light and should blink or close their eyes in response to light. However, this is not associated with strabismus. An absent red reflex or white areas over the pupils, not strabismus, may indicate congenital cataracts. Most neonates cannot focus well or accommodate for distance immediately after birth.

🔑 CN: Health promotion and maintenance; CL: Apply

30. **3.** A single crease across the palm (simian crease) is most commonly associated with chromosomal abnormalities, notably Down syndrome. Deep creases across the soles of the feet are a normal finding in a term neonate. Frequent sneezing in a term neonate is normal. This occurs because the neonate is a nose breather and sneezing helps to clear the nares. An absence of lanugo on the skin of a term neonate is a normal finding.

🔑 CN: Reduction of risk potential; CL: Analyze

31. **1, 5, 6.** Phenylketonuria, an inherited autosomal recessive disorder, involves the body's inability to metabolize the amino acid phenylalanine. A diet low

in phenylalanine must be followed. Such foods as meats, eggs, and milk are high in phenylalanine. Assistance from a dietitian is commonly necessary to keep phenylalanine levels low and to provide the essential amino acids necessary for cell function and tissue growth. With autosomal recessive disorders, future children will have a 25% chance of having the disease, a 50% chance of carrying the disease, and a 25% chance of being free of the disease. If a diet low in phenylalanine is followed until brain growth is complete (sometime in adolescence), the child should achieve normal intelligence.

CN: Health promotion and maintenance; CL: Evaluate

32. 1. Periods of apnea lasting longer than 20 seconds, mild cyanosis, and a heart rate of less than 100 bpm (bradycardia) are associated with a potentially life-threatening event and subsequent respiratory arrest. The neonate needs further evaluation by the HCP. Pneumonia is associated with tachycardia, anorexia, malaise, cyanosis, diminished breath sounds, and crackles. Intraventricular hemorrhage is associated with prematurity. Assessment findings include bulging fontanelles and seizures. Epiglottitis is a bacterial form of croup. Assessment findings include inspiratory stridor, cough, and irritability. It occurs most commonly in children age 3 to 7 years.

CN: Reduction of risk potential; CL: Analyze

33. 4. Normally, the anterior fontanelle closes between ages 12 and 18 months. Premature closure (craniosynostosis or premature synostosis) prevents proper growth and expansion of the brain, resulting in an intellectual disability. The posterior fontanel typically closes by ages 2 to 3 months.

CN: Health promotion and maintenance; CL: Apply

34. 2. Corneas of unequal size should be reported because this may indicate congenital glaucoma. An absence of tears is common because the neonate's lacrimal glands are not yet functioning. The neonate's pupils normally constrict when a bright light is focused on them. The finding implies that light perception and visual acuity are present, as they should be after birth. A red circle on the pupils is seen when a penlight or ophthalmoscope's light shines onto the retina and is a normal finding. Called the red reflex, this indicates that the light is shining onto the retina.

CN: Reduction of risk potential; CL: Analyze

35. 3. At 24 hours of age, the neonate is probably in a state of deep sleep, as evidenced by the closed eyes, lack of eye movements, normal skin color, and normal heart rate and respiratory rate. Jitteriness, a high-pitched cry, and tremors are associated with drug withdrawal. The first period of reactivity occurs in the first 30 minutes after birth, evidenced by alertness, sucking sounds, and rapid heart rate and respiratory rate. There is no evidence to suggest respiratory distress because the neonate's respiratory rate of 35 breaths/min is normal.

CN: Health promotion and maintenance; CL: Analyze

36. 4. The condition in which the urinary meatus is located on the ventral surface of the penis, termed *hypospadias*, occurs in 1 of every 500 male infants. Circumcision is delayed until the condition is corrected surgically, usually between 6 and 12 months of age. Phimosis is an inability to retract the prepuce at an age when it should be retractable or by age 3 years. Phimosis may necessitate circumcision or surgical intervention. Hydrocele is a painless swelling of the scrotum that is common in neonates. It is not a contraindication for circumcision. Epispadias occurs when the urinary meatus is located on the dorsal surface of the penis. It is extremely rare and is commonly associated with bladder exstrophy.

CN: Reduction of risk potential; CL: Analyze

The Preterm Neonate

37. 1, 3, 4, 5. Holding a neonate skin to skin with a caregiver has been shown to enhance bonding, improve physiologic stability, decrease length of stay, and improve breastfeeding. Research has not shown an increase in IQ as a developmental outcome. The experience is usually limited to 1 to 2 hours, two to three times per day.

CN: Health promotion and maintenance; CL: Apply

38. 4. When receiving oxygen by mask, the neonate is placed on the back with the neck slightly extended, in the "sniffing" or neutral position. This position optimizes lung expansion and places the upper respiratory tract in the best position for receiving oxygen. Placing a small rolled towel under the neonate's shoulders helps extend the neck properly without overextending it. Once stabilized and transferred to an isolette in the intensive care unit, the neonate can be positioned in the prone position, which allows for lung expansion in the oxygenated environment. Placing the neonate on the left side does not allow for maximum lung expansion. Also, slightly flexing the neck interferes with opening the airway. Placing the neonate on the back with the head turned to the left side does not allow for lung expansion. Placing the neonate on the abdomen interferes with proper positioning of the oxygen mask.

  CN: Physiological adaptation; CL: Apply

39. 1. Chest compressions should be alternated with ventilation to ensure breathing and circulation. Two fingers or two thumbs encircling hands, not the palm of the hand, are used to compress a neonate's sternum. The chest is compressed 100 to 120 times per minute. The proper technique recommended by the Neonatal Resuscitation Program is to use enough pressure to depress the sternum to a depth of approximately one-third of the anterior-posterior diameter of the chest.

  CN: Physiological adaptation; CL: Apply

40. 1. Whenever oxygen is administered, it should be humidified to prevent drying of the nasal passages and mucous membranes. Because the neonate is under a radiant warmer, a stocking cap is not necessary. Temperature, continuously monitored by a skin probe attached to the radiant warmer, is recorded every 30 to 60 minutes initially. Although the oxygen concentration in the hood requires close monitoring and measurement of blood gases, checking the blood glucose level is not necessary.

  CN: Physiological adaptation; CL: Apply

41. 3. The neonate is at high risk for sepsis due to exposure to the birth parent's infection. Temperature instability in a neonate at 38 weeks' gestation is an early sign of sepsis. Other signs include tachycardia, decreased muscle tone, acidosis, apnea, respiratory distress, hypotension, poor feeding behaviors, vomiting, and diarrhea. Late signs of infection include jaundice, seizures, enlarged liver and spleen, respiratory failure, and shock. Alkalosis is not typically seen in neonates who develop sepsis. Acidosis and respiratory distress may develop unless treatment such as antibiotics is started. A positive Babinski reflex is a normal finding and does not need to be reported.

  CN: Reduction of risk potential; CL: Analyze

42. 1. With an absent apical pulse left of the midclavicular line accompanied by cyanosis, grunting, and diminished breath sounds, the neonate is most likely experiencing pneumothorax. Pneumothorax occurs when alveoli are overdistended and subsequently the lung collapses, compressing the heart and lung and compromising the venous return to the right side of the heart. This condition can be confirmed by x-ray. An echocardiogram would be indicated if the chest x-ray did not reveal a respiratory cause for the problem or suggested a cardiac problem. Repositioning the infant may open the airway, but until the pneumothorax is resolved, the other symptoms will continue. Endotracheal intubation would be indicated if the infant's respiratory status continued to deteriorate, but placing the child on mechanical ventilation without decompressing the pneumothorax would likely worsen the newborn's status.

  CN: Physiological adaptation; CL: Analyze

43. 2. RDS, previously called *hyaline membrane disease*, is a developmental condition involving a decrease in lung surfactant that leads to improper expansion of the lung alveoli. Surfactant contains a group of surface-active phospholipids, of which one component—lecithin—is the most critical for alveolar stability. Surfactant production peaks at about 35 weeks' gestation. This syndrome primarily attacks preterm neonates, though it can also affect term and postterm neonates. Altered somatotropin secretion is associated with growth disorders such as gigantism or dwarfism. Altered testosterone secretion is associated with masculinization. Altered progesterone secretion is associated with spontaneous abortion during pregnancy.

  CN: Physiological adaptation; CL: Apply

44. 2. RDS is a developmental condition that primarily affects preterm infants before 35 weeks' gestation because of inadequate lung development from deficient surfactant production. The development of placenta previa has little correlation with the development of RDS. Although excessive analgesia can depress the neonate's respiratory condition if it is given shortly before birth, the scenario presents no information that this has occurred. The neonate's sluggish respiratory activity postpartum is not the likely cause of RDS but may be a sign that the neonate has the condition.

  CN: Reduction of risk potential; CL: Analyze

45. 3. Oxygen should be humidified before administration to help prevent drying of the mucous membranes in the respiratory tract. Drying impedes the normal functioning of cilia in the respiratory tract and predisposes to mucous membrane irritation. Humidification of oxygen does not promote expansion of the immature lungs. Expansion is promoted by placing the infant in a prone position or providing the preterm infant with surfactant medication. Humidified oxygen does not prevent viral or bacterial pneumonia. In fact, in some nurseries, *Staphylococcus aureus* has been detected in moist environments and on the hands and nails of staff members, predisposing the neonate to pneumonia. Humidified oxygen does not improve blood circulation in the cardiac system.

🔑 CN: Physiological adaptation; CL: Apply

46. 4. Many intensive care units that care for high-risk neonates recommend that the birth parent pump their breasts, store the milk, and bring it to the unit so the neonate can be fed with it, even if the neonate is being fed by gavage. As soon as the neonate has developed a coordinated suck-and-swallow reflex, breastfeeding can begin. Secretory immunoglobulin A, found in breast milk, is an important immunoglobulin that can provide immunity to the mucosal surfaces of the gastrointestinal tract. It can protect the neonate from enteric infections, such as those caused by *Escherichia coli* and *Shigella* species. Some studies have also shown that breastfed preterm neonates maintain transcutaneous oxygen pressure and body temperature better than bottle-fed neonates. There is some evidence that breast milk can decrease the incidence of necrotizing enterocolitis. The preterm neonate does not need additional fat in the diet. However, some neonates may need an increased caloric intake. In such cases, breast milk can be fortified with an additive to provide additional calories. Neonates who are receiving oxygen can breastfeed. During feedings, supplemental oxygen can be delivered by nasal cannula.

🔑 CN: Health promotion and maintenance; CL: Apply

47. 1. ROP, previously called *retrolental fibroplasia*, is associated with multiple risk factors, including high arterial blood oxygen levels, prematurity, and very low birth weight (1500 g [1.5 kg]). In the early acute stages of ROP, the neonate's immature retinal vessels constrict. If vasoconstriction is sustained, vascular closure follows, and irreversible capillary endothelial damage occurs. Normal room air is at 21%. Acidosis, not alkalosis, is commonly seen in preterm neonates, but this is not related to the development of ROP. Phototherapy is not related to the development of ROP. However, during phototherapy, the neonate's eyes should be constantly covered to prevent damage from the lights.

🔑 CN: Reduction of risk potential; CL: Apply

48. 1. Because the retina may become detached with ROP, laser therapy has been used successfully in some medical centers to treat ROP. Antiinflammatory eye drops may be used to treat seasonal allergies. ROP is not associated with glaucoma, so frequent testing is not necessary. Because the vessels of the eye are affected and not the corneas, corneal transplantation is not used.

🔑 CN: Physiological adaptation; CL: Apply

49. 1. Neonates who weigh less than 1500 g (1.5 kg) or who are born earlier than 34 weeks' gestation are susceptible to IVH. Cranial ultrasound scanning can confirm the diagnosis. The spinal fluid will show an increased number of red blood cells. Arterial blood gas specimen collection is done to evaluate the neonate's oxygen saturation level. Skull radiographs are not commonly used because of the danger of radiation. Additionally, computed tomography scans have replaced the use of skull x-ray films because they can provide more definitive results. Complete blood count specimen collection is usually performed to determine the hemoglobin, hematocrit, and white blood cell count. The results are not specific for IVH.

🔑 CN: Reduction of risk potential; CL: Apply

50. 3. A common finding of IVH is a bulging fontanelle. The most common site of hemorrhage is the periventricular subependymal germinal matrix, where there is a rich blood supply and where the capillary walls are thin and fragile. Rapid volume expansion, hypercarbia, and hypoglycemia contribute to the development of IVH. Other common manifestations include neurologic signs such as hypotonia, lethargy, temperature instability, nystagmus, apnea, bradycardia, decreased hematocrit, and increasing hypoxia. Seizures also may occur. Hyperbilirubinemia refers to an increase in bilirubin in the blood and may be seen if bleeding was severe.

🔑 CN: Physiological adaptation; CL: Analyze

51. 2, 3, 4, 5. Nonnutritive sucking has been seen in infants as early as 28 weeks, and ultrasound examinations have shown thumb sucking in utero even earlier. Nonnutritive sucking encourages sucking behaviors that help a baby maintain the sucking reflex needed for subsequent breast- or bottle-feedings. Nonnutritive sucking promotes digestion by stimulating secretions of gastrointestinal peptides that help with gastric emptying. Nonnutritive sucking has a calming effect that improves physiological stability. When it takes place during tube feedings, it helps the newborn make the association between sucking and the sensation of a full stomach. Improved digestion and physiological stability lead to improved weight gain. Sucking on a pacifier during a tube feeding does not lead to improved swallowing of feedings because milk is delivered directly into the stomach.

🔑 CN: Basic care and comfort; CL: Apply

52. **4.** Indications of NEC include abdominal distention with gastric retention and vomiting. Other signs may include lethargy, irritability, positive blood culture in stool, absent or diminished bowel sounds, apnea, diarrhea, metabolic acidosis, and unstable temperature. A gastric residual of 1 mL is not significant. Jaundice of the face and chest is associated with the neonate's immature liver function and increased bilirubin, not NEC. Typically with NEC, the neonate would exhibit absent or diminished bowel sounds, not increased peristalsis.

CN: Physiological adaptation; CL: Analyze

53. **2.** BPD is a chronic illness that may require prolonged hospitalization and permanent assisted ventilation. The disease typically occurs in compromised very-low-birth-weight neonates who require oxygen therapy and assisted ventilation for treatment of respiratory distress syndrome. The cause is multifactorial, and the disease has four stages. The neonate's activities may be limited by the disease. Antibiotics may be prescribed, and bronchodilators may be used, but these medications will not cure the chronic disease state. Seizure activity is associated with periventricular-intraventricular hemorrhage, not BPD.

CN: Physiological adaptation; CL: Evaluate

54. **4.** The client data support the diagnosis of pneumothorax, which would be confirmed with a chest x-ray. Pneumothorax is an accumulation of air in the thoracic cavity between the parietal and visceral pleurae and requires immediate removal of the accumulated air. Resolution is initiated with the insertion of a chest tube connected to continuous negative pressure. The neonate does not need to be placed on a ventilator unless there is evidence of severe respiratory distress. The goal of treatment is to reinflate the collapsed lung. Administering bronchodilators through the nares or suctioning the neonate's nares would do nothing to aid in lung reinflation.

CN: Physiological adaptation; CL: Analyze

55. **3.** Decreased protein or hypoproteinemia is a sign of overhydration, which can lead to patent ductus arteriosus or congestive heart failure. Bulging fontanelles, decreased serum sodium, decreased urine specific gravity, and decreased hematocrit are other signs of overhydration. Hypernatremia (increased serum sodium concentration) or increased urine specific gravity would suggest dehydration, not overhydration. Polycythemia evidenced by an elevated hematocrit would suggest hypoxia or congenital heart disorder.

CN: Reduction of risk potential; CL: Analyze

56. **0.6 mL.** Medication safety is enhanced with the use of standardized concentrations and dosing protocols. The standardized concentration of epinephrine used for neonatal resuscitation is 1 mg per 10 mL. Standard dosing regimens are in milliliters per kilogram, with acceptable ranges of 0.1 to 0.3 mL/kg. A prescribed dose of 0.2 mL/kg for a 3000-g (3-kg) infant equals 0.06 mL.

CN: Pharmacological and parenteral therapies; CL: Apply

The Post-term Neonate

57. **4.** Increased respiratory rate and tremors are indicative of hypoglycemia, which commonly affects the post-term neonate because of depleted glycogen stores. There is no indication that the neonate has ineffective airway clearance, which would be evidenced by excessive amounts of mucus or visualization of meconium on the vocal cords. Lethargy, not tremors, would suggest infection or hyperthermia. Furthermore, the post-term neonate typically has difficulty maintaining temperature, resulting in hypothermia, not hyperthermia. Decreased cardiac output is not indicated, particularly because the neonate was born by cesarean birth, which is not considered a difficult birth.

CN: Health promotion and maintenance; CL: Analyze

58. **2.** A loose, watery stool in the diaper is indicative of diarrhea and needs immediate attention. The infant may become severely dehydrated quickly because of the higher percentage of water content per body weight in the neonate, compared with the adult. Frequent hiccups are considered normal in a neonate and do not warrant additional investigation. Pink papular vesicles (erythema toxicum) on the face are considered normal in a neonate and disappear without treatment. Dry, peeling skin is normal in a post-term neonate.

CN: Health promotion and maintenance; CL: Analyze

59. **2, 3, 4.** Holding the neonate steady and in the proper position will help ensure a safe and accurate lumbar puncture. The neonate is usually held in a "C" position to open the spaces between the vertebral column. This position puts the neonate at risk for airway obstruction. Thus, ensuring the patency of the airway is the first priority, and the nurse should observe the neonate for adequate ventilation. Maintaining a sterile field is important to avoid infection in the neonate. It is not necessary to administer antibiotics or obtain a serum glucose level during the procedure.

CN: Safety and infection control; CL: Analyze

60. **4.** The priority problem for the neonate with probable MAS is impaired gas exchange related to the effects of respiratory distress. Obstruction of the airways may be complete or partial. Meconium aspiration may lead to pneumonia or pneumothorax. Establishing an adequate respiration rate is the primary goal. Impaired skin integrity is a concern, but establishing and maintaining an airway and gas exchange is always the priority. Hypoglycemia tends to be a problem for large-for-gestational-age babies, not hyperglycemia. If the parents do not express interest or concern for the neonate, risk for impaired parent-child attachment may be appropriate once the airway is established.

CN: Physiological adaptation; CL: Analyze

61. **1, 4, 5.** The pneumothorax may affect cardiac output, thus affecting perfusion and causing a decrease in blood pressure and changes in color from pallor to cyanosis. As the neonate attempts to compensate, bradycardia or tachycardia may be exhibited. A change in temperature and urinary output are very late signs of decompensation.

CN: Physiological adaptation; CL: Analyze

The Neonate Who Needs Phototherapy

62. **1.** Bruising causes red blood cell (RBC) destruction. A byproduct of RBC hemolysis is bilirubin, and thus infants who have significant bruising will have increased levels of bilirubin. The hematocrit may be decreased even if bruising is not increased. Bruising will have no effect on the BUN. Bruising in term infants does not affect potassium levels.

CN: Physiological adaptation; CL: Analyze

63.

Actions to Take	Possible Conditions	Parameters to Monitor
Obtain a bilirubin level	Neonatal jaundice	Intake and output
Provide lactation support		Color

This newborn is most likely experiencing neonatal jaundice as evidenced by visible jaundice and history of cephalohematoma. There is no evidence of dehydration as having one to two wet diapers and some weight loss are normal findings on day 1. A respiratory rate of 30 to 60 breaths/min and patterns of rapid breathing followed by pauses of 5 to 10 seconds are also normal newborn findings. Temperature instability is a sign of infection, but temperatures of 97.8°F (36.5°C) to 99°F (37.2°C) are normal. Obtaining a bilirubin level is indicated to determine if phototherapy is needed. Lactation support should be provided to increase breastfeeding frequency, which will aid in bilirubin excretion. There is no need for a supplement or a complete blood count at this point. A routine pulse oximeter reading may be needed based on protocol, but it is not needed based on the newborn's condition. The nurse should monitor the newborn's color and intake and output to determine if the interventions are effective. The nurse will continue to obtain routine vital signs, but these assessments provide very little information about the infant's bilirubin levels.

CJ: Standalone bowtie; CL: Create

64. **1, 3, 5.** For phototherapy to be effective, the skin needs to be exposed to the light waves to allow for the conversion of bilirubin to water-soluble isomers that are excreted without further metabolism by the liver. Eye protection is necessary to prevent retinal damage. As infants are usually dressed only in a diaper for maximum skin exposure to the light, thermoregulation is a concern. The infants can be too cool or potentially overheat if the phototherapy lights are not positioned correctly. Most often parents are allowed to hold their infants for feeding; there is usually a 30-minute time limit. For the phototherapy to be effective, the baby must be under the lights except for feedings. Water supplementation is not indicated as the baby needs the calories and nutrients that breast milk or formula provide. Extra water feedings will not prevent hyperbilirubinemia or decrease total serum bilirubin levels.

CN: Physiological adaptation; CL: Create

65. **2.** Jaundice that appears before 24 hours of age is considered pathologic. Jaundice appears when bilirubin levels reach 5 to 7 mg/dL (85.5 to 120 μmol). The health care provider should be notified for intervention to prevent kernicterus. This disease process can cause lifelong central nervous system damage. Disregarding the finding or waiting to report the finding will delay treatment and potentially cause permanent harm to the infant. Providing an extra feeding will have no effect on the hyperbilirubinemia that is causing the jaundice.

CN: Management of care; CL: Analyze

66. **1.** Kernicterus is a consequence of elevated bilirubin levels that can have lifelong central nervous effects. This is a true statement. Infants that have elevated bilirubin levels need close monitoring until the bilirubin levels fall. Placing the infant in the sunlight may cause thermoregulation issues such as overheating. Infants will burn very easily in the sun. Bilirubin levels peak at 72 to 120 hours of age. If a baby is

discharged at 3 days, the baby may need follow-up until the peak has been determined and the levels fall. Exclusive breastfeeding is a risk factor for an infant developing severe hyperbilirubinemia.

🔑 CN: Physiological adaptation; CL: Evaluate

67. **2.** Jaundice progresses in a cephalocaudal manner. The jaundice increased from the nipple line to the umbilicus, which indicates that the bilirubin levels are increasing in this infant. Continued assessment is necessary to monitor the rise in bilirubin levels with the potential need for phototherapy to prevent possible kernicterus.

🔑 CN: Reduction of risk potential; CL: Analyze

68. **1.** To prevent eye damage from phototherapy, the eyes must remain covered at all times while under the lights. The eye patches can be removed when the neonate is held out of the lights by the parents for feeding. Instead of a regular diaper, a "string" diaper or disposable face mask may be used to help contain loose stools, while allowing maximum skin exposure. Feeding formula or breast milk every 2 to 3 hours is recommended to prevent hypoglycemia and to encourage gastrointestinal motility. Because the phototherapy lights can overheat the neonate, the temperature should be checked by the axillary route every 2 to 4 hours.

🔑 CN: Physiological adaptation; CL: Apply

69. **4.** An absent Moro reflex, lethargy, opisthotonos, and seizures are symptoms of bilirubin encephalopathy, which, though rare, can be life-threatening. Bronze discoloration of the skin and maculopapular chest rash are normal findings caused by the phototherapy. They will disappear once the phototherapy is discontinued. A urine specific gravity of 1.001 to 1.020 is normal in term neonates.

🔑 CN: Reduction of risk potential; CL: Analyze

The Neonate with Risk Factors

70. **2.** Epinephrine is given for severe bradycardia and hypotension. An expected outcome would be an increased heart rate to a normal range. Epinephrine decreases renal blood flow, so a decrease in urine output would be expected. Epinephrine also stimulates alpha- and beta-adrenergic receptors, which do not offer pain relief or sedation.

🔑 CN: Pharmacological and parenteral therapies; CL: Evaluate

71. **4.** Neonates who are sick do not have the physical resources or energy to respond to all elements of the environment. The use of a constant touch provides comfort and only requires one response to a stimulus. To comfort a sick neonate, the care provider applies gentle, constant physical support or touch. Toys for distraction are not developmentally appropriate for a neonate. Sick neonates react to any stimulus; in responding, the sick neonate may have increased energy demands and increased oxygen requirements. A musical mobile may be too much audio stimulation and thus increases energy and oxygen demands. Repetitive touching with a hand going off and on the neonate, as with stroking or patting, requires the neonate to respond to every touch, thus increasing energy and oxygen demands.

🔑 CN: Basic care and comfort; CL: Analyze

72. **2.** The recommended pulse oximetry reading in a full-term neonate is 95% to 100%. The saturation reading of only 75% is an indication that the neonate is not adequately oxygenating in room air. Providing supplemental oxygen will increase the neonate's oxygen saturation. Increasing the IV rate will not improve the oxygen saturation. Documenting the finding and taking no action is not appropriate with a saturation of 75%. Wrapping and increasing the body temperature of the neonate may increase the saturation reading only if it is inaccurate due to cold extremities. Caution must be used because overheating a neonate can be harmful.

🔑 CN: Reduction of risk potential; CL: Analyze

73. **4.** Neonates with heart failure may need calorie-dense formula to provide extra calories for growth. Fluids should not be restricted because the nutritional requirements are based on calories per ounce of formula. Decreasing fluid intake will decrease the calories needed for growth. These neonates may have limited energy because of their heart condition, but they have a high caloric need to stimulate proper growth and development. The sodium level should be at a normal level to ensure adequate fluid and electrolyte balance unless prescribed by the health care provider.

🔑 CN: Health promotion and maintenance; CL: Create

74. **1.** The indication for the use of indomethacin is to close a patent ductus arteriosus. Adverse effects include decreased renal blood flow, platelet dysfunction with coagulation defects, decreased gastrointestinal motility, and an increase in necrotizing enterocolitis. Thus, increased bleeding time, decreased gastrointestinal function, and decreased renal output would be expected outcomes after the administration of indomethacin.

🔑 CN: Pharmacological and parenteral therapies; CL: Evaluate

75. 1. To ensure client safety, the nurse should first write the results on the medical record, then read them back to the caller, and wait for the caller to confirm that the nurse has understood the results. Using scrap paper increases the risk for losing the results as well as transcription errors. The nurse may receive results by telephone, and while electronic transfer to the client's medical record is appropriate, the nurse can also accept the telephone results if the laboratory has called the results to the nursery. Sending client information via email is unacceptable due to potential security and privacy issues.

CN: Safety and infection control; CL: Apply

76. 1, 3, 4. Hemolytic disease of the newborn can happen when a birth parent and baby have different blood types or Rh factors. Hemolytic disease of the newborn occurs most commonly when the parent is Rh negative and the infant is Rh positive. About 13% of Caucasians, 7% to 8% of people of African descent, and 1% of people of Asian descent are Rh negative. Rh-positive cells enter the parent's Rh-negative bloodstream, and in a response to the birth parent's immune system, they produce antibodies to the infant's Rh-positive cells. In a subsequent pregnancy, the antibodies cross the placenta to the Rh-positive fetus and begin the destruction of Rh-positive cells through hemolysis. This results in severe fetal anemia. Hemolytic disease does not happen when the infant is Rh negative. The infant does make antibodies to the birth parent's blood.

CN: Physiological adaptation; CL: Apply

77. 3. The problem of Rh sensitivity arises when the birth parent's blood develops antibodies after fetal red blood cells enter the maternal circulation. In cases of Rh sensitivity, this usually does not occur until after the first pregnancy. Hence, hemolytic disease of the newborn is rare in a primiparous client. A mismatched blood transfusion in the past or an unrecognized spontaneous abortion could also result in hemolytic disease because the transfusion or abortion would have the same effects on the client. The statement about the other baby having a different father may be true. However, if both fathers were Rh positive, sensitization could occur. Most birth parents do not have immunity against the antibodies formed when Rh-positive cells enter the bloodstream. Antibodies are not neutralized by the birth parent's system.

CN: Reduction of risk potential; CL: Evaluate

78. 2. The Rh-sensitized neonate generally does not have problems related to polycythemia. Therefore, the client needs additional teaching. In general, moderate-to-severe Rh sensitization can cause anemia, enlarged spleen, and cardiac decompensation. Cardiac decompensation (as in heart failure) occurs because of severe anemia. Anemia is caused by the destruction of red blood cells by antibodies as the severity of hemolytic disease of the neonate increases. Splenic enlargement is caused by the excessive destruction of fetal red blood cells.

CN: Physiological adaptation; CL: Evaluate

79. 4. A direct Coombs test is also known as a *direct antiglobulin test* (*DAT*). The test is done on umbilical cord blood to detect maternal antibodies coating the neonate's red blood cells. Rho(D) immune globulin doses are determined by the amount of Rh-positive neonatal blood found in the birth parent after birth. Hematocrit is used to detect anemia. A direct Coombs test does not measure bilirubin but may help explain the underlying cause of increased bilirubin levels.

CN: Reduction of risk potential; CL: Apply

80. 3. An exchange transfusion is done to reduce the blood concentration of bilirubin and correct the anemia. The exchange transfusion does not replenish the white blood cells or restore the fluid and electrolyte balance. The neonate's Rh-positive blood is replaced by Rh-negative blood.

CN: Reduction of risk potential; CL: Apply

81. 2. The organ most susceptible to damage from uncontrolled hemolytic disease is the brain. Bilirubin levels increase as the red blood cells are destroyed. Bilirubin crosses the blood-brain barrier and damages the cells of the central nervous system. This condition, called *kernicterus*, is potentially fatal. Although the kidneys, lungs, and liver may be affected by increased bilirubin levels, the brain will sustain the most life-threatening injury.

CN: Reduction of risk potential; CL: Apply

82. 2. Glucose crosses the placenta, but insulin does not. Hence, a high maternal blood glucose level causes a high fetal blood glucose level. This causes the fetal pancreas to secrete more insulin. At birth, the neonate loses the maternal glucose source but continues to produce much insulin, which commonly causes a drop in blood glucose levels (hypoglycemia), usually 30 to 60 minutes after birth. Most neonates do not develop hypoglycemia if their birth parents are not insulin dependent unless they are preterm. Therefore, hypoglycemia is not a normal response as the neonate transitions to extrauterine life.

CN: Reduction of risk potential; CL: Analyze

83. 1. This neonate has a birth parent with diabetes who tends to have higher calcium levels, which can cause secondary hypoparathyroidism in their neonates. This lack of calcium may be the cause of the tremors and jitteriness of this neonate, and a serum calcium level should be obtained. Other factors contributing to hypocalcemia in neonates include hypophosphatemia from tissue metabolism, vitamin D antagonism from increased cortisol levels, and decreased serum magnesium levels. Beginning IV glucose based on a normal infant glucose level would have no benefit. Rechecking the neonate's temperature is a precaution that can be taken to assure that it is within normal limits, but it is not the action to take first. Refeeding the infant who has a normal newborn blood glucose level is not appropriate.

CN: Management of care; CL: Analyze

84. 4. Hypoglycemia is caused by the rapid depletion of glucose stores. In addition, neonates born to birth parents with insulin-dependent diabetes are about seven times more likely to experience respiratory distress syndrome than neonates born to birth parents without diabetes. This neonate should be closely monitored for symptoms of hypoglycemia and respiratory distress. Neonates of birth parents with diabetes commonly have polycythemia, not anemia. Anemia and hemolytic disease are associated with erythroblastosis fetalis. Persistent pulmonary hypertension is associated with meconium aspiration syndrome.

CN: Reduction of risk potential; CL: Apply

85. 2. Manifestations of opiate withdrawal in the neonate, known as *neonatal abstinence syndrome* (*NAS*), include increased central nervous system irritability, which can manifest as a high-pitched cry. Sluggishness or lethargy are not symptoms of NAS. Metabolic, vasomotor, and respiratory disturbances seen with NAS involve tachycardia and fever, not bradycardia or fever. These signs usually appear within 72 hours and persist for several days.

CN: Reduction of risk potential; CL: Analyze

86. 1. Neonates experiencing opiate withdrawal have gastrointestinal problems similar to those of adults withdrawing from opiates. Diarrhea, not constipation, is typically seen in these neonates. Infants going through opiate withdrawal frequently demonstrate excessive sucking, but their suck is often uncoordinated. Other gastrointestinal symptoms can include vomiting, drooling, regurgitation, and anorexia.

CN: Reduction of risk potential; CL: Evaluate

87. 1. A neonate undergoing cocaine withdrawal is irritable, often restless, difficult to console, and often in need of increased activity. It is commonly helpful to swaddle the neonate tightly with a blanket, offer a pacifier, and cuddle and rock the neonate. Offering extra nourishment is not advised because overfeeding tends to increase gastrointestinal problems such as vomiting, regurgitation, and diarrhea. Environmental stimuli such as bright lights and loud noises should be kept to a minimum to decrease agitation. Minimizing touching of the neonate to only when they are crying will not aid the bonding process between birth parent and neonate. Frequent holding and touching are permissible.

CN: Reduction of risk potential; CL: Analyze

88. 4. New recommendations state that virologic diagnostic testing at birth should be considered for infants at high risk for HIV infection, but it may take several months before an accurate diagnosis can be made. New guidelines suggest that infants should be tested at 2 to 3 weeks, at 1 to 2 months, and at 4 to 6 months. It is estimated that 15% to 30% of all HIV-positive birth parents without treatment will give birth to HIV-positive infants. With appropriate drug intervention to the parent during pregnancy, 95% of these neonates can be born unaffected. An enlarged liver at birth is associated with erythroblastosis fetalis, not HIV infection. Virologic testing, such as deoxyribonucleic acid polymerase chain reaction, viral culture, or ribonucleic acid plasma assay, can diagnose HIV infection by 6 months of age and commonly in the first month.

CN: Reduction of risk potential; CL: Apply

89. 4. Breast milk has been found to contain the retrovirus HIV. In general, birth parents are discouraged from breastfeeding if they are HIV positive because of the risk for possible transmission of the virus if the neonate is HIV negative. Breast milk does contain some immunoglobulins, but it does not protect the neonate from HIV infection.

CN: Health promotion and maintenance; CL: Create

90. 1. Newborns are typically bathed 2 to 4 hours after birth when their temperatures have had time to stabilize, but early/immediate bathing is recommended for the infants of HIV-positive birth parents to decrease blood exposure. Placing the neonate under the radiant warmer for the vitamin K injection is not necessary unless the neonate's temperature is subnormal. Washing the injection site with povidone-iodine is not recommended and may increase the risk for possible allergy to iodine preparations. The first dose of zidovudine is given when the newborn is 6 to 12 hours old, but vitamin K is recommended to be given within an hour of birth to be most effective. Therefore, the vitamin K should not be delayed.

CN: Safety and infection control; CL: Analyze

91. 3. Symptoms of infection in a neonate include subtle behavioral changes, such as lethargy and irritability, and color changes such as pallor or cyanosis. Other symptoms include temperature instability, poor feeding, gastrointestinal disorders, hyperbilirubinemia, and apnea. An elevated WBC count, possibly as high as 30,000 cells/mm^3 (30 × 10^9/L) or more, may be normal during the first 24 hours. An apical heart rate of 132 bpm is normal. Warm, moist skin is not a typical sign of infection in neonates.

CN: Health promotion and maintenance; CL: Analyze

92. 3. The parents of a neonate with an infection should be allowed to participate in daily care as long as they use good handwashing technique. This includes touching and holding the neonate. It is not necessary for parents to wear protective gear near the isolation incubator. Restricting parental visits has not been shown to have any effect on the infection rate and may have detrimental effects on the neonate's psychological development. Normally, the neonate does not need to be isolated. The baby will not spread sepsis via respiratory droplets to the parents, so it is not necessary for the parents to wear a mask.

CN: Safety and infection control; CL: Apply

93. 3. On the initial visit, the parents may be shocked, fearful, and anxious. Nursing care should include spending time with the parents to allow them to express their emotions. The nurse should initially emphasize the neonate's normal characteristics. After the parents have had sufficient time to adjust to the neonate's special needs, surgical interventions can be discussed. Telling the parents that this is not a life-threatening defect or that everything will be all right after the surgery is not helpful. Doing so discounts their feelings. Reassuring the parents about the success rate of the surgery can be done once the parents have had time to adjust to the neonate and express their emotions.

CN: Psychosocial integrity; CL: Analyze

94. 1. It is not necessary to clean the mouth of an infant with an unrepaired cleft palate after each feeding. The neonate needs to be fed in an upright position to prevent aspiration. The neonate with a cleft lip and palate commonly swallows large amounts of air during feeding. Therefore, the neonate needs to be burped frequently to help eliminate the air and decrease the risk for regurgitation. The neonate with a cleft lip and palate should be fed with a special soft nipple that fills the cleft and facilitates sucking.

CN: Reduction of risk potential; CL: Evaluate

95. 4. The long-term prognosis for neonates with FAS is poor. Symptoms of withdrawal include tremors, sleeplessness, seizures, abdominal distention, hyperactivity, and inconsolable crying. Symptoms of withdrawal commonly occur within 6 to 12 hours or, at the latest, within the first 3 days of life. The neonate with FAS is usually growth deficient at birth. Most neonates with FAS have an intellectual disability that ranges from mild to severe. The facial deformities associated with FAS, such as short palpebral fissures, epicanthal folds, a broad nasal bridge, a flattened midface, and a short, upturned nose, are not easily corrected with plastic surgery.

CN: Reduction of risk potential; CL: Create

96. 3. Neurologic disorders are common in neonates with FAS. Speech and language disorders and hyperactivity are common manifestations of central nervous system dysfunction. Mild-to-severe intellectual disability and feeding problems also are common. Delayed growth and development are expected. These neonates feed poorly and commonly have persistent vomiting until age 6 to 7 months. These neonates do not have a 70% mortality rate, and there is no treatment for FAS, but early intervention improves client outcomes.

CN: Reduction of risk potential; CL: Apply

97. 4. Changes seen in the facial features of newborns with fetal alcohol syndrome remain that way. These include epicanthal folds, whorls, irregular hair, cleft lip or palate, small teeth, and lack of philtrum. Newborns with fetal alcohol syndrome are usually difficult to calm and frequently cry for long periods of time. Parents do need assistance with caring for themselves and their infants, particularly with continued alcohol use. A supportive family or a support system is essential. The problems seen with this newborn do not go away; they remain with the infant throughout life and are compounded when the child begins to develop mentally.

CN: Health promotion and maintenance; CL: Evaluate

98. **1.** The parents need to know that the neonate will be kept on NPO status and will receive intravenous therapy before surgery. After surgery, feeding will depend on the neonate's condition. Total parenteral nutrition may be prescribed after surgery, but not before. Breastfeeding may be started after surgery if the neonate's condition is stable. The parent can pump the breasts until that time.

CN: Reduction of risk potential; CL: Apply

99. **1, 2, 4.** The major goals for the neonate include preventing hypothermia, maintaining fluid and electrolyte balance, and preventing infection. Pain medication will be needed after surgery but is not typically needed before the procedure. In many cases, surgery is done very soon after birth, so while developmental care is important, it should be addressed after the closure of the abdominal wall defect.

CN: Reduction of risk potential; CL: Create

100. **2.** After a neonate is diagnosed with a birth defect, parents often go through stages of grief similar to those they would have if they had lost the child. The physical appearance of the anomaly and the life-threatening nature of the disorder may be shocking to the parents. The parents may hesitate to form a bond with the neonate because of the guarded prognosis. Denial would be evidenced if the parents acted as if nothing were wrong. Depression would be evidenced by parental statements involving sadness or a sense of finality. Anger would be evidenced if the parents attempted to blame someone, such as health care personnel, for the neonate's condition.

CN: Psychosocial integrity; CL: Analyze

101. **2.** Marked visible peristaltic waves in the abdomen and projectile vomiting are signs of pyloric stenosis. If the condition progresses without surgical intervention, the neonate will become dehydrated and develop metabolic alkalosis. Signs of esophageal atresia include coughing and regurgitation with feedings. Diaphragmatic hernia, a life-threatening event in which the abdominal contents herniate into the thoracic cavity, may be evidenced by breath sounds being heard over the abdomen and significant respiratory distress with cyanosis. Signs of hiatal hernia include vomiting, failure to thrive, and short periods of apnea.

CN: Reduction of risk potential; CL: Analyze

102. **3.** With a patent ductus arteriosus, a cardiac defect marked by a failure of the patent ductus arteriosus to close completely at birth, blood from the aorta flows into the pulmonary arteries to be reoxygenated in the lungs and returned to the left atrium and ventricle. The effect of this altered circulation includes increased workload on the left side of the heart and increased pulmonary vascular congestion. Term infants commonly have no symptoms, but a loud, machinery-like murmur may be heard throughout systole and diastole. This murmur may be accompanied by a suprasternal thrill, and the heart may be enlarged. Decreased cardiac output with faint peripheral pulses, poor peripheral perfusion, feeding difficulties, and severe congestive heart failure are symptoms associated with severe aortic stenosis. With this defect, the aortic valve is thickened and rigid, leading to decreased cardiac output and reduced myocardial blood flow. Profound cyanosis over most of the body, fatigue on exertion, feeding difficulties, and chronic hypoxemia are associated with tetralogy of Fallot. With this defect, malalignment of the ventricular system results in nonrestricted ventral septal defects, pulmonic stenosis, overriding of the aorta, and hypertrophy of the left ventricle. The heart appears boot shaped. A harsh systolic murmur with a palpable thrill is associated with truncus arteriosus. It is marked by an incomplete division of the great vessel. This is caused by a ventral septal defect. Bounding pulses and a widening pulse pressure may also be present.

CN: Reduction of risk potential; CL: Analyze

103. **1.** Coarctation of the aorta accounts for 5% to 7% of congenital heart disease. There is localized constriction of the aorta, at or near the insertion site of the ductus arteriosus, that increases afterload and decreases cardiac output. The infant with coarctation of the aorta presents with symptoms of poor lower body perfusion, weak lower extremity pulses, and congestive heart failure, including respiratory distress. The child with a partial atrioventricular septal defect may be asymptomatic at birth. The symptoms in a child with a complete defect depend on the pulmonary artery pressure. The child with pulmonary atresia has profound (complete) cyanosis. Transposition of the great arteries is associated with complete cyanosis during the first few hours of life.

CN: Reduction of risk potential; CL: Analyze

104. **3.** The neonate is experiencing quiet tachypnea with central cyanosis, which is a sign of possible congenital heart disease, so notifying the HCP is the correct answer. The baby is showing no signs of increased work of breathing, except increased respiratory rate. Breath sounds are clear; therefore, suctioning is not necessary and may cause further distress because of the trauma to the nasal passage. Changing the neonate's position would have no impact on the cyanosis. Encouraging the baby to cry would increase the distress by decreasing oxygen consumption.

🗝️ CJ: Standalone trend; CL: Analyze

105. 4. The next nursing action in this situation would be to assess the blood pressure in all four extremities and compare the findings. A difference of 15 mm Hg in the systolic blood pressure between the arms and legs is an indication of a narrowed aorta. This could be an emergency, and the HCP needs to be notified as soon as the blood pressure data have been collected. Generally, prescribing an HCP consult is not a nursing function. Placing the neonate in reverse Trendelenburg will only decrease the perfusion to the lower extremities.

🗝️ CN: Physiological adaptation; CL: Analyze

106. 4. Further assessment for signs of distress is necessary. At 4 hours of age, a transient murmur may be heard as the fetal shunts are closing. This is a normal finding. If no other distress is noted, the HCP does not need to be called. Results can be noted on the medical record. Further assessment is needed to know if continuing routine care and feeding are appropriate and safe for the neonate. Oxygen is only needed if the infant was manifesting low oxygen saturations or signs of distress.

🗝️ CN: Physiological adaptation; CL: Analyze

107.

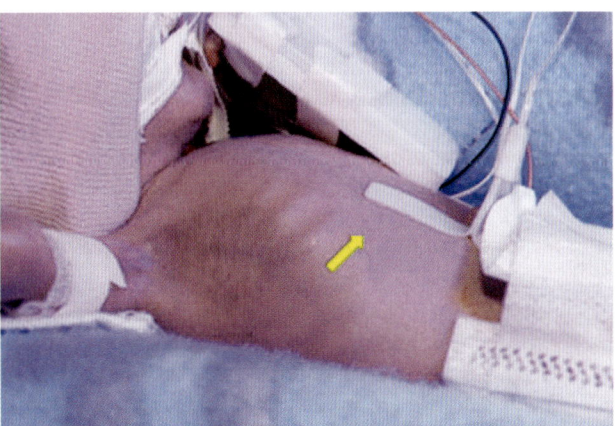

Subcostal retractions are noted under the rib cage. Intercostal retractions are noted between the ribs. Suprasternal retractions are found above the sternum, and the substernal retractions are found below the sternum.

🗝️ CN: Physiological adaptation; CL: Apply

Managing Care, Quality, and Safety of Neonatal Clients

108.

STEP 1

 Nurse's Notes

Day 2 0700:
S: A 2-day-old term newborn is breastfeeding.
B: The neonate was born by spontaneous vaginal birth to a primigravid parent with opioid use disorder who used opioids during pregnancy. The neonate's Apgar scores were 9 and 10. The birth weight was 3100 g (3.1 kg).
A: The neonate's vital signs are temperature (T) 99.5°F (37.5°C); heart rate (HR) 140 bpm; and respiration rate (RR) 62 breaths/min. The neonate is irritable with moderate tremors when disturbed and regurgitates two to three times with feedings. Today's weight is 2950 g (2.9 kg).
R: The baby has routine orders and needs to be reassessed.

Fever instability, a respiratory rate greater than 60 breaths/min, irritability, moderate tremors, and frequent regurgitation are all symptoms of neonatal abstinence syndrome or withdrawal symptoms associated with maternal substance use disorder. A normal newborn heart rate ranges from 110 to 160 bpm. The weight loss of up to 10% of the birth weight is an expected finding.

🗝️ CJ: Case study; Step 1: Recognize cues; CL: Analyze

109.

STEP 2

Findings	CNS Dysfunction	Metabolic, Vasomotor, and Respiratory Disturbances	Gastrointestinal Dysfunction
Fever		X	
Respiratory rate		X	
Irritability	X		
Moderate tremors	X		
Frequent regurgitation			X

Neonatal abstinence syndrome manifests in three categories: CNS dysfunction; metabolic, vasomotor, and respiratory disturbances, and gastrointestinal dysfunction. CNS dysfunction includes tremors and irritability. Other CNS symptoms include a high-pitched cry, hyperactive reflexes, hypertonia, sleep disturbances, and seizures. Fever and tachypnea are categorized as metabolic, vasomotor, and respiratory disturbances. Other symptoms of this category are yawning, sneezing, sweating, apnea, mottling, and nasal flaring. Spitting up frequently is a gastrointestinal dysfunction symptom. Poor feeding, frequent loose stools, projectile vomiting, and frantic sucking are other signs of gastrointestinal dysfunction.

  CJ: Case study; Step 2: Analyze cues; CL: Analyze

110.

STEP 3

0/1 *The nurse is most concerned that the client has* **neonatal abstinence syndrome**. *The nurse should take immediate actions to prevent the complications of* **seizure** *and* **dehydration**.

A history of maternal opioid use with CNS dysfunction (tremors and irritability), metabolic, vasomotor, and respiratory disturbances (fever and tachypnea), and gastrointestinal dysfunction (regurgitation) are most consistent with neonatal abstinence syndrome. While the possibility of a commitment infection causing the fever, tachypnea, and irritability should be ruled out, the nurse should prioritize preventing the most common serious risks, seizure and dehydration. Hyperbilirubinemia and respiratory arrest are less common complications.

  CJ: Case study; Step 3: Prioritize hypothesis; CL: Create

111.

STEP 4

 1, 2, 4, 5, 6, 7. Rooming in has been shown to significantly decrease the need for pharmacological therapy in clients experiencing neonatal abstinence syndrome. Other comfort measures include organizing care to avoid overstimulation, gentle rocking, nonnutritive sucking with a pacifier, and safe swaddling. Breastfeeding should be encouraged. Dim rather than bright lighting is desirable. Side positioning is discouraged as it increases the risk for sudden infant death syndrome.

  CJ: Case study; Step 4: Generate solutions; CL: Analyze

112.

STEP 5

0/1

Possible Findings	Indicated	Contraindicated
Negative maternal urine toxicology at birth	X	
Positive maternal human immunodeficiency virus (HIV) diagnosis		X
Maternal referral to an addiction counselor	X	
Previous maternal history of hepatitis A	X	
Need to give the newborn a PRN dose of morphine	X	
Positive meconium drug screen for opioids	X	
Maternal use of an illicit street drug		X

Birth parents with opioid use disorder who have no additional risk factors and are otherwise compliant with treatment may be encouraged to breastfeed. HIV crosses into breast milk; therefore, HIV-positive birth parents in developed countries should be advised not to breastfeed. Recommendations in developing countries with inconsistent water supplies to mix formula may vary. Exposure to an illicit street drug, such as cocaine, in breast milk presents an unacceptable health risk to a newborn. Breastfeeding parents with a history of opioid use disorder who test negative at birth and enter treatment programs can breastfeed if they remain compliant with treatment. Hepatitis A is transmitted via the oral-fecal route and is not a contraindication to breastfeeding. A positive meconium screen for opioids reflects many weeks of fetal development and does not. Breastfeeding has been shown to reduce the need for medications in newborns with neonatal abstinence syndrome and may help reduce the need for additional PRN morphine doses. A positive meconium drug screen for opioids indicates exposure in utero in the latter part of pregnancy and is consistent with the birth parent's history.

 CJ: Case study; Step 5: Take action; CL: Apply

113.

STEP 6

−/+ 1, 3, 4, 5, 6. One of the goals of the treatment of a neonate with neonatal abstinence syndrome is to allow the newborn to function as a normal neonate. The typical weight gain for a newborn after the initial weight loss is 15 mg/kg a day. Typical newborn behaviors include breastfeeding every 2 to 3 hours and sleeping between feedings. The empowerment of parents is important to the newborn's optimal long-term outcomes. This includes ensuring they can provide care and comfort and that they agree to the plan of care. An infant on 0.09 mg/kg of morphine still needs to be weaned off the medication before discharge.

  CJ: Case study; Step 6: Evaluate outcomes; CL: Evaluate

114. **−/+ 1, 3, 5.** Many of the circulatory transitions that infants make after birth are normal for a period of time and become abnormal as the infant ages. Tracking output is important as newborns are expected to void and stool at least once during the first 24 hours of life. Birth weight is recorded to determine if the baby is appropriate for gestational age. Birth weight changes will be measured daily. Pathology of hyperbilirubinemia is determined by when jaundice appears and acceptable levels are age dependent. The length of labor and the parent's marital status have no influence on the assessment of the infant.

  CN: Management of care; CL: Analyze

115. 3. The nurse should make rounds and first assess the neonate with the respiratory rate of 62 breaths/min. The respiratory rate is out of the normal range and needs reevaluation. The nurse should next assess the newborn with a borderline low temperature to determine if the newborn's body temperature is increasing. The newborn who is LGA still has 15 minutes before being due for the feeding, and much can be accomplished by the nurse in that time. A 36-week newborn weighing 2270 g (2.27 kg) will need to be fed on time to maintain the blood glucose level.

🗝️ CN: Management of care; CL: Analyze

116. 3. A temperature of 96.6°F (35.9°C) and jitteriness are signs of hypoglycemia in the newborn. The nurse must first obtain a heel-stick blood sample for blood glucose. Breastfeeding, preferably skin to skin, should be initiated immediately following the heel-stick puncture to treat the suspected hypoglycemia. The HCP can be notified once the blood glucose value is known and the baby is successfully breastfeeding. Normal newborn temperature ranges from 97.7°F (36.5°C) to 99.1°F (37.3°C). A temperature of 96.6°F (35.9°C) is low, another sign of hypoglycemia; however, breastfeeding takes precedence over the radiant heater. Also, breastfeeding via skin-to-skin contact has been found as the most effective way to maintain a newborn's temperature.

🗝️ CN: Management of care; CL: Analyze

117. 2. The birth parent demonstrates signs of a full bladder and vaginal bleeding and requires assistance with bladder emptying and uterine massage to assess the origin of the bleeding. The newborn requires further assessment because turning dusky when quiet and a respiration rate of 70 breaths/min indicate the beginning signs of respiratory distress and require prompt intervention. All other parents are recovering normally. While bilateral crackles in a newborn could indicate excessive fluid, a pink color indicates the infant is maintaining oxygenation. Normal respiration is 30 to 60 breaths/min. Although a respiratory rate of 67 breaths/min is slightly elevated, the baby is not demonstrating any other signs of respiratory distress. Acrocyanosis (bluish hands and feet) is a normal newborn finding and shows the ability to maintain oxygenation. Respirations of 70 breaths/min and intermittent expiratory grunting would indicate close observation but do not require immediate intervention if the infant is pink. The last newborn is maintaining oxygenation, with respirations just slightly above normal. Periodic breathing, featuring pauses in breathing that last less than 15 seconds, is a normal newborn finding.

🗝️ CN: Management of care; CL: Analyze

118. -/+ **2, 3, 4, 5.** A hospital-specific security system is the standard of care to prevent neonatal abduction. The bulb syringe should be visible and easily accessible to both the parent and the nurse in case of choking. Someone should remain in the room who is able to safely care for the infant. This may be the birth parent or a family member if the birth parent is physically not able to care for the infant. The infant should be lying on the back or side, rather than the abdomen to prevent sudden infant death syndrome ("back to sleep"). Infant falls from a parent's bed are a serious safety problem. The infant should be in the birth parent's arms or in the crib rather than lying on a bed, even with the side rails up, as an infant can slip through the rails. A sleeping parent is not aware of the status of the infant who can easily fall out of their arms; the infant can be in the birth parent's arms only if they are awake.

🗝️ CN: Safety and infection control; CL: Evaluate

119. 2. The blood glucose of 25 mg/dL (1.38 mmol/L) is the most critical. Glucose is the only fuel that the brain can use. It is important to protect the central nervous system, and levels of less than 30 mg/dL (1.7 mmol/L) in the first 6 hours of a neonate's life indicate hypoglycemia. Increased respiratory secretions is a normal finding in the second period of reactivity. A temperature of 97.4°F (36.4°C) is only slightly low for a neonate at this age. Ninety-five percent of all neonates will void at least once in the first 24 hours. This is not unusual at this age.

🗝️ CN: Management of care; CL: Analyze

120. 4, 1, 3, 2. Based on the report given by the preceding nurse, the nurse should plan to prioritize all clients and first make rounds on the client needing the highest level of nursing care. The nurse can then make rounds on all other clients. The nurse can then check for new prescriptions and, finally, inspect the room in which the next client will be admitted to be sure all of the equipment is available.

🗝️ CN: Management of care; CL: Analyze

121. -/+ **2, 4, 5.** The role of the UAP allows this member of the health care team to take the vital signs of clients and record feedings, voids, and stools of infants according to hospital guidelines. The newborn assessment is completed by a licensed care provider as is the tube feeding. Bathing of the newborn is within the scope of practice for the UAP, but the initial assessment of the patency of the gastrointestinal tract, which is initiated by the first feeding, is within the scope of licensed care providers. If there is a tracheoesophageal fistula, this is the time when it may become evident.

🗝️ CN: Management of care; CL: Apply

The Nursing Care of Children

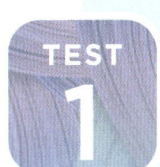

TEST 1

Health Promotion

- Health Promotion of the Infant and Family
- Health Promotion of the Toddler and Family
- Health Promotion of the Preschooler and Family
- Health Promotion of the School-Age Child and Family
- Health Promotion of the Adolescent and Family
- Health Promotion in Children with Down Syndrome (Trisomy 21)
- Common Childhood and Adolescent Health Problems
- Managing Care, Quality, and Safety of Children
- Answers, Rationales, and Test-Taking Strategies

Health Promotion of the Infant and Family

1. The nurse assesses an 8-month-old child's language development. Which finding would the nurse consider to be typical language development?
   ☐ 1. saying "dada" to father and "mama" to mother
   ☐ 2. saying three other words besides "mama" and "dada"
   ☐ 3. saying "dada" and "mama" nonspecifically
   ☐ 4. saying "mama" and "dada" while pointing to the parent

2. The nurse performs a developmental screening on an 8-month-old child. The nurse should refer the family to the health care provider (HCP) if the child was unable to demonstrate which gross motor ability?
   ☐ 1. standing momentarily without holding onto furniture
   ☐ 2. standing unsupported for long periods of time
   ☐ 3. stooping to recover an object on the ground
   ☐ 4. sitting without support for long periods of time

3. The nurse is teaching the parents of an 8-month-old about what the child should eat. The nurse should include which information points in the teaching plan?
   ☐ 1. Vegetables should be introduced before fruits when the infant is 6 months old.
   ☐ 2. Solid foods should not be introduced until the infant is 10 months old.
   ☐ 3. Iron-fortified cereals should not be introduced until the infant is 8 months old.
   ☐ 4. Formula can be changed to whole milk when the infant is 12 months old.

4. A 10-month-old child looks for objects that have been removed from their view. How does the nurse explain the finding to the parents?
   ☐ 1. The child is showing typical neuromuscular development.
   ☐ 2. The child's curiosity has increased.
   ☐ 3. The child understands objects are there even though the child cannot see them.
   ☐ 4. The child's long-term memory has increased.

5. The nurse performs a head-to-toe assessment on a 2-month-old infant. Which structure should be closed by the time the infant is 2 months old?

   ☐ 1. A
   ☐ 2. B
   ☐ 3. C
   ☐ 4. D

6. The parents of a 3-week-old healthy newborn ask the nurse why their child is intermittently cross-eyed. What is the nurse's **best** response?
   ☐ 1. "An eye patch may be necessary to correct your child's vision."
   ☐ 2. "Your child will likely need an ophthalmology consult."
   ☐ 3. "It is normal to have eye-crossing in the newborn period."
   ☐ 4. "Surgery may be necessary to correct your child's vision."

7. A parent brings a 4-month-old to the clinic for a regular well visit and expresses concern that the infant is not developing appropriately. Which finding in the infant would indicate the need for further developmental screening?
   ☐ 1. has no interest in peekaboo games
   ☐ 2. does not turn front to back
   ☐ 3. does not babble
   ☐ 4. does not sit without support

8. The nurse assesses a 6-month-old child for vaccination readiness. Which finding would **most** likely indicate the need to delay administering the diphtheria, tetanus, and acellular pertussis (DTaP) vaccine?
   ☐ 1. family history of sudden infant death syndrome (SIDS)
   ☐ 2. temperature of 101.3°F (38.5°C) following the 4-month vaccinations
   ☐ 3. acute bilateral ear infection
   ☐ 4. living with a family member who is immunosuppressed

9. The parents of a 9-month-old bring the infant to the clinic for a regular checkup. The infant has received no immunizations. Which vaccine if prescribed would the nurse question?
   ☐ 1. diphtheria, tetanus, and acellular pertussis (DTaP)
   ☐ 2. *Haemophilus influenzae* type B (Hib)
   ☐ 3. measles, mumps, and rubella (MMR)
   ☐ 4. inactivated influenza (Flu)

10. The nurse assesses the development of a 1-month-old infant. Which skills should the nurse ask the parent if the infant is able to demonstrate?
    ☐ 1. smile and laugh out loud
    ☐ 2. roll from their back to their side
    ☐ 3. hold a rattle briefly
    ☐ 4. lift their head from the prone position

11. The parent of a 6-month-old reports starting the child on 2% milk. What should the nurse ask the parent **first**?
    ☐ 1. "Do you think your baby will be fine with this milk?"
    ☐ 2. "Is it possible for you to switch your baby to whole milk?"
    ☐ 3. "Can you tell me more about the reason you switched your baby to 2% milk?"
    ☐ 4. "You cannot switch to 2% milk right now. Did your pediatrician tell you to do this?"

12. The nurse notes that an infant stares at an object placed in their hand and takes it to their mouth, coos and gurgles when talked to, and sustains part of their own weight when held in a standing position. The nurse correctly interprets these findings as characteristic of an infant at which age?
    ☐ 1. 2 months
    ☐ 2. 4 months
    ☐ 3. 7 months
    ☐ 4. 9 months

13. An 8-month-old infant is seen in the well-child clinic for a routine checkup. The nurse should expect the infant to be able to do which task(s)? Select all that apply.
    - ☐ 1. saying "mama" and "dada" with specific meaning
    - ☐ 2. feeding self with a spoon
    - ☐ 3. playing peekaboo
    - ☐ 4. walking independently
    - ☐ 5. stacking two blocks
    - ☐ 6. transferring an object from hand to hand

14. The parent of a 9-month-old infant is concerned that the infant's front soft spot is still open. What should the nurse tell the parent?
    - ☐ 1. "I will measure your baby's head to see if it is a normal size."
    - ☐ 2. "Your infant will need to be referred for more testing."
    - ☐ 3. "You should contact your health care provider immediately."
    - ☐ 4. "This is normal because this soft spot usually closes between 12 and 18 months."

15. The parent of a 9-month-old expresses concern that the baby "is developing slowly." The nurse is concerned about a developmental delay when finding the baby is unable to accomplish which skill?
    - ☐ 1. vocalizing single syllables
    - ☐ 2. standing alone
    - ☐ 3. building a tower of two cubes
    - ☐ 4. drinking from a cup with little spilling

16. The nurse assesses infant development at a well-child clinic. Which infant **most** needs a developmental referral for a gross motor delay?
    - ☐ 1. 2-month-old who does not roll over
    - ☐ 2. 4-month-old who does not sit without support
    - ☐ 3. 6-month-old who does not crawl
    - ☐ 4. 9-month-old who does not stand holding on

17. The nurse implements strategies to reduce pain associated with vaccinations. Which intervention should the nurse employ?
    - ☐ 1. Use a 5/8-inch (1.6-cm) needle.
    - ☐ 2. Simultaneously administer vaccines at separate sites with a second nurse.
    - ☐ 3. Aspirate to verify needle placement.
    - ☐ 4. Tell the parent to breastfeed right before the vaccines are administered.

Health Promotion of the Toddler and Family

18. An uncle is shopping for a toy to give their niece. They have no children of their own and ask a neighbor, a nurse, what would be the **most** appropriate toy to give a 15-month-old child. Which toy should the nurse recommend to facilitate learning and development?
    - ☐ 1. stuffed animal
    - ☐ 2. music box
    - ☐ 3. push-pull toy
    - ☐ 4. nursery mobile

19. A 2-year-old child tells their parent they are afraid to go to sleep because "the monsters will get me." What should the nurse tell the parent to do? Select all that apply.
    - ☐ 1. Allow the child to sleep with their parents in their bed whenever they are afraid.
    - ☐ 2. Increase the child's activity before they go to bed so they eventually fall asleep from being tired.
    - ☐ 3. Read a story to the child before bedtime, and allow them to have a cuddly animal or a blanket.
    - ☐ 4. Allow the child to stay up an hour later with the family until they fall asleep.
    - ☐ 5. Reassure the child that they are safe and nothing will bother them while in their own bed
    - ☐ 6. Tell the child that they are safe because you have destroyed the monsters.

20. A 2-year-old child always puts their teddy bear at the head of the bed before they go to sleep. The parents ask the nurse if this behavior is normal. The nurse should explain to the parents that toddlers use ritualistic patterns to establish which factor?
    - ☐ 1. a sense of identity
    - ☐ 2. control over adults in their environment
    - ☐ 3. sequenced patterns of learning behavior
    - ☐ 4. a sense of security

21. A parent asks if they should begin toilet training their 2-year-old child. Which development would be necessary for toilet training readiness for a toddler? Select all that apply.
    - ☐ 1. adequate neuromuscular development for sphincter control
    - ☐ 2. appropriate chronological age
    - ☐ 3. ability to communicate the need to use the toilet
    - ☐ 4. desire to please the parents
    - ☐ 5. ability to play with other 2-year-olds

22. A parent of a toilet-trained 3-year-old expresses concern over their child's bed-wetting while hospitalized. What should the nurse tell the parent?
    ☐ 1. "Your child was too immature to be toilet trained. In a few months, your child should be old enough."
    ☐ 2. "Children are afraid in the hospital and frequently wet their bed."
    ☐ 3. "It is very common for children to regress when they are in the hospital."
    ☐ 4. "This is normal. Your child probably received too much fluid the night before."

23. The nurse is to obtain a urine specimen from a toddler hospitalized with a urinary tract infection. In what order should the nurse perform the following steps? Place in order from first to last. All options must be used.

    | 1. Cleanse the genital area. |
    | 2. Apply gloves. |
    | 3. Offer fluids. |
    | 4. Apply a collection bag. |
    | |
    | |
    | |
    | |

24. A parent brings in an 18-month-old to the clinic because the child "eats ashes, crayons, and paper." Which information about the toddler should the nurse assess **first**?
    ☐ 1. evidence of eruption of large teeth
    ☐ 2. amount of attention from the parent
    ☐ 3. any changes in the home environment
    ☐ 4. intake of a soft, low-roughage diet

25. The nurse performs a well-child checkup on a 2-year-old at the clinic. Which skill should the nurse expect the child to be able to perform?
    ☐ 1. riding a tricycle
    ☐ 2. tying their shoelaces
    ☐ 3. kicking a ball forward
    ☐ 4. using blunt scissors

26. A 2-year-old child brought to the clinic by their parents is uncooperative when the nurse tries to look in their ears. What should the nurse try **first**?
    ☐ 1. Ask another nurse to assist.
    ☐ 2. Allow a parent to assist.
    ☐ 3. Wait until the child calms down.
    ☐ 4. Restrain the child's arms.

27. The nurse observes a parent instilling ear drops prescribed twice a day for a 2-year-old. The nurse decides that the teaching about positioning the pinna for instillation of the drops is effective when the parent pulls the toddler's pinna in which direction?
    ☐ 1. up and forward
    ☐ 2. up and backward
    ☐ 3. down and forward
    ☐ 4. down and backward

28. The parent asks the nurse for advice about discipline for their 18-month-old child. Which discipline strategy should the nurse suggest that the parent use?
    ☐ 1. reprimand
    ☐ 2. spanking
    ☐ 3. reasoning
    ☐ 4. time-out

29. The nurse assesses a toddler for pain. Which method would be the **most** appropriate?
    ☐ 1. Ask the child about the pain.
    ☐ 2. Observe the child for restlessness.
    ☐ 3. Use a numeric rating pain scale.
    ☐ 4. Assess for changes in vital signs.

Health Promotion of the Preschooler and Family

30. The parent of a 4-year-old expresses concern that the child may be hyperactive. The parent describes the child as always in motion, constantly dropping and spilling things. Which action would be appropriate at this time?
    ☐ 1. Determine whether there have been any changes at home.
    ☐ 2. Explain that this is not unusual behavior.
    ☐ 3. Explore the possibility that the child is being abused.
    ☐ 4. Suggest that the child be seen by a pediatric neurologist.

31. The parent of a preschooler reports that the child creates a scene every night at bedtime. What is the **best** course of action?
    ☐ 1. Allow the child to stay up later one or two nights a week.
    ☐ 2. Establish a set bedtime, and follow a routine.
    ☐ 3. Encourage active play before bedtime.
    ☐ 4. Give the child a cookie if bedtime is pleasant.

32. The parents of a preschooler ask the nurse how to handle their child's temper tantrums. Which technique(s) should the nurse include in the teaching plan? Select all that apply.
    ☐ 1. putting the child in "time-out"
    ☐ 2. ignoring the child
    ☐ 3. putting the child to bed
    ☐ 4. spanking the child
    ☐ 5. trying to reason with the child

33. After teaching a group of parents of preschoolers attending a well-child clinic about oral hygiene and tooth brushing, the nurse determines that the teaching has been successful when the parents state that children can begin to brush their teeth without supervision at which age?
☐ 1. 3 years
☐ 2. 5 years
☐ 3. 7 years
☐ 4. 9 years

34. After having a blood sample drawn, a 5-year-old child insists that the site be covered with a bandage. When the parent tries to remove the bandage before leaving the office, the child screams that all the blood will come out. The nurse encourages the parent to leave the bandage in place and tells the parent that the child's reaction is based on which factor?
☐ 1. fearing another procedure
☐ 2. lacking understanding of body integrity
☐ 3. expressing severe pain
☐ 4. attempting to regain control

Health Promotion of the School-Age Child and Family

35. The nurse takes the blood pressure of a preschool child. To determine if the blood pressure is normal, the nurse compares the results with percentiles for systolic and diastolic blood pressure. What other information does the nurse need to graph the blood pressure? Select all that apply.
☐ 1. age
☐ 2. body mass index (BMI)
☐ 3. sex
☐ 4. height
☐ 5. occipital frontal circumference (OFC)
☐ 6. weight

36. A nurse is assessing the growth and development of a 10-year-old. What is the expected behavior of this child?
☐ 1. enjoys physical demonstrations of affection
☐ 2. is selfish and insensitive to the welfare of others
☐ 3. is uncooperative in play and school
☐ 4. has a strong sense of justice and fair play

37. The nurse conducts a wellness screening on a 9-year-old client. Which finding **most** suggests that the client has typical social development?
☐ 1. thinks independently
☐ 2. is able to organize and plan
☐ 3. has a best friend
☐ 4. enjoys active play

38. A 10-year-old child proudly tells the nurse that brushing and flossing their teeth is their responsibility. How does the nurse interpret the statement?
The child:
☐ 1. is too young to be given this responsibility.
☐ 2. is most likely capable of this responsibility.
☐ 3. should have assumed this responsibility much sooner.
☐ 4. is probably just exaggerating the responsibility.

39. A parent tells the nurse that their 8-year-old child is continually telling jokes and riddles to the point of driving the other family members crazy. The nurse should explain this behavior is a sign of which factor?
☐ 1. inadequate parental attention
☐ 2. mastery of language ambiguities
☐ 3. inappropriate peer influence
☐ 4. excessive television watching

40. A parent asks the nurse about their 9-year-old child's apparent need for between-meal snacks, especially after school. What information should the nurse include in the teaching plan?
The child:
☐ 1. does not need to eat between-meal snacks.
☐ 2. should eat the snacks the parent thinks are appropriate.
☐ 3. should help with preparing their own snacks.
☐ 4. will instinctively select nutritional snacks.

41. The nurse compares a child's height and weight with standard growth charts and finds the child to be in the 50th percentile for height and in the 25th percentile for weight, similar to the last visit. How does the nurse interpret the child's growth pattern?
☐ 1. typical height and weight
☐ 2. overweight for height
☐ 3. underweight for height
☐ 4. abnormal in height

42. The nurse reviews the growth pattern of a 3-year-old female child at a well-child checkup.

Flow Sheet

Age	Height	Weight	Body Mass Index (BMI)	BMI-for-Age
2 years/2 months	36 inches (91 cm)	32 lb (14.5 kg)	17.4	74th
2 years/7 months	37 inches (94 cm)	33.5 lb (15.2 kg)	17.2	78th
3 years	38.5 inches (98 cm)	36.5 lb (16.6 kg)	17.3	85th

➤ Complete the following sentences by using the list of options.

The nurse determines that the toddler is [healthy weight / overweight / obese]

The most appropriate intervention is to [continue routine growth monitoring. / discuss healthy eating and activity guidelines. / discuss weight-loss strategies.]

Health Promotion of the Adolescent and Family

43. The nurse is assessing an 11-year-old girl using the Tanner staging of puberty. Which finding indicates preadolescent development of the breasts?
  ☐ 1.
  ☐ 2.
  ☐ 3.
  ☐ 4.

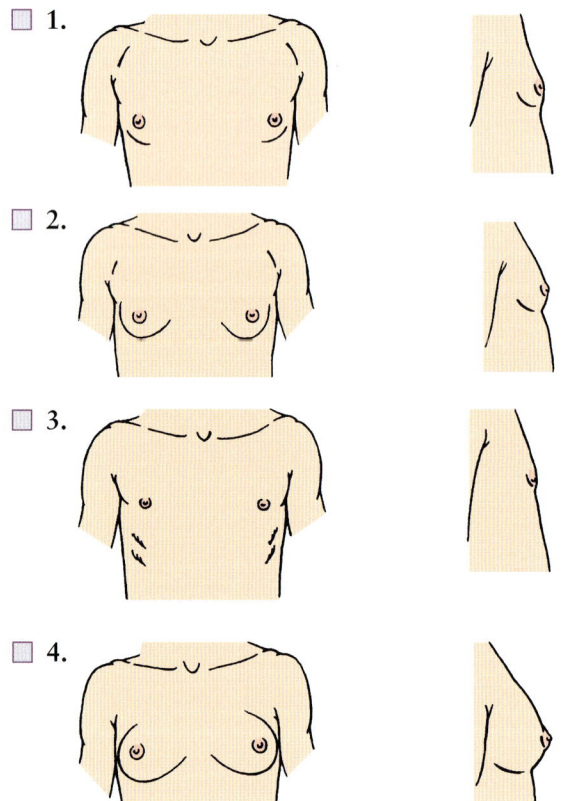

44. The parents of a 12-year-old girl ask why their child, who is not sexually active, should receive the human papillomavirus (HPV) vaccine. What should the nurse tell the parents?
  ☐ 1. "The vaccine is most effective against cervical cancer if given before becoming sexually active."
  ☐ 2. "Parents are never sure when their child might become sexually active."
  ☐ 3. "HPV is most common in teens and women in their late 20s."
  ☐ 4. "If your child is sexually assaulted, they may be exposed to HPV."

45. A 16-year-old female client who has been confined to a wheelchair since early childhood has lately been acting rebellious and rude. The client's parents ask the nurse, "Are all adolescents like this?" The nurse should respond with which statement?
  ☐ 1. "Yes, although your child's behaviors are more like those of an adolescent boy."
  ☐ 2. "No. Your child must need some help in dealing with their feelings."
  ☐ 3. "Your child's behavior seems to be typical adolescent behavior. Let us talk more about it."
  ☐ 4. "Your child's behavior results from feelings about their disability: ignore it."

46. The parents of an adolescent are concerned their child seems to need 9 hours of sleep a night. What should the nurse tell the parents?
☐ 1. "As long as they seem otherwise well, this sounds like a typical teenager."
☐ 2. "Adolescents need only 8 hours of sleep a night; anything over this is excessive."
☐ 3. "Your child is probably engaged in too many activities and is wearing themself out."
☐ 4. "The side effect of many drugs is sleepiness."

47. An adolescent tells the nurse that they would like to use tampons during their period. What should the nurse do **first**?
☐ 1. Assess the client's usual menstrual flow pattern.
☐ 2. Determine whether the client is sexually active.
☐ 3. Provide information about preventing toxic shock syndrome.
☐ 4. Refer the client to a specialist in adolescent gynecology.

48. Several high-school seniors are referred to the nurse because of suspected alcohol misuse. When the nurse assesses the situation, what would be **most** important to determine?
☐ 1. what they know about the legal implications of drinking
☐ 2. the type of alcohol they usually drink
☐ 3. the reasons they choose to use alcohol
☐ 4. when and with whom they use alcohol

Health Promotion of Children with Down Syndrome (Trisomy 21)

49. The parent of an adolescent girl with Down syndrome tells the nurse that their daughter recently stated that they have a boyfriend. The parent is concerned that their daughter might become pregnant. Which is the **most** appropriate suggestion made by the nurse?
☐ 1. "I understand your concern; you may want to start your child on long-acting contraception."
☐ 2. "Women with Down syndrome are infertile, so you do not need to worry about getting pregnant."
☐ 3. "I understand your concern; you may want to enroll your child in an abstinence program."
☐ 4. "I know it may be difficult, but you may want to suggest that your child break off the relationship."

50. A nurse is assessing a child with trisomy 21 who has a mild intellectual disability. The **best** indication of how this child is progressing can be obtained by observing in which social setting?
☐ 1. at school with their teacher
☐ 2. at home with their family
☐ 3. in the clinic with their parent
☐ 4. playing soccer with their friends

51. The nurse plans care with the parents of a child with trisomy 21. The nurse should help the parents establish which goal?
☐ 1. Encourage self-care skills in the child.
☐ 2. Teach the child something new each day.
☐ 3. Encourage more lenient behavior limits for the child.
☐ 4. Achieve age-appropriate social skills.

52. The nurse discusses with parents how best to raise the IQ of their child with Down syndrome. Which intervention would be **most** appropriate?
☐ 1. Serve hearty, nutritious meals.
☐ 2. Give vasodilator medications as prescribed.
☐ 3. Let the child play with more able children.
☐ 4. Provide stimulating, nonthreatening life experiences.

53. The nurse develops a teaching plan for the parents of a child with trisomy 21. The nurse focuses on activities to increase which factor for the parents?
☐ 1. affection for their child
☐ 2. responsibility for their child's welfare
☐ 3. understanding of their child's disability
☐ 4. confidence in their ability to care for their child

Common Childhood and Adolescent Health Problems

54. The nurse gives anticipatory guidance to the parents of an 8-month-old infant. Which finding(s) would indicate the parents need further teaching about preventing childhood accidents? Select all that apply.
☐ 1. placing a fire screen in front of the fireplace
☐ 2. placing a car seat in a front-seat, front-facing position
☐ 3. inspecting toys for loose parts
☐ 4. placing toxic substances out of reach or in a locked cabinet
☐ 5. checking the wheels on infant walkers for damage

55. A nurse is assessing the growth and development of a 14-year-old boy. The client reports that their 13-year-old sister is 2 inches (5 cm) taller than them. What information should the nurse provide about growth spurts in adolescent boys compared with growth spurts in adolescent girls? They occur:
☐ 1. at about the same time.
☐ 2. about 2 years earlier.
☐ 3. about 2 years later.
☐ 4. about 1 year earlier.

56. The parents of a 15-year-old state that their child is moody and rude. What should the nurse advise the parents to do?
☐ 1. Restrict their child's activities.
☐ 2. Discuss their feelings with their child.
☐ 3. Obtain family counseling.
☐ 4. Talk to other parents of adolescents.

57. Which statement by a parent whose child was just diagnosed with pediculosis capitis (head lice) demonstrates an understanding of the safety and efficacy of the common medications used to treat the infection?
☐ 1. "I am going to request a prescription for lindane because it works the best."
☐ 2. "After I shampoo, I will use the special comb to get the nits out."
☐ 3. "Most over-the-counter lice treatments are 100% effective at killing all the eggs."
☐ 4. "I can give a second treatment the next day if any lice remain."

58. A parent asks, "Can I get head lice too?" The nurse indicates that adults can also be infested with head lice but that pediculosis is more common among school-age children, primarily for what reason?
☐ 1. An immunity to pediculosis usually is established by adulthood.
☐ 2. School-age children tend to be more neglectful of frequent handwashing.
☐ 3. Pediculosis usually is spread by close contact with children with head lice.
☐ 4. The skin of adults is more capable of resisting the invasion of lice.

59. The nurses teaches parents about the cause of ringworm of the scalp (tinea capitis). Which statement by a parent would indicate that teaching had been successful?
☐ 1. "It results from overexposure to the sun."
☐ 2. "It is caused by infestation with a mite."
☐ 3. "It is a fungal infection of the scalp."
☐ 4. "It is an allergic reaction."

60. Griseofulvin was prescribed to treat a child's ringworm of the scalp. The nurse instructs the parents to use the medication for several weeks for which reason?
☐ 1. A sensitivity to the drug is less likely if it is used over a period of time.
☐ 2. Fewer side effects occur as the body slowly adjusts to a new substance over time.
☐ 3. Fewer allergic reactions occur if the drug is maintained at the same level long-term.
☐ 4. The growth of the causative organism into new cells is prevented with long-term use.

61. A parent asks the nurse, "How did my children get pinworms?" The nurse explains that pinworms are **most** commonly spread by which route?
☐ 1. food
☐ 2. hands
☐ 3. animals
☐ 4. toilet seats

62. A parent asks the nurse how to care for a child with chickenpox. What should the nurse include in the plan of care? Select all that apply.
☐ 1. Use over-the-counter aspirin for fever.
☐ 2. Encourage oatmeal baths.
☐ 3. Keep fingernails short.
☐ 4. Avoid overheating.
☐ 5. Do not return to school until all lesions have crusted over.

63. A parent states that a health care provider described their child as having 20/60 vision, and the parent asks the nurse what this means. The nurse responds based on the interpretation that the child is experiencing which condition?
☐ 1. a loss of approximately one-third of visual acuity
☐ 2. ability to see at 60 feet what they should see at 20 feet
☐ 3. ability to see at 20 feet what they should see at 60 feet
☐ 4. visual acuity three times better than average

64. The nurse discusses the eating habits of school-age children with their parents. The nurse should explain that eating habits are **most** influenced by which factor?
☐ 1. food preferences of their peers
☐ 2. smell and appearance of foods offered
☐ 3. examples provided by parents at mealtimes
☐ 4. parental encouragement to eat nutritious foods

65. The nurses discusses the onset of pubescence with parents. The nurse should explain that pubescence occurs at what time?
☐ 1. same age for both boys and girls
☐ 2. 1 to 2 years earlier in boys than in girls
☐ 3. 1 to 2 years earlier in girls than in boys
☐ 4. 3 to 4 years later in boys than in girls

66. A parent has heard that several adolescents have been diagnosed with mononucleosis. The parent asks the nurse what precautions should be taken to prevent this from occurring in their teen. What instructions should the nurse give the parent?
☐ 1. Tell the teen to avoid sharing food and drinks.
☐ 2. Sterilize the teen's eating utensils before they are reused.
☐ 3. Wash the teen's linens separately in hot, soapy water.
☐ 4. Have the teen vaccinated for mononucleosis.

67. A parent asks the nurse how they would know if their child had developed mononucleosis. The nurse explains that in addition to fatigue, which symptom would be **most** common?
☐ 1. liver tenderness
☐ 2. enlarged lymph glands
☐ 3. persistent nonproductive cough
☐ 4. a blush-like generalized skin rash

Managing Care, Quality, and Safety of Children

68. A 17-year-old high school senior calls the clinic because they think they might have gonorrhea. The client wants to be seen but wants assurances that no one will know. Which is the **most** appropriate response by the nurse?
☐ 1. "Because you are underage, we will need your parent's consent to treat you."
☐ 2. "We can treat you without your parents' consent, but they have the right to review your medical record."
☐ 3. "We can see you without your parents' consent but have to report any positive results to the public health department."
☐ 4. "We can see you, treat any infections, and will not share your results with anyone."

69. A parent brings a 5-year-old child to a weekend vaccination clinic to prepare for school entry. The nurse notes that the child has not had any vaccinations since 4 months of age. What is the **best** way for the nurse to determine how to catch up the child's vaccinations?
☐ 1. Contact the child's health care provider (HCP) during office hours.
☐ 2. Review nationally published immunization guidelines.
☐ 3. Read each vaccine's manufacturer's insert.
☐ 4. Ask a local pharmacist on duty.

70. A 13-month-old child has a febrile seizure 3 weeks after the administration of the chickenpox vaccine. What is the **best** action for the nurse to take?
☐ 1. Recognize that the events are unrelated.
☐ 2. Report the event through an immunization surveillance system.
☐ 3. Explain to the parents that this is a rare but acceptable risk.
☐ 4. Refer the child to a neurologist.

71. A child who is 18 months of age is brought to the emergency department by their babysitter. The babysitter states, "The baby fell from the sofa an hour ago and has not been the same since." On questioning, the babysitter appears to be unsure of the time of the incident and other facts related to it. Which question would be **most** effective in obtaining more information about the child's injuries?
☐ 1. "Why did you leave the child alone on the couch?"
☐ 2. "Have you taken a course in safe babysitting?"
☐ 3. "Tell me what was happening before the baby fell."
☐ 4. "Where are the baby's parents? Do they know this happened?"

72. | STEP 1 |

The nurse is performing a well-child checkup in the clinic on a 9-month-old male infant.

> Highlight the findings that require follow-up. Answer choices have been underlined.

Nurse's Notes

The infant was brought by a parent for a well-child visit. The client was last seen at the 2-month visit in April and was noted to have typical development. The parent reported that the family had immigration issues but now they feel safe bringing the infant to the clinic again. The baby is still breastfeeding four times daily as well as eating cereal and drinking juice twice a day. The parent is worried because the infant has just become very afraid of strangers, points all of the time, and is constantly putting things in their mouth. The client sits unsupported and has just started to crawl. The client's last immunizations were at the 2-month visit. Vital signs are temperature 97.6°F (36.4°C), heart rate 110 bpm, and respiration rate 30 breaths/min. The weight and height are in the 10th percentile, similar to the last visit.

Nurse's Notes

The infant was brought by a parent for a well-child visit. The client was last seen at the 2-month visit in April and was noted to have typical development. The parent reported that the <u>family had immigration issues</u> but now they feel safe bringing the infant to the clinic again. The baby is still breastfeeding four times daily as well as eating cereal and <u>drinking juice twice a day</u>. The parent is worried because the <u>infant has just become very afraid of strangers</u>, <u>points all of the time</u>, and <u>is constantly putting things in their mouth</u>. The client sits unsupported and has just started to crawl. <u>The client's last immunizations were at the 2-month visit</u>. <u>Vital signs are temperature 97.6°F (36.4°C), heart rate 110 bpm, and respiration rate 30 breaths/min</u>. <u>The weight and height are in the 10th percentile</u>, <u>similar to the last visit</u>.

73. STEP 2

The nurse is performing a well-child checkup in the clinic on a 9-month-old male infant.

Nurse's Notes

The infant was brought by a parent for a well-child visit. The client was last seen at the 2-month visit in April and was noted to have typical development. The parent reported that the family had immigration issues but now they feel safe bringing the infant to the clinic again. The baby is still breastfeeding four times daily as well as eating cereal and drinking juice twice a day. The parent is worried because the infant has just become very afraid of strangers, points all of the time, and is constantly putting things in their mouth. The client sits unsupported and has just started to crawl. The client's last immunizations were at the 2-month visit. Vital signs are temperature 97.6°F (36.4°C), heart rate 110 bpm, and respiration rate 30 breaths/min. The weight and height are in the 10th percentile, similar to the last visit.

Flow Sheet

Birth Immunizations	2-month Immunizations
Hepatitis B (Hep B)	Hep B
	Diphtheria, tetanus, acellular pertussis (DTaP)
	Haemophilus influenzae (Hib)
	Pneumococcal conjugate vaccine (PCV13)
	Inactivated polio (IPV)

The nurse reviews the client's flow sheet immunization record.

➤ The nurse determines that the delayed immunization status put the infant at risk for which disease(s)? Select all that apply.

☐	1. Hepatitis B
☐	2. Pertussis
☐	3. Measles
☐	4. *H. influenzae*
☐	5. Chickenpox
☐	6. Influenza
☐	7. Pneumococcal pneumonia
☐	8. Polio
☐	9. Rubella

74. STEP 3

The nurse is performing a well-child checkup in the clinic on a 9-month-old male infant.

Nurse's Notes

The infant was brought by a parent for a well-child visit. The client was last seen at the 2-month visit in April and was noted to have typical development. The parent reported that the family had immigration issues but now they feel safe bringing the infant to the clinic again. The baby is still breastfeeding four times daily as well as eating cereal and drinking juice twice a day. The parent is worried because the infant has just become very afraid of strangers, points all of the time, and is constantly putting things in their mouth. The client sits unsupported and has just started to crawl. The client's last immunizations were at the 2-month visit. Vital signs are temperature 97.6°F (36.4°C), heart rate 110 bpm, and respiration rate 30 breaths/min. The weight and height are in the 10th percentile, similar to the last visit.

Flow Sheet

Birth Immunizations	2-month Immunizations
Hepatitis B (Hep B)	Hep B
	Diphtheria, tetanus, acellular pertussis (DTaP)
	Haemophilus influenzae (Hib)
	Pneumococcal conjugate vaccine (PCV13)
	Inactivated polio (IPV)

➤ Based on the immunization history, the nurse determines that the infant is at the **highest** risk for developing which two serious complications of vaccine-preventable diseases?

☐	1. Dehydration
☐	2. Liver failure
☐	3. Paralysis
☐	4. Pneumonia
☐	5. Meningitis

75. STEP 4

The nurse is performing a well-child checkup in the clinic on a 9-month-old male infant.

Nurse's Notes

The infant was brought by a parent for a well-child visit. The client was last seen at the 2-month visit in April and was noted to have typical development. The parent reported that the family had immigration issues but now they feel safe bringing the infant to the clinic again. The baby is still breastfeeding four times daily as well as eating cereal and drinking juice twice a day. The parent is worried because the infant has just become very afraid of strangers, points all of the time, and is constantly putting things in their mouth. The client sits unsupported and has just started to crawl. The client's last immunizations were at the 2-month visit. Vital signs are temperature 97.6°F (36.4°C), heart rate 110 bpm, and respiration rate 30 breaths/min. The weight and height are in the 10th percentile, similar to the last visit.

Flow Sheet

Birth Immunizations	2-month Immunizations
Hepatitis B (Hep B)	Hep B
	Diphtheria, tetanus, acellular pertussis (DTaP)
	Haemophilus influenzae (Hib)
	Pneumococcal conjugate vaccine (PCV13)
	Inactivated polio (IPV)

Orders

Give today:
- Hep B
- DTaP
- Hib
- PCV13
- IPV
- Inactivated influenza

The nurse receives orders to administer vaccines per a catch-up schedule.

➤ For each possible intervention, click to specify whether the intervention is indicated or not indicated.

Possible Intervention	Indicated	Not Indicated
Provide vaccine information in the native language	○	○
Obtain parental consent	○	○
Screen for previous reactions	○	○
Mix vaccines in the same syringe	○	○
Administer all recommended vaccines on the same day	○	○
Record the vaccine lot number and manufacturer	○	○

76. STEP 5

The nurse is performing a well-child checkup in the clinic on a 9-month-old male infant.

Nurse's Notes

The infant was brought by a parent for a well-child visit. The client was last seen at the 2-month visit in April and was noted to have typical development. The parent reported that the family had immigration issues but now they feel safe bringing the infant to the clinic again. The baby is still breastfeeding four times daily as well as eating cereal and drinking juice twice a day. The parent is worried because the infant has just become very afraid of strangers, points all of the time, and is constantly putting things in their mouth. The client sits unsupported and has just started to crawl. The client's last immunizations were at the 2-month visit. Vital signs are temperature 97.6°F (36.4°C), heart rate 110 bpm, and respiration rate 30 breaths/min. The weight and height are in the 10th percentile, similar to the last visit.

Flow Sheet

Birth Immunizations	2-month Immunizations
Hepatitis B (Hep B)	Hep B
	Diphtheria, tetanus, acellular pertussis (DTaP)
	Haemophilus influenzae (Hib)
	Pneumococcal conjugate vaccine (PCV13)
	Inactivated polio (IPV)

Orders

Give today:
- Hep B
- DTaP
- Hib
- PCV13
- IPV
- Inactivated influenza

➤ Which action(s) should the nurse take to reduce the pain associated with vaccination? Select all that apply.

☐	1. Have the birth parent breastfeed.
☐	2. Inject vaccines rapidly without aspiration.
☐	3. Inject the most painful vaccine last.
☐	4. Partially insert the needle into muscle.
☐	5. Use tactile stimulation near the injection site.
☐	6. Use topical anesthetics.
☐	7. Give vaccines at the same location.

77. STEP 6

The nurse is performing a well-child checkup in the clinic on a 9-month-old male infant.

Nurse's Notes

The infant was brought by a parent for a well-child visit. The client was last seen at the 2-month visit in April and was noted to have typical development. The parent reported that the family had immigration issues but now they feel safe bringing the infant to the clinic again. The baby is still breastfeeding four times daily as well as eating cereal and drinking juice twice a day. The parent is worried because the infant has just become very afraid of strangers, points all of the time, and is constantly putting things in their mouth. The client sits unsupported and has just started to crawl. The client's last immunizations were at the 2-month visit. Vital signs are temperature 97.6°F (36.4°C), heart rate 110 bpm, and respiration rate 30 breaths/min. The weight and height are in the 10th percentile, similar to the last visit.

Flow Sheet

Birth Immunizations	2-month Immunizations
Hepatitis B (Hep B)	Hep B
	Diphtheria, tetanus, acellular pertussis (DTaP)
	Haemophilus influenzae (Hib)
	Pneumococcal conjugate vaccine (PCV13)
	Inactivated polio (IPV)

Orders

Give today:

- Hep B
- DTaP
- Hib
- PCV13
- IPV
- Inactivated influenza

The nurse performs a follow-up call the day after vaccination.

➤ For each possible finding, indicate if the finding would **most** indicate a minor vaccine reaction, a moderate-to-severe reaction, or an unrelated reaction.

Possible Finding	Minor Vaccine Reaction	Moderate-to-Severe Vaccine reaction	Unrelated Reaction
Rhinitis	○	○	○
Redness at the injection site	○	○	○
Nonstop crying for 3 hours	○	○	○
Fever of 102.5°F (39.1°C)	○	○	○
Loss of appetite	○	○	○
Hives	○	○	○
Slight swelling of one leg	○	○	○

Answers, Rationales, and Test-Taking Strategies

*The answers and rationales for each question follow below, along with keys (🔑) to the client need (CN) and cognitive level (CL) for each question. In addition, questions that measure clinical judgment will be coded (CJ). As you check your answers, use the **Content Mastery and Test-Taking Skill Self-Analysis** worksheet (tear-out worksheet in the back of the book) to identify the reason(s) for not answering the questions correctly. For additional information about test-taking skills and strategies for answering questions, refer to pages 12–51 in Part 1 of this book.*

Health Promotion of the Infant and Family

1. **3.** It is important for the nurse to assist parents in assessing speech development in their child so that developmental delays can be identified early. At 8 months of age, the child should say "mama" and "dada" nonspecifically and imitate speech sounds. Children cannot say "dada" or "mama" specifically or use more than three words until they are about 12 months of age. A child cannot respond to specific commands or point to objects when requested until about 17 months of age.

    🔑 CN: Health promotion and maintenance; CL: Apply

2. **4.** According to the Denver Developmental Screening Examination, a child of 8 months should sit without support for long periods of time. An 8-month-old child does not have the ability to stand without hanging onto a stationary object for support. Their muscles are not developed enough to support all their weight without assistance. Their balance has not developed to the point that they can stand and stoop over to reach an object.

    🔑 CN: Health promotion and maintenance; CL: Analyze

3. **4.** Infants should be kept on formula or breast milk until 1 year of age. The protein in cow's milk is harder to digest than the protein found in formula. It does not matter in what order fruits and vegetables are introduced as long as the foods are introduced slowly. Solids are introduced into the infant's diet around 4 to 6 months, after the extrusion reflex has diminished and when the child will accept new textures. Iron deficiency develops in term infants between 4 and 6 months when the prenatal iron stores are depleted. Fortified cereals can be added to the infant's diet at 4 to 6 months to prevent iron deficiency anemia.

    🔑 CN: Health promotion and maintenance; CL: Apply

4. **3.** Understanding object permanence means that the child is aware of the existence of objects that are covered or displaced. Neuromuscular development and curiosity are not associated with the principle of object permanence. Object permanence reflects short-term memory, not long-term memory.

    🔑 CN: Health promotion and maintenance; CL: Apply

5. **3.** The posterior fontanelle should be closed by age 2 months. The anterior fontanelle and sagittal and frontal sutures should be closed by age 18 months.

    🔑 CN: Health promotion and maintenance; CL: Apply

6. **3.** During the first few months of life, an infant's eyes may wander and appear to be crossing. As the eye muscles mature, between 2 and 3 months of age, both eyes will focus on the same thing. No intervention is necessary, as crossing of the eyes is normal in the first few months of life.

    🔑 CN: Health promotion and maintenance; CL: Apply

7. **3.** By the end of 3 months, infants should babble. The lack of babbling suggests a language delay and warrants further investigation. Infants typically would begin playing peekaboo around 7 months. The ability to roll front to back typically occurs at 5 months. Sitting unsupported is expected at 6 months.

    🔑 CN: Health promotion and maintenance; CL: Analyze

8. **3.** Vaccination in the presence of a moderate-to-severe infection, with or without fever, increases the risk for injury and decreases the chance of mounting good immunity. An acute bilateral ear infection would constitute a moderate infection or illness. There is currently no evidence to suggest vaccines increase the risk for SIDS. A mild temperature may be expected with the DTaP vaccine. A temperature higher than 105°F (40.5°C) within 48 hours of vaccination would warrant caution. The DTaP vaccine is not a live vaccine. No special precautions are needed regarding immunosuppressed family members.

    🔑 CN: Reduction of risk potential; CL: Analyze

9. **3.** The MMR vaccine is a live vaccine. Neither the American Academy of Pediatrics nor the Public Health Agency of Canada recommends routine vaccination with the MMR vaccine (either alone or combined with the varicella vaccine) to children younger than 12 months. The DTaP, Hib, and influenza vaccines are all indicated.

    CN: Health promotion and maintenance; CL: Analyze

10. **4.** A 1-month-old infant is usually able to lift the head from a prone position. The full-term infant with no complications has probably been able to do this since birth. Smiling and laughing is expected behavior at 2 to 3 months. Rolling from back to side and holding a rattle are characteristics of a 4-month-old.

    CN: Health promotion and maintenance; CL: Analyze

11. **3.** The American Academy of Pediatrics and Canadian Pediatric Society recommend that infants remain on iron-fortified formula or breast milk until 1 year of age. The nurse needs to first assess if the parent switched the baby prematurely because of a lack of information or lack of resources. Then appropriate teaching or referrals may be determined. At 1 year of age, the infant may be switched to whole milk, which has a higher fat content than 2%. A higher fat content is needed for brain growth. Demanding clients change behaviors without addressing the cause is unlikely to produce desired results.

    CN: Health promotion and maintenance; CL: Analyze

12. **2.** Holding the head erect when sitting, staring at an object placed in the hand, taking the object to the mouth, cooing and gurgling, and sustaining part of their body weight when in a standing position are behaviors characteristic of a 4-month-old infant. A 2-month-old typically vocalizes, follows objects to the midline, and smiles. A 7-month-old typically is able to sit without support, turn toward the voice, and transfer objects from hand to hand. Usually, a 9-month-old can crawl, stand while holding on, and initiate speech sounds.

    CN: Health promotion and maintenance; CL: Analyze

13. **3, 6.** Typical abilities demonstrated by 8-month-old infants include playing peekaboo and transferring objects from one hand to another. The ability to say "dada" and "mama" is more typical of 10-month-old infants. Infants usually are at least 12 months old when they achieve the ability to walk independently. Infants who are 15 months old commonly can feed themselves with a spoon and stack two blocks.

    CN: Health promotion and maintenance; CL: Analyze

14. **4.** The anterior fontanelle, commonly known as the *soft spot*, closes between 12 to 18 months in most infants. The nurse normally measures an infant's occipital frontal circumference at each well-child visit. This action alone does not relieve the parent's concerns. Referrals would be indicated for premature or delayed closures of the fontanelle, especially if there were other abnormal findings. Closure of the anterior fontanelle by 12 months can only be expected to occur in approximately a third of all infants.

    CN: Health promotion and maintenance; CL: Analyze

15. **1.** Typically, a 9-month-old infant should have been voicing single syllables since 6 months of age. The absence of this finding would be a cause for concern. An infant usually is able to stand alone at about 10 months of age. An infant usually is able to build a tower of two cubes at about 15 months of age. An infant usually is able to drink from a cup with little spilling at about 15 months of age.

    CN: Health promotion and maintenance; CL: Analyze

16. **4.** More than 90% of 9-month-olds are able to stand holding onto objects. Rolling over is expected at 4 to 6 months, and sitting without support is expected at 6 months. Crawling is expected at 9 months.

    CN: Health promotion and maintenance; CL: Analyze

17. **2.** Simultaneous injection reduces the anxiety related to anticipation of the next injection. Needle length must be long enough to deposit the vaccine into the muscle. A 5/8-inch (1.6-cm) needle is appropriate for newborns but is not long enough for infants older than 1 month or other children. Aspirating for blood return does not confirm needle placement. Breastfeeding during vaccinations, not before, has been found to reduce pain.

    CN: Basic care and comfort; CL: Apply

Health Promotion of the Toddler and Family

18. **3.** A push-pull toy will aid in the development of gross motor skills and muscle development. A stuffed animal is age appropriate for a toddler but

is not the toy to promote development. A music box and nursery mobile are most appropriate to stimulate development of an infant.

🗝️ CN: Health promotion and maintenance; CL: Apply

19. 🔲 **3, 5.** Behavior problems related to sleep and rest are common in young children. Consistent rituals around bedtime help to create an easier transition from waking to sleep. Parents can give reassurance that the child's bed is a safe place. Allowing a child to sleep with their parents commonly creates more problems for the family and child and does not alleviate the problem or foster autonomy. Increasing activity before bedtime does not alleviate the separation anxiety in the toddler and causes further anxiety. Allowing them to stay up later than their normal time for bed will increase their anxiety, make it more difficult to fall asleep, and do nothing to lessen the fear. Telling the child that the monster has been destroyed supports the belief in the imaginary creature and typically delays bedtime instead of providing comfort.

🗝️ CN: Psychosocial integrity; CL: Apply

20. 4. Toddlers establish ritualistic patterns to feel secure, despite inconsistencies in their environment. Establishing a sense of identity is the developmental task of the adolescent. The toddler's developmental task is to use rituals and routines to help make autonomy easier to accomplish. Ritualistic patterns involve patterns of behavior, but they are not utilized to develop learning behaviors.

🗝️ CN: Psychosocial integrity; CL: Apply

21. 🔲 **1, 3, 4.** Readiness for toilet training is based on neurologic, psychological, and physical developmental readiness. The nurse can introduce concepts of readiness for toilet training and encourage parents to look for adaptive and psychomotor signs such as the ability to walk well, balance, climb, sit in a chair, dress oneself, please the parent, and communicate awareness of the need to urinate or defecate. Chronological age is not an indicator for toilet training. Two-year-old children engage in parallel play, which is not an indicator of readiness for toilet training.

🗝️ CN: Health promotion and maintenance; CL: Apply

22. 3. A child will regress to behavior used in an earlier stage of development to cope with a perceived threatening situation. Readiness for toilet training should be based on neurologic, physical, and psychological development, not the age of the child. Children are afraid of hospitalization, but bed-wetting is a compensatory mechanism done to regress to a previous stage of development that is more comfortable and secure for the child. Telling the parent that bed-wetting is related to fluid intake does not provide an adequate explanation for the underlying regression to an earlier stage of development.

🗝️ CN: Psychosocial integrity; CL: Analyze

23. 3, 2, 1, 4. When obtaining a urine specimen from an infant, the nurse assists the client to drink fluids 30 to 60 minutes prior to specimen collection so the client voids as soon as possible after the collection bag is applied. Next, the nurse applies gloves and then cleanses the genital area with sterile water to prevent contamination of the urine. Finally, the nurse applies the collection bag and then removes the bag when the specimen is obtained.

🗝️ CN: Safety and infection control; CL: apply

24. 3. A craving to eat nonfood substances is known as *pica*. Toddlers use oral gratification as a means to cope with anxiety. Therefore, the nurse should first assess whether the child is experiencing any change in the home environment that could cause anxiety. Teething or the eruption of large teeth and the amount of attention from the parent are unlikely causes of pica. Nutritional deficiencies, especially iron deficiency, were once thought to cause pica, but research has not substantiated this theory. A soft, low-roughage diet is an unlikely cause.

🗝️ CN: Physiological adaptation; CL: Analyze

25. 3. A 2-year-old child usually can kick a ball forward. Riding a tricycle is characteristic of a 3-year-old child. Tying shoelaces is a behavior to be expected of a 5-year-old child. Using blunt scissors is characteristic of a 3-year-old child.

🗝️ CN: Health promotion and maintenance; CL: Analyze

26. 2. Parents can be asked to assist when their child becomes uncooperative during a procedure. Most commonly, the child's difficulty in cooperating is caused by fear. In most situations, the child will feel more secure with a parent present. Other methods, such as asking another nurse to assist or waiting until the child calms down, may be necessary, but obtaining a parent's assistance is the recommended first action. Restraints should be used only as a last resort after all other attempts have been made to encourage cooperation.

🗝️ CN: Health promotion and maintenance; CL: Analyze

27. 4. In a child younger than 3 years of age, the pinna is pulled back and down because the auditory canals are almost straight in children. In children over age 3 years through adulthood, the pinna is pulled up and backward because the auditory canals are directed inward, forward, and down.

🔑 CN: Pharmacological and parenteral therapies; CL: Evaluate

28. 4. Time-out is the most appropriate discipline for toddlers. It helps to remove them from the situation and allows them to regain control. Structuring interactions with 3-year-olds helps minimize unacceptable behavior. This approach involves setting clear and reasonable rules and calling attention to unacceptable behavior as soon as it occurs. Reprimanding a young child can reinforce undesirable behavior over time because it provides attention. Physical punishment, such as spanking, has limited effectiveness and serious negative effects. Reasoning is more appropriate for older children, such as preschoolers and those older, especially when moral issues are involved. Unfortunately, reasoning combined with scolding often takes the form of shame or criticism, and children take such remarks seriously, believing that they are "bad."

🔑 CN: Health promotion and maintenance; CL: Analyze

29. 2. Toddlers usually express pain through such behaviors as restlessness, facial grimaces, irritability, and crying. It is not particularly helpful to ask toddlers about pain. In most instances, they would be unable to understand or describe the nature and location of their pain because of their lack of verbal and cognitive skills. However, preschool and older children have the verbal and cognitive skills to be able to respond appropriately. While the FACES pain scale can be used in young children, numeric rating pain scales are more appropriate for children who are of school age or older. Changes in vital signs occur as a result of pain, but behavioral changes usually are noticed first.

🔑 CN: Physiological adaptation; CL: Analyze

Health Promotion of the Preschooler and Family

30. 2. Preschool-age children have been described as powerhouses of gross motor activity who seem to have endless energy. A limitation of their motor ability is that in moving as quickly as they do, they are not always able to judge distances, nor are they able to estimate the amount of strength and balance needed for activities. As a result, they have frequent mishaps. This level of activity typically is not associated with changes at home. However, if the behavior intensifies, a referral to a pediatric neurologist would be appropriate. Children who have been abused usually demonstrate withdrawn behaviors, not endless energy.

🔑 CN: Health promotion and maintenance; CL: Analyze

31. 2. Bedtime is often a problem with preschoolers. Recommendations for reducing conflicts at bedtime include establishing a set bedtime, having a dependable routine, such as story reading, and conveying the expectation that the child will comply. Allowing the child to stay up late one or two nights interferes with establishing needed bedtime rituals. Excitement, such as active play, just before bedtime should be avoided because it stimulates the child, making it difficult for the child to calm down and prepare for sleep. Using food such as a cookie as a reward if bedtime is pleasant should be avoided because it places too much importance on food. Other rewards, such as stickers, could be used as an alternative.

🔑 CN: Health promotion and maintenance; CL: Analyze

32. 1, 2. Some parents find that putting the child in time-out until control is regained is very effective. Others find that ignoring the behaviors works just as well with their child. Both suggestions are appropriate to include in the teaching plan. Spanking the child is never an option. Attempting to reason with a child having a temper tantrum does not work because the child is out of control. A more appropriate time to discuss it with the child is when the child regains control.

🔑 CN: Health promotion and maintenance; CL: Apply

33. 3. Children younger than 7 years do not have the manual dexterity needed for tooth brushing. Therefore, parents need to supervise and assist with the task until that time.

🔑 CN: Health promotion and maintenance; CL: Evaluate

34. 2. The preschool-age child does not have an accurate concept of skin integrity and can view medical and surgical treatments as hostile invasions that can destroy or damage the body. The child does not understand that exsanguinations will not occur from the injection site. Here, the child is verbalizing a fear consistent with their developmental age. The child would most likely verbalize concerns about not wanting another procedure or exhibit other symptoms associated with pain if those were the underlying issues. If control was the main issue, the child would try to control more than just the bandage removal.

🗝 CN: Psychosocial integrity; CL: Analyze

Health Promotion of the School-Age Child and Family

35. **1, 3, 4.** Blood pressure percentiles for children are referenced by age, sex, and height. Measurements at or above the 95th percentile are considered indicative of hypertension. Weight and elevated BMI contribute to hypertension but are not used to define it. The OFC is not routinely measured in children over 2 years of age and is not used to reference blood pressure readings.

🗝 CN: Health promotion and maintenance; CL: Analyze

36. **4.** School-age children are concerned about justice and fair play. They become upset when they think someone is not playing fair. Physical affection makes them embarrassed and uncomfortable. They are concerned about others and are cooperative in play and school.

🗝 CN: Health promotion and maintenance; CL: Analyze

37. **3.** During the school-age years, children learn to socialize with children of the same age. The "best friend" stage, which occurs around 9 or 10 years of age, is important in providing a foundation for self-esteem and later relationships. Thinking independently, organizing, and planning are cognitive skills. Active play relates to motor skills.

🗝 CN: Health promotion and maintenance; CL: Analyze

38. **2.** Children are capable of mastering the skills required for flossing when they reach 9 years of age. At this age, many children are able to assume responsibility for personal hygiene. The client is not too young to assume this responsibility, and they should not have been expected to assume this responsibility much earlier. It is not likely that they are exaggerating; this is expected behavior at this age.

🗝 CN: Health promotion and maintenance; CL: Analyze

39. **2.** School-age children delight in riddles and jokes. Mastery of the ambiguities of language and of sentence structure allows the school-age child to manipulate words, and telling riddles and jokes is a way of practicing this skill. Children who suffer from inadequate attention from parents tend to demonstrate abnormal behavior. Peer influence is less important to school-age children, and while the child may learn the joke from a friend, they are telling the joke to master language. Watching television does not influence the extent of joke telling.

🗝 CN: Health promotion and maintenance; CL: Analyze

40. **3.** Snacks are necessary for school-age children because of their high energy level. School-age children are in a stage of cognitive development in which they can learn to categorize or classify and can also learn cause and effect. By preparing their own snacks, children can learn the basics of nutrition (such as what carbohydrates are and what happens when they are eaten). The parent and child should make the decision about appropriate foods together. School-age children learn to make decisions based on information, not instinct. Some knowledge of nutrition is needed to make appropriate choices.

🗝 CN: Health promotion and maintenance; CL: Analyze

41. **1.** The values of height and weight percentiles are usually similar for an individual child. Measurements between the fifth and 95th percentiles are considered normal. Marked discrepancies identify overweight or underweight children.

🗝 CN: Health promotion and maintenance; CL: Analyze

42. **0/1** The nurse determines that the toddler is overweight. The most appropriate action is to **discuss healthy eating and activity guidelines.**

Growth for children 2 years of age and up should be monitored using the BMI-for-age growth charts. Weights falling between the fifth percentile and the 85th percentile are considered healthy. Weights between the 85th to less than the 95th percentile are classified as overweight. Weights equal to or greater than the 95th percentile are classified as obese. The child has just become overweight. The best intervention is to promote healthy eating and activity to help slow weight gain and help the child grow into a healthy weight. These recommendations include limiting sugary beverages and reducing screen time. Weight loss is rarely indicated for children under 6 and must be medically supervised. The child would not be due for another well-child visit for another year. Continuing routine monitoring without discussing healthy eating and physical activity guidelines put the child at risk for becoming obese.

🗝 CJ: Standalone trend; CL: Create

Health Promotion of the Adolescent and Family

43. 3. This figure indicates elevation of the papilla, without breast buds, considered stage 1 and typical of a preadolescent. Figure 1 shows stage 2, breast bud enlargement; there is elevation of the breast and the diameter of the areola has increased. Figure 2 shows stage 3, enlargement of the breast and areola. Figure 4 shows stage 4, in which there is projection of the areola and papilla to form a secondary mound above the level of the breast.

CN: Physiological adaptation; CL: Analyze

44. 1. Vaccines are preventative in nature and ideally given before exposure. Focusing on the benefits of cancer prevention is most appropriate, as opposed to discussing with parents the potential that their child may become sexually active without their knowledge. It is true that HPV is most common in adolescents and women in their late 20s, but parents still may not perceive that their child is at risk. Discussing the possibility of exposure through assault raises fears and does not focus on prevention.

CN: Health promotion and maintenance; CL: Apply

45. 3. It is normal behavior for adolescents to assert independence and begin to separate from their parents; the behavior is not changed by their child's disability, nor is it unique to a girl. The nurse offers reassurance to the parents and then opens the conversation for additional discussion.

CN: Health promotion; CL: Analyze

46. 1. Many teenagers feel fatigued from a combination of fast-food diets, many activities, and a rapid growth spurt; this is normal behavior, and the nurse should explain possible reasons for the sleep pattern. Adolescents typically need 8.5 to 9.5 hours of sleep. There are no data to suggest that activities are tiring for this teenager. It is not appropriate to suggest the child is taking drugs based on the question the parents are asking the nurse.

CN: Health Promotion; CL: Analyze

47. 3. The nurse should provide the adolescent with information about toxic shock syndrome because of the identified relationship between tampon use and the syndrome's development. Additionally, about 95% of cases of toxic shock syndrome occur during menses. Most adolescent females can use tampons safely if they change them frequently. Using tampons is not related to menstrual flow or sexual activity. There is no need to refer the girl to a gynecologist; a nurse can provide health teaching about tampon use.

CN: Reduction of risk potential; CL: Analyze

48. 3. Information about why adolescents choose to use alcohol or other drugs can be used to determine whether they are becoming responsible users or problem users. The senior students likely know the legal implications of drinking, and the nurse will establish a more effective relationship with the students by understanding their motivations for use. The type of alcohol and when and with whom they are using it are not the first data to obtain when assessing the situation.

CN: Health promotion and maintenance; CL: Analyze

Health Promotion of Children with Down Syndrome (Trisomy 21)

49. 1. Children with Down syndrome range from having severe intellectual disability to having low-average intelligence. Thus, the adolescent's ability to make informed choices regarding sexual activity is limited. Long-acting contraception, such as an intrauterine device or a progestin implant, greatly reduces the risk for unwanted pregnancy. Most women with Down syndrome are fertile; however, children born to women with Down syndrome often have congenital defects. An abstinence program may not be effective because of the intellectual level of children with Down syndrome. Suggesting that the adolescent break off the relationship does not ensure that they will.

CN: Health promotion and maintenance; CL: Analyze

50. 1. Watching the child relate to their teacher and schoolwork is the best indication of how they are progressing. School involves interacting with persons who are not relatives and places the child in a situation that is not totally familiar. Observing the client in situations with family and friends shows social relationships but does not indicate how the child is learning new intellectual skills.

CN: Health promotion and maintenance; CL: Evaluate

51. 1. The goal in working with children with intellectual disabilities is to train them to be as independent as possible, focusing on developmental skills. The child may not be capable of learning something new every day, but they do need to repeat what has been taught previously. Rather than encouraging more lenient behavior limits, the parents need to be strict and consistent when setting limits for the child. Most children with Down syndrome are unable to achieve age-appropriate social skills because of their disability. Rather, they are taught socially appropriate behaviors.

CN: Health promotion and maintenance; CL: Analyze

52. 4. Nonthreatening experiences that are stimulating and interesting to the child have been observed to help raise IQ. Practices such as serving nutritious meals or letting the child play with more able children have not been supported by research as beneficial in increasing intelligence. Vasodilator medications act to increase oxygenation to the tissues, including the brain. However, these medications do not increase the child's IQ.

CN: Health promotion and maintenance; CL: Analyze

53. 4. When the nurse is teaching the parents of a child with trisomy 21, also known as *Down syndrome*, activities should focus on increasing the parents' confidence in their ability to care for their child. The parents must continue to work daily with their child. Most parents feel affection and a sense of responsibility for their child regardless of the child's limitations. Parents usually understand the child's disability on the cognitive level but have difficulty accepting it on the emotional level. As the parents' confidence in their caring abilities increases, their understanding of the child's disability also increases on all levels.

CN: Psychosocial integrity; CL: Analyze

Common Childhood and Adolescent Health Problems

54. 2, 5. It is recommended that children up to 2 years of age ride in a rear-facing car seat. Walkers are a leading cause of injuries in babies, so health and safety experts strongly discourage their use. The middle of the back seat is considered the safest area of the car. Burns are a major cause of childhood accidents, and using fire screens in front of fireplaces can help prevent children from getting too close to a fire in a fireplace. Toys that contain loose parts or plastic eyes that can be swallowed or aspirated by small children should be avoided. Parents should inspect all toys for these parts before giving one to a child. Poisonings are most commonly caused by improper storage of a toxic substance. Keeping toxic substances in a childproof container in a locked cabinet and continually observing the child's activities can prevent most poisonings.

CN: Safety and infection control; CL: Evaluate

55. 3. Adolescent boys lag about 2 years behind adolescent girls in growth. Most girls are 1 to 2 inches (3 to 5 cm) taller than boys at the beginning of adolescence but tend to stop growing approximately 2 to 3 years after menarche with the closure of the epiphyseal lines of the long bones.

CN: Health promotion and maintenance; CL: Apply

56. 2. Parents need to discuss with their adolescent how they perceive their behavior and how they feel about it. Moodiness is characteristic of adolescents. The adolescent may have a reason for or not be aware of their behavior. Restricting the adolescent's activities will not change their mood or the way they respond to others. It may increase their unacceptable responses. Counseling may not be needed at this time if the parents are open to communicating and listening to the adolescent. Talking to other parents may be of some help, but what is helpful to others may not be helpful to their child.

CN: Health promotion and maintenance; CL: Analyze

57. 2. The makers of many of the pediculicides recommend manual removal of the nits following treatment with an extra–fine-tooth comb. None of the pediculicides are 100% effective in killing all the eggs. The FDA has issued a warning regarding the use of lindane because of the potential for neurotoxicity. Clients are treated with lindane only when the benefits outweigh the risks. Lice treatments may be repeated in 7 to 10 days; the next day is too soon.

CN: Health promotion; CL: Analyze

58. 3. Lice are spread by close personal contact and by contact with infested clothing, bed and bathroom linens, and combs and brushes. Lice are more common in school-age children than in adults because of the close contact in school or at sleepovers and the common practice of sharing possessions. Lice are not commonly spread by hand contact. There is no immunity conferred by having head lice. Adults can have head lice, particularly if they come in close contact with their children's infested clothing or linens.

CN: Physiological adaptation; CL: Apply

59. 3. Ringworm of the scalp is caused by a fungus of the dermatophyte group of the species. Overexposure to the sun would result in sunburn. Mites, such as chiggers or ticks, produce bites on the skin, resulting in inflammation. An allergic reaction commonly is manifested by hives, rash, or anaphylaxis.

🔑 CN: Physiological adaptation; CL: Evaluate

60. 4. Griseofulvin is an antifungal agent that acts by binding to the keratin that is deposited in the skin, hair, and nails as they grow. This keratin is then resistant to the fungus. But as the keratin is normally shed, the fungus enters new, uninfected cells unless drug therapy continues. Long-term administration of griseofulvin does not prevent sensitivity or allergic reactions. As the body adjusts to a new substance over time, side effects are variable and do not necessarily decrease.

🔑 CN: Pharmacological and parenteral therapies; CL: Apply

61. 2. The adult pinworm emerges from the rectum and colon at night onto the perianal area to lay its eggs. Itching and scratching introduce the eggs to the hands, from where they can easily reinfect the child or infect others. Nightclothes and bed linens can be sources of infection. The eggs can also be transmitted by dust in the home. Although transmission through contaminated food and water supplies is possible, it is rare. Contaminated animals can spread histoplasmosis and salmonella. The spread of infections by toilet seats has not been supported by research.

🔑 CN: Physiological adaptation; CL: Apply

62. ⊟ 2, 3, 4, 5. The care of a child with chickenpox focuses on keeping the child comfortable and preventing infection in the lesions. Oatmeal baths may ease severe itching. Keeping fingernails short reduces trauma from scratching and helps prevent skin infections. Overheating can make itching worse. Children may return to school once all lesions have crusted over. The use of aspirin in children with chickenpox is contraindicated because it has been linked to Reye syndrome.

🔑 CN: Basic care and comfort; CL: Analyze

63. 3. A child with 20/60 vision sees at 20 feet what those with 20/20 vision see at 60 feet. Visual acuity of 20/200 is considered to be the boundary of legal blindness.

🔑 CN: Physiological adaptation; CL: Analyze

64. 3. Although children may be influenced by their peers and the smell and appearance of foods may be important, children are most likely to be influenced by the example and atmosphere provided by their parents. Coaxing and badgering a child to eat most likely will aggravate poor eating habits.

🔑 CN: Health promotion and maintenance; CL: Apply

65. 3. Girls experience the onset of puberty about 1 to 2 years earlier than boys. The reason for this is not understood.

🔑 CN: Health promotion and maintenance; CL: Apply

66. 1. The cause of infectious mononucleosis is thought to be the Epstein-Barr virus. The virus is believed to be spread only by direct intimate contact. No precautionary measures for the general public are recommended to prevent mononucleosis. However, it is recommended that sharing food items and kissing be avoided with persons known to have mononucleosis. There currently is no vaccine for the disease.

🔑 CN: Physiological adaptation; CL: Analyze

67. 2. Mononucleosis usually has an insidious onset, with fatigue and the inability to maintain usual activity levels as the most common symptoms. The lymph nodes are typically enlarged, and the spleen also may be enlarged. Fever and a sore throat often accompany mononucleosis. A persistent nonproductive cough can follow an upper respiratory tract infection. A blush-like generalized skin rash is more characteristic of rubella.

🔑 CN: Physiological adaptation; CL: Analyze

Managing Care, Quality, and Safety of Children

68. 3. While some areas may specify a minimum age for treatment (usually 12 to 14 years), generally adolescents have the right to seek treatment for sexually transmitted infections without their parents' permission. These medical records are not shared with parents without the client's permission. However, adolescents must be made aware that certain infections, including gonorrhea, must be reported by law to public health agencies. Partner notification will also take place, but methods vary.

🔑 CN: Management of care; CL: Apply

69. 2. National advisory committees on immunization practices review vaccination evidence and update recommendations yearly. Current vaccination catch-up schedules are readily available on their websites. The lack of vaccinations is a strong

226 The Nursing Care of Children

indicator that the child probably does not have an HCP. Even if the client had a provider, however, that person might be difficult to reach on a weekend during the time frame of a vaccination clinic. If consulted, the pharmacist would most likely have to review the latest guidelines that are equally available to the nurse. Reading each of the manufacturer's inserts for multiple vaccines would be time consuming, and synthesis of the information could possibly lead to errors.

🗝 CN: Management of care; CL: Apply

70. 2. Any unusual event that occurs after the administration of a vaccine should be reported through an immunization surveillance system, especially if it happens within 1 month of the administration. In the United States, the immunization surveillance system is the Vaccine Adverse Event Reporting System (VAERS). In Canada, it is the Canadian Adverse Events Following Immunization Surveillance System (CAEFISS). A high fever, with or without a seizure, that occurs within 6 weeks of vaccination may have been caused by the vaccine. A febrile seizure is considered a moderate reaction that warrants caution with future chickenpox vaccination. A single febrile seizure does not require referral to a neurologist.

🗝 CN: Safety and infection control; CL: Analyze

71. 3. An open-ended question is apt to supply more information when a person is under stress and easily susceptible to being influenced by the question. The other questions are direct and only require an answer with limited information.

🗝 CN: Management of care; CL: Analyze

72.

STEP 1

−/+ **Nurse's Notes**

> The infant was brought by a parent for a well-child visit. The client was last seen at the 2-month visit in April and was noted to have typical development. The parent reported that the ==family had immigration issues== but now they feel safe bringing the infant to the clinic again. The baby is still breastfeeding four times daily as well as eating cereal and ==drinking juice twice a day==. The parent is worried because the ==infant has just become very afraid of strangers==, ==points all of the time==, and ==is constantly putting things in their mouth==. The client sits unsupported and has just started to crawl. ==The client's last immunizations were at the 2-month visit==. Vital signs are temperature 97.6°F (36.4°C), heart rate 110 bpm, and respiration rate 30 breaths/min. The weight and height are in the 10th percentile, similar to the last visit.

Juice should only be offered in limited amounts because it adds calories without the nutrition that comes in formula or breastmilk. Immunizations are a key activity at well-child checkups. Infants typically receive vaccinations at 2-, 4-, and 6-month visits. Since the last vaccines were at the 2-month visit, the infant is at risk for several vaccine-preventable diseases. Other findings show typical development. A 9-month-old infant typically shows stranger anxiety, and they may point as a way of communicating. They explore the world through their mouth. Sitting unsupported and crawling are normal gross motor findings. The vital signs typical for this age are a temperature between 97.4°F and 99.5°F (36.3°C and 37.5°C) axillary, a heart rate between 100 and 160 bpm, and a respiration rate between 24 and 30 breaths/min. Growth is best understood over time. Typical growth patterns are expected to follow growth percentiles. Following up on immigration status is not necessary and may lead to suspicion of health care providers.

🗝 CJ: Case study; Step 1: Recognize cues; CL: Analyze

73.

STEP 2

−/+ **1, 2, 4, 6, 7, 8.** Most immunizations take more than one dose to give optimal protection. The infant has not yet been vaccinated for seasonal influenza, which is recommended to begin at 6 months of age. The infant has had only one dose of DTaP, H. influenzae, PCV13, and IPV when they would have been expected to have two to three of each, leaving the infant at risk for those diseases. The infant still needs a third dose of the hep B vaccine to complete the series. The infant is not behind on immunization for measles, rubella, and chickenpox, which are given as a live vaccine after the child's first birthday.

🗝 CJ: Case study; Step 2: Analyze cues; CL: Analyze

74.

STEP 3

0/1 **4, 5.** Pneumococcus, pertussis, H. influenzae, and seasonal influenza all can lead to pneumonia. H. influenza and pneumococcus also carry the risk for meningitis. Dehydration in children is most associated with gastroenteritis. Liver failure can be a complication of hepatitis B, but the infant is at lower risk for this disease because they have had two immunizations for this disease. Paralysis is uniquely associated with polio, which is extremely rare in developed countries.

🗝 CJ: Case study; Step 3: Prioritize hypothesis; CL: Analyze

75.

STEP 4

0/1

Possible Intervention	Indicated	Not Indicated
Provide vaccine information in the native language	X	
Obtain parental consent	X	
Screen for previous reactions	X	
Mix vaccines in the same syringe		X
Administer all recommended vaccines on the same day	X	
Record the vaccine lot number and manufacturer	X	

Best practices in patient education include providing information in a client's native language. Obtaining written parental consent is necessary before giving vaccines. Vaccines can be given in the presence of mild disease. Therefore, it is only necessary to screen for moderate or severe illness. It is important to ask parents about any previous reactions to vaccines to ensure there were no allergic reactions or life-threatening reactions. Although there are commercially available combination vaccines available, the nurse should never mix two different vaccines in the same syringe. A general principle of vaccination is that all preparations may be given on the same day. Postponing the needed immunizations until another appointment leaves the child at risk for contracting diseases. When recording vaccine information in the medical record, the nurse must document the manufacturer, lot number, and expiration date along with the site of administration.

CJ: Case study; Step 4: Generate solutions; CL: Apply

76.

STEP 5

−/+ 1, 2, 3, 5, 6. Having the birth parent breastfeed is an effective pain management strategy when administering vaccines. Injecting vaccines rapidly without aspiration is recommended to reduce the time the needle is in the muscle. Research suggests that pain increases from the first to the second injection and giving the least painful vaccine first can decrease the overall pain associated with giving multiple injections. In general, the DTaP vaccine is considered less painful than the PCV13 vaccine. Pain is reduced with intramuscular injections when the needle is inserted into muscle. Inserting a needle part way risks injecting medication into subcutaneous tissues. Tactile stimulation near the injection site confuses nerves so pain is less sharp. Prescription topical creams that contain lidocaine or prilocaine can reduce vaccine pain but should be placed 20 to 60 minutes in advance to be effective. When multiple injections are needed, they should be given at least 2 cm apart and not at the exact same site.

CJ: Case study; Step 5: Take action; CL: Apply

77.

STEP 6

0/1

Possible Finding	Minor Vaccine Reaction	Moderate-to-Severe Vaccine reaction	Unrelated Reaction
Rhinitis			X
Redness at the injection site	X		
Nonstop crying for 3 hours		X	
Fever of 102.5°F (39.1°C)	X		
Loss of appetite	X		
Hives		X	
Slight swelling of one leg	X		

All vaccines carry the risk for local reactions, including soreness, redness, and swelling of the injection site. When vaccines are given in the anterolateral thigh, some leg swelling may be present. Low-grade fevers, fussiness, and loss of appetite are common minor reactions. Nonstop crying for 3 hours and a temperature over 105°F (40.5°C) indicate that the infant is having a severe vaccine reaction. The presence of hives suggests the possibility of an allergic reaction. The presence of rhinitis suggests the infant may be developing an upper respiratory infection, which is not associated with vaccination.

CJ: Case study; Step 6: Evaluate outcomes; CL: Evaluate

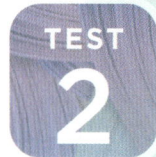

TEST 2 — The Child with Respiratory Health Problems

- The Client with Tonsillitis
- The Client with Otitis Media
- The Client with Foreign Body Aspiration
- The Client with Asthma
- The Client with Cystic Fibrosis and Bronchopneumonia
- The Client with Sudden Infant Death Syndrome
- The Client Who Requires Immediate Care and Cardiopulmonary Resuscitation
- The Client with Croup
- The Client with Bronchiolitis or Pharyngitis
- Managing Care, Quality, and Safety of Children with Respiratory Health Problems
- Answers, Rationales, and Test-Taking Strategies

The Client with Tonsillitis

1. The nurse is inspecting a child's throat (see figure). How should the nurse proceed with the throat examination?

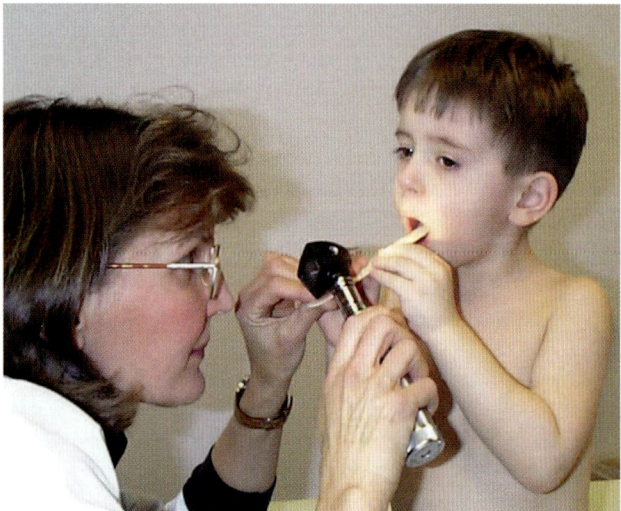

- ☐ 1. Remove the tongue blade from the child's hands after they have experienced what it feels like in their mouth.
- ☐ 2. Ask the child to hold the tongue blade with both hands in their lap while the nurse uses another tongue blade.
- ☐ 3. Have the parent hold the child with arms restrained.
- ☐ 4. Guide the tongue blade while the child is holding it to depress the tongue to visualize the throat.

2. The nurse has identified a problem of anxiety for a 4-year-old preparing for a tonsillectomy. What should the nurse tell the child?
- ☐ 1. "You will not have so many sore throats after your tonsils are removed."
- ☐ 2. "The doctor will put you to sleep so you do not feel anything."
- ☐ 3. "Show me how to give the doll an IV."
- ☐ 4. "When it is done, you will wake up from a nap and get to see your mommy"

3. The nurse cares for a 5-year-old child after a tonsillectomy and adenoidectomy. Which finding should alert the nurse to suspect early hemorrhage?
- ☐ 1. drooling of bright red secretions
- ☐ 2. pulse rate of 95 bpm
- ☐ 3. vomiting of 25 mL of dark brown emesis
- ☐ 4. blood pressure of 95/56 mm Hg

4. A nurse is teaching the parents of a preschooler about the possibility of postoperative hemorrhage after a tonsillectomy and adenoidectomy. When should the nurse explain that the risk for bleeding is the **greatest**?
- ☐ 1. 1 to 3 days after surgery
- ☐ 2. 4 to 6 days after surgery
- ☐ 3. 7 to 10 days after surgery
- ☐ 4. 11 to 14 days after surgery

The Client with Otitis Media

5. A toddler is scheduled to have tympanostomy tubes inserted. When the nurse is approaching the toddler for the first time, which should the nurse do?
   ☐ 1. Talk to the parent first so the toddler can get used to the new person.
   ☐ 2. Hold the toddler so they become more comfortable.
   ☐ 3. Walk over and pick the toddler up right away so the parent can relax.
   ☐ 4. Pick up the toddler and take the child to the play area so the parent can rest.

6. The nurse provides discharge teaching to the parent of a toddler after insertion of bilateral tympanostomy tubes. Which instructions should the nurse include in the child's discharge plan for the parents?
   ☐ 1. Insert ear plugs into the canals when the child bathes.
   ☐ 2. Gently clean the ear canal with cotton swabs.
   ☐ 3. Administer antibiotics daily while the tubes are in place.
   ☐ 4. Disregard any drainage from the ear after 1 week.

7. The nurse caring for a 3-year-old with otitis media notes that the client has an allergy to amoxicillin that causes wheezing. Which prescription should the nurse question?
   ☐ 1. azithromycin
   ☐ 2. cephalexin
   ☐ 3. trimethoprim-sulfamethoxazole
   ☐ 4. cefdinir

The Client with Foreign Body Aspiration

8. The nurse teaches the parents of a toddler about commonly aspirated foods. Which food, if identified by the parents as easily aspirated, would indicate the need for additional teaching?
   ☐ 1. popcorn
   ☐ 2. raw vegetables
   ☐ 3. round candy
   ☐ 4. crackers

9. A toddler who has been treated for a foreign body aspiration begins to fuss and cry when the parents attempt to leave the hospital for an hour. As the nurse tries to take the child out of the crib, the child pushes the nurse away. The nurse interprets this behavior as indicating which stage of separation anxiety?
   ☐ 1. protest
   ☐ 2. despair
   ☐ 3. regression
   ☐ 4. detachment

10. The nurse teaches the three cardinal signs of choking and total airway blockage to the parents of a toddler who was treated for a foreign body obstruction. When asked to repeat the signs, the parents identify "turn blue" and "cannot speak." What third sign would the parents identify if teaching was successful?
    ☐ 1. vomits
    ☐ 2. gasps
    ☐ 3. gags
    ☐ 4. collapses

11. The parent of a 2-year-old phones the emergency department on a Sunday evening and informs the nurse that their child has a bead stuck in their nose. What is the **most** appropriate recommendation made by the nurse?
    ☐ 1. "Try to remove the bead at home as soon as possible; you might try using a pair of tweezers."
    ☐ 2. "Be sure to take your child to the pediatrician in the morning so the pediatrician can remove the bead in the office."
    ☐ 3. "You should bring your child to the emergency department tonight so the bead can be removed as soon as possible."
    ☐ 4. "Ask your child to blow their nose several times; this should dislodge the bead."

The Client with Asthma

12. An 11-year-old child is admitted for treatment of an asthma attack. Which finding(s) would indicate **immediate** intervention is needed? Select all that apply.
    ☐ 1. thin, copious mucous secretions
    ☐ 2. productive cough
    ☐ 3. intercostal retractions
    ☐ 4. respiratory rate of 20 breaths/min
    ☐ 5. peak flow 85% of personal best
    ☐ 6. difficulty talking

13. A 12-year-old child with asthma wants to exercise. Which activity should the nurse suggest to improve breathing?
    ☐ 1. soccer
    ☐ 2. swimming
    ☐ 3. track
    ☐ 4. gymnastics

14. STEP 1

The nurse cares for a 5-year-old male client in the emergency department with an acute asthma attack.

Nurse's Notes

0900:
Accompanied by a parent, the child presented to the emergency department with respiratory distress. The parent reported that the client has had rhinorrhea and a dry cough for 2 days. The client has a history of mild expressive language delay but no other major medical history, no known allergies, and no home medication use. Social history includes living in a large urban area with two younger siblings and a parent who smokes one pack of cigarettes a day. The family has a cat. The child has wheezing upon expiration and labored breathing and appears mildly anxious. Vital signs are 97.4°F (36.3°C); pulse 142 bpm; respiration rate 40 breaths/min; blood pressure 110/50 mm Hg; pulse oximetry 95% on room air; and weight 79.2 lb (36 kg).

➤ Which finding(s) would need **immediate** follow-up? Select all that apply.

- [ ] 1. Breath sounds
- [ ] 2. Language delay
- [ ] 3. Temperature
- [ ] 4. Heart rate
- [ ] 5. Respiration rate
- [ ] 6. Blood pressure
- [ ] 7. Oxygen saturation

15. STEP 2

The nurse cares for a 5-year-old male client in the emergency department with an acute asthma attack.

Nurse's Notes

0900:
Accompanied by a parent, the child presented to the emergency department with respiratory distress. The parent reported that the client has had rhinorrhea and a dry cough for 2 days. The client has a history of mild expressive language delay but no other major medical history, no known allergies, and no home medication use. Social history includes living in a large urban area with two younger siblings and a parent who smokes one pack of cigarettes a day. The family has a cat. The child has wheezing upon expiration and labored breathing and appears mildly anxious. Vital signs are 97.4°F (36.3°C); pulse 142 bpm; respiration rate 40 breaths/min; blood pressure 110/50 mm Hg; pulse oximetry 95% on room air; and weight 79.2 lb (36 kg).

➤ For each potential assessment the nurse can make, indicate if the information is helpful or not helpful to assess the child's level of asthma severity.

Potential Assessment	Helpful	Not Helpful
History of school absenteeism	○	○
Home living environment	○	○
History of meconium ileus	○	○
Peak flow meter levels	○	○
Ability to speak	○	○

16. STEP 3

The nurse cares for a 5-year-old male client in the emergency department with an acute asthma attack.

Nurse's Notes

0900:
Accompanied by a parent, the child presented to the emergency department with respiratory distress. The parent reported that the client has had rhinorrhea and a dry cough for 2 days. The client has a history of mild expressive language delay but no other major medical history, no known allergies, and no home medication use. Social history includes living in a large urban area with two younger siblings and a parent who smokes one pack of cigarettes a day. The family has a cat. The child has wheezing upon expiration and labored breathing and appears mildly anxious. Vital signs are 97.4°F (36.3°C); pulse 142 bpm; respiration rate 40 breaths/min; blood pressure 110/50 mm Hg; pulse oximetry 95% on room air; and weight 79.2 lb (36 kg).

0915:
A peak expiratory flow of less than 50% is anticipated for age and gender. The client is speaking in short phrases only.

Orders

- Apply oxygen for saturation below 94%.
- Obtain a sputum culture.
- Administer albuterol via a nebulizer hourly three times and then every 3 hours.
- Obtain a chest x-ray.
- Administer 30 mg of prednisolone orally now.
- Transfer the client to the pediatric unit.
- Initiate asthma education.

The nurse receives orders.

➢ Highlight the two interventions the nurse should prioritize to address the client's condition.

Orders

Apply oxygen for saturation below 94%.

Obtain a sputum culture.

Administer albuterol via a nebulizer hourly three times and then every 3 hours.

Obtain a chest x-ray.

Administer 30 mg of prednisolone orally now.

Transfer the client to the pediatric unit.

Initiate asthma education.

17. STEP 4

The nurse cares for a 5-year-old male client in the emergency department with an acute asthma attack.

Nurse's Notes

0900:
Accompanied by a parent, the child presented to the emergency department with respiratory distress. The parent reported that the client has had rhinorrhea and a dry cough for 2 days. The client has a history of mild expressive language delay but no other major medical history, no known allergies, and no home medication use. Social history includes living in a large urban area with two younger siblings and a parent who smokes one pack of cigarettes a day. The family has a cat. The child has wheezing upon expiration and labored breathing and appears mildly anxious. Vital signs are 97.4°F (36.3°C); pulse 142 bpm; respiration rate 40 breaths/min; blood pressure 110/50 mm Hg; pulse oximetry 95% on room air; and weight 79.2 lb (36 kg).

0915:
A peak expiratory flow of less than 50% is anticipated for age and gender. The client is speaking in short phrases only.

Orders

- Apply oxygen for saturation below 94%.
- Obtain a sputum culture.
- Administer albuterol via a nebulizer hourly three times and then every 3 hours.
- Obtain a chest x-ray.
- Administer 30 mg of prednisolone orally now.
- Transfer the client to the pediatric unit.
- Initiate asthma education.

The client is given albuterol and prednisolone and stabilized in the emergency department before being transferred to the pediatric unit. The receiving nurse reviews the client's orders.

➢ What topic(s) should the nurse plan to address during asthma education? Select all that apply.

☐	1. creating an action plan
☐	2. knowing dietary sodium restrictions
☐	3. recognizing the importance of vaccinations
☐	4. understanding maintenance and rescue medications
☐	5. promoting physical activity
☐	6. reducing exposure to germs
☐	7. testing siblings for asthma
☐	8. understanding triggers

18. STEP 5

The nurse cares for a 5-year-old male client in the emergency department with an acute asthma attack.

Nurse's Notes

0900:
Accompanied by a parent, the child presented to the emergency department with respiratory distress. The parent reported that the client has had rhinorrhea and a dry cough for 2 days. The client has a history of mild expressive language delay but no other major medical history, no known allergies, and no home medication use. Social history includes living in a large urban area with two younger siblings and a parent who smokes one pack of cigarettes a day. The family has a cat. The child has wheezing upon expiration and labored breathing and appears mildly anxious. Vital signs are 97.4°F (36.3°C); pulse 142 bpm; respiration rate 40 breaths/min; blood pressure 110/50 mm Hg; pulse oximetry 95% on room air; and weight 79.2 lb (36 kg).

0915:
A peak expiratory flow of less than 50% is anticipated for age and gender. The client is speaking in short phrases only.

Orders

- Apply oxygen for saturation below 94%.
- Obtain a sputum culture.
- Administer albuterol via a nebulizer hourly three times and then every 3 hours.
- Obtain a chest x-ray.
- Administer 30 mg of prednisolone orally now.
- Transfer the client to the pediatric unit.
- Initiate asthma education.

The health care provider has indicated that the child will go home on albuterol nebulizer treatments. The nurse begins teaching the family about the medication.

➢ For each possible action, specify if it is appropriate or not appropriate to teach the family about albuterol nebulizer treatments.

Possible Actions	Appropriate to Teach	Not Appropriate to Teach
Understand that nervousness and shakiness are common side effects of albuterol.	○	○
Monitor the child for symptoms of nausea and vomiting.	○	○
Have the child rinse their mouth after administration to prevent thrush.	○	○
Know that the nebulizer apparatus is single use and must be discarded after each use.	○	○
Plan for treatments to take about 5 minutes to complete.	○	○
Have the child breathe normally when the nebulizer treatment is being administered.	○	○

19. STEP 6

The nurse cares for a 5-year-old male client in the emergency department with an acute asthma attack.

Nurse's Notes

0900:
Accompanied by a parent, the child presented to the emergency department with respiratory distress. The parent reported that the client has had rhinorrhea and a dry cough for 2 days. The client has a history of mild expressive language delay but no other major medical history, no known allergies, and no home medication use. Social history includes living in a large urban area with two younger siblings and a parent who smokes one pack of cigarettes a day. The family has a cat. The child has wheezing upon expiration and labored breathing and appears mildly anxious. Vital signs are 97.4°F (36.3°C); pulse 142 bpm; respiration rate 40 breaths/min; blood pressure 110/50 mm Hg; pulse oximetry 95% on room air; and weight 79.2 lb (36 kg).

0915:
A peak expiratory flow of less than 50% is anticipated for age and gender. The client is speaking in short phrases only.

Orders

- Apply oxygen for saturation below 94%.
- Obtain a sputum culture.
- Administer albuterol via a nebulizer hourly three times and then every 3 hours.
- Obtain a chest x-ray.
- Administer 30 mg of prednisolone orally now.
- Transfer the client to the pediatric unit.
- Initiate asthma education.

➤ For each finding, specify if the parent's statement indicates the asthma teaching has been effective or ineffective.

Parent Statement	Effective	Ineffective
"I need to keep the family cat out of my child's bed."	○	○
"I need to find more sanitary housing since our building has a persistent problem with cockroaches."	○	○
"I need to quit my job to manage my child's asthma."	○	○
"I plan to attend smoking cessation classes."	○	○
"I will try to keep our emergency department visits to once every 3 months."	○	○
"I will monitor my child for viral illnesses as I know this can trigger asthma symptoms."	○	○

20. The nurse assesses a toddler in the emergency department. Which assessment finding(s) should lead the nurse to suspect that the toddler is experiencing respiratory distress? Select all that apply.
   ☐ 1. coughing
   ☐ 2. respiratory rate of 35 breaths/min
   ☐ 3. heart rate of 95 bpm
   ☐ 4. restlessness
   ☐ 5. malaise
   ☐ 6. diaphoresis

21. A child who uses an inhaled bronchodilator only when needed for asthma has a best peak expiratory flow rate of 270 L per minute. The child's current peak flow reading is 180 L per minute. How does the nurse interpret this reading?
   ☐ 1. The child's asthma is under good control, so the routine treatment plan should continue.
   ☐ 2. The child needs to use short-acting, inhaled beta-2 agonist medication.
   ☐ 3. This is a medical emergency requiring a trip to the emergency department for treatment.
   ☐ 4. The child needs to use inhaled cromolyn sodium.

22. An adolescent with chest pain goes to the nurse. The nurse determines that the teenager has a history of asthma but has had no problems for years. What should the nurse do **next**?
   ☐ 1. Call the adolescent's parent.
   ☐ 2. Have the adolescent lie down for 30 minutes.
   ☐ 3. Obtain a peak flow reading.
   ☐ 4. Have the teen take two puffs of a short-acting bronchodilator.

23. A 7-year-old child with a history of asthma controlled without medications is referred to the school nurse by the teacher because of persistent coughing. What should the nurse do **first**?
   ☐ 1. Obtain the child's heart rate.
   ☐ 2. Give the child an as-needed (PRN) nebulizer treatment.
   ☐ 3. Call a parent to obtain more information.
   ☐ 4. Have a parent come and pick up the child.

24. The nurse develops a teaching plan for the parent of an asthmatic child concerning measures to reduce allergic triggers. Which suggestion should the nurse include?
☐ 1. Have the child bring their own pillow when sleeping away from home.
☐ 2. If using bunk beds, have the child sleep on the bottom.
☐ 3. Use a scented room deodorizer to keep the room fresh.
☐ 4. Vacuum the carpet once or twice a week.

25. A child with asthma states, "I want to play some sports like my friends. What can I do?" The nurse responds to the child based on the understanding of which information?
☐ 1. Physical activities are inappropriate for children with asthma.
☐ 2. Children with asthma must be excluded from team sports.
☐ 3. Vigorous physical exercise frequently precipitates an asthmatic episode.
☐ 4. Most children with asthma can participate in sports if the asthma is controlled.

The Client with Cystic Fibrosis and Bronchopneumonia

26. A child with cystic fibrosis does not like taking a pancreatic enzyme supplement with meals and snacks. The parent does not like to force the child to take the supplement. What is the **most** important reason for the child to take the pancreatic enzyme supplement with meals and snacks?
☐ 1. The child will become dehydrated if the supplement is not taken with meals and snacks.
☐ 2. The child needs these pancreatic enzymes to help the digestive system absorb fats, carbohydrates, and proteins.
☐ 3. The child needs the pancreatic enzymes to aid in liquefying mucus to keep the lungs clear.
☐ 4. The child will experience severe diarrhea if the supplement is not taken as prescribed.

27. An adolescent with cystic fibrosis has been hospitalized several times. On the latest admission, the client has labored respirations, fatigue, malnutrition, and failure to thrive. Which initial nursing action is **most** important?
☐ 1. placing the client on bed rest and obtaining a prescription for a blood gas analysis
☐ 2. implementing a high-calorie, high-protein, low-fat, vitamin-enriched diet and pancreatic granules
☐ 3. applying an oximeter and initiating respiratory therapy
☐ 4. inserting an intravenous (IV) line and initiating antibiotic therapy

28. A child with cystic fibrosis is receiving gentamicin. Which nursing action is **most** important?
☐ 1. monitoring intake and output
☐ 2. obtaining daily weights
☐ 3. monitoring the client for indications of constipation
☐ 4. obtaining stool samples to test for occult blood

29. The nurse develops the plan of care for a child with cystic fibrosis (CF) who is scheduled to receive postural drainage. The nurse should anticipate performing postural drainage at which times?
☐ 1. after meals
☐ 2. before meals
☐ 3. after rest periods
☐ 4. before inhalation treatments

30. The nurse assesses the results of a gentamicin trough blood level for an adolescent with cystic fibrosis who has been treated with gentamicin several times over the last year. The drug level is high. What is the nurse's **primary** concern?
☐ 1. The child may develop liver dysfunction.
☐ 2. The child may experience hearing loss.
☐ 3. The medication may have been administered incorrectly.
☐ 4. The child may need to have a different antibiotic.

31. The nurse includes recreational therapy in the plan of care for a 3-year-old child hospitalized with pneumonia and cystic fibrosis. What toy is the best choice for the child?
☐ 1. 100-piece jigsaw puzzle
☐ 2. child's favorite doll
☐ 3. fuzzy stuffed animal
☐ 4. scissors, paper, and paste

32. The nurse assesses a parent's understanding of the pathophysiology of cystic fibrosis (CF). Which factor, if described by the parents, indicates understanding the underlying problem of the disease?
☐ 1. an abnormality in the body's mucus-secreting glands
☐ 2. formation of fibrous cysts in various body organs
☐ 3. failure of the pancreatic ducts to develop properly
☐ 4. reaction to the formation of antibodies against streptococcus

33. The nurse creates a plan of care for a child with cystic fibrosis who has ineffective airway clearance related to increased pulmonary secretions and inability to expectorate. Which outcome criterion should the nurse develop?
☐ 1. respiratory rate and rhythm within the expected range
☐ 2. absence of chills and fever
☐ 3. ability to engage in age-related activities
☐ 4. ability to tolerate usual diet without vomiting

34. A school-age client with cystic fibrosis asks the nurse what sports they can become involved in as they become older. What is the **best** information for the nurse to provide about sports and cystic fibrosis?
☐ 1. "The best sport is one that you will enjoy and do regularly."
☐ 2. "Swimming is the best exercise for anyone with cystic fibrosis."
☐ 3. "You should avoid contact sports where you might experience a blow to the chest."
☐ 4. "Indoor sports have lower risks of infection than outdoor sports."

The Client with Sudden Infant Death Syndrome

35. The nurse creates a teaching plan for parents on how to reduce the risk for sudden infant death syndrome (SIDS). What measure(s) should the nurse include in the teaching plan? Select all that apply.
☐ 1. Maintain a smoke-free environment.
☐ 2. Use a wedge for side-lying positions.
☐ 3. Breastfeed the baby.
☐ 4. Place the baby on their back to sleep.
☐ 5. Use bumper pads over the bed rails.
☐ 6. Have the baby sleep in the parent's bed.

36. The nurse assesses clients' risk for sudden infant death syndrome (SIDS). Which client is **most** at risk for SIDS?
☐ 1. infant who is 3 months old
☐ 2. 2-year-old who has apnea lasting up to 5 seconds
☐ 3. firstborn child whose parents are in their early 40s
☐ 4. 6-month-old who has had two bouts of pneumonia

37. Parents bring their infant to the emergency department because the child has stopped breathing. A nurse obtains a brief history of events occurring before and after the parents found the infant not breathing. Which question should the nurse ask the parents **first**?
☐ 1. "Was the infant sleeping while wrapped in a blanket?"
☐ 2. "Was the infant lying on their stomach?"
☐ 3. "What did the infant look like when you found the child?"
☐ 4. "When had you last checked on the infant?"

38. The nurse plans to do a home visit with the parents of an infant who died of sudden infant death syndrome (SIDS) at home. When should the nurse visit the parents?
☐ 1. a few days after the funeral
☐ 2. 2 weeks after the funeral
☐ 3. as soon as the parents are ready to talk
☐ 4. as soon after the infant's death as possible

The Client Who Requires Immediate Care and Cardiopulmonary Resuscitation

39. The nurse finds a child who is not breathing. The nurse has someone activate the emergency medical system and then does what **first**?
☐ 1. Clear the airway.
☐ 2. Begin mouth-to-mouth resuscitation.
☐ 3. Initiate oxygen therapy.
☐ 4. Start chest compressions.

40. The nurse begins cardiopulmonary resuscitation (CPR) on a 5-year-old unresponsive client. When the emergency response team arrives, the child continues to have no respiratory effort but has a heart rate of 50 bpm with cyanotic legs. What should the team do **next**?
☐ 1. Continue administering breaths with a bag-mask device without compressions.
☐ 2. Suspend CPR briefly to apply defibrillation patches.
☐ 3. Begin two-person CPR at a ratio of two breaths to 15 compressions.
☐ 4. Begin two-person CPR at a ratio of two breaths to 30 compressions.

41. As part of a health education program, the nurse teaches a group of parents cardiopulmonary resuscitation (CPR). The nurse determines that the teaching has been effective when a parent makes which statement about providing CPR to a child?
☐ 1. "If I am by myself, I should call for help before starting CPR."
☐ 2. "I should compress a child's chest using two to three fingers."
☐ 3. "I should deliver chest compressions at a rate of 100 per minute."
☐ 4. "If I cannot get the breaths to make the chest rise, I should administer abdominal thrusts."

42. The nurse assesses the effectiveness of external chest compressions during cardiopulmonary resuscitation (CPR). Which finding indicates that the chest compressions are effective?
☐ 1. mottling of the skin
☐ 2. pupillary dilation
☐ 3. palpable pulse
☐ 4. cool, dry skin

43. A nurse walks into the room just as a 10-month-old infant places an object in his mouth and starts to choke. After opening the infant's mouth, what should the nurse do **next** to clear the airway?
☐ 1. Use blind finger sweeps.
☐ 2. Deliver back slaps and chest thrusts.
☐ 3. Apply four subdiaphragmatic abdominal thrusts.
☐ 4. Attempt to visualize the object.

44. A young child has had a cardiac arrest, and the rapid response team has been activated. The nurse arrives in the client's room and observes a licensed practical/vocational nurse (LPN/VN) administering CPR to the child (see figure). What should the nurse do to assist the LPN/VN with CPR?

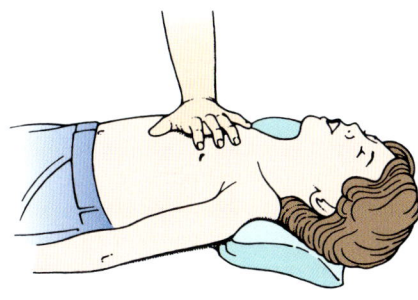

☐ 1. Take over rescue breaths with a rate of 1 breath per 5 compressions using a bag-mask device while the LPN/VN continues compressions.
☐ 2. Take over compressions using one hand while the LPN/VN uses a mask device to administer rescue breaths.
☐ 3. Take over rescue breaths using a rate of 2 breaths per 15 compressions using a bag-mask device while the LPN/VN delivers compressions.
☐ 4. Take over compressions at 80 compressions a minute while the LPN/VN uses a bag-mask device to administer rescue breaths.

45. The nurses teaches the parents of an infant how to perform back slaps to dislodge a foreign body. What should the nurse tell the parents to use to deliver the blows?
☐ 1. palm of the hand
☐ 2. heel of the hand
☐ 3. fingertips
☐ 4. entire hand

46. While the nurse is delivering abdominal thrusts to a 6-year-old who is choking on a foreign body, the child begins to cry. What should the nurse do **next**?
☐ 1. Tap or gently shake the shoulders.
☐ 2. Deliver back slaps.
☐ 3. Perform a blind finger sweep of the mouth.
☐ 4. Observe the child closely.

The Client with Croup

47. The parent of a 16-month-old child calls the clinic because the child has a low-grade fever, cold symptoms, and a hoarse cough. What should the nurse suggest that the parent do?
☐ 1. Offer extra fluids frequently.
☐ 2. Bring the child to the clinic immediately.
☐ 3. Count the child's respiratory rate.
☐ 4. Use a hot air vaporizer.

48. A 21-month-old child admitted with the diagnosis of croup now has a respiratory rate of 48 breaths/min, a heart rate of 120 bpm, and a temperature of 100.8°F (38.2°C) rectally. The nurse is having difficulty calming the child. What should the nurse do **next**?
☐ 1. Administer acetaminophen.
☐ 2. Notify the health care provider (HCP) immediately.
☐ 3. Allow the toddler to continue to cry.
☐ 4. Offer clear fluids every few minutes.

The Client with Bronchiolitis or Pharyngitis

49. A child has viral pharyngitis. What should the nurse advise the parents to do? Select all that apply.
☐ 1. Use a cool mist vaporizer.
☐ 2. Offer a soft-to-liquid diet.
☐ 3. Administer amoxicillin.
☐ 4. Administer acetaminophen.
☐ 5. Place the child on secretion precautions.

50. An infant is being treated at home for bronchiolitis. What should the nurse teach the parent about home care? Select all that apply.
☐ 1. offering small amounts of fluids frequently
☐ 2. allowing the infant to sleep prone
☐ 3. calling the clinic if the infant vomits
☐ 4. writing down how much the infant drinks
☐ 5. performing chest physiotherapy every 4 hours
☐ 6. watching for difficulty breathing

51. In preparation for discharge, the nurse teaches the parent of an infant diagnosed with bronchiolitis about the condition and its treatment. Which statement by the parent indicates successful teaching?
☐ 1. "I need to be sure to take my child's temperature every day."
☐ 2. "I hope I do not get a cold from my child."
☐ 3. "Next time my child gets a cold I need to listen to the chest."
☐ 4. "I need to wash my hands more often."

52. The nurse creates a teaching care plan to prevent the transmission of respiratory syncytial virus (RSV). What information should the nurse include? Select all that apply.
☐ 1. The virus can be spread by direct contact.
☐ 2. The virus can be spread by indirect contact.
☐ 3. Palivizumab is recommended to prevent RSV for all toddlers in daycare.
☐ 4. The virus is typically contagious for 3 weeks.
☐ 5. Older children seldom spread RSV.
☐ 6. Frequent handwashing helps reduce the spread of RSV.

Managing Care, Quality, and Safety of Children with Respiratory Health Problems

53. A charge nurse is making assignments for a group of children on a pediatric unit. Which client should the nurse **most** avoid assigning the same nurse caring for a 2-year-old with respiratory syncytial virus (RSV)?
☐ 1. an 18-month-old with RSV
☐ 2. a 9-year-old 8 hours post appendectomy
☐ 3. a 1-year-old with a heart defect
☐ 4. a 6-year-old with sickle cell crisis

54. The nurse observes an 18-month-old who has been admitted with a respiratory tract infection and is drooling (see figure). What should the nurse do **first**?

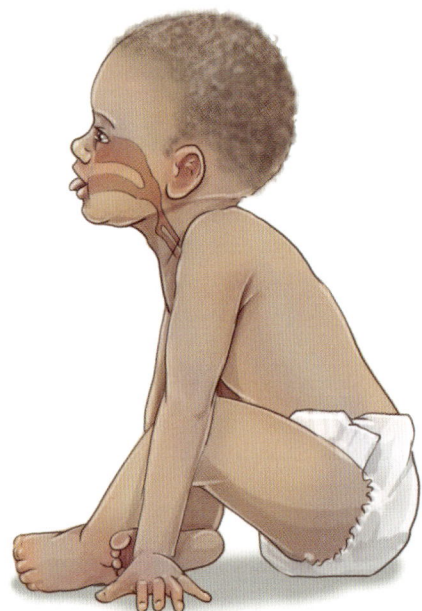

☐ 1. Position the child supine.
☐ 2. Call the rapid response team.
☐ 3. Suction the airway.
☐ 4. Administer oxygen.

55. A nurse administers cefazolin instead of ceftriaxone to an 8-year-old with pneumonia. The client has suffered no adverse effects. The nurse tells the charge nurse of the incident but fears disciplinary action from reporting the error. What should the charge nurse tell the nurse?
☐ 1. "If you do not report the error, I will have to."
☐ 2. "Reporting the error helps to identify system problems to improve client safety."
☐ 3. "Notify the client's health care provider to see if they want this reported."
☐ 4. "This is not a serious mistake, so reporting it will not affect your position."

56. A 12-year-old with cystic fibrosis is being treated in the hospital for pneumonia. The health care provider (HCP) is calling in a telephone prescription for ampicillin. The nurse should take which actions? Select all that apply.
☐ 1. Ask the unit clerk to listen on the speakerphone with the nurse and write down the prescription.
☐ 2. Ask the HCP to come to the hospital and write the prescription on the medical record.
☐ 3. Repeat the prescription to the HCP.
☐ 4. Ask the HCP to confirm that the prescription is correct as understood by the nurse.
☐ 5. Ask the nursing supervisor to cosign the telephone prescription as transcribed by the nurse.

57. The triage nurse in the emergency department must prioritize the children waiting to be seen. Which child is in the **greatest** need of emergency medical treatment?
☐ 1. a 6-year-old with a fever of 104°F (40°C), a muffled voice, no spontaneous cough, and drooling
☐ 2. a 3-year-old with a fever of 100°F (37.8°C), a barky cough, and mild intercostal retractions
☐ 3. a 4-year-old with a fever of 101°F (38.3°C), a hoarse cough, inspiratory stridor, and restlessness
☐ 4. a 13-year-old with a fever of 104°F (40°C), chills, and a cough with thick yellow secretions

58. A 6-month-old on the pediatric floor has a respiratory rate of 68, mild intercostal retractions, and oxygen saturation of 89%. The infant has not been feeding well for the last 24 hours and is restless. Using the situation, background, assessment, and recommendation (SBAR) technique for communication, the nurse calls the health care provider (HCP) with the recommendation for which treatment?
☐ 1. starting oxygen
☐ 2. providing sedation
☐ 3. transferring to pediatric intensive care
☐ 4. prescribing a chest CT scan

59. A child with cystic fibrosis has been admitted to the pediatric unit. What type of diet should the nurse request for the client?
☐ 1. high-fat, high-carbohydrate
☐ 2. high-calorie, high-protein
☐ 3. high-calorie, high-carbohydrate
☐ 4. high-carbohydrate, high-protein

Answers, Rationales, and Test-Taking Strategies

*The answers and rationales for each question follow below, along with keys (🗝) to the client need (CN) and cognitive level (CL) for each question. In addition, questions that measure clinical judgment will be coded (CJ). As you check your answers, use the **Content Mastery and Test-Taking Skill Self-Analysis** worksheet (tear-out worksheet in the back of the book) to identify the reason(s) for not answering the questions correctly. For additional information about test-taking skills and strategies for answering questions, refer to pages 12–51 in Part 1 of this book.*

The Client with Tonsillitis

1. **4.** If the child does not stick out their tongue so the nurse can visualize the throat, it is appropriate to use a tongue blade. Having the child participate by holding the tongue blade while the nurse guides it to facilitate visualization of the throat is the appropriate technique. It is not useful to remove the tongue blade or have the child hold it because the nurse will need to use the tongue blade to depress the tongue. It is preferable to engage the child's cooperation before asking the parent to restrain the child.

    🗝 CN: Health promotion and maintenance; CL: Apply

2. **4.** When preparing a child for a procedure the nurse should use neutral words, focus on sensory experiences, and emphasize the positive aspects at the end. Being reunited with parents would be considered a pleasurable event. Children this age fear bodily harm. To reduce anxiety, the nurse should use the word "fixed" instead of "removed" to describe what is being done to the tonsils. Using the terms "put to sleep" and "IV" may be threatening. Saying that the child will wake up from a nap is less scary Additionally, directing a play experience to focus on IV insertion may be counterproductive as the child may have little recollection of this aspect of the procedure.

    🗝 CN: Psychosocial integrity; CL: Analyze

3. **1.** After a tonsillectomy and adenoidectomy, drooling bright red blood is considered an early sign of hemorrhage. Often, because of discomfort in the throat, children tend to avoid swallowing; instead, they drool. Frequent swallowing would also be an indication of hemorrhage because the child attempts to clear the airway of blood by swallowing. Secretions may be slightly blood-tinged because of a small amount of oozing after surgery. However, bright red secretions indicate bleeding. A pulse rate of 95 bpm is within the normal range for a 5-year-old child, as is a blood pressure of 95/56 mm Hg. A small amount of blood that is partially digested, and therefore dark brown, is often present in postoperative emesis.

    🗝 CN: Reduction of risk potential; CL: Analyze

4. **3.** The risk for hemorrhage from a tonsillectomy is greatest when the tissue begins sloughing and the scabs fall off. This typically happens 7 to 10 days after a tonsillectomy.

    🗝 CN: Safety and infection control; CL: Apply

The Client with Otitis Media

5. **1.** Toddlers should be approached slowly because they are wary of strangers and need time to get used to someone they do not know. The best approach is to ignore them initially and to focus on talking to the parents. The child will likely resist being held by a stranger, so the nurse should not pick up or hold the child until the child indicates a readiness to be approached or the parent indicates that it is okay.

    🗝 CN: Health promotion and maintenance; CL: Analyze

6. **1.** Placing ear plugs in the ears will prevent contaminated bath water from entering the middle ear through the tympanostomy tube and causing an infection. Inserting cotton swabs into the ear canal is not recommended. Antibiotics may be given for a short period after insertion and are appropriate only when an ear infection is present. Tympanostomy tubes may remain in place for several years. It is not necessary to administer antibiotics continuously to a child with a tympanostomy tube. Drainage from the ear may be a sign of a middle ear infection and should be reported to the health care provider.

    🗝 CN: Reduction of risk potential; CL: Apply

7. **2.** Cephalexin is a first-generation cephalosporin. Because clients with a history of anaphylaxis to penicillin, or related antibiotics, have an increased risk for having a cross-reaction to first-generation cephalosporin, the nurse should question a prescription for cephalexin. Azithromycin is not usually considered to be a first-line antibiotic for ear infections in pediatric clients but is effective in pediatric clients with an allergy to amoxicillin. Trimethoprim-sulfamethoxazole is effective

against middle ear infections and can be used effectively in pediatric clients with an allergy to amoxicillin. Second- and third-generation cephalosporins, like cefdinir, do not have the same rates of cross-sensitivities to penicillins as first-generation cephalosporin and may be prescribed for pediatric clients with an allergy to amoxicillin.

CN: Management of care; CL: Analyze

The Client with Foreign Body Aspiration

8. 4. Crackers, because they crumble and easily dissolve, are not commonly aspirated. Because children commonly eat popcorn hulls or pieces that have not popped, popcorn can be easily aspirated. Toddlers frequently do not chew their food well, making raw vegetables a commonly aspirated food. Round candy is often difficult to chew and comes in large pieces, making it easily aspirated.

CN: Health promotion and maintenance; CL: Evaluate

9. 1. Young children have specific reactions to separation and hospitalization. In the protest stage, the toddler physically and verbally attacks anyone who attempts to provide care. Here, the child is fussing and crying and visibly pushes the nurse away. In the despair stage, the toddler becomes withdrawn and obviously depressed (e.g., not engaging in play activities and sleeping more than usual). Regression is a return to a developmentally earlier phase because of stress or crisis (e.g., a toddler who could feed themself before this event is not doing so now). Denial or detachment occurs if the toddler's stay in the hospital without the parent is prolonged because the toddler settles into hospital life and denies the parents' existence (e.g., not reacting when the parents come to visit).

CN: Psychosocial integrity; CL: Analyze

10. 4. The three cardinal signs indicating that a child is truly choking and requires immediate lifesaving interventions include an inability to speak, blue color (cyanosis), and collapse. Vomiting does not occur while a child is unable to breathe. Once the object is dislodged, however, vomiting may occur. Gasping, a sudden intake of air, indicates that the child is still able to inhale. When a child is choking, air is not being exchanged, so gagging will not occur.

CN: Reduction of risk potential; CL: Evaluate

11. 3. The bead should be removed by a health care professional as soon as possible to prevent the risk for aspiration and tissue necrosis. Unskilled individuals should not attempt to remove an object from the nose as they may push the object further, increasing the risk for aspiration. Two-year-old children are not skilled at blowing their nose and may breathe in, further increasing the risk for aspiration.

CN: Management of care; CL: Analyze

The Client with Asthma

12. 3, 6. Intercostal retractions indicate an increase in respiratory effort, which is a sign of respiratory distress. Having difficulty walking or talking is a sign the child has severe shortness of breath and needs immediate attention. During an asthma attack, secretions are thick, the cough is tight, and respiration is difficult (and shortness of breath may occur). If mucous secretions are copious but thin, the client can expectorate them, which indicates an improvement in the condition. If the cough is productive, it means the bronchospasms and the inflammation have been resolved to the extent that the mucus can be expectorated. A respiratory rate of 20 breaths/min would be considered normal, and no intervention would be needed. Peak flows of 80% to 100% of personal best indicate that the asthma is well controlled.

CN: Physiological adaptation; CL: Analyze

13. 2. Swimming is appropriate for this child because it requires controlled breathing, assists in maintaining cardiac health, enhances skeletal muscle strength, and promotes ventilation and perfusion. Stop-and-start activities, such as soccer, track, and gymnastics, commonly trigger symptoms in asthmatic clients.

CN: Health promotion and maintenance; CL: Analyze

14.

STEP 1

1, 4, 5. Expiratory wheezing in asthma is a hallmark assessment sign. Wheezing is heard as it becomes more difficult to force air through the narrowed lumens of bronchioles that are inflamed, swollen, and filled with mucus. Dyspnea, tachypnea (respiration rate greater than 30 breaths/min), and tachycardia (heart rate higher than 140 bpm) result as the air is being pushed forcibly past obstructed bronchioles. The temperature and blood pressure are within normal limits for a 5-year-old. An oxygen saturation of 95% or higher in room air is normal. A language delay does not require emergency care.

CJ: Case study; Step 1: Recognize cues; CL: Analyze

15.

STEP 2

Potential Assessment	Helpful	Not Helpful
History of school absenteeism	X	
Home living environment	X	
History of meconium ileus		X
Peak flow meter levels	X	
Ability to speak	X	

Asthma is a primary cause of school absenteeism, and missing school could indicate the problem has been more persistent. A home environment with environmental allergens such as smoking or cockroaches may trigger an asthma exacerbation. A peak flow meter is utilized to assess expiratory flow during attacks and can be done daily from home to help identify when extra asthma management interventions are needed. The inability to speak signals severe respiratory distress. The presence of meconium ileus is common in newborns with cystic fibrosis, not asthma.

CJ: Case study; Step 2: Analyze cues; CL: Analyze

16.

STEP 3

Orders

Apply oxygen for saturation below 94%.

Obtain a sputum culture.

Administer albuterol via a nebulizer hourly three times and then every 3 hours.

Obtain a chest x-ray

Administer 30 mg of prednisolone orally now.

Transfer the client to the pediatric unit.

Initiate asthma education.

A child with acute asthma exacerbation in the emergency department setting should promptly receive an inhaled bronchodilator such as albuterol and an oral or intravenous corticosteroid. Asthma is a disease of inadequate ventilation, not oxygenation. The child has a normal oxygen saturation given their condition, and oxygen administration is not a top priority. The child did not present with a fever or infectious prodrome, so a sputum culture and an x-ray can be done after giving the medications. The child can be transferred to the pediatric unit after the medications have been given. Asthma education can take place on the pediatric unit.

CJ: Case study; Step 3: Prioritize hypothesis; CL: Apply

17.

STEP 4

1, 3, 4, 5, 6, 8. Comprehensive asthma education includes discussing maintenance and rescue medications and having an action plan of what to do for various symptoms. Ways to stay physically active should be discussed, including the possible need to use an inhaler before engaging in exercise. Respiratory illnesses can trigger attacks, so the nurse should discuss ways to prevent infection, such as handwashing to reduce exposure to germs and keeping up to date with vaccinations, especially those for influenza and COVID-19. The family should be taught to monitor factors that trigger an attack, such as environmental factors, and attempt to reduce those triggers. There are no sodium restrictions with asthma. It is not necessary to test siblings for asthma.

CJ: Case study; Step 4: Generate solutions; CL: Apply

18.

STEP 5

Possible Actions	Appropriate to Teach	Not Appropriate to Teach
Understand that nervousness and shakiness are common side effects of albuterol.	X	
Monitor the child for symptoms of nausea and vomiting.	X	
Have the child rinse their mouth after administration to prevent thrush.		X
Know that the nebulizer apparatus is single use and must be discarded after each use.		X
Plan for treatments to take about 5 minutes to complete.		X
Have the child breathe normally when the nebulizer treatment is being administered.	X	

Nervousness, shakiness, nausea, and vomiting are common side effects of albuterol. The child should be monitored closely to prevent aspiration during treatment. When the nebulizer is no longer aerosolizing, the medication is complete. The length of a nebulizer may vary by vendor, so 5 minutes is not always the length of time for treatment. The child should be instructed to breathe normally during administration of the nebulizer. The apparatus should not be thrown out after single use as a nebulizer can be rinsed with water and is reusable. The child does not need to rinse their mouth after administration of albuterol, but rinsing would be recommended after inhaled steroids.

CJ: Case study; Step 5: Take action; CL: Apply

19.

STEP 6

Parent Statement	Effective	Ineffective
"I need to keep the family cat out of my child's bed."	X	
"I need to find more sanitary housing since our building has a persistent problem with cockroaches."	X	
"I need to quit my job to manage my child's asthma."		X
"I plan to attend smoking cessation classes."	X	
"I will try to keep our emergency department visits to once every 3 months."		X
"I will monitor my child for viral illnesses as I know this can trigger asthma symptoms."	X	

Teaching has been effective if the parent verbalizes the need to avoid common triggers, including viral illness, environmental tobacco smoke, pollution, cats, and indoor allergens such as dust mites, mice, and cockroaches. The goal of asthma management is to have symptom-free periods that allow for optimal quality of life to avoid emergency department visits and hospital admissions. A parent does not need to quit their job to manage their child's asthma, but it is important to involve teachers in the child's individualized asthma action plan to prevent exacerbations.

CJ: Case study; Step 6: Evaluate outcomes; CL: Evaluate

20. **1, 2, 4, 6.** Coughing, especially at night and in the absence of an infection, is a common symptom of asthma. Early signs of respiratory distress include restlessness, tachypnea, tachycardia, and diaphoresis. Other signs also include hypertension, nasal flaring, grunting, wheezing, and intercostal retractions. A heart rate of 95 bpm is normal for a toddler. Malaise typically does not indicate respiratory distress.

CN: Physiological adaptation; CL: Analyze

21. 2. The peak flow of 180 L per minute is in the yellow zone, or 50% to 80% of the child's personal best. This means that the child's asthma is not well controlled, thereby necessitating the use of a short-acting beta-2 agonist medication to relieve the bronchospasm. A peak flow reading of greater than 80% of the child's personal best (in this case, 220 L per minute or better) would indicate that the child's asthma is in the green zone or under good control. A peak flow reading in the red zone, or less than 50% of the child's personal best (135 L per minute or less), would require notification of the health care provider or a trip to the emergency department. Cromolyn sodium is not used for short-term treatment of acute bronchospasm. It is used as part of a long-term therapy regimen to help desensitize mast cells and thereby help prevent symptoms.

CN: Reduction of risk potential; CL: Evaluate

22. 3. Problems of chest pain in children and adolescents are rarely cardiac. With a history of asthma, the most likely cause of the chest pain is related to the asthma. Therefore, the nurse should check the adolescent's peak flow reading to evaluate the status of the airflow. Calling the adolescent's parent would be appropriate, but this would be done after the nurse obtains the peak flow reading and additional assessment data. Having the adolescent lie down may be an option, but more data need to be collected to help establish a possible cause. Because the adolescent has not experienced any asthma problems for a long time, it would be inappropriate for the nurse to administer a short-acting bronchodilator at this time.

CN: Reduction of risk potential; CL: Analyze

23. 3. Because persistent coughing may indicate an asthma attack and a 7-year-old child would be able to provide only minimal history information, it would be important to obtain information from the parent. Although determining the child's heart rate is an important part of the assessment, it would be done after the history is obtained. More information needs to be obtained before giving the child a nebulizer treatment. Although it may be necessary for the parent to come and pick up the child, a thorough assessment including history information should be obtained first.

CN: Reduction of risk potential; CL: Analyze

24. 1. Down pillows and exposure to dust mites are common allergic triggers. The family can reduce exposure to bedding-related allergens during travel or sleepovers by having the child bring a pillow from home. Typically, the child with asthma should sleep in the top bunk bed to minimize the risk for exposure to dust mites. The risk for exposure to dust mites increases when the child sleeps in the bottom bunk bed because dust mites fall from the top bed, settling in the bottom bed. Scented sprays should be avoided because they may trigger an asthmatic episode. Ideally, carpeting should be avoided in the home if the child has asthma. However, if it is present, carpeting in the child's room should be vacuumed often, possibly daily, to remove dust mites and dust particles.

CN: Reduction of risk potential; CL: Apply

25. 4. Physical activities are beneficial to asthmatic children, physically and psychosocially. Most children with asthma can engage in school and sports activities that are geared to the child's condition and within the limits imposed by the disease. The coach and other team members need to be aware of the child's condition and know what to do in case an attack occurs. Those children who have exercise-induced asthma usually use a short-acting bronchodilator before exercising.

🔑 CN: Health promotion and maintenance; CL: Apply

The Client with Cystic Fibrosis and Bronchopneumonia

26. 2. The child must take the pancreatic enzyme supplement with meals and snacks to help absorb nutrients so he can grow and develop normally. In cystic fibrosis, the normally liquid mucus is tenacious and blocks three digestive enzymes from entering the duodenum and digesting essential nutrients. Without the supplemental pancreatic enzyme, the child will have voluminous, foul, fatty stools due to the undigested nutrients and may experience developmental delays due to malnutrition. Dehydration is not a problem related to cystic fibrosis. The pancreatic enzymes have no effect on the viscosity of the tenacious mucus. Diarrhea is not caused by failing to take the pancreatic enzyme supplement.

🔑 CN: Pharmacological and parenteral therapies; CL: Apply

27. 3. Clients with cystic fibrosis commonly die from respiratory problems. The mucus in the lungs is tenacious and difficult to expel, leading to lung infections and interference with oxygen and carbon dioxide exchange. The client will likely need supplemental oxygen and respiratory treatments to maintain adequate gas exchange, as identified by the oximeter reading. The child will be on bed rest due to respiratory distress. However, although blood gases will probably be prescribed, the oximeter readings will be used to determine oxygen deficit and are therefore more of a priority. A diet high in calories, proteins, and vitamins with pancreatic granules added to all foods ingested will increase nutrient absorption and help treat the malnutrition; however, this intervention is not the priority at this time. Inserting an IV to administer antibiotics is important and can be done after ensuring adequate respiratory function.

🔑 CN: Physiological adaptation; CL: Analyze

28. 1. Monitoring intake and output is the most important nursing action when administering an aminoglycoside, such as gentamicin, because a decrease in output is an early sign of renal damage. Daily weight monitoring is not indicated when the client is receiving an aminoglycoside. Constipation and bleeding are not adverse effects of aminoglycosides.

🔑 CN: Pharmacological and parenteral therapies; CL: Analyze

29. 2. Postural drainage, which aids in mobilizing the thick, tenacious secretions commonly associated with CF, is usually performed before meals to avoid the possibility of vomiting or regurgitating food. Although the child with CF needs frequent rest periods, this is not an important factor in scheduling postural drainage. However, the nurse would not want to interrupt the child's rest period to perform the treatment. Inhalation treatments are usually given before postural drainage to help loosen secretions.

🔑 CN: Reduction of risk potential; CL: Apply

30. 2. When given for an extended period of time, aminoglycoside antibiotics can cause permanent hearing loss. The high trough level may indicate that the child has decreased kidney function and is not clearing the drug out of their system efficiently. Although hepatotoxicity has been shown in isolated reports, changes in liver function resolve rapidly once gentamicin is stopped. Errors in medication administration can cause abnormal lab test results, but the child's clinical history and frequency of gentamicin use support an elevated blood level. The lab result indicates that the dose of gentamicin may need to be decreased.

🔑 CN: Reduction of risk potential; CL: Analyze

31. 2. The child's favorite doll would be a good choice of toys. The doll provides support and is familiar to the child. Although a 3-year-old may enjoy puzzles, a 100-piece jigsaw puzzle is too complicated for an ill 3-year-old child. In view of the child's lung pathology, a fuzzy stuffed animal would not be advised because of its potential as a reservoir for dust and bacteria, possibly predisposing the child to additional respiratory problems. Scissors, paper, and paste are not appropriate for a 3-year-old unless the child is supervised closely.

🔑 CN: Health promotion and maintenance; CL: Apply

32. 1. CF is characterized by a dysfunction in the body's mucus-producing exocrine glands. The mucus secretions are thick and sticky rather than thin and slippery. The mucus obstructs the bronchi, bronchioles, and pancreatic ducts. Mucus plugs in the pancreatic ducts can prevent pancreatic digestive enzymes from reaching the small intestine, resulting in poor digestion and poor

244   The Nursing Care of Children

absorption of various food nutrients. Fibrous cysts do not form in various organs. CF is an autosomal recessive inherited disorder and does not involve any reaction to the formation of antibodies against streptococcus.

 CN: Physiological adaptation; CL: Evaluate

33. 1. After treatment, the client outcome would be that respiratory status would be within normal limits, as evidenced by a respiratory rate and rhythm within the expected range. The absence of chills and fever, though related to an underlying problem causing the respiratory problem (e.g., the infection), does not specifically relate to the respiratory problem of ineffective airway clearance. The child's ability to engage in age-related activities may provide some evidence of improved respiratory status; however, this outcome criterion is more directly related to activity intolerance. Although the child's ability to tolerate their usual diet may indirectly relate to respiratory function, this outcome is more specifically related to imbalanced nutrition that may or may not be related to the child's respiratory status.

 CN: Physiological adaptation; CL: Evaluate

34. 1. Responses to physical activity among children with cystic fibrosis vary greatly; therefore, plans of care must be individualized. Selecting a sport that the child likes and will do regularly is most important because children with CF who exercise regularly have better health and quality of life. Many children with CF tolerate and enjoy swimming, but some children do not. There are no universal recommendations that children with CF should not engage in contact sports. There is evidence to suggest that clients who exercise indoors are at greater risk for infection compared with those who exercise outdoors.

 CN: Health promotion and maintenance; CL: Analyze

The Client with Sudden Infant Death Syndrome

35. -/+ **1, 3, 4.** Exposure to environmental tobacco increases the risk for SIDS. Sleeping on the back and breastfeeding both decrease the risk for SIDS. The side-lying position is not recommended for sleep. It is recommended that babies be dressed in sleepers and that cribs are free of blankets, pillows, bumper pads, and stuffed animals. Co-bedding with parents is not recommended as parents may roll on the child.

 CN: Safety and infection control; CL: Apply

36. 1. The highest incidence of SIDS occurs in infants between the ages of 2 and 4 months. About 90% of SIDS occurs before the age of 6 months. Apnea lasting longer than 20 seconds has also been associated with a higher incidence of SIDS. SIDS occurs with higher frequency in families where a child in the family has already died of SIDS, but the age of the parents has not been shown to contribute to SIDS. A respiratory infection such as pneumonia has not been shown to cause a higher incidence of SIDS.

 CN: Health promotion and maintenance; CL: Analyze

37. 3. Because this is an especially disturbing and upsetting time for the parents, they must be approached in a sensitive manner. Asking what the infant looked like when found allows the parents to verbalize what they saw and felt, thereby helping to minimize their feelings of guilt without implying any blame, neglect, wrongdoing, or abuse. Asking if the child was wrapped in a blanket or lying on their stomach, or when the parents last checked on the infant, implies that the parents did something wrong or failed in their care of the infant, thus blaming them for the event.

 CN: Physiological adaptation; CL: Analyze

38. 4. The community health nurse should visit as soon after the death as possible because the parents may need help to deal with the sudden, unexpected death of their infant. Parents often have a great deal of guilt in these situations and need to express their feelings to someone who can provide counseling.

 CN: Psychosocial integrity; CL: Analyze

The Client Who Requires Immediate Care and Cardiopulmonary Resuscitation

39. 4. The current cardiopulmonary resuscitation (CPR) guidelines call for a CAB approach (chest compressions first, then airway and breathing). When breathlessness is determined, the priority nursing action is checking a pulse and beginning compressions. After 30 compressions, the nurse opens the airway and gives two breaths. Oxygen therapy would not be initiated at this time because the child is not breathing. Also, administering oxygen therapy would interfere with providing mouth-to-mouth resuscitation.

 CN: Physiological adaptation; CL: Analyze

40. 3. CPR is done on children with a heart rate of less than 60 bpm and signs of poor perfusion. Rescuers should use a 15:2 compression-to-ventilation ratio for two-rescuer CPR for a child. Breaths without compressions are indicated only for respiratory arrests where the heart rate remains above 60 bpm. The automated external defibrillator (AED) should be used as soon as it is ready, but rescuers should not discontinue compressions until the device is ready for use. The ratio for two-person CPR in adults is 30:2.

   CN: Physiological adaptation; CL: Analyze

41. **3.** To maintain the best perfusion, it is recommended that compressions be given at a rate of 100 per minute in a ratio of 30 compressions to two breaths for one-rescuer CPR. Children still are more likely to have had a respiratory arrest than a cardiac arrest and are more likely to respond to opening the airway and rescue breaths. Therefore, it is recommended that unless the collapse was witnessed, a sole rescuer should attempt five cycles of CPR before leaving to call for help. Using two to three fingers for chest compressions is recommended for infant CPR only. Abdominal thrusts are no longer recommended for unconscious victims.

   CN: Physiological adaptation; CL: Evaluate

42. **3.** With CPR, the effectiveness of external chest compressions is indicated by palpable peripheral pulses, the disappearance of mottling and cyanosis, the return of pupils to normal size, and warm, dry skin. To determine whether the person with cardiopulmonary arrest has resumed spontaneous breathing and circulation, chest compressions must be stopped for 5 seconds at the end of the first minute and every few minutes thereafter.

   CN: Physiological adaptation; CL: Evaluate

43. **2.** The nurse should use mechanical force—back slaps and chest thrusts—when attempting to dislodge the object. Blind finger sweeps are not appropriate in infants and children because the foreign body may be pushed back into the airway. Subdiaphragmatic abdominal thrusts are not used for infants age 1 year or younger because of the risk for injury to abdominal organs. If the object is not visible when the child's mouth is open, time is wasted in looking for it. Action is required to dislodge the object as quickly as possible.

   CN: Reduction of risk potential; CL: Apply

44. **3.** The nurse should first obtain a bag-mask device and assist with CPR by giving breaths at a rate of two breaths for every 15 compressions. The LPN/VN is using the correct technique by using one hand on the chest to administer chest compressions. The heel of both hands is used for older children and adolescents. The compression rate is at least 100 per minute.

   CN: Management of care; CL: Apply

45. **2.** Back slaps are delivered rapidly and forcefully with the heel of the hand between the infant's shoulder blades. Slowly delivered back slaps are less likely to dislodge the object. Using the heel of the hand allows more force to be applied than when using the palm or the whole hand, increasing the likelihood of loosening the object. The fingertips would be used to deliver chest compressions to an infant younger than 1 year of age.

   CN: Physiological adaptation; CL: Apply

46. **4.** Crying indicates that the airway obstruction has been relieved. No additional thrusts are needed. However, the child needs to be observed closely for complications, including respiratory distress. Tapping or shaking the shoulders is used initially to determine unresponsiveness in someone who appears unconscious. Delivering chest or back slaps could jeopardize the child's now-patent airway. Because the obstruction has been relieved, there is no need to sweep the child's mouth. Additionally, blind finger sweeps are contraindicated because the object may be pushed further back, possibly causing a complete airway obstruction.

   CN: Physiological adaptation; CL: Analyze

The Client with Croup

47. **1.** The toddler is exhibiting cold symptoms. A hoarse cough may be part of the upper respiratory tract infection. The best suggestion is to have the parent offer the child additional fluids at frequent intervals to help keep secretions loose and membranes moist. There is no evidence presented to suggest that the child needs to be brought to the clinic immediately. Although having the parent count the child's respiratory rate may provide some additional information, it may lead the parent to suspect that something is seriously wrong, possibly leading to undue anxiety. A hot air vaporizer is not recommended. However, a cool mist vaporizer would cause vasoconstriction of the respiratory passages, making it easier for the child to breathe and loosening secretions.

   CN: Physiological adaptation; CL: Analyze

48. **2.** The nurse may be having difficulty calming the child because the child is experiencing increasing respiratory distress. The normal respiratory rate for a 21-month-old is 25 to 30 breaths/min. The child's respiratory rate is 48 breaths/min. Therefore, the HCP needs to be notified immediately. Typically, acetaminophen is not given to a child unless the temperature is 101°F (38.6°C) or higher. Letting the toddler cry is inappropriate with croup because crying increases respiratory distress. Offering fluids every few minutes to a toddler experiencing increasing respiratory distress would do little, if anything, to calm the child. Also, the child would have difficulty coordinating breathing and swallowing, possibly increasing the risk for aspiration.

CN: Physiological adaptation; CL: Analyze

The Client with Bronchiolitis or Pharyngitis

49. 1, 2, 4. Viral pharyngitis is treated with symptomatic, supportive therapy. Treatment includes the use of a cool mist vaporizer, feeding a soft or liquid diet, and administration of acetaminophen for comfort. Viral infections do not respond to antibiotic administration. The child does not need to be on secretion precautions because viral pharyngitis is not contagious.

CN: Psychosocial integrity; CL: Analyze

50. 1, 6. An infant with bronchiolitis will have increased respirations and will tire more quickly, so it is best and easiest for the infant to take fluids more often in smaller amounts. The parents also would be instructed to watch for signs of increased difficulty breathing, which signal possible complications. Healthy infants and even those with bronchiolitis should sleep in the supine position. Calling the clinic for an episode of vomiting would not be necessary. However, the parents would be instructed to call if the infant cannot keep down any fluids for a period of more than 4 hours. Parents would not need to record how much the infant drinks. Chest physiotherapy is not indicated because it does not help and further irritates the infant.

CN: Basic care and comfort; CL: Apply

51. 4. Handwashing is the best way to prevent respiratory illnesses and the spread of disease. Bronchiolitis, a viral infection primarily affecting the bronchioles, causes swelling and mucus accumulation of the lumina and subsequent hyperinflation of the lung with air trapping. It is transmitted primarily by direct contact with respiratory secretions as a result of eye-to-hand or nose-to-hand contact or from contaminated fomites. Therefore, handwashing minimizes the risk for transmission. Taking the child's temperature is not appropriate in most cases. As long as the child is getting better, taking the temperature will not be helpful. The parent's statement that they hope they do not get a cold from their child does not indicate an understanding of what to do after discharge. For most parents, listening to the child's chest would not be helpful because the parents would not know what they were listening for. Rather, watching for an increased respiratory rate, fever, or evidence of poor eating or drinking would be more helpful in alerting the parent to potential illness.

CN: Physiological adaptation; CL: Evaluate

52. 1, 2, 6. RSV can be spread through direct contact such as kissing the face of an infected person, and it can be spread through indirect contact by touching surfaces covered with infected secretions. Handwashing is one of the best ways to reduce the risk for disease transmission. Palivizumab can prevent severe RSV infections but is only recommended for the most at-risk infants and children. RSV is typically contagious for 3 to 8 days. RSV frequently manifests in older children as cold-like symptoms. Infected school-age children frequently spread the virus to other family members.

CN: Safety and infection control; CL: Apply

Managing Care, Quality, and Safety of Children with Respiratory Health Problems

53. 3. RSV may be spread through both direct and indirect contact. While contact and standard precautions should be employed, a measure to further decrease the risk for nosocomial infections is to avoid assigning the same nurse caring for an RSV client to a client at risk for infection. A private room is preferred, but if this is not an option, the nurse should understand that children 2 years of age and younger are most at risk for RSV, especially if they have other chronic problems such as a heart defect. From an infection control perspective, pairing two clients with RSV is ideal. RSV infections are less likely to pose a serious problem in older children.

CN: Safety and infection control; CL: Analyze

54. 2. The nurse should suspect epiglottitis in any young child with a respiratory infection who sits leaning forward with an open mouth and protruding tongue and is drooling. Epiglottitis is a medical emergency. The rapid response team

should be notified to secure the airway. While waiting for the team, the child should remain sitting upright to facilitate breathing; complete obstruction may occur if the child is placed prone or becomes agitated. Therefore, it is important to avoid any procedures that upset the child such as suctioning or applying oxygen.

CN: Reduction of risk potential; CL: Analyze

55. 2. Client safety is enhanced when the emphasis on medication errors is to determine the root cause. All errors should be reported so systems can identify patterns that contribute to errors. Here, the similar names probably contributed to the error. The nurse who commits the error knows all the relevant information and is in the best position to report it. While the health care provider (HCP) should be notified, it is a nursing responsibility to report errors, not an HCP's choice. Relating mistakes to a nurse's position focuses on personal blame.

CN: Safety and infection control; CL: Analyze

56. 3, 4. To ensure client safety in obtaining telephone prescriptions, the prescription must be received by a registered nurse (RN). The nurse should write the prescription, read the prescription back to the HC, and receive confirmation from the HCP that the prescription is correct. It is not necessary to ask the unit clerk to listen to the prescription, to require the HCP to come to the hospital to write the prescription on the medical record, or to have the nursing supervisor cosign the telephone prescription.

CN: Safety and infection control; CL: Analyze

57. 1. This child is exhibiting signs and symptoms of epiglottitis, which is a medical emergency because of the risk for complete airway obstruction. The 3- and 4-year-olds are exhibiting signs and symptoms of croup. Symptoms often diminish after the child has been taken out in the cool night air. If symptoms do not improve, the child may need a single dose of dexamethasone. Fever should also be treated with antipyretics. The 13-year-old is exhibiting signs and symptoms of bronchitis. Treatment includes rest, antipyretics, and hydration.

CN: Management of care; CL: Analyze

58. 1. The infant is experiencing signs and symptoms of respiratory distress indicating the need for oxygen therapy. Sedation will not improve the infant's respiratory distress and would likely cause further respiratory depression. If the infant's respiratory status continues to decline, they may need to be transferred to the pediatric intensive care unit. Oxygen should be the priority as it may improve the infant's respiratory status. A chest CT is not indicated. However, a CXR would be another appropriate recommendation for this infant.

CN: Safety and infection control; CL: Apply

59. 2. A high-calorie, high-protein diet is necessary to ensure adequate growth. Some children require up to two times the recommended daily allowance of calories (increased calorie diet includes foods high in fat and balanced carbohydrates). Pancreatic enzyme activity is lost, and malabsorption of fats, proteins, and carbohydrates occurs.

CN: Management of care; CL: Apply

TEST 3: The Child with Cardiovascular and Hematologic Health Problems

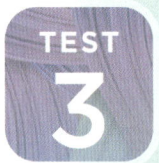

- The Client Undergoing a Cardiac Catheterization
- The Client with a Congenital Heart Defect
- The Client with Rheumatic Fever
- The Client with Kawasaki Disease
- The Client with Sickle Cell Anemia
- The Client with Iron-Deficiency Anemia
- The Client with Hemophilia
- The Client with Leukemia
- Managing Care, Quality, and Safety of Children with Cardiovascular and Hematologic Health Problems
- Answers, Rationales, and Test-Taking Strategies

The Client Undergoing a Cardiac Catheterization

1. The nurse caring for a 7-year-old child who has undergone a cardiac catheterization 2 hours ago finds the dressing and bed saturated with blood. What should the nurse do **first**?
   - ☐ 1. Assess the vital signs.
   - ☐ 2. Reinforce the dressing.
   - ☐ 3. Apply pressure just above the catheter insertion site.
   - ☐ 4. Notify the health care provider (HCP).

2. A preschool-age child has been scheduled for a cardiac catheterization. What should the nurse do to help prepare the family for the procedure?
   - ☐ 1. Advise the family to bring the child to the hospital for a tour a week in advance.
   - ☐ 2. Explain that the child will need a large bandage after the procedure.
   - ☐ 3. Discourage bringing favorite toys that might become associated with pain.
   - ☐ 4. Explain that the child may get up as soon as the vital signs are stable.

3. The nurse provides preprocedural teaching to the parents of a child with a ventricular septal defect who is scheduled for a cardiac catheterization. The nurse should explain that this procedure involves the use of which technique?
   - ☐ 1. ultra-high-frequency sound waves
   - ☐ 2. catheter placed in the right femoral vein
   - ☐ 3. cutdown procedure to place a catheter
   - ☐ 4. general anesthesia

4. The nurse develops the discharge teaching plan for the parents of a child who has undergone a cardiac catheterization for a ventricular septal defect. Which information should the nurse expect to include?
   - ☐ 1. restriction of the child's activities for the next 3 weeks
   - ☐ 2. use of sponge baths until the stitches are removed
   - ☐ 3. use of prophylactic antibiotics before receiving any dental work
   - ☐ 4. maintenance of a pressure dressing until a return visit with the health care provider

The Client with a Congenital Heart Defect

5. The nurse plans the discharge teaching for a 3-month-old infant with a cardiac defect who is to receive digoxin. What information should the nurse include in the plan? Select all that apply.
   - ☐ 1. Give the medication at regular intervals.
   - ☐ 2. Mix the medication with a small volume of breast milk or formula.
   - ☐ 3. Repeat the dose one time if the child vomits immediately after administration.
   - ☐ 4. Notify the health care provider (HCP) of poor feeding or vomiting.
   - ☐ 5. Make up any missed doses as soon as realized.
   - ☐ 6. Notify the HCP if more than two consecutive doses are missed.

6. The nurse is caring for a 2-day-old neonate in the postanesthesia care unit 30 minutes after surgical correction for the cardiac defect transposition of the great vessels. Which finding would alert the nurse to notify the health care provider (HCP)?
   ☐ 1. oxygen saturation of 90%
   ☐ 2. pale pink extremities
   ☐ 3. warm, dry skin
   ☐ 4. femoral pulse of 90 bpm

7. The nurse is caring for a newborn with a large ventricular septal defect. The client has undergone pulmonary artery banding. Which assessment finding **best** indicates that the pulmonary artery band is functioning effectively?
   ☐ 1. Capillary refill is less than 3 seconds.
   ☐ 2. Urine output is greater than 1 mL/kg per hour.
   ☐ 3. Breath sounds are clear and equal bilaterally.
   ☐ 4. Radial pulses are bounding.

8. A child diagnosed with tetralogy of Fallot becomes upset, cries, and thrashes around when a blood specimen is obtained. The child becomes cyanotic, and the respiratory rate increases to 44 breaths/min. Which action should the nurse do **first**?
   ☐ 1. Obtain a prescription for sedation for the child.
   ☐ 2. Assess for an irregular heart rate and rhythm.
   ☐ 3. Explain to the child that it will only hurt for a short time.
   ☐ 4. Place the child in a knee-to-chest position.

9. The nurse teaches a preschool-age child how to perform coughing and deep-breathing exercises before corrective surgery for tetralogy of Fallot. Which teaching and learning principles should the nurse address **first**?
   ☐ 1. organizing information to be taught in a logical sequence
   ☐ 2. arranging to use actual equipment for demonstrations
   ☐ 3. building the teaching on the child's current level of knowledge
   ☐ 4. presenting the information in order from simplest to most complex

10. The nurse assesses a child after heart surgery to correct tetralogy of Fallot. Which finding would the nurse report to the health care provider as an indication that the client has low cardiac output?
    ☐ 1. bounding pulses and mottled skin
    ☐ 2. altered level of consciousness and thready pulse
    ☐ 3. capillary refill of 2 seconds and blood pressure of 96/67 mm Hg
    ☐ 4. extremities warm to the touch and pale skin

11. The nurses manages the care of a child with congestive heart failure (CHF) caused by pulmonary stenosis. Which intervention is the **highest priority** for the therapeutic management of the CHF?
    ☐ 1. educating the family about the signs and symptoms of infection
    ☐ 2. administering enoxaparin to improve left ventricular contractility
    ☐ 3. assessing heart rate and blood pressure every 2 hours
    ☐ 4. administrating furosemide to decrease systemic venous congestion

12. An infant weighing 19.8 lb (9 kg) is in the pediatric intensive care unit following arterial switch surgery. In the past hour, the infant has had 16 mL of urine output. Which action should the nurse take?
    ☐ 1. Notify the health care provider (HCP) immediately.
    ☐ 2. Record the urine output in the medical record.
    ☐ 3. Administer a fluid bolus immediately.
    ☐ 4. Assess for other signs of hypervolemia.

13. A child has had open heart surgery to repair a tetralogy of Fallot with a patch. Which instructions should the nurse give to the parents?
    ☐ 1. Notify all health care providers (HCPs) before invasive procedures for the next 6 months.
    ☐ 2. Maintain adequate hydration of at least 10 glasses of water a day.
    ☐ 3. Provide frequent rest periods and naps during the first 4 weeks.
    ☐ 4. Restrict the ingestion of bananas and citrus fruit.

14. After undergoing a tetralogy of Fallot repair, a preschool child is transferred to the pediatric floor. Which intervention does the nurse tell the family to expect?
    ☐ 1. a reduced sodium diet
    ☐ 2. an activity restriction for several days
    ☐ 3. assignment to an isolation room
    ☐ 4. limiting visitation to parents only

15. After surgery to correct a tetralogy of Fallot, the child's parents express concern to the nurse that their 4-year-old child wants to be held more frequently than usual. What does the nurse recommend?
    ☐ 1. introducing a new skill
    ☐ 2. beginning play therapy
    ☐ 3. encouraging the behavior
    ☐ 4. having the volunteer hold the child

16. The parent of a child hospitalized with tetralogy of Fallot tells the nurse that the child's 3-year-old sibling has become quiet and shy and demonstrates more than a usual amount of genital curiosity since this child's hospitalization. What should the nurse tell the parent?
    ☐ 1. "This behavior is very typical for a 3-year-old."
    ☐ 2. "This may be how your child expresses feeling a need for attention."
    ☐ 3. "This may be an indication that your child may have been sexually abused."
    ☐ 4. "This may be a sign of depression in your child."

The Client with Rheumatic Fever

17. An adolescent client is admitted with a diagnosis of rheumatic fever and is on bed rest. The client has a sore throat. Their joints are painful and swollen. They have a red rash on their trunk and are experiencing aimless movements of their extremities. Use the chart below to determine what the nurse should do **first**.

    Vital Signs

Time	0800	1200
Temperature	39°C	37°C
Respirations	25	26
Apical heart rate	120	160
Blood pressure	120/90	130/95

    ☐ 1. Report the heart rate to the health care provider (HCP).
    ☐ 2. Apply lotion to the rash.
    ☐ 3. Splint the joints to relieve the pain.
    ☐ 4. Request a prescription to treat the elevated temperature.

18. The nurse plans the care for a child with rheumatic fever in the acute phase. What is the **most** important action for the nurse to teach the parents to monitor the child's progress?
    ☐ 1. listening to bilateral breath sounds
    ☐ 2. monitoring the child's pulse
    ☐ 3. observing closely for abnormal movements
    ☐ 4. recording the child's input and output

19. A school-age client with rheumatic fever is on long-term aspirin therapy. Which client statement **most** indicates that the client is experiencing a serious adverse reaction to aspirin?
    ☐ 1. "I hear ringing in my ears."
    ☐ 2. "I put lotion on my itchy skin."
    ☐ 3. "My stomach hurts after I take that medicine."
    ☐ 4. "These pills make me cough."

20. A school-age child has been put on an activity restriction during the acute phase of rheumatic fever. Which outcome indicates that the activity restriction has been effective?
    ☐ 1. The joints are free from permanent injury.
    ☐ 2. The resting heart rate is between 60 and 100 bpm.
    ☐ 3. The child exhibits a decrease in chorea movements.
    ☐ 4. The subcutaneous nodules over the joints are no longer palpable.

21. The nurse assesses a child with rheumatic fever. Which initial physical finding indicates the development of carditis in a child with rheumatic fever?
    ☐ 1. heart murmur
    ☐ 2. low blood pressure
    ☐ 3. irregular pulse
    ☐ 4. anterior chest wall pain

22. The health care provider (HCP) prescribes pulse assessments through the night for a school-age child with rheumatic fever who has a daytime heart rate of 120 bpm. The nurse explains to the parent that this is to evaluate if the elevated heart rate is caused by which factor?
    ☐ 1. the morning digitalis dose
    ☐ 2. routine activity during waking hours
    ☐ 3. a warmer daytime environment
    ☐ 4. normal variations in day and evening hours

23. The nurse plans the care of a child with rheumatic fever. Which action should the nurse perform to help alleviate a child's joint pain associated with rheumatic fever?
    ☐ 1. Maintain the joints in an extended position.
    ☐ 2. Apply gentle traction to the child's affected joints.
    ☐ 3. Support proper alignment with rolled pillows.
    ☐ 4. Use a bed cradle to keep linens off joints.

The Client with Kawasaki Disease

24. The nurse develops the plan of care for a newly admitted 2-year-old child with the diagnosis of Kawasaki disease (KD). Which intervention should be the **priority**?
  ☐ 1. taking vital signs every 6 hours
  ☐ 2. monitoring intake and output every hour
  ☐ 3. minimizing skin discomfort
  ☐ 4. providing passive range-of-motion exercises

25. A school-age child has been diagnosed with Kawasaki disease. What teaching should the nurse provide the family about the pharmacologic management of Kawasaki disease?
  ☐ 1. Inactivated vaccines are permissible while receiving intravenous (IV) immunoglobulin for Kawasaki disease.
  ☐ 2. The benefits of taking aspirin for Kawasaki disease outweigh the risk for Reye's syndrome.
  ☐ 3. Corticosteroids are often needed to control inflammation in Kawasaki disease.
  ☐ 4. Platelet infusions are needed with Kawasaki disease to prevent internal bleeding.

26. A 16-month-old child diagnosed with Kawasaki disease (KD) is very irritable, refuses to eat, and exhibits peeling skin on the hands and feet. What should the nurse do **first**?
  ☐ 1. Apply lotion to the hands and feet.
  ☐ 2. Offer foods the toddler likes.
  ☐ 3. Engage the child in quiet activities.
  ☐ 4. Encourage the parents to get some rest.

27. The nurse prepares discharge instructions for the parents of a 12-month-old child diagnosed with Kawasaki disease (KD) following treatment with intravenous immunoglobulin (IVIG). Which information should the nurse include in the discharge instructions?
  ☐ 1. Offer the child extra fluids every 2 hours for 2 weeks.
  ☐ 2. Take the child's temperature daily for several days.
  ☐ 3. Check the child's blood pressure daily until the follow-up appointment.
  ☐ 4. Call the health care provider if the irritability lasts for 2 more weeks.

The Client with Sickle Cell Anemia

28. The nurse is teaching the parents of a child with sickle cell disease. What information should the nurse give the family on how to prevent sickle cell crisis?
  ☐ 1. Exercise in cool temperatures.
  ☐ 2. Drink at least 8 cups (about 2 L) of fluids per day.
  ☐ 3. Avoid contact sports.
  ☐ 4. Take antiinflammatory medications before exercising.

29. The nurse admits a 1-year-old child to the hospital with the diagnosis of sickle cell crisis. The nurse explains to the parents that which condition leads to local tissue damage during a sickle cell crisis?
  ☐ 1. autoimmune reaction complicated by hypoxia
  ☐ 2. lack of oxygen in the red blood cells
  ☐ 3. obstruction to circulation
  ☐ 4. elevated serum bilirubin concentration

30. The parents of a child with sickle cell disease ask the nurse why their child's hemoglobin was normal at birth but now the child has S hemoglobin. Which response by the nurse is appropriate?
  ☐ 1. "The placenta prevents the passage of the hemoglobin S from the birth parent to the fetus."
  ☐ 2. "The red bone marrow does not begin to produce hemoglobin S until several months after birth."
  ☐ 3. "Antibodies transmitted from you to the fetus provide the newborn with temporary immunity."
  ☐ 4. "The newborn has a high concentration of fetal hemoglobin in the blood for some time after birth."

31. At a wellness check, the nurse monitors the routine laboratory values of an asymptomatic school-age client with sickle cell anemia. The reports reveal that the child has a hemoglobin of 10 g/100 mL (100 g/1 L). The nurse plans the client's care based on which interpretation of the hemoglobin level?
  ☐ 1. The child will most likely need a blood transfusion for the low hemoglobin.
  ☐ 2. This hemoglobin level is a typical finding in children with this disease.
  ☐ 3. The folic acid dose may need to be increased to improve hemoglobin production.
  ☐ 4. Additional tests are needed to determine if a sequestration crisis is causing the low hemoglobin.

32. The nurse cares for a 17-year-old male client on day 2 of hospitalization for a sickle cell crisis.

Flow Sheet

Laboratory Test	Value	Reference Range
White blood cells	16 × 10³ cells/mm³ (16 × 10⁹/L)	4.5–10.5 × 10³ cells/mm³ (4.5–10.5 × 10⁹/L)
Hemoglobin	10.1 mg/dL (101 g/L)	Ages 16–18: 11.1–15.7 g/dL (111–157 g/L)
Hematocrit	30.3% (0.30 proportion of 1)	In adolescents age 16–18 years, the value is 34%–44% (0.34–0.44 proportion of 1)

Day 2

0800:
The client was admitted with pain in the abdomen and upper thighs, but this morning, the client also reports pain in their chest. The client rates the chest pain as a 3, down from a 7 on a 0-to-10 scale after receiving intravenous (IV) morphine 30 minutes ago. The client has a peripheral IV of 5% dextrose in 0.45% normal saline (D5/½NS) infusing into the left hand at 150 mL per hour. Vital signs are temperature 100.4°F (38°C), pulse 100 bpm; respiration rate 22 breaths/min; and blood pressure 122/74 mm Hg. The pulse oximetry reading was 93% on room air but increased to 95% after the client was placed on 2 L of oxygen via nasal cannula.

The nurse updates the plan of care after reviewing the morning lab test results and assessment data.

➤ Complete the diagram by specifying the condition the client is most likely experiencing, two actions to take immediately, and two parameters the nurse should monitor to assess the client's progress.

Action to Take	Potential Conditions	Parameters to Monitor
Obtain a chest x-ray	Potential Conditions	Intake and output
Increase the morphine	Aplastic crisis	Oxygen saturation
Begin incentive spirometry	Vaso-occlusive crisis	Peripheral pulse
Administer a fluid bolus	Splenic sequestration	Pulmonary function
Transfuse packed cells		Pain level

The Client with Iron-Deficiency Anemia

33. The nurse evaluates the understanding of parents of a 12-month-old with iron-deficiency anemia of how to administer iron supplements. Which action(s) would indicate the parents are correctly administering the iron supplements? Select all that apply.
☐ 1. administering iron supplements in combination with fruit juice
☐ 2. scheduling iron supplements with meals
☐ 3. verbalizing the need to report dark stools
☐ 4. brushing the child's teeth after administering the iron supplements
☐ 5. decreasing the dietary intake of foods fortified with iron

34. During a health history, the nurse learns that a pediatric client seldom eats foods high in iron. Which physical assessment finding(s) would suggest that the child has developed iron-deficiency anemia? Select all that apply.
☐ 1. decreased heart rate
☐ 2. pale skin
☐ 3. swollen tongue
☐ 4. systolic murmur
☐ 5. yellowed sclera

35. The nurse completes a health history on a toddler at a wellness check. Which statement by the parent of a toddler **most** suggests that the child is at risk for iron-deficiency anemia?
☐ 1. "They drink over four glasses of milk per day."
☐ 2. "They must drink over 10 oz (300 mL) of apple juice per day."
☐ 3. "They refuse to eat more than two different kinds of vegetables."
☐ 4. "They do not like meat, but they will eat small amounts of it."

36. The nurse performs dietary teaching to the parents of a child with iron-deficiency anemia. Which foods should the nurse encourage a parent to offer to a child with iron-deficiency anemia?
☐ 1. cereal, milk, and yellow vegetables
☐ 2. potato, peas, and chicken
☐ 3. macaroni, cheese, and ham
☐ 4. pudding, green vegetables, and rice

The Client with Hemophilia

37. The nurse prepares to draw blood from a child with hemophilia. What is the **most** appropriate method to use?
☐ 1. Use finger punctures for lab draws.
☐ 2. Prepare to administer platelets.
☐ 3. Apply heat to the extremity before venipunctures.
☐ 4. Schedule all labs to be drawn at one time.

38. A diagnosis of hemophilia A is confirmed in an infant. Which instruction should the nurse provide the parents as the infant becomes more mobile and starts to crawl?
☐ 1. Administer one-half of a children's aspirin for a temperature higher than 101°F (38.3°C).
☐ 2. Sew thick padding into the elbows and knees of the child's clothing.
☐ 3. Check the color of the child's urine every day.
☐ 4. Expect the eruption of the primary teeth to produce moderate to severe bleeding.

39. A child with hemophilia presents with a burning sensation in the knee and reluctance to move the body part. The nurse collaborates with the care team to provide factor replacement and implements which intervention?
☐ 1. administers an aspirin-containing compound
☐ 2. institutes rest, ice, compression, and elevation (RICE)
☐ 3. begins physical therapy with active range of motion
☐ 4. initiates skin traction immobilization

40. The nurse creates a teaching plan for the family of a child with hemophilia who receives recombinant antihemophilic factor. Which problem is **most** important for the nurse to teach the family to report **immediately**?
☐ 1. yellowing of the skin
☐ 2. constipation
☐ 3. abdominal distention
☐ 4. hives

41. The parent tells the nurse they are afraid to allow their child with hemophilia to participate in sports because of the danger of injury and bleeding. After explaining that physical fitness is important for children with hemophilia, which activity should the nurse suggest as ideal? Select all that apply.
☐ 1. snow skiing
☐ 2. swimming
☐ 3. basketball
☐ 4. gymnastics
☐ 5. walking
☐ 6. bicycling

The Client with Leukemia

42. An adolescent client is admitted to the hospital with the diagnosis of acute lymphocytic leukemia. Which finding requires the **most** urgent nursing intervention?
☐ 1. fatigue and anorexia
☐ 2. fever and petechiae
☐ 3. swollen neck lymph glands and lethargy
☐ 4. enlarged liver and spleen

43. A school-age client with leukemia is receiving cyclophosphamide. The nurse should assess the client for which adverse effect of cyclophosphamide?
☐ 1. photosensitivity
☐ 2. ataxia
☐ 3. cystitis
☐ 4. cardiac arrhythmias

44. After the nurse teaches the parent of a child newly diagnosed with leukemia about the disease, which description if given by the parent **best** indicates an understanding of the nature of leukemia?
☐ 1. "Leukemia is an infection resulting in increased white blood cell production."
☐ 2. "Leukemia is a type of cancer characterized by an increase in immature white blood cells."
☐ 3. "Leukemia is an inflammation associated with enlargement of the lymph nodes."
☐ 4. "Leukemia is an allergic disorder involving increased circulating antibodies in the blood."

45. The nurse reviews the laboratory report of a 7-year-old child with leukemia (see exhibit). What does the nurse determine is the **priority** problem for this client?

Laboratory Results

Test	Traditional Units	SI Units	Normal Range
White blood cell (WBC) count	6.5×10^3 cells/mm^3	6.5×10^9/L	4.5–10.5 $\times 10^3$ cells/mm^3 (4.5–10.5 $\times 10^9$/L)
Platelet count	40,000/mm^3	40×10^9/L	Children: 150,000–450,000/mm^3 (150–450 $\times 10^9$/L)
Hematocrit	41.2%	0.412 proportion of 1.0	In children age 6–16 years, the value is 32%–42% (0.32–0.42 proportion of 1.0)

☐ 1. activity intolerance
☐ 2. risk for bleeding
☐ 3. impaired tissue perfusion
☐ 4. risk for infection

46. The nurse teaches the family of a child with leukemia about preventing infections. How should the nurse explain to the parents why their child is at risk for infections?
    ☐ 1. "Abnormal platelets lead to bruising and bleeding."
    ☐ 2. "There are an insufficient number of circulating white blood cells."
    ☐ 3. "The number of red blood cells is inadequate for carrying oxygen."
    ☐ 4. "Immature white blood cells are incapable of handling an infectious process."

47. The nurse is caring for a child with leukemia. Which beverage should the nurse plan to give the child to relieve nausea?
    ☐ 1. orange juice
    ☐ 2. weak tea
    ☐ 3. plain water
    ☐ 4. carbonated soda

48. The nurse treats pain in a child with leukemia. Which medication prescription should the nurse question?
    ☐ 1. hydromorphone
    ☐ 2. acetaminophen with codeine
    ☐ 3. ibuprofen
    ☐ 4. hydrocodone

49. The nurses teaches a child with leukemia about a scheduled bone marrow aspiration. The nurse determines that the teaching has been successful when the child identifies which place as the site for the aspiration?
    ☐ 1. right lateral side of the right wrist
    ☐ 2. middle of the chest
    ☐ 3. distal end of the thigh
    ☐ 4. back of the hipbone

50. The nurse and parents plan for the discharge of a child with leukemia who is receiving dactinomycin and vincristine. Which intervention should the nurse include in the teaching plan?
    ☐ 1. Encourage increased fluid intake.
    ☐ 2. Keep the child out of the sun.
    ☐ 3. Monitor the child's heart rate.
    ☐ 4. Observe the child for memory loss.

51. After doing well for a period of time, a child with leukemia develops an overwhelming infection. The child's death is imminent. Which statement offers the nurse the **best** guide in making plans to assist the parents in dealing with their child's imminent death?
    ☐ 1. Knowing that the prognosis is poor helps prepare parents for the death of children.
    ☐ 2. Parents are especially grieved when a child does well at first but then declines rapidly.
    ☐ 3. Parents' trust in health care personnel is most often destroyed by a death that is considered untimely.
    ☐ 4. It is more difficult for parents to accept the death of an older child than that of a toddler.

52. A school-age child with leukemia is taking immunosuppressive drugs. What health maintenance recommendation should the nurse include in the teaching plan?
    ☐ 1. Monitor the child's temperature at school.
    ☐ 2. Avoid any live attenuated vaccines.
    ☐ 3. Take daily vitamin and mineral supplements.
    ☐ 4. Stay away from other children.

53. A nurse is proving anticipatory guidance to the family of a school-age child with acute lymphocytic leukemia. Which recommendation should the nurse make?
    ☐ 1. participating in homeschooling for 2 years
    ☐ 2. avoiding all athletic activities
    ☐ 3. encouraging trips to the shopping mall
    ☐ 4. being treated as "normal" as much as possible

54. The nurse assesses a child with leukemia. Which sign(s) or symptom(s) would lead the nurse to suspect the client has thrombocytopenia? Select all that apply.
    ☐ 1. fever
    ☐ 2. petechiae
    ☐ 3. epistaxis
    ☐ 4. anorexia
    ☐ 5. bone pain
    ☐ 6. dyspnea

Managing Care, Quality, and Safety of Children with Cardiovascular and Hematologic Health Problems

55. A transfusion of packed red blood cells has been prescribed for a 1-year-old with sickle cell anemia. The infant has a 25-gauge IV infusing dextrose with sodium and potassium. Using the situation, background, assessment, and recommendation (SBAR) method of communication, the nurse contacts the health care provider and makes which recommendation?
    ☐ 1. starting a second IV with a 22-gauge catheter to infuse normal saline with the blood
    ☐ 2. using the existing IV, but changing the fluids to normal saline for the transfusion
    ☐ 3. replacing the IV with a 22-gauge catheter to infuse the prescribed fluids
    ☐ 4. starting a second IV with a 25-gauge catheter to infuse normal saline with the transfusion

56. An infant has been transferred from the intensive care unit to the pediatric floor after undergoing surgery to correct a heart defect. Which task(s) could the registered nurse (RN) delegate to the licensed practical/vocational nurse (LPN/VN)? Select all that apply.
☐ 1. administering oral medications
☐ 2. administering intravenous (IV) push morphine
☐ 3. obtaining vital signs
☐ 4. providing morning hygiene
☐ 5. obtaining circulation checks
☐ 6. providing discharge teaching

57. The nurse assists with conscious sedation of a school-age client undergoing a bone marrow biopsy. What is the nurse's **most** important responsibility during the procedure?
☐ 1. administering the topical anesthetic
☐ 2. keeping the parents informed
☐ 3. monitoring the client
☐ 4. recording the procedure

58. The nurse transfers a child who has had open heart surgery from the intensive care unit to the pediatric unit. The child's blood pressure has been fluctuating but has been stable during the last 2 hours. What information should the nurse include in the handoff report? Select all that apply.
☐ 1. medications being used
☐ 2. current vital signs
☐ 3. potential for blood pressure to drop
☐ 4. drip rate for the intravenous infusion
☐ 5. time of the most recent dose of pain medication
☐ 6. medications given during surgery

59. A school-age client with hemophilia A has fallen and badly bruised their knee. Which action should the nurse do **first** to manage the client's hemarthrosis?
☐ 1. Use active range of motion to prevent immobility.
☐ 2. Apply cold packs to promote vasoconstriction.
☐ 3. Apply pressure and immobilize the joint.
☐ 4. Notify the health care provider (HCP) of the injury.

60. The nurse completes discharge teaching with the family of an 8-week-old infant with congenital heart disease. What is the **most** important information for the nurse to convey regarding feeding?
☐ 1. Allow the infant 1 hour to complete each feeding.
☐ 2. Position the infant in an upright position after each feeding.
☐ 3. Give feedings per nasogastric tube to conserve energy.
☐ 4. Provide a higher calorie formula or fortified breast milk.

Answers, Rationales, and Test-Taking Strategies

*The answers and rationales for each question follow below, along with keys (🔑) to the client need (CN) and cognitive level (CL) for each question. In addition, questions that measure clinical judgment will be coded (CJ). As you check your answers, use the **Content Mastery and Test-Taking Skill Self-Analysis** worksheet (tear-out worksheet in the back of the book) to identify the reason(s) for not answering the questions correctly. For additional information about test-taking skills and strategies for answering questions, refer to pages 12–51 in Part 1 of this book.*

The Client Undergoing a Cardiac Catheterization

1. 3. Direct pressure is the first measure that should be used to control bleeding. Taking the vital signs will not control the bleeding. This should be done while another person is being sent to notify the HCP. The dressing can be reinforced after the bleeding has been contained.

🔑 CN: Reduction of risk potential; CL: Analyze

2. 2. The catheter insertion site will be covered with a bandage. This is important for preschool children to know as they are very concerned about bodily harm. The best time to prepare a preschool child for an invasive procedure is the night before. Bringing a favorite toy to the hospital will help decrease the child's anxiety. To prevent bleeding, the child will be expected to keep the extremity straight for 4 to 6 hours after the procedure, either in bed or on the parent's lap.

🔑 CN: Psychosocial integrity; CL: Analyze

3. 2. In children, cardiac catheterization usually involves a right-sided approach because septal defects permit entry into the left side of the heart. The catheter is usually inserted into the femoral vein through a percutaneous puncture. A cutdown procedure is rarely used. Echocardiography involves the use of ultra-high-frequency sound waves. The catheterization is usually performed under local, not general, anesthesia with sedation.

🔑 CN: Reduction of risk potential; CL: Apply

4. 3. Prophylactic antibiotics are suggested for children with heart defects before dental work is done to reduce the risk for bacterial infection. Typically, activities are not restricted after cardiac catheterization. A percutaneous approach is used to insert the catheter, so stitches are not necessary. Showering or bathing is allowed as usual. The pressure dressing will be removed before the child is discharged.

🗝️ CN: Reduction of risk potential; CL: Apply

The Client with a Congenital Heart Defect

5. -/+ **1, 4, 6.** To achieve optimal therapeutic levels, digoxin should be given at regular intervals without variation, usually every 12 hours. Vomiting and poor feeding are signs of toxicity. If more than two consecutive doses are missed, interventions may be needed to assure therapeutic drug levels. The medication should not be mixed with any other fluid as refusal may result in an inaccurate intake of the medication. Taking makeup doses, or taking the medication at times other than scheduled, may adversely affect serum levels.

🗝️ CN: Pharmacological and parenteral therapies; CL: Apply

6. **4.** The normal pulse rate in a neonate is 120 to 160 bpm. Therefore, a femoral pulse rate of 90 bpm is too low. Diminished peripheral pulses, coolness and mottling of the extremities, delayed capillary refill, hypotension, and decreased urine output are indicative of low cardiac output and poor perfusion. The neonate may be experiencing a complication of the surgery, such as blood loss or leaking of fluid into the interstitial space. The surgeon should be notified immediately to correct the diminished pulse, through either medications or transfusions. An oxygen saturation between 85% and 100% is considered normal. The surgeon does not need to be notified unless the oxygen saturation falls below 85%. Pale pink extremities are considered a normal finding. If mottling or cyanosis develops, the surgeon should be notified immediately. Warm, dry skin is also a normal finding. If the skin becomes cool or appears cyanotic, the surgeon should be notified.

🗝️ CN: Reduction of risk potential; CL: Analyze

7. **3.** Pulmonary artery banding is a palliative treatment used in pediatric clients with congenital cardiac defects with increased pulmonary blood flow. The pulmonary artery band reduces excessive pulmonary blood flow and protects the lungs from irreversible damage. When the pulmonary artery band is functioning properly, the lungs should no longer be receiving an increased amount of blood flow, which would be reflected in clear and equal breath sounds. A capillary refill of less than 3 seconds and a urine output greater than 1 mL/kg per hour reflect adequate peripheral perfusion. Bounding radial pulses suggest increased pulmonary blood flow.

🗝️ CN: Physiological adaptation; CL: Evaluate

8. **4.** The child is experiencing a tet spell, also known as a *hypoxic episode*. Therefore, the nurse should place the child in a knee-to-chest position. Flexing the legs reduces venous flow of blood from the lower extremities and reduces the volume of blood being shunted through the interventricular septal defect and the overriding aorta in the child with tetralogy of Fallot. As a result, the blood then entering the systemic circulation has higher oxygen content, and dyspnea is reduced. Flexing the legs also increases vascular resistance and pressure in the left ventricle. An infant often assumes a knee-to-chest position in the crib, or the parent learns to put the infant over their shoulder while holding the child in a knee-to-chest position to relieve dyspnea. If this position is ineffective, the child may need a sedative. Once the child is in the position, the nurse may assess for an irregular heart rate and rhythm. Explaining to the child that it will only hurt for a short time does nothing to alleviate the hypoxia.

🗝️ CN: Physiological adaptation; CL: Analyze

9. **3.** Before developing any teaching program for a child, the nurse's first step is to assess the child to determine what is already known. Most older preschool children have some understanding of a condition present since birth. However, the child's interest will soon be lost if familiar material is repeated too often. The nurse can then organize the information in a sequence because there are several steps to be demonstrated. These exercises do not require the use of equipment. The nurse should judge the amount and complexity of the information to be provided based on the child's current knowledge and response to teaching.

🗝️ CN: Psychosocial integrity; CL: Analyze

10. **2.** With a low cardiac output and subsequent poor tissue perfusion, signs and symptoms would include pale, cool extremities; cyanosis; weak, thready pulses; delayed capillary refill; and a decrease in the level of consciousness.

🗝️ CN: Physiological adaptation; CL: Analyze

11. **4.** Pulmonary stenosis can cause right-sided CHF, resulting in venous congestion. Removing accumulated fluid is a primary goal of treatment in right-sided CHF. Furosemide is used to reduce venous congestion. It is important to educate the family about the signs and symptoms of CHF, but treating the client's CHF is the priority. Enoxaparin is an anticoagulant and will not help improve left

ventricular contractility. It is important to assess vital signs frequently in a child with CHF, but assessments do not treat the problem.

- CN: Physiological adaptation; CL: Apply

12. 2. Urine output for an infant weighing 19.8 lb (9 kg) should be 1 mL/kg per hour. A urine output of 16 mL is more than adequate for 1 hour, so the nurse should record the output in the medical record. There is no reason to notify the HCP regarding adequate urine output. The infant has adequate output, so there is no need for a fluid bolus. A fluid bolus could also cause the infant to become fluid overloaded, increasing the workload on the heart. There is no information in the question indicating that the child is hypervolemic.

- CN: Physiological adaptation; CL: Analyze

13. 1. Children who have undergone open heart surgery with a patch are at risk for infection, especially subacute bacterial endocarditis (SBE), for the first 6 months following surgery. The newest evidence-based guidelines suggest that once the patch has epithelialized, these precautions are no longer necessary. Therefore, parents are instructed about SBE precautions, including the need to notify HCPs before invasive procedures so antibiotics can be prescribed for that time period. Having the child drink a very large amount of water may lead to fluid overload. Children gear their rest schedule to their activities, making it unnecessary to schedule frequent rest periods. Bananas and citrus fruit are high in potassium, but there is no evidence provided that the child has an elevated serum potassium level that requires restriction.

- CN: Physiological adaptation; CL: Analyze

14. 1. Because of the hemodynamic changes that occur with open heart surgery, particularly with septal defects, transient congestive heart failure may develop. Therefore, the child's sodium intake typically is restricted to 2 to 3 g a day. Activity restrictions are inappropriate. Typically, the child is encouraged to walk the halls and unit. The risk for infection after the repair is the same as that for any postoperative client; therefore, isolation is not necessary. The child may be placed in a room with other children who are not contagious. Visitors are not restricted unless the pediatric unit has restrictive visiting policies.

- CN: Physiological adaptation; CL: Analyze

15. 2. The child is exhibiting regression. During periods of stress, children frequently revert to behaviors that were comforting in earlier developmental stages; play therapy is one way to help the child cope with the stress. Teaching a new skill most likely would add more stress. Parents should be instructed to praise positive behaviors and ignore regressive behaviors rather than calling attention to them through encouragement or discouragement. Having someone else hold the child does not encourage coping with the stress or promoting appropriate development.

- CN: Psychosocial integrity; CL: Analyze

16. 2. According to Erikson, the central psychosocial task of a preschooler is to develop a sense of initiative versus guilt. Any environmental situation may affect the child. In this situation, the sibling is probably feeling less attention from the parent and trying to resolve the conflict in an inappropriate way. Three-year-old children are usually active and outgoing. These behaviors represent a change. The data are not sufficient to suggest the child has been exposed to a sexual experience. Symptoms of depression would include withdrawal and fatigue.

- CN: Psychosocial integrity; CL: Analyze

The Client with Rheumatic Fever

17. 1. The child's heart rate of 150 bpm is significantly above its rate at the time of their admission. The nurse must notify the HCP. The increase in heart rate may indicate carditis, a possible complication of rheumatic fever that can cause serious and lifelong effects on the heart. The HCP will intervene with medication and cardiac monitoring. While lotion may provide comfort, the most important action for the nurse is to notify the HCP of the increased heart rate. Splinting will not help the inflammation that is causing the painful joints. The joint pain will migrate and subside with time. The temperature is not elevated at this time and does not require intervention.

- CN: Physiological adaptation; CL: Analyze

18. 2. Tachycardia is associated with inflammation of the heart in rheumatic fever. Improvements in pulse rate are an indication that inflammation is decreasing. The nurse should teach the parents to monitor the child's pulse. Preferably the pulse is taken apically for a full minute. The pulse may be prescribed during sleep and wake times to determine activity tolerance. It is unnecessary to teach parents to monitor breath sounds or intake and output. The parents should report if the child develops purposeless movements, but the presence or absence of chorea is not the primary indicator of how rheumatic fever is progressing.

- CN: Physiological adaptation; CL: Apply

19. 1. Tinnitus is an adverse effect of prolonged aspirin therapy, and the child should be examined by a health care provider for hearing loss. Itchy skin commonly accompanies the rash associated with rheumatic fever, and the nurse can encourage lotion use. The nurse teaches clients to take aspirin with food or milk to avoid abdominal discomfort. The nurse can also address the fact that coughing after ingesting aspirin can be caused by inadequate fluid intake during administration.

CN: Pharmacological and parenteral therapies; CL: Analyze

20. 2. During the acute phase of rheumatic fever, the heart is inflamed, and every effort is made to reduce the work of the heart. Bed rest with limited activity is necessary to prevent heart failure. Therefore, the most reliable indicator that activity restriction has been effective is a resting heart rate between 60 and 100 bpm, which is normal for a 7-year-old child. No permanent damage to the joints occurs with rheumatic fever. The chorea movements associated with rheumatic fever are self-limited and usually disappear in 1 to 3 months. They are unrelated to activity restrictions. Subcutaneous nodules that occur over joint surfaces also resolve over time with no treatment. Therefore, they are not appropriate for evaluating the effectiveness of activity restrictions.

CN: Physiological adaptation; CL: Evaluate

21. 1. In rheumatic fever, the connective tissue of the heart becomes inflamed, leading to carditis. The most common signs of carditis are heart murmurs, tachycardia during rest, cardiac enlargement, and changes in the electrical conductivity of the heart. Heart murmurs are present in about 75% of all clients during the first week of carditis and in 85% of clients by the third week. Signs of carditis do not include hypotension or chest pain. The client may have a rapid pulse, but it is usually not irregular.

CN: Physiological adaptation; CL: Analyze

22. 2. An above-average pulse rate that is out of proportion to the degree of activity is an early sign of heart failure in a client with rheumatic fever. The sleeping pulse is used to determine whether the mild tachycardia persists during sleep (inactivity) or whether it is a result of daytime activities. The environmental temperature would need to be quite warmer before it could influence the heart rate. Digitalis lowers the heart rate, so the rate would be decreased during the daytime.

CN: Reduction of risk potential; CL: Analyze

23. 4. For a child with arthritis associated with rheumatic fever, the joints are usually so tender that even the weight of bed linens can cause pain. The use of a bed cradle is recommended to help remove the weight of the linens on painful joints. Joints need to be maintained in good alignment, not positioned in extension, to ensure that they remain functional. Applying gentle traction to the joints is not recommended because traction is usually used to relieve muscle spasms, which are not typically associated with rheumatic fever. Supporting the body in good alignment and changing the client's position are recommended, but these measures are not likely to relieve pain.

CN: Basic care and comfort; CL: Analyze

The Client with Kawasaki Disease

24. 2. Cardiac status must be monitored carefully in the initial phase of KD because the child is at high risk for congestive heart failure (CHF). Therefore, the nurse needs to assess the child frequently for signs of CHF, which would include respiratory distress and decreased urine output. Vital signs would be obtained more often than every 6 hours because of the risk for CHF. Although minimizing skin discomfort would be important, it does not take priority over monitoring the child's hourly intake and output. Passive range-of-motion exercises would be done if the child develops arthritis.

CN: Physiological adaptation; CL: Analyze

25. 2. Vasculitis in Kawasaki disease can lead to life-threatening complications such as myocardial infarction and aneurysms. High doses of aspirin or nonsteroidal antiinflammatory drugs (NSAIDs) are frequently prescribed to control fever, inflammation, and platelet aggregation. Although Reye's syndrome has been associated with the use of aspirin in children with viral infections, the same risk has not been found with aspirin use and Kawasaki disease. IV immunoglobulin provides a passive immunity that reduces the ability of a client to develop active immunity from vaccination. Therefore, routine vaccination should be delayed. Corticosteroids are contraindicated with Kawasaki disease because they have been associated with aneurysm formation. Platelet infusions are not part of Kawasaki treatment as medications are needed to reduce platelet aggregation.

CN: Pharmacologic and parental therapies; CL: Apply

26. 3. One of the characteristics of children with KD is irritability. They are often inconsolable. Engaging the child in quiet activities helps calm the child and reduces the workload of the heart. Although peeling of the skin occurs with KD, the child's irritability takes priority over applying lotion to the hands and feet. Children with KD usually are not hungry and do not eat well regardless of what is served. There is no indication that the parents need rest. Additionally, in this situation, the child takes priority over the parents.

    CN: Physiological adaptation; CL: Analyze

27. 2. The child' temperature should be taken daily for several days after discharge because children who develop a fever may require a second IVIG treatment. Offering the child fluids every 2 hours is not necessary. Doing so increases the child's risk for CHF. Checking the child's blood pressure at home usually is not included as part of the discharge instructions because by the time of discharge the child is considered stable and the risk for cardiac problems is minimal. Most children with KD recover fully. Irritability may last for 2 months after discharge.

    CN: Physiological adaptation; CL: Apply

The Client with Sickle Cell Anemia

28. 2. Increasing fluid intake and being well hydrated will help prevent cell stasis in the small vessels. Restricting fluids causes stasis of red blood cells and promotes obstruction and increases the chance of sickling with hypoxia and pain in the part that is involved. Clients with sickle cell disease should avoid exercising in cool temperatures or swimming in cold water. While contact sports are not recommended because of bleeding risks, they do not cause sickle crisis. Taking an antiinflammatory medication before exercising does not prevent sickle cell crisis.

    CN: Health promotion and maintenance; CL: Analyze

29. 3. Characteristic sickle cells tend to cause "log jams" in capillaries. This results in poor circulation to local tissues, leading to ischemia and necrosis. The basic defect in sickle cell disease is an abnormality in the structure of the red blood cells. The erythrocytes are sickle shaped, rough in texture, and rigid. Sickle cell disease is an inherited disease, not an autoimmune reaction. Elevated serum bilirubin concentrations are associated with jaundice, not sickle cell disease.

    CN: Physiological adaptation; CL: Apply

30. 4. Sickle cell disease is an inherited disease that is present at birth. However, 60% to 80% of a newborn's hemoglobin is fetal hemoglobin, which has a structure different from that of hemoglobin S or hemoglobin A. Sickle cell symptoms usually occur about 4 months after birth, when hemoglobin S begins to replace the fetal hemoglobin. The gene for sickle cell disease is transmitted at the time of conception, not passed through the placenta. Some hemoglobin S is produced by the fetus near term. The fetus produces all its own hemoglobin from the earliest production in the first trimester. Passive immunity conferred by maternal antibodies is not related to sickle cell disease, but this transmission of antibodies is important to protect the infant from various infections during early infancy.

    CN: Physiological adaptation; CL: Apply

31. 2. Between crises, hemoglobin levels between 6 and 9 g/100 mL (60 to 90/L) are typical for children with sickle cell anemia. The decision to transfuse a child must be weighed against the risks. Transfusions are most often considered to treat life-threatening sickle cell complications, to keep hemoglobin S levels within a desired range, or as prophylaxis before surgery. Oral folic acid is frequently prescribed to rebuild hemolyzed red blood cells. It would be appropriate for the nurse to verify that the client was taking folic acid as prescribed before making any further interpretations. Clients with sequestration crisis present with pain and signs and symptoms of hypovolemia.

    CN: Reduction of risk potential; CL: Analyze

32.

Action to Take	Potential Conditions	Parameters to Monitor
Obtain a chest x-ray	Acute chest syndrome	Oxygen saturation
Begin incentive spirometry		Pain level

The fever, elevated white blood cell count, respiratory distress, and new onset of chest pain suggest the client has acute chest syndrome (ACS). This complication happens when blood flow to the lungs is blocked and frequently follows a vaso-occlusive pain crisis. Severe anemia would signal a splenic sequestration or an aplastic crisis. The nurse should obtain a chest x-ray to confirm the diagnosis of ACS. Incentive spirometry should be used aggressively to prevent further atelectasis. Antibiotics are also typically prescribed in children. Increasing the morphine is not necessary as the teen is receiving relief with the current dose. Administering a fluid bolus could lead to pulmonary edema. The target hemoglobin range for a child with sickle cell anemia is 10 to 11 mg/dL (100 to 111 g/L). A transfusion is not needed if the client can wean off oxygen. The client presented with low oxygen saturation and chest pain. The nurse should monitor those parameters to determine if treatments have been effective for the ACS. Pulmonary functions are not needed at this time. Although the nurse should routinely monitor intake and output and peripheral pulses, these metrics provide more information about circulatory status than respiratory status.

: Standalone bowtie; CL: Create

The Client with Iron-Deficiency Anemia

33. 1, 4. Parent teaching concerning a child with iron-deficiency anemia should include directions about giving iron combined with fruit juice, in divided doses, between meals, and with a dropper for a 12-month-old or through a straw for older toddlers. Iron stains teeth, so brushing the teeth and administering liquid iron through a dropper or straw are necessary to prevent staining the teeth. Iron should not be given with milk, antacids, or tea and should be administered on an empty stomach. Iron will cause the stool to become black or green, which is normal and does not need to be reported. However, light-colored stools indicate the iron is not being absorbed and should be reported.

CN: Pharmacological and parenteral therapies; CL: Evaluate

34. 2, 3, 4. Pale skin is one of the most common physical findings associated with iron-deficiency anemia. Lower levels of myoglobin lead to soreness and swelling of the tongue. Low levels of hemoglobin force the heart to work harder to pump blood. Tachycardia and systolic murmurs may result. Anemia presents as an elevated heart rate, not a decreased one. Yellowed sclera is consistent with hemolytic anemia.

CN: Physiological adaptation; CL: Analyze

35. 1. Milk is a poor source of iron. Toddlers should have between two and three servings of milk per day. Iron-deficiency anemia can be caused when excessive milk intake of more than 32 oz (1 L)/day intake displaces iron-rich food in the diet. While 10 oz (300 mL) is the recommended daily limit for apple juice, it does contain more iron than milk. Food preferences vary among children. It is acceptable for the child to refuse foods as long as the diet is balanced and contains adequate calories.

CN: Basic care and comfort; CL: Analyze

36. 2. Potatoes, peas, chicken, green vegetables, and fortified cereal contain significant amounts of iron and therefore would be recommended. Milk and yellow vegetables are not good iron sources. Rice by itself also is not a good source of iron. Macaroni, cheese, and ham are not high in iron. Although pudding (made with fortified milk) and green vegetables contain some iron, the better diet has protein and iron from the chicken and potato.

CN: Basic care and comfort; CL: Apply

The Client with Hemophilia

37. 4. Coordinating labs to minimize sticks reduces trauma and the risk for bleeding. Fingersticks in general are more painful and associated with more bleeding than venipunctures. In hemophilia, platelets are typically normal. Heat would increase vasodilatation and increase bleeding.

CN: Reduction of risk potential; CL: Apply

38. 2. As the hemophilic infant begins to acquire motor skills, falls and bumps increase the risk for bleeding. Such injuries can be minimized by padding vulnerable joints. Aspirin is contraindicated because of its antiplatelet properties, which increase the infant's risk for bleeding. Because genitourinary bleeding is not a typical problem in children with hemophilia, urine testing is not indicated. Although some bleeding may occur with tooth eruption, it does not normally cause moderate to severe bleeding episodes in children with hemophilia.

CN: Safety and infection control; CL: Analyze

39. 2. The child is displaying symptoms of bleeding in the joint, and factor replacement is indicated. The RICE method is used as a supportive measure to help control the bleeding. Aspirin-containing compounds contribute to bleeding and should never be used to control pain. Physical therapy is instituted after acute bleeding to prevent further damage. Orthopedic traction is considered in some rare cases during the rehabilitation phase, but not the acute phase.

CN: Physiological adaptation; CL: Analyze

40. 4. Administration of antihemolytic factor (recombinant) is a biosynthetic preparation of factor VIII that carries the risk for severe allergic reaction. Signs include hives, difficulty breathing, tachycardia, chills, and fever. Originally, factor VIII preparations were derived from large pools of human plasma and carried the risk for hepatitis, but recombinant preparations do not. Antihemolytic factor (recombinant) is not associated with constipation or abdominal distention.

CN: Pharmacological and parenteral therapies; CL: Analyze

41. 🔁 **2, 5, 6.** Swimming is an ideal activity for a child with hemophilia because it is a noncontact sport. Walking and bicycling are also noncontact physical activities that do not place excessive strain on joints. Such activities strengthen the muscles surrounding joints and help control bleeding in these areas. Noncontact sports also enhance general mental and physical well-being. Falls and subsequent injury to the child may occur with snow skiing. Basketball is a contact sport and therefore increases the child's risk for injury. Gymnastics is a very strenuous sport. Gymnasts frequently have muscle and joint injuries that result in bleeding episodes.

🔑 CN: Health promotion and maintenance; CL: Apply

The Client with Leukemia

42. **2.** Fever and petechiae associated with acute lymphocytic leukemia indicate suppression of normal white blood cells and thrombocytes by the bone marrow and put the client at risk for other infections and bleeding. The nurse should initiate infection control and safety precautions to reduce these risks. Fatigue is a common symptom of leukemia due to red blood cell suppression. Although the client should be told about the need for rest and meal planning, such teaching is not the priority intervention. Swollen glands and lethargy may be uncomfortable, but they do not require immediate intervention. An enlarged liver and spleen require safety precautions that prevent injury to the abdomen; however, these precautions are not the priority.

🔑 CN: Reduction of risk potential; CL: Analyze

43. **3.** Cystitis is a potential adverse effect of cyclophosphamide. The client should be monitored for pain during urination. Photosensitivity, ataxia, and cardiac arrhythmias are not adverse effects associated with cyclophosphamide.

🔑 CN: Pharmacological and parenteral therapies; CL: Analyze

44. **2.** Leukemia is a neoplastic, or cancerous, disorder of blood-forming tissues that is characterized by a proliferation of immature white blood cells. Leukemia is not an infection, inflammation, or allergic disorder.

🔑 CN: Physiological adaptation; CL: Evaluate

45. **2.** A normal platelet count is 150,000 to 400,000/mm³ (150 to 400 × 10⁹/L). A platelet count of 40,000/mm³ (40 × 10⁹/L) is low and puts the child at risk for injury, bruising, and bleeding. A hematocrit level of 41.2% (0.41 proportion of 1.0) is normal; therefore, the child will have adequate oxygenation and tissue perfusion. The WBC count of 6500/mm³ (6.5 × 10⁹/L) is normal; therefore, the child has no increase in risk for infection.

🔑 CN: Reduction of risk potential; CL: Analyze

46. **4.** In leukemia, although there is an increased number of immature white blood cells, these cells are unable to combat infection. A lack of mature white blood cells puts a child with leukemia at risk for infection. The major morbidity and mortality factor associated with leukemia is an infection resulting from the presence of granulocytopenia. Decreased red blood cells are not directly caused by infection. While platelets play a role in the body's response to infection; bleeding does not directly cause infections.

🔑 CN: Reduction of risk potential; CL: Apply

47. **4.** Carbonated beverages ordinarily are best tolerated when a child feels nauseated. Many children find cola drinks especially easy to tolerate, but noncola beverages are also recommended. Orange juice usually is not tolerated well because of its high acid content. Tea may also be too acidic, and many children do not like tea. Water does not relieve nausea.

🔑 CN: Basic care and comfort; CL: Apply

48. **3.** Ibuprofen prolongs bleeding time and is contraindicated in clients with leukemia. Nonnarcotic drugs other than ibuprofen or aspirin, such as acetaminophen, may be prescribed to control pain and may be used in combination with codeine or hydrocodone if the pain is more severe. Hydromorphone may also be used for severe pain.

🔑 CN: Pharmacological and parenteral therapies; CL: Analyze

49. **4.** Although bone marrow specimens may be obtained from various sites, the most commonly used site in children is the posterior iliac crest, the back of the hipbone. This area is close to the body's surface but removed from vital organs. The area is large, so specimens can easily be obtained. For infants, the proximal tibia and the posterior iliac crest are used. The middle of the chest or sternum is the usual site for bone marrow aspiration in an adult. The wrist, chest, and thigh are not sites from which to obtain bone marrow specimens.

🔑 CN: Reduction of risk potential; CL: Evaluate

50. **1.** Dactinomycin and vincristine both cause nausea and vomiting. Oral fluids are encouraged, and antiemetics are given to prevent dehydration. Avoiding sun exposure is not necessary because photosensitivity is not associated with these drugs.

Heart rate changes and memory issues also are not associated with either of these two drugs.

🔑 CN: Pharmacological and parenteral therapies; CL: Analyze

51. 2. It has been found that parents are more grieved when optimism is followed by defeat. The nurse should recognize this when planning various ways to help the parents of a dying child. It is not necessarily true that knowing about a poor prognosis for years helps prepare parents for a child's death. Death is still a shock when it occurs. Trust in health care personnel is not necessarily destroyed when a death is untimely if the family views the personnel as having done all that was possible. It is not more difficult for parents to accept the death of an older child than that of a younger child.

🔑 CN: Psychosocial integrity; CL: Analyze

52. 2. Children who are immunosuppressed should not receive any live attenuated vaccines. Clients who are immunosuppressed and are given live attenuated vaccines such as measles, mumps, rubella, and oral polio vaccine can develop severe forms of the diseases for which they are being immunized, which can result in death. Inactivated vaccines may be given if necessary, but the client is not able to adequately produce needed antibodies, and it is recommended that immunizations be delayed for 3 months after the immunosuppressive drugs have been discontinued. It is unnecessary to monitor the child's temperature at school unless the child shows symptoms of an illness. Vitamin and mineral supplements are not normally given in conjunction with immunosuppressive drugs. When the client is immunosuppressed, the client should avoid only persons who have an infection.

🔑 CN: Health promotion and maintenance; CL: Analyze

53. 4. Any child with a chronic illness should be treated as normally as possible. Unless the child has severe bone marrow depression, they should be allowed to go to school with others and can go to the mall. If the child is in remission, athletic activities are allowed.

🔑 CN: Health promotion and maintenance; CL: Analyze

54. -/+ 2, 3. Children with acute lymphocytic leukemia have a reduced platelet count (thrombocytopenia), a reduced red blood cell count (anemia), and a reduced white blood cell count (neutropenia) because of the unrestricted proliferation of immature white blood cells. Chemotherapy is used to treat leukemia and contributes to thrombocytopenia, neutropenia, and anemia. Clients with thrombocytopenia are at risk for bleeding. Petechiae (small red or purple spots on the skin) and epistaxis (nose bleeds) are both signs of bleeding. A fever is a result of a decreased white blood cell count. Anorexia and dyspnea (shortness of breath) are a result of a decreased red blood cell count. Bone pain is a result of stress on the bone related to the unrestricted proliferation of the leukemic blast cells.

🔑 CN: Physiological adaptation; CL: Analyze

Managing Care, Quality, and Safety of Children with Cardiovascular and Hematologic Health Problems

55. 2. The best evidence indicates that a catheter as small as 27 gauge may safely be used for transfusion in children, but blood must be infused with normal saline, not dextrose. A 1-year-old should be able to maintain their blood glucose for the 2-hour duration of the infusion without the need for a second IV.

🔑 CN: Management of care; CL: Analyze

56. -/+ 1, 3, 4. The RN's scope of practice includes assessment, planning, implementation, and evaluation. Only aspects of care implementation may be delegated to the LPN/VN, and the exact skills that may be delegated vary by state and institution. In general, LPN/VNs have been trained to perform the tasks of administering oral medications, performing hygiene, and recording the intake and output. LPN/VNs may also take vital signs to gather data, but the nurse must interpret the data. Administering IV morphine requires an assessment of the client's respiratory status before, during, and after the procedure. Circulation checks are assessments the RN should complete.

🔑 CN: Management of care; CL: Analyze

57. 3. During conscious sedation, the client may lose protective reflexes, and adequate respiratory and cardiac function may be impaired. At every procedure, there must be one health care professional whose sole responsibility is to monitor the client. Topical agents must be given in advance of the procedure to be effective. During the procedure, the nurse would not leave the child to speak with the parents. While the procedure would be documented according to the facility's protocols, proper monitoring of the client is the intervention most associated with reducing risks.

🔑 CN: Reduction of risk potential; CL: Apply

58. -/+ 1, 2, 3, 4, 5. The report made when nurses are "handing off" a client from one nursing unit to another must include information about the condition of the client, the potential for changes in the client's condition, the client's current medications, and the care and services received. It is not necessary to know what medications were given in surgery to provide safe care at this point.

🗝 CN: Safety and infection control; CL: Analyze

59. 3. Application of pressure and immobilization of the affected limb are the first priority. Pressure is required to stop the bleeding, and immobilization aids in reducing swelling and pain. Active range of motion is recommended after the bleeding is controlled. The application of cold packs can be helpful in diminishing swelling and pain. Cold packs will also promote vasoconstriction, which can help reduce the bleeding. The HCP should be informed of the bleeding episode after initial measures to control the bleeding are implemented.

🗝 CN: Management of care; CL: Analyze

60. 4. Infants with congenital heart disease often have difficulty feeding and gaining weight. They will tire quickly during the feeding. Most will do well with smaller, more frequent feedings. An infant with a congenital heart defect should not be given more than 20 minutes per feeding. Fortified breast milk or a high-calorie formula will help the infant gain weight and conserve energy. Prolonging the feeding to an hour will merely tire the infant. Positioning the infant in an upright position is recommended for infants with gastrointestinal reflux. Some infants with a congenital heart defect may not consume adequate amounts of calories through breast- or bottle-feeding and may require supplemental feeding through a nasogastric tube; however, nasogastric tube feedings are not necessary for all infants with congenital heart defects.

🗝 CN: Management of care; CL: Analyze

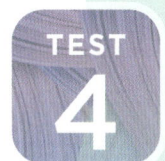

TEST 4: The Child with Health Problems of the Gastrointestinal Tract

- The Client with Cleft Lip and Palate
- The Client with Tracheoesophageal Fistula
- The Client with an Anorectal Anomaly
- The Client with Pyloric Stenosis
- The Client with Intussusception
- The Client with Inguinal Hernia
- The Client with Hirschsprung's Disease
- The Client with Diarrhea, Gastroenteritis, or Dehydration
- The Client with Appendicitis
- Managing Care, Quality, and Safety of Children with Health Problems of the Gastrointestinal Tract
- Answers, Rationales, and Test-Taking Strategies

The Client with Cleft Lip and Palate

1. The nurse is caring for an infant with an unrepaired cleft lip and palate. Which measure would be **most** effective in helping to retain oral feedings?
   - ☐ 1. Burp the infant at frequent intervals.
   - ☐ 2. Feed the infant small amounts at one time.
   - ☐ 3. Place the end of the nipple far to the back of the infant's tongue.
   - ☐ 4. Maintain the infant in a supine position while feeding.

2. The nurse teaches the parent of an infant who has had a surgical repair for a cleft lip about the use of elbow restraints at home. The nurse determines that the teaching has been successful when the parent makes which statement?
   - ☐ 1. "We will only remove the restraints one at a time to check the skin under them for redness."
   - ☐ 2. "We will keep the restraints on during the day while they are awake, but take them off when we put them to bed at night."
   - ☐ 3. "After we get home, we will not have to use the restraints because our child does not suck on their hands or fingers."
   - ☐ 4. "We will be sure to keep the restraints on all the time until we come to see the primary care provider for a follow-up visit."

3. The parent of an infant with a cleft lip asks when the repair will be scheduled. What is the nurse's **best** response?
   - ☐ 1. at birth
   - ☐ 2. during the first 6 months of life
   - ☐ 3. between the ages of 6 months and 1 year
   - ☐ 4. after 1 year of age

4. The nurse cares for a toddler on the second postoperative day after repair of a cleft palate. What should the nurse use to feed the toddler?
   - ☐ 1. cup
   - ☐ 2. straw
   - ☐ 3. rubber-tipped syringe
   - ☐ 4. large-holed nipple

The Client with Tracheoesophageal Fistula

5. The parents report that their 1-day-old is drooling and having choking episodes with excessive amounts of mucus and color changes, especially during feedings. The nurse should contact the health care provider to further assess the baby and request which prescription?
   - ☐ 1. a lactation consultation
   - ☐ 2. an arterial blood gas test
   - ☐ 3. an x-ray for nasogastric tube placement
   - ☐ 4. a serum blood glucose assessment

6. The parents of a child with a tracheoesophageal fistula express feelings of guilt about their baby's anomaly. Which approach by the nurse would **best** support the parents?
    ☐ 1. helping the parents accept their feelings as a normal reaction
    ☐ 2. explaining that the parents did nothing to cause the newborn's defect
    ☐ 3. encouraging the parents to concentrate on planning their baby's care
    ☐ 4. urging the parents to visit their newborn as often as possible

7. The nurse teaches the parents of a neonate diagnosed with a tracheoesophageal fistula (TEF) about this anomaly. The nurse determines that the teaching was successful when the parent describes the condition in which way?
    ☐ 1. "The muscle below the stomach is too tight, causing the baby to vomit forcefully."
    ☐ 2. "There is a blind upper pouch and an opening from the esophagus into the airway."
    ☐ 3. "The lower bowel is lacking certain nerves to allow normal function."
    ☐ 4. "A part of the bowel is on the outside without anything covering it."

8. The nurse maintains the airway of an infant with a tracheoesophageal fistula (TEF). Which finding would **most** indicate that the infant needs suctioning?
    ☐ 1. barking cough
    ☐ 2. substernal retractions
    ☐ 3. decreased activity level
    ☐ 4. increased respiratory rate

9. The nurse is administering bolus gastrostomy feedings to an infant after surgery to correct a tracheoesophageal fistula (TEF). What should the nurse do to prevent air from entering the stomach once the syringe barrel is attached to the gastrostomy tube?
    ☐ 1. Unclamp the tube after pouring the complete amount of formula to be administered into the syringe barrel.
    ☐ 2. Pour all of the formula to be administered into the syringe barrel after opening the clamp.
    ☐ 3. Maintain a continuous flow of formula down the side of the syringe barrel once the clamp is opened.
    ☐ 4. Allow a small amount of formula to enter the stomach before pouring more formula into the syringe barrel.

10. A newborn who had a surgical repair of a tracheoesophageal fistula (TEF) is started on oral feedings. What should the nurse include in the teaching plan for the parent about oral feedings?
    ☐ 1. They are better tolerated when larger but less frequent feedings are offered.
    ☐ 2. They should be offered on a feeding schedule to help the infant accept the feedings more readily.
    ☐ 3. They are best accepted by the infant when offered by the same nurse or by the infant's parent.
    ☐ 4. They are best planned in conjunction with observations of the infant's behavioral cues.

The Client with an Anorectal Anomaly

11. After completing diagnostic testing, the surgeon has scheduled a newborn with the diagnosis of an imperforate anus for surgery the next day. The infant's parents do not want the surgery to take place unless the infant has first been baptized. What should the nurse ask the parents?
    ☐ 1. "Are you worried your baby might die?"
    ☐ 2. "How can I arrange the baptism?"
    ☐ 3. "Do you want to speak with the social worker?"
    ☐ 4. "Would you prefer to wait for the surgery?"

12. The nurse completes an assessment on a newborn with an anorectal malformation. Which finding(s) would the nurse expect to assess in a newborn diagnosed with an anorectal malformation? Select all that apply.
    ☐ 1. abdominal distention
    ☐ 2. loose stools
    ☐ 3. vomiting
    ☐ 4. meconium in the urine
    ☐ 5. meconium stools

13. The nurse performs discharge teaching with the parents of a neonate who has successfully undergone surgery to repair a low anorectal anomaly. Which parent statement about the child's prognosis indicates teaching has been successful? "My child:
    ☐ 1. will need to wear protective pads until puberty."
    ☐ 2. will need extra fluids to prevent constipation."
    ☐ 3. will probably always need a high-fiber diet."
    ☐ 4. has a good chance of being potty trained."

14. The parent of a neonate scheduled for gastrointestinal surgery asks the nurse how newborns respond to painful stimuli. What is the nurse's **best** response?
    - ☐ 1. "Newborns cry and cannot be distracted to stop crying."
    - ☐ 2. "When faced with pain, newborns try to roll away from it."
    - ☐ 3. "Newborns typically move their whole body in response to pain."
    - ☐ 4. "Pain causes the newborn to withdraw the affected part."

15. The nurse develops the plan of care for a neonate who was diagnosed with an anorectal malformation and who subsequently underwent surgery. What intervention would be **most** helpful in facilitating parent-infant bonding?
    - ☐ 1. explaining to the parents that they can visit at any time
    - ☐ 2. encouraging the parents to hold their infant
    - ☐ 3. asking the parents to help monitor the infant's intake and output
    - ☐ 4. helping the parents plan for their infant's discharge

The Client with Pyloric Stenosis

16. A 4-week-old infant admitted with a diagnosis of hypertrophic pyloric stenosis presents with a history of vomiting. The nurse should anticipate that the infant's vomitus would contain gastric contents and which other body substances?
    - ☐ 1. bile and streaks of blood
    - ☐ 2. mucus and stool
    - ☐ 3. mucus and streaks of blood
    - ☐ 4. stool and bile

17. The nurse admits an infant with pyloric stenosis to the hospital. Which aspect of the plan of care should the nurse implement **first**?
    - ☐ 1. Weigh the infant.
    - ☐ 2. Begin an intravenous infusion.
    - ☐ 3. Switch the infant to an oral electrolyte solution.
    - ☐ 4. Orient the parent to the hospital unit.

18. The nurse teaches the parent of an infant with pyloric stenosis about the condition. Which cause, if stated by the parent, indicates effective teaching?
    - ☐ 1. "an enlarged muscle below the stomach"
    - ☐ 2. "a telescoping of the large bowel into the smaller bowel"
    - ☐ 3. "a result of giving the baby more formula than is necessary"
    - ☐ 4. "a genetically smaller stomach than normal"

19. A newborn admitted with pyloric stenosis is lethargic and has poor skin turgor. The health care provider (HCP) has prescribed intravenous fluids of dextrose water with sodium and potassium. The baby's admission potassium level is 3.4 mEq/L (3.4 mmol/L). What should the nurse do **first**?
    - ☐ 1. Notify the HCP.
    - ☐ 2. Administer the prescribed fluids.
    - ☐ 3. Verify that the infant is urinating.
    - ☐ 4. Have the potassium level redrawn.

20. After undergoing surgical correction of pyloric stenosis, an infant is returned to the room in stable condition. While standing by the crib, the parent says, "Perhaps if I had brought my baby to the hospital sooner, the surgery could have been avoided." What is the nurse's **best** response?
    - ☐ 1. "Surgery is the most effective treatment for pyloric stenosis."
    - ☐ 2. "Try not to worry; your baby will be fine."
    - ☐ 3. "Do you feel that this problem indicates that you are not a good parent?"
    - ☐ 4. "Do you think that earlier hospitalization could have avoided surgery?"

21. After surgery to correct pyloric stenosis, the nurse instructs the parents about the postoperative feeding schedule for their infant. The parents exhibit understanding of these instructions when they state that they can start feeding the child within which time frame?
    - ☐ 1. 6 hours
    - ☐ 2. 8 hours
    - ☐ 3. 10 hours
    - ☐ 4. 12 hours

22. Which behavior exhibited by the parent of an infant with pyloric stenosis should the nurse correctly interpret as a positive indication of parental coping?
    - ☐ 1. telling the nurse that they have to get away for a while
    - ☐ 2. discussing the infant's care realistically
    - ☐ 3. repeatedly asking if their child is normal
    - ☐ 4. exhibiting fear that they will disturb the infant

23. A 6-month-old has had a pyloromyotomy to correct a pyloric stenosis. Three days after surgery, the parents have placed their infant in their own infant seat (see figure). What should the nurse do?

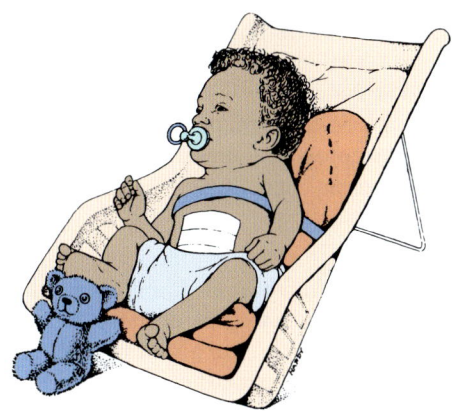

☐ 1. Reposition the infant to the left side.
☐ 2. Ask the parents to put the infant back in their crib.
☐ 3. Remind the parents that the infant cannot use a pacifier now.
☐ 4. Tell the parents they have positioned their infant correctly.

The Client with Intussusception

24. The nurse assesses a 4-month-old infant diagnosed with possible intussusception. The nurse should expect the parent to relate which information about the infant's crying and episodes of pain?
☐ 1. constant accompanied by leg extension
☐ 2. intermittent with knees drawn to the chest
☐ 3. shrill during ingestion of solids
☐ 4. intermittent while being held in the parent's arms

25. The nurse obtains the nursing history from the parent of an infant with suspected intussusception. Which question would be **most** helpful for the nurse to ask?
☐ 1. "What do the stools look like?"
☐ 2. "When was the last time your child urinated?"
☐ 3. "Is your child eating normally?"
☐ 4. "Has your child had any episodes of vomiting?"

26. A nasogastric tube inserted during surgical correction of an infant's intussusception is no longer freely removing gastric secretions. What should the nurse do **next**?
☐ 1. Verify the tube placement.
☐ 2. Irrigate the tube.
☐ 3. Increase the level of suction.
☐ 4. Rotate the tube.

27. The nurse assesses an infant who has had surgery to correct an intussusception and is now at risk for the development of a paralytic ileus postoperatively. Which assessment should be the **priority**?
☐ 1. measurement of urine specific gravity
☐ 2. auscultation of bowel sounds
☐ 3. inspection of the first stool passed
☐ 4. measurement of gastric output

The Client with Inguinal Hernia

28. The nurse assesses an infant with a suspected inguinal hernia. Which finding would be **most** concerning?
☐ 1. The inguinal swelling is reddened, and the abdomen is distended.
☐ 2. The infant is irritable, and a thickened spermatic cord is palpable.
☐ 3. The inguinal swelling can be reduced, and the infant has stool in their diaper.
☐ 4. The infant's diaper is wet with urine, and the abdomen is nontender.

29. Preoperatively, the nurse develops a plan to prepare a 7-month-old infant psychologically for a scheduled herniorrhaphy the next day. Which intervention should the nurse expect to implement to accomplish this goal?
☐ 1. explaining the preoperative and postoperative procedures to the parent
☐ 2. having the parent stay with the infant
☐ 3. making sure the infant's favorite toy is available
☐ 4. allowing the infant to play with surgical equipment

30. A parent asks, "How should I bathe my baby now that they have had surgery for an inguinal hernia?" Which instruction should the nurse give the parent?
☐ 1. "Clean only their face and diaper area for the next 2 weeks."
☐ 2. "Use sterile sponges to cleanse the inguinal incision until healed."
☐ 3. "Give them a sponge bath daily for 1 week."
☐ 4. "Let them take a full tub bath daily."

The Client with Hirschsprung's Disease

31. The nurse completes a physical assessment of a 4-month-old infant with Hirschsprung's disease. Which finding would the nurse **most** likely find?
☐ 1. scaphoid-shaped abdomen
☐ 2. weight less than expected for height and age
☐ 3. cyanosis of the fingers and toes
☐ 4. hyperactive deep tendon reflexes

32. An infant diagnosed with Hirschsprung's disease is scheduled to receive a temporary colostomy. When the nurse is initially discussing the diagnosis and treatment with the parents, which action by the nurse would be **most** appropriate?
☐ 1. assessing the adequacy of their coping skills
☐ 2. reassuring them that their child will be fine
☐ 3. encouraging them to ask questions
☐ 4. giving them printed material on the procedure

33. The nurse teaches the parents of an infant diagnosed with Hirschsprung's disease about the disease. The nurse determines that the parents understand the diagnosis when the parent makes which statement?
☐ 1. "There are congenital polyps obstructing the colon."
☐ 2. "A section of the colon is constricted."
☐ 3. "The nerves at the end of the large colon are missing."
☐ 4. "There is a weakened area in the colon that is inflamed."

34. The nurse develops the preoperative plan of care for an infant with Hirschsprung's disease. Which intervention should the nurse include?
☐ 1. administering a tap water enema
☐ 2. inserting a gastrostomy tube
☐ 3. restricting oral intake to clear liquids
☐ 4. using povidone-iodine solution to prepare the perineum

35. The nurse is showing the parent of a child with Hirschsprung's disease where the aganglionic area is located. Identify the area the nurse should point out as being aganglionic.

36. An infant diagnosed with Hirschsprung's disease undergoes surgery with the creation of a temporary colostomy. Which statement by the parent regarding the colostomy indicates the need for further teaching?
☐ 1. "The colostomy is only temporary to relieve the obstruction."
☐ 2. "The colostomy will give time for the nerves to return to normal."
☐ 3. "The colostomy may include two separate abdominal openings."
☐ 4. "Right after the procedure, the stoma may appear bruised."

37. When teaching the parent of an infant who has received a temporary colostomy for treatment of Hirschsprung's disease about how the stoma should normally appear, the nurse should include which description of the stoma's appearance in the teaching?
☐ 1. becoming dark brown in 2 months
☐ 2. staying deep red in color
☐ 3. changing to several shades of pink
☐ 4. turning almost purple in color

38. The nurse teaches the parent of an infant with Hirschsprung's disease who received a temporary colostomy about the types of foods the infant will be able to eat. Which diet would the nurse recommend?
☐ 1. high-fiber diet
☐ 2. low-fat diet
☐ 3. high-residue diet
☐ 4. regular diet

39. A child with Hirschsprung's disease is to be discharged 1 or 2 days after a colostomy takedown surgery. After teaching the infant's parents about the overall effects of their infant's surgery, the nurse determines that the teaching has been effective when the parents make which statement?
☐ 1. "Their abdomen will be large for a while."
☐ 2. "Toilet training may be difficult."
☐ 3. "We need to limit their intake of dairy products."
☐ 4. "We will give them vitamin supplements until they are an adolescent."

40. A parent of a 7-year-old child with Hirschsprung's disease and chronic constipation asks about increasing dietary fiber in the child's diet. Which food could the nurse recommend?
☐ 1. fruit juice
☐ 2. white bread
☐ 3. popcorn
☐ 4. pancakes

The Client with Diarrhea, Gastroenteritis, or Dehydration

41. A nurse is caring for a 10-month-old weighing 17.6 lb (8 kg) who was admitted for dehydration. The infant has an IV of 5% dextrose in 0.45% saline infusing at the maintenance rate of 100 mL/kg per day for children weighing 22 lb (10 kg) or less. The infant has vomited five times in the last 3 hours and has had no wet diapers in the last 8 hours. The nurse informs the health care provider. Which prescription should the nurse question?
    ☐ 1. Increase the intravenous fluids to 45 mL per hour for 24 hours.
    ☐ 2. Keep the infant on nothing-by-mouth (NPO) status while vomiting persists.
    ☐ 3. Administer a 10 mL/kg fluid bolus of dextrose 25%.
    ☐ 4. Maintain strict intake and output (I&O), weighing all diapers.

42. The nurse cares for an infant with diarrhea. Which sign(s) or symptom(s) would suggest that an infant is dehydrated? Select all that apply.
    ☐ 1. tacky mucous membranes
    ☐ 2. sunken anterior fontanelle
    ☐ 3. frothy saliva
    ☐ 4. restlessness
    ☐ 5. increased urine output

43. A child is admitted with a tentative diagnosis of shigella. The nurse performs which intervention(s)? Select all that apply.
    ☐ 1. Assess the child for nausea and vomiting.
    ☐ 2. Collect a stool specimen for white blood cells (WBCs).
    ☐ 3. Place the child on airborne precautions.
    ☐ 4. Monitor the child for signs and symptoms of dehydration.
    ☐ 5. Initiate an intake and output record.

44. The nurse assesses a preschooler with gastroenteritis. Which finding would **most** likely alert the nurse to the possibility that a preschooler is experiencing moderate dehydration?
    ☐ 1. deep, rapid respirations
    ☐ 2. diaphoresis
    ☐ 3. absence of tear formation
    ☐ 4. decreased urine specific gravity

45. The nurses assess an 8-month-old infant admitted with severe diarrhea. Which finding does the nurse recognize as being **most** significant?
    ☐ 1. bowel sounds every 5 seconds
    ☐ 2. pale yellow urine
    ☐ 3. normal skin elasticity
    ☐ 4. depressed anterior fontanelle

46. The nurse creates a monitoring plan for an infant with severe diarrhea. Which assessment would be the **most** important for the nurse to include in the plan of care?
    ☐ 1. monitoring the total 8-hour formula intake
    ☐ 2. weighing the infant each day
    ☐ 3. checking the anterior fontanelle every shift
    ☐ 4. monitoring abdominal skin turgor every shift

47. The health care provider prescribes an intravenous infusion of 5% dextrose in 0.45% saline to be infused at 2 mL/kg per hour in an infant who weighs 9 lb (4.1 kg). How many milliliters per hour of the solution should the nurse infuse? Round to one decimal place.
    _____ mL per hour.

48. A 3-year-old with dehydration has vomited 3 times in the last hour and continues to have frequent diarrhea stools. The child was admitted 2 days ago with gastroenteritis caused by rotavirus. The child weighs 48.5 lb (22 kg), has a normal saline lock in their right hand, and has had 30 mL of urine output in the last 4 hours. Using the situation-background-assessment-recommendation (SBAR) technique for communication, the nurse calls the health care provider with the recommendation for which prescription?
    ☐ 1. giving a dose of loperamide
    ☐ 2. starting a fluid bolus of normal saline
    ☐ 3. beginning an intravenous (IV) antibiotic
    ☐ 4. establishing an indwelling catheter

49. The nurse cares for a 6-month-old infant hospitalized with severe diarrhea. Which intervention would be **most** appropriate for the nurse to teach the parent to help comfort their infant who is fussy?
    ☐ 1. offering a pacifier
    ☐ 2. placing a mobile above the crib
    ☐ 3. sitting at the crib side talking to the infant
    ☐ 4. turning the television on to cartoons

50. The nurse admits an infant to the hospital with a diagnosis of gastroenteritis. What would the nurse identify as a **priority** nursing problem for the infant?
    ☐ 1. pain related to repeated episodes of vomiting
    ☐ 2. deficient fluid volume related to excessive losses from severe diarrhea
    ☐ 3. impaired parenting related to infant's loss of fluid
    ☐ 4. impaired urinary elimination related to increased fluid intake feeding pattern

51. The nurse teaches the parent of an infant hospitalized with gastroenteritis about the next step of the treatment plan once the infant's condition has been controlled. The nurse determines that the parent understands when they explain that which intervention will occur with their infant?
    ☐ 1. The infant will receive clear liquids for a period of time.
    ☐ 2. Formula and juice will be offered.
    ☐ 3. Blood will be drawn daily to test for anemia.
    ☐ 4. The infant will be allowed to go to the playroom.

52. The parent of a toddler who has just been admitted with severe dehydration secondary to gastroenteritis says that they cannot stay with their child because they have to take care of their other children at home. Which of the responses by the nurse would be **most** appropriate?
    ☐ 1. "You really shouldn't leave right now. Your child is very sick."
    ☐ 2. "I understand, but feel free to visit or call anytime to see how your child is doing."
    ☐ 3. "It's really not necessary to stay with your child. We will take very good care of them."
    ☐ 4. "Can you find someone to stay with your children? Your child needs you here."

53. A 9-month-old is admitted because of dehydration. How should the nurse go about accurately monitoring fluid intake and output? Select all that apply.
    ☐ 1. weighing and recording all wet diapers
    ☐ 2. changing breast feedings to bottle-feedings
    ☐ 3. obtaining an accurate daily weight
    ☐ 4. restricting fluids prior to weighing the child
    ☐ 5. obtaining an accurate stool count

54. The health care provider prescribes intravenous (IV) fluid replacement therapy with potassium chloride to be added for a child with severe gastroenteritis. Before the nurse hangs the IV fluids with potassium chloride, which assessment would be **most** important?
    ☐ 1. ability to void
    ☐ 2. passage of stool today
    ☐ 3. baseline electrocardiogram
    ☐ 4. serum calcium level

55. The nurse cares for a child with severe gastroenteritis who has been receiving intravenous therapy for the past several hours. Which finding would alert the nurse to suspect that a child may be developing circulatory overload?
    ☐ 1. a drop in blood pressure
    ☐ 2. change to slow, deep respirations
    ☐ 3. auscultation of moist crackles
    ☐ 4. marked increase in urine output

56. A child undergoes rehydration therapy after having diarrhea and dehydration. A nurse is teaching the child's parents about dietary management after rehydration. The nurse understands that the teaching plan has been successful when the parents tell the nurse that they will follow which type of diet?
    ☐ 1. regular
    ☐ 2. clear liquid
    ☐ 3. full liquid
    ☐ 4. soft

57. The nurse obtains a history from the parents of a child diagnosed with diarrhea due to *Salmonella*. The nurse should ask the parents if the child has been exposed to which possible source of infection?
    ☐ 1. nonrefrigerated custard
    ☐ 2. a pet canary
    ☐ 3. undercooked eggs
    ☐ 4. unwashed fruit

58. On a home visit following discharge from the hospital after treatment for severe gastroenteritis, the parent tells the nurse that a toddler answers "No!" and is difficult to manage. After discussing this further with the parent, the nurse explains that the child's behavior is **most** likely the result of which factor?
    ☐ 1. beginning leadership skills
    ☐ 2. inherited personality trait
    ☐ 3. expression of individuality
    ☐ 4. usual lack of interest in everything

59. The parent of a toddler hospitalized for episodes of diarrhea reports that when the toddler cannot have things the way they want, they throw their legs and arms around, scream, and cry. The parent says, "I don't know what to do!" After the nurse teaches the parent about ways to manage this behavior, which statement by the parent indicates that the nurse's teaching was successful?
    ☐ 1. "Next time my child screams and throws their legs, I'll ignore the behavior."
    ☐ 2. "I'll allow them to have what they want once in a while."
    ☐ 3. "I'll explain why they cannot have what they want."
    ☐ 4. "When they behave like this, I'll tell them that they are being a bad child."

60. The parent of a toilet-trained toddler who was admitted to the hospital for severe gastroenteritis and subsequent dehydration and is now at home asks the nurse why the child still wets the bed. What would be the nurse's **best** response?
☐ 1. "Regression is common, and it takes time for them to return to their former behavior."
☐ 2. "The stress of hospitalization is hard for many children, but usually they have no problems when they return home."
☐ 3. "After returning home from being hospitalized, children still feel they should be the center of attention."
☐ 4. "Children do not feel comfortable in their home surroundings once they return home from being hospitalized."

The Client with Appendicitis

61. An adolescent is being seen in the clinic for abdominal pain with a fever. In what order should the nurse assess the abdomen? All options must be used.

1. auscultate
2. inspect
3. palpate
4. percuss

62. STEP 1

A 10-year-old female client presents to the emergency department with abdominal pain.

Admission Note

1130:
The client has been vomiting for 2 days. They report generalized abdominal pain with rebound tenderness when palpated by the health care provider, and they rate their pain as an 8 on a 0 to 10 scale. The client has a history of COVID-19 infection 6 months ago with minor symptoms and a past hospitalization for a right supracondylar fracture with surgical pin placement 4 months ago following a fall from a trampoline. All immunizations are up to date. Vital signs are temperature (T) 103°F (39.4°C); pulse (P) 144 bpm; respiration rate (RR) 32 breaths/min; blood pressure (BP) 110/60 mm Hg; and oxygenation 96% on room air.

➢ Click to highlight the findings that require follow-up. Answer choices have been underlined.

Admission Note

1130:
The client has been <u>vomiting for 2 days</u>. They report <u>generalized abdominal pain with rebound tenderness</u> when palpated by the health care provider, and they <u>rate their pain as an 8 on a 0 to 10 scale</u>. The client has a history of <u>COVID-19 infection 6 months ago</u> with minor symptoms and a <u>past hospitalization for a right supracondylar fracture with surgical pin placement</u> 4 months ago following a fall from a trampoline. All immunizations are up to date. Vital signs are <u>temperature (T) 103°F (39.4°C)</u>; <u>pulse (P) 144 bpm</u>; <u>respiration rate (RR) 32 breaths/min</u>; <u>blood pressure (BP) 110/60 mm Hg</u>; and <u>oxygenation 96% on room air</u>.

63. STEP 2

A 10-year-old female client presents to the emergency department with abdominal pain.

Admission Note

1130:
The client has been vomiting for 2 days. They report generalized abdominal pain with rebound tenderness when palpated by the health care provider, and they rate their pain as an 8 on a 0 to 10 scale. The client has a history of COVID-19 infection 6 months ago with minor symptoms and a past hospitalization for a right supracondylar fracture with surgical pin placement 4 months ago following a fall from a trampoline. All immunizations are up to date. Vital signs are temperature (T) 103°F (39.4°C); pulse (P) 144 bpm; respiration rate (RR) 32 breaths/min; blood pressure (BP) 110/60 mm Hg; and oxygenation 96% on room air.

➤ What additional assessment(s) should the nurse obtain to help determine the client's appendicitis risk? Select all that apply.

- ☐ 1. Abdominal ultrasound
- ☐ 2. Bowel movement characteristics
- ☐ 3. Bowel sounds
- ☐ 4. Complete blood count
- ☐ 5. Fecal occult blood
- ☐ 6. Pain at McBurney's point
- ☐ 7. Stool cultures

64. STEP 3

A 10-year-old female client presents to the emergency department with abdominal pain.

Admission Note

1130:
The client has been vomiting for 2 days. They report generalized abdominal pain with rebound tenderness when palpated by the health care provider, and they rate their pain as an 8 on a 0 to 10 scale. The client has a history of COVID-19 infection 6 months ago with minor symptoms and a past hospitalization for a right supracondylar fracture with surgical pin placement 4 months ago following a fall from a trampoline. All immunizations are up to date. Vital signs are temperature (T) 103°F (39.4°C); pulse (P) 144 bpm; respiration rate (RR) 32 breaths/min; blood pressure (BP) 110/60 mm Hg; and oxygenation 96% on room air.

Diagnostics

Laboratory Test	Results	Reference Range
White blood cell count	21×10^3 cells/mm³ (21×10^9/L)	$4.5–10.5 \times 10^3$ cells/mm³ ($4.5–10.5 \times 10^9$/L)
Hemoglobin	14 g/dL (140 g/L)	Ages 6–16 years: 10.3–14.9 g/dL (103–149 g/L)
Hematocrit	42% (0.42 proportion of 1.0)	Ages 6–16 years: 32%–42% (0.32–0.42 proportion of 1.0)

Radiology:
Abdominal ultrasound shows an inflamed appendix.

➤ Additional assessment data are obtained, and the client receives the diagnosis of appendicitis.

Complete the sentence from the list of word choices.

The client's top risk if treatment is delayed is

_____ .

Word Choices

bleeding

bowel necrosis

hypovolemic shock

peritonitis

65. STEP 4

A 10-year-old female client presents to the emergency department with abdominal pain.

Admission Note

1130:
The client has been vomiting for 2 days. They report generalized abdominal pain with rebound tenderness when palpated by the health care provider, and they rate their pain as an 8 on a 0-to-10 scale. The client has a history of COVID-19 infection 6 months ago with minor symptoms and a past hospitalization for a right supracondylar fracture with surgical pin placement 4 months ago following a fall from a trampoline. All immunizations are up to date. Vital signs are temperature (T) 103°F (39.4°C); pulse (P) 144 bpm; respiration rate (RR) 32 breaths/min; blood pressure (BP) 110/60 mm Hg; and oxygenation 96% on room air.

Diagnostics

Laboratory Test	Results	Reference Range
White blood cell count	21×10^3 cells/mm^3 (21×10^9/L)	$4.5–10.5 \times 10^3$ cells/mm^3 ($4.5–10.5 \times 10^9$/L)
Hemoglobin	14 g/dL (140 g/L)	Ages 6–16 years: 10.3–14.9 g/dL (103–149 g/L)
Hematocrit	42% (0.42 proportion of 1.0)	Ages 6–16 years: 32%–42% (0.32–0.42 proportion of 1.0).

Radiology:
Abdominal ultrasound shows an inflamed appendix

The nurse prepares the client for an appendectomy.

➤ For each possible intervention, select if the intervention is anticipated or not anticipated to prepare the client for surgery.

Intervention	Anticipated	Not Anticipated
Administer antibiotics	○	○
Apply a heating pad	○	○
Insert a peripheral IV	○	○
Insert a nasogastric tube	○	○
Obtain a urine specimen	○	○
Position the client supine	○	○

66. STEP 5

The nurse cares for a 10-year-old female client following surgery for appendicitis.

Admission Note

1130:
The client has been vomiting for 2 days. They report generalized abdominal pain with rebound tenderness when palpated by the health care provider, and they rate their pain as an 8 on a 0 to 10 scale. The client has a history of COVID-19 infection 6 months ago with minor symptoms and a past hospitalization for a right supracondylar fracture with surgical pin placement 4 months ago following a fall from a trampoline. All immunizations are up to date. Vital signs are temperature (T) 103°F (39.4°C); pulse (P) 144 bpm; respiration rate (RR) 32 breaths/min; blood pressure (BP) 110/60 mm Hg; and oxygenation 96% on room air.

Diagnostics

Laboratory Test	Results	Reference Range
White blood cell count	21×10^3 cells/mm³ (21×10^9/L)	$4.5–10.5 \times 10^3$ cells/mm³ ($4.5–10.5 \times 10^9$/L)
Hemoglobin	14 g/dL (140 g/L)	Ages 6–16 years: 10.3–14.9 g/dL (103–149 g/L)
Hematocrit	42% (0.42 proportion of 1.0)	Ages 6–16 years: 32%–42% (0.32–0.42 proportion of 1.0)

Radiology:
Abdominal ultrasound shows an inflamed appendix.

Orders

Diagnosis: Appendectomy for a ruptured appendix

1. Vital signs once every hour for 4 hours, and then every 4 hours
2. Bathroom privileges
3. Strict intake and output (I&O)
4. Diet of clear liquids
5. Incentive spirometry hourly while awake for 24 hours
6. Penrose drain management
7. IV lactated Ringer's solution at 75 mL per hour
8. Piperacillin and tazobactam 3 g IV every 8 hours
9. Morphine 4 mg/mL, give 3 mg IV every 3 hours as needed for moderate to severe pain

---

The nurse reviews the orders and prepares to give the client morphine for pain.

➤ What step(s) should the nurse take to administer the IV morphine? Select all that apply.

☐ 1. Prepare 0.3 mL of morphine for administration.
☐ 2. Have a second nurse witness medication waste.
☐ 3. Administer morphine IV push over 1 minute.
☐ 4. Place the client on a cardiorespiratory/oxygen saturation monitor.
☐ 5. Assess the client's pain with the Faces, Legs, Activity, Cry, Consolability (FLACC) scale.

67. STEP 6

The nurse cares for a 10-year-old female client following surgery for appendicitis.

Admission Note

1130:
The client has been vomiting for 2 days. They report generalized abdominal pain with rebound tenderness when palpated by the health care provider, and they rate their pain as an 8 on a 0 to 10 scale. The client has a history of COVID-19 infection 6 months ago with minor symptoms and a past hospitalization for a right supracondylar fracture with surgical pin placement 4 months ago following a fall from a trampoline. All immunizations are up to date. Vital signs are temperature (T) 103°F (39.4°C); pulse (P) 144 bpm; respiration rate (RR) 32 breaths/min; blood pressure (BP) 110/60 mm Hg; and oxygenation 96% on room air.

Postoperative day 2, 0700:
Vital signs are T 101°F (38.3°C); P 156 bpm; RR 50 breaths/min; BP 78/40 mm Hg; and oxygenation 95% on room air. Capillary refill is 4 seconds. Urine output is 0.3 mL/kg per hour. The client appears lethargic but is taking clear liquids. IV lactated Ringer's solution is still infusing at 76 mL per hour in the left arm. There was 5 mL of serosanguinous drainage from the Penrose drain. The client has been taking 3 mg of IV morphine every 3 hours.

Diagnostics

Laboratory Test	Results	Reference Range
White blood cell count	21×10^3 cells/mm^3 (21×10^9/L)	4.5–10.5×10^3 cells/mm^3 (4.5–10.5×10^9/L)
Hemoglobin	14 g/dL (140 g/L)	Ages 6–16 years: 10.3–14.9 g/dL (103–149 g/L)
Hematocrit	42% (0.42 proportion of 1.0)	Ages 6–16 years: 32%–42% (0.32–0.42 proportion of 1.0)

Radiology:
Abdominal ultrasound shows an inflamed appendix.

Orders

Diagnosis: Appendectomy for a ruptured appendix

1. Vital signs once every hour for 4 hours, and then every 4 hours
2. Bathroom privileges
3. Strict intake and output (I&O)
4. Diet of clear liquids
5. Incentive spirometry hourly while awake for 24 hours
6. Penrose drain management
7. IV lactated Ringer's solution at 75 mL per hour
8. Piperacillin and tazobactam 3 g IV every 8 hours
9. Morphine 4 mg/mL, give 3 mg IV every 3 hours as needed for moderate to severe pain

---

The nurse reviews the change-of-shift report for a 10-year-old client 1 day after surgery for a ruptured appendix.

➢ Highlight the findings from the underlined terms that indicate the client's status is deteriorating. Answer choices have been underlined.

Nurses' Note

Postoperative day 2, 0700
Vital signs are <u>T 101°F (38.3°C)</u>; <u>P 156 bpm</u>; <u>RR 50 breaths/min</u>; <u>BP 78/40 mm Hg</u>; and <u>oxygenation 95%</u> on room air. <u>Capillary refill is 4 seconds.</u> <u>Urine output is 0.3 mL/kg per hour.</u> The <u>client appears lethargic</u> but is taking clear liquids. IV lactated Ringer's solution is still infusing at 76 mL per hour in the left arm. There was <u>5 mL of serosanguinous drainage from the Penrose drain</u>. The client has been <u>taking 3 mg of IV morphine every 3 hours</u>.

68. A pediatric client with suspected appendicitis presents with a fever and abdominal pain. Which area should the nurse assess to determine if the pain is localized at McBurney's point?

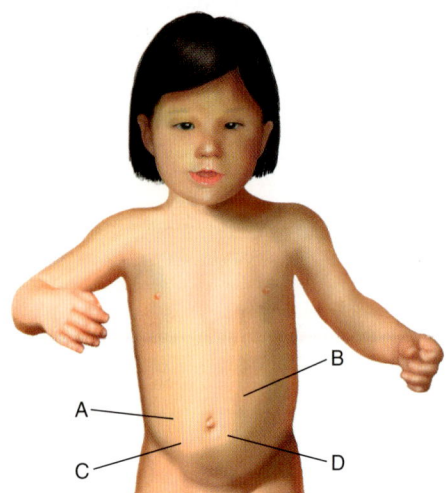

☐ 1. A
☐ 2. B
☐ 3. C
☐ 4. D

69. A child is admitted with constipation and a diagnosis of possible appendicitis. The child is in acute pain. Which nursing intervention(s) would be appropriate before surgery to decrease pain? Select all that apply.
☐ 1. Offer an ice pack.
☐ 2. Apply a heating pad.
☐ 3. Have the client assume a position of comfort.
☐ 4. Limit the client's activity.
☐ 5. Request a prescription for a cathartic.

70. A 10-year-old client underwent an appendectomy 24 hours ago. They are awake, alert, and oriented. The client tells the nurse they are experiencing pain. They have a prescription for morphine 1 to 2 mg as needed for pain. What is the **priority** nursing action in managing the child's pain?
☐ 1. Change the child's position in bed.
☐ 2. Determine the severity of the pain.
☐ 3. Administer 1 mg morphine as prescribed.
☐ 4. Perform a head-to-toe assessment.

71. A typically developing preschool child is experiencing pain after an appendectomy. Which data collection tool is the **most** appropriate for the nurse to use to assess the pain?
☐ 1. visual analog scale
☐ 2. faces, legs, activity, cry, consolability (FLACC) scale
☐ 3. numerical pain scale
☐ 4. FACES pain rating scale

72. A 7-year-old client had an appendectomy on November 12. They have had pain for the last 24 hours. There is a prescription to administer acetaminophen with codeine every 3 to 4 hours as needed. The nurse is beginning the shift, and the child is requesting pain medication. The nurse reviews the chart below for pain history. Based on the information in the medical record, what should the nurse do **next**?

Nurses' Notes		
Date	Time	Progress Notes
11/12	1600	Tylenol with Codeine given PO. FACES pain scale changed from 5 to 2 within 15 minutes.
11/12	1800	Tylenol with Codeine given PO. FACES pain scale changed from 5 to 2.
11/12	2130	Tylenol with Codeine given PO. FACES pain scale changed from 5 to 2.
11/13	0100	Tylenol with Codeine given PO. FACES pain scale changed from 4 to 1.
11/13	0700	Client rates pain on FACES pain scale as 4.

☐ 1. Administer the acetaminophen with codeine.
☐ 2. Distract the child by giving them breakfast.
☐ 3. Instruct the child to take deep breaths and blow their pain away.
☐ 4. Assess the child again in 1 hour.

73. The nurse obtains the initial health history from a 10-year-old child with abdominal pain and suspected appendicitis. Which question would be **most** helpful in eliciting data to help support the diagnosis?
☐ 1. "Where did the pain start?"
☐ 2. "What did you do for the pain?"
☐ 3. "How often do you have a bowel movement?"
☐ 4. "Is the pain continuous, or does it let up?"

74. The nurse develops the plan of care for a school-age child with a suspected diagnosis of appendicitis who has severe abdominal pain. The nurse should expect to include which measure in the child's plan of care?
☐ 1. application of a heating pad
☐ 2. insertion of a rectal tube
☐ 3. application of an ice bag
☐ 4. administration of an intravenous narcotic

75. The nurse assesses a male adolescent with severe abdominal pain. Which assessment finding should alert the nurse to suspect appendicitis?
☐ 1. The abdomen appears slightly rounded.
☐ 2. Bowel sounds are heard twice in 2 minutes.
☐ 3. All four abdominal quadrants reveal tympany.
☐ 4. The client demonstrates a cremasteric reflex.

76. An adolescent client scheduled for an emergency appendectomy is to be transferred directly from the emergency department to the operating room. Which statement by the client should the nurse interpret as **most** significant?
    ☐ 1. "All of a sudden, it does not hurt at all."
    ☐ 2. "The pain is centered around my navel."
    ☐ 3. "I feel like I am going to throw up."
    ☐ 4. "It hurts when you press on my stomach."

77. A nurse admits a pediatric client weighing 11.6 kg at the time of surgery for appendicitis. The nurse reviews the unit's standing prescription for intravenous (IV) fluids rates (see exhibit). At what hourly rate would the nurse set the IV pump? Round to whole numbers.

    Prescriptions
    ☐ 1. Start an IV of lactated Ringer's solution.
    ☐ 2. Run infusion at 4 mL per hour for each of the first 10 kg, then 2 mL per hour for each kilogram past 10 kg; 100 mL/kg for the first 10 kg, and 50 mL for each kilogram past 10 kg.

78. The nurse admits an adolescent client to the pediatric unit following an appendectomy. After obtaining the vital signs and pain ratings, what should be the **priority** assessment for the nurse to make?
    ☐ 1. the dressings on the surgical sites
    ☐ 2. intravenous fluid infusion site
    ☐ 3. nasogastric (NG) tube function
    ☐ 4. bowel sounds

79. An adolescent who has had an appendectomy and developed peritonitis has nausea. Which intervention should the nurse do **first**?
    ☐ 1. Administer an antiemetic.
    ☐ 2. Irrigate the nasogastric (NG) tube.
    ☐ 3. Notify the surgeon.
    ☐ 4. Take the blood pressure.

80. When developing the postoperative plan of care for an adolescent who has undergone an appendectomy for a ruptured appendix, the nurse should expect to place the client in which position during the early postoperative period?
    ☐ 1. semi-Fowler's
    ☐ 2. supine
    ☐ 3. lithotomy
    ☐ 4. prone

81. The nurse cares for an adolescent who has just returned to their room after an open appendectomy. What would the nurse expect as a normal response from an adolescent?
    ☐ 1. "I will need plastic surgery for this scar."
    ☐ 2. "I am worried about the size of my scar."
    ☐ 3. "I do not want to have any pain."
    ☐ 4. "What will my friends say about the scar?"

82. The nurse cares for an adolescent after an appendectomy. Which client action would the nurse judge to be a healthy coping behavior?
    ☐ 1. insisting on wearing a T-shirt and gym shorts rather than pajamas
    ☐ 2. avoiding interactions with other adolescents on the nursing unit
    ☐ 3. refusing to fill out the menu and allowing the nurse to do so
    ☐ 4. not taking telephone calls from friends so they can rest

83. The nurse prepares to teach an adolescent scheduled for an appendectomy about what to expect. The adolescent says, "I would rather look this up on the internet." What should the nurse do?
    ☐ 1. Explain that completing a teaching checklist is required by the hospital.
    ☐ 2. Help the client find information on the internet.
    ☐ 3. Provide the client with written information instead.
    ☐ 4. Explain that information found on the internet cannot be trusted.

Managing Care, Quality, and Safety of Children with Health Problems of the Gastrointestinal Tract

84. The health care team has noticed an increase in intravenous (IV) infiltrations on the pediatric floor. As part of a "Plan, Do, Study, Act" quality improvement plan, the team should perform the actions in which order? All options must be used.

    | 1. Analyze the data. |
    | 2. Decide to monitor IV gauges. |
    | 3. Perform chart audits. |
    | 4. Write a new IV insertion policy. |
    | |
    | |
    | |
    | |

85. The nurse works with the health care team to establish a policy regarding sleep positions for infants with gastroesophageal reflux. What information should the nurse search for **first**?
    ☐ 1. policies from other hospitals
    ☐ 2. data from retrospective studies
    ☐ 3. published national standards
    ☐ 4. expert opinions

86. The nurse is assisting another member of the health care team who is placing a peripherally inserted central catheter in a 10-year-old with peritonitis from a ruptured appendix. The family is present in the treatment room to support the child. The nurse observes that the other team member has contaminated a sterile glove. What should the nurse do **next**?
    ☐ 1. Discuss the incident with the team member after the event.
    ☐ 2. Report the incident to the nursing unit manager.
    ☐ 3. Tell the team member the glove is contaminated.
    ☐ 4. Ask the family to leave before confronting the team member.

87. The hospital is responding to a mass casualty disaster with adult and pediatric victims. What should the charge nurse on the pediatric floor do after reallocating staff?
    ☐ 1. Ask parents to leave to free up areas for incoming victims.
    ☐ 2. Review the census for candidates for early discharge.
    ☐ 3. Initiate paper charting backup.
    ☐ 4. Change taking all vital signs to every 8 hours.

88. Eight hours ago, an infant with Hirschsprung's disease had surgery to create a colostomy. Which finding should alert the nurse to notify the health care provider (HCP) **immediately**?
    ☐ 1. 3-cm increase in abdominal circumference
    ☐ 2. periods of occasional fussiness
    ☐ 3. absence of bowel sounds since surgery
    ☐ 4. appearance of a bright red stoma

Answers, Rationales, and Test-Taking Strategies

*The answers and rationales for each question follow below, along with keys (🔑) to the client need (CN) and cognitive level (CL) for each question. In addition, questions that measure clinical judgment will be coded (CJ). As you check your answers, use the **Content Mastery and Test-Taking Skill Self-Analysis** worksheet (tear-out worksheet in the back of the book) to identify the reason(s) for not answering the questions correctly. For additional information about test-taking skills and strategies for answering questions, refer to pages 12–51 in Part 1 of this book.*

The Client with Cleft Lip and Palate

1. **1.** An infant with a cleft lip and palate typically swallows large amounts of air while being fed and therefore should be burped frequently. The soft palate defect allows air to be drawn into the pharynx with each swallow of formula. The stomach becomes distended with air, and regurgitation, possibly with aspiration, is likely if the infant is not burped frequently. Feeding frequently, even in small amounts, would not prevent the swallowing of large amounts of air. A nipple placed in the back of the mouth is likely to cause the infant to gag and aspirate. Holding the infant in a supine position during feedings can also lead to regurgitation and aspiration of formula. The infant should be fed in an upright position.

   🔑 CN: Basic care and comfort; CL: Analyze

2. **1.** To keep the infant from disturbing the suture line by placing fingers or other objects in the mouth, either intentionally or accidentally, the restraints should be in place at all times. They should be removed for a short period, however, so that the underlying skin can be checked for any redness or breakdown. The best approach is to remove one restraint, complete the inspection, and reapply before checking the other arm. While the restraints are removed, the parents should be instructed to manually restrain the hands and arms.

   🔑 CN: Safety and infection control; CL: Evaluate

3. **2.** Cleft lips are typically repaired during the first 6 months of life. This allows the child to form a better seal around the nipple of a bottle for feeding and strengthens muscles needed for speech. If the surgery is delayed until after 6 months, the child may have possible dental issues and problems with sucking. The repair is not done at birth because the infant must first gain weight to safely undergo

surgery. The palate should be closed by 18 months to protect the formation of tooth buds and allow the infant to develop more normal speech patterns.

CN: Management of care; CL: Analyze

4. 1. A cup is the preferred drinking or eating utensil after repair of a cleft palate. At the age when repair is done, the child is ordinarily able to drink from a cup. Using a cup avoids having to place a utensil in the mouth, which would increase the potential for injury to the suture lines.

CN: Physiological adaptation; CL: Analyze

The Client with Tracheoesophageal Fistula

5. 3. The drooling and excessive mucus production are highly suggestive of a tracheoesophageal fistula (TEF). The initial diagnosis is made when a nasogastric tube cannot be passed to the stomach. A lactation consultation would be warranted only after determining feedings were safe to continue. While cyanosis can be a sign of sepsis and hypoglycemia, it is most likely related to the excessive secretions and airway patency. A blood gas test may be needed, but only after ruling out a TEF.

CN: Management of care; CL: Analyze

6. 1. The parents of children born with defects often have feelings of guilt and ask what they might have done to cause the condition or how they might have avoided it. It is important to allow parents to express their feelings and accept these feelings as normal reactions. Explaining that the parents are not at fault would not be appropriate until they have dealt with their feelings of guilt. Encouraging long-term planning generally is of little benefit to parents who are emotionally distraught. Additionally, the parents may interpret this as ignoring their feelings and confirming that they played a role in causing their child's anomaly. Urging the parents to visit their infant as often as possible would generally be of little help and could appear to the parents as though they are being "talked out" of their feelings.

CN: Psychosocial integrity; CL: Analyze

7. 2. Although a TEF can include several different structural anomalies, the most common type involves a blind upper pouch and a fistula from the esophagus into the trachea. Other types include a blind pouch at the end of the esophagus with no connection to the trachea and a normal trachea and esophagus with an opening that connects them. A tightened muscle below the stomach and projectile vomiting of normal amounts of formula are characteristic of pyloric stenosis. Aganglionic megacolon is a lack of autonomic parasympathetic ganglion cells in a portion of the lower intestine. Gastroschisis occurs when the bowel herniates through a defect in the abdominal wall and no membrane covers the exposed bowel.

CN: Physiological adaptation; CL: Evaluate

8. 2. With a TEF, an overflow of secretions into the larynx leads to laryngospasm. This obstruction to inspiration stimulates the strong contraction of accessory muscles of the thorax to assist the diaphragm in breathing. This produces substernal retractions. The laryngospasm that occurs with a TEF resolves quickly when secretions are removed from the oropharynx area. A barking cough is related to a relatively constant laryngeal narrowing, usually caused by edema seen with croup. It is not an indication of the need to suction. A decreased activity level and an increased respiratory rate in an infant with a TEF are usually the result of hypoxia, a relatively long-term and constant phenomenon in infants with a TEF.

CN: Physiological adaptation; CL: Analyze

9. 1. The best way to prevent air from entering the stomach when performing a bolus feeding on an infant through a gastrostomy tube is to open the clamp after all the formula has been placed in the syringe barrel. Doing so prevents air from mixing with the formula and thus being introduced into the stomach. Pouring all the formula into the barrel after opening the clamp, maintaining a continuous flow of formula down the side of the barrel after unclamping the tube, and allowing a small amount of formula to enter the stomach before adding more formula to the barrel permit air to enter the stomach.

CN: Reduction of risk potential; CL: Apply

10. 4. When initiating oral feedings after surgical repair of a TEF, it is best to follow a plan of care in conjunction with observation of the infant's needs and behavior, known as *cue-based feedings*. When the nurse follows a strict feeding schedule that overlooks the infant's readiness, plans are likely to be unsatisfactory and are more likely to meet the nurse's needs rather than the infant's needs. After a surgical procedure, infants initially tolerate small amounts of fluids offered more frequently better than larger amounts offered less often. Smaller amounts cause less bloating as the infant becomes used to feeding again. Although infants accept feedings more readily from their parent or from someone who feeds the infant repeatedly, the priority is to meet the infant's nutritional needs based on the infant's behavior.

CN: Basic care and comfort; CL: Apply

The Client with an Anorectal Anomaly

11. 2. The nurse should honor the parent's belief system and help arrange to have the infant baptized. This may be done through the hospital's chaplaincy department or by the family's clergy. The parents may indeed be worried that the infant may die during surgery. Having the infant baptized would help address the family's spiritual needs. At this time, there is an immediate need for chaplaincy, not social service. While surgery may be postponed briefly, the infant cannot begin feeding until an outlet for stool has been established. Therefore, it is not advisable to postpone the surgery for a prolonged period of time.

CN: Psychosocial integrity; CL: Analyze

12. -/+ 1, 3, 4. Anorectal malformations present with a lack of stool or evidence of meconium in the urine through a fistula. Meconium is not found in the stool. Because stool does not pass, abdominal distention and vomiting occur.

CN: Physiological adaptation; CL: Analyze

13. 4. Children who undergo surgical correction for low anorectal anomalies as infants usually are continent. Fecal continence can be expected after successful correction of anal membrane atresia. Therefore, this child probably has a good chance of being potty trained and will not need to wear protective pads. Extra fluids and a high-fiber diet are not required to prevent constipation. Children with high anorectal anomalies may or may not achieve continence.

CN: Physiological adaptation; CL: Evaluate

14. 3. The neonate responds to pain with total body movement and brief, loud crying that ceases with distraction. After the age of 6 months, an infant reacts to pain with intense physical resistance and tries to escape by rolling away. A toddler reacts to pain by withdrawing the affected part.

CN: Basic care and comfort; CL: Apply

15. 2. Encouraging the parents to hold their neonate promotes parent-infant attachment. Parent-infant bonding is based on a relationship that begins when the parent first touches the infant. Both the parents and the infant have predictable steps that they go through in this process. Explaining that the parents can visit at any time promotes bonding only if they do visit with, talk to, and hold the newborn. Asking the parents to help monitor intake and output at this time may be too anxiety producing, thus interfering with bonding. Helping the parents plan for the infant's discharge involves them in the newborn's care and is important. However, it is not the first step in the development of bonding.

CN: Psychosocial integrity; CL: Analyze

The Client with Pyloric Stenosis

16. 3. The vomitus of an infant with hypertrophic pyloric stenosis contains gastric contents, mucus, and streaks of blood. The vomitus does not contain bile or stool because the pyloric constriction is proximal to the ampulla of Vater.

CN: Physiological adaptation; CL: Analyze

17. 1. Unless the infant is in hypovolemic shock, obtaining a baseline weight is an important first action because the weight is used to calculate the child's fluid and electrolyte needs. The intravenous fluid rate and the amounts of electrolytes to be added to the fluid are based on the infant's weight. The weight also helps determine the infant's degree of dehydration. The intravenous infusion is initiated once the weight has been obtained. The child with pyloric stenosis typically experiences vomiting and is at risk for fluid volume deficit and metabolic acidosis. As a result, oral food and fluids are withheld, and the infant is allowed nothing by mouth. Fluid replacement is given intravenously. Orientation can wait until treatment is underway.

CN: Physiological adaptation; CL: Analyze

18. 1. Pyloric stenosis involves hypertrophy of the pylorus muscle distal to the stomach and obstruction of the gastric outlet resulting in vomiting, metabolic acidosis, and dehydration. Telescoping of the bowel is called intussusception. Overfeeding, feeding too quickly, or underfeeding is not associated with pyloric stenosis. The stomach is obstructed, but it is not smaller than normal.

CN: Physiological adaptation; CL: Evaluate

19. 3. Normal serum potassium levels are 3.5 to 4.5 mEq/L (3.5 to 4.5 mmol/L). Elevated potassium levels can cause life-threatening cardiac arrhythmias. The nurse must verify that the client has the ability to clear potassium through urination before administering the drug. Infants with pyloric stenosis frequently have low potassium levels due to vomiting. A level of 3.4 mEq/L (3.4 mmol/L) is not unexpected and should be corrected with the prescribed fluids. The lab value does not need to be redrawn as the findings are consistent with the infant's condition.

CN: Pharmacological and parenteral therapies; CL: Analyze

20. 4. Restating or rephrasing a parent's response provides the opportunity for clarification and validation. It also helps to focus on what the parent is saying and address their concerns and feelings. Although surgery is the most effective treatment for pyloric stenosis, stating this ignores the parent's feelings and does not give them an opportunity to express them. Telling the parent not to worry also ignores the parent's feelings. Additionally, this type of statement gives the parent premature reassurance, which may turn out to be false. Asking the parent if they think the problem indicates that they are not a good parent implies such an idea. It does not allow the parent to express their concerns and feelings and therefore is not a therapeutic response.

CN: Psychosocial integrity; CL: Analyze

21. 1. Clear liquids containing glucose and electrolytes are usually prescribed 4 to 6 hours after surgery. If significant vomiting does not occur, formula or breast milk then can be gradually substituted for clear liquids until the infant is taking normal feedings.

CN: Physiological adaptation; CL: Evaluate

22. 2. The parents' ability to verbalize the infant's care realistically indicates that they are working through their fears and concerns. This behavior demonstrates an understanding of the infant's condition and needs. Without further data, the fact that the parents have to get away could be interpreted as ineffective coping, possibly suggesting that they are unable to handle the situation. Continuing to ask about the child's general condition even after answers have been given does not suggest effective coping. The parents are demonstrating that they are unsure of themselves as parents or are hoping for positive information. Exhibiting fear that they will disturb the infant does not suggest effective coping. This behavior indicates that they are uncertain or lack knowledge about infants.

CN: Psychosocial integrity; CL: Analyze

23. 4. Following pyloromyotomy, the infant should be positioned with the head elevated and slightly on the right side to promote gastric emptying; the parents have positioned their infant correctly. The infant should be positioned on the right side, not the left side. When the child is in a crib, the head can be elevated, and the infant can be propped on the right side. The infant can use a pacifier if needed.

CN: Basic care and comfort; CL: Evaluate

The Client with Intussusception

24. 2. The infant with intussusception experiences acute episodes of colic-like abdominal pain. Typically, the infant screams and draws the knees to the chest. Between these episodes of acute abdominal pain, the infant appears comfortable and normal. Feeding does not precipitate episodes of pain. Additionally, a 4-month-old infant typically would not be ingesting solid foods. Pain exhibited by crying that occurs when the infant is placed in a reclining position, as in the parent's arms, is not associated with intussusception. This type of cry may indicate that the infant wants attention, wants to be held, or needs to have a diaper change.

CN: Physiological adaptation; CL: Analyze

25. 1. For the infant with intussusception, stools characteristically have the appearance of currant jelly because of the intestinal inflammation and hemorrhage resulting from intestinal obstruction. These stools occur later in the course of the disease process. Questions that focus on urination, vomiting, and food intake do not elicit information about the effects of intussusception.

CN: Physiological adaptation; CL: Analyze

26. 1. The first action is to check the placement of the tube to ensure that it is in the correct position. To check tube position, the nurse should aspirate the tube with a syringe. A return of gastric contents indicates that the end of the tube is in the stomach. Another method is to inject a small amount of air while auscultating with a stethoscope over the epigastric area. The tube is irrigated only after the position of the tube is confirmed. The suction level should not be increased because doing so could damage the mucosa. Rotating the tube could irritate or traumatize the nasal mucosa.

CN: Reduction of risk potential; CL: Analyze

27. 2. Development of a paralytic ileus postoperatively is a functional obstruction of the bowel. Bowel sounds initially may be hyperactive, but then they diminish and cease. Measurement of urine specific gravity provides information about fluid and electrolyte status. The first stool and the amount of gastric output provide information about the return of gastric function.

CN: Physiological adaptation; CL: Analyze

The Client with Inguinal Hernia

28. 1. Abdominal distention and redness of the inguinal swelling are significant findings. Their presence in conjunction with area tenderness and inability to reduce the hernia indicate an incarcerated hernia. An incarcerated hernia can lead to strangulation, necrosis, and gangrene of the bowel. Other findings associated with strangulation include irritability, anorexia, and difficulty in defecation. A strangulated hernia necessitates immediate surgical intervention. The ability to reduce the hernia and normal stooling do not indicate it is incarcerated. Irritability is nonspecific and could be caused by various factors. A palpable, thickened spermatic cord on the affected side is diagnostic of inguinal hernia and would be an expected finding. A wet diaper indicates that urine is being excreted, a finding unrelated to inguinal hernia.

CN: Physiological adaptation; CL: Analyze

29. 2. The best way to prepare a 7-month-old infant psychologically for surgery is to have the primary caretaker stay with the child. Infants in the second 6 months of life commonly develop separation anxiety. Therefore, the priority in this case is to support the child by having the parent present. Teaching the parent what to expect may decrease their anxiety; this is important because infants sense anxiety and distress in parents, but the priority in this case is to have the parent present. Actual play and acting out life experiences are appropriate for preschool-age children. Allowing an infant to play with surgical equipment would be inappropriate and dangerous.

CN: Psychosocial integrity; CL: Analyze

30. 3. The incision must be kept as clean and dry as possible. Therefore, daily sponge baths are given for about 1 week postoperatively. The infant can have more than just the face and diaper area cleaned following surgery. Because this type of surgery results in a wound that heals through primary intention, the skin will heal and cover the wound in 2 to 3 days. Therefore, it is not necessary to use sterile gauze to cleanse the incision; clean technique is acceptable. Because the incision must be kept clean and dry, full tub baths are inappropriate.

CN: Reduction of risk potential; CL: Analyze

The Client with Hirschsprung's Disease

31. 2. Infants with Hirschsprung's disease typically display failure to thrive, with poor weight gain due to malabsorption of nutrients. Therefore, the nurse would expect to see a child who weighs less than that expected for height and age. A distended, rather than a scaphoid-shaped, abdomen would be noted. Cyanosis of fingers and toes is associated with congenital heart disease. Hyperactive deep tendon reflexes are associated with upper motor neuron problems, such as cerebral palsy.

CN: Physiological adaptation; CL: Analyze

32. 3. By encouraging parents to ask questions during information-sharing sessions, the nurse can clarify misconceptions and determine the parents' understanding of information. A better understanding of what is happening allows the parents to feel some control over the situation. Assessing the adequacy of the parents' coping skills is important but secondary to encouraging them to express their concerns. The questions they ask and their interactions with the nurse may provide clues to the adequacy of their coping skills. The nurse should never give false reassurance to parents. At this point, there is no way for the nurse to know whether the child will be fine. Written materials are appropriate for augmenting the nurse's verbal communication. However, these are secondary to encouraging questions.

CN: Psychosocial integrity; CL: Analyze

33. 3. The primary defect in Hirschsprung's disease is an absence of autonomic parasympathetic ganglion cells in the distal portion of the colon. Thus, the nerves at the end of the large colon are missing. Constipation is caused by decreased peristalsis, not a physical obstruction like polyps. The colon typically enlarges, giving rise to the name "megacolon" versus being constricted. Weakened areas of the colon are associated with diverticulosis. The absence of a rectal opening refers to an imperforate anus. A tube between the trachea and esophagus refers to a tracheoesophageal fistula. The presence of a tight muscle below the stomach refers to pyloric stenosis.

CN: Physiological adaptation; CL: Evaluate

34. 3. Before intestinal surgery, dietary intake is limited to clear liquids for 24 to 48 hours. A clear liquid diet meets the child's fluid needs and avoids the formation of fecal material in the intestine. Typically, repeated saline enemas, not tap water enemas, are given to empty the bowel. Soapsuds enemas are contraindicated for infants, as are tap water enemas. A nasogastric tube may be inserted for gastric decompression. Insertion of a gastrostomy tube is outside the scope of nursing practice. Because the perineal area is not involved in the surgery, it does not need to be prepared.

CN: Physiological adaptation; CL: Apply

35. In most instances, the absence of ganglionic innervation occurs in the lower portion of the sigmoid colon just above the anus.

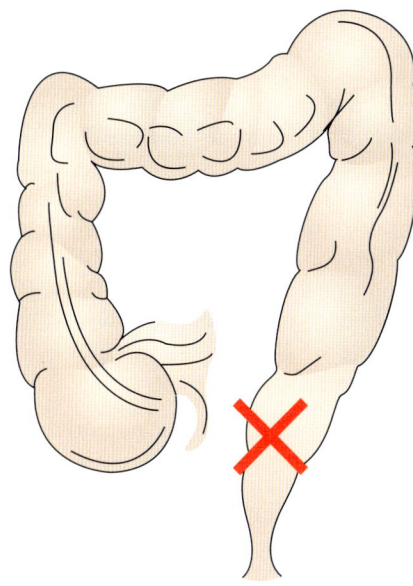

🔑 CN: Physiological adaptation; CL: Apply

36. 2. The goal of the surgery is to remove the aganglionic portion of the intestine. The remaining intestines should have normal innervation. Colostomies are used to relieve the obstruction and allow the remaining intestines to return to normal size. A temporary loop or double-barreled colostomy has stomas for both the proximal and distal portion of the bowel. The final surgical repair is usually done when the infant is around 20 lb (9.1 kg). A new stoma is frequently swollen and bruised after surgery.

🔑 CN: Physiological adaptation; CL: Evaluate

37. 2. Typically, the stoma should remain deep red in color as long as the infant has the colostomy. A dark red to purplish color may indicate impaired circulation to the stoma.

🔑 CN: Physiological adaptation; CL: Apply

38. 4. A regular diet would be recommended for the child with a colostomy; no special diet is needed. A high-fiber diet is not necessary. Fat is necessary for brain growth in the first year of life. A high-residue diet would result in bulkier stools and increased gas production, which will collect in the colostomy bag. Therefore, a high-residue diet is not indicated.

🔑 CN: Basic care and comfort; CL: Apply

39. 2. Toilet training is commonly more difficult for children who have undergone surgery for Hirschsprung's disease than it is for other children. This is because of the trauma to the area and the associated psychological implications. Abdominal distention is an early sign of infection, and therefore the parents need to report it to the health care provider. Typically, dietary restrictions are not required, but fiber is encouraged. Usually, the infant is placed on an age-appropriate diet. Vitamin supplementation is not necessary if the infant's dietary intake is adequate.

🔑 CN: Physiological adaptation; CL: Evaluate

40. 3. Popcorn is high in fiber. Foods high in fiber help the bowels move. Constipation may be managed initially with increased fiber and fluids. White bread, fruit juice, and pancakes are foods that are not high in fiber.

🔑 CN: Health promotion and maintenance; CL: Analyze

The Client with Diarrhea, Gastroenteritis, or Dehydration

41. 3. The infant needs a fluid bolus. A fluid bolus should consist of an isotonic fluid such as normal saline or lactated Ringer's. Dextrose 25% is not an appropriate bolus for dehydrated children because it could cause a fluid shift that may result in cerebral edema and death; thus, the nurse should question the prescription. D5W0.45% normal saline is an appropriate IV fluid for infants. The rate is 1.5 times maintenance for this child and is appropriate for the first 24 hours if the child is dehydrated. Once hydration is adequate, the infant's IV rate should be reduced to a maintenance rate. Vomiting is persistent, so it is appropriate for the child to be NPO. Strict I&O is an appropriate prescription for all dehydrated children.

🔑 CN: Safety and infection control; CL: Analyze

42. 1, 2, 4. Diarrhea in infants is a serious condition as it can proceed rapidly to dehydration. Clinical signs of dehydration are irritability and restlessness, weakness, stupor, loss of body weight, poor skin turgor, and sunken fontanelles. The urine output is decreased in dehydrated infants. The saliva decreases with dehydration and is not frothy.

🔑 CN: Physiologic adaptation; CL: Analyze

43. 1, 2, 4, 5. Shigella is caused by the *Shigella* organism. Clinical manifestations of shigella include fever, nausea and vomiting, some cramping, headache, seizures, rectal prolapse, and loose, watery stools containing pus, mucus, and blood. The nurse should assess the child for these symptoms on an ongoing basis. Shigella is spread via direct contact with the organism, which is found in the stool. A stool specimen will show increased numbers of WBCs, blood, and mucus. Vomiting and loose stools can result in severe dehydration and electrolyte imbalance. Thus, the nurse should record intake, output, and daily weights. There is no need for strict isolation; masks are not needed as shigella is not transmitted by airborne methods.

🔑 CN: Physiological adaptation; CL: Analyze

44. 3. The absence of tears is typically found when moderate dehydration is observed as the body attempts to conserve fluids. Other typical findings associated with moderate dehydration include a dry mouth, sunken eyes, poor skin turgor, and an increased pulse rate. Deep, rapid respirations are associated with severe dehydration. Decreased perspiration, not diaphoresis, would be seen with moderate dehydration. The specific gravity of urine increases with decreased output in the presence of dehydration.

🔑 CN: Reduction of risk potential; CL: Analyze

45. 4. An infant with severe diarrhea will experience some degree of dehydration. In an 8-month-old child, the anterior fontanelle has not closed. Therefore, a depressed anterior fontanelle would be an important finding. Additionally, the infant would exhibit dry mucous membranes, lethargy, hyperactive bowel sounds, dark urine, and sunken eyeballs. Skin turgor would be decreased or delayed (e.g., slow to return when pinched). Bowel sounds every 5 seconds would not be considered abnormal for an infant.

🔑 CN: Reduction of risk potential; CL: Analyze

46. 2. Because an infant experiencing severe diarrhea is at high risk for a fluid volume deficiency, the nurse needs to evaluate the infant's fluid balance status by weighing the infant at least every day. Body weight is the best indicator of hydration status because a higher proportion of an infant's body weight is water, compared with an adult. Initially, the infant with severe diarrhea is not allowed liquids but is given fluids intravenously. Therefore, monitoring the oral intake of formula is inappropriate. Although checking the anterior fontanelle for depression or bulging provides information about hydration status, this method is not considered the best indicator of the infant's fluid balance. Monitoring skin turgor can provide information about fluid volume status. The abdomen is commonly used to assess skin turgor in an infant because it is a large surface area and can be accessed quickly. However, weight is the best indicator of fluid balance.

🔑 CN: Physiological adaptation; CL: Analyze

47. 8.2 mL per hour

$$4.1 \text{ kg} \times 2 \text{ mL/kg} = 8.2 \text{ mL/h}$$

🔑 CN: Pharmacological and parenteral therapies; CL: Apply

48. 2. The child is dehydrated, is not able to retain oral fluids, and continues to have diarrhea. A normal saline bolus should be given followed by maintenance of IV fluids. Antidiarrheal medications are not recommended for children and will prolong the illness. The child has gastroenteritis caused by a viral illness. IV antibiotics are not indicated for viral illnesses. Maintaining strict intake and output is important in all children with gastroenteritis.

🔑 CN: Reduction of risk potential; CL: Apply

49. 1. Typically, an infant hospitalized with severe diarrhea receives fluid replacement intravenously rather than orally. Oral fluids and food are usually withheld. Although activities such as placing a mobile over the crib, speaking to the infant, or turning on the television may provide distraction for or help in calming the infant, a fussy infant receiving nothing by mouth is usually best comforted by providing a pacifier to satisfy sucking needs.

🔑 CN: Health promotion and maintenance; CL: Analyze

50. 2. Given this infant's history of gastroenteritis, the priority problem would be fluid volume deficit. With gastroenteritis, vomiting and diarrhea occur, leading to the loss of fluids. This loss of fluids is problematic in infants because a higher proportion of their body weight is water. Pain is not a priority problem, though the nurse should continue to assess the infant for pain. There are no data to indicate impaired parenting. Impaired urinary elimination is related to the infant's fluid volume deficit resulting from vomiting and diarrhea associated with gastroenteritis. If the infant's fluid volume deficit is not corrected, this nursing diagnosis may become the priority.

🔑 CN: Physiological adaptation; CL: Analyze

51. 1. The usual way to treat an infant hospitalized with gastroenteritis is to keep the infant on nothing-by-mouth status to rest the gastrointestinal tract. The resulting fluid volume deficit is treated with intravenous fluids. When the infant's condition is controlled (e.g., when vomiting subsides), clear liquids are then started slowly. Formula and juice will be started once the infant's vomiting has subsided and the infant has demonstrated the ability to tolerate clear liquids for a period of time. In this situation, there is no need to test the infant's blood every day for anemia. Most likely, the infant's serum electrolyte levels would be monitored closely. Typically, an infant is placed in a private room because gastroenteritis is most commonly caused by a virus that is easily transmitted to others.

CN: Physiological adaptation; CL: Evaluate

52. 2. The nurse's best course of action would be to support the parent. This is best done by conveying understanding and encouraging the parent to visit or call. Telling the parent that they should not leave and that the child is very sick is critical and insensitive. Additionally, it implies guilt should the parent leave. Commenting that the child does not need anyone is not appropriate or true. Toddlers, in particular, need family members present because of the stresses associated with hospitalization. They experience separation anxiety, a normal aspect of development, and need constancy in their environment. Asking the parent to find someone else to stay with their other children is inappropriate. The children at home also need the support of the parent or other family members to minimize the disruptions in family life resulting from the toddler's hospitalization and to maintain consistency.

CN: Psychosocial integrity; CL: Analyze

53. 1, 3, 5. Accurate intake and output recording includes noting all intake, including intravenous fluids; noting output, such as emesis and stool; weighing diapers; measuring weight daily; measuring urine specific gravity; monitoring serum electrolytes; and monitoring for signs of dehydration. Children who are dehydrated must receive sufficient fluid intake, but having a breastfeeding child switch to bottle-feeding will not promote intake. Restricting fluids just prior to weighing the child will not alter the accuracy of the weight, and the nurse should continue to encourage fluids for this dehydrated child.

CN: Management of care; CL: Analyze

54. 1. Potassium chloride is readily excreted in the urine. Before hanging IV fluids with potassium chloride, the nurse should ascertain whether the child can void; if not, potassium chloride may build up in the serum and cause hyperkalemia. An electrocardiogram could be done during intravenous potassium replacement therapy to evaluate for these changes. Having a stool daily is important, but because potassium is primarily excreted in the urine, the child's ability to void must be verified. Serum calcium levels do not indicate the child's ability to tolerate potassium replacement.

CN: Pharmacological and parenteral therapies; CL: Analyze

55. 3. An early sign of circulatory overload is moist rales or crackles heard when auscultating over the chest wall. Elevated blood pressure, engorged neck veins, a wide variation between fluid intake and output (with a higher intake than output), shortness of breath, increased respiratory rate, dyspnea, and cyanosis occur later.

CN: Reduction of risk potential; CL: Analyze

56. 1. Dietary management following rehydration for diarrhea and mild dehydration would include offering the child a regular diet. Following rehydration, there is no need for the child to be on a special diet, such as a clear liquid, full liquid, or soft diet.

CN: Basic care and comfort; CL: Evaluate

57. 3. Diarrhea related to *Salmonella* bacilli is commonly spread by raw or undercooked fowl and eggs, pet turtles, and kittens. Food poisoning caused by *Staphylococcus* species is commonly spread by inadequately cooked or refrigerated custards, cream fillings, or mayonnaise. Psittacosis, a respiratory illness, may be spread by canaries. Contaminated, unwashed fruit is associated with typhoid fever (caused by *Salmonella typhi*), a disorder rarely seen in the United States.

CN: Physiological adaptation; CL: Analyze

58. 3. The "no" behavior demonstrated by a toddler is typical of this age group as the child attempts to be self-assertive as an individual. The negativism does not demonstrate an inherited personality trait or disinterest. Rather, it reflects the developmental task of establishing autonomy. The toddler is attempting to exert control over the environment. It is too early to assess leadership qualities in a toddler.

CN: Health promotion and maintenance; CL: Analyze

59. 1. The child is demonstrating behavior associated with temper tantrums, which are relatively frequent normal occurrences during toddlerhood as the child attempts to develop a sense of autonomy. The development of autonomy requires opportunities for the child to make decisions and express individuality. Ignoring the outbursts is probably the best strategy. Doing so avoids rewarding the behavior and helps the child to learn limits, promoting the development of self-control. However, the parent should intervene in a temper tantrum if the child is likely to injure themselves. Allowing the child to have what they want occasionally would typically add to the problems associated with temper tantrums because doing so rewards the behavior and prevents the child from developing self-control. Toddlers do not possess the capacity to understand explanations about behavior. Expressing disappointment in the child's behavior or telling them that they are being bad reinforces feelings of guilt and shame, thus interfering with the child's ability to develop a sense of autonomy.

CN: Health promotion and maintenance; CL: Evaluate

60. **1.** Hospitalization is a traumatic time for a child, and it takes some time to readjust to the home environment. The child may regress at home for a period until they feel comfortable. Children normally do not dislike their home environment; in fact, they usually are eager to get home to familiar surroundings where they feel safe.

CN: Health promotion and maintenance; CL: Analyze

The Client with Appendicitis

61. **2, 1, 4, 3.** The nurse should first inspect the abdomen for abnormalities. Auscultation should be done before percussion and palpation as vigorous touching may disturb the intestines. Percussion is next. Palpation is the last step as it is most likely to cause pain.

CN: Basic care and comfort; CL: Apply

62.

STEP 1

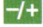

Admission Note

1130
The client has been vomiting for 2 days. They report generalized abdominal pain with rebound tenderness when palpated by the health care provider, and they rate their pain as an 8 on a 0 to 10 scale. The client has a history of COVID-19 infection 6 months ago with minor symptoms and a past hospitalization for a right supracondylar fracture with surgical pin placement 4 months ago following a fall from a trampoline. All immunizations are up to date. Vital signs are temperature (T) 103°F (39.4°C); (P) pulse 144 bpm; (RR) respiration rate 32 breaths/min; blood pressure (BP) 110/60 mm Hg; and oxygenation 96% on room air.

A child with new onset of fever, nausea, vomiting, and generalized abdominal pain rated as an 8 on a 10-point scale should be further assessed for abdominal infections, including appendicitis. Tachycardia (heart rate greater than 140 bpm) and tachypnea (respiration rate greater than 30 breaths/min) often accompany fever in children. Rebound tenderness occurs when a child feels relatively mild pain when the abdomen is palpated but develops acute pain once an examiner's hand is withdrawn. This is due to abdominal contents shifting and is associated with peritonitis. The child's history of a broken arm and minor COVID-19 symptoms are irrelevant to the current situation. Blood pressure and oxygen saturation are normal findings for a 10-year-old.

CJ: Case study; Step 1: Recognize cues; CL: Analyze

63.

STEP 2

1, 2, 3, 4, 6. An abdominal ultrasound can be used to visualize a swollen appendix. Clients can report constipation or diarrhea with appendicitis. Bowel sounds are typically reduced with appendicitis and may be absent if peritonitis is present. A complete blood count will most likely reveal leukocytosis with appendicitis. Pain initially presents as diffuse and gradually becomes localized to the right lower quadrant. The point of sharpest pain is often one-third of the way between the anterior superior iliac crest and the umbilicus, called *McBurney's point*. Occult fecal blood is used to determine cancer risk. Stool cultures are used to determine the source of infection with gastroenteritis.

CJ: Case study; Step 2: Analyze cues; CL: Apply

64.

STEP 3

The client's top risk if treatment is delayed is **peritonitis**.

The appendix is likely to rupture if surgery is delayed, and infection can spread in the abdomen, causing peritonitis. Antibiotics should be initiated preoperatively to help decrease the risk of widespread infection. The risk for bleeding tends to be greater after surgery. A ruptured appendix can be associated with bowel necrosis, but this complication is much rarer than peritonitis or abscesses. IV fluids will be given before surgery, which helps mitigate the risk of hypovolemic shock.

CJ: Case study; Step 3: Prioritize hypothesis; CL: Analyze

65.

STEP 4

Intervention	Anticipated	Not Anticipated
Administer antibiotics	X	
Apply a heating pad		X
Insert a peripheral IV	X	
Insert a nasogastric tube		X
Obtain a urine specimen	X	
Position the client supine		X

The nurse anticipates giving antibiotics preoperatively based on the client's elevated white blood cell count and peritonitis risk. Routine preoperative care includes obtaining a urinalysis and inserting an IV. The use of a heating pad is contraindicated because it can cause the appendix to rupture. If a nasogastric tube is needed, it will be placed in surgery when the child is anesthetized. The child should be placed in a semi-Fowler's position to increase comfort and ease of breathing and to facilitate drainage should the appendix rupture.

🔑 CJ: Case study; Step 4: Generate solutions; CL: Apply

66.
STEP 5

2, 4. The ordered dose of morphine will be less than a full vial. Disposal of waste of a controlled substance should be witnessed by two licensed health care providers. Children receiving narcotics are at high risk for respiratory suppression. Thus, their cardiorespiratory and oxygen saturation status should be continuously monitored.

The correct dose of morphine for this child is 0.75 mL. If morphine is given via IV push, it must be given slowly over at least 5 minutes to decrease the risk of respiratory depression. A preferable method is to administer the drug on a syringe pump. The FLACC pain scale is a behavioral scale to assess pain for younger children when a child cannot give input. The 0-to-10 pain numeric intensity scale was used before surgery and would be preferred for a 10-year-old who can provide a subjective rating.

🔑 CJ: Case study; Step 5: Take action; CL: Apply

67.
STEP 6

> **Nurses' Note**
>
> **Postoperative day 2, 0700**
> Vital signs are T 101°F (38.3°C); P 156 bpm; RR 50 breaths/min; BP 78/40 mm Hg; and oxygenation 95% on room air. Capillary refill is 4 seconds. Urine output is 0.3 mL/kg per hour. The client appears lethargic but is taking clear liquids. IV lactated Ringer's solution is still infusing at 76 mL per hour in the left arm. There was 5 mL of serosanguinous drainage from the Penrose drain. The client has been taking 3 mg of IV morphine every 3 hours.

A ruptured appendix followed by an invasive appendectomy and subsequent peritonitis can result in bacteremia. Sepsis is the systemic response to bacteremia and is characterized by fever, tachycardia, tachypnea, and urine output less than 1 mL/kg per hour in a pediatric patient. The clinical presentation will also include a change in the level of activity or consciousness. As the sepsis progresses, perfusion decreases, as evidenced by a prolonged capillary refill time (greater than 3 seconds) and falling blood pressure.

An oxygen saturation of 95% in room air is a normal finding. A Penrose drain with 5 mL of serosanguinous drainage is expected during the initial postoperative period. Requiring pain medication every 3 hours on postoperative day 1 is expected.

🔑 CJ: Case study; Step 6: Evaluate outcomes; CL: Evaluate

68. 3. Appendicitis starts as vague abdominal pain. As the disease progresses over the course of a few hours, the pain localizes at McBurney's point midway between the right iliac crest and the umbilicus.

🔑 CN: Reduction of risk potential; CL: Apply

69. 1, 3, 4. Cold is a vasoconstrictor and supplies some degree of anesthesia. The child is usually more comfortable on their side with their legs flexed to take the strain off the inflamed appendix. Limiting the child's activity puts less stress on the inflamed appendix and lessens the discomfort. Heat increases circulation to an area, causing more engorgement and pain and, possibly, rupture of the appendix. Heat is contraindicated in any situation where rupture or perforation is a possibility. A cathartic is contraindicated when appendicitis is suspected. Increasing peristalsis can cause the appendix to rupture.

🔑 CN: Physiological adaptation; CL: Analyze

70. 2. The child is in pain and needs intervention, but before the nurse can determine how to proceed, it is essential to know the severity of the client's pain score to determine whether to give 1 or 2 mg of morphine. In addition, the nurse cannot evaluate the effectiveness of the pain medication if there is no pain score prior to administering the medication. Changing the child's position and administering pain medication may be helpful to relieve the child's pain, but the nurse must first know the severity of the pain before determining the appropriate intervention. The nurse must perform a head-to-toe assessment, but it is not the priority in managing the child's pain.

🔑 CN: Basic care and comfort; CL: Analyze

71. 4. The nurse should use the FACES pain rating scale for children age 3 years or older. The visual analog and numerical scales are used preferred with adults or older children who count well. The FLACC scale is a behavioral scale that is appropriate for very small children or nonverbal children.

🔑 CN: Basic care and comfort; CL: Analyze

72. 1. The nurse should administer the acetaminophen with codeine because the client indicates they are having pain. Although the child reports less severe pain, they are still experiencing pain. The nurse will also want the child to have less pain because they will need to be more active during the day. Assessing the child later will likely cause the pain to have increased and be more difficult to manage. While distraction is appropriate for short-term pain, such as from a needlestick or pain that the child might be able to manage themself, postoperative pain should be relieved with medication.

🔑 CN: Basic care and comfort; CL: Analyze

73. 1. The most helpful question would be to determine the location of the pain when it started. The pain associated with appendicitis usually begins in the periumbilical area and then progresses to the right lower quadrant. After the nurse has determined the location of the pain, asking about what was done for the pain would be appropriate. Asking about the child's usual bowel movement pattern is a general question unrelated to the child's condition. Children with appendicitis may have diarrhea or constipation. Additionally, knowledge about the child's usual pattern would not be a priority because a child with appendicitis typically is not hospitalized long enough to reestablish the normal pattern. Although the characteristics of the pain are important, asking if the pain is continuous or intermittent is vague and general because the pain could be associated with numerous conditions. With appendicitis, the client's pain may begin as intermittent, but it eventually becomes continuous.

CN: Physiological adaptation; CL: Analyze

74. **3.** Application of an ice bag may help relieve pain by decreasing circulation to the area. A heating pad is contraindicated because heat may increase circulation to the appendix, possibly leading to rupture. Rectal tubes are contraindicated because they stimulate bowel motility and can exacerbate abdominal pain. Also, they would be ineffective because an accumulation of gas in the lower bowel is not likely to be the cause of the child's discomfort. Because narcotics can mask the child's symptoms, such as pain and discomfort, and they also decrease bowel motility, they are not given until after a definitive diagnosis has been made.

CN: Physiological adaptation; CL: Apply

75. **2.** Manifestations of appendicitis include decreased or absent bowel sounds. Normally, bowel sounds are heard every 10 to 30 seconds. Therefore, bowel sounds heard twice in 2 minutes suggest appendicitis. Normally, the contour of the male adolescent abdomen is flat to slightly rounded, and tympany is typically heard when auscultating over most of the abdomen. A cremasteric reflex is normal for male adolescents.

CN: Physiological adaptation; CL: Analyze

76. **1.** Sudden relief of pain in a client with appendicitis may indicate that the appendix has ruptured. Rupture relieves the pressure within the appendix but spreads the infection to the peritoneal cavity. Periumbilical pain (pain centered around the navel), vomiting, and abdominal tenderness on palpation are common findings associated with appendicitis.

CN: Physiological adaptation; CL: Analyze

77. **43 mL per hour.** Fluid needs are calculated for the first 10 kg at 4 mL/kg per hour. The next 1.6 kg are calculated at 2 mL/kg per hour.

(10 kg × 4 mL/kg per hour) + (1.6 kg × 2 mL/kg per hour) =
= 40 mL per hour + 3.2 mL per hour
= 43.2 mL per hour.
Round to 43 mL per hour per rounding instructions.

CN: Pharmacological and parenteral therapies; CL: Apply

78. **1.** The priority assessment after an appendectomy would be the dressing over the surgical site to determine whether there is any drainage or bleeding. If the procedure was done laparoscopically, there may be more than one incision. Any surgical dressings should be clean, dry, and intact. Once the dressing has been assessed, the nurse would assess the intravenous infusion site, and assess the NG tube to be sure it is functioning. Finally, the nurse would assess the bowel sounds, expecting them to be absent or greatly diminished.

CN: Physiological adaptation; CL: Analyze

79. **2.** After an appendectomy, the client who develops peritonitis typically has an NG tube in place. When a client has nausea, the nurse would first check to ensure that the NG tube is functioning correctly because the client's nausea may be related to a blockage of the NG tube. If the tube is clogged, it can be irrigated with normal saline. An antiemetic may be given, but only after the nurse has determined that the NG tube is functioning properly. Postoperative prescriptions usually include an antiemetic. Typically, the nurse would notify the surgeon if the client did not obtain relief from irrigation of the NG tube or administration of a prescribed antiemetic. Although taking the client's blood pressure is an important postoperative nursing activity, it is unrelated to relieving the client's nausea.

CN: Physiological adaptation; CL: Analyze

80. **1.** After an appendectomy for a ruptured appendix, assuming semi-Fowler's or a right side-lying position helps localize the infection. These positions promote drainage from the peritoneal cavity and decrease the incidence of subdiaphragmatic abscesses.

CN: Physiological adaptation; CL: Analyze

81. **2.** Adolescents are concerned about the immediate state and functioning of their bodies. The adolescent needs to know whether any changes (e.g., illness, trauma, surgery) will alter their lifestyle or interfere with their quest for physical perfection. Having a scar may be devastating to the adolescent. The need for plastic surgery cannot be determined at this point. The adolescent has just returned from surgery and has yet to see the scar. Healing has yet to occur. Typically, scars

become smaller and fade over time. The desire for no pain is unrealistic. Although adolescents are worried about pain and how they will respond, they typically are discharged within 24 hours after an appendectomy with pain well controlled by oral analgesics. The immediate concern of adolescents is the state and functioning of their bodies. After concerns about themselves, then adolescents are concerned about their peer group and their responses. Although friends' responses will matter, this concern would be more common later in the course of the adolescent's recovery.

 CN: Health promotion and maintenance; CL: Analyze

82. 1. Adolescents struggle for independence and identity, needing to feel in control of situations and conform to peers. Control and conformity are often manifested in appearance, including clothing, and this carries over into the hospital experience. An adolescent feels best when they are able to look and act as they normally do, for example, wearing a T-shirt and gym shorts. Adolescents normally want to interact with peers and commonly seek every opportunity to do so. Avoiding other adolescents on the nursing unit or not taking phone calls from friends might suggest ineffective coping behavior. Refusing to fill out the menu and allowing the nurse to do so demonstrate dependent behavior, not a healthy coping mechanism.

 CN: Psychosocial integrity; CL: Analyze

83. 2. Part of providing client-centered care is to honor the client's preferred method of learning. The nurse should help the adolescent find accurate information about the procedure. By assisting with the information search, the nurse can verify learning. Teaching straight from a checklist does not encourage customization. If the client has requested to use the internet, it is unlikely that written information will be read. While it is true that some information on the internet is not accurate, the nurse can take this opportunity to help the client learn how to determine if a source is reliable.

 CN: Psychosocial integrity; CL: Analyze

Managing Care, Quality, and Safety of Children with Health Problems of the Gastrointestinal Tract

84. 2, 3, 1, 4. Deciding what to study and how to do it is part of the planning process. Collecting data through chart audits is part of the "do" phase. Once the chart audits are complete, the data may be "studied" or analyzed. The final step of the process, or the "act" phase, is to determine what should be done, which may include writing a new policy.

 CN: Reduction of risk potential; CL: Analyze

85. 3. Published national standards are based on the best evidence and, when available, should serve as the foundation for nursing unit policies. Policies from other hospitals may or may not be evidence based. Retrospective studies and expert opinions should only be used to form policy when data from experimental studies or national standards are not available.

 CN: Reduction of risk potential; CL: Analyze

86. 3. It is the responsibility of all health care members to protect the client. The team member may honestly not have realized that the glove was contaminated. Therefore, the nurse needs to alert the team member to the situation. Waiting until after the procedure to address the problem puts the child at unnecessary risk for infection. Asking the parents to leave could invoke anxiety in both the child and the parents. Alerting the team member does not need to be confrontational. If done with a calm approach, the result is most likely to be gratitude instead of embarrassment.

 CN: Reduction of risk potential; CL: Analyze

87. 2. The charge nurse can anticipate needing beds for incoming victims. Any client who can go home should go home. Parents are a child's primary caregivers and should not be asked to leave. If computers were not affected by the disaster, charting in the electronic health record is safer. Some routine procedures are altered during a disaster, but clients who are unstable will still need frequent assessments; reducing vital sign frequency must be considered on a case-to-case basis.

 CN: Management of care; CL: Analyze

88. 1. Abdominal circumference is measured to monitor for abdominal distention. An increase of 3 cm in 8 hours would require notification of the HCP because it would indicate a substantial degree of abdominal distention, possibly from fluid or gas accumulation. Normally, after surgery, an infant experiences occasional periods of fussiness. However, as long as the infant is able to be quiet by themselves or with the aid of a pacifier, the HCP does not need to be contacted. The absence of bowel sounds would be expected after surgery because of the effects of anesthesia. It takes approximately 48 hours for gastric motility to resume. New stomas are typically bright red or pink.

 CN: Reduction of risk potential; CL: Analyze

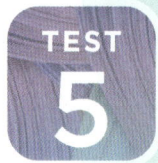

TEST 5: The Child with Health Problems Involving Ingestion, Nutrition, or Diet

- The Client with Toxic Substance Ingestion
- The Client with Lead Poisoning
- The Client with Celiac Disease
- The Client with Phenylketonuria
- The Client with Colic
- The Client with Obesity
- The Client with Food Sensitivity
- The Client with Failure to Thrive
- Managing Care, Quality, and Safety of Children with Health Problems Involving Ingestion, Nutrition, or Diet
- Answers, Rationales, and Test-Taking Strategies

The Client with Toxic Substance Ingestion

1. A toddler is brought to the emergency department after ingesting an undetermined amount of drain cleaner. The nurse should expect to implement which intervention **first**?
   - ☐ 1. administering an emetic
   - ☐ 2. securing the airway
   - ☐ 3. performing gastric lavage
   - ☐ 4. inserting an indwelling urinary catheter

2. The nurse cares for a child after the acute stage following ingestion of drain cleaner. The nurse should be alert for the development of which likely complication?
   - ☐ 1. tracheal stenosis
   - ☐ 2. tracheal varices
   - ☐ 3. esophageal strictures
   - ☐ 4. esophageal diverticula

3. The parents of a preschooler suspect that the child has recently ingested a large amount of acetaminophen. The child does not appear in immediate distress. The nurse should anticipate doing which intervention in order of priority, from first to last? All options must be used.

| 1. Draw acetaminophen serum levels. |
| 2. Determine the time and amount of drug ingested. |
| 3. Administer acetylcysteine intravenously. |
| 4. Administer activated charcoal. |
| |
| |
| |
| |

4. The nurse develops the plan of care for a toddler with an acetaminophen overdose. Which intervention should the nurse expect to include as part of the initial treatment?
☐ 1. frequent serum drug levels
☐ 2. gastric lavage
☐ 3. tracheostomy
☐ 4. electrocardiogram

5. The nurse assesses a preschooler brought by their parents to the emergency department after ingestion of kerosene. The nurse should be alert for which complication?
☐ 1. uremia
☐ 2. hepatitis
☐ 3. carditis
☐ 4. pneumonitis

The Client with Lead Poisoning

6. In an initial screening for lead poisoning, a toddler is found to have a minimally elevated lead level. What is the **most** important action the nurse should take?
☐ 1. Arrange a follow-up appointment in 6 months.
☐ 2. Obtain a consultation for chelation therapy.
☐ 3. Educate parents on ways to reduce lead in the environment.
☐ 4. Assure the parents this is not an unexpected finding.

7. The nurse teaches the parent of a toddler diagnosed with lead poisoning about the importance of adherence to the treatment plan. What should the nurse include as the **most** serious complication if the condition goes untreated?
☐ 1. liver cirrhosis
☐ 2. stunted growth
☐ 3. neurologic deficits
☐ 4. heart failure

8. The nurse is teaching dietary interventions to the parents of a child with an elevated blood lead level (EBLL). The nurse recognizes the need for more teaching when the parent makes which statement?
☐ 1. "Diets high calcium help prevent lead from depositing in the body."
☐ 2. "The body is less likely to absorb lead if iron intake is high."
☐ 3. "Adequate intake of vitamin A helps keep lead out of fatty tissues."
☐ 4. "Vitamin C deficiencies increase the risk for lead toxicity."

The Client with Celiac Disease

9. The nurse is conducting a health history on a school-age child. Which parent statement would suggest to the nurse that a child may have celiac disease?
☐ 1. "Their urine is so dark in color."
☐ 2. "Their stools are large and smelly."
☐ 3. "Their belly is so small."
☐ 4. "They are so short."

10. The nurse assesses a child with celiac disease. The nurse would **most** likely note which physical finding?
☐ 1. enlarged liver
☐ 2. protuberant abdomen
☐ 3. tender inguinal lymph nodes
☐ 4. periorbital edema

11. The nurse is teaching the parent of a child with celiac disease about dietary management. Which statement by the parent indicates successful teaching?
"I will:
☐ 1. feed my child foods that contain wheat products."
☐ 2. be sure to give my child lots of milk."
☐ 3. plan to feed my child foods that contain rice."
☐ 4. be sure my child gets oatmeal every day."

12. The nurse is teaching the parent of a preschool-age child with celiac disease about a gluten-free diet. The nurse determines that teaching has been successful when the parent tells the nurse they will prepare which breakfast for the child?
☐ 1. eggs and orange juice
☐ 2. wheat toast and grape jelly
☐ 3. oatmeal and skim milk
☐ 4. rye toast and peanut butter

13. The nurse teaches a parent about caring for a 12-month-old child newly diagnosed with celiac disease. Which food would be **most** appropriate to include in the child's diet?
☐ 1. oatmeal
☐ 2. pancakes
☐ 3. rice cereal
☐ 4. waffles

The Client with Phenylketonuria

14. The nurse prepares to obtain a neonatal screening test for phenylketonuria (PKU). The nurse understands that the neonate must have been fed what to ensure reliable results?
☐ 1. iron-rich formula
☐ 2. nothing by mouth for 4 hours before the test
☐ 3. initial formula or breast milk at least 24 hours before the test
☐ 4. glucose water

15. The nurse takes a diet history from the parent of a 7-year-old child with phenylketonuria. A report of an intake of which food should cause the nurse to gather additional information?
☐ 1. diet cola
☐ 2. carrots
☐ 3. orange juice
☐ 4. bananas

16. The nurse teaches the parent of a child diagnosed with phenylketonuria (PKU) about its transmission. The nurse should understand which factor as the basis for the discussion?
☐ 1. chromosome translocation
☐ 2. chromosome deletion
☐ 3. autosomal recessive gene
☐ 4. X-linked recessive gene

17. A newborn diagnosed with phenylketonuria (PKU) is placed on a low-phenylalanine formula. The parent asks the nurse how long their infant will need to have a dietary restriction. Which response would be **most** appropriate?
☐ 1. "Your baby needs to stay on low-phenylalanine formula until they are taking solid foods well."
☐ 2. "Once your child has stopped growing, they can come off the phenylalanine restricted diet."
☐ 3. "Your child can switch to a regular diet when phenylalanine levels remain normal for 6 months."
☐ 4. "Most likely your child will need to follow a low-phenylalanine diet for the rest of their life."

18. Even though several teaching sessions have been documented in the client's health record, the parent asks the nurse again what caused their child's phenylketonuria (PKU). Which statement would **best** reflect the nurse's interpretation of why the parent keeps asking for information they have already received?
☐ 1. Because the child's condition is chronic, parents commonly want very detailed explanations about the causes of and treatments for their child's disease.
☐ 2. Parents of a chronically ill child commonly require a long time to work through the grieving process for their child's disease.
☐ 3. Parents commonly test health workers' knowledge about the causes of and treatments for their child's disease.
☐ 4. Parents commonly deal with their guilt about possibly causing their child's disease by asking challenging questions.

The Client with Colic

19. A parent reports that they think their infant has colic. Which information should the nurse obtain **next** from the parent?
☐ 1. the type of formula the infant is taking
☐ 2. the infant's crying pattern
☐ 3. the infant's sleep position
☐ 4. the position of the infant during burping

20. The parents of a child with colic are asked to describe the infant's bowel movements. Which description should the nurse expect?
☐ 1. soft, yellow stools
☐ 2. frequent watery stools
☐ 3. ribbon-like stools
☐ 4. foul-smelling stools

21. The parent tells the nurse that the diagnosis of colic upsets them because they know the infant will continue to have colicky pain. Which response by the nurse would be **most** appropriate?
☐ 1. "I know that your baby's crying upsets you, but they need your undivided attention for the next few months."
☐ 2. "It can be difficult to listen to your baby cry so loud and so long, so try to make sure that you get some free time."
☐ 3. "It must be distressing to see your baby in pain, but at least they do not have an intestinal obstruction."
☐ 4. "The next 3 months will be a difficult time for you, but your baby will outgrow the colic by this time."

22. The nurse teaches a parent about feeding an infant with colic. The nurse determines that the parent has understood the teaching when the nurse observes the parent doing which action?
☐ 1. holding the infant prone while feeding
☐ 2. holding the infant in their lap to burp
☐ 3. placing the infant prone after the feeding
☐ 4. burping the infant during and after the feeding

The Client with Obesity

23. An 8-year-old is found to have a body mass index (BMI) for age at the 90th percentile at a well-child checkup. What action should the take?
☐ 1. Assess the child for the presence of diabetes or metabolic syndrome.
☐ 2. Recommend the child be reweighed in 1 year.
☐ 3. Refer the child to a pediatric weight loss specialist.
☐ 4. Recommend the child participate in a commercial diet program.

24. A parent brings a 7-month-old infant to the well-baby clinic for a check-up. The parent feeds the infant formula whenever the infant is hungry but is concerned that the infant is overweight. What instructions should the nurse give the parent?
    ☐ 1. Give the infant 2% milk formula, and add vitamins.
    ☐ 2. Use skim milk because it is high in protein and lower in calories.
    ☐ 3. Decrease the amount of formula feedings to 16 oz (480 mL) daily and supplement with juice and water.
    ☐ 4. Bring a 3-day record of the infant's intake back for further evaluation.

25. The nurse is providing nutrition counseling for an obese adolescent. What is the **most** effective way for the nurse to obtain a nutrition history from this client?
    ☐ 1. Ask the client what they know about good nutrition.
    ☐ 2. Tell the client to list what they plan to eat for the next 24 hours.
    ☐ 3. Ask the client what they ate yesterday if it was a typical day.
    ☐ 4. Telephone the parent, and ask what the client ate yesterday.

26. The nurse counsels an obese adolescent. The nurse should advise the client that which complication is the **most** common?
    ☐ 1. lifelong obesity
    ☐ 2. gastrointestinal problems
    ☐ 3. orthopedic problems
    ☐ 4. psychosocial problems

27. The nurse develops a teaching plan for the parent of an infant about introducing solid foods into the diet. The nurse should expect to include which measure in the plan to help prevent obesity?
    ☐ 1. decreasing the amount of formula or breast milk intake as solid food intake increases
    ☐ 2. introducing the infant to the taste of vegetables by mixing them with formula or breast milk
    ☐ 3. mixing cereal and fruit in a bottle when offering solid food for the first few times
    ☐ 4. thin cereal with juice during the first several months

28. A pregnant parent who has brought their toddler to the clinic for a checkup asks the nurse how they can keep their next baby from becoming obese. The parent plans to bottle-feed the next child. Which information should the nurse include in the teaching plan to help the parent avoid over nourishing the infant?
    ☐ 1. recognizing clues indicating that the baby is full
    ☐ 2. establishing a regular feeding schedule
    ☐ 3. supplementing feedings with sterile water
    ☐ 4. adding more water than directed when preparing formula

The Client with Food Sensitivity

29. During a school party, a child with a known food allergy has an itchy throat, is wheezing, and is not feeling "quite right." The nurse should do what in order from first to last? All options must be used.

    | 1. Administer the child's epinephrine. |
    | 2. Assess vital signs. |
    | 3. Position to facilitate breathing. |
    | 4. Send someone to activate the emergency medical system (EMS). |
    | 5. Notify the parents. |

30. The nurse teaches the parents of a child with lactose intolerance about the disorder. The nurse determines that the teaching was effective when the parent uses which statement to describe the condition?
    "Lactose intolerance refers to:
    ☐ 1. the lack of an enzyme to break down lactose."
    ☐ 2. an allergy to lactose found in milk."
    ☐ 3. an inability to digest proteins completely."
    ☐ 4. an inability to digest fats completely."

31. The breastfeeding parent of a 1-month-old diagnosed with cow's milk sensitivity asks the nurse what they should do about feeding their infant. Which recommendation would be **most** appropriate?
    ☐ 1. "Continue to breastfeed, but eliminate all milk products from your own diet."
    ☐ 2. "Discontinue breastfeeding, and start using a predigested formula."
    ☐ 3. "Limit breastfeeding to once per day, and begin feeding an iron-fortified formula."
    ☐ 4. "Change to a soy-based formula exclusively, and begin solid foods."

32. The nurse teaches the parents of a preschool child diagnosed with lactose intolerance how to incorporate dairy products into their child's diet. Which statement by the parent reflects the need for more teaching?
  ☐ 1. "My child should limit milk consumption to one small glass at a time."
  ☐ 2. "It is best to drink milk alone, not with meals."
  ☐ 3. "Eating hard cheese, cottage cheese, or yogurt may cause fewer symptoms than drinking milk."
  ☐ 4. "Using lactase enzymes or milk products containing lactase may help decrease gas."

The Client with Failure to Thrive

33. The nurse is inserting a nasogastric tube in an infant to administer feedings. In the figure below, indicate the location for the correct placement of the distal end of the tube.

34. The nurse formulates a plan of care to address negative feeding patterns for a 5-month-old infant diagnosed with failure to thrive. To meet the short-term outcomes of the infant's plan of care, the nurse should expect to implement which intervention(s)? Select all that apply.
  ☐ 1. Observe the parent-child interactions.
  ☐ 2. Instruct the parents on proper feeding techniques.
  ☐ 3. Give the infant high-calorie formula.
  ☐ 4. Provide support to decrease parental anxiety.
  ☐ 5. Allow the infant to sit in a highchair during feedings.

35. The health care team determines that the family of an infant with failure to thrive who is to be discharged will need follow-up care. Which approach would be the **most** effective method of follow-up?
  ☐ 1. daily phone calls from the hospital nurse
  ☐ 2. enrollment in community parenting classes
  ☐ 3. twice-weekly clinic appointments
  ☐ 4. weekly visits by a community health nurse

Managing Care, Quality, and Safety of Children with Health Problems Involving Ingestion, Nutrition, or Diet

36. The nurse provides intermittent nasogastric feedings to an infant with failure to thrive. Which method is preferred to confirm tube placement before each feeding?
  ☐ 1. obtaining a bedside chest x-ray
  ☐ 2. verifying that the gastric pH is less than 5.5
  ☐ 3. auscultating the stomach while instilling an air bolus
  ☐ 4. comparing the tube insertion length with a standardized chart

37. The nurse conducts a parent workshop about measures to prevent lead poisoning in children. The nurse should identify which preventive measure as being the **most** effective?
  ☐ 1. condemning old housing developments
  ☐ 2. educating the public on common sources of lead
  ☐ 3. conducting workshops on the importance of good nutrition
  ☐ 4. keeping pregnant women out of old homes that are being remodeled

38. A child with a nut allergy presents with a severe reaction for the third time in 3 months. The parent says, "I'm having trouble with the food labels." What should the nurse do **first**?
  ☐ 1. Assess the parent's ability to read.
  ☐ 2. Refer the client to the dietician.
  ☐ 3. Notify the health care provider (HCP).
  ☐ 4. Obtain a social service consult.

39. During an admission history, the parents of a pediatric client explain that the family is Jewish and follows a kosher diet. Which food items would **most likely** be appropriate for the client?
  ☐ 1. sausage and pepperoni pizza and a glass of milk
  ☐ 2. bacon and eggs and a glass of orange juice
  ☐ 3. chicken, a cup of fruit, and a glass of water
  ☐ 4. turkey sandwich and a glass of milk

Answers, Rationales, and Test-Taking Strategies

*The answers and rationales for each question follow below, along with keys (🔑) to the client need (CN) and cognitive level (CL) for each question. In addition, questions that measure clinical judgment will be coded (CJ). As you check your answers, use the **Content Mastery and Test-Taking Skill Self-Analysis** worksheet (tear-out worksheet in the back of the book) to identify the reason(s) for not answering the questions correctly. For additional information about test-taking skills and strategies for answering questions, refer to pages 12–51 in Part 1 of this book.*

The Client with Toxic Substance Ingestion

1. **2.** Drain cleaner almost always contains lye, which can burn the mouth, pharynx, and esophagus on ingestion. The nurse would be prepared to assist with procedures to secure the airway, which may include intubation or performing a tracheostomy. An emetic is contraindicated because, as the substance burns on ingestion, so too would it burn when vomiting. Additionally, the mucosa becomes necrotic, and vomiting could lead to perforations. Gastric lavage is contraindicated because the mucosa is burned from the ingestion of the caustic lye, causing necrosis. Gastric lavage also could lead to perforation of the necrotic mucosa. Insertion of an indwelling urinary catheter would be indicated after the measures to remove the caustic substance have been started.

    🔑 CN: Reduction of risk potential; CL: Apply

2. **3.** As the burn from the lye ingestion heals, scar tissue develops and can lead to esophageal strictures, a common complication of lye ingestion. Tracheal stenosis would occur if the child had vomited and aspirated. Tracheal varices do not commonly occur after the ingestion of lye or other substances. Although very rare, esophageal diverticula may occur. Diverticula are commonly found in the colon of adults.

    🔑 CN: Physiological adaptation; CL: Analyze

3. **2, 4, 1, 3.** The nurse should first attempt to determine exactly when and how much acetaminophen the parents think the child has taken. Determining the time of ingestion helps establish the immediate care and when lab values should be drawn. Gastric decontamination with activated charcoal is used within 4 hours of ingestion to bind the drug and help prevent toxic serum levels. Serum blood levels should be done after the gastric decontamination but preferably not too soon after ingestion since levels drawn before 4 hours may not reflect maximum serum concentrations and will need to be repeated. The decision to administer acetylcysteine and prevent liver damage is based on serum levels.

    🔑 CN: Pharmacological and parenteral therapies; CL: Analyze

4. **2.** Initial management of a child who has ingested a large amount of acetaminophen would include inducing vomiting or performing gastric lavage with or without activated charcoal to aid in the removal of the substance. Frequent blood level determinations may be obtained during the follow-up phase, but they are not done as part of the initial treatment. Tracheostomy is not typically part of the initial treatment for acetaminophen overdose. However, it may be necessary later if respiratory distress develops. Acetaminophen primarily affects the liver, not the heart. Therefore, an electrocardiogram would not be considered part of the initial treatment plan.

    🔑 CN: Reduction of risk potential; CL: Apply

5. **4.** Chemical pneumonitis is the most common complication of ingestion of hydrocarbons, such as those found in kerosene. The pneumonitis is caused by irritation from the hydrocarbons aspirated into the lungs. Uremia is the result of renal insufficiency, which causes nitrogenous waste products to build up in the blood rather than being excreted. Hepatitis is caused by a viral infection. Carditis in a preschooler may be the result of rheumatic fever.

    🔑 CN: Physiological adaptation; CL: Analyze

The Client with Lead Poisoning

6. **3.** Treatment for children with minimally elevated lead levels should include family lead education, follow-up testing, and a social service consultation if needed. Waiting 6 months for a follow-up screening is too long because the effects of lead are irreversible. Oral chelation therapy is not begun until levels approach high levels, 45 mcg/dL (2.2 μmol/L). There is no such thing as a "normal" lead level because there is no beneficial action in the body.

    🔑 CN: Safety and infection control; CL: Analyze

7. **3.** The most serious and irreversible consequence of lead poisoning is neurologic changes leading to an intellectual disability. It can be expected if lead poisoning is long-standing and goes untreated. Lead poisoning also affects the hematologic and renal systems. Cirrhosis is the end stage of several

chronic liver diseases, such as biliary atresia and hepatitis. Lead poisoning is not associated with stunted growth. Chronic illnesses, such as cystic fibrosis, cause slowing of the growth velocity. Heart failure is associated with congenital heart disease and rheumatic fever.

🔑 CN: Physiological adaptation; CL: Apply

8. 3. Vitamin A is not known to play a significant role in preventing EBLL. Calcium intake inhibits lead absorption. Children with EBLL levels often are anemic. While this relationship is not well understood, iron supplementation has been shown to improve developmental outcomes. Vitamin C improves iron absorption. Increased vitamin intake is associated with decreased EBLL levels.

🔑 CN: Health promotion and maintenance; CL: Evaluate

The Client with Celiac Disease

9. 2. Celiac disease is a disorder involving intolerance to the protein gluten, which is found in wheat, rye, oats, and barley. The stools of a child with celiac disease are characteristically malodorous, pale, large (bulky), and soft (loose). Excessive flatus is common, and bouts of diarrhea may occur. Dark urine is commonly associated with concentrated urine, such as when a child has dehydration. The belly of a child with celiac disease, a malabsorption disorder, typically is protuberant. A small belly may be associated with a child who is thin. Short stature is not associated with this malabsorption disorder.

🔑 CN: Physiological adaptation; CL: Analyze

10. 2. The intestines of a child with celiac disease fill with accumulated undigested food and flatus, causing the characteristic protuberant abdomen. Celiac disease is not usually associated with any liver dysfunction, including poor liver functioning leading to liver enlargement. Tender inguinal lymph nodes are often associated with an infection. Periorbital edema, swelling around the eyes, is associated with nephritis.

🔑 CN: Physiological adaptation; CL: Analyze

11. 3. Damage to the intestinal mucosa in celiac disease is caused by gliadin, a part of the gluten protein found in wheat, rye, barley, and oats. Foods containing these grains must be eliminated entirely from the diet of children with celiac disease. Foods containing rice and corn are a good substitute. Although an adequate intake of milk is important for any child, children with celiac disease do not need an increased milk intake.

🔑 CN: Physiological adaptation; CL: Evaluate

12. 1. Children with celiac disease cannot digest the protein in common grains such as wheat, rye, and oats. Eggs and orange juice would be appropriate foods.

🔑 CN: Basic care and comfort; CL: Evaluate

13. 3. The child with celiac disease should not eat foods containing wheat, oats, rye, or barley. Pancakes and waffles are made from flour that typically is derived from wheat and therefore should be avoided. Foods containing rice, such as rice cereal, or corn are appropriate. Pancakes and waffles are made from flour that typically is derived from wheat and therefore should be avoided.

🔑 CN: Physiological adaptation; CL: Analyze

The Client with Phenylketonuria

14. 3. PKU is an autosomal recessive disorder involving the absence of an enzyme needed to metabolize the essential amino acid phenylalanine to tyrosine. To ensure reliable results, the neonate must have ingested sufficient protein, such as breast milk or formula, for at least 24 hours. Testing the infant before that time, excessive vomiting, or poor intake can yield false-negative results. The infant does not need to fast 4 hours before the test. A loading dose of glucose water does not affect test values.

🔑 CN: Reduction of risk potential; CL: Evaluate

15. 1. Foods with low phenylalanine levels include vegetables, fruits, and juices. Foods high in phenylalanine include meats and dairy products, which must be restricted or eliminated. Diet colas contain more phenylalanine than the fruits listed.

🔑 CN: Physiological adaptation; CL: Analyze

16. 3. PKU is caused by an inborn error of metabolism. It is an autosomal recessive disorder that inhibits the conversion of phenylalanine to tyrosine. A form of Down syndrome, trisomy 21, is an example of a disorder caused by chromosomal translocation. Cri du chat is an example of a disorder caused by chromosomal deletion. Hemophilia A is an example of a disorder caused by an X-linked recessive gene.

🔑 CN: Physiological adaptation; CL: Apply

17. 4. Clients with PKU have better cognitive outcomes and long-term health when they remain on a low-phenylalanine diet their entire life. Clients who follow the PKU diet will not get enough essential nutrients from food. They will

have to drink a special formula for the rest of their lives, but older children and adults will drink a different formula than infants and toddlers. Older treatment plans permitted adolescents to come off the diet once they had stopped growing but advised female clients that they had to resume the diet before conception to lower risks to the fetus. It is now understood that rising phenylalanine levels in adolescents and young adults are associated with decreased mental well-being. The safe amount of dietary phenylalanine that clients with PKU can tolerate varies over time. Clients who stay on the diet will need regular phenylalanine monitoring for the rest of their lives.

CN: Physiological adaptation; CL: Analyze

18. **2.** PKU is considered a chronic illness. Parents typically grieve about the loss of health in their child afflicted with a chronic disease. Many times, they repeat questions, as though trying to deny what is really happening. This type of behavior represents an attempt to integrate the experience and their feelings with their self-image as they pass through the grieving process. Asking for detailed explanations, testing the competence of health workers, and expressing impatience with health workers may explain the parents' behavior, but viewing the behavior as a part of the grieving process is the most plausible explanation.

CN: Psychosocial integrity; CL: Analyze

The Client with Colic

19. **2.** Information on the crying pattern of the infant is most helpful in confirming the diagnosis of colic. Typically, the colic attack begins abruptly, with the infant crying loudly and continuously, possibly for hours. The attack may end when the child becomes exhausted. The child also may attain some relief after passing stool or flatus. Often, in an attempt to alleviate the infant's crying, parents try to feed the infant, resulting in overfeeding, leading to discomfort and distention. Asking about the type of formula, sleep position, or position for burping will not provide sufficient information to confirm the diagnosis of colic. However, the nurse can obtain additional information after determining the nature of the crying pattern.

CN: Physiological adaptation; CL: Analyze

20. **1.** Infants with colic usually pass normal stools, typically soft and yellowish. Frequent watery stools might indicate diarrhea. Ribbon-like stools are suggestive of a narrowing of the colon or the rectum. Foul-smelling stools by themselves are related to diet. When other symptoms such as large size and protuberant abdomen are present, malabsorption may be possible.

CN: Physiological adaptation; CL: Analyze

21. **2.** The nurse needs to provide the parents with support because of the infant's crying. The parents are stressed and need to be encouraged to get out of the house and arrange for some free time. Although infants need lots of attention and care for the first few months, they do not need the parent's undivided attention. Comparing colic with other problems is inappropriate. Parents have the right to be upset. Although colic usually disappears spontaneously by age 3 months, the nurse should not make any guarantees.

CN: Psychosocial integrity; CL: Analyze

22. **4.** Infants with colic should be burped frequently during and after the feeding. Much of the discomfort of colic appears to be associated with the presence of air in the stomach and the intestines. Frequent burping helps to relieve the air. Infants with colic should be held fairly upright while being fed, to help air rise. The preferred position for burping the infant with colic is to hold the infant at the parent's shoulder so that the infant's abdomen lies on the shoulder. This position causes more pressure to be exerted on the infant's abdomen, leading to a more forceful burp. The child should be placed in an infant seat after feedings.

CN: Physiological adaptation; CL: Evaluate

The Client with Obesity

23. **1.** Children age 2 to 20 years with a BMI for age at the 90th percentile are considered overweight. The nurse should assess the child for related complications, including type 2 diabetes and metabolic syndrome, before creating a plan of care. If no other risk factors are present, the family should receive counseling on lifestyle modifications to slow the child's weight gain until an appropriate height for weight is attained. Without intervention, the child may become obese. A health care provider who specializes in pediatric weight loss should be considered when the child is obese and has complicating factors. Commercial diet programs alone do not include the necessary monitoring for children and thus are rarely appropriate.

CN: Management of care; CL: Analyze

24. 4. A 3-day diet history is the best way to accurately assess the child's intake. Children under age 1 year should not drink cow's milk because of the risk for allergy. Children over age 1 year should drink whole milk because skim milk and 2% milk do not contain all the essential fatty acids needed by young children. It is unknown at this time how much formula the child is actually taking, but an infant should not have more than 6 oz (177.4 mL) of juice per day, and additional water is usually not necessary. If an infant is taking no more than 32 oz (946 mL) of formula per day and is eating some baby food and cereal, additional fluids and frequent feeding should not be necessary.

CN: Health promotion and maintenance; CL: Analyze

25. 3. A 24-hour recall history is the best method to obtain a dietary history from an adolescent. Open-ended questions tend not to provide sufficient details for a nutrition history. Asking what the client plans to eat in the future gives the client an opportunity to report the "right" answer. The nurse obtains the information directly from the client; asking the parent has the potential to undermine trust.

CN: Health promotion; CL: Apply

26. 1. The most common complication of adolescent obesity is its persistence into adulthood. The incidence of gastrointestinal and orthopedic problems, such as Legg-Calvé-Perthes disease and genu valgum (knock knees), is greater for obese adolescents; however, they are not the most common complication. Although psychosocial problems do occur, they are not the most common complication.

CN: Reduction of risk potential; CL: Apply

27. 1. Decreasing the amount of formula given as the infant begins to take solids helps prevent excess caloric intake. Because the infant is receiving calories from solid foods, the formula no longer needs to provide the infant's total caloric requirements. Mixing vegetables with formula or breast milk does not allow the child to become accustomed to new textures or tastes. Solid foods should be given with a spoon, not in a bottle. Using a bottle with food allows the infant to ingest more food than is needed. Juice has very little nutritional value compared with formula or breast milk and contributes to obesity. The nurse should advise parents not to give juice to children under the age of 1 year. After 1 year of age, juice intake should be limited to 1 serving or less a day.

CN: Basic care and comfort; CL: Apply

28. 1. Infants generally do not overeat unless they are urged to do so. Parents should watch for clues indicating that the infant is full—for example, stopping sucking and pushing the nipple out of the mouth. Bottle-feeding instead of breastfeeding is more likely to lead to excessive caloric intake. A demand schedule, rather than a regulated schedule, allows the infant to regulate intake according to individual needs. Normally, giving an infant a regular supplementation of water is unnecessary; the infant's sucking needs can be met by providing a pacifier. Adding more water to the formula than as directed decreases the caloric intake and also places the infant at risk for hyponatremia due to decreased sodium and increased water intake.

CN: Basic care and comfort; CL: Analyze

The Client with Food Sensitivity

29. 4, 1, 3, 2, 5. The child is exhibiting signs of anaphylaxis. The principles of emergency management involve activating EMS when an emergency is first realized. The nurse then follows the priorities of Circulation, Airway, Breathing (C, A, B). The epinephrine should then be given to reduce airway constriction and prevent cardiovascular collapse. The child should be assisted into the most comfortable position to facilitate breathing, usually with the head elevated. Then the nurse can take the child's vital signs to assess the effectiveness of the treatment. Lastly, the nurse should notify the family.

CN: Physiological adaptation; CL: Analyze

30. 1. Lactose intolerance is not an allergy. Rather, it is caused by the lack of the digestive enzyme lactase. This enzyme, found in the intestines, is necessary for the digestion of lactose, the primary carbohydrate in cow's milk. Protein and fat digestion are not affected.

CN: Physiological adaptation; CL: Evaluate

31. 1. Parents of infants with a cow's milk allergy can continue to breastfeed if they eliminate cow's milk from their diet. It is important to encourage birth parents to continue to breastfeed because breast milk is usually the least allergic and most easily digested food for an infant. In addition, the infant is able to obtain protein through the birth parent's milk. If the parent stops breastfeeding, a predigested protein hydrolysate formula would be the first choice. An iron-fortified formula is a cow's milk-based formula. A soy-based formula is not used because approximately 20% of infants with cow's milk sensitivity are also sensitive to soy. Solid foods are not introduced until the infant is 4 to 6 months of age.

CN: Basic care and comfort; CL: Analyze

32. **2.** Children with lactose intolerance often tolerate small amounts of dairy products better when they are consumed at mealtime with other foods. Most people with lactose intolerance can consume 2 to 4 oz (60 to 120 mL) of milk at a time without symptoms. Larger quantities are more likely to cause gas and bloating. Cheeses contain less lactose than milk and may be better tolerated. Yogurt also contains enzymes that are activated in the duodenum that substitute for natural lactase. Taking supplemental enzymes or drinking lactase-treated milk may also substitute for natural lactase.

CN: Basic care and comfort; CL: Analyze

The Client with Failure to Thrive

33. The nasogastric tube should reside in the stomach. The site placement can be verified by inserting 3 to 5 mL of air in the tube and auscultating the infant's abdomen for the sound of air. The nurse should then aspirate the injected air and a small amount of stomach contents and then test the contents for acidity.

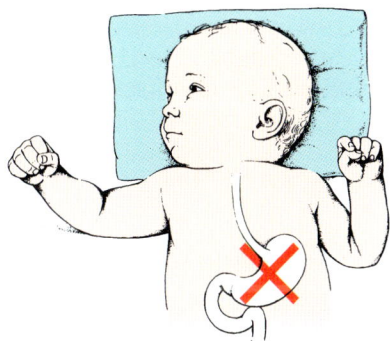

CN: Safety and infection control; CL: Apply

34. **1, 2, 4.** Consistency to build trust is important when caring for infants with failure to thrive. Parents can best provide consistency. Therefore, the nurse should instruct the parent on proper feeding techniques and observe the feeding to provide support. The parent-child interactions should be monitored before, during, and after feedings. The nurse should especially be alert for increases in parental anxiety that affect the parent and child and provide extensive support to alleviate anxiety related to slow weight gain. Because there is no organic reason for the failure to thrive, it should not be necessary to increase the formula's calorie content. A 5-month-old infant is too young to be expected to sit in a highchair for feedings and should still be bottle-fed.

CN: Physiological adaptation; CL: Analyze

35. **4.** The most effective follow-up care would occur in the home environment. The community health nurse can be supportive of the parents and will be able to observe parent-infant interactions in a natural environment. The community health nurse can evaluate the infant's progress in gaining weight, offer suggestions to the parents, and help the family solve problems as they arise.

CN: Physiological adaptation; CL: Analyze

Managing Care, Quality, and Safety of Children with Health Problems Involving Ingestion, Nutrition, or Diet

36. **2.** For children receiving intermittent gavage feedings, the best method to verify the tube placement before each feeding is to aspirate a small amount of gastric contents to verify that the pH is acidic. A pH of 5.5 or less should indicate correct placement in most babies. Depending on the type of feeding tube used, an x-ray may be used to confirm the original tube placement, but use before every feeding would expose the child to unnecessary radiation. Air boluses are misleading because placement in the esophagus or respiratory tract may make the same sound in small infants. Charts might be helpful in determining initial tube insertion length but do not substitute for nursing assessments.

CN: Reduction of risk potential; CL: Apply

37. **2.** Public education about the sources of lead that could cause poisoning has been found to be the most effective measure to prevent lead poisoning. This includes recent efforts to alert the public to lead in certain types of window blinds. Condemning old housing developments has been ineffective because lead paint still exists in many other dwellings. Providing education about good nutrition, though important, is not an effective preventive measure. Pregnant women and children should not remain in an older home that is being remodeled because they may breathe in lead in the dust, but this is not the most effective preventive measure.

CN: Safety and infection control; CL: Analyze

38. **1.** Three severe reactions in 3 months indicate a serious problem with adhering to the prevention plan. The nurse should first determine if the parent can actually read the label. The underlying problem may be that the parent is visually impaired or unable to read. The parent's reading level determines what additional support is needed. Referrals to social services or a dietician may be indicated, but the nurse does not yet have enough information about the problem. The nurse would communicate with the HCP after assessing the situation to recommend referrals.

🔑 CN: Management of care; CL: Analyze

39. 3. The kosher diet includes meat and fowl that are butchered using only humane methods. Meat and dairy may not be eaten together. Pigs are considered unclean and may not be eaten as part of a kosher diet. Chicken is kosher as long as it is butchered humanely. Fruits and vegetables are considered kosher as long as they are free from insects.

🔑 CN: Psychosocial integrity; CL: Apply

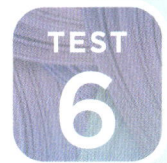

TEST 6: The Child with Health Problems of the Urinary System

- The Client with Cryptorchidism
- The Client with Hydrocele
- The Client with Hypospadias
- The Client with Urinary Tract Infection
- The Client with Glomerulonephritis
- The Client with Nephrotic Syndrome
- The Client with Acute or Chronic Renal Failure
- The Client with Wilms' Tumor
- Managing Care, Quality, and Safety of Children with Health Problems of the Urinary System
- Answers, Rationales, and Test-Taking Strategies

The Client with Cryptorchidism

1. The nurse prepares to examine a 6-week-old infant's scrotal sac and testes for possible undescended testes. Which action would be **most** important for the nurse to do?
   - ☐ 1. Check the diaper for recent urination.
   - ☐ 2. Give the infant a pacifier.
   - ☐ 3. Ensure that the room is kept warm.
   - ☐ 4. Tap lightly on the left inguinal ring.

2. While the nurse is examining the infant for the presence of testes, the parent paces around the room shaking their head. Which statement would be the **most** appropriate response by the nurse?
   - ☐ 1. "I am sure everything will work out for the best, and they will be fine."
   - ☐ 2. "You seem upset; please tell me how you are feeling."
   - ☐ 3. "Don't worry; the testes will probably descend on their own."
   - ☐ 4. "Would you like to talk with a parent of a child who has the same problem?"

3. The nurse assesses an infant with an undescended testis. The nurse should be alert for which symptom?
   - ☐ 1. abnormal lower extremity reflexes
   - ☐ 2. history of frequent emesis
   - ☐ 3. bulging in the inguinal area
   - ☐ 4. poor weight gain

4. The nurse develops the preoperative teaching plan for a 14-month-old child with an undescended testis who is scheduled to have surgery. Which method is **most** appropriate?
   - ☐ 1. Tell the child that their penis and scrotum will be "fixed."
   - ☐ 2. Explain to the parents how the defect will be corrected.
   - ☐ 3. Tell the child that they will not see any incisions after surgery.
   - ☐ 4. Use an anatomically correct doll to show the child what will be "fixed."

5. An adolescent with a history of surgical repair for an undescended testis comes to the clinic for a sports physical. Which anticipatory guidance for the parents and adolescent is **most** important?
   - ☐ 1. the adolescent's sterility
   - ☐ 2. the adolescent's future plans
   - ☐ 3. technique for monthly testicular self-examinations
   - ☐ 4. need for a lot of psychological support

The Client with Hydrocele

6. During a clinic visit, the parent of an infant with hydrocele states that the infant's scrotum is smaller now than when born. After teaching the parent about the infant's condition, which statement by the parent indicates that the teaching has been effective?
☐ 1. "I guess keeping their bottom elevated has helped."
☐ 2. "Massaging the groin area is working."
☐ 3. "It seems like the fluid is being reabsorbed."
☐ 4. "Keeping my child quiet and in an infant seat has helped."

7. Shortly after an infant is returned to their room following hydrocele repair, the infant's parent approaches the nurse in the hall to report that the child's scrotum looks swollen and bruised. Which response by the nurse would be **most** appropriate?
☐ 1. "Let me see if the surgeon has prescribed acetaminophen for your child. If they did, I'll get it right away."
☐ 2. "Can you wait in the room? Then you can ask me any questions when I get there."
☐ 3. "What you are describing is unusual after this type of surgery. I will let the surgeon know."
☐ 4. "This is normal after this type of surgery. Let's look at it together just to be sure."

The Client with Hypospadias

8. The parents of a neonate with hypospadias and chordee wish to have them circumcised. Which explanation should the nurse incorporate into the discussion with the parents concerning the recommendation to delay circumcision?
☐ 1. The associated chordee is difficult to remove during circumcision.
☐ 2. The foreskin is used to repair the deformity surgically.
☐ 3. The meatus can become stenosed, leading to urinary obstruction.
☐ 4. The infant's penis is too small to safely circumcise.

9. The nurse is caring for an infant with hypospadias. Identify the area where the nurse would assess for this condition.

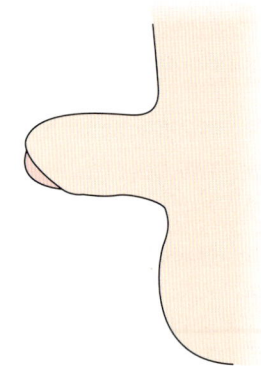

10. After teaching the parents about the urethral catheter placed after surgical repair of their child's hypospadias, the nurse determines that the teaching was successful when the parent states that the catheter in their child's penis accomplishes which goal?
☐ 1. decreases pain at the surgical site
☐ 2. keeps the new urethra from closing
☐ 3. measures their urine correctly
☐ 4. prevents bladder spasms

11. While assessing the penis of a child who has had surgery to repair hypospadias, the nurse observes the appearance of the penis. The nurse should report which aspect to the surgeon?
☐ 1. swollen
☐ 2. dusky blue at the tip
☐ 3. somewhat misshapen
☐ 4. pink

12. The nurse develops the teaching plan for the parents of a 12-month-old infant with hypospadias and chordee repair. What information is **most** important to include?
☐ 1. Assist the child to become familiar with their dressings so they will leave them alone.
☐ 2. Encourage the child to ambulate as soon as possible by using a favorite push toy.
☐ 3. Force fluids to at least 2500 mL a day by offering their favorite juices.
☐ 4. Prevent the child from disrupting the catheters by using soft restraints if needed.

The Client with Urinary Tract Infection

13. A teenage girl has been diagnosed with a urinary tract infection. The nurse recognizes the need for teaching when the client makes which statement?
☐ 1. "I will not take bubble baths."
☐ 2. "I will drink plenty of water."
☐ 3. "I can drink coffee."
☐ 4. "I can drink cranberry juice."

14. A preschool-age client with a history of urinary reflux had bilateral urethral implant surgery 2 days ago. Which assessment finding is **most** concerning?
☐ 1. intermittent bladder spasms
☐ 2. small amounts of blood-tinged urine
☐ 3. decreased oral intake
☐ 4. continuous drainage from an indwelling catheter

15. The health care provider (HCP) has prescribed a sterile urine specimen for a 3-year-old boy with a history of recurrent urinary tract infections. The family is upset because the last time the child was catheterized, the procedure was very painful and traumatic. What is the nurse's **best** response?
☐ 1. "I'll request a prescription for a sedative to help them relax."
☐ 2. "I can't do anything to reduce the pain, but you can hold your child during the procedure."
☐ 3. "I'll get a prescription for a numbing lubricant to make the procedure more comfortable."
☐ 4. "I can apply a topical anesthetic 20 minutes before placing the catheter."

16. A recent history of which problem should alert the nurse to gather additional information about the possibility of a urinary tract infection in a toddler with a fever? Select all that apply.
☐ 1. irritability
☐ 2. swollen lymph glands
☐ 3. skin rash
☐ 4. vomiting
☐ 5. abdominal distention

17. A parent of a child with a urinary tract infection calls the clinic and explains, "I'm concerned because my child refuses to obey me concerning the preventions you told me about. My child refuses to take the medication unless I buy them a present. I don't want to use discipline because of the illness, but I'm worried about the behavior." Which response by the nurse is **best**?
☐ 1. "I sympathize with your difficulties, but just ignore the behavior for now."
☐ 2. "I understand it's hard to discipline a child who is ill, but things need to be kept as normal as possible."
☐ 3. "I understand that things are difficult for you right now, but your child is ill and deserves special treatment."
☐ 4. "I understand your concern, but this type of behavior happens all the time; your child will get over it when feeling better."

18. A nurse is teaching the parents of a child diagnosed with a urinary tract infection secondary to vesicoureteral reflux. How should the nurse explain how the reflux contributes to the infection?
☐ 1. "It prevents complete emptying of the bladder."
☐ 2. "It causes urine backflow into the kidney."
☐ 3. "It results in painful bladder spasms."
☐ 4. "It causes painful urination."

The Client with Glomerulonephritis

19. The nurse requests a dinner tray for an adolescent with glomerulonephritis with severe hypertension. Which meal would be **most** appropriate?
☐ 1. egg noodles, hamburger, canned peas, milk
☐ 2. baked ham, baked potato, pear, canned carrots, milk
☐ 3. baked chicken, rice, green beans, orange juice
☐ 4. hot dog on a bun, corn chips, pickle, cookie, milk

20. A school-age child with glomerulonephritis reports a headache and blurred vision. What **immediate** action should the nurse take?
☐ 1. Put the client to bed.
☐ 2. Obtain the child's blood pressure.
☐ 3. Notify the health care provider (HCP).
☐ 4. Administer acetaminophen.

21. A school-age client admitted to the hospital because of decreased urine output and periorbital edema is diagnosed with acute poststreptococcal glomerulonephritis. Which assessment gives the nurse the **best** indication of the child's fluid balance?
☐ 1. Assess vital signs every 4 hours.
☐ 2. Monitor intake and output every 12 hours.
☐ 3. Obtain daily weight measurements.
☐ 4. Draw serum electrolyte levels daily.

22. The nurse develops the plan of care for a school-age child with acute poststreptococcal glomerulonephritis who has a fluid restriction of 1000 mL a day. Which fluid should the nurse consider as **most** appropriate for the client's condition and effective for preventing excessive thirst?
☐ 1. diet cola
☐ 2. ice chips
☐ 3. lemonade
☐ 4. tap water

23. The nurse is planning interventions for a school-age child hospitalized with acute poststreptococcal glomerulonephritis in need of diversional activity. Which activity is **most** likely to meet the child's social needs?
    ☐ 1. playing a card game with someone the same age
    ☐ 2. putting together a puzzle with parent
    ☐ 3. playing video games with a 4-year-old
    ☐ 4. watching a movie with a younger sibling

24. A school-age child hospitalized with acute poststreptococcal glomerulonephritis during the acute stage has elevated blood pressure and low urine output for 14 hours. What should the nurse do **next**?
    ☐ 1. Assess the child's neurologic status.
    ☐ 2. Encourage the child to drink more water.
    ☐ 3. Advise the child to eat a low-sodium breakfast.
    ☐ 4. Help the client ambulate in the hallway.

25. The nurse reviews the medical record of an adolescent with a history of losing weight and fatigue who has been admitted to the hospital with a diagnosis of stage I chronic renal failure (see exhibit).

Intake and Output	
Day 1: Intake 1850 mL	Output 1550 mL
Day 2: Intake 2200 mL	Output 1150 mL

    Based on these findings, what action should the nurse take?
    ☐ 1. Continue monitoring intake and output.
    ☐ 2. Notify the health care provider (HCP).
    ☐ 3. Restrict the client's fluids.
    ☐ 4. Increase the client's fluids.

26. A parent of a child with acute poststreptococcal glomerulonephritis (APSGN) asks how a strep infection caused the child to have a kidney problem. What is the nurse's **best** response?
    ☐ 1. "The streptococcal infection spread through the bloodstream to your child's kidneys."
    ☐ 2. "Your child made excessive antibodies to fight the infection that are now attacking the kidneys."
    ☐ 3. "By-products of immune complexes that fought the infection are depositing in the kidneys."
    ☐ 4. "The strep infection weakened your child's immune system, making them susceptible to a secondary infection."

The Client with Nephrotic Syndrome

27. A child with nephrosis is taking prednisone. The nurse should teach the caregivers to report which adverse effect(s)? Select all that apply.
    ☐ 1. increased urinary output
    ☐ 2. hematemesis
    ☐ 3. respiratory infection
    ☐ 4. bleeding gums
    ☐ 5. vision problems

28. The nurse is caring for a 5-year-old boy who is taking prednisolone for nephrotic syndrome. The child is at the 75th percentile for height and has a blood pressure of 114/73 mm Hg. The nurse compares the reading with the below blood pressure levels for boys' age and height percentiles.

    The nurse determines that the blood pressure represents a change and notifies the health care provider of which assessment?

Age Percentile	Systolic BP Reading ←Percentile for Height→							Diastolic BP Reading ←Percentile for height→						
	5th	10th	25th	50th	75th	90th	95th	5th	10th	25th	50th	75th	90th	95th
50th	90	91	93	95	96	98	9 8	50	51	52	53	54	55	55
90th	104	105	106	108	110	111	112	65	66	67	68	69	69	70
95th	108	109	110	112	114	115	116	69	70	71	72	73	74	74
99th	115	116	118	120	121	123	123	77	78	79	80	81	81	82

    ☐ 1. hypotension
    ☐ 2. prehypertension
    ☐ 3. hypertension
    ☐ 4. hypertension stage II

29. The charge nurse reviews the laboratory results of a child admitted with nephrotic syndrome with a nurse new to the pediatric unit. The nurse is aware that teaching is required when the new nurse states that which finding is expected with nephrotic syndrome?
    ☐ 1. hyperalbuminemia
    ☐ 2. elevated triglycerides
    ☐ 3. elevated cholesterol
    ☐ 4. proteinuria

30. The nurse teaches the parent of a toddler diagnosed with nephrotic syndrome about the disease. Which statement by the parent indicates that they understood the nurse's teaching about this disease?
    ☐ 1. "My child really likes chips and bologna. I guess we'll have to find something else."
    ☐ 2. "We will have to encourage lots of liquids. Did you say about 17 cups (4 L) every day?"
    ☐ 3. "We worry about the surgery. Do you think we should do a direct donation of blood?"
    ☐ 4. "We understand the need for antibiotics. I just wish the antibiotics could be given by mouth."

31. A toddler diagnosed with nephrotic syndrome has a fluid volume excess related to fluid accumulation in the tissues. Which measure should the nurse anticipate including in the child's plan of care?
☐ 1. Limit visitors to 2 to 3 hours a day.
☐ 2. Maintain strict bed rest.
☐ 3. Test urine specific gravity every shift.
☐ 4. Weigh the child before breakfast.

32. The parent of a toddler with nephrotic syndrome asks the nurse what can be done about the child's swollen eyes. Which is the **best** measure that the nurse should suggest?
☐ 1. Apply cool compresses to the child's eyes.
☐ 2. Elevate the head of the child's bed.
☐ 3. Apply eye drops every 8 hours.
☐ 4. Limit the child's television watching.

33. The nurse implements interventions for decreasing fluid retention in a child with nephrotic syndrome. Which finding indicates that the interventions have been effective?
☐ 1. decreased abdominal girth
☐ 2. increased caloric intake
☐ 3. increased respiratory rate
☐ 4. decreased heart rate

34. The toddler with nephrotic syndrome exhibits generalized edema. Which measure should the nurse institute for this child with impaired skin integrity related to edema?
☐ 1. Ambulate every shift while awake.
☐ 2. Apply lotion on opposing skin surfaces.
☐ 3. Apply powder to skinfolds.
☐ 4. Separate opposing skin surfaces with a soft cloth.

35. A child with nephrosis is placed on prednisone. The dose is 2 mg/kg a day to be administered twice a day. The child weighs 25 lb (11.3 kg). How many milligrams will the child receive at each dose? Record your answer using one decimal place.

_____ mg.

36. The toddler with nephrotic syndrome responds to treatment and is ready to go home. When helping the family plan for home care, the nurse should include which instruction in the teaching?
☐ 1. Administer pain medication as needed.
☐ 2. Keep the child away from others with an infection.
☐ 3. Notify the health care provider (HCP) if there is an increase in the child's urine output.
☐ 4. Administer acetaminophen daily.

The Client with Acute or Chronic Renal Failure

37. The nurse is planning care with the parents of a child who requires continuous peritoneal dialysis. Which finding should be discussed with the health care provider (HCP)?
☐ 1. The family lives a long distance from the medical facility.
☐ 2. The child attends a large public school.
☐ 3. The child reports having a previous surgery for a ruptured appendix.
☐ 4. The family feels the child cannot self-regulate to wake at night and change bags.

38. The nurse teaches the family of a school-age child with acute renal failure about continuous ambulatory peritoneal dialysis. Which statement indicates that the family needs more teaching about peritoneal dialysis?
☐ 1. "Dialysate bags should be weighed before filling and after draining."
☐ 2. "Sterile technique must be used when changing dialysate bags."
☐ 3. "Our child should remain quiet during the dialysate dwell stage."
☐ 4. "We will instill dialysate at bedtime using a peritoneal dialysis machine."

39. The nurse assists a parent in performing daily peritoneal dialysis and catheter exit site care for the first time for a child with chronic renal failure. Which information would be an important step to emphasize to the parent?
☐ 1. Apply an occlusive dressing after cleaning the site.
☐ 2. Change the dressing when the peritoneal space is dry.
☐ 3. Examine the site for signs of infection while cleaning the area.
☐ 4. Pull on the catheter to hold taut while cleaning the skin.

40. The nurse develops the family discharge teaching plan for a child with chronic renal failure. The nurse should emphasize restriction of which nutrient?
☐ 1. ascorbic acid
☐ 2. calcium
☐ 3. magnesium
☐ 4. phosphorus

41. The nurse implements a plan targeted at maintaining a positive self-concept in an adolescent with renal failure. Which behavior by the adolescent would indicate that the plan is working?
☐ 1. reports of headaches, abdominal pain, and nausea
☐ 2. insistence on making diet choices even if the foods chosen are restricted
☐ 3. verbalization of plans to quit all after-school activities when returning home
☐ 4. demonstration of a desire to do the dressing changes and take care of the medications

42. The nurse creates a diet plan with the family of a child with acute renal failure. Which diet plan would be **most** appropriate for the child?
☐ 1. high carbohydrate and protein
☐ 2. high fat and carbohydrate
☐ 3. low fat and protein
☐ 4. low carbohydrate and fat

43. An adolescent with chronic renal failure is scheduled to go home with a peritoneal dialysis catheter in place. When developing the discharge teaching plan for the client and the family focusing on psychosocial needs, the nurse should include which area as a **priority**?
☐ 1. advantages of limiting social activities and contacts for the first few months
☐ 2. not disclosing information about the peritoneal dialysis to people outside the family
☐ 3. possible effect on body image of the presence of an abdominal catheter
☐ 4. importance of relying on parents to do the dialysis and dressing changes

44. During a home visit, the public health nurse assesses the peritoneal catheter exit site of a child with chronic renal failure. Which finding should lead the nurse to determine that the child has an infection?
☐ 1. dialysate leakage
☐ 2. granulation tissue
☐ 3. increased time for drainage
☐ 4. tissue swelling

45. The nurse teaches the parent of a young child with a peritoneal catheter about the signs and symptoms of peritonitis. The nurse determines that the parent has understood the teaching when they identify which finding as an important sign?
☐ 1. cloudy dialysate drainage return
☐ 2. distended abdomen
☐ 3. shortness of breath
☐ 4. weight gain of 3 lb (1.36 kg) in 2 days

46. The parent of a child with chronic renal failure who is receiving peritoneal dialysis at home asks the nurse what they can do if both inflow and drain times are increased. Which instructions would be **most** appropriate for the nurse to include when responding to the parent?
☐ 1. Assess the child for constipation.
☐ 2. Decrease the amount of dialysate infused for each dwell.
☐ 3. Incorporate the increased inflow and drain times into the dialysis schedule.
☐ 4. Monitor the child for shoulder pain during inflow and drain times.

47. The nurse determines that the parent understands the diet restrictions for a child with chronic renal failure who is receiving peritoneal dialysis when the parent reports providing a diet involving which components?
☐ 1. sodium and water restrictions
☐ 2. high protein and carbohydrates
☐ 3. high potassium and iron
☐ 4. protein and phosphorous restrictions

The Client with Wilms' Tumor

48. A toddler receiving chemotherapy after surgery for a Wilms' tumor has developed neutropenia. The parent is trying to encourage the child to eat by bringing extra foods to the room. Which food would the nurse discourage for this child?
☐ 1. fudge
☐ 2. French fries
☐ 3. fresh strawberries
☐ 4. a milkshake

49. The nurse assesses a toddler diagnosed with a Wilms' tumor. What should the nurse avoid?
☐ 1. measuring the child's chest circumference
☐ 2. palpating the child's abdomen
☐ 3. placing the child in an upright position
☐ 4. measuring the child's occipitofrontal circumference

50. The nurse does postoperative teaching with the parent of a child with Wilms' tumor. Which parental statement indicates that the parent understands what *stage II tumor* means?
☐ 1. "The tumor has extended beyond the kidney but was completely removed."
☐ 2. "Although the tumor was in the kidney, it has spread to the lung, liver, and bone."
☐ 3. "The tumor has extended outside the kidney to the lungs and the liver."
☐ 4. "The tumor was solely located in the kidney, but it was totally removed."

51. A child diagnosed with Wilms' tumor undergoes successful surgery for removal of the diseased kidney. When the child returns to the room, the nurse should place the child in which position?
☐ 1. modified Trendelenburg
☐ 2. lateral recumbent
☐ 3. semi-Fowler's
☐ 4. supine

52. The nurse assesses a child who had a nephrectomy for a Wilms' tumor. The nurse should assess the child postoperatively for which early sign of a complication?
☐ 1. increased abdominal distention
☐ 2. elevated blood pressure
☐ 3. increased respiratory rate
☐ 4. increased urine output

53. The nurse develops the discharge plan for a child who had a nephrectomy for a Wilms' tumor. The nurse identifies outcomes to prevent damage to the child's remaining kidney and to accomplish which goal?
☐ 1. Minimize pain.
☐ 2. Prevent dependent edema.
☐ 3. Prevent urinary tract infection.
☐ 4. Minimize sodium intake.

Managing Care, Quality, and Safety of Children with Health Problems of the Urinary System

54. The nurse reads the new medication prescriptions for a 4-year-old child with nephrotic syndrome (see exhibit).
What action should the nurse take?

Prescriptions

- D/C prednisolone 40 mg PO Daily
- Prednisolone 30 mg PO QOD

☐ 1. Discontinue the prednisolone 40 mg, and give the 30-mg dose today.
☐ 2. Check the medication record first to see when the last dose of prednisolone was given.
☐ 3. Start the 30-mg dose tomorrow.
☐ 4. Contact the prescriber for clarification.

Answers, Rationales, and Test-Taking Strategies

The answers and the rationales for each question follow below, along with keys (🔑) to the client need (CN) and cognitive level (CL) for each question. In addition, questions that measure clinical judgment will be coded (CJ). As you check your answers, use the **Content Mastery and Test-Taking Skill Self-Analysis** *worksheet (tear-out worksheet in the back of the book) to identify the reason(s) for not answering the questions correctly. For additional information about test-taking skills and strategies for answering questions, refer to pages 12–51 in Part 1 of this book.*

The Client with Cryptorchidism

1. 3. A cold environment can cause the testes to retract. Cold and touch stimulate the cremasteric reflex, which causes a normal retraction of the testes toward the body. Therefore, the nurse should warm the hands and make sure that the environment also is warm. Checking the diaper for urination provides information about the infant's voiding and urinary function, not information about the testes. Giving the infant a pacifier may help calm the infant and possibly make the examination easier, but the concern here is with the temperature of the environment. Tapping on the inguinal ring would not be helpful in assessing the infant.

🔑 CN: Health promotion and maintenance; CL: Analyze

2. 2. The nurse needs more information about the parent's perceptions and feelings before providing any information or taking action. Determining the exact nature of the parent's concern rather than making an assumption about it is essential. Therefore, the nurse should identify what is observed and ask the parent how they are feeling. Telling the parent that everything will be fine or not to worry is inappropriate and provides false reassurance. It also devalues the parent's concern. Later on, it may be appropriate for the parent to talk to another parent of a child with the same problem for support.

🔑 CN: Psychosocial integrity; CL: Analyze

3. 3. When an anomaly is found in one system, such as the genitourinary system, that system requires a more focused assessment to reveal other conditions that also may be occurring. A bulging in the inguinal area may suggest an inguinal hernia. Also, hydrocele or an upper urinary tract anomaly may occur on the same side as the undescended testis. A neuromuscular problem, not a genitourinary problem such as undescended testes, would most likely be the cause of abnormal lower extremity reflexes. A history of frequent emesis may be caused by pyloric stenosis or viral gastroenteritis. Poor weight gain might suggest a metabolic or a feeding problem.

CN: Health promotion and maintenance; CL: Analyze

4. **2.** Preoperative teaching would be directed at the parents because the child is too young to understand the teaching. Telling the child that their penis and scrotum will be "fixed," telling the child they will not see incisions after surgery, and using a doll to illustrate the surgery are appropriate interventions for a preschool-age child.

CN: Psychosocial integrity; CL: Apply

5. **3.** Because the incidence of testicular cancer is increased in adulthood among children who have had undescended testes, it is extremely important to teach the adolescent how to perform the testicular self-examination monthly. The undescended testicle is removed to reduce the risk for cancer in that testicle. Removal of a testis would not necessarily make the adolescent sterile because the other testicle remains. Although discussing the adolescent's future plans is important, it is not the priority at this time. Because the adolescent has been dealing with the situation for a long time, the need for a sports physical at this time should not be a cause of emotional distress requiring a lot of psychological support.

CN: Health promotion and maintenance; CL: Analyze

The Client with Hydrocele

6. **3.** A hydrocele is a collection of fluid in the tunica vaginalis of the testicle or along the spermatic cord that results from a patent processus vaginalis. As fluid is being absorbed, scrotal size decreases. Elevation of the infant's bottom, massage, or keeping the infant quiet or in an infant seat would have no effect on promoting fluid reabsorption in hydrocele.

CN: Physiological adaptation; CL: Evaluate

7. **4.** Some swelling and bruising are normal postoperatively. By assessing the area with the parent, the nurse is conveying acceptance of the parent's concern. In addition, the nurse needs to inspect the area to determine if what the parent is describing is accurate. Doing so also provides an opportunity for teaching. Acetaminophen is commonly administered for fever or pain relief, but this medication does not treat swelling. Asking the parent to wait in the child's room ignores the parent's concerns. There is no need to notify the surgeon at this time.

CN: Psychosocial integrity; CL: Analyze

The Client with Hypospadias

8. **2.** The condition in which the urethral opening is on the ventral side of the penis or below the glans penis is referred to as *hypospadias*. *Chordee* refers to a ventral curvature of the penis that results from a fibrous band of tissue that has replaced normal tissue. Circumcision is delayed because the foreskin, which is removed with a circumcision, often is used to reconstruct the urethra. The chordee is corrected when the hypospadias is repaired. Circumcision is performed at the same time. Urethral meatal stenosis, which can occur in circumcised infants, results from meatal ulceration, possibly leading to urinary obstruction. It is not associated with hypospadias or circumcision. The reason for delaying circumcision is related to correcting the position of the meatus and is not related to penis size.

CN: Reduction of risk potential; CL: Apply

9. In hypospadias, the urethral opening is on the ventral side of the penis.

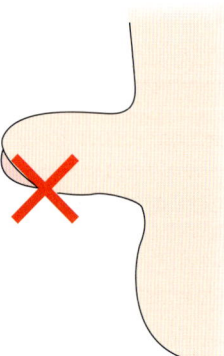

CN: Physiological adaptation; CL: Apply

10. **2.** The main purpose of the urethral catheter is to maintain the patency of the reconstructed urethra. The catheter prevents the new tissue inside the urethra from healing on itself. However, the urethral catheter can cause bladder spasms. Recently, stents have been used instead of catheters. The urethral catheter will have no effect on the child's pain level. In fact, because bladder

spasms are associated with its use, the child's problems of pain may actually increase. Urine output can be measured through the suprapubic catheter because it provides an alternative route for urinary elimination, thus keeping the bladder empty and pressure free.

🔑 CN: Reduction of risk potential; CL: Evaluate

11. 2. A dusky blue color at the tip of the penis may indicate a problem with circulation, and the nurse should notify the surgeon. Following surgery, it is normal for the penis to be swollen and pink. The penis may be misshapen and is unlikely to look normal even after reconstruction.

🔑 CN: Physiological adaptation; CL: Analyze

12. 4. The most important consideration for a successful outcome of this surgery is maintenance of the catheters or stents. A 12-month-old infant likes to explore their environment but must be prevented from manipulating their dressings or catheters through the use of soft restraints. Allowing the infant to become familiar with the dressings will not prevent them from pulling at them. After surgery, the child is allowed limited activity, possibly while sitting on the parent's lap. A 12-month-old infant may or may not be walking. If the client is, most likely they will be clumsy and possibly injure themself. Although increasing fluids is important, 2500 mL a day is an excessive amount for a 12-month-old. Fluid requirements would be 115 mL/kg.

🔑 CN: Physiological adaptation; CL: Analyze

The Client with Urinary Tract Infection

13. 3. Drinking coffee and other beverages that contain caffeine can irritate the bladder and should be avoided. Bubble baths, bath oils, and hot tubs can irritate the urethra and perineal area. Drinking plenty of water will keep urine flushed through the bladder. Cranberry juice helps to acidify the urine.

🔑 CN: Health promotion and maintenance; CL: Evaluate

14. 3. Children with bilateral ureteral implants often have pain with urination due to bladder spasms. Some children will avoid drinking to avoid the pain associated with urination, thus putting the child at risk for dehydration. Intermittent bladder spasms are common after ureteral reimplant surgery and can be treated with oxybutynin to decrease discomfort. Small amounts of blood-tinged urine, bladder spasms, urinary frequency, and urinary incontinence are common following ureteral reimplant surgery.

🔑 CN: Physiological adaptation; CL: Analyze

15. 3. Two percent lidocaine lubricants have been found to significantly reduce the pain of urinary catheter insertion in children. If the unit does not have a standing protocol to use the lubricant, the nurse should request a prescription. A sedative would carry with it additional risks that could be avoided with the use of other methods to reduce pain. The parents should be encouraged to hold the child in addition to other pain relief methods. Frequent urination would make the use of topical anesthetics that must be left in place for a period of time impractical.

🔑 CN: Basic care and comfort; CL: Analyze

16. ➕ **1, 4.** Infants and toddlers with urinary tract infections frequently are fussy and irritable because they are in pain. Other associated signs and symptoms include decreased appetite and vomiting. The presence of swollen lymph glands (lymphadenopathy) is unrelated to urinary tract infections. Lymphadenopathy is associated with a systemic infection or possibly cancer. Skin rash is associated with exposure to allergens or irritants (e.g., poison ivy or harsh soaps); prolonged contact with urine (e.g., diaper dermatitis); or illnesses such as measles, rheumatic fever, or juvenile rheumatoid arthritis. Abdominal distention is associated with gastrointestinal disorders.

🔑 CN: Physiological adaptation; CL: Analyze

17. 2. To ensure appropriate psychosocial development, a child needs to have normal patterns maintained as much as possible during illness. It is tempting to give ill children special treatment and to relax discipline. However, family routines and discipline should be kept as normal as possible. The child needs to know the limits to ensure feelings of security. When they are ill, children commonly attempt to stretch the rules and limits. If this occurs, returning to the previous well-behavior patterns will take time.

🔑 CN: Health promotion and maintenance; CL: Analyze

18. 1. The reason that urinary tract infections are a problem in children with vesicoureteral reflux is that urine flows back up the ureter, past the incompetent valve, and back into the bladder after the child has finished voiding. This incomplete emptying of the bladder results in stasis of urine, providing a good medium for bacterial growth and subsequent infection. Vesicoureteral reflux does not cause bladder spasms or painful urination.

However, the child may experience painful urination with a urinary tract infection.

🔑 CN: Physiological adaptation; CL: Apply

The Client with Glomerulonephritis

19. 3. The best selection of food would include no added salt or salty food. Because sodium cannot be excreted due to the oliguria and to avoid increasing the hypertension, a low-salt diet is recommended. Most canned foods have sodium added as a preservative. Ham, hot dogs, canned peas, canned carrots, corn chips, pickles, and milk are high in sodium.

🔑 CN: Health promotion and maintenance; CL: Analyze

20. 2. Hypertension occurs with acute glomerulonephritis. The symptoms of headache and blurred vision may indicate elevated blood pressure. Hypertension in acute glomerulonephritis occurs because of the inability of the kidneys to remove fluid and sodium; the fluid is reabsorbed, causing fluid volume excess. The nurse must verify that these symptoms are due to hypertension. Calling the HCP before confirming the cause of the symptoms would not facilitate the treatment. Putting the client to bed may help treat the elevated blood pressure, but first the nurse must establish that high blood pressure is the cause of the symptoms. Administering acetaminophen for high blood pressure is not recommended.

🔑 CN: Physiological adaptation; CL: Analyze

21. 3. The child with acute poststreptococcal glomerulonephritis experiences a problem with renal function that ultimately affects fluid balance. While intake and output, electrolytes, and vital signs all provide information about fluid status, weight is the best indicator of fluid balance.

🔑 CN: Physiological adaptation; CL: Analyze

22. 2. The most appropriate and effective choice would be ice chips because they help moisten the mouth and lips while keeping fluid intake low. However, ice chips must still be counted as intake with the fluid restriction. Sweet beverages, such as diet cola or lemonade, commonly increase thirst. Tap water effectively relieves thirst but does not help keep fluid intake low.

🔑 CN: Physiological adaptation; CL: Analyze

23. 1. Generally, school-age children enjoy activities with their peers first, then family members, and lastly younger children. School-age children like to be busy but also to accomplish something. This helps to meet their task of industry versus inferiority, feeling good about what they are able to accomplish.

🔑 CN: Health promotion and maintenance; CL: Analyze

24. 1. The nurse should assess the child's neurologic status because hypertensive encephalopathy is a major potential complication of the acute phase of glomerulonephritis. Seizure precautions also should be instituted. Hypertensive encephalopathy can result in transient loss of vision, hemiparesis, disorientation, and grand mal seizures. Encouraging the child to drink more water is inappropriate because the child has had a low urine output for 14 hours. Typically, in this situation, fluids would be restricted. Although a low-sodium diet is encouraged, it is not the priority action at this time. Initially, bed rest, not ambulation, is advocated during the acute phase of glomerulonephritis.

🔑 CN: Reduction of risk potential; CL: Analyze

25. 2. The nurse would expect a person with a normal glomerular filtration rate (GFR) to have approximately equal inputs and outputs. Chronic renal failure has five stages. In stage I, the GFR is approximately greater than or equal to 90 mL/min/1.73 m^2. In stage II, the GFR decreases to approximately 60 to 89 mL/min/1.73 m^2. The decreased urine output may indicate worsening disease and should be reported. Assessing the client's intake and output is still important, but notifying the provider is the priority. Fluids are restricted based on decreased sodium. Clients are encouraged to drink to thirst. Therefore, there is not enough information to suggest increasing or restricting fluids.

🔑 CN: Physiological adaptation; CL: Analyze

26. 3. APSGN is an immune complex disease. Large antigen-antibody complexes are formed that deposit in the glomerular capillary loops, leading to obstruction. APSGN is considered an autoimmune disorder, not an infection. Antibodies do not attack the kidneys in this disorder.

🔑 CN: Physiologic adaptation; CL: Analyze

The Client with Nephrotic Syndrome

27. -/+ **2, 3, 5.** Adverse effects of steroid therapy include edema of the face and trunk, increased susceptibility to infection, gastric and intestinal mucosal bleeding, sodium and water retention, and hypertension. Steroid therapy can also cause vision problems. Urinary output is decreased due to the retention of sodium. Bleeding gums do not result from steroids.

🗝 CN: Pharmacological and parenteral therapies; CL: Apply

28. 3. Readings at or above the 95th percentile are considered indicative of hypertension. Here, both the systolic and diastolic readings are at the 95th percentile for a boy who is at the 75th percentile for height. This blood pressure may be a side effect of the medication or part of the disease process and needs to be reported. The charts do not define hypotension. Readings below the 90th percentile are considered normal. Blood pressures at the 90th percentile but below the 95th are considered prehypertension. Blood pressures at the 99th percentile are considered stage II hypertension and are most likely to need antihypertensive medications.

🗝 CN: Reduction of risk potential; CL: Analyze

29. 1. The child with nephrotic syndrome would present with hypoalbuminemia not hyperalbuminemia due to a decrease of albumin in the bloodstream and an increase in glomerular permeability. Nephrotic syndrome is characterized by edema, massive proteinuria, hypoalbuminemia, hypoproteinemia, hyperlipidemia, and altered immunity.

🗝 CN: Reduction of risk potential; CL: Evaluate

30. 1. Children with nephrotic syndrome usually require sodium restriction. Because potato chips and bologna are high in sodium, the parent's statement about finding something else reflects an understanding of this need. Although fluid intake is not restricted in children with nephrotic syndrome, 17 cups (4 L) is an excessive amount for a toddler. The typical fluid requirement for a toddler is 115 mL/kg. Surgical intervention and antibiotic therapy are not parts of the treatment plan for nephrotic syndrome.

🗝 CN: Physiological adaptation; CL: Evaluate

31. 4. The best indicator of fluid balance is weight. Therefore, daily weight measurements help determine fluid losses and gains. Although limiting visitors to 2 to 3 hours per day or maintaining strict bed rest would help ensure that the child gets adequate rest, this is unrelated to the child's fluid balance. In nephrotic syndrome, urine is tested for protein, not specific gravity.

🗝 CN: Physiological adaptation; CL: Analyze

32. 2. The child's swollen eyes are caused by fluid accumulation. Elevating the head of the bed allows gravity to increase the downward flow of fluids in the body, away from the face. Applying cool compresses or eye drops or limiting television may be comforting but will not relieve the swelling.

🗝 CN: Physiological adaptation; CL: Analyze

33. 1. Fluid accumulates in the abdomen and interstitial spaces as a result of hydrostatic pressure changes. Increased abdominal fluid is evidenced by an increase in abdominal girth. Therefore, decreased abdominal girth is a sign of reduced fluid in the third spaces and tissues. When fluid accumulates in the abdomen and interstitial spaces, the child does not feel hungry and does not eat well. Although increased caloric intake may indicate decreased intestinal edema, it is not the best and most accurate indicator of fluid retention. An increased respiratory rate may be an indication of increased fluid in the abdomen (ascites) causing pressure on the diaphragm. Heart rate usually stays in the normal range even with excessive fluid volume.

🗝 CN: Physiological adaptation; CL: Evaluate

34. 4. Placing soft cloth between opposing skin surfaces absorbs moisture and keeps the area dry, thus preventing any further breakdown. A child with nephrotic syndrome and severe edema is usually maintained on bed rest; therefore, ambulation is not appropriate. Applying lotion or powder to edematous surfaces that touch increases moisture and can lead to maceration, causing further breakdown.

🗝 CN: Basic care and comfort; CL: Analyze

35. 11.3 mg

11.3 kg × 2 mg = 22.7 mg/day

22.7 mg ÷ 2 = 11.3 mg per dose

🗝 CN: Pharmacological and parenteral therapies; CL: Apply

36. 2. A child recovering from nephrotic syndrome should be protected from infection. Therefore, the nurse would teach the parents to keep the child away from others with an infection. Because pain is not associated with this disorder, pain medication typically is not needed. The HCP should be notified if urine output decreases, not increases. In children recovering from nephrotic syndrome, there is no reason to administer acetaminophen daily.

🗝 CN: Reduction of risk potential; CL: Analyze

The Client with Acute or Chronic Renal Failure

37. 3. A client who has had a ruptured appendix may have peritoneal scarring that may alter the effectiveness of treatment. Living a long distance from a medical facility is typically a reason to select peritoneal dialysis. Attending a large school is not a problem, but the school nurse needs to be included as part of the health care team. Typically, the treatment schedule can be planned to allow for uninterrupted sleep at night.

CN: Management of care; CL: Analyze

38. 3. One of the advantages of using continuous ambulatory peritoneal dialysis is that clients have more mobility. Fluid is manually filled into the abdomen and dwells for 3 to 6 hours. During the dwell phase, the client may be mobile and participate in activities. The fluid is manually drained into the dialysate bag by gravity after the dwell phase. Dialysate bags are weighed before filling and after draining to determine the amount of fluid removal. All forms of peritoneal dialysis carry the risk for infection, so sterile technique must be maintained with catheter care, dressing changes, and dialysate bag changes. A peritoneal dialysis machine is used with continuous cyclical peritoneal dialysis. This method is done at night and requires that the client remain in bed.

CN: Physiological adaptation; CL: Evaluate

39. 3. Until it heals, the catheter exit site is particularly vulnerable to invasion by pathogenic organisms. Therefore, the site must be monitored for signs of infection. An occlusive dressing is not needed because there is no danger of air being sucked in or out of the peritoneal space. Furthermore, the catheter used is designed with a cuff so that the skin grows around the catheter, sealing off the area. Site care may be done at any time, but the child may experience abdominal discomfort if the peritoneal space is dry during site care. Holding the catheter taut or pulling on it may cause irritation of the skin at the exit site, which could lead to infection.

CN: Safety and infection control; CL: Analyze

40. 4. With minimal or absent kidney function, the serum phosphate level rises, and the ionized calcium level falls in response. This causes increased secretion of parathyroid hormone, which releases calcium from the bones. Therefore, the intake of foods high in phosphorus is restricted. Because renal failure results in decreased erythropoietin production, an increase in ascorbic acid intake is needed. Because magnesium is minimally affected by renal failure, its intake need not be restricted.

CN: Physiological adaptation; CL: Apply

41. 4. Demonstration of desire to do the dressing changes and manage medications implies compliance with the medical regimen and acceptance of the condition, thereby indicating a positive self-image. Diffuse somatic symptoms could indicate anxiety or problems with coping, which could have a negative effect on self-concept. Insistence on choosing restricted foods implies that the adolescent has not accepted the diagnosis and is noncompliant, possibly indicating a negative self-concept. Social withdrawal from activities may indicate depression, possibly negatively affecting the self-concept.

CN: Physiological adaptation; CL: Evaluate

42. 2. The child with acute renal failure needs extra calories to reduce tissue catabolism, metabolic acidosis, and uremia. Using a high-fat and high-carbohydrate diet helps supply the necessary extra calories. If the child is able to tolerate oral foods, concentrated food sources that are high in carbohydrates and fat but low in protein, potassium, and sodium may be provided.

CN: Physiological adaptation; CL: Apply

43. 3. For an adolescent, body image is a major concern. The presence of an abdominal catheter can greatly affect the client's body image. The adolescent needs opportunities to discuss feelings about altered body image due to the catheter. Adolescents need to be with their peers and maintain social activities and contacts to meet the developmental tasks of this age group. The adolescent client may choose to confide in friends for both psychological health and physical safety. Because peers are most important to adolescents, they will confide in their peers before confiding in family members. Another major developmental need of the adolescent is achieving independence. Relying on the parents would interfere with the adolescent's ability to do so.

CN: Psychosocial integrity; CL: Analyze

44. 4. Tissue swelling, pain, redness, and exudate indicate infection. Dialysate leakage is associated with improper catheter function, incomplete healing at the insertion site, or excessive instillation of dialysate. Granulation tissue indicates healing around the exit site, not infection. Increased time for drainage may indicate that the tube is kinked, suggesting an obstruction.

CN: Reduction of risk potential; CL: Analyze

45. **1.** Normally, dialysate drainage return should be clear. With peritonitis, large numbers of bacteria, white blood cells, and fibrin cause the dialysate to appear cloudy. Abdominal distention is unrelated to peritonitis. However, it might suggest an obstruction. Weight gain and shortness of breath are associated with fluid excess, not infection.

CN: Physiological adaptation; CL: Evaluate

46. **1.** Accumulation of hard stool in the bowel can cause the distended intestine to block the holes of the catheter. Consequently, the dialysate cannot flow freely through the catheter. Decreasing the dialysate infusion may make the dialysis less effective. Altering fluid, electrolyte, and waste product removal can cause fluid and electrolyte imbalance and increased levels of blood urea nitrogen and creatinine. Incorporating the increased times into the dialysis may make the dialysis less effective because fewer cycles can be scheduled. Shoulder pain, which may occur occasionally, can be caused by air in the peritoneal space and diaphragmatic irritation. However, it is unrelated to inflow and drain times.

CN: Physiological adaptation; CL: Analyze

47. **4.** Regulation of the diet is the most effective means, besides dialysis, for reducing renal excretion. Dietary phosphorus is restricted, which reduces the protein load on the kidneys. Clients are also given substances to bind phosphorus in the intestines to prevent absorption. Limited protein in the diet should include foods high in essential amino acids. Foods high in fat and carbohydrate are used to increase caloric intake. Sodium and water may not be restricted because of the continual loss of sodium and water through the dialysate. Iron-rich foods are commonly high in protein.

CN: Physiological adaptation; CL: Evaluate

The Client with Wilms' Tumor

48. **3.** When a client receiving chemotherapy develops neutropenia, eating uncooked fruits and vegetables may pose a health risk due to possible bacterial contamination. All other foods are either cooked or pasteurized and would not produce a health risk.

CN: Safety and infection control; CL: Apply

49. **2.** The abdomen of the child with Wilms' tumor should not be palpated because of the danger of disseminating tumor cells. Techniques such as measuring the occipitofrontal circumference (which is done in children younger than 18 months of age because the anterior fontanelle closes between 12 and 18 months of age), upright positioning, and measuring chest circumference are not necessarily contraindicated; however, the child with Wilms' tumor should always be handled gently and carefully.

CN: Physiological adaptation; CL: Analyze

50. **1.** A stage II tumor is one that extends beyond the kidney but is completely resected. The tumor staging is verified during surgery to maximize treatment protocols. The following criteria for staging are commonly used: *stage I*, tumor is limited to the kidney and completely resected; *stage II*, tumor extends beyond the kidney but is completely resected; *stage III*, residual nonhematogenous tumor is confined to the abdomen; *stage IV*, hematogenous metastasis occurs, with deposits beyond stage III (lung, bone and brain, liver); and *stage V*, bilateral renal involvement is present at diagnosis.

CN: Physiological adaptation; CL: Evaluate

51. **3.** The child who has undergone abdominal surgery is usually placed in a semi-Fowler's position to facilitate draining of abdominal contents and promote pulmonary expansion. The modified Trendelenburg position is used for clients in shock. The lateral recumbent position is likely to be uncomfortable for this child because of the large transabdominal incision. The supine position, without the head elevated, puts the child at increased risk for aspiration.

CN: Reduction of risk potential; CL: Analyze

52. **1.** Children who have undergone abdominal surgery are at risk for intestinal obstruction from a dynamic ileus. Indications of intestinal obstruction include abdominal distention, decreased or absent bowel sounds, and vomiting. Later signs of intestinal obstruction include tachycardia, fever, hypotension, increased respirations, shock, and decreased urinary output.

CN: Reduction of risk potential; CL: Analyze

53. **3.** Because the child has only one kidney, measures should be recommended to prevent urinary tract infection and injury to the remaining kidney. Severe pain and dependent edema are not associated with surgery for Wilms' tumor. Dietary sodium is not restricted because the function of the remaining kidney is not impaired.

CN: Reduction of risk potential; CL: Analyze

Managing Care, Quality, and Safety of Children with Health Problems of the Urinary System

54. 4. There are many problems with this medication prescription. The abbreviation *QOD* is ambiguous and open to various interpretations. The abbreviation *D/C* may be interpreted as "discontinue" or "discharge." The prescriber should have specifically stated when to start the lower dose because the nurse could reason beginning the medication that day, the next, or even the day after that. The only safe thing to do is call for clarification.

CN: Safety and infection control; CL: Analyze

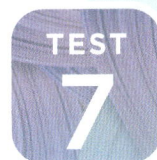

TEST 7: The Child with Neurologic Health Problems

- The Client with Myelomeningocele
- The Client with Hydrocephalus
- The Client with a Seizure Disorder
- The Client with Meningitis
- The Client with Near-Drowning
- The Client with Guillain-Barré Syndrome (Infectious Polyneuritis)
- The Client with a Head Injury
- The Client with a Brain Tumor
- The Client with a Spinal Cord Injury
- Managing Care, Quality, and Safety of Children with Neurologic Health Problems
- Answers, Rationales, and Test-Taking Strategies

The Client with Myelomeningocele

1. Parents bring a 10-month-old boy with myelomeningocele and hydrocephalus with a ventriculoperitoneal shunt to the emergency department. The client's symptoms include vomiting, poor feeding, lethargy, and irritability. What intervention(s) by the nurse would be **most** appropriate? Select all that apply.
   - ☐ 1. Weigh the child.
   - ☐ 2. Listen to bowel sounds.
   - ☐ 3. Palpate the posterior fontanelle.
   - ☐ 4. Obtain vital signs.
   - ☐ 5. Assess the pitch and quality of the child's cry.

2. The nurse positions a neonate with an unrepaired myelomeningocele. Which position is **most** appropriate?
   - ☐ 1. supine with the hips at 90-degree flexion
   - ☐ 2. right side-lying position with the knees flexed
   - ☐ 3. prone with the hips in abduction
   - ☐ 4. supine in semi-Fowler position with the chest and abdomen elevated

3. The nurse assesses an infant with a myelomeningocele. Which finding should be reported to the health care provider as a sign of increased intracranial pressure?
   - ☐ 1. minimal lower extremity movement
   - ☐ 2. a high-pitched cry
   - ☐ 3. overflow voiding only
   - ☐ 4. a fontanelle that bulges with crying

4. The nurse develops the plan of care for an infant diagnosed with myelomeningocele and the parents who have just been informed of the infant's diagnosis. The nurse should include which action as the **priority** when the parents visit the infant for the first time?
   - ☐ 1. Emphasize the infant's normal and positive features.
   - ☐ 2. Encourage the parents to discuss their fears and concerns.
   - ☐ 3. Reinforce the health care provider's (HCP's) explanation of the defect.
   - ☐ 4. Have the parents feed their infant.

5. The birth parent of an infant with myelomeningocele asks if the child is likely to have any other defects. The nurse responds based on the understanding that myelomeningocele is commonly associated with which disorder?
   - ☐ 1. excessive cerebrospinal fluid within the cranial cavity
   - ☐ 2. abnormally small head
   - ☐ 3. congenital absence of the cranial vault
   - ☐ 4. overriding of the cranial sutures

6. The parents of an infant with myelomeningocele ask the nurse about their child's future mental ability. What is the nurse's **best** response?
   ☐ 1. "About one-third have an intellectual disability, but it is too early to tell about your child."
   ☐ 2. "Intellectual disabilities occur in about two-thirds of these children, and you will know soon if this will occur."
   ☐ 3. "Your child will probably be of normal intelligence since they demonstrate signs of it now."
   ☐ 4. "You will need to talk with the health care provider (HCP) about that, but you can ask later."

7. The nurse places an infant with myelomeningocele in an isolette bed shortly after birth. The nurse should use which indicator as the **best** way to determine the effectiveness of this intervention?
   ☐ 1. The partial pressure of arterial oxygen remains between 94 and 100 mm Hg.
   ☐ 2. The axillary temperature remains between 97°F and 98°F (36.1°C and 36.7°C).
   ☐ 3. The bilirubin level remains stable.
   ☐ 4. Weight increases by about 30 g (1 oz) per day.

8. The nurse cares for an infant after surgical repair of a myelomeningocele. Which position should the nurse use to prevent musculoskeletal deformity in the infant?
   ☐ 1. Place the feet in flexion.
   ☐ 2. Allow the hips to be abducted.
   ☐ 3. Maintain the knees in the neutral position.
   ☐ 4. Place the legs in adduction.

9. The nurse develops the discharge plan for the parents of an infant who has undergone a myelomeningocele repair. What information is **most** important for the nurse to include?
   ☐ 1. a list of available hospital services
   ☐ 2. schedule for daily home health care
   ☐ 3. chaplain referral for psychological support
   ☐ 4. daily care required by the infant

10. The nurse performs discharge teaching with the parent of an infant with a repaired upper lumbar myelomeningocele. Which statement indicates that the parent understands the nurse's teaching?
    ☐ 1. "I can apply a heating pad to the lower back."
    ☐ 2. "I will be sure to keep my child away from other children."
    ☐ 3. "I will call the health care provider (HCP) if their urine has a funny smell."
    ☐ 4. "I will prop my child on pillows to keep them from rolling over."

11. A preschooler with a history of repaired lumbar myelomeningocele is in the emergency department with wheezing and skin rash. Which question should the nurse ask the parent **first**?
    ☐ 1. "Is your child taking any medications?"
    ☐ 2. "Who brought your child to the emergency department?"
    ☐ 3. "Is your child allergic to bananas or any other food?"
    ☐ 4. "What are you doing to treat your child's skin rash?"

The Client with Hydrocephalus

12. The nurse completes an assessment of an infant in the outpatient clinic. Which clinical manifestation(s) would lead the nurse to suspect an infant has hydrocephaly? Select all that apply.
    ☐ 1. depressed fontanelle
    ☐ 2. headache
    ☐ 3. vomiting
    ☐ 4. low-pitched cry
    ☐ 5. irritability
    ☐ 6. pupillary changes

13. The nurse assesses a 2-month-old infant with hydrocephalus and a ventriculoperitoneal shunt. The nurse obtains the infant's vital signs. To obtain the **most** significant information about the child's status, which assessment should the nurse make **next**?

    ☐ 1. status of the posterior fontanelle
    ☐ 2. pupillary reaction to light
    ☐ 3. occipital frontal head circumference
    ☐ 4. presence of the primitive reflex

14. The nurse is providing postoperative care for an infant who had a ventriculoperitoneal shunt placed to correct hydrocephalus. Which clinical finding warrants **immediate** intervention?
    ☐ 1. abdominal distention
    ☐ 2. lethargy
    ☐ 3. facial edema
    ☐ 4. headache

15. The nurse provides postoperative care to a child after insertion of a ventriculoperitoneal shunt. Which action is **most** indicated?
☐ 1. Administer narcotics for pain control.
☐ 2. Check the urine for glucose and protein.
☐ 3. Monitor for increased temperature.
☐ 4. Test cerebrospinal fluid leakage for protein.

16. A nurse evaluates discharge teaching as successful when the parents of a school-age child with a ventriculoperitoneal shunt insertion identify which sign as signaling a blocked shunt?
☐ 1. decreased urine output with stable intake
☐ 2. tense fontanelle and increased head circumference
☐ 3. elevated temperature and reddened incisional site
☐ 4. irritability and increasing difficulty with eating

The Client with a Seizure Disorder

17. STEP 1

The parent brings a 15-month-old male client to the pediatrician's office after a possible febrile seizure.

> **Nurse's Notes**
>
> **0800:**
> The parent reports that the toddler was a vaginal birth and was born 1 week before the due date. Immunizations were administered last week and are now up to date. The client is still bottle-feeding, sleeps through the night, and is generally a happy toddler. Last night, the client developed a fever of 102.5°F (39.2°C) that came down with acetaminophen. This morning, the parent reported seeing the toddler have 20 seconds of eye twitching and rhythmical bilateral movements of the upper extremities. When it stopped, they brought the client to the office to be evaluated. Vital signs are temperature 104°F (40.0°C); heart rate 130 bpm; respiration rate 30 breaths/min; blood pressure 100/60 mm Hg; and pulse oximetry 95%.

➤ Highlight the findings that require follow-up. Answer choices have been underlined.

> **Nurse's Notes**
>
> **0800:**
> The parent reports that the toddler was a vaginal birth and was born 1 week before the due date. <u>Immunizations were administered last week</u> and are now up to date. The <u>client is still bottle-feeding</u>, sleeps through the night, and is generally a happy toddler. Last night, the client developed a fever of 102.5°F (39.2°C) that came down with acetaminophen. This morning, the parent reported seeing the toddler have <u>20 seconds of eye twitching and rhythmical bilateral movements of the upper extremities.</u> When it stopped, they brought the client to the office to be evaluated. Vital signs are <u>temperature 104°F (40.0°C)</u>; <u>heart rate 130 bpm</u>; <u>respiration rate 30 breaths/min</u>; blood pressure 100/60 mm Hg; and pulse oximetry 95%.

18. STEP 2

The parent brings a 15-month-old male client to the pediatrician's office after a possible febrile seizure.

> **Nurse's Notes**
>
> **0800:**
> The parent reports that the toddler was a vaginal birth and was born 1 week before the due date. Immunizations were administered last week and are now up to date. The client is still bottle-feeding, sleeps through the night, and is generally a happy toddler. Last night, the client developed a fever of 102.5°F (39.2°C) that came down with acetaminophen. This morning, the parent reported seeing the toddler have 20 seconds of eye twitching and rhythmical bilateral movements of the upper extremities. When it stopped, they brought the client to the office to be evaluated. Vital signs are temperature 104°F (40.0°C); heart rate 130 bpm; respiration rate 30 breaths/min; blood pressure 100/60 mm Hg; and pulse oximetry 95%.

➤ What assessment(s) would be critical in determining the infant's risk for a subsequent seizure? Select all that apply.

☐ 1. family history of febrile seizures
☐ 2. recent trauma to the head
☐ 3. limp and flaccid appearance after the seizure
☐ 4. known maternal infection
☐ 5. height in centimeters
☐ 6. prolonged time between maternal membrane rupture and delivery
☐ 7. recent possibility of poisoning

19. STEP 3

The parent brings a 15-month-old male client to the pediatrician's office after a possible febrile seizure.

Nurse's Notes

0800:
The parent reports that the toddler was a vaginal birth and was born 1 week before the due date. Immunizations were administered last week and are now up to date. The client is still bottle-feeding, sleeps through the night, and is generally a happy toddler. Last night, the client developed a fever of 102.5°F (39.2°C) that came down with acetaminophen. This morning, the parent reported seeing the toddler have 20 seconds of eye twitching and rhythmical bilateral movements of the upper extremities. When it stopped, they brought the client to the office to be evaluated. Vital signs are temperature 104°F (40.0°C); heart rate 130 bpm; respiration rate 30 breaths/min; blood pressure 100/60 mm Hg; and pulse oximetry 95%.

Flow Sheet Immunization Record

Vaccine	Birth	2-month	4-month	6-month	12-month	15-month
Hepatitis B	Dose 1	Dose 2		Dose 3		Dose 4
Diphtheria, tetanus, and pertussis		Dose 1	Dose 2	Dose 3		Dose 4
Haemophilus influenzae type b		Dose 1	Dose 2	Dose 3		Dose 4
Pneumococcal conjugate		Dose 1	Dose 2	Dose 3	Dose 4	
Inactivated polio		Dose 1	Dose 2			Dose 3
Hepatitis A					Dose 1	
Measles, mumps, rubella						Dose 1
Varicella						Dose 1

The nurse reviews the immunization record from last week.

➤ Select **two** priorities for the care of this client.

☐	1. ruling out causes of the seizure other than fever
☐	2. preventing future fevers
☐	3. stopping future vaccination for measles, mumps, and rubella
☐	4. teaching parent first aid for seizures
☐	5. arranging developmental testing

20. STEP 4

The parent brings a 15-month-old male client to the pediatrician's office after a possible febrile seizure.

Nurse's Notes

0800:
The parent reports that the toddler was a vaginal birth and was born 1 week before the due date. Immunizations were administered last week and are now up to date. The client is still bottle-feeding, sleeps through the night, and is generally a happy toddler. Last night, the client developed a fever of 102.5°F (39.2°C) that came down with acetaminophen. This morning, the parent reported seeing the toddler have 20 seconds of eye twitching and rhythmical bilateral movements of the upper extremities. When it stopped, they brought the client to the office to be evaluated. Vital signs are temperature 104°F (40.0°C); heart rate 130 bpm; respiration rate 30 breaths/min; blood pressure 100/60 mm Hg; and pulse oximetry 95%.

0820:
The toddler experienced a 30-second tonic-clonic seizure involving all four extremities.

Flow Sheet Immunization Record

Vaccine	Birth	2-month	4-month	6-month	12-month	15-month
Hepatitis B	Dose 1	Dose 2		Dose 3		Dose 4
Diphtheria, tetanus, and pertussis		Dose 1	Dose 2	Dose 3		Dose 4
Haemophilus influenzae type b		Dose 1	Dose 2	Dose 3		Dose 4
Pneumococcal conjugate		Dose 1	Dose 2	Dose 3	Dose 4	
Inactivated polio		Dose 1	Dose 2			Dose 3
Hepatitis A					Dose 1	
Measles, mumps, rubella						Dose 1
Varicella						Dose 1

The toddler experiences another seizure during the office visit. The health care provider decides to admit the toddler for diagnostic testing. The nurse calls the report to the receiving unit.

➤ Which diagnostic test(s) should the receiving nurse be prepared to include in parent teaching? Select all that apply.

- [ ] 1. electroencephalogram (EEG)
- [ ] 2. chest x-ray
- [ ] 3. serum electrolytes
- [ ] 4. cerebrospinal fluid (CSF) analysis
- [ ] 5. serum type and cross to determine blood type
- [ ] 6. computerized tomography (CT) scan
- [ ] 7. gentamicin trough level

21. STEP 5

A 15-month-old toddler is admitted to the pediatric unit after a possible febrile seizure.

Nurse's Notes

0800:
The parent reports that the toddler was a vaginal birth and was born 1 week before the due date. Immunizations were administered last week and are now up to date. The client is still bottle-feeding, sleeps through the night, and is generally a happy toddler. Last night, the client developed a fever of 102.5°F (39.2°C) that came down with acetaminophen. This morning, the parent reported seeing the toddler have 20 seconds of eye twitching and rhythmical bilateral movements of the upper extremities. When it stopped, they brought the client to the office to be evaluated. Vital signs are temperature 104°F (40.0°C); heart rate 130 bpm; respiration rate 30 breaths/min; blood pressure 100/60 mm Hg; and pulse oximetry 95%.

0820:
The toddler experienced a 30-second tonic-clonic seizure involving all four extremities.

Flow Sheet
Immunization Record

Vaccine	Birth	2-month	4-month	6-month	12-month	15-month
Hepatitis B	Dose 1	Dose 2		Dose 3		Dose 4
Diphtheria, tetanus, and pertussis		Dose 1	Dose 2	Dose 3		Dose 4
Haemophilus influenzae type b		Dose 1	Dose 2	Dose 3		Dose 4
Pneumococcal conjugate		Dose 1	Dose 2	Dose 3	Dose 4	
Inactivated polio		Dose 1	Dose 2			Dose 3
Hepatitis A					Dose 1	
Measles, mumps, rubella						Dose 1
Varicella						Dose 1

Orders

1. Nursing
   - seizure precautions
   - diet as tolerated
   - vital signs every 4 hours
2. Medications
   - acetaminophen 80-mg suppository. Give 1 per rectum every 6 hours as needed (PRN) for fever *or*
   - acetaminophen 160-mg/5-mL suspension. Give 5 mL orally (PO) every 4 hours PRN for fever *or*
   - ibuprofen 100-mg/5-mL oral suspension. Give 5 mL every 6 to 8 hours PRN for fever
   - may alternate acetaminophen with ibuprofen every 3 hours
3. Diagnostics
   - CBC and electrolytes
   - EEG
   - CT scan
   - CSF culture

The nurse receives admission orders for the 15-month-old with a probable febrile seizure. The infant's admitting temperature is 104°F (40.0°C), and the infant is irritable.

➤ Which intervention(s) should the nurse take to reduce the fever quickly? Select all that apply.

- ☐ 1. Sponge the child with tepid water.
- ☐ 2. Apply cool washcloths on the child's forehead or axillary or groin area.
- ☐ 3. Put the child in a tub of water.
- ☐ 4. Put the child in an alcohol bath.
- ☐ 5. Administer ibuprofen suspension orally.
- ☐ 6. Administer an acetaminophen suppository.

22. STEP 6

A 15-month-old toddler is admitted to the pediatric unit after a possible febrile seizure.

Nurse's Notes

0800:
The parent reports that the toddler was a vaginal birth and was born 1 week before the due date. Immunizations were administered last week and are now up to date. The client is still bottle-feeding, sleeps through the night, and is generally a happy toddler. Last night, the client developed a fever of 102.5°F (39.2°C) that came down with acetaminophen. This morning, the parent reported seeing the toddler have 20 seconds of eye twitching and rhythmical bilateral movements of the upper extremities. When it stopped, they brought the client to the office to be evaluated. Vital signs are temperature 104°F (40.0°C); heart rate 130 bpm; respiration rate 30 breaths/min; blood pressure 100/60 mm Hg; and pulse oximetry 95%.

0820:
The toddler experienced a 30-second tonic-clonic seizure involving all four extremities.

Flow Sheet — Immunization Record

Vaccine	Birth	2-month	4-month	6-month	12-month	15-month
Hepatitis B	Dose 1	Dose 2		Dose 3		Dose 4
Diphtheria, tetanus, and pertussis		Dose 1	Dose 2	Dose 3		Dose 4
Haemophilus influenzae type b		Dose 1	Dose 2	Dose 3		Dose 4
Pneumococcal conjugate		Dose 1	Dose 2	Dose 3	Dose 4	
Inactivated polio		Dose 1	Dose 2			Dose 3
Hepatitis A					Dose 1	
Measles, mumps, rubella						Dose 1
Varicella						Dose 1

Orders

1. Nursing
   - seizure precautions
   - diet as tolerated
   - vital signs every 4 hours
2. Medications
   - acetaminophen 80-mg suppository. Give 1 per rectum every 6 hours as needed (PRN) for fever *or*
   - acetaminophen 160-mg/5-mL suspension. Give 5 mL orally (PO) every 4 hours PRN for fever *or*
   - ibuprofen 100-mg/5-mL oral suspension. Give 5 mL every 6 to 8 hours PRN for fever
   - may alternate acetaminophen with ibuprofen every 3 hours
3. Diagnostics
   - CBC and electrolytes
   - EEG
   - CT scan
   - CSF culture

The diagnosis of febrile seizures is confirmed. The nurse completes discharge teaching.

➤ Which parent statement(s) would indicate effective teaching? Select all that apply.

- ☐ 1. "Febrile seizures cannot be prevented, but they are outgrown."
- ☐ 2. "If my infant has one seizure and then another, I will put them in the car and bring them to the emergency department."
- ☐ 3. "If my child starts to have a seizure at home, I will move away furniture or any sharp objects."
- ☐ 4. "If my child starts to have a seizure, I will not put anything in their mouth."
- ☐ 5. "My child might have blue extremities during the seizure."
- ☐ 6. "If my child needs acetaminophen, I will put it in their bottle to disguise the taste."

23. After the nurse instructs a group of schoolteachers about seizures, the teachers role-play a scenario involving a child experiencing a generalized tonic-clonic seizure. Which action, when performed **first**, indicates that the nurse's teaching has been successful?
- ☐ 1. Ask the other children what happened before the seizure.
- ☐ 2. Move the child to the nurse's office for privacy.
- ☐ 3. Remove any nearby objects that could harm the child.
- ☐ 4. Place a padded tongue blade between the child's teeth.

24. A nurse is developing a plan of care with the parents of a school-age client diagnosed with a seizure disorder. What instructions should the nurse give the parents to promote the client's growth and development?
- ☐ 1. The child will need activity limitation and will be unable to perform as well as their peers.
- ☐ 2. There is potential for a learning disability, and the child may need tutoring to reach their grade level.
- ☐ 3. The child will likely have normal intelligence and be able to attend regular school.
- ☐ 4. There will be problems associated with social stigma, and parents should consider home-schooling.

25. The telehealth nurse obtains a history from a parent of a toddler. Which finding should alert the nurse to suspect that the child has had a febrile seizure?
    ☐ 1. The child has had a low-grade fever for several weeks.
    ☐ 2. The family history is negative for convulsions.
    ☐ 3. The seizure resulted in respiratory arrest.
    ☐ 4. The seizure occurred when the child had a respiratory infection.

26. The nurse teaches the parents of a child with febrile seizures about nonpharmacologic methods to lower temperature. Which statement by the parents indicates successful teaching?

    "We will:
    ☐ 1. add extra blankets when they say they are cold."
    ☐ 2. wrap them in a blanket if they start shivering."
    ☐ 3. make the bath water cold enough to make them shiver."
    ☐ 4. use a solution of half alcohol and half water when sponging them."

27. An adolescent girl with a seizure disorder controlled with phenytoin and carbamazepine asks the nurse about getting married and having children. Which response by the nurse would be **most** appropriate?
    ☐ 1. "You probably should not consider having children until your seizures are cured."
    ☐ 2. "Your children will not necessarily have an increased risk for a seizure disorder."
    ☐ 3. "When you decide to have children, talk to the health care provider (HCP) about changing your medication."
    ☐ 4. "Women who have seizure disorders commonly have a difficult time conceiving."

28. The nurse performs medication teaching with an adolescent with a seizure disorder who is receiving valproic acid. The nurse should instruct the client to **immediately** report which sign or symptom to the health care provider (HCP)?
    ☐ 1. diarrhea
    ☐ 2. loss of appetite
    ☐ 3. jaundice
    ☐ 4. sore throat

The Client with Meningitis

29. A 3-month-old infant with meningococcal meningitis has just been admitted to the pediatric unit. Which nursing intervention has the **highest priority**?
    ☐ 1. instituting droplet precautions
    ☐ 2. administering acetaminophen
    ☐ 3. obtaining history information from the parents
    ☐ 4. orienting the parents to the call bell

30. During the acute stage of meningitis, a 3-year-old child is restless and irritable. Which intervention would be **most** appropriate to institute?
    ☐ 1. limiting conversation with the child
    ☐ 2. keeping extraneous noise to a minimum
    ☐ 3. allowing the child to play in the bathtub
    ☐ 4. performing treatments quickly

31. The nurse assesses a child with meningitis. Which finding would lead the nurse to suspect that the child has developed disseminated intravascular coagulation?
    ☐ 1. hemorrhagic skin rash
    ☐ 2. edema
    ☐ 3. cyanosis
    ☐ 4. dyspnea on exertion

32. When interviewing the parents of a toddler, the nurse should suspect pneumococcal meningitis if there is a history of which illness?
    ☐ 1. bladder infection
    ☐ 2. middle ear infection
    ☐ 3. fractured clavicle
    ☐ 4. septic arthritis

33. A preschooler with pneumococcal meningitis is receiving intravenous antibiotic therapy. When discontinuing the intravenous therapy, the nurse allows the child to apply a dressing to the area where the catheter is removed. The nurse's rationale for doing so is based on the interpretation that a child in this age group needs to accomplish which goal?
    ☐ 1. Trust those caring for her.
    ☐ 2. Find diversional activities.
    ☐ 3. Protect the image of an intact body.
    ☐ 4. Relieve the anxiety of separation from home.

34. A child with meningitis is to receive 1000 mL of dextrose 5% in normal saline over 12 hours. At what rate in milliliters per hour should the nurse set the pump? Round your answer to the nearest whole number.

    _____ mL per hour

35. The nurse implements the plan of care for a child with bacterial meningitis. Which intervention(s) would the nurse plan to implement? Select all that apply.
☐ 1. administration of intravenous (IV) antibiotics
☐ 2. IV fluids at 1½ times maintenance
☐ 3. decreasing environmental stimuli
☐ 4. neurologic checks every 4 hours
☐ 5. administration of IV anticonvulsants

36. The nurse is monitoring an infant with meningitis for signs of increased intracranial pressure (ICP). The nurse should assess the infant for which sign(s) or symptom(s)? Select all that apply.
☐ 1. irritability
☐ 2. headache
☐ 3. mood swings
☐ 4. bulging fontanelle
☐ 5. emesis

37. A hospitalized preschooler with meningitis who is to be discharged becomes angry when the discharge is delayed. Which play activity would be **most** appropriate at this time?
☐ 1. reading the child a story
☐ 2. painting with watercolors
☐ 3. pounding on a pegboard
☐ 4. stacking a tower of blocks

The Client with Near-Drowning

38. The nurse is admitting a toddler with the diagnosis of near-drowning in a neighbor's heated swimming pool to the emergency department. The nurse should assess the child for which complication?
☐ 1. hypothermia
☐ 2. hypoxia
☐ 3. fluid aspiration
☐ 4. cutaneous capillary paralysis

39. The nurse is caring for a lethargic but arousable preschooler who is a victim of a near-drowning accident. What should the nurse do **first**?
☐ 1. Administer oxygen.
☐ 2. Institute rewarming.
☐ 3. Prepare for intubation.
☐ 4. Start an intravenous (IV) infusion.

40. The parents of a child tell the nurse that they feel guilty because their child almost drowned. Which remark by the nurse would be **most** appropriate?
☐ 1. "I can understand why you feel guilty, but these things happen."
☐ 2. "Tell me a little bit more about your feelings of guilt."
☐ 3. "You should not have taken your eyes off of your child."
☐ 4. "You should focus on the fact that your child will be all right."

The Client with Guillain-Barré Syndrome (Infectious Polyneuritis)

41. The nurse assesses a school-age child in the clinic who has a sore throat, muscle tenderness, and arms feeling weak and is generally not feeling well. Which is the **most** important assessment for the nurse to make?
☐ 1. difficulty swallowing
☐ 2. diet intake for the last 24 hours
☐ 3. exposure to illnesses
☐ 4. difficulty urinating

42. The nurse cares for a school-age child admitted to the pediatric unit with the diagnosis of Guillain-Barré syndrome. Which action should be the **priority**?
☐ 1. Assess the child's ability to follow simple commands.
☐ 2. Evaluate the child's bilateral muscle strength.
☐ 3. Make a game of range-of-motion exercises.
☐ 4. Provide the child with a diversional activity.

43. The nurse asks a school-age child with Guillain-Barré syndrome to cough and also assesses the child's speech for decreased volume and clarity. The underlying rationale for these assessments is to determine which finding?
☐ 1. inflammation of the larynx and epiglottis
☐ 2. increased intracranial pressure
☐ 3. involvement of facial and cranial nerves
☐ 4. regression to an earlier developmental phase

44. A 9-year-old child with Guillain-Barré syndrome requires mechanical ventilation. Which action should the nurse take?
☐ 1. Maintain the child in a supine position to prevent unnecessary nerve stimulation.
☐ 2. Transfer the child to a bedside chair three times a day to prevent postural hypotension.
☐ 3. Engage the child in vigorous passive range-of-motion exercises to prevent loss of muscle function.
☐ 4. Turn the child slowly and gently from side to side to prevent respiratory complications.

45. The parent brings a child to the clinic after discharge from the hospital for Guillain-Barré syndrome. Which statement by the parent indicates that the discharge plan is being followed?
☐ 1. "My child and their sibling argue all day."
☐ 2. "I have to bribe them to do their exercises."
☐ 3. "I take them to the pool where it is possible to exercise with other children."
☐ 4. "My child has missed a few therapy sessions because they often are asleep."

The Client with a Head Injury

46. A 12-year-old child has had a traumatic head injury from playing in a football game. The client is admitted to the emergency department and transferred to the pediatric intensive care unit. The client has an IV of dextrose 5% in water at 21 mL per hour and nasal oxygen at 2 L per minute. The nurse is assessing the child at the beginning of the shift (2300 hours) and reviews the Glasgow Coma Scale flow sheet below. The nurse notes that the child responds to pain, is making incomprehensible sounds, and has abnormal flexion of the limbs. What should the nurse do **first**?

Flow Sheet

Glasgow Coma Score		
Test	Score	Client Response
Eye Opening		
Spontaneously	4	Opens eyes spontaneously
To Speech	3	Opens eyes to verbal commands
To Pain	2	Opens eyes to pain stimulus
None	1	Doesn't open eyes in response to stimulus
Motor Response		
Obeys	6	Reacts to verbal command
Localizes	5	Identifies localized pain
Withdraws	4	Flexes and withdraws from painful stimulus
Abnormal Flexion	3	Assumes a decorticate position
Abnormal Extension	2	Assumes a decerebrate position
None	1	No response; lies flaccid
Verbal Response		
Oriented	5	Is oriented and converses
Confused	4	Is oriented and confused
Inappropriate Words	3	Replies randomly with incorrect words
Incomprehensible	2	Moans or screams
None	1	No response

Date	Time	Progress Notes
11/13	1700	GCS = 13
11/13	1800	GCS = 12
11/13	1900	GCS = 13
11/13	2000	GCS = 11
11/13	2100	GCS = 10
11/13	2200	GCS = 9

☐ 1. Notify the health care provider (HCP).
☐ 2. Lower the head of the bed.
☐ 3. Increase the rate of nasal oxygen.
☐ 4. Increase the rate of the IV infusion.

47. A school-age child with a severe head injury is unconscious and has coarse breath sounds, a temperature of 39°C (102.2°F), a heart rate of 70 bpm, a blood pressure of 130/60 mm Hg, and an intracranial pressure (ICP) of 36 mm Hg. Which action should the nurse perform **first**?
☐ 1. Administer prescribed intravenous (IV) mannitol.
☐ 2. Suction the child.
☐ 3. Encourage the parent to talk to the child.
☐ 4. Administer prescribed rectal acetaminophen.

48. The nurse is inserting a nasogastric (NG) tube in a child admitted with head trauma. The nurse should explain to the parents that the NG tube will be used for what purpose?
☐ 1. Administer medications.
☐ 2. Decompress the stomach.
☐ 3. Obtain gastric specimens for analysis.
☐ 4. Provide adequate nutrition.

49. A nasogastric tube is prescribed to be inserted for a child with severe head trauma. Diagnostic testing reveals that the child has a basilar skull fracture. What should the nurse do **next**?
☐ 1. Ask for the prescription to be changed to an oral gastric tube.
☐ 2. Attempt to place the tube into the duodenum.
☐ 3. Test the gastric aspirate for blood.
☐ 4. Use extra lubrication when inserting the nasogastric tube.

50. The parents of a child in a coma with a serious head injury ask the nurse if the child is going to be all right. Which response by the nurse would be **most** appropriate?
☐ 1. "Children usually do not do very well after head injuries like this."
☐ 2. "Children usually recover rapidly from head injuries."
☐ 3. "It is hard to tell this early, but we will keep you informed of the progress."
☐ 4. "That is something you will have to talk to the health care provider (HCP) about."

51. A parent of a child with a moderate head injury asks the nurse, "How will you know if my child is getting worse?" The nurse should tell the parents that the **best** indicator of the child's brain function is which factor?
☐ 1. vital signs
☐ 2. level of consciousness (LOC)
☐ 3. reactions of the pupils
☐ 4. motor strength

52. The nurse develops the plan of care for a child who is unconscious after a serious head injury. The nurse would expect to place the child in which position?
☐ 1. prone with hips and knees slightly elevated
☐ 2. lying on the side, with the head of the bed elevated
☐ 3. lying on the back, in the Trendelenburg position
☐ 4. in the semi-Fowler position, with arms at the side

53. The health care provider has prescribed intravenous mannitol for a child with a head injury. The **best** indicator that the drug has been effective is which assessment finding?
☐ 1. increased urine output
☐ 2. improved level of consciousness
☐ 3. decreased intracranial pressure (ICP)
☐ 4. decreased edema

54. The nurse assigned to telephone triage returns the call of a parent whose teenager experienced a hard tackle last night. The parent reports, "They seemed dazed after it happened, and the coach had them sit out the rest of the game, but they're fine now." What is the **most** appropriate instruction for the nurse to give?
☐ 1. "Take your child immediately to the emergency department."
☐ 2. "Your child can't return to play until they have been evaluated by a health care provider (HCP)."
☐ 3. "If your child seems fine now and has had no other symptoms, it probably was not a concussion."
☐ 4. "Watch your child closely, and call us back if you see any changes."

55. The nurse reviews the history of a child with a concussion. Which finding(s) should be considered risk factors that may complicate recovery from a concussion? Select all that apply.
☐ 1. asthma
☐ 2. attention deficit hyperactivity disorder (ADHD)
☐ 3. depression
☐ 4. migraines
☐ 5. obesity
☐ 6. previous concussion

56. A 3-year-old is recovering from a concussion. The persistence of which finding would the nurse consider as being a normal finding for a 3-year-old?
☐ 1. lack interest in favorite toys
☐ 2. change in eating habits
☐ 3. inability to hop
☐ 4. increased temper tantrums

57. The nurse teaches an adolescent about returning to school after a concussion. Which statement by the client reflects the need for more teaching?
☐ 1. "I should limit my activities that require concentration."
☐ 2. "I must slowly return to my previous activity level as my symptoms improve."
☐ 3. "My symptoms may reemerge with exertion."
☐ 4. "Time is the most important factor in my recovery."

The Client with a Brain Tumor

58. A child with a brain tumor has a decreased respiratory rate and is less responsive to verbal commands than they were when the nurse assessed the client the previous hour. What should the nurse do **next**?
☐ 1. Raise the head of the bed.
☐ 2. Notify the health care provider (HCP).
☐ 3. Turn the client to the side
☐ 4. Obtain an oximeter reading.

59. The nurse reviews the labs for a preschool-age client with a neuroblastoma who has been receiving chemotherapy for the last 4 weeks.

Laboratory Report		
Test	Results	Reference range
Hematocrit	36.8% (0.37)	Males: 42%–52% (0.42–0.52); Females: 35%–47% (0.35–0.47)
Hemoglobin	12.5 g/dL (125 g/L)	Males: 14–17.4 g/dL (140–174 g/L); Females: 12–16 g/dL (120–160 g/L)
WBC	2 x 10^3/mm^3 (2 x 10^9/L)	4.5–10.5 x 10^3 cells/mm^3 (4.5–10.5 x 10^9/L)
Platelets	150,000/mm^3 (150 x 10^9/L)	140,000–400,000/μL (140–400 x 10^9/L).

Based on the child's lab values, what is the **highest priority** nursing intervention?
☐ 1. Encourage meticulous handwashing by the client and visitors.
☐ 2. Prepare to give the child a transfusion of platelets.
☐ 3. Encourage mouth care with a soft toothbrush.
☐ 4. Prepare to give the child a transfusion of packed red blood cells.

60. A school-age child is admitted to the hospital with the diagnosis of probable infratentorial brain tumor. During the child's admission to the pediatric unit, which action should the nurse anticipate taking **first**?
☐ 1. Eliminate the child's anxiety.
☐ 2. Implement seizure precautions.
☐ 3. Introduce the child to other clients of the same age.
☐ 4. Prepare the child and parents for diagnostic procedures.

61. The nurse is giving care to an infant with a brain tumor. The nurse observes the infant arches their back (see figure). What action should the nurse take **first**?

☐ 1. Notify the health care provider (HCP).
☐ 2. Stroke the back to release the arching.
☐ 3. Pad the side rails of the crib.
☐ 4. Place the child prone.

62. The nurse is assessing a child diagnosed with a brain tumor. Which sign(s) or symptom(s) should the nurse expect the child to demonstrate? Select all that apply.
☐ 1. head tilt
☐ 2. vomiting
☐ 3. polydipsia
☐ 4. lethargy
☐ 5. increased appetite
☐ 6. increased pulse

63. The nurse care for a child following a craniotomy for an infratentorial brain tumor. The nurse should place the child in which position to prevent undue strain on the sutures?
☐ 1. prone
☐ 2. semi-Fowler
☐ 3. side-lying
☐ 4. Trendelenburg

64. A child who was intubated after a craniotomy now shows signs of decreased level of consciousness. The health care provider (HCP) prescribes manual hyperventilation to keep the partial pressure of arterial carbon dioxide ($PaCO_2$) between 25 and 29 mm Hg and the partial pressure of arterial oxygen (PaO_2) between 80 and 100 mm Hg. The nurse interprets this prescription based on the understanding that this action will accomplish which goal?
☐ 1. Decrease intracranial pressure.
☐ 2. Ensure a patent airway.
☐ 3. Lower the arousal level.
☐ 4. Produce hypoxia.

65. The nurse notes clear drainage on the child's dressing and bed linen after a craniotomy for a brain tumor. Which action should the nurse do **first**?
☐ 1. Change the dressing.
☐ 2. Elevate the head of the bed.
☐ 3. Test the fluid for glucose.
☐ 4. Notify the health care provider (HCP).

66. An 8-year-old child does well after infratentorial tumor removal and is transferred back to the pediatric unit. Although the client had been told about having their head shaved for surgery, they are very upset. After exploring the child's feelings, the nurse should take which action?
☐ 1. Ask the child if they would like to wear a hat.
☐ 2. Reassure the child that their hair will grow back.
☐ 3. Explain to the child's parents that the reaction is normal.
☐ 4. Suggest that the parents buy the child a wig as a surprise.

67. The nurse discusses home care with the parent of a school-age child who has had a craniotomy for a brain tumor. Which statement made by the parent would warrant further exploration by the nurse?
☐ 1. "After this, I will never let them out of my sight again."
☐ 2. "I hope that my child can go back to school soon."
☐ 3. "I wonder how long it will be before they can ride their bike."
☐ 4. "My child's best friend is eager to see them; I hope they won't be upset."

The Client with a Spinal Cord Injury

68. A nurse, who witnesses an adolescent being thrown from a motorcycle, stops to help. The adolescent reports that they are unable to move their legs. While waiting for the emergency medical service to arrive, what should the nurse do?
☐ 1. Flex the adolescent's knees to relieve stress on their back.
☐ 2. Leave the adolescent as they are, staying close by.
☐ 3. Remove the adolescent's helmet as soon as possible.
☐ 4. Assess the adolescent for abdominal trauma.

69. An adolescent sustains a T3 spinal cord injury. After insertion of an intravenous line, a nasogastric tube, and an indwelling urinary catheter, the adolescent is admitted to the intensive care unit. What should the nurse do **next** when assessment reveals that the adolescent's feet and legs are cool to the touch?
☐ 1. Cover the adolescent's legs with blankets.
☐ 2. Report this finding to the health care provider (HCP) immediately.
☐ 3. Reposition the adolescent's legs.
☐ 4. Lay the adolescent flat to aid circulation.

70. The nurse evaluates the care of an adolescent with a recent spinal cord injury. Which finding should lead the nurse to determine that spinal shock was resolving?
☐ 1. atonic urinary bladder
☐ 2. flaccid paralysis
☐ 3. hyperactive reflexes
☐ 4. widened pulse pressure

71. A school-age client with a spinal cord injury is moved to the rehabilitation unit. The nurse notes that the child tends to refuse to cooperate in care and to be hostile. The nurse interprets this behavior as indicative of which response?
☐ 1. a stage of grief reaction
☐ 2. a phase of rebellion
☐ 3. a reaction to sensory overload
☐ 4. a response to too much attention

72. Two months after an adolescent's thoracic spinal cord injury, the client has a pounding headache. The nurse notes that the client's arms and face are flushed and they are diaphoretic. What should the nurse do **next**?
☐ 1. Check the patency of the urinary catheter.
☐ 2. Lower the adolescent's head below their knees.
☐ 3. Place the adolescent flat on their back.
☐ 4. Prepare to administer epinephrine subcutaneously.

Managing Care, Quality, and Safety of Children with Neurologic Health Problems

73. The nurse is admitting a child who has been diagnosed with bacterial meningitis to the pediatric unit. The nurse should implement which type of isolation?
☐ 1. standard or routine precautions
☐ 2. contact precautions
☐ 3. airborne precautions
☐ 4. droplet precautions

74. A multidisciplinary team is updating recommendations to reduce medication errors on the pediatric unit. Which strategy, if suggested by the team to reduce medication errors, would the nurse question?
☐ 1. Increase the number of steps in the medication administration procedure.
☐ 2. Avoid using parenteral syringes when administering liquid oral medications.
☐ 3. Limit the size of intravenous (IV) fluid bags that can be hung on small children.
☐ 4. Reduce the available concentrations or dose strengths of high-alert medications to the minimum.

75. The health care provider (HCP) prescribes carbamazepine extended release for a client with cerebral palsy who also has a seizure disorder. The client has a gastrostomy feeding tube, and carbamazepine is on the hospital's "no crush" list. What should the nurse do to administer the medication?
☐ 1. Cut the medication into four pieces.
☐ 2. Dissolve the medication in 30 mL of juice.
☐ 3. Ask the pharmacist for an oral suspension.
☐ 4. Contact the HCP to change the prescription.

76. When making rounds on the pediatric neurology unit, the nurse manager notes that when giving IV medications many of the staff nurses are disconnecting the flush syringe first and then clamping the intermittent infusion device. The nurse is concerned that the nurses do not understand the benefits of positive pressure technique and turbulence flow flush in preventing clots. After the nurse manager discusses the problem with the staff educator, which intervention would be the **most** effective way to improve the nursing practice?
☐ 1. Create a poster presentation on the topic with a required posttest.
☐ 2. Send a group email discussing the importance of clamping the device first.
☐ 3. Ask each nurse if they are aware that their practice is not current.
☐ 4. Post an evidence-based article on the unit.

328 The Nursing Care of Children

77. The emergency department nurse has admitted an infant with bulging fontanelles, setting sun eyes, and lethargy. Which diagnostic procedure would be **contraindicated** in this infant?
☐ 1. lumbar puncture
☐ 2. magnetic resonance imaging
☐ 3. arterial blood draw
☐ 4. computerized tomography scan

78. A 7-year-old with a history of tonic-clonic seizures has been actively seizing for 10 minutes. The child weighs 48.5 lb (22 kg) and currently has an IV of D5 NS + 20 mEq KCl/L running at 60 mL per hour. The vital signs are temperature 100.4°F (38°C); heart rate 120 bpm; respiratory rate 28 breaths/min; and oxygen saturation 92%. Using the SBAR (situation-background-assessment-recommendation) technique for communication, the nurse calls the health care provider with the recommendation for which medication?
☐ 1. rectal diazepam
☐ 2. IV lorazepam
☐ 3. rectal acetaminophen
☐ 4. IV fosphenytoin

Answers, Rationales, and Test-Taking Strategies

*The answers and the rationales for each question follow below, along with keys (🔑) to the client need (CN) and cognitive level (CL) for each question. In addition, questions that measure clinical judgment will be coded (CJ). As you check your answers, use the **Content Mastery and Test-Taking Skill Self-Analysis** worksheet (tear-out worksheet in the back of the book) to identify the reason(s) for not answering the questions correctly. For additional information about test-taking skills and strategies for answering questions, refer to pages 12–51 in Part 1 of this book.*

The Client with Myelomeningocele

1. -/+ **1, 2, 4, 5.** Common shunt complications are obstruction, infection, and disconnection of the tubing. The signs presented by the child indicate increased intracranial pressure from a shunt malfunction, which could be caused by an infection, such as peritonitis or meningitis. By listening to bowel sounds, the nurse will note if peritonitis might be a possibility. Intracranial pressure manifests as a bulging or taut anterior fontanel, but the posterior fontanel is typically closed. Obtaining vital signs would assess for signs of infection, such as elevated temperature or, possibly, the Cushing triad (elevated blood pressure, slow pulse, and depressed respirations). A high-pitched cry is a sign of increased intracranial pressure. Weighing the child, while it would not help identify the cause of the problem, would help determine the severity of the dehydration from vomiting.

🔑 CN: Physiological adaptation; CL: Analyze

2. 3. Before surgery, the infant is kept flat in the prone position to decrease tension on the sac. This allows for optimal positioning of the hips, knees, and feet because orthopedic problems are common. The supine position is unacceptable because it causes pressure on the defect. Flexing the knees when side-lying will increase tension on the sac, as will placing the infant in semi-Fowler position, even though the chest and abdomen are elevated.

🔑 CN: Physiological adaptation; CL: Analyze

3. 2. A Chiari malformation obstructs the flow of cerebral spinal fluid resulting in hydrocephalus. This is a common problem in infants with myelomeningocele and will require surgical intervention with a shunt. A high-pitched cry is one sign of increased intracranial pressure that may indicate the presence of a Chiari malformation and requires further evaluation. Minimal movement of the lower extremities is an expected finding associated with spinal cord damage. Overflow voiding comes from a neurogenic bladder, not increased intracranial pressure. It is normal for the fontanelle to bulge with crying.

🔑 CN: Physiological adaptation; CL: Analyze

4. 1. The parents should see the neonate as soon as possible because the longer they must wait to see the neonate, the more anxiety they will feel. Because the parents are acutely aware of the deficit, the nurse should emphasize the neonate's normal and positive features during the visit. All parents, but especially those with a child who has a disability or defect, need to hear positive comments and comments that reflect how the infant is normal. Although the parents need to discuss their fears and concerns, the priority on the first visit is to emphasize the neonate's normal and positive features. Reinforcing the HCP's explanation of the defect may be necessary later. Reinforcing the explanation at this initial visit emphasizes the defect, not the child. The parents should spend time with or care for the neonate after birth because parent-infant contact is necessary for attachment. The parents cannot feed the neonate before the defect is repaired because the repair typically occurs within 24 hours. The infant will be prone in an isolette bed or warmed and watched closely. However, the parents can fondle and stroke the neonate.

~ CN: Psychosocial integrity; CL: Analyze

5. 1. Excessive cerebrospinal fluid in the cranial cavity, called *hydrocephalus*, is the most common anomaly associated with myelomeningocele. Microcephaly, an abnormally small head, is associated with maternal exposure to rubella or cytomegalovirus. Anencephaly, a congenital absence of the cranial vault, is a different type of neural tube defect. Overriding of the sutures, possibly a normal finding after vaginal birth, is not associated with myelomeningocele.

~ CN: Physiological adaptation; CL: Apply

6. 1. Approximately one-third of infants diagnosed with myelomeningocele have an intellectual disability, but the degree of disability is variable, and it is difficult to predict intellectual functioning in neonates. The parents are asking for an answer now and should not be told to talk with the HCP later.

~ CN: Physiological adaptation; CL: Analyze

7. 2. The nurse places the neonate with myelomeningocele in an Isolette shortly after birth to help to maintain the infant's temperature. Because of the defect, the neonate cannot be bundled in blankets. Therefore, it may be difficult to prevent cold stress. The Isolette can be maintained at higher than room temperature, helping to maintain the temperature of a neonate who cannot be dressed or bundled. Body temperature readings, not arterial oxygen levels, are the best indicator. Typically, an infant loses 5% to 10% of body weight before beginning to regain the weight.

~ CN: Reduction of risk potential; CL: Analyze

8. 2. Because of the potential for hip dislocation, the neonate's legs should be slightly abducted, hips maintained in slight to moderate abduction, and feet maintained in a neutral position. The infant's knees are flexed to help maintain the hips in abduction.

~ CN: Reduction of risk potential; CL: Analyze

9. 4. The most important aspect of the discharge plan is to ensure that the parents understand what the daily care of their infant involves and to provide teaching related to carrying out this daily care. In addition to the routine care required by the infant, care also may include physical therapy to the lower extremities. Providing a list of available hospital services may be helpful to the parents, but it is not the most important aspect to include in the discharge plan. Usually, home health care is not needed because the parents are able to care for their child. A referral for counseling is initiated whenever the need arises, not just at discharge.

~ CN: Reduction of risk potential; CL: Analyze

10. 3. Children with a myelomeningocele are prone to urinary tract infections (UTIs), and foul-smelling urine is one symptom of a UTI. Because of the level of defect, the child may be insensitive to pressure or heat. Using a heating pad may lead to thermal injury because the child may not be able to sense if the pad is too hot. Keeping the child away from other children is unnecessary and can retard social development. Using pillows as props increases the risk for sudden infant death syndrome.

~ CN: Safety and infection control; CL: Evaluate

11. 3. Children with myelomeningocele are at high risk for the development of latex allergy because of repeated exposure to latex products during surgery and bladder catheterizations. Cross-reactions to food items such as bananas, kiwi, chestnuts, and avocados also occur. These allergic reactions vary in severity ranging from mild (such as sneezing) to severe anaphylaxis. While the child could have allergies to medications that caused the wheezing, latex and food allergies are more common. Asking about the skin rash is not a priority when a child is wheezing. Who brought the child to the emergency department is irrelevant at this time.

~ CN: Reduction of risk potential; CL: Analyze

The Client with Hydrocephalus

12. -/+ 3, 5, 6. Hydrocephaly is a block in the flow of cerebral spinal fluid. Hydrocephaly results in increased intracranial pressure (ICP). Vomiting, irritability, bulging fontanelle, and pupillary changes are all signs of increased intracranial pressure in an infant. A depressed fontanelle could be an indication of dehydration, not increased intracranial pressure. A headache may be present in an infant with increased ICP; however, the infant has no way of communicating this to the nurse or parent. A headache is an indication of increased ICP in a verbal child. A high-pitched cry is indicative of infants with increased intracranial pressure.

~ CN: Physiological adaptation; CL: Analyze

13. 3. Measuring the occipital frontal head circumference over time is the most obvious way to monitor if hydrocephalus is worsening or improving in an infant. The infant exhibits sunsetting of the eyes, which is a sign of hydrocephalus. Pupillary reactions may be decreased or unequal, but these measurements do not give as much information about changes in the infant's status. The posterior fontanelle usually closes by 2 months in a typically developing infant. Finding the posterior fontanelle still open in an infant with hydrocephalus would not be unexpected and would not necessarily be an indicator of the severity of the disorder. A finding of primitive reflexes in a 3-month-old infant would be an expected finding.

🗝️ CN: Reduction of risk potential; CL: Apply

14. 1. Abdominal distension in a pediatric client with a ventriculoperitoneal shunt can be an indication of peritonitis and requires intervention. Lethargy may be present for several days following surgery for a ventriculoperitoneal shunt. Facial and eye edema is common during the postoperative period and can be reduced by utilizing a cold compress on the eyes. Infants commonly have pain in the postoperative period that should be treated with analgesic medication; however, infants cannot convey that they specifically have a headache.

🗝️ CN: Management of care; CL: Analyze

15. 3. Monitoring the temperature allows the nurse to assess for infection, the most common and the most hazardous postoperative complication after ventriculoperitoneal shunt placement. Typically, pain after insertion of a ventriculoperitoneal shunt is mild, requiring the use of mild analgesic medication. Usually, narcotics are not administered because they alter the level of consciousness, making assessment of cerebral function difficult. Neither proteinuria nor glycosuria is associated with shunt placement. Cerebrospinal fluid leakage commonly occurs with a head injury. It is not usually associated with shunt placement.

🗝️ CN: Reduction of risk potential; CL: Analyze

16. 4. In a school-age child, irritability, lethargy, vomiting, difficulty with eating, and decreased level of consciousness are signs of increased intracranial pressure caused by a blocked shunt. Decreased urine output with stable fluid intake indicates fluid loss from a source other than the kidneys. A tense fontanelle and increased head circumference would be signs of a blocked shunt in an infant. Elevated temperature and redness around incisions might suggest an infection.

🗝️ CN: Reduction of risk potential; CL: Evaluate

The Client with a Seizure Disorder

17.

STEP 1

-/+ **Nurse's Notes**

0800:
The parent reports that the toddler was a vaginal birth and was born 1 week before the due date. Immunizations were administered last week and are now up to date. The client is still bottle-feeding, sleeps through the night, and is generally a happy toddler. Last night, the client developed a fever of 102.5°F (39.2°C) that came down with acetaminophen. This morning, the parent reported seeing the toddler have 20 seconds of eye twitching and rhythmical bilateral movements of the upper extremities. When it stopped, they brought the client to the office to be evaluated. Vital signs are temperature 104°F (40.0°C); heart rate 130 bpm; respiration rate 30 breaths/min; blood pressure 100/60 mm Hg; and pulse oximetry 95%.

A seizure is an involuntary contraction of muscle caused by abnormal electrical brain discharges, and 5% of children will have at least one seizure by the time they reach adulthood. Febrile seizures are associated with high fever (102°F to 104°F [38.9°C to 40.0°C]) and are caused by a sudden spike in temperature, not a gradual incline. A transient rash, fever, and subsequent seizure may develop 5 to 12 days after vaccine administration. A febrile seizure is usually a generalized tonic-clonic pattern that commonly includes eye twitching and rhythmical movements and lasts 15 seconds to 2 minutes. A normal heart rate for a toddler is 80 to 130 bpm and a normal respiration rate is 20 to 30 breaths/min. The heart rate and respiration rate are on the high end of the normal range, which is expected when a child is febrile. Blood pressure, oxygen saturation, and blood sugar values remain within normal limits. A 15-month-old child who was born 1 week early via a vaginal birth, eagerly takes a bottle, and sleeps through the night is exhibiting expected findings for their age.

🗝️ CJ: Case study; Step 1: Recognize cues; CL: Analyze

18.

STEP 2

-/+ **1, 2, 3, 7.** With febrile seizures, there is usually a positive family history. Although 50% of all seizures in children are idiopathic, they can be attributed to infection, tumor growth, or trauma to the head. Further history-taking should include any potential trauma to the head as a 15-month-old should have reached the developmental milestone of being able to walk independently but also lacking coordination with the potential for falling and bumping their head. Head trauma could also be associated with child maltreatment and should be screened accordingly. During the postictal phase or recovery phase of a seizure, the child enters into a sound sleep and will appear limp and flaccid.

The possibility of accidental poisoning for an ambulatory, curious child has to be considered in any child who has a first seizure. It is not necessary to determine maternal infections or the length of a maternal membrane rupture as the neonatal period has ended and such criteria would not apply. A viral invasion such as herpes or cytomegalovirus should be considered if seizures persist. Although the height of a child is nice to know, it is irrelevant to determine the child's subsequent risk for another seizure.

CJ: Case study; Step 2: Analyze cues; CL: Analyze

19.
STEP 3

0/1 1, 4. The diagnosis of febrile seizure is most often based on history. The child's medical history needs to be reviewed to exclude other risk factors for epilepsy. The workup should then focus on what caused the fever to determine if there is an underlying infection that needs treating. The younger a child is when the febrile seizure occurs, the more likely the child will experience a second one. Care should focus on teaching the parent how to manage seizures at home. Febrile seizures are benign and outgrown by the age of 6. Febrile seizures cannot be prevented. Fevers serve a physiological function in fighting disease. Trying to prevent future fevers is not advisable or practical. Vaccination with the live measles, mumps, and rubella vaccine can cause a fever 5 to 12 days after the first dose and carries a small risk for a febrile seizure. The second dose of the vaccine is not due until the child is older, between 4 and 6 years of age when the child is at a lower risk for a febrile seizure. The child can continue with the recommended vaccine schedule. There is no indication that the child is not developing normally and needs developmental testing.

CJ: Case study; Step 3: Prioritize hypothesis; CL: Analyze

20.
STEP 4

−/+ 1, 3, 4, 6. An EEG is obtained to record the irregular electrical activity across the surface of the brain associated with seizure disorders. Patients may be awake or asleep during an EEG, and it may include a video recording. Serum electrolytes may demonstrate hypoglycemia, hyponatremia, or hypernatremia, all of which can cause seizures in children. A lumbar puncture may be ordered to complete a cerebrospinal fluid analysis, which may identify bleeding into the CSF, or a bacterial organism, which may include a diagnosis of meningitis. A meningeal infection is very serious and potentially contagious. A CT scan uses multiple x-ray beams that pass through the brain at different angles. A CT scan differentiates tissue density to assess for blood, CSF, or other abnormalities such as blood clots and tumors. The infant does not present with any respiratory physiology, and therefore a chest x-ray is not indicated. Similarly, a gentamicin level is not indicated because the child is not yet on antibiotics. A serum type and cross to determine blood type is not indicated because it is unlikely the child will need a blood transfusion following a seizure.

CJ: Case study; Step 4: Generate solutions; CL: Apply

21.
STEP 5

−/+ 1, 2, 6. After a febrile seizure subsides, the parents or nurse should sponge the child with tepid water or apply cool washcloths on the child's forehead or the axillary or groin area to reduce the fever quickly. An acetaminophen suppository may be given rectally at the appropriate dose based on the child's weight. The child should not be put in a bathtub of water because it would be easy for the child to slip under the water should a second seizure occur. Cold water is contraindicated because extreme cooling causes shock to an immature nervous system or shivering, which will cause the temperature to rise. An alcohol bath can be absorbed by the skin, or the fumes can be inhaled in toxic amounts, further compounding the child's problems. Oral medications such as ibuprofen should not be given as the child will be in a drowsy or postictal state after the seizure, and this creates a risk for aspiration.

CJ: Case study; Step 5: Take action; CL: Apply

22.
STEP 6

−/+ 1, 3, 4, 5. There is no major prevention strategy to recommend to prevent febrile seizures, but the nurse should reassure the family that the condition is outgrown by the time the child turns 6 years of age. Safety is a priority whether a child has a seizure at home or in the acute care setting. Nearby sharp objects should be removed, and the child should be lowered to the floor. No objects should be placed in the mouth as teeth may break, posing an aspiration risk. Slight cyanosis, or bluish extremities, may occur during the tonic and clonic phases. This is a normal finding and should resolve when the seizure stops. If a child has one seizure followed by another (status epilepticus) the infant may need oxygen or advanced treatment to stop the seizures, and 911 should be called. A child's medication should not be put in the bottle because if the child does not finish the bottle, it is difficult to ascertain how much of the medicine was taken and absorbed. The medication should be administered orally by itself.

CJ: Case study; Step 6: Evaluate outcomes; CL: Evaluate

23. 3. During a generalized tonic-clonic seizure, the priority is to keep the child safe and protect the child by removing any nearby objects that could cause injury. Although obtaining information about events surrounding the seizure is important, this information can be obtained later once the child's safety is ensured. During a seizure, the child should not be moved. Although providing privacy is important, the child's safety is the priority. During a seizure, nothing should be forced into the client's mouth because this can cause severe damage to the teeth and mouth.

🔑 CN: Physiological adaptation; CL: Evaluate

24. 3. Most children who develop seizures after infancy are intellectually normal. A child with a seizure disorder needs the same experiences and opportunities to develop intellectual, emotional, and social abilities as any other child. Activity limitation is not needed. Learning disabilities are not associated with seizures. The child is able to attend public school, and social stigma is a rarity.

🔑 CN: Health promotion and maintenance; CL: Apply

25. 4. Most febrile seizures occur in the presence of an upper respiratory infection, otitis media, or tonsillitis. Febrile seizures typically occur during a temperature rise rather than after prolonged fever. There appears to be increased susceptibility to febrile seizures within families. Infrequently, febrile seizures may lead to respiratory arrest.

🔑 CN: Physiological adaptation; CL: Analyze

26. 2. Shivering, the body's defense against rapid temperature decrease, increases body temperature. Therefore, the parents need to take measures to stop the shivering (and the resulting increase in body temperature) by increasing the room temperature or the temperature of the child's immediate environment (such as with blankets) until the shivering stops. Then, attempts are made to lower the temperature more slowly. Shivering does not necessarily correlate with being cold. Alcohol, a toxic substance, can be absorbed through the skin. Its use is to be avoided.

🔑 CN: Physiological adaptation; CL: Evaluate

27. 3. Phenytoin sodium is a known teratogenic agent, causing numerous fetal problems. Therefore, the adolescent should be advised to talk to the HCP to see if changing the medication is possible. Additionally, anticonvulsant requirements usually increase during pregnancy. Seizures can be controlled but cannot be cured. There is a familial tendency for seizure disorders. Seizure disorders and infertility are not related.

🔑 CN: Pharmacological and parenteral therapies; CL: Analyze

28. 3. A toxic effect of valproic acid is liver toxicity, which may manifest with jaundice and abdominal pain. If jaundice occurs, the client needs to notify the HCP as soon as possible. Diarrhea and sore throat are not common side effects of this drug. Increased appetite is common with this drug.

🔑 CN: Pharmacological and parenteral therapies; CL: Analyze

The Client with Meningitis

29. 1. Instituting droplet precautions is the priority for a newly admitted infant with meningococcal meningitis. Acetaminophen may be prescribed, but administering it does not take priority over instituting droplet precautions. Obtaining history information and orienting the parents to the call bell takes place after droplet precautions have been implemented, but before the nurse leaves the room.

🔑 CN: Safety and infection control; CL: Apply

30. 2. A child in the acute stage of meningitis is irritable and hypersensitive to loud noise and light. Therefore, extraneous noise should be minimized and bright lights avoided as much as possible. There is no need to limit conversations with the child. However, the nurse should speak in a calm, gentle, reassuring voice. The child needs gentle and calm bathing. Because of the acuteness of the infection, sponge baths would be more appropriate than tub baths. Although treatments need to be completed as quickly as possible to prevent overstressing the child, they should be performed carefully and at a pace that avoids sudden movements to prevent startling the child and subsequently increasing intracranial pressure.

🔑 CN: Basic care and comfort; CL: Analyze

31. 1. Disseminated intravascular coagulation is characterized by skin petechiae and a purpuric skin rash caused by spontaneous bleeding into the tissues. An abnormal coagulation phenomenon causes the condition. Heparin therapy is often used to interrupt the clotting process. Edema would suggest a fluid volume excess. Cyanosis would indicate decreased tissue oxygenation. Dyspnea on exertion would suggest respiratory problems, such as pulmonary edema.

🔑 CN: Physiological adaptation; CL: Analyze

32. 2. Organisms that cause bacterial meningitis, such as pneumococci or meningococci, are commonly spread in the body by vascular dissemination from a middle ear infection. Meningitis may also be a direct extension from the paranasal and mastoid sinuses. The causative organism is pneumococcus. A chronically draining ear is also frequently found. Bladder infections commonly are caused by *Escherichia coli*, unrelated to the development of pneumococcal meningitis. Pneumococcal meningitis is unrelated to a fractured clavicle or to septic arthritis, which is commonly caused by *Staphylococcus aureus*, group A streptococci, or *Haemophilus influenzae*.

CN: Physiological adaptation; CL: Analyze

33. **3.** Preschool-age children worry about having an intact body and become fearful of any threat to body integrity. Allowing the child to participate in required care helps protect their image of an intact body. Development of trust is the task typically associated with infancy. Additionally, allowing the child to apply a dressing over the intravenous insertion site is unrelated to the development of trust. Finding diversional activities is not a priority need for a child in this age group. Separation anxiety is more common in toddlers than in preschoolers.

CN: Health promotion and maintenance; CL: Apply

34. 83 mL per hour

1000 mL ÷ 12 h = 83 mL/h

CN: Pharmacological and parenteral therapies; CL: Apply

35. **1, 3, 4.** Antibiotics are indicated for the treatment of bacterial meningitis. Clients with bacterial meningitis often have increased intracranial pressure (ICP). It is necessary to maintain adequate hydration. However, infusing fluids at 1½ maintenance can increase ICP, further risking neurologic damage due to cerebral edema. Most children with meningitis are sensitive to sound, light, and stimulation. Decreasing environmental stimuli and keeping the room dim and quiet are essential. Frequent neurologic checks are necessary to monitor any changes in the child's level of consciousness. Anticonvulsants are not indicated unless the child experiences seizures as a result of the meningitis.

CN: Physiological adaptation; CL: Apply

36. **1, 4, 5.** Irritability, bulging fontanelle, and emesis are all signs of increased ICP in an infant. A headache may be present in an infant with increased ICP; however, the infant has no way of communicating this to the parent. A headache is an indication of increased ICP in a verbal child. An infant cannot exhibit mood swings; this is indicative of increased ICP in a child or adolescent.

CN: Reduction of risk potential; CL: Apply

37. **3.** The child is angry and needs a positive outlet for the expression of feelings. An emotionally tense child with pent-up hostilities needs a physical activity that will release energy and frustration. Pounding on a pegboard offers this opportunity. Listening to a story does not allow the child to express emotions. It also places the child in a passive role and does not allow the child to deal with feelings in a healthy and positive way. Activities such as painting and stacking a tower of blocks require concentration and fine movements, which could add to their frustration. However, if the child then knocks the tower over, doing so may help to dispel some of the anger.

CN: Health promotion and maintenance; CL: Analyze

The Client with Near-Drowning

38. **2.** Hypoxia is the primary problem because it results in brain cell damage. Irreversible brain damage occurs after 4 to 6 minutes of submersion. Hypothermia occurs rapidly in infants and children because of their large body surface area. Hypothermia is more of a problem when the child is in cold water. Although fluid aspiration occurs in most drownings and results in atelectasis and pulmonary edema, further aggravating hypoxia, hypoxia is the primary problem. Cutaneous capillary paralysis is not a problem.

CN: Physiological adaptation; CL: Analyze

39. **1.** Near-drowning victims typically suffer hypoxia and mixed acidosis. The priority is to restore oxygenation and prevent further hypoxia. Here, the client has blunted sensorium but is not unconscious; therefore, delivery of supplemental oxygen with a mask is appropriate. Warming protocols and fluid resuscitation will most likely be needed to help correct acidosis, but these interventions are secondary to oxygen administration. Intubation is required if the child is comatose, shows signs of airway compromise, or does not respond adequately to more conservative therapies.

CN: Physiological adaptation; CL: Analyze

40. **2.** Guilt is a common parental response. The parents need to be allowed to express their feelings openly in a nonthreatening, nonjudgmental atmosphere. Telling the parents that these things happen does not allow them to verbalize their feelings. Telling the parents that they should not have taken their eyes off the child blames them, possibly further contributing to their guilt. Telling the parents that they should not feel guilty denies the parents' feelings of guilt and is inappropriate. Telling the parents that they are lucky that the child will be okay does not remove the feelings of guilt.

CN: Psychosocial integrity; CL: Analyze

The Client with Guillain-Barré Syndrome (Infectious Polyneuritis)

41. 1. The child is exhibiting symptoms associated with Guillain-Barré syndrome (infectious polyneuritis). Most children with sore throat have some difficulty swallowing, so it is important for the nurse to determine the extent of difficulty to aid in determining what action is necessary. Typically, a sore throat precedes paralysis in clients with Guillain-Barré syndrome. Muscle tenderness is an initial symptom. Distal muscle weakness follows proximal muscle weakness, ultimately progressing to paralysis. Diet history and difficulty urinating will not contribute to an assessment of the cause of a sore throat or difficulty swallowing. After determining the extent of difficulty swallowing, the nurse can obtain information about exposure to illness.

🔑 CN: Health promotion and maintenance; CL: Analyze

42. 2. With Guillain-Barré syndrome, progressive ascending paralysis occurs. Therefore, the nurse should assess the child's muscle strength bilaterally to determine the extent of involvement and progression of the illness. Assessing the child's ability to follow simple commands evaluates brain function. Range-of-motion exercises are an important part of treatment, but they are not a priority initially. Although the child may need diversional activities later, they also are not an initial priority.

🔑 CN: Physiological adaptation; CL: Analyze

43. 3. In a child with Guillain-Barré syndrome, decreased volume and clarity of speech and decreased ability to cough voluntarily indicate ascending progression of neural inflammation, specifically affecting the cranial nerves. Inflammation of the larynx and epiglottis is manifested by hoarseness, stridor, and dyspnea. A child with laryngeal inflammation still retains the ability to cough. Irritability, behavior changes, headache, and vomiting are common signs of increased intracranial pressure in a school-age child. Regression would be manifested by being more dependent and less able to care for self.

🔑 CN: Physiological adaptation; CL: Apply

44. 4. Even in the absence of respiratory problems or distress, the child must be turned frequently to help prevent the cardiopulmonary complications associated with immobility, such as atelectasis and pneumonia. Maintaining the child in a supine position is unnecessary. Doing so does not prevent unnecessary nerve stimulation. In addition, maintaining a supine position may lead to stasis of secretions, placing the child at risk for pneumonia. Transferring the child to a chair will not prevent postural hypotension. However, doing so will increase vascular tone and help prevent respiratory and skin complications. During the acute disease phase, vigorous physiotherapy is contraindicated because the child may experience muscle pain and be hypersensitive to touch. Careful and gentle handling is essential.

🔑 CN: Physiological adaptation; CL: Analyze

45. 3. Developmentally appropriate activities and therapeutic play should be used as rehabilitation modalities. Taking the child to the pool to exercise with other children indicates that the child is participating in exercise as well as engaging with other children, thus fostering development. Arguing with the sibling does not address the discharge plan. Inappropriate rewards or threats should not be used to coerce a child into compliance. Although the parent is attempting to comply with the discharge plan, bribery is an inappropriate technique to foster compliance. Missing therapy sessions delays recovery. The parents need to help set the child's schedule to ensure that the client gets adequate rest to be able to follow the treatment plan.

🔑 CN: Physiological adaptation; CL: Evaluate

The Client with a Head Injury

46. 1. This client is experiencing neurologic changes consistent with increasing intracranial pressure (ICP). The nurse should first notify the HCP. The HCP may intubate the child to ensure a patent airway. The nurse should not lower the head of the bed as this will cause increased ICP. The nurse should ensure an adequate fluid balance. The HCP will likely prescribe hypertonic saline to draw fluid from the brain.

🔑 CN: Management of care; CL: Analyze

47. 1. An ICP level higher than 15 mm Hg is abnormal. This child's vital signs indicate increased ICP. Mannitol is an osmotic diuretic and will decrease the child's ICP. Suctioning the child will increase the ICP. Encouraging the parent to talk to the child may be comforting but will not decrease the ICP. The priority for this child is decreasing the ICP to avoid further brain injury. The fever is likely due to the head injury and will not decrease with acetaminophen. A cooling blanket is the most effective means of reducing a fever in a client with a head injury.

🔑 CN: Reduction of risk potential; CL: Apply

The Child with Neurologic Health Problems 335

48. 2. For the child with serious head trauma, a nasogastric tube is inserted initially to decompress the stomach and prevent vomiting and aspiration. Medications would be administered intravenously in the initial period. The tube will not be used to obtain gastric specimens. Nutrition is not a priority initially. Later on, the tube may be used to administer feedings.

   CN: Reduction of risk potential; CL: Apply

49. 1. Because a basilar skull fracture can involve the frontal and ethmoid bones, inserting a nasogastric tube carries the risk for introducing the tube into the cranial cavity through the fracture. An oral gastric tube is preferred for a client with a basilar skull fracture. The tube would not be placed into the duodenum. Gastric aspirate is not routinely tested for blood unless there is an indication to suggest bleeding, such as a decreasing hemoglobin level or visible blood in the drainage.

   CN: Reduction of risk potential; CL: Analyze

50. 3. As a rule, children demonstrate more rapid and complete recovery from coma than adults. However, it is extremely difficult to predict a specific outcome. Reassuring the parents that they will be kept informed helps open lines of communication and establish trust. Telling the parents that children do not do well would be extremely negative, destroying any hope that the parents might have. Telling the parents that children recover rapidly may give the parents false hopes. Telling the parents to talk to the HCP ignores the parents' concerns and interferes with trust building.

   CN: Physiological adaptation; CL: Analyze

51. 2. The LOC is the best indicator of brain function. If the child's condition deteriorates, the nurse would notice changes in LOC before any other changes and should notify the health care provider that these changes are occurring. Changes in vital signs and pupils typically follow changes in LOC. Motor strength is primarily assessed as a voluntary function. With changes in LOC, there may be motor changes.

   CN: Physiological adaptation; CL: Apply

52. 2. The unconscious child is positioned to prevent aspiration of saliva and minimize intracranial pressure. The head of the bed should be elevated, and the child should be in either the semiprone or the side-lying position. Lying prone with hips and knees slightly elevated increases intracranial pressure, as does lying on the back in the Trendelenburg position. The semi-Fowler position with arms at the side is not the best choice.

   CN: Physiological adaptation; CL: Analyze

53. 3. Mannitol is an osmotic diuretic used to reduce ICP. The use of the drug is controversial and should be reserved for clients who do not respond to other treatments or when brain herniation is likely. Children this sick should be on ICP monitoring. The best indicator that the drug has produced the desired results is a reduction in the ICP. Improved levels of consciousness should follow reduced ICP. While the drug will cause increased urine output, that measurement in and of itself does not indicate successful treatment. Because the drug is being used for head injuries and not to improve urine output in acute renal failure, the child may not have visible edema.

   CN: Pharmacological and parenteral therapies; CL: Evaluate

54. 2. Appearing dazed or stunned after a head injury is a symptom of a concussion. Concussion care includes removing the athlete from play and having the injury evaluated. Athletes should not return to play until they have been cleared by an HCP. Concussions require ongoing monitoring. Since the client has no signs of deterioration in neurologic function, it may best be provided by an HCP, who will follow him over time, rather than through an emergency department.

   CN: Reduction of risk potential; CL: Apply

55. 2, 3, 4, 6. Concussion recovery can be complicated by any previous brain injury, such as a previous concussion. Recovery can also be complicated by the presence of other neurologic problems, such as migraines, ADHD, and depression. Asthma and obesity have not been linked to concussion recovery.

   CN: Risk reduction; CL: Analyze

56. 3. The inability to hop is not concerning because it is a milestone for a 4-year-old, not a 3-year-old. Lack of interest in toys, changes in eating habits, and increased temper tantrums that persist for several weeks all require an evaluation by a neurologist or other specialist.

   CN: Physiologic adaptation; CL: Analyze

57. 4. While recovery from a concussion takes time, adequate rest and limiting exertion facilitate recovery. Both physical and cognitive exertion can cause the reemergence of symptoms and delay recovery. As symptoms resolve, clients may slowly return to previous levels of activity.

   CN: Risk reduction; CL: Evaluate.

The Client with a Brain Tumor

58. 2. A decreasing level of consciousness, decerebrate positioning, or the Cushing triad (elevated systolic blood pressure, decreased pulse, and decreased respiratory rate) indicates that there is pressure on the brain stem and the client could require intubation and cardiac resuscitation unless the HCP can prescribe a medication or surgical procedure to reduce the intracranial pressure. Raising the head of the bed could offer some reduction in the intracranial pressure by increasing venous blood return from the head, but it is not the priority at this time. Turning the client to the side is a measure taken when there is an impending risk for a seizure. The impending risk for seizure is not as great as the potential for respiratory arrest. An oximeter would measure the oxygen level in the blood but not necessarily in the brain.

CN: Physiological adaptation; CL: Analyze

59. 1. A WBC count of 2000 mm³ (2×10^9/L) is low and increases the risk for infection. Meticulous handwashing is a universal precaution and the first line of defense in combating infection. A platelet count of 150,000/μL (150×10^9/L) is normal, so there is no need for a platelet transfusion. Mouth care will help decrease the risk for infection. However, handwashing is the priority as it will have the greatest impact on diminishing the risk for infection. A hemoglobin level of 12.5 g/dL (125 g/L) and hematocrit reading of 36.8% (0.37) are within normal range, so there is no need to transfuse packed red blood cells.

CN: Reduction of risk potential; CL: Analyze

60. 4. When a brain tumor is suspected, the child and parents are likely to be very apprehensive and anxious. It is unrealistic to expect to eliminate their fears; rather, the nurse's goal is to decrease them. Preparing both the child and family during hospitalization can help them cope with some of their fears. Although the nurse may be able to decrease some of the child's anxiety, it would be impossible to eliminate it. Children with infratentorial tumors seldom have seizures, so seizure precautions are not indicated. Although introducing the child to other children is a positive action, this action would be more appropriate once the nurse has decreased some of the child's and parents' anxiety by preparing them.

CN: Psychosocial integrity; CL: Analyze

61. 1. The infant has opisthotonos, an indication of brain stem herniation; the nurse should notify the HCP immediately and have resuscitation equipment ready. Stroking the back will not relieve the herniation or release the arching. Although the infant may also have a seizure, and padded side rails will prevent injury, the first action is to notify the HCP. Placing the child in a prone position will not relieve the herniation or release the arching.

CN: Management of care; CL: Analyze

62. 1, 2, 4. Head tilt, vomiting, and lethargy are classic signs assessed in a child with a brain tumor. Clinical manifestations are the result of the location and size of the tumor. Polydipsia is rare with a brain tumor. It is more often a sign of diabetes insipidus following a closed head injury. Increased appetite occurs during a growth spurt and is not necessarily a sign of a brain tumor. Increased pulse is a nonspecific sign and can occur with many illnesses, cardiac anomalies, fever, or exercise. Slow heart rate is more associated with increased intracranial pressure seen with brain tumors

CN: Physiological adaptation; CL: Analyze

63. 3. After surgery for an infratentorial tumor, the child is usually positioned flat on either side, with the head and neck in midline and the body slightly extended. Pillows against the back, not the head, help maintain position. Such a position helps avoid pressure on the operative site. Placing the child in a prone or semi-Fowler position will cause pressure on the operative site. The Trendelenburg position is usually contraindicated because keeping the head below the level of the heart increases intracranial pressure as well as the risk for hemorrhage.

CN: Physiological adaptation; CL: Analyze

64. 1. Hypercapnia, hypoxia, and acidosis are potent cerebral vasodilating mechanisms that can cause increased intracranial pressure. Lowering the carbon dioxide level and increasing the oxygen level through hyperventilation is the most effective short-term method of reducing intracranial pressure. Although ensuring a patent airway is important, this is not accomplished by manual hyperventilation. Manual hyperventilation does not lower the arousal level; in fact, the arousal level may increase. Manual hyperventilation is used to reduce hypoxia, not produce it.

CN: Reduction of risk potential; CL: Evaluate

65. 3. Glucose in this clear, colorless fluid indicates the presence of cerebrospinal fluid. Excessive fluid leakage should be reported to the HCP. The nurse should not change the dressing of a client who underwent a postoperative craniotomy unless instructed to do so by the surgeon. Ordinarily, the head of the bed would not be elevated because this would put pressure on the sutures. The nurse should notify the HCP after testing the fluid for glucose.

🗝️ CN: Reduction of risk potential; CL: Analyze

66. 1. It is not uncommon for a child to be concerned about a change in appearance when the entire head or only part of the head has been shaved. The child should be encouraged to participate in decisions about care when possible. Asking the client if they would like to wear a hat is one way to encourage this participation. Reassuring the child that their hair will grow back does not address the immediate change in appearance, and it ignores the child's current feelings. Explaining that this type of reaction is normal does not address the child's feelings. The child needs to be able to express feelings and be involved in care as much as possible. Buying the child a wig as a surprise does not address the child's feelings and does not allow them to participate in decision-making. Rather, the parents should ask the child if they would like a wig and then work with the child to determine what kind of wig they would like.

🗝️ CN: Psychosocial integrity; CL: Analyze

67. 1. Parents of a child who has undergone neurosurgery can easily become overprotective. Yet, the parents must foster independence in the convalescing child. It is important for the child to resume age-appropriate activities, and parents play an important role in encouraging this. Statements about going back to school would be expected. Parents want the child to return to normal activities after a serious illness or injury as a sign that the child is doing well.

🗝️ CN: Psychosocial integrity; CL: Evaluate

The Client with a Spinal Cord Injury

68. 2. The adolescent's signs and symptoms suggest a spinal cord injury. A client with suspected spinal cord injury should not be moved until the spine has been immobilized. Removing the helmet could further aggravate a spinal cord injury. The nurse could assess for abdominal trauma, but only if it can be done without moving the adolescent.

🗝️ CN: Reduction of risk potential; CL: Analyze

69. 1. In spinal cord injury, temperature regulation is lost below T3. Body temperature must be maintained by adjusting room temperature or bed linens, such as covering the client's legs with blankets. Coolness of the extremities is an expected finding. Therefore, it is not necessary to notify the HCP immediately. Repositioning the client's legs does not alleviate the temperature regulation problem and could be harmful, considering the client's diagnosis. Moving the legs before the spine is stabilized could lead to further cord damage. Laying the client flat will not increase the warmth of the legs and feet.

🗝️ CN: Physiological adaptation; CL: Analyze

70. 3. Spinal shock causes a loss of reflex activity below the level of the injury, resulting in bladder atony and flaccid paralysis. When the reflex arc returns, it tends to be overactive, resulting in spasticity. The reflexes and bladder become hypertonic during this phase of spinal shock resolution; sensation does not return. A widened pulse pressure is not associated with the resolution of spinal shock.

🗝️ CN: Physiological adaptation; CL: Evaluate

71. 1. After a catastrophic injury, individuals commonly experience grief. Initially, the person experiences denial, the most common response. With gradual awareness of the situation, anger commonly occurs. The child is demonstrating anger, not rebellion, as they gradually become aware of their situation. Rebellion is the child's way to maintain autonomy and individuality. It is a reaction to rigid rules. Examples include refusing to follow a treatment protocol when the child had no input and running away. Sensory overload would cause the child to be irritable and tired and to have difficulty sleeping. Too much attention usually would lead to irritability, difficulty sleeping, and mood swings.

🗝️ CN: Psychosocial integrity; CL: Analyze

72. 1. The adolescent is exhibiting signs of autonomic dysreflexia, a generalized sympathetic response usually caused by bladder or bowel distention. Immediate treatment involves eliminating the cause. Because bladder distention is a common cause of this problem, the nurse should immediately determine the patency of the indwelling (Foley) catheter. Lowering the head below the knees would increase the blood pressure and is contraindicated because of the spinal cord injury. Lying flat will not decrease blood pressure. Epinephrine is contraindicated because it elevates blood pressure and therefore can exacerbate the problem.

🗝️ CN: Physiological adaptation; CL: Analyze

Managing Care, Quality, and Safety of Children with Neurologic Health Problems

73. 4. Bacterial meningitis is caused by one of three organisms, *Haemophilus influenzae* type b, *Neisseria meningitidis*, or *Streptococcus pneumoniae*. All three organisms may be transmitted through contact with respiratory droplets. These droplets are heavy and typically fall within 3 feet (91.4 cm) of the client. Droplet precautions require, in addition to standard (routine) precautions, that health care providers wear masks when coming into close contact with the client. Standard or routine precautions, previously referred to as universal precautions, are general measures used for all clients. Contact precautions are used when direct or indirect contact with the client causes disease transmission. Gowns and gloves are needed but not masks. Airborne precautions differ from droplet precautions in that the particles are smaller and may stay suspended in the air for longer periods. These clients require negative pressure rooms, and all health care workers must wear respirators.

CN: Safety and infection control; CL: Apply

74. 1. Any time steps are added to the medication administration process, there is one more place where an error might occur. Using only oral syringes to administer oral medications reduces the chance that the medication will be given intravenously. The use of smart pumps alone is not enough to prevent IV fluid administration. An additional measure that pediatric floors can institute to prevent accidental fluid overload is to use smaller IV fluid bags, such as 250 mL. Whenever a medication comes in multiple concentrations and doses, there is a risk for administering the wrong dose.

CN: Safety and infection control; CL: Analyze

75. 4. The coating on an extended-release medication helps assure slow absorption of the medication. If the nurse crushes the medication, the medication may enter the client's system too quickly and result in toxic levels. The only appropriate action is to contact the prescriber and ask that the prescription be changed. Cutting the medication or trying to dissolve a whole tablet would have similar results as crushing it. Carbamazepine comes as an oral suspension, but it is not extended release. Therefore, a prescription would be needed to address dosing if switching to this form.

CN: Safety and infection control; CL: Analyze

76. 1. A poster presentation is an eye-catching way to disseminate information that can be used to educate nurses on all shifts. The addition of the posttest will verify that the poster information has been received. Because of the large volume of emails the typical employee receives, information sent this way might be overlooked. If several nurses are observed not using the most current practice, it is quite possible that many more do not understand it. Thus, a larger-scale plan is needed. Posting an article will not assure that the information is read.

CN: Reduction of risk potential; CL: Apply

77. 1. The child is exhibiting signs and symptoms of increased intracranial pressure (ICP). A lumbar puncture is contraindicated in children with increased ICP due to the risk for herniation. Magnetic resonance imaging and a computerized tomography scan are indicated in children with suspected increased ICP. Radiology studies will allow visualization of the cause of the increased ICP, such as inflammation, a tumor, or hemorrhage. An arterial blood draw is not indicated in this client. However, there is no contraindication for performing an arterial blood draw on a child with increased ICP.

CN: Reduction of risk potential; CL: Analyze

78. 2. IV lorazepam is the benzodiazepine of choice for treating prolonged seizure activity. IV benzodiazepines act to potentiate the action of the gamma-aminobutyric acid (GABA) neurotransmitter, stopping seizure activity. If an IV is not available, rectal diazepam is the benzodiazepine of choice. The child does have a low-grade fever; however, this is likely caused by excessive motor activity. The primary goal for the child is to stop the seizure in order to reduce neurologic damage. Benzodiazepines are used for the initial treatment of prolonged seizures. Once the seizure has ended, a loading dose of fosphenytoin is given.

CN: Pharmacological and parenteral therapies; CL: Apply

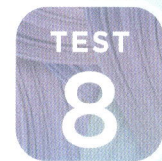

TEST 8: The Child with Musculoskeletal Health Problems

- The Client with Torticollis, Legg-Calvé-Perthes Disease, and Musculoskeletal Dysfunction
- The Client with Cerebral Palsy
- The Client with Duchenne Muscular Dystrophy
- The Client with Developmental Dysplasia of the Hip
- The Client with Congenital Clubfoot
- The Client with Juvenile Idiopathic Arthritis
- The Client with a Fracture
- The Client with Osteomyelitis
- The Client with Scoliosis
- Managing Care, Quality, and Safety of Children with Musculoskeletal Health Problems
- Answers, Rationales, and Test-Taking Strategies

The Client with Torticollis, Legg-Calvé-Perthes Disease, and Musculoskeletal Dysfunction

1. The nurse plans the discharge of a newborn diagnosed with torticollis (wry neck). Which action should the nurse take?
   - ☐ 1. Teach the parent the side effects of botulinum toxin.
   - ☐ 2. Coordinate outpatient physical therapy.
   - ☐ 3. Verify the date for corrective surgery.
   - ☐ 4. Demonstrate the use of positioning wedges for sleep.

2. A child who limps and has pain has been found to have Legg-Calvé-Perthes disease. What should the nurse expect to include in the child's plan of care?
   - ☐ 1. initiation of pain control measures, especially at night when acute
   - ☐ 2. promotion of ambulation despite the child's discomfort in the affected hip
   - ☐ 3. prevention of flexion in the affected hip and knee
   - ☐ 4. avoidance of weight-bearing on the head of the affected femur

3. The nurse plans home care for a child with Legg-Calvé-Perthes disease. What should be the **primary** focus for family teaching?
   - ☐ 1. need for intake of protein-rich foods
   - ☐ 2. gentle stretching exercises for both legs
   - ☐ 3. management of the corrective appliance
   - ☐ 4. relaxation techniques for pain control

4. At the 2-week well-child visit, a parent states, "My baby seems to keep their head tilted to the right." Which area should the nurse further assess?
   - ☐ 1. anterior fontanelle
   - ☐ 2. cervical vertebrae
   - ☐ 3. trapezius muscle
   - ☐ 4. sternocleidomastoid muscle

5. An adolescent is on the football team and practices in the morning and afternoon before school starts for the year. The temperature on the field has been high. The school nurse has been called to the practice field because the adolescent is now reporting that they have muscle cramps, nausea, and dizziness. Which action should the school nurse do **first**?
   - ☐ 1. Administer cold water with ice cubes.
   - ☐ 2. Take the adolescent's temperature.
   - ☐ 3. Elevate the child's legs.
   - ☐ 4. Move the adolescent to a cool environment.

The Client with Cerebral Palsy

6. During a developmental screening, the nurse finds that a toddler child with cerebral palsy has arrested social and language development. What should the nurse tell the family?
   - ☐ 1. "This is a sign the cerebral palsy is progressing."
   - ☐ 2. "Your child has reached their maximum language abilities."
   - ☐ 3. "I need to refer you for more developmental testing."
   - ☐ 4. "We need to modify your therapy plan."

7. A child with spastic cerebral palsy is to begin botulinum toxin type A injections. Which treatment goal(s) should the health care team set for the child related to botulinum toxin? Select all that apply.
   ☐ 1. improved nutritional status
   ☐ 2. decreased pain from spasticity
   ☐ 3. improved motor function
   ☐ 4. enhanced self-esteem
   ☐ 5. reduced caregiver strain
   ☐ 6. decreased speech impediments

8. The nurse assesses a parent's understanding of cerebral palsy (CP). The nurse determines that the parent has an accurate understanding of CP when they describe it as a term applied to impaired movement resulting from which factor?
   ☐ 1. injury to the cerebrum caused by a viral infection
   ☐ 2. malformed blood vessels in the ventricles caused by inheritance
   ☐ 3. nonprogressive brain damage caused by injury
   ☐ 4. inflammatory brain disease caused by metabolic imbalances

9. The nurse conducts a developmental screening of a 15-month-old child with cerebral palsy. Which milestones would the nurse expect a typically developing toddler of this age to have achieved?
   ☐ 1. walking up steps
   ☐ 2. using a spoon
   ☐ 3. copying a circle
   ☐ 4. putting a block in a cup

10. The parent asks the nurse whether a child with hemiparesis due to spastic cerebral palsy will be able to walk normally because they can pull to a standing position. Which response by the nurse would be **most** appropriate?
    ☐ 1. "Ask your health care provider what they think at your next appointment."
    ☐ 2. "Being able to pull to a stand really only tells us the client's upper-body strength is good."
    ☐ 3. "It is difficult to predict, but their ability to bear weight is a positive factor."
    ☐ 4. "If the client really wants to walk, and works hard, they probably will eventually."

11. The nurse assesses a family's ability to cope with their child's cerebral palsy. Which action should alert the nurse to the possibility of their inability to cope with the disease?
    ☐ 1. limiting interaction with extended family and friends
    ☐ 2. learning measures to meet the child's physical needs
    ☐ 3. requesting teaching about cerebral palsy in general
    ☐ 4. seeking advice on coping on social media

The Client with Duchenne Muscular Dystrophy

12. The parent of a child with Duchenne muscular dystrophy asks about the chance that a next child will have the disease. What should the nurse tell the parent?
    ☐ 1. "Sons have a 50% chance of being affected."
    ☐ 2. "Daughters have a 1 in 4 chance of being carriers."
    ☐ 3. "Each child has a 1 in 4 chance of developing the disease."
    ☐ 4. "Each child has a 50% chance of being a carrier."

13. A nurse is making an initial visit to a family with a preschool child with early Duchenne muscular dystrophy. Which assessment is an expected finding in this child?
    ☐ 1. contractures of the large joints
    ☐ 2. enlarged calf muscles
    ☐ 3. difficulty riding a tricycle
    ☐ 4. atrophied muscles

14. The nurse observes as a child with Duchenne muscular dystrophy attempts to rise from a sitting position on the floor. After attaining a kneeling position, the child "walks" their hands up to their legs to stand. The nurse documents this as which sign?
    ☐ 1. Galeazzi's sign
    ☐ 2. Goodell's sign
    ☐ 3. Goodenough's sign
    ☐ 4. Gower's sign

15. The nurse develops the plan of care for a child with early Duchenne muscular dystrophy. What is the **priority** goal for this client?
    ☐ 1. Encourage early wheelchair use.
    ☐ 2. Foster social interactions.
    ☐ 3. Maintain function of unaffected muscles.
    ☐ 4. Prevent circulatory impairment.

16. When interacting with the parent of a child who has Duchenne muscular dystrophy, the nurse observes behavior indicating that the parent may feel guilty about the child's condition. The nurse interprets this behavior as guilt stemming from which factor?
    ☐ 1. the terminal nature of the disease
    ☐ 2. the dependent behavior of the child
    ☐ 3. the genetic mode of transmission
    ☐ 4. the sudden onset of the disease

17. The nurse teaches the parent of a young child with Duchenne muscular dystrophy about the disease and its management. Which statement by the parent indicates successful teaching?
☐ 1. "My child will probably be unable to walk independently by the time they are 9 to 11 years old."
☐ 2. "Muscle relaxants are effective for some children; I hope they can help my child."
☐ 3. "When my child is a little older, they can have surgery to improve their ability to walk."
☐ 4. "I need to help my child be as active as possible to prevent progression of the disease."

The Client with Developmental Dysplasia of the Hip

18. The nurse is assessing the infant shown in the figure. On observing the client from this angle, the nurse should document that this infant has which finding?

☐ 1. Ortolani "click"
☐ 2. limited abduction
☐ 3. Galeazzi's sign
☐ 4. asymmetric gluteal folds

19. The nurse teaches the parents of an infant with developmental dysplasia of the hip how to handle their child in a Pavlik harness. Which care is **most** appropriate?
☐ 1. Fit the diaper under the straps.
☐ 2. Leave the harness off while the infant sleeps.
☐ 3. Check for skin redness under straps every other day.
☐ 4. Put powder on the skin under the straps every day.

20. The nurse develops the teaching plan for the parents of a child needing a Pavlik harness. What should be the nurse's **initial** step?
☐ 1. Assess the parents' current coping strategies.
☐ 2. Determine the parents' knowledge about the device.
☐ 3. Provide the parents with written instructions.
☐ 4. Give the parents a list of community resources.

21. The nurse creates a teaching plan for the family of an older infant who has had a spica cast applied for developmental dysplasia of the hip. Which information should the nurse include when describing the abduction stabilizer bar?
☐ 1. It can be adjusted to a position of comfort.
☐ 2. It is used to lift the child.
☐ 3. It adds strength to the cast.
☐ 4. It is necessary to turn the child.

22. A parent asks the nurse about using a car seat for a toddler who is in a hip spica cast. What should the nurse tell the parent?
☐ 1. "You can use a seat belt because of the spica cast."
☐ 2. "You will need a specially designed car seat for your toddler."
☐ 3. "You can still use the car seat you already have."
☐ 4. "You will need to get a special release from the police so that a car seat will not be needed."

The Client with Congenital Clubfoot

23. The nurse is discharging a newborn with clubfoot who has had a cast applied. The nurse should provide additional teaching to the parents if they make which statement?
☐ 1. "I should call if I see changes in the color of the toes under the cast."
☐ 2. "I should use a pillow to elevate my child's foot as they sleep."
☐ 3. "My baby will need a series of casts to fix their foot."
☐ 4. "Having a cast should not prevent me from holding my baby."

24. The parents of a neonate born with congenital clubfoot express feelings of helplessness and guilt and are exhibiting anxiety about how the neonate will be treated. Which action by the nurse would be **most** appropriate initially?
☐ 1. Ask them to share these concerns with the health care provider (HCP).
☐ 2. Arrange a meeting with other parents whose infants have had successful clubfoot treatment.
☐ 3. Discuss the problem with the parents and the current feelings that they are experiencing.
☐ 4. Suggest that they make an appointment to talk things over with a counselor.

25. The nurse teaches the parents of an infant with clubfoot requiring application of a plaster cast how to care for the cast. Which statement would indicate that the parents have understood the teaching?
    ☐ 1. "If the cast becomes soiled, we will clean it with soap and water."
    ☐ 2. "We will elevate the leg with the cast on pillows so the leg is above heart level."
    ☐ 3. "We will check the color and temperature of the toes of the casted leg frequently."
    ☐ 4. "The petals on the edge of the cast can be removed after the first 24 hours."

The Client with Juvenile Idiopathic Arthritis

26. The parent of a preschool-age child with a tentative diagnosis of juvenile idiopathic arthritis (JIA) asks about a test to definitively diagnose JIA. What should the nurse tell the parent?
    ☐ 1. "The latex fixation test is diagnostic."
    ☐ 2. "An increased erythrocyte sedimentation rate is diagnostic."
    ☐ 3. "A positive synovial fluid culture is diagnostic."
    ☐ 4. "No specific laboratory test is diagnostic."

27. The parents of a child just diagnosed with juvenile idiopathic arthritis (JIA) tell the nurse that the diagnosis frightens them because they know nothing about the prognosis. What information should the nurse include when teaching the parents about the disease?
    ☐ 1. The more joints affected, the more severe the disease will be.
    ☐ 2. Many affected children go into long remissions but have severe deformities.
    ☐ 3. The disease usually progresses to crippling rheumatoid arthritis.
    ☐ 4. Most affected children recover completely within a few years.

28. The parent of a preschool child with juvenile idiopathic arthritis (JIA) is worried that their child will have to stop attending preschool because of the illness. Which response by the nurse would be **most** appropriate?
    ☐ 1. "It may be difficult for your child to attend school because of the side effects of the medications they will be prescribed."
    ☐ 2. "Your child should be encouraged to attend school, but they will need extra time to work out early morning stiffness."
    ☐ 3. "You should keep your child at home from school whenever they experience discomfort or pain in their joints."
    ☐ 4. "Your child will probably need to wear splints and braces so that their joints will be supported properly."

29. A preschool-age child with juvenile idiopathic arthritis (JIA) has become withdrawn, and the parent asks the nurse what they should do. Which suggestion by the nurse would be **most** appropriate?
    ☐ 1. Introduce the child to other children their age who also have JIA.
    ☐ 2. Tell the parent to spend extra time with the child and less time with their other children.
    ☐ 3. Recommend that the parent send the child to see a counselor for therapy.
    ☐ 4. Encourage the parent to be supportive and understanding of the child.

30. The nurse develops the teaching plan for the parents of a child with juvenile idiopathic arthritis who is being treated with naproxen. What information should the nurse include?
    ☐ 1. An anti-inflammatory effect will occur in approximately 8 weeks.
    ☐ 2. Within 24 hours, the child will have anti-inflammatory relief.
    ☐ 3. The nurse should be called before giving the child any over-the-counter medications.
    ☐ 4. If a dose is forgotten or missed, that dose is not made up.

The Client with a Fracture

31. A school-age child has 5 lb (2.27 kg) of Buck extension traction on their left leg. What finding(s) should the nurse assess the child for? Select all that apply.
    ☐ 1. dryness of the skin, by removing the foam wraps and boot
    ☐ 2. alignment of the shoulder, hips, and knees
    ☐ 3. frayed rope near pulleys
    ☐ 4. correct amount of traction weight on fracture
    ☐ 5. pressure on the coccyx

32. A pediatric client has just had a plaster cast placed on their lower left leg. Which action should the nurse take to provide safe cast care?
    ☐ 1. Petal the cast as soon as it is put on.
    ☐ 2. Keep the child in the same position for 24 hours until the cast is dry.
    ☐ 3. Use only the palms of the hand when handling the cast.
    ☐ 4. Notify the health care provider (HCP) if the client feels heat.

33. The nurse is explaining the nature of the fracture to the parents of a school-age client who has a greenstick fracture. Which drawing should the nurse choose to explain the fracture to the parents?
☐ 1.
☐ 2.
☐ 3.
☐ 4.

34. A pediatric client is given morphine for postoperative pain following a fracture repair. As the nurse is assessing the client for pain 4 hours later, their parent leaves the room, and the child begins to cry. What assessment does the nurse make about the child's pain?
☐ 1. not in pain because the crying began after the parent leaves
☐ 2. less tolerant of pain because they are upset
☐ 3. in pain because they are crying
☐ 4. not in pain because they were medicated 4 hours ago

35. An adolescent client is having surgery to repair a fractured left femur. As a part of the preoperative safety checklist, what should the nurse do?
☐ 1. Ask the teen to point to the surgery site.
☐ 2. Verify that the site, side, and level are marked.
☐ 3. Ask the parents if they have signed the operative permit.
☐ 4. Restate the surgery risks to the parents.

36. A child is admitted from the operating room to the pediatric unit with a fracture of the femur and skeletal traction. What should the nurse assess **first**?
☐ 1. the pull of traction on the pin
☐ 2. the elastic bandage
☐ 3. the pin sites for signs of infection
☐ 4. the dressings for tightness

37. The nurse is caring for a child in Bryant traction (see figure). What action should the nurse take?

☐ 1. Adjust the weights on the legs until the buttocks rest on the bed.
☐ 2. Provide frequent skin care.
☐ 3. Place a pillow under the buttocks.
☐ 4. Remove the elastic leg wraps every 8 hours for 10 minutes.

38. A preschooler with a fractured femur of the left leg in traction tells the nurse that their leg hurts. It is too early for pain medication. What is the **first** action the nurse should take?
☐ 1. Place a pillow under the child's buttocks to provide support.
☐ 2. Remove the weight from the left leg.
☐ 3. Assess the feet for signs of neurovascular impairment.
☐ 4. Reposition the pulleys so the traction is looser.

39. The nurse in the emergency department is caring for a preschool-age child with a fractured humerus. The child is crying and screaming, "I hate you!" Which action would be **most** appropriate?
☐ 1. Tell the parents they will need to wait out in the lobby.
☐ 2. Ask the charge nurse to assign this client to another nurse.
☐ 3. Reassure the parents that this is normal behavior under the circumstances.
☐ 4. Ask the parents to discipline the child so that the team can treat her.

40. After a plaster cast has been applied to the arm of a child with a fractured right humerus, the nurse completes discharge teaching. The nurse should evaluate the teaching as successful when the birth parent agrees to seek medical advice if the child experiences which symptom?
☐ 1. inability to extend the fingers on the right hand
☐ 2. vomiting after the cast is applied
☐ 3. coolness and dampness of the cast after 5 hours
☐ 4. fussiness with statements that the cast is heavy

41. The nurse teaches the parent of a child who has a new cast for a fractured radius about home care. Which intervention does the nurse recommend for the first few days at home?
  ☐ 1. Use a hair dryer to dry the cast more quickly.
  ☐ 2. Have the child refrain from strenuous activities.
  ☐ 3. Watch the child wiggle their fingers once a day.
  ☐ 4. Administer acetaminophen every 8 to 12 hours for discomfort.

42. While assessing a 3-year-old child who has had an injury to the leg, has pain, and refuses to walk, the nurse notes that the child's left thigh is swollen. What should the nurse do **next**?
  ☐ 1. Assess the neurologic status of the toes.
  ☐ 2. Determine the circulatory status of the upper thigh.
  ☐ 3. Obtain the child's vital signs.
  ☐ 4. Notify the health care provider (HCP) immediately.

43. The nurse anticipates that a preschool-age child in traction will need diversion. What should the nurse offer the child?
  ☐ 1. a video game
  ☐ 2. blocks
  ☐ 3. hand puppets
  ☐ 4. remote-controlled car

44. The child in a new hip spica cast seems to be adjusting to the cast, except that after each meal the child tells the nurse that the cast is too tight. What should the nurse plan to do?
  ☐ 1. Administer a laxative before each meal.
  ☐ 2. Offer smaller, more frequent meals.
  ☐ 3. Give the child a mechanical soft diet.
  ☐ 4. Offer the child more fruits and grains.

45. The nurse is measuring a child for crutches. What factor(s) should the nurse consider? Select all that apply.
  ☐ 1. type of gait child will be using
  ☐ 2. degree of child's elbow flexion
  ☐ 3. space above the crutch to the child's axilla
  ☐ 4. weight of the child
  ☐ 5. whether the child has to use the stairs

The Client with Osteomyelitis

46. The nurse completes an admission assessment of a child admitted to the pediatric unit with osteomyelitis of the left tibia. When assessing the area over the tibia, the nurse understands that which finding is expected?
  ☐ 1. diffuse tenderness
  ☐ 2. decreased pain
  ☐ 3. increased warmth
  ☐ 4. localized edema

47. A child is to receive intravenous (IV) antibiotics for osteomyelitis. Before the initial dose of antibiotics can be given, the nurse confirms that a blood sample for which test has been drawn?
  ☐ 1. creatinine
  ☐ 2. culture
  ☐ 3. hemoglobin
  ☐ 4. white blood cell count

48. A child is being treated with vancomycin 40 mg/kg per day intravenously divided into three doses for osteomyelitis. The health care provider (HCP) has prescribed drug protocol management by pharmacy and a trough vancomycin level 30 minutes before the third dose scheduled for 0900 hours. The laboratory report returns before the third dose:

Laboratory Results			
Time	Test	Results	Normal Range
0830	Vancomycin	7 mcg/mL (4.8 µmol/L)	10–15 mcg/mL (6.9–10.4 µmol/L)

What action should the nurse take?
  ☐ 1. Administer the 0900 dose.
  ☐ 2. Notify the HCP.
  ☐ 3. Notify the pharmacist.
  ☐ 4. Draw a peak drug level.

49. The nurse is caring for a child with osteomyelitis who will be receiving high-dose intravenous antibiotic therapy for 3 to 4 weeks. What should the nurse plan to monitor?
  ☐ 1. blood glucose level
  ☐ 2. thrombin times
  ☐ 3. urine glucose level
  ☐ 4. urine specific gravity

50. The nurse creates a plan of care to meet the developmental needs of an 8-year-old child who is confined to home with osteomyelitis. What goal should the nurse include in the care plan?
  ☐ 1. Encourage the child to communicate with schoolmates.
  ☐ 2. Encourage the parents to stay with the child.
  ☐ 3. Allow siblings to visit freely throughout the day.
  ☐ 4. Talk to the child about their interests twice daily.

51. A child with newly diagnosed osteomyelitis has nausea and vomiting. The parent wishes to give the child ginger cookies to help control the nausea. What should the nurse tell the parents?
  ☐ 1. "You can try them and see how they do."
  ☐ 2. "I will need to get a prescription."
  ☐ 3. "Your child needs medication for the vomiting."
  ☐ 4. "We discourage the use of home remedies in children."

The Client with Scoliosis

52. When assessing an adolescent for scoliosis, the nurse should ask the client to perform which action(s)? Select all that apply.
☐ 1. Stand straight with their arms at their side.
☐ 2. Bend forward at the waist with arms hanging freely.
☐ 3. Lie flat on the floor and extend the legs straight from the trunk.
☐ 4. Sit in a chair while lifting the feet and legs to a right angle with the trunk.
☐ 5. Stand against a wall while pressing the length of the back against the wall.

53. The nurse teaches a family about the correct use of a Boston brace to treat scoliosis. The nurse determines teaching has been effective when the child and family state they will remove the brace at which times?
☐ 1. when bathing, for about 1 hour per day
☐ 2. while eating, for a total of 3 hours a day
☐ 3. during school, for about 8 hours a day
☐ 4. when sleeping, for a total of 10 hours a day

54. The nurse teaches the child with scoliosis being treated with a Boston brace about exercises. The nurse explains that the exercises are performed primarily for what reason?
☐ 1. to decrease back muscle spasms
☐ 2. to improve the brace's traction effect
☐ 3. to prevent spinal contractures
☐ 4. to strengthen the back and abdominal muscles

55. A pediatric client with scoliosis has to wear a brace. The nurse should develop a teaching plan with the client to include which instruction?
☐ 1. Wear the brace during waking hours.
☐ 2. Use lotions to relieve skin irritations.
☐ 3. Wear a form-fitting t-shirt under the brace.
☐ 4. Bathe the skin under the brace once per week.

Managing Care, Quality, and Safety of Children with Musculoskeletal Health Problems

56. A child with spastic cerebral palsy receiving intrathecal baclofen therapy is admitted to the pediatric floor with vomiting and dehydration. The family tells the nurse that they were scheduled to refill the baclofen pump today but had to cancel the appointment when the child became ill. Which action should the nurse take?
☐ 1. Explain that the medication should be discontinued during illness.
☐ 2. Arrange for the pump to be refilled in the hospital.
☐ 3. Reschedule the pump refill for the day of discharge.
☐ 4. Instruct caregivers to call for a refill when the low-volume alarm sounds.

57. The nurse on the pediatric floor is working on a team that includes a licensed practical/vocational nurse (LPN/VN). Which procedure(s) can the nurse working on a pediatric floor safely assign to the LPN/VN? Select all that apply.
☐ 1. refilling a baclofen pump
☐ 2. administering gastrostomy tube feedings
☐ 3. inserting hearing aids
☐ 4. giving an intravenous (IV) push medication
☐ 5. calling the morning blood sugars to the health care provider (HCP)

58. A school-age child with juvenile idiopathic arthritis (JIA) is being admitted to the hospital for evaluation of progressively increasing symptoms. The child weighs 60 lb (27 kg) and is 50 inches (127 cm) tall. The nurse is reconciling the medications the parent brought from home with the medications prescribed. What should the nurse do? (See chart.)

Prescriptions	
Home Medication	Prescribed Medication
Ibuprofen tablet, 200 mg orally (PO) four times a day (for arthritis), purchased over the counter	Ibuprofen tablet, 200 mg PO four times a day
Cetirizine hydrochloride tablet, 10 mg PO daily (for allergies), purchased over the counter	Methotrexate tablet, 10 mg PO every Monday

☐ 1. Have the family give the child cetirizine daily using the medication they have from home.
☐ 2. Explain the need to limit over-the-counter medications while in the hospital.
☐ 3. Request a cetirizine prescription from the health care provider (HCP).
☐ 4. Contact the HCP to question the methotrexate.

59. A preschool-age child presents to the emergency department. The client's parent tearfully reports that the child was on their shoulders in the driveway playing when the child began to fall. The parent grabbed the client by the leg, swinging them toward the grass to avoid landing on the pavement. As the parent swung the client, the client hit their head on the driveway and twisted their right leg. After a complete examination, it is determined that the client has a skull fracture and a spiral fracture of the femur. Which action should the nurse take?
☐ 1. Restrict the parent's visitation.
☐ 2. Notify the police immediately.
☐ 3. Refer the parent for parenting classes.
☐ 4. Record the parent's story in the medical record.

60. STEP 1

The nurse cares for an adolescent, male client admitted to the pediatric unit from surgery following long cast placement for a right upper tibial fracture.

Nurse's Notes

1615:
The cast is intact, and the toes are pink and warm to touch. Capillary refill is less than 2 seconds. The client states it hurts to wiggle their toes and rates their pain as a 7 on a scale of 0 to 10. The client's leg is elevated. The client is medicated with 1 mg morphine via intravenous (IV) push. Bowel sounds are present. Ringer's lactate solution is infusing at a rate of 120 mL per hour in the left arm. Vital signs are temperature (T) 99.0°F (37.2°C); pulse (P) 96 bpm; respiration rate (RR) 14 breaths/min; blood pressure (BP) 128/80 mm Hg; and pulse oximetry 97% on room air.

1645:
The cast is intact, and swelling in the right foot has increased. The toes are pink. Capillary refill is less than 3 seconds. The client states they are unable to wiggle their toes. The client rates their pain as an 8 on a scale of 0 to 10 and describes the pain as continuous, deep, and throbbing. The leg is elevated. Bowel sounds are present. The client reports mild nausea. Ringer's lactate solution is infusing at a rate of 120 mL per hour in the left arm. The client has not voided yet. Vital signs are T 99.3°F (37.4°C); P 100 bpm; RR 16 breaths/min; BP 132/84 mm Hg; and pulse oximetry 98% on room air.

➤ Which assessment(s) need **immediate** follow-up? Select all that apply.

- ☐ 1. Circulation
- ☐ 2. Edema
- ☐ 3. Movement
- ☐ 4. Nausea
- ☐ 5. Pain
- ☐ 6. Urinary output
- ☐ 7. Vital signs

61. STEP 2

The nurse cares for an adolescent, male client admitted to the pediatric unit from surgery following long cast placement for a right upper tibial fracture.

Nurse's Notes

1615:
The cast is intact, and the toes are pink and warm to touch. Capillary refill is less than 2 seconds. The client states it hurts to wiggle their toes and rates their pain as a 7 on a scale of 0 to 10. The client's leg is elevated. The client is medicated with 1 mg morphine via intravenous (IV) push. Bowel sounds are present. Ringer's lactate solution is infusing at a rate of 120 mL per hour in the left arm. Vital signs are temperature (T) 99.0°F (37.2°C); pulse (P) 96 bpm; respiration rate (RR) 14 breaths/min; blood pressure (BP) 128/80 mm Hg; and pulse oximetry 97% on room air.

1645:
The cast is intact, and swelling in the right foot has increased. The toes are pink. Capillary refill is less than 3 seconds. The client states they are unable to wiggle their toes. The client rates their pain as an 8 on a scale of 0 to 10 and describes the pain as continuous, deep, and throbbing. The leg is elevated. Bowel sounds are present. The client reports mild nausea. Ringer's lactate solution is infusing at a rate of 120 mL per hour in the left arm. The client has not voided yet. Vital signs are T 99.3°F (37.4°C); P 100 bpm; RR 16 breaths/min; BP 132/84 mm Hg; and pulse oximetry 98% on room air.

➤ For each client finding below, specify if the finding is consistent with the complication of compartment syndrome, deep vein thrombosis (DVT), or hypovolemic shock. Each finding may support more than one complication.

	Compartment Syndrome	DVT	Hypovolemic Shock
Delayed capillary refill	☐	☐	☐
Throbbing pain	☐	☐	☐
Swelling	☐	☐	☐
Impaired movement	☐	☐	☐

Note: Each column must have at least one response option selected.

62. STEP 3

The nurse cares for an adolescent, male client admitted to the pediatric unit from surgery following long cast placement for a right upper tibial fracture.

Nurse's Notes

1615:
The cast is intact, and the toes are pink and warm to touch. Capillary refill is less than 2 seconds. The client states it hurts to wiggle their toes and rates their pain as a 7 on a scale of 0 to 10. The client's leg is elevated. The client is medicated with 1 mg morphine via intravenous (IV) push. Bowel sounds are present. Ringer's lactate solution is infusing at a rate of 120 mL per hour in the left arm. Vital signs are temperature (T) 99.0°F (37.2°C); pulse (P) 96 bpm; respiration rate (RR) 14 breaths/min; blood pressure (BP) 128/80 mm Hg; and pulse oximetry 97% on room air.

1645:
The cast is intact, and swelling in the right foot has increased. The toes are pink. Capillary refill is less than 3 seconds. The client states they are unable to wiggle their toes. The client rates their pain as an 8 on a scale of 0 to 10 and describes the pain as continuous, deep, and throbbing. The leg is elevated. Bowel sounds are present. The client reports mild nausea. Ringer's lactate solution is infusing at a rate of 120 mL per hour in the left arm. The client has not voided yet. Vital signs are T 99.3°F (37.4°C); P 100 bpm; RR 16 breaths/min; BP 132/84 mm Hg; and pulse oximetry 98% on room air.

➤ Complete the sentences from the list of drop-down options.

The priority intervention for this client is to [restore volume. / decrease compression. / administer anticoagulants.]

Delayed treatment can lead to the serious complication of [cardiac arrest. / tissue necrosis. / pulmonary embolism.]

63. STEP 4

The nurse cares for an adolescent, male client admitted to the pediatric unit from surgery following long cast placement for a right upper tibial fracture.

Nurse's Notes

1615:
The cast is intact, and the toes are pink and warm to touch. Capillary refill is less than 2 seconds. The client states it hurts to wiggle their toes and rates their pain as a 7 on a scale of 0 to 10. The client's leg is elevated. The client is medicated with 1 mg morphine via intravenous (IV) push. Bowel sounds are present. Ringer's lactate solution is infusing at a rate of 120 mL per hour in the left arm. Vital signs are temperature (T) 99.0°F (37.2°C); pulse (P) 96 bpm; respiration rate (RR) 14 breaths/min; blood pressure (BP) 128/80 mm Hg; and pulse oximetry 97% on room air.

1645:
The cast is intact, and swelling in the right foot has increased. The toes are pink. Capillary refill is less than 3 seconds. The client states they are unable to wiggle their toes. The client rates their pain as an 8 on a scale of 0 to 10 and describes the pain as continuous, deep, and throbbing. The leg is elevated. Bowel sounds are present. The client reports mild nausea. Ringer's lactate solution is infusing at a rate of 120 mL per hour in the left arm. The client has not voided yet. Vital signs are T 99.3°F (37.4°C); P 100 bpm; RR 16 breaths/min; BP 132/84 mm Hg; and pulse oximetry 98% on room air.

The nurse notifies the orthopedic surgeon about the change in the client's condition. The orthopedic surgeon wants to attempt conservative treatment.

➤ For each intervention, indicate if the intervention is anticipated or not indicated.

Intervention	Anticipated	Not Indicated
Splint the cast on each side	☐	☐
Cut the undercast padding	☐	☐
Elevate the leg above heart level	☐	☐
Insert a tissue-pressure monitoring device	☐	☐
Administer narcotic analgesic medication	☐	☐
Reassess in 2 hours	☐	☐

64. STEP 5

The client's condition does not improve. The client must undergo an emergency fasciotomy for compartment syndrome.

Nurse's Notes

1615:
The cast is intact, and the toes are pink and warm to touch. Capillary refill is less than 2 seconds. The client states it hurts to wiggle their toes and rates their pain as a 7 on a scale of 0 to 10. The client's leg is elevated. The client is medicated with 1 mg morphine via intravenous (IV) push. Bowel sounds are present. Ringer's lactate solution is infusing at a rate of 120 mL per hour in the left arm. Vital signs are temperature (T) 99.0°F (37.2°C); pulse (P) 96 bpm; respiration rate (RR) 14 breaths/min; blood pressure (BP) 128/80 mm Hg; and pulse oximetry 97% on room air.

1645:
The cast is intact, and swelling in the right foot has increased. The toes are pink. Capillary refill is less than 3 seconds. The client states they are unable to wiggle their toes. The client rates their pain as an 8 on a scale of 0 to 10 and describes the pain as continuous, deep, and throbbing. The leg is elevated. Bowel sounds are present. The client reports mild nausea. Ringer's lactate solution is infusing at a rate of 120 mL per hour in the left arm. The client has not voided yet. Vital signs are T 99.3°F (37.4°C); P 100 bpm; RR 16 breaths/min; BP 132/84 mm Hg; and pulse oximetry 98% on room air.

Orders

Morphine sulfate 5 mg/mL (150 mg in 30 mL) per patient-controlled analgesia (PCA) pump.
- Loading dose 5 to 10 mg
- Client dose 1 mg
- Lockout 10 minutes
- 4-hour limit 30 mg

The client returns to the pediatric unit with new postoperative orders.

➤ What does the nurse teach the client about using a PCA pump? Select all that apply.

☐ 1. Press the button attached to the pump to give yourself pain medicine.
☐ 2. There are safety controls in place to prevent you from getting too much pain medicine.
☐ 3. You will need to be on an oxygen saturation monitor while you are using a PCA pump.
☐ 4. You are less likely to have constipation using a PCA pump than getting morphine in larger doses.
☐ 5. If you push the button and do not feel better in 10 minutes, call your nurse.
☐ 6. Your parent can push the button for you while you are sleeping.

65. STEP 6

The nurse cares for an adolescent, male client on the pediatric unit who has undergone an emergency right tibial fasciotomy for compartment syndrome.

Nurse's Notes

1615:
The cast is intact, and the toes are pink and warm to touch. Capillary refill is less than 2 seconds. The client states it hurts to wiggle their toes and rates their pain as a 7 on a scale of 0 to 10. The client's leg is elevated. The client is medicated with 1 mg morphine via intravenous (IV) push. Bowel sounds are present. Ringer's lactate solution is infusing at a rate of 120 mL per hour in the left arm. Vital signs are temperature (T) 99.0°F (37.2°C); pulse (P) 96 bpm; respiration rate (RR) 14 breaths/min; blood pressure (BP) 128/80 mm Hg; and pulse oximetry 97% on room air.

1645:
The cast is intact, and swelling in the right foot has increased. The toes are pink. Capillary refill is less than 3 seconds. The client states they are unable to wiggle their toes. The client rates their pain as an 8 on a scale of 0 to 10 and describes the pain as continuous, deep, and throbbing. The leg is elevated. Bowel sounds are present. The client reports mild nausea. Ringer's lactate solution is infusing at a rate of 120 mL per hour in the left arm. The client has not voided yet. Vital signs are T 99.3°F (37.4°C); P 100 bpm; RR 16 breaths/min; BP 132/84 mm Hg; and pulse oximetry 98% on room air.

Postoperative Day 2, 0800:
The right leg is in a splint at heart level. The saline dressing is intact. The right leg remains swollen. The toes are pink and warm to touch; capillary refill is less than 2 seconds; the pedal pulse is +1; and the client can wiggle their toes. The client is using the maximum dose of morphine and has an average pain rating of 2 on a 10-point scale. The client's urine is brown, and the morning creatine kinase level is elevated. Other lab test results are within normal limits. The client has started taking PO fluids. An IV of Ringer's lactate is infusing at 120 mL per hour in the left arm. Vital signs are T 99.9°F (37.7°C); P 96 bpm; RR 16 breaths/min; BP 128/80 mm Hg; and pulse oximetry 97% in room air.

Orders

Morphine sulfate 5 mg/mL (150 mg in 30 mL) per patient-controlled analgesia (PCA) pump.
- Loading dose 5 to 10 mg
- Client dose 1 mg
- Lockout 10 minutes
- 4-hour limit 30 mg

The nurse assesses the adolescent on postoperative day 2 after a right tibial fasciotomy.

➢ Complete the sentences from the list of drop-down options.

The nurse is concerned that the client is developing the complication of [infection / muscle necrosis / nerve damage]

as evidenced by the client's [swelling / urine / pain]

and [temperature. / lab results. / pulses.]

Answers, Rationales, and Test-Taking Strategies

The answers and the rationales for each question follow below, along with keys (🔑) to the client need (CN) and cognitive level (CL) for each question. In addition, questions that measure clinical judgment will be coded (CJ). As you check your answers, use the Content Mastery and Test-Taking Skill Self-Analysis worksheet (tear-out worksheet in the back of the book) to identify the reason(s) for not answering the questions correctly. For additional information about test-taking skills and strategies for answering questions, refer to pages 12–51 in Part 1 of this book.

The Client with Torticollis, Legg-Calvé-Perthes Disease, and Musculoskeletal Dysfunction

1. **2.** Physical therapy is the most important part of the child's plan of care. Most cases of torticollis respond to gentle stretching exercises, which the parents perform daily. Regular physical therapy is needed to monitor the infant's progress. Botulinum toxin injections are not approved for children under the age of 2 years and would not be an appropriate first-line treatment for an infant. Surgery is only done if physical therapy is not successful after several months. The use of wedges to position children during sleep is not recommended because they increase the risk for sudden infant death syndrome (SIDS).

   🔑 CN: Management of care; CL: Apply

2. **4.** Legg-Calvé-Perthes disease, also known as *coxa plana* or *osteochondrosis*, is characterized by aseptic necrosis at the head of the femur when the blood supply to the area is interrupted. Avoidance of weight-bearing is especially important to prevent the head of the femur from leaving the acetabulum, thus preventing hip dislocation. Devices such as an abduction brace, a leg cast, or a harness sling are used to protect the affected joint while revascularization and bone healing occur. Surgical procedures are used in some cases. Although pain control measures may be appropriate, pain is not necessarily more acute at night. Initial therapy involves rest and non–weight-bearing to help restore motion. Preventing flexion is not necessary.

   🔑 CN: Physiological adaptation; CL: Apply

3. **3.** Because most of the child's care takes place at home, the primary focus of family teaching would be on the care and management of the corrective device. Devices such as an abduction brace, a leg cast, or a harness sling are used to protect the affected joint while revascularization and bone healing occur. As long as the child is eating a well-balanced diet, there is no need for an intake of protein-rich foods. The parents can encourage range of motion in the unaffected leg, but motion in the affected leg is limited until it heals. Once therapy has been initiated, pain is usually not a problem. The key is management of the corrective device.

   🔑 CN: Reduction of risk potential; CL: Analyze

4. **4.** The parent is describing symptoms consistent with torticollis, or wry neck syndrome. With this musculoskeletal disorder, the sternocleidomastoid muscle shortens, causing the infant to drop the head toward the affected muscle and tilt the chin upward in the opposite direction. Frequently, a lump may be felt in the affected muscle. Palpating the fontanelle is done to assess neurologic status, not musculoskeletal status. Torticollis does not involve the cervical vertebrae or trapezius muscle.

   🔑 CN: Physiological adaptation; CL: Analyze

5. **4.** The adolescent is most likely experiencing heat exhaustion or heat collapse, which are common after vigorous exercise in a hot environment. Symptoms result from loss of fluids and include nausea, vomiting, dizziness, headache, and thirst. Treatment consists of moving the adolescent to a cool environment and giving cool liquids. Cool liquids are easier to drink than cold liquids. Taking the adolescent's temperature would be appropriate once these actions have been completed. However, the adolescent's temperature is likely to be normal or only mildly elevated. Elevating the child's legs is a measure that is used to treat dizziness, but it should only be implemented after the child has been moved to a cooler environment.

   🔑 CN: Basic care and comfort; CL: Analyze

The Client with Cerebral Palsy

6. **3.** It is important to identify primary developmental delays in children with cerebral palsy and to prevent secondary and tertiary delays. The arrested development is worrisome and requires further investigation. It is possible the lack of development indicates hearing loss, or it may be a sign of autism. The brain damage caused by

cerebral palsy is not progressive. The brain of a young child is quite plastic; assuming that the child's development has peaked at age 3 would be a serious mistake. The therapy plan will need to be modified, but a better understanding of the underlying problem will lead to the greatest chance of creating a successful therapy plan.

CN: Health promotion and maintenance; CL: Analyze

7. 2, 3, 4, 5. Botulinum toxin injections can be used to improve many aspects of quality of life for a child with cerebral palsy. The injections can help decrease pain from spasticity. Injections improve motor status by reducing rigidity and allowing for more effective physical therapy to improve range of motion. Decreased spasms enhance self-esteem. Improved motor status facilitates the ability to provide some aspects of care, especially transfers. Botulinum does not significantly affect nutritional status or speech.

CN: Management of care; CL: Apply

8. 3. The term *cerebral palsy* refers to a group of nonprogressive disorders of upper motor neuron impairment that result in motor dysfunction due to injury. In addition, a child may have speech or ocular difficulties, seizures, hyperactivity, or cognitive impairment. The condition of congenital malformed blood vessels in the ventricles is known as *arteriovenous malformations*. Viral infection and metabolic imbalances do not cause CP.

CN: Physiological adaptation; CL: Evaluate

9. 4. Delay in achieving developmental milestones is a characteristic of children with cerebral palsy. Ninety percent of typically developing 15-month-old children can put a block in a cup. Walking up steps typically is accomplished at 18 to 24 months. A child usually can use a spoon at 18 months. The ability to copy a circle is achieved at approximately 3 to 4 years of age.

CN: Health promotion and maintenance; CL: Analyze

10. 3. The nurse needs to respond honestly to the parent. Most children with hemiparesis due to spastic cerebral palsy can walk because the motor deficit is usually greater in the upper extremity. There is no need to refer the parent to the health care provider. Pulling to a stand requires both upper body and lower body strength. The will to walk is important, but without neurologic stability, the child may be unable to do so.

CN: Physiological adaptation; CL: Analyze

11. 1. Limited interaction or lack of interaction with friends and family may lead the nurse to suspect a possible problem with the family's ability to cope with others' reactions and responses to a child with cerebral palsy. Learning measures to meet the child's physical needs demonstrates some understanding and acceptance of the disease. Requesting teaching about the disease suggests curiosity or a desire for understanding, thus demonstrating that the family is dealing with the situation. Participating in social media may serve as a form of support and can be a healthy coping mechanism.

CN: Psychosocial integrity; CL: Evaluate

The Client with Duchenne Muscular Dystrophy

12. 1. Duchenne muscular dystrophy is an X-linked recessive disorder. The gene is transmitted through female carriers to affected sons 50% of the time. Daughters have a 50% chance of being carriers.

CN: Physiological adaptation; CL: Apply

13. 3. Usually, the first clinical manifestations of Duchenne muscular dystrophy include difficulty with typical age-appropriate physical activities such as running, riding a tricycle, and climbing stairs. Contractures of the large joints typically occur much later in the disease process. Occasionally, enlarged calves may be noted, but they are not typical findings in a child with Duchenne muscular dystrophy. Muscular atrophy and the development of small, weak muscles are later signs.

CN: Physiological adaptation; CL: Analyze

14. 4. With the Gower's sign, the child walks the hands up the legs in an attempt to stand, a common approach used by children with Duchenne muscular dystrophy when rising from a sitting to a standing position. *Galeazzi's sign* refers to the shortening of the affected limb in congenital hip dislocation. *Goodell's sign* refers to the softening of the cervix, considered a sign of probable pregnancy. *Goodenough's sign* refers to a test of mental age.

CN: Physiological adaptation; CL: Analyze

15. 3. The primary nursing goal is to maintain function in unaffected muscles for as long as possible. There is no effective treatment for childhood muscular dystrophy. Children who remain active can forestall being confined in a wheelchair. Remaining active also minimizes the risk for social isolation. Preventing rather than encouraging wheelchair use by maintaining function for as long as possible is an appropriate nursing goal. Children with muscular dystrophy become socially isolated as their condition deteriorates and they can no longer keep up with friends. Maintaining function helps prevent social isolation. Circulatory impairment is not associated with muscular dystrophy.

 CN: Physiological adaptation; CL: Analyze

16. 3. The guilt that birth parents of children with muscular dystrophy commonly experience usually results from the fact that the disease is genetic and the birth parent transmitted the defective gene. Although many children die from the disease, the disease is considered chronic and progressive. As the disease progresses, the child becomes more dependent. However, guilt typically stems from the knowledge that the birth parent transmitted the disease to their child rather than the dependency of the child. The disease onset is usually gradual, not sudden.

 CN: Psychosocial integrity; CL: Analyze

17. 1. Muscular dystrophy is a progressive disease. Children who are affected by this disease usually are unable to walk independently by age 9 to 11 years. There is no effective treatment for childhood muscular dystrophy. Although children who remain active can avoid wheelchair confinement for a longer period, activity does not prevent disease progression.

 CN: Physiological adaptation; CL: Evaluate

The Client with Developmental Dysplasia of the Hip

18. 4. This infant with congenital hip dysplasia has asymmetric gluteal folds. The Ortolani "click" occurs when the nurse feels the femur sliding into the acetabulum with a click. Limited abduction may be observed during an attempt to abduct the infant's thighs. Galeazzi's sign reveals femoral foreshortening and is observed by flexing the thighs.

 CN: Health promotion and maintenance; CL: Analyze

19. 1. The Pavlik harness is worn over a diaper. Knee socks are also worn to prevent the straps and foot and leg pieces from rubbing directly on the skin. For maximum results, the infant needs to wear the harness continuously. The skin should be inspected several times a day, not every other day, for signs of redness or irritation. Lotions and powders are to be avoided because they can cake and irritate the skin.

 CN: Reduction of risk potential; CL: Analyze

20. 2. Assessing the learner's knowledge level is the initial step in any teaching plan to promote the maximum amount of learning. This assessment also provides the nurse with a starting point for teaching. Assessing coping strategies can provide important information to the development of the teaching plan but is not the initial step. Giving parents written instructions or a list of community resources is appropriate once the parents' knowledge level has been determined and teaching has begun.

 CN: Reduction of risk potential; CL: Apply

21. 3. The abduction bar is incorporated into the cast to increase the cast's strength and maintain the legs in alignment. The bar cannot be removed or adjusted unless the cast is removed, and a new cast is applied. The bar should never be used to lift or turn the client because doing so may weaken the cast.

 CN: Reduction of risk potential; CL: Analyze

22. 2. The toddler in a hip spica cast needs a specially designed car seat. The one that the parent already has will not be appropriate because of the need for the car seat to accommodate the cast and abductor bar.

 CN: Safety and infection control; CL: Analyze

The Client with Congenital Clubfoot

23. 2. Elevating the extremity at different points during the day is helpful to prevent edema, but pillows should not be used in the crib because they increase the risk for sudden infant death syndrome (SIDS). A change in the color of the toes is a sign of impaired circulation and requires medical evaluation. Children typically need a series of 5 to 10 casts to correct the deformity. Infants with clubfeet still need frequent holding like any other newborn.

 CN: Safety and infection control; CL: Evaluate

24. 3. When an infant is born with an unexpected anomaly, parents are faced with questions, uncertainties, and possible disappointments. They may feel inadequate, helpless, and anxious. The nurse can help the parents initially by assessing their concerns and providing appropriate information to help them clarify or resolve the immediate problems. Referring the parents to the HCP is not necessary at this time. The nurse can assist the parents by listening to their concerns. Having them talk with other parents would be helpful a little bit later once the nurse assesses their concerns and discusses the problem and the parents' current feelings. If the parents continue to have difficulties expressing and working through their feelings, referral to a counselor would be appropriate.

CN: Psychosocial integrity; CL: Analyze

25. **3.** A cast that is too tight can cause a tourniquet effect, compromising the neurovascular integrity of the extremity. Manifestations of neurovascular impairment include pain, edema, pulselessness, coolness, altered sensation, and inability to move the distal exposed extremity. The toes of the casted extremity should be assessed frequently to evaluate for changes in neurovascular integrity. Wetting a plaster cast with water and soap softens the plaster, which may alter the cast's effectiveness. There is no reason to elevate the casted extremities when a child with clubfoot is being treated with nonsurgical measures. The legs would be elevated if swelling were present. Petals, which are applied to cover the rough edges of the cast, are to be left in place to minimize the risk for skin irritation from the cast edges.

CN: Reduction of risk potential; CL: Evaluate

The Client with Juvenile Idiopathic Arthritis

26. **4.** The nurse's response to the parent is based on the knowledge that there is no definitive test for JIA. The latex fixation test, which is commonly used to diagnose arthritis in adults, is negative in 90% of children. The erythrocyte sedimentation rate may or may not be increased during active disease. This test identifies the presence of inflammation only. Synovial fluid cultures are done to rule out septic arthritis, not to diagnose JIA.

CN: Reduction of risk potential; CL: Analyze

27. **1.** With JIA, the more joints affected, the more severe the disease is likely to be and the less likely the symptoms will totally resolve. Approximately one-third of the children will continue to have the disease into adulthood, and approximately one-sixth will experience severe, crippling deformities.

CN: Physiological adaptation; CL: Apply

28. **2.** Socialization is important for this preschool-age child, and activity is important to maintain function. Because children with JIA commonly experience most problems in the early morning after arising, they need more time to "warm up." Adverse effects may or may not occur. The child's normal routine needs to be maintained as much as possible. Although splints and braces may be needed, they are worn during periods of rest, not activity, to maintain function.

CN: Physiological adaptation; CL: Analyze

29. **4.** Because the child is dealing with grief and loss associated with a chronic illness, parents need to be supportive and understanding. The child needs to feel valued and worthwhile. Introducing the child to others of the same age who also have JIA most probably would be ineffective because preschoolers are developmentally egocentric. Although the child needs to feel valued, the birth parent spending more time with the child and less time with their other children is inappropriate because the child with JIA may experience secondary gain from the illness if the family interaction patterns are altered. Also, this action reinforces the child's withdrawal behavior. Psychological counseling is not needed at this time because the child's reaction is normal.

CN: Psychosocial integrity; CL: Analyze

30. **3.** The first group of drugs typically prescribed is the nonsteroidal anti-inflammatory drugs, which include naproxen. Once therapy is started, it takes hours or days for relief from pain to occur. However, it takes 3 to 4 weeks for the anti-inflammatory effects to occur, including a reduction in swelling and less pain with movement. Naproxen is included in only a few over-the-counter medications, but aspirin is in several. The family should check with the nurse before giving any over-the-counter medications. Toxicity or gastrointestinal bleeding may occur when nonsteroidal anti-inflammatory drugs are combined. The missed dose will need to be made up to maintain the serum level and the therapeutic effectiveness of the drug.

CN: Pharmacological and parenteral therapies; CL: Apply

The Client with a Fracture

31. **2, 3, 4, 5.** Buck traction provides skin traction that keeps the extremity in straight alignment and can be observed by noting a straight line formed between the shoulder, hips, and knees. The rope must be intact to maintain the prescribed traction

from the weights. The correct amount of traction must be maintained to keep the fractured femur in correct alignment. Because the client is in a recumbent position, the nurse should also inspect the skin on the back and buttocks for integrity. The nurse should not remove the client's wraps and boot unless they have a health care provider's prescription to do so.

CN: Physiological adaptation; CL: Analyze

32. 3. The wet plaster cast should be handled using only the palms of the hands to prevent indentations of the cast surface. Petaling a cast should be done only when the edges of the cast are rough and are causing irritation to the client's skin. The nurse should not keep the child in the same position until the cast is dry. Doing so would prohibit proper toileting and elimination and would produce undue pressure on the coccyx. The cast typically emits heat as it dries, so notifying an HCP is not necessary in this instance. If needed, a fan can be used to circulate the room air.

CN: Health promotion and maintenance; CL: Evaluate

33. 3. The nurse should show the parents the figure of the greenstick fracture as noted in answer 3 in which the fracture does not completely cross through the bone. Answer 1 is a plastic deformation, or a bend in the bone. Answer 1 is a buckle. Answer 4 is a complete fracture.

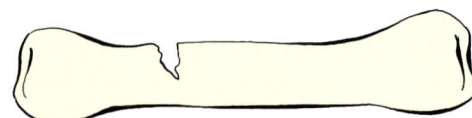

CN: Physiological adaptation; CL: Analyze

34. 2. Emotional or physical stress lowers a person's tolerance of pain. The parent's presence may have distracted the client, and when the parent left, it caused the client to focus on the pain they were having. Crying does not automatically indicate pain. The nurse must further assess the client for pain. Although an analgesic medication was given 4 hours before, pain may be present.

CN: Physiological adaptation; CL: Analyze

35. 2. As part of a surgery safety checklist, the nurse must verify that the site, side, and level are marked. Pointing to the area is not sufficient identification of the surgery site. The nurse must verify the form has been signed by reviewing the form. The surgeon holds primary responsibility for explaining the risks of surgery.

CN: Safety and infection control; CL: Analyze

36. 1. Skeletal traction applies the pull directly to the skeletal structure by tongs, pin, or wire. The nurse should assess the pull of the traction on the pin first. This is critical to the success of the traction. Once this is assessed, the pin sites are assessed for signs of infection. The dressings would be examined after the pull of the traction, neurovascular status, and pin sites were assessed. The elastic wrap is used to anchor skin traction nonadherent straps, not skeletal traction.

CN: Reduction of risk potential; CL: Analyze

37. 2. The traction is positioned correctly; the nurse should provide frequent skin care to the back and shoulder areas. The hips and buttocks should be lifted off the bed to provide countertraction; the nurse should not adjust the weights. The nurse should not place a pillow under the buttocks as this would prevent countertraction. The elastic wraps should remain on the legs unless removal is prescribed by the health care provider.

CN: Physiological adaptation; CL: Analyze

38. 3. The nurse should assess the client frequently for signs of neurovascular impairment of the feet, such as pallor, coldness, numbness, or tingling. Pillows are not placed under the buttocks because the pillows would alter the alignment of the traction. Weights provide traction and should not be removed. Pulleys help maintain optimal alignment of the traction and therefore should be left alone.

CN: Basic care and comfort; CL: Analyze

39. 3. Explaining to the parents that this is a normal reaction under the circumstances is most appropriate. The child's outburst is related to the child's fears of the unknown. The child is scared and anxious and needs the parents for support. Asking the parents to wait outside would only add to the child's fear and anxiety. The reaction is normal for a child that age and does not usually call for a change in staff assignments. Asking the parents to discipline their child for the child's behavior is inappropriate. The nurse needs to handle the situation.

CN: Health promotion and maintenance; CL: Analyze

40. 1. Inability to extend the fingers of the involved arm may indicate neurologic impairment caused by pressure on soft tissue. It is not unusual for a child to vomit after experiencing a traumatic injury. It may take up to 72 hours for a plaster cast to dry. Until the cast dries, the dampness causes the sensation of coolness. The cast will seem heavy until the child adjusts to the extra weight.

The child may exhibit fussiness (such as whining, crying, or clinging) as a result of numerous causes, such as placement of the cast, the hospital experience, or pain. These reactions are normal and do not warrant medical advice.

CN: Reduction of risk potential; CL: Evaluate

41. 2. For the first few days after application of a plaster or fiberglass cast, the child should not engage in strenuous activities, to minimize swelling that would cause the cast to become too tight. Using a hair dryer to complete the drying of the cast is not encouraged because the hair dryer only dries the outside of the cast. Movement and sensation of the fingers need to be checked several times a day for the first few days. Typically, the parent would be instructed to administer acetaminophen every 4 to 6 hours, not every 8 to 12 hours, for discomfort.

CN: Reduction of risk potential; CL: Analyze

42. 1. Because the nurse suspects a possible fracture based on the child's presentation, assessing the neurologic and circulatory status of the toes, the tissues distal to the fracture, is important. Soft tissue contusions, which accompany femur fractures, can result in severe hemorrhage into the tissue and subsequent circulatory and neurologic impairment. Once this information has been obtained, vital signs can be assessed, and the nurse can notify the HCP and report the findings. In fractures, circulation impairment will occur distal to the injury.

CN: Physiological adaptation; CL: Analyze

43. 3. Hand puppets would enable a 3-year-old child in traction to act out feelings within the constraints imposed by the traction. A 3-year-old needs creative play. The video game would make the child too active in bed and does not meet the child's developmental need for creative play. Blocks would be more appropriate for a younger child. Remote-controlled cars are appropriate for older children but can present a fall risk to others if used in a hospital.

CN: Health promotion and maintenance; CL: Analyze

44. 2. A hip spica cast encircles the abdomen. When the child eats a large meal, abdominal pressure increases, causing the cast to feel tight. Therefore, the nurse should plan to offer smaller, more frequent meals to minimize abdominal distention. If the child's appetite were decreased in conjunction with a feeling of fullness, the nurse might suspect that the child was becoming constipated and plan to use laxatives or a higher-fiber diet. A mechanical soft diet is indicated when the child has difficulty chewing food adequately. Giving the child more fruits and grains would contribute to abdominal distention and problems with the cast tightness after eating.

CN: Reduction of risk potential; CL: Analyze

45. -/+ 2, 3. To ensure the proper fit of crutches, the child's elbow flexion should be 20 degrees, and the area above the top of the crutch to the child's axilla should be 1 to 1.5 inches (2.5 to 3.8 cm). The type of gait, the weight of the child, and the use of stairs are not factors in the measurement.

CN: Reduction of risk potential; CL: Apply

The Client with Osteomyelitis

46. 3. Findings associated with osteomyelitis commonly include pain over the area, increased warmth, localized tenderness, and diffuse swelling over the involved bone. The area over the affected bone is red.

CN: Physiological adaptation; CL: Analyze

47. 2. Cultures are used to determine exactly what organism is causing the inflammation. From the culture, sensitivities to various antibiotics may be determined. If the antibiotics are given before obtaining the culture, the antibiotics may inhibit the growth of the organism in the culture medium. This may lead to a delay in the most appropriate treatment. Unless a child has a known renal problem, baseline creatinine levels are not typically needed. However, levels may be needed during treatment depending on the medication. A complete blood count with hemoglobin and a white blood cell count is typically prescribed for any suspected infection, but these tests do not identify the causative organism.

CN: Reduction of risk potential; CL: Apply

48. 3. The vancomycin level is not therapeutic and will need to be adjusted. Drug management by the pharmacy is prescribed. Thus, the nurse should notify the pharmacist to adjust the dose. This is very frequently done in institutions with pediatric clinical pharmacists. Giving subtherapeutic doses may prolong care. If needed, the pharmacist would notify the HCP. Peak levels are not prescribed for this client.

CN: Pharmacological and parenteral therapies; CL: Analyze

49. 4. Long-term, high-dose antibiotic therapy can adversely affect renal, hepatic, and hematopoietic function. Urine specific gravity would provide valuable information about the kidneys' ability to concentrate or dilute urine, thereby suggesting renal impairment. Blood glucose levels reveal how well the client's body is using glucose. Thrombin times reveal information about the clotting mechanism. Urine glucose levels reveal information about the body's use and excretion of glucose.

CN: Pharmacological and parenteral therapies; CL: Analyze

50. 1. Encouraging contact with schoolmates allows the school-age child to maintain and develop socialization with peers, an important developmental task of this age group. Although having family visits and interacting with the child are important, they do not meet the child's developmental needs. Talking to the child about their interests is important, but encouraging contact with schoolmates is crucial to maintain and develop socialization with peers.

CN: Health promotion and maintenance; CL: Apply

51. 1. Some clients find ginger cookies or "snaps" help relieve nausea. Ginger, in small doses such as would be found in the cookies, has few side effects. There is no reason that the parent should not try this dietary intervention; however, the nurse must monitor the client's response. If the child has a diet as tolerated prescription, there is no need for an additional prescription. Ultimately, the child may need an antiemetic medication, but dietary strategies are often successful in treating vomiting related to osteomyelitis. Making a universal statement disregarding home remedies is not a client-centered approach.

CN: Physiological adaptation; CL: Analyze

The Client with Scoliosis

52. -/+ **1, 2.** Scoliosis is a lateral deviation of the spine. It is assessed by first asking the client to stand straight while looking for limp length discrepancy. Then the client bends forward at the waist with their arms hanging freely as the nurse looks for lateral curvature of the spine and a rib hump. The other positions will not reveal deviation of the spine.

CN: Health promotion and maintenance; CL: Analyze

53. 1. One of the most effective spinal braces for correcting scoliosis, the Boston brace should be worn for at least 16 to 23 hours a day, except when carrying out personal hygiene measures.

CN: Reduction of risk potential; CL: Evaluate

54. 4. Exercises are prescribed for the child with scoliosis wearing a Boston brace to help strengthen spinal and abdominal muscles and provide support. Typically, children wearing a Boston brace do not have muscle spasms. Performing exercises provides no effect on the brace's traction ability. Spinal contractures do not occur when a Boston brace is worn.

CN: Physiological adaptation; CL: Apply

55. 3. A form-fitting t-shirt can be worn under the brace to prevent skin irritation and collect perspiration. Braces are worn 23 hours each day. Lotions may cause irritation and should not be used. The skin under the brace should be bathed daily to help prevent irritation from the brace. The brace can be removed for bathing so all the skin can be bathed.

CN: Physiological adaptation; CL: Apply

Managing Care, Quality, and Safety of Children with Musculoskeletal Health Problems

56. 2. To prevent baclofen withdrawal, pump refills are scheduled several days before anticipated low-volume alarms. The nurse should make it a high priority to have the pump refilled as soon as possible. Discontinuing baclofen suddenly can result in a high fever, muscle rigidity, change in level of consciousness, and even death. Waiting until the child leaves the hospital for a refill may lead to a low dose or withdrawal. Waiting for the low-volume alarm puts the client at risk because medication and team members who can refill the pump may not be readily available under all circumstances.

CN: Management of care; CL: Analyze

57. -/+ **2, 3.** In general, LPN/VNs may perform skills related to feeding, oral medication administration, and activities of daily living, such as insertion of a hearing aid. Refilling a baclofen pump constitutes administering an intrathecal medication and is beyond the scope of practice for LPN/VNs in most areas. Some institutions allow LPN/VNs to give IV push medicines; however, special training is required. Communicating with the HCP would require discussion of the client's assessments and evaluations, which fall under the RN scope of practice.

🔑 CN: Management of care; CL: Analyze

58. 3. If the child was taking cetirizine for allergies, the nurse should contact the HCP for a prescription to continue the medication in the hospital. The provider should either prescribe the medication or provide a valid reason to discontinue its use. Advising the family to take a home supply of medications increases the risk for adverse reactions because the provider would be unaware of potential medication interactions. Many allergy medications that formerly required a prescription are now available over the counter, and because parents use them, the nurse should be aware of the interactions and risks. The nurse does not need to question the methotrexate prescription as this medication is being added to treat the JIA.

🔑 CN: Safety and infection control; CL: Analyze

59. 4. The parent's story is consistent with the injuries incurred by the child; therefore, the nurse should document the cause of injury. There is no need to restrict the parent's visitation because the injuries sustained by the child are consistent with the explanation given. The police only need to be notified if there is suspicion of child abuse. The injuries incurred by this child appear to be accidental. There is no need to refer the parent for parenting classes. The parent appears to be upset about the accident and will not likely repeat such reckless behavior. However, the nurse should educate the parent regarding child safety.

🔑 CN: Management of care; CL: Analyze

60.

STEP 1

–/+ 1, 2, 3, 5. Neurovascular assessment after a fracture focuses on the "five P's:" pain, pulselessness, pallor, paresthesia, and paralysis. While the extremity is still pink, capillary refill is delayed, and the edema suggests venous congestion. Severe pain that did not respond to medication and an inability to move the toes are serious signs of nerve involvement. Mild nausea after surgery is not unexpected. Urinary retention is not a problem unless it persists for more than 8 hours. The vital signs are within normal limits, though increasing pulse, respiratory rate, and pain may be related to the pain.

🔑 CJ: Case study; Step 1: Recognize cues; CL: Analyze

61.

STEP 2

–/+

	Compartment Syndrome	DVT	Hypovolemic Shock
Delayed capillary refill	X	X	X
Throbbing pain	X		
Swelling	X	X	
Impaired movement	X		

Compartment syndrome, DVT, and shock all involve alterations in perfusion that can manifest as delayed (greater than 2 seconds) capillary refill. With compartment syndrome and DVT, the delayed capillary refill would most likely be present in the affected extremity, whereas with hypovolemic shock, impaired circulation would most likely be bilateral. Throbbing, unrelenting pain that is out of proportion to the injury is characteristic of the ischemic pain seen with compartment syndrome. Characteristic DVT pain is described as cramping or soreness and tends to be episodic. Impaired venous return can cause edema with both a DVT and compartment syndrome. Swelling is seldom present with hypovolemic shock. Paralysis is a characteristic finding of nerve involvement with compartment syndrome.

🔑 CJ: Case study; Step 2: Analyze cues; CL: Analyze

62.

STEP 3

0/1 *The priority intervention for this client is to* **decrease compression**. *Delayed treatment can lead to the serious complication of* **tissue necrosis**.

The client is exhibiting signs of compartment syndrome, which happens when excessive pressure builds up in an area of the body encased by bone or fascia. Injuries, including fractures, are common causes of compartment syndrome, but the problem can also be caused by treatments to treat injuries such as casting. Relieving pressure is the priority when treating compartment syndrome because the pressure impairs circulation. Compartment syndrome is a medical emergency. Untreated complications can include permanent muscle or nerve damage, tissue necrosis, and even the need for amputation. Restoring volume is the primary treatment for hypovolemic shock, which can lead to cardiac arrest. Here, increasing volume without relieving the compression is unlikely to be effective. Anticoagulant therapy is the primary treatment for DVT, which can lead to pulmonary embolism. DVT is characterized by intermittent or cramping pain; it seldom causes paralysis, and it is much more likely to occur later in the client's recovery.

🔑 CJ: Case study; Step 3: Prioritize hypothesis; CL: Analyze

63.

STEP 4

0/1

Intervention	Anticipated	Not Indicated
Splint the cast on each side	X	
Cut the undercast padding	X	
Elevate the leg above heart level		X
Insert a tissue-pressure monitoring device	X	
Administer narcotic analgesic medication	X	
Reassess in 2 hours		X

The immediate management of acute compartment syndrome (ACS) involves relieving all external pressure on the compartment. The orthopedic surgeon may bivalve the cast by splinting it lengthwise on either side. The undercast padding should also be removed. The limb should be placed at heart level, which helps edema but avoids reductions in arterial inflow that can exacerbate limb ischemia when a limb is elevated. Direct measures of compartment pressure should be obtained by the health care provider. One method involves inserting a wick catheter into the muscle compartment connected to a pressure manometer. Narcotic analgesic medication should be given to help treat the ischemic pain. The client must be monitored closely. If no improvement is seen with conservative treatment in 1 hour, surgical treatment with a fasciotomy is indicated.

 CJ: Case study; Step 4: Generate solutions; CL: Apply

64.

STEP 5

1, 2, 3, 5. When teaching a client about PCA use, the nurse should tell the client that pressing the button delivers a dose of pain medication. The pump has 4-hour dose limits and time lockouts to help prevent a client from receiving too much medication. The risk for sedation remains a possibility when giving narcotics with a PCA, but it is lower than giving larger doses of morphine via IV push. The respiratory status of clients should be monitored closely, which can be facilitated with the use of continuous pulse oximetry. If a client pushes the button and gets no relief, the nurse should be notified. There may be a problem with the IV site, the equipment, or the client status. Constipation is a common side effect of opioids regardless of the route of administration. Clients should be taught that no one should push the PCA button for them. If friends or family begin to push the button as a way of helping, the risk for oversedation increases.

CJ: Case study; Step 5: Take action; CL: Apply

65.

STEP 6

0/1 The nurse is concerned that the client is developing the complication of **muscle necrosis** based on the **urine** and **lab results**.

Muscle necrosis is one of the most common complications following a fasciotomy. Serum creatine kinase rises when muscle tissue is damaged. Muscles release myoglobin, leading to dark urine from myoglobinuria. Permanent muscle damage and severe kidney damage may follow. Swelling is expected on the second day after a fasciotomy. The slight elevation of temperature without changes in the complete blood count or wound site does not suggest the presence of infection. While the client is using the maximum pain medication on day 2, the pain is controlled, the pedal pulses are present, and the client can move the toes indicating there has been some neurovascular improvement.

CJ: Case study; Step 6: Evaluate outcomes; CL: Evaluate

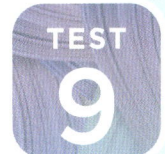

TEST 9

The Child with Dermatologic and Endocrine Health Problems

- The Client with Skin Disorders
- The Client with Burns
- The Client with a Thyroid Problem
- The Client with Insulin-Dependent Diabetes Mellitus
- Client with a Sex or Growth Hormone Problem
- Managing Care, Quality, and Safety of Children with Dermatologic and Endocrine Health Problems
- Answers, Rationales, and Test-Taking Strategies

The Client with Skin Disorders

1. A 17-year-old female client with severe nodular acne is considering treatment with isotretinoin. What does the nurse instruct the client to do prior to beginning the medication?
   - ☐ 1. Enroll in a risk management plan.
   - ☐ 2. Have proof of a mental health evaluation.
   - ☐ 3. Begin an effective form of birth control with the first dose.
   - ☐ 4. Temporarily give up sports.

2. The nurse teaches an adolescent about measures to improve facial acne. The nurse should give the client what instruction(s) about skin care? Select all that apply.
   - ☐ 1. Wash the face twice a day with mild soap and water.
   - ☐ 2. Remove whiteheads and comedones after washing the face with antibacterial soap.
   - ☐ 3. Apply vitamin E ointment twice daily to the affected skin.
   - ☐ 4. Apply tretinoin daily in the morning, and expose the face to the sun.
   - ☐ 5. Wash the hands after eating greasy foods.

3. A 9-month-old infant with eczema has lesions that are secondarily infected. Which recommendation is the **most** appropriate to help the parents best meet the needs of the child?
   - ☐ 1. Prevent siblings from being in close contact.
   - ☐ 2. Send the child to daycare as usual.
   - ☐ 3. Play video games for several hours each evening.
   - ☐ 4. Play with the child every day.

4. A school-age child brought to the clinic with several superficial sores on the front of the left leg is diagnosed with impetigo. Which instructions should the nurse give the parent?
   - ☐ 1. Wash the child's legs once a day with mild soap.
   - ☐ 2. Cover the sores with loose gauze.
   - ☐ 3. Allow the child to go back to school after 24 hours of treatment.
   - ☐ 4. Have the child return in 1 week for a follow-up examination.

5. The nurse develops a teaching plan for the parent of a toddler diagnosed with scabies. What information should the nurse expect to include?
   - ☐ 1. Disinfect all hard surfaces in the home.
   - ☐ 2. Hold the child frequently.
   - ☐ 3. Itching should cease in a few days.
   - ☐ 4. Treat the entire family.

The Client with Burns

6. A school-age child has just spilled hot liquid on their arm, and a 4-inch (10-cm) area on the forearm is severely burned. The client's parent calls the emergency department. What should the nurse advise the parent to do?
   - ☐ 1. Keep the child warm.
   - ☐ 2. Cover the burned area with an antibiotic cream.
   - ☐ 3. Apply cool water to the burned area.
   - ☐ 4. Call 911 to transport the child to the hospital.

7. A school-age child who has received burns over 60% of their body is to receive 2000 mL of intravenous fluid over the next 8 hours. At what rate (in milliliters per hour) should the nurse set the infusion pump? Round your answer to a whole number.

_____ mL per hour.

8. A school-age child with burns becomes angry and combative when it is time to change the dressings and apply mafenide acetate. Which intervention would be **most** appropriate to institute?
- ☐ 1. Ensure parental support during the dressing changes.
- ☐ 2. Allow the child to assist in removing the dressings and applying the cream.
- ☐ 3. Give the child permission to cry during the procedure.
- ☐ 4. Allow the child to schedule the time for dressing changes.

9. A school-age child with burns on the trunk and arms has no appetite. The nurse and the parent develop a plan of care to stimulate the child's appetite. Which suggestion made by the parent would indicate the need for additional teaching?
- ☐ 1. deciding that the parent will feed the child
- ☐ 2. withholding dessert and treats unless meals are eaten
- ☐ 3. offering the child finger foods that the child likes
- ☐ 4. serving smaller and more frequent meals

10. The nurse teaches the parent of a child with severe burns about the importance of specific nutritional support in burn management. The nurse recognizes the need for more teaching if the parent selects which food for their child?
- ☐ 1. bacon, lettuce, and tomato sandwich; milk; and celery and carrot sticks
- ☐ 2. cheeseburger; cottage cheese and pineapple salad; chocolate milk; and a brownie
- ☐ 3. chicken nuggets; orange and grapefruit sections; and a vanilla milkshake
- ☐ 4. beef, bean, and cheese burrito; a banana; fruit-flavored yogurt; and skim milk

11. The nurse is caring for a child with moderate burns from the waist down. Which measure should the nurse implement when positioning the child?
- ☐ 1. Place the child in a position of comfort.
- ☐ 2. Allow the child to lie on the abdomen.
- ☐ 3. Ensure the application of leg splints.
- ☐ 4. Have the child flex the hips and knees.

The Client with a Thyroid Problem

12. An adolescent is to receive radioactive iodine for Graves' disease. Which statement by the client reflects the need for more teaching?
- ☐ 1. "I plan to spend more time using social media since I have to keep several feet (meters) from my friends for 3 days."
- ☐ 2. "Taking radioactive iodine will not affect my ability to have children in the future."
- ☐ 3. "The advantage of radioactive iodine is that I will not need future medication for my disease."
- ☐ 4. "I should try to use a separate bathroom from the rest of my family for several days."

13. The nurse completes an assessment of an infant at the well-child clinic. Which clinical manifestation(s) would lead the nurse to suspect that an infant has hypothyroidism? Select all that apply.
- ☐ 1. cool extremities
- ☐ 2. increased appetite
- ☐ 3. muscle weakness
- ☐ 4. lethargy
- ☐ 5. tachycardia
- ☐ 6. bulging eyes

14. The nurse teaches the family of a child with newly diagnosed hyperthyroidism about home care. What instruction should the nurse give the family?
- ☐ 1. Keep their home warmer than usual.
- ☐ 2. Encourage plenty of outdoor activities.
- ☐ 3. Promote interactions with one friend instead of groups.
- ☐ 4. Limit bathing to prevent skin irritation.

15. A school-age child has been diagnosed with Graves' disease and is to start drug therapy. Which instruction should the nurse include in the teaching plan for the child's parent and teacher?
- ☐ 1. Continue with the same amount of schoolwork and homework.
- ☐ 2. Understand that mood swings are rare with this disorder.
- ☐ 3. Limit the amount of food that is offered to the child.
- ☐ 4. Provide the child with a calm, nonstimulating environment.

The Client with Insulin-Dependent Diabetes Mellitus

16. A student with type 1 diabetes tells the nurse they are feeling light-headed. The student's blood sugar is 60 mg/dL (3.3 mmol/L). Using the 15-15 rule, the nurse should perform which action to treat the blood glucose?
Administer:
☐ 1. 15 mL of juice, and give another 15 mL in 15 minutes.
☐ 2. 15 g of carbohydrate, and retest the blood sugar in 15 minutes.
☐ 3. 15 g of carbohydrate and 15 g of protein.
☐ 4. 15 oz of juice, and retest in 15 minutes.

17. An overweight adolescent has been diagnosed with type 2 diabetes. What should the nurse do to increase the client's self-efficacy to manage the disease?
☐ 1. Provide the client with a written daily food and exercise plan.
☐ 2. Discuss eliminating junk food in the home with the parents.
☐ 3. Arrange for the school nurse to weigh the child weekly.
☐ 4. Utilize a peer with type 2 diabetes to role model lifestyle changes.

18. After 6 months of treatment with diet and exercise, an adolescent with type 2 diabetes still has a fasting blood glucose level of 140 mg/dL (7.8 mmol/L). The health care provider has decided to begin metformin. The client asks how the medication works. The nurse should tell the client that the medicine decreases glucose production and performs which other function?
☐ 1. replaces natural insulin
☐ 2. helps the body make more insulin
☐ 3. increases insulin sensitivity
☐ 4. decreases carbohydrate adsorption

19. The nurse is evaluating a child's skills in self-administering insulin (see figure). What should the nurse do?

☐ 1. Have the child use both hands on the syringe.
☐ 2. Ask the child to place the needle at a 45-degree angle.
☐ 3. Tell the child to use a site lower on their thigh.
☐ 4. Remind the child to rotate sites.

20. An adolescent client is using glargine and lispro to manage type 1 diabetes. The nurse reviews the prescription for sliding scale lispro (see exhibit).

Lispro
Lispro subcutaneous: give units according to a sliding scale:
• Blood glucose 70 to 75 mg/dL (3.9 to 8.3 mmol/L) = 0 units
• 151 to 200 mg/dL (8.4 to 11.1 mmol/L) = 1 unit
• 201 to 250 mg/dL (11.2 to 13.9 mmol/L) = 2 units
• 251 to 300 mg/dL (13.9 to 16.7 mmol/L) = 3 units
• 301 to 350 mg/dL (17 to 19.4 mmol/L) = 4 units
• Call for a blood glucose level higher than 350 mg/dL (19.4 mmol/L)
• In addition, give 1 unit for every 15 g of carbohydrate.

The morning blood glucose level is 202 mg/dL (11.2 mmol/L), and the client is going to eat two carbohydrate exchanges. The nurse has the client administer how many units of lispro? Round your answer to a whole number

_____ units.

21. A nurse is teaching a school-age child with diabetes and their parents about managing diabetes during illness. The nurse determines that the parents understand the instruction when they indicate that they will make which treatment plan modification on days when the child is ill?
☐ 1. holding all carbohydrate-containing foods
☐ 2. increasing the frequency of blood glucose monitoring
☐ 3. decreasing the sliding scale insulin
☐ 4. monitoring morning ketone levels

22. The nurse talks to an adolescent about how they can tell their friends about their new diagnosis of diabetes. Which behavior by the adolescent indicates that the adolescent has responded positively to the discussion?
☐ 1. The client asks the nurse for material on diabetes for a school paper.
☐ 2. The client introduces the nurse to their friends as "the one who taught me all about my diabetes."
☐ 3. The client says, "I will try to tell my friends, but they will probably quit hanging out with me."
☐ 4. The client asks their friends what they think about someone who has a lifelong illness.

23. An adolescent with insulin-dependent diabetes is being taught the importance of rotating the sites of insulin injections. The nurse should judge that the teaching was successful when the adolescent identifies which complication that can result from using the same site?
☐ 1. destruction of the fat tissue and poor absorption
☐ 2. damage to nerves and painful neuritis
☐ 3. thickening of the subcutis and too-rapid insulin uptake
☐ 4. development of resistance to insulin and need for increased amounts

24. STEP 1

A 9-year-old child with a history of type 1 diabetes is brought to the school nurse's office by the gym teacher.

Nurse's Notes

0900:
The client was playing basketball when the teacher noted that the client became sweaty and confused. The client was out of school yesterday for flulike symptoms but came to school today because they were afebrile. The client has a 3-year history of type 1 diabetes that they manage with two planned injections a day of premixed 30% regular and 70% NPH, which they took this morning at 0600. The client takes additional regular insulin as needed. The client's blood glucose ran high yesterday while they were sick, and they needed two extra doses of regular insulin. The client's morning blood glucose was 120 mg/dL (6.7 mmol/L) before breakfast.

➤ Which three findings are **most** significant?

☐ 1. Diaphoresis
☐ 2. Increased regular insulin use yesterday
☐ 3. Morning blood glucose
☐ 4. Regular insulin today
☐ 5. NPH insulin today
☐ 6. Recent illness
☐ 7. Confusion

25. STEP 2

A 9-year-old child with a history of type 1 diabetes is brought to the school nurse's office by the gym teacher.

Nurse's Notes

0900:
The client was playing basketball when the teacher noted that the client became sweaty and confused. The client was out of school yesterday for flulike symptoms but came to school today because they were afebrile. The client has a 3-year history of type 1 diabetes that they manage with two planned injections a day of premixed 30% regular and 70% NPH, which they took this morning at 0600. The client takes additional regular insulin as needed. The client's blood glucose ran high yesterday while they were sick, and they needed two extra doses of regular insulin. The client's morning blood glucose was 120 mg/dL (6.7 mmol/L) before breakfast.

➤ For each possible finding below, indicate if the finding is consistent with the condition of hypoglycemia, hyperglycemia, or dehydration. Each finding may support more than one condition.

Assessment Findings	Hypoglycemia	Hyperglycemia	Dehydration
Diaphoresis	☐	☐	☐
Tachycardia	☐	☐	☐
Confusion	☐	☐	☐

Note: Each column must have at least one response option selected.

26. STEP 3

A 9-year-old child with a history of type 1 diabetes is brought to the school nurse's office by the gym teacher.

Nurse's Notes

0900:
The client was playing basketball when the teacher noted that the client became sweaty and confused. The client was out of school yesterday for flulike symptoms but came to school today because they were afebrile. The client has a 3-year history of type 1 diabetes that they manage with two planned injections a day of premixed 30% regular and 70% NPH, which they took this morning at 0600. The client takes additional regular insulin as needed. The client's blood glucose ran high yesterday while they were sick, and they needed two extra doses of regular insulin. The client's morning blood glucose was 120 mg/dL (6.7 mmol/L) before breakfast.

➤ Complete the following sentence by using the list of options.

The client is most likely demonstrating symptoms of [hypoglycemia. / hyperglycemia. / dehydration.]

Left untreated, the child is most at risk for developing the serious complication of [seizure. / cardiac arrest. / shock.]

27. STEP 4

A 9-year-old child with a history of type 1 diabetes is brought to the school nurse's office by the gym teacher.

Nurse's Notes

0900:
The client was playing basketball when the teacher noted that the client became sweaty and confused. The client was out of school yesterday for flulike symptoms but came to school today because they were afebrile. The client has a 3-year history of type 1 diabetes that they manage with two planned injections a day of premixed 30% regular and 70% NPH, which they took this morning at 0600. The client takes additional regular insulin as needed. The client's blood glucose ran high yesterday while they were sick, and they needed two extra doses of regular insulin. The client's morning blood glucose was 120 mg/dL (6.7 mmol/L) before breakfast.

0910:
The client's blood glucose level is 65 mg/dL (3.6 mmol/L).

The nurse obtains a blood glucose level and implements the emergency management plan for mild to moderate hypoglycemia.

➤ For each possible intervention, identify whether the intervention is essential or nonessential.

Possible Interventions	Essential	Nonessential
Activate the emergency medical response system.	○	○
Check the client's blood pressure.	○	○
Give 15 g of quick-acting glucose.	○	○
Recheck the blood glucose level 15 minutes after treatment.	○	○
Call the parents.	○	○
Observe the client in the nurse's office for 4 hours.	○	○

28. STEP 5

A 9-year-old child with a history of type 1 diabetes is brought to the school nurse's office by the gym teacher.

Nurse's Notes

0900:
The client was playing basketball when the teacher noted that the client became sweaty and confused. The client was out of school yesterday for flulike symptoms but came to school today because they were afebrile. The client has a 3-year history of type 1 diabetes that they manage with two planned injections a day of premixed 30% regular and 70% NPH, which they took this morning at 0600. The client takes additional regular insulin as needed. The client's blood glucose ran high yesterday while they were sick, and they needed two extra doses of regular insulin. The client's morning blood glucose was 120 mg/dL (6.7 mmol/L) before breakfast.

0910:
The client's blood glucose level is 65 mg/dL (3.6 mmol/L).

The nurse prepares to give the client a simple fast-acting carbohydrate.

➤ Which option(s) would be appropriate to give the client? Select all that apply.

- ☐ 1. 0.5 L of regular soda
- ☐ 2. 15 mL of honey
- ☐ 3. 150 mL of fruit juice
- ☐ 4. 240 mL of low-fat milk
- ☐ 5. 4 glucose tablets
- ☐ 6. 125-g (full-size) chocolate candy bar

29. STEP 6

A 9-year-old child with a history of type 1 diabetes is brought to the school nurse's office by the gym teacher.

Nurse's Notes

0900:
The client was playing basketball when the teacher noted that the client became sweaty and confused. The client was out of school yesterday for flulike symptoms but came to school today because they were afebrile. The client has a 3-year history of type 1 diabetes that they manage with two planned injections a day of premixed 30% regular and 70% NPH, which they took this morning at 0600. The client takes additional regular insulin as needed. The client's blood glucose ran high yesterday while they were sick, and they needed two extra doses of regular insulin. The client's morning blood glucose was 120 mg/dL (6.7 mmol/L) before breakfast.

0910:
The client's blood glucose level is 65 mg/dL (3.6 mmol/L).

0925:
The client's blood glucose level is 65 mg/dL (3.6 mmol/L) after drinking 150 mL of fruit juice. The client reports a headache, and their speech is slurred. The client refuses to take more fluids. Slight twitching is noted in the extremities.

➢ Which finding(s) would indicate that the client is developing severe hypoglycemia? Select all that apply.

☐ 1. Repeat blood glucose level of 65 mg/dL (3.6 mmol/L)
☐ 2. Refusal to eat or drink
☐ 3. Development of a headache
☐ 4. Slurred speech
☐ 5. Twitching movements

The Client with a Sex or Growth Hormone Problem

30. An adolescent has been diagnosed with polycystic ovarian syndrome (PCOS). Which statement by the adolescent indicates the need for more teaching?
☐ 1. "High levels of male hormones contribute to my PCOS."
☐ 2. "I am at risk for type 2 diabetes."
☐ 3. "Maintaining a healthy weight is an important part of my treatment plan."
☐ 4. "Untreated PCOS will make getting pregnant impossible."

31. An adolescent female client suspects that they might have polycystic ovarian syndrome (PCOS). Which symptom(s) would be consistent with PCOS? Select all that apply.
☐ 1. primary amenorrhea
☐ 2. obesity
☐ 3. increased body hair
☐ 4. acne
☐ 5. darkened skin in body fold
☐ 6. enlarged breast

32. An adolescent client with polycystic ovarian syndrome (PCOS) has been placed on metformin. The nurse determines the client needs more teaching about metformin if they state the medication helps achieve which outcome?
☐ 1. reduced androgen levels
☐ 2. normalization of the menstrual cycle
☐ 3. increased insulin levels
☐ 4. reduced blood glucose levels

33. The nurse reviews the stature for age growth chart (see exhibit) on a 12-year-old female client. The child is not showing the development of secondary sexual characteristics and has not started their menses. What hypothesis does the nurse make about the assessment data?

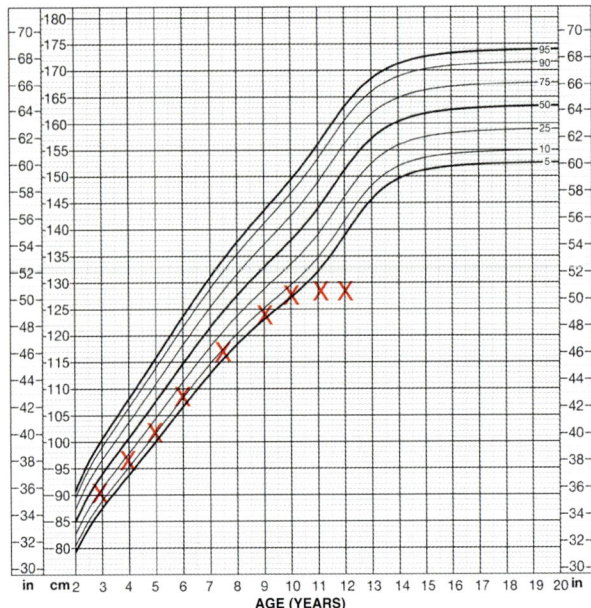

   ☐ 1. The client is experiencing delayed puberty.
   ☐ 2. A referral is needed to rule out Turner's syndrome.
   ☐ 3. The client should be evaluated for Klinefelter's syndrome.
   ☐ 4. The growth pattern is typical just prior to puberty.

34. The interdisciplinary plan of care for a 6-year-old female client with Turners syndrome includes beginning treatment with the recombinant growth hormone (GH) somatropin. What information does the nurse teach the family about somatropin?
   ☐ 1. Injections are best given early in the morning when hormone levels peak.
   ☐ 2. Radiographs are needed before beginning therapy.
   ☐ 3. Supplemental glucocorticoid therapy will help build lean muscle mass.
   ☐ 4. Treatment begins with weekly injections until a therapeutic response is seen.

35. An adolescent female with Turner's syndrome tells the nurse, "I do better with family activities. I just don't fit in with the other girls." Which intervention is **most** needed?
   ☐ 1. Encourage establishing friendships with girls of their own age.
   ☐ 2. Praise the client for establishing trusting relationships with their family.
   ☐ 3. Provide more information on treatment options for Turner's syndrome.
   ☐ 4. Suggest the client join a Turner's syndrome support group.

36. The nurse conducts a well-child visit on a 7-year-old female client with a body mass index (BMI) for age at the 99th percentile. Which finding(s) would suggest that the child may have signs or symptoms of precocious puberty? Select all that apply.
   ☐ 1. Development of breast buds
   ☐ 2. Presence of underarm hair
   ☐ 3. Growing 2.5 inches (6.35 cm) in 1 year
   ☐ 4. Mild facial acne
   ☐ 5. Adult body odor

Managing Care, Quality, and Safety of Children with Dermatologic and Endocrine Health Problems

37. The parent of a 17-year-old client who is hospitalized for complications related to type 1 diabetes requests to review the adolescent's medical record. The client reported receiving mental health counseling during their admission history but did not want their parent to know. The nurse is uncertain of how to protect the adolescent's privacy and accommodate the parent's request. Who is the **most** appropriate person to consult?
   ☐ 1. unit nurse manager
   ☐ 2. health care provider (HCP)
   ☐ 3. organization's privacy officer
   ☐ 4. customer service representative

38. The charge nurse on the pediatric floor has assigned a 6-year-old girl with newly diagnosed type 1 diabetes and an 8-year-old girl recovering from ketoacidosis to the same semiprivate room. The 6-year-old's birth parent is upset because the parent staying with the other child is male, and the girl's parent believes the arrangement violates their social norms. What should the nurse do?
   ☐ 1. Explain to the parents that this room arrangement facilitates teaching.
   ☐ 2. Reassign the children to different rooms.
   ☐ 3. Offer the parent another place to sleep.
   ☐ 4. Refer the parent to the customer service representative.

39. A school-age client with type 1 diabetes is sick with the flu. What information should the nurse convey to the parent of the child regarding diabetes management during illness? Select all that apply.
  ☐ 1. Blood glucose needs to be checked more frequently during illness.
  ☐ 2. Children require less insulin when they are sick with the flu.
  ☐ 3. Urine ketones should be checked if the blood glucose is elevated.
  ☐ 4. The intake of fluids high in carbohydrates should be increased to prevent diarrhea.
  ☐ 5. The health care provider should be called if the child cannot think clearly.

40. The nurse manages the care of a pediatric client admitted to the emergency department with severe diabetic ketoacidosis (DKA). Which nursing intervention should be done **first**?
  ☐ 1. Begin an insulin drip to lower the client's blood glucose level.
  ☐ 2. Correct any fluid deficit using an isotonic saline solution.
  ☐ 3. Draw a blood glucose level and a serum electrolyte panel.
  ☐ 4. Secure the client's airway to ensure adequate ventilation.

41. The parent of a school-age client with diabetes tells the nurse that they do not want the school to know about their child's condition. Which is the nurse's **best** response?
  ☐ 1. "Our office will not discuss your child's diabetes with the school without your written permission."
  ☐ 2. "What is it that concerns you about having the school know about your child's condition?"
  ☐ 3. "It would be fine not to tell your child's friends, but the teacher must know."
  ☐ 4. "To keep your child safe, it is necessary for all adults in the school to know about the condition."

42. The nurse reviews the plan of care of an adolescent client with diabetes using an insulin pump. This is the second visit that the client has come without their parent. The client's hemoglobin A1C and blood glucose levels are normal. The client reports that they are playing a sport and they have not had any hypoglycemic episodes. Which factor does the nurse determine is the **best** indicator that the client is transitioning to independent self-management?
  ☐ 1. managing an insulin pump
  ☐ 2. attending health care appointments alone
  ☐ 3. having normal hemoglobin A1C and blood glucose levels
  ☐ 4. playing sports without hypoglycemic episodes

Answers, Rationales, and Test-Taking Strategies

*The answers and rationales for each question follow below, along with keys (🗝) to the client need (CN) and cognitive level (CL) for each question. In addition, questions that measure clinical judgment will be coded (CJ). As you check your answers, use the **Content Mastery and Test-Taking Skill Self-Analysis** worksheet (tear-out worksheet in the back of the book) to identify the reason(s) for not answering the questions correctly. For additional information about test-taking skills and strategies for answering questions, refer to pages 12–51 in Part 1 of this book.*

The Client with Skin Disorders

1. 1. Because of the risk for birth defects with isotretinoin, risk management plans require all clients to meet certain requirements to obtain the medication. Providers are advised to closely monitor clients for signs of depression, but a mental health evaluation is not universally required. It is not sufficient to begin a single form of an effective method of birth control with the first dose of the medication. Women of childbearing age must use two forms of effective birth control for 1 month before, during, and 1 month after taking the drug. Isotretinoin may cause muscle aches, and extreme exercise should be avoided, but general participation in sports should be considered on an individual basis.

🗝 CN: Safety and infection control; CL: Analyze

2. -/+ 1, 5. Washing the face once or twice a day with a mild soap removes fatty acids from the skin. Acne is an inflammation of the sebaceous glands that produce sebum. Washing the face with mild soap and water keeps the sebaceous glands from becoming plugged. While dietary intake of greasy foods is not associated with increased acne, touching the face after eating greasy foods can add additional oil to the skin. Excessive washing or squeezing the eruptions can cause rupture of these glands, spreading the sebum and causing further inflammation. Applying vitamin E to the lesions does not reduce the inflammation and, due to the greasiness of the preparation, may plug the ducts. Isotretinoin should be applied at night. Exposure to the sun can result in sunburn and an increased risk for skin cancer and should be avoided. Sunscreen with a sun protection factor of at least 15 must be applied before the client can be exposed to the sun.

🗝 CN: Physiological adaptation; CL: Analyze

3. **4.** The parents can best meet the needs of their 9-month-old infant by playing with the child every day. All infants need time with their parents to develop trust and thus attain optimal development. The parents of a child with a chronic problem may need more guidance to meet the child's needs because of the focus on medical problems. The child's lesions are secondarily infected and therefore should not be contagious. Siblings do not need to stay away. Even with lesions that are infected, the child can still attend daycare, but the child needs attention from the parents as well. Playing video games for several hours is not appropriate for a 9-month-old infant.

   🗝 CN: Health promotion and maintenance; CL: Analyze

4. **3.** Impetigo involving several superficial lesions is usually treated topically, including washing the affected areas, removing crusts, and applying antibiotic ointment several times a day. The child can return to daycare or school after being treated for 24 hours. The lesions do not need to be covered, and they can remain open to the air. There is no need for follow-up unless the lesions have not resolved or have become more severe.

   🗝 CN: Physiological adaptation; CL: Analyze

5. **4.** Scabies is caused by the scabies mite, *Sarcoptes scabiei*. The mite burrows into the stratum corneum of the epidermis, where the female deposits eggs and fecal material. These burrows are linear. Scabies is highly contagious. The length of time from infestation to physical symptoms is 30 to 60 days, so everyone in close contact with the child will need to be treated. The bed linens and the child's clothing should be washed in hot water and dried on the hot setting. Disinfect all hard surfaces to prevent the spread of scabies. The child should be held minimally until treatment is completed. Family members should wash their hands after contact with the child. Itching lasts for 2 to 3 weeks until the stratum corneum is replaced.

   🗝 CN: Safety and infection control; CL: Apply

The Client with Burns

6. **3.** To prevent further injury to the skin, the parent should apply cool water to the burn site. Doing so causes vasoconstriction, retards further damage to tissues, and decreases fluid loss. Keeping the child warm promotes vasodilation, increases fluid loss, and decreases blood pressure and, thus, circulation to the area. Applying ointment to the burn is contraindicated because it does not allow healing to occur and may need to be removed in the hospital. Only a clean cloth should be used to cover the wound to prevent contamination or decrease pain or chilling. If only the arm is burned, a call to 911 for emergency care is not necessary, but the parent should seek health care services immediately.

   🗝 CN: Health promotion and maintenance; CL: Analyze

7. 250 mL per hour

   $$2{,}000 \text{ mL} \div 8\text{h} = 250 \text{ mL/h}$$

   🗝 CN: Pharmacological and parenteral therapies; CL: Apply

8. **2.** Expressions of anger and combativeness are often the result of loss of control and a feeling of powerlessness. Some control over the situation is regained by allowing the child to participate in care. Although having parental support during the dressing changes may be helpful, this action does nothing to allow the child control. Giving the child permission to cry may help with verbalizing feelings, but doing so does nothing to provide the child with control over the situation. Although allowing the child to determine the time for dressing changes may provide a sense of control over the situation, doing so is inappropriate because the dressing changes need to be performed as prescribed to ensure effectiveness and healing.

   🗝 CN: Physiological adaptation; CL: Analyze

9. **2.** Withholding certain foods until the child complies is punitive and rarely successful. Allowing the parent to feed the child, serving smaller and more frequent meals, and offering finger foods are all acceptable interventions for a 5-year-old child. This is true whether the child is well or ill.

   🗝 CN: Basic care and comfort; CL: Evaluate

10. **1.** Hypoproteinemia is common after severe burns. The child's diet should be high in protein to compensate for protein loss and to promote tissue healing. The child will also require a diet that is high in calories and rich in iron. The menu of bacon, lettuce, and tomato sandwich; milk; and celery sticks is lacking in sufficient protein and calories.

    🗝 CN: Physiological adaptation; CL: Evaluate

11. **3.** A child with moderate burns is at high risk for contractures. A position of comfort would encourage contracture formation. Therefore, splints need to be applied to maintain proper positioning and joint function, thereby preventing contractures and loss of function. Allowing the

child to lie on the abdomen or with the hips and knees flexed often encourages contracture formation.

🗝️ CN: Reduction of risk potential; CL: Analyze

The Client with a Thyroid Problem

12. 3. Most clients will need lifelong thyroid replacement after treatments with radioactive iodine. Most clients are treated as outpatients. To reduce the risk for exposure to radioactivity to others, clients are advised to avoid public places for at least 1 day and maintain a prudent distance from others for 2 to 3 days. Additionally, clients are advised to avoid close contact with pregnant women and children for 5 to 11 days. The use of radioiodine to treat Graves' disease has not been found to affect long-term fertility. Clients are taught not to share food, utensils, and towels. Use of a private bathroom is desirable. Clients are also instructed to flush the toilet more than one time after each use.

🗝️ CN: Safety and infection control; CL: Evaluate

13. -/+ 1, 2, 3, 4. Hypothyroidism is a disorder in which the levels of active thyroid hormone are decreased. Clinical manifestations include cool extremities, mottling, lethargy, constipation, muscle weakness, and a hoarse cry. Hyperthyroidism occurs when thyroid hormone levels are increased. Clinical manifestations include increased appetite, goiter, irritability, prominent eyes, and tachycardia.

🗝️ CN: Physiological adaptation; CL: Analyze

14. 3. Children with hyperthyroidism experience emotional lability that may strain interpersonal relationships. Focusing on one friend is easier than adapting to group dynamics until the child's condition improves. Because of their high metabolic rate, children with hyperthyroidism feel too warm. Bright sunshine may be irritating because of disease-related ophthalmopathy. Sweating is common, and bathing should be encouraged.

🗝️ CN: Physiological adaptation; CL: Analyze

15. 4. Because it takes approximately 2 weeks before the response to drug treatment occurs, much of the child's care focuses on managing the child's physical symptoms. Signs and symptoms of the disorder include an inability to sit still or concentrate, increased appetite with weight loss, emotional lability, and fatigue. Nursing care is directed toward ensuring that the parent and teacher know how to handle the child and suggesting a shortened school day, a nonstimulating environment, and decreased stress and workload. The child should be encouraged to eat a well-balanced diet.

🗝️ CN: Physiological adaptation; CL: Apply

The Client with Insulin-Dependent Diabetes Mellitus

16. 2. The 15-15 rule is a general guideline for treating hypoglycemia where the client consumes 15 g of carbohydrate and repeats testing the blood sugar in 15 minutes. Fifteen grams of carbohydrate equals 60 calories and is roughly equal to ½ cup (120 mL) of juice or soda, six to eight Life Savers, or a tablespoon of honey or sugar. The general recommendation is if the blood sugar is still low, the client may repeat the sequence. Fifteen milliliters of juice would only provide 8 calories. This would not be sufficient carbohydrates to treat the hypoglycemia. Protein does not treat insulin-related hypoglycemia; however, a protein-starch snack may be offered after the blood glucose improves. Fifteen ounces of juice would be approximately 440 mL—almost four times the recommended 4 oz (120 mL) of juice.

🗝️ CN: Physiological adaptation; CL: Analyze

17. 4. Self-efficacy, or the belief that one can act in a way to produce a desired outcome, can be promoted through the observation of role models. Peers are particularly effective role models because clients can more readily identify with them and believe they are capable of similar behaviors. Providing a written plan alone does not promote self-efficacy. Having parents eliminate junk food and having the school nurse weigh the adolescent can be part of the plan, but these actions do not empower the client.

🗝️ CN: Management of care; CL: Analyze

18. 3. Metformin is currently approved by the Food and Drug Administration and Health Canada to treat type 2 diabetes in children. The medication decreases glucogenesis in the liver and increases insulin sensitivity in the peripheral tissues. Only insulin can actually replace insulin. This treatment is reserved for clients with type 1 diabetes or those with type 2 who do not respond to diet, exercise, and an oral diabetic agent. Other oral medications used to treat diabetes augment insulin production or decrease carbohydrate absorption, but those medications are primarily used in adults.

🗝️ CN: Pharmacological and parenteral therapies; CL: Apply

19. 4. The child is using the correct injection technique, and the nurse can remind the child to rotate sites. The nurse should also reinforce that the child has used the correct technique and praise the child for doing so. If the child can manipulate the plunger of the syringe with one hand, this is appropriate. Insulin is administered at a 90-degree angle as shown. The child should identify appropriate sites on the thighs as one handbreadth below the hip and above the knee; the child is using appropriate sites.

CN: Health promotion and maintenance; CL: Apply

20. Four units. Each carbohydrate food exchange has 15 g of carbohydrate. Two units are needed to cover the current blood glucose, and 2 units are needed to cover the anticipated carbohydrate intake.

CN: Pharmacological and parenteral therapies; CL: Apply

21. 2. During an illness, cells become more insulin resistant, increasing the risk for hyperglycemia. Clients are advised to check their blood glucose more frequently, as often as every 2 to 3 hours. Clients should continue to take their insulin and are likely to need more during illness to achieve a normal blood glucose level. Simple carbohydrates are often the nutrient source best tolerated if nausea is present, and clients must consume sufficient amounts of carbohydrates to prevent burning fat. Clients are advised that they should check blood or urine ketones every 4 hours to ensure they are not developing ketoacidosis.

CN: Physiological adaptation; CL: Evaluate

22. 2. The ability to talk about their diabetes indicates that the adolescent feels good enough about themself to share their problem with their peers. Asking for reference material does not specifically indicate that the client's self-esteem has improved or that they have accepted their diagnosis. Saying that their friends will probably desert them if the client tells them about the illness indicates that the adolescent still needs to work on their self-esteem and their feelings about the disease. Asking friends what they think of someone with a lifelong illness would not indicate that the nurse's interventions targeted toward improving self-esteem have been successful. Rather, this statement demonstrates the adolescent's uncertainty about themself.

CN: Psychosocial integrity; CL: Evaluate

23. 1. Repeated use of the same injection site can result in atrophy of the fat in the subcutaneous tissue and lead to poor insulin absorption. The neuritis that develops from diabetes is related to microvascular changes that occur. Subcutaneous tissue may thicken and harden, but this leads to decreased, not rapid, insulin absorption. Resistance to insulin is caused by an immune response to the insulin protein.

CN: Pharmacological and parenteral therapies; CL: Evaluate

24.

STEP 1

–/+ **1, 4, 7.** The most significant findings are the sudden development of diaphoresis and confusion while engaging in exercise and the use of regular insulin that peaks 2 to 3 hours after injection. The timing of the symptoms coincides with the peaks of regular insulin taken this morning but would not be associated with regular insulin taken the day before. An insulin reaction from the intermediate-acting NPH would not be expected until 4 to 12 hours after injection. Children typically need increased insulin when they are ill, but this morning's blood glucose was normal.

CJ: Case study; Step 1: Recognize cues; CL: Analyze

25.

STEP 2

Assessment Findings	Hypoglycemia	Hyperglycemia	Dehydration
Diaphoresis	X		
Tachycardia	X	X	X
Confusion	X	X	X

Diaphoresis is a unique symptom of hypoglycemia. The skin is dry with hyperglycemia, which can lead to dehydration. All problems can cause tachycardia and confusion. Confusion from hypoglycemia is most related to brain deprivation of glucose that comes on rapidly. Confusion from hyperglycemia tends to come on more slowly and is complicated by perfusion problems that are associated with dehydration.

CJ: Case study; Step 2: Analyze cues; CL: Analyze

26.

STEP 3

0/1 The client is most likely demonstrating symptoms of **hypoglycemia**. Left untreated, the child is most at risk for developing the serious complication of **seizure**.

Regular insulin peaks 2 to 4 hours after injection, and the symptoms came on suddenly during exercise, suggesting the child is most likely experiencing hypoglycemia. Untreated neurologic symptoms will worsen, leading to unconsciousness, seizure, and coma. Hyperglycemia comes on more slowly. Untreated hyperglycemia can lead to ketoacidosis and life-threatening dehydration.

CJ: Case study; Step 3: Prioritize hypothesis; CL: Analyze

27.

STEP 4

0/1

Possible Interventions	Essential	Nonessential
Activate the emergency medical response system.		X
Obtain the client's blood pressure.		X
Give 15 g of quick-acting glucose.	X	
Recheck the blood glucose level 15 minutes after treatment.	X	
Call the parents.	X	
Observe the client in the nurse's office for 4 hours.		X

Checking the blood glucose level is essential to determine the severity of the hypoglycemia, which may in turn guide treatment. The 15-15 rule is used to guide treatment in clients with hypoglycemia who are conscious. The rule involves oral intake of approximately 15 g of carbohydrate followed by rechecking the glucose in 15 minutes. The nurse should take emergency actions to treat the hypoglycemia and notify parents of any emergency action taken at the earliest possible convenience. Students with diabetes should have an emergency management plan. Activating the emergency medical response system is not necessary if the client responds to treatment. Hemodynamic changes associated with hypoglycemia may cause shifts in blood pressure, but while the client is still alert, there is no clear need to check the client's blood pressure. The client can be observed for an hour and be encouraged to eat a snack or meal. If the blood glucose remains stable, they should be allowed to return to class.

🔑 CJ: Case study; Step 4: Generate solutions; CL: Apply

28.

STEP 5

−/+ 2, 3, 4, 5. To treat hypoglycemia in a client able to safely intake oral sources, the nurse gives a quick-acting glucose product equal to 1 carbohydrate exchange (12 to 15 g of carbohydrate) or the amount specified in the emergency care plan. Food options that equal 1 carbohydrate exchange include: 15 mL of honey, 120 to 180 mL of juice, and 240 mL of low-fat milk. Four glucose tablets also provide 12 to 15 g of glucose. A full-size candy bar and 0.5 L of soda are not ideal because each has substantially more than 15 g of carbohydrate and can lead to overcorrection and too high blood sugar.

🔑 CJ: Case study; Step 5: Take action; CL: Apply

29.

STEP 6

−/+ 2, 4, 5. Refusal to eat or drink, slurred speech, and twitching movements are symptoms of severe hypoglycemia. At this point in treatment, the child needs immediate treatment with glucagon and advanced medical care. The nurse administers the glucagon if available and stays with the client while having someone else call emergency medical services. If the client's blood glucose does not rise after the first treatment with 15 g of glucose, treatment may be repeated if the client's status has not changed. The development of a headache is common even with mild to moderate hypoglycemia.

🔑 CJ: Case study; Step 6: Evaluate outcomes; CL: Evaluate

The Client with a Sex or Growth Hormone Problem

30. 4. While pregnancy may be difficult for some clients, the nurse must work to prevent the false conception that a sexually active teen with PCOS does not need to use a reliable form of birth control. PCOS is associated with high levels of androgens and excessive insulin. It is the excess insulin that is thought to increase androgen production. Clients with PCOS are at risk for type 2 diabetes. Initial treatment focuses on weight management and exercise. These measures often reduce insulin production and restore normal menstrual cycles.

🔑 CN: Physiologic adaptation; CL: Evaluate

31. −/+ 2, 3, 4, 5. PCOS is associated with obesity, increased body or facial hair (hirsutism), acne, and darkening of the skin usually in body folds (acanthosis nigricans). When a female has never had a menstrual cycle, it is referred to as *primary amenorrhea*. PCOS is associated with irregular menstrual cycles, secondary amenorrhea, or both, not primary amenorrhea. High androgen levels frequently lead to decreased versus enlarged breast size.

🔑 CN: Physiologic adaptation; CL: Analyze

32. 3. Metformin works by decreasing the production of glucose in the liver and improving insulin sensitivity. These two mechanisms reduce insulin and blood glucose level. Reducing insulin levels reduces androgens and helps restore menstruation.

🔑 CN: Pharmacology and parental therapies; CL: Evaluate

33. 2. Growth in girls continues through puberty and does not stop until 2 years after menses begins. Arrested growth without signs of secondary sexual characteristics is consistent with the genetic disorder Turner's syndrome, which is characterized by short stature and nonfunctioning ovaries. Once diagnosed, treatment involves estrogen therapy and possibly growth hormone. Klinefelter's syndrome is a genetic disorder that occurs when a boy is born with an extra copy of the X chromosome. The diagnosis of delayed puberty is not made until a female does not have breasts by the age of 13 or does not begin menses by the age of 16.

🔑 CN: Health Promotion and Maintenance; CL: Apply

34. 2. Radiographs of the wrist and hips are done to determine bone age before beginning GH therapy. Bone x-rays are recommended at least annually thereafter during treatment. GH treatment typically ends when the child achieves a bone age of 14 years. Injections are best given at night when GH naturally peaks. Glucocorticoid steroids may interfere with GH. Therefore, parents need to be advised to tell all health care providers their child is on GH. To be most effective, injections are needed at least 2 to 3 times a week. In some cases, GH may be given daily.

🔑 CN Pharmacological and parental therapies; CL: Apply

35. 1. Adolescents with Turner's syndrome often display immature behaviors and are at risk for anxiety, depression, and social withdrawal. They tend to begin dating at a later age than other girls, which can make them feel more left out in a gathering of peers. The nurse can best support the development of long-term social functioning by encouraging clients with Turner's syndrome to establish healthy friendships with other children the same age and participate in age-appropriate social activities. Praising how the client has established family relationships does not help the client with the next level of developmental tasks and preparation for independence. The client is not demonstrating a knowledge deficit to suggest more treatment information is needed. Clients with Turner's syndrome may benefit from a support group, but these groups would not be as effective in promoting normal social development as interacting with other peers.

🔑 CN: Health Promotion and Maintenance; CL: Apply

36. -/+ 1, 2, 4, 5. When puberty begins before age 8 in girls and before age 9 in boys, it is considered precocious puberty. Being obese increases the risk for developing precocious puberty. Other possible causes include tumors, brain injuries, or hormonal disorders. Breast development in girls is typically one of the first signs of puberty and normally begins between 8 and 11. Underarm hair, acne, and adult body odor all signal the beginning of puberty. Growing 2 to 2.5 inches (5.08 to 6.35 cm) in a year is a typical growth pattern for a school-age child.

🔑 CN: Health Promotion and Maintenance; CL: Analyze

Managing Care, Quality, and Safety of Children with Dermatologic and Endocrine Health Problems

37. 3. Confidentiality legislation specifies that institutions designate a "privacy officer" who is responsible for developing and implementing privacy policies. This would be the very best resource for the nurse to contact. Depending on the nurse manager's experience, they may or may not know the answer and may have to consult the privacy officer. While HCPs would have an understanding of confidentiality laws, it is unlikely they understand the specifics of nursing policies. Customer service representatives typically address client concerns. At this time, the family has not voiced a concern.

🔑 CN: Management of care; CL: Apply

38. 2. Sleeping in the same room with a person of the opposite sex may be viewed as a violation of norms by persons of conservative faiths. If at all possible, the charge nurse should reassign the family to a different room. While it makes sense to have two clients with similar educational needs in the same room, it is likely that the arrangement would be distressing enough to create a learning barrier. Offering the parent another place to sleep deprives the child of their parent at night. The customer service representative would only need to be involved if it became impossible to accommodate the parent's needs.

🔑 CN: Management of care; CL: Analyze

39. -/+ 1, 3, 5. Blood sugar levels can go up during the flu; therefore, blood glucose levels should be monitored every 3 to 4 hours during flu. Because glucose levels are higher when a client has the flu, clients should continue to take diabetes medications as prescribed. If the blood sugar level is over 240 mg/dL (13.32 mmol/L), ketones should be checked. If ketones are present, the client should be encouraged to drink calorie-free fluids and eat small meals. The health care provider should be contacted if the client cannot think clearly as confusion can be a sign of diabetic ketoacidosis.

🔑 CN: Management of care; CL: Analyze

40. 4. Treating pediatric clients with severe DKA is a medical emergency; therefore, attending to the airway, breathing, and circulation is the first priority. Once the airway is secured, the health care team should estimate the level of dehydration and begin replacement fluids of normal saline. An insulin drip should be started after the initial 1 to 2 hours of treatment at a rate of 0.1 units/kg per hour. Blood glucose should be tested every 1 to 2 hours until the client is stable; then it should be tested every 6 hours. Additionally, serum electrolytes should be drawn every 1 to 2 hours until the client is stable and then every 4 to 6 hours.

🔑 CN: Management of care; CL: Analyze

41. 2. The nurse's first response should be to obtain more information about the parent's concerns. The nurse can then facilitate a dialogue that will help the parent weigh their concerns against the potential risks to the child's safety. It is true that the nurse would not discuss a client's medical condition with a school without permission, but this statement does facilitate discussion. It is also true that the child may have a diabetic reaction anywhere at school, and it is advisable that their teacher, classmates, and other adults know about their diabetes to help the client; however, it is ultimately the client and their parents who will make the decision about informing the school. Dictating to the parent does not explain any rationale for the necessity of sharing the information.

🔑 CN: Safety and infection control; CL: Analyze

42. 2. During adolescence, the responsibility for chronic disease management is shared. As clients transition to adulthood, they assume more responsibility for their care. Attending appointments alone shows that the client is developing the decision-making skills needed to interact with the health care team without parental assistance. School-age children are often able to manage an insulin pump because they have developed the logical reasoning required to follow protocols. Having normal hemoglobin A1C and blood glucose levels is positive, but the nurse does not know what role the parents may have played in the client's management. The nurse would also not know if a coach or trainer played a significant role in reminding the client to monitor glucose needs during sports.

🔑 CN: Management of care; CL: Analyze

3

The Nursing Care of Adults with Medical and Surgical Health Problems

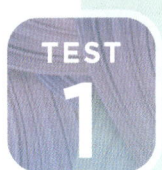

TEST 1 — The Adult with Cardiac Health Problems

- The Adult with Acute Coronary Syndromes
- The Adult with Heart Failure
- The Adult with Valvular Heart Disease
- The Adult with Hypertension
- The Adult with Atrial Fibrillation and Other Dysrhythmias
- The Adult Requiring Rapid Response or Cardiopulmonary Resuscitation
- Managing Care, Quality, and Safety for Adults with Cardiac Health Problems

The Adult with Acute Coronary Syndromes

1. A client returns from a left heart catheterization. The right groin was used for catheter access. To evaluate distal blood flow, the nurse should palpate the pulse on this client at which location?
☐ 1. anterior to the right tibia
☐ 2. dorsal surface of the right foot
☐ 3. posterior to the right knee
☐ 4. right midinguinal area

2. A client is to have a treadmill stress test. Prior to the stress test, the nurse reviews the results of the laboratory reports. The nurse should report which elevated laboratory value to the health care provider (HCP) before the stress test?
☐ 1. cholesterol level
☐ 2. erythrocyte sedimentation rate
☐ 3. prothrombin time
☐ 4. troponin level

3. A client has chest pain rated at 8 on a 10-point visual analog scale and is receiving intravenous nitroglycerin. The 12-lead electrocardiogram reveals ST elevation in the inferior leads, and troponin levels are elevated. What should the nurse do **first**?
☐ 1. Monitor urine output.
☐ 2. Limit visitors.
☐ 3. Teach the client how to manage pain.
☐ 4. Notify the health care provider.

4. A client with chest pain is prescribed intravenous nitroglycerin. Which finding is of **greatest** concern for the nurse initiating the nitroglycerin drip?
☐ 1. Serum potassium is 3.5 mEq/L (3.5 mmol/L).
☐ 2. Blood pressure is 88/46 mm Hg.
☐ 3. ST elevation is present on the electrocardiogram.
☐ 4. Heart rate is 61 bpm.

5. The nurse is caring for a client diagnosed with an anterior myocardial infarction (MI) 2 days ago. Upon assessment, the nurse identifies a systolic murmur at the apex. What should the nurse do **first**?
   - ☐ 1. Assess for changes in vital signs.
   - ☐ 2. Draw blood for an arterial blood gas test.
   - ☐ 3. Evaluate heart sounds with the client leaning forward.
   - ☐ 4. Obtain a 12-lead electrocardiogram (ECG).

6. A client with acute chest pain is receiving IV morphine sulfate. Which effect(s) of morphine would be expected? Select all that apply.
   - ☐ 1. reduces myocardial oxygen consumption
   - ☐ 2. promotes reduction in respiratory rate
   - ☐ 3. prevents ventricular remodeling
   - ☐ 4. reduces blood pressure and heart rate
   - ☐ 5. reduces anxiety and fear

7. A client is receiving an intravenous (IV) infusion of heparin sodium at 1200 units per hour. The dilution is 25,000 units per 500 mL. How many milliliters per hour will this client receive? Round your answer to a whole number.

   _____ mL per hour.

8. An older adult has chest pain and shortness of breath. The health care provider (HCP) prescribes nitroglycerin tablets. What should the nurse instruct the client to do?
   - ☐ 1. Put the tablet under the tongue until it is absorbed.
   - ☐ 2. Swallow the tablet with 120 mL of water.
   - ☐ 3. Chew the tablet until it is dissolved.
   - ☐ 4. Place the tablet between the cheek and gums until it disappears.

9. The nurse has completed an assessment of a client with a decreased cardiac output. Which findings should receive the **highest priority**?
   - ☐ 1. blood pressure of 110/62 mm Hg, atrial fibrillation with a heart rate of 82 bpm, and bilateral basilar crackles
   - ☐ 2. confusion, urine output of 15 mL over the last 2 hours, and orthopnea
   - ☐ 3. oxygen saturation measured by pulse oximetry 92% on 2 L via nasal cannula, respiration rate of 20 breaths/min, and 1+ edema of the lower extremities
   - ☐ 4. weight gain of 2.2 lb (1 kg) in 3 days, blood pressure of 130/80 mm Hg, and mild dyspnea with exercise

10. The nurse notices that a client's heart rate decreases from 63 bpm to 50 bpm on the monitor. What should the nurse do **first**?
    - ☐ 1. Administer atropine 0.5 mg via intravenous (IV) push.
    - ☐ 2. Auscultate for abnormal heart sounds.
    - ☐ 3. Prepare for transcutaneous pacing.
    - ☐ 4. Take the client's blood pressure.

11. The nurse is preparing a client for a cardiac angiogram. What action(s) should the nurse take? Select all that apply.
    - ☐ 1. Determine if the client has an allergy to liquid contrast material.
    - ☐ 2. Inform the client that an intravenous infusion will be started before the procedure.
    - ☐ 3. Remind the client to have nothing to eat or drink 8 hours before the procedure.
    - ☐ 4. Instruct the client to remain still during the procedure.
    - ☐ 5. Explain that the client will receive a fast-acting acting anesthetic.

12. An adult comes into the emergency department with crushing substernal chest pain that radiates to the shoulder and left arm. The admitting diagnosis is acute myocardial infarction. Prescriptions include oxygen by nasal cannula at 4 L per minute, a complete blood count, a chest radiograph, a 12-lead electrocardiogram (ECG), and 2 mg of morphine sulfate given intravenously. What should the nurse do **first**?
    - ☐ 1. Administer the morphine.
    - ☐ 2. Obtain a 12-lead ECG.
    - ☐ 3. Obtain the blood work.
    - ☐ 4. Order the chest radiograph.

13. An older adult had a myocardial infarction (MI) 4 days ago. At 0930, the client's blood pressure is 102/64 mm Hg. After reviewing the client's progress notes (see chart), what should the nurse do first?

Nurse's Notes	
Date	1/10
Time	0030
Urinary output for the last 4 hours	90 mL
Capillary refill	>3 seconds
Blood pressure	128/82 mm Hg
Extremities	Cool

    - ☐ 1. Give a fluid challenge/bolus.
    - ☐ 2. Notify the health care provider (HCP).
    - ☐ 3. Assist the client to walk.
    - ☐ 4. Administer furosemide as prescribed.

14. The nurse has administered a thrombolytic drug to the client who is experiencing a myocardial infarction (MI) and who has premature ventricular contractions. The nurse is evaluating the effectiveness of this drug. Which is the expected outcome of the drug?
    - ☐ 1. Promote hydration.
    - ☐ 2. Dissolve clots.
    - ☐ 3. Prevent kidney failure.
    - ☐ 4. Treat dysrhythmias.

15. The nurse is assessing a client who has had a myocardial infarction (MI). The nurse notes the cardiac rhythm on the monitor (see the electrocardiogram [ECG] strip). What should the nurse do **first**?

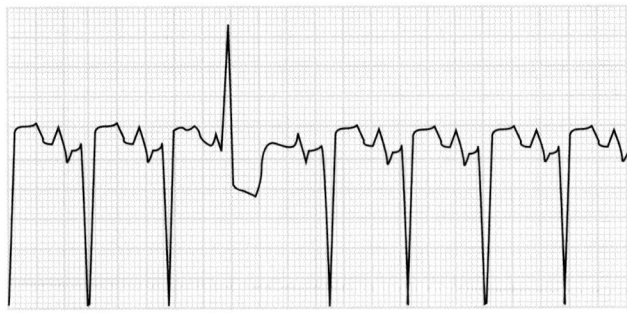

☐ 1. Notify the health care provider (HCP).
☐ 2. Call the rapid response team.
☐ 3. Assess the client for changes in the rhythm.
☐ 4. Administer lidocaine as prescribed.

16. The nurse is assessing a client who has had a stent inserted in a coronary artery via the right femoral artery. The client is receiving intravenous heparin sodium at 1000 units per hour. During the second post-procedure check, the nurse notes that the puncture site at the groin has begun to steadily ooze blood. What should the nurse do **first**?
☐ 1. Don gloves and apply direct pressure over the site.
☐ 2. Observe and document the bleeding.
☐ 3. Notify the health care provider (HCP).
☐ 4. Prepare protamine sulfate for intravenous administration.

17. A client admitted for a myocardial infarction (MI) develops cardiogenic shock. An arterial line is inserted. Which prescription from the health care provider should the nurse verify before implementing?
☐ 1. Call for urine output less than 30 mL per hour for 2 consecutive hours.
☐ 2. Administer metoprolol 5 mg via intravenous (IV) push.
☐ 3. Prepare for a pulmonary artery catheter insertion.
☐ 4. Titrate dobutamine to keep systolic blood pressure higher than 100 mm Hg.

18. The nurse is caring for a 75-year-old male admitted to the outpatient surgical center at 0845 for a hernia repair scheduled for 1030. The client has a history of myocardial infarction.

Progress Notes

Vital Signs	Time		
	0900	0915	0930
Heart rate	70 bpm	75 bpm	110 bpm
Blood pressure systolic	110 mm Hg	100 mm Hg	90 mm Hg
Blood pressure diastolic	70 mm Hg	65 mm Hg	60 mm Hg
Respiration rate	20 breaths/min	26 breaths/min	28 breaths/min
Temperature	98.6°F (37°C)	98.6°F (37°C)	
Oxygen saturation	96%	93%	91%

The nurse is reviewing the progress notes.

➢ Which information should the nurse report to the health care provider **immediately**? Select all that apply.

☐ 1. Heart rate
☐ 2. Blood pressure
☐ 3. Respiratory rate
☐ 4. Temperature
☐ 5. Oxygen saturation
☐ 6. Type of surgery scheduled
☐ 7. History of myocardial infarction
☐ 8. Time of scheduled surgery

19. The health care provider prescribes continuous intravenous (IV) nitroglycerin infusion for a client who has had a myocardial infarction. What should the nurse do to ensure the safe administration of this drug?
☐ 1. Use an infusion pump for the medication.
☐ 2. Take the blood pressure every 4 hours.
☐ 3. Monitor urine output hourly.
☐ 4. Obtain serum potassium levels daily.

20. The client is admitted to the telemetry unit because of chest pain. The client has polysubstance abuse disorder, and the nurse assesses that the client is anxious and irritable and has moist skin. What should the nurse do in order of priority from first to last? All options must be used.

| 1. Obtain a history of which drugs the client has used recently. |
| 2. Administer the prescribed dose of morphine. |
| 3. Position electrodes on the chest. |
| 4. Take vital signs. |
| |
| |
| |
| |

21. A client is scheduled for insertion of a coronary stent with right groin access. Which teaching point(s) should the nurse include in this client's preoperative teaching plan? Select all that apply.
☐ 1. "If you have a hearing aid, you will need to remove it before leaving for the procedure."
☐ 2. "If you have chest pain during this procedure, please tell the staff when or if this should occur."
☐ 3. "The stitches at your right groin will be able to be removed in 7 to 10 days after the procedure."
☐ 4. "You will be given general anesthesia and will be asleep throughout this procedure."
☐ 5. "You will need to remain flat during the procedure and for 3 to 6 hours after the procedure."
☐ 6. "You will need to keep your right leg in a flexed position for 1 to 2 hours after the procedure."

22. The nurse is assessing a client who has had a myocardial infarction. The nurse notes the cardiac rhythm shown on the electrocardiogram strip. How should the nurse interpret this rhythm strip?

☐ 1. atrial fibrillation
☐ 2. ventricular tachycardia
☐ 3. premature ventricular contractions
☐ 4. sinus tachycardia

23. While caring for a client who has sustained a myocardial infarction (MI), the nurse notes eight premature ventricular contractions (PVCs) in 1 minute on the cardiac monitor. The client is receiving an intravenous (IV) infusion of 5% dextrose in water (D_5W) at 125 mL per hour and oxygen at 2 L per minute. What should the nurse do first?
☐ 1. Increase the IV infusion rate to 150 mL per hour.
☐ 2. Notify the health care provider (HCP).
☐ 3. Increase the oxygen concentration to 4 L per minute.
☐ 4. Administer a prescribed analgesic medication.

24. The nurse is planning care for a client on the second day of hospitalization after a myocardial infarction (MI). Which is an expected outcome of care at this time?
☐ 1. The client continues to have severe chest pain.
☐ 2. The client can identify risk factors for MI.
☐ 3. The client participates in a cardiac rehabilitation walking program.
☐ 4. The client can perform personal self-care activities without pain.

25. The nurse is administering furosemide as an intravenous infusion. Which is an expected outcome?
☐ 1. increased blood pressure
☐ 2. increased urine output
☐ 3. decreased pain
☐ 4. decreased premature ventricular contractions

26. A client is hospitalized for a myocardial infarction. The nurse is teaching the client to do ankle pumps. What is the expected outcome of this exercise?
☐ 1. Prepare the client for ambulation.
☐ 2. Promote urinary and intestinal elimination.
☐ 3. Prevent thrombophlebitis and blood clot formation.
☐ 4. Decrease the likelihood of pressure ulcer formation.

27. The nurse is assisting the client during the acute phase of myocardial infarction (MI) in making a meal plan. Which is the **most** appropriate diet for this client?
    ☐ 1. liquids as desired
    ☐ 2. small, easily digested meals
    ☐ 3. three regular meals per day
    ☐ 4. nothing by mouth

28. The nurse is caring for a client who recently experienced a myocardial infarction and has been started on clopidogrel. The nurse should develop a teaching plan that includes which point(s)? Select all that apply.
    ☐ 1. to report unexpected bleeding or bleeding that lasts a long time
    ☐ 2. to take clopidogrel with food
    ☐ 3. to understand that the client may bruise more easily and may experience bleeding gums
    ☐ 4. to know that clopidogrel works by preventing platelets from sticking together and forming a clot
    ☐ 5. to drink a glass of water after taking clopidogrel

29. The nurse is assessing clients in a community outreach program. Which client is at the **greatest** risk for coronary artery disease (CAD)?
    ☐ 1. a 32-year-old woman with mitral valve prolapse who quit smoking 10 years ago
    ☐ 2. a 43-year-old man with a family history of CAD and a cholesterol level of 158 mg/dL (8.8 mmol/L)
    ☐ 3. a 56-year-old man with a high-density lipoprotein (HDL) level of 60 mg/dL (3.3 mmol/L) who takes atorvastatin
    ☐ 4. a 65-year-old woman who is obese with a low-density lipoprotein (LDL) level of 188 mg/dL (10.4 mmol/L)

30. The client has been managing angina episodes with nitroglycerin. Which finding indicates that the therapeutic effect of the drug has been achieved?
    ☐ 1. decreased chest pain
    ☐ 2. increased blood pressure
    ☐ 3. decreased blood pressure
    ☐ 4. decreased heart rate

31. The nurse is teaching a client who has had a myocardial infarction about using nitroglycerin spray. Which information should the nurse include in the teaching plan? Select all that apply.
    ☐ 1. "Spray the medication under your tongue as soon as you have chest pain."
    ☐ 2. "Swallow the medication as soon as you have sprayed it in your mouth."
    ☐ 3. "Store the medication in the refrigerator when not in use."
    ☐ 4. "Shake the medication container before using."
    ☐ 5. "If the chest pain continues after two sprays of the medication, wait 5 minutes, and use one more spray."
    ☐ 6. "Call 911 if chest pain continues after 10 minutes of using the third spray."

32. A client has risk factors for coronary artery disease, including smoking cigarettes, eating a diet high in saturated fat, and leading a sedentary lifestyle. Which coaching strategies from the nurse will be **most** effective in assisting the client to improve their health?
    ☐ 1. explaining how the risk factors lead to poor health
    ☐ 2. withholding praise until the client changes the risky behavior
    ☐ 3. helping the client establish a wellness vision to reduce the health risks
    ☐ 4. instilling mild fear into the client about the potential outcomes of the risky health behaviors

33. The nurse is evaluating a client who received tissue plasminogen activator (t-PA) following a myocardial infarction (MI). What is the expected outcome of this drug?
    ☐ 1. Control chest pain.
    ☐ 2. Reduce coronary artery vasospasm.
    ☐ 3. Control the dysrhythmia associated with MI.
    ☐ 4. Revascularize the blocked coronary artery.

34. The nurse is monitoring a client who is receiving tissue plasminogen activator (t-PA). The nurse should assess the client for which changes?
    ☐ 1. cardiac arrhythmias
    ☐ 2. hypertension
    ☐ 3. seizure
    ☐ 4. hypothermia

35. A middle-age client with a history of hypertension reports having "indigestion." The nurse connects the client to a cardiac monitor, which reveals eight premature ventricular contractions per minute. What should the nurse do **next**?
    ☐ 1. Call the health care provider (HCP).
    ☐ 2. Start an intravenous (IV) infusion.
    ☐ 3. Obtain a portable chest radiograph.
    ☐ 4. Draw blood for laboratory studies.

36. Following a diagnosis of angina pectoris, a client reports being unable to walk up two flights of stairs without pain. What should the nurse instruct the client to do?
    ☐ 1. Climb the steps early in the day.
    ☐ 2. Rest for at least an hour before climbing the stairs.
    ☐ 3. Take a nitroglycerin tablet before climbing the stairs.
    ☐ 4. Lie down after climbing the stairs.

37. A client who experiences angina has been told to follow a low-cholesterol diet. Which meal would be **best**?
    ☐ 1. hamburger, salad, and a milkshake
    ☐ 2. baked liver, green beans, and coffee
    ☐ 3. spaghetti with tomato sauce, salad, and coffee
    ☐ 4. fried chicken, green beans, and skim milk

38. The nurse is preparing the client who has unstable angina for discharge to home. Which symptom should the nurse teach the client to report **immediately** to the health care provider?
  ☐ 1. a change in the pattern of the chest pain
  ☐ 2. pain during sexual activity
  ☐ 3. pain during an argument
  ☐ 4. pain during or after a physical activity

39. The nurse is caring for a client who has just returned from having a percutaneous transluminal balloon angioplasty with femoral artery access. In which order, from first to last, should the nurse obtain information about the client? All options must be used.

1. vital signs and oxygen saturation
2. pedal pulses
3. color and sensation of extremity
4. catheterization site

40. A client has a throbbing headache when nitroglycerin is taken for angina. What should the nurse instruct the client to do?
  ☐ 1. Take acetaminophen or ibuprofen.
  ☐ 2. Limit the frequency of using nitroglycerin.
  ☐ 3. Take the nitroglycerin with a few glasses of water.
  ☐ 4. Rest in a supine position to minimize the headache.

41. The nurse is teaching a client with unstable angina to use sublingual nitroglycerin tablets when chest pain occurs. What should the nurse tell the client?
  ☐ 1. "Sit down, and then take one tablet every 2 to 5 minutes until the pain stops."
  ☐ 2. "Sit down, and then take one tablet and rest for 15 minutes. Call the health care provider (HCP) if pain persists after 15 minutes."
  ☐ 3. "Sit down, and then take one tablet; if the pain persists, take two additional tablets in 5 minutes. Call the HCP if the pain persists after 15 minutes."
  ☐ 4. "Sit down, and then take one tablet. If pain persists after 5 minutes, call 911."

42. A client with angina is taking nifedipine. What instruction should the nurse give the client?
  ☐ 1. Monitor blood pressure monthly.
  ☐ 2. Perform daily weights.
  ☐ 3. Inspect the gums daily.
  ☐ 4. Limit intake of green leafy vegetables.

43. The nurse is preparing a client who had a myocardial infarction for discharge. What instruction(s) should the nurse give the client who will be starting a prescription for simvastatin 40 mg per day? Select all that apply.
  ☐ 1. "Take once a day in the morning."
  ☐ 2. "If you miss a dose, take it when you remember it."
  ☐ 3. "Limit greens such as lettuce in the diet to prevent bleeding."
  ☐ 4. "Be sure to take the pill with food."
  ☐ 5. "Report muscle pain or tenderness to your health care provider (HCP)."
  ☐ 6. "Continue to follow a diet that is low in saturated fats."

The Adult with Heart Failure

44. The health care provider has prescribed captopril, furosemide, and metoprolol for a 78-year-old male with systolic heart failure. The client's blood pressure is 136/82 mm Hg, and the heart rate is 65 bpm. Prior to medication administration at 0900, the nurse reviews the following lab tests (see chart). What should the nurse do **first**?

Laboratory Results		
Test	Results	Normal Range
Sodium	140 mEq/L (140 mmol/L)	Adults: 135–145 mEq/L (135–145 mmol/L)
Potassium	6.8 mEq/L (6.8 mmol/L)	Adults: 3.5–5.2 mEq/L (3.5–5.2 mmol/L)
Blood urea nitrogen (BUN)	18 mg/dL (6.4 mmol/L)	8–20 mg/dL (2.9–7.5 mmol/L)
Creatinine	1.0 mg/dL (76.3 μmol/L)	Men: 0.9–1.3 mg/dL (80–115 μmol/L).
Hemoglobin	12 g/dL (120 g/L)	Men: 14–17.4 g/dL (140–174 g/L)
Hematocrit	37% (0.37)	Men: 42%–52% (0.42–0.52 proportion of 1.0)

  ☐ 1. Administer the medications.
  ☐ 2. Call the health care provider (HCP).
  ☐ 3. Withhold the captopril.
  ☐ 4. Question the metoprolol dose.

45. A client was admitted with an exacerbation of heart failure breath at 0200. At 0700, which information is **most** important for the nurse who admitted the client to communicate during the hand-off of care report to the nurse who will next take care of the client?
☐ 1. admission weight of 210 lb (95 kg)
☐ 2. elevated B-type natriuretic peptide of 600 pg/mL
☐ 3. reaching 250 mL by incentive spirometer
☐ 4. urinary output of 120 mL

46. A client with chronic heart failure has atrial fibrillation and is taking warfarin. What should the nurse tell the client about the expected outcome of this drug?
☐ 1. "This medication will decrease the extra fluid your heart is circulating."
☐ 2. "This medication will improve the work of your heart."
☐ 3. "This medication will prevent a clot from forming."
☐ 4. "This medication will regulate the rhythm of your heart."

47. A client with heart failure is taking furosemide, digoxin, and potassium chloride. The client has nausea, blurred vision, headache, and weakness. The nurse notes that the client is confused. The telemetry strip shows first-degree atrioventricular block. What other information should the nurse obtain **next**?
☐ 1. potassium levels
☐ 2. digoxin levels
☐ 3. fluid balance
☐ 4. evidence of pulmonary edema

48. The nurse is conducting a focused assessment for a client with left-sided heart failure. Which finding(s) would be concerning? Select all that apply.
☐ 1. dyspnea
☐ 2. jugular vein distention (JVD)
☐ 3. crackles
☐ 4. right upper quadrant pain
☐ 5. oliguria
☐ 6. decreased oxygen saturation levels

49. Which finding(s) would indicate that a client with a history of left-sided heart failure is developing pulmonary edema? Select all that apply.
☐ 1. distended jugular veins
☐ 2. dependent edema
☐ 3. anorexia
☐ 4. coarse crackles
☐ 5. tachycardia

50. An older adult with a history of heart failure is admitted to the emergency department with pulmonary edema. During admission, what should the nurse assess **first**?
☐ 1. blood pressure
☐ 2. skin breakdown
☐ 3. serum potassium level
☐ 4. urine output

51. The nurse is caring for an older adult with mild dementia who has been admitted with heart failure. What nursing care will be helpful for this client in reducing potential confusion related to hospitalization and change in routine? Select all that apply.
☐ 1. Reorient frequently to time, place, and situation.
☐ 2. Put the client in a quiet room furthest from the nursing station.
☐ 3. Perform necessary procedures quickly.
☐ 4. Arrange for familiar pictures or special items at the bedside.
☐ 5. Limit the client's visitors.
☐ 6. Spend time with the client, establishing a trusting relationship.

52. Furosemide 40 mg intravenous push is prescribed. Furosemide 10 mg/mL is available. How much should the nurse administer? Round your answer to a whole number.

_____ mL.

53. Which position is **best** for a client with heart failure who has orthopnea?
☐ 1. semisitting (low Fowler position) with the legs elevated on pillows
☐ 2. lying on the right side (semi-prone) with a pillow between the legs
☐ 3. sitting upright (high Fowler position) with the legs resting on the mattress
☐ 4. lying on the back with the head lowered (Trendelenburg position) and the legs elevated

54. The nurse is administering furosemide intravenously to a client with heart failure. How soon after administration should the nurse begin to see evidence of the drug's desired effect?
☐ 1. 5 to 10 minutes
☐ 2. 30 to 60 minutes
☐ 3. 2 to 4 hours
☐ 4. 6 to 8 hours

55. The nurse teaches a client with heart failure to take oral furosemide in the morning. What is the expected outcome for taking this drug in the morning? The client will:
☐ 1. avoid concentrated urine.
☐ 2. prevent the risk for falling.
☐ 3. limit the excretion of electrolytes.
☐ 4. obtain more sleep.

56. The nurse is assessing a client with a known history of chronic heart failure. Which finding indicates poor perfusion to the tissues?
☐ 1. blood pressure of 102/64 mm Hg
☐ 2. cool, pale extremities
☐ 3. heart rate of 104 bpm
☐ 4. shortness of breath when supine

57. The nurse is teaching a client with heart failure about taking digoxin. Which sign of digoxin toxicity should the nurse include in the teaching plan?
☐ 1. rash over the chest and back
☐ 2. increased appetite
☐ 3. visual disturbances such as seeing yellow spots
☐ 4. elevated blood pressure

58. A client is receiving a loop diuretic. Which food(s) should the nurse encourage the client to eat to prevent potassium loss? Select all that apply.
☐ 1. angel food cake
☐ 2. banana
☐ 3. dried fruit
☐ 4. orange juice
☐ 5. peppers

59. The nurse is admitting an older adult to the hospital. The echocardiogram report revealed left ventricular enlargement. The nurse notes 2+ pitting edema in the ankles when getting the client into bed. Based on this finding, what should the nurse do **first**?
☐ 1. Assess respiratory status.
☐ 2. Draw blood for laboratory studies.
☐ 3. Insert a Foley catheter.
☐ 4. Weigh the client.

60. The nurse is teaching a client with heart failure how to avoid complications and future hospitalizations. The client has understood the instruction when the client identifies which potential complication(s)? Select all that apply.
☐ 1. becoming increasingly short of breath at rest
☐ 2. weight gain of 2 lb (0.9 kg) or more in 1 day
☐ 3. high intake of sodium for breakfast
☐ 4. having to sleep sitting up in a reclining chair
☐ 5. weight loss of 2 lb (0.9 kg) in 1 day

The Adult with Valvular Heart Disease

61. A client has returned from the cardiac catheterization laboratory after a balloon valvuloplasty for mitral stenosis. Which finding requires **immediate** nursing action?
☐ 1. There is a low, grade 1 intensity mitral regurgitation murmur.
☐ 2. The oxygen saturation (SpO$_2$) is 94% on 2 L of oxygen via nasal cannula.
☐ 3. The client has become more somnolent.
☐ 4. The urine output decreased from 60 mL per hour to 40 mL over the last hour.

62. A client with diabetes who has been maintained on metformin has been scheduled for a cardiac catheterization. The nurse should verify that the health care provider (HCP) has written which prescription for taking the metformin before the procedure?
☐ 1. Increase the amount of protein in the diet the day before.
☐ 2. Withhold the metformin.
☐ 3. Administer the metformin with only a sip of water.
☐ 4. Give the metformin before breakfast.

63. A client with aortic stenosis has increasing dyspnea and dizziness. Identify the area where the nurse would place the stethoscope to assess a murmur from aortic stenosis.

64. A client is scheduled for a cardiac catheterization. The nurse should perform which preprocedural task(s)? Select all that apply.
☐ 1. Verify the client has stopped taking anticoagulants if instructed by the health care provider.
☐ 2. Check for iodine sensitivity.
☐ 3. Verify that written consent has been obtained.
☐ 4. Withhold food and oral fluids before the procedure.
☐ 5. Insert a urinary drainage catheter.

65. The nurse is assessing a client who has returned to the cardiac step-down unit following a cardiac catheterization. Which information about the client should the nurse obtain **first**?
☐ 1. Lab value results
☐ 2. Neurologic status
☐ 3. Puncture site appearance
☐ 4. Skin warmth and turgor

66. A client experiences dizziness 5 minutes after the start of an intravenous (IV) infusion of lidocaine hydrochloride. The nurse should further assess the client for which symptoms?
    ☐ 1. palpitations
    ☐ 2. tinnitus
    ☐ 3. urinary frequency
    ☐ 4. lethargy

67. A pulmonary artery catheter is inserted in a client with severe mitral stenosis and regurgitation. The nurse administers furosemide and nitroprusside as prescribed. The nurse notices a sudden drop in the pulmonary artery diastolic pressure and pulmonary artery wedge pressure. What should the nurse assess **next**?
    ☐ 1. 12-lead ECG
    ☐ 2. blood pressure
    ☐ 3. lung sounds
    ☐ 4. urine output

68. A client has mitral stenosis and will have a valve replacement. The nurse is instructing the client about health maintenance prior to surgery. Inability to follow which prescription would pose the **greatest** health hazard to this client at this time?
    ☐ 1. medication therapy
    ☐ 2. diet modification
    ☐ 3. activity restrictions
    ☐ 4. dental care

69. A client who has undergone a mitral valve replacement has had a mediastinal chest tube inserted. The client has persistent bleeding from the sternal incision during the early postoperative period. What action(s) should the nurse take? Select all that apply.
    ☐ 1. Administer warfarin.
    ☐ 2. Check the postoperative complete blood count (CBC), international normalized ratio (INR), partial thromboplastin time (PTT), and platelet levels.
    ☐ 3. Confirm the availability of blood products.
    ☐ 4. Monitor the mediastinal chest tube drainage.
    ☐ 5. Start a dopamine drip for a systolic blood pressure of less than 100 mm Hg.

70. The nurse is changing a client's dressing after coronary artery bypass surgery. Which nursing action will be **most** helpful in preventing infection?
    ☐ 1. Wash the hands before changing the dressing.
    ☐ 2. Clean the incisional area with an antiseptic.
    ☐ 3. Use prepackaged sterile dressings to cover the incision.
    ☐ 4. Place soiled dressings in a hazardous waste container.

71. Good dental care is an important measure in reducing the risk for endocarditis. What information about dental care should the nurse include in the teaching plan for a client with mitral stenosis? Select all that apply.
    ☐ 1. Brush the teeth at least twice a day.
    ☐ 2. Avoid using an electric toothbrush.
    ☐ 3. Take an antibiotic before oral surgery.
    ☐ 4. Floss the teeth at least once a day.
    ☐ 5. Have regular dental checkups.
    ☐ 6. Rinse the mouth with an antibiotic mouthwash once a day.

72. The nurse is preparing the client for discharge after mitral valve replacement surgery. Which activity should the client avoid until after the 1-month postdischarge appointment with the surgeon?
    ☐ 1. showering
    ☐ 2. lifting anything heavier than 10 lb (4.5 kg)
    ☐ 3. a program of gradually progressive walking
    ☐ 4. light housework

73. Three days after mitral valve replacement surgery, the client tells the nurse there is a "clicking" noise coming from the chest incision. The nurse's response should reflect the understanding that the client may be experiencing:
    ☐ 1. anxiety related to altered body image.
    ☐ 2. depression related to altered health status.
    ☐ 3. altered tissue perfusion.
    ☐ 4. lack of knowledge regarding the postoperative course.

The Adult with Hypertension

74. The health care provider (HCP) has prescribed metoprolol for a client with stage 2 hypertension who has been initially treated with furosemide and ramipril. The nurse should evaluate the client for which expected therapeutic effect of the metoprolol?
    ☐ 1. decrease in heart rate
    ☐ 2. lessening of fatigue
    ☐ 3. improvement in blood sugar levels
    ☐ 4. increase in urine output

75. A client is taking clonidine for treatment of hypertension. The nurse should teach the client about which common adverse effect(s) of this drug? Select all that apply.
    ☐ 1. dry mouth
    ☐ 2. hyperkalemia
    ☐ 3. impotence
    ☐ 4. pancreatitis
    ☐ 5. sleep disturbance

76. A client with hypertensive emergency is being treated with sodium nitroprusside. In a dilution of 50 mg/250 mL, how many micrograms of sodium nitroprusside are in each milliliter? Round your answer to a whole number.

_____ mcg.

77. The nurse is discussing medications with a client with hypertension who has a prescription for furosemide daily. Which comment by the client indicates the client needs further education?
☐ 1. "I know I shouldn't drive after taking my furosemide."
☐ 2. "I should be careful not to stand up too quickly when taking furosemide."
☐ 3. "I should take the furosemide in the morning instead of before bed."
☐ 4. "I need to be sure to also take the potassium supplement that the doctor prescribed along with my furosemide."

78. The nurse is teaching a client with hypertension how to prevent orthostatic hypotension. What information should the nurse give the client? Select all that apply.
☐ 1. Plan regular times for taking medications.
☐ 2. Arise slowly from bed.
☐ 3. Avoid standing still for long periods.
☐ 4. Avoid excessive alcohol intake.
☐ 5. Avoid hot baths.

79. The nurse is teaching a client with hypertension about taking atenolol. What should the nurse instruct the client to do?
☐ 1. Avoid sudden discontinuation of the drug.
☐ 2. Monitor the blood pressure annually.
☐ 3. Follow a 2-g sodium diet.
☐ 4. Discontinue the medication if severe headaches develop.

80. The nurse teaches a client who has recently been diagnosed with hypertension about following a low-calorie, low-fat, low-sodium diet. Which menu selection would **best** meet the client's needs?
☐ 1. mixed green salad with blue cheese dressing, crackers, and cold cuts
☐ 2. ham sandwich on rye bread and an orange
☐ 3. baked chicken, an apple, and a slice of white bread
☐ 4. hot dogs, baked beans, and celery and carrot sticks

81. A client who has diabetes is taking metoprolol for hypertension. What should the nurse instruct the client to do? Select all that apply.
☐ 1. Take the tablets with food at the same time each day.
☐ 2. Avoid crushing or chewing the tablets.
☐ 3. Notify the health care provider (HCP) if the pulse is 82 bpm.
☐ 4. Have a blood glucose level drawn every 6 to 12 months during therapy.
☐ 5. Use an appropriate decongestant if needed.
☐ 6. Report any fainting spells to the HCP.

82. A client diagnosed with primary (essential) hypertension is taking chlorothiazide. The nurse determines that teaching about this medication is effective when the client makes which statement(s)? Select all that apply.
☐ 1. "I'll weigh myself at the same time each day."
☐ 2. "I won't drink alcoholic beverages while on this medication."
☐ 3. "I'll reduce salt intake in my diet."
☐ 4. "If I have severe dizziness, I'll reduce my dosage."
☐ 5. "If I have prolonged exposure to sunlight, I'll use sunscreen."
☐ 6. "I'll take the drug before I go to bed."

83. Which would be **most** helpful when coaching a client to stop smoking?
☐ 1. Review the negative effects of smoking on the body.
☐ 2. Discuss the effects of passive smoking on environmental pollution.
☐ 3. Establish the client's daily smoking pattern.
☐ 4. Explain how smoking worsens high blood pressure.

84. The nurse is making a discharge plan with an obese client with hypertension who smokes. What is the **most** important long-term goal for this client?
☐ 1. Take medications as prescribed.
☐ 2. Stop smoking.
☐ 3. Make a commitment to long-term lifestyle changes.
☐ 4. Lose weight.

The Adult with Atrial Fibrillation and Other Dysrhythmias

85. Cardiac telemetry shows that a client who is up to the bathroom has converted from normal sinus rhythm with a rate of 72 bpm to atrial fibrillation with a ventricular response rate of 100 bpm. In what order from first to last should the nurse perform these interventions? All options must be used.

| 1. Assess vital signs. |
| 2. Assist the client to the bed. |
| 3. Initiate intravenous (IV) access. |
| 4. Obtain a stat 12-lead electrocardiogram. |
| |
| |
| |

86. A client admitted to the telemetry unit with newly diagnosed atrial fibrillation has been started on warfarin. What should the nurse instruct the client to do when taking this medication? Select all that apply.
☐ 1. Avoid injury to prevent bruising.
☐ 2. Be careful using a razor or fingernail clippers.
☐ 3. Report any change in color of urine or stool.
☐ 4. Floss the teeth deep into the gums.
☐ 5. Avoid taking the medication if the pulse is below 60 bpm.

87. The nurse is planning care for a client with a newly diagnosed cardiac dysrhythmia. Which laboratory value(s) should the nurse review when developing the care plan? Select all that apply.
☐ 1. blood urea nitrogen (BUN) of 20 mg/dL (7.14 mmol/L)
☐ 2. hematocrit of 40% (0.40 proportion of 1.0)
☐ 3. sodium of 124 mEq/L (124 mmol/L)
☐ 4. potassium of 3.1 mEq/L (3.10 mmol/L)
☐ 5. hemoglobin of 14 g/dL (140 g/L)
☐ 6. calcium of 8.5 mEq/L (2.13 mmol/L)
☐ 7. prothrombin time (PT) of 12 seconds with an international normalized ratio (INR) of 1

88. Six hours after pacemaker insertion, a client reports the sudden onset of chest pain and shortness of breath with a drop in oxygen saturation (SpO$_2$) from 98% on 2 L per minute of oxygen to 90% on 2 L per minute of oxygen. Which action should the nurse take **first**?
☐ 1. Assess the client's breath sounds and chest movement.
☐ 2. Notify the health care provider to obtain a chest x-ray.
☐ 3. Check the client's blood pressure and heart rate.
☐ 4. Assess the incision site for redness, pain, drainage, or swelling.

89. A client suddenly develops paroxysmal supraventricular tachycardia (PSVT) at a rate of 180 bpm. Current vital signs are a blood pressure of 90/45 mm Hg, a heart rate of 180 bpm, a respiration rate of 30 breaths/min, and an oxygen saturation of 90% on room air. The client is diaphoretic and reports dizziness. What should the nurse do **first**?
☐ 1. Ask the client about current caffeine use.
☐ 2. Administer atropine per agency protocol.
☐ 3. Prepare a defibrillator for synchronized cardioversion.
☐ 4. Start cardiopulmonary resuscitation (CPR).

90. A client admitted with normal sinus rhythm converts to the following rhythm on the cardiac monitor.

For which symptom(s) should the nurse assess the client? Select all that apply.
☐ 1. carotid bruit
☐ 2. light-headedness
☐ 3. nausea
☐ 4. palpitations
☐ 5. shortness of breath
☐ 6. systolic murmur

91. A nurse hears an irregular heart rate of 110 bpm when auscultating a client's chest. The client also has new-onset shortness of breath. Which action should the nurse take **next**?
☐ 1. Check the availability of medication to relieve anxiety.
☐ 2. Recheck the pulse later in the shift.
☐ 3. Obtain a prescription for a stat electrocardiogram.
☐ 4. Call the radiology service to obtain a stat chest x-ray.

92. A client is admitted to the hospital for evaluation of recurrent episodes of ventricular tachycardia as observed on Holter monitoring. The client is scheduled for electrophysiology studies (EPS) the following morning. Which statement should the nurse include in a teaching plan for this client?
☐ 1. "You'll continue to take your medications until the morning of the test."
☐ 2. "You might be sedated during the procedure and won't remember what's happened."
☐ 3. "This test is a noninvasive method of determining the effectiveness of your medication regimen."
☐ 4. "During the procedure, the health care provider will insert a special wire to increase the heart rate and produce the irregular beats that caused your signs and symptoms."

93. The nurse is palpating the radial pulse of a client who has atrial fibrillation. Which finding should the nurse report to the health care provider (HCP)?
☐ 1. two regular beats followed by one irregular beat
☐ 2. an irregular rhythm with a pulse rate higher than 100 bpm
☐ 3. a pulse rate below 60 bpm
☐ 4. a weak, thready pulse

94. The nurse is teaching a client about self-care following the placement of a permanent pacemaker in the client's left upper chest. Which information should the nurse include in the teaching plan? Select all that apply.
   ☐ 1. Take and record the daily pulse rate.
   ☐ 2. Avoid air travel because of airport security alarms.
   ☐ 3. Immobilize the affected arm for 4 to 6 weeks.
   ☐ 4. Avoid using a microwave oven.
   ☐ 5. Avoid lifting anything heavier than 3 lb (1.36 kg).

95. A client has been admitted to the coronary care unit. The nurse observes third-degree heart block at a rate of 35 bpm on the client's cardiac monitor. The client has a blood pressure of 90/60 mm Hg. What should the nurse do **first**?
   ☐ 1. Prepare for transcutaneous pacing.
   ☐ 2. Prepare to defibrillate the client at 200 J.
   ☐ 3. Administer an intravenous lidocaine infusion.
   ☐ 4. Schedule the operating room for the insertion of a permanent pacemaker.

96. A client has atrial fibrillation and a heart rate of 165 bpm. In which order from first to last should the nurse implement these prescriptions from the health care provider? All options must be used.

| 1. Administer oxygen via nasal cannula. |
| 2. Gather supplies for insertion of an intravenous (IV) line. |
| 3. Place the client on a cardiac monitor (ECG). |
| 4. Obtain vital signs, including blood pressure, pulse, respiration rate, temperature, and oxygen saturation. |

97. A client is scheduled for the insertion of an implantable cardioverter-defibrillator (ICD). The spouse expresses anxiety about what would happen if the device discharges during physical contact. What should the nurse tell the spouse?
   ☐ 1. Physical contact should be avoided whenever possible.
   ☐ 2. They will not feel the countershock.
   ☐ 3. The shock would feel like a "tingle," but it would not cause any harm.
   ☐ 4. A warning device sounds before the countershock, so there is time to move away.

98. An older adult is admitted to the telemetry unit for placement of a permanent pacemaker because of sinus bradycardia. What is a **priority** goal for the client within 24 hours after insertion of a permanent pacemaker?
   ☐ 1. Maintain skin integrity.
   ☐ 2. Maintain cardiac conduction stability.
   ☐ 3. Decrease cardiac output.
   ☐ 4. Increase activity level.

99. A client who had a permanent pacemaker implanted 2 days earlier is being discharged from the hospital. What evidence will indicate to the nurse that the client understands the discharge plan?
   ☐ 1. The client selects a low-cholesterol diet to control coronary artery disease.
   ☐ 2. The client states a need for bed rest for 1 week after discharge.
   ☐ 3. The client verbalizes safety precautions needed to prevent pacemaker malfunction.
   ☐ 4. The client explains the signs and symptoms of myocardial infarction (MI).

100. An older adult is admitted to the emergency department at 2000 hours with syncope, shortness of breath, and reported palpitations (see nurse's notes below). At 2015, the nurse places the client on the electrocardiogram (ECG) monitor and identifies the following rhythm (see below). What should the nurse do? Select all that apply.

Nurse's Notes	
Admitted to emergency department	2000
Pulse	150
Blood pressure	90/62 mm Hg
Oxygen saturation	92% on room air
Respiratory rate	22
Progress notes	Client has shortness of breath and states, "My heart is jumping out of my chest and hurts some. I am having trouble catching my breath. I don't want to faint again."

☐ 1. Apply oxygen.
☐ 2. Prepare to defibrillate the client.
☐ 3. Monitor vital signs.
☐ 4. Have the client sign consent for cardioversion as prescribed.
☐ 5. Teach the client about warfarin treatment and the need for frequent blood testing.
☐ 6. Draw blood for a complete blood count (CBC) and thyroid function study.

The Adult Requiring Rapid Response or Cardiopulmonary Resuscitation

101. The nurse is observing the client's monitor and notes third-degree heart block. What should the nurse do **first**?
☐ 1. Call a code.
☐ 2. Begin cardiopulmonary resuscitation (CPR).
☐ 3. Place transcutaneous pacing pads on the client.
☐ 4. Prepare for defibrillation.

102. The nurse observes the cardiac rhythm (see below) for a client who is being admitted with a myocardial infarction. What should the nurse do **first**?

☐ 1. Prepare for immediate cardioversion.
☐ 2. Begin cardiopulmonary resuscitation (CPR).
☐ 3. Check for a pulse.
☐ 4. Prepare for immediate defibrillation.

103. A client who has been given cardiopulmonary resuscitation is admitted to the emergency department. What is the **most** effective way for the nurse to quickly determine if this client has adequate oxygenation?
☐ 1. There is a pulse.
☐ 2. Pupils are reacting to light.
☐ 3. Mucous membranes are pink.
☐ 4. Systolic blood pressure is at least 80 mm Hg.

104. The nurse administers amiodarone to a client with a dysrhythmia. Which finding indicates the drug is having the desired effect?
☐ 1. The ventricular rate is increasing.
☐ 2. The absent pulse is now palpable.
☐ 3. The number of premature ventricular contractions is decreasing.
☐ 4. The fine ventricular fibrillation changes to coarse ventricular fibrillation.

105. The nurse is giving rescue breaths to a client who just had a cardiac arrest while a team member performs chest compressions. The chest wall fails to rise after the team has been performing cardiopulmonary resuscitation for 30 seconds. What should the nurse do **next**?
☐ 1. Try using a bag mask device.
☐ 2. Decrease the rate of compressions.
☐ 3. Intubate the client.
☐ 4. Reposition the airway.

106. The nurse is giving rescue breaths during cardiopulmonary resuscitation (CPR). How will the nurse evaluate that the client is exhaling?
☐ 1. observing normal relaxation of the chest
☐ 2. giving gentle pressure from the rescuer's hand on the upper chest
☐ 3. noting the depth of pressure of cardiac compressions
☐ 4. turning the client's head to the side

107. The rapid response team has been called to manage an unwitnessed cardiac arrest in a client's hospital room. How long should the nurse estimate the maximum time a person can be without cardiopulmonary function and still not experience permanent brain damage?
☐ 1. 1 to 2 minutes
☐ 2. 4 to 6 minutes
☐ 3. 8 to 10 minutes
☐ 4. 12 to 15 minutes

108. A nurse is helping a client who is suspected of choking. When should the nurse perform the Heimlich maneuver?
☐ 1. The victim starts to become cyanotic.
☐ 2. The victim cannot speak due to airway obstruction.
☐ 3. The victim can make only minimal vocal noises.
☐ 4. The victim is coughing vigorously.

109. The nurse is performing the Heimlich maneuver on a conscious adult victim. What landmark should the nurse use to deliver the inward and upward thrusts?
☐ 1. above the umbilicus
☐ 2. at the level of the xiphoid process
☐ 3. over the victim's midabdominal area
☐ 4. below the xiphoid process and above the umbilicus

110. The nurse notices on the cardiac monitor that the client has started having premature ventricular contractions every other beat. What should the nurse do **first**?
☐ 1. Activate the rapid response team.
☐ 2. Assess the client's orientation and vital signs.
☐ 3. Call the health care provider (HCP).
☐ 4. Administer a bolus of lidocaine.

111. A client returns to the nursing unit after undergoing successful synchronized cardioversion using transthoracic chest wall patches. What should the nurse assess when the client returns to the room? Select all that apply.
☐ 1. vital signs
☐ 2. skin of the chest wall
☐ 3. arterial puncture site
☐ 4. level of consciousness
☐ 5. cardiac rhythm

112. The nurse is preparing to defibrillate a client on a cardiac monitor who is in ventricular fibrillation (see photo). What should the nurse do?

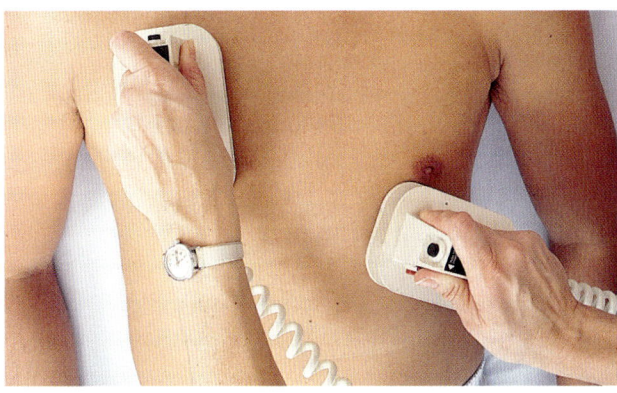

☐ 1. Move the paddle in the nurse's left hand to the midline.
☐ 2. Move the paddle in the nurse's right hand to above the client's nipple.
☐ 3. Grasp the handles of the paddles to allow visibility of the black markings on the paddle.
☐ 4. After pressing the charge button and calling "all clear," push the shock button.

113. The nurse is caring for a client who has become unresponsive. The blood pressure is 80/40 mm Hg, and oxygen saturation (SpO$_2$) is 90% on a 50% partial rebreather mask. What should the nurse do **next**?
☐ 1. Begin chest compressions.
☐ 2. Call the rapid response team.
☐ 3. Remove the family from the room.
☐ 4. Ventilate the client with a bag mask device.

Managing Care, Quality, and Safety for Adults with Cardiac Health Problems

114. A nurse working the day shift on a cardiac unit receives the shift report. At the conclusion of the shift report, it is 0730. Put the clients in the order from first to last in which the nurse should plan to assess them. All options must be used.

1. Client 1: Admitted yesterday morning with hypokalemia. Awaiting repeat electrolyte lab results drawn at 0600.

2. Client 2: Experienced chest pain at 0630. Pain resolved after two sublingual nitroglycerin tablets.

3. Client 3: Scheduled for oral antihypertensive medications at 0900. Incontinent of urine during the night.

4. Client 4: Scheduled for coronary artery bypass surgery at 0800. The client's family is in the client's room.

115. The unlicensed assistive personnel (UAP) reports to the nurse that a client is "feeling short of breath." The client's blood pressure was 124/78 mm Hg 2 hours ago with a heart rate of 82 bpm; the UAP reports that blood pressure is now 84/44 mm Hg with a heart rate of 54 bpm, and the client stated, "I just don't feel good." What action(s) should the nurse take? Select all that apply.
  ☐ 1. Confirm the client's vital signs, and complete a quick assessment.
  ☐ 2. Inform the charge nurse of the change in condition, and initiate the hospital's rapid/emergency response team.
  ☐ 3. Make a quick check on other assigned clients before spending the amount of time required to take care of this client.
  ☐ 4. Position the client in semi-Fowler position.
  ☐ 5. Stay with the client, and reassure them.
  ☐ 6. Call the health care provider (HCP), and report the situation using SBAR (situation, background, assessment, recommendation) format.

116. The nurse is caring for a 72-year-old female client with heart failure whose blood pressure and weight are being monitored remotely. The client takes ramipril 5 mg twice a day and is on a 2-mg sodium diet.

The nurse reviews the client's record for the last 3 days.

Flow Sheet

	Day 1	Day 2	Day 3
Weight	160 lb (72 kg)	162 lb (73 kg)	165 lb (74 kg)
Blood pressure	120/80 mm Hg	130/88 mm Hg	140/90 mm Hg

➤ The nurse calls the client to follow up. Which information will be most helpful to determine the reason for the change in weight and blood pressure? Select all that apply.
  ☐ 1. How the client is feeling
  ☐ 2. If the client has shortness of breath
  ☐ 3. When the client last calibrated the scales
  ☐ 4. The client's daily fluid intake
  ☐ 5. How many times a day the client voids
  ☐ 6. When the client took the last dose of ramipril
  ☐ 7. Did the client use the same arm for taking the blood pressure

117. The nurse is tracking data on a group of clients with heart failure who have been discharged from the hospital and are being followed at a clinic. Which data are the **best** indicators that nursing interventions of monitoring and teaching have been effective?
☐ 1. Ninety percent of clients have not gained weight.
☐ 2. Seventy-five percent of the clients viewed the educational DVD.
☐ 3. Eighty percent of the clients reported that they are taking their medications.
☐ 4. Five percent of the clients required hospitalization in the last 90 days.

118. The nurse in the intensive care unit is giving a report to the nurse in a cardiac step-down unit about a client who had coronary artery bypass surgery. Which is the **most** effective way to assure essential information about the client is reported?
☐ 1. Give the report face to face with both nurses in a quiet room.
☐ 2. Audiotape the report for future reference and documentation.
☐ 3. Use a printed checklist with information individualized for the client.
☐ 4. Document essential transfer information in the client's medical record.

119. The nurse is caring for a group of clients on a medical-surgical nursing unit. Which task(s) could the nurse delegate to unlicensed assistive personnel (UAP)? Select all that apply.
☐ 1. Assess pedal pulses on a client who just returned from a cardiac angiogram.
☐ 2. Administer oxygen via nasal cannula to a client with a saturation of 89%.
☐ 3. Administer acetaminophen to a client with a pain level of 5 on a scale of 0 to 10.
☐ 4. Perform vital signs and oxygen saturation on a client returning from the catheterization lab.
☐ 5. Obtain intake and output on a client experiencing heart failure.

120. The nurse is caring for a group of clients. Which client should the nurse see **first**?
☐ 1. a client with a history of sinus tachycardia who is to receive a beta-blocker
☐ 2. a client with stable angina who took one sublingual nitroglycerine tablet 30 minutes ago
☐ 3. a client who underwent placement of a coronary artery stent 30 minutes ago
☐ 4. a client with new-onset atrial fibrillation who has a heart rate of 95 bpm

Answers, Rationales, and Test-Taking Strategies

*The answers and the rationales for each question follow below, along with keys (🔑) to the client need (CN) and cognitive level (CL) for each question. In addition, questions that measure clinical judgment will be coded (CJ). As you check your answers, use the **Content Mastery and Test-Taking Skill Self-Analysis** worksheet (tear-out worksheet in the back of the book) to identify the reason(s) for not answering the questions correctly. For additional information about test-taking skills and strategies for answering questions, refer to pages 12–51 in Part 1 of this book.*

The Adult with Acute Coronary Syndromes

1. 2. To best monitor that the client's circulation remains intact, the dorsal surface of the right foot should be palpated. When the left side of the heart is catheterized, the cannula enters via an artery. In this instance, the right femoral artery was accessed. While all options assess arterial points of the right leg, the dorsal surface of the right foot (the pedal pulse) is the most distal. If this pulse point is present and unchanged from before the procedure, the other pulse points should also be intact.

🔑 CN: Physiological adaptation; CL: Apply

2. 4. The elevated troponin level should be reported to the HCP before the stress test because this change indicates myocardial damage. Sending the client to walk on a treadmill for stress testing would be contraindicated with evidence of recent myocardial injury and could further extend the damage. The other blood levels are helpful but not critical to this client's welfare at this point in time.

🔑 CN: Reduction of risk potential; CL: Analyze

3. 4. The nurse should first contact the HCP and report the level of pain and recommend pain management that would help decrease myocardial oxygen demand. The nurse should monitor fluid status, but this is not the priority. The nurse can begin teaching the client about health management once the client is stable and amenable to teaching. Visitation should be based on client comfort and maintaining a calm environment.

🔑 CN: Physiological adaptation; CL: Synthesize

4. **2.** Nitroglycerin is a vasodilator that will lower blood pressure. The client is having chest pain, and the ST elevation indicates injury to the myocardium, which may benefit from nitroglycerin. The potassium and heart rate are within normal range.

🗝️ CN: Pharmacological and parenteral therapies; CL: Analyze

5. **1.** The nurse should first obtain vital signs because changes in the vital signs will reflect the severity of the sudden drop in cardiac output: a decrease in blood pressure, an increase in the heart rate, and an increase in the respiration rate. Infarction of the papillary muscles is a potential complication of an MI, causing ineffective closure of the mitral valve during systole. Mitral regurgitation results when the left ventricle contracts and blood flows backward into the left atrium, which is heard at the fifth intercostal space at the left midclavicular line. The murmur worsens during expiration and in the supine or left-side position and can best be heard when the client is in these positions, not with the client leaning forward. A 12-lead ECG views the electrical activity of the heart; an echocardiogram views valve function.

🗝️ CN: Physiological adaptation; CL: Synthesize

6. 🔢 **1, 4, 5.** Morphine sulfate acts as an analgesic and sedative. It also reduces myocardial oxygen consumption, blood pressure, and heart rate. Morphine also reduces anxiety and fear because of its sedative effects and by slowing the heart rate. It can depress respirations; however, such an effect may lead to hypoxia, which should be avoided in the treatment of chest pain. Angiotensin-converting enzyme inhibitor drugs, not morphine, may help prevent ventricular remodeling.

🗝️ CN: Pharmacological and parenteral therapies; CL: Evaluate

7. **24 mL per hour**

First, calculate how many units are in each milliliter of the medication:

$$\frac{25{,}000 \text{ units}}{500 \text{ mL}} = \frac{50 \text{ units}}{1 \text{ mL}}$$

Next, calculate how many milliliters the client receives per hour:

$$\frac{1{,}200 \text{ units}}{1 \text{ hour}} \div \frac{50 \text{ units}}{1 \text{ mL}}$$

$$= \frac{\cancel{1{,}200}^{24} \text{ units}}{1 \text{ hour}} \times \frac{1 \text{ mL}}{\cancel{50}_{1} \text{ units}} = 24 \text{ mL/h}$$

🗝️ CN: Pharmacological and parenteral therapies; CL: Apply

8. **1.** The client is having symptoms of a myocardial infarction. The first action is to prevent platelet formation and block prostaglandin synthesis. The client should place the tablet under the tongue and wait until it is absorbed. Nitroglycerin tablets are not effective if chewed, swallowed, or placed between the cheek and gums.

🗝️ CN: Pharmacological and parenteral therapies; CL: Apply

9. **2.** Low urine output and confusion are signs of decreased tissue perfusion. Orthopnea is a sign of left-sided heart failure. Crackles, edema, and weight gain should be monitored closely, but these levels are not as high a priority. With atrial fibrillation, there is a loss of atrial kick, but the blood pressure and heart rate are stable.

🗝️ CN: Physiological adaptation; CL: Analyze

10. **4.** The nurse should first assess the client's tolerance to the drop in heart rate by checking the blood pressure and level of consciousness and determining if atropine is needed. If the client is symptomatic, atropine and transcutaneous pacing are interventions for symptomatic bradycardia. Once the client is stable, further physical assessments can be done.

🗝️ CN: Physiological adaptation; CL: Synthesize

11. 🔢 **1, 2, 3, 4.** When preparing the client for a cardiac angiogram, the nurse should determine if the client has an allergy to the liquid contrast medium used in the procedure. Contrast dyes contain iodine, and the administration of a dye could lead to an anaphylactic response in clients who are allergic to the dye. An intravenous infusion will be started before the procedure to administer the contrast dye. The client should not eat or drink for 8 hours prior to the procedure. The client may experience a flushing sensation, but this is a normal response and does not indicate a life-threatening reaction. The client may receive light sedation, but not an anesthetic as the client must be awake to follow instructions. The client should be instructed to remain still during the procedure.

🗝️ CN: Reduction of risk potential; CL: Apply

12. **1.** Although obtaining the ECG, chest radiograph, and blood work are all important, the nurse's priority action should be to relieve the crushing chest pain. Therefore, administering morphine sulfate is the priority action.

🗝️ CN: Physiological adaptation; CL: Synthesize

13. **2.** All of the 1200-hour assessments are signs of decreased cardiac output and can be an ominous sign in a client who has recently experienced an

MI; the nurse should notify the HCP of these changes. Cardiac output and blood pressure may continue to fall to dangerous levels, which can induce further coronary ischemia and extension of the infarct. Although the client is currently hypotensive, giving a fluid challenge/bolus can precipitate an increased workload on a damaged heart and extend the myocardial infarction. Exercise or walking for this client will increase both the heart rate and stroke volume, both of which will increase cardiac output, but the increased cardiac output will increase oxygen needs, especially in the heart muscle, and can induce further coronary ischemia and extension of the infarct. The client is hypotensive. Although the client has decreased urinary output, this is the body's response to a decreasing cardiac output, and it is not appropriate to administer furosemide.

CN: Physiological adaptation; CL: Synthesize

14. 2. Thrombolytic drugs are administered within the first 6 hours after the onset of an MI to lyse clots and reduce the extent of myocardial damage.

CN: Pharmacological and parenteral therapies; CL: Evaluate

15. 3. The client is experiencing a single premature ventricular contraction (PVC). PVCs are characterized by a QRS of longer than 0.12 seconds and by a wide, notched, or slurred QRS complex. There is no P wave related to the QRS complex, and the T wave is usually inverted. PVCs are potentially serious and can lead to ventricular fibrillation or cardiac arrest when they occur more than 6 to 10 times an hour in clients with myocardial infarction. The nurse should continue to monitor the client and note if the PVCs are increasing. It is not necessary to notify the HCP or call the rapid response team at this point. Lidocaine is not indicated from the data on this ECG.

CN: Reduction of risk potential; CL: Synthesize

16. 1. The nurse should first don gloves and apply direct pressure over the site to stop blood loss from the femoral artery. Although the nurse will later observe the site for further bleeding and record the extent of bleeding, this is not the first action that is needed. If the bleeding cannot be controlled, the HCP who performed the procedure should be contacted, but first, an attempt to manually stop the bleeding with direct pressure is warranted. Protamine sulfate is the antidote for heparin sodium, but this is not an initial action to control the bleeding.

CN: Reduction of risk potential; CL: Synthesize

17. 2. Metoprolol is indicated in the treatment of hemodynamically stable clients with an acute MI to reduce cardiovascular mortality. Cardiogenic shock causes severe hemodynamic instability, and a beta-blocker will further depress myocardial contractility. The metoprolol should be discontinued. The decrease in cardiac output will impair perfusion to the kidneys. Cardiac output, hemodynamic measurements, and appropriate interventions can be determined with a pulmonary artery catheter. Dobutamine will improve contractility and increase the cardiac output that is depressed in cardiogenic shock.

CN: Physiological adaptation; CL: Synthesize

18. 1, 2, 3, 5, 7. The client's heart rate, blood pressure, respiration rate, and oxygen saturation indicate the client's vital signs are changing rapidly, and the nurse should report them to the surgeon immediately. The client is going into cardiogenic shock. The nurse should report that the client has a history of myocardial infarction. The client's temperature is within normal limits. It is not necessary to report the type of surgery or the time that it is scheduled.

CJ: Standalone trend; CL: Analyze

19. 1. IV nitroglycerin infusion requires an infusion pump for precise control of the medication. Blood pressure monitoring would be done with a continuous system and more frequently than every 4 hours. Hourly urine outputs are not always required. Obtaining serum potassium levels is not associated with nitroglycerin infusion.

CN: Pharmacological and parenteral therapies; CL: Synthesize

20. 3, 4, 2, 1. The nurse should first connect the client to the monitor by attaching the electrodes. Electrocardiography can be used to identify myocardial ischemia and infarction, rhythm and conduction disturbances, chamber enlargement, electrolyte imbalances, and the effects of drugs on the client's heart. The nurse next obtains vital signs to establish a baseline. Next, the nurse should administer the morphine; morphine is the drug of choice in relieving myocardial infarction pain; it may cause a transient decrease in blood pressure. When the client is stable, the nurse can obtain a history of the client's drug use.

CN: Reduction of risk potential; CL: Synthesize

21. 2, 5. It is important for clients to wear hearing aids to this procedure so that they can hear the questions posed to them by the health care team. Chest pain often occurs when the balloon within the stent is inflated and deployed into the coronary artery. It is expected and brief but should still be reported by the client. During the procedure and for a prescribed amount of time after the procedure, the client will need to remain flat in bed with the right leg straight, not flexed, to prevent bleeding from the access site. The site is not routinely stitched. It is a puncture rather than an incision requiring sutures. The client may be given intravenous medication to help with comfort, but the client is kept awake to answer questions and to hear instructions and explanations. General anesthesia is not given.

CN: Reduction of risk potential; CL: Create

22. 4. Sinus tachycardia is characterized by normal conduction and a regular rhythm, but with a rate exceeding 100 bpm. A P wave precedes each QRS, and the QRS is usually normal.

CN: Reduction of risk potential; CL: Analyze

23. 2. PVCs are often a precursor of life-threatening arrhythmias, including ventricular tachycardia and ventricular fibrillation. An occasional PVC is not considered dangerous, but if PVCs occur at a rate greater than five or six per minute in a client who has experienced an MI, the HCP should be notified immediately. More than six PVCs per minute is considered serious and usually calls for decreasing ventricular irritability by administering medications such as lidocaine hydrochloride. Increasing the IV infusion rate would not decrease the number of PVCs. Increasing the oxygen concentration should not be the nurse's first course of action; rather, the nurse should notify the HCP promptly. Administering a prescribed analgesic medication would not decrease ventricular irritability.

CN: Physiological adaptation; CL: Synthesize

24. 4. By day 2 of hospitalization after an MI, clients are expected to be able to perform personal care without chest pain. Severe chest pain should not be present on day 2 after an MI. Day 2 of hospitalization may be too soon for clients to be able to identify risk factors for MI or to begin a walking program; however, the client may be sitting up in a chair as part of the cardiac rehabilitation program.

CN: Physiological adaptation; CL: Evaluate

25. 2. Furosemide is a loop diuretic that acts to increase urine output. Furosemide does not increase blood pressure, decrease pain, or decrease arrhythmias.

CN: Pharmacological and parenteral therapies; CL: Evaluate

26. 3. Encouraging the client to move the legs while in bed is a preventive strategy taught to all clients who are hospitalized and on bed rest to promote venous return. The muscular action aids in venous return and prevents venous stasis in the lower extremities. These exercises are not intended to prepare the client for ambulation. These exercises are not associated with promoting urinary and intestinal elimination. These exercises are not performed to decrease the risk for pressure ulcer formation.

CN: Physiological adaptation; CL: Apply

27. 2. Recommended dietary principles in the acute phase of MI include avoiding large meals because small, easily digested foods are better tolerated. Fluids are given according to the client's needs, and sodium restrictions may be prescribed, especially for clients with manifestations of heart failure. Cholesterol restrictions may be prescribed as well. Clients are not prescribed diets of liquids only or restricted to nothing by mouth unless their condition is very unstable.

CN: Physiological adaptation; CL: Apply

28. 1, 3, 4. Clopidogrel is generally well absorbed and may be taken with or without food; it should be taken at the same time every day, and, while food may help prevent potential gastrointestinal upset, food has no effect on the absorption of the drug. Bleeding is the most common adverse effect of clopidogrel; the client must understand the importance of reporting any unexpected, prolonged, or excessive bleeding, including blood in urine or stool. Increased bruising and bleeding gums are possible side effects of clopidogrel; the client should be aware of this possibility. Clopidogrel is an antiplatelet agent used to prevent clot formation in clients who have experienced or are at risk for myocardial infarction, ischemic stroke, peripheral artery disease, or acute coronary syndrome. It is not necessary to drink a glass of water after taking clopidogrel.

CN: Pharmacological and parenteral therapies; CL: Create

29. 4. The woman who is 65 years old, overweight, and with an elevated LDL level is at the greatest risk for CAD. Total cholesterol higher than 200 mg/dL (11.1 mmol/L); LDL higher than 100 mg/dL (5.5 mmol/L); HDL lower than 40 mg/dL (2.2 mmol/L) in men; HDL lower than 50 mg/dL (2.8 mmol/L) in women; men 45 years and older; women 55 years and older; smoking; and obesity increase the risk for CAD. Atorvastatin reduces LDL and decreases the risk for CAD. The combination of being postmenopausal, having obesity, and having a high LDL level places this client at greatest risk.

CN: Health promotion and maintenance; CL: Analyze

30. **1.** Nitroglycerin acts to decrease myocardial oxygen consumption. Vasodilation makes it easier for the heart to eject blood, resulting in decreased oxygen needs. Decreased oxygen demand reduces pain caused by heart muscle not receiving sufficient oxygen. While blood pressure may decrease ever so slightly due to the vasodilation effects of nitroglycerin, it is only secondary and not related to the angina the client is experiencing. Increased blood pressure would mean the heart would work harder, increasing oxygen demand and thus angina. Decreased heart rate is not an effect of nitroglycerin.

    CN: Pharmacological and parenteral therapy; CL: Evaluate

31. **1, 5, 6.** The nurse should instruct the client to spray the nitroglycerin under the tongue at the first sign of chest pain. If pain continues after using two doses of the medication, wait 5 minutes, and administer one more spray. If the chest pain continues after 10 minutes, the client should call 911 and seek emergency assistance. The client should not swallow the medication. The medication should be stored at room temperature away from heat and light, not in the refrigerator. It is not necessary to shake the medication container before use.

    CN: Pharmacological and parenteral therapies; CL: Synthesize

32. **3.** In health coaching, unlike traditional client education techniques in which the nurse provides information, the goal of coaching is to encourage the client to explore the reasons for the behavior and establish a vision for health behavior and the way they can make changes to improve health behavior and reduce or eliminate health risks. When coaching a client, the nurse does not provide information, withhold praise, or instill fear.

    CN: Health promotion and maintenance; CL: Synthesize

33. **4.** The thrombolytic agent t-PA, administered intravenously, lyses the clot blocking the coronary artery. The drug is most effective when administered within the first 6 hours after the onset of an MI. The drug does not reduce coronary artery vasospasm; nitrates are used to promote vasodilation. Arrhythmias are managed by antiarrhythmic drugs. Surgical approaches are used to open the coronary artery and reestablish a blood supply to the area.

    CN: Pharmacological and parenteral therapies; CL: Apply

34. **1.** Cardiac arrhythmias are commonly observed with the administration of t-PA. Cardiac arrhythmias are associated with reperfusion of the cardiac tissue. Hypotension is commonly observed with the administration of t-PA. Seizures and hypothermia are not generally associated with reperfusion of the cardiac tissue.

    CN: Reduction of risk potential; CL: Synthesize

35. **2.** Advanced cardiac life support recommends that at least one or two IV lines be inserted in one or both of the antecubital spaces. Calling the HCP, obtaining a portable chest radiograph, and drawing blood for the laboratory are important but secondary to starting the IV line.

    CN: Physiological adaptation; CL: Synthesize

36. **3.** Nitroglycerin may be used prophylactically before stressful physical activities such as stair climbing to help the client remain pain free. Climbing the stairs early in the day would have no impact on decreasing pain episodes. Resting before or after an activity is not as likely to help prevent an activity-related pain episode.

    CN: Reduction of risk potential; CL: Synthesize

37. **3.** Pasta, tomato sauce, salad, and coffee would be the best selection for the client following a low-cholesterol diet. Hamburgers, milkshakes, liver, and fried foods tend to be high in cholesterol.

    CN: Basic care and comfort; CL: Apply

38. **1.** The client should report a change in the pattern of chest pain. It may indicate the increasing severity of coronary artery disease. Pain occurring during stress or sexual activity would not be unexpected, and the client may be instructed to take nitroglycerin to prevent this pain. Pain during or after an activity such as lawn mowing also would not be unexpected; the client may be instructed to take nitroglycerin to prevent this pain or may be restricted from doing such activities.

    CN: Reduction of risk potential; CL: Apply

39. **1, 2, 4, 3.** When a client returns from having a transluminal balloon angioplasty with femoral access, the nurse should first obtain baseline vital signs and oxygen saturation to determine evidence of bleeding or decreased tissue perfusion. The nurse should next assess the pedal pulses to determine if the client has adequate peripheral tissue perfusion. Next, the nurse should inspect the catheterization site and then determine the color and sensation in the affected leg.

    CN: Physiologic integrity; CL: Analyze

40. 1. Headache is a common side effect of nitroglycerin that can be alleviated with aspirin, acetaminophen, or ibuprofen. The sublingual nitroglycerin needs to be absorbed in the mouth, which will be disrupted with drinking. Lying flat will increase blood flow to the head and may increase pain and exacerbate other symptoms, such as shortness of breath.

CN: Pharmacological and parenteral therapy; CL: Synthesize

41. 4. The nurse should instruct the client that the correct protocol for using sublingual nitroglycerin involves immediate administration when chest pain occurs. Sublingual nitroglycerin appears in the bloodstream within 2 to 3 minutes and is metabolized within about 10 minutes. The client should sit down and place the tablet under the tongue. If the chest pain is not relieved within 5 minutes, the client should call 911. Although some HCPs may recommend taking a second or third tablet spaced 5 minutes apart and then calling for emergency assistance, it is not appropriate to take two tablets at once. Nitroglycerin acts within 2 to 3 minutes, and the client should not wait 15 minutes to take further action. The client should call 911 to obtain emergency help rather than calling the HCP.

CN: Pharmacological and parenteral therapies; CL: Synthesize

42. 3. The client taking nifedipine should inspect the gums daily to monitor for gingival hyperplasia. This is an uncommon adverse effect but one that requires monitoring and intervention if it occurs. The client taking nifedipine might be taught to monitor blood pressure, but more often than monthly. These clients would not generally need to perform daily weights or limit intake of green leafy vegetables.

CN: Pharmacological and parenteral therapies; CL: Synthesize

43. 2, 5, 6. Simvastatin is used in combination with diet and exercise to decrease elevated total cholesterol. The client should take simvastatin in the evening, and the nurse should instruct the client that if a dose is missed, it should be taken as soon as remembered, but it should not be taken at the same time as the next scheduled dose. It is not necessary to take the pill with food. The client does not need to limit greens (limiting greens is appropriate for clients taking warfarin), but the nurse should instruct the client to avoid grapefruit and grapefruit juice, which can increase the amount of the drug in the bloodstream. A serious side effect is myopathy, and the client should report muscle pain or tenderness to the HCP.

CN: Pharmacology; CL: Create

The Adult with Heart Failure

44. 3. The nurse should withhold the dose of captopril; captopril is an angiotensin-converting enzyme (ACE) inhibitor, and a side effect of the medication is hyperkalemia. The BUN and creatinine levels, which are normal, should be viewed prior to administration since renal insufficiency is another potential side effect of an ACE inhibitor. The heart rate is within normal limits. The nurse should question the dose of metoprolol if the client's heart rate indicates bradycardia. The hemoglobin and hematocrit are normal for a woman. The nurse should report the high potassium level and that the captopril was withheld.

CN: Pharmacological and parenteral therapies; CL: Synthesize

45. 4. The urinary output is less than the expected minimum of 30 mL per hour, and if the urinary output does not increase, the nurse who will next care for the client should report the decreased urinary output to the health care provider. An elevated B-type natriuretic peptide level is expected with acute heart failure. The level that the client can reach with the incentive spirometer is good to know, but it is not the most essential finding to report at this time. The admission weight is helpful only if a prior or baseline weight is also provided.

CN: Management of care; CL: Synthesis

46. 3. Warfarin is an anticoagulant, which is used in the treatment of atrial fibrillation and decreased left ventricular ejection fraction (less than 20%) to prevent thrombus formation and the release of emboli into the circulation. The client may also take other medication as needed to manage the heart failure. Warfarin does not reduce circulatory load or improve myocardial workload. Warfarin does not affect cardiac rhythm.

CN: Reduction of risk potential; CL: Evaluate

47. 2. Early symptoms of digoxin toxicity include anorexia, nausea, and vomiting. Visual disturbances can also occur, including double or blurred vision and visual halos. Hypokalemia is a common cause of digoxin toxicity associated with arrhythmias because low serum potassium can enhance ectopic pacemaker activity. Although vomiting can lead to a fluid deficit, given the client's history, the vomiting is likely due to the adverse effects of digoxin toxicity. Pulmonary edema is manifested by dyspnea and coughing.

CN: Pharmacological and parenteral therapies; CL: Analyze

48. **1, 3, 5, 6.** Dyspnea, crackles, oliguria, and decreased oxygen saturation are signs and symptoms related to pulmonary congestion and inadequate tissue perfusion associated with left-sided heart failure. JVD and right upper quadrant pain along with ascites and edema are usually associated with congestion of the peripheral tissues and viscera in right-sided heart failure.

  CN: Physiological adaptation; CL: Apply

49. **4, 5.** Signs of pulmonary edema are identical to those of acute heart failure. Signs and symptoms are generally apparent in the respiratory system and include coarse crackles, severe dyspnea, and tachypnea. Severe tachycardia occurs due to sympathetic stimulation in the presence of hypoxemia. Blood pressure may be decreased or elevated, depending on the severity of the edema. Jugular vein distention, dependent edema, and anorexia are symptoms of right-sided heart failure.

  CN: Physiological adaptation; CL: Analyze

50. **1.** It is a priority to assess blood pressure first because people with pulmonary edema typically experience severe hypertension that requires early intervention. The client probably does not have skin breakdown, but when the client is stable and the nurse obtains a complete health history, the nurse should inspect the client's skin for any signs of breakdown; however, when the client is stable, the nurse should inspect the skin. Potassium levels are not the first priority. The nurse should monitor urine output after the client is stable.

  CN: Reduction of risk potential; CL: Analyze

51. **1, 4, 6.** It is not unusual for the older adult client to become somewhat confused when "relocated" to the hospital, and this may be more difficult for those with known dementia. Frequent reorientation delivered patiently and calmly along with placing familiar items nearby so the client can see them may help decrease confusion related to hospitalization. Establishing a trusting relationship is important with every client but may be more so with this client. Putting the client in a room further from the nursing station may decrease extra noise for the client but will also make it more difficult to observe the client and maintain a safe environment. Procedures should be explained to the client prior to proceeding and should not be rushed. Visits by family and friends may help keep the client oriented.

  CN: Basic care and comfort; CL: Synthesize

52. **4 mL.** Desired amount (D) divided by what is available (H) times quantity (Q) = amount to administer. D = 40 mg divided by H = 10 mg/mL equals 40 divided by 10 = 4 mL.

  CN: Pharmacological and parenteral therapies; CL: Apply

53. **3.** Sitting almost upright in bed with the feet and legs resting on the mattress decreases venous return to the heart, thus reducing myocardial workload. Also, the sitting position allows maximum space for lung expansion. The low Fowler position would be used if the client could not tolerate the high Fowler position for some reason. Lying on the right side would not be a good position for the client with heart failure. The client with heart failure would not tolerate the Trendelenburg position.

  CN: Physiological adaptation; CL: Synthesize

54. **1.** After intravenous injection of furosemide, diuresis normally begins in about 5 minutes and reaches its peak within about 30 minutes. Medication effects last 2 to 4 hours. When furosemide is given intramuscularly or orally, drug action begins more slowly and lasts longer than when it is given intravenously.

  CN: Pharmacological and parenteral therapies; CL: Evaluate

55. **4.** When diuretics are given early in the day, the client will void frequently during the daytime hours and will not need to void frequently during the night. Therefore, the client will be able to sleep more. The client may be at risk for falling, and the nurse should instruct all clients to rise from a sitting or lying position slowly, but the primary reason for taking the drug in the morning is to limit the number of times the client would need to void during the night if the drug were taken at bedtime. Taking furosemide in the morning has no effect on concentrating the urine or preventing electrolyte imbalances.

  CN: Pharmacological and parenteral therapies; CL: Apply

56. **2.** In heart failure, the heart is unable to adequately meet the body's metabolic demands; in an attempt to supply major organs, less blood is circulated to extremities, leaving them cool, pale, and potentially cyanotic. A blood pressure of 102/64 mm Hg is lower than average, but it may be normal for this client and would not indicate poor perfusion of tissues. It is not unusual for the client with heart failure to have a slightly elevated heart rate (unless taking medications to lower the heart rate) because the increased rate may help compensate for reduced stroke volume (and therefore, decreased cardiac output). Shortness of breath may occur with heart failure as a result of poor pumping action of the heart that allows fluid to accumulate in the lungs; however, it is not an indicator of peripheral perfusion.

CN: Physiological adaptation; CL: Analysis

57. 3. Colored vision and seeing yellow spots are symptoms of digoxin toxicity. Abdominal pain, anorexia, nausea, and vomiting are other common symptoms of digoxin toxicity. Additional signs of toxicity include arrhythmias, such as atrial fibrillation or bradycardia. Rash, increased appetite, and elevated blood pressure are not associated with digoxin toxicity.

CN: Pharmacological and parenteral therapies; CL: Apply

58. 2, 3, 4. Hypokalemia is a side effect of loop diuretics. Bananas, dried fruit, and oranges are examples of food high in potassium. Angel food cake and peppers are low in potassium.

CN: Pharmacological and parenteral therapies; CL: Apply

59. 1. The ankle edema suggests fluid volume overload. The nurse should assess the respiratory rate, lung sounds, and oxygen saturation (SpO$_2$) to identify any signs of respiratory symptoms of heart failure requiring immediate attention. The nurse can then draw blood for laboratory studies, insert the Foley catheter, and weigh the client.

CN: Physiological adaptation; CL: Synthesize

60. 1, 2, 4. If the client will call the health care provider (HCP) when there is increasing shortness of breath, weight gain over 2 lb (0.9 kg) in 1 day, and a need to sleep sitting up, this indicates an understanding of the teaching because these signs and symptoms suggest worsening of the client's heart failure. Although the client will most likely be placed on a sodium-restricted diet, the client would not need to notify the HCP if they had consumed a high-sodium breakfast. Instead, the client would need to be alert for possible signs and symptoms of worsening heart failure and work to reduce sodium intake for the rest of that day and in the future.

CN: Reduction of risk potential; CL: Evaluate

The Adult with Valvular Heart Disease

61. 3. A complication of balloon valvuloplasty is emboli resulting in a stroke. The client's increased drowsiness should be evaluated. Some degree of mitral regurgitation is common after the procedure. The oxygen status and urine output should be monitored closely but do not warrant concern.

CN: Reduction of risk potential; CL: Synthesize

62. 2. The nurse should verify that the HCP has requested to withhold the metformin prior to any procedure requiring dye such as a cardiac catheterization because of the increased risk for lactic acidosis. Additionally, the drug will usually be withheld for up to 48 hours following a procedure involving dye while it clears the client's system. The HCP may prescribe sliding scale insulin during this time if needed. Regardless of how or when the medication is administered, the medication should be withheld. The amount of protein in the client's diet prior to the cardiac catheterization has no correlation with the medication or the test.

CN: Pharmacological and parenteral therapies; CL: Synthesize

63. To assess a murmur from aortic stenosis, the stethoscope is placed at the second intercostal space to the right of the sternum; (1) location, (2) the pulmonic valve area, (3) Erb's point, (4) tricuspid valve area, and (5) mitral valve area.

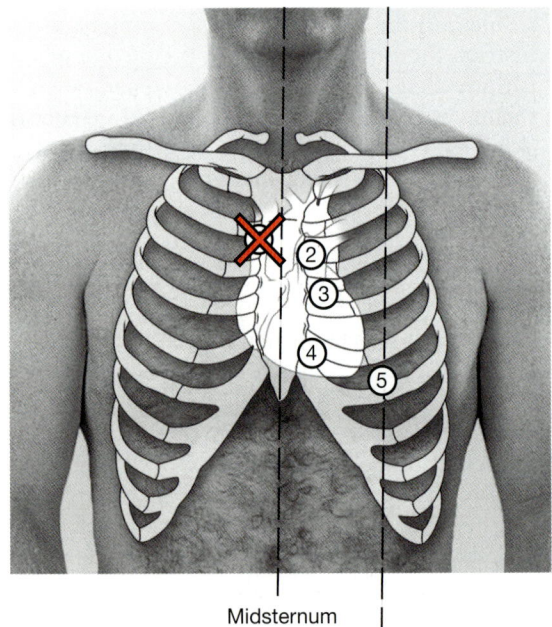

CN: Physiological adaptation; CL: Apply

64. 1, 2, 3, 4. For clients scheduled for cardiac catheterization, it is important to assess for iodine sensitivity, verify written consent, and instruct the client to take nothing by mouth for 6 to 18 hours before the procedure. If the client is taking anticoagulant drugs, the nurse should ask the client if the health care provider has given instructions to withhold these medications. Oral medications are withheld unless specifically prescribed. A urinary drainage catheter is rarely required for this procedure.

🗝️ CN: Reduction of risk potential;
CL: Apply

65. 3. Assessment of circulatory status, including observation of the puncture site, is of primary importance after cardiac catheterization. Laboratory values and skin warmth and turgor are important to monitor but are not the most important initial nursing assessment. Neurologic assessment every 15 minutes is not required.

🗝️ CN: Reduction of risk potential;
CL: Analyze

66. 2. Common adverse effects of lidocaine hydrochloride include dizziness, tinnitus, blurred vision, tremors, numbness and tingling of extremities, excessive perspiration, hypotension, seizures, and, finally, coma. Cardiac effects include slowed conduction and cardiac arrest. Palpitations, urinary frequency, and lethargy are not considered typical adverse reactions to lidocaine.

🗝️ CN: Pharmacological and parenteral therapies; CL: Analyze

67. 2. The nurse should immediately assess the blood pressure since nitroprusside and furosemide can cause severe hypotension from a decrease in preload and afterload. If the client is hypotensive, the nitroprusside dose should be reduced or discontinued. Urine output should then be monitored to make sure there is adequate renal perfusion. A 12-lead ECG is performed if the client experiences chest pain. A reduction in pulmonary artery pressures should improve the pulmonary congestion and lung sounds.

🗝️ CN: Physiological adaptation;
CL: Synthesize

68. 1. Preoperatively, anticoagulants may be prescribed for the client with advanced valvular heart disease to prevent emboli. Postoperatively, all clients with mechanical valves and some clients with bioprosthesis are maintained indefinitely on anticoagulant therapy. Adhering strictly to a dosage schedule and observing specific precautions are necessary to prevent hemorrhage or thromboembolism. Some clients are maintained on lifelong antibiotic prophylaxis to prevent the recurrence of rheumatic fever. Episodic prophylaxis is required to prevent infective endocarditis after dental procedures or upper respiratory, gastrointestinal, or genitourinary tract surgery. Diet modification, activity restrictions, and dental care are important; however, they do not have as much significance postoperatively as medication therapy does.

🗝️ CN: Reduction of risk potential;
CL: Evaluate

69. -/+ 2, 3, 4. The hemoglobin and hematocrit should be assessed to evaluate blood loss. An elevated INR and PTT and decreased platelet count increase the risk for bleeding. The client may require blood products depending on the lab values and severity of bleeding; therefore, the availability of blood products should be confirmed by calling the blood bank. Close monitoring of blood loss from the mediastinal chest tubes should be done. Warfarin is an anticoagulant that will increase bleeding. Anticoagulation should be held at this time. Information is needed on the type of valve replacement. For a mechanical heart valve, the INR is kept at 2 to 3.5. Tissue valves do not require anticoagulation. Dopamine should **not** be initiated if the client is hypotensive from hypovolemia. Fluid volume assessment should always be done first. Volume replacement should be initiated in a hypovolemic client before starting an inotrope such as dopamine.

🗝️ CN: Physiological adaptation;
CL: Synthesize

70. 1. Many factors help prevent wound infections, including washing hands carefully, using sterile prepackaged supplies and equipment, cleaning the incisional area well, and disposing of soiled dressings properly. However, most authorities say that the single most effective measure in preventing wound infections is to wash the hands carefully before and after changing dressings. Careful handwashing is also important in reducing other infections often acquired in hospitals, such as urinary tract and respiratory tract infections.

🗝️ CN: Reduction of risk potential;
CL: Synthesize

71. -/+ 1, 4, 5. Daily dental care including brushing the teeth twice a day and flossing once a day and frequent checkups by a dentist who is informed about the client's condition are required to maintain good oral health. The client can use a regular toothbrush; it is not necessary to avoid the use of an electric toothbrush. Taking antibiotics prior to certain dental procedures is recommended only if the client has a prosthetic valve or a heart transplant. It is not necessary to use an antibiotic mouthwash.

🗝️ CN: Health promotion and maintenance;
CL: Create

72. 2. Most cardiac surgical clients have median sternotomy incisions, which take about 3 months to heal. Measures that promote healing include avoiding heavy lifting, performing muscle reconditioning exercises, and using caution when driving. Showering or bathing is allowed as long as the incision is well approximated with no open areas or drainage. Activities should be gradually resumed on discharge.

CN: Safety and infection control; CL: Evaluate

73. 1. Verbalized concerns from this client may stem from anxiety over the changes in the body after open-heart surgery. Although the client may experience depression related to altered health status or may have a lack of knowledge regarding the postoperative course, the client is pointing out the changes in the body image. The client is not concerned about altered tissue perfusion.

CN: Psychosocial integrity; CL: Analyze

The Adult with Hypertension

74. 1. The effect of a beta-blocker is a decrease in heart rate, contractility, and afterload, which leads to a decrease in blood pressure. The client may have an initial increase in fatigue when starting the beta-blocker. The mechanism of action does not improve blood sugar or urine output.

CN: Pharmacological and parenteral therapies; CL: Evaluate

75. -/+ 1, 3, 5. Clonidine is a central-acting adrenergic antagonist. It reduces sympathetic outflow from the central nervous system. Dry mouth, impotence, and sleep disturbances are possible adverse effects. Hyperkalemia and pancreatitis are not anticipated with the use of this drug.

CN: Pharmacological and parenteral therapies; CL: Apply

76. 200 mcg

First, calculate the number of milligrams per milliliter:

$$0.2 \text{ mg} \times \frac{1,000 \text{ mcg}}{1 \text{ mg}} = 200 \text{ mcg}$$

Next, calculate the number of micrograms in each milliliter:

$$\frac{1,200 \text{ units}}{1 \text{ hour}} \div \frac{50 \text{ units}}{1 \text{ mL}}$$

$$= \frac{\overset{24}{\cancel{1,200}} \text{ units}}{1 \text{ hour}} \times \frac{1 \text{ mL}}{\underset{1}{\cancel{50}} \text{ units}} = 24 \text{ mL/h}$$

CN: Pharmacological and parenteral therapies; CL: Apply

77. 1. Furosemide is a diuretic often prescribed for clients with hypertension or heart failure; the drug should not affect a client's ability to drive safely. Furosemide may cause orthostatic hypotension, and clients should be instructed to be careful when changing from supine to sitting to standing position. Diuretics should be taken in the morning if possible to prevent sleep disturbance due to the need to get up to void. Furosemide is a loop diuretic that is not potassium sparing; clients should take potassium supplements as prescribed and have their serum potassium levels checked at prescribed intervals.

CN: Pharmacological and parenteral therapies; CL: Evaluate

78. -/+ 2, 3. Changing positions slowly and avoiding long periods of standing may limit the occurrence of orthostatic hypotension. Scheduling regular medication times is important for blood pressure management, but this aspect is not related to the development of orthostatic hypotension. Excessive alcohol intake and hot baths are associated with vasodilation.

CN: Reduction of risk potential; CL: Create

79. 1. Atenolol is a beta-adrenergic antagonist indicated for the management of hypertension. Sudden discontinuation of this drug is dangerous because it may exacerbate symptoms. The medication should not be discontinued without a prescription. Blood pressure needs to be monitored more frequently than annually in a client who is newly diagnosed and treated for hypertension. Clients are not usually placed on a 2-g sodium diet for hypertension.

CN: Pharmacological and parenteral therapies; CL: Synthesize

80. 3. Processed and cured meat products, such as cold cuts, ham, and hot dogs, are all high in fat and sodium and should be avoided on a low-calorie, low-fat, low-salt diet. Dietary restrictions of all types are complex and difficult to implement with clients who are basically without symptoms.

CN: Basic care and comfort; CL: Apply

81. -/+ 1, 2, 4, 6. Metoprolol is a beta-adrenergic blocker indicated for hypertension, angina, and myocardial infarction. The tablets should be taken with food at the same time each day; they should not be chewed or crushed. The HCP should be notified if the pulse falls below 50 bpm for several days. Blood glucose should be checked regularly during therapy since increased episodes of hypoglycemia may occur. It may mask evidence of hypoglycemia such as palpitations, tachycardia, and tremor. The use of any over-the-counter decongestants, asthma and cold remedies, and herbal preparations must be avoided. Fainting spells may occur due to exercise or stress, and the dosage of the drug may need to be reduced or discontinued.

 CN: Pharmacological and parenteral therapies; CL: Create

82. -/+ **1, 2, 3, 5.** Chlorothiazide causes increased urination and decreased swelling (if there is edema) and weight loss. It is important to check and record weight two to three times per week at the same time of day with a similar amount of clothing. Clients should not drink alcoholic beverages or take other medications without the approval of the health care provider (HCP). Reducing sodium intake in the diet helps diuretic drugs be more effective and allows smaller doses to be taken. Smaller doses are less likely to cause adverse effects, and therefore excessive table salt, as well as salty foods, should be avoided. Chlorothiazide is a diuretic that is prescribed for lower blood pressure and may cause dizziness and faintness when the client stands up suddenly. This can be prevented or decreased by changing positions slowly. If dizziness is severe, the HCP must be notified. Diuretics may cause sensitivity to sunlight, hence the need to avoid prolonged exposure to sunlight, use sunscreens, and wear protective clothing. Chlorothiazide causes increased urination and must be taken early in the day to decrease nighttime trips to the bathroom. Fewer bathroom trips mean less interference with sleep and less risk for falls. The client should not change the dosage without consulting the HCP.

 CN: Pharmacological and parenteral therapies; CL: Evaluate

83. 3. A plan to reduce or stop smoking begins with establishing the client's personal daily smoking pattern and activities associated with smoking. It is important that the client understands the associated health and environmental risks, but this knowledge has not been shown to help clients change their smoking behavior.

 CN: Psychosocial integrity; CL: Synthesize

84. 3. In most instances, clients with hypertension require lifelong treatment, and their hypertension cannot be managed successfully without changes in health behavior. The client must first commit to making these long-term changes. The changes will involve taking medications, stopping smoking, and losing weight, but the client must first accept the need for lifelong management and establish a vision and plan to control the hypertension.

 CN: Psychosocial integrity; CL: Synthesize

The Adult with Atrial Fibrillation and Other Dysrhythmias

85. 2, 1, 3, 4. To decrease myocardial workload and promote timely intervention, the client should be assisted to the bed. Assessing vital signs provides the data needed to determine client tolerance. Early initiation of IV access will enable timely medication administration if it is urgently needed. Although a 12-lead electrocardiogram is needed, it can be obtained after the IV is initiated.

 CN: Physiological adaptation; CL: Synthesize

86. -/+ **1, 2, 3.** Warfarin is an anticoagulant used in clients with atrial fibrillation to reduce the risk for stroke or systemic embolization and, therefore, will put the client at risk for bleeding. The nurse should instruct the client to watch for signs of bleeding and prevent bruising. While good oral hygiene remains important, the nurse would advise against vigorous flossing and irritating the gums as it may increase the risk for bleeding. Warfarin does not affect the heart rate.

 CN: Pharmacological and parenteral therapies; CL: Synthesis

87. -/+ **3, 4, 6.** Because abnormalities in electrolytes are likely to affect the depolarization and repolarization of cardiac cells, it is most important for the nurse to monitor sodium, potassium, and calcium levels. The blood urea nitrogen is within normal range. Hemoglobin and hematocrit are not generally associated with cardiac dysrhythmias; the hemoglobin is within normal range. The PT and INR would be monitored closely on a client taking warfarin, not necessarily a client with cardiac dysrhythmia; the PT and INR are within normal range.

 CN: Physiological adaptation; CL: Synthesis

88. 1. The client is showing signs of pneumothorax, a potential complication of pacemaker placement. The nurse should immediately assess the client's breath sounds and chest movement as this information will be important to share with the health care provider when notified. Assessing the insertion site and the client's blood pressure and pulse are important, but the nurse should first perform a focused respiratory assessment.

 CN: Physiological adaptation; CL: Synthesis

89. 3. The nurse first should prepare the defibrillator for synchronized cardioversion. The client is experiencing PSVT with a heart rate of 180 bpm. PSVT with a heart rate of 180 bpm causes a decrease in cardiac output. The client's vital signs and symptoms reveal the client is becoming hemodynamically unstable and require immediate intervention. Atropine is not a treatment for PSVT. CPR is not indicated for PSVT. Caffeine use can contribute to PSVT, but the client requires defibrillation now.

🗝️ CN: Physiological adaptation; CL: Analysis

90. 🔢 **2, 4, 5.** This electrocardiogram strip indicates the client has atrial fibrillation. There is no P wave and PR interval; these are replaced with fine wavy lines. In atrial fibrillation, the ventricular rate may be normal, slow, or fast. Clients with atrial fibrillation may have palpitations secondary to a fast and irregular atrial rhythm. Because atrial fibrillation also may result in a sudden decrease in cardiac output, the client may also experience light-headedness and shortness of breath. A carotid bruit, nausea, and a systolic murmur are not manifestations of new-onset atrial fibrillation.

🗝️ CN: Physiological adaptation; CL: Analyze

91. 3. The nurse should contact the health care provider to request a stat electrocardiogram to verify the change in rhythm. The cardiac rhythm and fast heart rate may predispose the client to decreased cardiac output. Administering an antianxiety medication may calm the client but does not effectively treat the problem of an irregular rhythm. Rechecking the pulse later leaves the problem unaddressed. A chest x-ray may be helpful, but it is not the priority at this time.

🗝️ CN: Physiological adaptation; CL: Synthesis

92. 4. The purpose of EPS is to study the heart's electrical system. During this invasive procedure, a special wire is introduced into the heart to produce dysrhythmia. To prepare for this procedure, the client should be NPO for 6 to 8 hours before the test, and all antiarrhythmic medications are held for at least 24 hours before the test to study the dysrhythmia without the influence of medications. Because the client's verbal responses to the rhythm changes are extremely important, sedation is avoided if possible.

🗝️ CN: Physiological integrity; CL: Create

93. 2. Characteristics of atrial fibrillation include a pulse rate higher than 100 bpm, a totally irregular rhythm, and no definite P waves on the electrocardiogram. During assessment, the nurse is likely to note the irregular rate and should report it to the HCP. A weak, thready pulse is characteristic of a client in shock. Two regular beats followed by an irregular beat may indicate a premature ventricular contraction.

🗝️ CN: Reduction of risk potential; CL: Analyze

94. 🔢 **1, 5.** The nurse must teach the client how to take and record the pulse daily. The client should be instructed to avoid lifting the operative-side arm above shoulder level for 1 week after insertion. It takes up to 2 months for the incision site to heal and for full range of motion to return. The client should avoid heavy lifting until approved by the health care provider. The pacemaker metal casing does not set off airport security alarms, so there are no travel restrictions. Prolonged immobilization is not required. Microwave ovens are safe to use and do not alter pacemaker function.

🗝️ CN: Physiological adaptation; CL: Create

95. 1. Transcutaneous pacemaker therapy provides an adequate heart rate to a client in an emergency situation. Defibrillation and a lidocaine infusion are not indicated for the treatment of third-degree heart block. Transcutaneous pacing is used temporarily until a transvenous or permanent pacemaker can be inserted.

🗝️ CN: Physiological adaptation; CL: Synthesize

96. 1, 3, 4, 2. Because atrial fibrillation causes a decrease in cardiac output, the heart rate increases in response to this drop. As a result of an increased heart rate, the oxygen demands of the heart increase. It is important for oxygen to be administered first to help compensate for the increased oxygen demand and cardiac workload. Placing the client on a cardiac monitor will help confirm a diagnosis of atrial fibrillation. Performing vital signs will determine the client's response to the abnormal rhythm and responses to treatment. If the rhythm is determined to be atrial fibrillation, it will be necessary for an IV to be inserted so medication can be administered.

🗝️ CN: Physiological integrity; CL: Synthesize

97. 3. The spouse can have physical contact with the client, but if the ICD were to discharge while the spouse had contact with the client, the spouse would feel a "tingle" but would not be harmed. There is no warning device on the ICD.

🗝️ CN: Health promotion and maintenance; CL: Synthesize

98. 2. Maintaining cardiac conduction stability to prevent arrhythmias is a priority immediately after artificial pacemaker implantation. The client should have continuous electrocardiographic monitoring until proper pacemaker functioning is verified. Skin integrity, while important, is not an immediate concern. The pacemaker is used to increase heart rate and cardiac output, not decrease it. The client should limit activity for the first 24 to 48 hours after pacemaker insertion. The client should also restrict movement of the affected extremity for 24 hours.

🔑 CN: Physiological adaptation; CL: Synthesize

99. **3.** Education is a major component of the discharge plan for a client with an artificial pacemaker. The client with a permanent pacemaker needs to be able to state specific information about safety precautions, such as to refrain from lifting more than 3 lb (1.35 kg) or stretching and bending. The client should know how to count the pulse and do so daily or as instructed by the health care provider. The client will not necessarily be placed on a low-cholesterol diet. The client should resume activities and does not need to remain on bed rest. The client should know the signs and symptoms of an MI but is not at risk because of the pacemaker.

🔑 CN: Physiological adaptation; CL: Evaluate

100. **1, 3, 4.** The client has atrial fibrillation and will have an irregular pulse and will commonly be tachycardic, with rapid ventricular responses (heart rates) typically in the 110 to 140 bpm range, but rarely over 150 to 170 bpm. The goal of treatment is the restoration of sinus rhythm. With a heart rate higher than 150 bpm and symptoms such as shortness of breath, dizziness, syncope, and chest pain, synchronized cardioversion will most likely be the treatment of choice. With more controlled heart rates and more minor signs and symptoms, chemical conversion with drugs such as diltiazem and digoxin prior to other interventions such as synchronized cardioversion with appropriate anticoagulation may be attempted. Because of the decreased cardiac output, monitoring is essential. Obtaining consent for cardioversion requires a prescription from a health care provider, but with the current heart rate, having cardioversion is a very strong possibility for this client. Defibrillation is used for ventricular fibrillation, not atrial fibrillation. Teaching the client about warfarin will be a possibility but not an immediate intervention. Clients in continued atrial fibrillation usually require some form of anticoagulation. Drawing labs for CBCs to detect anemia or infection, thyroid function studies (to determine thyrotoxicosis, a rare, but not-to-be-missed cause, especially in older adults), serum electrolytes, and blood urea nitrogen/creatinine (looking for electrolyte disturbances or renal failure) are commonly drawn for to determine the cause of atrial fibrillation; they are not an immediate action.

🔑 CN: Physiological adaptation; CL: Synthesize

The Adult Requiring Rapid Response or Cardiopulmonary Resuscitation

101. **3.** Transcutaneous pads should be placed on the client with a third-degree heart block. For a client who is symptomatic, transcutaneous pacing is the treatment of choice. The hemodynamic stability and pulse should be assessed prior to calling a code or initiating CPR. Defibrillation is performed for ventricular fibrillation or ventricular tachycardia with no pulse.

🔑 CN: Management of care; CL: Synthesize

102. **3.** This electrocardiogram strip indicates the client has ventricular tachycardia. The nurse should first check the client for the presence of a pulse. The presence of a pulse determines the treatment for ventricular tachycardia. It is also important to assess the client's heart rate and level of consciousness. Cardioversion may be used to treat hemodynamically unstable tachycardias. Assessment of instability is required before cardioversion. It is not appropriate to begin CPR unless the pulse is absent. Defibrillation is used to treat ventricular fibrillation or pulseless ventricular tachycardia.

🔑 CN: Physiological adaptation; CL: Synthesize

103. **2.** Pupillary reaction is the best indication of whether oxygenated blood has been reaching the client's brain. Pupils that remain widely dilated and do not react to light may indicate a lack of oxygenation and that serious brain damage may have occurred. The pulse rate may be normal, mucous membranes may still be pink, and systolic blood pressure may be 80 mm Hg or higher, yet there can be inadequate oxygenation to the brain.

🔑 CN: Reduction of risk potential; CL: Evaluate

104. **3.** Amiodarone is used for the treatment of premature ventricular contractions, ventricular tachycardia with a pulse, atrial fibrillation, and atrial flutter. Amiodarone is not used as initial therapy for a pulseless dysrhythmia.

🔑 CN: Pharmacological and parenteral therapies; CL: Evaluate

105. **4.** If the chest wall is not rising with rescue breaths, the head should be repositioned first to ensure that the airway is adequately opened. A bag mask device allows for delivery of 100% oxygen but is difficult to manage if there is just one rescuer; ideally, two persons are used to operate the bag mask device, one to maintain the

106. 1. The exhalation phase of ventilation is a passive activity that occurs during CPR as part of the normal relaxation of the victim's chest. No action by the rescuer is necessary.

CN: Reduction of risk potential; CL: Apply

107. 2. After a person is without cardiopulmonary function for 4 to 6 minutes, permanent brain damage is almost certain. To prevent permanent brain damage, it is important to begin cardiopulmonary resuscitation promptly after cardiopulmonary arrest.

CN: Reduction of risk potential; CL: Apply

108. 2. The Heimlich maneuver should be administered only to a victim who cannot make *any* sounds due to airway obstruction. If the victim can whisper words or cough, some air exchange is occurring, and the emergency medical system should be called instead of attempting the Heimlich maneuver. Cyanosis may accompany or follow choking; however, the Heimlich maneuver should only be initiated when the victim cannot speak.

CN: Reduction of risk potential; CL: Apply

109. 4. The thrusts should be delivered below the xiphoid process, but above the umbilicus, to minimize the risk for internal injuries.

CN: Reduction of risk potential; CL: Apply

110. 2. The priority action is to assess the client and determine whether the rhythm is life-threatening. More information, including vital signs, should be obtained, and the nurse should notify the HCP. A bolus of lidocaine may be prescribed to treat this arrhythmia. This is not a code-type situation unless the client has been determined to be in a life-threatening situation.

CN: Physiological adaptation; CL: Synthesize

111. 1, 2, 4, 5. Vital signs give an important initial assessment of this client's status. The client may experience burns from the patches and current used for the cardioversion. Therefore, it is important to assess the skin of the chest wall for redness or burns. Because conscious sedation is used for this procedure, assessing the client's level of consciousness also is an important initial step. Attaching the client to cardiac monitoring is also important to assess rhythm abnormalities. There is no arterial puncture associated with the procedure.

CN: Reduction of risk potential; CL: Synthesize

112. 4. The paddles are in the correct position. The nurse can push the shock button to defibrillate the client.

CN: Physiological adaptation; CL: Apply

113. 2. The rapid response team should be called immediately to evaluate and treat the client. There is no indication at this time for manual ventilations or chest compressions. If the family is not interfering in client care, it can be reassuring to the family to see that all possible care is being provided.

CN: Management of care; CL: Synthesize

Managing Care, Quality, and Safety for Adults with Cardiac Health Problems

114. 2, 4, 3, 1. Even though the chest pain experienced by client 2 is resolved, it was recent and requires reassessment. Client 4 is scheduled to leave for major surgery very soon. The nurse should check this client and the client's chart and make certain that everything is ready so as to not delay the surgery. Client 3 has scheduled medications for blood pressure control. While the client is not experiencing any acute problems, this medication should be administered as scheduled. Client 1 is stable at this time and can be seen last.

CN: Management of care; CL: Create

115. 1, 2, 4, 5, 6. The nurse must have assessment data and verify vital signs if necessary to determine the action that is required. If there is a significant change in the client's condition, the charge nurse should be notified to help the nurse with both this client and the nurse's other assigned clients if necessary; most acute care facilities have a rapid response team that can also help assess and intervene with basic standing prescriptions if necessary. Positioning the client in semi-Fowler's is a nursing action that may assist in breathing and relieve shortness of breath. It is important for the nurse to reassure the client by staying calm and remaining with the client. The nurse must notify the HCP about the change in the client's condition; the nurse must have all information available and present it in a concise and accurate manner using SBAR format including a recommendation for treatment if indicated. The nurse should stay with this client and delegate checking on other assigned clients to the charge nurse or UAP.

 CN: Management of care; CL: Synthesize

116. -/+ **2, 6.** The nurse should conduct a focused assessment to quickly determine the reason for the client's change in weight and blood pressure. The client has gained 5 lb (2.3 kg) in 3 days, and the blood pressure has increased over the last 3 days. The client is exhibiting signs of heart failure, and if the client is short of breath, this is another sign. The nurse should determine if the client is taking the prescribed medications, and if the client is not taking the medication as prescribed to manage the heart failure, the nurse should obtain additional information to find out why the client is not taking the medication. Asking how the client is feeling is too general; a more focused question will quickly determine the client's current health status. The client should calibrate the scales periodically, but the rapid weight gain along with the increased blood pressure is likely not due to the scales, fluid intake, or the arm used to take the blood pressure. The client is not taking a diuretic and likely has an intake and output within normal limits.

 CJ: Standalone trend; CL: Apply

117. 4. The goals of managing clients outside of the hospital are for the clients to maintain health and prevent readmission; thus, interventions, such as monitoring and teaching, appear to have contributed to the low readmission rate in this group of clients. Although it is important that clients view educational material, continue to take their medication, and avoid gaining weight, the primary indicator of the effectiveness of the program is the lack of rehospitalization.

 CN: Management of care; CL: Evaluate

118. 3. Using an individualized, printed checklist ensures that all key information is reported; the checklist can then serve as a record to which nurses can refer later. Giving a verbal report leaves room for error in memory; using an audiotape or a medical record requires nurses to spend unnecessary time retrieving information.

 CN: Management of care; CL: Evaluate

119. -/+ **4, 5.** Performing vital signs and obtaining intake and output are tasks that can be delegated to UAP. Assessing pedal pulses and administering medications and oxygen are skills that require nursing judgment.

 CN: Management of care; CL: Analyze

120. 3. The client who has just returned from having a stent placed in a coronary artery should be seen first. The nurse should assess this client to establish a baseline. Risks associated with a stent placement include reocclusion, cardiac tamponade, dysrhythmias, bleeding, and thrombosis. Although a new onset of atrial fibrillation is a concern, this client's heart rate is less than 100 bpm and is not showing signs of being hemodynamically unstable. A client with a history of sinus rhythm who will receive a beta-blocker is not a higher priority. While a client with stable angina who took sublingual nitroglycerine 30 minutes ago will need to be assessed frequently, there is no evidence to suggest this client is currently experiencing chest pain.

 CN: Management of care; CL: Analysis

TEST 2: The Adult with Vascular Disease

- The Adult with Peripheral Artery Disease
- The Adult with Peripheral Vascular Disease Having an Amputation
- The Adult with an Aneurysm
- The Adult with Raynaud Phenomenon
- The Adult with Peripheral Venous Disease: Thrombophlebitis, Deep Vein Thrombosis, and Embolus Formation
- The Adult with Varicose Veins
- The Adult with Stasis Ulcers
- Managing Care, Quality, and Safety for Adults with Vascular Disease
- Answers, Rationales, and Test-Taking Strategies

The Adult with Peripheral Artery Disease

1. The nurse is developing a teaching plan for a client with arterial insufficiency. What information should the nurse include in the plan? Select all that apply.
   - ☐ 1. Avoid smoking and exposure to the cold.
   - ☐ 2. Take acetaminophen if experiencing pain at night.
   - ☐ 3. Take aspirin or clopidogrel as prescribed.
   - ☐ 4. Use additional bedclothes at night.
   - ☐ 5. Wear tight socks to keep the feet warm.

2. A client is admitted for a revascularization procedure for arteriosclerosis in the left iliac artery. What should the nurse do to promote circulation in the extremities?
   - ☐ 1. Position the client on a firm mattress.
   - ☐ 2. Keep the involved extremity warm with blankets.
   - ☐ 3. Position the left leg at or below the body's horizontal plane.
   - ☐ 4. Encourage the client to raise and lower the leg four times every hour.

3. A sedentary, middle-age client with obesity is recovering from surgery to remove an embolus in the right iliac artery. The nurse should develop a discharge plan with the client that will focus on participating in which activities? Select all that apply.
   - ☐ 1. aerobic activity
   - ☐ 2. strength training
   - ☐ 3. weight control
   - ☐ 4. stress management
   - ☐ 5. wearing supportive athletic shoes

4. The nurse is assessing the pulse of a client with aortoiliac disease. On the illustration below, indicate the pulse site that will give the nurse the **most** useful data.

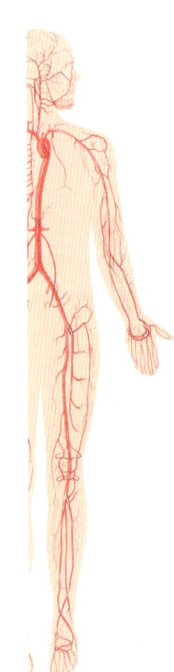

5. The nurse is assessing a 48-year-old client with a history of smoking. The client, who exercises regularly, reports having pain in the calf during exercise that disappears at rest. Which finding indicates that the nurse should further assess the client?
☐ 1. heart rate of 57 bpm
☐ 2. oxygen saturation (SpO$_2$) of 94% on room air
☐ 3. blood pressure of 134/82 mm Hg
☐ 4. ankle-brachial index of 0.65

6. A client with peripheral artery disease has undergone a right femoral-popliteal bypass graft. The blood pressure has decreased from 124/80 mm Hg to 88/62 mm Hg. What should the nurse assess **first**?
☐ 1. intravenous (IV) fluid infusion rate
☐ 2. pedal pulses
☐ 3. nasal cannula flow rate
☐ 4. capillary refill

7. A client taking warfarin has dry skin due to decreased arterial blood flow. What should the nurse instruct the client to do? Select all that apply.
☐ 1. Apply lanolin or petroleum jelly to intact skin.
☐ 2. Follow a reduced-calorie, reduced-fat diet.
☐ 3. Inspect the involved areas daily for new ulcerations.
☐ 4. Limit activities of daily living (ADLs).
☐ 5. Use an electric razor to shave.

8. The nurse is caring for a client with peripheral artery disease who has recently been prescribed clopidogrel. Which statement by the client indicates that the nurse should continue giving information to the client about this medication?
☐ 1. "I shouldn't be surprised if I bruise easier or if my gums bleed a little when brushing my teeth."
☐ 2. "It doesn't really matter if I take this medicine with or without food, whatever works best for my stomach."
☐ 3. "I should stop taking my medicine if it makes me feel weak and dizzy."
☐ 4. "The doctor prescribed this medicine to make my platelets less likely to stick together and help prevent clots from forming."

9. A client is receiving cilostazol for peripheral artery disease causing intermittent claudication. Which statement by the client indicates to the nurse that this medication is effective?
☐ 1. "I am having fewer aches and pains."
☐ 2. "I do not have headaches anymore."
☐ 3. "I am able to walk further without leg pain."
☐ 4. "My toes are turning grayish-black in color."

10. The client with peripheral artery disease reports both legs hurt when walking. What should the nurse instruct the client to do?
☐ 1. Avoid walking when the pain occurs.
☐ 2. Rest frequently with the legs elevated.
☐ 3. Wear support stockings.
☐ 4. Enroll in a supervised exercise training program.

11. The nurse is assessing a client with peripheral artery insufficiency. On the illustration below, where should the nurse palpate the client's pulse to identify tibioperoneal artery involvement on the right side of the body?

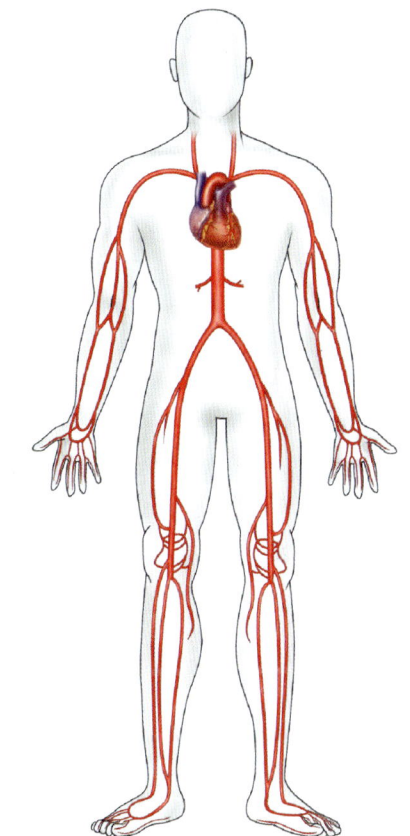

12. The nurse is obtaining the pulse of a client who had femoral-popliteal bypass surgery 6 hours ago (see below). Which assessment provides the **most** accurate information about the client's postoperative status?

☐ 1.
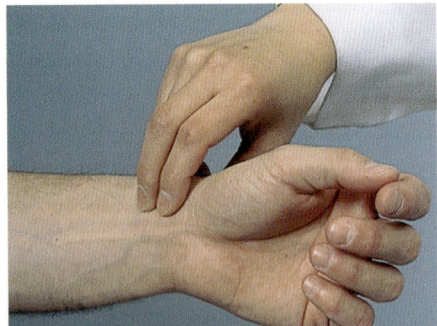

☐ 2.
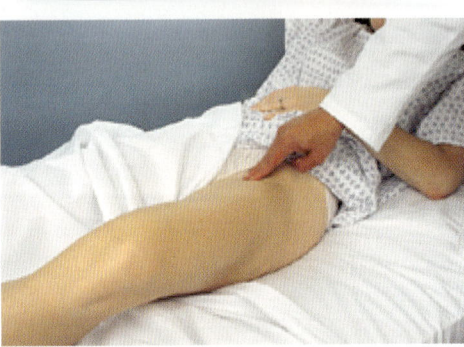

☐ 3.
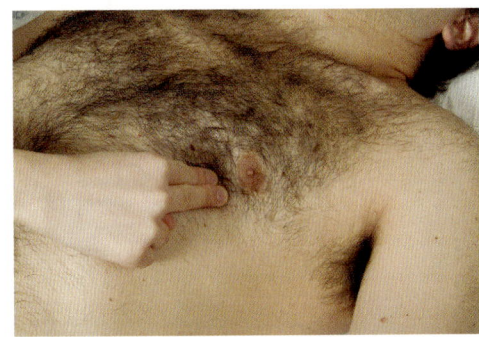

☐ 4.
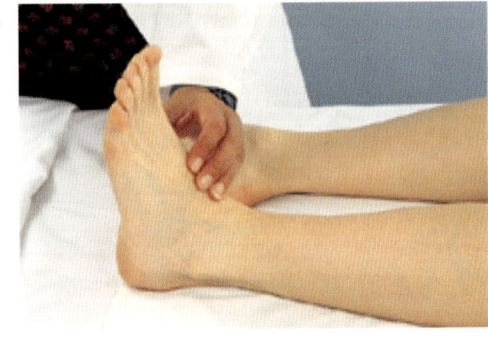

13. The nurse is assessing the lower extremities of a client with peripheral artery disease. Which finding(s) would be expected? Select all that apply.
☐ 1. hairy legs
☐ 2. mottled skin
☐ 3. pink skin
☐ 4. coolness
☐ 5. moist skin

14. The nurse is not able to palpate the left pedal pulses of a client with peripheral artery disease. What should the nurse do **first**?
☐ 1. Auscultate the pulses with a stethoscope.
☐ 2. Call the health care provider (HCP).
☐ 3. Use a Doppler ultrasound device.
☐ 4. Inspect the lower left extremity.

15. The nurse is assessing an individual with peripheral artery disease. Which finding indicates complete arterial obstruction in the lower left leg?
☐ 1. aching pain in the left calf
☐ 2. burning pain in the left calf
☐ 3. numbness and tingling in the left leg
☐ 4. coldness of the left foot and ankle

16. A client has returned to the surgical care unit after having femoral-popliteal bypass grafting. Place in order from first to last the findings the nurse should assess for this client. All options must be used.

| 1. postoperative pain |
| 2. peripheral pulses |
| 3. urine output |
| 4. incision site |
| |
| |
| |
| |

17. The nurse is assessing a client who has a history of peripheral artery disease. The nurse observes that the left great toe is black. The nurse determines that the black color is caused by which factor?
☐ 1. atrophy
☐ 2. contraction
☐ 3. gangrene
☐ 4. rubor

18. A client has peripheral artery disease of both lower extremities. The client tells the nurse, "I've really tried to manage my condition well." Which example indicates the client is using appropriate care management strategies?
☐ 1. The client rests with the legs elevated above the level of the heart.
☐ 2. The client walks slowly but steadily for 30 minutes twice a day.
☐ 3. The client limits activity to walking around the house.
☐ 4. The client wears antiembolism stockings at all times when out of bed.

19. A client is scheduled to have an arteriogram. During the arteriogram, the client reports having nausea, tingling, and dyspnea. What should the nurse do **first**?
- ☐ 1. Administer epinephrine.
- ☐ 2. Inform the health care provider (HCP).
- ☐ 3. Administer oxygen.
- ☐ 4. Inform the client that the procedure is almost over.

20. A client who has been diagnosed with peripheral artery disease (PVD) is being discharged. What statement by the client indicates the client needs further instruction?
- ☐ 1. "I won't use a heating pad."
- ☐ 2. "I'll sit in a chair with both of my legs on the floor."
- ☐ 3. "I'll wear leather shoes when I'm out of bed.
- ☐ 4. "I should wipe any injury with iodine on a cotton ball."

21. A client with peripheral artery disease has femoral-popliteal bypass surgery. What goal should the nurse establish with the client **immediately** after surgery?
- ☐ 1. Maintain circulation.
- ☐ 2. Prevent infection.
- ☐ 3. Relieve pain.
- ☐ 4. Provide education.

22. The nurse is instructing a client who is at risk for peripheral artery disease on how to use knee-length elastic stockings (support hose). What instruction(s) should the nurse include in the teaching plan? Select all that apply.
- ☐ 1. Apply the elastic stockings before getting out of bed.
- ☐ 2. Remove the stockings if swelling occurs.
- ☐ 3. Remove the stockings every 8 hours, elevate the feet, and reapply in 15 minutes.
- ☐ 4. Once the stockings have been pulled over the calf, roll the remaining stocking down to make a cuff.
- ☐ 5. Keep the stockings in place for 48 hours, and reapply using a clean pair of stockings.

23. A client is scheduled to undergo right axillary-to-axillary artery bypass surgery tomorrow. Before surgery, what action should the nurse take?
- ☐ 1. Assess the temperature in the right arm.
- ☐ 2. Monitor the radial pulse in the right arm.
- ☐ 3. Protect the right arm from cold.
- ☐ 4. Avoid using the right arm for venipuncture.

24. One goal in caring for a client with arterial occlusive disease is to promote vasodilation in the affected extremity. What should the nurse instruct the client to do to achieve this goal?
- ☐ 1. Avoid eating low-fat foods.
- ☐ 2. Elevate the legs above the heart.
- ☐ 3. Stop smoking.
- ☐ 4. Jog daily.

25. The nurse is caring for a client with peripheral artery disease (PAD) who has just returned from having a percutaneous transluminal balloon angioplasty. Which of these findings require **immediate** action from the nurse?
- ☐ 1. a change in the intensity of the pulse from the baseline
- ☐ 2. pain "2 out of 10" at the catheterization site
- ☐ 3. shiny skin and a hairless appearance on the affected leg
- ☐ 4. the presence of an ulcer on the limb of the catheterization site

26. The nurse is developing a care plan for a client who had a left femoral-popliteal bypass yesterday. Which instruction(s) should be included in the care plan? Select all that apply.
- ☐ 1. Turn frequently, and use pillows to support the incision.
- ☐ 2. Encourage the client to change positions frequently to prevent atelectasis.
- ☐ 3. Place the left leg in a knee-flexed position to promote oxygenation.
- ☐ 4. Place the client in a supine position, and elevate the leg above the heart to prevent edema.
- ☐ 5. Encourage the client to walk short distances to promote circulation.
- ☐ 6. Encourage the client to maintain bed rest to prevent stress on the suture line.

27. A client with peripheral artery disease has been prescribed diltiazem. To determine the effectiveness of this medication, the nurse should evaluate the client for which intended outcome?
- ☐ 1. decreased anxiety
- ☐ 2. prolonged sleep
- ☐ 3. cooler extremities
- ☐ 4. improved blood flow

28. A client is receiving cilostazol for intermittent claudication. What should the nurse ask the client to determine the effectiveness of the drug?
- ☐ 1. "Do you have less pain in the legs?"
- ☐ 2. "Can you wiggle your toes?"
- ☐ 3. "Are you urinating more frequently?"
- ☐ 4. "Do you experience less dizziness?"

29. A client with peripheral artery disease is recovering from surgery to insert an aortofemoral-popliteal bypass graft. When developing a postoperative education plan, the nurse understands that which question will provide the **most** helpful information?
- ☐ 1. "How did you manage your health before admission?"
- ☐ 2. "How far could you walk without pain before surgery?"
- ☐ 3. "What is your home environment like?"
- ☐ 4. "Do you have problems with urine retention?"

30. A client with peripheral artery disease and a history of hypertension is to be discharged on a low-fat, low-cholesterol, low-sodium diet. Which should be the nurse's **first** step in planning the dietary instructions?
    ☐ 1. Determine the client's knowledge level about cholesterol.
    ☐ 2. Ask the client to name foods high in fat, cholesterol, and salt.
    ☐ 3. Explain the importance of complying with the diet.
    ☐ 4. Assess the family's food preferences.

The Adult with Peripheral Vascular Disease Having an Amputation

31. While the nurse is providing preoperative teaching for a client with peripheral vascular disease who is to have a below-the-knee amputation, the client says, "I hate the idea of being an invalid after they cut off my leg." What would be the nurse's **most** therapeutic response?
    ☐ 1. "Focusing on using your one good leg will make your recovery easier."
    ☐ 2. "Tell me more about how you are feeling."
    ☐ 3. "We will talk more about this after your surgery."
    ☐ 4. "You are fortunate to have a spouse who can take care of you."

32. The client asks the nurse, "Why can't the doctor tell me exactly how much of my leg they're going to take off? Don't you think I should know that?" What information should the nurse use to answer the client's question?
    The decision about the level of the amputation depends on:
    ☐ 1. the need to remove as much of the leg as possible.
    ☐ 2. the adequacy of the blood supply to the tissues.
    ☐ 3. the ease with which a prosthesis can be fitted.
    ☐ 4. the method used to fit a prosthesis.

33. A client has undergone an amputation of three toes and a femoral-popliteal bypass. The nurse should teach the client that after surgery, which leg position is contraindicated while sitting in a chair?
    ☐ 1. crossing the legs
    ☐ 2. elevating the legs
    ☐ 3. flexing the ankles
    ☐ 4. extending the knees

34. The nurse is assessing a client after an above-the-knee amputation and notes that blood has saturated through the distal part of the dressing. What should the nurse do **immediately**?
    ☐ 1. Apply a tourniquet.
    ☐ 2. Assess vital signs.
    ☐ 3. Call the health care provider (HCP).
    ☐ 4. Elevate the involved extremity with a large pillow.

35. The client has had a below-the-knee amputation secondary to arterial occlusive disease. The nurse is instructing the client about residual limb care. Which statement by the client indicates that the client understands how to implement the plan of care?
    ☐ 1. "I should inspect the incision carefully when I change the dressing every other day."
    ☐ 2. "I should wash the incision, dry it, and apply moisturizing lotion daily."
    ☐ 3. "I should rewrap the stump as often as needed."
    ☐ 4. "I should elevate the stump on pillows to decrease swelling."

The Adult with an Aneurysm

36. The nurse is developing a discharge teaching plan for a client who had a graft insertion for an abdominal aortic aneurysm 4 days ago. The nurse reviews the client's chart for information about the client's history. See the chart below.

History and Physical
1. Smokes four cigars a month.
2. Vital signs: blood pressure, ranges from 150/76–170/98 mm Hg; heart rate, 90–100 bpm; respirations, 12–18 bpm; temperature, 99.9°F (37.8°C).
3. +1 bilateral ankle edema.

    Based on the data and expected outcomes, what should the nurse emphasize in the teaching plan?
    ☐ 1. food intake
    ☐ 2. fluid volume
    ☐ 3. skin integrity
    ☐ 4. tissue perfusion

37. A client is admitted with a 6.5-cm thoracic aneurysm. The nurse records findings from the initial assessment in the client's chart, as shown below.

Vital Signs	
Date	05/07
Time	1000
Blood pressure	160/90 mm Hg
Heart rate	74 bpm
Respiratory rate	20/min

    At 1030, the client has sharp midchest pain after having a bowel movement. What should the nurse do **first**?
    ☐ 1. Assess the client's vital signs.
    ☐ 2. Administer pain medication as prescribed.
    ☐ 3. Assess the client's neurologic status.
    ☐ 4. Contact the health care provider (HCP).

38. A client with an enlarged abdominal aorta admitted to the emergency department has severe back pain, nausea, blood pressure of 90/40 mm Hg, a heart rate of 128 bpm, and a respiration rate of 28 breaths/min. In which order from first to last should the nurse implement these prescriptions? All options must be used.

1. Monitor intake and output.

2. Establish an intravenous infusion.

3. Administer pain medication.

4. Insert a nasogastric tube.

39. A client with a ruptured aneurysm is to have surgery to insert a graft. The surgeon has explained the procedure to the client, but the client is not ready to sign the surgical consent form. What should the nurse do **next**?
 ☐ 1. Notify the surgeon.
 ☐ 2. Ask if the client wants to speak with a religious advisor.
 ☐ 3. Cancel the surgery.
 ☐ 4. Ask if the client wants to speak with someone else about the surgery.

40. A client had a repair of a thoracoabdominal aneurysm 2 days ago. Which finding should the nurse consider unexpected and report to the health care provider **immediately**?
 ☐ 1. abdominal pain at 5 on a scale of 0 to 10 for the last 2 days
 ☐ 2. heart rate of 100 bpm after ambulating 200 feet (0.06 km)
 ☐ 3. urine output of 2000 mL in 24 hours
 ☐ 4. weakness and numbness in the lower extremities

41. A client is admitted to the emergency department with severe abdominal pain. A radiograph reveals a large abdominal aortic aneurysm. What is the nurse's **primary** goal at this time?
 ☐ 1. Maintain circulation.
 ☐ 2. Manage pain.
 ☐ 3. Prepare the client for emergency surgery.
 ☐ 4. Teach postoperative breathing exercises.

42. A client has sudden, severe pain in the back and chest, accompanied by shortness of breath. The client describes the pain as a "tearing" sensation. The health care provider suspects the client is experiencing a dissecting aortic aneurysm. The nurse should assess the client for which potential complication of a dissecting aneurysm?
 ☐ 1. cardiac tamponade
 ☐ 2. stroke
 ☐ 3. pulmonary edema
 ☐ 4. myocardial infarction

43. The nurse is planning care for a client who has just returned to the medical-surgical unit following repair of an aortic aneurysm. The nurse should assess which effect of the surgery **first**?
 ☐ 1. decreased urinary output
 ☐ 2. electrolyte imbalance
 ☐ 3. anxiety
 ☐ 4. wound infection

44. A client underwent surgery to repair an abdominal aortic aneurysm. The surgeon made an incision that extends from the xiphoid process to the pubis. At 1200 hours 2 days after surgery, the client has abdominal distention. The nurse checks the progress notes in the client's medical record, as shown below.

Nurse's Notes		
Date	Time	Progress Notes
07/07	2200	The client is receiving D$_5$W 1000 mL every 8 h. The NG tube is attached to low suction and draining well. The client has been NPO except ice chips. The client has had 10 mg morphine for pain at 0600.

What is **most** likely contributing to the client's abdominal distention?
 ☐ 1. nasogastric (NG) tube
 ☐ 2. ice chips
 ☐ 3. intravenous (IV) fluid intake
 ☐ 4. morphine

45. A client is discharged after an aortic aneurysm repair with a synthetic graft to replace part of the aorta. The nurse should instruct the client to notify the health care provider (HCP) before having which procedure?
 ☐ 1. blood drawn
 ☐ 2. an intravenous (IV) line inserted
 ☐ 3. tooth extraction
 ☐ 4. an x-ray examination

46. The nurse is assessing a client who had an abdominal aortic aneurysm repair 2 hours ago. Which finding warrants further evaluation?
 ☐ 1. absent bowel sounds and mild abdominal distension
 ☐ 2. a blood urea nitrogen (BUN) level of 26 mg/dL (26 mmol/L) and creatinine level of 1.2 mg/dL (1.2 μmol/L)
 ☐ 3. an arterial blood pressure of 80/50 mm Hg
 ☐ 4. +1 pedal pulses in the bilateral lower extremities

47. The nurse is planning care for a client who had an abdominal aortic aneurysm repair 3 days ago. The nurse is reviewing the progress notes below.

Nurse's Notes

Date	Time	Progress Notes
2/20	0900	Temperature is 98.2°F (36.8 C); Pulse is 138; BP is 86/44 mm Hg; CVP is 2 mm Hg
2/20	1100	Urine output is 20 mL/h for the last 2 hours; Hgb is 7.8 g/dL, IV of D51/2 normal saline is infusing at 7t cc/h

Two units of packed red blood cells (PRBCs) have been prescribed for transfusion. What should the nurse do **first**?
☐ 1. Administer furosemide.
☐ 2. Increase the drip rate of intravenous (IV) fluids.
☐ 3. Initiate a dopamine drip.
☐ 4. Transfuse PRBCs.

The Adult with Raynaud Phenomenon

48. A client has been diagnosed with Raynaud phenomenon on the tip of the nose and fingertips. The health care provider has prescribed reserpine to determine if the client will obtain relief. The client often works outside in cold weather and also smokes two packs of cigarettes per day. The nurse should include which instruction(s) in the discharge plan for this client? Select all that apply.
☐ 1. Stop smoking.
☐ 2. Wear a face covering and gloves in the winter.
☐ 3. Place fingertips in cool water to rewarm them.
☐ 4. Find employment that can be done in a warm environment.
☐ 5. Report signs of orthostatic hypotension.

49. A nurse assesses a client with Raynaud phenomenon involving the right hand. The nurse records the information in the progress notes, as shown below. From these findings, what should the nurse **first** instruct the client how to manage?

Nurse's Notes

Date	Time	Progress Notes
06/10	1500	The client has a palpable but faint right radial pulse. Capillary refill on all five digits < 8s. No observable swelling. The client is reporting numbness in the tips of all five digits. The skin is warm, dry, and red.

☐ 1. acute pain
☐ 2. numbness
☐ 3. lack of circulation
☐ 4. potential for skin breakdown

50. A client has Raynaud phenomenon. What information should the nurse include in a teaching plan about managing an attack? Select all that apply.
☐ 1. Go to a warm room.
☐ 2. Move the fingers and toes.
☐ 3. Place hands under hot, running water.
☐ 4. Massage the fingers and toes.
☐ 5. Place hands under the armpits.

51. A client with Raynaud phenomenon has a skin ulcer on the forearm. The skin surrounding the ulcer is dry. The health care provider prescribed nitroglycerine cream. What should the nurse instruct the client about the purpose of nitroglycerine?
☐ 1. It treats pain.
☐ 2. It prevents infection.
☐ 3. It promotes healing.
☐ 4. It softens the surrounding skin.

52. The nurse is teaching a client who has been diagnosed with Raynaud phenomenon how to prevent a vasospastic attack. What information should the nurse include in the teaching plan? Select all that apply.
☐ 1. Avoid sudden changes in temperatures.
☐ 2. Wear hand splints to limit constricting movements of the fingers.
☐ 3. Wear warm clothing when the temperature gets below 50°F (10°C).
☐ 4. Use gloves when handling ice or frozen foods.
☐ 5. Limit stressful situations.

53. A client with Raynaud phenomenon is prescribed diltiazem. The nurse should assess the client for which intended outcome of this drug?
☐ 1. increased heart rate
☐ 2. less pain in extremities
☐ 3. fewer episodes of numbness in the fingers
☐ 4. lower serum calcium levels

54. A client with Raynaud phenomenon is considering having a sympathectomy. What information should the nurse give the client about this surgery?

A sympathectomy is performed:
☐ 1. in the early stages of the disease to prevent further circulatory disturbances.
☐ 2. when the disease is controlled by medication.
☐ 3. when the client is unable to control stress-related vasospasm.
☐ 4. when other treatment alternatives have not been effective.

The Adult with Peripheral Venous Disease: Thrombophlebitis, Deep Vein Thrombosis, and Embolus Formation

55. The nurse reviews the laboratory results from a female client admitted with deep vein thrombosis. The client is receiving intravenous heparin. Based on the client's current laboratory values, what should the nurse do?

Laboratory Results

Test	Result	Normal Range
Hemoglobin	12 g/dL (120 g/L)	Women: 12–16 g/dL (120–160 g/L)
Hematocrit	40%	Women: 36%–48% (0.36–0.48 proportion of 1.0)
Platelet count	165,000 mm³ (165 × 10⁹/L)	Adults: 140,000–400,000/μL (140–400 × 10⁹/L)
Activated partial thromboplastin time (aPTT)	65 seconds (control 26 seconds)	30–40 seconds
Prothrombin time (PT)	11.0 seconds	11–13 seconds
International normalized ratio (INR)	1.1	2.0–3.0
Blood urea nitrogen (BUN)	19 mg/dL (6.78 mmol/L)	8–20 mg/dL (2.9–7.5 mmol/L)
Creatinine	1.0 mg/dL (76.3 μmol/L)	Women: 0.6–1.1 mg/dL (53–97 μmol/L)
Aspartate aminotransferase (AST)	25 IU/L (0.42 μkat/L)	10–36 units/L (0.17–0.60 μkat/L)
Alanine transaminase (ALT)	30 IU/L (0/5 μkat/L)	Levels of 7–35 units/L (0.12–0.60 μkat/L) are normal for female clients

☐ 1. Notify the health care provider (HCP) about the increased liver enzymes.
☐ 2. Encourage the client to drink 3500 mL of fluids daily.
☐ 3. Monitor oxygen saturation levels every 4 hours.
☐ 4. Maintain the current rate of the heparin infusion.

56. A client is being treated for deep vein thrombosis (DVT) in the left femoral artery. The health care provider (HCP) has prescribed 60 mg of enoxaparin subcutaneously. Before administering the drug, the nurse checks the client's laboratory results, noted below.

Laboratory Results

Test	Result	Normal Range
Prothrombin time	12.5 seconds	11–13 seconds
International normalized ratio (INR)	2.0 (2.0)	2.0–3.0
Platelet count	50,000 μL (50 × 10⁹/L)	Adults: 140,000–400,000/μL (140–400 × 10⁹/L)

Based on these results, what should the nurse do?
☐ 1. Contact the pharmacist for a lower dose of the medication.
☐ 2. Administer the medication as prescribed.
☐ 3. Assess the client for signs of bruising on the extremities.
☐ 4. Withhold the dose of the medication, and contact the health care provider (HCP).

57. A client with deep vein thrombosis suddenly develops dyspnea, tachypnea, and chest discomfort. What should the nurse do **first**?
☐ 1. Elevate the head of the bed 30 to 45 degrees.
☐ 2. Encourage the client to cough and deep breathe.
☐ 3. Auscultate the lungs to detect abnormal breath sounds.
☐ 4. Contact the health care provider (HCP).

58. A client with a recent diagnosis of deep vein thrombosis (DVT) has sudden-onset shortness of breath and chest pain that increases with a deep breath. What should the nurse do **first**?
☐ 1. Assess the oxygen saturation.
☐ 2. Call the health care provider (HCP).
☐ 3. Administer morphine sulfate, 2 mg intravenously (IV).
☐ 4. Perform range-of-motion exercises in the involved leg.

59. The nurse is caring for a client with venous thrombosis of the left lower extremity. To prevent further tissue damage, the nurse should observe the client for which finding?
☐ 1. blood pressure and heart rate changes
☐ 2. gradual or acute loss of sensory and motor function
☐ 3. metabolic acidosis
☐ 4. swelling in the left lower extremity

60. The nurse is instructing a client who had knee surgery 2 days ago about taking rivaroxaban to prevent deep vein thrombosis. Which information should the nurse include in the teaching plan? Select all that apply.
☐ 1. "You may bleed more easily."
☐ 2. "You should not play contact sports."
☐ 3. "You will need to have prothrombin levels checked regularly."
☐ 4. "Tell your health care provider (HCP) if you have increased urination."
☐ 5. "Continue to take your medication until the HCP tells you otherwise."

61. A client with venous thrombus reports having pain in the legs. What should the nurse do **first**?
☐ 1. Elevate the foot of the bed.
☐ 2. Elevate the legs by using a pillow under the knees.
☐ 3. Encourage adequate fluid intake.
☐ 4. Massage the lower legs.

62. A 45-year-old client had a complete abdominal hysterectomy with bilateral salpingo-oophorectomy 2 days ago. The client's abdominal dressing is dry and intact. While sitting up in the chair, the client has severe pain and numbness in their left leg. What should the nurse do **first**?
☐ 1. Administer pain medication.
☐ 2. Assess edema in the left leg.
☐ 3. Assess the color and temperature of the left leg.
☐ 4. Encourage the client to change their position.

63. A client who is being discharged after hospitalization for thrombophlebitis will be riding home in a car. During the 2-hour ride, what should the nurse advise the client to do?
☐ 1. Perform arm circles.
☐ 2. Do ankle pumps.
☐ 3. Elevate the legs.
☐ 4. Lay flat in the back seat.

64. A client with a cerebral embolus is receiving intravenous (IV) recombinant tissue-type plasminogen activator (rt-PA). The nurse should evaluate the client for which expected therapeutic outcomes of this drug therapy?
☐ 1. improved cerebral perfusion
☐ 2. decreased vascular permeability
☐ 3. dissolved emboli
☐ 4. prevention of cerebral hemorrhage

65. A client who weighs 187 lb (85 kg) has a prescription to receive enoxaparin 1 mg/kg. This drug is available in a concentration of 30 mg/0.3 mL. What dose would the nurse administer in milliliters? Record your answer to two decimal points.
_____ mL.

66. The health care provider (HCP) prescribed knee-high sequential compression devices. The client reports new pain localized in the right calf area. The nurse notes the area is reddened and warm to touch. What should the nurse do **first**?
☐ 1. Offer analgesics as prescribed, and apply the compression devices.
☐ 2. Leave the compression devices off, and contact the HCP to report the assessment findings.
☐ 3. Massage the area of discomfort before applying the compression devices.
☐ 4. Leave the compression devices off, and report assessment findings to the oncoming shift.

67. A client is receiving an intravenous (IV) infusion of 5% dextrose in water (D_5W). The skin around the IV insertion site is red, warm to touch, and painful. What should the nurse do **first**?
☐ 1. Administer acetaminophen.
☐ 2. Change the D_5W to normal saline.
☐ 3. Discontinue the IV.
☐ 4. Place a warm compress on the area.

68. The nurse is planning care for a client on complete bed rest. To prevent venous thrombosis, the nurse should include which measure(s) in the plan of care? Select all that apply.
☐ 1. turning every 2 hours
☐ 2. performing passive and active range-of-motion exercises
☐ 3. using thromboembolic disease (TED) support hose
☐ 4. maintaining the client in the supine position
☐ 5. increasing fluid intake to 3500 mL/day

69. A client is admitted with left lower leg pain, a positive Homans sign, and a temperature of 100.4°F (38°C). What additional sign should the nurse assess?
☐ 1. aortic aneurysm
☐ 2. deep vein thrombosis (DVT) in the left leg
☐ 3. intravenous (IV) drug abuse disorder
☐ 4. intermittent claudication

70. A client is admitted with a diagnosis of thrombophlebitis and deep vein thrombosis of the right leg. A loading dose of heparin has been given in the emergency department, and intravenous (IV) heparin will be continued for the next several days. What should the nurse include in the plan of care for this client?
☐ 1. administering aspirin as prescribed
☐ 2. encouraging green leafy vegetables in the diet
☐ 3. monitoring the client's prothrombin time (PT)
☐ 4. monitoring the client's activated partial thromboplastin time (aPTT) and international normalized ratio (INR)

71. A client has had abdominal surgery. What should the nurse do to prevent deep vein thrombosis (DVT)?
☐ 1. Limit fluids to 1000 mL in 24 hours.
☐ 2. Encourage deep breathing.
☐ 3. Assist the client to remain sedentary.
☐ 4. Use pneumatic compression stockings.

72. A client diagnosed with deep vein thrombosis has heparin sodium infusing at 1500 units per hour. The concentration of heparin is 25,000 units/500 mL. If the infusion remains at the same rate for a full 12-hour shift, how many milliliters of fluid will infuse? Round your answer to a whole number.
_____ mL.

73. A client weighs 300 lb (136 kg) and has a history of deep vein thrombosis and thrombophlebitis. When coaching a client about behaviors to maintain health, the nurse determines that the client has understood the instructions when the client makes which statement?
☐ 1. "I'll limit exercise that involves walking."
☐ 2. "I'll try to lose weight by following a reduced-calorie, balanced diet."
☐ 3. "I'll perform leg lifts every 4 hours to strengthen hamstring muscles."
☐ 4. "I'll wear knee-high stockings, rolled at the top to hold the stockings up."

74. Which instruction(s) should the nurse include when developing a teaching plan for a client being discharged from the hospital on anticoagulant therapy after having deep vein thrombosis (DVT)? Select all that apply.
☐ 1. Check urine for bright blood and a dark smoky color.
☐ 2. Walk daily as a good exercise.
☐ 3. Use garlic and ginger, which may decrease bleeding time.
☐ 4. Perform foot/leg exercises and walk around the airplane cabin when on long flights.
☐ 5. Prevent DVT because of the risk for pulmonary emboli.
☐ 6. Avoid surface bumps because the skin is prone to injury.

75. A client has an emergency embolectomy for an embolus in the femoral artery. After the client returns from the recovery room, in what order, from first to last, should the nurse provide care? All options must be used.

| 1. Administer pain medication. |
| 2. Draw blood for laboratory studies. |
| 3. Regulate the intravenous (IV) infusion. |
| 4. Monitor the pulses. |
| 5. Inspect the dressing. |
| |
| |
| |
| |
| |

76. A client with deep vein thrombosis has been receiving warfarin for 2 months. The client is to go to an anticoagulant monitoring laboratory every 3 weeks. The last visit to the laboratory was 2 weeks ago. The client reports bleeding gums, increased bruising, and dark stools. What should the nurse instruct the client to do?
☐ 1. Decrease the dose of the warfarin.
☐ 2. Return to the laboratory for analysis of prothrombin times.
☐ 3. Decrease the amount of vitamin K in the diet.
☐ 4. Notify the health care provider (HCP) about the bleeding.

The Adult with Varicose Veins

77. A client is talking with the nurse about unsightly varicose veins and their discomfort. What information should the nurse provide to the client?
☐ 1. Avoid walking to reduce discomfort.
☐ 2. Keep the legs elevated when sitting or lying down.
☐ 3. Undergo sclerotherapy for cosmetic improvement.
☐ 4. Contact a surgeon to perform a femoral-popliteal bypass graft.

78. The nurse is teaching a group of clients about the risks for varicose veins. Which client is at risk for varicose veins?
    ☐ 1. a client who has had a cerebrovascular accident
    ☐ 2. a client who has had anemia
    ☐ 3. a client who has had thrombophlebitis
    ☐ 4. a client who has had transient ischemic attacks

79. A client is to have sclerotherapy to treat varicose veins. What information about the procedure should the nurse include in the teaching plan for this client?
    ☐ 1. It causes the veins to fade and disappear.
    ☐ 2. It ensures that varicosities will not occur again.
    ☐ 3. It requires a short hospitalization for complete recovery.
    ☐ 4. It results in bruising lasting for 2 weeks.

80. A client with clinical obesity who has moderately painful varicose veins chooses self-care options for managing the varicosities. The nurse should coach the client to follow which health care practice(s)? Select all that apply.
    ☐ 1. Lose weight.
    ☐ 2. Wear compression stockings.
    ☐ 3. Apply lotion to the veins.
    ☐ 4. Elevate the legs.
    ☐ 5. Sleep with pillows under the knees.

The Adult with Stasis Ulcers

81. A well-nourished client is admitted with a stasis ulcer. The nurse assesses the ulcer and finds excavation of the skin surface as a result of sloughing of inflammatory necrotic tissue. The health care provider has prescribed the ulcer to be flushed with a fibrinolytic agent. Which goal(s) would be appropriate for this client? Select all that apply.
    ☐ 1. Increase oxygen to the tissues.
    ☐ 2. Prevent direct trauma to the ulcer.
    ☐ 3. Improve nutrition.
    ☐ 4. Prevent infection.
    ☐ 5. Reduce pain.

82. A client has had a stasis ulcer of the left ankle with 2+ pitting edema for 2 years. The client is taking chlorothiazide. What should the nurse evaluate to determine the effectiveness of this drug?
    ☐ 1. improved capillary circulation
    ☐ 2. decreased blood pressure
    ☐ 3. wound healing
    ☐ 4. absence of infection

83. The nurse assesses a client with a 5-inch × 2-inch (12.7-cm × 5-cm) stasis ulcer just above the left malleolus. The wound is open with irregular, reddened, swollen edges, and there is a moderate amount of yellowish-tan drainage coming from the wound. The client verbalizes pressure-type pain and rates the discomfort at 7 on a scale of 0 to 10. What is the **primary** nursing goal for this client?
    ☐ 1. administering prescribed analgesics
    ☐ 2. applying lanolin lotions to the left ankle stasis ulcer
    ☐ 3. encouraging the client to sit up in a chair four times per day
    ☐ 4. keeping the pressure of bed linens off the area

84. In preparation for being discharged home, the nurse is teaching a client with a chronic right ankle stasis ulcer about wound care. What statement by the client indicates a need for further teaching?
    ☐ 1. "I'll make an appointment with a physical therapist."
    ☐ 2. "I'll apply a home herb mixture to the wound to promote healing."
    ☐ 3. "I'll be patient with the healing process."
    ☐ 4. "I'll eat a balanced diet."

Managing Care, Quality, and Safety for Adults with Vascular Disease

85. The nurse has received a change-of-shift report about clients. Which client should the nurse assess **first**?
    ☐ 1. a client with chronic heart failure with right upper quadrant fullness
    ☐ 2. a client in atrial fibrillation with a heart rate of 90 bpm with a "fluttering" feeling
    ☐ 3. a client with peripheral artery disease (PAD) just returning from an angiogram
    ☐ 4. a client who had coronary artery bypass surgery 2 days ago and who reports having incisional pain of "3" out of "10"

86. A client with a history of hypertension and peripheral vascular disease underwent an aortobifemoral bypass graft. Preoperative medications included pentoxifylline, metoprolol, and furosemide. On postoperative day 1, the 1200 vital signs are as follows: temperature 98.9°F (37.2°C), heart rate 132 bpm, respiratory rate 20 breaths/min, and blood pressure 126/78 mm Hg. Urine output is 50 to 70 mL per hour. The hemoglobin and the hematocrit are stable. The medications have not been prescribed for administration after surgery. Using the SBAR (Situation-Background-Assessment-Recommendation) technique for communication, the nurse contacts the health care provider (HCP) and recommends to:
    ☐ 1. continue the pentoxifylline.
    ☐ 2. increase the intravenous (IV) fluids.
    ☐ 3. restart the metoprolol.
    ☐ 4. resume the furosemide.

87. The nurse is planning care for a client who underwent abdominal aortic aneurysm repair 2 days ago. The pain medication and the use of relaxation and imagery techniques are not relieving the client's pain, and the client refuses to get out of bed to ambulate as prescribed. The nurse contacts the health care provider (HCP), explains the situation, and provides information about the drug dose, the frequency of administration, the client's vital signs, and the client's score on the pain scale. The nurse requests a prescription for a different, or stronger, pain medication. The HCP tells the nurse that the current prescription for pain medication is sufficient for this client and that the client will feel better in several days. What should the nurse do **next**?
☐ 1. Explain to the HCP that the current pain medication and other strategies are not helping the client and it is making it difficult for the client to ambulate as prescribed.
☐ 2. Ask the surgical resident to prescribe a stronger pain medication.
☐ 3. Wait until the next shift, and ask the nurse on that shift to contact the HCP.
☐ 4. Report the incident to the team leader.

88. The nurse is making the client assignment for a group of clients. The personnel include the registered nurse (RN), a licensed practical/vocational nurse (LPN/VN), and an unlicensed assistive personnel (UAP). Which client would the nurse assign to the LPN/VN?
☐ 1. a client who is undergoing femoropopliteal bypass graft surgery this morning and needs the preoperative checklist completed
☐ 2. a stable client with thrombophlebitis of the lower left extremity with limited mobility and requiring a complete bed bath
☐ 3. a client with a palpable abdominal mass, painful lower extremities, and a decreasing blood pressure
☐ 4. a client with intermittent claudication who needs frequent assistance with getting out of bed and ambulating

89. The nurse is obtaining a blood sample for a partial thromboplastin time test prescribed for a client who is taking heparin. It is 0500 when drawing the blood. What should the nurse do? Select all that apply.
☐ 1. Awaken the client.
☐ 2. Check the armband for the client identification number, and compare it with the prescription.
☐ 3. Label the sample vial in front of the client.
☐ 4. Verify the room number with the room assignment.
☐ 5. Ask the client to state their name.

90. A client has acute arterial occlusion. The health care provider has prescribed intravenous (IV) heparin. What should the nurse do **before** starting the medication?
☐ 1. Review the blood coagulation laboratory values.
☐ 2. Test the client's stools for occult blood.
☐ 3. Count the client's apical pulse for 1 minute.
☐ 4. Check the 24-hour urine output record.

91. The nurse is caring for a client who has a below-the-knee amputation. The client has been somewhat confused since returning from surgery last evening but has no history of falls. The client is receiving intravenous (IV) antibiotics intermittently through a peripheral IV and has prescriptions to be up with physical therapy only. Using the Morse Fall Risk Scale (see scale), what is this client's total score and risk level?

Morse Fall Risk/Scale

Item	Scale	Scoring
1. History of falling, immediate or within 3 months	No 0 Yes 25	
2. Secondary diagnosis	No 0 Yes 15	
3. Ambulatory aid 　Bed rest/nurse assist 　Crutches/cane/walker 　Furniture	 0 15 30	
4. IV/heparin lock	No 0 Yes 20	
5. Gait/transferring 　Normal/bed rest/immobile 　Weak 　Impaired	 0 10 20	
6. Mental status 　Oriented to own ability 　Forgets limitations	 0 15	

☐ 1. 20, low risk
☐ 2. 30, medium risk
☐ 3. 40, medium risk
☐ 4. 50, high risk

Answers, Rationales, and Test-Taking Strategies

The answers and rationales for each question follow below, along with keys (🗝) to the client need (CN) and cognitive level (CL) for each question. As you check your answers, use the **Content Mastery and Test-Taking Skill Self-Analysis** worksheet (tear-out worksheet in the back of the book) to identify the reason(s) for not answering the questions correctly. For additional information about test-taking skills and strategies for answering questions, refer to pages 12–51 in Part 1 of this book.

The Adult with Peripheral Artery Disease

1. **1, 3, 4.** Smoking and exposure to the cold cause vasoconstriction and should be avoided. Aspirin and clopidogrel should be taken as prescribed for the antiplatelet properties. Using extra bedclothes at night provides warmth, which increases vasodilation. The presence of pain should be investigated as it could indicate increasing arterial insufficiency. Tight socks should be avoided as they could impair circulation.

   🗝 CN: Health promotion and maintenance; CL: Synthesis

2. **3.** Keeping the involved extremity at or below the body's horizontal plane will facilitate tissue perfusion and prevent tissue damage. The nurse should avoid placing the affected extremity on a hard surface, such as a firm mattress, to avoid pressure ulcers. In addition, the involved extremity should be free from heavy overlying bed linens. The nurse should handle the involved extremity gently to prevent friction or pressure. Raising the leg would cause occlusion to the iliac artery, which is contrary to the goal to promote arterial circulation.

   🗝 CN: Physiological adaptation; CL: Analyze

3. **1, 3.** Discharge teaching begins when the client enters the hospital. One of the risk factors for clot formation is a sedentary lifestyle, and the client should engage in daily aerobic activity, such as biking or swimming (non–weight-bearing). The client is also overweight and should plan to control the weight through dietary counseling or attending weight management programs in the community. Strength training is beneficial because it increases strength and lean body mass, but it does not help prevent vascular disease. Stress management is not a focus based on the client's needs at this time. It is not necessary to wear special supportive shoes; comfortable shoes for walking are adequate.

   🗝 CN: Health promotion and maintenance; CL: Create

4. The nurse should assess the femoral artery. Weak or absent femoral pulses are symptomatic of aortoiliac disease.

   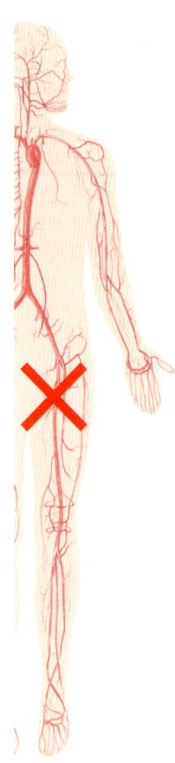

   🗝 CN: Physiological adaptation; CL: Analyze

5. **4.** An ankle-brachial index of 0.65 suggests moderate arterial vascular disease in a client who is experiencing intermittent claudication. A Doppler ultrasound is indicated for further evaluation. The bradycardic heart rate is acceptable in an athletic client with normal blood pressure. The SpO_2 is acceptable; the client has a smoking history.

   🗝 CN: Physiological adaptation; CL: Analyze

6. **2.** With each set of vital signs, the nurse should assess the dorsalis pedis and posterior tibial pulses. The nurse needs to ensure adequate perfusion to the lower extremity with the drop in blood pressure. IV fluids, the nasal cannula setting, and capillary refill are important to assess; however, the priority is to determine the cause of the drop in blood pressure and that adequate perfusion through the new graft is maintained.

   🗝 CN: Reduction of risk potential; CL: Analyze

7. ➕ **1, 2, 3, 5.** Maintaining skin integrity is important in preventing chronic ulcers and infections. The client should be taught to inspect the skin daily. The client should reduce weight to promote circulation; a diet lower in calories and fat is appropriate. Because the client is receiving warfarin, the client is at risk for bleeding from cuts. To decrease the risk for cuts, the nurse should suggest that the client use an electric razor. A client with decreased arterial blood flow should be encouraged to participate in ADLs and to consult an exercise physiologist for an exercise program that enhances the aerobic capacity of the body.

🔑 CN: Health promotion and maintenance; CL: Analyze

8. 3. Weakness, dizziness, and headache are common adverse effects of clopidogrel, and the client should report these to the health care provider (HCP) if they are problematic; to decrease the risk for clot formation, the drug must be taken regularly and should not be stopped or taken intermittently. The main adverse effect of clopidogrel is bleeding, which often occurs as increased bruising or bleeding when brushing teeth. Clopidogrel is well absorbed, and while food may help decrease potential gastrointestinal upset, the drug may be taken with or without food. Clopidogrel is an antiplatelet agent used to prevent clot formation in clients who have experienced or are at risk for myocardial infarction, ischemic stroke, peripheral artery disease, or acute coronary syndrome.

🔑 CN: Pharmacological and parenteral therapies; CL: Evaluate

9. 3. Cilostazol is indicated for management of intermittent claudication. Symptoms usually improve within 2 to 4 weeks of therapy. Intermittent claudication prevents clients from walking for long periods. Cilostazol inhibits platelet aggregation induced by various stimuli and improves blood flow to the muscles, allowing the client to walk long distances without pain. Peripheral artery disease causes pain mainly in the leg muscles. "Aches and pains" does not specify exactly where the pain is occurring. Headaches may occur as a side effect of this drug, and the client should report this information to the health care provider. Peripheral artery disease causes decreased blood supply to the peripheral tissues and may cause gangrene of the toes; the drug is effective when the toes are warm to the touch and the color of the toes is similar to the color of the body.

🔑 CN: Pharmacological and parenteral therapies; CL: Evaluate

10. 4. Decreased blood flow is a common characteristic of all peripheral artery disease. When the demand for oxygen to the working muscles becomes greater than the supply, pain is the outcome. The nurse should suggest that the client enroll in a supervised exercise training program that will assist the client to gradually increase walking distances without pain. Not walking and resting will not increase blood flow to the legs. Support stockings may be prescribed, but the client should improve the capacity to walk and obtain exercise.

🔑 CN: Reduction of risk potential; CL: Apply

11. The nurse palpates the dorsalis pedis; if the pulse is obtained in that artery, the tibioperoneal artery is patent.

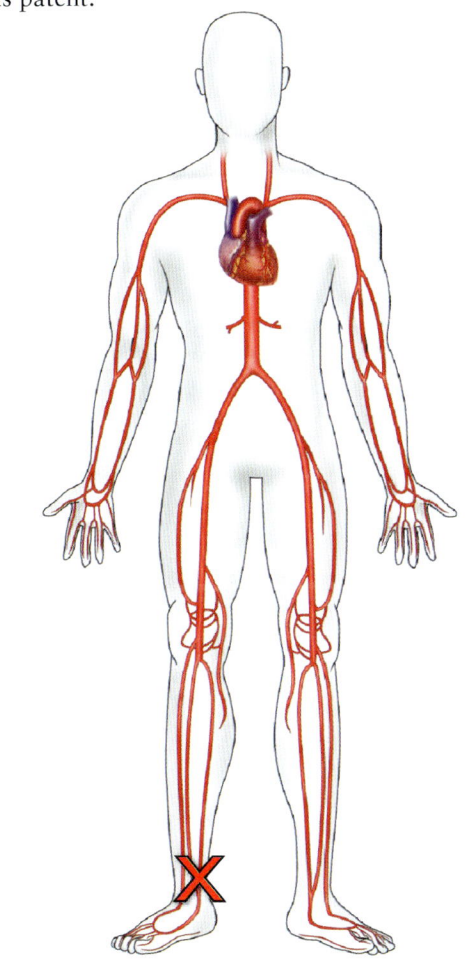

12. 4.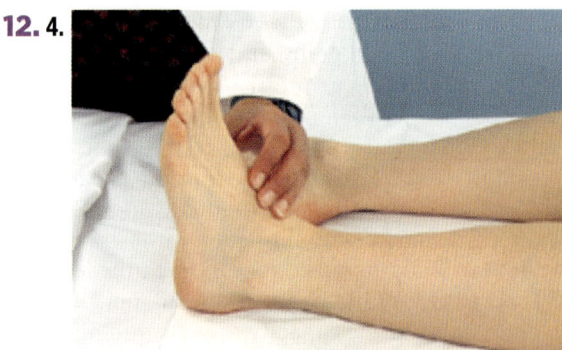

    The presence of a strong dorsalis pedis pulse indicates that there is circulation to the extremity distal to the surgery, indicating that the graft between the femoral and popliteal artery is allowing blood to circulate effectively. Option 1 shows the nurse obtaining the radial pulse; option 2 shows the femoral pulse, which is proximal to the surgery site and will not indicate circulation distal to the surgery site. Option 3 shows the nurse obtaining an apical pulse.

    CN: Reduction of risk potential; CL: Analyze

13. 2, 4. The reduction of blood flow to a specific area results in decreased oxygen and nutrients. As a result, the skin may appear mottled. The skin will also be cool to the touch. Loss of hair and dry skin are other signs that the nurse may observe in a client with peripheral artery disease of the lower extremities.

    CN: Reduction of risk potential; CL: Analyze

14. 3. When pedal pulses are not palpable, the nurse should obtain a Doppler ultrasound device. Auscultation is not likely to be helpful if the pulse is not palpable. Inspection of the lower extremity can be done simultaneously when palpating, but the nurse should first try to locate a pulse by Doppler. Calling the HCP may be necessary if there is a change in the client's condition.

    CN: Physiological adaptation; CL: Analyze

15. 4. Coldness in the left foot and ankle is consistent with complete arterial obstruction. Other expected findings would include paralysis and pallor. Aching pain, a burning sensation, or numbness and tingling are earlier signs of tissue hypoxia and ischemia and are commonly associated with incomplete obstruction.

    CN: Physiological adaptation; CL: Analyze

16. 2, 4, 3, 1. Because assessment of the presence and quality of the pedal pulses in the affected extremity is essential after surgery to make sure that the bypass graft is functioning, this step should be done **first**. The nurse should next ensure that the dressing is intact and then that the client has adequate urine output. Lastly, the nurse should determine the client's level of pain.

    CN: Physiological adaptation; CL: Analyze

17. 3. The term *gangrene* refers to blackened, decomposing tissue that is devoid of circulation. Chronic ischemia and death of the tissue can lead to gangrene in the affected extremity. Injury, edema, and decreased circulation lead to infection, gangrene, and tissue death. Atrophy is the shrinking of tissue, and contraction is joint stiffening secondary to disuse. The term *rubor* denotes a reddish color of the skin.

    CN: Physiological adaptation; CL: Analyze

18. 2. Slow, steady walking is a recommended activity for clients with peripheral vascular disease because it stimulates the development of collateral circulation. The client with PVD should not remain inactive. Elevating the legs above the heart or wearing antiembolism stockings is a strategy for alleviating venous congestion and may worsen peripheral artery disease.

    CN: Basic care and comfort; CL: Evaluate

19. 2. Clients may have an immediate or a delayed reaction to the radiopaque dye. The HCP should be notified immediately because the symptoms suggest an allergic reaction. Treatment may involve administering oxygen and epinephrine. Explaining that the procedure is over does not address the current symptoms.

    CN: Physiological adaptation; CL: Analyze

20. 4. The client should avoid using iodine or over-the-counter medications. Iodine is a highly toxic solution. An individual who has known PVD should be seen by a health care provider for treatment to avoid infection. The client with PVD should avoid heating pads and crossing the legs and should wear leather shoes. A heating pad can cause injury, which, because of the decreased blood supply, can be difficult to heal. Crossing the legs can further impede blood flow. Leather shoes provide better protection.

    CN: Health promotion and maintenance; CL: Evaluate

21. 1. Maintaining circulation in the affected extremity after surgery is the focus of care. The graft can become occluded, and the client must be assessed frequently to determine whether the graft is patent. Preventing infection and relieving pain are important but are secondary to maintaining graft

patency. Education should have taken place in the preoperative phase and then continued during the recovery phase.

   CN: Physiological adaptation; CL: Analyze

22. **1, 3.** Elastic stockings (support hose) are used to promote circulation by preventing the pooling of blood in the feet and legs. The stockings should be applied in the morning before the client gets out of bed. The stockings should be applied smoothly to avoid wrinkles, but the top should not be rolled down to avoid constriction of circulation. The stockings should be removed every 8 hours, and the client should elevate the legs for 15 minutes and reapply the stockings. Clean stockings should be applied daily or as needed.

   CN: Health promotion and maintenance; CL: Create

23. **4.** If surgery is scheduled, the nurse should avoid venipunctures in the affected extremity. The goal should be to prevent unnecessary trauma and possible infection in the affected arm. Disruptions in skin integrity and even minor skin irritations can cause the surgery to be canceled. The nurse can continue to monitor the temperature and radial pulse in the affected arm; however, doing so is not the priority. Keeping the client warm is important, but it is not the priority at this time.

   CN: Reduction of risk potential; CL: Analyze

24. **3.** Nicotine causes vasospasm and impedes blood flow. Stopping smoking is the most significant lifestyle change the client can make. The client should eat low-fat foods as part of a balanced diet. The legs should not be elevated above the heart because this will impede arterial flow. The legs should be in a slightly dependent position. Jogging is not necessary and probably is not possible for many clients with arterial occlusive disease. A rehabilitation program that includes daily walking is suggested.

   CN: Health promotion and maintenance; CL: Analyze

25. **1.** A change in the intensity of a pulse may be indicative of arterial closure and warrants immediate attention; the nurse should notify the health care provider immediately. A pain level of 2 out of 10 is not uncommon from the catheter insertion site, especially after the placement of a stent. Shiny and hairless skin is expected in clients with PAD. A client undergoing a catheterization may experience pain at the catheterization site as large-bore sheaths are placed in the femoral artery. Because people with PAD have poor circulation in their lower extremities, they can develop leg ulcers. However, it is unlikely that the percutaneous transluminal balloon angioplasty caused this.

   CN: Physiological adaptation; CL: Analyze

26. **1, 2, 5.** Turning frequently promotes circulation, and using pillows for support will prevent stress on the suture line. Short periods of different leg/body positions will not impair postoperative oxygen levels. The client should only be in a knee-flexed position when walking and not at rest. Prolonged sitting is discouraged because it may cause pain and edema. It is not recommended that the leg be placed in a dependent position as this promotes edema. Placing a client in a supine position with the leg elevated above the heart is recommended only if the client develops edema.

   CN: Physiological adaptation; CL: Analyze

27. **4.** Diltiazem is a calcium channel blocker that blocks the influx of calcium into the cell. The primary use of diltiazem for this client is to promote vasodilation and prevent spasms of the arteries so blood, oxygen, and nutrients can reach the muscle and tissues. Diltiazem is not an antianxiety agent and does not promote sleep. It also does not cause vasoconstriction, which would cause coolness in the extremities, and it is contraindicated for the client with peripheral vascular disease.

   CN: Pharmacological and parenteral therapies; CL: Evaluate

28. **1.** Cilostazol improves blood flow, and the client should have improved circulation in the legs as evidenced by less pain. The client does not have nerve impairment and should be able to wiggle the toes. Urination is not improved by taking cilostazol. Dizziness is a side effect of the drug, not an intended outcome.

   CN: Pharmacological and parenteral therapies; CL: Evaluate

29. **1.** Assessing the individual's health behavior before surgery will help the nurse and client develop strategies to manage the postoperative course. Asking open-ended questions will elicit the most helpful information. The client's ability to walk will be improved after surgery. The client should report any changes in urination, but urinary retention is not expected before or after surgery.

   CN: Health promotion and maintenance; CL: Create

30. **4.** Before beginning dietary interventions, the nurse must assess the client's pattern of food intake, lifestyle, food preferences, and ethnic, cultural, and financial influences. With this information, the

nurse can then discuss the client's knowledge about cholesterol and foods high in fat, cholesterol, and sodium and coach the client about the importance of following the diet plan.

CN: Basic care and comfort; CL: Analyze

The Adult with Peripheral Vascular Disease Having an Amputation

31. 2. Encouraging the client who is undergoing amputation to verbalize feelings is the **most** therapeutic nursing intervention. By eliciting concerns, the nurse may be able to provide information to help the client cope. The nurse should avoid value-laden responses, such as "You will still have one good leg," which may make the client feel guilty or hostile and block further communication. The nurse should not ignore the client's expressed concerns, nor should the nurse reinforce the client's concern about invalidism and dependency or assume that the client's spouse is willing to care for them.

CN: Psychosocial integrity; CL: Analyze

32. 2. The level of amputation commonly cannot be accurately determined until surgery, when the surgeon can directly assess the adequacy of the circulation of the residual limb. A longer residual limb facilitates prosthesis fitting and will make it easier for the client to walk. However, although these aspects will be considered in the final decision, they are not the primary factors influencing the decision. The method used to fit the prosthesis is not a factor in determining the level of the amputation.

CN: Physiological adaptation; CL: Analyze

33. 1. Leg crossing is contraindicated because it causes adduction of the hips and decreases the flow of blood into the lower extremities. This may result in increased pressure in the graft in the affected leg. Elevating the legs, flexing the ankles, and extending the knees are not necessarily contraindicated.

CN: Reduction of risk potential; CL: Analyze

34. 2. The client should be evaluated for hemodynamic stability and the extent of bleeding before calling the HCP. Direct pressure can be used before applying a tourniquet if there is significant bleeding. To avoid flexion contractures, which can delay rehabilitation, elevation of the surgical limb is contraindicated.

CN: Reduction of risk potential; CL: Analyze

35. 3. The purpose of wrapping the residual limb is to shape the residual limb to accept a prosthesis and bear weight. The compression bandaging should be worn at all times for many weeks after surgery and should be reapplied as needed to keep it free of wrinkles and snug. The dressing should be changed daily to allow for inspection of the stump incision. No lotions should be applied to the stump unless specifically prescribed by the health care provider. The stump should not be elevated on pillows because this will contribute to the formation of flexion contractures. Contractures will prevent the client from wearing a prosthesis and ambulating.

CN: Physiological adaptation; CL: Evaluate

The Adult with an Aneurysm

36. 4. The underlying pathophysiology in this client is atherosclerosis. The findings from the assessment indicate the risk factors of smoking and high blood pressure. Therefore, tissue perfusion is a priority for health-promoting education. The data do not support education that focuses on food or fluid intake. Although edema is a potential problem and could contribute to poor skin integrity, the edema will likely be resolved by the aneurysm repair.

CN: Physiological adaptation; CL: Analyze

37. 1. The size of the thoracic aneurysm is rather large, so the nurse should anticipate rupture. A sudden incidence of pain may indicate leakage or rupture. The blood pressure and heart rate will provide useful information in assessing for hypovolemic shock. The nurse needs more data before initiating other interventions. After assessment of vital signs, neurologic status, and pain, the nurse can then contact the HCP.

CN: Physiological adaptation; CL: Analyze

38. 2, 4, 3, 1. The data suggest an abdominal aortic aneurysm that is leaking or rupturing. When implementing the prescriptions, the nurse should **first** establish an intravenous infusion with a large-bore needle for immediate volume replacement. Next, the nurse should insert the nasogastric tube to relieve the nausea and vomiting and decompress the stomach. The nurse next should administer pain medication. Last, the nurse should monitor intake and output; with hypovolemia, the urine output will be diminished.

CN: Physiological adaptation; CL: Analyze

39. 4. There may be many reasons why the client has doubts about the surgery and is not ready to sign the surgical consent. The nurse should assist the client in obtaining information that will help the client make the decision to have surgery by offering to have the client talk with family members or others who can offer support to the client. The nurse should not contact the surgeon or cancel the surgery until the client has had time to consider the decision. Unless the client requests to speak with a religious advisor or the chaplain, it is not necessary at this time to refer the client to the chaplain.

CN: Psychosocial integrity; CL: Analyze

40. 4. One of the complications of a thoracoabdominal aneurysm repair is spinal cord injury. Therefore, it is important for the nurse to assess for signs and symptoms of neurologic changes at and below the site where the aneurysm was repaired. The client is expected to have moderate pain following surgery. An elevated heart rate is expected after physical exertion. It is important to monitor urine output following aneurysm surgery, but a urine output of 2000 mL in 24 hours is adequate following surgery.

CN: Reduction of risk potential; CL: Analyze

41. 3. The primary goal is to prepare the client for emergency surgery. The goal would be to prevent rupture of the aneurysm and potential death. Circulation is maintained unless the aneurysm ruptures. When the client is prepared for surgery, the nurse should place the client in a recumbent position to promote circulation, teach the client about postoperative breathing exercises, and administer pain medication if prescribed.

CN: Physiological adaptation; CL: Analyze

42. 1. Cardiac tamponade is a life-threatening complication of a dissecting thoracic aneurysm. The sudden, painful "tearing" sensation is typically associated with the sudden release of blood, and the client may experience cardiac arrest. Stroke, pulmonary edema, and myocardial infarction are not common complications of a dissecting aneurysm.

CN: Physiological adaptation; CL: Apply

43. 1. Following surgical repair of an aortic aneurysm, there is a potential for an alteration in renal perfusion, manifested by decreased urine output. The altered renal perfusion may be related to renal artery embolism, prolonged hypotension, or prolonged aortic cross-clamping during surgery. Electrolyte imbalance and anxiety do not present an imminent risk for this client; signs of wound infection are generally not evident immediately following surgery, but the nurse should monitor the incision on an ongoing basis.

CN: Physiological adaptation; CL: Analyze

44. 4. The client is experiencing paralytic ileus. One of the adverse effects of morphine used to manage pain is decreased gastrointestinal motility. Bowel manipulation and immobility also contribute to a postoperative ileus. Insertion of an NG tube generally prevents a postoperative ileus. The ice chips and IV fluids will not affect the ileus.

CN: Basic care and comfort; CL: Analyze

45. 3. The client with a synthetic graft may need to be treated with prophylactic antibiotics before undergoing major dental work and should notify the HCP before any such procedure. Prophylactic antibiotic treatment reduces the danger of systemic infection caused by bacteria from the oral cavity. Venous access for drawing blood, IV line insertion, and x-rays do not contribute to the risk for infection.

CN: Pharmacological and parenteral therapies; CL: Analyze

46. 3. A blood pressure of 80/50 mm Hg in a client who has just had surgical repair of an abdominal aortic aneurysm warrants further evaluation as this indicates decreased perfusion to the brain, heart, and kidneys. A BUN level of 26 mg/dL (26 mmol/L) and a creatinine level of 1.2 mg/dL (1.2 μmol/L) are normal findings. While +1 pedal pulses may be an abnormal finding, it is not uncommon, and it is important to compare this finding with previous assessments and note if this is a change in the strength of the pedal pulses. Absent bowel sounds and mild abdominal distension are expected for a client immediately following surgery. However, this finding should be monitored as it could indicate a paralytic ileus.

CN: Physiological adaptation; CL: Analyze

47. 4. A blood transfusion is required postoperatively with significant blood loss from surgery or bleeding. Data from the progress notes indicate the client is hypovolemic and has a low hemoglobin level, which warrants transfusion at this time rather than IV fluids. The nurse must continue to assess the client for signs of bleeding. Correction of hypovolemia precedes a dopamine infusion. The transfusion should improve the hemodynamics, and the hemoglobin and hematocrit are reassessed after the transfusion. The client has a fluid volume deficit, so furosemide is not needed at this time.

CN: Pharmacological and parenteral therapies; CL: Analyze

The Adult with Raynaud Phenomenon

48. 1, 2, 5. Vasospastic disorder (Raynaud disease) is a form of intermittent arteriolar vasoconstriction that results in coldness; pain; pallor of the fingertips, toes, or tip of the nose; and a rebound circulation with redness and pain. The nurse should instruct the client to stop smoking because nicotine is a vasoconstrictor. An adverse effect of reserpine is orthostatic hypotension. The client should report dizziness and low blood pressure as it may be necessary to consider stopping the drug. The client should prevent vasoconstriction by covering affected parts when in cold environments. The nurse can teach the client to rewarm exposed extremities by using warm water or placing them next to the body, such as under the axilla. It is not realistic to ask this client to change jobs at this time.

 CN: Health promotion and maintenance; CL: Create

49. 2. The client has numbness in the fingertips, and the nurse should **first** help the client regain sensory perception and discuss strategies for the prevention of injury. The client does not have acute pain. The client does have adequate circulation and is not at risk for skin breakdown at this time.

 CN: Physiological adaptation; CL: Analyze

50. 1, 2, 4, 5. When the client with Raynaud disease is having a vasospastic attack, the nurse can teach the client to go to a warmer room, move the fingers and toes to improve circulation, massage the extremities to promote circulation, and put the hands under the armpits to take advantage of body heat. The client should not put the hands or fingers under hot water as there is a risk for burns. If necessary, the client can warm the hands and fingers under slightly warm water.

 CN: Health promotion and maintenance; CL: Create

51. 3. The nurse should instruct the client with Raynaud disease that the nitroglycerine cream is used to promote healing by promoting vasodilation. The drug is not used in this instance to treat pain. The drug does not have properties to treat infection or soften the skin.

 CN: Pharmacological and parenteral therapies; CL: Apply

52. 1, 3, 4, 5. The nurse should instruct the client to prevent vasospastic attacks by avoiding extreme temperature changes; using gloves when handling frozen foods or ice; wearing clothing that will keep the client warm; and avoiding stressful situations. The client does not need to wear hand splints.

 CN: Health promotion and maintenance; CL: Create

53. 3. Calcium channel blockers are first-line drug therapy for the treatment of vasospasms with Raynaud phenomenon when other therapies are ineffective. Diltiazem relaxes smooth muscles and improves peripheral perfusion, thereby reducing finger numbness. Diltiazem reduces the heart rate; it does not increase it. Diltiazem does not directly reduce pain, but it does improve circulation. Decreasing calcium levels is not the intended outcome of diltiazem.

 CN: Pharmacological and parenteral therapies; CL: Evaluate

54. 4. Sympathectomy is scheduled only after other treatment alternatives have been explored and have failed. Medication and stress management are beneficial strategies to prevent advancement of the disease process. If the disease is controlled by medication, there is no reason for surgery.

 CN: Physiological adaptation; CL: Apply

The Adult with Peripheral Venous Disease: Thrombophlebitis, Deep Vein Thrombosis, and Embolus Formation

55. 4. An aPTT of 65 seconds is considered therapeutic with a control of 30 seconds. Therapeutic levels for heparin are 1.5 to 2.5 times the control, which would make the therapeutic level between 45 and 75 seconds. The nurse should continue the infusion at the current rate and continue to monitor the client. The liver enzymes (AST, ALT) are within normal range; it is not necessary to notify the HCP. The BUN and creatinine levels are within normal limits; the client does not need to increase fluid intake beyond 3000 mL. The hemoglobin and hematocrit are within normal limits; it is not necessary to obtain frequent oxygen saturation levels.

 CN: Reduction of risk potential; CL: Synthesis

56. 4. Based on the laboratory findings, the prothrombin time and the INR are at acceptable anticoagulation levels for the treatment of DVT. However, the platelets are below the acceptable level. Clients taking enoxaparin are at risk for thrombocytopenia. Because of the low platelet level, the nurse should contact the HCP before administering the next dose. The nurse should not administer the drug until the HCP has been contacted. The HCP, not the pharmacist, will decide the dose of the enoxaparin. The decision about administering the drug will be based on laboratory results, not evidence of bruising or bleeding.

 CN: Pharmacological and parenteral therapies; CL: Analyze

57. 1. Elevating the head of the bed facilitates

breathing because the lungs are able to expand as the diaphragm descends. Coughing and deep breathing do not alleviate the symptoms of a pulmonary embolus, nor does lung auscultation. The HCP must be kept informed of changes in a client's status, but in this case, the priority is alleviating the symptoms.

CN: Reduction of risk potential; CL: Analyze

58. 1. A client with DVT is at high risk for a pulmonary embolism from an embolus traveling to the lung. Sudden onset of symptoms and worsening chest pain with a deep breath suggest a pulmonary embolism. The nurse assesses the client and obtains oxygen saturation levels prior to calling the HCP and administering morphine. Range of motion is a preventive measure for DVT and is not appropriate that this time.

CN: Reduction of risk potential; CL: Analyze

59. 2. Acute arterial occlusion is a sudden interruption of blood flow. The interruption can be the result of complete or partial obstruction. Acute pain, loss of sensory and motor function, and a pale, mottled, numb extremity are the most dramatic and observable changes that indicate a life-threatening interruption of tissue perfusion. Blood pressure and heart rate changes may be associated with the acute pain episode. Metabolic acidosis is a complication of irreversible ischemia. Swelling may result but may also indicate venous stasis or arterial insufficiency.

CN: Physiological adaptation; CL: Analyze

60. 1, 2, 5. The nurse should instruct the client who is taking oral rivaroxaban that the client will bleed more easily and should avoid contact sports that could cause bruising or injury and continue to take the medication until the HCP indicates otherwise. It is not necessary for the client to have prothrombin time checks because rivaroxaban does not act on the clotting process in this way. The client should report a decrease in urination as this may be a sign of kidney disease, which can be a side effect of rivaroxaban.

CN: Health promotion and maintenance; CL: Create

61. 1. Venous stasis can increase pain. Therefore, proper positioning in bed with the foot of the bed elevated or when sitting up in a chair can help promote venous drainage, reduce swelling, and reduce the amount of pain the client might experience. Placing a pillow under the knees causes flexion of the joint, resulting in a dependent position of the lower leg and causing a decrease in blood flow. Fluids are encouraged to maintain normal fluid and electrolyte balance but do little to relieve pain. Therapeutic massage to the legs is discouraged because of the danger of breaking up the clot.

CN: Basic care and comfort; CL: Analyze

62. 3. The client is likely suffering from an embolus as a result of abdominal surgery. The nurse should inspect the left leg for color and temperature changes associated with tissue perfusion. Administering pain medication without gathering more information about the pain can mask important signs and symptoms. Although assessing for edema is important, it is not critical to this situation. Encouraging the client to change their position does not adequately address the need for gathering more data.

CN: Reduction of risk potential; CL: Analyze

63. 2. Performing active ankle and foot range-of-motion exercises periodically during the ride home will promote muscular contraction and provide support to the venous system. It is the muscular action that facilitates blood return from the lower extremities, especially when in the dependent position. Arm circle exercises will not promote circulation in the leg. The client does not need to elevate the legs as long as the client does not occlude blood flow to the legs and does the leg exercises. It is not necessary to lay flat in the back seat because the client is able to sit in the car safely.

CN: Reduction of risk potential; CL: Analyze

64. 3. Thrombolytic agents such as streptokinase are used for clients with a history of thrombus formation, cerebrovascular accidents, and chronic atrial fibrillation. The thrombolytic agents act by dissolving emboli. Thrombolytic agents do not directly improve perfusion or increase vascular permeability, nor do they prevent cerebral hemorrhage.

CN: Pharmacological and parenteral therapies; CL: Evaluate

65. **0.85 mL.** The prescription is for the client to receive enoxaparin 1 mg/kg. Therefore, the client is to receive 85 mg. The desired dose in milliliters then can be calculated by using the formula of desired dose (D) divided by dose or strength of dose on hand (H) times volume (V).

$$85 (mg) \times 0.3 \text{ mL} = 25.5 \text{ mg/mL}$$

$$25.5 \text{ mg} \div 30 = 0.85 \text{ mL}$$

CN: Pharmacological and parenteral therapies; CL: Apply

66. 2. Localized pain, tenderness, redness, and warmth may be symptoms of deep vein thrombosis (DVT), information the nurse should report to the HCP; the compression devices should not be applied until further evaluation is completed as intermittent compression may dislodge a thrombus. Massaging the area may dislodge a thrombus and is not recommended. The nurse may offer as-needed (PRN) analgesics if the client requires pain management, but the compression devices should not be applied until further evaluation is completed. Diagnosis and treatment of DVT should be discussed with the HCP as soon as possible; the nurse should not wait until the next shift to report findings as a DVT can become life-threatening if a thrombus travels to the lung and becomes a pulmonary embolus.

CN: Reduction of risk potential; CL: Analyze

67. 3. The nurse's first action should be to discontinue the IV. The nurse should restart the IV elsewhere and then apply a warm compress to the affected area. The nurse should administer acetaminophen or an antiinflammatory agent only if prescribed by the health care provider (HCP). The type of infusion cannot be changed without an HCP's prescription, and such a change would not help in this case.

CN: Reduction of risk potential; CL: Analyze

68. -/+ 1, 2, 3, 5. Bed rest and immobilization are associated with decreased blood flow and venous pooling in the lower extremities. The nurse should turn the client every 1 to 2 hours, use passive and active range-of-motion exercises, and apply TED hose to help prevent venous stasis in the lower extremities. The client should increase fluid intake to prevent hypercoagulability of the blood. Keeping the client in the supine position would contribute to venous stasis.

CN: Reduction of risk potential; CL: Create

69. 2. The client demonstrates classic symptoms of DVT, and the nurse should continue to assess the client. Signs and symptoms of an aortic aneurysm include abdominal pain and a pulsating abdominal mass. Clients with IV substance abuse disorder demonstrate confusion and decreased levels of consciousness. Claudication is intermittent pain in the leg.

CN: Psychosocial integrity; CL: Analyze

70. 4. Heparin dosage is usually determined by the health care provider based on the client's aPTT and INR laboratory values. Therefore, the nurse monitors these values to prevent complications. Administering aspirin when the client is on heparin is contraindicated. Green leafy vegetables are high in vitamin K and therefore are not recommended for clients receiving heparin. Monitoring of the client's PT is done when the client is receiving warfarin sodium.

CN: Pharmacological and parenteral therapies; CL: Create

71. 4. The use of pneumatic compression stockings is an intervention used to prevent DVT. Other strategies include early ambulation, leg exercises if the client is confined to bed, adequate fluid intake, and administering anticoagulant medication as prescribed. Deep breathing would be encouraged postoperatively, but it does not prevent DVT.

CN: Health promotion and maintenance; CL: Analyze

72. 360 mL

$25,000 \text{ U} / 500 \text{ mL} = 50 \text{ U} / \text{mL}$

$1 \text{ mL} / 50 \text{ U} \times 1500 \text{ U} / \text{h} = 30 \text{ mL} / \text{h} \times 12 \text{ h}$
$= 360 \text{ mL}$

CN: Pharmacological and parenteral therapies; CL: Apply

73. 2. The client is at risk for the development of varicose veins. Therefore, prevention is key in the treatment plan. Maintaining an ideal body weight is the goal. To achieve this, the client should consume a balanced diet and participate in a regular exercise program. Performing leg lifts improves muscle strength, but it is more important for the client to increase exercise by walking. Wearing support stockings is helpful to promote circulation, but the client should not roll the stockings at the top to hold the stockings up as this will decrease circulation at the knees.

CN: Reduction of risk potential; CL: Evaluate

74. -/+ 1, 2, 4, 5, 6. Clients with resolving DVT being sent home on anticoagulant therapy need instructions about assessing and preventing bleeding episodes and preventing a recurrence of DVT. Blood in the urine (hematuria) is often one of the first symptoms of anticoagulant overdose. Fresh blood in the urine is red; however, blood in the urine may also be a dark smoky color. Daily ambulation is an excellent activity to keep the venous blood circulating and thus prevent blood clots from forming in the lower extremities. Garlic and ginger increase the bleeding time and should not be used when a client is on anticoagulant therapy. Clients who have had previous DVTs should avoid activities that cause stagnation and pooling of venous blood. Prolonged sitting coupled with a change in air pressure without foot or leg exercises or ambulation in the cabin are activities that prevent venous return. Instructing the client about prevention measures is important because clients with DVT are at high risk for pulmonary emboli (PE), which can be fatal. The client can be taught risk factors for DVT and PE. In addition, recommendations for the prevention of these events also are standard protocol in practice and should be shared with the client for home care purposes. Older adults should be monitored closely for bleeding because the skin becomes thinner and the capillaries become more fragile with the aging process.

CN: Health promotion and maintenance; CL: Create

75. **4, 5, 3, 1, 2.** The nurse should first monitor the popliteal and the pedal pulses in the affected extremity after arterial embolectomy. Monitoring peripheral pulses below the site of occlusion checks the arterial circulation in the involved extremity. The nurse should next inspect the dressing to be sure that the client is not bleeding at the surgical site. The nurse should next regulate the IV infusion to prevent fluid overload. Then the nurse should assess pain and administer pain medications as prescribed. Last, the nurse can obtain blood for laboratory studies.

CN: Physiological adaptation; CL: Analyze

76. **2.** These symptoms suggest that the client is receiving too much warfarin; the client should return to the laboratory and have a blood sample drawn to determine the prothrombin levels and have the dosage of warfarin adjusted. The diet can influence clotting, but the client needs to first have the prothrombin levels checked. It is not necessary to contact the HCP; the client should return to the laboratory first, and the results of the prothrombin time will be reported to the HCP.

CN: Pharmacological and parenteral therapies; CL: Evaluate

The Adult with Varicose Veins

77. **2.** The nurse instructs the client to elevate the legs to improve venous return and alleviate discomfort. Walking is encouraged to increase venous return. Sclerotherapy or laser treatment is done for cosmetic reasons, but it does not improve circulation. Surgery may be performed for severe venous insufficiency or recurrent thrombophlebitis in the varicosities. A femoral-popliteal bypass graft is a surgical intervention for arterial disease.

CN: Health promotion and maintenance; CL: Analyze

78. **3.** Secondary varicosities can result from previous thrombophlebitis of the deep femoral veins, with subsequent valvular incompetence. Cerebrovascular accidents, anemia, and transient ischemic attacks are not associated with an increased risk for varicose veins.

CN: Health promotion and maintenance; CL: Analyze

79. **1.** Sclerotherapy involves injecting small- and medium-sized varicose veins with a solution that scars and closes those veins. In a few weeks, the veins should fade and disappear. This procedure does not require anesthesia and can be done in a health care provider's office. Varicose veins can reoccur regardless of the procedure. Bruising is more likely following vein stripping or catheter-assisted procedures.

CN: Physiological adaptation; CL: Application

80. **1, 2, 4.** To manage varicose veins, the nurse should coach the client to lose weight to relieve pressure on the veins, wear compression stockings to promote circulation, and elevate the legs when sitting or lying down. Applying lotion to the veins will keep the skin moist, but it does not promote venous circulation. Pillows under the knees will obstruct circulation.

CN: Health promotion and maintenance; CL: Create

The Adult with Stasis Ulcers

81. **1, 2, 4, 5.** The underlying pathophysiology in stasis ulcers of the skin surface is a result of inadequate oxygen and other nutrients to the tissues because of edema and decreased circulation. The nurse should first initiate care that will increase oxygen and improve tissue integrity. It is also important to prevent trauma to the tissues and prevent infections, which result from decreased microcirculation that limits the body's response to infection. Stasis ulcers are painful. The nurse can administer prescribed analgesics 30 minutes before changing the dressing. There is no indication that the client's overall nutrition needs to be improved.

CN: Physiological adaptation; CL: Create

82. **1.** The result of chronic venous stasis is swelling and edema and superficial varicose veins. Diuretics will help reduce the swelling, thus improving capillary circulation. Although diuretics may decrease blood pressure, that is not the intended outcome of this drug. The nurse should teach the client to prevent infection and monitor wound healing, but these are not the primary outcomes of chlorothiazide.

CN: Pharmacological and parenteral therapies; CL: Evaluate

83. **4.** The nurse should keep bed linens off of the stasis ulcer to decrease the amount of pressure that the linens exert upon the lower extremity and prevent further tissue breakdown. Administering prescribed analgesics would be an intervention for reducing the pain. Applying lanolin lotions to the left ankle ulcer will not promote healing. Encouraging the client to sit up in a chair four times per day is an intervention to promote activity. The nurse would elevate the involved extremity while the client is sitting up to reduce venous stasis and capillary pressure.

CN: Basic care and comfort; CL: Analyze

84. **2.** The nurse should first determine how the client will apply an herb mixture to the ulcer. The nurse should then encourage the client to consult the health care provider because home remedies may be beneficial or may interfere with the medical treatment plan. In many cultures, home remedies are commonly used and may be helpful. The nurse must be sensitive to these traditions and cultural beliefs. The other statements demonstrate that the client understands the plan of care for the ulcer.

CN: Pharmacological and parenteral therapies; CL: Evaluate

Managing Care, Quality, and Safety for Adults with Vascular Disease

85. **3.** It is important for the nurse to assess the client with PAD returning from an angiogram. It will be important to make baseline assessments on this client. A client with atrial fibrillation with a heart rate of 90 bpm is not an abnormal finding. A "fluttering feeling" is expected in a client with atrial fibrillation. A client with heart failure experiencing right upper quadrant fullness does not require urgent attention; the client might be experiencing signs and symptoms of hepatomegaly.

CN: Management of care; CL: Analyze

86. **3.** The client is experiencing rebound tachycardia because of the abrupt withdrawal of the beta-blocker. The beta-blocker should be restarted because of the tachycardia, history of hypertension, and the desire to reduce the risk for postoperative myocardial morbidity. The bypass surgery should correct the claudication and the need for pentoxifylline. The furosemide and increasing fluids are not indicated since the client's urine output and blood pressure are satisfactory and there is no indication of bleeding. The nurse should also determine the potassium level before starting the furosemide.

CN: Management of care; CL: Analyze

87. **1.** The nurse is the client's advocate in planning for pain relief. When presented with a communications conflict, the nurse should first restate the concern, providing as much information as needed. If the HCP still does not offer an acceptable solution for pain management, the nurse can then discuss the situation with the hospitalist on the team and report the incident to the team leader. Waiting until the next shift to handle the problem does not contribute to the goal of managing the client's pain.

CN: Management of care; CL: Analyze

88. **1.** The LPN/VN can complete the assessment sheet and care for the client before surgery. Clients who are stable and require complete care or frequent assistance with basic care needs along with vital signs and intake and output recordings can be assigned to a UAP. An unstable client requiring critical assessments receives care from the RN.

CN: Management of Care; CL: Analyze

89. **1, 2, 3, 5.** When obtaining blood samples, the nurse must use two acceptable sources of identification (the client states their name; the nurse verifies the client's name and the identification number of the armband); verifying a room number is not acceptable as clients can be easily reassigned to other rooms. The client must be awake to state their name. Blood samples must be labeled in front of the client.

CN: Safety and infection control; CL: Analyze

90. **1.** Before starting a heparin infusion, the nurse needs to know the client's baseline blood coagulation values (hematocrit, hemoglobin, and red blood cell and platelet counts). In addition, the partial thromboplastin time should be monitored closely during the process. The client's stools would be tested only if internal bleeding is suspected. Although monitoring vital signs such as apical pulse is important in assessing potential signs and symptoms of hemorrhage or potential adverse reactions to the medication, vital signs are not the most important data to collect before administering the heparin. Intake and output are not important assessments for heparin administration unless the client has fluid and volume problems or kidney disease.

🔑 CN: Reduction of risk potential; CL: Analyze

91. 4. Several variables make this client a high fall risk, including a secondary diagnosis of diabetes (15); intermittent IV antibiotics (20); and mental status changes (15) possibly due to anesthesia, pain, or recent limb loss. This client's assessment may change as the effects of anesthesia wear off, pain is controlled, and the client becomes accustomed to ambulating with a prosthesis. Because assessments may be continually changing, in most acute care facilities, a fall risk assessment is completed every 24 hours and sometimes every shift.

🔑 CN: Safety and infection control; CL: Apply

TEST 3: The Adult with Hematologic Health Problems

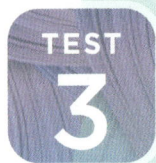

- The Adult with Red Blood Cell Disorders
- The Adult with Platelet Disorders
- The Adult with White Blood Cell Disorders
- The Adult with Lymphoma
- The Adult with Cardiogenic, Hypovolemic, or Septic Shock
- Managing Care, Quality, and Safety for Adults with Hematologic Health Problems
- Answers, Rationales, and Test-Taking Strategies

The Adult with Red Blood Cell Disorders

1. The nurse is assisting with a bone marrow aspiration and biopsy. In which order, from first to last, should the nurse complete these tasks? All options must be used.

1. Position the client in a side-lying position.
2. Clean the skin with an antiseptic solution.
3. Verify the client has signed an informed consent.
4. Apply ice to the biopsy site.

2. A client with iron deficiency anemia is refusing to take the prescribed oral iron medication because the medication is causing nausea; the client is also constipated. What action(s) should the nurse take? Select all that apply.
☐ 1. Suggest that the client use ginger when taking the medication.
☐ 2. Ask the client what is causing the nausea.
☐ 3. Tell the client to use stool softeners to minimize constipation.
☐ 4. Offer to administer the medication by intramuscular injection.
☐ 5. Suggest that the client take the iron with orange juice.

3. A client is to have a transfusion of packed red blood cells from a designated donor. The client asks if any diseases can be transmitted by this donor. The nurse should inform the client that which disease(s) can be transmitted by a designated donor? Select all that apply.
☐ 1. Epstein-Barr virus
☐ 2. human immunodeficiency virus (HIV)
☐ 3. cytomegalovirus (CMV)
☐ 4. hepatitis A
☐ 5. malaria

4. The nurse is preparing to teach a client with iron deficiency anemia about the diet to follow after discharge. Which food should be included in the diet?
☐ 1. eggs
☐ 2. lettuce
☐ 3. citrus fruits
☐ 4. cheese

5. The nurse is teaching the client with vitamin B_{12} deficiency about ways to increase the dietary intake of vitamin B_{12}. Which foods would provide the **best** supply of vitamin B_{12}?
☐ 1. whole grains
☐ 2. green leafy vegetables
☐ 3. meats and dairy products
☐ 4. broccoli and Brussels sprouts

6. The nurse is developing a teaching plan for the client with aplastic anemia. Which is **most** important to include in the plan?
☐ 1. Eat animal protein and dark green, leafy vegetables every day.
☐ 2. Avoid exposure to others with acute infections.
☐ 3. Practice yoga and meditation to decrease stress and anxiety.
☐ 4. Get 8 hours of sleep at night, and take naps during the day.

7. A client had a resection of the terminal ileum 3 years ago. While obtaining a health history and conducting a physical assessment, the nurse finds that the client is experiencing weakness, shortness of breath, and a sore tongue. Which additional information from the client indicates a need for client teaching?
   ☐ 1. "I have been drinking plenty of fluids."
   ☐ 2. "I have been gargling with warm salt water for my sore tongue."
   ☐ 3. "I have regular bowel movements on most days."
   ☐ 4. "I take a vitamin B$_{12}$ tablet every day."

8. A client who follows a vegetarian diet was referred to a dietitian for nutritional counseling for anemia. Which client outcome indicates that the client needs further nutritional counseling?
   ☐ 1. The client adds dried fruit to cereal and baked goods.
   ☐ 2. The client cooks tomato-based foods in iron pots.
   ☐ 3. The client drinks coffee or tea with meals.
   ☐ 4. The client adds vitamin C to all meals.

9. A client was admitted to the hospital with iron deficiency anemia and blood-streaked emesis. Which question is **most** appropriate for the nurse to ask in determining the extent of the client's activity intolerance?
   ☐ 1. "What daily activities were you able to do 6 months ago compared with the present?"
   ☐ 2. "How long have you had this problem?"
   ☐ 3. "Have you been able to keep up with all your usual activities?"
   ☐ 4. "Are you more tired now than you used to be?"

10. A health care provider (HCP) prescribes vitamin B$_{12}$ for a client with pernicious anemia. Which site(s) are appropriate for the nurse to administer vitamin B$_{12}$ to an adult? Select all that apply.
    ☐ 1. median cutaneous
    ☐ 2. greater femur trochanter
    ☐ 3. acromion muscle
    ☐ 4. ventrogluteal
    ☐ 5. upper back
    ☐ 6. dorsogluteal

11. The nurse is administering an injection of vitamin B$_{12}$. In which position should the nurse place the client to decrease discomfort when injecting the medication into the ventrogluteal site?
    ☐ 1. lying on the side with legs extended
    ☐ 2. lying on the abdomen with toes pointed inward
    ☐ 3. leaning over the edge of a low table with hips flexed
    ☐ 4. standing upright with the feet one shoulder-width apart

12. A client is admitted to the emergency department after falling down a flight of stairs at home. The client's vital signs are stable, and the history states that the client had a gastric stapling 2 years ago. The client jokes about being clumsy lately and tripping over things. The nurse should gather additional information by asking the client which question(s)? Select all that apply.
    ☐ 1. "Are you experiencing numbness in your extremities?"
    ☐ 2. "How much vitamin B$_{12}$ are you getting?"
    ☐ 3. "Are you feeling depressed?"
    ☐ 4. "Do you feel safe at home?"
    ☐ 5. "Are you getting sufficient iron in your diet?"

13. A client has fatigue, a temperature of 99.5°F (37.5°C), yellow-tinged skin and sclera, and dark urine. The client's hemoglobin is 9 g/dL (90 g/L), and the hematocrit is 49% (0.49 proportion of 1.0). What should the nurse do **first**?
    ☐ 1. Start an intake and output record.
    ☐ 2. Place the client on bed rest.
    ☐ 3. Initiate contact precautions.
    ☐ 4. Keep the client out of sunlight.

14. The nurse is administering a cephalosporin to a client. The nurse should monitor the client for which finding?
    ☐ 1. drug-induced hemolytic anemia
    ☐ 2. purpura
    ☐ 3. infectious emboli
    ☐ 4. ecchymosis

15. A client with pernicious anemia is receiving vitamin B$_{12}$. The nurse should evaluate the client for which expected outcome of vitamin B$_{12}$ administration?
    ☐ 1. increased energy
    ☐ 2. healed tongue and lips
    ☐ 3. absence of paresthesia
    ☐ 4. improved clotting time

16. A client with pernicious anemia asks why it is necessary to take vitamin B$_{12}$ injections forever. Which is the nurse's **best** response?
    ☐ 1. "The reason for your vitamin deficiency is an inability to absorb the vitamin because the stomach is not producing sufficient acid."
    ☐ 2. "The reason for your vitamin deficiency is an inability to absorb the vitamin because the stomach is not producing sufficient amounts of a factor that allows the vitamin to be absorbed."
    ☐ 3. "The reason for your vitamin deficiency is an excessive excretion of the vitamin because of kidney dysfunction."
    ☐ 4. "The reason for your vitamin deficiency is an increased requirement for the vitamin because of rapid red blood cell production."

17. The nurse is assessing a client's activity tolerance. Which report from a treadmill test indicates an abnormal response?
- ☐ 1. heart rate increased by 20 bpm immediately after the activity
- ☐ 2. respiratory rate decreased by 5 breaths/min
- ☐ 3. diastolic blood pressure increased by 7 mm Hg
- ☐ 4. pulse rate within 6 bpm of resting pulse after 3 minutes of rest

18. Three days following surgery, the client's hematocrit decreased from 36% (0.36 proportion of 1.0) to 34% (0.34 proportion of 1.0), and the red blood cell (RBC) count and hemoglobin value remained stable at 4.5 million/μL (4.5×10^{12}/L) and 11.9 g/dL (119 g/L), respectively. What should the nurse do **next**?
- ☐ 1. Check the dressing and drains for frank bleeding.
- ☐ 2. Call the health care provider (HCP).
- ☐ 3. Continue to monitor vital signs.
- ☐ 4. Start oxygen at 2 L per minute via nasal cannula.

19. The nurse is administering packed red blood cells (PRBCs) to a client. What should the nurse do **first**?
- ☐ 1. Discontinue the intravenous (IV) catheter if a blood transfusion reaction occurs.
- ☐ 2. Administer the PRBCs through a percutaneously inserted central catheter line with a 20-gauge needle.
- ☐ 3. Flush PRBCs with 5% dextrose and 0.45% normal saline solution.
- ☐ 4. Stay with the client during the first 15 minutes of infusion.

20. The nurse is preparing a client with sickle cell anemia for discharge. What information should the nurse include in the teaching plan? Select all that apply.
- ☐ 1. Drink plenty of fluids when outside in hot weather.
- ☐ 2. Avoid being in high altitudes where less oxygen is available.
- ☐ 3. Be aware that since the client is homozygous for HbS, they carry the sickle cell trait.
- ☐ 4. Know that pregnancy with sickle cell disease increases the risk for a crisis.
- ☐ 5. Avoid flying on commercial airlines.

21. The nurse is teaching a client newly diagnosed with hemochromatosis about reducing the risk for complications. Which information should the nurse include in the teaching plan? Select all that apply.
- ☐ 1. "You should not take any iron supplements."
- ☐ 2. "Read labels on multivitamins, and do not use them if they contain iron."
- ☐ 3. "Increase the amount of vitamin C in your diet by drinking more orange juice."
- ☐ 4. "Try to increase your fluid intake to 3500 mL per day."
- ☐ 5. "You should not have drinks or medications containing alcohol."

22. A client is having a blood transfusion reaction. What must the nurse do in order of **priority** from first to last? All options must be used.

1. Notify the health care provider (HCP) and blood bank.
2. Complete the appropriate transfusion reaction form(s).
3. Stop the transfusion.
4. Keep the intravenous (IV) line open with normal saline infusion.

23. A client is receiving 2 units of packed red blood cells (PRBCs). Which safety measure(s) should the nurse implement? Select all that apply.
- ☐ 1. Verify that the ABO and Rh of the two units are the same.
- ☐ 2. Infuse a unit of PRBCs in less than 4 hours.
- ☐ 3. Stop the transfusion if a reaction occurs, but keep the line open.
- ☐ 4. Take vital signs every 15 minutes while the unit is transfusing.
- ☐ 5. Inspect the blood bag for leaks, abnormal color, and clots.
- ☐ 6. Use a 22-gauge catheter for optimal flow of a blood transfusion.

24. A client who had received 25 mL of packed red blood cells (PRBCs) has low back pain and pruritus. After stopping the infusion, the nurse should take what action **next**?
    ☐ 1. Administer a prescribed antihistamine and antipyretic.
    ☐ 2. Collect blood and urine samples, and send them to the lab.
    ☐ 3. Administer prescribed diuretics.
    ☐ 4. Administer prescribed vasopressors.

25. A client is to receive epoetin injections. What laboratory value should the nurse review before giving the injection?
    ☐ 1. hematocrit
    ☐ 2. partial thromboplastin time
    ☐ 3. hemoglobin concentration
    ☐ 4. prothrombin time

26. A client is to begin intravenous (IV) erythropoietin therapy. What action(s) should the nurse take? Select all that apply.
    ☐ 1. Check the hemoglobin levels before administering subsequent doses.
    ☐ 2. Shake the vial thoroughly to mix the concentrated white, milky solution.
    ☐ 3. Keep the multidose vial refrigerated between scheduled twice-a-day doses.
    ☐ 4. Administer the medication through the IV line without other medications.
    ☐ 5. Adjust the initial doses according to the client's changes in blood pressure.
    ☐ 6. Instruct the client to avoid driving and performing hazardous activities during the initial treatment.

27. A client is afraid of receiving vitamin B_{12} injections because of potential toxic reactions. Which is the nurse's **best** response to relieve these fears?
    ☐ 1. "Vitamin B_{12} will cause ringing in the ears before a toxic level is reached."
    ☐ 2. "Vitamin B_{12} may cause a very mild rash initially."
    ☐ 3. "Vitamin B_{12} causes mild nausea but nothing toxic."
    ☐ 4. "Vitamin B_{12} is generally free of toxicity because it is water soluble."

28. A client with iron deficiency anemia is having trouble selecting food from the hospital menu. Which food(s) should the nurse suggest to meet the client's need for iron? Select all that apply.
    ☐ 1. eggs
    ☐ 2. brown rice
    ☐ 3. dark green vegetables
    ☐ 4. tea with sugar
    ☐ 5. oatmeal

29. A client with macrocytic anemia has a burn on the foot and reports watching television while lying on a heating pad. Which action should the nurse take **first**?
    ☐ 1. Assess for potential abuse.
    ☐ 2. Check for diminished sensations.
    ☐ 3. Document the findings.
    ☐ 4. Clean and dress the area.

30. The nurse is assessing a client who has aplastic anemia. Which finding indicates the client has physiologic changes as a result of the disease?
    ☐ 1. bleeding tendencies
    ☐ 2. decreased intake and output
    ☐ 3. loss of peripheral sensation
    ☐ 4. frequent diarrhea

The Adult with Platelet Disorders

31. The nurse is to administer subcutaneous heparin to an underweight older adult. What should the nurse consider when administering this medication? Select all that apply.
    ☐ 1. It is administered in the anterior area of the iliac crest.
    ☐ 2. The onset is immediate.
    ☐ 3. A 27-gauge, 5/8-inch (1.6-mm) needle should be used.
    ☐ 4. Cephalosporin potentiates the effects of heparin.
    ☐ 5. The dose should be verified with another nurse according to agency policy.

32. A client with a platelet disorder has a platelet count of 31,000/µL (31×10^9/L). What should the nurse instruct the client to do?
    ☐ 1. Pad sharp surfaces to avoid minor trauma when walking.
    ☐ 2. Assess for spontaneous petechiae in the extremities.
    ☐ 3. Wear a mask when in crowds of people.
    ☐ 4. Check for blood in the urine.

33. A female client with a history of systemic lupus erythematosus was admitted with a severe viral respiratory tract infection and diffuse petechiae. Based on these data, what recent information about the client should the nurse assess further?
    ☐ 1. quality and quantity of food intake
    ☐ 2. type and amount of fluid intake
    ☐ 3. extent of weakness and fatigue
    ☐ 4. length and amount of menstrual flow

34. A client with thrombocytopenia has a severe headache. The nurse should interpret this finding as resulting from which underlying cause?
    ☐ 1. stress of the disease
    ☐ 2. cerebral bleeding
    ☐ 3. migraine headache
    ☐ 4. sinus congestion

35. The nurse is teaching the client with a platelet disorder about signs of bleeding. What statement from the client indicates the client has understood the teaching?
☐ 1. "Petechiae are large, red skin bruises."
☐ 2. "Ecchymoses are large, purple skin bruises."
☐ 3. "Purpura is an open cut on the skin."
☐ 4. "Abrasions are small pinpoint red dots on the skin."

36. A client with a platelet disorder has a platelet count of less than 150,000/μL (150 × 10⁹/L). The nurse should instruct the client to avoid which activity?
☐ 1. walking for more than 10 minutes
☐ 2. straining to have a bowel movement
☐ 3. visiting with young children
☐ 4. sitting in the semi-Fowler position

37. A client who is taking aspirin caplets develops prolonged bleeding from a superficial skin injury on the forearm. The nurse should tell the client to do which action **first**?
☐ 1. Place the forearm under a running stream of lukewarm water.
☐ 2. Pat the injury with a dry washcloth.
☐ 3. Wrap the entire forearm from the wrist to the elbow.
☐ 4. Apply an ice pack for 20 minutes.

38. A client with thrombocytopenia has developed a hemorrhage. The nurse should assess the client for which finding?
☐ 1. tachycardia
☐ 2. bradycardia
☐ 3. decreased partial pressure of carbon dioxide (PaCO₂)
☐ 4. narrowed pulse pressure

39. The client with idiopathic thrombocytopenic purpura (ITP) asks the nurse why it is necessary to take steroids. The nurse should base the response on which information?
☐ 1. Steroids destroy the antibodies and prolong the life of platelets.
☐ 2. Steroids neutralize the antigens and prolong the life of platelets.
☐ 3. Steroids increase phagocytosis and increase the life of platelets.
☐ 4. Steroids alter the spleen's recognition of platelets and increase the life of platelets.

40. A client with a platelet disorder is to be discharged with a prescription for prednisone. Which statement indicates that the client understands how to take the medication?
☐ 1. "I need to take the medicine in divided doses at morning and bedtime."
☐ 2. "I am to take 40 mg of prednisone for 2 months and then stop."
☐ 3. "I need to wear or carry identification that I am taking prednisone."
☐ 4. "I will take the medication on an empty stomach."

41. When teaching a client older than age 50 who is receiving long-term prednisone therapy, the nurse should make which suggestion?
☐ 1. Take the prednisone with food.
☐ 2. Take over-the-counter antiemetics.
☐ 3. Exercise three to four times a week.
☐ 4. Eat foods that are low in potassium.

42. The nurse is preparing a teaching plan about increased exercise for a female client who is receiving long-term corticosteroid therapy. What type of exercise is **most** appropriate for this client?
☐ 1. floor exercises
☐ 2. stretching
☐ 3. running
☐ 4. walking

43. The nurse is teaching a female client with a history of acquired thrombocytopenia about how to prevent and control hemorrhage. Which statement indicates that the client needs further instruction?
☐ 1. "I can apply direct pressure over small cuts for at least 5 to 10 minutes to stop a venous bleed."
☐ 2. "I can count the number of tissues saturated to detect blood loss during a nosebleed."
☐ 3. "I can take hormones to decrease blood loss during menses."
☐ 4. "I can count the number of sanitary napkins to detect excess blood loss during menses."

44. A client has been on long-term prednisone therapy. What food source(s) should the nurse instruct the client to be sure to include in the diet to counteract the adverse effects of the drug? Select all that apply.
☐ 1. carbohydrates
☐ 2. protein
☐ 3. saturated fat
☐ 4. potassium
☐ 5. calcium
☐ 6. vitamin D

45. The nurse has received a bag of platelets from the pharmacy and is preparing to administer them to a client. Which finding indicates the nurse should the nurse contact the pharmacist?
☐ 1. The platelet bag is cold.
☐ 2. The platelet bag is 2 days old.
☐ 3. The platelet bag is at room temperature.
☐ 4. The platelet bag is 12 hours old.

46. The nurse is preparing to administer platelets. What should the nurse do **first**?
☐ 1. Check the ABO compatibility.
☐ 2. Administer the platelets slowly.
☐ 3. Gently rotate the bag.
☐ 4. Use a whole-blood tubing set.

47. A client is scheduled for an elective splenectomy. What is the **last** thing the nurse should determine before the client goes to surgery? The client has:
☐ 1. voided completely.
☐ 2. signed the consent.
☐ 3. vital signs recorded.
☐ 4. a name band on their wrist.

48. The nurse is receiving a client from the postanesthesia care unit after a splenectomy. After obtaining vital signs, what information should the nurse obtain **next**?
☐ 1. the presence of nasogastric drainage
☐ 2. the amount of urine drainage from the urinary catheter
☐ 3. the presence of blood or drainage on the dressing
☐ 4. the client's pain level

49. A client who had a splenectomy yesterday has a nasogastric (NG) tube. What should the nurse assess to determine the effectiveness of the NG tube?
☐ 1. depth of diaphragmatic breathing
☐ 2. amount of blood draining from the tube
☐ 3. absence of abdominal distention
☐ 4. normal pH of gastric contents

50. A client who had a splenectomy is being discharged. What should the nurse teach the client to do?
☐ 1. Refrain from driving a car for 6 weeks.
☐ 2. Alternate rest and activity.
☐ 3. Make an appointment for the staples to be removed.
☐ 4. Report early signs of infection.

51. The nurse is assessing a client at risk for acute disseminated intravascular coagulation (DIC). Which finding indicates the client is showing an early sign of DIC?
☐ 1. severe shortness of breath
☐ 2. bleeding without history or cause
☐ 3. orthopnea
☐ 4. hematuria

52. The nurse is planning care for a client with disseminated intravascular coagulation (DIC)? Which action is contraindicated?
☐ 1. treating the underlying cause
☐ 2. administering heparin
☐ 3. administering warfarin sodium
☐ 4. replacing depleted blood products

53. A client with disseminated intravascular coagulation develops clinical manifestations of microvascular thrombosis. What signs should the nurse report to the health care provider (HCP)?
☐ 1. hemoptysis
☐ 2. focal ischemia
☐ 3. petechiae
☐ 4. hematuria

The Adult with White Blood Cell Disorders

54. A client is diagnosed with infectious mononucleosis. The white blood cell count is 19,000/µL (19 × 10⁹/L). The client has a streptococcal throat infection, enlarged spleen, and aching muscles. Which instruction(s) should the nurse include in discharge planning with the client? Select all that apply.
☐ 1. Stay on bed rest until the temperature is normal.
☐ 2. Gargle with warm saline while the throat is irritated.
☐ 3. Increase intake of fluids until the infection subsides.
☐ 4. Wear a mask if others are present.
☐ 5. Avoid contact sports while the spleen is enlarged.

55. A client who had an exploratory laparotomy 3 days ago now has a white blood cell (WBC) count of 15,000 µL (15 × 10⁹/L). For which clinical finding(s) of this laboratory report should the nurse assess the client? Select all that apply.
☐ 1. swelling around the incision
☐ 2. redness around the incision
☐ 3. elevated temperature
☐ 4. nonproductive cough
☐ 5. weak pedal pulses

56. The nurse is developing a care plan with a client who has leukemia. What instruction(s) should the nurse include in the plan? Select all that apply.
☐ 1. Monitor temperature and report elevation.
☐ 2. Recognize signs and symptoms of infection.
☐ 3. Avoid crowds.
☐ 4. Maintain the integrity of skin and mucous membranes.
☐ 5. Take a baby aspirin each day.

57. A client with neutropenia has an absolute neutrophil count (ANC) of 900/µL (0.9 × 10⁹/L). The nurse teaches the client to prevent which risk for neutropenia?
☐ 1. bleeding
☐ 2. infection
☐ 3. hemorrhagic stroke
☐ 4. sickle cell crisis

58. The nurse is taking care of a client with neutropenia. Which nursing action is **most** important in preventing cross-contamination?
☐ 1. changing gloves immediately after use
☐ 2. standing 2 feet (61 cm) from the client
☐ 3. speaking minimally when in the room
☐ 4. wearing protective coverings

59. The nurse is preparing the client with neutropenia for discharge to home. What should the nurse teach the client to avoid?
☐ 1. using suppositories or enemas
☐ 2. using a high-efficiency particulate air (HEPA) filter mask
☐ 3. performing perianal care after every bowel movement
☐ 4. performing oral care after every meal

60. A client with granulocytopenia has many visitors. What is the **most** important thing the nurse should tell the visitors to do to prevent infection?
☐ 1. Visit only if they do not have a cold.
☐ 2. Wash their hands.
☐ 3. Leave the children at home.
☐ 4. Avoid kissing the client.

61. A nurse is obtaining consent for a bone marrow aspiration. Which action(s) should the nurse take? Select all that apply.
☐ 1. Witness the client signing the consent form.
☐ 2. Evaluate that the client understands the procedure.
☐ 3. Explain the risks of the procedure to the client.
☐ 4. Verify that the client is signing the consent form of their own free will.
☐ 5. Determine that the client understands postprocedure care.

62. A client is about to undergo bone marrow aspiration of the sternum. What should the nurse tell the client?
☐ 1. "You may feel a solution being wiped over your entire front from your neck down to your navel and out to your shoulders."
☐ 2. "You will not feel the local anesthetic being applied because it will be sprayed on."
☐ 3. "You will feel a pulling type of discomfort for a few seconds."
☐ 4. "After the needle is removed, you will feel a bandage being applied around your chest."

63. Twenty-four hours after a bone marrow aspiration, the nurse is evaluating the client's postprocedure status. Which outcome is expected?
☐ 1. The client maintains bed rest.
☐ 2. There is redness and swelling at the aspiration site.
☐ 3. The client requests a strong analgesic for pain.
☐ 4. There is no bleeding at the aspiration site.

64. A client states, "I don't want any more tests. Who cares what kind of leukemia I have? I just want to be treated now." Which is the nurse's **best** response?
☐ 1. "I am sure you are frustrated and want to be well now."
☐ 2. "Your treatment can be more effective if it is based on more specific information about your disease."
☐ 3. "These tests are necessary, and the health care provider has ordered them for you."
☐ 4. "I understand how you feel."

65. A client is in the induction stage of treatment for leukemia. The nurse should ask the family to remove which items they have brought into the room?
☐ 1. a prayer book
☐ 2. a picture
☐ 3. a bouquet of flowers
☐ 4. a hairbrush

66. The nurse is teaching the client who is undergoing induction therapy for leukemia. The nurse realizes the client needs additional instruction when the client makes which statement?
☐ 1. "I will pace my activities with rest periods."
☐ 2. "I cannot wait to get home to my cat!"
☐ 3. "I will use a warm saline gargle instead of brushing my teeth."
☐ 4. "I must report a temperature of 100°F (37.7°C)."

67. A client with chronic myelogenous leukemia is taking imatinib. The nurse should instruct the client to report which adverse effect of this drug?
☐ 1. edema
☐ 2. numbness and tingling in extremities
☐ 3. bloody stools
☐ 4. persistent cough

68. A client with acute lymphocytic leukemia is receiving vincristine. Prior to infusing the drug, the nurse administers diphenhydramine. What should the nurse tell the client about the purpose of taking diphenhydramine?
☐ 1. Diphenhydramine promotes sleep while the vincristine is infusing.
☐ 2. Diphenhydramine decreases the incidence of a reaction to the vincristine.
☐ 3. Diphenhydramine potentiates the action of the vincristine.
☐ 4. Diphenhydramine reduces anxiety associated with the vincristine infusion.

69. A nurse is administering an intravenous (IV) antineoplastic agent when the client says, "My arm is burning by the IV site." What should the nurse do **first**?
☐ 1. Slow the infusion rate and check the IV site.
☐ 2. Tell the client to take a deep breath.
☐ 3. Stop infusing the medication.
☐ 4. Place a warm, moist pack on the IV site area.

70. A client who is receiving a blood transfusion suddenly experiences chills and a temperature of 101°F (38°C). The client also has a headache and appears flushed. In what order, from first to last, should the nurse perform the actions? All options must be used.

1. Obtain a blood culture from the client.

2. Send the blood bag and administration set to the blood bank.

3. Stop the blood infusion.

4. Infuse normal saline to keep the vein open.

☐

☐

☐

☐

71. A client undergoing antineoplastic therapy is prescribed subcutaneous epoetin. What indicates to the nurse that the drug has been effective?
☐ 1. Biopsies no longer show malignancy.
☐ 2. Hemoglobin levels rise.
☐ 3. Nausea and vomiting stop.
☐ 4. A scan shows tumor shrinkage.

72. The nurse is planning care for a client with acute myeloid leukemia (AML). What is an appropriate goal for this client?
☐ 1. Prevent cardiac arrhythmias.
☐ 2. Prevent liver failure.
☐ 3. Prevent renal failure.
☐ 4. Prevent hemorrhage.

73. The client with acute lymphocytic leukemia (ALL) is at risk for infection. What action should the nurse take?
☐ 1. Place the client in a private room.
☐ 2. Have the client wear a mask.
☐ 3. Have staff wear gowns and gloves.
☐ 4. Restrict visitors.

74. The nurse is planning care for a client with acute leukemia who has mucositis. What should the nurse advise the client to use for mouth care?
☐ 1. lemon-glycerin swabs
☐ 2. a commercial mouthwash
☐ 3. normal saline
☐ 4. a commercial toothpaste and brush

75. An adult client with acute leukemia and the health care team establish goals of improved tidal volume and activity tolerance. Which action(s) would be **most** helpful in attaining these goals? Select all that apply.
☐ 1. increasing fluids to 3000 mL every 24 hours
☐ 2. walking to increase the number of steps each day
☐ 3. sitting in a chair to read or watch television
☐ 4. taking deep breaths while sitting or lying in bed
☐ 5. using a stationary bicycle to increase elevation and time

76. The nurse is evaluating the client's understanding of combination chemotherapy. Which statement by the client about the reasons for using combination chemotherapy indicates the need for **further** explanation?
☐ 1. "Combination chemotherapy is used to interrupt cell growth cycle at different points."
☐ 2. "Combination chemotherapy is used to destroy cancer cells and treat side effects simultaneously."
☐ 3. "Combination chemotherapy is used to decrease resistance."
☐ 4. "Combination chemotherapy is used to minimize the toxicity from using high doses of a single agent."

77. In providing care to a client with leukemia who has developed thrombocytopenia, the nurse is assessing the client for bleeding. Which are the most common site(s) for bleeding that the nurse should assess? Select all that apply.
☐ 1. biliary system
☐ 2. gastrointestinal tract
☐ 3. brain and meninges
☐ 4. pulmonary system
☐ 5. integumentary system

78. The nurse is placing a client with severe neutropenia on neutropenic precautions. The nurse should tell the client that neutropenic precautions will prevent the spread of organisms in which way?
☐ 1. preventing the spreading of organisms to the client from sources outside the client's environment
☐ 2. limiting the transfer of organisms from the client to health care personnel and visitors
☐ 3. disposing of contaminated materials in marked containers
☐ 4. keeping the client's linens and personal items in the room

The Adult with Lymphoma

79. The nurse is developing a care plan for a client who has had radiation therapy for Hodgkin lymphoma. What is the **primary** goal of care for this client?
    ☐ 1. Maintain fluid balance.
    ☐ 2. Obtain sufficient exercise.
    ☐ 3. Prevent infection.
    ☐ 4. Avoid depression.

80. A client with a suspected diagnosis of Hodgkin disease is to have a lymph node biopsy. What should the nurse make sure that personnel involved with the procedure do?
    ☐ 1. Maintain sterile technique.
    ☐ 2. Use a mask, gloves, and a gown when assisting with the procedure.
    ☐ 3. Send the specimen to the laboratory when someone is available to take it.
    ☐ 4. Ensure that all instruments used are placed in a sealed and labeled container.

81. A client with Hodgkin disease undergoes an excisional cervical lymph node biopsy under local anesthesia. After the procedure, what does the nurse assess **first**?
    ☐ 1. vital signs
    ☐ 2. the incision
    ☐ 3. the airway
    ☐ 4. neurologic signs

82. The nurse is assessing a client with Hodgkin disease. Which finding is concerning?
    ☐ 1. herpes zoster infections
    ☐ 2. discolored teeth
    ☐ 3. hemorrhage
    ☐ 4. hypercellular immunity

83. A client with Hodgkin disease develops B symptoms. Which symptom is a manifestation of B symptoms?
    ☐ 1. a low-grade fever (temperature lower than 100°F [37.8°C])
    ☐ 2. a weight loss of 5% or less of body weight
    ☐ 3. night sweats
    ☐ 4. not progressing to an advanced stage

84. The nurse is developing a discharge plan with a client who is receiving chemotherapy to treat lymphoma. What should the nurse include in the plan?
    ☐ 1. Wear a mask when in crowded, enclosed areas.
    ☐ 2. Rest as needed.
    ☐ 3. Avoid people with colds or flu.
    ☐ 4. Decrease the protein in your diet.
    ☐ 5. Contact the health care provider (HCP) if a fever develops.

85. The client asks the nurse to explain what it means that Hodgkin disease is diagnosed at stage 1A. What should the nurse explain about the involvement of the disease?
    ☐ 1. involvement of a single lymph node
    ☐ 2. involvement of two or more lymph nodes on the same side of the diaphragm
    ☐ 3. involvement of lymph node regions on both sides of the diaphragm
    ☐ 4. diffuse disease of one or more extralymphatic organs

86. A client is undergoing a bone marrow aspiration and biopsy. The client is very worried about the procedure. What should the nurse do to prepare the client for the procedure?
    ☐ 1. Allow the client's family to stay as long as possible.
    ☐ 2. Listen as the client expresses concerns.
    ☐ 3. Encourage the client to take slow, deep breaths to relax.
    ☐ 4. Suggest the client request the health care provider prescribe a sedative.

87. The nurse explains to the client with Hodgkin disease that a bone marrow biopsy will be taken after the aspiration. What should the nurse explain about the biopsy?
    ☐ 1. "Your biopsy will be performed before the aspiration because enough tissue may be obtained so that you will not have to go through the aspiration."
    ☐ 2. "You will feel a pressure sensation when the biopsy is taken but should not feel actual pain; if you do, tell the health care provider so that you can be given extra numbing medicine."
    ☐ 3. "You may hear a crunch as the needle passes through the bone, but when the biopsy is taken, you will feel a suction-type pain that will last for just a moment."
    ☐ 4. "You will be shaved and cleaned with an antiseptic agent, after which the health care provider will inject a needle without making an incision to aspirate out the bone marrow."

88. A client with advanced Hodgkin disease is admitted to hospice because death is imminent. What is the most important nursing goal at this time?
    ☐ 1. Reduce the client's fear of pain.
    ☐ 2. Support the client's wish to discontinue further therapy.
    ☐ 3. Prevent feelings of isolation.
    ☐ 4. Help the client overcome feelings of social inadequacy.

89. The client is a survivor of non-Hodgkin lymphoma. Which statement indicates the client needs additional information?
- ☐ 1. "Regular screening is very important for me."
- ☐ 2. "The survivor rate is directly proportional to the incidence of second malignancy."
- ☐ 3. "The survivor rate is indirectly proportional to the incidence of second malignancy."
- ☐ 4. "It is important for survivors to know the stage of the disease and their current treatment plan."

The Adult with Cardiogenic, Hypovolemic, or Septic Shock

90. The nurse is planning care for a client who is in cardiogenic shock following a myocardial infarction. What is the **most** important goal of nursing care for this client?
- ☐ 1. Prevent fluid overload.
- ☐ 2. Improve cardiac output.
- ☐ 3. Ensure adequate tissue perfusion.
- ☐ 4. Monitor for vasoconstriction of vascular beds.

91. A client has a traumatic injury to the leg and has a blood loss of about 15%. Which finding is **most** concerning for this client?
- ☐ 1. heart rate less than 60 bpm
- ☐ 2. respiratory rate of 4 breaths/min
- ☐ 3. pupils unequally dilated
- ☐ 4. systolic blood pressure less than 90 mm Hg

92. The nurse is evaluating the effectiveness of fluid replacement for a client in hypovolemic shock. Which finding is the **best** indication that fluid replacement is adequate?
- ☐ 1. urine output greater than 30 mL per hour
- ☐ 2. systolic blood pressure higher than 110 mm Hg
- ☐ 3. diastolic blood pressure higher than 90 mm Hg
- ☐ 4. respiratory rate of 20 breaths/min

93. The nurse is assessing a client whose blood pressure is dropping and heart rate and respiratory rate are increasing. Which finding indicates the client is at risk for hypovolemic shock?
- ☐ 1. severe hemorrhage
- ☐ 2. antigen-antibody reaction
- ☐ 3. gram-negative bacteria
- ☐ 4. massive vasodilation

94. The nurse is administering an intravenous (IV) infusion of packed red blood cells and normal saline solution to a client who is in hemorrhagic shock. Which is a **priority** for the nurse to assess for this client?
- ☐ 1. fluid balance
- ☐ 2. anaphylactic reaction
- ☐ 3. pain
- ☐ 4. altered level of consciousness

95. A client who is in hypovolemic shock and not responding to fluid replacement has a prescription for an intravenous (IV) infusion of dopamine hydrochloride at 5 mcg/kg/min. To determine that the drug is having the desired effect, what should the nurse assess?
- ☐ 1. increased renal and mesenteric blood flow
- ☐ 2. increased cardiac output
- ☐ 3. vasoconstriction
- ☐ 4. reduced preload and afterload

96. A client is receiving dopamine hydrochloride to manage cardiogenic shock. What action should the nurse take?
- ☐ 1. Administer pain medication concurrently.
- ☐ 2. Monitor blood pressure continuously.
- ☐ 3. Evaluate arterial blood gases at least every 2 hours.
- ☐ 4. Monitor for signs of infection.

97. When assessing a client for early septic shock, the nurse should assess the client for which finding?
- ☐ 1. cool, clammy skin
- ☐ 2. warm, flushed skin
- ☐ 3. increased blood pressure
- ☐ 4. hemorrhage

98. The nurse is planning care for an older adult with an indwelling catheter who is at risk for septic shock. Which nursing action will be **most** important for this client?
- ☐ 1. administering intravenous (IV) fluid replacement therapy as prescribed
- ☐ 2. obtaining vital signs every 4 hours
- ☐ 3. monitoring red blood cell counts for elevation
- ☐ 4. using aseptic technique when caring for the catheter

99. An older adult client with chronic obstructive pulmonary disease (COPD) is admitted to the emergency department because of rapid-onset confusion. The client's spouse tells the nurse the client has a urinary tract infection but became confused 2 hours ago. The client's vital signs are now heart rate 98 bpm; respiratory rate 24 breaths/min; and blood pressure 95/68 mm Hg. Which information from the admission history is **most** concerning?
- ☐ 1. The client is an older adult.
- ☐ 2. The client has COPD.
- ☐ 3. The client is confused.
- ☐ 4. The client has a urinary tract infection.

100. The nurse is assessing a client with septic shock. Which finding is an indication of a complication of septic shock?
  ☐ 1. anaphylaxis
  ☐ 2. acute respiratory distress syndrome (ARDS)
  ☐ 3. chronic obstructive pulmonary disease (COPD)
  ☐ 4. mitral valve prolapse

Managing Care, Quality, and Safety for Adults with Hematologic Health Problems

101. A nurse is taking care of two clients who are receiving transfusions of packed red blood cells at the same time. The first client's blood pressure dropped from the preoperative value of 120/80 mm Hg to a postoperative value of 100/50 mm Hg. The second client is hospitalized because they developed dehydration and anemia following pneumonia. After checking the patency of their intravenous (IV) lines and vital signs, the nurse should perform which action **next**?
  ☐ 1. Call for both clients' blood transfusions at the same time.
  ☐ 2. Ask another nurse to verify the compatibility of both units at the same time.
  ☐ 3. Call for and hang the first client's blood transfusion.
  ☐ 4. Ask another nurse to call for and hang the blood for the second client.

102. When a blood transfusion is terminated following a reaction, what action(s) must the nurse take? Select all that apply.
  ☐ 1. Send freshly collected urine samples to the laboratory.
  ☐ 2. Return the remainder of the blood component unit to the blood bank.
  ☐ 3. Return the intravenous administration set to the blood bank.
  ☐ 4. Alert the risk management department about the incident.
  ☐ 5. Report the incident to the infection control manager.

103. The nurse is administering a medication to a client with myeloid leukemia and does not know the use, dose, or side effects. To obtain the **most** up-to-date information about this drug, the nurse should perform which action?
  ☐ 1. Check a commercially published drug guide.
  ☐ 2. Read a pharmacology textbook.
  ☐ 3. Consult the drug guide provided by the clinical agency.
  ☐ 4. Review information at the drug manufacturer's website.

104. The charge nurse on a hematology/oncology unit is reviewing the policy for using abbreviations with the staff. The charge nurse should emphasize which information about why dangerous abbreviations need to be eliminated? Select all that apply.
  ☐ 1. to ensure efficient and accurate communication
  ☐ 2. to prevent medication errors
  ☐ 3. to ensure client safety
  ☐ 4. to make it easier for clients to understand the medication prescriptions
  ☐ 5. to make data entry into a computerized health record easier

105. The nurse is delegating the care of a client with neutropenia who is in isolation to an unlicensed assistive personnel (UAP). What information should the nurse give the UAP about the care of this client?
  ☐ 1. listening and responding to the client's feelings of concern
  ☐ 2. completing the client's care in a calm, unhurried manner
  ☐ 3. completing all of the client's care for the shift at one time
  ☐ 4. instructing the client to dispose of tissues used after blowing the nose

Answers, Rationales, and Test-Taking Strategies

*The answers and rationales for each question follow below, along with keys (🔑) to the client need (CN) and cognitive level (CL) for each question. In addition, questions that measure clinical judgment will be coded (CJ). As you check your answers, use the **Content Mastery and Test-Taking Skill Self-Analysis** worksheet (tear-out worksheet in the back of the book) to identify the reason(s) for not answering the questions correctly. For additional information about test-taking skills and strategies for answering questions, refer to pages 12–51 in Part 1 of this book.*

The Adult with Red Blood Cell Disorders

1. 3, 1, 2, 4. First, the nurse must verify that the client has voluntarily signed a consent form before the procedure begins and check that the client understands the procedure. The nurse then positions the client in a side-lying, or *lateral decubitus*, position with the affected side up. Then, the nurse should clean the skin site and surrounding area with an antiseptic solution before the health care provider numbs the site and collects the specimen. When the procedure is finished, the nurse must apply ice to the biopsy site to reduce pain.

CN: Management of care; CL: Analyze

2. **-/+ 1, 2, 5.** Nausea and vomiting are common adverse effects of oral iron preparations. The nurse should first ask the client why the client does not want to take the oral medication and then suggest ways to decrease nausea and vomiting. Ginger may help minimize nausea, and the client can try this remedy and evaluate its effectiveness. Iron should be taken on an empty stomach but can be taken with orange juice. The client can evaluate if this helps the nausea. Stool softeners should not be used in clients with iron deficiency anemia. Instead, constipation can be prevented by following a high-fiber diet. Administering iron intramuscularly is done only if other approaches are not effective.

CN: Health promotion and maintenance; CL: Analyze

3. **-/+ 1, 2, 3.** Using designated donors does not decrease the risk for contracting infectious diseases, such as the Epstein-Barr virus, HIV, or CMV. Hepatitis A is transmitted by the oral-fecal route, not the blood route; however, hepatitis B and C can be contracted from a designated donor. Malaria is transmitted by mosquitoes.

CN: Safety and infection control; CL: Apply

4. **1.** For the client with iron deficiency anemia, a rich source of iron is needed in the diet, and eggs are high in iron. Other foods high in iron include organ and muscle (dark) meats; shellfish, shrimp, and tuna; enriched, whole-grain, and fortified cereals and breads; legumes, nuts, dried fruits, and beans; oatmeal; and sweet potatoes. Dark green, leafy vegetables and citrus fruits are good sources of vitamin C. Cheese is a good source of calcium.

CN: Reduction of risk potential; CL: Apply

5. **3.** Good sources of vitamin B_{12} include meats and dairy products. Whole grains are a good source of thiamine. Green, leafy vegetables are good sources of niacin, folate, and carotenoids (precursors of vitamin A). Broccoli and Brussels sprouts are good sources of ascorbic acid (vitamin C).

CN: Reduction of risk potential; CL: Apply

6. **2.** Clients with aplastic anemia are severely immunocompromised and at risk for infection and possible death related to bone marrow suppression and pancytopenia. Strict aseptic technique and reverse isolation are important measures to prevent infection. Although diet, reduced stress, and rest are valued in supporting health, the potentially fatal consequence of an acute infection places it as a priority for teaching the client about health maintenance. Animal meat and dark green leafy vegetables, good sources of vitamin B_{12} and folic acid, should be included in the daily diet. Yoga and meditation are good complementary therapies to reduce stress. Eight hours of rest and naps are good for spacing and pacing activity and rest.

CN: Reduction of risk potential; CL: Analyze

7. **4.** Vitamin B_{12} combines with intrinsic factor in the stomach and is then carried to the ileum, where it is absorbed into the bloodstream. In this situation, vitamin B_{12} cannot be absorbed regardless of the amount of oral intake of sources of vitamin B_{12}, such as animal protein or vitamin B_{12} tablets. Vitamin B_{12} needs to be injected every month because the ileum has been surgically removed. Warm salt water is used to soothe sore mucous membranes. Crohn disease and a small-bowel resection may cause several loose stools a day, but the client does not report having this problem.

CN: Physiological adaptation; CL: Analyze

8. **3.** Coffee and tea increase gastrointestinal motility and inhibit the absorption of nonheme iron. Clients are instructed to add dried fruits to dishes at every meal because dried fruits are a nonheme or nonanimal iron source. Cooking in iron cookware, especially acid-based foods such as tomatoes, adds iron to the diet. Clients are instructed to add a rich supply of vitamin C to every meal because the absorption of iron is increased when food with vitamin C or ascorbic acid is consumed.

CN: Reduction of risk potential; CL: Evaluate

9. **1.** It is difficult to determine activity intolerance without objectively comparing activities from one time frame to another. Because iron deficiency anemia can occur gradually and individual endurance varies, the nurse can best assess the client's activity tolerance by asking the client to compare activities 6 months ago and at present. Asking a client how long a problem has existed is a very open-ended question that allows for too much subjectivity for any definition of the client's activity tolerance. Also, the client may not even identify that a "problem" exists. Asking if the client is staying abreast of usual activities addresses whether the tasks were completed, not the tolerance of the client while the tasks were being completed or the resulting condition of the client after the tasks were completed. Asking the

client about being more tired now than usual does not address activity tolerance. Tiredness is a subjective evaluation and again can be distorted by factors such as the gradual onset of the anemia or the endurance of the individual.

🗝 CN: Reduction of risk potential; CL: Analyze

10. −/+ **4, 6.** A client with pernicious anemia has lost the ability to absorb vitamin B_{12} either because of the lack of an acidic gastric environment or the lack of the intrinsic factor. Vitamin B_{12} must be administered by a deep intramuscular route. The ventrogluteal and dorsogluteal locations are the most acceptable sites for a deep intramuscular injection. The other sites are not acceptable.

🗝 CN: Pharmacological and parenteral therapies; CL: Apply

11. **2.** To promote comfort when injecting at the ventrogluteal site, the position of choice is with the client lying on the abdomen with toes pointed inward. This positioning promotes muscle relaxation, which decreases the discomfort of making an injection into a tense muscle. Lying on the side with legs extended will not provide the greatest muscle relaxation. Leaning over the edge of a table with the hips flexed and standing upright with the feet apart will increase muscular tension.

🗝 CN: Physiological adaptation; CL: Apply

12. −/+ **1, 2, 3, 4.** The nurse should ask the client about symptoms related to pernicious anemia because the client had the stomach stapled 2 years ago and shows no history of supplemental vitamin B_{12}. Numbness and tingling relate to a loss of intrinsic factor from the gastric stapling. Intrinsic factor is necessary for the absorption of vitamin B_{12}. The nurse should suspect pernicious anemia if the client is not taking supplemental vitamin B_{12}. Other signs and symptoms of pernicious anemia include cognitive problems and depression. The nurse also should ask about the client's support at home in case the fall was not an accident. Pernicious anemia is not related to the dietary intake of iron.

🗝 CN: Pharmacological and parenteral therapies; CL: Analyze

13. **1.** The nurse should prepare to start an intake and output record because the client is exhibiting clinical manifestations of anemia with jaundice and is demonstrating a fluid imbalance. The client does not need to be on bed rest at this point. The client is not contagious and does not require contact precautions. The changes in the color of the skin and urine are related to the jaundice and will not be affected by sunlight.

🗝 CN: Physiological adaptation; CL: Analyze

14. **1.** Drug-induced hemolytic anemia is acquired, antibody-mediated, red blood cell destruction precipitated by medications, such as cephalosporins, sulfa drugs, rifampin, methyldopa, procainamide, quinidine, and thiazides. Purpura is a condition with various manifestations characterized by hemorrhages into the skin, mucous membranes, internal organs, and other tissues. Infectious emboli are clumps of bacteria present in blood or lymph. Ecchymoses are skin discolorations due to extravasations of blood into the skin or mucous membranes.

🗝 CN: Reduction of risk potential; CL: Analyze

15. **3.** Pernicious anemia is caused by a lack of vitamin B_{12}. Primary symptoms include neuropathy with paresthesia of the hands and feet. The nurse assesses the client to determine the effectiveness of the monthly dose of vitamin B_{12}, which is to reverse the deficiency and the related symptoms. Improved energy is associated with treatment for iron deficiency anemia. Healing of cracked lips and tongue is an outcome of taking folic acid for folic acid deficiency. Delayed clotting time is associated with hemophilia; the clotting time is not affected by vitamin B_{12}.

🗝 CN: Pharmacological and parenteral therapies; CL: Evaluate

16. **2.** Most clients with pernicious anemia have deficient production of intrinsic factor in the stomach. Intrinsic factor attaches to the vitamin in the stomach and forms a complex that allows the vitamin to be absorbed in the small intestine. The stomach is producing enough acid, there is not an excessive excretion of the vitamin, and there is not a rapid production of red blood cells in this condition.

🗝 CN: Physiological adaptation; CL: Analyze

17. **2.** The normal physiologic response to activity is an increased metabolic rate over the resting basal rate. The decrease in the respiratory rate indicates that the client is not strong enough to complete the mechanical cycle of respiration needed for gas exchange. The postactivity pulse is expected to increase immediately after activity but by no more than 50 bpm if it is strenuous activity. The diastolic blood pressure is expected to rise but by no more than 15 mm Hg. The pulse returns to within 6 bpm of the resting pulse after 3 minutes of rest.

🗝 CN: Physiological adaptation; CL: Evaluate

18. **3.** The nurse should continue to monitor the client because this value reflects a normal physiologic response. The HCP does not need to be called, and oxygen does not need to be started based

on these laboratory findings. Immediately after surgery, the client's hematocrit reflects a falsely high value related to the body's compensatory response to the stress of sudden loss of fluids and blood. Activation of the intrinsic pathway and the renin-angiotensin cycle via antidiuretic hormone produces vasoconstriction and retention of fluid for the first 1 to 2 days postoperatively. By the second or third day, this response decreases, and the client's hematocrit level is more reflective of the number of RBCs in the plasma. Fresh bleeding is a less likely occurrence on the third postoperative day but is not impossible; however, the nurse should have expected to see a decrease in the RBC count and hemoglobin value accompanying the hematocrit.

CN: Physiological adaptation; CL: Analyze

19. 4. The most likely time for a blood transfusion reaction to occur is during the first 15 minutes or first 50 mL of the infusion. If a blood transfusion reaction does occur, it is imperative to keep an established IV line so that medication can be administered to prevent or treat cardiovascular collapse in case of anaphylaxis. PRBCs should be administered through a 19-gauge or larger needle; a peripherally inserted central catheter line is not recommended to avoid a slow flow. RBCs will hemolyze in dextrose or lactated Ringer's solution and should be infused with only normal saline solution.

CN: Pharmacological and parenteral therapies; CL: Analyze

20. -/+ 1, 2, 4. The nurse should teach the client to drink plenty of fluids to avoid becoming dehydrated. The client should avoid being in high altitudes, such as mountains above 5000 feet (1524 m) where less oxygen is available, which may precipitate a sickle cell crisis. The nurse should alert young women with sickle cell anemia that pregnancy increases the risk for a crisis. People who are homozygous for HbS have sickle cell anemia; the heterozygous form is the sickle cell carrier trait. A client with sickle cell anemia may fly on commercial airlines; the airplane is pressurized and has an adequate oxygen level.

CN: Health promotion and maintenance; CL: Analyze

21. -/+ 1, 2, 5. Hemochromatosis is a hereditary disease that causes the body to absorb increased amounts of iron from food, which can lead to liver and heart disease. The primary treatment is periodic removal of blood. To avoid complications, the nurse should instruct the client to not take iron supplements, vitamins with iron, or vitamin C. The client should not increase the amount of vitamin C in the diet because vitamin C promotes the absorption of iron. The client should not drink alcoholic beverages to prevent liver damage. It is not necessary to increase fluids in the diet, but the client should not become dehydrated.

CN: Health promotion and maintenance; CL: Analyze

22. 3, 4, 1, 2. When the client is having a blood transfusion reaction, the nurse should first stop the transfusion and then keep the IV open with a normal saline infusion. Next, the nurse should notify the HCP and blood bank and then complete the required form(s) regarding the transfusion reaction.

CN: Physiological adaptation; CL: Analyze

23. -/+ 2, 3, 5. The American Association of Blood Banks and Canadian Blood Services recommend that two qualified people, such as two registered nurses, compare the name and number on the identification bracelet with the tag on the blood bag. Verifying that the two units are the same is not a recommendation. Rather, the verification is always with the client, not with bags of blood. A unit of blood should infuse in 4 hours or less to avoid the risk for septicemia since no preservatives are used. When a blood transfusion reaction occurs, the blood transfusion should be stopped immediately, but the IV line should be kept open so that emergency medications and fluids can be administered.

The unit of PRBCs should be inspected for contamination by looking for leaks, abnormal color, clots, and excessive air bubbles. When a unit of PRBCs is being transfused, vital signs are assessed before the transfusion begins, after the first 15 minutes, and then every hour until 1 hour after the transfusion has been completed. When PRBCs are being administered, a 20-gauge or larger needle is needed to avoid destroying the RBCs passing through the lumen and to allow for maximal flow rate.

CN: Pharmacological and parenteral therapies; CL: Analyze

24. 2. ABO- and Rh-incompatible blood causes an antigen-antibody reaction that produces hemolysis or agglutination of RBCs. At the first indication of any sign or symptom of reaction, the blood transfusion is stopped. Blood and urine samples are obtained from the client and sent to the lab along with the remaining untransfused blood. Hemoglobin in the urine and blood samples taken at the time of the reaction provides evidence of a hemolytic blood transfusion reaction.

Antihistamine, aspirin, diuretics, and vasopressors may be administered with different types of transfusion reactions.

🗝 CN: Reduction of risk potential; CL: Analyze

25. 1. Epoetin is a recombinant DNA form of erythropoietin, which stimulates the production of red blood cells and therefore causes the hematocrit to rise. The partial thromboplastin time, hemoglobin level, and prothrombin time are not monitored for this drug.

🗝 CN: Pharmacological and parenteral therapies; CL: Analyze

26. -/+ 4, 5, 6. Erythropoietin is administered to decrease the need for blood transfusions by stimulating red blood cell (RBC) production. The medication should be administered through the IV line without other medications to avoid a reaction. The hematocrit, a simple measurement of the percentage of RBCs in the total blood volume, is used to monitor this therapy. When initiating IV erythropoietin therapy, the nurse should monitor the hematocrit level so that it rises no more than four points in any 2-week period. In addition, the initial doses of erythropoietin are adjusted according to the client's changes in blood pressure. The nurse should tell the client to avoid driving and performing hazardous activities during the initial treatment because of the possibility for dizziness and headaches secondary to the adverse effect of hypertension. The hematocrit, not the hemoglobin level, is used for monitoring the effectiveness of therapy. The vial of erythropoietin should not be shaken because it may be biologically inactive. The solution should not be used if it is discolored. The nurse should not reenter the vial once it has been entered; it is a single-use vial. All the remaining erythropoietin should be discarded because it does not contain preservatives.

🗝 CN: Pharmacological and parenteral therapies; CL: Analyze

27. 4. Vitamin B_{12} is a water-soluble vitamin. When water-soluble vitamins are taken in excess of the body's needs, they are filtered through the kidneys and excreted. Vitamin B_{12} is considered to be nontoxic. Adverse reactions that have occurred are believed to be related to impurities or to the preservative in B_{12} preparations. Ringing in the ears, rash, and nausea are not considered to be related to vitamin B_{12} administration.

🗝 CN: Pharmacological and parenteral therapies; CL: Analyze

28. -/+ 1, 2, 3, 5. Eggs are a source of iron, but they may not be well absorbed. Brown rice is a source of iron from plant sources (nonheme iron). Other sources of nonheme iron are whole-grain cereals and breads, dark green vegetables, legumes, nuts, dried fruits (apricots, raisins, dates), oatmeal, and sweet potatoes. Tea contains tannin, which combines with nonheme iron, preventing its absorption.

🗝 CN: Physiological adaptation; CL: Apply

29. 2. Macrocytic anemias can result from deficiencies in vitamin B_{12} or ascorbic acid. Only vitamin B_{12} deficiency causes diminished sensations of peripheral nerve endings. The nurse should assess for peripheral neuropathy and instruct the client in self-care activities for the diminished sensation of heat and pain (e.g., using a heating pad at a lower heat setting, making frequent checks to protect against skin trauma). The burn could be related to abuse, but this conclusion would require more supporting data. The findings should be documented, but the nurse would want to address the client's sensations first. The decision of how to treat the burn should be determined by the health care provider.

🗝 CN: Reduction of risk potential; CL: Analyze

30. 1. Aplastic anemia decreases the bone marrow production of red blood cells, white blood cells, and platelets. The client is at risk for bruising and bleeding tendencies. A change in the client's intake and output is important, but an assessment for the potential for bleeding takes priority. Change in the peripheral nervous system is a priority problem specific to clients with vitamin B_{12} deficiency. Change in bowel function is not associated with aplastic anemia.

🗝 CN: Physiological adaptation; CL: Analyze

The Adult with Platelet Disorders

31. -/+ 1, 3, 4, 5. Underweight older adults may have little subcutaneous tissue, so the area around the anterior iliac crest is a suitable site for these clients. The nurse should use a 27-gauge, 5/8-inch (1.6-cm) needle. Cephalosporin and penicillin potentiate the effects of heparin. Some agency medication safety policies require that two nurses check the dose because a dose error could cause bleeding. The onset of heparin is not immediate when given subcutaneously.

🗝 CN: Pharmacological and parenteral therapies; CL: Apply

32. 1. A client with a platelet count of 30,000 to 50,000/μL (30 to 50 × 10^9/L) is susceptible to bruising with minor trauma. Padding areas that the client might bump, scratch, or hit may help prevent minor trauma. A platelet count of 15,000 to 30,000/μL (15 to 30 × 10⁹/L) may result in spontaneous petechiae and bruising, especially on the extremities. Padding measures would still be used, but the focus would be on assessing for new spontaneous petechiae. Although the client should use precautions to prevent infection, the white blood cell count is not affected, and the client does not need to wear a mask when in areas where there are large numbers of people who are sources of potential infection. With a count below 20,000/μL (20 × 10⁹/L), the client is at risk for spontaneous bleeding from the mucous membranes and intracranial bleeding.

CN: Reduction of risk potential; CL: Analyze

33. 4. A recent viral infection in a female client between the ages of 20 and 30 with a history of systemic lupus erythematosus and an insidious onset of diffuse petechiae are hallmarks of idiopathic thrombocytopenic purpura. It is important to ask whether the client's recent menses have been lengthened or are heavier. Determining the client's ability to clot can help determine their risk for increased bleeding tendency until a platelet count is drawn. Petechiae are not caused by poor nutrition. Because of poor food and fluid intake or weakness and fatigue, the client may have gotten bruises from falling or bumping into things, but not petechiae.

CN: Reduction of risk potential; CL: Analyze

34. 2. When the platelet count is very low, red blood cells leak out of the blood vessels and into the tissue. If the blood pressure is elevated and the platelet count falls to less than 15,000/μL (15 × 10⁹/L), internal bleeding in the brain can occur. A severe headache occurs from meningeal irritation when blood leaks out of the cerebral vasculature. When a client has thrombocytopenia, the nurse should always assess for cerebral bleeding by checking vital signs and performing neurologic checks. Headaches can be caused by stress, migraines, and sinus congestion. However, the concern here is the risk for internal bleeding into the brain.

CN: Health promotion and maintenance; CL: Analyze

35. 2. Large, purplish skin lesions caused by hemorrhage are called *ecchymoses*. Petechiae are small, flat, red pinpoint lesions. Numerous petechiae result in a reddish, bruised appearance called *purpura*. An abrasion is a wound caused by scraping.

CN: Health promotion and maintenance; CL: Evaluate

36. 2. When the platelet count is less than 150,000/μL (150 × 10⁹/L), prolonged bleeding can occur from trauma, injury, or strain such as with the Valsalva maneuver. Clients should avoid any activity that causes straining to evacuate the bowel. Clients can ambulate, but pointed or sharp surfaces should be padded. Clients can visit with their families but should avoid any scratches, bumps, or scrapes. Clients can sit in a semi-Fowler position but should change positions to promote circulation and check for petechiae.

CN: Health promotion and maintenance; CL: Analyze

37. 4. Aspirin has an antiplatelet effect, and bleeding time can consequently be prolonged. Intermittent use of ice packs to the site may stop the bleeding; ice causes blood vessels to vasoconstrict. Use of lukewarm water, patting the injury, and wrapping the entire forearm do not promote vasoconstriction to stop bleeding.

CN: Pharmacological and parenteral therapies; CL: Analyze

38. 1. The nurse should assess the client who is bleeding for tachycardia because the heart beats faster to compensate for decreased circulating volume and decreased numbers of oxygen-carrying red blood cells. The degree of cardiopulmonary distress and anemia will be related to the amount of hemorrhage that occurred and the period of time over which it occurred. Bradycardia is a late symptom of hemorrhage; it occurs after the client is no longer able to compromise and is debilitated further into shock. If bradycardia is left untreated, the client will die from cardiovascular collapse. Decreased $PaCO_2$ is a late symptom of hemorrhage, after transport of oxygen to the tissue has been affected. A narrowed pulse pressure is not an early sign of hemorrhage.

CN: Physiological adaptation; CL: Analyze

39. 4. ITP is treated with steroids to suppress the splenic macrophages from phagocytizing the antibody-coated platelets, which are recognized as foreign bodies, so that the platelets live longer. The steroids also suppress the binding of the autoimmune antibody to the platelet surface. Steroids do not destroy the antibodies on the platelets, neutralize antigens, or increase phagocytosis.

CN: Pharmacological and parenteral therapies; CL: Apply

40. 3. The client needs to wear or carry information containing the name of the drug, dosage, health care provider and contact information, and emergency instructions because additional corticosteroid drug therapy would be needed during emergency situations. Prednisone should be taken in the morning because it can cause insomnia and because exogenous corticosteroid suppression of the adrenal cortex is less when it is administered in the morning. Prednisone must never be stopped suddenly. It must be tapered off to allow for the adrenal cortex to recover from drug-induced atrophy so that it can resume its function. Prednisone should be taken with food or milk to prevent stomach irritation.

CN: Pharmacological and parenteral therapies; CL: Evaluate

41. 1. Nausea, vomiting, and peptic ulcers are gastrointestinal adverse effects of prednisone, so it is recommended that clients take the prednisone with food. In some instances, the client may be advised to take a prescribed antacid prophylactically. The client should never take over-the-counter drugs without notifying the health care provider (HCP) who prescribed the prednisone. The client should ask the HCP about the amount and kind of exercise because of the need to establish baseline physical values before starting an exercise program and because of the increased potential for comorbidity with increasing age. The client should eat foods that are high in potassium to prevent hypokalemia.

CN: Pharmacological and parenteral therapies; CL: Analyze

42. 4. The best exercise for female clients who are on long-term corticosteroid therapy is a low-impact, weight-bearing exercise, such as walking or weight lifting. Floor exercises do not provide for weight bearing. Stretching is appropriate but does not offer sufficient weight bearing. Running provides for weight bearing but is hard on the joints and may cause bleeding.

CN: Pharmacological and parenteral therapies; CL: Analyze

43. 2. The client needs further teaching if they think that the number of tissues saturated represents all of the blood lost during a nosebleed. During a nosebleed, a significant amount of blood can be swallowed and go undetected. It is important that clients with severe thrombocytopenia do not take a nosebleed lightly. Clients with thrombocytopenia can apply pressure for 5 to 10 minutes over a small, superficial cut. Clients with thrombocytopenia can take hormones to suppress menses and control menstrual blood loss. Clients can also count the number of saturated sanitary napkins to approximate blood loss during menses. Some authorities estimate that a completely soaked sanitary napkin holds 50 mL.

CN: Reduction of risk potential; CL: Evaluate

44. 2, 4, 5, 6. Adverse effects of prednisone are weight gain, retention of sodium and fluids with hypertension and cushingoid features, a low serum albumin level, suppressed inflammatory processes with masked symptoms, and osteoporosis. A diet high in protein, potassium, calcium, and vitamin D is recommended. Carbohydrates would elevate glucose and further compromise a client's immune status. Saturated fat does not counteract the adverse effects of steroids such as prednisone.

CN: Pharmacological and parenteral therapies; CL: Analyze

45. 1. Platelets cannot survive cold temperatures. The platelets should be stored at room temperature and last for no more than 5 days.

CN: Pharmacological and parenteral therapies; CL: Analyze

46. 3. The bag containing platelets needs to be gently rotated to prevent clumping. ABO compatibility is not a necessary requirement, but human leukocyte antigen (HLA) matching of lymphocytes may be completed to avoid the development of anti-HLA antibodies when multiple platelet transfusions are necessary. Platelets should be administered as fast as can be tolerated by the client to avoid aggregation. Most institutions use tubing made especially for platelets instead of tubing made for blood and blood products.

CN: Pharmacological and parenteral therapies; CL: Analyze

47. 3. An elective surgical procedure is scheduled in advance so that all preparations can be completed ahead of time. The vital signs are the final check that must be completed before the client leaves the room so that continuity of care and assessment is provided. The first assessment that will be completed in the preoperative holding area or operating room will be the client's vital signs. The client should have emptied the bladder before receiving preoperative medications so that the bladder is empty when it is time for transport into the operating room. The client should have signed the consent before the transport time so that if there were any questions or concerns, there was time to meet with the surgeon. Also, the consent form must be signed before any sedative medications are given. The client's name band should be placed as soon as the client arrives in the perioperative setting, and it remains in place through discharge.

CN: Physiological adaptation; CL: Analyze

48. 3. After a splenectomy, the client is at high risk for hypovolemia and hemorrhage. The dressing should be checked often; if drainage is present, a circle should be drawn around the drainage and the time noted to help determine how fast bleeding is occurring. The nasogastric tube should be connected, but this can wait until the dressing has been checked. A urinary catheter is not needed. The last pain medication administered and the client's current pain level should be communicated in the hand-off-of-care report. Checking for hemorrhage is a greater priority than assessing pain level.

CN: Physiological adaptation; CL: Analyze

49. 3. A splenectomy may involve manipulation of the upper abdominal organs, such as the diaphragm, stomach, liver, spleen, and small intestines. Manipulation of these organs and resulting inflammation lead to a slowed peristalsis. An NG tube is placed to decrease abdominal distention in the immediate postoperative phase. The NG tube does not affect the depth of diaphragmatic breathing. The NG tube drains gastric contents and air in the stomach; it is not in the operative site and therefore cannot be used to irrigate it, and there should not be bloody drainage. The gastric juices are not checked as an indicator that peristalsis has returned, and the pH should be normal; instead, bowel sounds are auscultated in all four quadrants to indicate the return of peristalsis.

CN: Physiological adaptation; CL: Apply

50. 4. Clients who have had a splenectomy are especially prone to infection. The reduction of immunoglobulin M leaves the client particularly at risk for immunologic deficiency infections. All clients who have had major abdominal surgery usually receive discharge instructions not to drive because the stomach muscles are not strong enough to brake hard or quickly after the abdominal muscles have been separated. All clients need to pace activity and rest when going home after major surgery. Rest and sleep allow the growth hormone to repair the tissue, and activity allows the energy and strength to build endurance and muscle strength. An appointment is usually made to see the surgeon in the office 1 week after discharge for follow-up and to remove sutures or staples if this has not already been done.

CN: Reduction of risk potential; CL: Analyze

51. 2. There is no well-defined sequence for acute DIC other than that the client starts bleeding without a history or cause and does not stop bleeding. Later signs may include severe shortness of breath, hypotension, pallor, petechiae, hematoma, orthopnea, hematuria, vision changes, and joint pain.

CN: Physiological adaptation; CL: Analyze

52. 3. DIC has not been found to respond to oral anticoagulants such as warfarin sodium. Treatments for DIC are controversial but include treating the underlying cause, administering heparin, and replacing depleted blood products.

CN: Pharmacological and parenteral therapies; CL: Analyze

53. 2. Clinical manifestations of microvascular thrombosis are those that represent a blockage of blood flow and oxygenation to the tissue that results in the eventual death of the organ. Examples of microvascular thrombosis include acute respiratory distress syndrome, focal ischemia, superficial gangrene, oliguria, azotemia, cortical necrosis, acute ulceration, delirium, and coma. Hemoptysis, petechiae, and hematuria are signs of hemorrhage.

CN: Physiological adaptation; CL: Analyze

The Adult with White Blood Cell Disorders

54. 1, 2, 3, 5. The nurse should teach this client to stay on bed rest as long as there is a fever, gargle with warm saline, and increase oral fluids to prevent dehydration from the elevated temperature. The client with an enlarged spleen should avoid contact sports because of the increased risk for injury due to the enlargement. The client does not need to wear a mask but should observe handwashing procedures.

CN: Basic care and comfort; CL: Create

55. 1, 2, 3. The client has an elevated WBC count. A normal WBC count is 4300 to 10,800 μL (4.3 to 10.8 × 10⁹/L). The client is at risk for infection, and the nurse should assess the client for inflammation around the incision site, redness at the incision site, and elevated temperature. The client should be encouraged to cough and deep breathe, and it is unlikely that a cough is related to an incisional infection. Weak pedal pulses are not indications of an infection, but the nurse should report this finding if it persists.

CN: Physiological adaptation; CL: Analyze

56. 1, 2, 3, 4. Nursing care of a client with leukemia includes managing and preventing infection, maintaining the integrity of skin and mucous membranes, instituting measures to prevent bleeding, and monitoring for bleeding. Aspirin is an anticoagulant; bleeding tendencies, such as petechiae, ecchymosis, epistaxis, gingival bleeding, and retinal hemorrhages, are likely due to thrombocytopenia.

CN: Reduction of risk potential; CL: Create

57. 2. A client is at moderate risk for infection when the ANC is less than 1000/μL (1×10^9/L). The client does not have a platelet disorder and is not at risk for bleeding or hemorrhagic stroke. The client does not have sickle cell anemia and is not at risk for a crisis.

🔑 CN: Physiological adaptation; CL: Analyze

58. 1. Bedside rails, call bells, drug administration controls operated by the client, and other surface areas are frequently touched by caregivers with used gloves. Changing gloves immediately after use protects the client from contamination by organisms. Cross-contamination is a break in technique of serious consequence to the severely compromised client. Standing 2 feet (61 cm) from the client, speaking minimally, and wearing protective covering shirts are not required in standard interventions for risk for infection.

🔑 CN: Safety and infection control; CL: Analyze

59. 1. The neutropenic client is at risk for infection, especially bacterial infection of the respiratory and gastrointestinal tracts. Breaks in the mucous membranes, such as those that could be caused by the insertion of a suppository or enema tube, would be a break in the first line of the body's defense and a direct port of entry for infection. The client with neutropenia is encouraged to wear a HEPA filter mask and to use an incentive spirometer for pulmonary hygiene. The client needs to know the importance of completing meticulous total body hygiene daily, including perianal care after every bowel movement, to decrease the flora at normal body orifices. The client also needs to know the importance of performing oral care after every meal and every 4 hours while the client is awake to decrease the bacterial buildup in the oropharynx.

🔑 CN: Health promotion and maintenance; CL: Analyze

60. 2. Washing hands before, during, and after care has a significant effect on reducing infections. It is advisable to avoid introducing a cold or children's germs and to avoid kissing the client, but the primary prevention technique is handwashing.

🔑 CN: Health promotion and maintenance; CL: Analyze

61. ➕ **1, 2, 4, 5.** The nurse can serve as a witness for consent for procedures. The nurse also ascertains whether the client has an understanding that is consistent with the procedure listed on the form, determines that the client is signing the consent of their own free will, and determines that the client understands postprocedure care. The nurse's role does not include explaining the risks of the procedure; that responsibility belongs to the person who is to perform the procedure, such as the health care provider.

🔑 CN: Management of care; CL: Analyze

62. 3. As the bone marrow is being aspirated, the client will feel a suction or pulling type of sensation or discomfort that lasts a few seconds. A systemic premedication may be given to decrease this discomfort. A small area over the sternum is cleaned with an antiseptic. It is unnecessary to paint the entire anterior chest. The local anesthetic is injected through the subcutaneous tissue to numb the tissue for the larger-bore needle that is used for aspiration and biopsy. After the needle is removed, pressure is held over the aspiration site for 5 to 10 minutes to achieve hemostasis. A small dressing is applied; a large pressure dressing, such as an Ace bandage, would restrict the expansion of the lungs and is not used.

🔑 CN: Psychosocial adaptation; CL: Apply

63. 4. After a bone marrow aspiration, the puncture site should be checked every 10 to 15 minutes for bleeding. For a short period after the procedure, bed rest may be prescribed. Signs of infection, such as redness and swelling, are not anticipated at the aspiration site. A mild analgesic may be prescribed for pain, but if the client has pain longer than 24 hours, the nurse should assess the client for internal bleeding or increased pressure at the puncture site, which may be the cause of the pain, and should consult the health care provider.

🔑 CN: Physiological adaptation; CL: Evaluate

64. 2. The nurse is an advocate for the client with leukemia who can be empowered with knowledge of the treatment. Immunologic, cytogenic, morphologic, histochemical, and other means are used to identify cell subtypes and stages of leukemia cell development for very specific and optimal treatment. The nurse should not label the client's feelings, such as frustration or being emotional; only the client can identify their own feelings. Chastising the client is not helpful. It disavows the client's emotional state and responses to the diagnosis and involved treatment. Unless nurses have had leukemia, they cannot possibly know how the client feels even though they may be trying to offer empathy.

🔑 CN: Psychosocial adaptation; CL: Analyze

65. 3. The induction phase of chemotherapy is an aggressive treatment to kill leukemia cells. The client is severely immunocompromised and severely at risk for infection. Flowers, herbs, and plants should be avoided during this time. The client's prayer book, pictures, and other personal belongings can be cleaned before being brought into the room to prevent the client from coming into contact with pathogenic and nonpathogenic organisms.

CN: Safety and infection control; CL: Analyze

66. 2. The nurse identifies that the client does not understand that contact with animals must be avoided because they carry infection and the induction therapy will destroy the client's white blood cells (WBCs). The induction therapy will cause anemia, and the client will experience fatigue and will have to pace activities with rest periods. Platelet production will be decreased, and the client will be at risk for bleeding tendencies; oral hygiene will have to be provided by using a warm saline gargle instead of brushing the teeth and gums. The client will be at risk for infection owing to the decrease in WBC production and should report a temperature of 100°F (37.8°C) or higher.

CN: Safety and infection control; CL: Evaluate

67. 1. Imatinib works by inhibiting the proliferation of abnormal cells. Adverse effects include edema and gastrointestinal irritation. The typical effects of this drug do not include numbness and tingling, bloody stools, or persistent cough. If the client has these symptoms, they may relate to disease occurrence or recurrence.

CN: Pharmacological and parenteral therapies; CL: Apply

68. 2. Diphenhydramine is an antihistamine. This drug helps reduce the incidence of an allergic response by blocking the release of histamine. Diphenhydramine also possesses anticholinergic effects and can reduce the incidence of nausea and vomiting for clients receiving chemotherapy. Although diphenhydramine may promote sleep, it is not the primary reason for its administration in this instance. Diphenhydramine will not reduce anxiety or potentiate the action of the vincristine.

CN: Pharmacological and parenteral therapies; CL: Apply

69. 3. Antineoplastic agents can cause severe tissue damage if they extravasate; therefore, the nurse should immediately stop the infusion. The correct dose should be verified before starting the infusion. After stopping the infusion, the nurse should notify the health care provider. If extravasation has occurred, it may be appropriate to apply ice packs to the site. Ice packs cause desired vasoconstriction; warm, moist packs cause vasodilation. Ice packs should not remain in place for more than 15 to 20 minutes because rebound vasodilation can occur; the ice packs are removed for a short time and then reapplied as needed.

CN: Pharmacological and parenteral therapies; CL: Analyze

70. 3, 4, 1, 2. The client is experiencing a septic reaction to the blood transfusion. The nurse first stops the infusion and notifies the health care provider and blood bank; then, the nurse uses an infusion of normal saline to keep the vein open and follows by obtaining a sample of the client's blood for a blood culture. Lastly, the nurse sends the blood bag and the administration set to the blood bank for culture.

CN: Pharmacological and parenteral therapies; CL: Analyze

71. 2. Epoetin stimulates erythropoiesis and the production of red blood cells. This is important for clients taking antineoplastics because they often experience bone marrow depression as a side effect of antineoplastic therapy. Epoetin does not affect tissue malignancy or tumor size. Nausea and vomiting are commonly associated with antineoplastics, but these are treated with antiemetics.

CN: Pharmacological parenteral therapies; CL: Evaluate

72. 4. Bleeding and infection are the major complications and causes of death for clients with AML. Bleeding is related to the degree of thrombocytopenia, and infection is related to the degree of neutropenia. Cardiac arrhythmias rarely occur as a result of AML. Liver or renal failure may occur, but neither is a major cause of death in AML.

CN: Reduction of risk potential; CL: Analyze

73. 1. Clients with ALL are at risk for infection due to granulocytopenia. The nurse should place the client in a private room. Strict handwashing procedures should be enforced and will be the most effective way to prevent infection. It is not necessary to have the client wear a mask. The client is not contagious, and the staff does not need to wear gloves. The client can have visitors; however, they should be screened for infection and use handwashing procedures.

CN: Physiological adaptation; CL: Analyze

74. 3. Simple rinses with saline or a baking soda and water solution are effective and moisten the oral mucosa. Commercial mouthwashes and lemon glycerin swabs contain glycerin and alcohol, which are drying to the mucosa and should be avoided. Brushing after each meal is recommended, but every 4 hours may be too traumatic. During acute leukemia, the neutrophil and platelet counts are often low, and a soft-bristle toothbrush, instead of the client's usual brush, should be used to prevent bleeding gums.

🔑 CN: Reduction of risk potential; CL: Analyze

75. **2, 4, 5.** The client with acute leukemia experiences fatigue and deconditioning. To improve tidal volume, the nurse can encourage the client to take deep breaths while sitting or lying with the goal of increasing the depth and duration of the breath each time. The client should also increase activity tolerance. The client can do this by walking or using a stationary bike with the goal of increasing the activity. These exercises also help the client increase tidal volume. Although drinking fluids and sitting rather than lying down are helpful, it is not necessary to increase the fluid intake to 3000 mL a day or spend much time sitting.

🔑 CN: Reduction of risk potential; CL: Analyze

76. **2.** Combination chemotherapy does not mean two groups of drugs, one to kill the cancer cells and one to treat the adverse effects of the chemotherapy. Combination chemotherapy means that multiple drugs are given to interrupt the cell growth cycle at different points, decrease resistance to a chemotherapy agent, and minimize the toxicity associated with the use of a high dose of a single agent (i.e., by using multiple agents with different toxicities).

🔑 CN: Pharmacological and parenteral therapies; CL: Evaluate

77. **2, 3, 4.** Thrombocytopenia (a low platelet count) leaves the client at risk for a potentially life-threatening spontaneous hemorrhage in the gastrointestinal, respiratory, and intracranial cavities. The biliary and integumentary systems are not common sites for bleeding when the client has thrombocytopenia.

🔑 CN: Physiological adaptation; CL: Analyze

78. **1.** The primary purpose of neutropenic precautions is to reduce the transmission of organisms to the client from sources outside the client's environment, not to reduce the transfer of organisms from the client to others. It is not necessary to place items in specially marked containers or to keep the client's linens and personal items in the room.

🔑 CN: Safety and infection control; CL: Apply

The Adult with Lymphoma

79. **3.** The client with Hodgkin lymphoma who has had radiation therapy is prone to infection; therefore, the primary goal is to prevent infection. The nurse instructs the client to perform frequent hand hygiene, avoid crowded areas, and report a temperature over 100°F (37.7°C). Maintaining fluid balance, exercising, and maintaining mental health are also important, but these are not primary goals at this time.

🔑 CN: Safety and infection control; CL: Analyze

80. **1.** The nurse must ensure that sterile technique is used when a biopsy is obtained because the client is at high risk for infection. In most cases, a lymph node biopsy is sent immediately to the laboratory once it is placed in a specific solution in a closed container. It is not necessary to wear a gown and mask when obtaining the specimen. It is not necessary to use special handling procedures for the instruments used.

🔑 CN: Management of care; CL: Apply

81. **3.** Assessing for an open airway is always first. The procedure involves the neck; the anesthesia may have affected the swallowing reflex, or the inflammation may have closed in on the airway, leading to ineffective air exchange. Once a patent airway is confirmed and an effective breathing pattern established, the circulation is checked. Vital signs and the incision are assessed as soon as possible, but only after it is established that the airway is patent and the client is breathing normally. A neurologic assessment is completed as soon as possible after other important assessments.

🔑 CN: Physiological adaptation; CL: Analyze

82. **1.** Herpes zoster infections are common in clients with Hodgkin disease. Discoloring of the teeth is not related to Hodgkin disease but rather to the ingestion of iron supplements or some antibiotics such as tetracycline. Mild anemia is common in Hodgkin disease, but the platelet count is not affected until the tumor has invaded the bone marrow. A cellular immunity defect occurs in Hodgkin disease in which there is little or no reaction to skin sensitivity tests. This is called *anergy*.

🔑 CN: Physiological adaptation; CL: Analyze

83. **3.** A temperature higher than 100.4°F (38°C), profuse night sweats, and an unintentional weight loss of 10% of body weight represent the cluster of clinical manifestations known as the *B symptoms*. Forty percent of clients with Hodgkin disease have B symptoms, and B symptoms are more common in the advanced stages of the disease.

🔑 CN: Physiological adaptation; CL: Analyze

84. **1, 2, 3, 5.** The nurse should teach the client to wear a mask when planning to be in crowded or enclosed spaces, such as when grocery shopping or going to a movie. The client should get as much rest as needed, avoid people who have a cold or the flu, and report a fever to the HCP. It is not necessary to decrease the amount of protein in the diet, but rather, the client should eat a well-balanced diet. The client may need to change some foods if they experience side effects of the chemotherapy and may need to obtain more calories.

CN: Health promotion and maintenance; CL: Create

85. **1.** In the staging process, the designations A and B signify that symptoms were or were not present when Hodgkin disease was found, respectively. The Roman numerals I through IV indicate the extent and location of involvement of the disease. Stage I indicates involvement of a single lymph node; stage II, two or more lymph nodes on the same side of the diaphragm; stage III, lymph node regions on both sides of the diaphragm; and stage IV, diffuse disease of one or more extralymphatic organs.

CN: Physiological adaptation; CL: Apply

86. **4.** Administering a sedative prior to a bone marrow aspiration and biopsy is common preparation for the procedure, and the nurse can suggest that the client request a sedative if it has not been prescribed. Encouraging the client to take slow, deep breaths may be helpful, but a sedative may be more helpful during the uncomfortable parts of the procedure to decrease the stress response of tightening and tensing the muscles. Allowing the client's family to stay may be appropriate if the family has a calming effect on the client *prior* to the procedure, but they will not be able to be present during the procedure. The nurse should listen while the client expresses concerns, but this may not be sufficient for calming the client during the procedure.

CN: Psychosocial adaptation; CL: Analyze

87. **2.** A biopsy needle is inserted through a separate incision in the anesthetized area. The client will feel a pressure sensation when the biopsy is taken but should not feel actual pain. The client should be instructed to inform the health care provider (HCP) if pain is felt so that more anesthetic agent can be administered to keep the client comfortable. The biopsy is performed after the aspiration and from a slightly different site so that the tissue is not disturbed by either test. The client will feel a suction-type pain for a moment when the aspiration is being performed, not the biopsy. A small incision is made for the biopsy to accommodate the larger-bore needle. This may require a stitch.

CN: Psychosocial adaptation; CL: Analyze

88. **3.** Terminally ill clients most often describe feelings of isolation because they tend to be ignored, they are often left out of conversations (especially those dealing with the future), and they sense the attitudes of discomfort that many people feel in their presence. Helpful nursing measures include taking the time to be with the client, offering opportunities to talk about feelings, and answering questions honestly.

CN: Psychosocial adaptation; CL: Analyze

89. **2.** It is incorrect that the survivor rate is directly proportional to the incidence of second malignancy. The survivor rate is indirectly proportional to the incidence of second malignancy, and regular screening is very important to detect a second malignancy, especially acute myeloid leukemia or myelodysplastic syndrome. Survivors should know the stage of the disease and their current treatment plan so that they can remain active participants in their health care.

CN: Physiological adaptation; CL: Evaluate

The Adult with Cardiogenic, Hypovolemic, or Septic Shock

90. **2.** The most important goal of nursing care and collaborative management for the client in cardiogenic shock is to maintain adequate cardiac function. Inotropic drugs such as dopamine are prescribed to improve cardiac function. Fluid deficit, not fluid overload, occurs when clients are in shock; inadequate tissue perfusion typically occurs in hemorrhagic shock. The nurse should monitor clients in cardiogenic shock for signs of fluid imbalances and vasoconstriction, but the priority is to maintain cardiac function.

CN: Physiological adaptation; CL: Analyze

91. **4.** Typical signs and symptoms of hypovolemic shock include systolic blood pressure less than 90 mm Hg, narrowing pulse pressure, tachycardia, tachypnea, cool and clammy skin, decreased urine output, and mental status changes, such as irritability or anxiety. Unequal dilation of the pupils is related to central nervous system injury or possibly to a previous history of eye injury.

CN: Physiological adaptation; CL: Analyze

92. **1.** Urine output provides the most sensitive indicator of the client's response to therapy for hypovolemic shock. Urine output should be consistently greater than 35 mL per hour. Blood pressure is a more accurate reflection of the adequacy of vasoconstriction than of tissue perfusion. Respiratory rate is not a sensitive indicator of fluid balance in a client recovering from hypovolemic shock.

🔑 CN: Pharmacological and parenteral therapies; CL: Evaluate

93. 1. Causes of hypovolemic shock include external fluid loss, such as hemorrhage; internal fluid shifting, such as ascites and severe edema; and dehydration. Massive vasodilation is the initial phase of vasogenic or distributive shock, which can be further subdivided into three types of shock: septic, neurogenic, and anaphylactic. A severe antigen-antibody reaction occurs in anaphylactic shock. Gram-negative bacterial infection is the most common cause of septic shock. Loss of sympathetic tone (vasodilation) occurs in neurogenic shock.

🔑 CN: Physiological adaptation; CL: Analyze

94. 2. The client who is receiving a blood product requires an astute assessment for signs and symptoms of allergic reaction and anaphylaxis, including pruritus (itching), urticaria (hives), facial or glottal edema, and shortness of breath. If such a reaction occurs, the nurse should stop the transfusion immediately, but leave the IV line intact, and notify the health care provider. Usually, an antihistamine (such as diphenhydramine hydrochloride) is administered. Epinephrine and corticosteroids may be administered in severe reactions. Fluid balance is not an immediate concern during blood administration. The administration should not cause pain unless it is extravasating out of the vein, in which case the IV administration should be stopped. The administration of a unit of blood should not affect the level of consciousness.

🔑 CN: Pharmacological and parenteral therapies; CL: Analyze

95. 2. At medium doses (4 to 8 mcg/kg/min), dopamine hydrochloride slightly increases the heart rate and improves contractility to increase cardiac output and improve tissue perfusion. When given at low doses (0.5 to 3.0 mcg/kg/min), dopamine increases renal and mesenteric blood flow. At high doses (8 to 10 mcg/kg/min), dopamine produces vasoconstriction, which is an undesirable effect. Dopamine is not given to affect preload and afterload.

🔑 CN: Pharmacological and parenteral therapies; CL: Evaluate

96. 2. The client who is receiving dopamine hydrochloride requires continuous blood pressure monitoring with an invasive or noninvasive device. The nurse may titrate the intravenous infusion to maintain a systolic blood pressure of 90 mm Hg. Administration of a pain medication concurrently with dopamine hydrochloride, which is a potent sympathomimetic with dose-related alpha-adrenergic agonist, beta 1-selective adrenergic agonist, and dopaminergic blocking effects, is not an essential nursing action for a client who is in shock with already low hemodynamic values. Arterial blood gas concentrations should be monitored according to the client's respiratory status and acid-base balance status and are not directly related to the dopamine hydrochloride dosage. Monitoring for signs of infection is not related to the nursing action for the client receiving dopamine hydrochloride.

🔑 CN: Pharmacological and parenteral therapies; CL: Analyze

97. 2. Warm, flushed skin from a high cardiac output with vasodilation occurs in warm shock or the hyperdynamic phase (first phase) of septic shock. Other signs and symptoms of early septic shock include fever with restlessness and confusion; normal or decreased blood pressure with tachypnea and tachycardia; increased or normal urine output; and nausea and vomiting or diarrhea. Cool, clammy skin occurs in the hypodynamic or cold phase (later phase). Hemorrhage is not a factor in septic shock.

🔑 CN: Physiological adaptation; CL: Analyze

98. 4. Maintaining asepsis of indwelling urinary catheters is essential to prevent infection. Preventing septic shock is a major focus of nursing care because the mortality rate for septic shock is as high as 90% particularly in clients who are younger than age 2 or older than age 65. Administering IV fluid replacement therapy, obtaining vital signs every 4 hours, and monitoring red blood cell counts for an increase are not measures to prevent septic shock.

🔑 CN: Safety and infection control; CL: Analyze

99. 4. The client's history and the current vital signs indicate the client is likely experiencing septic shock. Septic shock is caused by the body's response to an infection. The nurse is concerned because the client has a urinary tract infection, which can trigger septic shock. Older adults are at greater risk for septic shock, and confusion can be a sign of shock, but the most significant contributing factor to septic shock is a urinary tract infection. The client's history of COPD, while important, is not the most concerning at this time.

🔑 CN: Safety and infection control; CL: Analyze

100. **2.** ARDS is a complication associated with septic shock. ARDS causes respiratory failure and may lead to death, even after the client has recovered from shock. Anaphylaxis is a type of distributive or vasogenic shock. COPD is a functional category of pulmonary disease that consists of persistent obstruction of bronchial air flow and involves chronic bronchitis and chronic emphysema. Mitral valve prolapse is a condition in which the mitral valve is pushed back too far during ventricular contraction.

CN: Physiological adaptation;
CL: Analyze

Managing Care, Quality, and Safety for Adults with Hematologic Health Problems

101. **3.** When two clients are to receive blood at the same time, the nurse should call for and hang the clients' transfusions separately to avoid error. The nurse should call for and hang the first client's blood first because this client has experienced a change in blood pressure over a short period of time. The nurse should next call and hang the second client's blood transfusion as there is no indication that this client is unstable at this time. The nurse should not call for both units of transfusions at the same time due to the increased risk for misidentification. The nurse should not verify the compatibility of both units at the same time due to the increased risk for misidentification. It is not necessary to involve two nurses because the second client can wait until the nurse has time to hang the blood.

CN: Management of care; CL: Analyze

102. **1, 2, 3, 4.** If a blood transfusion is terminated, the nurse must send a freshly collected blood sample to the blood bank and a urine sample to the laboratory; the nurse must also send the blood component unit with the attached administration set and completed transfusion reaction form to the blood bank. It is not necessary to inform the infection control manager, but the risk management department should be notified because a transfusion reaction may be a significant liability issue.

CN: Reduction of risk potential;
CL: Analyze

103. **3.** The most current pharmacology information is found in the clinical agency's drug guide, which may be available on electronic sources that are frequently updated and can be transmitted to a handheld device or by logging into the internet or hospital's intranet, if available. A commercially published drug guide and pharmacology textbooks are outdated once published and, therefore, may not have current information. The manufacturer's website has the potential for bias.

CN: Management of care; CL: Apply

104. **1, 2, 3.** Abbreviations can be misinterpreted, and all health care professionals should avoid the use of easily misunderstood abbreviations. The purpose of avoiding abbreviations is not to make it easier for clients to understand the medication prescriptions or to make data entry easier.

CN: Management of care; CL: Analyze

105. **4.** The most common source of infection and microbial colonization in neutropenic clients is their own nonpathogenic normal flora. Attention to personal hygiene, such as oral, pulmonary, urinary, and rectal care, is essential. It is important to acknowledge the client's concerns and fears and to provide organized, calm, compassionate care, but it is more important to teach the client how to prevent an infection that could be life-threatening.

CN: Health promotion and maintenance;
CL: Analyze

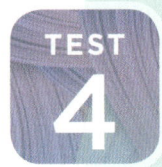

TEST 4

The Adult with Respiratory Health Problems

- The Adult with an Upper Respiratory Tract Infection
- The Adult Undergoing Nasal Surgery
- The Adult with Cancer of the Larynx
- The Adult with Pneumonia
- The Adult with Tuberculosis
- The Adult with Chronic Obstructive Pulmonary Disease
- The Adult with Asthma
- The Adult with Lung Cancer
- The Adult with Chest Trauma
- The Adult with Acute Respiratory Distress Syndrome
- Managing Care, Quality, and Safety of Adults with Respiratory Health Problems
- Answers, Rationales, and Test-Taking Strategies

The Adult with an Upper Respiratory Tract Infection

1. A nurse is teaching a client about taking antihistamines. Which information should the nurse include in the teaching plan? Select all that apply.
   ☐ 1. Operating machinery and driving may be dangerous while taking antihistamines.
   ☐ 2. Continue taking antihistamines even if a nasal infection develops.
   ☐ 3. The effect of antihistamines is not felt until a day later.
   ☐ 4. Do not use alcohol with antihistamines.
   ☐ 5. Increase fluid intake to 2000 mL a day.

2. A nurse instructs a client with allergic rhinitis about the correct technique for using an intranasal inhaler. Which statement indicates that the client understands the instructions?
   ☐ 1. "I should limit the use of the inhaler to early morning and bedtime."
   ☐ 2. "It is important to not shake the canister because that can damage the spray device."
   ☐ 3. "I should hold one nostril closed while I insert the spray into the other nostril."
   ☐ 4. "The inhaler tip is inserted into the nostril and pointed toward the inside nostril wall."

3. The nurse is evaluating the effectiveness of a teaching plan for a client recovering from an upper respiratory tract infection. Which is an expected outcome of the plan?

   The client will:
   ☐ 1. maintain a fluid intake of 800 mL every 24 hours.
   ☐ 2. have a temperature below 100°F (37.8°C).
   ☐ 3. cough productively without chest discomfort.
   ☐ 4. experience less nasal obstruction and discharge.

4. The nurse teaches the client how to instill nose drops. Which technique is correct?
   ☐ 1. The client uses sterile technique when handling the dropper.
   ☐ 2. The client blows the nose gently before instilling drops.
   ☐ 3. The client uses a new dropper for each instillation.
   ☐ 4. The client sits in a semi-Fowler position for 2 minutes.

5. The nurse should include which instruction(s) in the teaching plan for a client with chronic sinusitis? Select all that apply.
   ☐ 1. Avoid the use of caffeinated beverages.
   ☐ 2. Perform postural drainage every day.
   ☐ 3. Take a hot shower in the morning and evening.
   ☐ 4. Report a temperature of 102°F (38.9°C) or higher.
   ☐ 5. Limit fluid intake to 1000 mL per 24 hours.

6. A client with allergic rhinitis asks the nurse what to do to decrease rhinorrhea. Which instruction would be appropriate for the nurse to give the client?
   ☐ 1. "Use your nasal decongestant spray regularly to help clear your nasal passages."
   ☐ 2. "Ask the health care provider for antibiotics. Antibiotics will help decrease the secretion."
   ☐ 3. "It is important to increase your activity. A daily brisk walk will help promote drainage."
   ☐ 4. "Keep a diary of when your symptoms occur. This can help you identify what precipitates your attacks."

7. The health care provider has prescribed guaifenesin 300 mg four times a day. The dosage strength of the liquid is 200 mg/5 mL. How many milliliters should the nurse administer for each dose? Record your answer using one decimal place.
   _____ mL.

8. The health care provider has prescribed pseudoephedrine. The nurse should instruct the client about which possible adverse effect of this drug?
   ☐ 1. constipation
   ☐ 2. bradycardia
   ☐ 3. diplopia
   ☐ 4. restlessness

The Adult Undergoing Nasal Surgery

9. A health care provider (HCP) has just inserted nasal packing for a client with epistaxis. The client is taking ramipril for hypertension. What should the nurse instruct the client to do?
   ☐ 1. Use 81 mg of aspirin daily for relief of discomfort.
   ☐ 2. Omit the next dose of ramipril.
   ☐ 3. Remove the packing if there is difficulty swallowing.
   ☐ 4. Avoid rigorous aerobic exercise.

10. A client had surgery for a deviated nasal septum. Which finding indicates that bleeding is occurring even if the nasal drip pad remains dry and intact?
    ☐ 1. nausea
    ☐ 2. repeated swallowing
    ☐ 3. increased respiratory rate
    ☐ 4. increased pain

11. A client who has undergone outpatient nasal surgery is ready for discharge and has nasal packing in place. What should the nurse instruct the client to do?
    ☐ 1. Avoid activities that elicit the Valsalva maneuver.
    ☐ 2. Take aspirin to control nasal discomfort.
    ☐ 3. Avoid brushing the teeth until the nasal packing is removed.
    ☐ 4. Apply heat to the nasal area to control swelling.

12. The nurse is evaluating the client's understanding of home care instructions following nasal surgery. Which statement indicates to the nurse that a client has understood the discharge instructions?
    ☐ 1. "I should not shower until my packing is removed."
    ☐ 2. "I will take stool softeners and modify my diet to prevent constipation."
    ☐ 3. "Coughing every 2 hours is important to prevent respiratory complications."
    ☐ 4. "It is important to blow my nose each day to remove the dried secretions."

13. The nurse is giving preoperative instructions to a client who will be undergoing rhinoplasty. What should the nurse tell the client?
    ☐ 1. "After surgery, nasal packing will be in place for 7 to 10 days."
    ☐ 2. "Normal saline nose drops will need to be administered preoperatively."
    ☐ 3. "The results of the surgery will be immediately obvious postoperatively."
    ☐ 4. "Do not take aspirin-containing medications for 2 weeks before surgery."

14. A client has had surgery for a deviated nasal septum. The client has returned from the postanesthesia care unit. What should the nurse do **first**?
    ☐ 1. Assess the client's pain.
    ☐ 2. Inspect the area for periorbital ecchymosis.
    ☐ 3. Assess respiratory status.
    ☐ 4. Measure intake and output.

15. After nasal surgery, the client expresses concern about how to decrease facial pain and swelling while recovering at home. Which instruction would be **most** effective for decreasing pain and edema?
    ☐ 1. Take analgesics every 4 hours around the clock.
    ☐ 2. Use corticosteroid nasal spray as needed to control symptoms.
    ☐ 3. Use a bedside humidifier while sleeping.
    ☐ 4. Apply cold compresses to the area.

16. A client is being discharged with nasal packing in place. What should the nurse instruct the client to do?
    ☐ 1. Perform frequent mouth care.
    ☐ 2. Use normal saline nose drops daily.
    ☐ 3. Sneeze and cough with the mouth closed.
    ☐ 4. Gargle every 4 hours with salt water.

17. The nurse is teaching a client how to manage a nosebleed. What instruction should the nurse give the client?
    ☐ 1. "Tilt your head backward, and pinch your nose."
    ☐ 2. "Lie down flat, and place an ice compress over the bridge of the nose."
    ☐ 3. "Blow your nose gently with your neck flexed."
    ☐ 4. "Sit down, lean forward, and pinch the soft portion of your nose."

18. A client had posterior packing inserted to control a severe nosebleed. After insertion of the packing, the nurse should observe the client for which finding?
☐ 1. vertigo
☐ 2. Bell's palsy
☐ 3. hypoventilation
☐ 4. loss of gag reflex

The Adult with Cancer of the Larynx

19. A client has had a radical neck dissection for laryngeal cancer. Which action is the **priority** for nursing care immediately following this surgery?
☐ 1. maintaining complete bed rest until postsurgical swelling decreases
☐ 2. taking vital signs once a shift until the client is stable
☐ 3. determining if the client can swallow
☐ 4. suctioning the laryngectomy tube as often as needed

20. A client who has had a total laryngectomy appears withdrawn and depressed. The client keeps the curtain drawn, refuses visitors, and indicates a desire to be left alone. Which nursing intervention would be **most** therapeutic for the client?
☐ 1. discussing the behavior with the spouse to determine the cause
☐ 2. exploring future plans
☐ 3. respecting the need for privacy
☐ 4. encouraging expression of feelings nonverbally and in writing

21. The nurse is suctioning a client who had a laryngectomy. What is the **maximum** amount of time the nurse should suction the client?
☐ 1. 10 seconds
☐ 2. 20 seconds
☐ 3. 25 seconds
☐ 4. 30 seconds

22. The nurse is suctioning a tracheostomy for a client who had the tracheostomy tube placed 3 days ago. Which is the correct procedure for suctioning at this time?
☐ 1. Use a sterile catheter each time the client is suctioned.
☐ 2. Clean the catheter in sterile water after each use, and reuse for no longer than 8 hours.
☐ 3. Protect the catheter in sterile packaging between suctioning episodes.
☐ 4. Use a clean catheter with each suctioning, and disinfect it in hydrogen peroxide between uses.

23. The client with a laryngectomy does not want to be observed by the family because the opening in the throat is "disgusting." How should the nurse respond to the client?
☐ 1. Initiate teaching about the care of a stoma.
☐ 2. Explain that the stoma will not always look as it does now.
☐ 3. Inform the client of the benefits of family support at this time.
☐ 4. Explore why the client believes the stoma is "disgusting."

24. The nurse team leader is making rounds and observes a client who had a tracheostomy tube inserted 2 days ago (see figure). The nursing policy manual recommends the use of the gauze pad. What should the nurse do?

☐ 1. Make sure the gauze pad is dry and the client is in a comfortable position.
☐ 2. Ask the unlicensed assistive personnel to tie the tracheostomy tube ties in the back of the client's neck.
☐ 3. Reposition the gauze pad around the stoma with the open end downward.
☐ 4. Ask a registered nurse to change the ties and position another gauze pad around the stoma.

25. The nurse is assessing a client who has had hoarseness for more than 2 weeks. What action should the nurse take?
☐ 1. Refer the client to a health care provider for a prescription for an antibiotic.
☐ 2. Instruct the client to gargle with salt water at home.
☐ 3. Assess the client for dysphagia.
☐ 4. Instruct the client to take a throat analgesic.

26. A client has just returned from the postanesthesia care unit after undergoing a laryngectomy. Which instruction should the nurse include in the plan of care?
☐ 1. Maintain the head of the bed at 30 to 40 degrees.
☐ 2. Teach the client how to use esophageal speech.
☐ 3. Initiate small feedings of soft foods.
☐ 4. Irrigate drainage tubes as needed.

27. The nurse is making a discharge plan for a client recovering from a total laryngectomy. What is an expected outcome?

The client will:
☐ 1. regain the ability to taste and smell food.
☐ 2. demonstrate appropriate care of the gastrostomy tube.
☐ 3. communicate feelings about body image changes.
☐ 4. demonstrate sterile suctioning technique for stoma care.

28. The nurse is developing a discharge teaching plan for a client who underwent a laryngectomy 3 days ago. What information should the nurse include in the plan?
☐ 1. Perform mouth care every morning and evening.
☐ 2. Provide adequate humidity in the home.
☐ 3. Maintain a soft, bland diet.
☐ 4. Limit physical activity to shoulder and neck exercises.

The Adult with Pneumonia

29. The nurse is caring for a client with bacterial pneumonia. The effectiveness of the client's oxygen therapy can be **best** determined by which indicator of oxygenation?
☐ 1. absence of cyanosis
☐ 2. client's respiratory rate
☐ 3. arterial blood gas (ABG) values
☐ 4. client's level of consciousness

30. A client admitted with pneumonia and dementia has attempted several times to pull out the IV and Foley catheter. After trying other options, the nurse obtains a prescription for bilateral soft wrist restraints. Which nursing action is **most** appropriate?
☐ 1. Perform circulation checks to bilateral upper extremities each shift.
☐ 2. Attach the ties of the restraints to the bed frame.
☐ 3. Reevaluate the need for restraints and document weekly.
☐ 4. Ensure the restraint prescription has been signed by the health care provider (HCP) within 72 hours.

31. An older adult is admitted to the hospital with a diagnosis of bacterial pneumonia. While obtaining the client's health history, the nurse learns that the client has osteoarthritis, follows a vegetarian diet, and is very concerned with cleanliness. Which client information would **most** likely be a predisposing factor for the diagnosis of pneumonia?
☐ 1. age
☐ 2. osteoarthritis
☐ 3. vegetarian diet
☐ 4. daily bathing

32. A client with bacterial pneumonia is to be started on intravenous antibiotics. The nurse should verify that which diagnostic test has been completed before administering the antibiotic?
☐ 1. urinalysis
☐ 2. sputum culture
☐ 3. chest radiograph
☐ 4. red blood cell count

33. A client with bacterial pneumonia is receiving an aminoglycoside antibiotic. To ensure safe use of the drug, the nurse should monitor which laboratory value?
☐ 1. serum sodium
☐ 2. serum potassium
☐ 3. serum creatinine
☐ 4. serum calcium

34. A client with pneumonia has a temperature of 102.6°F (39.2°C), is diaphoretic, and has a productive cough. The client is able to ambulate. What should the nurse do?
☐ 1. Change the client's position every 4 hours.
☐ 2. Use nasotracheal suctioning to clear secretions.
☐ 3. Change the bedsheets frequently.
☐ 4. Offer the use of a bedpan every 2 hours.

35. A client with pneumonia has pleuritic chest pain. Which action should the nurse take to help the client manage the pain?
☐ 1. Encourage the client to breathe shallowly.
☐ 2. Have the client practice abdominal breathing.
☐ 3. Offer the client incentive spirometry.
☐ 4. Teach the client to splint the rib cage when coughing.

36. The nurse administers two 325-mg aspirin every 4 hours to a client with pneumonia. The nurse should evaluate the outcome of administering the drug by assessing the client for which finding(s)? Select all that apply.
☐ 1. decreased pain when breathing
☐ 2. prolonged clotting time
☐ 3. decreased temperature
☐ 4. decreased respiratory rate
☐ 5. increased ability to expectorate secretions

37. The nurse is assessing a client with pneumonia. Which change in the client's mental status is concerning at this time?
- ☐ 1. coma
- ☐ 2. apathy
- ☐ 3. irritability
- ☐ 4. depression

38. The nurse is assessing a client who is being treated for bacterial pneumonia. Which is an expected finding for this client?
- ☐ 1. a respiratory rate of 25 to 30 breaths/min
- ☐ 2. the ability to perform activities of daily living without dyspnea
- ☐ 3. a maximum loss of 5 to 10 lb (2 to 5 kg) of body weight
- ☐ 4. chest pain that is minimized by splinting the rib cage

The Adult with Tuberculosis

39. A client newly diagnosed with tuberculosis (TB) is being admitted with the prescription for "isolation precautions for tuberculosis." The nurse should assign the client to which type of room?
- ☐ 1. a room at the end of the hall for privacy
- ☐ 2. a private room to implement airborne precautions
- ☐ 3. a room near the nurses' station to ensure confidentiality
- ☐ 4. a room with windows to allow sunlight

40. The nurse is reviewing the history and physical and health care provider prescriptions on the medical record of a newly admitted client.

History and Physical	
Subjective:	19-year-old reports a constant cough for the past "few weeks" with "dark" sputum for the past few days. Has night sweats, 10-lb (4.5-kg) weight loss in the past month, and "always" being tired. Client took one acetaminophen about an hour prior to arrival.
Objective:	
Blood pressure	120/64 mm Hg
Heart rate	84/reg
Respiratory rate	26/unlabored/slight wheezing in right lower lobe posteriorly
O_2 Saturation	92%
Temperature	99.9°F (37.7°C) oral
Skin	Warm, slightly diaphoretic
Nonproductive cough at this time	
Assessment:	Possible respiratory infection
Health care provider prescriptions	
	Chest x-ray
	Sputum specimen
	Oxygen at 2 L per nasal cannula

What should the nurse do **first**?
- ☐ 1. Initiate airborne precautions.
- ☐ 2. Apply 2 L of oxygen via nasal cannula.
- ☐ 3. Collect a sputum sample.
- ☐ 4. Reassess vital signs.

41. A client is receiving streptomycin to treat tuberculosis. What should the nurse evaluate to determine an adverse effect of the drug?
- ☐ 1. decreased serum creatinine
- ☐ 2. difficulty swallowing
- ☐ 3. hearing loss
- ☐ 4. IV infiltration

42. The nurse is reconciling the prescriptions for a client diagnosed recently with pulmonary tuberculosis who is being admitted to the hospital for a total hip replacement (see medication prescription sheet). The client asks if it is necessary to take all of these medications while in the hospital. What should the nurse tell the client?

Prescriptions
- isoniazid (INH), 300 mg PO daily
- Rifampin, 600 mg PO daily
- Pyridoxine (vitamin B_6), 10 mg PO daily
- ethambutol, 400 mg PO daily
- pyrazinamide, 1.5 g PO daily

☐ 1. "I'll ask your health care provider (HCP) to review the prescriptions for a duplication between isoniazid and ethambutol."
☐ 2. "I can't discontinue any of these drugs until you can eat solid foods."
☐ 3. "I'll ask the pharmacist to check for drug interactions between the rifampin and isoniazid."
☐ 4. "It's important to continue to take the medications because the combination of drugs prevents bacterial resistance."

43. The client with tuberculosis is to be discharged home with nursing follow-up. Which aspect of nursing care will have the **highest priority**?
☐ 1. offering the client emotional support
☐ 2. teaching the client about the disease and its treatment
☐ 3. coordinating various agency services
☐ 4. assessing the client's environment for sanitation

44. The nurse is reading the results of a tuberculin skin test (see figure). How should the nurse interpret the results?

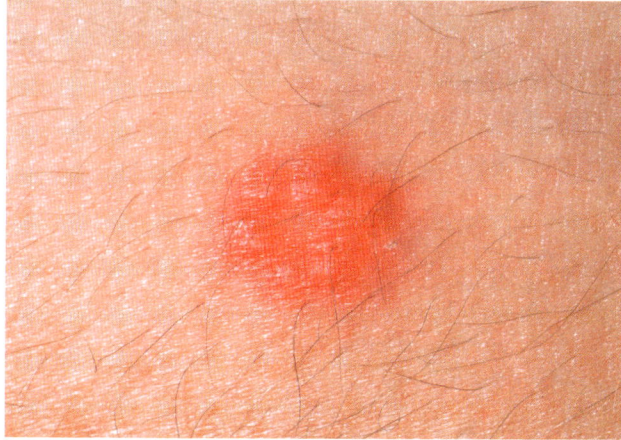

☐ 1. negative
☐ 2. needing to be repeated
☐ 3. positive
☐ 4. false

45. The nurse is preparing to administer a Mantoux test. Which technique is correct?
☐ 1. Hold the needle and syringe almost parallel to the client's skin.
☐ 2. Pinch the skin when inserting the needle.
☐ 3. Aspirate before injecting the medication.
☐ 4. Massage the site after injecting the medication.

46. A client had a Mantoux test result of an 8-mm induration. When should the nurse interpret the test as positive?

The client:
☐ 1. lives in a long-term care facility.
☐ 2. has no known risk factors.
☐ 3. is immunocompromised.
☐ 4. works as a health care provider in a hospital.

47. Prior to discharging a client diagnosed with tuberculosis, the nurse is determining if others in the home are at risk for contracting the disease. Which of these family members who have been exposed to tuberculosis would be at **highest** risk for contracting the disease?
☐ 1. 45-year-old parent
☐ 2. 17-year-old adolescent
☐ 3. 8-year-old child
☐ 4. 76-year-old grandparent

48. The nurse is teaching a client who has been diagnosed with tuberculosis how to avoid spreading the disease to family members. Which statement(s) would indicate that the client has understood the nurse's instructions? Select all that apply.
☐ 1. "I will need to dispose of my old clothing when I return home."
☐ 2. "I should always cover my mouth and nose when sneezing."
☐ 3. "It is important that I isolate myself from family when possible."
☐ 4. "I should use paper tissues to cough in and dispose of them promptly."
☐ 5. "I will avoid crowds."

49. A client has a positive reaction to the Mantoux test. How should the nurse interpret this reaction?

The client has:
☐ 1. active tuberculosis.
☐ 2. been exposed to *Mycobacterium tuberculosis*.
☐ 3. developed resistance to tubercle bacilli.
☐ 4. developed passive immunity to tuberculosis.

50. A client with tuberculosis is taking isoniazid (INH). What should the nurse instruct the client to do to help prevent the development of peripheral neuropathies?
☐ 1. Adhere to a low-cholesterol diet.
☐ 2. Supplement the diet with pyridoxine (vitamin B_6).
☐ 3. Get extra rest.
☐ 4. Avoid excessive sun exposure.

51. The nurse is instructing a sexually active female who is taking isoniazid (INH). What should the nurse tell the client?
INH:
☐ 1. increases the risk for vaginal infection.
☐ 2. has mutagenic effects on ova.
☐ 3. decreases the effectiveness of hormonal contraceptives.
☐ 4. inhibits ovulation.

52. Clients who have had active tuberculosis are at risk for recurrence. Which condition increases that risk?
☐ 1. cool and damp weather
☐ 2. active exercise and exertion
☐ 3. physical and emotional stress
☐ 4. rest and inactivity

53. The nurse is conducting a community assessment for areas of risk for tuberculosis. In which areas of the United States and Canada is the incidence of tuberculosis **highest**?
☐ 1. rural farming areas
☐ 2. inner-city areas
☐ 3. areas where clean water standards are low
☐ 4. suburban areas with significant industrial pollution

54. A client who has been diagnosed with tuberculosis has been placed on drug therapy. The medication regimen includes rifampin. Which instruction(s) should the nurse give the client about the potential adverse effects of rifampin? Select all that apply.
☐ 1. Have eye examinations every 6 months.
☐ 2. Maintain follow-up monitoring of liver enzymes.
☐ 3. Decrease protein intake in the diet.
☐ 4. Avoid alcohol intake.
☐ 5. The urine may have an orange color.

55. The nurse is providing follow-up care to a client with tuberculosis who does not regularly take the prescribed medication. Which nursing action would be **most** appropriate for this client?
☐ 1. Ask the client's spouse to supervise the daily administration of the medications.
☐ 2. Visit the client weekly to verify compliance with taking the medication.
☐ 3. Notify the health care provider (HCP) of the client's noncompliance, and request a different prescription.
☐ 4. Remind the client that tuberculosis can be fatal if it is not treated promptly.

The Adult with Chronic Obstructive Pulmonary Disease

56. A client with newly diagnosed chronic obstructive disease is to be discharged home with oxygen per nasal prongs. Which teaching point(s) should the nurse include in this client's discharge plan? Select all that apply.
☐ 1. Apply petroleum jelly on lips and nose to prevent dryness and irritation.
☐ 2. Avoid areas where people are smoking cigarettes or cigars.
☐ 3. Increase oxygen flow at night during hours of sleep.
☐ 4. Place gauze between the ears and oxygen tubing to prevent skin irritation.
☐ 5. Request a large, pressurized oxygen tank for use during car travel.
☐ 6. Avoid using a microwave oven when using oxygen.

57. The nurse is developing a teaching plan for the client newly diagnosed with chronic obstructive pulmonary disease (COPD). Which information should be included in the plan? Select all that apply.
☐ 1. Pulmonary rehabilitation programs offer very little benefit.
☐ 2. Pneumococcal vaccination is contraindicated for clients with lung disease.
☐ 3. High humidity increases the effort of breathing.
☐ 4. A bronchodilator with a metered-dose inhaler should be readily available.
☐ 5. Smoking cessation is important to slow or stop disease progression.

58. A nurse is assessing a client with chronic emphysema. Which finding requires **immediate** intervention?
☐ 1. using pursed-lip breathing and prolonged expiration
☐ 2. circumoral cyanosis
☐ 3. crackles auscultated posteriorly halfway up the left lung
☐ 4. appearance of a "barrel chest"

59. The nurse is assessing a client with chronic obstructive pulmonary disease. Which finding requires **immediate** intervention?
☐ 1. distant heart sounds
☐ 2. diminished lung sounds
☐ 3. inability to speak
☐ 4. pursed-lip breathing

60. The nurse is instructing a client with chronic obstructive pulmonary disease on how to do pursed-lip breathing. In which order from first to last should the nurse explain the steps to the client? All options must be used.

1. "Breathe in normally through your nose for two counts (while counting to yourself, one, two)."

2. "Relax your neck and shoulder muscles."

3. "Pucker your lips as if you were going to whistle."

4. "Breathe out slowly through pursed lips for four counts (while counting to yourself, one, two, three, four)."

61. The nurse reviews an arterial blood gas report for a client with chronic obstructive pulmonary disease (COPD). The results are as follows: pH 7.35; partial pressure of arterial carbon dioxide ($PaCO_2$) 62 mm Hg (8.25 kPa); partial pressure of arterial oxygen (PaO_2) 70 mm Hg (9.31 kPa); and bicarbonate (HCO_3^-) 34 mEq/L (34 mmol/L). What should the nurse do **first**?
☐ 1. Apply a 100% nonrebreather mask.
☐ 2. Assess the vital signs.
☐ 3. Reposition the client.
☐ 4. Prepare for intubation.

62. The nurse is developing a discharge plan with a client with chronic obstructive pulmonary disease (COPD). What information should the nurse include in the plan?

People with COPD:
☐ 1. develop respiratory infections easily.
☐ 2. usually maintain their current status.
☐ 3. require less supplemental oxygen.
☐ 4. show permanent improvement.

63. The client with chronic obstructive pulmonary disease is taking theophylline. The nurse should instruct the client to report which sign(s) of theophylline toxicity? Select all that apply.
☐ 1. nausea
☐ 2. vomiting
☐ 3. seizures
☐ 4. insomnia
☐ 5. vision changes

64. Which statement indicates that the client with chronic obstructive pulmonary disease (COPD) who has been discharged to home understands the care plan?

The client:
☐ 1. plans to avoid direct contact with family and friends.
☐ 2. can state actions to reduce pain.
☐ 3. will use oxygen via a nasal cannula at 5 L per minute.
☐ 4. agrees to call the health care provider (HCP) if dyspnea on exertion increases.

65. The nurse is conducting a wellness class about how to decrease the risk for developing chronic obstructive pulmonary disease (COPD). Which is the **most** important point the nurse should emphasize?
☐ 1. Participate regularly in aerobic exercises.
☐ 2. Maintain a high-protein diet.
☐ 3. Avoid exposure to people with known respiratory infections.
☐ 4. Abstain from cigarette smoking.

66. The nurse is instructing the client with chronic obstructive pulmonary disease to do pursed-lip breathing. What is the expected outcome of this exercise?
☐ 1. improved oxygen intake
☐ 2. deeper diaphragmatic breathing
☐ 3. stronger intercostal muscles
☐ 4. better elimination of carbon dioxide

67. The nurse is developing a care plan with a client with chronic obstructive pulmonary disease (COPD). Which is the **priority** goal?
☐ 1. maintaining functional ability
☐ 2. minimizing chest pain
☐ 3. increasing carbon dioxide levels in the blood
☐ 4. treating infectious agents

68. When teaching a client with chronic obstructive pulmonary disease to conserve, what instruction should the nurse give the client about breathing when lifting heavy objects?

Lift the object by:
☐ 1. inhaling through an open mouth.
☐ 2. exhaling through pursed lips.
☐ 3. exhaling but before inhaling.
☐ 4. taking a deep breath and holding it.

69. The nurse is teaching a client with chronic obstructive pulmonary disease (COPD) to assess for signs and symptoms of right-sided heart failure. Which signs and symptoms should be included in the teaching plan?
☐ 1. clubbing of nail beds
☐ 2. hypertension
☐ 3. peripheral edema
☐ 4. increased appetite

70. The nurse is assessing the respiratory status of a client who is experiencing an exacerbation of chronic obstructive pulmonary disease (COPD) secondary to an upper respiratory tract infection. Which finding is expected?
☐ 1. normal breath sounds
☐ 2. prolonged inspiration
☐ 3. normal chest movement
☐ 4. coarse crackles and rhonchi

71. A client with chronic obstructive pulmonary disease (COPD) is experiencing dyspnea and has a low partial pressure of arterial oxygen (PaO₂) level. The nurse plans to administer oxygen as prescribed. Which statement is true concerning oxygen administration to a client with COPD?
☐ 1. High oxygen concentrations will cause coughing and dyspnea.
☐ 2. High oxygen concentrations may inhibit the hypoxic stimulus to breathe.
☐ 3. Increased oxygen use will cause the client to become dependent on oxygen.
☐ 4. Administration of oxygen is contraindicated in clients who are using bronchodilators.

72. The nurse is teaching the client with chronic obstructive pulmonary disease (COPD) about obtaining the best nutrition. Which diet would be **best** for this client?
☐ 1. low-fat, low-cholesterol diet
☐ 2. bland, soft diet
☐ 3. low-sodium diet
☐ 4. high-calorie, high-protein diet

73. The nurse administers theophylline to a client. When evaluating the effectiveness of this medication, what is an expected outcome?
☐ 1. suppression of the client's respiratory infection
☐ 2. decrease in bronchial secretions
☐ 3. less difficulty breathing
☐ 4. thinning of tenacious, purulent sputum

74. The nurse is planning to teach a client with chronic obstructive pulmonary disease how to cough effectively. Which instruction should be included?
☐ 1. Take a deep abdominal breath, bend forward, and cough three or four times on exhalation.
☐ 2. Lie flat on the back, splint the thorax, take two deep breaths, and cough.
☐ 3. Take several rapid, shallow breaths, and then cough forcefully.
☐ 4. Assume a side-lying position, extend the arm over the head, and alternate deep breathing with coughing.

75. **STEP 1**

The nurse is caring for a 68-year-old female client in the emergency department with increased shortness of breath, cough, and sputum production.

▸ Highlight the findings that require follow-up. Answer choices have been underlined.

Nurse's Notes

Today: 1500
The client has not been able to take the daily medications and has shortness of breath when ambulating due to worsening respiratory symptoms and fatigue. The client has a history of smoking one pack of cigarettes per day for 35 years, has been diagnosed with chronic obstructive pulmonary disease (COPD), and uses 2 L per minute of oxygen via nasal cannula and continuous positive airway pressure (CPAP) overnight for obstructive sleep apnea. The client also has hypertension, depression, and anxiety. The client is wheezing with diminished breath sounds on auscultation, performing pursed-lip breathing using accessory muscles, and coughing thick, yellow sputum.
Vital signs are temperature (T) 100.4 °F (38.0°C); heart rate (HR) 112 bpm; blood pressure (BP) 150/90 mm Hg; respiration rate (RR) 18 breaths/min; and oxygen saturation 90% on 2 L per minute via nasal cannula.

Nurse's Notes

Today: 1500
The client has not been able to take the daily medications and has shortness of breath when ambulating due to worsening respiratory symptoms and fatigue. The client has a history of smoking one pack of cigarettes per day for 35 years, has been diagnosed with chronic obstructive pulmonary disease (COPD), and uses 2 L per minute of oxygen via nasal cannula and continuous positive airway pressure (CPAP) overnight for obstructive sleep apnea. The client also has hypertension, depression, and anxiety. The client is <u>wheezing</u> with <u>diminished breath sounds</u> on auscultation, <u>performing pursed-lip breathing using accessory muscles</u>, and <u>coughing thick, yellow sputum</u>.
Vital signs are <u>temperature (T) 100.4 °F (38.0°C); heart rate (HR) 112 bpm; blood pressure (BP) 150/90 mm Hg; respiration rate (RR) 18 breaths/min;</u> and <u>oxygen saturation 90% on 2 L per minute via nasal cannula</u>.

76. STEP 2

The nurse is caring for a 68-year-old female older adult in the emergency department with increased shortness of breath, cough, and sputum production.

Nurse's Notes

Today: 1500
The client has not been able to take the daily medications and has shortness of breath when ambulating due to worsening respiratory symptoms and fatigue. The client has a history of smoking one pack of cigarettes per day for 35 years, has been diagnosed with chronic obstructive pulmonary disease (COPD), and uses 2 L per minute of oxygen via nasal cannula and continuous positive airway pressure (CPAP) overnight for obstructive sleep apnea. The client also has hypertension, depression, and anxiety. The client is wheezing with diminished breath sounds on auscultation, performing pursed-lip breathing using accessory muscles, and coughing thick, yellow sputum. Vital signs are temperature (T) 100.4°F (38.0°C); heart rate (HR) 112 bpm; blood pressure (BP) 150/90 mm Hg; respiration rate (RR) 18 breaths/min; and oxygen saturation 90% on 2 L per minute via nasal cannula. An intravenous infusion of 5% dextrose with normal saline (D5NS) was started at 125 mL per hour.

➢ Complete the following sentence by choosing from the list of options.

The nurse is **most** concerned about the client's [COPD; anxiety; use of continuous positive airway pressure (CPAP),]

as evidenced by the client's [temperature of 100.4°F (38.0°C); respiratory rate of 18 breaths/min; heart rate of 112 bpm, and oxygen saturation of 90%.]

77. STEP 3

An older adult presents to the emergency department with increased shortness of breath, cough, and sputum production.

Nurse's Notes

Today: 1500
The client has not been able to take the daily medications and has shortness of breath when ambulating due to worsening respiratory symptoms and fatigue. The client has a history of smoking one pack of cigarettes per day for 35 years, has been diagnosed with chronic obstructive pulmonary disease (COPD), and uses 2 L per minute of oxygen via nasal cannula and continuous positive airway pressure (CPAP) overnight for obstructive sleep apnea. The client also has hypertension, depression, and anxiety. The client is wheezing with diminished breath sounds on auscultation, performing pursed-lip breathing using accessory muscles, and coughing thick, yellow sputum.
Vital signs are temperature (T) 100.4°F (38.0°C); heart rate (HR) 112 bpm; blood pressure (BP) 150/90 mm Hg; respiration rate (RR) 18 breaths/min; and oxygen saturation 90% on 2 L per minute via nasal cannula.
An intravenous infusion of 5% dextrose with normal saline (D5NS) was started at 125 mL per hour per health care provider's orders.

1600:
The client was transferred to intermediate care.

The client was transferred to intermediate care, and the nurse is reviewing the health care provider's orders.

➢ Identify the four orders the nurse should implement **immediately** to the box on the right.

☐ 1. Obtain a sputum culture.
☐ 2. Administer a beta-blocker.
☐ 3. Administer mucolytics.
☐ 4. Provide a recliner.
☐ 5. Administer acetaminophen 325 mg, 2 tablets every 4 to 6 hours, for a temperature above 101°F (38.3°C).
☐ 6. Provide chest physical therapy.
☐ 7. Place the client on telemetry.

78. STEP 4

The nurse is caring for an older adult with COPD in an intermediate care unit.

Nurse's Notes

Today: 1500
The client has not been able to take the daily medications and has shortness of breath when ambulating due to worsening respiratory symptoms and fatigue. The client has a history of smoking one pack of cigarettes per day for 35 years, has been diagnosed with chronic obstructive pulmonary disease (COPD), and uses 2 L per minute of oxygen via nasal cannula and continuous positive airway pressure (CPAP) overnight for obstructive sleep apnea. The client also has hypertension, depression, and anxiety. The client is wheezing with diminished breath sounds on auscultation, performing pursed-lip breathing using accessory muscles, and coughing thick, yellow sputum.
Vital signs are temperature (T) 100.4°F (38.0°C); heart rate (HR) 112 bpm; blood pressure (BP) 150/90 mm Hg; respiration rate (RR) 18 breaths/min; and oxygen saturation 90% on 2 L per minute via nasal cannula.
An intravenous infusion of 5% dextrose with normal saline (D5NS) was started at 125 mL per hour per healthcare provider's orders.

1600:
The client was transferred to intermediate care.

1800:
Telemetry reports changes in the client's vital signs: T 101.0°F (38.3°C); HR 120 to 130 bpm on telemetry; BP 100/60 mm Hg; RR 28 breaths/min; and oxygen saturation 83% on 2 L per minute via nasal cannula.

➢ For each potential intervention, specify if the intervention is indicated, not indicated, or contraindicated.

Intervention	Indicated	Not Indicated	Contraindicated
Transfer to the intensive care unit	○	○	○
Increase oxygen to 6 L per minute	○	○	○
Increase intravenous fluids to 150 mL per hour	○	○	○
Administer acetaminophen	○	○	○
Notify the health care provider (HCP)	○	○	○

79. STEP 5

The nurse is planning care for a client with COPD.

Nurse's Notes

Today: 1500
The client has not been able to take the daily medications and has shortness of breath when ambulating due to worsening respiratory symptoms and fatigue. The client has a history of smoking one pack of cigarettes per day for 35 years, has been diagnosed with chronic obstructive pulmonary disease (COPD), and uses 2 L per minute of oxygen via nasal cannula and continuous positive airway pressure (CPAP) overnight for obstructive sleep apnea. The client also has hypertension, depression, and anxiety. The client is wheezing with diminished breath sounds on auscultation, performing pursed-lip breathing using accessory muscles, and coughing thick, yellow sputum.
Vital signs are temperature (T) 100.4°F (38.0°C); heart rate (HR) 112 bpm; blood pressure (BP) 150/90 mm Hg; respiration rate (RR) 18 breaths/min; and oxygen saturation 90% on 2 L per minute via nasal cannula.
An intravenous infusion of 5% dextrose with normal saline (D5NS) was started at 125 mL per hour per healthcare provider's orders.

1600:
The client was transferred to intermediate care.

1800:
Telemetry reports changes in the client's vital signs: T 101.0°F (38.3°C); HR 120 to 130 bpm on telemetry; BP 100/60 mm Hg; RR 28 breaths/min; and oxygen saturation 83% on 2 L per minute via nasal cannula.

➢ For each potential intervention, indicate whether the intervention is indicated, not indicated, or contraindicated.

Intervention	Indicated	Not Indicated	Contraindicated
Administer bronchodilators	○	○	○
Replace electrolytes	○	○	○
Increase oxygen to 6 L per minute	○	○	○
Offer smoking cessation education	○	○	○
Order chest physical therapy	○	○	○
Check immunizations	○	○	○
Position the client supine in bed	○	○	○

80. **STEP 6**

The nurse is preparing the client for discharge to home.

Nurse's Notes

Today: 1500
The client has not been able to take the daily medications and has shortness of breath when ambulating due to worsening respiratory symptoms and fatigue. The client has a history of smoking one pack of cigarettes per day for 35 years, has been diagnosed with chronic obstructive pulmonary disease (COPD), and uses 2 L per minute of oxygen via nasal cannula and continuous positive airway pressure (CPAP) overnight for obstructive sleep apnea. The client also has hypertension, depression, and anxiety. The client is wheezing with diminished breath sounds on auscultation, performing pursed-lip breathing using accessory muscles, and coughing thick, yellow sputum.
Vital signs are temperature (T) 100.4°F (38.0°C); heart rate (HR) 112 bpm; blood pressure (BP) 150/90 mm Hg; respiration rate (RR) 18 breaths/min; and oxygen saturation 90% on 2 L per minute via nasal cannula.
An intravenous infusion of 5% dextrose with normal saline (D5NS) was started at 125 mL per hour per healthcare provider's orders.

1600:
The client was transferred to intermediate care.

1800:
Telemetry reports changes in the client's vital signs: T 101.0°F (38.3°C); HR 120 to 130 bpm on telemetry; BP 100/60 mm Hg; RR 28 breaths/min; and oxygen saturation 83% on 2 L per minute via nasal cannula.

▸ For each assessment finding, specify if the client's condition has improved, has not changed, or has declined.

Assessment Finding	Improved	Not Changed	Declined
Can walk to the bathroom without shortness of breath	○	○	○
Sputum culture negative for bacteria	○	○	○
Needs 2 L of oxygen per nasal cannula at night	○	○	○
Requires CPAP at night	○	○	○
Decreased sputum production	○	○	○
Lungs clear on auscultation	○	○	○

The Adult with Asthma

81. The nurse observes a client using a metered-dose inhaler (MDI) to aid in the management of asthma. Which action(s) would indicate that the client needs further instruction? Select all that apply.
☐ 1. shakes the MDI before using
☐ 2. exhales before starting to use the MDI
☐ 3. inspires rapidly when dispensing the medication from the MDI
☐ 4. holds the breath for 3 seconds after inhaling with the MDI
☐ 5. cleans the inhaler and canister in soapy water before using again in rapid succession

82. A client with a history of asthma is admitted to the emergency department. The nurse notes that the client is dyspneic, with a respiratory rate of 35 breaths/min, nasal flaring, and use of accessory muscles. Auscultation of the lung fields reveals greatly diminished breath sounds. What should the nurse do **first**?
☐ 1. Initiate oxygen therapy as prescribed, and reassess the client in 10 minutes.
☐ 2. Draw blood for an arterial blood gas test.
☐ 3. Encourage the client to relax and breathe slowly through the mouth.
☐ 4. Administer bronchodilators as prescribed.

83. A client is experiencing an acute asthmatic attack. Prior to treatment with levalbuterol, the client's respirations were 40 breaths/min, pulse was 132 bpm, oxygen saturation was 86% on room air, and there was audible wheezing. Which finding indicates achievement of the desired outcome of asthma treatment?
☐ 1. decreased peak expiratory flow (PEF) rate
☐ 2. wheezing inaudible with diminished breath sounds
☐ 3. pulse 96 bpm and percutaneous oxygen saturation (SpO_2) 92% on room air
☐ 4. inspiratory cycle twice as long as the expiratory cycle

84. For a client with asthma, the health care provider (HCP) prescribes albuterol, two puffs twice a day via a metered-dose inhaler (MDI), and beclomethasone, two puffs twice a day via MDI. How should the nurse instruct the client to administer these drugs?
☐ 1. "Take the medications 1 hour apart, two times a day."
☐ 2. "Take the albuterol first, and follow with beclomethasone two times a day."
☐ 3. "Take the albuterol on awakening, and alternate the medications every 4 hours."
☐ 4. "Take the beclomethasone inhaler first, and follow with albuterol."

85. A client experiencing a severe asthma attack has the following arterial blood gas results: pH 7.33; partial pressure of arterial carbon dioxide (PaCO₂) 48 mm Hg (6.4 kPa); partial pressure of arterial oxygen (PaO₂) 58 mm Hg (7.7 kPa); and bicarbonate (HCO₃⁻) 26 mEq/L (26 mmol/L). Which prescription should the nurse implement **first**?
☐ 1. albuterol nebulizer
☐ 2. chest x-ray
☐ 3. ipratropium inhaler
☐ 4. sputum culture

86. The nurse is instructing a client with acute asthma who is undergoing short-term corticosteroid therapy. The nurse should tell the client that steroids will have which expected outcome?
☐ 1. Promote bronchodilation.
☐ 2. Act as an expectorant.
☐ 3. Have an antiinflammatory effect.
☐ 4. Prevent the development of respiratory infections.

87. The nurse is teaching the client how to use a metered-dose inhaler (MDI) to administer a corticosteroid. Which observation indicates that the client is using the MDI correctly? Select all that apply.

The client:
☐ 1. holds the inhaler upright.
☐ 2. tilts the head down while inhaling the medicine.
☐ 3. waits 5 minutes between puffs.
☐ 4. rinses the mouth with water following administration.
☐ 5. lies supine for 15 minutes following administration.

88. A client is prescribed metaproterenol via a metered-dose inhaler, two puffs every 4 hours. The nurse should instruct the client to report which adverse effect?
☐ 1. irregular heartbeat
☐ 2. constipation
☐ 3. pedal edema
☐ 4. decreased pulse rate

89. A client who has been taking flunisolide nasal spray, two inhalations a day, for treatment of asthma has painful, white patches in the mouth. What should the nurse tell the client?
☐ 1. "This is an anticipated adverse effect of your medication. It should go away in a couple of weeks."
☐ 2. "You are using your inhaler too much, and it has irritated your mouth."
☐ 3. "You have developed a fungal infection from your medication. It will need to be treated with an antifungal agent."
☐ 4. "Be sure to brush your teeth and floss daily. Good oral hygiene will treat this problem."

90. A nurse is teaching a client to use a metered-dose inhaler (MDI) to administer bronchodilator medication. Indicate the correct order of the steps from first to last the client should take to use the MDI appropriately. All options must be used.

1. Shake the inhaler immediately before use.
2. Hold the breath for 10 seconds, and then exhale.
3. Activate the MDI on inhalation.
4. Breathe out through the mouth.

91. The nurse is preparing a client with asthma for discharge to home. Which instruction(s) should the nurse include in the discharge teaching plan? Select all that apply.
☐ 1. Incorporate physical exercise as tolerated into the daily routine.
☐ 2. Monitor peak flow numbers after meals and at bedtime.
☐ 3. Eliminate stressors in the work and home environment.
☐ 4. Use melatonin to ensure uninterrupted sleep at night.
☐ 5. Avoid smoke-filled rooms.

92. The nurse is teaching a client with asthma to avoid situations that will precipitate an asthma attack. Which situation should the nurse instruct the client to avoid?
☐ 1. occupational exposure to toxins
☐ 2. Valsalva maneuver
☐ 3. exposure to cigarette smoke
☐ 4. exercising in cold temperatures

93. The nurse is assessing a client with asthma. Which finding would **most** likely indicate the presence of a respiratory infection?
☐ 1. cough productive of yellow sputum
☐ 2. bilateral expiratory wheezing
☐ 3. chest tightness
☐ 4. respiratory rate of 30 breaths/min

The Adult with Lung Cancer

94. The nurse has assisted the health care provider at the bedside with the insertion of a left subclavian, triple lumen catheter in a client admitted with lung cancer. Suddenly, the client becomes restless and tachypneic. What should the nurse do **next**?
☐ 1. Assess breath sounds.
☐ 2. Remove the catheter.
☐ 3. Insert a peripheral IV.
☐ 4. Reposition the client.

95. A client who has been recently extubated has shortness of breath. The nurse reports the client's discomfort and the results of the recently prescribed arterial blood gas analysis to the health care provider (HCP). After reviewing the report of the complete blood count (CBC; see the laboratory report below), the nurse should also report which result to the HCP?

Laboratory Results

Complete Blood Count (CBC) with Differential			
Test Result	Current Results	Previous Results	Reference Range
White Blood Count (WBC)	$3.6 \times 10^3/mm^3$ ($3.6 \times 10^9/L$)	$3.4 \times 10^3/mm^3$ ($3.4 \times 10^9/L$)	$4.5 - 10.5 \times 10^3$ cells/mm^3 ($4.5 - 10.5 \times 10^9/L$)
Red Blood Count (RBC)	$3.20 \times 10^6/mm^3$ ($3.2 \times 10^{12}/L$)	$3.6 \times 10^6/mm^3$ ($3.6 \times 10^{12}/L$)	4.2 – 5.4 million/μL ($4.2 - 5.4 \times 10^{12}/L$)
Hemoglobin (Hgb)	9.6 g/dL (96 g/L)	10.5 g/dL (105 g/L)	12 to 16 g/dL (120 to 160 g/L)
Hematocrit (Hct)	30.5% (0.31)	32.6% (0.33)	In adult men, the value is 42% to 52% (0.42 to 0.52).
Platelets	302,000/μL ($302 \times 10^9/L$)	300,000/μL ($300 \times 10^9/L$)	Adults, 140,000 to 400,000/μL (140 to 400 $\times 10^9/L$).
Polys (neutrophils)	36%	34%	45%–76%
Lymphocytes	68%	70%	17%–44%
Monocytes	7%	8%	3%–10%
Eosinophils	2%	3%	0%–4%
Basophils	0.6%	0.6%	0.2%
Polys (absolute)	$0.34 \times 10^3/mm^3$	$0.36 \times 10^3/mm^3$	$1.8–7.8 \times 10^3/mm^3$
Lymphocytes (absolute)	$1.0 \times 10^3/mm^3$	$1.0 \times 10^3/mm^3$	$0.7–4.5 \times 10^3/mm^3$
Monocytes (absolute)	$0.1 \times 10^3/mm^3$	$0.1 \times 10^3/mm^3$	$0.1–1.0 \times 10^3/mm^3$
Eosinophils (absolute)	$0.1 \times 10^3/mm^3$	$0.1 \times 10^3/mm^3$	$0.0–0.4 \times 10^3/mm^3$
Basophils (absolute)	$0.0 \times 10^3/mm^3$	$0.0 \times 10^3/mm^3$	$0.0–0.2 \times 10^3/mm^3$
Hemoglobin A1c			
Test Results	Current Results	Previous Results	Reference Interval
HA1c	7.4%		<7%
Prothrombin			
Test Results	Current Results	Previous Results	Reference Interval
PT	13s	12s	10–12 s

☐ 1. prothrombin time (PT)
☐ 2. hemoglobin and hematocrit
☐ 3. monocytes
☐ 4. platelets

96. A client diagnosed with lung cancer is to have a left lower lobectomy. The nurse should assess the client for which factor that **increases** the client's risk for developing postoperative pulmonary complications?
☐ 1. Height is 5 feet, 7 inches (170.2 cm), and weight is 110 lb (49.9 kg).
☐ 2. The client tends to avoid verbalizing their real feelings.
☐ 3. The client ambulates and can climb one flight of stairs without dyspnea.
☐ 4. The client is 58 years of age.

97. The nurse is preparing a client for surgery and notices that the client looks sad. The client says, "I'm scared of having cancer. It's so horrible, and I brought it on myself. I should have quit smoking years ago." What would be the nurse's **best** response to the client?
☐ 1. "It's okay to be scared. What is it about cancer that you are afraid of?"
☐ 2. "It's normal to be scared. I would be, too. We will help you through it."
☐ 3. "Don't be so hard on yourself. You don't know if your smoking caused the cancer."
☐ 4. "Do you feel guilty because you smoked?"

98. A client who underwent a left lower lobectomy has been out of surgery for 48 hours. The client is receiving morphine sulfate via a patient-controlled analgesia (PCA) system and reports having pain in the left thorax that worsens when coughing. After checking the PCA system, what should the nurse do **next**?
☐ 1. Let the client rest so the client is not stimulated to cough.
☐ 2. Encourage the client to take deep breaths to help control the pain.
☐ 3. Reassure the client that the machine is working and will administer medication to relieve the pain.
☐ 4. Obtain a more detailed assessment of the client's pain using a pain scale.

99. The nurse is developing a discharge plan with a client who has had a lobectomy for treatment of lung cancer. To evaluate the client's understanding of the plan, what should the nurse ask the client to identify?
☐ 1. the support available to assist the client at home
☐ 2. the distance the client lives from the hospital
☐ 3. the client's ability to do home blood pressure monitoring
☐ 4. the client's knowledge of the causes of lung cancer

100. After a thoracotomy, the nurse instructs the client to perform deep-breathing exercises. What is an expected outcome of these exercises?
☐ 1. The elevated diaphragm enlarges the thorax and increases the lung surface available for gas exchange.
☐ 2. There is increased blood flow to the lungs to allow them to recover from the trauma of surgery.
☐ 3. The rate of airflow to the remaining lobe is controlled so that it will not become hyperinflated.
☐ 4. The alveoli expand and increase the lung surface available for ventilation.

101. Following a thoracotomy, the client reports a pain rating of 9 on a 10-point scale. What should the nurse do 30 minutes after administering the highest dose of the prescribed pain medication?
☐ 1. Reposition the client.
☐ 2. Reassess the client.
☐ 3. Reassure the client.
☐ 4. Readjust the pain medication dosage as needed.

102. While assessing a thoracotomy incisional area from which a chest tube exits, the nurse feels a crackling sensation under the fingertips along the entire incision. What should the nurse do **next**?
☐ 1. Lower the head of the bed, and call the health care provider (HCP).
☐ 2. Prepare a tracheotomy tray.
☐ 3. Mark the area with a skin pencil at the outer periphery of the crackling.
☐ 4. Turn off the suction of the chest drainage system.

103. The nurse is teaching a client to deep breathe effectively after a lobectomy. What should the nurse instruct the client to do?
☐ 1. Contract the abdominal muscles; take a slow, deep breath through the nose; hold it for 3 to 5 seconds; and then exhale.
☐ 2. Contract the abdominal muscles, take a deep breath through the mouth, and exhale slowly as if trying to blow out a candle.
☐ 3. Relax the abdominal muscles; take a slow, deep breath through the nose; and hold it for 3 to 5 seconds.
☐ 4. Relax the abdominal muscles, take a deep breath through the mouth, and exhale slowly over 10 seconds.

104. The nurse is teaching the client who has undergone chest surgery about exercises to prevent shoulder ankylosis. What information should the nurse give the client?
☐ 1. Turn from side to side.
☐ 2. Raise and lower the head.
☐ 3. Raise the arm on the affected side over the head.
☐ 4. Flex and extend the elbow on the affected side.

105. A client has a chest tube and water seal drainage system. What should the nurse do to ensure safe and effective use of the drainage system?
☐ 1. Verify that the air vent on the water seal drainage system is capped when the suction is off.
☐ 2. Strip the chest drainage tubes at least every 4 hours if excessive bleeding occurs.
☐ 3. Ensure that the chest tube is clamped when moving the client out of the bed.
☐ 4. Make sure that the drainage apparatus is always below the client's chest level.

106. A client has a chest tube attached to a water-seal drainage system, and the nurse notes that the fluid in the chest tube and in the water seal column has stopped fluctuating. How should the nurse interpret this finding?
☐ 1. The lung has fully expanded.
☐ 2. The lung has collapsed.
☐ 3. The chest tube is in the pleural space.
☐ 4. The mediastinal space has decreased.

107. The nurse observes a constant gentle bubbling in the water seal column of a water seal chest drainage system. What should the nurse do **next**?
☐ 1. Continue monitoring as usual; this is expected.
☐ 2. Check the connectors between the chest and drainage tubes and where the drainage tube enters the chest drainage system.
☐ 3. Decrease the suction, and continue observing the system for changes in bubbling during the next several hours.
☐ 4. Notify the health care provider (HCP).

108. A client who underwent a lobectomy and has a water seal chest drainage system is breathing with a little more effort and at a faster rate than 1 hour ago. The client's pulse rate is also increased. What should the nurse do **next**?
☐ 1. Check the tubing to ensure that the client is not lying on it or kinking it.
☐ 2. Increase the suction.
☐ 3. Lower the drainage bottles 2 to 3 feet (61 to 91.4 cm) below the level of the client's chest.
☐ 4. Ensure that the chest tube has two clamps on it to prevent air leaks.

109. The nurse is assessing a client who has a chest tube connected to a water seal chest tube drainage system. According to the illustration shown, what should the nurse do?

☐ 1. Clamp the chest tube near the insertion site to prevent air from entering the pleural cavity.
☐ 2. Notify the health care provider (HCP) of the amount of chest tube drainage.
☐ 3. Add water to maintain the water seal.
☐ 4. Lower the drainage system to maintain gravity flow.

110. The nurse is preparing to assist with the removal of a chest tube. Which dressing is appropriate at the site from which the chest tube is removed?
☐ 1. adhesive strips
☐ 2. petrolatum gauze
☐ 3. dry 4 × 4 gauze
☐ 4. moist saline

The Adult with Chest Trauma

111. The nurse is assessing a client admitted to the emergency department with a chest injury. Which finding is **most** concerning?
☐ 1. diminished bilateral breath sounds
☐ 2. muffled heart sounds
☐ 3. respiratory distress
☐ 4. tracheal deviation

112. A nurse is to administer 10 mg of morphine sulfate to a client with three fractured ribs. The available concentration for this drug is 15 mg/mL. How many milliliters should the nurse administer? Round to one decimal point.

_____ mL.

113. A young adult is admitted to the emergency department after an automobile accident. The client has severe pain in the right chest from contact with the steering wheel. What should the nurse do **first**?
☐ 1. Reduce the client's anxiety.
☐ 2. Maintain adequate oxygenation.
☐ 3. Decrease chest pain.
☐ 4. Maintain adequate circulating volume.

114. A client with rib fractures and a pneumothorax has a chest tube inserted that is connected to a water seal chest tube drainage system. The nurse notes that the fluid in the water seal column is fluctuating with each breath that the client takes. What is the significance of this fluctuation?
☐ 1. An obstruction is present in the chest tube.
☐ 2. The client is developing subcutaneous emphysema.
☐ 3. The chest tube system is functioning properly.
☐ 4. There is a leak in the chest tube system.

115. For a client with rib fractures and a pneumothorax, the health care provider prescribes morphine sulfate, 1 to 2 mg per hour, given intravenously (IV) as needed for pain. The nursing care goal is to provide adequate pain control so that the client can breathe effectively. Which finding indicates the goal has been met?
☐ 1. pain rating of 0 to 2 on a scale of 0 to 10 by the client
☐ 2. decreased client anxiety
☐ 3. respiratory rate of 26 breaths/min
☐ 4. partial pressure of arterial oxygen (PaO_2) of 70 mm Hg (9.31 kPa)

116. A client undergoes surgery to repair lung injuries. Postoperative prescriptions include the transfusion of one unit of packed red blood cells at a rate of 60 mL per hour. How long will this transfusion take to infuse?
☐ 1. 2 hours
☐ 2. 4 hours
☐ 3. 6 hours
☐ 4. 8 hours

117. A client has been in an automobile accident, and the nurse is assessing the client for possible pneumothorax. What finding should the nurse immediately report to the health care provider?
☐ 1. sudden, sharp chest pain
☐ 2. wheezing breath sounds over the affected side
☐ 3. hemoptysis
☐ 4. cyanosis

118. A client is undergoing a thoracentesis. What should the nurse monitor the client for during and immediately after the procedure? Select all that apply.
☐ 1. pneumothorax
☐ 2. subcutaneous emphysema
☐ 3. tension pneumothorax
☐ 4. pulmonary edema
☐ 5. infection

119. When assessing a client with chest trauma, the nurse notes that the client is taking small breaths at first, then bigger breaths, and then a couple of small breaths, then 10 to 20 seconds of no breaths. How should the nurse record the breathing pattern?
☐ 1. Cheyne-Stokes respiration
☐ 2. hyperventilation
☐ 3. obstructive sleep apnea
☐ 4. Biot respiration

The Adult with Acute Respiratory Distress Syndrome

120. The nurse has placed the intubated client with acute respiratory distress syndrome (ARDS) in the prone position for 30 minutes. Which factor(s) would require the nurse to discontinue prone positioning and return the client to the supine position? Select all that apply.
☐ 1. The family is coming in to visit.
☐ 2. The client has increased secretions requiring frequent suctioning.
☐ 3. The percutaneous oxygen saturation (SpO_2) and partial pressure of arterial oxygen (PaO_2) have decreased.
☐ 4. The client is tachycardic with a drop in blood pressure.
☐ 5. The face has increased skin breakdown and edema.

121. The nurse is positioning a client with acute respiratory distress syndrome (ARDS) who is receiving mechanical ventilation. To improve oxygenation, which is the **best** position for this client?
☐ 1. supine
☐ 2. semi-Fowler
☐ 3. lateral side
☐ 4. prone

122. A client with acute respiratory distress syndrome (ARDS) has fine crackles at the lung bases, and the respirations are shallow at a rate of 28 breaths/min. The client is restless and anxious. In addition to monitoring the arterial blood gas results, what should the nurse do? Select all that apply.
☐ 1. Monitor serum creatinine and blood urea nitrogen levels.
☐ 2. Administer a sedative.
☐ 3. Keep the head of the bed flat.
☐ 4. Administer humidified oxygen.
☐ 5. Auscultate the lungs.

123. The nurse is planning care for a client with a crushing chest injury. The client is in an intensive care unit, and the client's vital signs have not stabilized. Which finding puts the client at risk for acute respiratory distress syndrome (ARDS)?
    ☐ 1. history of smoking
    ☐ 2. low serum potassium
    ☐ 3. hypercapnia
    ☐ 4. hypovolemia

124. The nurse is conducting a focused assessment for a client at risk for acute respiratory distress syndrome (ARDS). Which finding indicates the client is becoming hypoxemic?
    ☐ 1. elevated carbon dioxide level
    ☐ 2. hypoxia not responsive to oxygen therapy
    ☐ 3. metabolic acidosis
    ☐ 4. severe, unexplained electrolyte imbalance

125. A client with acute respiratory distress syndrome is showing signs of increased dyspnea. The nurse reviews a report of blood gas values (see report of laboratory results).

    Laboratory Results

Blood Chemistry	Result
pH	7.35
$PaCO_2$	25 mm Hg (3.3 kPa)
HCO_3^-	22 mEq/L (22 mmol/L)
PaO_2	95 mm Hg (12.6 kPa)

    Which finding is concerning?
    ☐ 1. pH
    ☐ 2. partial pressure of carbon dioxide ($PaCO_2$)
    ☐ 3. bicarbonate (HCO_3^-)
    ☐ 4. partial pressure of arterial oxygen (PaO_2)

126. A client with acute respiratory distress syndrome is on a ventilator. The client's peak inspiratory pressures and spontaneous respiratory rate are increasing, and the partial pressure of arterial oxygen (PaO_2) is not improving. Using the SBAR (Situation-Background-Assessment-Recommendation) technique for communication, the nurse calls the health care provider (HCP). What recommendation should the nurse give to the HCP?
    ☐ 1. initiating intravenous sedation
    ☐ 2. starting a high-protein diet
    ☐ 3. providing pain medication
    ☐ 4. increasing the ventilator rate

127. A client, diagnosed with acute pancreatitis 5 days ago, is experiencing respiratory distress. Which finding should the nurse report to the health care provider (HCP)?
    ☐ 1. arterial oxygen level of 46 mm Hg (6.1 kPa)
    ☐ 2. respirations of 12 breaths/min
    ☐ 3. lack of adventitious lung sounds
    ☐ 4. oxygen saturation of 96% on room air

128. A client has the following arterial blood gas values: pH 7.52; partial pressure of arterial oxygen (PaO_2) 50 mm Hg (6.7 kPa); partial pressure of carbon dioxide ($PaCO_2$) 28 mm Hg (3.72 kPa); HCO_3^- 24 mEq/L (24 mmol/L). Based upon the client's PaO_2, which nursing clinical judgment should the nurse make?
    ☐ 1. The client is severely hypoxic.
    ☐ 2. The oxygen level is low but poses no risk for the client.
    ☐ 3. The client's PaO_2 level is within normal range.
    ☐ 4. The client requires oxygen therapy with very low oxygen concentrations.

129. The nurse is planning care for a client with acute respiratory distress. Which action will be most helpful to promote effective airway clearance?
    ☐ 1. Administer oxygen every 2 hours.
    ☐ 2. Turn the client every 4 hours.
    ☐ 3. Administer sedatives to promote rest.
    ☐ 4. Suction if cough is ineffective.

Managing Care, Quality, and Safety of Adults with Respiratory Health Problems

130. A nurse has received a report on four clients. Which client would the nurse visit **first**?
    ☐ 1. a client with congestive heart failure (CHF) who has gained 2 lb (0.91 kg) overnight
    ☐ 2. a client with tuberculosis who raised 50 mL of sanguineous sputum over the past 2 hours
    ☐ 3. a client with *Clostridium difficile* who continues to have loose, foul-smelling stools
    ☐ 4. a client with chronic obstructive pulmonary disease (COPD) whose last report of oxygen saturation was 91%

131. A client with chronic obstructive pulmonary disease (COPD) has a signed living will with a do not resuscitate (DNR) request. While the spouse was visiting the client, the client had a cardiac arrest. The spouse requested the client be resuscitated immediately. When the nurse hesitated to start resuscitation procedures, the spouse threatened to sue the hospital. What should the nurse do? Select all that apply.
    ☐ 1. Call the code for fear of being sued by the spouse.
    ☐ 2. Carry out the written DNR request and client wishes.
    ☐ 3. Calmly remind the spouse of the client's wishes and DNR request.
    ☐ 4. Notify the nurse manager of the situation.
    ☐ 5. Call the chaplain to come and remain with the spouse.
    ☐ 6. Notify the health care provider (HCP).

132. The nurse has received a change of shift report on clients. Which client should the nurse assess **first**?
    ☐ 1. a client with chronic obstructive pulmonary disease (COPD) with a partial pressure of carbon dioxide ($PaCO_2$) of 56 mm Hg who is being discharged home on oxygen
    ☐ 2. a client with asthma with respirations of 36 breaths/min whose wheezing has diminished
    ☐ 3. a client with asthma who has a heart rate of 90 bpm and whose beta-blocker is scheduled to be administered now
    ☐ 4. a client who is scheduled for an angiogram now and is ready to be transported

133. The nurse is caring for a group of clients on a pulmonary unit. The nurse can delegate which task to unlicensed assistive personnel (UAP)?
    ☐ 1. assisting a client with adjusting their nasal cannula
    ☐ 2. adjusting flow rates based on client responses
    ☐ 3. monitoring a client for adverse effects of oxygen therapy
    ☐ 4. assessing a client for the best method of oxygen delivery

134. A confused client with carbon monoxide poisoning experiences dizziness when ambulating to the bathroom. What should the nurse do?
    ☐ 1. Put all four side rails up on the bed.
    ☐ 2. Ask the unlicensed assistive personnel (UAP) to place restraints on the client's upper extremities.
    ☐ 3. Request that the client's roommate put the call light on when the client is attempting to get out of bed.
    ☐ 4. Check on the client at regular intervals to ascertain the need to use the bathroom.

135. The nurse is admitting a client with suspected tuberculosis to the hospital. The nurse should institute which type of precautions for this client?
    ☐ 1. standard precautions
    ☐ 2. contact precautions
    ☐ 3. droplet precautions
    ☐ 4. airborne precautions

136. A client has developed hospital-acquired pneumonia. When preparing to administer cephalexin 500 mg, the nurse notices that the pharmacy sent cefazolin. What should the nurse do? Select all that apply.
    ☐ 1. Administer the cefazolin.
    ☐ 2. Verify the medication prescription as written by the health care provider.
    ☐ 3. Contact the pharmacy and speak to a pharmacist.
    ☐ 4. Request that cephalexin be sent promptly.
    ☐ 5. Return the cefazolin to the pharmacy.

137. A nurse receives the taped change-of-shift report for assigned clients and prioritizes client rounds. In what order from first to last should the nurse assess these clients? All options must be used.

1. a client who has an endotracheal tube and who will be transferred to a long-term respiratory care unit that day
2. a client with type 2 diabetes who had a cerebrovascular accident 4 days ago
3. a client with cellulitis of the left lower extremity with a fever of 100.8°F (38.2°C)
4. a client receiving intravenous (IV) dextrose 5% in water (D5W) at 125 mL per hour with 75 mL remaining

138. The nurse is a member of a team that is planning a client-centered, community-based approach to care for clients with chronic obstructive pulmonary disease. In which area(s) should the team focus on improving the quality of care and delivery? Select all that apply.
    ☐ 1. the community
    ☐ 2. clinical information systems
    ☐ 3. delivery system design
    ☐ 4. administrative leadership
    ☐ 5. acute care setting

139. The nurse is caring for a client admitted for pneumonia with a history of hypertension and heart failure. The client has reported at least one fall in the last 3 months. The client may ambulate with assistance, has a saline lock in place, and has demonstrated appropriate use of the call light to request assistance. Using the Morse Fall Scale (see chart), what is this client's total score and risk level?

Morse Fall Risk/Scale

Item	Scale	Scoring
History of falling, immediate or within 3 months	No 0 Yes 25	
Secondary diagnosis	No 0 Yes 15	

Ambulatory aid
  Bed rest/nurse assist
  Crutches/cane/walker
  Furniture
	
	0
	15
	30	

IV/heparin lock	No 0 Yes 20	

Gait/transferring
  Normal/bed rest/immobile
  Weak
  Impaired
	
	0
	10
	20	

Mental status
  Oriented to own ability
  Forgets limitations
	
	0
	15	

☐ 1. 20, low risk
☐ 2. 30, medium risk
☐ 3. 40, medium risk
☐ 4. 60, high risk

140. The nurse is caring for a client who has been placed on droplet precautions. Which protective gear is required to take care of this client? Select all that apply.
☐ 1. gloves
☐ 2. gown
☐ 3. surgical mask
☐ 4. glasses
☐ 5. respirator

141. While making rounds, the nurse finds a client with chronic obstructive pulmonary disease sitting in a wheelchair, slumped over a lunch tray. After determining the client is unresponsive and calling for help, what should the nurse do **next**?
☐ 1. Push the "code blue" (emergency response) button.
☐ 2. Call the rapid response team.
☐ 3. Open the client's airway.
☐ 4. Call for a defibrillator.

142. The nurse is caring for a client with pneumonia who is confused about time and place and has intravenous (IV) fluids infusing. Despite the nurse's attempt to reorient the client and then provide a distraction, the client has begun to pull at the IV tubing. After increasing the frequency of observation, in which order should the nurse implement interventions to ensure the client's safety? All options must be used.

1. Review the client's medications for interactions that may cause or increase confusion.
2. Assess the client's respiratory status, including oxygen saturation.
3. Ensure the client does not need toileting or pain medications.
4. Contact the health care provider, and request a prescription for soft wrist restraints.

143. The nurse's assignment consists of four clients. After the nurse receives the shift report, in which order from first to last should the nurse assess these clients? All options must be used.

1. an 85-year-old client with bacterial pneumonia, a temperature of 102.2°F (42°C), and shortness of breath
2. a 60-year-old client with chest tubes who is 2 days postoperative following a thoracotomy for lung cancer and is requesting something for pain
3. a 35-year-old client with suspected tuberculosis who has a cough
4. a 56-year-old client with emphysema who has a scheduled dose of a bronchodilator due to be administered, with no report of acute respiratory distress

144. The nurse is caring for a 74-year-old female client who has been admitted to the medical-surgical unit with bacterial pneumonia.

Nurse's Notes

1200: The client is restless and diaphoretic. The client's respirations are labored. The nurse reviews the vital signs record.

Vital Signs

Time	0800	1000	1200
Temperature	100.9°F (38.3°C)		101.8°F (38.8°C)
Pulse	90 bpm	104 bpm	118 bpm
Respirations	16 bpm	18 bpm	24 bpm
Blood Pressure	112/74 mm Hg	110/68 mm Hg	116/78 mm Hg
O₂ Saturation	93%	92%	92%

Which action(s) should the nurse take? Select all that apply.
1. Ensure the client stays in bed with one pillow under their head.
2. Obtain an accurate measure of urine output.
3. Increase oral fluids to 1200 mL every 8 hours.
4. Use a cool, moist cloth to wipe areas of diaphoresis.
5. Notify the health care provider.
6. Administer acetaminophen as prescribed.
7. Initiate oxygen per nasal cannula at 2 L per minute as prescribed.

Answers, Rationales, and Test-Taking Strategies

*The answers and rationales for each question follow below, along with keys ( ) to the client need (CN) and cognitive level (CL) for each question. In addition, questions that measure clinical judgment will be coded (CJ). As you check your answers, use the **Content Mastery and Test-Taking Skill Self-Analysis** worksheet (tear-out worksheet in the back of the book) to identify the reason(s) for not answering the questions correctly. For additional information about test-taking skills and strategies for answering questions, refer to pages 12–51 in Part 1 of this book.*

The Adult with an Upper Respiratory Tract Infection

1. **1, 4, 5.** Antihistamines have an anticholinergic action and a drying effect and reduce nasal, salivary, and lacrimal gland hypersecretion (runny nose, tearing, and itching eyes). An adverse effect is drowsiness, so operating machinery and driving are not recommended. There is also an additive depressant effect when alcohol is combined with antihistamines, so alcohol should be avoided during antihistamine use. The client should ensure adequate fluid intake of at least 2000 mL (about eight glasses) per day because of the drying effect of the drug. Antihistamines have no antibacterial action and are not used to treat nasal infections. The effect of antihistamines is prompt, not delayed.

    CN: Pharmacological and parenteral therapies; CL: Create

2. **3.** When using an intranasal inhaler, it is important to close off one nostril while inhaling the spray into the other nostril to ensure the best inhalation of the spray. The use of the inhaler is not limited to mornings and bedtime. The canister should be shaken immediately before use. The inhaler tip should be inserted into the nostril and pointed toward the outside nostril wall to maximize inhalation of the medication.

    CN: Pharmacological and parenteral therapies; CL: Evaluate

3. **4.** A client recovering from an upper respiratory tract infection should report decreasing or no nasal discharge and obstruction. Daily fluid intake should be increased to more than 1 L every 24 hours to liquefy secretions. The temperature should be below 100°F (37.8°C) with no chills or

diaphoresis. A productive cough with chest pain indicates a pulmonary infection, not an upper respiratory tract infection.

🔑 CN: Physiological adaptation; CL: Evaluate

4. 2. The client should blow the nose before instilling nose drops. Instilling nose drops is a clean technique. The dropper should be cleaned after each administration, but it does not need to be changed. The client should assume a position that will allow the medication to reach the desired area; this is usually a supine position.

🔑 CN: Pharmacological and parenteral therapies; CL: Evaluate

5. -/+ 3, 4. The client with chronic sinusitis should be instructed to take hot showers in the morning and evening to promote drainage of secretions. There is no need to limit caffeine intake. Performing postural drainage will inhibit the removal of secretions, not promote it. Clients should elevate the head of the bed to promote drainage. Clients should report all temperatures higher than 100.4°F (38°C) because a temperature that high can indicate infection. The client should increase, not limit, fluid intake; a 24-hour fluid intake of 2000 to 3000 mL would be appropriate.

🔑 CN: Reduction of risk potential; CL: Analyze

6. 4. It is important for clients with allergic rhinitis to determine the precipitating factors so that they can be avoided. Keeping a diary can help identify these triggers. Nasal decongestant sprays should not be used regularly because they can cause a rebound effect. Antibiotics are not appropriate for allergic rhinitis because an infection is not present. Increasing activity will not control the client's symptoms; in fact, walking outdoors may increase them if the client is allergic to pollen.

🔑 CN: Health promotion and maintenance; CL: Analyze

7. **7.5 mL**

$300 \text{ mg}/X = 200 \text{ mg}/5 \text{ mL}$
$X = 7.5 \text{ mL}.$

🔑 CN: Pharmacological and parenteral therapies; CL: Apply

8. 4. Adverse effects of pseudoephedrine are experienced primarily in the cardiovascular system and through sympathetic effects on the central nervous system (CNS). The most common CNS adverse effects include restlessness, dizziness, tension, anxiety, insomnia, and weakness. Common cardiovascular adverse effects include tachycardia, hypertension, palpitations, and arrhythmias. Constipation and diplopia are not adverse effects of pseudoephedrine. Tachycardia, not bradycardia, is an adverse effect of pseudoephedrine.

🔑 CN: Pharmacological and parenteral therapies; CL: Analyze

The Adult Undergoing Nasal Surgery

9. 4. Epistaxis, or nosebleed, is a common, sudden emergency. Commonly, no apparent explanation for the bleeding is known. With significant blood loss, systemic symptoms, such as vertigo, increased pulse, shortness of breath, decreased blood pressure, and pallor, will occur. Because aerobic exercise may increase blood pressure and increased blood pressure can cause epistaxis, the client with hypertension should avoid it. Aspirin inhibits platelet aggregation, reducing the ability of the blood to clot. The client should continue to take their antihypertension medication, ramipril. Posterior nasal packing should be left in place for 1 to 3 days.

🔑 CN: Health promotion and maintenance; CL: Analyze

10. 2. Because of the dense nasal packing, bleeding may not be apparent through the nasal drip pad. Instead, the blood may run down the throat, causing the client to swallow frequently. The back of the throat, where the blood will be apparent, can be assessed with a flashlight. An accumulation of blood in the stomach can cause nausea and vomiting, but nausea would not be the initial indicator of bleeding. An increased respiratory rate occurs in shock but is not an early sign of bleeding in a client who has undergone nasal surgery. Increased pain warrants further assessment but is not an indicator of bleeding.

🔑 CN: Reduction of risk potential; CL: Analyze

11. 1. The client should be instructed to avoid any activities that cause the Valsalva maneuver (e.g., constipation, vigorous coughing, exercise) to reduce bleeding and stress on suture lines. The client should not take aspirin because of its antiplatelet properties, which may cause bleeding. Oral hygiene is important to rid the mouth of old dried blood and to enhance the client's appetite. Cool compresses, not heat, should be applied to decrease swelling and control discoloration of the area.

🔑 CN: Health promotion; CL: Create

12. 2. Constipation can cause straining during defecation, which can induce bleeding. Showering is not contraindicated. The client should take measures to prevent coughing, which can cause bleeding. The client should avoid blowing the nose for 48

hours after the packing is removed. Thereafter, the client should blow the nose gently, using the open-mouth technique to minimize bleeding in the surgical area.

🗝️ CN: Physiological adaptation; CL: Evaluate

13. 4. Aspirin-containing medications should be discontinued for 2 weeks before surgery to decrease the risk for bleeding. Nasal packing is usually removed the day after surgery. Normal saline nose drops are not routinely administered preoperatively. The results of the surgery will not be obvious immediately after surgery because of edema and ecchymosis.

🗝️ CN: Reduction of risk potential; CL: Create

14. 3. Immediately after nasal surgery, ineffective breathing patterns may develop as a result of the nasal packing and nasal edema. Nasal packing may dislodge, leading to obstruction. Assessing for airway obstruction is a priority. Assessing for pain is important, but it is not as high a priority as assessment of the airways. It is too early to detect ecchymosis. Measuring intake and output is not typically a priority nursing assessment after nasal surgery.

🗝️ CN: Physiological adaptation; CL: Analyze

15. 4. Applying cold compresses helps to decrease facial swelling and pain from edema. Analgesics may decrease pain, but they do not decrease edema. A corticosteroid nasal spray would not be administered postoperatively because it can impair healing. The use of a bedside humidifier promotes comfort by providing moisture for nasal mucosa, but it does not decrease edema.

🗝️ CN: Basic care and comfort; CL: Analyze

16. 1. Frequent mouth care is important to provide comfort and encourage eating. Mouth care promotes moist mucous membranes. Nose drops cannot be used with nasal packing in place. When sneezing and coughing, the client should do so with the mouth open to decrease the chance of dislodging the packing. Gargling should not be attempted with packing in place.

🗝️ CN: Basic care and comfort; CL: Create

17. 4. The client should assume a sitting position and lean forward. Firm pressure should be applied to the soft portion of the nose for approximately 10 minutes. Tilting the head backward can cause the client to swallow blood, which can obscure the amount of bleeding and also can lead to nausea. Ice compresses may be applied, but the client should not lie flat. Blowing the nose is to be avoided because it can increase bleeding.

🗝️ CN: Reduction of risk potential; CL: Analyze

18. 3. Posterior packing may alter the respiratory status of the client, especially in older adult clients, causing hypoventilation. Clients should be observed carefully for changes in the level of consciousness, respiratory rate, and heart rate and rhythm after the insertion of the packing. Vertigo does not occur as a result of the insertion of posterior packing. Bell's palsy, a disorder of the seventh cranial nerve, is not associated with epistaxis or nasal packing. Loss of the gag reflex does not occur as a result of the insertion of posterior packing.

🗝️ CN: Reduction of risk potential; CL: Analyze

The Adult with Cancer of the Larynx

19. 4. The nurse must maintain patency of the airway with frequent suctioning of the laryngectomy tube that can become occluded from secretions, blood, and mucus plugs. Once the client is hemodynamically stable, getting out of bed should be encouraged to prevent postoperative complications. Vital signs should be monitored more frequently in a postoperative client. A swallow study is done approximately 5 to 7 days after surgery, prior to starting oral intake.

🗝️ CN: Physiological adaptation; CL: Analyze

20. 4. The client has undergone body changes and permanent loss of verbal communication. The client may feel isolated and insecure. The nurse can encourage them to express their feelings and use this information to develop an appropriate plan of care. Discussing the client's behavior with their spouse may not reveal their feelings. Exploring future plans is not appropriate at this time because more information about the client's behavior is needed before proceeding to this level. The nurse can respect the client's need for privacy while also encouraging them to express their feelings.

🗝️ CN: Psychosocial adaptation; CL: Analyze

21. 1. A client should be suctioned for no longer than 10 seconds at a time. Suctioning for longer than 10 seconds may reduce the client's oxygen level so much that the client becomes hypoxic.

🗝️ CN: Reduction of risk potential; CL: Apply

22. 1. The recommended technique is to use a sterile catheter each time the client is suctioned. There is a danger of introducing organisms into the respiratory tract when strict aseptic technique is not used. Reusing a suction catheter is not consistent with aseptic technique. The nurse does not use a clean catheter when suctioning a tracheostomy or a laryngectomy; it is a sterile procedure.

🔑 CN: Reduction of risk potential; CL: Apply

23. 4. Changes in body image are expected after a laryngectomy, and the nurse should first explore what is upsetting the client the most at this time. Many clients are concerned about how their family members will respond to the physical changes that have occurred as a result of a laryngectomy, but discussing the importance of family support is not helpful; instead, the nurse should allow the client to communicate any negative feelings or concerns that exist because of the surgery. The client's feelings are not related to a knowledge deficit, and therefore, it is too early to begin teaching about stoma care. It is also not helpful to offer reassurances about the change in appearance; the client will require time to adjust to the changed body image.

🔑 CN: Psychosocial adaptation; CL: Analyze

24. 1. The tracheostomy tube, ties, and gauze pad are positioned correctly; the nurse team leader should be sure the client is comfortable. The tracheostomy tube ties should be tied in a square knot on the side of the neck and alternate sides of the neck when the ties are changed. The full part of the gauze square should be placed under the tracheostomy tube to absorb drainage. There is no indication the ties need to be changed; an additional gauze pad is not necessary; if necessary, the current gauze square should be changed rather than adding an additional pad.

🔑 CN: Basic care and comfort; CL: Evaluate

25. 3. Hoarseness occurring longer than 2 weeks is a warning sign of laryngeal cancer. The nurse should first assess other signs, such as a lump in the neck or throat, persistent sore throat or cough, earache, pain, and difficulty swallowing (dysphagia). Gargling with salt water may lead to increased irritation. There is no indication of infection warranting an antibiotic. An oral analgesic would provide only temporary relief of discomfort if hoarseness were accompanied by a sore throat.

🔑 CN: Physiological adaptation; CL: Analyze

26. 1. Immediately after surgery, the client should be maintained in a position with the head of the bed elevated 30 to 40 degrees (semi-Fowler position) to decrease tissue edema, facilitate breathing, and decrease pain related to edema formation. Immediately postoperatively, the client should be provided alternative means of communicating, such as a communication board. As healing progresses and edema subsides, a speech therapist should work with the client to explore various voice restoration options, such as the use of a voice prosthesis, electrolarynx, artificial larynx, or esophageal speech. Food is not initiated in the immediate postoperative phase; enteral feedings are usually used to meet nutritional needs until edema subsides. Irrigation of the drainage tubes is an inappropriate action.

🔑 CN: Physiological adaptation; CL: Analyze

27. 3. It is important that the client be able to communicate their feelings about the body image changes that have occurred as a result of surgery. Open communication helps promote adjustment. The client may not regain the ability to taste and smell food because of no longer breathing through the nose or because of radiation therapy treatments, or both. A gastrostomy tube would not typically be placed after a total laryngectomy, nor would it be necessary for the client to demonstrate sterile suctioning technique for stoma care. The client would use clean technique.

🔑 CN: Physiological adaptation; CL: Evaluate

28. 2. Adequate humidity should be provided in the home to help keep secretions moist. A bedside humidifier is recommended. A high fluid intake is also important to liquefy secretions. Mouth care is important to prevent drying of mucous membranes and should be performed frequently throughout the day, especially before and after meals, to help stimulate the appetite. The client may eat any food that can be chewed and swallowed comfortably. The client may resume physical activity as tolerated.

🔑 CN: Reduction of risk potential; CL: Analyze

The Adult with Pneumonia

29. 3. The client's ABG levels are the most sensitive indicator of the effectiveness of the client's oxygen therapy. Cyanosis is a late sign of decreased oxygenation and is not a reliable indicator. The client's respiratory rate and level of consciousness may be altered because of other problems not related to the client's oxygenation.

🔑 CN: Physiological adaptation; CL: Evaluate

30. 2. Restraints should be secured to the bed frame, not the side rails, to ensure that the side rails can be raised and lowered safely. Circulation checks, reevaluating the need for restraints, and

476 The Nursing Care of Adults with Medical and Surgical Health Problems

documentation should be done every 1 to 2 hours. Medical restraint prescriptions must be renewed and signed by an HCP every 24 hours.

CN: Safety and infection control; CL: Analyze

31. 1. The client's age is a predisposing factor for pneumonia; pneumonia is more common in older or debilitated clients. Other predisposing factors include smoking, upper respiratory tract infections, malnutrition, immunosuppression, and the presence of a chronic illness. Osteoarthritis, a nutritionally sound vegetarian diet, and frequent bathing are not predisposing factors for pneumonia.

CN: Reduction of risk potential; CL: Analyze

32. 2. A sputum specimen is obtained for culture to determine the causative organism. After the organism is identified, an appropriate antibiotic can be prescribed. Beginning antibiotic therapy before obtaining the sputum specimen may alter the results of the test. Urinalysis, a chest radiograph, and a red blood cell count do not need to be obtained before the initiation of antibiotic therapy for pneumonia.

CN: Reduction of risk potential; CL: Apply

33. 3. It is essential to monitor serum creatinine in the client receiving an aminoglycoside antibiotic because of the potential for this type of drug to cause acute tubular necrosis. Aminoglycoside antibiotics do not affect serum sodium, potassium, or calcium levels.

CN: Pharmacological and parenteral therapies; CL: Analyze

34. 3. Frequent changes of the bedsheets are appropriate for this client because of the diaphoresis. Diaphoresis produces general discomfort, and the client should be kept dry to promote comfort and prevent skin irritation. The client should change position every 2 hours. Nasotracheal suctioning is not indicated with the client's productive cough. The client can ambulate to the bathroom, but the nurse should offer assistance as needed.

CN: Basic care and comfort; CL: Analyze

35. 4. The pleuritic pain is triggered by chest movement and is particularly severe during coughing. Splinting the chest wall will help reduce the discomfort of coughing. Deep breathing is essential to prevent further atelectasis. Abdominal breathing is not as effective in decreasing pleuritic chest pain as is splinting of the rib cage. Incentive spirometry facilitates effective deep breathing but does not decrease pleuritic chest pain.

CN: Physiological adaptation; CL: Analyze

36. 1, 3. Aspirin is administered to clients with pneumonia because it is an analgesic that helps control chest discomfort and an antipyretic that helps reduce fever. Aspirin has an anticoagulant effect, but that is not the reason for prescribing it for a client with pneumonia, and the use of the drug will be short term. Aspirin does not affect the respiratory rate and does not facilitate the expectoration of secretions.

CN: Pharmacological and parenteral therapies; CL: Evaluate

37. 3. Clients who are experiencing hypoxia characteristically exhibit irritability, restlessness, or anxiety as initial mental status changes. As the hypoxia becomes more pronounced, the client may become confused and combative. Coma is a late clinical manifestation of hypoxia. Apathy and depression are not symptoms of hypoxia.

CN: Physiological adaptation; CL: Analyze

38. 2. An expected outcome for a client recovering from pneumonia would be the ability to perform activities of daily living without experiencing dyspnea. A respiratory rate of 25 to 30 breaths/min indicates the client is experiencing tachypnea, which would not be expected on recovery. A weight loss of 5 to 10 lb (2.27 to 4.53 kg) is undesirable; the expected outcome would be to maintain a normal weight. A client who is recovering from pneumonia should experience decreased or no chest pain.

CN: Management of care; CL: Evaluate

The Adult with Tuberculosis

39. 1. Implementing airborne precautions for possible TB requires a private room assignment. In addition to isolating the client by using a private room, engineering controls can help prevent the spread of TB; a room at the end of the hall will aid in controlling airflow direction and can prevent contamination of air in adjacent areas. Confidentiality is provided for every client, regardless of the client's room location. Sunlight is not a component of isolation precautions.

CN: Physiological adaptation; CL: Apply

40. 1. There is a high risk and potential for tuberculosis, and airborne precautions should be implemented immediately to prevent the spread of infection. After initiating precautions, the nurse can start the oxygen, check the vital signs, and collect the sputum specimen.

CN: Safety and infection control; CL: Analyze

41. 3. Streptomycin can cause toxicity to the eighth cranial nerve, which is responsible for hearing, balance, and body position sense. Nephrotoxicity is a side effect that would be indicated with an increase in creatinine. Streptomycin does not cause difficulty in swallowing. Streptomycin is given via intramuscular injection.

  CN: Pharmacological and parenteral therapies; CL: Analyze

42. 4. The nurse should tell the client that it is necessary to take all of these medications because combination drug therapy prevents bacterial resistance; they will be administered throughout the hospitalization to maintain blood levels. The HCP will review the prescriptions per hospital policy because the client is being admitted to the hospital; there is no duplication between any of the drugs being prescribed for this client. It is not necessary to ask the pharmacist to check for drug interactions as these drugs are commonly used together.

  CN: Pharmacologic and parenteral therapy; CL: Analyze

43. 2. Ensuring that the client is well educated about tuberculosis is the highest priority. Education of the client and family is essential to help the client understand the need for completing the prescribed drug therapy to cure the disease. Offering the client emotional support, coordinating various agency services, and assessing the environment may be part of the care for the client with tuberculosis; however, these interventions are of less importance than education about the disease process and its treatment.

  CN: Safety and infection control; CL: Analyze

44. 3. The tuberculin test is positive. The test should be interpreted 2 to 3 days after administering the purified protein derivative (PPD) by measuring the size of the firm, raised area (induration). Positive responses indicate that the client may have been exposed to the tuberculosis bacteria. A negative response is indicated by the absence of a firm, raised area, or an area that is less than 5 mm in diameter. Since the test is positive, it is not necessary to redo the test. The test is positive, not false.

  CN: Reduction of risk potential; CL: Analyze

45. 1. The Mantoux test is administered via intradermal injection. The appropriate technique for an intradermal injection includes holding the needle and syringe almost parallel to the client's skin, keeping the skin slightly taut when the needle is inserted, and inserting the needle with the bevel side up. There is no need to aspirate, a technique that assesses for incorrect placement in a blood vessel when giving an intradermal injection. The injection site is not massaged.

  CN: Pharmacological and parenteral therapies; CL: Apply

46. 3. An induration (a palpable, raised, hardened area of skin) of more than 5 to 15 mm (depending upon the person's risk factors) after injection of 10 Mantoux units is considered a positive result, indicating tuberculosis (TB) infection. An induration of more than 5 mm is found in HIV-positive individuals; those with recent contact with persons with TB; persons with nodular or fibrotic changes on chest x-ray consistent with old, healed TB; persons with organ transplants; and persons who are immunosuppressed. An induration of more than 10 mm is positive, and the client may be a recent arrival (less than 5 years) from a country with a high incidence of TB; a person with injection drug use disorder; a resident or an employee of high-risk congregate settings (e.g., prisons, long-term care facilities, hospitals, homeless shelters); or mycobacteriology lab personnel. An induration of more than 10 mm is also considered positive in persons with clinical conditions that place them at high risk (e.g., diabetes, prolonged corticosteroid therapy, leukemia, end-stage renal disease, chronic malabsorption syndromes, low body weight), a child younger than 4 years of age, or a child or adolescent exposed to adults in high-risk categories.

  CN: Reduction of risk potential; CL: Analyze

47. 4. Older adults are believed to be at higher risk for contracting tuberculosis because of decreased immunocompetence. Other high-risk populations in the United States and Canada include the urban poor, clients with AIDS, and minority groups.

  CN: Safety and infection control; CL: Analyze

48. 2, 4. When the nurse is teaching the client how to avoid the transmission of tubercle bacilli, it is important for the client to understand that the organism is transmitted by droplet infection. Therefore, covering the mouth and nose when sneezing and using paper tissues to cough in with prompt disposal indicates that the client has understood the nurse's instructions about preventing the spread of airborne droplets. It is not essential to discard clothing, nor does the client need to be isolated from family members. The client does not need to avoid crowds.

  CN: Safety and infection control; CL: Evaluate

49. **2.** A positive Mantoux skin test indicates that the client has been exposed to tubercle bacilli. Exposure does not necessarily mean that active disease exists. A positive Mantoux test does not mean that the client has developed resistance. Unless involved in treatment, the client may still develop active disease at any time. Immunity to tuberculosis is not possible.

🗝️ CN: Reduction of risk potential; CL: Analyze

50. **2.** INH competes for the available vitamin B_6 in the body and leaves the client at risk for the development of neuropathies related to vitamin deficiency. Supplemental vitamin B_6 is routinely prescribed. Following a low-cholesterol diet, getting extra rest, and avoiding excessive sun exposure will not prevent the development of peripheral neuropathies.

🗝️ CN: Pharmacological and parenteral therapies; CL: Analyze

51. **3.** INH interferes with the effectiveness of hormonal contraceptives, and female clients of birth age should be counseled to use an alternative form of birth control while taking the drug. INH does not increase the risk for vaginal infection, nor does it affect the ova or ovulation.

🗝️ CN: Pharmacological and parenteral therapies; CL: Apply

52. **3.** Tuberculosis can be controlled but never completely eradicated from the body. Periods of intense physical or emotional stress increase the likelihood of recurrence. Clients should be taught to recognize the signs and symptoms of a potential recurrence. Weather and activity levels are not related to recurrences of tuberculosis.

🗝️ CN: Physiological adaptation; CL: Analyze

53. **2.** Statistics show that of the four geographic areas described, most cases of tuberculosis are found in inner-core residential areas of large cities, where health and sanitation standards tend to be low. Substandard housing, poverty, and crowded living conditions also generally characterize these city areas and contribute to the spread of the disease. Farming areas have a low incidence of tuberculosis. Variations in water standards and industrial pollution are not correlated to tuberculosis incidence.

🗝️ CN: Safety and infection control; CL: Analyze

54. -/+ **2, 4, 5.** A potential adverse effect of rifampin is hepatotoxicity. Clients should be instructed to avoid alcohol while taking rifampin and keep follow-up appointments for periodic monitoring of liver enzyme levels to detect liver toxicity. Rifampin causes the urine to turn an orange color, and the client should understand that this is normal. It is not necessary to restrict protein intake in the diet or have the eyes examined due to rifampin therapy.

🗝️ CN: Pharmacological and parenteral therapies; CL: Create

55. **1.** Directly observed therapy (DOT) can be implemented with clients who are not compliant with drug therapy. In DOT, a responsible person, who may be a family member or an HCP, observes the client taking the medication. Visiting the client, changing the prescription, or threatening the client will not ensure compliance if the client will not or cannot follow the prescribed treatment.

🗝️ CN: Pharmacological and parenteral therapies; CL: Analyze

The Adult with Chronic Obstructive Pulmonary Disease

56. -/+ **2, 4.** Close proximity to smoking, fire, and small electrical appliances can be a fire hazard and should be avoided. The use of gauze is helpful in preventing skin irritation from the constant pressure and friction of the oxygen tubing. Typically, oxygen needs are lower at rest and during sleep. Increasing oxygen flow should be done at the discretion of the prescribing health care provider and not the client. Water-soluble lubricants are considered safer than petroleum-based lubricants. Small liquid oxygen tanks are easier to transport during travel than pressurized tanks. The use of microwave ovens for cooking is considered safe for those using supplemental oxygen.

🗝️ CN: Reduction of risk potential; CL: Create

57. -/+ **3, 4, 5.** High humidity has been shown to increase the work of breathing. Carrying a metered-dose inhaler can facilitate early intervention if bronchospasm and shortness of breath should occur. Smoking cessation is difficult to achieve but very important in preventing COPD progression. Pulmonary rehabilitation programs are a great source of support for health promotion and maintenance for clients with COPD. Both the pneumococcal and influenza vaccines can help protect against respiratory infections.

🗝️ CN: Reduction of risk potential; CL: Create

58. **3.** Crackles auscultated in the lung field indicate excessive fluid, a problem that requires immediate intervention. Pursed-lip breathing and a prolonged expiratory phase, circumoral cyanosis, and increased anterior-posterior diameter of the chest (resulting in "barrel chest") are not unusual findings for clients with emphysema.

CN: Physiological adaptation; CL: Analyze

59. 3. Inability to speak could indicate respiratory distress. Pursed-lip breathing, while it is an abnormal finding, is not indicative of respiratory distress. Distant heart sounds could indicate heart failure but are not indicative of any distress. Diminished lung sounds may be normal for this client and do not require immediate intervention.

CN: Physiological adaptation; CL: Analyze

60. 2, 1, 3, 4. The nurse should first instruct the client to relax the neck and the shoulders and then take several normal breaths. After taking a breath in, the client should pucker the lips and finally breathe out through pursed lips.

CN: Health promotion and maintenance; CL: Apply

61. 2. Clients with chronic COPD have CO_2 retention, and the respiratory drive is stimulated when the PaO_2 decreases. The heart rate, respiratory rate, and blood pressure should be evaluated to determine if the client is hemodynamically stable. Symptoms, such as dyspnea, should also be assessed. After assessing the vital signs, the nurse should assist the client as needed to assume the most comfortable position for breathing. Oxygen supplementation, if indicated, should be titrated upward in small increments. There is no indication that the client is experiencing respiratory distress requiring intubation.

CN: Physiological adaptation; CL: Analyze

62. 1. A client with COPD is at high risk for the development of respiratory infections. COPD is slowly progressive; therefore, maintaining the current status and establishing a goal that the client will require less supplemental oxygen are unrealistic expectations. Treatment may slow the progression of the disease, but permanent improvement is highly unlikely.

CN: Management of care; CL: Analyze

63. 1, 2, 3, 4. The therapeutic range for serum theophylline is 10 to 20 mcg/mL (55.5 to 111 μmol/L). At higher levels, the client will experience signs of toxicity such as nausea, vomiting, seizures, and insomnia. The nurse should instruct the client to report these signs and to keep appointments to have theophylline blood levels monitored. If the theophylline level is below the therapeutic range, the client may be at risk for more frequent exacerbations of the disease.

CN: Pharmacological and parenteral therapies; CL: Apply

64. 4. Increasing dyspnea on exertion indicates that the client may be experiencing complications of COPD. Therefore, the client should notify the HCP. It is not necessary to avoid being around others. Pain is not a common symptom of COPD. Clients with COPD use low-flow oxygen supplementation (1 to 2 L per minute) to avoid suppressing the respiratory drive, which, for these clients, is stimulated by hypoxia.

CN: Management of care; CL: Evaluate

65. 4. Cigarette smoking is the primary cause of COPD. Other risk factors include exposure to environmental pollutants and chronic asthma. Participating in an aerobic exercise program, although beneficial, will not decrease the risk for COPD. Insufficient protein intake and exposure to people with respiratory infections do not increase the risk for COPD.

CN: Health promotion and maintenance; CL: Analyze

66. 4. Pursed-lip breathing prolongs exhalation and prevents air trapping in the alveoli, thereby promoting carbon dioxide elimination. By prolonging exhalation and helping the client relax, pursed-lip breathing helps the client learn to control the rate and depth of respiration. Pursed-lip breathing does not promote the intake of oxygen, strengthen the diaphragm, or strengthen intercostal muscles.

CN: Physiological adaptation; CL: Evaluate

67. 1. A priority goal for the client with COPD is to manage the signs and symptoms of the disease process so as to maintain the client's functional ability. Chest pain is not a typical symptom of COPD. The carbon dioxide concentration in the blood is increased to an abnormal level in clients with COPD; it would not be a goal to increase the level further. Preventing infection would be a goal of care for the client with COPD.

CN: Basic care and comfort; CL: Analyze

68. 2. Exhaling requires less energy than inhaling. Therefore, lifting while exhaling saves energy and reduces perceived dyspnea. Pursing the lips prolongs exhalation and provides the client with more control over breathing. Lifting after exhaling but before inhaling is similar to lifting with the breath held. This should not be recommended because it is similar to the Valsalva maneuver, which can stimulate cardiac arrhythmias.

CN: Basic care and comfort; CL: Analyze

69. 3. Right-sided heart failure is a complication of COPD that occurs because of pulmonary hypertension. The signs and symptoms of right-sided heart failure include peripheral edema, jugular venous distention, hepatomegaly, and weight gain due to increased fluid volume. Clubbing of nail beds is associated with conditions of chronic hypoxemia. Hypertension is associated with left-sided heart failure. Clients with heart failure have decreased appetites.

CN: Physiological adaptation; CL: Analyze

70. 4. Exacerbations of COPD are commonly caused by respiratory infections. Coarse crackles and rhonchi would be auscultated as air moves through airways obstructed with secretions. In COPD, breath sounds are diminished because of an enlarged anteroposterior diameter of the chest. Expiration, not inspiration, becomes prolonged. Chest movement is decreased as lungs become overdistended.

CN: Physiological adaptation; CL: Analyze

71. 2. Clients who have a long history of COPD may retain carbon dioxide (CO_2). Gradually, the body adjusts to the higher CO_2 concentration, and the high levels of CO_2 no longer stimulate the respiratory center. The major respiratory stimulant then becomes hypoxemia. Administration of high concentrations of oxygen eliminates this respiratory stimulus and leads to hypoventilation. Oxygen can be drying if it is not humidified, but it does not cause coughing and dyspnea. Increased oxygen use will not create an oxygen dependency; clients should receive oxygen as needed. Oxygen is not contraindicated with the use of bronchodilators.

CN: Physiological adaptation; CL: Apply

72. 4. The client should eat high-calorie, high-protein meals to maintain nutritional status and prevent weight loss that results from the increased work of breathing. The client should be encouraged to eat small, frequent meals. A low-fat, low-cholesterol diet is indicated for clients with coronary artery disease. The client with COPD does not necessarily need to follow a sodium-restricted diet, unless otherwise medically indicated. There is no need for the client to eat bland, soft foods.

CN: Basic care and comfort; CL: Analyze

73. 3. Theophylline is a bronchodilator that is administered to relax airways and decrease dyspnea. Theophylline is not used to treat infections and does not decrease or thin secretions.

CN: Pharmacological and parenteral therapies; CL: Evaluate

74. 1. The goal of effective coughing is to conserve energy, facilitate the removal of secretions, and minimize airway collapse. The client should assume a sitting position with the feet on the floor if possible. The client should bend forward slightly and, using pursed-lip breathing, exhale. After resuming an upright position, the client should use abdominal breathing to inhale slowly and deeply. After repeating this process three or four times, the client should take a deep abdominal breath, bend forward, and cough three or four times upon exhalation ("huff" cough). Lying flat does not enhance lung expansion; sitting upright promotes full expansion of the thorax. Shallow breathing does not facilitate the removal of secretions, and forceful coughing promotes the collapse of airways. A side-lying position does not allow for adequate chest expansion to promote deep breathing.

CN: Basic care and comfort; CL: Create

75.

STEP 1

Nurse's Notes

Today: 1500
The client has not been able to take the daily medications and has shortness of breath when ambulating due to worsening respiratory symptoms and fatigue. The client has a history of smoking one pack of cigarettes per day for 35 years, has been diagnosed with chronic obstructive pulmonary disease (COPD), and uses 2 L per minute of oxygen via nasal cannula and continuous positive airway pressure (CPAP) overnight for obstructive sleep apnea. The client also has hypertension, depression, and anxiety. The client is <u>wheezing</u> with <u>diminished breath sounds</u> on auscultation, <u>performing pursed-lip breathing using accessory muscles</u>, and <u>coughing thick, yellow sputum</u>. Vital signs are <u>temperature (T) 100.4°F (38.0°C)</u>; <u>heart rate (HR) 112 bpm</u>; <u>blood pressure (BP) 150/90 mm Hg</u>; respiration rate (RR) 18 breaths/min; and <u>oxygen saturation 90% on 2 L per minute via nasal cannula</u>.

The client is demonstrating signs that indicate a worsening of respiratory status for a client with COPD: wheezing, diminished breath sounds, pursed-lip breathing using accessory muscles, and coughing up thick, yellow sputum. The client also has an elevated temperature and heart rate. These indicate the nurse should follow up with the client. The respiratory rate is within the normal range, and the oxygen saturation on 2 L per minute via nasal cannula is in the low range of normal.

CJ: Case study; Step 1: Recognize cues; CL: Understand

76.
STEP 2

0/1 *The nurse is most concerned about the exacerbation of **COPD** as evidenced by the client's temperature of 100.4°F (38.0°C).*

The nurse should identify the client's presentation as an exacerbation of COPD and should be concerned about a fever, which may indicate an infection. The client does have a history of anxiety; a respiratory rate of 18 breaths/min is stable; the client uses continuous positive pressure (CPAP); but there is no indication that there is a problem with use. Thus, these findings are not the main concern at this time. The client's elevated blood pressure may be due to the client not taking their medication and will require follow-up. The heart rate is elevated, likely due to the increased temperature; the oxygen saturation is low, but within normal range.

🗝️ CJ: Case study; Step 2: Analyze cues; CL: Analyze

77.
STEP 3

−/+ **1, 2, 3, 7.** The nurse should first obtain a sputum culture to rule out infection, administer a beta-blocker to manage the client's hypertension, administer mucolytics to thin the mucus (making it less thick and easier to cough up), and place the client on telemetry to monitor the client's cardiac rhythm. After completing these orders, the nurse can assist the client to a recliner, which will provide support for deep breathing, and order the physical therapy. The client does not have a temperature above 101°F (38.3°C).

🗝️ CJ: Case study; Step 3: Prioritize hypothesis; CL: Create

78.
STEP 4

0/1

Intervention	Indicated	Not Indicated	Contraindicated
Transfer to the intensive care unit		X	
Increase oxygen to 6 L per minute			X
Increase intravenous fluids to 150 mL per hour			X
Administer acetaminophen	X		
Notify the health care provider (HCP)	X		

The nurse should first notify the HCP because the client's vital signs indicate an increased temperature, which may be indicative of an infection. The blood pressure has dropped, and with an increase in the heart rate and respiratory rate, it could be indicative of septic shock. The nurse can also administer acetaminophen as prescribed for the temperature above 101°F (38.3°C). The client is in an intermediate care unit where the health care providers can manage changes in vital signs and initiating a transfer to an intensive care unit is not indicated. Increasing intravenous fluids requires an HCP's order.

🗝️ CJ: Case study; Step 4: Generate solutions; CL: Analyze

79.
STEP 5

0/1

Intervention	Indicated	Not Indicated	Contraindicated
Administer bronchodilators	X		
Replace electrolytes		X	
Increase oxygen to 6 L per minute			X
Offer smoking cessation education	X		
Order chest physical therapy	X		
Check immunizations	X		
Position the client supine in bed			X

The nurse should administer the bronchodilators to open up the airways to improve breathing. It is not indicated for the client to have electrolytes replaced at this time as there is no evidence of abnormal laboratory values or that the client is at risk for arrhythmias. It is contraindicated to increase the oxygen to 6 L per minute because increasing the oxygen can lead to oxygen toxicity or atelectasis. Cigarette smoking is the most significant contributing factor to developing COPD; thus, the nurse should plan to provide smoking cessation education. Chest physical therapy will help with mucus clearance. The nurse should check the client's immunization record to be sure the client is up to date with influenza and pneumococcal vaccines, which are recommended for adults, particularly those with chronic lung conditions such as COPD. A supine position is contraindicated as the client will have difficulty expanding the chest; the nurse should place the client in a position with the head of the bed elevated to support breathing effort.

🗝️ CJ: Case study; Step 5: Take action; CL: Apply

80.

Assessment Finding	Improved	Not Changed	Declined
Can walk to the bathroom without shortness of breath	X		
Sputum culture negative for bacteria	X		
Needs 2 L of oxygen per nasal cannula at night		X	
Requires CPAP at night		X	
Decreased sputum production	X		
Lungs clear on auscultation	X		

STEP 6

The client can now walk to the bathroom without becoming short of breath. The nurse can advise the client to increase the amount of walking as strength improves. The client's sputum production has decreased and is negative for bacteria; the client will continue the prescription for oral antibiotics at home until completed. The client continues to have COPD and sleep apnea and will use oxygen and CPAP at home. The nurse can advise the client to continue to use a recliner or elevate the head of the bed to make breathing easier.

CJ: Case study; Step 6: Evaluate outcomes; CL: Evaluate

The Adult with Asthma

81. 3, 4, 5. Utilization of an MDI requires the following actions: shaking the MDI before use; exhaling prior to dispensing the medication; taking a deep breath to ensure the medication is distributed in the lungs and holding it for 10 seconds or as long as possible to disperse the medication into the lungs; and allowing 30 seconds between puffs to provide an adequate amount of inhalation medication. The client should rinse the plastic parts of the MDI and wipe them dry; the canister should not become wet.

CN: Pharmacological and parenteral therapies; CL: Evaluate

82. 4. In an acute asthma attack, diminished or absent breath sounds can be an ominous sign that indicates a lack of air movement in the lungs and impending respiratory failure. The client requires immediate intervention with inhaled bronchodilators, intravenous (IV) corticosteroids, and, possibly, IV theophylline. Administering oxygen and reassessing the client 10 minutes later would delay needed medical intervention, as would drawing blood for an arterial blood gas analysis. It would be futile to encourage the client to relax and breathe slowly without providing the necessary pharmacologic intervention.

CN: Management of care; CL: Analyze

83. 3. Quick-acting bronchodilators are used in acute asthma to improve airflow and relieve symptoms; following treatment, tachycardia resolves as gas exchange and work of breathing are improved. SpO_2 and PEF rates improve, and wheezing from a constricted airway resolves. The normal inspiratory to expiratory ratio is 1:2.

CN: Physiological adaptation; CL: Evaluate

84. 2. The nurse instructs the client to administer the bronchodilator first (the beta-2 agonist always leads) to open the airway and allow for improved delivery of the corticosteroid to the lung tissue, which follows after 1 minute between puffs. Using a spacer device with an MDI provides the best delivery of medication to the lungs.

CN: Pharmacological and parenteral therapies; CL: Analyze

85. 1. The arterial blood gas reveals respiratory acidosis with hypoxia. A quick-acting bronchodilator, albuterol, should be administered via a nebulizer to improve gas exchange. Ipratropium is a maintenance treatment for bronchospasm that can be used with albuterol. A chest x-ray and a sputum sample can be obtained once the client is stable.

CN: Physiological adaptation; CL: Analyze

86. 3. Corticosteroids have an antiinflammatory effect and act to decrease edema in the bronchial airways and decrease mucus secretion. Corticosteroids do not have a bronchodilator effect, act as expectorants, or prevent respiratory infections.

CN: Pharmacological and parenteral therapies; CL: Evaluate

87. 1, 4. The client should shake the inhaler and hold it upright when administering the drug. The head should be tilted back slightly. The client should wait about 30 seconds between puffs. The mouth should be rinsed following the use of a corticosteroid MDI to decrease the likelihood of developing an oral infection. The client does not need to lie supine; instead, the client will likely be able to breathe more freely if sitting upright.

CN: Pharmacological and parenteral therapies; CL: Evaluate

88. 1. Irregular heartbeats should be reported promptly to the care provider. Metaproterenol may cause irregular heartbeat, tachycardia, or anginal pain because of its adrenergic effect on beta-adrenergic receptors in the heart. It is not recommended for use in clients with known cardiac disorders. Metaproterenol does not cause constipation, pedal edema, or bradycardia.

🔑 CN: Pharmacological and parenteral therapies; CL: Analyze

89. **3.** Use of oral inhalant corticosteroids such as flunisolide can lead to the development of oral thrush, a fungal infection. Once developed, thrush must be treated by antifungal therapy; it will not resolve on its own. Fungal infections can develop even without overuse of the corticosteroid inhaler. Although good oral hygiene can help prevent the development of a fungal infection, it cannot be used alone to treat the problem.

🔑 CN: Pharmacological and parenteral therapies; CL: Analyze

90. **1, 4, 3, 2.** When using inhalers, clients should first shake the inhaler to activate the MDI and then breathe out through the mouth. Next, the client should activate the MDI while inhaling, hold the breath for 5 to 10 seconds, and then exhale normally.

🔑 CN: Pharmacological and parenteral therapies; CL: Apply

91. **1, 5.** Physical exercise is beneficial and should be incorporated as tolerated into the client's schedule. The client should also avoid areas with smoke because smoke is a trigger for an asthma attack. Peak flow numbers should be monitored daily, usually in the morning (before taking medication). Peak flow does not need to be monitored after each meal. Stressors in the client's life should be modified but cannot be totally eliminated. Although adequate sleep is important, it is not recommended that a drug such as melatonin or sedatives be routinely taken to induce sleep.

🔑 CN: Reduction of risk potential; CL: Create

92. **3.** A common precipitator of asthma attacks is exposure to cigarette and cigar smoke. The client should avoid being in environments where there is exposure to smoke. Environmental exposure to toxins or heavy particulate matter can trigger asthma attacks; however, far fewer asthmatics are exposed to such toxins than are exposed to smoke. The Valsalva maneuver (holding the breath while defecating or bearing down) is associated with causing cardiac arrhythmias. Rarely, asthmatic attacks are triggered by exercising in cold weather.

🔑 CN: Health promotion and infection control; CL: Analyze

93. **1.** A cough that produces yellow sputum is the most likely indicator of a respiratory infection. The other signs and symptoms—wheezing, chest tightness, and increased respiratory rate—are all findings associated with an asthma attack and do not necessarily mean an infection is present.

🔑 CN: Physiological adaptation; CL: Analyze

The Adult with Lung Cancer

94. **1.** The nurse should first assess for bilateral breath sounds since a complication of central line insertion is a pneumothorax, which would cause an increase in respiratory rate and a drop in oxygen, causing irritability. The nurse should also assess blood pressure and heart rate for the complication of bleeding. A chest x-ray will be performed to determine correct placement and complications. A central line was most likely placed because peripheral IV access was not available or adequate for the client. Repositioning may be considered after assessments are done.

🔑 CN: Physiological adaptation; CL: Analyze

95. **2.** The nurse should review the CBC with differential to evaluate the client's hemoglobin and hematocrit, which are abnormal and should be reported to the HCP. Anemia leads to decreased oxygen-carrying capacity of the blood. A client unable to compensate for the anemia may experience a profound sense of dyspnea. There has been a significant drop in the hemoglobin and hematocrit since the previous report, and these should be reported to the HCP. The monocytes are within normal range. A1C is a laboratory test evaluating glycosylated hemoglobin and is in the normal range. This test is used to diagnose diabetes or monitor diabetic glucose control over time. PT is a coagulation study reflecting liver function and clotting time and is in the normal range.

🔑 CN: Management of care; CL: Analyze

96. **1.** Risk factors for postoperative pulmonary complications include malnourishment, which is indicated by this client's height and weight. It is thought that emotional responses can affect overall health; however, not verbalizing one's feelings is not a contributing factor in postoperative pulmonary complications. The client's current activity level and age do not place them at increased risk for complications.

🔑 CN: Physiological adaptation; CL: Analyze

97. **1.** Acknowledging the basic feeling the client expresses—fear—and asking an open-ended question are actions that allow the client to explain any fears. The other options dismiss the client's feelings and may give false reassurance or label the client's feelings. The client should be encouraged to explore feelings about a cancer diagnosis.

🔑 CN: Psychosocial adaptation; CL: Analyze

98. 4. Systematic pain assessment is necessary for adequate pain management in the postoperative client. Guidelines from a variety of health care agencies and nursing groups recommend that institutions adopt a pain assessment scale to assist in facilitating pain management. Even though the client is receiving morphine sulfate by PCA, and the pump is working, the nurse should continue to assess the client. The concern is not to eliminate coughing but to control pain adequately. Coughing is necessary to prevent postoperative atelectasis and pneumonia. Breathing exercises may help control pain in some circumstances; however, most clients with thoracic surgery require parenteral opioid analgesics in the early postoperative period. Although it is necessary that the PCA device be checked periodically, reassuring the client is not sufficient, so further assessment is needed.

CN: Basic care and comfort; CL: Analyze

99. 1. Because clients are discharged as soon as possible from the hospital, it is essential to evaluate the support they have to assist them with self-care at home. The distance the client lives from the hospital is not a critical factor in discharge planning. There are no data indicating that home blood pressure monitoring is needed. Knowledge of the causes of lung cancer, though important, is not the most essential area to evaluate given the client's postoperative status.

CN: Reduction of risk potential; CL: Analyze

100. 4. Deep breathing helps prevent microatelectasis and pneumonitis and also helps force air and fluid out of the pleural space into the chest tubes. More than half of the ventilatory process is accomplished by the rise and fall of the diaphragm. The diaphragm is the major muscle of respiration; deep breathing causes it to descend, not elevate, thereby increasing the ventilating surface. Deep breathing increases blood flow to the lungs; however, the primary reason for deep breathing is to expand alveoli and prevent atelectasis. The remaining lobe naturally hyperinflates to fill the space created by the resected lobe. This is an expected phenomenon.

CN: Physiological adaptation; CL: Evaluate

101. 2. It is essential that the nurse evaluate the effects of pain medication after the medication has had time to act; reassessment is necessary to determine the effectiveness of the pain management plan. Although it is prudent to check for discomfort related to positioning when assessing the client's pain, repositioning the client immediately after administering pain medication is not necessary. Verbally reassuring the client after administering pain medication may be useful to help instill confidence in the treatment plan; however, it is not as important as evaluating the effectiveness of the medication. Readjusting the pain medication dosage as needed according to the client's condition is essential, but the effectiveness of the medication must be evaluated first.

CN: Physiological adaptation; CL: Analyze

102. 3. This crackling sensation is subcutaneous emphysema. Subcutaneous emphysema is not an unusual finding and is not dangerous if confined, and the nurse should mark the area to detect if the area is expanding. Progression can be serious, especially if the neck is involved; a tracheotomy may be needed at that point. If emphysema progresses noticeably within 1 hour, the HCP should be notified. Lowering the head of the bed will not arrest the progress or provide any further information. A tracheotomy tray would be useful if subcutaneous emphysema progresses to the neck. Subcutaneous emphysema may progress if the chest drainage system does not adequately remove air and fluid; therefore, the system should not be turned off.

CN: Physiological adaptation; CL: Analyze

103. 1. The recommended procedure for teaching clients postoperatively to deep breathe includes contracting (pulling in) the abdominal muscles and taking a slow, deep breath through the nose. This breath is held for 3 to 5 seconds, which facilitates alveolar ventilation by improving the inspiratory phase of ventilation. Exhaling slowly as if trying to blow out a candle is a technique used in pursed-lip breathing to facilitate exhalation in clients with chronic obstructive pulmonary disease. It is recommended that the abdominal muscles be contracted, not relaxed, to promote deep breathing. The client should breathe through the nose.

CN: Health promotion and maintenance; CL: Analyze

104. 3. A client who has undergone chest surgery should be taught to raise the arm on the affected side over the head to help prevent shoulder ankylosis. This exercise helps restore normal shoulder movement, prevents stiffening of the shoulder joint, and improves muscle tone and power. Turning from side to side, raising and lowering the head, and flexing and extending the elbow on the affected side do not exercise the shoulder joint.

CN: Basic care and comfort; CL: Analyze

105. 4. The drainage apparatus is always kept below the client's chest level to prevent the backflow of fluid into the pleural space. The air vent must always be open in the closed chest drainage system to allow air from the client to escape. Stripping a chest tube causes excessive negative intrapleural pressure and is not recommended. Clamping a chest tube when moving a client is not recommended.

CN: Physiological adaptation; CL: Analyze

106. 1. Cessation of fluid fluctuation in the tubing can mean one of several things: the lung has fully expanded, and negative intrapleural pressure has been reestablished; the chest tube is occluded; or the chest tube is not in the pleural space. Fluid fluctuation occurs because during inspiration, intrapleural pressure exceeds the negative pressure generated in the water seal system. Therefore, drainage moves toward the client. During expiration, the pleural pressure exceeds that generated in the water seal system, and fluid moves away from the client. When the lung is collapsed or the chest tube is in the pleural space, fluid fluctuation is likely to be noted. The chest tube is not inserted in the mediastinal space.

CN: Physiological adaptation; CL: Analyze

107. 2. There should never be constant bubbling in the water seal system; normally, the bubbling is intermittent. Constant bubbling in the water seal bottle indicates an air leak, which means that less negative pressure is being exerted on the pleural space. Decreasing the suction will not reduce the leak. It is not necessary to notify the HCP until the system has been checked and the problem identified.

CN: Physiological adaptation; CL: Analyze

108. 1. In this case, there may be some obstruction to the flow of air and fluid out of the pleural space, causing air and fluid to collect and build up pressure. This prevents the remaining lung from reexpanding and can cause a mediastinal shift to the opposite side. The nurse's first response is to assess the tubing for kinks or obstruction. Increasing the suction is not done without a health care provider's prescription. The normal position of the drainage bottles is 2 to 3 feet (61 to 91.4 cm) below chest level. Clamping the tubes obstructs the flow of air and fluid out of the pleural space and should not be done.

CN: Physiological adaptation; CL: Analyze

109. 4. To promote chest tube drainage, the drainage system must be lower than the client's lungs. The amount of drainage is not abnormal; it is not necessary to notify the HCP. The nurse should chart the amount and color of drainage every 4 to 8 hours. The chest tube does not need to be clamped; the tubing connection is intact. There is sufficient water to maintain a water seal.

CN: Physiological adaptation; CL: Analyze

110. 2. Gauze saturated with petrolatum is placed over the site to make an airtight seal to prevent air leakage during the healing process. Dry or wet dressings or adhesive strips are not used. An airtight dressing is needed until the insertion site is healed.

CN: Management of care; CL: Apply

The Adult with Chest Trauma

111. 3. Respiratory distress or arrest is a universal finding of a tension pneumothorax. Unilateral, diminished, or absent breath sounds is a common finding. Tracheal deviation is an inconsistent and late finding. Muffled heart sounds are suggestive of pericardial tamponade.

CN: Physiological adaptation; CL: Analyze

112. **0.7 mL**

$$10 \text{ mg} : X \text{ mL} = 15 \text{ mg} : 1 \text{ mL}$$
$$15 \text{ mg} \times X \text{ mL} = 10 \text{ mg} \times 1 \text{ mL}$$
$$15X = 10$$
$$X = 0.6667$$
$$X = 0.67 \text{ mL}$$

CN: Pharmacological and parenteral therapies; CL: Apply

113. 2. Blunt chest trauma may lead to respiratory failure, and maintenance of adequate oxygenation is the priority for the client. Decreasing the client's anxiety is related to maintaining effective respirations and oxygenation. Although pain is distressing to the client and can increase anxiety and decrease respiratory effectiveness, pain control is secondary to maintaining oxygenation. Maintaining adequate circulatory volume is also secondary to maintaining adequate oxygenation.

CN: Physiological adaptation; CL: Analyze

114. 3. Fluctuation of fluid in the water seal column with respirations indicates that the system is functioning properly. If an obstruction were present in the chest tube, fluid fluctuation would be absent. Subcutaneous emphysema occurs when air pockets can be palpated beneath the client's skin around the chest tube insertion site. A leak in the system is indicated when continuous bubbling occurs in the water seal column.

🗝 CN: Physiological adaptation; CL: Analyze

115. **1.** If the client reports no pain, then the objective of adequate pain relief has been met. Decreased anxiety is not related only to pain control; it could also be related to other factors. A respiratory rate of 26 breaths/min is not within normal limits, nor is the PaO_2 of 70 mm Hg (9.31 kPa), but these values are not measures of pain relief.

🗝 CN: Physiological adaptation; CL: Evaluate

116. **2.** One unit of packed red blood cells is about 250 mL. If the blood is delivered at a rate of 60 mL per hour, it will take about 4 hours to infuse the entire unit. The transfusion of a single unit of packed red blood cells should not exceed 4 hours to prevent the growth of bacteria and minimize the risk for septicemia.

🗝 CN: Pharmacological and parenteral therapies; CL: Apply

117. **1.** Pneumothorax signs and symptoms include sudden, sharp chest pain, tachypnea, and tachycardia. The nurse should report these to the health care provider (HCP). Other signs and symptoms include diminished or absent breath sounds over the affected lung, anxiety, and restlessness. Hemoptysis and cyanosis are not typically present with a pneumothorax.

🗝 CN: Physiological adaptation; CL: Analyze

118. –/+ **1, 2, 3, 4.** Following a thoracentesis, the nurse should assess the client for possible complications of the procedure such as pneumothorax, tension pneumothorax, and subcutaneous emphysema, which can occur because of the needle entering the chest cavity. Pulmonary edema could occur if a large volume was aspirated causing a significant mediastinal shift. Although infection is a possible complication, signs of infection will not be evident immediately after the procedure.

🗝 CN: Reduction of risk potential; CL: Analyze

119. **1.** Cheyne-Stokes respiration is defined as a regular cycle that starts with normal breaths, which increase and then decrease followed by a period of apnea. It can be related to heart failure or dysfunction of the respiratory center of the brain. Hyperventilation is associated with an increased rate and depth of respirations. Obstructive sleep apnea is recurring episodes of upper airway obstruction and reduced ventilation. Biot respiration, also known as "cluster breathing," is periods of normal respirations followed by varying periods of apnea.

🗝 CN: Reduction of risk potential; CL: Analyze

The Adult with Acute Respiratory Distress Syndrome

120. –/+ **3, 4, 5.** The prone position is used to improve oxygenation, ventilation, and perfusion. The importance of placing clients with ARDS in prone positioning should be explained to the family. The positioning allows for the mobilization of secretions, and the nurse can provide suctioning. Clinical judgment must be used to determine the length of time in the prone position. If the client's hemodynamic status, oxygenation, or skin is compromised, the client should be returned to the supine position for evaluation. Facial edema is expected with the prone position, but the skin breakdown is of concern.

🗝 CN: Physiological adaptation; CL: Analyze

121. **4.** Prone positioning is used to improve oxygenation in clients with ARDS who are receiving mechanical ventilation. The positioning allows for the recruitment of collapsed alveolar units, improvement in ventilation, reduction in shunting, mobilization of secretions, and improvement in functional reserve capacity. When the client is supine, side-to-side repositioning should be done every 2 hours with the head of the bed elevated at least 30 degrees.

🗝 CN: Physiological adaptation; CL: Analyze

122. –/+ **1, 4, 5.** ARDS may cause renal failure and superinfection, so the nurse should monitor urine output and urine chemistries. Treatment of hypoxemia can be complicated because changes in lung tissue leave less pulmonary tissue available for gas exchange, thereby causing inadequate perfusion. Humidified oxygen may be one means of promoting oxygenation. The client has crackles in the lung bases, so the nurse should continue to assess breath sounds. Sedatives should be used with caution in clients with ARDS. The nurse should try other measures to relieve the client's restlessness and anxiety. The head of the bed should be elevated to 30 degrees to promote chest expansion and prevent atelectasis.

🗝 CN: Management of care; CL: Create

123. **4.** One of the major risk factors for the development of ARDS is hypovolemic shock. Adequate fluid replacement is essential to minimize this risk. A history of smoking is not a direct risk factor for ARDS. A low serum potassium level and hypercapnia are not risk factors for ARDS.

🗝 CN: Reduction of risk potential; CL: Analyze

124. **2.** A hallmark of early ARDS is refractory hypoxemia. The client's partial pressure of arterial oxygen (PaO_2) level continues to fall, despite higher concentrations of administered oxygen. Elevated carbon dioxide and metabolic acidosis occur late in the disorder. Severe electrolyte imbalances are not indicators of ARDS.

🗝 CN: Physiological adaptation; CL: Analyze

125. **2.** The normal range for $PaCO_2$ is 35 to 45 mm Hg (4.7 to 6 kPa). Thus, this client's $PaCO_2$ level is low. The client is experiencing respiratory alkalosis (carbonic acid deficit) due to hyperventilation. The nurse should report this finding to the health care provider (HCP) because it requires intervention. The increase in ventilation decreases the $PaCO_2$ level, which leads to decreased carbonic acid and alkalosis. The HCO_3 level is normal in uncompensated respiratory alkalosis along with the normal PaO_2 level. Normal serum pH is 7.35 to 7.45; in uncompensated respiratory alkalosis, the serum pH is greater than 7.45.

🗝 CN: Reduction of risk potential; CL: Analyze

126. **1.** The client may be fighting the ventilator breaths. Sedation is indicated to improve compliance with the ventilator in an attempt to lower peak inspiratory pressures. The workload of breathing does indicate the need for increased protein calories; however, this will not correct the respiratory problems with high pressures and respiratory rate. There is no indication that the client is experiencing pain. Increasing the rate on the ventilator is not indicated with the client's increased spontaneous rate.

🗝 CN: Physiological adaptation; CL: Analyze

127. **1.** Manifestations of adult respiratory distress syndrome (ARDS) secondary to acute pancreatitis include respiratory distress, tachypnea, dyspnea, fever, dry cough, fine crackles heard throughout lung fields, possible confusion and agitation, and hypoxemia with an arterial oxygen level below 50 mm Hg. The nurse should report the arterial oxygen level of 46 mm Hg (6.1 kPa) to the HCP. A respiratory rate of 12 breaths/min is normal and not considered a sign of respiratory distress. Adventitious lung sounds, such as crackles, are typically found in clients with ARDS. Oxygen saturation of 96% is satisfactory and does not represent hypoxemia or low arterial oxygen saturation.

🗝 CN: Physiologic adaptation; CL: Analyze

128. **1.** Normal PaO_2 level ranges from 80 to 100 mm Hg (10.7 to 13.3 kPa). When PaO_2 falls to 50 mm Hg (6.7 kPa), the nurse should be alert for signs of hypoxia and impending respiratory failure. An oxygen level this low poses a severe risk for respiratory failure. The client will require oxygenation at a concentration that maintains the PaO_2 at 55 to 60 mm Hg (7.3 to 8 kPa) or more.

🗝 CN: Physiological adaptation; CL: Analyze

129. **4.** The nurse should suction the client if the client is not able to cough up secretions and clear the airway. Administering oxygen will not promote airway clearance. The client should be turned every 2 hours to help move secretions; every 4 hours is not often enough. Administering sedatives to promote rest is contraindicated in acute respiratory distress because sedatives can depress respirations.

🗝 CN: Physiological adaptation; CL: Analyze

Managing Care, Quality, and Safety of Adults with Respiratory Health Problems

130. **2.** Sanguineous or bloody sputum (hemoptysis) is a sign of possible hemorrhage and may indicate vessel damage in the lungs; the nurse should assess this client first. The nurse should next evaluate the client with CHF and weight gain for additional signs of heart failure. Loose stools are expected for a client with C. difficile, and the nurse can delegate care to an unlicensed assistive personnel and follow up with this client later to determine the character and frequency of the stools. The client with COPD has an oxygen saturation that is within acceptable levels at this time, and the nurse can assess this client last.

🗝 CN: Management of care; CL: Synthesis

131. **−/+ 2, 3, 4, 5, 6.** The nurse's role is to carry out the client's written wishes as indicated in the DNR and living will, and the nurse should calmly remind the spouse of the client's wishes. The nurse next should notify the HCP who will determine that the client has died. The HCP also should reaffirm the client's wishes with the spouse.

Chaplains are an important resource for families at times of loss. They will remain with the families if they wish and attend to their needs. The nurse manager needs to be notified of the spouse's statement in order to notify risk management of a potential legal concern. Not carrying out the client's written directions and wishes places the nurse and the facility under legal liability.

CN: Management of care; CL: Synthesis

132. 2. Respirations of 36 breaths/min and diminished wheezing are indicative of respiratory distress. This finding takes precedence over a client scheduled for an angiogram, a client with a heart rate of 90 bpm needing a scheduled beta-blocker, and a client with a PaO_2 of 56 mm Hg, which is indicated for a client being discharged home on oxygen.

CN: Management of care; CL: Analyze

133. 1. UAP can assist a client with the adjustment of their oxygen delivery device. Making adjustments based on client responses, monitoring for adverse effects, and assessing the best methods of oxygen delivery are skills that require nursing judgments and can only be performed by a nurse.

CN: Management of care; CL: Analyze

134. 4. Confusion and vertigo are risk factors for falls. Measures must be taken to minimize the risk for injury. The nurse or UAP should check on the client regularly to determine needs regarding elimination. Restraints, including bed rails and extremity restraints, should be used only to ensure the person's safety or the safety of others, and there must be a written prescription from a health care provider before using them. The nurse should never ask the roommate of a client to be responsible for the client's safety.

CN: Safety and infection control; CL: Analyze

135. 4. Airborne precautions prevent the transmission of infectious agents that remain infectious over long distances when suspended in the air (e.g., *Mycobacterium tuberculosis*, measles, varicella virus [chickenpox], and possibly SARS-CoV). The preferred placement is in an isolation single-client room that is equipped with special air handling and ventilation. A negative pressure room, or an area that exhausts room air directly outside or through HEPA filters, should be used if recirculation is unavoidable. While standard precautions such as hand hygiene and wearing gloves and a gown are important, they are not sufficient to prevent the transmission of tuberculosis. Contact precautions are used with clients with known or suspected infections who present an increased risk for contact transmission. Droplet precautions are intended to prevent the transmission of pathogens spread through close respiratory or mucous membrane contact with respiratory secretions. Because these pathogens do not remain infectious over long distances in a health care facility, special air handling and ventilation are not required to prevent droplet transmission.

CN: Safety and infection control; CL: Analyze

136. -/+ 2, 3, 4, 5. One of the "five rights" of drug administration is "right medication." Cefazolin was not the medication prescribed. The pharmacist is a professional resource and serves as a check to ensure that clients receive the right medication. Returning unwanted medications to the pharmacy will decrease the opportunity for a medication error by the nurse who follows the current nurse.

CN: Pharmacological and parenteral therapies; CL: Analyze

137. 1, 3, 4, 2. Because two major complications of endotracheal tube intubation, inadvertent extubation and aspiration, can be catastrophic events, assessment of this client is the first priority. Cellulitis is a serious infection as there is inflammation of subcutaneous tissues; third spacing of fluid may promote the formation of a fluid volume deficit, which can be exacerbated by the fever due to insensible fluid loss. The nurse should assess this client next to determine current vital signs and fluid status. The nurse should assess the client with the IV fluids next because the new bag of fluids will need to be hung in 30 to 40 minutes. IV therapy necessitates that the client is assessed for signs and symptoms of adequate hydration (moist mucous membranes, elastic skin turgor, vital signs within normal limits, adequate urine output, and level of consciousness within normal limits), and the IV access site needs to be assessed. From the information provided, there is no indication that the client who had the cerebrovascular accident is unstable. Thus, this client is the last priority for assessment.

CN: Management of care; CL: Analyze

138. -/+ 1, 2, 3. The process of changing a health care system from an acute care model to a community-based care model uses continuous quality improvement methods. The goal is to improve the health of chronically ill clients. Areas for improvement include health systems, delivery system design, decision support, clinical information systems, self-management support, and the community. This system requires health care services that are client centered and coordinated among members of the health care team and the client and the family. These changes do not focus on the administrative leadership or the care in the acute care setting alone.

🔑 CN: Management of care; CL: Analyze

139. **4.** Several factors designate this client as a high fall risk based on the Morse Fall Scale: history of falling (25), secondary diagnosis (15), plus IV access (20). The client's total score is 60. There is also concern that the client's gait is at least weak if not impaired due to hospitalization for pneumonia, which may add to the client's fall risk. After evaluating the client's risk, the nurse must develop a plan and take action to maximize the client's safety.

🔑 CN: Safety and infection control; CL: Analyze

140. −/+ **1, 2, 3, 4.** Gloves, a gown, a surgical mask, and eye protection/glasses are worn to protect health care workers and help prevent the spread of infection when clients are placed in droplet isolation. Because droplets are too heavy to be airborne, a respirator is not required when caring for a client in droplet precautions.

🔑 CN: Safety and infection control; CL: Apply

141. **3.** The nurse has already called for help and established unresponsiveness, so the first action is to open the client's airway; opening the airway may result in spontaneous breathing and will help the nurse determine whether or not further intervention is required. Pushing the "code blue" button may not be the appropriate action if the client is breathing and becomes responsive once the airway is open. A quick assessment upon opening the client's airway will help the nurse determine if the rapid response team is needed. Calling for a defibrillator may not be the necessary or appropriate action once the client's airway has been opened.

🔑 CN: Safety and infection control; CL: Analyze

142. **2, 3, 1, 4.** The nurse should first assess the client's respiratory status to determine if there is a physiological reason for the client's confusion. Other physiological factors to assess include pain and elimination. Safety needs including medication interactions should then be evaluated. Requesting restraints to maintain client safety should be used as a last resort.

🔑 CN: Safety and infection control; CL: Analyze

143. **1, 2, 4, 3.** The older adult client with pneumonia, an elevated temperature, and shortness of breath is the most acutely ill client described and should be the client with the highest priority. The elevated temperature and the shortness of breath can lead to a decrease in the client's oxygen levels and can predispose the client to dehydration and confusion. Then the nurse should assess the client with the thoracotomy who is requesting pain medication and administer any needed medication. The client with emphysema should be the next priority so that the bronchodilator can be administered on schedule as close as possible. The nurse would then assess the client with suspected tuberculosis and a cough.

🔑 CN: Management of care; CL: Analyze

144. −/+ **2, 3, 4, 5, 6.** The client's condition is worsening as evidenced by the diaphoresis that puts the client at risk for dehydration and the increase in heart rate, respiration rate, and blood pressure because of the increase in temperature and the infection in the lungs. The nurse should initiate accurate intake and output records to monitor fluid deficit and ensure the client obtains at least 1200 mL of fluids in 8 hours. The nurse can make the client comfortable using a cool, moist cloth in areas of diaphoresis. The nurse should administer the acetaminophen to reduce the temperature and notify the health care provider of the changes in vital signs. The client should not remain in bed and can ambulate with assistance or sit in a chair; the head of the bed can be elevated; these actions will encourage deep breathing and support lung expansion. The client's oxygen saturation, while slightly declining, is still within normal limits.

🔑 CJ: Standalone trend; CL: Analyze

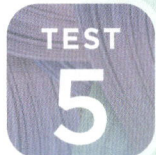

TEST 5: The Adult with Upper Gastrointestinal Tract Health Problems

- The Adult with Disorders of the Oral Cavity
- The Adult with Peptic Ulcer Disease
- The Adult with Cancer of the Stomach
- The Adult with Gastroesophageal Reflux Disease
- Managing Care, Quality, and Safety of Adults with Upper Gastrointestinal Tract Health Problems
- Answers, Rationales, and Test-Taking Strategies

The Adult with Disorders of the Oral Cavity

1. A nurse is caring for a client who has just returned from surgery to treat a fractured mandible. The jaws are wired. What should the nurse do if the client begins to vomit?
   - ☐ 1. Administer an antiemetic as prescribed.
   - ☐ 2. Cut the wires, and assist the client to expectorate.
   - ☐ 3. Have the client sit up, bend over, and spit into an emesis basin.
   - ☐ 4. Insert a suction tube to clear the vomitus from the oral cavity.

2. The nurse is teaching a client with stomatitis about managing oral discomfort. Which instruction is **most** appropriate?
   - ☐ 1. Drink hot tea at frequent intervals.
   - ☐ 2. Gargle with an antiseptic mouthwash.
   - ☐ 3. Use an electric toothbrush.
   - ☐ 4. Eat a soft, bland diet.

3. A client who has a history of bacterial endocarditis is scheduled to have oral surgery to remove a tooth. What should the nurse instruct the client to do?
   - ☐ 1. Gargle with a saline solution before the appointment.
   - ☐ 2. Rinse the mouth with mouthwash the night before and the day of the surgery.
   - ☐ 3. Contact the health care provider (HCP) to request a sedative.
   - ☐ 4. Be sure the dentist prescribes a prophylactic antibiotic before the oral surgery.

4. Amoxicillin trihydrate 300 mg oral (PO) has been prescribed for a client with an oral infection. The medication is available in a liquid suspension that is available as 250 mg/5 mL. How many milliliters should the nurse administer? Record your answer using a whole number.

   _____ mL.

5. During the assessment of a client's mouth, the nurse notes the absence of saliva. The client reports having pain behind the ear. The client has been nothing-by-mouth (NPO) for several days but now can have liquids. What should the nurse do **next**?
   - ☐ 1. Request a prescription for an antifungal mouthwash.
   - ☐ 2. Instruct the client to brush the gums as well as the teeth.
   - ☐ 3. Encourage the client to suck on hard candy.
   - ☐ 4. Give the client a hydrogen peroxide–based mouthwash.

6. The nurse is preparing a community presentation on oral cancer. Which is a **primary** risk factor for oral cancer that the nurse should emphasize in the presentation?
   - ☐ 1. use of alcohol
   - ☐ 2. frequent use of mouthwash
   - ☐ 3. lack of vitamin B_{12}
   - ☐ 4. lack of regular teeth cleaning by a dentist

7. A client has early signs of oral cancer. What should the nurse include in a focused assessment? Select all that apply.
   - ☐ 1. an infection or inflammation in the mouth
   - ☐ 2. lost the sense of taste
   - ☐ 3. difficulty swallowing
   - ☐ 4. significant weight loss
   - ☐ 5. changes in the frequency of urination
   - ☐ 6. numbness of the tongue

8. Following surgery to set a fractured mandible, the client has swelling at the surgery site. What is the **priority** goal of nursing care?
   - ☐ 1. Prevent nausea and vomiting.
   - ☐ 2. Maintain a patent airway.
   - ☐ 3. Provide frequent oral hygiene.
   - ☐ 4. Establish a way for the client to communicate.

The Adult with Peptic Ulcer Disease

9. A client is admitted to the hospital after vomiting bright red blood and is diagnosed with a bleeding duodenal ulcer. The client develops a sudden, sharp pain in the midepigastric region along with a rigid, boardlike abdomen. After obtaining the client's vital signs, what should the nurse do **next**?
☐ 1. Administer pain medication as prescribed.
☐ 2. Raise the head of the bed.
☐ 3. Prepare to insert a nasogastric tube.
☐ 4. Notify the health care provider (HCP).

10. The nurse is obtaining a nursing history from a client with a suspected gastric ulcer. Which sign(s) or symptom(s) should the nurse assess? Select all that apply.
☐ 1. epigastric pain at night
☐ 2. relief of epigastric pain after eating
☐ 3. vomiting
☐ 4. weight loss
☐ 5. melena

11. The nurse is caring for a client who has had a gastroscopy. Which finding(s) indicate that the client is developing a complication related to the procedure? Select all that apply.

The client:
☐ 1. has a sore throat.
☐ 2. has a temperature of 100°F (37.8°C).
☐ 3. appears drowsy following the procedure.
☐ 4. has epigastric pain.
☐ 5. experiences hematemesis.

12. A client admitted to the hospital with peptic ulcer disease tells the nurse about having black, tarry stools. What should the nurse do?
☐ 1. Encourage the client to increase fluid intake.
☐ 2. Advise the client to avoid iron-rich foods.
☐ 3. Place the client on contact precautions.
☐ 4. Report the finding to the health care provider (HCP).

13. A client with peptic ulcer disease is taking cimetidine. What is the expected outcome of this drug?
☐ 1. Heal the ulcer.
☐ 2. Protect the ulcer surface from acids.
☐ 3. Reduce acid concentration.
☐ 4. Limit gastric acid secretion.

14. A client with a peptic ulcer reports epigastric pain that frequently causes the client to wake up during the night. The nurse should instruct the client to take which action(s)? Select all that apply.
☐ 1. Obtain adequate rest to reduce stimulation.
☐ 2. Eat small, frequent meals throughout the day.
☐ 3. Take all medications on time as prescribed.
☐ 4. Sit up for 1 hour when awakened at night.
☐ 5. Stay away from crowded areas.

15. A client with peptic ulcer disease is taking omeprazole over the counter to relieve symptoms of stomach pain. The nurse should instruct the client that long-term use of this drug is a risk for which complication?
☐ 1. gastric bleeding
☐ 2. hip fracture
☐ 3. anemia
☐ 4. dizziness

16. The nurse is teaching a client with a peptic ulcer about the diet that should be followed after discharge. What types of food should the nurse suggest the client include in the diet?
☐ 1. bland foods
☐ 2. high-protein foods
☐ 3. any foods that are tolerated
☐ 4. a glass of milk with each meal

17. A client is diagnosed with peptic ulcer disease caused by *Helicobacter pylori* infection. The client is following a 2-week drug regimen that includes clarithromycin along with omeprazole and amoxicillin. How should the nurse instruct the client to take these medications?
☐ 1. Alternate the use of the drugs.
☐ 2. Take the drugs at different times during the day.
☐ 3. Discontinue all drugs if nausea occurs.
☐ 4. Take the drugs for the entire 2-week period.

18. A client with peptic ulcer disease is admitted to the hospital for a gastric resection. The client reports a sudden sharp pain in the midepigastric area that radiates to the shoulder. What should the nurse do **first**?
☐ 1. Establish an intravenous (IV) line.
☐ 2. Administer pain medication.
☐ 3. Notify the surgeon.
☐ 4. Call for a stat electrocardiogram (ECG).

19. A client is to take one daily dose of ranitidine at home to treat a peptic ulcer. Which response from the client indicates that the client understands how to take the medication?
"I'll take the drug:
☐ 1. before meals."
☐ 2. with meals."
☐ 3. at bedtime."
☐ 4. when pain occurs."

20. A client has been taking aluminum hydroxide 30 mL six times per day at home to treat a peptic ulcer. The client has been unable to have a bowel movement for 3 days. What should the nurse determine is the **most** likely cause of the client's constipation?
☐ 1. The client has not been including enough fiber in the diet.
☐ 2. The client needs to increase daily exercise.
☐ 3. The client is experiencing an adverse effect of aluminum hydroxide.
☐ 4. The client has developed a gastrointestinal obstruction.

The Adult with Cancer of the Stomach

21. The nurse is assessing a client who is being admitted to the hospital with upper gastrointestinal (GI) bleeding. Which finding(s) are significant? Select all that apply.
☐ 1. dry, flushed skin
☐ 2. decreased urine output
☐ 3. tachycardia
☐ 4. widening pulse pressure
☐ 5. rapid respirations
☐ 6. thirst

22. A client with cancer of the stomach had a total gastrectomy 2 days earlier. Which finding indicates the client is ready to try a liquid diet?

The client:
☐ 1. is hungry.
☐ 2. took pain medication 2 hours ago.
☐ 3. has frequent bowel sounds.
☐ 4. has had a bowel movement.

23. Within 6 hours following a subtotal gastrectomy, the drainage from the client's nasogastric (NG) tube is bright red. What should the nurse do **first**?
☐ 1. Clamp the NG tube.
☐ 2. Remove the existing NG tube.
☐ 3. Irrigate the NG tube with iced saline.
☐ 4. Chart the finding in the client's medical record.

24. Since receiving a diagnosis of stomach cancer, a client has been having trouble sleeping and is frequently preoccupied with thoughts about how life will change. The client says, "I wish my life could stay the same." The nurse determines that the client is experiencing which problem?
☐ 1. having difficulty coping
☐ 2. experiencing a sleep disorder
☐ 3. going through a grieving process
☐ 4. showing signs of anxiety disorder

25. A client has had a subtotal gastrectomy and has a nasogastric tube with intermittent suction. Twenty-four hours after the surgery, the drainage in the client's nasogastric tube is dark brown. What should the nurse do?
☐ 1. Reassure the client that this is normal drainage.
☐ 2. Irrigate the nasogastric tube.
☐ 3. Notify the health care provider (HCP).
☐ 4. Discontinue the suction.

26. Following a subtotal gastrectomy, a client has a nasogastric (NG) tube connected to low suction. What should the nurse do?
☐ 1. Irrigate the tube with 30 mL of sterile water every hour, if needed.
☐ 2. Reposition the tube if it is not draining well.
☐ 3. Monitor the client for nausea, vomiting, and abdominal distention.
☐ 4. Change to high suction if the drainage is sluggish on low suction.

27. A client who is recovering from gastric surgery is receiving intravenous (IV) fluids to be infused at 100 mL per hour. The IV tubing delivers 15 gtt/mL. The nurse should infuse the solution at a flow rate of how many drops per minute to ensure that the client receives 100 mL per hour? Record your answer using a whole number.

_____ gtt/min.

28. The client has just returned to the nursing unit following a gastrectomy. The nurse should place the client in which position?
☐ 1. prone
☐ 2. supine
☐ 3. low Fowler
☐ 4. lateral recumbent

29. The nurse is teaching a client who had a gastrectomy how to reduce the risk for dumping syndrome. What should the nurse teach the client to do?
☐ 1. Sit upright for 30 minutes after meals.
☐ 2. Drink liquids with meals, avoiding caffeine.
☐ 3. Avoid milk and other dairy products.
☐ 4. Decrease the carbohydrate content of meals.

30. A client who is recovering from a subtotal gastrectomy experiences dumping syndrome and is to eat six small meals a day. The client asks the nurse, "When will I be able to eat three meals a day again like I used to?" Which response by the nurse is **most** appropriate?
☐ 1. "Eating six meals a day is time-consuming, isn't it?"
☐ 2. "You will have to eat six small meals a day for the rest of your life."
☐ 3. "You will be able to tolerate three meals a day before you are discharged."
☐ 4. "Most clients can resume their normal meal patterns in about 6 to 12 months."

31. After a gastric resection for a malignant tumor, a client is scheduled to undergo radiation therapy. What is the **most** important information the nurse should include in the discharge teaching plan?
☐ 1. how to maintain adequate nutrition
☐ 2. what do for alopecia
☐ 3. how to exercise to attain activity goals
☐ 4. where to access community resources

32. One month following a subtotal gastrectomy for cancer, the nurse is evaluating the nursing care goal related to improved nutrition. What indicates that the client has attained the goal?

The client:
☐ 1. has regained weight loss.
☐ 2. has resumed their normal dietary intake of three meals a day.
☐ 3. has controlled nausea and vomiting through regular use of antiemetics.
☐ 4. has achieved adequate nutritional status through oral or parenteral feedings.

The Adult with Gastroesophageal Reflux Disease

33. A client is experiencing gastroesophageal reflux. What should the nurse teach the client about managing reflux?
☐ 1. Limit caffeine intake to two cups of coffee per day.
☐ 2. Do not lie down for 2 hours after eating.
☐ 3. Follow a low-protein diet.
☐ 4. Take medications with milk to decrease irritation.

34. The client is scheduled to have an upper gastrointestinal tract series of x-rays. Following the x-rays, what should the nurse instruct the client to do?
☐ 1. Take a laxative.
☐ 2. Follow a clear liquid diet.
☐ 3. Administer an enema.
☐ 4. Take an antiemetic.

35. A client who has been diagnosed with gastroesophageal reflux disease (GERD) has heartburn. To decrease the heartburn, the nurse should instruct the client to **eliminate** which item from the diet?
☐ 1. lean beef
☐ 2. air-popped popcorn
☐ 3. hot chocolate
☐ 4. raw vegetables

36. The client with gastroesophageal reflux disease (GERD) has a chronic cough. The nurse should further assess the client for which other possible problem?
☐ 1. development of laryngeal cancer
☐ 2. irritation of the esophagus
☐ 3. esophageal scar tissue formation
☐ 4. aspiration of gastric contents

37. The health care provider (HCP) has prescribed bethanechol for a client with gastroesophageal reflux disease (GERD). The nurse should assess the client for which adverse effect?
☐ 1. constipation
☐ 2. urinary urgency
☐ 3. hypertension
☐ 4. dry oral mucosa

38. The nurse is developing a care management plan with a client who has been diagnosed with gastroesophageal reflux disease (GERD). What should the nurse instruct the client to do? Select all that apply.
☐ 1. Avoid a diet high in fatty foods.
☐ 2. Avoid beverages that contain caffeine.
☐ 3. Eat three meals a day, with the largest meal being at dinner in the evening.
☐ 4. Avoid all alcoholic beverages.
☐ 5. Lie down after consuming each meal for 30 minutes.
☐ 6. Use over-the-counter (OTC) antisecretory agents rather than prescriptions.

39. The nurse is obtaining a health history from a client who has a sliding hiatal hernia associated with reflux. The nurse should ask the client about the presence of which symptom?
☐ 1. heartburn
☐ 2. jaundice
☐ 3. anorexia
☐ 4. stomatitis

40. The nurse is obtaining a health history for an adult with a possible hiatal hernia. Which is a risk factor for this client that would **most** likely contribute to the development of a hiatal hernia?
☐ 1. having a sedentary desk job
☐ 2. being 5 feet, 3 inches tall (160 cm) and weighing 190 lb (86.2 kg)
☐ 3. using laxatives frequently
☐ 4. being 40 years old

41. The nurse is developing a teaching plan with a client who has a hiatal hernia. What action should the nurse take that would be **most** helpful in promoting behavior changes for this client?
☐ 1. Introduce the client to other people who are successfully managing their care.
☐ 2. Include the client's daughter in the teaching so that they can help implement the plan.
☐ 3. Ask the client to identify other situations in which the client changed health care habits.
☐ 4. Provide reassurance that the client will be able to implement all aspects of the plan successfully.

42. The client has been taking magnesium hydroxide (milk of magnesia) to control symptoms of a hiatal hernia. The nurse should assess the client for which condition that is **most** commonly associated with the ongoing use of magnesium-based antacids?
☐ 1. anorexia
☐ 2. weight gain
☐ 3. diarrhea
☐ 4. constipation

43. The nurse is teaching a client about managing a hiatal hernia. Which lifestyle modification should the nurse encourage the client with a hiatal hernia to include in activities of daily living?
☐ 1. engaging in daily aerobic exercise
☐ 2. eliminating smoking and alcohol use
☐ 3. balancing activity and rest
☐ 4. avoiding high-stress situations

44. The nurse is developing a teaching plan for the client with a hiatal hernia. Asking the client about which work-related factors would be **most** helpful when teaching this client?
☐ 1. number and length of breaks
☐ 2. body mechanics used in lifting
☐ 3. temperature in the work area
☐ 4. cleaning solvents used

45. The nurse is instructing the client about health maintenance activities to help control symptoms from a hiatal hernia. Which statement would indicate that the client has understood the instructions?
☐ 1. "I will avoid lying down after a meal."
☐ 2. "I can still enjoy my potato chips and cola at bedtime."
☐ 3. "I wish I did not have to give up swimming."
☐ 4. "If I wear a girdle, I will have more support for my stomach."

46. The nurse is teaching the client with a hiatal hernia about taking metoclopramide hydrochloride. Which medication should the client avoid while taking this drug?
☐ 1. antacids
☐ 2. antihypertensives
☐ 3. anticoagulants
☐ 4. central nervous system depressants

47. A client is taking cimetidine to treat a hiatal hernia. The nurse should evaluate the client to determine whether the drug has been effective in preventing which health problem?
☐ 1. esophageal reflux
☐ 2. dysphagia
☐ 3. esophagitis
☐ 4. ulcer formation

48. The client asks the nurse if surgery is needed to correct a hiatal hernia. Which reply by the nurse would be **most** accurate?
☐ 1. "Surgery is usually required, though medical treatment is attempted first."
☐ 2. "Hiatal hernia symptoms can usually be successfully managed with diet modifications, medications, and lifestyle changes."
☐ 3. "Surgery is not performed for this type of hernia."
☐ 4. "A minor surgical procedure to reduce the size of the diaphragmatic opening will probably be planned."

Managing Care, Quality, and Safety of Adults with Upper Gastrointestinal Tract Health Problems

49. A client has returned from surgery during which the jaws were wired as treatment for a fractured mandible. The client is in stable condition. The nurse is instructing the unlicensed assistive personnel (UAP) on how to properly position the client. Which instruction about positioning would be appropriate for the nurse to give the UAP?
☐ 1. Keep the client in a side-lying position with the head slightly elevated.
☐ 2. Do not reposition the client without the assistance of a registered nurse (RN).
☐ 3. The client can assume any position that is comfortable.
☐ 4. Keep the client's head elevated on two pillows at all times.

50. The nurse has been assigned to provide care for four clients. In what order, from first to last, should the nurse assess these clients? All options must be used.

1. a client awaiting surgery for a hiatal hernia repair at 1100
2. a client with suspected gastric cancer who is on nothing-by-mouth (NPO) status for tests
3. a client with peptic ulcer disease experiencing a sudden onset of acute stomach pain
4. a client who is requesting pain medication 2 days after surgery to repair a fractured jaw

51. The nurse is caring for a client who has just had an upper gastrointestinal (GI) endoscopy. The client's vital signs must be taken every 30 minutes for 2 hours after the procedure. The nurse assigns an unlicensed assistive personnel (UAP) to take the vital signs. One hour later, the UAP reports the client, who was previously afebrile, has developed a temperature of 101.8°F (38.8°C). What should the nurse do **next**?
☐ 1. Promptly assess the client for potential perforation.
☐ 2. Tell the assistant to change thermometers and retake the temperature.
☐ 3. Plan to give the client acetaminophen to lower the temperature.
☐ 4. Ask the UAP to bathe the client with tepid water.

52. Which hospitalized client is at risk for developing parotitis?
☐ 1. a 50-year-old client with nausea and vomiting who is on nothing-by-mouth status
☐ 2. a 75-year-old client with diabetes who has ill-fitting dentures
☐ 3. an 80-year-old client who has poor oral hygiene and is dehydrated
☐ 4. a 65-year-old client with lung cancer who has a feeding tube in place

53. The nurse instructs the unlicensed assistive personnel (UAP) on how to provide oral hygiene for clients who cannot perform this task for themselves. Which technique should the nurse ask the UAP to incorporate into the client's daily care?
    ☐ 1. Assess the oral cavity each time mouth care is given and record observations.
    ☐ 2. Use a soft toothbrush to brush the client's teeth after each meal.
    ☐ 3. Swab the client's tongue, gums, and lips with a soft foam applicator every 2 hours.
    ☐ 4. Rinse the client's mouth with mouthwash several times a day.

54. The nurse is developing standards of care for a client with gastroesophageal reflux disease and wants to review current evidence for practice. Which resource will provide the **most** helpful information?
    ☐ 1. a review in the Cochrane Library
    ☐ 2. a literature search in a database, such as the Cumulative Index to Nursing and Allied Health Literature (CINAHL)
    ☐ 3. an online nursing textbook
    ☐ 4. the policy and procedure manual at the health care agency

55. The nurse in the intensive care unit is giving a hand-off of care report to the nurse in the postsurgical unit about a client who had a gastrectomy. What is the **most** effective way for the nurse to assure essential information about the client is reported?
    ☐ 1. Give the report face to face with both nurses in a quiet room.
    ☐ 2. Audiotape the report for future reference and documentation.
    ☐ 3. Use a checklist with information individualized for the client.
    ☐ 4. Document essential transfer information in the client's electronic health record.

56. A nurse is delegating activities to unlicensed assistive personnel (UAP). Which action(s) can be appropriately delegated? Select all that apply.
    ☐ 1. Assist a client with oral care prior to breakfast.
    ☐ 2. Ask about the location, quality, and radiation of pain.
    ☐ 3. Observe and document the effect of medication after it is administered by the nurse.
    ☐ 4. Measure and record intake and output throughout the shift.
    ☐ 5. Determine if the client is oriented to person, place, and time, and report findings to the nurse.
    ☐ 6. Change a simple dry dressing on a client's coccyx while bathing.

57. The nurse is making staffing assignments. Which client can be assigned to an unlicensed assistive personnel (UAP)?
    ☐ 1. a client with stomatitis who requires instruction about mouth care before discharge
    ☐ 2. a client who is having radiation for cancer of the stomach and is to have the radiation site bathed with warm water, followed by an application of a moisturizer
    ☐ 3. a client who had a gastric resection and has a nasogastric tube draining bright red blood
    ☐ 4. a client who had abdominal surgery and requires wet-to-dry dressing changes

Answers, Rationales, and Test-Taking Strategies

*The answers and rationales for each question follow below, along with keys (🔑) to the client need (CN) and cognitive level (CL) for each question. In addition, questions that measure clinical judgment will be coded (CJ). As you check your answers, use the **Content Mastery and Test-Taking Skill Self-Analysis** worksheet (tear-out worksheet in the back of the book) to identify the reason(s) for not answering the questions correctly. For additional information about test-taking skills and strategies for answering questions, refer to pages 12–51 in Part 1 of this book.*

The Adult with Disorders of the Oral Cavity

1. **3.** Following surgery for a fractured mandible, the client's jaws will be wired. The nurse should be prepared to intervene quickly in case the client develops respiratory distress or begins to choke or vomit. If the client begins to vomit, the nurse should assist the client to a sitting position and have the client bend over and expectorate the emesis into an emesis basin. Wire cutters or scissors should always be available in case the wires need to be cut in a medical emergency, but they are only used if the client cannot breathe or is choking. Suction equipment should be available to help clear the client's airway if necessary, but this is not the first course of action. The nurse should administer the antiemetic if the client reports nausea, but the drug will not be effective if the client is already vomiting.

    🔑 CN: Safety and infection control; CL: Apply

2. **4.** Clients with stomatitis (inflammation of the mouth) have significant discomfort, which impacts their ability to eat and drink. They will be most comfortable eating soft, bland foods and avoiding temperature extremes in their food and liquids. Gargling with an antiseptic mouthwash will be irritating to the mucosa. Mouth care should include gentle brushing with a soft toothbrush and flossing.

    CN: Basic care and comfort; CL: Analyze

3. **4.** Clients who are at risk for developing infective endocarditis due to cardiac conditions such as a history of bacterial endocarditis must take prophylactic antibiotics before any dental procedure that may cause bleeding. Gargling with saline or using mouthwash is not sufficient to prevent infection. The client will not need a sedative prior to the surgery.

    CN: Reduction of risk potential; CL: Analyze

4. **6 mL.** To administer 300 mg PO, the nurse will need to administer 6 mL. The following formula is used to calculate the correct dosage:

    300 mg/X mL = 250 mg/5 mL.

    CN: Pharmacological and parenteral therapies; CL: Apply

5. **3.** The lack of saliva, pain near the area of the ear, and the prolonged NPO status of the client are indications that the client may be developing parotitis, or inflammation of the parotid gland. Parotitis usually develops with dehydration combined with poor oral hygiene or when clients have been NPO for an extended period. Preventive measures include the use of sugarless hard candy or gum to stimulate saliva production, adequate hydration, and frequent mouth care. The client does not have indications of stomatitis (inflammation of the mouth), which produces excessive salivation and a sore mouth. The client does not have indications of oral candidiasis (thrush), which causes bluish-white mouth lesions, and the nurse does not need to request a prescription for an antifungal mouthwash. There are no indications that the client has gingivitis, which can be recognized by the inflamed gingiva and bleeding that occur during toothbrushing, and while the client should brush the teeth and gums, increasing salivation to prevent parotitis is the priority at this time.

    CN: Basic care and comfort; CL: Analyze

6. **1.** Chronic and excessive use of alcohol can lead to oral cancer. Smoking and the use of smokeless tobacco are other significant risk factors. Additional risk factors include chronic irritation such as a broken tooth or ill-fitting dentures, poor dental hygiene, overexposure to the sun (lip cancer), and syphilis. Use of mouthwash, lack of vitamin B_{12}, and lack of regular teeth cleaning appointments have not been implicated as primary risk factors for oral cancer.

    CN: Health promotion and maintenance; CL: Analyze

7. **-/+ 1, 3, 4, 6.** The nurse is conducting a focused assessment of the client's mouth and ability to obtain nutrition. Therefore, the nurse focuses on inspecting the mouth for infection or inflammation, determining if the client has difficulty swallowing, and assuring nutrition by noting weight loss. A sign of oral cancer is numbness of the tongue; losing a sense of taste is not an early sign of oral cancer. Urinary output, while important, is not a part of a focused assessment for this health problem.

    CN: Reduction of risk potential; CL: Analyze

8. **2.** The priority of care in the immediate postoperative phase is to maintain a patent airway. The nurse should observe the client carefully for signs of respiratory distress. If the client becomes nauseated, antiemetics should be administered to decrease the chance of vomiting with obstruction of the airway and aspiration of vomitus. Providing frequent oral hygiene and an alternative means of communication are important aspects of nursing care, but maintaining a patent airway is most important.

    CN: Physiological adaptation; CL: Analyze

The Adult with Peptic Ulcer Disease

9. **4.** The client is experiencing a perforation of the ulcer, and the nurse should notify the HCP immediately. The body reacts to the perforation of an ulcer by immobilizing the area as much as possible. This results in boardlike abdominal rigidity, usually with extreme pain. Perforation is a medical emergency requiring immediate surgical intervention because peritonitis develops quickly after perforation. Administering pain medication is not the first action, though the nurse should later institute measures to relieve pain. Elevating the head of the bed will not minimize the perforation. A nasogastric tube may be used following surgery.

    CN: Physiological adaptation; CL: Analyze

10. **-/+ 3, 4, 5.** Vomiting and weight loss are common with gastric ulcers. The client may also have blood

in the stools (melena) from gastric bleeding. Clients with a gastric ulcer are most likely to have a burning epigastric pain that occurs about 1 hour after eating. Eating frequently aggravates the pain. Clients with duodenal ulcers are more likely to have pain that occurs during the night and is frequently relieved by eating.

CN: Physiological adaptation; CL: Analyze

11. 2, 4, 5. Following a gastroscopy, the nurse should monitor the client for complications, which include perforation and the potential for aspiration. An elevated temperature, epigastric pain, or the vomiting of blood (hematemesis) are all indications of a possible perforation and should be reported promptly. A sore throat is a common occurrence following a gastroscopy. Clients are usually sedated to decrease anxiety, and the nurse would anticipate that the client will be drowsy following the procedure.

CN: Reduction of risk potential; CL: Analyze

12. 4. Black, tarry stools are an important warning sign of bleeding in peptic ulcer disease. Digested blood in the stool causes it to be black; the odor of the stool is very offensive. The nurse should instruct the client to report the incidence of black stools promptly to the HCP. Increasing fluids or avoiding iron-rich foods will not change the stool color or consistency if the stools contain digested blood. Until other information is available, it is not necessary to initiate contact precautions.

CN: Reduction of risk potential; CL: Analyze

13. 4. Histamine-2 (H_2) receptor antagonists, such as cimetidine, reduce gastric acid secretion. Antisecretory drugs, or proton pump inhibitors, such as omeprazole, help ulcers heal quickly in 4 to 8 weeks. Cytoprotective drugs, such as sucralfate, protect the ulcer surface against acid, bile, and pepsin. Antacids reduce acid concentration and help reduce symptoms.

CN: Pharmacological and parenteral therapies; CL: Evaluate

14. 1, 2, 3, 4. The nurse should encourage the client to reduce stimulation that may enhance gastric secretion. The nurse can also advise the client to utilize health practices that will prevent recurrences of ulcer pain, such as avoiding fatigue and eliminating smoking. Eating small, frequent meals helps to prevent gastric distention if not actively bleeding and decreases distention and release of gastrin. Medications should be administered promptly to maintain optimum levels. After awakening during the night, the client should eat a small snack and return to bed, keeping the head of the bed elevated for an hour after eating. It is not necessary to stay away from crowded areas.

CN: Physiological adaptation; CL: Analyze

15. 2. Long-term use of proton pump inhibitors such as omeprazole is a risk factor for fractures, particularly in the hip, spine, and wrist, and the nurse should instruct the client about this risk, particularly if the client is taking the drug in high doses. This drug does not contribute to gastric bleeding, anemia, or dizziness.

CN: Pharmacological and parenteral therapies CL: Analyze

16. 3. Diet therapy for ulcer disease is a controversial issue. There is no scientific evidence that diet therapy promotes healing. Most clients are instructed to follow a diet that they can tolerate. There is no need for the client to ingest only a bland or high-protein diet. Milk may be included in the diet, but it is not recommended in excessive amounts.

CN: Basic care and comfort; CL: Apply

17. 4. The use of the triple-therapy approach to the *H. pylori* infection has proved effective; therefore, the nurse advises the client to take the drugs as prescribed for the duration of the prescription. The nurse instructs the client to avoid alternating the use of the drugs and to take all medication at the same time, three times a day unless otherwise noted by the health care provider (HCP). Drugs have very few side effects; however, the nurse instructs the client to continue taking medications and contact the HCP if adverse effects occur.

CN: Pharmacological and parenteral therapies; CL: Analyze

18. 3. The sharp, sudden midepigastric pain indicates the client may have a perforated ulcer. The nurse notifies the surgeon and may then obtain prescriptions for pain medication and IV fluids. It is not necessary to first obtain an ECG because the pain from ulcer perforation is different from that of chest pain that may indicate coronary artery syndrome (crushing pain radiating to the jaw).

CN: Physiological adaptation; CL: Analyze

19. 3. Ranitidine blocks the secretion of hydrochloric acid. Clients who take only one daily dose of ranitidine are usually advised to take it at bedtime to inhibit the nocturnal secretion of acid. Clients who take the drug twice a day are advised to take it in the morning and at bedtime. It is not necessary to take the drug before meals. The client should take the drug regularly, not just when pain occurs.

🔑 CN: Pharmacological and parenteral therapies; CL: Evaluate

20. 3. It is most likely that the client is experiencing an adverse effect of the antacid. Antacids with aluminum salt products, such as aluminum hydroxide, form insoluble salts in the body. These precipitate and accumulate in the intestines, causing constipation. Increasing dietary fiber intake or daily exercise may be a beneficial lifestyle change for the client but is not likely to relieve constipation caused by the aluminum hydroxide. Constipation, in isolation from other symptoms, is not a sign of a bowel obstruction.

🔑 CN: Pharmacological and parenteral therapies; CL: Analyze

The Adult with Cancer of the Stomach

21. −/+ 2, 3, 5, 6. The client who is experiencing upper GI bleeding is at risk for developing hypovolemic shock from blood loss. Therefore, the signs and symptoms the nurse should expect to find are those related to hypovolemia, including decreased urine output, tachycardia, rapid respirations, and thirst. The client's skin would be cool and clammy, not dry, and flushed. The client would also be likely to develop hypotension, which would lead to a narrowing pulse pressure, not a widening pulse pressure.

🔑 CN: Physiological adaptation; CL: Analyze

22. 3. The client can begin eating with a liquid diet when bowel sounds return, usually in 2 to 3 days. The client may be hungry but cannot have oral fluids or foods until intestinal motility has been established. The client may continue to have postoperative pain for several days; because receiving a liquid diet does not depend on the client being pain free, the nurse can continue to offer pain medication. The client does not have to experience a bowel movement to receive fluids and food.

🔑 CN: Physiological adaptation; CL: Analyze

23. 4. NG drainage is expected to be bright red during the first 12 hours after surgery and then darken within 24 hours. The nurse notes the color of the drainage on the medical record and then monitors the change of color of the drainage throughout the immediate postoperative period. To prevent stress on the suture line, NG suction is applied, and patency of the tube is maintained. Removal of the NG tube may traumatize the surgical site. The NG tube is irrigated only if the health care provider prescribes irrigation because there is a danger of injury to the suture line; saline at room temperature is usually prescribed.

🔑 CN: Physiological adaptation; CL: Analyze

24. 3. The client is going through the grieving process as they adjust to the diagnosis. There are no indications of inadequate coping as the client is able to verbalize concerns. The client may be having thoughts about their new health status, but there is no indication that the client has a sleep disorder or has signs of an anxiety disorder.

🔑 CN: Physiological adaptation; CL: Apply

25. 1. About 12 to 24 hours after a subtotal gastrectomy, gastric drainage is normally brown, which indicates digested blood; the nurse can reassure the client that this is a normal color. The nasogastric tube does not need to be irrigated as it is draining normally. It is not necessary to notify the HCP unless the drainage contains bright red blood. The nurse should continue the suction until the HCP indicates to discontinue, usually when the drainage has stopped.

🔑 CN: Physiological adaptation; CL: Analyze

26. 3. Nausea, vomiting, or abdominal distention indicates that gas and secretions are accumulating within the gastric pouch due to impaired peristalsis or edema at the operative site and may indicate that the drainage system is not working properly. Saline is used to irrigate NG tubes. Hypotonic solutions such as water increase electrolyte loss. In addition, a health care provider's (HCP) prescription is needed to irrigate the NG tube because this procedure could disrupt the suture line. After gastric surgery, only the surgeon repositions the NG tube because of the danger of rupturing or dislodging the suture line. The amount of suction varies with the type of tube used and is prescribed by the HCP. High suction may create too much tension on the gastric suture line.

🔑 CN: Reduction of risk potential; CL: Analyze

27. 25 gtt/min. To administer IV fluids at 100 mL per hour using tubing that has a drip factor of 15 gtt/mL, the nurse should use the following formula: 100 mL/60 minutes × 15 gtt/1 mL = 25 gtt/min.

🔑 CN: Pharmacological and parenteral therapies; CL: Apply

28. 3. A client who has had abdominal surgery is best placed in a low Fowler position postoperatively. This positioning relaxes abdominal muscles and provides for maximum respiratory and cardiovascular function. The prone, supine, or lateral recumbent position would not be tolerated by a client who has had abdominal surgery, nor do those positions support respiratory or cardiovascular functioning.

🔑 CN: Physiological adaptation; CL: Analyze

29. **4.** Carbohydrates are restricted, but protein, including meat and dairy products, is recommended because it is digested more slowly. Lying down for 30 minutes after a meal is encouraged to slow the movement of the food bolus. Fluids are restricted to reduce the bulk of food. There is no need to avoid caffeine.

🔑 CN: Basic care and comfort; CL: Analyze

30. **4.** The symptoms related to dumping syndrome that occur after a gastrectomy usually disappear by 6 to 12 months after surgery. Most clients can begin to resume normal meal patterns after signs of the dumping syndrome have stopped. Acknowledging that eating six meals a day is time-consuming does not address the client's question and makes an assumption about the client's concerns. It is not necessarily true that a six-meal-a-day dietary pattern will be required for the rest of the client's life. Clients will not be able to eat three meals a day before hospital discharge.

🔑 CN: Physiological adaptation; CL: Analyze

31. **1.** Clients who have had gastric surgery are prone to postoperative complications, such as dumping syndrome and postprandial hypoglycemia, which can affect nutritional intake. Vitamin absorption can also be an issue, depending on the extent of the gastric surgery. Radiation therapy to the upper gastrointestinal area also can affect nutritional intake by causing anorexia, nausea, and esophagitis. The client would not be expected to develop alopecia. Exercise and activity levels as well as access to community resources are important teaching areas, but nutritional intake is a priority need.

🔑 CN: Reduction of risk potential; CL: Analyze

32. **4.** An appropriate expected outcome is for the client to achieve optimal nutritional status through the use of oral feedings or total parenteral nutrition (TPN). TPN may be used to supplement oral intake, or it may be used alone if the client cannot tolerate oral feedings. The client would not be expected to regain lost weight within 1 month after surgery or to tolerate a normal dietary intake of three meals a day. Nausea and vomiting would not be considered an expected outcome of gastric surgery, and regular use of antiemetics would not be anticipated.

🔑 CN: Physiological adaptation; CL: Evaluate

The Adult with Gastroesophageal Reflux Disease

33. **2.** The nurse should instruct the client to not lie down for about 2 hours after eating to prevent reflux. Caffeinated beverages decrease pressure in the lower esophageal sphincter, and milk increases gastric acid secretion, so these beverages should be avoided. The client is encouraged to follow a high-protein, low-fat diet and avoid foods that are irritating.

🔑 CN: Reduction of risk potential; CL: Analyze

34. **1.** The client should take a laxative after an upper gastrointestinal series to stimulate a bowel movement. This examination involves the administration of barium, which must be promptly eliminated from the body because it may harden and cause an obstruction. A clear liquid diet would have no effect on stimulating the removal of the barium. The client should not have nausea, and an antiemetic would not be necessary; additionally, the antiemetic will decrease peristalsis and increase the likelihood of eliminating the barium. An enema would be ineffective because the barium is too high in the gastrointestinal tract.

🔑 CN: Reduction of risk potential; CL: Analyze

35. **3.** With GERD, eating substances that decrease lower esophageal sphincter pressure causes heartburn. A decrease in the lower esophageal sphincter pressure allows gastric contents to reflux into the lower end of the esophagus. Foods that can cause a decrease in esophageal sphincter pressure include fatty foods, chocolate, caffeinated beverages, peppermint, and alcohol. A diet high in protein and low in fat is recommended for clients with GERD. Lean beef, popcorn, and raw vegetables would be acceptable.

🔑 CN: Physiological adaptation; CL: Analyze

36. **4.** Clients with GERD can develop pulmonary symptoms, such as coughing, wheezing, and dyspnea, that are caused by the aspiration of gastric contents. GERD does not predispose the client to the development of laryngeal cancer. Irritation of the esophagus and esophageal scar tissue formation can develop as a result of GERD. However, GERD is more likely to cause painful and difficult swallowing.

🔑 CN: Physiological adaptation; CL: Analyze

37. **2.** Bethanechol, a cholinergic drug, may be used in GERD to increase lower esophageal sphincter pressure and facilitate gastric emptying. Cholinergic adverse effects may include urinary urgency, diarrhea, abdominal cramping, hypotension, and increased salivation. To avoid these adverse effects, the client should be closely monitored to establish the minimum effective dose.

🔑 CN: Pharmacological and parenteral therapies; CL: Analyze

38. −/+ **1, 2, 4.** No specific diet is necessary, but foods that cause reflux are avoided, including fatty foods (which decrease the rate of gastric emptying) and foods that decrease lower esophageal sphincter pressure such as chocolate, peppermint, coffee, and tea. The client should also avoid alcohol. The client should not lie down for 3 to 4 hours after eating. Antisecretory agents decrease the secretion of hydrochloric acid by the stomach; some are available in both OTC and prescription formulations, but the OTC preparations have lower drug dosages compared with prescription drugs. Cimetidine, ranitidine, famotidine, and nizatidine are available in both formulations.

🔑 CN: Physiological adaptation; CL: Analyze

39. **1.** Heartburn, the most common symptom of a sliding hiatal hernia, results from reflux of gastric secretions into the esophagus. Regurgitation of gastric contents and dysphagia are other common symptoms. Jaundice, which results from a high concentration of bilirubin in the blood, is not associated with hiatal hernia. Anorexia is not a typical symptom of a hiatal hernia. Stomatitis is inflammation of the mouth.

🔑 CN: Physiological adaptation; CL: Analyze

40. **2.** Any factor that increases intra-abdominal pressure, such as obesity, can contribute to the development of a hiatal hernia. Other factors include abdominal straining, frequent heavy lifting, and pregnancy. Hiatal hernia is also associated with older age and occurs in women more frequently than in men. Having a sedentary desk job, using laxatives frequently, or being 40 years old is not likely to be a contributing factor in the development of a hiatal hernia.

🔑 CN: Health promotion and maintenance; CL: Analyze

41. **3.** Self-responsibility is the key to individual health maintenance. Using examples of situations in which the client has demonstrated self-responsibility can be reinforcing and supporting. The client has ultimate responsibility for personal health habits. Meeting other people who are managing their care and involving family members can be helpful, but individual motivation is more important. Reassurance can be helpful but is less important than individualization of care.

🔑 CN: Health promotion and maintenance; CL: Analyze

42. **3.** The magnesium salts in magnesium hydroxide are related to those found in laxatives and may cause diarrhea. Aluminum salt products can cause constipation. Many clients find that a combination product is required to maintain normal bowel elimination. The use of magnesium hydroxide does not cause anorexia or weight gain.

🔑 CN: Pharmacological and parenteral therapies; CL: Analyze

43. **2.** Smoking and alcohol use both reduce esophageal sphincter tone and can result in reflux. They therefore should be avoided by clients with hiatal hernia. Daily aerobic exercise, balancing activity and rest, and avoiding high-stress situations may increase the client's general health and well-being, but they are not directly associated with hiatal hernia.

🔑 CN: Health promotion and maintenance; CL: Analyze

44. **2.** Bending, especially after eating, can cause gastroesophageal reflux. Lifting heavy objects increases intra-abdominal pressure. Assessing the client's lifting techniques enables the nurse to evaluate the client's knowledge of factors contributing to hiatal hernia and how to prevent complications. The number and length of breaks, the temperature in the work area, and the cleaning solvents used are not directly related to the treatment of hiatal hernia.

🔑 CN: Health promotion and maintenance; CL: Create

45. **1.** A client with a hiatal hernia should avoid the recumbent position immediately after meals to minimize gastric reflux. Bedtime snacks, as well as high-fat foods and carbonated beverages, should be avoided. Excessive vigorous exercise also should be avoided, especially after meals, but there is no reason why the client must give up swimming. Wearing tight, constrictive clothing such as a girdle can increase intra-abdominal pressure and thus lead to reflux of gastric juices.

🔑 CN: Basic care and comfort; CL: Evaluate

46. **4.** Metoclopramide hydrochloride can cause sedation. Alcohol and other central nervous system depressants add to this sedation. A client who is taking this drug should be cautioned to avoid driving or performing other hazardous activities for a few hours after taking the drug.

Clients may take antacids, antihypertensives, and anticoagulants while on metoclopramide.

CN: Pharmacological and parenteral therapies; CL: Analyze

47. **3.** Cimetidine is a histamine receptor antagonist that decreases the quantity of gastric secretions. It may be used in hiatal hernia therapy to prevent or treat the esophagitis and heartburn associated with reflux. Cimetidine is not used to prevent reflux, dysphagia, or ulcer development.

CN: Pharmacological and parenteral therapies; CL: Apply

48. **2.** Most clients can be treated successfully with a combination of diet restrictions, medications, weight control, and lifestyle modifications. Surgery to correct a hiatal hernia, which commonly produces complications, is performed only when medical therapy fails to control the symptoms.

CN: Reduction of risk potential; CL: Analyze

Managing Care, Quality, and Safety of Adults with Upper Gastrointestinal Tract Health Problems

49. **1.** Immediately after surgery, the client should be placed on the side with the head slightly elevated. This position helps facilitate the removal of secretions and decreases the likelihood of aspiration should vomiting occur. An RN does not need to be present to reposition the client unless the client's condition warrants the presence of the nurse. Although it is important to elevate the head, there is no need to keep the client's head elevated on two pillows unless that position is comfortable for the client.

CN: Reduction of risk potential; CL: Analyze

50. **3, 4, 2, 1.** The client with peptic ulcer disease who is experiencing a sudden onset of acute stomach pain should be assessed first by the nurse. The sudden onset of stomach pain could be indicative of a perforated ulcer, which would require immediate medical attention. It is also important for the nurse to thoroughly assess the nature of the client's pain. The client with the fractured jaw is experiencing pain and should be assessed next. The nurse should then assess the client who is NPO for tests to ensure NPO status and comfort. Last, the nurse can assess the client before surgery.

CN: Management of care; CL: Analyze

51. **1.** A sudden spike in temperature following an endoscopic procedure may indicate perforation of the GI tract. The nurse should promptly conduct a further assessment of the client, looking for further indicators of perforation, such as a sudden onset of acute upper abdominal pain; a rigid, boardlike abdomen; and developing signs of shock. Telling the assistant to change thermometers is not an appropriate action and only further delays the appropriate action of assessing the client. The nurse would not administer acetaminophen without further assessment of the client or without a health care provider's prescription; a suspected perforation would require that the client be placed on nothing-by-mouth status. Asking the assistant to bathe the client before any assessment by the nurse is inappropriate.

CN: Management of care; CL: Analyze

52. **3.** Parotitis is inflammation of the parotid gland. Although any of the clients listed could develop parotitis, given the data provided, the one most likely to develop parotitis is the older adult client who is dehydrated with poor oral hygiene. Any client who experiences poor oral hygiene is at risk for developing parotitis. To help prevent parotitis, it is essential for the nurse to ensure the client receives oral hygiene at regular intervals and has an adequate fluid intake.

CN: Reduction of risk potential; CL: Analyze

53. **2.** A soft toothbrush should be used to brush the client's teeth after every meal and more often as needed. Mechanical cleaning is necessary to maintain oral health, stimulate gingiva, and remove plaque. Assessing the oral cavity and recording observations are the responsibilities of the nurse, not of the UAP. Swabbing with a safe foam applicator does not provide enough friction to clean the mouth. Mouthwash can be a drying irritant and is not recommended for frequent use.

CN: Basic care and comfort; CL: Analyze

54. **1.** The Cochrane Library provides systematic reviews of health care interventions and will provide the best resource for evidence for nursing care. The CINAHL offers keyword searches to published articles in nursing and allied health literature, but not reviews. A nursing textbook has information about nursing care, which may include evidence-based practices, but textbooks may not have the most up-to-date information. While the policy and procedure manual may be based on evidence-based practices, the most current practices will be found in evidence-based reviews of literature.

CN: Management of care; CL: Apply

55. 3. Using a checklist assures that all key information is reported; the checklist can then serve as a record to which nurses can refer later. Giving a verbal report leaves room for error in memory; using an audiotape or an electronic health record requires nurses to spend unnecessary time retrieving information.

　CN: Management of care; CL: Apply

56. -/+ **1, 4.** Although the nurse is still responsible for following up to make sure oral care is completed and accurate intake and output is ongoing, these are appropriate tasks to delegate to UAP. Evaluating the level of consciousness (orientation), pain, and the effect of medications given by the nurse requires nursing judgment and should not be delegated to UAP. Although UAP often assist clients with bathing, dressing changes are not delegated to UAP as the wound should be assessed by a nurse while changing the dressing.

　CN: Management of care; CL: Analyze

57. 2. The care of the client who is having radiation treatments and who requires skin care at the site that involves bathing and application of a nonmedicated moisturizer is within the scope of practice for the UAP. Discharge planning, assessing drainage, and changing wet-to-dry dressings are nursing care activities that must be performed by a licensed nurse.

　CN: Management of care; CL: Analyze

TEST 6: The Adult with Lower Gastrointestinal Tract Health Problems

- The Adult with Cancer of the Colon
- The Adult with Hemorrhoids
- The Adult with an Ileostomy
- The Adult with an Intestinal Obstruction
- The Adult Receiving Total Parenteral Nutrition
- The Adult with Diverticular Disease
- The Adult with Appendicitis
- The Adult with an Inguinal Hernia
- Managing Care, Quality, and Safety for Adults with Lower Gastrointestinal Tract Health Problems
- Answers, Rationales, and Test-Taking Strategies

The Adult with Cancer of the Colon

1. A client refuses to look at or care for their colostomy. Which statement by the nurse would be **most** appropriate?
   - ☐ 1. "It's been 4 days since your surgery, and you'll soon be discharged. You have to learn to care for your colostomy before you leave the hospital."
   - ☐ 2. "I think we will need to teach your spouse to care for your colostomy if you are not going to be able to do it."
   - ☐ 3. "I understand how you are feeling. It is important for you to feel attractive, and you think having a colostomy changes your attractiveness."
   - ☐ 4. "I can see that you are upset. Would you like to share your concerns with me?"

2. The nurse is conducting a wellness program for adults about cancer. The nurse should teach clients about which potential risk factor for the development of colon cancer?
   - ☐ 1. chronic constipation
   - ☐ 2. long-term use of laxatives
   - ☐ 3. history of smoking
   - ☐ 4. history of inflammatory bowel disease

3. A client had a colon resection yesterday. The client's hemoglobin reading was 14.1 g/dL (141 g/L) yesterday, and today it is 7.2 g/dL (72 g/L). The client's oxygen saturation is 87%. After reviewing the chart (see chart) and notifying the health care provider, the nurse should do which action **first**?

   Prescriptions
   - 1000 mL normal saline every 8 hours at 125 gtt/h
   - Vital signs every 4 hours
   - Morphine sulfate 10 mg IV every 4 hours as needed for pain
   - Nothing by mouth
   - Oxygen 2 to 4 L/min per mask

   - ☐ 1. Take vital signs every hour.
   - ☐ 2. Increase the saline infusion to 150 gtt/h.
   - ☐ 3. Administer oxygen at 2 L per minute.
   - ☐ 4. Determine when pain medication was last administered.

4. A client with colon cancer is having a barium enema. The nurse should instruct the client to take which type of medication after the procedure is completed?
   ☐ 1. laxative
   ☐ 2. anticholinergic
   ☐ 3. antacid
   ☐ 4. demulcent

5. A client has a nasogastric tube inserted at the time of an abdominal-perineal resection with a permanent colostomy for colon cancer. When should the nurse tell the client that the tube will **most** likely be removed?
   ☐ 1. The client no longer has nausea and vomiting.
   ☐ 2. Mucus from passes from the rectum.
   ☐ 3. Gas and fecal material pass from the colostomy.
   ☐ 4. There is absence of stomach drainage for 24 hours.

6. A client with colon cancer has an abdominal-perineal resection with a colostomy. To promote hygiene following surgery, the nurse should take which action?
   ☐ 1. Maintain the client in a semi-Fowler's position.
   ☐ 2. Assist the client with warm sitz baths.
   ☐ 3. Administer 30 mL of milk of magnesia to stimulate peristalsis.
   ☐ 4. Remove the ostomy pouch as needed so the stoma can be assessed.

7. The nurse assesses the client's stoma during the initial postoperative period. What observation should the nurse report to the health care provider (HCP) **immediately**?

   The stoma:
   ☐ 1. is slightly edematous.
   ☐ 2. is dark red to purple.
   ☐ 3. oozes a small amount of blood.
   ☐ 4. does not expel stool.

8. The nurse is changing the client's colostomy bag and dressing. What observation will indicate to the nurse that the client is ready to participate in self-care?

   The client:
   ☐ 1. asks if the health care provider (HCP) will change the dressing soon.
   ☐ 2. asks about the supplies used during the dressing change.
   ☐ 3. inquires about who will change the dressing at home.
   ☐ 4. is upset about the way the night nurse changed the dressing.

9. The nurse is instructing the client with a new colostomy about protecting the skin around the colostomy. Which skin barrier should the nurse tell the client is **best** to apply around the colostomy?
   ☐ 1. adhesive skin barrier
   ☐ 2. petroleum jelly
   ☐ 3. cornstarch
   ☐ 4. antiseptic cream

10. The nurse is teaching the client who has a colostomy about diet management. Which information should the nurse discuss with the client?
    ☐ 1. Avoid foods containing roughage.
    ☐ 2. Liquids are best limited to prevent diarrhea.
    ☐ 3. Experiment to find what diet works best.
    ☐ 4. Follow a high-fiber diet.

11. The nurse is teaching a client who is recovering from an abdominal-perineal resection with a colostomy about health promotion. What is an expected outcome for a client during the first 2 weeks after surgery?
    ☐ 1. maintaining a fluid intake of 3000 mL a day
    ☐ 2. eliminating fiber from the diet
    ☐ 3. limiting physical activity to light exercise
    ☐ 4. accepting that sexual activity will be diminished

12. A client with colon cancer has developed ascites. The nurse should conduct a focused assessment for which additional sign(s) or symptom(s)? Select all that apply.
    ☐ 1. respiratory distress
    ☐ 2. bleeding
    ☐ 3. fluid and electrolyte imbalance
    ☐ 4. weight gain
    ☐ 5. infection

13. A client has 4000 mL excess fluid removed via paracentesis. When the nurse weighs the client after the procedure, how many kilograms is an expected weight loss? Record your answer in whole numbers.

    _____ kg.

14. Two days following a colon resection, an older adult client shows new-onset confusion. When contacting the health care provider, the nurse should make which recommendation?
    ☐ 1. "Do you want to request a computed tomography scan to rule out stroke?"
    ☐ 2. "May we have a prescription for restraining this client?"
    ☐ 3. "Shall I collect and send a urine sample for culture and sensitivity?"
    ☐ 4. "Would you like a stat potassium level done?"

15. The nurse is caring for a 70-year-old male client after a colectomy. The client received chemotherapy before surgery and has hypertension and diabetes mellitus. Which factor(s) would put this client at risk for sepsis? Select all that apply.
☐ 1. age of 70
☐ 2. abdominal surgery
☐ 3. sex
☐ 4. diabetes mellitus
☐ 5. weight

The Adult with Hemorrhoids

16. A 36-year-old female client has been diagnosed with hemorrhoids. Which factor in the client's history would **most** likely be a primary cause of the hemorrhoids?
☐ 1. the client's age
☐ 2. three vaginal births
☐ 3. the client's job as a schoolteacher
☐ 4. varicosities in the client's legs

17. The nurse is teaching a client who has had a hemorrhoidectomy about postoperative care at home. The nurse should tell the client not to use sitz baths until at least 12 hours postoperatively to avoid causing which complication?
☐ 1. bleeding
☐ 2. rectal spasm
☐ 3. urine retention
☐ 4. constipation

18. The nurse teaches a client who has had rectal surgery the proper timing for a cleansing sitz bath. What will indicate to the nurse that the client has understood when to take the sitz bath? The client will take the sitz bath:
☐ 1. first thing each morning.
☐ 2. as needed for discomfort.
☐ 3. after a bowel movement.
☐ 4. at bedtime.

The Adult with Ulcerative Colitis

19. A client who is experiencing an exacerbation of ulcerative colitis is receiving intravenous (IV) fluids that are to be infused at 125 mL per hour. The IV tubing delivers 15 gtt/mL. How quickly should the nurse infuse the fluids in drops per minute to infuse the fluids at the prescribed rate? Record your answer using a whole number.

_____ gtt/min.

20. The nurse is planning care for a client who is being treated for an exacerbation of ulcerative colitis. Which goal is the **priority**?
☐ 1. promoting self-care and independence
☐ 2. managing diarrhea
☐ 3. maintaining adequate nutrition
☐ 4. promoting rest and comfort

21. The client with an exacerbation of ulcerative colitis is to be on bed rest with bathroom privileges. What will indicate to the nurse that being on bed rest has had the desired outcome?

The client has:
☐ 1. not fallen.
☐ 2. slowed intestinal peristalsis.
☐ 3. slept through the night.
☐ 4. minimized stress.

22. A client has had an exacerbation of ulcerative colitis with cramping and diarrhea persisting longer than 1 week. The nurse should assess the client for which complication?
☐ 1. heart failure
☐ 2. deep vein thrombosis
☐ 3. hypokalemia
☐ 4. hypocalcemia

23. A client who has ulcerative colitis says to the nurse, "I can't take this anymore; I'm constantly in pain, and I can't leave my room because I need to stay by the toilet. I don't know how to deal with this." Based on these comments, what judgment should the nurse make about what the client is experiencing?
☐ 1. extreme fatigue
☐ 2. disturbed thought
☐ 3. a sense of isolation
☐ 4. difficulty coping

24. A client newly diagnosed with ulcerative colitis who has been placed on steroids asks the nurse why steroids are prescribed. What should the nurse tell the client?
☐ 1. "Ulcerative colitis can be cured by the use of steroids."
☐ 2. "Steroids are used in severe flare-ups because they can decrease the incidence of bleeding."
☐ 3. "Long-term use of steroids will prolong periods of remission."
☐ 4. "The side effects of steroids outweigh their benefits to clients with ulcerative colitis."

25. A client who has ulcerative colitis has persistent diarrhea and has lost 12 lb (5.5 kg) since the exacerbation of the disease. Which approach will be **most** effective in helping the client meet nutritional needs and allow healing?
☐ 1. continuous enteral feedings
☐ 2. following a high-calorie, high-protein diet
☐ 3. total parenteral nutrition (TPN)
☐ 4. eating six small meals a day

26. A client with ulcerative colitis is to take sulfasalazine. Which instruction(s) should the nurse give the client about taking this medication at home? Select all that apply.
☐ 1. Drink enough fluids to maintain a urine output of at least 1200 to 1500 mL a day.
☐ 2. Discontinue therapy if symptoms of acute intolerance develop, and notify the health care provider (HCP).
☐ 3. Stop taking the medication if the urine turns orange-yellow.
☐ 4. Avoid activities that require alertness.
☐ 5. If a dose is missed, skip it and continue with the next dose.

27. The nurse has a prescription to administer sulfasalazine 2 g. The medication is available in 500-mg tablets. How many tablets should the nurse administer?

_____ tablets.

28. The nurse is instructing the client with ulcerative colitis about the best diet to maintain nutrition for tissue healing while avoiding foods that will exacerbate ulceration. Which diet would be **most** appropriate?
☐ 1. high-calorie, low-protein
☐ 2. high-protein, low-residue
☐ 3. low-fat, high-fiber
☐ 4. low-sodium, high-carbohydrate

The Adult with an Ileostomy

29. The nurse is teaching a client how to care for an ileostomy. The client asks the nurse how long to wear the pouch before changing it. What should the nurse tell the client?
☐ 1. "The pouch is changed only when it leaks."
☐ 2. "You can wear the pouch for about 4 to 7 days."
☐ 3. "You should change the pouch every evening before bedtime."
☐ 4. "It depends on your activity level and your diet."

30. A client is scheduled for an ileostomy. Which would be **most** helpful in preparing the client psychologically for the surgery?
☐ 1. Include family members in preoperative teaching sessions.
☐ 2. Encourage the client to ask questions about managing an ileostomy.
☐ 3. Provide a brief, thorough explanation of all preoperative and postoperative procedures.
☐ 4. Invite a member of the ostomy association to visit the client.

31. The nurse is preparing a client for an ileostomy. Two weeks before the surgery, the nurse should instruct the client to take which action?
☐ 1. Stop taking drugs that will interfere with clotting.
☐ 2. Follow a low-residue diet.
☐ 3. Limit fluids to 1000 mL a day.
☐ 4. Report having a temperature above 99°F (37.2°C).

32. The nurse is planning care for a client who had surgery 24 hours ago to create an ileostomy. Which goal has the **highest priority**?
☐ 1. providing relief from constipation
☐ 2. assisting the client with self-care activities
☐ 3. maintaining fluid and electrolyte balance
☐ 4. minimizing odor formation

33. The client asks the nurse, "Is it really possible to lead a normal life with an ileostomy?" Which action by the nurse would be the **most** effective to address this question?
☐ 1. Have the client talk with a member of the clergy about these concerns.
☐ 2. Tell the client to worry about those concerns after surgery.
☐ 3. Arrange for a person with an ostomy to visit the client preoperatively.
☐ 4. Notify the health care provider (HCP) of the client's question.

34. Three weeks after the client has had an ileostomy, the nurse is following up with instructions on using a skin barrier around the stoma. How will the nurse determine that the client has been applying the skin barrier correctly?
☐ 1. There is no odor from the stoma.
☐ 2. The client is adequately hydrated.
☐ 3. There is no skin irritation around the stoma.
☐ 4. The client only changes the ostomy pouch once a day.

35. The nurse is teaching a client about managing an ileostomy. What observation should the nurse instruct the client with an ileostomy to report **immediately**?
☐ 1. passage of liquid stool from the stoma
☐ 2. occasional presence of undigested food in the effluent
☐ 3. absence of drainage from the ileostomy for 6 or more hours
☐ 4. temperature of 99.8°F (37.7°C)

36. The nurse finds the client who has had an ileostomy crying. The client explains to the nurse, "I'm upset because I know I won't be able to have children now that I have an ileostomy." Which response by the nurse is **best**?
☐ 1. "Many women with ileostomies decide to adopt. Perhaps you could consider that option?"
☐ 2. "Having an ileostomy doesn't necessarily mean that you can't have children. Let's talk about your concerns."
☐ 3. "I can understand your reasons for being upset. Having children must be important to you."
☐ 4. "I'm sure you will adjust to this situation with time. Try not to be too upset."

37. Which statement about ileostomy care indicates that the client understands the discharge instructions?
☐ 1. "I should be able to resume weight lifting in 2 weeks."
☐ 2. "I can return to work in 2 weeks."
☐ 3. "I need to drink at least 3000 mL a day of fluid."
☐ 4. "I will need to avoid getting my stoma wet while bathing."

38. A client with a well-managed ileostomy has the sudden onset of abdominal cramps, vomiting, and watery discharge from the ileostomy. What should the nurse tell the client to do?
☐ 1. Take an antiemetic.
☐ 2. Increase fluid intake to 3 L per day.
☐ 3. Use 30 mL of milk of magnesia daily.
☐ 4. Notify the health care provider (HCP).

The Adult with an Intestinal Obstruction

39. A nurse is assessing a client who has been admitted with a diagnosis of an obstruction in the small intestine. The nurse should assess the client for which sign(s) or symptom(s)? Select all that apply.
☐ 1. projectile vomiting
☐ 2. significant abdominal distention
☐ 3. copious diarrhea
☐ 4. rapid onset of dehydration
☐ 5. increased bowel sounds

40. A client is admitted with a bowel obstruction. The client has nausea, vomiting, and crampy abdominal pain. The health care provider (HCP) has written the following prescriptions: for the client to be up ad lib, have narcotics for pain, have a nasogastric tube inserted if needed, and for intravenous (IV) Ringer's lactate and hyperalimentation fluids. What should the nurse do in order of priority from first to last? All options must be used.

1. Assist with ambulation to promote peristalsis.
2. Insert a nasogastric tube.
3. Administer IV Ringer's lactate.
4. Start an infusion of hyperalimentation fluids.

41. The health care provider (HCP) prescribes intestinal decompression with a Cantor tube for a client with an intestinal obstruction. What should the nurse evaluate to determine the effectiveness of intestinal decompression?
☐ 1. Intestinal fluid and gas have been removed.
☐ 2. The client has had a bowel movement.
☐ 3. The client's urinary output is adequate.
☐ 4. The client can sit up without pain.

42. The client has had a nasoenteric tube inserted. The nurse should place the client in which position?
☐ 1. supine
☐ 2. right side-lying
☐ 3. semi-Fowler's
☐ 4. upright in a bedside chair

43. The client with an intestinal obstruction continues to have acute pain even though the nasoenteric tube is patent and draining. What should the nurse do **first**?
☐ 1. Reassure the client that the nasoenteric tube is functioning.
☐ 2. Assess the client for signs of peritonitis.
☐ 3. Administer an opioid as prescribed.
☐ 4. Reposition the client on the left side.

44. Before a client undergoes abdominal surgery for an intestinal obstruction, the nurse monitors the client's urine output and finds that the total output for the past 2 hours was 35 mL. The nurse then assesses the client's total intake and output over the last 24 hours and notes 2000 mL of intravenous fluid for intake, 500 mL of drainage from the nasogastric tube, and 700 mL of urine, for a total output of 1200 mL. How should the nurse interpret these findings?
    ☐ 1. decreased renal function
    ☐ 2. the nasogastric tube not draining well
    ☐ 3. extension of the obstruction
    ☐ 4. inadequate fluid replacement

The Adult Receiving Total Parenteral Nutrition

45. The nurse is changing the subclavian dressing of a client who is receiving total parenteral nutrition. When assessing the catheter insertion site, the nurse notes the presence of yellow drainage from around the sutures that are anchoring the catheter. What should the nurse do **first**?
    ☐ 1. Clean the insertion site and redress the area.
    ☐ 2. Document assessment findings in the client's chart.
    ☐ 3. Request a prescription to obtain a culture of the drainage.
    ☐ 4. Check the client's temperature.

46. The health care provider (HCP) has ordered total parenteral nutrition (TPN) for a client who has recently had a small and large bowel resection and who is currently not taking anything by mouth. What should the nurse do to safely administer the TPN?
    ☐ 1. Administer the TPN through a nasogastric or gastrostomy tube.
    ☐ 2. Handle the TPN using strict aseptic technique.
    ☐ 3. Auscultate for the presence of bowel sounds before administering the TPN.
    ☐ 4. Designate a peripheral intravenous (IV) site for TPN administration.

47. Using a sliding scale schedule, the nurse is preparing to administer an evening dose of regular insulin to a client who is receiving total parenteral nutrition (TPN). On which information should the nurse base the dosage?
    ☐ 1. glucometer reading of the client's glucose level obtained immediately before administering the insulin
    ☐ 2. fasting blood glucose level obtained earlier in the day
    ☐ 3. amount of TPN fluid the client has received since the last dose of insulin
    ☐ 4. client's dietary intake for the evening meal and snack

48. A nurse is assisting the health care provider (HCP) with the removal of a central venous access device (CVAD). What should the nurse do to prepare the client?
    ☐ 1. Turn the client to the left side.
    ☐ 2. Have the client exhale slowly and evenly.
    ☐ 3. Elevate the head of the bed.
    ☐ 4. Instruct the client to take a deep breath and hold it.

49. A client is receiving total parenteral nutrition (TPN) solution. The nurse should assess a client's ability to metabolize the TPN solution adequately by monitoring the client for which sign?
    ☐ 1. tachycardia
    ☐ 2. hypertension
    ☐ 3. elevated blood urea nitrogen concentration
    ☐ 4. hyperglycemia

50. A client is receiving total parenteral nutrition (TPN) through a central line. What should the nurse do to prevent complications associated with this infusion? Select all that apply.
    ☐ 1. Use aseptic technique for dressing changes.
    ☐ 2. Secure all connections of the system.
    ☐ 3. Keep the client in a supine position for 24 hours after insertion.
    ☐ 4. Cover the insertion site with a moisture-proof dressing.
    ☐ 5. Limit ambulation to walking to the bathroom.

51. A client is receiving total parenteral nutrition (TPN) therapy. Which finding should the nurse report to the health care provider?
    ☐ 1. glycosuria
    ☐ 2. a 1- to 2-lb (0.45- to 0.9-kg) weight gain
    ☐ 3. decreased appetite
    ☐ 4. elevated temperature

52. The nurse is assessing a client who is receiving an infusion of total parenteral nutrition (TPN). The infusion rate is now faster than prescribed. After adjusting the infusion rate, the nurse should assess the client for which adverse effect?
    ☐ 1. negative nitrogen balance
    ☐ 2. circulatory overload
    ☐ 3. hypoglycemia
    ☐ 4. hypokalemia

The Adult with Diverticular Disease

53. The nurse is teaching a client with diverticulosis about dietary management of the disease. Which food(s) should the nurse encourage the client to incorporate into their diet? Select all that apply.
    ☐ 1. bran cereal
    ☐ 2. broccoli
    ☐ 3. tomato juice
    ☐ 4. navy beans
    ☐ 5. cheese

54. A client is having an acute attack of diverticulitis. What should the nurse do **first**?
☐ 1. Prepare the client for a colonoscopy.
☐ 2. Encourage the client to eat a high-fiber diet.
☐ 3. Assess the client for signs of peritonitis.
☐ 4. Encourage the client to drink a glass of water every 2 hours.

55. The nurse is teaching a client about managing diverticulitis. The nurse should teach the client to integrate which measure into their daily routine?
☐ 1. using enemas to relieve constipation
☐ 2. decreasing fluid intake to increase the formed consistency of the stool
☐ 3. eating a high-fiber diet when symptomatic with diverticulitis
☐ 4. refraining from straining and lifting activities

56. The nurse is instructing a client with diverticulosis about appropriate self-care activities. Which comment(s) by the client would indicate effective teaching? Select all that apply.
☐ 1. "With careful attention to my diet, my diverticulosis can be cured."
☐ 2. "Using a cathartic laxative weekly is okay to control bowel movements."
☐ 3. "I should follow a diet that is high in fiber."
☐ 4. "It is important for me to drink at least 2000 mL of fluid every day."
☐ 5. "I should exercise regularly."

57. A client with diverticular disease is receiving psyllium hydrophilic mucilloid. Which response from the client indicates to the nurse that the drug is having the intended effect?
☐ 1. "I can pass stool without cramping."
☐ 2. "I have occasional diarrhea."
☐ 3. "My stool is firm."
☐ 4. "I don't expel gas."

58. A client with diverticulitis has developed peritonitis following diverticular rupture. When assessing the client, the nurse should perform which action? Select all that apply.
☐ 1. Percuss the abdomen to note tympany.
☐ 2. Percuss the liver to note lack of dullness.
☐ 3. Monitor the vital signs for fever.
☐ 4. Assess the presence of excessive thirst.
☐ 5. Auscultate bowel sounds to note frequency.

The Adult with Appendicitis

59. A nurse is providing wound care to a client 1 day after an appendectomy. A drain was inserted into the incisional site during surgery. What should the nurse do to provide wound care?
☐ 1. Remove the dressing, and leave the incision open to air.
☐ 2. Remove the drain if wound drainage is minimal.
☐ 3. Gently irrigate the drain to remove exudate.
☐ 4. Clean the area around the drain, moving away from the drain.

60. An adult with appendicitis has severe abdominal pain. Which action will be the **most** effective to assist the client to manage pain before surgery?
☐ 1. Place the client in semi-Fowler's position with the knee gatch raised.
☐ 2. Apply moist heat to the abdomen.
☐ 3. Teach the client to massage the painful area.
☐ 4. Provide distraction with music.

61. The nurse is instructing a client about postoperative care following a laparoscopic appendectomy. What information should the nurse include in the teaching plan? Select all that apply.
☐ 1. "Nausea, gas, and diarrhea are normal for several days."
☐ 2. "You can return to work in 1 to 3 weeks."
☐ 3. "Follow a low-residue diet until the incision has healed."
☐ 4. "Take a tub bath to relieve abdominal swelling."
☐ 5. "You can drive when you are not taking pain medications."

62. A client who had an open appendectomy for a perforated appendix has an incision secured with adhesive strips. What instruction should the nurse give the client about caring for the incision?
☐ 1. Remove the adhesive strips to cleanse the area.
☐ 2. Cover the adhesive strips with a dressing to protect the area.
☐ 3. Leave the adhesive strips in place until they fall off.
☐ 4. Place plastic wrap over the incision when taking a bath.

The Adult with an Inguinal Hernia

63. A client who has a history of an inguinal hernia is admitted to the hospital with sudden, severe abdominal pain, vomiting, and abdominal distention. The nurse should assess the client further for which complication?
☐ 1. peritonitis
☐ 2. incarcerated hernia
☐ 3. strangulated hernia
☐ 4. intestinal perforation

64. The nurse is providing discharge instructions for a client who had an inguinal herniorrhaphy. What information should the nurse give the client?
☐ 1. Cough and deep breathe every 2 hours.
☐ 2. Apply warm, moist heat to the groin.
☐ 3. Sneeze with the mouth closed.
☐ 4. Avoid lifting items weighing more than 5 lb (2.3 kg).

65. The nurse is assessing a male client who has an inguinal herniorrhaphy. The nurse should assess the male client carefully for which potential complication?
    ☐ 1. hypostatic pneumonia
    ☐ 2. deep vein thrombosis
    ☐ 3. paralytic ileus
    ☐ 4. urine retention

Managing Care, Quality, and Safety for Adults with Lower Gastrointestinal Tract Health Problems

66. A client has anemia resulting from bleeding from ulcerative colitis and is to receive two units of packed red blood cells (PRBCs). The client is receiving an infusion of total parenteral nutrition (TPN). In preparing to administer the PRBCs, the nurse should take which action to ensure client comfort and safety?
    ☐ 1. Discontinue the TPN infusion.
    ☐ 2. Start an intravenous (IV) infusion of normal saline.
    ☐ 3. Administer PRBCs in the same IV line as the TPN.
    ☐ 4. Wait until the TPN infusion is completed, and use the same IV line to infuse the PRBCs.

67. The nurse is assigning clients for the evening shift. Which client(s) would be appropriate for the nurse to assign to a licensed practical/vocational nurse (LPN/VN) to provide client care? Select all that apply.

    The client:
    ☐ 1. who is receiving total parenteral nutrition (TPN).
    ☐ 2. who had an inguinal hernia repair surgery 3 hours ago; vital signs are stable.
    ☐ 3. with an intestinal obstruction who needs a Cantor tube inserted.
    ☐ 4. with diverticulitis who needs teaching about take-home medications.
    ☐ 5. being treated for an exacerbation of ulcerative colitis who is ambulatory.

68. When the nurse is planning care for a client with ulcerative colitis who is experiencing an exacerbation of symptoms, which client care measure(s) can the nurse appropriately delegate to an unlicensed assistive personnel (UAP)? Select all that apply.
    ☐ 1. assessing the client's bowel sounds
    ☐ 2. providing skin care following bowel movements
    ☐ 3. evaluating the client's response to antidiarrheal medications
    ☐ 4. maintaining intake and output records
    ☐ 5. obtaining the client's weight

69. The nurse is caring for a client 1 day after having a colectomy. The client is lethargic and difficult to arouse; the temperature is 101.5°F (38.6°C), blood pressure is 92/36 mm Hg (mean arterial pressure [MAP 55 mm Hg]), and heart rate is 114 bpm, with a percutaneous oxygen saturation (SpO_2) of 88% on oxygen at 2 L per minute per nasal cannula (previously 94%). A saline lock has been established and is patent. Which prescription should the nurse implement **first**?
    ☐ 1. Obtain a stat portable chest x-ray.
    ☐ 2. Administer vancomycin intravenously.
    ☐ 3. Draw blood cultures.
    ☐ 4. Insert an indwelling urinary catheter.

70. The nurse is taking care of a client with *Clostridioides difficile*. To prevent the spread of infection, the nurse should take which action(s)? Select all that apply.
    ☐ 1. Wear a particulate respirator.
    ☐ 2. Wear sterile gloves when providing care.
    ☐ 3. Cleanse the hands with alcohol-based hand sanitizer.
    ☐ 4. Wash the hands with soap and water.
    ☐ 5. Wear a protective gown when in the client's room.

71. The nurse discovers that a client's TPN solution was running at an incorrect rate and is now 2 hours behind schedule. Which action is **most** appropriate for the nurse to take to correct the problem?
    ☐ 1. Readjust the solution to infuse the desired amount.
    ☐ 2. Continue the infusion at the current rate, but run the next bottle at an increased rate.
    ☐ 3. Double the infusion rate for 2 hours.
    ☐ 4. Notify the health care provider (HCP).

72. The nurse is to administer ampicillin 500 mg orally to a client with a ruptured appendix. The nurse checks the capsule in the client's medication box, which is located inside the client's room. The dosage of the medication is not labeled, but the nurse recognizes the color and shape of the capsule. What should the nurse do **next**?
    ☐ 1. Administer the medication to maintain blood levels of the drug.
    ☐ 2. Ask another registered nurse to verify that the capsule is ampicillin.
    ☐ 3. Contact the pharmacy to bring a properly labeled medication.
    ☐ 4. Notify the unit manager to report the problem.

73. On the second day following an abdominal-perineal resection, the nurse notes that the wound edges are not approximated and one-half of the incision has torn apart. What should the nurse do **first**?
☐ 1. Flush the wound with sterile water.
☐ 2. Apply an abdominal binder.
☐ 3. Cover the wound with a sterile dressing moistened with normal saline.
☐ 4. Apply strips of tape.

74. A client has received numerous different antibiotics and now is experiencing diarrhea. What type of precautions should the nurse institute?
☐ 1. airborne precautions
☐ 2. contact precautions
☐ 3. droplet precautions
☐ 4. standard precautions

75. The health care provider has prescribed ciprofloxacin for a client who takes warfarin. What should the nurse instruct the client to do? Select all that apply.
☐ 1. Take the medication with food.
☐ 2. Avoid exposure to sunlight.
☐ 3. Eliminate caffeine from the diet.
☐ 4. Report unusual bleeding.
☐ 5. Increase fluid intake to 3000 mL a day.

76. The nurse has completed the discharge process for a client, but the client has turned on the nurse call light, and on assessment, the nurse notices the client has indigestion, shortness of breath, and is diaphoretic and anxious. The client's blood pressure and heart rate are elevated. The nurse notifies the health care provider who tells the nurse to discharge the client. The nurse explains the situation again, but the health care provider hangs up. What should the nurse do next?
☐ 1. Contact the discharge coordinator to arrange for home health services.
☐ 2. Notify the charge nurse and request a second opinion.
☐ 3. Reassure the client that the health care provider is aware of the client's situation and discharge the client.
☐ 4. Notify the risk manager of the client's status before discharge.

Answers, Rationales, and Test-Taking Strategies

*The answers and rationales for each question follow below, along with keys (🗝) to the client need (CN) and cognitive level (CL) for each question. In addition, questions that measure clinical judgment will be coded (CJ). As you check your answers, use the **Content Mastery and Test-Taking Skill Self-Analysis** worksheet (tear-out worksheet in the back of the book) to identify the reason(s) for not answering the questions correctly. For additional information about test-taking skills and strategies for answering questions, refer to pages 12–51 in Part 1 of this book.*

The Adult with Cancer of the Colon

1. 4. It is important for the nurse to recognize that individuals go through a grieving process when adjusting to a colostomy. The nurse should be accepting and provide the client with opportunities to share concerns and feelings when ready. Lecturing the client about the need to learn how to care for the colostomy is not productive, nor is attempting to shame the client into caring for the colostomy by implying the spouse will have to provide the care if the client does not. It is not possible for the nurse to understand what the client is feeling.

🗝 CN: Psychosocial adaptation; CL: Analyze

2. 4. A history of inflammatory bowel disease is a risk factor for colon cancer. Other risk factors include age (older than 40 years), history of familial polyposis, colorectal polyps, and a high-fat or low-fiber diet.

🗝 CN: Reduction of risk potential; CL: Analyze

3. 3. This client has decreased oxygen saturation and also decreased hemoglobin, which puts the client at great risk for cardiac ischemia. The nurse should start the oxygen as prescribed. The nurse can take the vital signs more frequently once the oxygen flow has been started. It is not appropriate to increase the rate of the intravenous infusion, and it would be necessary to request a prescription to do so. After starting the oxygen, the nurse can ask the client about the current pain level.

🗝 CN: Physiological adaptation; CL: Analyze

4. 1. After a barium enema, a laxative is ordinarily prescribed. This is done to promote the elimination of barium. Retained barium predisposes the client to constipation and fecal impaction. Anticholinergic drugs decrease gastrointestinal motility. Antacids decrease gastric acid secretion. Demulcents soothe mucous membranes of the gastrointestinal tract and are used to treat diarrhea.

🔑 CN: Reduction of risk potential; CL: Analyze

5. 3. A sign indicating that a client's colostomy is open and ready to function is the passage of feces and flatus. When this occurs, gastric suction is ordinarily discontinued, and the client is allowed to start taking fluids and food orally. The absence of bowel sounds would indicate that the tube should remain in place because peristalsis has not yet returned.

🔑 CN: Physiological adaptation; CL: Analyze

6. 2. Appropriate nursing interventions after an abdominal-perineal resection with a colostomy include assisting the client with warm sitz baths three to four times a day to clean the perineal incision. The client will be more comfortable assuming a side-lying position because of the perineal incision. It would be inappropriate to administer milk of magnesia to stimulate colostomy activity. Stool passage will begin as peristalsis returns. It is not necessary or desirable to change the ostomy pouch daily to assess the stoma. The ostomy pouch should be transparent to allow easy observation of the stoma and drainage.

🔑 CN: Physiological adaptation; CL: Analyze

7. 2. A dark red to purple stoma indicates inadequate blood supply. Mild edema and slight oozing of blood are normal in the early postoperative period. The colostomy would typically not begin functioning until 2 to 4 days after surgery.

🔑 CN: Physiological adaptation; CL: Analyze

8. 2. A client who displays interest in the procedure and asks about supplies used for dressings may be ready to participate in self-care. Inquiring about when the HCP will change the dressing does not indicate the client's readiness to change the dressing, nor does asking about who will do the irrigation when the client is at home.

🔑 CN: Basic care and comfort; CL: Analyze

9. 1. An adhesive skin barrier is effective for protecting the skin around a colostomy to keep the skin healthy and prevent skin irritation from stoma drainage. Petroleum jelly, cornstarch, and antiseptic creams do not protect the skin adequately and may prevent an adequate seal between the skin and the colostomy bag.

🔑 CN: Basic care and comfort; CL: Apply

10. 3. It is best to adjust the diet of a client with a colostomy in a manner that suits the client rather than trying special diets. Severe restriction of roughage is not recommended. The client is encouraged to drink 2 to 3 L of fluid per day. A high-fiber diet may produce loose stools.

🔑 CN: Basic care and comfort; CL: Create

11. 1. An expected outcome is that the client will maintain a fluid intake of 3000 mL a day unless contraindicated. There is no need to eliminate fiber from the diet; the client can eat whatever foods are desired and avoid those that are bothersome. Physical activity does not need to be limited to light exercise. The client can resume normal activities as tolerated, usually within 6 to 8 weeks. The client's sexual activity may be affected, but it does not need to be diminished.

🔑 CN: Physiological adaptation; CL: Evaluate

12. -/+ **1, 3, 4.** Ascites limits the movement of the diaphragm leading to respiratory distress. Fluid shift from the intravascular space precipitates fluid and electrolyte imbalances. The client may gain weight due to the fluid gain, but weight loss may result in decreased albumin levels. Decreased albumin in the intravascular space results in decreased oncotic pressure, precipitating movement of fluid out of space. A client with ascites is not at increased risk for infection unless a peritoneal tap is done to remove fluid. The risk of bleeding is a result of alterations in liver enzymes affecting coagulation.

🔑 CN: Physiological adaptation; CL: Analyze

13. 4 kg. A liter of water weighs 1 kg. Therefore, the client should weigh 4 kg less than their preprocedure weight.

🔑 CN: Physiological adaptation; CL: Apply

14. 3. Sending a urine sample for culture and sensitivity is most warranted. An older adult often has confusion when experiencing a bladder infection. Although stroke is always a concern, particularly in an older adult, the presenting information most supports a bladder infection and perhaps early-onset urosepsis. Restraining the client may be needed at some point in time, but finding the cause of the client's new onset of confusion has the greatest priority. Potassium is usually related to cardiac rhythm irritability rather than confusion.

🔑 CN: Physiological adaptation; CL: Analysis

15. -/+ **1, 2, 4.** Known risk factors for sepsis include age (younger than 1 year and older than 65 years), chronic illness, and invasive procedures. Immunosuppression and malnourishment are also risk factors. There is no correlation between sex or age and risk for sepsis. Nurses must be aware of risk factors and monitor clients at risk closely for any signs of sepsis.

CN: Reduction of risk potential; CL: Apply

The Adult with Hemorrhoids

16. **2.** Hemorrhoids are associated with prolonged sitting or standing, portal hypertension, chronic constipation, and prolonged increased intra-abdominal pressure, as associated with pregnancy and the strain of vaginal birth. The client's job as a schoolteacher does not require prolonged sitting or standing. Age and leg varicosities are not related to the development of hemorrhoids.

CN: Reduction of risk potential; CL: Analyze

17. **1.** Applying heat during the immediate postoperative period may cause hemorrhage at the surgical site. Moist heat may relieve rectal spasms after bowel movements. Urine retention caused by reflex spasms may also be relieved by moist heat. Increasing fiber and fluid in the diet can help prevent constipation.

CN: Physiological adaptation; CL: Apply

18. **3.** Adequate cleaning of the anal area is difficult but essential. After rectal surgery, sitz baths assist in this process, so the client should take a sitz bath after a bowel movement. Other times are dictated by client comfort.

CN: Reduction of risk potential; CL: Evaluate

The Adult with Ulcerative Colitis

19. **31 gtt/min.** To administer IV fluids at 125 mL per hour using tubing that has a drip factor of 15 gtt/mL, the nurse should use the formula:

125 mL/60 min × 15 gtt/1 mL = 31 gtt/min

CN: Pharmacological and parenteral therapies; CL: Apply

20. **2.** Diarrhea is the primary symptom in an exacerbation of ulcerative colitis, and decreasing the frequency of stools is the first goal of treatment. The other goals are ongoing and will be best achieved by halting the exacerbation. The client may receive antidiarrheal agents, antispasmodic agents, bulk hydrophilic agents, or anti-inflammatory drugs.

CN: Physiological adaptation; CL: Analyze

21. **2.** Although bed rest does help conserve energy and promote comfort, falling is not a risk, and its primary purpose in this case is to help reduce the hypermotility of the colon. Remaining on bed rest does not by itself reduce stress, and if the client is having stress, the nurse can plan with the client to use strategies that will help the client manage the stress.

CN: Physiological adaptation; CL: Evaluate

22. **3.** Excessive diarrhea causes significant depletion of the body's stores of sodium and potassium as well as fluid. The client should be closely monitored for hypokalemia and hyponatremia. Ulcerative colitis does not place the client at risk for heart failure, deep vein thrombosis, or hypocalcemia.

CN: Reduction of risk potential; CL: Analyze

23. **4.** It is not uncommon for clients with ulcerative colitis to become apprehensive and have difficulty coping with the frequency of stools and the presence of abdominal cramping. During these acute exacerbations, clients need emotional support and encouragement to verbalize their feelings about their chronic health concerns and assistance in developing effective coping methods. The client has not expressed feelings of fatigue or isolation or demonstrated disturbed thought processes.

CN: Psychosocial adaptation; CL: Analyze

24. **2.** Steroids are effective in the management of the acute symptoms of ulcerative colitis. Steroids do not cure ulcerative colitis, which is a chronic disease. Long-term use is not effective in prolonging the remission and is not advocated. Clients should be assessed carefully for side effects related to steroid therapy, but the benefits of short-term steroid therapy usually outweigh the potential adverse effects.

CN: Pharmacological and parenteral therapies; CL: Apply

25. **3.** Food will be withheld from the client with severe symptoms of ulcerative colitis to rest the bowel. To maintain the client's nutritional status, the client will be started on TPN. Enteral feedings or dividing the diet into six small meals does not allow the bowel to rest. A high-calorie, high-protein diet will worsen the client's symptoms.

CN: Pharmacological and parenteral therapies; CL: Apply

26. **1, 2, 4.** Sulfasalazine may cause dizziness, and the nurse should caution the client to avoid driving or other activities that require alertness until response to medication is known. If symptoms of acute intolerance (cramping, acute abdominal pain, bloody diarrhea, fever, headache, rash) occur, the client should discontinue therapy and notify the HCP immediately. Fluid intake should be sufficient to maintain a urine output of at least 1200 to 1500 mL daily to prevent crystalluria and stone formation. The nurse can also inform the client that this medication may cause orange-yellow discoloration of urine and skin, which is not significant and does not require the client to stop taking the medication. The nurse should instruct the client to take missed doses as soon as remembered unless it is 1 hour before the next dose.

🔑 CN: Pharmacological and parenteral therapies; CL: Analyze

27. **4 tablets.** To administer 2 g sulfasalazine, the nurse will need to administer four tablets. The following formula is used to calculate the correct dosage:

The first step is to convert grams into milligrams:
$$1 \text{ g}/1000 \text{ mg} = 2 \text{ g}/X \text{ mg}$$
$$X = 2000 \text{ mg}$$
Then, $2000 \text{ mg}/X \text{ tablets} = 500 \text{ mg}/1 \text{ tablet}$
$$X = 4 \text{ tablets}$$

🔑 CN: Pharmacological and parenteral therapies; CL: Apply

28. **2.** Clients with ulcerative colitis should follow a well-balanced high-protein, high-calorie, low-residue diet, avoiding such high-residue foods as whole-wheat grains, nuts, and raw fruits and vegetables. Clients with ulcerative colitis need more protein for tissue healing and should avoid excess roughage. There is no need for clients with ulcerative colitis to follow low-sodium diets.

🔑 CN: Basic care and comfort; CL: Apply

The Adult with an Ileostomy

29. **2.** Unless the pouch leaks, the client can wear the ileostomy pouch for about 4 to 7 days. If leakage occurs, it is important to promptly change the pouch to avoid skin irritation. It is not necessary to change the pouch daily or in the evening. Diet and activity typically do not affect the schedule for changing the pouch.

🔑 CN: Health promotion and maintenance; CL: Analyze

30. **3.** Providing explanations of preoperative and postoperative procedures helps the client prepare and understand what to expect. It also provides an opportunity for the client to share concerns. Including family members in the teaching sessions is beneficial but does not focus on the client's psychological preparation. Encouraging the client to ask questions about managing the ileostomy may be rushing the client psychologically into accepting the change in body image and function. The client may need time to first handle the stress of surgery and then observe the care of the ileostomy by others before it is appropriate to begin discussing self-management. The nurse should gently explore whether the client is ready to ask questions about management throughout the hospitalization. The client should have the opportunity to express concerns and to agree to an ostomy association visitor before an invitation is extended.

🔑 CN: Psychosocial adaptation; CL: Analyze

31. **1.** The nurse should instruct the client to stop taking drugs that would interfere with clotting, such as aspirin or ibuprofen. The client should follow a high-fiber diet with increased fluids during the 2-week preoperative period. It is not necessary to limit fluids. The client does not need to report having a temperature above 99°F (37.2°C) to the health care provider (HCP) as this is within normal limits; however, if the temperature is higher, this could indicate an infection, and the client should notify the HCP.

🔑 CN: Pharmacological and parenteral therapies; CL: Apply

32. **3.** A high-priority outcome after ileostomy surgery is the maintenance of fluid and electrolyte balance. The client will experience continuous liquid to semiliquid stools. The client should be engaged in self-care activities, and minimizing odor formation is important; however, these goals do not take priority over maintaining fluid and electrolyte balance.

🔑 CN: Physiological adaptation; CL: Analyze

33. **3.** If the client agrees, having a visit by a person who has successfully adjusted to living with an ileostomy would be the most helpful measure. This would let the client see that typical activities of daily living can be pursued postoperatively. Someone who has felt some of the same concerns can answer the client's questions. A visit from the clergy may be helpful to some clients but would not provide this client with the information sought. Disregarding the client's concerns is not helpful. Although the HCP should know about the client's concerns, this in itself will not reassure the client about life after an ileostomy.

🔑 CN: Psychosocial adaptation; CL: Analyze

34. **3.** Because of high concentrations of digestive enzymes, ileostomy effluent is irritating to the skin and can cause excoriation and ulceration. Some form of protection must be used to keep the effluent from contacting the skin. A skin barrier does not decrease odor formation; odor is controlled by diet. The barrier does not affect the client's hydration status, and the nurse can encourage the client to have an adequate daily intake of fluids. Pouches are usually worn for 4 to 7 days before being changed.

    CN: Basic care and comfort; CL: Evaluate

35. **3.** Any sudden decrease in drainage or onset of severe abdominal pain should be reported to the health care provider immediately because it could mean that an obstruction has developed. The ileostomy drains liquid stool at frequent intervals throughout the day. Undigested food may be present at times. A temperature of 99.8°F (37.7°C) is not necessarily abnormal or a cause for concern.

    CN: Reduction of risk potential; CL: Analyze

36. **2.** The fact that the client has an ileostomy does not necessarily mean that they cannot get pregnant and give birth. It may be recommended, however, that the number of pregnancies be limited. Women of an age to give birth should be encouraged to discuss their concerns with their health care provider. Discussing their concerns about sexual functioning and pregnancy will help decrease fears and anxiety. Empathizing or telling the client that they can adopt does not address their concerns. The client's current fears may be based on erroneous understanding. Telling the client that they will adjust to the situation ignores their concerns.

    CN: Psychosocial adaptation; CL: Analyze

37. **3.** To maintain an adequate fluid balance, the client needs to drink at least 3000 mL a day. Heavy lifting should be avoided; the health care provider will indicate when the client can participate in sports again. The client will not resume working as soon as 2 weeks after surgery. Water does not harm the stoma, so the client does not have to worry about getting it wet.

    CN: Physiological adaptation; CL: Evaluate

38. **4.** The sudden onset of abdominal cramps, vomiting, and watery discharge with no stool from an ileostomy are likely indications of an obstruction. It is imperative that the HCP examine the client immediately. Although the client is vomiting, the client should not take an antiemetic until the HCP has examined the client. If an obstruction is present, ingesting fluids or taking milk of magnesia will increase the severity of symptoms. Oral intake is avoided when a bowel obstruction is suspected.

    CN: Health promotion and maintenance; CL: Analyze

The Adult with an Intestinal Obstruction

39. **1, 4, 5.** Signs and symptoms of intestinal obstructions in the small intestine may include projectile vomiting and rapidly developing dehydration and electrolyte imbalances. The client will also have increased bowel sounds that are usually high pitched and tinkling. The client would not normally have diarrhea and would have minimal abdominal distention. Pain is intermittent and relieved by vomiting. Intestinal obstructions in the large intestine usually evolve slowly and produce persistent pain, and vomiting is less common. Clients with a large intestine obstruction may develop obstipation and significant abdominal distention.

    CN: Physiological adaptation; CL: Analyze

40. **1, 3, 2, 4.** The nurse should first help the client ambulate to try to induce peristalsis; this may be effective and require the least amount of invasive procedures. Next, the nurse should initiate IV fluid therapy to correct fluid and electrolyte imbalances (sodium and potassium) with Ringer's lactate to correct the interstitial fluid deficit. Nasogastric decompression of the gastrointestinal tract to reduce gastric secretions and nasointestinal tubes may also be used as necessary. Lastly, hyperalimentation can be used to correct protein deficiency from chronic obstruction, paralytic ileus, or infection.

    CN: Physiological adaptation; CL: Analyze

41. **1.** Intestinal decompression is accomplished with a Cantor, Harris, or Miller-Abbott tube. These 6- to 10-foot (180- to 300-cm) tubes are passed into the small intestine to the obstruction. They remove accumulated fluid and gas, relieving the pressure. The client will not have an adequate bowel movement until the obstruction is removed. The pressure from the distended intestine should not obstruct urinary output. Although the client may be able to sit up more easily and the pain caused by the intestinal pressure will be less, these are not the primary indicators for successful intestinal decompression.

    CN: Physiological adaptation; CL: Evaluate

42. 2. The client is placed in a right side-lying position to facilitate movement of the mercury-weighted tube through the pyloric sphincter. After the tube is in the intestine, the client is turned from side to side or encouraged to ambulate to facilitate tube movement through the intestinal loops. Placing the client in the supine or semi-Fowler's position or having the client sitting out of bed in a chair will not facilitate tube progression.

CN: Reduction of risk potential; CL: Apply

43. 2. The client's pain may be indicative of peritonitis, and the nurse should assess for signs and symptoms, such as a rigid abdomen, elevated temperature, and increasing pain. Reassuring the client is important, but an accurate assessment of the client is essential. A full assessment should occur before pain relief measures are employed. Repositioning the client to the left side will not resolve the pain.

CN: Reduction of risk potential; CL: Analyze

44. 4. Considering that there is usually 1 L of insensible fluid loss, this client's output exceeds their intake (intake, 2000 mL; output, 2200 mL), indicating deficient fluid volume. The kidneys are concentrating urine in response to low circulating volume, as evidenced by a urine output of less than 30 mL an hour. This indicates that increased fluid replacement is needed. Decreased urine output can be a sign of decreased renal function, but the data provided suggest that the client is dehydrated. Pain does not affect urine output. There are no data to suggest that the obstruction has worsened.

CN: Reduction of risk potential; CL: Analyze

The Adult Receiving Total Parenteral Nutrition

45. 3. The nurse should first obtain a prescription to obtain a culture specimen. The presence of drainage is a potential indication of an infection, and the catheter may need to be removed. A culture specimen should be obtained and sent for analysis so that treatment can be promptly initiated. Since removing the catheter will be required in the presence of an infection, the nurse would not clean and redress the area. Although the body temperature may increase, indicating an infection, a culture needs to be obtained to identify the causative organism. After the culture report is obtained, the nurse should notify the health care provider and document all assessments and client care activities in the client's record.

CN: Safety and infection control; CL: Analyze

46. 2. TPN is a hypertonic, high-calorie, high-protein IV fluid that should be provided for clients who do not have functional gastrointestinal tract motility to better meet the metabolic needs of the client and to support optimal nutrition and healing. TPN is prescribed once daily, based on the client's current electrolyte and fluid balance, and must be handled with strict aseptic technique (due to the high glucose content, it is a perfect medium for bacterial growth). Also, because of the high tonicity, TPN must be administered through a central venous access, not a peripheral IV line. There is no specific need to auscultate for bowel sounds to determine whether TPN can safely be administered.

CN: Pharmacological and parenteral therapies; CL: Analyze

47. 1. When using a sliding scale insulin schedule, the nurse obtains a glucometer reading of the client's blood glucose level immediately before giving the insulin and bases the dosage on those findings. The fasting blood glucose level obtained earlier in the day is not relevant to an evening sliding scale insulin dosage. The nurse cannot calculate insulin dosage by assessing the amount of TPN intake or dietary intake.

CN: Pharmacological and parenteral therapies; CL: Analyze

48. 4. The client should be asked to perform the Valsalva maneuver (take a deep breath and hold it) during the insertion and removal of a CVAD. This increases central venous pressure during the procedure and prevents air embolism. Trendelenburg is the preferred position for CVAD insertion and removal. If not possible, a supine position is sufficient for CVAD removal. The client should hold their breath, not exhale.

CN: Physiological integrity; CL: Apply

49. 4. During TPN administration, the client should be monitored regularly for hyperglycemia. The client may require small amounts of insulin to improve glucose metabolism. The client should also be observed for signs and symptoms of hypoglycemia, which may occur if the body overproduces insulin in response to a high glucose intake or if too much insulin is administered to help improve glucose metabolism. Tachycardia or hypertension is not indicative of the client's ability to metabolize the solution. An elevated blood urea nitrogen concentration is indicative of renal status and fluid balance.

CN: Pharmacological and parenteral therapies; CL: Analyze

50. 1, 2, 4. Complications associated with the administration of TPN through a central line include infection and air embolism. To prevent these complications, strict aseptic technique is used for all dressing changes, the insertion site is covered with an air-occlusive dressing, and all connections of the system must be secure. Ambulation and activities of daily living are encouraged and not limited during the administration of TPN, and the client does not need to remain in a prone position immediately after the insertion of the central line.

🔑 CN: Pharmacological and parenteral therapies; CL: Analyze

51. 4. An elevated temperature can be an indication of an infection at the insertion site or in the catheter. Vital signs should be taken every 2 to 4 hours after initiation of TPN therapy to detect early signs of complications. Glycosuria is to be expected during the first few days of therapy until the pancreas adjusts by secreting more insulin. A gradual weight gain is to be expected as the client's nutritional status improves. Some clients experience a decreased appetite during TPN therapy.

🔑 CN: Reduction of risk potential; CL: Analyze

52. 2. A too rapid infusion of TPN solution can lead to circulatory overload. The client should be assessed carefully for indications of excess fluid volume. A negative nitrogen balance occurs in nutritionally depleted individuals, not when TPN fluids are administered in excess. When TPN is administered too rapidly, the client is at risk for receiving an excess of dextrose and electrolytes. Therefore, the client is at risk for hyperglycemia and hyperkalemia.

🔑 CN: Pharmacological and parenteral therapies; CL: Analyze

The Adult with Diverticular Disease

53. 1, 2, 4. Clients with diverticulosis are encouraged to follow a high-fiber diet. Bran, broccoli, and navy beans are foods high in fiber. Tomato juice and cheese are low-residue foods.

🔑 CN: Reduction of risk potential; CL: Apply

54. 3. The nurse should first assess the client for signs of peritonitis. Complications of diverticulitis include perforation with peritonitis, abscess, and fistula formation; bowel obstruction; ureteral obstruction; and bleeding. A computed tomography scan with oral contrast is the test of choice for diverticulitis. A client with acute diverticulitis does not receive a barium enema or colonoscopy because of the possibility of peritonitis and perforation. With acute diverticulitis, the goal of treatment is to allow the colon to rest and inflammation to subside. The client is kept on nothing-by-mouth (NPO) status; parenteral fluid therapy is provided.

🔑 CN: Physiological adaptation; CL: Analyze

55. 4. Clients with diverticular disease should refrain from any activities, such as lifting, straining, or coughing, that increase intra-abdominal pressure and may precipitate an attack. Enemas are contraindicated because they increase intestinal pressure. Fluid intake should be increased, rather than decreased, to promote soft, formed stools. A low-fiber diet is used when inflammation is present.

🔑 CN: Reduction of risk potential; CL: Analyze

56. 3, 4, 5. Clients who have diverticulosis should be instructed to maintain a diet high in fiber and, unless contraindicated, should increase their fluid intake to a minimum of 2000 mL/day. Participating in a regular exercise program is also strongly encouraged. Diverticulosis can be controlled with treatment but cannot be cured. Clients should be instructed to avoid the regular use of cathartic laxatives. Bulk laxatives and stool softeners may be helpful to maintain regularity and decrease straining.

🔑 CN: Reduction of risk potential; CL: Evaluate

57. 1. Diverticular disease is treated with a high-fiber diet and bulk laxatives such as psyllium hydrophilic mucilloid. Fiber decreases the intraluminal pressure and makes it easier for stool to pass through the colon. Bulk laxatives do not manage diarrhea or relieve gas formation. The stool should remain soft and easy to expel.

🔑 CN: Pharmacological and parenteral therapies; CL: Evaluate

58. 1, 2, 3, 5. Percussion will show resonance and tympany, indicating paralytic ileus. Lack of liver dullness may indicate free air in the abdomen. The client with peritonitis will have fever, tachypnea, and tachycardia. The abdomen becomes rigid with rebound tenderness, and there will be absent bowel sounds. The client will not demonstrate excessive thirst but may have anorexia, nausea, and vomiting as peristalsis decreases.

🔑 CN: Physiological adaptation; CL: Analyze

The Adult with Appendicitis

59. 4. The nurse should gently clean the area around the drain by moving in a circular motion away from the drain. Doing so prevents the introduction of microorganisms to the wound and drain site. The incision cannot be left open to air as long as the drain is intact. The nurse should note the amount and character of wound drainage, but the surgeon will determine when the drain should be removed. Surgical wound drains are not irrigated.

CN: Safety and infection control; CL: Analyze

60. 1. Appendicitis typically begins with periumbilical pain, followed by anorexia, nausea, and vomiting. The pain is persistent and continuous, eventually shifting to the right lower quadrant and localizing at McBurney's point (located halfway between the umbilicus and the right iliac crest). To relieve pain before surgery, the nurse assists the client into a comfortable position with the knees drawn to the chest and the head of the bed slightly elevated. The nurse may also administer analgesics and ice packs if prescribed; heat is avoided as heat may precipitate rupture of the appendix. The abdomen is not palpated or massaged more than necessary to avoid increasing the pain. Distraction with music may be helpful, but positioning, using ice packs, and analgesics are most effective.

CN: Basic care and comfort; CL: Analyze

61. 1, 2, 5. The nurse should instruct the client that nausea, abdominal distention from gas, and diarrhea are normal following an appendectomy. The client will be able to return to work and usual activities in 1 to 3 weeks. The client does not need to follow a low-residue diet but may prefer a bland diet if the client has nausea or an upset stomach. The client can drive if not taking pain medication. The client should not take a tub bath until the incision has healed.

CN: Health promotion and maintenance; CL: Analyze

62. 3. The adhesive strips should stay in place until they fall off. The client should not remove them to cleanse the area. It is not necessary to place an additional dressing over the adhesive strips. The client should not take a tub bath until the incision has healed.

CN: Reduction of risk potential; CL: Analyze

The Adult with an Inguinal Hernia

63. 3. The symptoms are indicative of a strangulated hernia. In a strangulated hernia, the hernia cannot be reduced back into the abdominal cavity. The intestinal lumen and the blood supply to the intestine are obstructed, causing an acute intestinal obstruction. Without immediate intervention, necrosis and gangrene may develop. Surgery is required to release the strangulation. Although many of these signs and symptoms are present with peritonitis or perforated bowel, abdominal rigidity, a cardinal sign of peritonitis and perforated bowel, is not mentioned. Therefore, the nurse would not immediately suspect these conditions. An incarcerated hernia is a hernia that is irreducible but has not necessarily resulted in an obstruction.

CN: Physiological adaptation; CL: Analyze

64. 4. The client is instructed to avoid lifting items heavier than 5 lb (2.3 kg) for 4 to 6 weeks after hernia repair. The client continues to take deep breaths and expand the lungs but is instructed to avoid coughing. Ice, rather than heat, is used to reduce scrotal swelling. The client is instructed to sneeze with the mouth open to avoid sudden stress on the sutures.

CN: Health promotion and adaptation; CL: Apply

65. 4. The most common complication after an inguinal hernia repair is the inability to void, especially in male clients. The nurse should evaluate the client carefully for urine retention. Hypostatic pneumonia, deep vein thrombosis, and paralytic ileus are potential postoperative problems with any surgical client but are not as likely to occur after an inguinal hernia repair as is urine retention.

CN: Reduction of risk potential; CL: Analyze

Managing Care, Quality, and Safety for Adults with Lower Gastrointestinal Tract Health Problems

66. 2. The nurse administers the PRBCs using a separate infusion line and appropriate tubing, with normal saline as the priming solution. It is not necessary to discontinue the TPN infusion or wait until the TPN infusion is completed.

CN: Pharmacological and parenteral therapies; CL: Analyze

67. -/+ **2, 5.** The nurse should consider client needs and scope of practice when assigning staff to provide care. The client who is recovering from inguinal hernia repair surgery and the client who is experiencing an exacerbation of ulcerative colitis are appropriate clients to assign to an LPN/VN as the care they require falls within the scope of practice for an LPN or a VN. It is not within the scope of practice for the LPN/VN to administer TPN, insert nasoenteric tubes, or provide client teaching related to medications.

CN: Management of care; CL: Analyze

68. -/+ **2, 4, 5.** The nurse can delegate the following basic care activities to the UAP: providing skin care following bowel movements, maintaining intake and output records, and obtaining the client's weight. Assessing the client's bowel sounds and evaluating the client's response to medication are registered nurse (RN) activities that cannot be delegated.

CN: Management of care; CL: Analyze

69. 3. This client has signs and symptoms of severe sepsis. Blood cultures should be drawn before administering the antibiotic (vancomycin), and the antibiotics should be administered within the first 45 minutes after recognition of these signs to try to prevent septic shock. Obtaining a chest x-ray and inserting a urinary catheter to accurately measure intake and output are also important actions, but they are not the first priority for this client.

CN: Reduction of risk potential; CL: Analyze

70. -/+ **4, 5.** *C. difficile* is an organism that has developed very resistant and highly morbid strains. Universal precautions, most importantly handwashing, wearing personal protective gear, and modest use of antibiotics, are critical actions for stopping the spread. *C. difficile* is not spread via the respiratory tract; therefore, a mask is not needed. Alcohol-based hand sanitizers do not kill the spores of *C. difficile*; soap and water must be used. Sterile gloves are not needed to provide care; clean gloves may be worn.

CN: Safety and infection control; CL: Analyze

71. 4. When TPN fluids are infused too rapidly or too slowly, the HCP should be notified. TPN solutions must be carefully and accurately infused. Rate adjustments should not be made without a written prescription from the HCP. Significant alterations in rate (10% increase or decrease) can result in fluctuations of blood glucose levels. Speeding up the solution can result in too much glucose entering the system.

CN: Pharmacological and parenteral therapies; CL: Analyze

72. 3. The nurse should contact the pharmacy directly and request that a properly labeled medication be provided. The nurse should not administer any drug that is not properly labeled, even if the nurse or another nurse recognizes the medication. It is not necessary to notify the unit manager at this point because the client needs to receive the antibiotic as soon as possible.

CN: Pharmacological and parenteral therapies; CL: Apply

73. 3. When dehiscence occurs, the nurse should immediately cover the wound with a sterile dressing moistened with normal saline. If the dehiscence is extensive, the incision must be resutured in surgery. Later, after the sutures are removed, additional support may be provided to the incision by applying strips of tape as directed by institutional policy or by the surgeon. An abdominal binder may also be utilized for additional support.

CN: Reduction of risk potential; CL: Analyze

74. 2. The nurse should initiate contact precautions to prevent bloodborne infection through percutaneous injury. Extreme care is essential when needles, scalpels, and other sharp objects are handled. Airborne precautions are required for clients with presumed or proven pulmonary tuberculosis, chickenpox, or other airborne pathogens. Contact precautions are used for organisms that are spread by skin-to-skin contact, such as antibiotic-resistant organisms or *Clostridioides difficile*. Droplet precautions are used for organisms such as influenza or *Neisseria meningitidis* that can be transmitted by close respiratory or mucous membrane contact with respiratory secretions. Standard precautions include handwashing and the use of a mask and gown.

CN: Safety and infection control; CL: Apply

75. -/+ **2, 4.** A black box warning for ciprofloxacin is that ciprofloxacin may increase the anticoagulant effects of warfarin. The nurse should instruct the client to report increased bleeding and to monitor the prothrombin time and the international normalized ratio closely. The client can take the drug with or without food. Although there is a drug-food interaction and taking ciprofloxacin may increase the stimulatory effect of caffeine, the client does not need to eliminate caffeine but should report signs of stimulant effect. Ciprofloxacin may cause photosensitivity reactions; the nurse must advise the client to avoid excessive sunlight or artificial ultraviolet light during therapy. Clients must be advised not to crush, split, or chew the extended-release tablets.

CN: Pharmacological and parenteral therapies; CL: Analyze

76. 2. A reasonable and prudent nurse would act as the client's advocate and question a prescription that places a client at risk. Consulting the charge nurse to assess the client, shifts responsibility to the next in command with higher authority and will validate the nurse's assessment. The client should not be discharged until the client is stable. Although the client may require home health services, the client is not ready for discharge at this time. It is not appropriate to notify the risk manager at this time, and if necessary, that would be the role of the charge nurse or nurse manager.

CN: Management of care; CL: Analyze

TEST 7

The Adult with Pancreatic and Biliary Tract Disorders

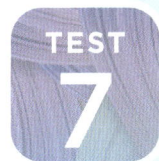

- The Adult with Cholecystitis
- The Adult with Pancreatitis
- The Adult with Viral Hepatitis
- The Adult with Cirrhosis
- Managing Care, Quality, and Safety of Adults with Biliary Tract Disorders
- Answers, Rationales, and Test-Taking Strategies

The Adult with Cholecystitis

1. A client has undergone a laparoscopic cholecystectomy. Which instruction should the nurse include in the discharge teaching?
   - ☐ 1. Empty the bile bag daily.
   - ☐ 2. Breathe deeply into a paper bag when nauseated.
   - ☐ 3. Keep adhesive dressings in place for 6 weeks.
   - ☐ 4. Report bile-colored drainage from any incision.

2. A client with acute cholecystitis has severe pain. Which prescription will be **most** effective in relieving the pain?
   - ☐ 1. infusing normal saline solution at 100 mL per hour
   - ☐ 2. administering morphine sulfate 10 mg intramuscularly every 3 to 4 hours
   - ☐ 3. receiving nothing by mouth (NPO)
   - ☐ 4. having a nasogastric tube connected to low intermittent suction

3. A client's stools are light gray in color. What additional information should the nurse obtain from the client? Select all that apply.
   - ☐ 1. intolerance to fatty foods
   - ☐ 2. fever
   - ☐ 3. jaundice
   - ☐ 4. respiratory distress
   - ☐ 5. pain at McBurney's point
   - ☐ 6. bleeding ulcer

4. A client has an open cholecystectomy with bile duct exploration. Following surgery, the client has a T-tube. What should the nurse do to determine the effectiveness of the T-tube?
   - ☐ 1. Irrigate the tube with 20 mL of normal saline every 4 hours.
   - ☐ 2. Unclamp the T-tube, and empty the contents every day.
   - ☐ 3. Assess the color and amount of drainage every shift.
   - ☐ 4. Monitor the incision sites for bile drainage.

5. At 0800, the nurse reviews the amount of T-tube drainage for a client who underwent an open cholecystectomy yesterday. After reviewing the output record (see chart), the nurse should perform which action **next**?

   Output Record

Time	T-Tube
1200	50 mL
1600	60 mL
2000	60 mL
0000	70 mL
0400	70 mL
0800	10 mL

   - ☐ 1. Report the 24-hour drainage amount at 1200.
   - ☐ 2. Clamp the T-tube.
   - ☐ 3. Evaluate the tube for patency.
   - ☐ 4. Irrigate the T-tube.

6. A client who had a cholecystectomy has a T-tube for drainage. The nurse measures the amount of bile drainage from the T-tube at the end of each shift. How should the nurse record the drainage?
   - ☐ 1. adding it to the client's urine output
   - ☐ 2. charting it separately on the output record
   - ☐ 3. adding it to the amount of wound drainage
   - ☐ 4. subtracting it from the total intake for each day

7. The nurse is caring for a client who had an open cholecystectomy 24 hours ago. The client's vital signs have been stable over the last 24 hours, with the most recent being temperature 98.6°F (37°C), blood pressure (BP) 118/76 mm Hg, respiratory rate (RR) 16 breaths/min, and heart rate (HR) 78 bpm, but these signs are now changing. Which set of vital signs indicates that the nurse should contact the health care provider (HCP)?
    ☐ 1. temperature 101.8°F (38.8°C); BP 140/86 mm Hg; HR 94 bpm; RR 24 breaths/min
    ☐ 2. temperature 100.7°F (38.2°C); BP 118/68 mm Hg; HR 84 bpm; RR 20 breaths/min
    ☐ 3. temperature 99.5°F (37.5°C); BP 126/80 mm Hg; HR 58 bpm; RR 16 breaths/min
    ☐ 4. temperature 97.5°F (36.4°C); BP 98/64 mm Hg; HR 98 bpm; RR 18 breaths/min

8. After a cholecystectomy, the client is to follow a low-fat diet. Which food would be **most** appropriate to include in a low-fat diet?
    ☐ 1. cheese omelet with onions
    ☐ 2. peanut butter on wheat toast
    ☐ 3. ham salad sandwich made with mayonnaise
    ☐ 4. roast beef sandwich with lettuce and tomato

9. A client with cholecystitis has severe pain unrelieved by ibuprofen. The client feels nauseated. The nurse obtains the following vital signs: temperature 101.1°F (38.4°C); pulse 114 bpm; respirations 22 breaths/min; and blood pressure 142/90 mm Hg. Using the SBAR (Situation-Background-Assessment-Recommendation) technique for communication, what should the nurse recommend to the health care provider for this client?
    ☐ 1. a medication for severe pain
    ☐ 2. a medication for increased temperature
    ☐ 3. a medication for elevated blood pressure
    ☐ 4. a medication for feelings of nausea

10. The nurse prepares to administer promethazine 35 mg intramuscularly prescribed as needed for a client with cholecystitis who has severe nausea. The ampule label reads that the medication is available in 25 mg/mL. How many milliliters should the nurse administer? Record your answer using one decimal place.

    _____ mL.

11. A client undergoes a laparoscopic cholecystectomy. Which instruction should the nurse give the client about a diet immediately after surgery?
    ☐ 1. "You can't eat or drink anything for 24 hours."
    ☐ 2. "You may resume your normal diet the day after your surgery."
    ☐ 3. "Start with liquids and see how you feel."
    ☐ 4. "You can progress from a liquid to a bland diet as tolerated."

12. The nurse is preparing a client for discharge. The client had a laparoscopic cholecystectomy and has sutures covered by a dressing. Which instruction should the nurse give this client?
    ☐ 1. "Avoid showering for 1 week after surgery."
    ☐ 2. "You can return to work within 1 week."
    ☐ 3. "Leave the dressing in place until seeing the surgeon at the postoperative visit."
    ☐ 4. "Use acetaminophen to control any fever."

13. A client who has had a laparoscopic cholecystectomy has adhesive strips over the puncture sites. When preparing the client for discharge, which client statement(s) would indicate that the teaching has been successful? Select all that apply.
    ☐ 1. "I can resume my normal diet when I feel ok."
    ☐ 2. "I need to avoid driving for about 4 weeks."
    ☐ 3. "I may experience some pain in my right shoulder."
    ☐ 4. "I should spend 2 to 3 days in bed before resuming activity."
    ☐ 5. "I can take a shower 2 days later."

14. Following an emergency cholecystectomy, the client has a Jackson-Pratt drain with closed suction. After 4 hours, the drainage unit is full. What should the nurse do?
    ☐ 1. Notify the surgeon.
    ☐ 2. Remove the drain and suction unit.
    ☐ 3. Check the dressing for bleeding.
    ☐ 4. Empty the drainage unit.

The Adult with Pancreatitis

15. The nurse is obtaining a health history for a client with pancreatitis. The does not drink alcohol because of religious convictions and becomes upset when the nurse asks about alcohol intake. What should the nurse tell the client about why this is an important question?
    ☐ 1. "There is a strong link between alcohol use and acute pancreatitis."
    ☐ 2. "Alcohol intake can interfere with the tests used to diagnose pancreatitis."
    ☐ 3. "Alcoholism is a major health problem, and all clients are questioned about alcohol intake."
    ☐ 4. "The health care provider (HCP) must obtain the pertinent facts, regardless of religious beliefs."

16. A client with acute pancreatitis has a blood pressure of 88/40 mm Hg, a heart rate of 128 bpm, respirations of 28 breaths/min, and Grey Turner sign. What prescription should the nurse implement **first**?
    ☐ 1. Initiate an intake/output record.
    ☐ 2. Place an intravenous (IV) line.
    ☐ 3. Position the client on the left side.
    ☐ 4. Insert a nasogastric tube.

17. When the nurse is providing care for a client hospitalized with acute pancreatitis who has severe abdominal pain, which nursing intervention(s) would be **most** appropriate for this client? Select all that apply.
   ☐ 1. Place the client in a side-lying position.
   ☐ 2. Administer morphine sulfate for pain as needed.
   ☐ 3. Maintain the client on a high-calorie, high-protein diet.
   ☐ 4. Monitor the client's respiratory status.
   ☐ 5. Obtain daily weights.

18. The nurse notes that a client with acute pancreatitis occasionally experiences muscle twitching and jerking. How should the nurse interpret the significance of these symptoms? The client:
   ☐ 1. may be developing hypocalcemia.
   ☐ 2. is experiencing a reaction to meperidine.
   ☐ 3. has a nutritional imbalance.
   ☐ 4. needs a muscle relaxant to promote rest.

19. A client is receiving propantheline bromide for the management of acute pancreatitis. Which finding would indicate that the nurse should discuss withholding the medication with the health care provider?
   ☐ 1. absent bowel sounds
   ☐ 2. increased urine output
   ☐ 3. diarrhea
   ☐ 4. decreased heart rate

20. The health care provider has prescribed pancreatic enzyme replacements for a client with chronic pancreatitis. When should the nurse tell the client about how to take them to obtain the **most** therapeutic effect?
   ☐ 1. three times daily between meals
   ☐ 2. with each meal and snack
   ☐ 3. in the morning and at bedtime
   ☐ 4. every 4 hours, at specified times

21. A client has chronic pancreatitis. What should the nurse teach the client to do to monitor the effectiveness of pancreatic enzyme replacement?
   ☐ 1. Record daily fluid intake.
   ☐ 2. Perform glucose fingerstick tests twice a day.
   ☐ 3. Observe stools for steatorrhea.
   ☐ 4. Test urine for ketones.

The Adult with Viral Hepatitis

22. The nurse is assessing a client with chronic hepatitis B who is receiving lamivudine. What information about the client is **most** important to communicate to the health care provider?
   ☐ 1. a 6.6-lb (3-kg) weight gain over 2 days
   ☐ 2. intermittent nausea
   ☐ 3. a temperature of 99°F (37.2°C) orally
   ☐ 4. constant fatigue

23. The nurse is assessing a client with hepatitis A and notices that the aspartate transaminase (AST) and alanine transaminase (ALT) lab values have increased. Which statement by the client indicates the need for further instruction by the nurse?
   ☐ 1. "I require increased periods of rest."
   ☐ 2. "I follow a low-fat, high-carbohydrate diet."
   ☐ 3. "I eat dry toast to relieve my nausea."
   ☐ 4. "I take acetaminophen for arthritis pain."

24. A client plans to travel to a country where hepatitis B is common. What should the nurse advise the client about the **most** effective way to prevent the disease?
   ☐ 1. Drink purified water.
   ☐ 2. Avoid crowded, enclosed spaces.
   ☐ 3. Complete the vaccination series.
   ☐ 4. Observe safe sex practices.

25. The nurse is assessing a client who is in the icteric phase of hepatitis A. Which is an expected finding?
   ☐ 1. tarry stools
   ☐ 2. yellowed sclerae
   ☐ 3. shortness of breath
   ☐ 4. light, frothy urine

26. The nurse is teaching an adult with intravenous substance use disorder about measures to avoid acquiring hepatitis A. What information should the nurse include in the instruction? Select all that apply.
   ☐ 1. observing proper handwashing technique
   ☐ 2. following safe syringe disposal procedures
   ☐ 3. obtaining a vaccination
   ☐ 4. wearing a mask when in crowds
   ☐ 5. using caution when eating fresh fruits and vegetables

27. A client with chronic hepatitis C is experiencing nausea, anorexia, and fatigue. During the health history, the client states that they are homosexual, drink one to two glasses of wine with dinner, take St. John's wort for a "bit of depression," and take acetaminophen for frequent headaches. What action(s) should the nurse take? Select all that apply.
   ☐ 1. Instruct the client that the wine with meals can be beneficial for cardiovascular health.
   ☐ 2. Instruct the client to ask the health care provider (HCP) about taking any other medications as they may interact with medications the client is currently taking.
   ☐ 3. Instruct the client to increase the protein in their diet and eat less frequently.
   ☐ 4. Advise the client of the need for additional testing for HIV.
   ☐ 5. Encourage the client to obtain sufficient rest.

28. The nurse is caring for a client recently diagnosed with hepatitis C. In reviewing the client's history, what information will be **most** helpful as the nurse develops a teaching plan?

The client:
☐ 1. has a history of exercise-induced asthma.
☐ 2. is a scientist and is frequently exposed to multiple chemicals.
☐ 3. traveled to Central America recently and ate uncooked vegetables.
☐ 4. has a known history of sexually transmitted disease.

29. The nurse is developing a teaching plan for a client with viral hepatitis. What information should the nurse include in the plan?
☐ 1. Obtain adequate bed rest.
☐ 2. Increase fluid intake.
☐ 3. Take antibiotic therapy as prescribed.
☐ 4. Drink 8 oz (240 mL) of an electrolyte solution every day.

30. The nurse is planning care for a client with hepatitis A. Information from which laboratory report will be helpful in planning care?
☐ 1. prolonged prothrombin time
☐ 2. decreased blood glucose level
☐ 3. elevated serum potassium level
☐ 4. decreased serum calcium level

31. The nurse develops a teaching plan for the client about how to prevent the transmission of hepatitis A. Which discharge instruction is appropriate for the client?
☐ 1. Spray the house to eliminate infected insects.
☐ 2. Tell family members to try to stay away from the client.
☐ 3. Ask family members to wash their hands frequently.
☐ 4. Disinfect all clothing and eating utensils.

32. The client with hepatitis A is experiencing fatigue, weakness, and a general feeling of malaise. The client tires rapidly during morning care. What is the **most** appropriate goal for this client?
☐ 1. Increase mobility.
☐ 2. Learn new self-care skills.
☐ 3. Adapt to new levels of energy.
☐ 4. Gradually increase activity tolerance.

33. The health care provider has prescribed interferon alfa-2b to treat a client with chronic hepatitis B. The nurse should assess the client for which common adverse effect?
☐ 1. retinopathy
☐ 2. constipation
☐ 3. flulike symptoms
☐ 4. hypoglycemia

34. The nurse is preparing a community education program about preventing hepatitis B infection. Which information should be incorporated into the teaching plan?
☐ 1. Hepatitis B is relatively uncommon among college students.
☐ 2. Frequent ingestion of alcohol can predispose an individual to the development of hepatitis B.
☐ 3. Good personal hygiene habits are most effective at preventing the spread of hepatitis B.
☐ 4. The use of a condom is advised for sexual intercourse.

35. The nurse is establishing goals for the client with hepatitis A. Which goal is appropriate?
☐ 1. Demonstrate a decrease in fluid retention related to ascites.
☐ 2. Verbalize the importance of reporting bleeding gums or bloody stools.
☐ 3. Limit the use of alcohol to two to three drinks per week.
☐ 4. Restrict activity to within the home to prevent disease transmission.

The Adult with Cirrhosis

36. A client had a liver biopsy 1 hour ago. What should the nurse do **first**?
☐ 1. Auscultate lung sounds.
☐ 2. Check for fever.
☐ 3. Obtain a complete blood count (CBC).
☐ 4. Apply packing to the biopsy site.

37. The nurse is assessing a client for ascites. Where does the nurse place the hands to percuss for the presence of fluid?

38. A client with cirrhosis is receiving lactulose. The nurse notes the client is more confused and has asterixis. What should the nurse do **next**?
☐ 1. Assess for gastrointestinal (GI) bleeding.
☐ 2. Withhold the lactulose.
☐ 3. Increase protein in the diet.
☐ 4. Monitor serum bilirubin levels.

39. The nurse is assessing a client with cirrhosis who has developed hepatic encephalopathy. The nurse should notify the health care provider of a decrease in which serum lab value that is a potential precipitating factor for hepatic encephalopathy?
☐ 1. aldosterone
☐ 2. creatinine
☐ 3. potassium
☐ 4. protein

40. A client has advanced cirrhosis of the liver. The client's spouse asks the nurse why the client's abdomen is swollen, making it very difficult to fasten their pants. How should the nurse respond to provide the **most** accurate explanation of the disease process?
☐ 1. "They must have been eating too many foods with salt in them. Salt pulls water with it."
☐ 2. "The swelling in the ankles must have moved up closer to their heart so the fluid circulates better."
☐ 3. "The client must have forgotten to take their daily water pill."
☐ 4. "Blood is not able to flow readily through the liver now, and the liver cannot make protein to keep fluid inside the blood vessels."

41. A nurse is developing a care plan for a client with hepatic encephalopathy. Which would be the goal(s) for the care for this client? Select all that apply.
☐ 1. Prevent constipation.
☐ 2. Administer lactulose to reduce blood ammonia levels.
☐ 3. Monitor coordination while walking.
☐ 4. Check the pupil reaction.
☐ 5. Provide food and fluids high in carbohydrates.
☐ 6. Encourage physical activity.

42. A client with cirrhosis begins to develop ascites. The health care provider prescribes spironolactone to treat the ascites. The nurse should monitor the client closely for which drug-related adverse effect?
☐ 1. constipation
☐ 2. hyperkalemia
☐ 3. irregular pulse
☐ 4. dysuria

43. A client with jaundice has pruritus and areas of irritation from scratching. What measure(s) can the nurse suggest the client use to prevent skin breakdown? Select all that apply.
☐ 1. Avoid lotions containing calamine.
☐ 2. Add baking soda to the water in a tub bath.
☐ 3. Keep nails short and clean.
☐ 4. Rub the skin when it itches with knuckles instead of nails.
☐ 5. Massage skin with alcohol.
☐ 6. Increase sodium intake in the diet.

44. The nurse is developing a health promotion plan with a client with cirrhosis. Which activity should the nurse suggest the client add to the daily routine at home?
☐ 1. Supplement the diet with daily multivitamins.
☐ 2. Abstain from drinking alcohol.
☐ 3. Take a sleeping pill at bedtime.
☐ 4. Limit contact with other people whenever possible.

45. The nurse is reviewing the chart information for a client with increased ascites. The data include: temperature 98.9°F (37.2°C); heart rate 118 bpm; shallow respirations 26 breaths/min; blood pressure 128/76 mm Hg; and percutaneous oxygen saturation (SpO_2) 89% on room air. What should the nurse do **first**?
☐ 1. Assess heart sounds.
☐ 2. Obtain a prescription for blood cultures.
☐ 3. Prepare for a paracentesis.
☐ 4. Raise the head of the bed.

46. The nurse is caring for a client with esophageal varices. The nurse should discuss which laboratory report finding with the health care provider (HCP)?
☐ 1. normal serum albumin
☐ 2. decreased ammonia
☐ 3. slightly decreased levels of calcium
☐ 4. elevated prothrombin time (PT)/international normalized ratio (INR)

47. A client with cirrhosis who has ascites receives 100 mL of 25% serum albumin intravenously. Which finding would indicate that the albumin is having its desired effect?
☐ 1. reduced ascites
☐ 2. increased serum albumin level
☐ 3. decreased anorexia
☐ 4. increased ease of breathing

48. The nurse is assessing a client with a Sengstaken-Blakemore tube. The oxygen saturation on pulse oximetry has dropped from 97% to 91%, and the respiratory rate has changed from 24 to 40 breaths/min. What should the nurse do in order from first to last? All options must be used.

1. Affirm airway obstruction by the tube.
2. Remove the tube.
3. Deflate the tube by cutting with bedside scissors.
4. Apply oxygen via face mask.

49. The nurse monitors a client with cirrhosis for the development of hepatic encephalopathy. Which is an indication that hepatic encephalopathy is developing?
☐ 1. decreased mental status
☐ 2. elevated blood pressure
☐ 3. decreased urine output
☐ 4. labored respirations

50. A client's serum ammonia level is elevated, and the health care provider prescribes 30 mL of lactulose. The nurse should assess the client for which expected effect of this drug?
☐ 1. increased urine output
☐ 2. improved level of consciousness
☐ 3. increased bowel movements
☐ 4. absence of nausea and vomiting

51. A client is to be discharged with a prescription for lactulose. The nurse teaches the client how to administer this medication. Which statement would indicate that the client has understood the information?

"I will:
☐ 1. take it with an antacid."
☐ 2. mix it with apple juice."
☐ 3. take it with a laxative."
☐ 4. mix the crushed tablets in some gelatin."

52. The nurse is providing discharge instructions for a client with cirrhosis. Which statement **best** indicates that the client has understood the teaching?
☐ 1. "I should eat a high-protein, high-carbohydrate diet to provide energy."
☐ 2. "It is safer for me to take acetaminophen for pain instead of aspirin."
☐ 3. "I should avoid constipation to decrease chances of bleeding."
☐ 4. "If I get enough rest and follow my diet, it's possible for my cirrhosis to be cured."

53. The nurse is preparing a client for a paracentesis. What should the nurse do?
☐ 1. Have the client void immediately before the procedure.
☐ 2. Place the client in a side-lying position.
☐ 3. Initiate an intravenous (IV) line to administer sedatives.
☐ 4. Place the client on nothing-by-mouth (NPO) status 6 hours before the procedure.

54. A client with ascites and peripheral edema is at risk for impaired skin integrity. To prevent skin breakdown, the nurse should perform which action?
☐ 1. Institute range-of-motion (ROM) exercises every 4 hours.
☐ 2. Massage the abdomen once a shift.
☐ 3. Use an alternating air pressure mattress.
☐ 4. Elevate the lower extremities.

Managing Care, Quality, and Safety of Adults with Biliary Tract Disorders

55. A client is admitted to the hospital with a diagnosis of hepatitis A. Which precautions should the health care team observe when caring for this client?
☐ 1. gowning when entering a client's room
☐ 2. wearing a mask when providing care
☐ 3. assigning the client to a private room
☐ 4. wearing gloves when giving direct care

56. The nurse has made rounds on a team of clients. The nurse should discuss which client with the health care provider (HCP)?
☐ 1. a client with cirrhosis who is depressed and has refused to eat for the past 2 days
☐ 2. a client with stable vital signs who has been receiving intravenous (IV) ciprofloxacin following a cholecystectomy for 1 day and has developed a rash on the chest and arms
☐ 3. a client with pancreatitis whose family requests to speak with the HCP regarding the treatment plan
☐ 4. a client with hepatitis whose pulse was 84 bpm and regular and is now 118 bpm and irregular

57. The nurse's assignment consists of four clients. From highest to lowest priority, in which order should the nurse assess the clients after receiving the morning report? All options must be used.

1. the client with cirrhosis who became confused and disoriented during the night
2. the client who is 1-day postoperative following a cholecystectomy and has a T-tube inserted
3. the client with acute pancreatitis who is requesting pain medication
4. the client with hepatitis B who has questions about discharge instructions

58. A client with hepatitis C has been admitted to the hospital. The nurse should institute which measure to prevent transmission of the hepatitis C virus to health care personnel?
☐ 1. administering hepatitis C vaccine to all health care personnel
☐ 2. decreasing contact with blood and blood-contaminated fluids
☐ 3. wearing gloves when emptying the bedpan
☐ 4. wearing a gown and mask when providing direct care

59. The nurse is taking care of a client who has an IV infusion pump. The pump alarm rings. What should the nurse do in order from first to last? All options must be used.

| 1. Silence the pump alarm. |
| 2. Determine if the infusion pump is plugged into an electrical outlet. |
| 3. Assess the client's access site for infiltration or inflammation. |
| 4. Assess the tubing for hindrances to flow of solution. |

Answers, Rationales, and Test-Taking Strategies

*The answers and rationales for each question follow below, along with keys (⚿) to the client need (CN) and cognitive level (CL) for each question. In addition, questions that measure clinical judgment will be coded (CJ). As you check your answers, use the **Content Mastery and Test-Taking Skill Self-Analysis** worksheet (tear-out worksheet in the back of the book) to identify the reason(s) for not answering the questions correctly. For additional information about test-taking skills and strategies for answering questions, refer to pages 12–51 in Part 1 of this book.*

The Adult with Cholecystitis

1. 4. There should be no bile-colored drainage coming from any of the incisions postoperatively. A laparoscopic cholecystectomy does not involve a bile bag. Breathing deeply into a paper bag will prevent a person from passing out due to hyperventilation; it does not alleviate nausea. If the adhesive dressings have not already fallen off, they are removed by the surgeon in 7 to 10 days, not 6 weeks.

⚿ CN: Management of care; CL: Create

2. 2. The client is in severe pain, and the nurse should administer the morphine to relieve the pain. The client will receive intravenous fluids to maintain fluid and electrolyte balance, but that will not relieve the pain. The client may be NPO and have a nasogastric tube to promote gastric decompression to prevent further gallbladder stimulation, but these are not sufficient to manage the pain.

⚿ CN: Pharmacologic and parenteral therapies; CL: Analyze

3. -/+ **1, 2, 3.** Bile is created in the liver, stored in the gallbladder, and released into the duodenum, giving stool its brown color. A bile duct obstruction can cause pale-colored stools. Other symptoms associated with cholelithiasis are right upper quadrant tenderness, fever from inflammation or infection, jaundice from elevated serum bilirubin levels, and nausea or right upper quadrant pain after a fatty meal. Pain at McBurney's point lies between the umbilicus and the right iliac crest and is associated with appendicitis. A bleeding ulcer produces black, tarry stools. Respiratory distress is not a symptom of cholelithiasis.

⚿ CN: Physiological adaptation; CL: Analyze

4. **3.** A T-tube is inserted in the common bile duct to maintain patency when there is a likelihood of edema. The tube remains in place until edema from the duct exploration subsides. The bile color should be gold to dark green, and the amount of drainage should be closely monitored to ensure tube patency. Irrigation is not routinely done unless it was prescribed using a smaller volume of fluid. The T-tube is not clamped in the early postoperative period to allow for continuous drainage. An open cholecystectomy has one right subcostal incision, whereas a laparoscopic cholecystectomy has multiple small incisions.

    CN: Physiological adaptation; CL: Evaluate

5. 0/1 **3.** The T-tube should drain approximately 300 to 500 mL in the first 24 hours, and after 3 to 4 days, the amount should decrease to less than 200 mL in 24 hours. With the sudden decrease in drainage at 0800, the nurse should immediately assess the tube for obstruction of flow that can be caused by kinks in the tube or the client lying on the tube. Clients with drainage color must also be assessed for signs of bleeding. The tube should not be irrigated or clamped without a prescription.

    CJ: Standalone trend; CL: Analyze

6. **2.** T-tube bile drainage is recorded separately on the output record. Adding the T-tube drainage to the urine output or wound drainage makes it difficult to accurately determine the amounts of bile, urine, or drainage. The client's total intake will be incorrect if drainage is subtracted from it.

    CN: Reduction of risk potential; CL: Apply

7. **1.** This client is exhibiting signs of sepsis, and the nurse should notify the HCP. The client has three signs indicating sepsis: temperature higher than 101.0°F (38.3°C) (or lower than 96.8°F [36°C]), HR greater than 90 bpm, and RR greater than 20 breaths/min. At least two of these variables are required to diagnose sepsis.

    CN: Physiological integrity; CL: Evaluate

8. **4.** Lean meats, such as beef, lamb, veal, and well-trimmed lean ham and pork, are low in fat. Rice, pasta, and vegetables are low in fat when not served with butter, cream, or sauces. Fruits are low in fat. The amount of fat allowed in a client's diet after a cholecystectomy will depend on the client's ability to tolerate fat. Typically, the client does not require a special diet but is encouraged to avoid excessive fat intake. A cheese omelet and peanut butter have high fat content. Ham salad is high in fat from the fat in a mayonnaise-based salad dressing.

    CN: Basic care and comfort; CL: Apply

9. **1.** The client has severe pain, and the nurse should contact the health care provider for pain medication. An opioid such as morphine is usually prescribed intravenously to manage severe pain. Elevation of the heart rate and blood pressure is likely due to the pain. The pain medication may also relieve the nausea.

    CN: Pharmacological and parenteral therapies; CL: Analyze

10. **1.4 mL.**

    The following formula is used to calculate the correct dosage:

    $$35 \text{ mg}/X \text{ mL} = 25 \text{ mg}/1 \text{ mL}$$
    $$X = 1.4 \text{ mL}$$

    CN: Pharmacological and parenteral therapies; CL: Apply

11. **3.** Immediately after surgery, the client can drink liquids. A light or regular diet can be resumed when the client can tolerate the liquids. There is no need for the client to remain on nothing-by-mouth status after surgery because peristaltic bowel activity should not be affected. The client will probably not be able to tolerate a full meal comfortably the day after surgery. There is no need for the client to stay on a bland diet after a laparoscopic cholecystectomy. The client should, however, avoid excessive fats.

    CN: Physiological adaptation; CL: Analyze

12. **3.** After a laparoscopic cholecystectomy when there are sutures covered by a dressing, the client should not remove dressings from the puncture sites but should wait until visiting the surgeon. The client may shower 48 hours after surgery. A client can return to work within 1 week, but only if approved by the surgeon and no strenuous activity is involved. The client should report any fever, which could be an indication of a complication.

    CN: Reduction of risk potential; CL: Analyze

13. -/+ **1, 3, 5.** Following a laparoscopic cholecystectomy, the client can resume a normal diet as tolerated. The client may experience right shoulder pain from the gas that was used to inflate the abdomen during surgery. The client can take a shower 48 hours after the surgery. The adhesive strips will fall off in about 10 days. The client can resume driving within 3 to 4 days following surgery as long as the client is not taking pain medication. There is no need for the client to maintain bed rest in the days following surgery. Light exercise such as walking can be resumed immediately.

    CN: Physiological adaptation; CL: Evaluate

14. **4.** Portable suction units should be emptied and drained every shift or when full. It is normal for the unit to fill within the first hours after surgery; the nurse does not need to contact the surgeon. There should not be bleeding on the dressing if the drainage system is emptied when full. The drain should not be removed until prescribed by the health care provider.

🔑 CN: Management of care; CL: Analyze

The Adult with Pancreatitis

15. **1.** Alcoholism is a major cause of acute pancreatitis in the United States and Canada. Because some clients are reluctant to discuss alcohol use, staff may inquire about it in several ways. Generally, alcohol intake does not interfere with the tests used to diagnose pancreatitis. Recent ingestion of large amounts of alcohol, however, may cause an increased serum amylase level. Large amounts of ethyl and methyl alcohol may produce an elevated urinary amylase concentration. All clients are asked about alcohol and drug use on hospital admission, but this information is especially pertinent for clients with pancreatitis. HCPs do need to seek facts, but this can be done while respecting the client's religious beliefs. Respecting religious beliefs is important in providing holistic client care.

🔑 CN: Health promotion and maintenance; CL: Apply

16. **2.** Grey Turner sign is a bluish discoloration in the flank area caused by retroperitoneal bleeding. The vital signs are showing hemodynamic instability. IV access should be obtained to provide immediate volume replacement. The urine output will provide information on the fluid status. A nasogastric tube is indicated for clients with uncontrolled nausea and vomiting or gastric distension. Repositioning the client may be considered for pain management once the client's vital signs are stable.

🔑 CN: Physiological adaptation; CL: Analyze

17. **1, 2, 4, 5.** The client with acute pancreatitis usually experiences severe abdominal pain. The client will likely receive an opioid such as morphine to treat the pain. Placing the client in a side-lying position relieves the tension on the abdominal area and promotes comfort. A semi-Fowler position is also appropriate. The nurse should also monitor the client's respiratory status because clients with pancreatitis are prone to develop respiratory complications. Daily weights are obtained to monitor the client's nutritional and fluid volume status. During the acute phase of the illness, when the client is experiencing pain, the pancreas is rested by withholding food and drink. When the diet is reintroduced, it is a high-carbohydrate, low-fat, bland diet.

🔑 CN: Physiological adaptation; CL: Analyze

18. **1.** Hypocalcemia develops in severe cases of acute pancreatitis. The exact cause is unknown. Signs and symptoms of hypocalcemia include jerking and muscle twitching, numbness of fingers and lips, and irritability. Meperidine may cause tremors or seizures as an adverse effect, but not muscle twitching. Muscle twitching is not caused by a nutritional deficit, nor does it indicate that the client needs a muscle relaxant.

🔑 CN: Reduction of risk potential; CL: Analyze

19. **1.** Propantheline is an anticholinergic, antispasmodic medication that decreases vagal stimulation and pancreatic secretions. It is contraindicated in paralytic ileus; therefore, the nurse should be concerned with the absent bowel sounds. Side effects are urinary retention, constipation, and tachycardia.

🔑 CN: Pharmacological and parenteral therapies; CL: Analyze

20. **2.** In chronic pancreatitis, destruction of pancreatic tissue requires pancreatic enzyme replacement. Pancreatic enzymes are prescribed to facilitate the digestion of proteins and fats and should be taken in conjunction with every meal and snack. Specified hours or limited times for administration are ineffective because the enzymes must be taken in conjunction with food ingestion.

🔑 CN: Pharmacological and parenteral therapies; CL: Apply

21. **3.** If the dosage and administration of pancreatic enzymes are adequate, the client's stool will be relatively normal. Any increase in odor or fat content would indicate the need for dosage adjustment. Stable body weight would be another indirect indicator. Fluid intake does not affect enzyme replacement therapy. If diabetes has developed, the client will need to monitor glucose levels. However, glucose and ketone levels are not affected by pancreatic enzyme therapy and would not indicate the effectiveness of the therapy.

🔑 CN: Pharmacological and parenteral therapies; CL: Evaluate

The Adult with Viral Hepatitis

22. **1.** The fluid weight gain is of concern since the drug should be used with caution with impaired renal function. Dosage adjustment may be needed with renal insufficiency since the drug is excreted in the urine. Nausea, minor temperature elevation, and fatigue are symptoms that should be monitored, but they are associated with hepatitis.

🗝 CN: Pharmacological and parenteral therapies; CL: Analyze

23. 4. Acetaminophen is toxic to the liver and should be avoided in a client with liver dysfunction. Increased periods of rest allow for liver regeneration. A low-fat, high-carbohydrate diet and dry toast to relieve nausea are appropriate.

🗝 CN: Health promotion and maintenance; CL: Evaluate

24. 3. The hepatitis B vaccine is the most effective way to prevent infection. The client must complete a series of three or four injections over a period of time for the vaccine to be effective. Hepatitis B is considered a sexually transmitted disease, and the client also should observe safe sex practices, but being vaccinated is most effective. Poor sanitary conditions contribute to the spread of hepatitis A and E, but the client should also avoid drinking liquids that are not bottled. It is not necessary to avoid crowds or closed-in areas.

🗝 CN: Reduction of risk potential; CL: Analyze

25. 2. Liver inflammation and obstruction block the normal flow of bile. Excess bilirubin turns the skin and sclerae yellow and the urine dark and frothy. Profound anorexia is also common. Tarry stools are indicative of gastrointestinal bleeding and would not be expected in hepatitis. Light- or clay-colored stools may occur in hepatitis owing to bile duct obstruction. Shortness of breath would be unexpected.

🗝 CN: Physiological adaptation; CL: Analyze

26. -/+ 1, 2, 3, 5. The client is at risk for having hepatitis C because of intravenous drug use. The main route of transmission for hepatitis A is the oral-fecal route; the disease can be prevented by good handwashing. The client should receive a vaccine for hepatitis A. The vaccine is administered in 2 doses 6 months apart. Percutaneous transmission is more common with hepatitis B, C, and D, but the client should follow safe needle and syringe precautions. Hepatitis A is not transmitted by droplet infection; the client does not need to wear a mask.

🗝 CN: Safety and infection control; CL: Analyze

27. -/+ 2, 4, 5. Clients with chronic hepatitis C should abstain from alcohol as it can speed cirrhosis and end-stage liver disease. Clients should also check with their HCPs before taking any nonprescription or prescription medications or herbal supplements. It is also important that clients who are infected with HCV be tested for HIV, as clients who have both HIV and HCV have a more rapid progression of liver disease than do those who have HCV alone. Clients with HCV and nausea should be instructed to eat four to five times a day to help reduce anorexia and nausea. The client should obtain sufficient rest to manage the fatigue.

🗝 CN: Physiologic adaptation; CL: Analyze

28. 4. Although primarily bloodborne, unprotected sex with multiple partners and a history of sexually transmitted disease are risk factors for transmission of the hepatitis C virus. Other risk factors include blood transfusions, past treatment with chronic hemodialysis, being a child born to a birth mother infected with hepatitis C virus, past or current intravenous drug use disorder, or needlestick injuries to health care workers. It is important for the nurse to be aware of the client's history to help determine the client's level of understanding of the disease, promote a healthy lifestyle, and discuss the role of viral transmission of the disease.

🗝 CN: Safety and infection control; CL: Analyze

29. 1. Treatment of hepatitis consists primarily of bed rest with bathroom privileges. Bed rest is maintained during the acute phase to reduce metabolic demands on the liver, thus increasing its blood supply and promoting liver cell regeneration. When activity is gradually resumed, the client should be taught to rest before becoming overly tired. Although adequate fluid intake is important, it is not necessary to force fluids to treat hepatitis. Antibiotics are not used to treat hepatitis. Electrolyte imbalances are not typical of hepatitis.

🗝 CN: Basic care and comfort; CL: Analyze

30. 1. The prothrombin time may be prolonged because of decreased absorption of vitamin K and decreased production of prothrombin by the liver. The client should be assessed carefully for bleeding tendencies. Blood glucose, serum potassium, and serum calcium levels are not affected by hepatitis.

🗝 CN: Reduction of risk potential; CL: Analyze

31. 3. The hepatitis A virus is transmitted via the fecal-oral route. It spreads through contaminated hands, water, and food, especially shellfish growing in contaminated water. Certain animal handlers are at risk for hepatitis A, particularly those handling primates. Frequent handwashing is probably the single most important preventive action. Insects do not transmit hepatitis A. Family members do not need to stay away from the client with hepatitis. It is not necessary to disinfect food and clothing.

🔑 CN: Safety and infection control; CL: Analyze

32. 4. The most appropriate goal for this client with hepatitis is to increase activity gradually as tolerated. Periods of alternating rest and activity should be included in the plan of care. There is no evidence that the client is physically immobile, is unable to provide self-care, or needs to adapt to new energy levels.

🔑 CN: Basic care and comfort; CL: Analyze

33. 3. Interferon alfa-2b most commonly causes flulike adverse effects, such as myalgia, arthralgia, headache, nausea, fever, and fatigue. Retinopathy is a potential adverse effect, but not a common one. Diarrhea may develop as an adverse effect. Clients are advised to administer the drug at bedtime and get adequate rest. Medications may be prescribed to treat the symptoms. The drug may also cause hematologic changes; therefore, laboratory tests such as a complete blood count and differential should be conducted monthly during drug therapy. Blood glucose laboratory values should be monitored for the development of hyperglycemia.

🔑 CN: Pharmacological and parenteral therapies; CL: Analyze

34. 4. Hepatitis B is spread through exposure to blood or blood products and through high-risk sexual activity. Hepatitis B is considered to be a sexually transmitted disease. High-risk sexual activities include sex with multiple partners, unprotected sex with an infected individual, male homosexual activity, and sexual activity with intravenous drug users. College students are at high risk for the development of hepatitis B and are encouraged to be immunized. Alcohol intake by itself does not predispose an individual to hepatitis B, but it can lead to high-risk behaviors such as unprotected sex. Good personal hygiene alone will not prevent the transmission of hepatitis B.

🔑 CN: Safety and infection control; CL: Create

35. 2. The client should be able to verbalize the importance of reporting any bleeding tendencies that could be the result of a prolonged prothrombin time. Ascites is not typically a clinical manifestation of hepatitis; it is associated with cirrhosis. Alcohol use should be eliminated for at least 1 year after the diagnosis of hepatitis to allow the liver time to fully recover. There is no need for a client to be restricted to the home because hepatitis is not spread through casual contact between individuals.

🔑 CN: Physiological adaptation; CL: Evaluate

The Adult with Cirrhosis

36. 1. Because the biopsy needle insertion site is close to the lung, there is a risk for lung puncture and pneumothorax; therefore, immediately after the procedure, the nurse should determine diminished or absent lung sounds in the right lung. Although fever indicates infection, a rise in temperature is not seen immediately. A CBC is warranted if the vital signs and client symptoms indicate potential hemorrhage. The needle insertion site is covered with a pressure dressing; there is no need for a dressing requiring packing.

🔑 CN: Safety and infection control; CL: Analyze

37. The nurse places the client in a supine position and percusses from the midline laterally and listens for a change from tympany from bowel gas to dullness, which indicates the presence of fluid.

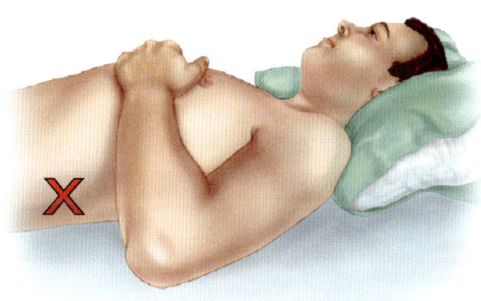

🔑 CN: Physiological adaptation; CL: Apply

38. 1. Clients with cirrhosis can develop hepatic encephalopathy caused by increased ammonia levels. Asterixis, a flapping tremor, is a characteristic symptom of increased ammonia levels. Bacterial action on increased protein in the bowel will increase ammonia levels and cause the encephalopathy to worsen. GI bleeding and protein consumed in the diet increase protein in the intestine and can elevate ammonia levels. Lactulose is given to reduce ammonia formation in the intestine and should not be held since neurologic symptoms are worsening. Bilirubin is associated with jaundice.

🔑 CN: Pharmacological and parenteral therapies; CL: Analyze

39. 3. Hypokalemia is a precipitating factor in hepatic encephalopathy. A decrease in creatinine results from muscle atrophy; an increase in creatinine would indicate renal insufficiency. With liver dysfunction, increased aldosterone levels are seen. A decrease in serum protein will decrease colloid osmotic pressure and promote edema.

 CN: Physiological adaptation; CL: Analyze

40. 4. Portal hypertension and hypoalbuminemia as a result of cirrhosis cause a fluid shift into the peritoneal space causing ascites. In a cardiac or kidney problem, not cirrhosis, sodium can promote edema formation and subsequent decreased urine output. Edema does not migrate upward toward the heart to enhance its circulation. Although diuretics promote the excretion of excess fluid, occasionally forgetting or omitting a dose will not yield the ascites found in cirrhosis of the liver.

 CN: Physiological adaptation; CL: Analyze

41. -/+ 1, 2, 3, 4, 5. Constipation leads to increased ammonia production. Lactulose is a hyperosmotic laxative that reduces blood ammonia by acidifying the colon contents, which retards the diffusion of nonionic ammonia from the colon to the blood while promoting its migration from the blood to the colon. Hepatic encephalopathy is considered a toxic or metabolic condition that causes cerebral edema; it affects a person's coordination and pupil reaction to light and accommodation. Food and fluids high in carbohydrates should be given because the liver is not synthesizing and storing glucose. Because exercise produces ammonia as a by-product of metabolism, physical activity should be limited, not encouraged.

 CN: Management of care; CL: Create

42. 2. Spironolactone is a potassium-sparing diuretic; therefore, clients should be monitored closely for hyperkalemia. Other common adverse effects include abdominal cramping, diarrhea, dizziness, headache, and rash. Constipation and dysuria are not common adverse effects of spironolactone. An irregular pulse is not an adverse effect of spironolactone but could develop if serum potassium levels are not closely monitored.

 CN: Pharmacological and parenteral therapies; CL: Analyze

43. -/+ 2, 3, 4. Baking soda baths can decrease pruritus. Keeping nails short and rubbing the area with knuckles can decrease breakdown when scratching. Calamine lotions help relieve itching. Alcohol will increase skin dryness. Sodium in the diet will increase edema and weaken skin integrity.

 CN: Basic care and comfort; CL: Create

44. 2. General health promotion measures include maintaining good nutrition, avoiding infection, and abstaining from alcohol. It is not necessary to take multivitamins if the client is obtaining adequate nutrition. Rest and sleep are essential, but an impaired liver may not be able to detoxify sedatives and barbiturates. Such drugs must be used cautiously, if at all, by clients with cirrhosis. The client does not need to limit contact with others but should exercise caution to stay away from ill people.

 CN: Health promotion and maintenance; CL: Analyze

45. 4. Elevating the head of the bed will allow for increased lung expansion by decreasing the ascites pressing on the diaphragm. The client requires reassessment. A paracentesis is reserved for symptomatic clients with ascites with impaired respiration or abdominal pain not responding to other measures such as sodium restriction and diuretics. There is no indication for blood cultures. Heart sounds are assessed with a routine physical assessment.

 CN: Physiological adaptation; CL: Analyze

46. 4. The client with esophageal varices is at even higher risk for bleeding with an elevated PT/INR. The nurse and HCP collaborate to prevent bleeding. The other laboratory findings are not as life-threatening. A decreased serum albumin can cause fluid to move into the interstitial tissues. Increased ammonia levels are toxic to the brain. Calcium loss is more common with pancreatitis.

 CN: Physiological adaptation; CL: Analyze

47. 1. Normal serum albumin is administered to reduce ascites. Hypoalbuminemia, a mechanism underlying ascites formation, results in decreased colloid osmotic pressure. Administering serum albumin increases the plasma colloid osmotic pressure, which causes fluid to flow from the tissue space into the plasma. Increased urine output is the best indication that the albumin is having the desired effect. An increased serum albumin level and increased ease of breathing may indirectly imply that the administration of albumin is effective in relieving the ascites. However, it is not as direct an indicator as increased urine output and reduced ascites. Anorexia is not affected by the administration of albumin.

 CN: Pharmacological and parenteral therapies; CL: Evaluate

48. 1, 3, 2, 4. The nurse should first assess the client to determine if the tube is obstructing the airway; assessment is done by assessing airflow.

Once the obstruction is established, the tube should be deflated and then quickly removed. A set of scissors should always be at the bedside to allow for emergency deflation of the balloon. Oxygen via face mask should then be applied once the tube is removed.

🗝 CN: Safety and infection control; CL: Analyze

49. 1. The client should be monitored closely for changes in mental status. Ammonia has a toxic effect on central nervous system tissue and produces an altered level of consciousness, marked by drowsiness and irritability. If this process is unchecked, the client may lapse into a coma. Increasing ammonia levels are not detected by changes in blood pressure, urine output, or respirations.

🗝 CN: Physiological adaptation; CL: Analyze

50. 3. Lactulose increases intestinal motility, thereby trapping and expelling ammonia in the feces. An increase in the number of bowel movements is expected.. Lactulose does not affect urine output. Any improvements in mental status would be the result of increased ammonia elimination, not a direct effect of the drug. Nausea and vomiting are not expected effects of lactulose.

🗝 CN: Pharmacological and parenteral therapies; CL: Apply

51. 2. The taste of lactulose is a problem for some clients. Mixing it with fruit juice, water, or milk can make it more palatable. Lactulose should not be given with antacids, which may inhibit its action. Lactulose should not be taken with a laxative because increased stooling is an adverse effect of the drug and would be potentiated by using a laxative. Lactulose comes in the form of syrup for oral or rectal administration.

🗝 CN: Pharmacological and parenteral therapies; CL: Evaluate

52. 3. Clients with cirrhosis should be instructed to avoid constipation and straining at stool to prevent hemorrhage. The client with cirrhosis has bleeding tendencies because of the liver's inability to produce clotting factors. A low-protein and high-carbohydrate diet is recommended. Clients with cirrhosis should not take acetaminophen, which is potentially hepatotoxic. Aspirin also should be avoided if esophageal varices are present. Cirrhosis is a chronic disease.

🗝 CN: Reduction of risk potential; CL: Evaluate

53. 1. Immediately before a paracentesis, the client should empty the bladder to prevent perforation. The client will be placed in a high Fowler position or seated on the side of the bed for the procedure. IV sedatives are not usually administered. The client does not need to be NPO.

🗝 CN: Reduction of risk potential; CL: Analyze

54. 3. Edematous tissue is easily traumatized and must receive meticulous care. An alternating air pressure mattress will help decrease pressure on the edematous tissue. ROM exercises are important to maintain joint function, but they do not necessarily prevent skin breakdown. When abdominal skin is stretched taut due to ascites, it must be cleaned very carefully. The abdomen should not be massaged. Elevation of the lower extremities promotes venous return and decreases swelling.

🗝 CN: Reduction of risk potential; CL: Analyze

Managing Care, Quality, and Safety of Adults with Biliary Tract Disorders

55. 4. Contact precautions are recommended for clients with hepatitis A. This includes wearing gloves for direct care. A gown is not required unless substantial contact with the client is anticipated. It is not necessary to wear a mask. The client does not need a private room unless incontinent of stool.

🗝 CN: Safety and infection control; CL: Create

56. 4. A change in a client's baseline vital signs should be brought to the HCP's attention immediately. In this case, the client's heart rate has increased, and the rhythm appears to have changed; the HCP may prescribe an electrocardiogram to determine if treatment is necessary. The nurse should also have a complete set of current vital signs as well as a physical assessment before providing the HCP information using the SBAR (Situation-Background-Assessment-Recommendation) format. The nutritional as well as psychological needs of a client must be addressed, but they are not the first priority. A rash that develops after a new antibiotic is started must be brought to the HCP's attention; however, this client is stable and is not the first priority. The nurse is responsible to facilitate discussion between the client, the client's family, and the HCP, but only after all of the immediate physical and psychological needs of all clients have been met.

🗝 CN: Reduction of risk potential; CL: Analyze

57. **1, 3, 2, 4.** The nurse should first assess the client with cirrhosis to ensure the client's safety and assess the client for the onset of hepatic encephalopathy. The nurse should then assess the client with acute pancreatitis who is requesting pain medication and administer the needed medication. The nurse should next assess the client who underwent a cholecystectomy and is 1 day postoperative to make sure that the T-tube is draining and that the client is performing postoperative breathing exercises. This client's safety is not at risk, and the client is not reporting having pain. The nurse can speak last with the client with hepatitis B who has questions about discharge instructions because this client's issues are not urgent.

CN: Management of care; CL: Analyze

58. **2.** Hepatitis C is usually transmitted through blood exposure or needlesticks. A hepatitis C vaccine is currently under development, but it is not available for use. The first line of defense against hepatitis B is the hepatitis B vaccine. Hepatitis C is not transmitted through feces or urine. Wearing a gown and mask will not prevent transmission of the hepatitis C virus if the caregiver comes in contact with infected blood or needles.

CN: Safety and infection control; CL: Apply

59. **1, 3, 4, 2.** Silencing the alarm will eliminate a stressor for the client and allow the nurse to focus on the task at hand. The nurse should then assess the access site to note if the needle is inserted in the vein or if there is tissue trauma, infiltration, or inflammation. Next, the nurse should check for kinks in the tubing. Finally, the nurse can plug the pump into the wall to allow the battery to become recharged.

CN: Pharmacological and parenteral therapies; CL: Analyze

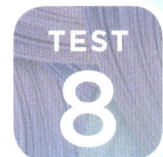

TEST 8

The Adult with Endocrine Health Problems

- The Adult with Disorders of the Thyroid
- The Adult with Diabetes Mellitus
- The Adult with Pituitary Adenoma
- The Adult with Addison's Disease
- The Adult with Cushing's Disease
- Managing Care, Quality, and Safety of Adults with Endocrine Health Problems
- Answers, Rationales, and Test-Taking Strategies

The Adult with Disorders of the Thyroid

1. The nurse is completing a health assessment of a client with suspected Grave's disease. When conducting a focused assessment, the nurse should assess the client for which finding?
☐ 1. anorexia
☐ 2. tachycardia
☐ 3. weight gain
☐ 4. cold skin

2. When conducting a health history with a young female client with thyrotoxicosis, the nurse should ask about which changes related to menstruation?
☐ 1. dysmenorrhea
☐ 2. metrorrhagia
☐ 3. oligomenorrhea
☐ 4. menorrhagia

3. A young female client is diagnosed with hypothyroidism. What information should the nurse obtain when conducting a focused assessment? Select all that apply.
☐ 1. rapid pulse
☐ 2. decreased energy and fatigue
☐ 3. weight gain of 10 lb (4.5 kg)
☐ 4. fine, thin hair with hair loss
☐ 5. constipation
☐ 6. menorrhagia

4. Propylthiouracil (PTU) is prescribed for a client with Grave's disease. Which symptom should the nurse teach the client to report?
☐ 1. sore throat
☐ 2. excessive menstruation
☐ 3. constipation
☐ 4. increased urine output

5. A client with thyrotoxicosis says to the nurse, "I'm so irritable. I'm having problems at work because I lose my temper very easily." Which response by the nurse would give the client the most accurate explanation of this behavior?

"You are experiencing:
☐ 1. temporary confusion brought on by your illness."
☐ 2. excess thyroid hormone in your system."
☐ 3. worry about the seriousness of your illness."
☐ 4. stress of trying to manage a career and cope with illness."

6. The nurse is evaluating a client with hyperthyroidism who is taking propylthiouracil (PTU) 100 mg a day in three divided doses for maintenance therapy. Which statement from the client indicates the drug is effective?
☐ 1. "I have excess energy throughout the day."
☐ 2. "I'm able to sleep and rest at night."
☐ 3. "I've lost weight since taking this medication."
☐ 4. "I perspire throughout the entire day."

7. A client with hyperthyroidism is to have a thyroidectomy. The health care provider (HCP) has prescribed propranolol. In reviewing the client's history, the nurse notes that the client has asthma. What should the nurse do next?
☐ 1. Take the client's pulse, and withhold the propranolol if the pulse is less than 100 bpm.
☐ 2. Count the client's respirations, and withhold the propranolol if the respirations are less than 20 breaths/min.
☐ 3. Contact the HCP, and discuss the prescription for propranolol because of the client's history of having asthma.
☐ 4. Instruct the client to make position changes slowly.

8. A client with Grave's disease has exophthalmos. What should the nurse teach the client to do to prevent corneal irritation?
☐ 1. Massage the eyes every 4 hours.
☐ 2. Instill an ophthalmic anesthetic as prescribed.
☐ 3. Wear dark-colored glasses when awake.
☐ 4. Cover both eyes with moistened gauze pads at night.

9. A client with hyperthyroidism is to be treated with radioactive iodine (RAI, I-131). Following treatment, what should the nurse teach the client to do?
☐ 1. Monitor for signs and symptoms of hyperthyroidism.
☐ 2. Rest for 1 week to prevent complications of the medication.
☐ 3. Take thyroxine replacement for the remainder of the client's life.
☐ 4. Assess for hypertension and tachycardia resulting from altered thyroid activity.

10. A client with a large goiter is scheduled for a subtotal thyroidectomy to treat thyrotoxicosis. Saturated solution of potassium iodide (SSKI) is prescribed preoperatively for the client. What should the nurse explain to the client about the expected outcome of using this drug?
The drug helps:
☐ 1. slow the progression of exophthalmos.
☐ 2. reduce the vascularity of the thyroid gland.
☐ 3. decrease the body's ability to store thyroxine.
☐ 4. increase the body's ability to excrete thyroxine.

11. A client with hyperthyroidism is to take saturated solution of potassium iodide (SSKI). What should the nurse do when administering this drug?
☐ 1. Pour the solution over ice chips.
☐ 2. Mix the solution with an antacid.
☐ 3. Dilute the solution with water or juice.
☐ 4. Mix the solution in pureed fruit.

12. Immediately following a thyroidectomy, the nurse asks the client to say "hello." The client moves their lips but is not able to speak the word. What should the nurse do **next**?
☐ 1. Give the client a sip of water.
☐ 2. Have the client take a deep breath and cough.
☐ 3. Notify the surgeon.
☐ 4. Check the client's pupillary response.

13. One day after a subtotal thyroidectomy, a client begins to have tingling in the fingers and toes. What should the nurse do **first**?
☐ 1. Encourage the client to flex and extend the fingers and toes.
☐ 2. Notify the health care provider (HCP).
☐ 3. Assess the client for thrombophlebitis.
☐ 4. Ask the client to speak.

14. The nurse is planning care for a client who is to have a subtotal thyroidectomy. Which medication should be available to provide emergency treatment if a client develops tetany?
☐ 1. sodium phosphate
☐ 2. calcium gluconate
☐ 3. echothiophate iodide
☐ 4. sodium bicarbonate

15. A client is diagnosed with hypothyroidism. What additional information should the nurse obtain when conducting a focused assessment?
☐ 1. tachycardia
☐ 2. weight gain
☐ 3. diarrhea
☐ 4. nausea

16. A client is being evaluated for hypothyroidism. To plan care, the nurse should ask the client about which sign or symptom?
☐ 1. corneal abrasion
☐ 2. weight loss
☐ 3. diarrhea
☐ 4. fatigue

17. A client with hypothyroidism has started to take thyroid hormone replacement therapy and asks the nurse about the reason for feeling sad and depressed. What should the nurse tell the client? "The feelings of sadness and depression are caused by:
☐ 1. the side effects of thyroid hormone replacement therapy and will diminish over time."
☐ 2. a condition unrelated to hypothyroidism and require follow-up."
☐ 3. having a chronic illness and are normal."
☐ 4. low thyroid hormone levels and will improve with replacement therapy."

18. The nurse is instructing the client with hypothyroidism who takes levothyroxine 100 mcg, digoxin, and simvastatin. The nurse judges that the teaching regarding the use of these medications is effective if the client will take:
☐ 1. the levothyroxine with breakfast and the other medications after breakfast.
☐ 2. the levothyroxine before breakfast and the other medications 4 hours later.
☐ 3. all medications together 1 hour after eating breakfast.
☐ 4. all medications before going to bed.

The Adult with Diabetes Mellitus

19. The nurse is teaching a client who has been newly diagnosed with type 2 diabetes. The nurse should begin the teaching process by asking which question?
☐ 1. "How much does your family need to be involved in learning about your condition?"
☐ 2. "What is required for your family to manage your symptoms?"
☐ 3. "What activities are most important for you to be able to maintain control of your diabetes?"
☐ 4. "What do you know about your medications and condition?"

20. The nurse is obtaining a health history from a client with type 2 diabetes mellitus who has been taking insulin for 20 years. Currently, the client reports having periods of hypoglycemia followed by periods of hyperglycemia. What should the nurse ask about the client's current management plan?
Is the client:
☐ 1. eating snacks between meals?
☐ 2. using an insulin pump?
☐ 3. injecting insulin at a site of lipodystrophy?
☐ 4. adjusting insulin according to blood glucose levels?

21. An adult with type 2 diabetes mellitus has been on nothing by mouth (NPO) status since 2200 in preparation for having a nephrectomy the next day. At 0600 on the day of surgery, the nurse reviews the client's medical record and laboratory results. Which finding should the nurse report to the health care provider?
☐ 1. urine output of 350 mL in 8 hours
☐ 2. urine specific gravity of 1.015
☐ 3. potassium of 4.0 mEq (4 mmol/L)
☐ 4. blood glucose of 140 mg/dL (7.8 mmol/L)

22. The nurse is checking the laboratory results of an adult female client with type 1 diabetes (see chart). What laboratory result indicates a problem that should be managed?

Laboratory Results

Test	Results	Normal Range
Blood glucose	192 mg/dL (10.7 mmol/L)	Adults: less than or equal to 110 mg/dL (less than or equal to 5.6 mmol/L)
Total cholesterol	180 mg/dL (4.7 mmol/L)	Adults: 140–199 mg/dL (3.63–5.15 mmol/L)
Hemoglobin	12.3 mg/dL (123 g/L)	Women: 12–16 g/dL (120–160 g/L)
Low-density lipoprotein cholesterol	125 mg/dL (3.2 mmol/L)	Optimal LDL levels are less than 100 mg/dL (less than 2.6 mmol/L)

☐ 1. blood glucose
☐ 2. total cholesterol
☐ 3. hemoglobin
☐ 4. low-density lipoprotein (LDL) cholesterol

23. A client with type 1 diabetes mellitus has diabetic ketoacidosis. Which finding has the **greatest** effect on fluid loss?
☐ 1. hypotension
☐ 2. decreased serum potassium level
☐ 3. rapid, deep respirations
☐ 4. warm, dry skin

24. A client is to receive glargine insulin in addition to a dose of aspart. When the nurse checks the blood glucose level at the bedside, it is higher than 200 mg/dL (11.1 mmol/L). How should the nurse administer the insulins?
☐ 1. Put air into the glargine insulin vial and then air into the aspart insulin vial, and draw up the correct dose of aspart insulin first.
☐ 2. Roll the glargine insulin vial, and then roll the aspart insulin vial. Draw up the longer-acting glargine insulin first.
☐ 3. Shake both vials of insulin before drawing up each dose in separate insulin syringes.
☐ 4. Put air into the glargine insulin vial, and draw up the correct dose in an insulin syringe; then with a different insulin syringe, put air into the aspart vial, and draw up the correct dose.

25. The client with type 2 insulin-requiring diabetes asks the nurse about having alcoholic beverages. Which is the **best** response by the nurse?
☐ 1. "You can have one or two drinks a day as long as you have something to eat with them."
☐ 2. "Alcohol is detoxified in the liver, so it's not a good idea for you to drink anything with alcohol."
☐ 3. "If you are going to have a drink, it's best to consume alcohol on an empty stomach."
☐ 4. "If you do have a drink, the blood glucose value may be elevated at bedtime, and you should skip having a snack."

26. An adult with type 2 diabetes is taking metformin 1000 mg two times every day. The client asks the nurse about having an alcoholic drink. Which statement indicates the client understands the interaction of alcohol and metformin?
☐ 1. "If I know I'll be having alcohol, I shouldn't take metformin."
☐ 2. "If my health care provider approves, I may drink alcohol with my metformin."
☐ 3. "Adverse effects I should watch for are feeling excessively energetic, unusual muscle stiffness, low back pain, and a rapid heartbeat."
☐ 4. "If I feel bloated, I should call my health care provider."

27. Before supper, an adult client who has type 2 diabetes and requires insulin tells the nurse about having tremors and being weak and anxious. What should the nurse do **next**?
☐ 1. Tell the client to lie down for 30 minutes.
☐ 2. Have the client drink a glass of milk or orange juice.
☐ 3. Contact the client's health care provider (HCP) to decrease the insulin dose.
☐ 4. Administer the next dose of insulin.

28. The health care provider (HCP) has prescribed insulin detemir for a client with type 2 diabetes requiring insulin. What should the nurse teach the client about this insulin?
☐ 1. "You may increase the carbohydrates in your diet when using this insulin."
☐ 2. "You do not need to rotate injection sites with this insulin."
☐ 3. "You do not mix insulin detemir; the solution is clear."
☐ 4. "You may refill the detemir insulin pen."

29. A nurse is evaluating the effectiveness of teaching a client about how to self-administer insulin. Which action indicates that additional teaching is necessary?
The client:
☐ 1. draws up the regular insulin first and then the NPH.
☐ 2. rotates sites from legs to arms.
☐ 3. identifies that the syringe is U-100.
☐ 4. waits 30 minutes to eat breakfast after injecting rapid-acting insulin.

30. A client with newly diagnosed type 1 diabetes is scheduled to receive regular insulin 10 units and NPH insulin 20 units every morning. When should the nurse schedule the administration of these medications?
☐ 1. regular insulin with breakfast; NPH after breakfast
☐ 2. both insulins 0.5 hours before breakfast
☐ 3. in two separate syringes with breakfast
☐ 4. NPH 1 hour before and regular 0.5 hours before breakfast

31. Which information should the nurse include when developing a teaching plan for a client newly diagnosed with type 2 diabetes mellitus? Select all that apply.
☐ 1. A major risk factor for complications is obesity and central abdominal obesity.
☐ 2. Supplemental insulin is mandatory for controlling the disease.
☐ 3. Exercise increases insulin resistance.
☐ 4. The primary nutritional source requiring monitoring in the diet is carbohydrates.
☐ 5. Annual eye and foot examinations are recommended by the American and Canadian Diabetes Associations.

32. The nurse is teaching a client with diabetes about foot care. What should the nurse instruct the client to do?
☐ 1. Avoid going barefoot.
☐ 2. Buy shoes a half size larger.
☐ 3. Cut toenails at angles.
☐ 4. Use heating pads for sore feet.

33. A client with type 1 diabetes mellitus asks the nurse to recommend something to remove corns from the toes. What should the nurse advise the client to do?
☐ 1. Apply high-quality corn plaster to the area.
☐ 2. Consult a health care provider (HCP) about removing the corns.
☐ 3. Apply iodine to the corns before peeling them off.
☐ 4. Soak the feet in borax solution to peel off the corns.

34. A client with diabetes mellitus presents to the clinic for a regular 3-month follow-up appointment. The nurse notes several small bandages covering cuts on the client's hands. The client says, "I'm so clumsy. I'm always cutting my finger cooking or burning myself on the iron." Which response by the nurse would be **most** appropriate?
☐ 1. "Wash all wounds in isopropyl alcohol."
☐ 2. "Keep all cuts clean and covered."
☐ 3. "Could you have your children do the cooking and ironing?"
☐ 4. "You really should be fine as long as you take your daily medication."

35. STEP 1

The nurse is caring for a 22-year-old adult male client in the emergency department.

Nurse's Notes

Today: 1030
The client ran out of insulin 3 days ago. The client has a medical history of type 1 diabetes and anxiety. They use the carbohydrate counting method for administering insulin, and they adjust the dose based on the premeal glucose ranges.

Vital signs are temperature 99.4°F (37.6°C); pulse 135 bpm; respiration rate 34 breaths/min; and blood pressure 130/83 mm Hg. Pulse oximetry shows an oxygen saturation of 98% on room air. The client is alert and oriented, but breathing appears deep and rapid with clear lung sounds. The client feels hot to the touch, has dry mucous membranes, and has a fruity odor to their breath. The client reports fatigue and nausea. The client's stat blood glucose level is 420 mg/dL (23.3 mmol/L).

➤ Highlight the findings below that require follow-up. Answer choices have been underlined.

Nurse's Notes

Today: 1030
The client ran out of insulin 3 days ago. The client has a medical history of type 1 diabetes and anxiety. They use the carbohydrate counting method for administering insulin, and they adjust the dose based on the premeal glucose ranges.

Vital signs are temperature 99.4°C (37.6°C); <u>pulse 135 bpm</u>; <u>respiration rate 34 breaths/min</u>; and <u>blood pressure 130/83 mm Hg</u>. Pulse oximetry shows an oxygen saturation of 98% on room air. The client is alert and oriented, but <u>breathing appears deep and rapid</u> with clear lung sounds. The client feels hot to the touch, has <u>dry mucous membranes</u>, and has a <u>fruity odor to their breath</u>. The client reports fatigue and nausea. The client's stat <u>blood glucose level is 420 mg/dL (23.3 mmol/L)</u>.

36. STEP 2

The nurse is caring for a 22-year old male client in the emergency department.

Nurse's Notes

Today: 1030
The client ran out of insulin 3 days ago. The client has a medical history of type 1 diabetes and anxiety. They use the carbohydrate counting method for administering insulin, and they adjust the dose based on the premeal glucose ranges.

Vital signs are temperature 99.4°F (37.6°C); pulse 135 bpm; respiration rate 34 breaths/min; and blood pressure 130/83 mm Hg. Pulse oximetry shows an oxygen saturation of 98% on room air. The client is alert and oriented, but breathing appears deep and rapid with clear lung sounds. The client feels hot to the touch, has dry mucous membranes, and has a fruity odor to their breath. The client reports fatigue and nausea. The client's stat blood glucose level is 420 mg/dL (23.3 mmol/L).

The nurse continues to gather information about the client.

➤ For each additional assessment, indicate if the information would be helpful or not helpful in determining the severity of the client's high blood sugar.

Assessment	Helpful	Not Helpful
Pulse oximetry	○	○
Urinalysis	○	○
Complete metabolic panel	○	○
Electrocardiogram (ECG)	○	○
Abdominal computed tomography (CT)	○	○

37. STEP 3

The nurse is caring for a 22-year-old male client in the emergency department.

Nurse's Notes

Today: 1030
The client ran out of insulin 3 days ago. The client has a medical history of type 1 diabetes and anxiety. They use the carbohydrate counting method for administering insulin, and they adjust the dose based on the premeal glucose ranges.

Vital signs are temperature 99.4°F (37.6°C); pulse 135 bpm; respiration rate 34 breaths/min; and blood pressure 130/83 mm Hg. Pulse oximetry shows an oxygen saturation of 98% on room air. The client is alert and oriented, but breathing appears deep and rapid with clear lung sounds. The client feels hot to the touch, has dry mucous membranes, and has a fruity odor to their breath. The client reports fatigue and nausea. The client's stat blood glucose level is 420 mg/dL (23.3 mmol/L).

The nurse is determining the client's priority problem.

➤ Complete the following sentence from the list of options.

The client's [neurologic assessment / gastrointestinal assessment / integumentary assessment]

is indicative that the client is at risk for [diabetic ketoacidosis. / hypoglycemia. / Addison's disease.]

38. STEP 4

The nurse is caring for a 22-year-old male client in the emergency department.

Nurse's Notes

Today: 1030
The client ran out of insulin 3 days ago. The client has a medical history of type 1 diabetes and anxiety. They use the carbohydrate counting method for administering insulin, and they adjust the dose based on the premeal glucose ranges.

Vital signs are temperature 99.4°F (37.6°C); pulse 135 bpm; respiration rate 34 breaths/min; and blood pressure 130/83 mm Hg. Pulse oximetry shows an oxygen saturation of 98% on room air. The client is alert and oriented, but breathing appears deep and rapid with clear lung sounds. The client feels hot to the touch, has dry mucous membranes, and has a fruity odor to their breath. The client reports fatigue and nausea. The client's stat blood glucose level is 420 mg/dL (23.3 mmol/L).

Orders

Time	Order
1050	Administer 10 units of regular insulin PIV
1050	Place an indwelling urinary catheter
1050	Administer 10 mEq/dL (10 mmol/L) of oral potassium
1050	Administer 1 L of 0.9% normal saline intravenously
1050	Obtain a hemoglobin A1C level
1050	Place a central line
1050	Obtain a chest x-ray
1050	Obtain a serum potassium level

The nurse receives orders from the health care provider.

➤ Identify the top three orders the nurse should perform **right away**.

- ☐ 1. Administer 10 units of regular insulin.
- ☐ 2. Place an indwelling urinary catheter.
- ☐ 3. Administer 10 mEq/dL (10 mmol/L) of oral potassium.
- ☐ 4. Administer 1 L of 0.9% normal saline intravenously.
- ☐ 5. Obtain a hemoglobin A1C level.
- ☐ 6. Place a central line.
- ☐ 7. Obtain a chest x-ray.
- ☐ 8. Obtain a serum potassium level.

39. STEP 5

The nurse is caring for a 22-year-old male client in the emergency department.

Nurse's Notes

Today: 1030
The client ran out of insulin 3 days ago. The client has a medical history of type 1 diabetes and anxiety. They use the carbohydrate counting method for administering insulin, and they adjust the dose based on the premeal glucose ranges.

Vital signs are temperature 99.4°F (37.6°C); pulse 135 bpm; respiration rate 34 breaths/min; and blood pressure 130/83 mm Hg. Pulse oximetry shows an oxygen saturation of 98% on room air. The client is alert and oriented, but breathing appears deep and rapid with clear lung sounds. The client feels hot to the touch, has dry mucous membranes, and has a fruity odor to their breath. The client reports fatigue and nausea. The client's stat blood glucose level is 420 mg/dL (23.3 mmol/L).

Orders

Time	Order
1050	Administer 10 units of regular insulin per IV
1050	Place an indwelling urinary catheter
1050	Administer 10 mEq/dL (10 mmol/L) of oral potassium
1050	Administer 1 L of 0.9% normal saline per IV
1050	Obtain a hemoglobin A1C level
1050	Place a central line
1050	Obtain a chest x-ray
1050	Obtain a serum potassium level

The nurse is administering 10 units of regular insulin to the client.

➤ For each step, specify if the step is appropriate or inappropriate for administering insulin.

Steps to Administering Insulin	Appropriate	Inappropriate
1. Verify with another nurse the type and dose of the insulin.	○	○
2. Verify two client identifiers before administration.	○	○
3. Shake the vial vigorously.	○	○
4. Rotate sites between legs and arms.	○	○
5. Place the insulin in the refrigerator after administering the dose.	○	○

40. STEP 6

The nurse is caring for a 22-year-old male client in the emergency department.

Nurse's Notes

Today: 1030
The client ran out of insulin 3 days ago. The client has a medical history of type 1 diabetes and anxiety. They use the carbohydrate counting method for administering insulin, and they adjust the dose based on the premeal glucose ranges.
Vital signs are temperature 99.4°F (37.6°C); pulse 135 bpm; respiration rate 34 breaths/min; and blood pressure 130/83 mm Hg. Pulse oximetry shows an oxygen saturation of 98% on room air. The client is alert and oriented, but breathing appears deep and rapid with clear lung sounds. The client feels hot to the touch, has dry mucous membranes, and has a fruity odor to their breath. The client reports fatigue and nausea. The client's stat blood glucose level is 420 mg/dL (23.3 mmol/L).

Orders

Time	Order
1050	Administer 10 units of regular insulin per IV
1050	Place an indwelling urinary catheter
1050	Administer 10 mEq/dL (10 mmol/L) of oral potassium
1050	Administer 1 L of 0.9% normal saline per IV
1050	Obtain a hemoglobin A1C level
1050	Place a central line
1050	Obtain a chest x-ray
1050	Obtain a serum potassium level

The nurse has administered the insulin as ordered.

➤ For each finding below, specify if the finding is a desired outcome or a side or adverse effect.

Client Finding	Desired Outcome	Side Effect or Adverse Effect
Respiratory rate of 26 breaths/min	○	○
Moist skin	○	○
Hypokalemia	○	○
Blood glucose level lower than 125 mg/dL (6.94 mmol/L)	○	○
Altered level of consciousness	○	○

---

41. A client with type 1 diabetes mellitus is admitted to the emergency department. Which respiratory pattern in a client with diabetes mellitus requires **immediate** action?
- ☐ 1. deep, rapid respirations with long expirations
- ☐ 2. shallow respirations alternating with long expirations
- ☐ 3. regular depth of respirations with frequent pauses
- ☐ 4. short expirations and inspirations

42. A client has been recently diagnosed with type 2 diabetes and is taking metformin two times per day, 1000 mg before breakfast and 1000 mg before supper. The client is experiencing diarrhea, nausea, vomiting, abdominal bloating, and anorexia on admission to the hospital. The admission prescriptions include metformin. What should the nurse do? Select all that apply.
- ☐ 1. Discontinue the metformin.
- ☐ 2. Administer glargine insulin rather than the metformin.
- ☐ 3. Inform the client that the adverse effects of diarrhea, nausea, and upset stomach gradually subside over time.
- ☐ 4. Assess the client's renal function.
- ☐ 5. Monitor the client's glucose value before each meal.

43. A client with type 2 diabetes has just started to take dulaglutide. The client reports having severe nausea. What should the nurse instruct the client to do to manage the nausea? Select all that apply.
☐ 1. Eat small meals more frequently.
☐ 2. Increase the fat content in the diet.
☐ 3. Drink ginger tea.
☐ 4. Stop using the drug.
☐ 5. Avoid fried foods.

44. A client is to use an insulin pen. Which action(s) would indicate the client is using the pen correctly? Select all that apply.
☐ 1. stores the unopened pens in the refrigerator
☐ 2. injects the insulin in sites around the abdomen
☐ 3. primes the pen by expelling any air
☐ 4. massages the site after injection
☐ 5. saves the needle for reuse

45. A client with type 2 insulin-requiring diabetes has the flu with nausea, body aches, and lack of appetite. The client's blood sugar is 180 mg/dL (10 mmol/L). The vital signs are temperature 101°F (38.3°C), pulse 88 bpm, and respirations 20 breaths/min. What should the nurse instruct the client to do? Select all that apply.
☐ 1. Stop taking insulin.
☐ 2. Check the blood sugar every 4 hours.
☐ 3. Drink 240 mL of fluids every hour.
☐ 4. Check the urine for ketones.
☐ 5. Take two 325-mg aspirin.

46. A client who uses an insulin pen asks the nurse how to dispose of the needles. The client's job requires frequent travel by airplane. What information should the nurse include in the teaching plan? Select all that apply.
☐ 1. At home, dispose of needles in a sharps container or solid plastic container.
☐ 2. Put three-quarters-full sharps containers in recycling bins for home waste management pick-up.
☐ 3. Carry a travel-size disposal container, and dispose of needles in the hotel recycling bin.
☐ 4. Follow Transportation Safety Agency (TSA) guidelines for labeling medications and safe disposal.
☐ 5. Wipe the needle with alcohol, wrap it in tissue, and discard it in a recycling container.

47. The health care provider has s prescribed exenatide for a client with type 2 diabetes mellitus. What should the nurse instruct the client to do? Select all that apply.
☐ 1. Review the one-time setup for each new pen.
☐ 2. Inject in the thigh, abdomen, or upper arm.
☐ 3. Administer the drug within 60 minutes before morning and evening meals.
☐ 4. Understand that there is a low incidence of hypoglycemia when exenatide is taken with insulin.
☐ 5. Take the dose of exenatide as soon as the client remembers a dose has been missed.

48. The nurse is administering the initial dose of rapid-acting insulin to a client with type 1 diabetes. At what time should the nurse assess the client for hypoglycemia?
☐ 1. 0.5 hours
☐ 2. 1 hour
☐ 3. 2 hours
☐ 4. 3 hours

49. The nurse notes grapefruit juice on the breakfast tray of a client with type 2 diabetes mellitus who is taking repaglinide. What should the nurse do **next**?
☐ 1. Contact the manager of the food and nutrition department.
☐ 2. Request that the dietitian discuss the drug-food interaction between repaglinide and grapefruit juice with the client.
☐ 3. Substitute a half grapefruit in place of the grapefruit juice.
☐ 4. Remove the grapefruit juice from the client's tray, and bring another juice of the client's preference.

50. The nurse is instructing a client with type 1 diabetes about how to reduce the risk for developing type 2 diabetes mellitus. What should the nurse instruct the client to do?
☐ 1. Stop smoking cigarettes.
☐ 2. Increase the amount of protein in the diet.
☐ 3. Maintain weight within normal limits.
☐ 4. Prevent hypertension.

51. The client with type 1 diabetes mellitus is taught to take isophane insulin suspension NPH at 1700 each day. The client should be instructed that the **greatest** risk for hypoglycemia will occur at about what time?
☐ 1. 1100, shortly before lunch
☐ 2. 1300, shortly after lunch
☐ 3. 1800, shortly after dinner
☐ 4. 0100, while sleeping

52. The nurse is developing a teaching plan with a client with type 2 diabetes about how to use an insulin pump. Which information should be included in the plan? Select all that apply.
☐ 1. The pump is more accurate than insulin injections.
☐ 2. The pump will need to be changed every 2 to 3 days.
☐ 3. The pump will need to be programmed for basal level insulin needs.
☐ 4. Use only long-acting insulin.
☐ 5. Continue to check blood glucose levels daily.
☐ 6. Increase the bolus dose if dietary intake has increased.
☐ 7. Information will need to be entered into the pump every day.

53. A nurse is teaching a client with type 1 diabetes mellitus who jogs daily about the preferred sites for insulin absorption. What is the **most** appropriate site for a client who jogs?
- ☐ 1. arms
- ☐ 2. legs
- ☐ 3. abdomen
- ☐ 4. iliac crest

54. A client with diabetes is taking insulin lispro injections. At what time should the nurse advise the client to eat?
- ☐ 1. within 10 to 15 minutes after the injection
- ☐ 2. 1 hour after the injection
- ☐ 3. at any time because timing meals with lispro injections is unnecessary
- ☐ 4. 2 hours before the injection

55. The nurse has instructed a client newly diagnosed with diabetes on how to self-inject insulin. Which is the **best** indicator that the client has learned how to give an insulin self-injection correctly?

The client can:
- ☐ 1. perform the procedure safely and correctly.
- ☐ 2. critique the nurse's performance of the procedure.
- ☐ 3. explain all steps of the procedure correctly.
- ☐ 4. obtain 100% correct answers on a posttest.

56. The nurse is instructing the client on insulin administration. The client is performing a return demonstration for preparing the insulin. The client's morning dose of insulin is 10 units of regular and 22 units of NPH. The nurse checks the dose accuracy with the client. The nurse determines that the client has prepared the correct dose when the syringe reads how many units? Record your answer using a whole number.
_____ **units.**

57. The nurse should teach a client with diabetes that which symptom is **most** indicative of hypoglycemia?
- ☐ 1. nervousness
- ☐ 2. anorexia
- ☐ 3. Kussmaul respirations
- ☐ 4. bradycardia

58. The nurse is assessing the client's understanding of the use of medications. Which medication may cause a complication with the treatment plan of a client with diabetes?
- ☐ 1. aspirin
- ☐ 2. steroids
- ☐ 3. sulfonylureas
- ☐ 4. angiotensin-converting enzyme (ACE) inhibitors

59. A client with diabetes begins to cry and says, "I just can't stand the thought of having to give myself a shot every day." What would be the **best** response by the nurse?
- ☐ 1. "If you don't give yourself your insulin shots, you'll be at greater risk for complications."
- ☐ 2. "We can teach a family member to give the shots so you won't have to do it."
- ☐ 3. "I can arrange to have a home care nurse give you the shots every day."
- ☐ 4. "What bothers you about giving yourself the insulin shots?"

The Adult with Pituitary Adenoma

60. A client is to have a transsphenoidal hypophysectomy to remove a large, invasive pituitary tumor. Where should the nurse tell the client the surgical incision will be made?
- ☐ 1. back of the mouth
- ☐ 2. high in the nares
- ☐ 3. sinus channel below the right eye
- ☐ 4. upper gingival mucosa in the space between the upper gums and lip

61. A client is to have a hypophysectomy. To minimize the risk for postoperative respiratory complications, the nurse should instruct the client to perform which action?
- ☐ 1. Limit the use of pain medications.
- ☐ 2. Turn the head from side to side.
- ☐ 3. Take deep breaths.
- ☐ 4. Clear the throat and cough.

62. A client underwent a transsphenoidal hypophysectomy 2 hours ago. The nurse should assess the client for which sign of a potential complication?
- ☐ 1. cerebrospinal fluid (CSF) leak
- ☐ 2. fluctuating blood glucose levels
- ☐ 3. Cushing's syndrome
- ☐ 4. cardiac arrhythmias

63. After undergoing a transsphenoidal hypophysectomy, a client has a cerebrospinal fluid (CSF) leak. The nurse should prepare the client for which treatment of the leak?
- ☐ 1. packing the nose with pressure dressings
- ☐ 2. returning the client to surgery to close the leak
- ☐ 3. maintaining bed rest with the head of the bed elevated to 30 degrees
- ☐ 4. administering high-dose corticosteroid therapy

64. A client is recovering from transsphenoidal hypophysectomy. What should the nurse instruct the client to do to ensure oral hygiene?
- ☐ 1. Rinse the mouth with saline.
- ☐ 2. Perform frequent toothbrushing.
- ☐ 3. Clean the teeth with an electric toothbrush.
- ☐ 4. Floss the teeth thoroughly.

65. A client has had a hypophysectomy. What sign of a potential complication should the nurse teach the client to report?
☐ 1. acromegaly
☐ 2. Cushing's disease
☐ 3. diabetes mellitus
☐ 4. hypopituitarism

66. The nurse is planning care for a client who had a hypophysectomy. The nurse reviews the client's lab reports and intake/output record. Which laboratory finding should the nurse report to the health care provider?
☐ 1. urine specific gravity less than 1.010
☐ 2. urine output between 5 to 40 L in 24 hours
☐ 3. blood glucose level of 300 mg/dL (16.7 mmol/L)
☐ 4. absence of glucose and ketones in the urine

67. A client with diabetes insipidus is receiving vasopressin. Which sign indicates that the drug is having the intended effect?
☐ 1. lower blood pressure
☐ 2. concentration of urine
☐ 3. normal insulin levels
☐ 4. improved glucose metabolism

68. Which statement indicates that the client with diabetes insipidus understands how to manage care? The client will:
☐ 1. maintain normal fluid and electrolyte balance.
☐ 2. select a diabetic diet correctly.
☐ 3. state dietary restrictions.
☐ 4. exhibit a serum glucose level within normal range.

The Adult with Addison's Disease

69. The nurse is instructing an 18-year-old college freshman with Addison's disease who is on the football team on how to adjust the dose of glucocorticoids. The nurse should explain that the client may need an increased dosage of glucocorticoids in which situation?
☐ 1. taking a test
☐ 2. gaining 4 lb (1.8 kg)
☐ 3. drinking a beer
☐ 4. working out at football practice

70. The nurse is assessing a client who is in addisonian crisis. Which goal is the **priority**?
☐ 1. controlling hypertension
☐ 2. preventing irreversible shock
☐ 3. preventing infection
☐ 4. relieving anxiety

71. The nurse is assessing a client who is in addisonian crisis. What is an expected finding?
☐ 1. fluid retention
☐ 2. pain
☐ 3. peripheral edema
☐ 4. hunger

72. A client with Addison's disease is taking corticosteroid replacement therapy. The nurse should instruct the client about which side effect(s) of corticosteroids? Select all that apply.
☐ 1. hyperkalemia
☐ 2. skeletal muscle weakness
☐ 3. mood changes
☐ 4. hypocalcemia
☐ 5. increased susceptibility to infection
☐ 6. hypotension

73. A client with Addison's disease has fluid and electrolyte loss due to inadequate fluid intake and fluid loss. As the client's oral intake increases, which fluids would be **most** appropriate?
☐ 1. milk and diet soda
☐ 2. water and eggnog
☐ 3. chicken broth and juice
☐ 4. coffee and milkshakes

74. The nurse is conducting discharge education with a client newly diagnosed with Addison's disease. Which information should be included in the client and family teaching plan? Select all that apply.
☐ 1. Addison's disease will resolve over a few weeks, requiring no further treatment.
☐ 2. Avoiding stress and maintaining a balanced lifestyle will minimize the risk for exacerbations.
☐ 3. Fatigue, weakness, dizziness, and mood changes need to be reported to the health care provider.
☐ 4. A medical identification bracelet should be worn.
☐ 5. Family members need to be informed about the warning signals of adrenal crisis.
☐ 6. Dental work or surgery will require adjustment of daily medication.

75. A client has been diagnosed with Addison's disease. The nurse should plan with the client to manage which effect of the disease?
☐ 1. weight gain
☐ 2. hunger
☐ 3. lethargy
☐ 4. muscle spasms

76. The nurse is developing a teaching plan with a client who is newly diagnosed with Addison's disease. Which topic is **most** important to include in the teaching plan?
☐ 1. the importance of watching for signs of hyperglycemia
☐ 2. the need to adjust the steroid dose based on dietary intake and exercise
☐ 3. to notify the health care provider (HCP) when the blood pressure is suddenly high
☐ 4. how to decrease the dose of the corticosteroids when the client experiences stress

77. A client with Addison's disease is taking glucocorticoids at home. Which statement indicates that the client understands how to take the medication?
    - ☐ 1. "Various circumstances increase the need for glucocorticoids, so I will need to adjust the dosage."
    - ☐ 2. "My need for glucocorticoids will stabilize, and I will be able to take a predetermined dose once a day."
    - ☐ 3. "Glucocorticoids are cumulative, so I will take a dose every third day."
    - ☐ 4. "I must take a dose every 6 hours to ensure consistent blood levels of glucocorticoids."

78. Cortisone acetate and fludrocortisone acetate are prescribed as replacement therapy for a client with Addison's disease. What administration schedule should be followed for this therapy?
    - ☐ 1. Take both drugs three times a day.
    - ☐ 2. Take the entire dose of both drugs first thing in the morning.
    - ☐ 3. Take all the fludrocortisone acetate and two-thirds of the cortisone acetate in the morning, and take the remaining cortisone acetate in the afternoon.
    - ☐ 4. Take half of each drug in the morning and the remaining half of each drug at bedtime.

79. The nurse is teaching a client with Cushing's disease about taking oral glucocorticoids. What information should the nurse give to the client about taking the medication?
    - ☐ 1. with a full glass of water
    - ☐ 2. on an empty stomach
    - ☐ 3. at bedtime to increase absorption
    - ☐ 4. with meals or with an antacid

80. The nurse is assessing a client with Addison's disease about taking a glucocorticoid replacement. Which is the best indicator that the medication is having the intended effect?
    - ☐ 1. skin turgor
    - ☐ 2. temperature
    - ☐ 3. thirst
    - ☐ 4. daily weight

81. The nurse is evaluating the outcome of the care plan for a client with Addison's disease. Which outcome indicated the care plan is effective?
    - ☐ **none.** The client:
    - ☐ 1. takes medication as prescribed.
    - ☐ 2. avoids stressful situations.
    - ☐ 3. follows a 2-g sodium diet.
    - ☐ 4. prevents hypertensive episodes.

82. A client with Addison's disease is concerned about the bronze color of their skin. What should the nurse tell the client about the cause of the bronze color?
    - ☐ 1. hypersensitivity to sun exposure
    - ☐ 2. increased serum bilirubin level
    - ☐ 3. adverse effects of the glucocorticoid therapy
    - ☐ 4. increased secretion of adrenocorticotropic hormone (ACTH)

The Adult with Cushing's Disease

83. A client diagnosed with Cushing's syndrome is admitted to the hospital and scheduled for a dexamethasone suppression test. What should the nurse do during this test?
    - ☐ 1. Collect a 24-hour urine specimen to measure serum cortisol levels.
    - ☐ 2. Administer 1 mg of dexamethasone orally at night, and obtain serum cortisol levels the next morning.
    - ☐ 3. Draw blood samples before and after exercise to evaluate the effect of exercise on serum cortisol levels.
    - ☐ 4. Administer an injection of adrenocorticotropic hormone (ACTH) 30 minutes before drawing blood to measure serum cortisol levels.

84. The nurse is assessing a client with Cushing's disease. Which finding is concerning?
    - ☐ 1. postprandial hypoglycemia
    - ☐ 2. hypokalemia
    - ☐ 3. hyponatremia
    - ☐ 4. decreased urine calcium level

85. The client with Cushing's disease needs to modify dietary intake to control symptoms. In addition to increasing protein, which strategy would be **most** appropriate?
    - ☐ 1. Increase calories.
    - ☐ 2. Restrict sodium.
    - ☐ 3. Restrict potassium.
    - ☐ 4. Reduce fat to 10%.

86. Bone resorption is a possible complication of Cushing's disease. To help the client prevent this complication, the nurse should make which recommendation to the client?
    - ☐ 1. Increase the amount of potassium in the diet.
    - ☐ 2. Maintain a regular program of weight-bearing exercise.
    - ☐ 3. Limit dietary vitamin D intake.
    - ☐ 4. Perform isometric exercises.

87. A client has an adrenal tumor and is scheduled for a bilateral adrenalectomy. During preoperative teaching, the nurse teaches the client how to do deep-breathing exercises after surgery. What should the nurse tell the client to do?
    - ☐ 1. "Sit in an upright position, and take a deep breath."
    - ☐ 2. "Hold your abdomen firmly with a pillow, and take several deep breaths."
    - ☐ 3. "Tighten your stomach muscles as you inhale, and breathe normally."
    - ☐ 4. "Raise your shoulders to expand your chest."

88. A client has had an adrenalectomy. What is the **priority** goal for this client in the first 24 hours after surgery?
☐ 1. beginning oral nutrition
☐ 2. promoting self-care activities
☐ 3. preventing adrenal crisis
☐ 4. ambulating in the hallway

89. A client undergoing a bilateral adrenalectomy has postoperative prescriptions for hydromorphone hydrochloride 2 mg to be administered subcutaneously every 4 hours as needed for pain. Why should the nurse administer hydromorphone in small doses?

A small dose is:
☐ 1. less likely to cause dependency.
☐ 2. less irritating to subcutaneous tissues in small doses.
☐ 3. as potent as morphine in larger doses.
☐ 4. excreted before accumulating in toxic amounts in the body.

90. The nurse is caring for a client who is scheduled for an adrenalectomy. Which drug may be included in the preoperative prescriptions to prevent addisonian crisis following surgery?
☐ 1. prednisone orally
☐ 2. fludrocortisone subcutaneously
☐ 3. spironolactone intramuscularly
☐ 4. methylprednisolone sodium succinate intravenously

91. A client who is recovering from a bilateral adrenalectomy has a patient-controlled analgesia (PCA) system with morphine sulfate. What should the nurse do to manage the safe administration of the morphine?
☐ 1. Observe the client at regular intervals for opioid addiction.
☐ 2. Encourage the client to reduce analgesic use and tolerate the pain.
☐ 3. Evaluate pain control at least every 2 hours.
☐ 4. Increase the amount of morphine if the client does not administer the medication.

92. A client has had a bilateral adrenalectomy. For which potential complication should the nurse assess the client?
☐ 1. postoperative confusion
☐ 2. delayed wound healing
☐ 3. pulmonary emboli
☐ 4. malnutrition

93. The client who has undergone a bilateral adrenalectomy is concerned about persistent body changes and unpredictable moods. What should the nurse teach the client about these changes?
☐ 1. The body changes are permanent, and the client will not be the same as before this condition.
☐ 2. The body and mood will gradually return to normal.
☐ 3. The physical changes are permanent, but the mood swings will disappear.
☐ 4. The physical changes are temporary, but the mood swings are permanent.

94. After a bilateral adrenalectomy for Cushing's disease, the client will receive periodic testosterone injections. What is the expected outcome of these injections?
☐ 1. balanced reproductive cycle
☐ 2. restored sodium and potassium balance
☐ 3. stimulated protein metabolism
☐ 4. stabilized mood swings

95. The nurse is developing a teaching plan with a client who had a bilateral adrenalectomy. What information should the nurse include in the plan?
☐ 1. The client will need steroid replacement for the rest of their life.
☐ 2. The client must decrease the dose of steroid medication carefully to prevent a crisis.
☐ 3. The client will require steroids only until their body can manufacture sufficient quantities.
☐ 4. The client will need to take steroids whenever their life involves physical or emotional stress.

Managing Care, Quality, and Safety of Adults with Endocrine Health Problems

96. The nurse is reviewing the postoperative prescriptions (see chart) just written by a health care provider (HCP) for a client with type 1 diabetes who has returned to the surgery floor from the recovery room following surgery for a left hip replacement. The client has a pain rating of 5 on a scale of 0 to 10. The hand-off report from the nurse in the recovery room indicated that the vital signs have been stable for the last 30 minutes. After obtaining the client's glucose level, the nurse should do what **first**?

Prescriptions
- Vital signs every 15 minutes for 4 hours, then every hour for 8 hours.
- Oxygen 2 L/min per nasal cannula.
- 1,000 mL NS every 8 hours.
- 10 mg morphine intramuscularly every 4 hours as needed.
- 10 U regular insulin stat.

☐ 1. Administer the morphine.
☐ 2. Contact the health care provider (HCP) to rewrite the insulin prescription.
☐ 3. Administer oxygen per nasal cannula at 2 L per minute.
☐ 4. Take the vital signs.

97. The nurse is receiving results of a blood glucose level from the laboratory over the telephone. What should the nurse do?
☐ 1. Write down the results, read back the results to the caller from the laboratory, and receive confirmation from the caller.
☐ 2. Repeat the results to the caller from the laboratory, write the results on scrap paper, and then transfer the results to the medical record.
☐ 3. Indicate to the caller that the nurse cannot receive results from lab tests over the telephone, and ask the lab to bring the written results to the nurses' station.
☐ 4. Request that the laboratory send the results by email to transfer to the client's medical record.

98. A client with type 1 diabetes is admitted to the emergency department with dehydration following the flu. The client has a blood glucose level of 325 mg/dL (18 mmol/L) and a serum potassium level of 3.5 mEq (3.5 mmol/L). The health care provider (HCP) has prescribed 1000 mL 5% dextrose in water to be infused every 8 hours. What should the nurse do before implementing the HCP's prescriptions? Contact the HCP and:
☐ 1. suggest adding potassium to the fluids.
☐ 2. request an increase in the volume of intravenous fluids.
☐ 3. verify the prescription for 5% dextrose in water.
☐ 4. determine if the client should be placed in isolation.

99. Glulisine insulin is prescribed to be administered to a client before each meal. To assist the day-shift nurse who is receiving the report, the night-shift nurse gives the morning dose of glulisine. When the day-shift nurse goes to the room of the client who requires glulisine, the nurse finds that the client is not in the room. The client's roommate tells the nurse that the client "went for a test." What should the nurse do **next**?
☐ 1. Bring a small glass of juice, and locate the client.
☐ 2. Call the client's health care provider (HCP).
☐ 3. Check the computerized care plan to determine what test was scheduled.
☐ 4. Send the nurse's assistant to the x-ray department to bring the client back to his room.

100. A client who has been diagnosed with type 1 diabetes has an insulin drip to aid in lowering the serum blood glucose level of 600 mg/dL (33.3 mmol/L). The client is also receiving ciprofloxacin intravenously (IV). The health care provider (HCP) prescribes discontinuation of the insulin drip. What should the nurse do **next**?
☐ 1. Discontinue the insulin drip, as prescribed.
☐ 2. Hang the next IV dose of antibiotic before discontinuing the insulin drip.
☐ 3. Inform the HCP that the client has not received any subcutaneous insulin yet.
☐ 4. Add glargine to the insulin drip before discontinuing it.

101. A nurse has just received a report on four clients. Which client should the nurse see **first**?
☐ 1. a client who underwent a thyroidectomy and has new-onset hoarseness
☐ 2. a client with Cushing's syndrome who has been noted to have a blood sugar level of 134 mg/dL (7.4 mmol/L)
☐ 3. a client in renal failure who has a laboratory report noting a creatinine level of 3.2 mg/dL (282.3 μmol/L)
☐ 4. a client who was diagnosed with ulcerative colitis and recently passed 100 mL of loose, bloody stools

Answers, Rationales, and Test-Taking Strategies

*The answers and rationales for each question follow below, along with keys (🗝) to the client need (CN) and cognitive level (CL) for each question. In addition, questions that measure clinical judgment will be coded (CJ). As you check your answers, use the **Content Mastery and Test-Taking Skill Self-Analysis** worksheet (tear-out worksheet in the back of the book) to identify the reason(s) for not answering the questions correctly. For additional information about test-taking skills and strategies for answering questions, refer to pages 12–51 in part 1 of this book.*

The Adult with Disorders of the Thyroid

1. **2.** Grave's disease, the most common type of thyrotoxicosis, is a state of hypermetabolism. The increased metabolic rate generates heat and produces tachycardia and fine muscle tremors. Anorexia is associated with hypothyroidism. Loss of weight, despite a good appetite and adequate caloric intake, is a common feature of hyperthyroidism. Cold skin is associated with hypothyroidism.

    🗝 CN: Physiological adaptation; CL: Analyze

2. **3.** A change in the menstrual interval, diminished menstrual flow (oligomenorrhea), or even the absence of menstruation (amenorrhea) may result from the hormonal imbalances of thyrotoxicosis. Oligomenorrhea in women and decreased libido and impotence in men are common features of thyrotoxicosis. Dysmenorrhea is painful menstruation. Metrorrhagia, blood loss between menstrual periods, is a symptom of hypothyroidism. Menorrhagia, excessive bleeding during menstrual periods, is a symptom of hypothyroidism.

    🗝 CN: Physiological adaptation; CL: Analyze

3. -/+ **2, 3, 5, 6.** Clients with hypothyroidism exhibit symptoms indicating a lack of thyroid hormone. Bradycardia, decreased energy and lethargy, memory problems, weight gain, coarse hair, constipation, and menorrhagia are common signs and symptoms of hypothyroidism.

    🗝 CN: Physiological adaptation; CL: Analyze

4. **1.** The most serious adverse effects of PTU are leukopenia and agranulocytosis, which usually occur within the first 3 months of treatment. The client should be taught to promptly report to the health care provider signs and symptoms of infection, such as a sore throat and fever. Clients having a sore throat and fever should have an immediate white blood cell count and differential performed, and the drug must be withheld until the results are obtained. Painful menstruation, constipation, and increased urine output are not associated with PTU therapy.

    🗝 CN: Pharmacological and parenteral therapies; CL: Analyze

5. **2.** A typical sign of thyrotoxicosis is irritability caused by the high levels of circulating thyroid hormones in the body. This symptom decreases as the client responds to therapy. Thyrotoxicosis does not cause confusion. The client may be worried about the illness, and stress may influence their mood; however, irritability is a common symptom of thyrotoxicosis, and the client should be informed of that fact rather than blamed.

    🗝 CN: Psychosocial integrity; CL: Analyze

6. **2.** PTU is a prototype of thioamide antithyroid drugs. It inhibits the production of thyroid hormones and peripheral conversion of T_4 to the more active T_3. A client taking this antithyroid drug should be able to sleep and rest well at night since the level of thyroid hormones is reduced in the blood. Excess energy throughout the day, loss of weight, and perspiring through the day are symptoms of hyperthyroidism indicating the drug has not produced its outcome.

    🗝 CN: Pharmacological and parenteral therapies; CL: Evaluate

7. **3.** Propranolol hydrochloride is a nonselective beta-blocker of both cardiac and bronchial adrenoreceptors, which competes with epinephrine and norepinephrine for available beta-receptor sites. Propranolol blocks the cardiac effects of beta-adrenergic stimulation; as a result, it reduces heart rate; a hypertensive effect is associated with decreased cardiac output. A contraindication of propranolol is bronchial asthma; propranolol can cause bronchiolar constriction even in normal clients. The nurse takes the apical pulse and blood pressure before administering propranolol. The medication is withheld if the heart rate is less than 60 bpm or the systolic blood pressure is less than 90 mm Hg.

    🗝 CN: Pharmacological and parenteral therapies; CL: Analyze

8. **3.** Treatment of mild ophthalmopathy that may accompany thyrotoxicosis includes measures such as wearing sunglasses to protect the eyes from corneal irritation. Treatment of ophthalmopathy should be performed in consultation with an ophthalmologist. Massaging the eyes will not help to protect the cornea. An ophthalmic anesthetic is used to

examine and possibly treat a painful eye, not protect the cornea. Covering the eyes with moist gauze pads is not a satisfactory nursing measure to protect the eyes of a client with exophthalmos because treatment is not focused on moisture to the eye but rather on protecting the cornea and optic nerve. In exophthalmos, the retrobulbar connective tissues and extraocular muscle volume are expanded because of fluid retention. The pressure is also increased.

🗝️ CN: Reduction of risk potential; CL: Analyze

9. 3. The client needs to be educated about the need for lifelong thyroid hormone replacement. Permanent hypothyroidism is the major complication of radioactive iodine treatment. Lifelong medical follow-up and thyroid replacement are warranted. The client needs to monitor for signs and symptoms of hypothyroidism, not hyperthyroidism. Resting for 1 week is not necessary. Hypertension and tachycardia are signs of hyperthyroidism, not hypothyroidism.

🗝️ CN: Pharmacological and parenteral therapies; CL: Analyze

10. 2. SSKI is frequently administered before a thyroidectomy because it helps decrease the vascularity of the thyroid gland. A highly vascular thyroid gland is very friable, a condition that presents a hazard during surgery. Preparation of the client for surgery includes depleting the gland of thyroid hormone and decreasing vascularity. SSKI does not decrease the progression of exophthalmos, and it does not decrease the body's ability to store thyroxine or increase the body's ability to excrete thyroxine.

🗝️ CN: Pharmacological and parenteral therapies; CL: Apply

11. 3. SSKI should be diluted well in milk, water, juice, or a carbonated beverage before administration to help disguise the strong, bitter taste. Also, this drug is irritating to the mucosa if taken undiluted. The client should sip the diluted preparation through a drinking straw to help prevent staining of the teeth. Pouring the solution over ice chips will not sufficiently dilute the SSKI or cover the taste. Antacids are not used to dilute or cover the taste of SSKI. Mixing in a puree would put the SSKI in contact with the teeth.

🗝️ CN: Pharmacological and parenteral therapies; CL: Apply

12. 3. The nurse first should notify the surgeon; the inability to speak may indicate laryngeal nerve damage. The client should not receive water until fully recovered from anesthesia. Coughing now will irritate the throat. The client is responsive, so a pupillary check would not be indicated as the immediate action.

🗝️ CN: Reduction of risk potential; CL: Analyze

13. 2. Tetany may occur after thyroidectomy if the parathyroid glands are accidentally injured or removed during surgery. This would cause a disturbance in serum calcium levels. An early sign of tetany is numbness and tingling of the fingers or toes and in the circumoral region. Tetany may occur from 1 to 7 days postoperatively. Late signs and symptoms of tetany include seizures, contraction of the glottis, and respiratory obstruction. The nurse should notify the HCP. Exercising the joints in the fingers and toes will not relieve the tetany. The client is not exhibiting signs of thrombophlebitis. There is no indication of nerve damage that would cause the client not to be able to speak.

🗝️ CN: Physiological adaptation; CL: Analyze

14. 2. The client with tetany has hypocalcemia, which is treated by administering an intravenous preparation of calcium, such as calcium gluconate or calcium chloride. Oral calcium is then necessary until normal parathyroid function returns. Sodium phosphate is a laxative. Echothiophate iodide is an eye preparation used as a miotic for an antiglaucoma effect. Sodium bicarbonate is a potent systemic antacid.

🗝️ CN: Pharmacological and parenteral therapies; CL: Apply

15. 2. Typical signs and symptoms of hypothyroidism include weight gain, fatigue, decreased energy, apathy, brittle nails, dry skin, cold intolerance, hair loss, constipation, and numbness and tingling in the fingers. Tachycardia is a sign of hyperthyroidism, not hypothyroidism. Diarrhea and nausea are not symptoms of hypothyroidism.

🗝️ CN: Physiological adaptation; CL: Analyze

16. 4. A major problem for the person with hypothyroidism is fatigue. Other signs and symptoms include lethargy, personality changes, generalized edema, impaired memory, slowed speech, cold intolerance, dry skin, muscle weakness, constipation, weight gain, and hair loss. Incomplete closure of the eyelids, hypermetabolism, and diarrhea are associated with hyperthyroidism.

🗝️ CN: Basic care and comfort; CL: Analyze

17. 4. Hypothyroidism may contribute to sadness and depression. This client needs to know that these feelings may be related to low thyroid hormone levels and may improve with treatment. Replacement therapy does not cause depression. Depression may accompany chronic illness, but it is not "normal."

🔑 CN: Psychosocial integrity; CL: Analyze

18. 2. Levothyroxine must be given at the same time each day on an empty stomach, preferably ½ to 1 hour before breakfast. Other medications may impair the action of levothyroxine absorption; the client should separate doses of other medications by 4 to 5 hours.

🔑 CN: Pharmacological and parenteral therapies; CL: Evaluate

The Adult with Diabetes Mellitus

19. 3. Empowerment is an approach to clinical practice that emphasizes helping people discover and use their innate abilities to gain mastery over their own condition. Empowerment means that individuals with a health problem have the tools, such as knowledge, control, resources, and experience, to implement and evaluate their self-management practices. Involvement of others, such as asking the client about family involvement, implies that the others will provide the direct care needed rather than the client. Asking the client what the client needs to know implies that the nurse will be the one to provide the information. Telling the client what is required does not provide the client with options or lead to empowerment.

🔑 CN: Health promotion and maintenance; CL: Analyze

20. 3. Lipodystrophy, specifically lipohypertrophy, involves swelling of the fat at the site of repeated injections, which can interfere with the absorption of insulin, resulting in erratic blood glucose levels. Because the client has been receiving insulin for many years, this is the most likely cause of poor control. Eating snacks between meals causes hyperglycemia. Adjusting insulin according to blood glucose levels would not cause hypoglycemia; it would cause normal glucose levels. Initiating an insulin pump would not, in itself, cause periods of hyperglycemia.

🔑 CN: Physiological Integrity; CL: Analyze

21. 4. The client's blood glucose level is elevated, beyond levels accepted for fasting; the normal blood glucose range is 70 to 120 mg/dL (3.9 to 6.7 mmol/L). The specific gravity is within normal range (1.001 to 1.030). Urine output should be 30 to 50 mL per hour; thus, 350 mL is a normal urinary output over 8 hours. The potassium level is normal.

🔑 CN: Reduction of risk potential; CL: Analyze

22. 1. The normal range for blood glucose is 70 to 100 mg/dL (3.9 to 5.6 mmol/L); the elevated blood glucose level indicates hyperglycemia. The hemoglobin is normal. The client's cholesterol and LDL levels are both normal. The nurse should determine if there are standing prescriptions for the hyperglycemia or notify the health care provider.

🔑 CN: Reduction of risk potential; CL: Analyze

23. 3. Due to the rapid, deep respirations, the client is losing fluid from vaporization from the lungs and skin (insensible fluid loss). Normally, about 900 mL of fluid is lost per day through vaporization. A decreased serum potassium level has no effect on insensible fluid loss. Hypotension occurs due to polyuria and inadequate fluid intake. It may decrease the flow of blood to the skin, causing the skin to be warm and dry.

🔑 CN: Reduction of risk potential; CL: Analyze

24. 4. Glargine is a long-acting recombinant human insulin analog. Glargine should not be mixed with any other insulin product. Insulins should not be shaken; instead, if the insulin is cloudy, roll the vial or insulin pen between the palms of the hands.

🔑 CN: Pharmacological and parenteral therapies; CL: Analyze

25. 1. A modest alcohol intake (1 to 2 drinks/day) may be incorporated into the nutrition plan for individuals who choose to drink. Alcohol is detoxified in the liver where glycogen reserves are stored and normally released in case of hypoglycemia. At the time alcohol is consumed, glucose values will likely rise because of the carbohydrate in the beer, wine, or mixed drinks; however, the later and more dangerous effect of alcohol is a hypoglycemic effect. Alcohol should be consumed with food; even if blood glucose values are elevated, the bedtime snack should not be skipped.

🔑 CN: Health promotion and maintenance; CL: Analyze

26. 1. Lactic acidosis is a rare but serious adverse effect of metformin when combined with alcohol use; half the cases are fatal. Ideally, one should stop metformin for 2 days before and 2 days after drinking alcohol. Signs and symptoms of lactic acidosis are weakness, fatigue, unusual muscle pain, dyspnea, unusual stomach discomfort, dizziness or light-headedness, and bradycardia or cardiac arrhythmias. Bloating is not an adverse effect of metformin.

CN: Pharmacological and parenteral therapies; CL: Evaluate

27. 2. Hypoglycemia is a blood glucose level below 70 mg/dL (3.9 mmol/L). The signs and symptoms of hypoglycemia include confusion, irritability, diaphoresis, tremors, hunger, weakness, and visual disturbances. Untreated hypoglycemia can progress to loss of consciousness, seizures, coma, and death. With effective treatment, hypoglycemia can usually be quickly reversed. If the client has manifestations of hypoglycemia and monitoring equipment is not available, hypoglycemia is assumed, and treatment is initiated. Hypoglycemia is treated by ingesting 10 to 15 g of simple (fast-acting) carbohydrates, such as 4 to 8 oz (118 to 236 mL) of fruit juice or regular (nondiet) soft drink or 8 oz (236 mL) of low-fat milk. The nurse can tell the client to eat the regularly scheduled meal or a snack that has protein, such as cheese or peanut butter, to prevent hypoglycemia from recurring. Without treating the possible hypoglycemia, the blood glucose level will go down even lower, and the client may lose consciousness, develop seizures, or go into a coma. Contacting the HCP would delay treating the possible hypoglycemia. Decreasing the insulin dose or increasing the meal plan may prevent episodes of hypoglycemia in the future. Administering insulin would cause the blood sugar to go even lower.

CN: Physiological adaptation; CL: Analyze

28. 3. Insulin detemir is used only if the solution appears clear and colorless with no visible particles. Insulin detemir is not diluted or mixed with any other insulin preparations. As with any insulin therapy, lipodystrophy may occur at the injection site and delay insulin absorption. Continuous rotation of the injection site within a given area may help to reduce or prevent this reaction. The client should continue to follow the prescribed diet and monitor glucose levels when taking insulin detemir. Insulin detemir is available in a prefilled insulin pen. When the insulin pen is empty, it may not be refilled; instead, the pen is discarded.

CN: Pharmacological and parenteral therapies; CL: Analyze

29. 4. The nurse instructs the client to not wait any longer than 5 to 15 minutes to eat after injecting rapid-acting insulin, which has an onset action of 5 minutes and a duration of 1 hour. The client is using the proper technique for mixing the insulins, rotating sites, and using the U-100 syringe.

CN: Pharmacological and parenteral therapies; CL: Evaluate

30. 2. Regular and NPH insulins are scheduled together one-half hour before breakfast. They do not need to be given separately or in different syringes.

CN: Pharmacological and parenteral therapies; CL: Apply

31. –/+ **1, 5.** Being overweight and having a large waist-hip ratio (central abdominal obesity) increase insulin resistance, making control of diabetes more difficult. The American and Canadian Diabetes Associations recommend a yearly referral to an ophthalmologist and podiatrist. Exercise and weight management decrease insulin resistance. Insulin is not always needed for type 2 diabetes; diet, exercise, and oral medications are the first-line treatment. The client must monitor all nutritional sources for a balanced diet—fats, carbohydrates, and protein.

CN: Reduction of risk potential; CL: Create

32. 1. The client with diabetes is prone to serious foot injuries secondary to peripheral neuropathy and decreased circulation. The client should be taught to avoid going barefoot to prevent injury. Shoes that do not fit properly should not be worn because they will cause blisters that can become nonhealing, serious wounds for the client with diabetes. Toenails should be cut straight across. A heating pad should not be used because of the risk for burns due to insensitivity to temperature.

CN: Reduction of risk potential; CL: Analyze

33. 2. A client with diabetes should be advised to consult an HCP or a podiatrist for corn removal because of the danger of traumatizing the foot tissue and the potential for the development of ulcers. A client with diabetes should never self-treat foot problems but should consult an HCP or a podiatrist.

CN: Reduction of risk potential; CL: Analyze

34. 2. Proper and careful first aid treatment is important when a client with diabetes has a skin cut or laceration. The skin should be kept supple and as free of organisms as possible. Washing and bandaging the cut will accomplish this. Washing wounds with alcohol is too caustic and drying to the skin. Having the children help is an unrealistic suggestion and does not educate the client about proper care of wounds. Tight control of blood glucose levels through adherence to the medication regimen is vitally important; however, it does not mean that careful attention to cuts can be ignored.

🔑 CN: Reduction of risk potential; CL: Analyze

35.

STEP 1

Nurse's Notes

Today: 1030

The client ran out of insulin 3 days ago. The client has a medical history of type 1 diabetes and anxiety. They use the carbohydrate counting method for administering insulin, and they adjust the dose based on the premeal glucose ranges.
  Vital signs are temperature 99.4°F (37.6°C); <mark>pulse 135 bpm</mark>; <mark>respiration rate 34 breaths/min</mark>; and <mark>blood pressure 130/83 mm Hg</mark>. Pulse oximetry shows an oxygen saturation of 98% on room air. The client is alert and oriented, but <mark>breathing appears deep and rapid</mark> with clear lung sounds. The client feels hot to the touch, has <mark>dry mucous membranes</mark>, and has a <mark>fruity odor to their breath</mark>. The client reports fatigue and nausea. The client's stat <mark>blood glucose level is 420 mg/dL (23.3 mmol/L)</mark>.

The client's blood glucose level is above 420 mg/dL (23.3 mmol/L) with a normal range of 70 to 100 mg/dL (3.9 to 5.5 mmol/L). The pulse and respiration rate are above normal limits. The client has rapid and labored breathing, dry mucous membranes, and breath with a fruity odor. These signs are indicative of diabetic ketoacidosis. The blood pressure is within normal limits.

🔑 CJ: Case study; Step 1: Recognize cues; CL: Apply

36.

STEP 2

Assessment	Helpful	Not Helpful
Pulse oximetry		X
Urinalysis	X	
Complete metabolic panel	X	
Electrocardiogram (ECG)		X
Abdominal computed tomography (CT)		X

A urinalysis should be used to check for glucose and ketones. A complete metabolic panel would be helpful to determine the client's potassium and glucose levels. A pulse oximetry reading for oxygen saturation is useful, but it does not help determine the severity of the client's high blood glucose. An ECG and an abdominal CT assessment are not necessary at this time as the client does not have chest pain or abdominal pain.

🔑 CJ: Case study; Step 2: Analyze cues; CL: Analyze

37.

STEP 3

R The client's **integumentary assessment** is indicative that the client is at risk for **diabetic ketoacidosis.**

The client's integumentary assessment reveals that the client has hot, dry skin and dry mucous membranes, indicating that the client's blood glucose is elevated. The neurologic assessment indicates the client is alert and oriented. Although the client has nausea, this does not put the client at risk for diabetic ketoacidosis.

🔑 CJ: Case study; Step 3: Prioritize hypothesis; CL: Analyze

38.

STEP 4

1, 4, 8. Right away, the nurse should administer 10 units of regular insulin, administer 1 L of 0.9% normal saline intravenously, and obtain a serum potassium level. The regular insulin will lower the blood sugar level. Intravenous normal saline is used to correct dehydration. Potassium levels would need to be monitored for potential hypokalemia caused by the high blood glucose levels, and the nurse should request the order for a serum potassium level. Placing an indwelling urinary catheter would be inappropriate for a client who can ambulate and urinate without assistance. There is no indication that the client needs oral potassium until laboratory reports are available. A hemoglobin A1C assessment would be appropriate for outpatient management, but at this time, it is unnecessary. A chest x-ray is not indicated at this time because of the deep respirations associated with Kussmaul breathing that are related to diabetic ketoacidosis.

🔑 CJ: Case study; Step 4: Generate solutions; CL: Create

39.

STEP 5

Steps to Administering Insulin	Appropriate	Inappropriate
1. Verify with another nurse the type and dose of the insulin.	X	
2. Verify two client identifiers before administration.	X	
3. Shake the vial vigorously.		X
4. Rotate sites between legs and arms.	X	
5. Place the insulin in the refrigerator after administering the dose.		X

The nurse should verify the type and dose of insulin with another nurse before administering the insulin. The nurse should verify two client identifiers before administering the insulin. The administration sites should be rotated to prevent lipodystrophy. The vial should be rolled between the hands and not shaken, as this can form air bubbles that may affect the amount of insulin withdrawn. The vial should not be returned to the refrigerator; the insulin should be kept at room temperature.

🔑 CJ: Case study; Step 5: Take action; CL: Apply

40.

Client Finding	Desired Outcome	Side Effect or Adverse Effect
Respiratory rate of 26 breaths/min	X	
Moist skin		X
Hypokalemia		X
Blood glucose level lower than 125 mg/dL (6.94 mmol/L)	X	
Altered level of consciousness		X

The *desired outcomes* for administering insulin to this client are to see the respiratory rate trending downward and a blood glucose level of less than 125 mg/dL. The client's respiratory rate and rhythm should begin to return to baseline as the blood glucose level begins to normalize. The nurse should also evaluate the client for potential *adverse effects* of the insulin. The blood glucose level could drop too low, causing signs of hypoglycemia, such as moist or clammy skin. The nurse also should evaluate the client for signs of hypokalemia because as the insulin draws the glucose into the cell, the potassium may follow and cause hypokalemia. An altered level of consciousness is also a concern because the insulin could lower the blood glucose too quickly, potentially causing increased intracranial pressure.

CJ: Case study; Step 6: Evaluate outcomes; CL: Evaluate

41. 1. Deep, rapid respirations with long expirations are indicative of Kussmaul respirations, which occur in metabolic acidosis. The respirations increase in rate and depth, and the breath has a "fruity" or acetonelike odor. This breathing pattern is the body's attempt to blow off carbon dioxide and acetone, thus compensating for the acidosis. The other breathing patterns listed are not related to ketoacidosis and would not compensate for the acidosis.

CN: Physiological adaptation; CL: Analyze

42. 3, 4, 5. The nurse may not discontinue a medication without a health care provider's prescription, and the nurse may not substitute one medication for another. Maximum doses may be better tolerated if given with meals. Before therapy begins, and at least annually thereafter, assess the client's renal function; if renal impairment is detected, a different antidiabetic agent may be indicated. To evaluate the effectiveness of therapy, the client's glucose value must be monitored regularly. The prescriber must be notified if the glucose value increases, despite therapy.

CN: Pharmacological and parenteral therapies; CL: Analyze

43. 1, 3, 5. Nausea is a common side effect when clients first start taking dulaglutide. To manage the nausea, the nurse can suggest that the client eat smaller meals more frequently, drink beverages with ginger in them, and avoid fried foods. The client should decrease the fat content in the diet. The client should not stop using the drug unless prescribed by the health care provider.

CN: Pharmacological and parenteral therapies; CL: Analyze

44. 1, 2, 3. Insulin pens should be stored in the refrigerator before use; once opened, they can be stored at a cool room temperature. The pen needs to be primed by expelling air before injecting the insulin. After the injection, the site can be patted, but not massaged. Needles cannot be reused; the client should remove the needle and place it in a hard plastic container for disposal.

CN: Pharmacologic and parenteral therapies; CL: Analyze

45. 2, 3. The nurse should instruct the client with insulin-requiring diabetes who has the flu to check the blood sugar every 4 hours. The client should try to drink 240 mL of fluids every hour. If the blood sugar levels become low, the client should drink liquids with sugar in them. The client should continue to take insulin. It is not necessary to check for ketones until the blood glucose level is above 240 mg/dL. The nurse cannot prescribe aspirin for this client. If the symptoms of the flu continue, the nurse should instruct the client to contact the health care provider.

CN: Health promotion and maintenance; CL: Analyze

46. 1, 3, 4. Used needles must be disposed of safely; local community, state, and home waste management services have different regulations about needle disposal. The nurse should instruct the client when at home to discard the needles in a sharps container or other plastic container and contact the local community or waste management services about where the containers used at home should be disposed of. When traveling, the client should carry a travel-size disposable container, bring it home, and discard it according to home disposal procedures. The client should not place the used needles in a hotel recycling bin unless they are approved containers. When traveling with insulin pens and needles, the client should follow TSA-approved procedures for labeling medications. The client should not touch the needle or wipe it with alcohol. All needles should be placed immediately in sharps containers.

CN: Pharmacologic and parenteral therapies; CL: Analyze

47. ✓ **1, 2, 3.** Client teaching includes reviewing the proper use and storage of the exenatide dosage pen, particularly the one-time setup for each new pen. The nurse should instruct the client to inject the drug in the thigh, abdomen, or upper arm. The drug should be administered within 60 minutes of the morning and evening meals; the client should not inject the drug after a meal. The nurse should review steps for managing hypoglycemia, especially if the client also takes a sulfonylurea or insulin. If a dose is missed, the client should resume treatment as prescribed, with the next scheduled dose.

🔑 CN: Pharmacological and parenteral therapies; CL: Analyze

48. **2.** Rapid-acting insulin has an onset in 15 minutes, peaks at 1 hour, and lasts for 3 to 4 hours. Rapid-acting insulin is administered right before or right after a meal. The nurse should assess the client for hypoglycemia 1 hour after administration of the drug.

🔑 CN: Pharmacological and parenteral therapies; CL: Apply

49. **4.** There is a drug-food interaction between repaglinide and grapefruit juice that may inhibit the metabolism of repaglinide; fresh grapefruit also interacts with repaglinide. It is not necessary for the dietitian to inform the client of the drug–food interaction first. Contacting the manager of the food and nutrition department is not an intervention that will bring about prompt removal of the juice.

🔑 CN: Pharmacological and parenteral therapies; CL: Analyze

50. **3.** The most important factor predisposing to the development of type 2 diabetes mellitus is obesity. Insulin resistance increases with obesity. Cigarette smoking is not a predisposing factor, but it is a risk factor that increases the complications of diabetes mellitus. If the client is following a diabetic diet and obtaining adequate sources of protein, it is not necessary to increase the protein in the diet. Hypertension is not a predisposing factor for type 2 diabetes, but it is a risk factor for developing complications of diabetes mellitus.

🔑 CN: Health promotion and maintenance; CL: Apply

51. **4.** The client with diabetes mellitus who is taking NPH insulin in the evening is most likely to become hypoglycemic shortly after midnight because this insulin peaks in 6 to 8 hours. The client should eat a bedtime snack to help prevent hypoglycemia while sleeping.

🔑 CN: Pharmacological and parenteral therapies; CL: Apply

52. ✓ **1, 2, 5, 6, 7.** An insulin pump is an alternative to daily injections of insulin, but it is not an option for everyone because using the pump requires the client to commit to maintaining it correctly. Using the pump is more accurate than giving injections, and there are fewer incidences of low blood glucose levels. The client will need to program the pump to deliver a steady dose of insulin (basal dose) and to handle increased glucose levels at meals (bolus doses). The nurse should instruct the client that the pump will need to be changed every few days. The client will need to check glucose levels daily and will need to monitor dietary intake and increase the bolus dose accordingly. The pump can be only used with rapid-acting and short-acting insulins. The client will need to enter information into the pump every day.

🔑 CN: Pharmacological and parenteral theapies; CL: Apply

53. **3.** If the client engages in an activity or exercise that focuses on one area of the body, that area may cause inconsistent absorption of insulin. A good regimen for a jogger is to inject the abdomen for 1 week and then rotate to the buttock. A jogger may have inconsistent absorption in the legs or arms with strenuous running. The iliac crest is not an appropriate site due to a lack of loose skin and subcutaneous tissue in that area.

🔑 CN: Pharmacological and parenteral therapies; CL: Apply

54. **1.** Insulin lispro begins to act within 10 to 15 minutes and lasts approximately 4 hours. A major advantage of lispro is that the client can eat almost immediately after the insulin is administered. The client needs to be instructed regarding the onset, peak, and duration of all insulin, as meals need to be timed with these parameters. Waiting 1 hour to eat may precipitate hypoglycemia. Eating 2 hours before the insulin lispro could cause hyperglycemia if the client does not have circulating insulin to metabolize the carbohydrate.

🔑 CN: Pharmacological and parenteral therapies; CL: Analyze

55. **1.** The nurse should judge that learning has occurred when the client can perform the procedure correctly, indicating both a cognitive understanding of the skill as well as being able to perform it correctly. Having the client critique a demonstration does not indicate the client can perform the skill. Explaining the steps demonstrates the acquisition of knowledge at the cognitive level only. A posttest does not indicate the degree to which the client has learned a psychomotor skill.

🔑 CN: Pharmacological and parenteral therapies; CL: Evaluate

56. **32 units.** Clients commonly need to mix insulin, requiring careful mixing and calculation. The total dosage is 10 units plus 22 units, for a total of 32 units.

🗝️ CN: Pharmacological and parenteral therapies; CL: Apply

57. 1. The four most commonly reported signs and symptoms of hypoglycemia are nervousness, weakness, perspiration, and confusion. Other signs and symptoms include hunger, incoherent speech, tachycardia, and blurred vision. Anorexia and Kussmaul respirations are clinical manifestations of hyperglycemia or ketoacidosis. Bradycardia is not associated with hypoglycemia; tachycardia is.

🗝️ CN: Health promotion and maintenance; CL: Apply

58. 2. Steroids can cause hyperglycemia because of their effects on carbohydrate metabolism, making diabetic control more difficult. Aspirin is not known to affect glucose metabolism. Sulfonylureas are oral hypoglycemic agents used in the treatment of diabetes mellitus. ACE inhibitors are not known to affect glucose metabolism.

🗝️ CN: Pharmacological and parenteral therapies; CL: Apply

59. 4. The best response is to allow the client to verbalize fears about performing self-injection. Tactics that increase fear, such as threatening the client about complications, are not effective in changing behavior. If possible, the client needs to be responsible for self-care, including giving self-injections. A nurse for home care visits is not justified if the client is capable of self-administration.

🗝️ CN: Psychosocial integrity; CL: Analyze

The Adult with Pituitary Adenoma

60. 4. With transsphenoidal hypophysectomy, the sella turcica is entered from below, through the sphenoid sinus. There is no external incision; the incision is made between the upper lip and gums.

🗝️ CN: Reduction of risk potential; CL: Apply

61. 3. Deep breathing is the best choice for helping prevent atelectasis. The client should be placed in the semi-Fowler position (or as prescribed) and taught deep breathing, sighing, mouth breathing, and how to avoid coughing. The client should receive sufficient medication to control postoperative pain. Frequent position changes help loosen lung secretions, but deep breathing is most important in preventing atelectasis. Coughing is contraindicated because it increases intracranial pressure and can cause cerebrospinal fluid to leak from the point at which the sella turcica was entered.

🗝️ CN: Reduction of risk potential; CL: Analyze

62. 1. A major focus of nursing care after transsphenoidal hypophysectomy is the prevention of and monitoring for a CSF leak. CSF leakage can occur if the patch or incision is disrupted. The nurse should monitor for signs of infection, including elevated temperature, increased white blood cell count, rhinorrhea, nuchal rigidity, and persistent headache. Hypoglycemia and adrenocortical insufficiency may occur. Monitoring for fluctuating blood glucose levels is not related specifically to transsphenoidal hypophysectomy. The client will be given intravenous fluids postoperatively to supply carbohydrates. Cushing's disease results from adrenocortical excess, not insufficiency. Monitoring for cardiac arrhythmias is important, but arrhythmias are not anticipated following a transsphenoidal hypophysectomy.

🗝️ CN: Reduction of risk potential; CL: Analyze

63. 3. If CSF leakage is suspected or confirmed, the client is treated initially with bed rest with the head of the bed elevated to decrease pressure on the graft site. Most leaks heal spontaneously, but occasionally, surgical repair of the site in the sella turcica is needed. Repacking the nose will not heal the leak at the graft site in the dura. The client will not be returned to surgery immediately because most leaks heal spontaneously. High-dose corticosteroid therapy is not effective in healing a CSF leak.

🗝️ CN: Physiological adaptation; CL: Apply

64. 1. After transsphenoidal surgery, the client must be careful not to disturb the suture line while healing occurs. Frequent oral care should be provided with rinses of saline, and the teeth may be gently cleaned with oral swabs. Frequent or vigorous toothbrushing or flossing is contraindicated because it may disturb or cause tension on the suture line.

🗝️ CN: Physiological adaptation; CL: Analyze

65. 4. Most clients who undergo adenoma removal experience a gradual return of normal pituitary secretion and do not experience complications. However, hypopituitarism can cause growth hormone, gonadotropin, thyroid-stimulating hormone, and adrenocorticotropic hormone deficits. The client should be taught to monitor for changes in mental status, energy level, muscle strength, and cognitive function. In adults, changes in sexual function, impotence, or decreased libido should be reported.

Acromegaly and Cushing's disease are conditions of hypersecretion. Diabetes mellitus is related to the function of the pancreas and is not directly related to the function of the pituitary.

🗝️ CN: Reduction of risk potential; CL: Analyze

66. **1.** Pituitary diabetes insipidus is a potential complication after pituitary surgery because of possible interference with the production of antidiuretic hormone (ADH). One major manifestation of diabetes insipidus is polyuria because lack of ADH results in insufficient water reabsorption by the kidneys. The polyuria leads to a decreased urine specific gravity (between 1.001 and 1.010). The client may drink and excrete 5 to 40 L of fluid daily. Diabetes insipidus does not affect metabolism. A blood glucose level higher than 300 mg/dL (16.7 mmol/L) is associated with impaired glucose metabolism or diabetes mellitus. Urine negative for sugar and ketones is normal.

🗝️ CN: Reduction of risk potential; CL: Analyze

67. **2.** The major characteristic of diabetes insipidus is decreased tubular reabsorption of water due to insufficient amounts of antidiuretic hormone (ADH). Vasopressin is administered to the client with diabetes insipidus because it has pressor and ADH activities. Vasopressin works to increase the concentration of the urine by increasing tubular reabsorption, thus preserving up to 90% water. Vasopressin is administered to the client with diabetes insipidus because it is a synthetic ADH. The administration of vasopressin results in increased tubular reabsorption of water, and it is effective for emergency treatment or daily maintenance of mild diabetes insipidus. Vasopressin does not lower blood pressure or affect insulin production or glucose metabolism.

🗝️ CN: Pharmacological and parenteral therapies; CL: Apply

68. **1.** Because diabetes insipidus involves the excretion of large amounts of fluid, maintaining normal fluid and electrolyte balance is a priority for this client. Special dietary programs or restrictions are not indicated in the treatment of diabetes insipidus. Serum glucose levels are priorities in diabetes mellitus but not in diabetes insipidus.

🗝️ CN: Physiological adaptation; CL: Evaluate

The Adult with Addison's Disease

69. **4.** Adrenal crisis can occur with physical stress, such as increased exercise, surgery, dental work, infection, flu, trauma, and pregnancy. In these situations, glucocorticoid and mineralocorticoid dosages are increased. The psychological stress of taking a test has less effect on corticosteroid need than physical stress. Modest alcohol consumption does not require an increased dose of corticosteroids. Weight loss, not gain, occurs with adrenal insufficiency. Psychological stress has less effect on corticosteroid need than physical stress.

🗝️ CN: Reduction of risk potential; CL: Analyze

70. **2.** Addison's disease is caused by a deficiency of adrenal corticosteroids and can result in severe hypotension and shock because of uncontrolled loss of sodium in the urine and impaired mineralocorticoid function. This results in loss of extracellular fluid and dangerously low blood volume. Glucocorticoids must be administered to reverse hypotension. Preventing infection is not an appropriate goal of care in this life-threatening situation. Relieving anxiety is appropriate when the client's condition is stabilized, but the calm, competent demeanor of the emergency department staff will be initially reassuring.

🗝️ CN: Physiological adaptation; CL: Analyze

71. **2.** Adrenal hormone deficiency can cause profound physiologic changes. The client may experience severe pain (headache, abdominal pain, back pain, or pain in the extremities). Inhibited gluconeogenesis commonly produces hypoglycemia, and impaired sodium retention causes decreased, not increased, fluid volume. Edema would not be expected. Gastrointestinal disturbances, including nausea and vomiting, are expected findings in Addison's disease, not hunger.

🗝️ CN: Physiological adaptation; CL: Analyze

72. -/+ **2, 3, 4, 5.** The long-term administration of corticosteroids in therapeutic doses often leads to serious complications or side effects. Corticosteroid therapy is not recommended for minor chronic conditions; the potential benefits of treatment must always be weighed against the risks. Hypokalemia may develop; corticosteroids act on the renal tubules to increase sodium reabsorption and enhance potassium and hydrogen excretion. Corticosteroids stimulate the breakdown of protein for gluconeogenesis, which can lead to skeletal muscle wasting. Central nervous system adverse effects are euphoria, headache, insomnia, confusion, and psychosis. The nurse watches for changes in mood and behavior, emotional stability, sleep pattern, and psychomotor activity, especially with long-term therapy. Hypocalcemia related to anti–vitamin D effect may occur. Corticosteroids cause atrophy of the lymphoid tissue, suppress cell-mediated immune responses, and decrease the production of antibodies. The nurse must be alert to the possibility of masked infection and delayed healing (antiinflammatory and immunosuppressive actions). Retention of sodium (and subsequently water) increases blood volume and, therefore, blood pressure.

🔑 CN: Pharmacological parenteral therapies; CL: Apply

73. 3. Electrolyte imbalances associated with Addison's disease include hypoglycemia, hyponatremia, and hyperkalemia. Regular salted (not low-salt) chicken or beef broth and fruit juices provide glucose and sodium to replenish these deficits. Diet soda does not contain sugar. Water could cause further sodium dilution. Coffee's diuretic effect would aggravate the fluid deficit. Milk contains potassium and sodium.

🔑 CN: Basic care and comfort; CL: Apply

74. -/+ 2, 3, 4, 5, 6. Addison's disease occurs when the client does not produce enough steroids from the adrenal cortex. Lifetime steroid replacement is needed. The client should be taught lifestyle management techniques to avoid stress and maintain rest periods. A medical identification bracelet should be worn, and the family should be taught signs and symptoms that indicate an impending adrenal crisis, such as fatigue, weakness, dizziness, or mood changes. Dental work, infections, and surgery commonly require an adjusted dosage of steroids.

🔑 CN: Health promotion and maintenance; CL: Create

75. 3. Although many of the disease signs and symptoms are vague and nonspecific, most clients experience lethargy and depression as early symptoms. Other early signs and symptoms include mood changes, emotional lability, irritability, weight loss, muscle weakness, fatigue, nausea, and vomiting. Most clients experience a loss of appetite. Muscles become weak, not spastic, because of adrenocortical insufficiency.

🔑 CN: Physiological adaptation; CL: Analyze

76. 1. Since Addison's disease can be life-threatening, treatment often begins with the administration of corticosteroids. Corticosteroids, such as prednisone, may be taken orally or intravenously, depending on the client. A serious adverse effect of corticosteroids is hyperglycemia. Clients do not adjust their steroid dose based on dietary intake and exercise; insulin is adjusted based on diet and exercise. Addisonian crisis can occur secondary to hypoadrenocorticism, resulting in a crisis situation of acute hypotension, not increased blood pressure. Addison's disease is a disease of inadequate adrenal hormone, and therefore the client will have an inadequate response to stress. If the client takes more medication than prescribed, there can be a potential increase in potassium depletion, fluid retention, and hyperglycemia. Taking less medication than was prescribed can trigger an addisonian crisis state, which is a medical emergency manifested by signs of shock.

🔑 CN: Pharmacological and parenteral therapies; CL: Analyze

77. 1. The need for glucocorticoids changes with circumstances. The basal dose is established when the client is discharged, but this dose covers only normal daily needs and does not provide for additional stressors. As the manager of the medication schedule, the client needs to know the signs and symptoms of excessive and insufficient dosages. Glucocorticoid needs fluctuate. Glucocorticoids are not cumulative and must be taken daily. They must never be discontinued suddenly; in the absence of endogenous production, addisonian crisis could result. Two-thirds of the daily dose should be taken at about 0800 and the remainder at about 1600. This schedule approximates the diurnal pattern of normal secretion, with the highest levels between 0400 and 0600 and lowest levels in the evening.

🔑 CN: Pharmacological and parenteral therapies; CL: Evaluate

78. 3. Fludrocortisone acetate can be administered once a day, but cortisone acetate administration should follow the body's natural diurnal pattern of secretion, in which greater amounts of cortisol are secreted during the daytime to meet the increased demand of the body. To mimic this pattern, baseline administration of cortisone acetate is typically 25 mg in the morning and 12.5 mg in the afternoon. Taking it three times a day would result in an excessive dose. Taking the drug only in the morning would not meet the needs of the body later in the day and evening.

🔑 CN: Pharmacological and parenteral therapies; CL: Apply

79. 4. Oral steroids can cause gastric irritation and ulcers and should be administered with meals, if possible, or otherwise with an antacid. Only instructing the client to take the medication with a full glass of water will not help prevent gastric complications from steroids. Steroids should never be taken on an empty stomach. Glucocorticoids should be taken in the morning, not at bedtime.

🔑 CN: Pharmacological and parenteral therapies; CL: Apply

80. 4. Measuring daily weight is a reliable, objective way to monitor fluid balance. Rapid variations in weight reflect changes in fluid volume, which suggests insufficient control of the disease and the need for more glucocorticoids in the client with Addison's disease. Nurses should instruct clients taking oral steroids to weigh themselves daily and to report any unusual weight loss or gain. Skin turgor testing does supply information about fluid status, but daily weight monitoring is more reliable. Temperature is not a direct measurement of fluid balance. Thirst is a nonspecific and very late sign of weight loss.

 CN: Pharmacological and parenteral therapies; CL: Evaluate

81. 1. Medication compliance is an essential part of the self-care required to manage Addison's disease. The client must learn to adjust the glucocorticoid dose in response to the normal and unexpected stresses of daily living. The nurse should instruct the client never to stop taking the drug without consulting the health care provider to avoid an addisonian crisis. Regularity in daily habits makes adjustment easier, but the client should not be encouraged to withdraw from normal activities to avoid stress. The client does not need to restrict sodium. The client is at risk for hyponatremia. Hypotension, not hypertension, is more common with Addison's disease.

 CN: Reduction of risk potential; CL: Evaluate

82. 4. Bronzing, or general deepening of skin pigmentation, is a classic sign of Addison's disease and is caused by melanocyte-stimulating hormone produced in response to increased ACTH secretion. The hyperpigmentation is typically found in the distal portion of extremities and in areas exposed to the sun. Additionally, areas that may not be exposed to the sun, such as the nipples, genitalia, tongue, and knuckles, become bronze colored. Treatment of Addison's disease usually reverses hyperpigmentation. Bilirubin level is not related to the pathophysiology of Addison's disease. Hyperpigmentation is not related to the effects of glucocorticoid therapy.

 CN: Physiological adaptation; CL: Apply

The Adult with Cushing's Disease

83. 2. When Cushing's syndrome is suspected, a 24-hour urine collection for free cortisol is performed. Levels of 50 to 100 mcg a day (1379 to 2756 mmol/L a day) in adults indicate Cushing's syndrome. If these results are borderline, a high-dose dexamethasone suppression test is done. The dexamethasone is given at 2300 to suppress the secretion of the corticotrophin-releasing hormone. A plasma cortisol sample is drawn at 0800. A normal cortisol level of less than 5 mcg/dL (140 mmol/L) indicates a normal adrenal response.

 CN: Management of care; CL: Apply

84. 2. Sodium retention is typically accompanied by potassium depletion. Hypertension, hypokalemia, edema, and heart failure may result from the hypersecretion of aldosterone. The client with Cushing's disease exhibits postprandial or persistent hyperglycemia. Clients with Cushing's disease have hypernatremia, not hyponatremia. Bone resorption of calcium increases the urine calcium level.

 CN: Reduction of risk potential; CL: Analyze

85. 2. A primary dietary intervention is to restrict sodium, thereby reducing fluid retention. Increased protein catabolism results in loss of muscle mass and necessitates supplemental protein intake. The client may be asked to restrict total calories to reduce weight. The client should be encouraged to eat potassium-rich foods because serum levels are typically depleted. Although reducing fat intake as part of an overall plan to restrict calories is appropriate, a fat intake of less than 20% of total calories is not recommended.

 CN: Basic care and comfort; CL: Analyze

86. 2. Osteoporosis is a serious outcome of prolonged cortisol excess because calcium is resorbed out of the bone. Regular daily weight-bearing exercise (e.g., brisk walking) is an effective way to drive calcium back into the bones. The client should also be instructed to have a dietary or supplemental intake of calcium of 1500 mg daily. Potassium levels are not relevant to the prevention of bone resorption. Vitamin D is needed to aid in the absorption of calcium. Isometric exercises condition muscle tone but do not build bones.

 CN: Reduction of risk potential; CL: Analyze

87. 2. Effective splinting for a high incision reduces stress on the incision line, decreases pain, and increases the client's ability to deep breathe effectively. Deep breathing should be done hourly by the client after surgery. Sitting upright ignores the need to splint the incision to prevent pain. Tightening the stomach muscles is not an effective strategy for promoting deep breathing. Raising the shoulders is not a feature of deep-breathing exercises.

 CN: Reduction of risk potential; CL: Apply

88. 3. The priority in the first 24 hours after adrenalectomy is to identify and prevent adrenal crisis. Monitoring of vital signs is the most important

evaluation measure. Hypotension, tachycardia, orthostatic hypotension, and arrhythmias can be indicators of pending vascular collapse and hypovolemic shock that can occur with an adrenal crisis. Beginning oral nutrition is important, but not necessarily in the first 24 hours after surgery, and it is not more important than preventing adrenal crisis. Promoting self-care activities is not as important as preventing adrenal crisis. Ambulating in the hallway is not a priority in the first 24 hours after adrenalectomy.

CN: Reduction of risk potential; CL: Analyze

89. 3. Hydromorphone hydrochloride is about five times more potent than morphine sulfate, from which it is prepared. Therefore, it is administered only in small doses. Hydromorphone hydrochloride can cause dependency in any dose; however, fear of dependency developing in the postoperative period is unwarranted. The dose is determined by the client's need for pain relief. Hydromorphone hydrochloride is not irritating to subcutaneous tissues. As with opioid analgesics, excretion depends on normal liver function.

CN: Pharmacological and parenteral therapies; CL: Apply

90. 4. A glucocorticoid preparation will be administered intravenously or intramuscularly in the immediate preoperative period to a client scheduled for an adrenalectomy. Methylprednisolone sodium succinate protects the client from developing acute adrenal insufficiency (addisonian crisis) that occurs as a result of the adrenalectomy. Spironolactone is a potassium-sparing diuretic. Prednisone is an oral corticosteroid. Fludrocortisone is a mineral corticoid.

CN: Pharmacological and parenteral therapies; CL: Apply

91. 3. Pain control should be evaluated at least every 2 hours for the client with a PCA system. Addiction is not a common problem for the postoperative client. A client should not be encouraged to tolerate pain; in fact, other nursing actions besides PCA should be implemented to enhance the action of opioids. One of the purposes of PCA is for the client to determine the frequency of administering the medication; the nurse should not interfere unless the client is not obtaining pain relief. The nurse should ensure that the client is instructed on the use of the PCA control button and that the button is always within reach.

CN: Pharmacological and parenteral therapies; CL: Analyze

92. 2. Persistent cortisol excess undermines the collagen matrix of the skin, impairing wound healing. It also carries an increased risk for infection and bleeding. The wound should be observed and documentation performed regarding the status of healing. Confusion and emboli are not expected complications after adrenalectomy. Malnutrition also is not an expected complication after adrenalectomy. Nutritional status should be regained postoperatively.

CN: Reduction of risk potential; CL: Analyze

93. 2. As the body readjusts to normal cortisol levels, mood and physical changes will gradually return to a normal state. The body changes are not permanent, and the mood swings should level off.

CN: Physiological adaptation; CL: Analyze

94. 3. Testosterone is an androgen hormone that is responsible for protein metabolism as well as maintenance of secondary sexual characteristics; therefore, it is needed by both males and females. Removal of both adrenal glands necessitates the replacement of glucocorticoids and androgens. Testosterone does not balance the reproductive cycle, stabilize mood swings, or restore sodium and potassium balance.

CN: Physiological adaptation; CL: Apply

95. 1. Bilateral adrenalectomy requires lifelong adrenal hormone replacement therapy. If unilateral surgery is performed, most clients gradually reestablish a normal secretion pattern. The client and family will require extensive teaching and support to maintain self-care management at home. Information on dosing, adverse effects, what to do if a dose is missed, and follow-up examinations is needed in the teaching plan. Although steroids are tapered when given for an intermittent or one-time problem, they are not discontinued when given to clients who have undergone bilateral adrenalectomy because the clients will not regain the ability to manufacture steroids. Steroids must be taken on a daily basis, not just during periods of physical or emotional stress.

CN: Physiological adaptation; CL: Analyze

Managing Care, Quality, and Safety of Adults with Endocrine Health Problems

96. 2. Insulin is on the list of error-prone medications, and the nurse should ask the HCP to rewrite the prescription to spell out the word "units" and to indicate the route by which the drug is to be administered. The nurse should contact the HCP immediately as the nurse is to administer the insulin now. The nurse can then also report the most current glucose level. While waiting for the insulin prescription to be rewritten, the nurse can administer the pain medication if needed, start the oxygen, and check the client's vital signs.

🗝 CN: Safety and infection control; CL: Analyze

97. 1. To assure client safety, the nurse first writes the results on the chart, then reads them back to the caller, and waits for the caller to confirm that the nurse has understood the results. The nurse may receive results by telephone; and although an electronic transfer to the client's medical record is appropriate, the nurse can also accept the telephone results if the laboratory has called the results to the nurses' station.

🗝 CN: Management of care; CL: Apply

98. 3. The client needs fluid volume replacement because of the dehydration. However, the nurse should verify the prescription for intravenous dextrose with the HCP due to the risk for hyperglycemia that dextrose would present when administered to a client with diabetes. The potassium level is within normal limits. The client does not have restrictions on oral fluids, and the nurse can encourage the client to drink fluids. The client does not need to be placed in isolation at this time.

🗝 CN: Physiological adaptation; CL: Analyze

99. 3. Glulisine is a rapid-acting insulin with an action onset of 15 minutes. The client could experience hypoglycemia with the insulin in the bloodstream and no breakfast. It is not necessary to call the client's HCP; the nurse should determine what test was scheduled and then locate the client and provide either breakfast or 4 oz (120 mL) of fruit juice. To bring the client back to the room would be wasting valuable time needed to prevent or correct hypoglycemia.

🗝 CN: Management of care; CL: Analyze

100. 3. Because subcutaneous administration of insulin has a slower rate of absorption than IV insulin, there must be an adequate level of insulin in the bloodstream before discontinuing the insulin drip; otherwise, the glucose level will rise. Adding an IV antibiotic has no influence on the insulin drip; it should not be piggy-backed into the insulin drip. Glargine cannot be administered IV and should not be mixed with other insulins or solutions.

🗝 CN: Pharmacological and parenteral therapies; CL: Analyze

101. 1. New onset of hoarseness following a thyroidectomy may be a sign of tracheal edema and impending airway obstruction, and the nurse should evaluate this client first. The client with Cushing's syndrome may have increased blood sugars associated with stress and hospitalization and will need further information to determine whether the blood sugar was obtained when the client was fasting. A client with renal failure would be expected to have an increase in creatinine, and the nurse can later follow up to compare this result with previous results. The client with ulcerative colitis will experience loose, bloody stools and needs to be continuously evaluated for amounts, but this is not the nurse's priority.

🗝 CN: Management of care; CL: Analyze

TEST 9

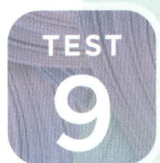

The Adult with Urinary Tract Health Problems

- The Adult with Cancer of the Bladder
- The Adult with Renal Calculi
- The Adult with Acute Kidney Injury (Acute Renal Failure)
- The Adult with Urinary Tract Infection
- The Adult with Pyelonephritis
- The Adult with Chronic Renal Failure
- The Adult with Urinary Incontinence
- Managing Care, Quality, and Safety of Adults with Urinary Tract Health Problems
- Answers, Rationales, and Test-Taking Strategies

The Adult with Cancer of the Bladder

1. A client has undergone a cystectomy and an ileal conduit diversion. What should the nurse include in the discharge instructions? Select all that apply.
   - ☐ 1. Drink at least 101 oz (3000 mL) of fluid each day.
   - ☐ 2. Minimize daily activities.
   - ☐ 3. Keep urine alkaline to prevent urinary tract infections.
   - ☐ 4. Avoid odor-producing foods, such as onions, fish, eggs, and cheese.
   - ☐ 5. Wear snug clothing over the stoma to encourage urine flow into the drainage bag.

2. A nurse is instructing a client with an ileal conduit about skin care around the stoma. What should the nurse tell the client about stoma care? Select all that apply.
   - ☐ 1. "The stoma will shrink to a normal size in 4 to 6 weeks."
   - ☐ 2. "You can take a shower or a bath with the appliance on or off."
   - ☐ 3. "You should wash around the stoma with an antibacterial soap."
   - ☐ 4. "You can use an electric razor to remove the hair around the stoma."
   - ☐ 5. "You should remove the collection bag every day to inspect the stoma for infection."

3. A client is admitted to the recovery room after cystoscopy with biopsy. Before discharging the client, what should the nurse determine?

   The client has:
   - ☐ 1. had a bowel movement.
   - ☐ 2. no pain.
   - ☐ 3. emptied the bladder.
   - ☐ 4. no blood in the urine.

4. The nurse is conducting a focused assessment for the client with suspected bladder cancer. What information should the nurse obtain when assessing this client?
   - ☐ 1. suprapubic pain
   - ☐ 2. painful voiding
   - ☐ 3. painless hematuria
   - ☐ 4. urine retention

5. The nurse is assessing a client who just had a cystoscopy. Which symptom indicates that a client has developed a complication?
   - ☐ 1. dizziness
   - ☐ 2. chills
   - ☐ 3. pink-tinged urine
   - ☐ 4. bladder spasms

6. If a client who had a cystoscopy 2 hours ago has lower abdominal pain, what action should the nurse take?
   - ☐ 1. Apply an ice pack to the pubic area.
   - ☐ 2. Massage the abdomen gently.
   - ☐ 3. Encourage the client to ambulate.
   - ☐ 4. Have the client sit in a tub of warm water.

7. A client who has been diagnosed with bladder cancer is scheduled for an ileal conduit. Prior to surgery, what comment by the client indicates that the client understands the procedure?
   - ☐ 1. "This is a temporary procedure that can be reversed later."
   - ☐ 2. "I will urinate through my rectum."
   - ☐ 3. "My urine will come out through an opening on my abdomen."
   - ☐ 4. "My urine will go from my bladder into a drainage bag."

8. After a client has surgery for an ileal conduit, the nurse should assess the client for the occurrence of which complication?
☐ 1. peritonitis
☐ 2. thrombophlebitis
☐ 3. ascites
☐ 4. inguinal hernia

9. The nurse is assessing the urine of a client who has had an ileal conduit and notes that there is a moderate amount of mucus in the urine. What should the nurse do **next**?
☐ 1. Change the appliance bag.
☐ 2. Notify the health care provider (HCP).
☐ 3. Obtain a urine specimen for culture.
☐ 4. Encourage a high fluid intake.

10. When teaching the client to care for an ileal conduit, the nurse instructs the client to empty the appliance frequently. Which outcome indicates that the client is following instructions?
☐ 1. The skin around the stoma is red.
☐ 2. The urine is a deep yellow.
☐ 3. There is no odor present.
☐ 4. The seal around the stoma is intact.

11. The nurse is instructing a client with an ileal conduit. What should the nurse instruct the client to do to prevent urine leakage when changing the appliance?
☐ 1. Insert a gauze wick into the stoma.
☐ 2. Close the opening temporarily with a cellophane seal.
☐ 3. Suction the stoma before changing the appliance.
☐ 4. Limit oral fluids for several hours before changing the appliance.

12. The client with an ileal conduit will be using a reusable appliance at home. The nurse should teach the client to clean the appliance routinely with which product?
☐ 1. baking soda
☐ 2. soap
☐ 3. hydrogen peroxide
☐ 4. alcohol

13. The nurse is evaluating the discharge teaching for a client who has an ileal conduit. Which statement(s) would indicate that the client has correctly understood the teaching? Select all that apply.
☐ 1. "If I limit my fluid intake, I won't have to empty my ostomy pouch as often."
☐ 2. "I can place an aspirin tablet in my pouch to decrease odor."
☐ 3. "I can usually keep my ostomy pouch on for 3 to 7 days before changing it."
☐ 4. "I must use a skin barrier to protect my skin from urine."
☐ 5. "I should empty my ostomy pouch of urine when it is full."

14. A client has an ileal conduit. Which solution will be useful to help control odor in the urine collecting bag after it has been cleaned?
☐ 1. salt water
☐ 2. vinegar
☐ 3. ammonia
☐ 4. bleach

15. A client who has a urinary diversion tells the nurse, "This urinary pouch is embarrassing. Everyone will know that I'm not normal. I don't see how I can go out in public anymore." What is an appropriate goal for the nurse to set with this client?
☐ 1. Manage anxiety about not being normal.
☐ 2. Learn how to care for the urinary diversion.
☐ 3. Overcome feelings of worthlessness.
☐ 4. Express fears about the urinary diversion.

16. The nurse teaches the client with a urinary diversion to attach the appliance to a standard urine collection bag at night. The intended outcome of the instruction is to prevent what occurrence?
☐ 1. urine reflux into the stoma
☐ 2. appliance separation
☐ 3. urine leakage
☐ 4. the need to restrict fluids

17. The nurse is teaching a client with an ileal conduit how to prevent a urinary tract infection. Which measure would be **most** effective?
☐ 1. Avoid people with respiratory tract infections.
☐ 2. Maintain a daily fluid intake of 68 to 101 oz (2000 to 3000 mL).
☐ 3. Use sterile technique to change the appliance.
☐ 4. Irrigate the stoma daily.

18. The nurse evaluates the effectiveness of the client's postoperative plan of care. Which outcome is expected for a client with an ileal conduit?

The client:
☐ 1. verbalizes the understanding that physical activity must be curtailed.
☐ 2. will place an aspirin in the drainage pouch to help control odor.
☐ 3. demonstrates how to catheterize the stoma.
☐ 4. will empty the drainage pouch frequently throughout the day.

19. A client is scheduled to undergo weekly intravesical chemotherapy for bladder cancer for 8 weeks. Which statement indicates that the client understands how to manage the urine as a biohazard?
☐ 1. "I'll void into a bedpan and then empty the urine into the toilet."
☐ 2. "I can disinfect the urine and toilet with bleach for 6 hours following a treatment."
☐ 3. "It's important to clean the bathroom daily with disinfectant wipes."
☐ 4. "I should use a separate bathroom from the rest of the family for the next 8 weeks."

20. A nurse is planning care for a client who underwent a percutaneous needle biopsy of the kidney. What should the nurse do **immediately** after the biopsy? Select all that apply.
☐ 1. Assess the biopsy site.
☐ 2. Take vital signs every hour.
☐ 3. Assess urine for hematuria.
☐ 4. Place the client in a prone position.
☐ 5. Assess the client for chest pain.

The Adult with Renal Calculi

21. A client had a percutaneous nephrolithotomy to remove a kidney stone. The client is being discharged with drainage tubes from the kidney. What should the nurse instruct the client to do after the procedure? Select all that apply.
☐ 1. Avoid heavy lifting for 2 to 4 weeks.
☐ 2. Return to work after 1 month.
☐ 3. Report fever or chills to the health care provider (HCP).
☐ 4. Go to the emergency department for bleeding from the drainage tubes.
☐ 5. Strain all urine, and report the presence of stones.

22. A client has renal colic due to renal lithiasis. What is the nurse's **priority** in managing care for this client?
☐ 1. Do not allow the client to ingest fluids.
☐ 2. Encourage the client to drink at least 17 oz (500 mL) of water each hour.
☐ 3. Request the central supply department to send supplies for straining urine.
☐ 4. Administer an opioid analgesic as prescribed.

23. A client is admitted to the hospital with a diagnosis of renal calculi. The client is experiencing severe flank pain and nausea; their temperature is 100.6°F (38.1°C). Which goal is a **priority** for this client?
☐ 1. Prevent urinary tract complications.
☐ 2. Manage nausea.
☐ 3. Relieve pain.
☐ 4. Maintain fluid and electrolyte balance.

24. The client is scheduled to have a kidney, ureter, and bladder (KUB) radiograph. What should the nurse explain to the client about this procedure?
☐ 1. Fluid and food will be withheld on the morning of the examination.
☐ 2. A tranquilizer will be given before the examination.
☐ 3. An enema will be given before the examination.
☐ 4. No special preparation is required for the examination.

25. In addition to nausea and severe flank pain, a female client with renal calculi has pain in the groin and bladder. What additional sign should the nurse assess?
☐ 1. nephritis
☐ 2. referred pain
☐ 3. urine retention
☐ 4. additional stone formation

26. The nurse is planning care for a client with pain associated with renal colic. Which nursing action will provide the **most** relief?
☐ 1. applying moist heat to the flank area
☐ 2. administering morphine
☐ 3. encouraging high fluid intake
☐ 4. maintaining complete bed rest

27. A client who has been diagnosed with renal calculi reports that the pain is intermittent and less colicky. Which nursing action is **most** important at this time?
☐ 1. Report hematuria to the health care provider.
☐ 2. Strain the urine carefully.
☐ 3. Administer morphine every 3 hours.
☐ 4. Apply warm compresses to the flank area.

28. The client is scheduled for an intravenous pyelogram (IVP) to determine the location of the renal calculi. Which action would be **most** important for the nurse to include in preparing the client for this test?
☐ 1. Ensure adequate fluid intake on the day of the test.
☐ 2. Prepare the client for the possibility of bladder spasms during the test.
☐ 3. Check the client's history for allergy to iodine.
☐ 4. Determine when the client last had a bowel movement.

29. A client had an intravenous pyelogram (IVP) 1 hour ago. What should the nurse include in the client's plan of care?
☐ 1. Maintain bed rest.
☐ 2. Encourage adequate fluid intake.
☐ 3. Assess for hematuria.
☐ 4. Administer a laxative.

30. A client has a ureteral catheter in place after renal surgery. What should the nurse do to provide safe care of the ureteral catheter?
☐ 1. Irrigate the catheter with 30 mL of normal saline every 8 hours.
☐ 2. Ensure that the catheter is draining freely.
☐ 3. Clamp the catheter every 2 hours for 30 minutes.
☐ 4. Ensure that the catheter drains at least 15 mL per hour.

31. Which would be the most appropriate measure for preventing the development of a paralytic ileus in a client who had renal surgery yesterday?
    1. Encourage the client to ambulate every 2 to 4 hours.
    2. Offer 3 to 4 oz (90 to 120 mL) of a carbonated beverage periodically.
    3. Administer a stool softener daily.
    4. Ensure 3000 mL of intravenous (IV) fluids in 24 hours.

32. The nurse is conducting a postoperative assessment of a client on the first day after renal surgery. The nurse should report which finding to the health care provider (HCP)?
    1. temperature: 99.8°F (37.7°C)
    2. urine output: 20 mL per hour
    3. absence of bowel sounds
    4. serosanguineous drainage on the dressing

33. A client with a history of renal calculi formation is being discharged after surgery to remove the calculus. What instruction should the nurse include in the client's discharge teaching plan?
    1. Increase daily fluid intake to at least 68 to 101 oz (2011 to 2987 mL).
    2. Strain all urine for 1 week.
    3. Eliminate dairy products from the diet.
    4. Follow measures to alkalinize the urine.

34. Allopurinol is prescribed for the client with renal calculi to take at home. The nurse should teach the client about which adverse effect of this medication?
    1. retinopathy
    2. maculopapular rash
    3. nasal congestion
    4. dizziness

35. The health care provider (HCP) has prescribed allopurinol for a client who has renal calculi. Which symptom(s) would indicate the client is experiencing adverse effects of this drug? Select all that apply.
    1. nausea
    2. rash
    3. constipation
    4. flushed skin
    5. bone marrow depression

The Adult with Acute Kidney Injury (Acute Renal Failure)

36. A client with acute kidney injury is to receive peritoneal dialysis. What should the nurse do to prepare the client for the procedure?
    1. Assess the dialysis access for a bruit and thrill.
    2. Insert an indwelling urinary catheter and drain all urine from the bladder.
    3. Ask the client to turn toward the left side.
    4. Warm the dialysis solution in the warmer.

37. A client has been admitted with acute kidney injury. What should the nurse do while admitting the client? Select all that apply.
    1. Elevate the head of the bed 30 to 45 degrees.
    2. Take vital signs.
    3. Establish an intravenous (IV) access site.
    4. Call the admitting health care provider (HCP) for prescriptions.
    5. Contact the hemodialysis unit.

38. A client with acute kidney injury has a serum potassium level of 6.5 mEq/L (6.5 mmol/L). The nurse should monitor the client for which potential complication?
    1. cardiac arrest
    2. pulmonary edema
    3. circulatory collapse
    4. hemorrhage

39. A client is in the oliguric phase of acute kidney injury. For which risk should the nurse assess the client?
    1. pulmonary edema
    2. metabolic alkalosis
    3. hypotension
    4. hypokalemia

40. A client in acute kidney injury has an external cannula inserted in the forearm for hemodialysis. Which nursing measure is appropriate for the care of this client?
    1. Use the unaffected arm for blood pressure measurements.
    2. Draw blood from the cannula for routine laboratory work.
    3. Percuss the cannula for bruits each shift.
    4. Inject heparin into the cannula each shift.

41. During dialysis, a client has disequilibrium syndrome. What should the nurse do first?
    1. Administer oxygen per nasal cannula.
    2. Slow the rate of dialysis.
    3. Reassure the client that the symptoms are normal.
    4. Place the client in a modified Trendelenburg position.

42. The nurse is reviewing laboratory values for a client who is receiving hemodialysis. Which values are an expected outcome of dialysis? Select all that apply.
    1. elevated serum creatinine level
    2. potassium within normal limits
    3. decreased hemoglobin concentration
    4. sodium levels within normal limits
    5. decreased red blood cells

43. The nurse is teaching a client who is receiving hemodialysis how to recognize infection in the shunt. What sign should the nurse tell the client to assess each day?
☐ 1. absence of a bruit
☐ 2. sluggish capillary refill time
☐ 3. coolness of the involved extremity
☐ 4. swelling at the shunt site

44. A client with acute kidney injury asks the nurse, "Will my kidneys ever function normally again?" What should the nurse tell the client?

"You will:
☐ 1. continue to improve over a period of weeks."
☐ 2. likely need dialysis."
☐ 3. improve when you have a kidney transplant."
☐ 4. have more kidney damage in several years."

The Adult with Urinary Tract Infection

45. A client with a urinary tract infection is to take nitrofurantoin four times each day. The client asks the nurse, "What should I do if I forget a dose?" What should the nurse tell the client?
☐ 1. "You can wait and take the next dose when it's due."
☐ 2. "Double the amount prescribed with your next dose."
☐ 3. "Take the prescribed dose as soon as you remember it, but if it's very close to the time for the next dose, delay that next dose."
☐ 4. "Tell your health care provider (HCP), who can then adjust your prescribed dose."

46. The nurse is planning care for a client with a catheter. What action(s) should the nurse take to prevent a catheter-associated urinary tract infection? Select all that apply.
☐ 1. Change the catheter daily.
☐ 2. Provide perineal care at least once a day.
☐ 3. Maintain a closed drainage system.
☐ 4. Encourage the client to drink 101 oz (3000 mL) fluids daily.
☐ 5. Recommend the health care provider prescribe antibiotics.

47. A nurse is assessing a client with a urinary tract infection who takes an antihypertensive drug. The nurse reviews the client's urinalysis results (see chart). What should the nurse do **next**?

Laboratory Results	
Test	Result
pH	6.8
Red blood cells	3 per high power field
Color	Yellow
Specific gravity	1.030

☐ 1. Encourage the client to increase fluid intake.
☐ 2. Withhold the next dose of antihypertensive medication.
☐ 3. Restrict the client's sodium intake.
☐ 4. Encourage the client to eat at least half of a banana per day.

48. A client has nephropathy. The health care provider (HCP) prescribes a 24-hour urine collection for creatinine clearance. Which action is necessary to ensure proper collection of the specimen?
☐ 1. Collect the urine in a preservative-free container, and keep it on ice.
☐ 2. Inform the client to discard the last voided specimen at the conclusion of urine collection.
☐ 3. Obtain a self-report of the client's weight before beginning the collection of urine.
☐ 4. Request a prescription for the insertion of an indwelling urinary catheter.

49. A client who weighs 207 lb (94.1 kg) is to receive 1.5 mg/kg of gentamicin sulfate intravenously three times each day. How many milligrams of medication should the nurse administer for each dose? Round to the nearest whole number.
_____ mg.

50. STEP 1

The nurse is caring for a 74-year-old female client admitted to the medical-surgical unit.

> **Nurse's Notes**
>
> **Today: 1800**
> A 74-year-old client is admitted to the medical-surgical unit from the health care provider's office. The client is alert and oriented to person, place, and time. The client is experiencing the urge to void as well as dysuria, which the client states is getting worse. The client also voids frequently and reports having a headache. Vital signs are temperature (T) 99.6°F (37.5°C); heart rate (HR) 106 bpm; respiration rate (RR) 25 breaths/min; blood pressure (BP) 116/62 mm Hg; and oxygen saturation 98% per pulse oximetry on room air. The client's adult child is on the way to the hospital.

➤ Highlight the findings that would require follow-up. Answer choices have been underlined.

> **Nurse's Notes**
>
> **Today: 1800**
> A 74-year-old client is admitted to the medical-surgical unit from the <u>health care provider's office</u>. The client is alert and oriented to person, place, and time. The client is experiencing the urge to void as well as <u>dysuria</u>, which the client states is getting worse. The client also <u>voids frequently</u> and <u>reports having a headache</u>. Vital signs are <u>temperature (T) 99.6°F (37.5°C)</u>; <u>heart rate (HR) 106 bpm</u>; <u>respiration rate (RR) 25 breaths/min</u>; <u>blood pressure (BP) 116/62 mm Hg</u>; and oxygen saturation 98% per pulse oximetry on room air. The client's adult child is on the way to the hospital.

51. STEP 2

The nurse is caring for a 74-year-old female client admitted to the medical-surgical unit.

> **Nurses' Notes**
>
> **Today: 1800**
> A 74-year-old client is admitted to the medical-surgical unit from the health care provider's office. The client is alert and oriented to person, place, and time. The client is experiencing the urge to void as well as dysuria, which the client states is getting worse. The client also voids frequently and reports having a headache. Vital signs are temperature (T) 99.6°F (37.5°C); heart rate (HR) 106 bpm; respiration rate (RR) 25 breaths/min; blood pressure (BP) 116/62 mm Hg; and oxygen saturation 98% per pulse oximetry on room air. The client's adult child is on the way to the hospital.

The nurse is analyzing the client's findings.

➤ For each finding below, specify if the findings are consistent with the disease process of a urinary tract infection, cerebrovascular accident, or urosepsis. Each finding may support more than one disease process.

Client Finding	Urinary Tract Infection	Cerebrovascular Accident	Urosepsis
1. Urinary frequency	☐	☐	☐
2. Dysuria	☐	☐	☐
3. Headache	☐	☐	☐
4. Altered mental status	☐	☐	☐
5. Elevated heart rate	☐	☐	☐
6. Fever	☐	☐	☐

Note: Each column must have at least one response option selected.

52. STEP 3

The nurse is caring for a 74-year-old female client admitted to the medical-surgical unit.

> **Nurses' Notes**
>
> **Today: 1800**
> A 74-year-old client is admitted to the medical-surgical unit from the health care provider's office. The client is alert and oriented to person, place, and time. The client is experiencing the urge to void as well as dysuria, which the client states is getting worse. The client also voids frequently and reports having a headache. Vital signs are temperature (T) 99.6°F (37.5°C); heart rate (HR) 106 bpm; respiration rate (RR) 25 breaths/min; blood pressure (BP) 116/62 mm Hg; and oxygen saturation 98% per pulse oximetry on room air. The client's adult child is on the way to the hospital.

The nurse is prioritizing the findings from the client's assessment. Based on the client's current clinical findings, the older adult client is at risk for developing [dehydration. / sepsis. / stroke.]

To encourage early recognition, the nurse should review the client's [urine output. / vital signs. / oxygen saturation.]

53. STEP 4

The nurse is caring for a 74-year-old female client admitted to the medical-surgical unit.

Nurses' Notes

Today: 1800
A 74-year-old client is admitted to the medical-surgical unit from the health care provider's office. The client is alert and oriented to person, place, and time. The client is experiencing the urge to void as well as dysuria, which the client states is getting worse. The client also voids frequently and reports having a headache. Vital signs are temperature (T) 99.6°F (37.5°C); heart rate (HR) 106 bpm; respiration rate (RR) 25 breaths/min; blood pressure (BP) 116/62 mm Hg; and oxygen saturation 98% per pulse oximetry on room air. The client's adult child is on the way to the hospital.

Today: 2000
The client is being monitored for a urinary tract infection with a risk for urosepsis. The client is alert and oriented to person, place, and time. Vital signs are T 99.8°F (37.9°C); HR 118 bpm; RR 28 breaths/min; BP 110/52 mm Hg; and oxygen saturation 97% per pulse oximetry on room air.

Laboratory Results

Labs	Value	Normal Range	Date	Time
Sodium	145 mg/dL (145 mmol/L)	Adults: 40–220 mEq/L/24 hours (40–220 mmol/24 hours)	Today	1500
Potassium	4.9 mEq/L	Adults: 25–125 mEq/24 hours (25–125 mmol/24 hours), varying with diet	Today	1500
Calcium	8.8 mg/dL (2.2 mmol/L)	Adults: 8.2–10.2 mg/dL (2.05–2.54 mmol/L)	Today	1500
Blood urea nitrogen	30 mg/dL (10.7 mmol/L)	8–20 mg/dL (2.9–7.5 mmol/L)	Today	1500
Creatinine	1.6 mg/dL (122 µmol/L)	Women: 0.6–1.1 mg/dL (53–97 µmol/L)	Today	1500
Glucose	125 mg/dL (6.9 mmol/L)	Adults: less than or equal to 110 mg/dL (less than or equal to 5.6 mmol/L)	Today	1500
White blood cells	15,500 mg/dL (15.5 × 10^9/L)	4.5–10.5 × 10^3 cells/mm^3 (4.5–10.5 × 10^9/L)	Today	1500
Hemoglobin	12.5 g/dL (125 g/L)	Women: 12–16 g/dL (120–160 g/L)	Today	1500
Hematocrit	37.2% (0.37 proportion of 1.0)	Women: 36%–48% (0.36–0.48 proportion of 1.0)	Today	1500
Lactic acid	2 mg/dL	0.5–1 mmol/L	Today	1500
Platelets	132,000/µL	Adults: 140,000–400,000/µL (140–400 × 10^9/L) 150,000 and 400,000 platelets per microliter.	Today	1500
Urinalysis: • Color • Blood • Specific gravity • Protein • Leukocyte • Nitrites	Cloudy Positive 1.035 < 1.030 Trace-none Positive negative Positive none	Yellow Negative <1.030 None Negative none	Today	1500

Orders

Perform in-and-out catheterization
Place an intravenous (IV) line
Administer 0.9% normal saline at 200 mL/h
Obtain blood cultures
Start vancomycin 500 mg via IV push
Order abdominal computed tomography (CT)

▶ The nurse reviews the laboratory results and receives orders from the health care provider. Which order(s) should the nurse question? Select all that apply.

☐ 1. Perform in-and-out catheterization.
☐ 2. Place an intravenous (IV) line.
☐ 3. Administer 0.9% normal saline at 200 mL/h.
☐ 4. Obtain blood cultures.
☐ 5. Start vancomycin 500 mg via IV push.
☐ 6. Order abdominal computed tomography (CT).

54. STEP 5

The nurse is caring for a 74-year-old female client admitted to the medical-surgical unit.

Nurses' Notes

Today: 1800
A 74-year-old client is admitted to the medical-surgical unit from the health care provider's office. The client is alert and oriented to person, place, and time. The client is experiencing the urge to void as well as dysuria, which the client states is getting worse. The client also voids frequently and reports having a headache. Vital signs are temperature (T) 99.6°F (37.5°C); heart rate (HR) 106 bpm; respiration rate (RR) 25 breaths/min; blood pressure (BP) 116/62 mm Hg; and oxygen saturation 98% per pulse oximetry on room air. The client's adult child is on the way to the hospital.

Today: 2000
The client is being monitored for a urinary tract infection with a risk for urosepsis. The client is alert and oriented to person, place, and time. Vital signs are T 99.8°F (37.9°C); HR 118 bpm, RR 28 breaths/min; BP 110/52 mm Hg; and oxygen saturation 97% per pulse oximetry on room air.

Laboratory Results

Labs	Value	Normal Range	Date	Time
Sodium	145 mg/dL (145 mmol/L)	Adults: 40–220 mEq/L/24 hours (40–220 mmol/24 hours)	Today	1500
Potassium	4.9 mEq/L	Adults: 25–125 mEq/24 hours (25–125 mmol/24 hours), varying with diet	Today	1500
Calcium	8.8 mg/dL (2.2 mmol/L)	Adults: 8.2–10.2 mg/dL (2.05–2.54 mmol/L)	Today	1500
Blood urea nitrogen	30 mg/dL (10.7 mmol/L)	8–20 mg/dL (2.9–7.5 mmol/L)	Today	1500
Creatinine	1.6 mg/dL (122 µmol/L)	Women: 0.6–1.1 mg/dL (53–97 µmol/L)	Today	1500
Glucose	125 mg/dL (6.9 mmol/L)	Adults: less than or equal to 110 mg/dL (less than or equal to 5.6 mmol/L)	Today	1500
White blood cells	15,500 mg/dL (15.5 × 10^9/L)	4.5–10.5 × 10^3 cells/mm^3 (4.5–10.5 × 10^9/L)	Today	1500
Hemoglobin	12.5 g/dL (125 g/L)	Women: 12–16 g/dL (120–160 g/L)	Today	1500
Hematocrit	37.2% (0.37 proportion of 1.0)	Women: 36%–48% (0.36–0.48 proportion of 1.0)	Today	1500
Lactic acid	2 mg/dL	0.5–1 mmol/L	Today	1500
Platelets	132,000/µL	Adults: 140,000–400,000/µL (140–400 × 10^9/L)	Today	1500
Urinalysis: • Color • Clarity • Blood • Specific gravity • Protein • Leukocyte • Nitrites	Amber Cloudy Positive Positive 1.035 Trace Positive Positive	Yellow Negative <1.030 None Negative none	Today	1500
Sodium	145 mg/dL (145 mmol/L)	Adults: 40–220 mEq/L/24 hours (40–220 mmol/24 hours)	Today	1500

Orders

Perform in-and-out catheterization

Place an intravenous (IV) line

Administer 0.9% normal saline at 200 mL/h

Obtain blood cultures

Start vancomycin 500 mg via IV push

Order abdominal computed tomography (CT)

➤ The nurse needs to place a Foley catheter to accurately monitor the client's intake and output. Identify the top three steps of the procedure that are essential to prevent a urinary tract infection in this client.

- ☐ 1. Insert the catheter into the urinary meatus until urine flow is observed.
- ☐ 2. Secure the catheter to the client's thigh.
- ☐ 3. Use sterile gloves.
- ☐ 4. Using antiseptic-soaked cotton balls, perform downward strokes to clean the labia minora.
- ☐ 5. Verify latex and iodine allergies.
- ☐ 6. Place a sterile fenestrated drape over the perineal area.

STEP 6

The nurse is caring for a 74-year-old female client admitted to the medical-surgical unit.

Nurses' Notes

Today: 1800
A 74-year-old client is admitted to the medical-surgical unit from the health care provider's office. The client is alert and oriented to person, place, and time. The client is experiencing the urge to void as well as dysuria, which the client states is getting worse. The client also voids frequently and reports having a headache. Vital signs are temperature (T) 99.6°F (37.5°C); heart rate (HR) 106 bpm; respiration rate (RR) 25 breaths/min; blood pressure (BP) 116/62 mm Hg; and oxygen saturation 98% per pulse oximetry on room air. The client's adult child is on the way to the hospital.

Today: 2000
The client is being monitored for a urinary tract infection with a risk for urosepsis. The client is alert and oriented to person, place, and time. Vital signs are T 99.8°F (37.9°C); HR 118 bpm, RR 28 breaths/min; BP 110/52 mm Hg; and oxygen saturation 97% per pulse oximetry on room air.

Three days later: 1600
The client was treated with fluids and antibiotics for a urinary tract infection and is soon going to be discharged. The client is alert and oriented to person, place, time, and situation. The client remains ambulatory with one-person assistance as this is the client's baseline. Vital signs are T 98.3°F (36.8°C); HR 87 bpm; RR 20 breaths/min; BP 120/65 mm Hg; and oxygen saturation 99% per pulse oximetry on room air.

Laboratory Results

Labs	Value	Normal Range	Date	Time
Sodium	145 mg/dL (145 mmol/L)	Adults: 40–220 mEq/L/24 hours (40–220 mmol/24 hours)	Today	1500
Potassium	4.9 mEq/L	Adults: 25–125 mEq/24 hours (25–125 mmol/24 hours), varying with diet	Today	1500
Calcium	8.8 mg/dL (2.2 mmol/L)	Adults: 8.2–10.2 mg/dL (2.05–2.54 mmol/L)	Today	1500
Blood urea nitrogen	30 mg/dL (10.7 mmol/L)	8–20 mg/dL (2.9–7.5 mmol/L)	Today	1500
Creatinine	1.6 mg/dL (122 µmol/L)	Women: 0.6–1.1 mg/dL (53–97 µmol/L)	Today	1500
Glucose	125 mg/dL (6.9 mmol/L)	Adults: less than or equal to 110 mg/dL (less than or equal to 5.6 mmol/L)	Today	1500
White blood cells	15,500 mg/dL (15.5 × 10^9/L)	4.5–10.5 × 10^3 cells/mm^3 (4.5–10.5 × 10^9/L)	Today	1500
Hemoglobin	12.5 g/dL (125 g/L)	Women: 12–16 g/dL (120–160 g/L)	Today	1500
Hematocrit	37.2% (0.37 proportion of 1.0)	Women: 36%–48% (0.36–0.48 proportion of 1.0)	Today	1500
Lactic acid	2 mg/dL	0.5–1 mmol/L	Today	1500
Platelets	132,000/µL	Adults: 140,000–400,000/µL (140–400 × 10^9/L)	Today	1500
Urinalysis: • Color • Clarity • Blood • Specific gravity • Protein • Leukocyte • Nitrites	Amber Cloudy Positive Positive 1.035 Trace Positive Positive	Yellow Negative <1.030 None Negative none	Today	1500
Sodium	145 mg/dL (145 mmol/L)	Adults: 40–220 mEq/L/24 hours (40–220 mmol/24 hours)	Today	1500

Orders

Perform in-and-out catheterization
Place an intravenous (IV) line
Administer 0.9% normal saline at 200 mL/h
Obtain blood cultures
Start vancomycin 500 mg via IV push
Order abdominal computed tomography (CT)

The nurse is instructing the client about how to prevent another urinary tract infection.

➤ Which statement(s) would indicate the client understands the instruction? Select all that apply.

☐ 1. "I will limit my fluids to 17 oz (500 mL) per day to decrease my chances of developing a urinary tract infection."
☐ 2. "I will add cranberry juice to my diet."
☐ 3. "I will ensure that I wipe from front to back after every urinary incident."
☐ 4. "I will increase my intake of caffeine to help my kidneys."
☐ 5. "If I need to utilize adult diapers, I need to check them every 2 hours."
☐ 6. "I will use the bathroom as soon as the need arises."
☐ 7. "I will take a bath every day to reduce bacteria buildup."

56. A client, who is a newlywed, is afraid to discuss their diagnosis of cystitis with their spouse. Which approach would be **best**?
☐ 1. Arrange a meeting with the client, their spouse, the health care provider (HCP), and the nurse.
☐ 2. Insist that the client talk with their spouse because good communication is necessary for a successful marriage.
☐ 3. Talk first with the spouse alone and then with both of them together to share the spouse's reactions.
☐ 4. Spend time with the client addressing their concerns and then, if the client requests, stay with the client while they talk with their spouse.

57. The nurse teaches a female client who has cystitis methods to relieve discomfort until the antibiotic takes effect. Which response by the client would indicate that they understand the nurse's instructions?

"I will:
☐ 1. place ice packs on my perineum."
☐ 2. take warm tub baths."
☐ 3. drink a cup of warm tea every hour."
☐ 4. void every 5 to 6 hours."

58. When teaching a client with a urinary tract infection about taking a prescribed antibiotic for 7 days, the nurse should tell the client to report which symptom(s) to the health care provider (HCP)? Select all that apply.
☐ 1. cloudy urine for the first few days
☐ 2. blood in the urine
☐ 3. rash
☐ 4. mild nausea
☐ 5. fever above 100°F (37.8°C)
☐ 6. urinating every 3 to 4 hours

59. A client has been prescribed nitrofurantoin for treatment of a lower urinary tract infection. Which instruction(s) should the nurse include when teaching the client about this medication? Select all that apply.
☐ 1. "Take the medication on an empty stomach."
☐ 2. "Your urine may become brown in color."
☐ 3. "Increase your fluid intake."
☐ 4. "Take the medication until your symptoms subside."
☐ 5. "Take the medication with an antacid to decrease gastrointestinal distress."

60. Nitrofurantoin, 75 mg four times per day, has been prescribed for a client with a lower urinary tract infection. The medication comes in an oral suspension of 25 mg/5 mL. How many milliliters should the nurse administer for each dose? Record your answer using a whole number.
_____ mL.

61. The nurse has taught a female client about preventing the recurrence of cystitis. Which statement indicates that further teaching is needed?

"I can:
☐ 1. go 8 to 10 hours without emptying my bladder."
☐ 2. take a tub bath every evening."
☐ 3. continue to drink herbal tea."
☐ 4. workout by lifting weights three times a week."

62. To prevent recurrence of cystitis, the nurse should plan to encourage a female client to include which measure in their daily routine?
☐ 1. wearing cotton underpants
☐ 2. increasing citrus juice intake
☐ 3. douching regularly with 0.25% acetic acid
☐ 4. using vaginal sprays

63. The nurse explains to the client the importance of drinking large quantities of fluid to prevent cystitis. How much fluid should the nurse tell the client to drink?
☐ 1. twice as much fluid as usual
☐ 2. at least 34 fl oz (1020 mL) more than usual
☐ 3. as much water or juice, as possible
☐ 4. at least 101 fl oz (3030 mL) of fluids daily

The Adult with Pyelonephritis

64. A client is at risk for acute pyelonephritis. The nurse should instruct the client about which health promotion behavior that will be **most** effective in preventing pyelonephritis?
☐ 1. Wash the perineum with warm water and soap, cleaning from front to back.
☐ 2. Treat fungal infections such as athlete's foot immediately.
☐ 3. Have a pneumonia immunization to prevent streptococcal infection.
☐ 4. Treat skin lesions with antibiotics, and cover any open lesions.

65. A client is diagnosed with acute pyelonephritis. What should the nurse instruct the client to do?
☐ 1. Empty the bladder every 2 to 3 hours.
☐ 2. Take bubble baths instead of showers.
☐ 3. Take antibiotics for the rest of the client's life.
☐ 4. Decrease fluid intake to 34 oz (1000 mL) per day.

66. The nurse is obtaining a health history for a client with possible pyelonephritis. Which factor would put the client at increased risk for pyelonephritis?
☐ 1. history of hypertension
☐ 2. intake of large quantities of cranberry juice
☐ 3. fluid intake of 68 oz (2000 mL) per day
☐ 4. history of diabetes mellitus

67. The client with pyelonephritis asks the nurse, "How will I know whether the antibiotics are treating my infection?" What should the nurse tell the client?
☐ 1. "After you take the antibiotics for 2 weeks, you won't have any infection."
☐ 2. "Your health care provider can tell by the color and odor of your urine."
☐ 3. "Your health care provider will take a urine culture."
☐ 4. "When your symptoms disappear, you'll know that your infection is gone."

68. The nurse is to administer 1200 mg of an antibiotic. The drug is prepared with 6 g of the drug in 2 mL of solution. The nurse should administer how many milliliters of the drug? Record your answer using one decimal point.
_____ mL.

69. The client with acute pyelonephritis wants to know the possibility of developing chronic pyelonephritis. The nurse's response is based on knowledge of which disorder that **most** commonly leads to chronic pyelonephritis?
☐ 1. acute pyelonephritis
☐ 2. recurrent urinary tract infections
☐ 3. acute renal failure
☐ 4. glomerulonephritis

70. A client is diagnosed with pyelonephritis. Which nursing action is a **priority**?
☐ 1. Monitor hemoglobin levels.
☐ 2. Insert a urinary catheter.
☐ 3. Stress the importance of the use of long-term antibiotics.
☐ 4. Ensure sufficient hydration.

The Adult with Chronic Renal Failure

71. A client with end-stage renal failure has an internal arteriovenous fistula in the left arm for vascular access during hemodialysis. What should the nurse instruct the client to do? Select all that apply.
☐ 1. Remind health care providers to draw blood from veins on the left side.
☐ 2. Avoid sleeping on the left arm.
☐ 3. Wear a wristwatch on the right arm.
☐ 4. Assess fingers on the left arm for warmth.
☐ 5. Obtain blood pressure (BP) from the left arm.

72. A client with end-stage chronic renal failure is admitted to the hospital with a serum potassium level of 7 mEq/L (7 mmol/L). In what order of priority from first to last should the nurse administer the prescriptions? All options must be used.

| 1. Administer insulin and glucose. |
| 2. Start an intravenous (IV) access site. |
| 3. Obtain a serum potassium level. |
| 4. Attach the client to a cardiac monitor. |

| |
| |
| |
| |

73. A client with chronic renal failure is receiving hemodialysis three times a week. What should the nurse do to protect the fistula?
☐ 1. Take the blood pressure in the arm with the fistula.
☐ 2. Report the loss of a thrill or bruit on the arm with the fistula.
☐ 3. Maintain a pressure dressing on the shunt.
☐ 4. Start a second intravenous (IV) line in the arm with the fistula.

74. A client with chronic renal failure who receives hemodialysis twice a week is experiencing severe nausea. What should the nurse advise the client to do to manage the nausea? Select all that apply.
☐ 1. Drink fluids before eating solid foods.
☐ 2. Have limited amounts of fluids only when thirsty.
☐ 3. Limit activity.
☐ 4. Keep all dialysis appointments.
☐ 5. Eat smaller, more frequent meals.

75. The nurse warms the dialysis solution before use in peritoneal dialysis. What is the expected outcome of warming the solution?
☐ 1. Encourage the removal of serum urea.
☐ 2. Force potassium back into the cells.
☐ 3. Add extra warmth to the body.
☐ 4. Promote abdominal muscle relaxation.

76. A client is receiving peritoneal dialysis. What should the nurse assess while the dialysis solution is dwelling in the client's abdomen?
☐ 1. Assess for urticaria.
☐ 2. Observe respiratory status.
☐ 3. Check capillary refill time.
☐ 4. Monitor electrolyte status.

77. A client is having peritoneal dialysis. During the exchange, the nurse observes that the solution draining from the client's abdomen is consistently blood tinged. The client has a permanent peritoneal catheter in place. What clinical judgment should the nurse make about the blood-tinged drainage?
- ☐ 1. It is expected with a permanent peritoneal catheter.
- ☐ 2. It indicates abdominal blood vessel damage.
- ☐ 3. It can indicate kidney damage.
- ☐ 4. It is caused by a too-rapid infusion of the dialysate.

78. A client undergoing long-term peritoneal dialysis at home is currently experiencing a reduced outflow from the dialysis catheter. To determine if the catheter is obstructed, what should the nurse ask the client about experiencing recently?
- ☐ 1. diarrhea
- ☐ 2. vomiting
- ☐ 3. flatulence
- ☐ 4. constipation

79. The nurse is planning care for a client receiving hemodialysis. Which should be included in the client's plan of care?
- ☐ 1. Limit the client's visitors.
- ☐ 2. Monitor the client's blood pressure.
- ☐ 3. Pad the side rails of the bed.
- ☐ 4. Keep the client on nothing-by-mouth (NPO) status.

80. The client performs self-peritoneal dialysis. What should the nurse teach the client about preventing peritonitis? Select all that apply.
- ☐ 1. Broad-spectrum antibiotics may be administered to prevent infection.
- ☐ 2. Antibiotics may be added to the dialysate to treat peritonitis.
- ☐ 3. Clean technique is permissible for the prevention of peritonitis.
- ☐ 4. Peritonitis is characterized by cloudy dialysate drainage and abdominal discomfort.
- ☐ 5. Peritonitis is the most common and serious complication of peritoneal dialysis.

81. The nurse is assessing a client who has just received peritoneal dialysis. For which symptom should the nurse assess the client?
- ☐ 1. hematuria
- ☐ 2. weight loss
- ☐ 3. hypertension
- ☐ 4. increased urine output

82. Aluminum hydroxide gel is prescribed for a client with chronic renal failure to take at home. What is the expected outcome of this drug?
- ☐ 1. relieving the pain of gastric hyperacidity
- ☐ 2. preventing Curling stress ulcers
- ☐ 3. binding phosphate in the intestine
- ☐ 4. reversing metabolic acidosis

83. The nurse teaches a client with chronic renal failure when to take aluminum hydroxide gel. Which statement indicates that the client understands the teaching?

"I'll take it:
- ☐ 1. every 4 hours around the clock."
- ☐ 2. between meals and at bedtime."
- ☐ 3. when I have an upset stomach."
- ☐ 4. with meals and bedtime snacks."

84. Which teaching approach for the client with chronic renal failure who has difficulty concentrating due to high uremia levels would be **most** appropriate?
- ☐ 1. Provide all needed teaching in one extended session.
- ☐ 2. Validate the client's understanding of the material frequently.
- ☐ 3. Conduct a one-on-one session with the client.
- ☐ 4. Use video clips to reinforce the material as needed.

85. The nurse is instructing a client with chronic renal failure to maintain adequate nutritional intake. Which diet would be **most** appropriate?
- ☐ 1. high-carbohydrate, high-protein
- ☐ 2. high-calcium, high-potassium, high-protein
- ☐ 3. low-protein, low-sodium, low-potassium
- ☐ 4. low-protein, high-potassium

86. The nurse is discussing concerns about sexual activity with a client with chronic renal failure. Which strategy would be **most** useful?
- ☐ 1. Help the client to accept that sexual activity will be decreased.
- ☐ 2. Suggest using alternative forms of sexual expression and intimacy.
- ☐ 3. Tell the client to plan rest periods after sexual activity.
- ☐ 4. Refer the client to a counselor.

The Adult with Urinary Incontinence

87. An older adult who lives alone has stress incontinence. What should the nurse teach the client to do to prevent incontinence? Select all that apply.
- ☐ 1. Ask someone else to lift heavy objects.
- ☐ 2. Refrain from drinking coffee or alcohol.
- ☐ 3. Perform perineal muscle exercises (i.e., Kegel exercises).
- ☐ 4. Apply estrogen cream to the urinary meatus after voiding.
- ☐ 5. Avoid jumping up and down.

88. A 45-year-old female client has stress incontinence. Which data from the client's history contributes **most** to the client's incontinence?
- ☐ 1. intake of 68 to 101 oz (2000 to 3000 mL) of fluid per day
- ☐ 2. history of three full-term pregnancies
- ☐ 3. age of 45 years
- ☐ 4. history of competitive swimming

89. The nurse is planning care for a client with stress incontinence. What goal is realistic for the nurse to establish with the client?
    ☐ 1. Help the client adjust to the frequent episodes of incontinence.
    ☐ 2. Eliminate all episodes of incontinence.
    ☐ 3. Prevent the development of urinary tract infections.
    ☐ 4. Decrease the number of incontinence episodes.

90. A client has urge incontinence. When obtaining the health history, the nurse should ask the client about which factor that could precipitate incontinence?
    ☐ 1. inability to empty the bladder
    ☐ 2. loss of urine when coughing
    ☐ 3. involuntary urination
    ☐ 4. frequent dribbling of urine

91. Which nursing action is **most** appropriate for a client who has urge incontinence?
    ☐ 1. Have the client urinate on a timed schedule.
    ☐ 2. Provide a bedside commode.
    ☐ 3. Administer prophylactic antibiotics.
    ☐ 4. Teach the client intermittent self-catheterization technique.

Managing Care, Quality, and Safety of Adults with Urinary Tract Health Problems

92. The nurse manager on the urology unit has employed three nurses from a culture that is different from that of most of the nurses and patients on this unit. Which strategy would help the newly employed nurses socialize into the team and promote the cultural competence of all of the nurses?
    ☐ 1. Create a staffing plan, placing one of the newly employed nurses on each shift.
    ☐ 2. Require newly employed nurses to speak English only when working.
    ☐ 3. Hold a culture-sharing session at monthly meetings.
    ☐ 4. Encourage the staff to invite the new nurses to meet their families.

93. The nurse manager is developing an assessment guide for clients on the urology unit. Which client is at **highest** risk for catheter-associated urinary tract infection (CAUTI)?
    ☐ 1. client with diabetes mellitus
    ☐ 2. client who had one course of antibiotic therapy
    ☐ 3. client with a family history of UTIs
    ☐ 4. client with a urinary calculus

94. A client is scheduled for an intravenous pyelogram. Before the procedure, the nurse learns that the client has a sensitivity to shellfish. What should the nurse do **next**?
    ☐ 1. Administer a cathartic to the client to empty the colon.
    ☐ 2. Administer an antiflatulent to the client to relieve gas.
    ☐ 3. Keep the client on nothing-by-mouth (NPO) status.
    ☐ 4. Notify the health care provider.

95. The nurse finds a container with the client's urine specimen sitting on a counter in the bathroom. The client states that the specimen has been sitting in the bathroom for at least 2 hours. What should the nurse do with the urine specimen?
    ☐ 1. Discard the urine, and obtain a new specimen.
    ☐ 2. Send the urine to the laboratory as quickly as possible.
    ☐ 3. Add fresh urine to the collected specimen, and send the specimen to the laboratory.
    ☐ 4. Refrigerate the specimen until it can be transported to the laboratory.

96. A client with early acute kidney injury has anemia, tachycardia, hypotension, and shortness of breath. The health care provider has prescribed 2 units of packed red blood cells (PRBCs). What should the nurse determine before initiating the blood transfusion? Select all that apply.
    ☐ 1. There is an intravenous (IV) access with the appropriate tubing and normal saline as the priming solution.
    ☐ 2. There is a signed informed consent for transfusion therapy.
    ☐ 3. Blood typing and cross-matching are documented in the medical record.
    ☐ 4. The vital signs have been taken and documented in accordance with facility policy and procedure.
    ☐ 5. There is a second unit of blood in the medication room.
    ☐ 6. The client has an identification bracelet.

97. The nurse is instructing the unlicensed assistive personnel (UAP) about the correct technique for obtaining a clean-catch urine culture from a female client. Which statement indicates that the UAP has understood the instructions:?

    "I will:
    ☐ 1. have the client completely empty their bladder into the specimen cup."
    ☐ 2. need to catheterize the client to get the urine specimen."
    ☐ 3. ask the client to clean their labia, void into the toilet, and then into the specimen cup."
    ☐ 4. obtain the specimen in the afternoon after the client has had plenty of fluids."

98. An older adult is admitted with new-onset confusion, headache, poor skin turgor, bounding pulse, and urinary incontinence and has been drinking copious amounts of water. Upon reviewing the lab results, the nurse discovers a sodium level of 122 mEq/L (122 mmol/L). A report to the health care provider (HCP) should include what recommendation(s)? Select all that apply.
    ☐ 1. fluid restriction
    ☐ 2. vital signs every 2 hours
    ☐ 3. bed alarm
    ☐ 4. Foley catheter
    ☐ 5. 2-g sodium diet

99. Which action(s) related to the care of a client with a Foley catheter would be appropriate for the nurse to delegate to the unlicensed assistive personnel (UAP)? Select all that apply.
    ☐ 1. Flush the catheter as needed to ensure patency.
    ☐ 2. Empty the drainage bag, and record output at specified times.
    ☐ 3. Apply a catheter-securing device to the client's leg.
    ☐ 4. Perform bladder irrigation as prescribed.
    ☐ 5. Provide a Foley catheter and perineal care each shift.
    ☐ 6. Ensure the urine drainage bag is below the level of the bladder at all times.

100. The client is to receive antibiotic intravenous (IV) therapy in the home. The nurse should develop a teaching plan to ensure that the client and family can manage the IV fluid and infusion correctly and avoid complications. What should the nurse instruct the client to do? Select all that apply.
    ☐ 1. Report signs of redness or inflammation at the site.
    ☐ 2. Wear sterile gloves to change the fluids.
    ☐ 3. Call the health care provider (HCP) for a temperature above 100°F (37.8°C).
    ☐ 4. Cleanse the port with alcohol wipes.
    ☐ 5. Place the IV bag on a table level with the client's arm.

101. Prior to discharging a client with end-stage cancer of the bladder from the hospital, the nurse should take which action(s)? Select all that apply.
    ☐ 1. Determine if the client is likely to become suicidal.
    ☐ 2. Give a list of the client's medications to the client before discharge.
    ☐ 3. Instruct the client to update information when medications are discontinued, doses are changed, or new medications are added.
    ☐ 4. Explain the need to carry medication information with the client at all times.
    ☐ 5. Instruct the client that the use of over-the-counter products need not be reported to the health care provider (HCP).

Answers, Rationales, and Test-Taking Strategies

The answers and rationales for each question follow below, along with keys (🔑) to the client need (CN) and cognitive level (CL) for each question. In addition, questions that measure clinical judgment will be coded (CJ). As you check your answers, use the **Content Mastery and Test-Taking Skill Self-Analysis** *worksheet (tear-out worksheet in the back of the book) to identify the reason(s) for not answering the questions correctly. For additional information about test-taking skills and strategies for answering questions, refer to pages 12–51 in Part 1 of this book.*

The Adult with Cancer of the Bladder

1. **1, 4.** An adequate fluid intake aids in the prevention of urinary calculi and infection. Odor-producing foods can produce offensive odors that may impact the client's lifestyle and relationships. Lack of activity leads to urinary stasis, which promotes urinary calculi development and infection. Acidic urine helps prevent urinary tract infections. Tight clothing over the stoma obstructs blood circulation and urine flow.

    🔑 CN: Reduction of risk potential; CL: Analyze

2. **1, 2, 4.** The nurse should instruct the client with an ileal conduit that the stoma will shrink in about 4 to 6 weeks. The client can take a shower or a bath with the collection pouch on or off. The client can shave the hair around the stoma using an electric razor to make it easier for the collection bag to adhere to the skin. The client should wash the skin around the stoma with water; it is not necessary to use antibacterial soap, and soap may cause the skin to become dry and irritated. The collection bag can remain in place for up to 7 days.

    🔑 CN: Physiological adaptation; CL: Evaluate

3. **3.** The nurse should verify that the client has voided before discharge to evaluate bladder function. Bowel function is not expected to be affected by this procedure. There may not be a need for pain medication immediately after the procedure and before discharge, but the nurse should assess the client's pain status and inform the client about the use and side effects of the medication. It is normal for the client to have hematuria because of the procedure.

    🔑 CN: Management of care; CL: Analyze

4. 3. Painless hematuria is the most common clinical finding in bladder cancer. Other symptoms include urinary frequency, dysuria, and urinary urgency, but these are not as common as hematuria. Suprapubic pain and urine retention do not occur in bladder cancer.

🔑 CN: Physiological adaptation; CL: Analyze

5. 2. Chills could indicate the onset of acute infection that can progress to septic shock. Dizziness would not be an anticipated symptom after a cystoscopy. Pink-tinged urine and bladder spasms are common after cystoscopy.

🔑 CN: Reduction of risk potential; CL: Analyze

6. 4. Lower abdominal pain after a cystoscopy is frequently caused by bladder spasms. Warm water can help relax muscles. Ice is not effective in relieving spasms. Massage and ambulation may increase bladder irritability.

🔑 CN: Basic care and comfort; CL: Analyze

7. 3. An ileal conduit is a permanent urinary diversion in which a portion of the ileum is surgically resected and one end of the segment is closed. The ureters are surgically attached to this segment of the ileum, and the open end of the ileum is brought to the skin surface of the abdomen to form the stoma. The client must wear a pouch to collect the urine that continually flows through the conduit. The bladder is removed during the surgical procedure, and the ileal conduit is not reversible. Diversion of urine to the sigmoid colon is called a *ureteroileosigmoidostomy*. An opening in the bladder that allows urine to drain externally is called a *cystostomy*.

🔑 CN: Reduction of risk potential; CL: Apply

8. 2. After pelvic surgery, there is an increased chance of thrombophlebitis owing to the pelvic manipulation that can interfere with circulation and promote venous stasis. Peritonitis is a potential complication of any abdominal surgery, not just pelvic surgery. Ascites is most frequently an indication of liver disease. Inguinal hernia may be caused by an increase in intra-abdominal pressure or a congenital weakness of the abdominal wall; ventral hernia occurs at the site of a previous abdominal incision.

🔑 CN: Reduction of risk potential; CL: Analyze

9. 4. Mucus is secreted by the intestinal segment used to create the conduit and is a normal occurrence. The client should be encouraged to maintain a large fluid intake to help flush the mucus out of the conduit. Because mucus in the urine is expected, it is not necessary to change the appliance bag or notify the HCP. The mucus is not an indication of an infection, so a urine culture is not necessary.

🔑 CN: Reduction of risk potential; CL: Analyze

10. 4. If the appliance becomes too full, it is likely to pull away from the skin completely or leak urine onto the skin; thus, if the seal is intact, the client is emptying the appliance regularly. The skin around the seal should not be red or irritated, which could indicate a leak. There will likely be an odor from the urine. Deep yellow urine indicates that the client should be increasing fluid intake.

🔑 CN: Physiological adaptation; CL: Evaluate

11. 1. Inserting a gauze wick into the stoma helps prevent urine leakage when changing the appliance. The stoma should not be sealed or suctioned. Oral fluids do not need to be avoided.

🔑 CN: Physiological adaptation; CL: Analyze

12. 2. A reusable appliance should be routinely cleaned with soap and water. Other products are not necessary and may damage the appliance or be caustic to the client's skin.

🔑 CN: Physiological adaptation; CL: Apply

13. ➖➕ **3, 4.** The client with an ileal conduit must learn self-care activities related to the care of the stoma and ostomy appliances. The client should be taught to increase their fluid intake to about 101 oz (3000 mL) a day and should not limit their intake. Adequate fluid intake helps flush mucus from the ileal conduit. The ostomy appliance should be changed approximately every 3 to 7 days and whenever a leak develops. A skin barrier is essential for protecting the skin from the irritation of the urine. An aspirin should not be used as a method of odor control because it can be an irritant to the stoma and lead to ulceration. The ostomy pouch should be emptied when it is one-third to one-half full to prevent the weight of the urine from pulling the appliance away from the skin.

🔑 CN: Reduction of risk potential; CL: Evaluate

14. 2. A distilled vinegar solution acts as a good deodorizing agent after an appliance has been cleaned well with soap and water. If the client prefers, a commercial deodorizer may be used. Salt solution does not deodorize. Ammonia and bleaching agents may damage the appliance.

🔑 CN: Basic care and comfort; CL: Apply

15. **4.** It is normal for clients to express fears and concerns about the body changes associated with a urinary diversion. Allowing the client time to verbalize concerns in a supportive environment and suggesting that they discuss these concerns with people who have successfully adjusted to ostomy surgery can help them begin coping with these changes in a positive manner. Although the client may be anxious about this situation and may be feeling worthless, the underlying problem is a disturbance in body image. There are no data to indicate that the client does not know how to care for the urinary diversion.

CN: Psychosocial integrity; CL: Analyze

16. **1.** The most important reason for attaching the appliance to a standard urine collection bag at night is to prevent urine reflux into the stoma and ureters, which can result in infection. Using a standard collection bag also keeps the appliance from separating from the skin and helps prevent urine leakage from an overly full bag, but the primary purpose is to prevent reflux of urine. A client with a urinary diversion should drink 68 to 101 oz (2000 to 3000 mL) of fluid each day; it would be inappropriate to suggest decreasing fluid intake.

CN: Physiological adaptation; CL: Apply

17. **2.** Maintaining a fluid intake of 68 to 101 oz (2000 to 3000 mL) a day is likely to be most effective in preventing urinary tract infections. A high fluid intake results in high urine output, which prevents urinary stasis and bacterial growth. Avoiding people with respiratory tract infections will not prevent urinary tract infections. Clean, not sterile, technique is used to change the appliance. An ileal conduit stoma is not irrigated.

CN: Physiological adaptation; CL: Analyze

18. **4.** It is important that the client empty the drainage pouch throughout the day to decrease the risk for leakage. The client does not normally need to curtail physical activity. Aspirin should never be placed in a pouch because aspirin can irritate or ulcerate the stoma. The client does not catheterize an ileal conduit stoma.

CN: Physiological adaptation; CL: Evaluate

19. **2.** After intravesical chemotherapy, the client must treat the urine as a biohazard; this involves disinfecting the urine and the toilet with household bleach for 6 hours following treatment. It is not necessary to use a bedpan and then empty the urine in the toilet; the client can use the toilet but must disinfect the urine with bleach. The bathroom does not need to be cleaned daily with disinfectant wipes. The client does not need to use a separate bathroom as long as the client's urine is disinfected with bleach.

CN: Physiological integrity; CL: Evaluate

20. **1, 3, 4.** The nurse should assess the biopsy site for bleeding and hematoma formation. The client should remain prone for 8 to 24 hours after the biopsy. A pressure dressing will aid in blood coagulation. Vital signs should be taken every 5 to 15 minutes for the first hour and then less often if the client is stable. The urine does not need to be collected and kept on ice. The nurse should collect serial urine specimens to assess for hematuria. A renal biopsy does not put the client at increased risk for chest pain.

CN: Reduction of risk potential; CL: Analyze

The Adult with Renal Calculi

21. **1, 3, 4.** Following percutaneous nephrolithotomy, the nurse should instruct the client to avoid lifting heavy objects for 2 to 4 weeks. The client should contact the HCP if they are having chills or fever. The client should go to the emergency department if there is bleeding from the drainage tubes. Usually, the client can return to work in a week. It is not necessary to strain the urine. The client will likely have x-rays or an ultrasound several weeks after the surgery to determine if there are other stones in the kidney.

CN: Health promotion and maintenance; CL: Analyze

22. **4.** If infection or blockage caused by calculi is present, a client can experience sudden severe pain in the flank area, known as *renal colic*. Pain from a kidney stone is considered an emergency situation and requires analgesic intervention. Withholding fluids will make urine more concentrated and stones more difficult to pass naturally. Forcing large quantities of fluid may cause hydronephrosis if urine is prevented from flowing past calculi. Straining urine for small stones is important but does not take priority over pain management.

CN: Management of care; CL: Analyze

23. **3.** The priority nursing goal for this client is to alleviate the pain, which can be excruciating. Prevention of urinary tract complications and alleviation of nausea are appropriate throughout the client's hospitalization, but relief of the severe pain is a priority. The client is at little risk for fluid and electrolyte imbalance.

CN: Physiological adaptation; CL: Analyze

24. **4.** A KUB radiographic examination ordinarily requires no preparation. It is usually done while the client lies supine and does not involve the use of radiopaque substances. It is not necessary for the client to withhold fluids; the client will not need to take a tranquilizer; an enema is not included in the preparation.

CN: Reduction of risk potential; CL: Apply

25. **2.** The pain associated with renal colic due to calculi is commonly referred to the groin and bladder in female clients and to the testicles in male clients. Nausea, vomiting, abdominal cramping, and diarrhea may also be present. Nephritis or urine retention is an unlikely cause of the referred pain. The type of pain described in this situation is unlikely to be caused by additional stone formation.

CN: Physiological adaptation; CL: Analyze

26. **2.** During episodes of renal colic, the pain is excruciating. It is necessary to administer opioid analgesics such as morphine to control the pain. Application of heat, encouraging high fluid intake, and limitation of activity are important interventions, but they will not relieve the renal colic pain.

CN: Reduction of risk potential; CL: Analyze

27. **2.** Intermittent pain that is less colicky indicates that the calculi may be moving along the urinary tract. Fluids should be encouraged to promote movement, and the urine should be strained to detect the passage of the stone. Hematuria is to be expected from the irritation of the stone. Analgesics should be administered when the client needs them, not routinely. Moist heat to the flank area is helpful when renal colic occurs, but it is less necessary as pain is lessened.

CN: Physiological adaptation; CL: Analyze

28. **3.** A client scheduled for an IVP should be assessed for allergies to iodine and shellfish. Clients with such allergies may be allergic to the IVP dye and be at risk for an anaphylactic reaction. Adequate fluid intake is important after the examination. Bladder spasms are not common during an IVP. Bowel preparation is important before an IVP to allow visualization of the ureters and bladder, but checking for allergies is most important.

CN: Reduction of risk potential; CL: Analyze

29. **2.** After an IVP, the nurse should encourage fluids to decrease the risk for renal complications caused by the contrast agent. There is no need to place the client on bed rest or administer a laxative. An IVP would not cause hematuria.

CN: Reduction of risk potential; CL: Analyze

30. **2.** The ureteral catheter should drain freely without bleeding at the site. The catheter is rarely irrigated, and any irrigation would be done by the health care provider (HCP). The catheter is never clamped. The client's total urine output (ureteral catheter plus voiding or indwelling urinary catheter output) should be at least 30 mL per hour.

CN: Reduction of risk potential; CL: Analyze

31. **1.** Ambulation stimulates peristalsis. A client with paralytic ileus is kept on nothing-by-mouth status until peristalsis returns. Carbonated beverages will increase gas and distention but will not stimulate peristalsis. A stool softener will not stimulate peristalsis. An IV fluid infusion is a routine postoperative prescription that does not have any effect on preventing paralytic ileus.

CN: Physiological adaptation; CL: Analyze

32. **2.** The decrease in urine output may reflect inadequate renal perfusion and should be reported immediately. Urine output of 30 mL per hour or greater is considered acceptable. A slight elevation in temperature is expected after surgery. Peristalsis returns gradually, usually on the second or third day after surgery. Bowel sounds will be absent until then. A small amount of serosanguineous drainage is to be expected.

CN: Physiological adaptation; CL: Analyze

33. **1.** A high daily fluid intake is essential for all clients who are at risk for calculi formation because it prevents urinary stasis and concentration, which can cause crystallization. Depending on the composition of the stone, the client also may be instructed to institute specific dietary measures aimed at preventing stone formation. Clients may need to limit purine, calcium, or oxalate. Urine may need to be either alkaline or acid. There is no need to strain urine.

CN: Basic care and comfort; CL: Analyze

34. **2.** Allopurinol is used to treat renal calculi composed of uric acid. Adverse effects of allopurinol include drowsiness, maculopapular rash, anemia, abdominal pain, nausea, vomiting, and bone marrow depression. Clients should be instructed to report rashes and unusual bleeding or bruising. Retinopathy, nasal congestion, and dizziness are not adverse effects of allopurinol.

CN: Pharmacological and parenteral therapies; CL: Analyze

35. **1, 2, 5.** Common adverse effects of allopurinol include gastrointestinal distress, such as anorexia, nausea, vomiting, and diarrhea. A rash is another potential adverse effect. A potentially life-threatening adverse effect is bone marrow depression. Constipation and flushed skin are not associated with this drug.

🔑 CN: Pharmacological and parenteral therapies; CL: Analyze

The Adult with Acute Kidney Injury (Acute Renal Failure)

36. 4. When the nurse is preparing a solution for a client with acute kidney injury receiving peritoneal dialysis, the solution should be warmed to body temperature in a warmer or with a heating pad; do not use the microwave. Cold dialysate increases discomfort. Assessment for a bruit and thrill is necessary with hemodialysis when the client has a fistula, graft, or shunt. An indwelling urinary catheter is not required for this procedure. The nurse should position the client in a supine or low Fowler position.

🔑 CN: Reduction of risk potential; CL: Analyze

37. 1, 2, 3, 4. When admitting a client with acute kidney injury (acute renal failure) the nurse should raise the head of the bed to promote ease of breathing. Respiratory manifestations of acute renal failure include shortness of breath, orthopnea, crackles, and the potential for pulmonary edema. Therefore, priority is placed on the facilitation of respiration. The nurse should assess the vital signs because the pulse and respirations will be elevated. Establishing a site for IV therapy will become important because fluids will be administered IV in addition to orally. The HCP will need to be contacted for further prescriptions; there is no need to contact the hemodialysis unit.

🔑 CN: Physiological adaptation; CL: Analyze

38. 1. Normal potassium levels range from 3.5 to 5.0 mEq/L (3.5 to 5.0 mmol/L). Hyperkalemia places the client at risk for serious cardiac arrhythmias and cardiac arrest. Therefore, the nurse should carefully monitor the client for cardiac arrhythmias and be prepared to treat cardiac arrest when caring for a client with hyperkalemia. Increased potassium levels do not result in pulmonary edema, circulatory collapse, or hemorrhage.

🔑 CN: Pharmacological and parenteral therapies; CL: Analyze

39. 1. Pulmonary edema can develop during the oliguric phase of acute renal failure because of decreased urine output and fluid retention. Metabolic acidosis develops because the kidneys cannot excrete hydrogen ions, and bicarbonate is used to buffer the hydrogen. Hypertension may develop as a result of fluid retention. Hyperkalemia develops as the kidneys lose the ability to excrete potassium.

🔑 CN: Physiological adaptation; CL: Analyze

40. 1. The unaffected arm should be used for blood pressure measurement. The external cannula must be handled carefully and protected from damage and disruption. In addition, a tourniquet or clamps should be kept at the bedside because dislodgment of the cannula would cause arterial hemorrhage. The arm with the cannula is not used for blood pressure measurement, intravenous therapy, or venipuncture. Patency is assessed by auscultating for bruits every shift. Heparin is not injected into the cannula to maintain patency. Because it is part of the general circulation, the cannula cannot be heparinized.

🔑 CN: Reduction of risk potential; CL: Analyze

41. 2. If disequilibrium syndrome occurs during dialysis, the most appropriate intervention is to slow the rate of dialysis. The syndrome is believed to result from too-rapid removal of urea and excess electrolytes from the blood; this causes transient cerebral edema, which produces the symptoms. Administration of oxygen and position changes do not affect the symptoms. It would not be appropriate to reassure the client that the symptoms are normal.

🔑 CN: Reduction of risk potential; CL: Analyze

42. 2, 5. Dialysis will clear metabolic waste products from the body and correct electrolyte imbalances, such as creatinine, potassium, and sodium level, and the client's lab values will be within normal range. Dialysis has no effect on hemoglobin levels because some red blood cells are injured during the procedure; dialysis aggravates a low hemoglobin concentration and may contribute to anemia.

🔑 CN: Reduction of risk potential; CL: Apply

43. 4. Signs and symptoms of an external access shunt infection include redness, tenderness, swelling, and drainage from around the shunt site. The absence of a bruit indicates closing of the shunt. Sluggish capillary refill time and coolness of the extremity indicate decreased blood flow to the extremity.

🔑 CN: Reduction of risk potential; CL: Analyze

44. 1. The kidneys have a remarkable ability to recover from serious insult. Recovery may take 3 to 12 months. The client should be taught how to recognize the signs and symptoms of decreasing renal function and to notify the health care provider if such problems occur. In a client who is recovering from acute renal failure, there is no need for renal transplantation or permanent hemodialysis. Chronic renal failure develops before end-stage renal failure.

🔑 CN: Physiological adaptation; CL: Apply

The Adult with Urinary Tract Infection

45. 3. Antibiotics have the maximum effect when the level of the medication in the blood is maintained, and the client should take the medication as soon as possible after missing a dose. Because nitrofurantoin is readily absorbed from the gastrointestinal tract and is primarily excreted in the urine, toxicity may develop by taking the dose too close to the time the next dose should be taken or doubling the dose. If possible, the client should not skip a dose if one dose is missed. It is not necessary to contact the HCP as the dosage does not need to be adjusted. The nurse can coach the client to set a timer or use a pill container with timed doses so that the client does not forget to take the medication.

🔑 CN: Pharmacological and parenteral therapies; CL: Analyze

46. 2, 3, 4. Catheter-associated urinary tract infection is the most frequent type of health care–acquired infection (HAI) and represents as much as 80% of HAIs in hospitals. The nurse should provide meticulous perineal care at least once a day, maintain a closed drainage system, and encourage the client to obtain an adequate fluid intake. It is not necessary to change the catheter daily. It is recommended that long-term use of an indwelling urinary catheter be evaluated carefully and other methods considered if the catheter will be in place longer than 2 weeks. It is not necessary to request a prescription for antibiotics as the client does not currently have an infection.

🔑 CN: Safety and infection control; CL: Analyze

47. 1. The client's urine specific gravity is elevated. Specific gravity is a reflection of the concentrating ability of the kidneys. This level indicates that the urine is concentrated. By increasing fluid intake, the urine will become more dilute. Antihypertensives do not make urine more concentrated unless there is a diuretic component within them. The nurse should not hold a dose of antihypertensive medication. Sodium tends to pull water with it; by restricting sodium, less water, not more, will be present. Bananas do not aid in the dilution of urine.

🔑 CN: Reduction of risk potential; CL: Analyze

48. 1. All urine for creatinine clearance determination must be saved in a container with no preservatives and refrigerated or kept on ice. The first urine voided at the beginning of the collection is discarded, not the last. A self-report of weight may not be accurate. It is not necessary to have an indwelling urinary catheter inserted for urine collection.

🔑 CN: Reduction of risk potential; CL: Apply

49. 141 mg

$$1.5\,mg \times 94.1 = 141.15 = 141\,mg$$

🔑 CN: Pharmacological and parenteral therapies; CL: Apply

50.

STEP 1

Nurses' Notes

Today: 1800
A 74-year-old client is admitted to the medical-surgical unit from the health care provider's office. The client is alert and oriented to person, place, and time. The client is experiencing the urge to void as well as dysuria, which the client states is getting worse. The client also voids frequently and reports having a headache. Vital signs are temperature (T) 99.6°F (37.5°C); heart rate (HR) 106 bpm; respiration rate (RR) 25 breaths/min; blood pressure (BP) 116/62 mm Hg; and oxygen saturation 98% per pulse oximetry on room air. The client's adult child is on the way to the hospital.

The client reports symptoms of urinary urgency, frequency, and dysuria, and these will require follow-up. The client also has a headache, which is concerning. The client's temperature, heart rate, and respiration rate are elevated, and the diastolic blood pressure may be low for this client and will require follow-up. The oxygen saturation is normal. The client is oriented to person, place, and time.

🔑 CJ: Case study; Step 1: Recognize cues; CL: Understand

51.

STEP 2

Client Finding	Urinary Tract Infection	Cerebrovascular Accident	Urosepsis
1. Urinary frequency	X		
2. Dysuria	X		X
3. Headache		X	
4. Altered mental status	X	X	X
5. Elevated heart rate		X	X
6. Fever	X		X

A client who may have a urinary tract infection may experience signs of urinary frequency, dysuria, elevated heart rate, altered mental status (in older adults), and a fever. If a urinary tract infection leads to urosepsis, clients may begin to experience urinary retention, dysuria, altered mental status, elevated heart rate, and fever. A client experiencing a cerebrovascular accident may experience a headache and altered mental status.

CJ: Case study; Step 2: Analyze cues; CL: Analyze

52.

STEP 3

The nurse is prioritizing the findings from the client's assessment. Based on the client's current clinical findings, the older adult client is at risk for developing **sepsis**. *To encourage early recognition, the nurse should review the client's* **vital signs**.

The nurse should recognize that the client is an older adult with a possible urinary tract infection, which may lead to urosepsis. The findings do not indicate the client is having a stroke or urinary infection. The nurse should prioritize early recognition by closely monitoring the client's vital signs, particularly an increasing heart rate and temperature. The oxygen saturation should not be affected at this point in the client's care.

CJ: Case study; Step 3: Prioritize hypothesis; CL: Analyze

53.

STEP 4

1, 5, 6. The nurse should verify that the health care provider intends for the client to have an in-and-out catheter as the client would need to have a Foley catheter to obtain an accurate assessment of urinary output due to the worsening condition related to urosepsis. Vancomycin should not be given via IV push, and an abdominal CT scan is not necessary at this time.

CJ: Case study; Step 4: Generate solutions; CL: Apply

54.

STEP 5

3, 4, 6. When placing a Foley catheter, it is essential to observe sterile technique to prevent infection. The nurse should take particular care to create a sterile field by placing the sterile fenestrated drape over the perineal area. The procedure should be performed using sterile gloves donned after obtaining equipment and positioning the client. The nurse should clean the labia minora with antiseptic-soaked swabs with downward strokes to avoid contamination from potential microbes. Although other steps also must be performed as a part of the procedure, they do not contribute to preventing infection.

CJ: Case study; Step 5: Take action; CL: Apply

55.

STEP 6

2, 3, 5, 6. The client understands that they should drink cranberry juice to maintain the pH of the urine and wipe from front to back after voiding or defecating. If the client continues to have frequency, they can use adult diapers, but they should inspect them every 2 hours and change as needed. The client should be aware of the need to urinate and get to the bathroom in time. The client should increase, not decrease, the intake of fluids to facilitate the flushing of bacteria. The client should also avoid caffeine; caffeine is a diuretic and will increase the need to void. The client should take showers because sitting in bathwater can allow bacteria to travel to the urethra easier.

CJ: Case study; Step 6: Evaluate outcomes; CL: Analysis

56. 4. As newlyweds, the client and their spouse need to develop a strong communication base. The nurse can facilitate communication by preparing and supporting the client. Given the situation, an interdisciplinary conference is inappropriate and would not promote intimacy for the client and their spouse. Insisting that the client talk with their spouse is not addressing their fears. Being present allows the nurse to facilitate the discussion of a difficult topic. Having the nurse speak first with the spouse alone shifts responsibility away from the couple.

CN: Psychosocial integrity; CL: Analyze

57. 2. Warm tub baths promote relaxation and help relieve urgency, discomfort, and spasm. Applying heat to the perineum is more helpful than cold because heat reduces inflammation. Although liberal fluid intake should be encouraged, caffeinated beverages, such as tea, coffee, and cola, can be irritating to the bladder and should be avoided. Voiding at least every 2 to 3 hours should be encouraged because it reduces urinary stasis.

CN: Basic care and comfort; CL: Evaluate

58. 2, 3, 5. The nurse should instruct the client to report signs of adverse reaction to the antibiotic or indications that the urinary tract infection is not clearing. Blood in the urine is not an expected outcome, a rash is an adverse response to the antibiotic, and an elevated temperature indicates a persistent infection. These signs should be reported to the HCP. Cloudy urine can be expected during the first few days of antibiotic treatment. Mild nausea is a side effect of antibiotic therapy, but it can be managed by eating small, frequent meals. Urinating every 3 to 4 hours or more is expected, particularly if the client is increasing the fluid intake as directed.

CN: Pharmacological and parenteral therapies; CL: Analyze

59. -/+ **2, 3.** Clients who are taking nitrofurantoin should be instructed to take the medication with meals and to increase their fluid intake to minimize gastrointestinal distress. The urine may become brown in color. Although this change is harmless, clients need to be prepared for this color change. The client should be instructed to take the full prescription and not to stop taking the drug because symptoms have subsided. The medication should not be taken with antacids as this may interfere with the drug's absorption.

CN: Pharmacological and parenteral therapies; CL: Analyze

60. **15 mL**

The following formula is used to calculate the correct dosage:

$$25\,mg / 5\,mL = 75\,mg / X\,mL$$
$$X = 15\,mL.$$

CN: Pharmacological and parenteral therapies; CL: Apply

61. 1. Stasis of urine in the bladder is one of the chief causes of bladder infection, and a client who voids infrequently is at greater risk for reinfection. A tub bath does not promote urinary tract infections as long as the client avoids harsh soaps and bubble baths. Scrupulous hygiene and liberal fluid intake (unless contraindicated) are excellent preventive measures, but the client also should be taught to void every 2 to 3 hours during the day. Drinking herbal tea or lifting weights are not risk factors for cystitis.

CN: Reduction of risk potential; CL: Analyze

62. 1. A woman can adopt several health-promotion measures to prevent the recurrence of cystitis, including avoiding too-tight pants, noncotton underpants, and irritating substances, such as bubble baths and vaginal soaps and sprays. Increasing citrus juice intake can be a bladder irritant. Regular douching is not recommended; it can alter the pH of the vagina, increasing the risk for infection.

CN: Health promotion and maintenance; CL: Analyze

63. 4. Instructions should be as specific as possible, and the nurse should avoid general statements such as "a lot." A specific goal is most useful. A mix of fluids will increase the likelihood of client compliance. It may not be sufficient to tell the client to drink twice as much as or 34 fl oz (1020 mL) more than they usually drink if their intake was inadequate to begin with.

CN: Basic care and comfort; CL: Apply

The Adult with Pyelonephritis

64. 1. Acute pyelonephritis usually begins with a bacterial infection of the lower urinary tract via the ascending urethral route; most infections are due to gram-negative bacilli, such as *Escherichia coli*, normally found in the gastrointestinal tract. Thorough perineal care using soap and warm water, and cleansing from front to back, decreases the likelihood that organisms will be introduced into the urinary tract and ascend upward toward the kidneys. Although preventing and treating all infections are appropriate actions, fungal infections from the feet and bacterial infections in the throat or skin are less likely to be immediate sources of infection, causing pyelonephritis.

CN: Health promotion and maintenance; CL: Analyze

65. 1. Pyelonephritis usually begins with colonization and infection of the lower urinary tract via the ascending urethral route, and the client should have an adequate intake of fluids to promote the flushing action of urination. Bubble baths and limiting fluid intake increase the risk for developing a urinary tract infection. Antibiotics should be used on a short-term basis because the risk for antibiotic resistance may lead to breakthrough infections with increasingly virulent pathogens.

CN: Health promotion and maintenance; CL: Analyze

66. 4. A client with a history of diabetes mellitus, urinary tract infections, or renal calculi is at increased risk for pyelonephritis. Others at high risk include pregnant women and people with structural alterations of the urinary tract. A history of hypertension may put the client at risk for kidney damage, but not kidney infection. Intake of large quantities of cranberry juice and a fluid intake of 68 oz (2000 mL) a day are not risk factors for pyelonephritis.

🗝 CN: Reduction of risk potential; CL: Analyze

67. 3. Antibiotics are usually prescribed for a 2- to 4-week period. A urine culture is needed to evaluate the effectiveness of antibiotic therapy. Urine must be examined microscopically to adequately determine the presence of bacteria; looking at the color of the urine or checking the odor is not sufficient. Symptoms usually disappear 48 to 72 hours after antibiotic therapy is started, but antibiotics may need to continue for up to 4 weeks.

🗝 CN: Pharmacological and parenteral therapies; CL: Evaluate

68. 0.4 mL

First, convert grams to milligram: 6 g = 6000 mg.

Next, set up a proportion:

$$6000 \text{ mg} / 2 \text{ mL} = 1200 \text{ mg} / X$$
$$X = (1200 / 6000) \times 2 \text{ mL}$$
$$X = 0.4 \text{ mL}.$$

🗝 CN: Pharmacologic and parenteral therapy; CL: Apply

69. 2. Chronic pyelonephritis is most commonly the result of recurrent urinary tract infections. Chronic pyelonephritis can lead to chronic renal failure. Single cases of acute pyelonephritis rarely cause chronic pyelonephritis. Acute renal failure is not a cause of chronic pyelonephritis. Glomerulonephritis is an immunologic disorder, not an infectious disorder.

🗝 CN: Physiological adaptation; CL: Apply

70. 4. The nurse should ensure the client has adequate hydration. A urinary catheter is discouraged because of the risk for urinary tract infection. Monitoring the hemoglobin level is not necessary for clients with pyelonephritis. Although antibiotics may be prescribed for long-term management and for chronic pyelonephritis, at this time, the nurse should focus on helping the client maintain hydration.

🗝 CN: Physiologic adaptation; CL: Analyze

The Adult with Chronic Renal Failure

71. -/+ **2, 3, 4.** The nurse instructs the client to protect the site of the fistula. The client should avoid pressure on the involved arm such as sleeping on it, wearing tight jewelry, or obtaining the BP. The client is also advised to assess the area distal to the fistula for adequate circulation, such as warmth and color. When the client is hospitalized, the nurse posts a sign on the client's bed not to draw blood or obtain BP on the left side; the client is also instructed to be sure that none of the health care team members do so.

🗝 CN: Physiological adaptation; CL: Analyze

72. 2, 4, 1, 3. The nurse first assures an IV access site in case the client has a respiratory or cardiac arrest. Next, the nurse monitors the client's heart rate and rhythm: Cardiovascular signs of elevated serum potassium levels are irregular, slow heart rate; decreased blood pressure; narrow, peaked T waves; widened QRS complexes, prolonged PR intervals, and flattened D waves; frequent ectopy; ventricular fibrillation; and ventricular standstill. The nurse then administers intravenous insulin and dextrose 50% in water (D50W), which have an immediate action to antagonize the effect of hyperkalemia on cardiac muscle. Last, the nurse obtains a blood sample to evaluate the effectiveness of the medication.

🗝 CN: Physiological adaptation; CL: Analyze

73. 2. The nurse must always auscultate for a bruit and palpate for a thrill in the arm with the fistula and promptly report the absence of either a thrill or bruit to the health care provider as it indicates an occlusion. The client should not have a pressure dressing on the shunt and should avoid wearing tight clothing or carrying heavy items such as a purse over the area of the shunt to avoid restricting blood flow in the shunt. No procedures such as IV access, blood pressure measurements, or blood draws are done on an arm with a fistula as they could damage the fistula.

🗝 CN: Physiological adaptation; CL: Analyze

74. -/+ **2, 4, 5.** To manage nausea, the nurse can advise the client to drink limited amounts of fluid only when thirsty and eat food before drinking fluids to alleviate dry mouth, and encourage strict follow-up for blood work, dialysis, and health care provider visits. Smaller, more frequent meals may help reduce nausea and facilitate medication-taking. The client should be as active as possible to avoid immobilization because it increases bone demineralization. The client should also maintain the dialysis schedule because the dialysis will remove wastes that can contribute to nausea.

🗝 CN: Physiological adaptation; CL: Analyze

75. 1. The main reason for warming the peritoneal dialysis solution is that the warm solution helps dilate peritoneal vessels, which increases urea clearance. Warmed dialyzing solution also contributes to client comfort by preventing chilly sensations, but this is a secondary reason for warming the solution. The warmed solution does not force potassium into the cells or promote abdominal muscle relaxation.

🗝️ CN: Reduction of risk potential; CL: Apply

76. 2. During dwell time, the dialysis solution is allowed to remain in the peritoneal cavity for the time prescribed by the health care provider (usually 20 to 45 minutes). During this time, the nurse should monitor the client's respiratory status because the pressure of the dialysis solution on the diaphragm can create respiratory distress. The dialysis solution would not cause urticaria or affect circulation to the fingers. The client's laboratory values are obtained before beginning treatment and are monitored every 4 to 8 hours during the treatment, not just during the dwell time.

🗝️ CN: Reduction of risk potential; CL: Analyze

77. 2. Because the client has a permanent catheter in place, blood-tinged drainage should not occur. Persistent blood-tinged drainage could indicate damage to the abdominal vessels, and the health care provider should be notified. The bleeding is originating in the peritoneal cavity, not the kidneys. Too-rapid infusion of the dialysate can cause pain, not blood-tinged drainage.

🗝️ CN: Reduction of risk potential; CL: Analyze

78. 4. Constipation may contribute to reduced urine outflow in part because peristalsis facilitates drainage outflow. For this reason, bisacodyl suppositories can be used prophylactically, even without a history of constipation. Diarrhea, vomiting, and flatulence typically do not cause decreased outflow in a peritoneal dialysis catheter.

🗝️ CN: Physiological integrity; CL: Analyze

79. 2. Because hypotension is a complication associated with peritoneal dialysis, the nurse records intake and output, monitors vital signs, and observes the client's behavior. The nurse also encourages visiting and other diversional activities. A client on peritoneal dialysis does not need to be placed in a bed with padded side rails or kept on NPO status.

🗝️ CN: Reduction of risk potential; CL: Analyze

80. ➕ **1, 2, 4, 5.** Broad-spectrum antibiotics may be administered to prevent infection when a peritoneal catheter is inserted for peritoneal dialysis. If peritonitis is present, antibiotics may be added to the dialysate. Aseptic technique is imperative. Peritonitis, the most common and serious complication of peritoneal dialysis, is characterized by cloudy dialysate drainage, diffuse abdominal pain, and rebound tenderness.

🗝️ CN: Safety and infection control; CL: Analyze

81. 2. Weight loss is expected because of the removal of fluid. The client's weight before and after dialysis is one measure of the effectiveness of treatment. Blood pressure usually decreases because of the removal of fluid. Hematuria would not occur after the completion of peritoneal dialysis. Dialysis only minimally affects the damaged kidneys' ability to manufacture urine.

🗝️ CN: Reduction of risk potential; CL: Evaluate

82. 3. A client in renal failure develops hyperphosphatemia that causes a corresponding excretion of the body's calcium stores, leading to renal osteodystrophy. To decrease this loss, aluminum hydroxide gel is prescribed to bind phosphates in the intestine and facilitate their excretion. Gastric hyperacidity is not necessarily a problem associated with chronic renal failure. Antacids will not prevent Curling stress ulcers and do not affect metabolic acidosis.

🗝️ CN: Pharmacological and parenteral therapies; CL: Evaluate

83. 4. Aluminum hydroxide gel is administered to bind the phosphates in ingested foods and must be given with or immediately after meals and snacks. There is no need for the client to take it on a 24-hour schedule. It is not administered to treat an upset stomach caused by hyperacidity in clients with chronic renal failure and therefore is not prescribed between meals.

🗝️ CN: Pharmacological and parenteral therapies; CL: Evaluate

84. 2. Uremia can cause decreased alertness, so the nurse needs to validate the client's comprehension frequently. Because the client's ability to concentrate is limited, short lessons are most effective. If family members are present at the sessions, they can reinforce the material. Written materials that the client can review are superior to videos because the client may not be able to maintain alertness during the viewing of the videotape.

🗝️ CN: Physiological adaptation; CL: Analyze

85. 3. Dietary management for clients with chronic renal failure is usually designed to restrict protein, sodium, and potassium intake. Protein intake is reduced because the kidney can no longer excrete the by-products of protein metabolism. The degree of dietary restriction depends on the degree of renal impairment. The client should also receive a high-carbohydrate diet along with appropriate vitamin and mineral supplements. Calcium requirements remain 1000 to 2000 mg a day.

CN: Basic care and comfort; CL: Analyze

86. 2. Altered sexual functioning commonly occurs in chronic renal failure and can stress marriages and relationships. Altered sexual functioning can be caused by decreased hormone levels, anemia, peripheral neuropathy, or medication. The client should not decrease or avoid sexual activity but instead should modify it. The client should rest before sexual activity. Unless the client provides additional information, it is not necessary to refer the client to counseling at this time.

CN: Psychosocial integrity; CL: Analyze

The Adult with Urinary Incontinence

87. 2, 3, 5. The nurse can teach the client that coffee and alcohol promote urination and should be eliminated from the diet. The client can perform perineal muscle exercises (Kegel exercises) to increase the tone of the urethral sphincters; the nurse teaches the client to perform the exercises in sets of at least 10 contractions, four to five times per day. The client also should avoid putting pressure on the bladder by jumping. Asking someone else to lift heavy loads may not always be practical. Applying estrogen cream to the urinary meatus after each intentional voiding can lead to urinary tract infections. Drug therapy has a very limited role in the management of stress urinary incontinence.

CN: Health promotion and maintenance; CL: Analyze

88. 2. The history of three pregnancies is most likely the cause of the client's current episodes of stress incontinence. The client's fluid intake, age, or history of swimming would not create an increase in intra-abdominal pressure.

CN: Reduction of risk potential; CL: Analyze

89. 4. The primary goal of nursing care is to decrease the number of incontinence episodes and the amount of urine expressed in an episode. Behavioral interventions (e.g., diet and exercise) and medications are the nonsurgical management methods used to treat stress incontinence. Without surgical intervention, it may not be possible to eliminate all episodes of incontinence. Helping the client adjust to incontinence is not treating the problem. Clients with stress incontinence are not prone to the development of urinary tract infections.

CN: Physiological adaptation; CL: Analyze

90. 3. A characteristic of urge incontinence is involuntary urination with little or no warning. The inability to empty the bladder is urine retention. Loss of urine when coughing occurs with stress incontinence. Frequent dribbling of urine is common in male clients after some types of prostate surgery or may occur in women after the development of a vesicovaginal or urethrovaginal fistula.

CN: Physiological adaptation; CL: Analyze

91. 1. Instructing the client to void at regularly scheduled intervals can help decrease the frequency of incontinence episodes. Providing a bedside commode does not decrease the number of incontinence episodes and does not help the client who leads an active lifestyle. Infections are not a common cause of urge incontinence, so antibiotics are not an appropriate treatment. Intermittent self-catheterization is appropriate for overflow or reflux incontinence but not urge incontinence because it does not treat the underlying cause.

CN: Physiological adaptation; CL: Analyze

Managing Care, Quality, and Safety of Adults with Urinary Tract Health Problems

92. 3. Cultural competence is necessary for all nurses to provide culturally appropriate care and meet the needs of a diverse client population. Allowing staff time to share individual culturally specific information provides the opportunity to learn from each other and form relationships. This strategy also facilitates nurse identification with personal cultural attributes. It is important to provide support to the nurses from different cultures. Assigning one nurse to each shift may undermine the initial goal and result in attrition. Restricting language to only English could decrease client satisfaction for those who also speak a similar language. Asking staff to invite new staff to after-work activities is not appropriate because not all staff may have time to participate in these activities and could result in decreased staff morale.

CN: Psychosocial integrity; CL: Analyze

93. 1. Clients who are immunosuppressed, have diabetes mellitus, or have undergone multiple courses of antibiotic therapy are prone to bacterial, fungal, and parasitic infections. Taking one course of antibiotic therapy or having a family history of UTIs does not place a client at high risk for the development of a CAUTI. A predisposing factor for a UTI is ongoing problems of urinary calculi; one calculus would not place a client at high risk.

CN: Management of care; CL: Analyze

94. 4. Sensitivity to shellfish or iodine may cause an anaphylactic reaction to the contrast material, which contains iodine. Administering a cathartic or antiflatulent will not prevent an anaphylactic reaction to the contrast material. Keeping a client on NPO status for 8 hours before the procedure is part of the usual preparation for such a procedure to prevent aspiration of food or fluids if the client vomits when lying on the x-ray table.

CN: Reduction of risk potential; CL: Analyze

95. 1. The appropriate action would be to discard the specimen and obtain a new one. Urine that is allowed to stand at room temperature will become alkaline, with multiplying bacteria. The specimen should be examined within 1 hour after urination.

CN: Reduction of risk potential; CL: Analyze

96. 1, 2, 3, 4, 6. Before prescribing and administering PRBCs, the nurse should assess the IV site to make sure it has an 18- to 20-gauge infusion set. The nurse should also ensure that normal saline solution is used to prime the tubing to prevent PRBCs from adhering to the tubing. The client must indicate informed consent for the procedure by signing the consent form. The client's blood must be typed to determine ABO blood typing and Rh factor and ensure that the client receives compatible blood. Cross-matching is done to detect the presence of recipient antibodies to the donor's minor antigens. Vital signs provide a baseline reference for continuous monitoring throughout the transfusion. An identification bracelet and red blood band are essential for client identification per facility policy. Two nurses must double-check the client's identification with the client listed on the unit of RBCs. The transfusion should be started within 30 minutes of the time that the PRBC unit is checked out of the blood bank. Thus, no blood should be kept in the medication room before transfusion.

CN: Safety and infection control; CL: Analyze

97. 3. The correct technique for a clean-catch urine culture specimen is to have the female client clean the labia from front to back, void into the toilet, and then void into the cup. The client does not need to fully empty their bladder into the cup. It is not necessary to catheterize the client to obtain the specimen. The first voided specimen of the day has the highest bacterial counts.

CN: Basic care and comfort; CL: Evaluate

98. 1, 2, 3, 4. The client is hyponatremic. When the nurse contacts the HCP, the nurse can recommend that the client be placed on fluid restrictions and that the vital signs should be taken every 2 hours. The nurse can request a bed alarm for the client's safety and a Foley catheter to prevent skin breakdown and facilitate accurate recording of intake and output. Restricting dietary sodium to 2 g may further exacerbate the hyponatremia. The nurse will also monitor for neurologic changes and inform the HCP immediately of any change or if the client becomes unable to take food/fluids by mouth.

CN: Management of care; CL: Analyze

99. 2, 3, 5, 6. While the scope of practice for a UAP may vary by state, province, or territory, as well as by place of employment, general duties include recording input and output, including emptying and recording urine output from a Foley catheter. A UAP with proper training may apply a securing device to maintain safety, provide regular Foley catheter and perineal care, and ambulate a client with a catheter, continually monitoring that the collection bag remains below the level of the bladder to help prevent infection. Activities such as irrigating or flushing a catheter should not be assigned to a UAP as these activities involve nursing assessment skills.

CN: Management of care; CL: Evaluate

100. 1, 3, 4. When IV therapy must be administered in the home setting, teaching is essential. Written instructions as well as demonstration and return demonstration help reinforce key points. The client or caregiver is responsible for adhering to the established plan of care that includes the treatment plan, monitoring plan, potential for complications, expected outcome/outcomes, potential adverse effects, and plan for communicating with the HCP. Periodic laboratory testing may be necessary to assess the effects of IV therapy and the client's progress. The client should report signs of redness or inflammation that could indicate infection and also report an elevated temperature. Before changing the fluids, the caregiver should cleanse the port with alcohol wipes. It is not necessary to use sterile gloves; the IV bag should be elevated to promote gravity flow.

CN: Reduction of risk potential; CL: Create

101. **1, 2, 3, 4.** To ensure client safety, the nurse should assess clients that might be at risk for suicide, such as those with end-stage cancer. The nurse should also communicate accurate medication information by explaining the importance of managing medication information to the client when they are discharged from the hospital or at the end of an outpatient encounter. Examples include instructing the client to give a list of medications to their HCP; to update the information when medications are discontinued, doses are changed, or new medications, including over-the-counter products, are added; and to carry medication information at all times in the event of emergency situations.

CN: Safety and infection control; CL: Application

TEST 10: The Adult with Reproductive Health Problems

- The Adult with a Vaginal Infection
- The Adult with Uterine Fibroids
- The Adult with Breast Cancer
- The Adult with Benign Prostatic Hypertrophy
- The Adult with a Sexually Transmitted Disease
- The Adult with Cancer of the Cervix
- The Adult with Cancer of the Ovaries
- The Adult with Testicular Disease
- The Adult with Cancer of the Prostate
- The Adult with Erectile Dysfunction
- Managing Care, Quality, and Safety of Adults with Reproductive Health Problems
- Answers, Rationales, and Test-Taking Strategies

The Adult with a Vaginal Infection

1. A young adult client tells the nurse they have a slightly yellow vaginal discharge. The nurse should tell the client to contact their health care provider (HCP) if they have which additional symptom(s)? Select all that apply.
   ☐ 1. vaginal discharge that has a fishy odor
   ☐ 2. starting their menstrual period
   ☐ 3. abdominal pain
   ☐ 4. a temperature above 101°F (38.3°C)
   ☐ 5. loss of appetite

2. A nurse is teaching a client how to prevent a vaginal infection. Which activity puts the client at risk for altering the normal pH of their vagina?
   ☐ 1. consuming over four cups of coffee per day
   ☐ 2. having sexual intercourse during the menstrual cycle
   ☐ 3. douching unless instructed to do so by the health care provider (HCP)
   ☐ 4. using tampons during the menstrual cycle

3. A client is prescribed oral metronidazole for the treatment of bacterial vaginosis. What should the nurse instruct the client to avoid during treatment and for 24 hours thereafter?
   ☐ 1. douching
   ☐ 2. sexual intercourse
   ☐ 3. hot tub baths
   ☐ 4. alcohol consumption

4. The nurse is obtaining a health history from an adult female client with vulvovaginal candidiasis. Which health problem(s) would put this client at risk for increased severity of the vulvovaginal candidiasis? Select all that apply.
   ☐ 1. uncontrolled diabetes
   ☐ 2. immunosuppression due to cancer
   ☐ 3. human immunodeficiency virus (HIV) infection
   ☐ 4. hypertension
   ☐ 5. asthma

5. A client taking oral contraceptives is placed on a 10-day course of antibiotics for an infection. Which instruction should the nurse include in the teaching plan?
   ☐ 1. "Use a barrier method of birth control for the rest of your cycle."
   ☐ 2. "You should stop taking the oral contraceptives while taking the antibiotic."
   ☐ 3. "Call your health care provider for increased hunger or fluid retention."
   ☐ 4. "Take the antibiotics 2 hours after the oral contraceptive."

6. A client is asking for information about using an intrauterine device (IUD). Which question when asked by the nurse would provide pertinent information on whether or not a client is a candidate for an IUD?
   ☐ 1. "Do you smoke?"
   ☐ 2. "Do you have hypertension?"
   ☐ 3. "How often do you have sex?"
   ☐ 4. "Are you in a monogamous relationship?"

The Adult with Uterine Fibroids

7. A 39-year-old female client has been experiencing intermittent vaginal bleeding for several months. The client's health care provider (HCP) tells the client that they have uterine fibroids and recommends an abdominal hysterectomy. When the client expresses fear about the surgery, what should the nurse do?
☐ 1. Reassure the client of their HCP's competence.
☐ 2. Give the client opportunities to express their fears.
☐ 3. Teach the client that fear impedes recovery.
☐ 4. Change the topic of conversation.

8. A female client with uterine fibroids has dysmenorrhea and menorrhagia. After reviewing the laboratory reports, the nurse should report which result(s) to the health care provider? Select all that apply.
☐ 1. hemoglobin, 9.0 g/dL (90 g/L)
☐ 2. hematocrit, 27.1% (0.27)
☐ 3. white blood cell count, 10,000 cells/mm³ (10 × 10⁹/L)
☐ 4. potassium, 4.0 mEq/L (4.0 mmol/L)
☐ 5. normocytic red blood cells

9. The client will have an abdominal hysterectomy tomorrow. Which information will be **most** important for the nurse to give to the client before admission to the hospital?
☐ 1. what to wear to the hospital
☐ 2. what they can eat and drink before admission
☐ 3. the type of pain medication that will be prescribed postoperatively
☐ 4. the amount of activity they can have after surgery

10. The nurse is witnessing a client's signature on the informed surgical consent for an abdominal hysterectomy. The nurse should be certain the client understands that what will be the outcome of this surgery?
☐ 1. decreased libido
☐ 2. infertility
☐ 3. depression
☐ 4. weight gain

11. The nurse is inserting a urinary catheter. Which is the correct order, from first to last, for proper placement of a urinary catheter? All options must be used.

| 1. Lubricate the catheter adequately with a water-soluble lubricant. |
| 2. Ensure free flow of urine. |
| 3. Insert the catheter far enough into the bladder to prevent trauma to the urethral tissue. |
| 4. Prepare a sterile field. |
| |
| |
| |
| |

12. After undergoing an abdominal hysterectomy, a client has gas pains. Which nursing action would **most** likely relieve the gas pains?
☐ 1. offering the client a hot beverage
☐ 2. providing extra warmth
☐ 3. applying a snugly fitting abdominal binder
☐ 4. helping the client walk

13. On the second postoperative day after an abdominal hysterectomy, a client develops a temperature of 100.4°F (38°C). What should the nurse do **first**?
☐ 1. Increase the number of wound dressing changes to minimize infection.
☐ 2. Obtain a culture and sensitivity study of the urine to determine the source of infection.
☐ 3. Ensure that the client takes at least 10 deep breaths every hour.
☐ 4. Change the site of the client's intravenous (IV) fluid catheter to reduce the risk for infection.

14. The nurse is changing the dressing of a client after an abdominal hysterectomy. If the dressing adheres to the client's incisional area, what should the nurse do?
☐ 1. Pull off the dressing quickly, and then apply slight pressure over the area.
☐ 2. Lift an easily moved portion of the dressing, and then remove it slowly.
☐ 3. Moisten the dressing with sterile normal saline solution, and then remove it.
☐ 4. Remove part of the dressing, and then remove the remainder gradually over several minutes.

15. A client with an abdominal hysterectomy is being prepared for discharge in the morning. The client has a special needs adult child who they care for at home. The nurse should discuss with the health care provider the need for a referral to which service?
☐ 1. home health care
☐ 2. social work
☐ 3. pastoral care
☐ 4. volunteer care

16. The nurse is developing a discharge plan with a client who has had an abdominal hysterectomy. Before implementing the plan, the nurse should perform which action **first**?
☐ 1. Have the client watch an educational video.
☐ 2. Assess the client's available social support system.
☐ 3. Call the social worker to evaluate the client.
☐ 4. Read the discharge instructions to the client.

17. A client who had a hysterectomy 2 hours ago is returning to the postsurgical unit from the recovery room. The nurse is assessing the client. The vital signs are temperature 99°F (37.2°C), pulse 98 bpm, respirations 20 breaths/min, and blood pressure 100/65 mm Hg. The urinary catheter is draining freely, and the client wants to try voiding without the catheter. The intravenous (IV) line is infusing at a keep-open rate. The perineal pad is saturated with bright red blood. The nurse reviews the progress notes from the recovery room (see notes).

Nurse's Notes		
Date	Time	Progress Notes
5/24	1145	Client ready for transfer to room. Vital signs T = 98.6°F (37°C), P = 78; R = 14, BP = 114/70, O₂ Sat of 95% per pulse oximetry; catheter to straight drainage; IV in left cephalic vein infusing at keep open rate; client awake and oriented ×3. Peri pad changed; moderately saturated.

What should the nurse do first?
☐ Change the perineal pad.
☐ Contact the surgeon.
☐ Increase the IV fluids.
☐ Remove the urinary catheter.

18. The nurse is preparing a client for discharge 2 days after an abdominal hysterectomy. The nurse should instruct the client to avoid which activity until recovery is complete?
☐ 1. swimming in a pool treated with chlorine for 6 weeks after surgery
☐ 2. walking at a leisurely pace for 30 minutes at least once a day
☐ 3. driving until the client can push the brake pedal without pain
☐ 4. lifting more than 2 lb (0.9 kg) until the abdominal incision has healed

19. A client who returned to the recovery room after a dilatation and curettage has the postoperative medication prescriptions shown in the medical record. What should the nurse do **next**?

Prescriptions
- Morphine sulfate 10 mg IM every 4 hours for severe pain
- Acetaminophen P.O. every 4 hours for pain
- Ibuprofen 800 mg P.O. every 4 hours for pain

☐ 1. Ask the client to rate the intensity of pain on a scale of 0 to 10, and administer the analgesia according to the intensity of the pain.
☐ 2. Administer the morphine first because the client had surgery today.
☐ 3. Administer the acetaminophen first, and if it does not relieve the pain in 2 hours, administer the morphine.
☐ 4. Administer the ibuprofen first, and if it does not relieve the pain, administer the morphine.

20. On the second day following an abdominal hysterectomy, a client reports they have had three brown, loose stools of a moderate amount. The morning medications include a prescription for 100 mg of docusate sodium daily or as needed. What should the nurse do **next**?
☐ 1. Administer the docusate sodium according to the prescription.
☐ 2. Ask the client if they are having gas pains or hunger.
☐ 3. Withhold the medication, and document the client's report of loose stools.
☐ 4. Administer the docusate sodium, and instruct the client to avoid high-fiber foods.

21. The nurse is teaching a 55-year-old woman who is just beginning menopause. Which information should the nurse include in the teaching plan? Select all that apply.
☐ 1. The average age of onset for menopause is 50 to 52 years.
☐ 2. Vaginal infections will increase.
☐ 3. Depression is very common as a result of menopause.
☐ 4. Hot flashes, especially at night, can occur in about 80% of women.
☐ 5. When periods become irregular, contraception is unnecessary.

The Adult with Breast Cancer

22. A nurse is palpating a female client's breast while assessing for breast disease. In which area of the breast are tumors **most** commonly found?

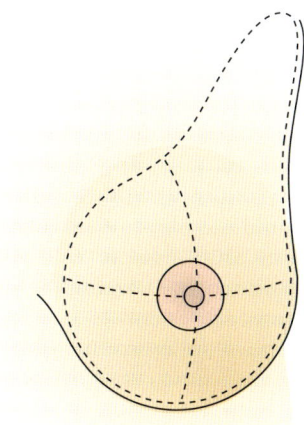

☐ 1. nipple
☐ 2. upper inner
☐ 3. upper outer
☐ 4. lower outer

23. A client states that they noticed their bra fits more snugly at certain times of the month. The client asks the nurse if this is a sign of breast disease. What should the nurse tell the client?
☐ 1. "Benign cysts tend to cause the breasts to vary in size."
☐ 2. "It's normal for the breasts to increase in size before menstruation begins."
☐ 3. "A change in breast size warrants further investigation."
☐ 4. "Differences in breast size are related to normal growth and development."

24. A 70-year-old client asks the nurse if they need to have a mammogram. Which is the nurse's **best** response?
☐ 1. "Having a mammogram when you are older is less painful."
☐ 2. "The incidence of breast cancer increases with age."
☐ 3. "We need to consider your family history of breast cancer first."
☐ 4. "It will be sufficient if you perform breast examinations monthly."

25. Before surgery for a modified radical mastectomy, a client is extremely anxious and asks many questions. Which approach offers the **best** guide for the nurse to answer these questions?
☐ 1. Tell the client as much as they want to know and can understand.
☐ 2. Postpone discussing the client's questions until they are convalescing.
☐ 3. Delay discussing the client's questions until their apprehension subsides.
☐ 4. Explain to the client that they should discuss their questions first with the health care provider.

26. Following a simple mastectomy, the nurse is totaling the amount of drainage in 24 hours from a suction drain in the incision. The nurse notes there is 200 mL of serosanguineous drainage for the first 24 hours. What should the nurse do?
☐ 1. Document the findings.
☐ 2. Notify the surgeon.
☐ 3. Remove the drain.
☐ 4. Place the client's arm in a dependent position.

27. The nurse is administering atropine sulfate to a client undergoing a modified radical mastectomy. What is the expected outcome of this drug?
☐ 1. Promote general muscular relaxation.
☐ 2. Decrease pulse and respiratory rates.
☐ 3. Decrease nausea.
☐ 4. Inhibit oral and respiratory secretions.

28. During the postoperative period after a modified radical mastectomy, the client confides in the nurse that they think they got breast cancer because they had an abortion and did not tell their spouse. What is the **best** response by the nurse?
☐ 1. "Cancer is not a punishment; it's a disease."
☐ 2. "You might feel better if you confided in your husband."
☐ 3. "Tell me more about your feelings about this."
☐ 4. "I can have the social worker talk to you if you would like."

29. The nurse is positioning a client following surgery for a right modified radical mastectomy with multiple lymph node excisions. The nurse should place the client's right arm in which position?
☐ 1. across the chest wall
☐ 2. at their side at the same level as their body
☐ 3. in the position that affords them the greatest comfort without placing pressure on the incision
☐ 4. on pillows, with their hand higher than their elbow and their elbow higher than their shoulder

30. A client develops lymphedema after a left mastectomy with lymph node dissection. The nurse should include which point(s) in the discharge teaching plan? Select all that apply.
☐ 1. Do not allow blood pressures or blood draws in the affected arm.
☐ 2. Avoid applying sunscreen on the left arm.
☐ 3. Use an electric razor for shaving.
☐ 4. Immobilize the left arm.
☐ 5. Elevate the left arm.
☐ 6. Perform hand pump exercises.

31. A client with breast cancer is prescribed tamoxifen 20 mg daily. The client states they do not like taking medicine and asks the nurse if the tamoxifen is worth taking. What should the nurse tell the client?
"This drug:
☐ 1. is part of your chemotherapy program."
☐ 2. has been found to decrease metastatic breast cancer."
☐ 3. will act as an estrogen in your breast tissue."
☐ 4. will prevent hot flashes since you cannot take hormone replacement."

32. A client undergoing chemotherapy after a modified radical mastectomy asks the nurse questions about a breast prosthesis and wigs. After answering the questions directly, the nurse should provide what additional information?
☐ 1. contact information for the breast cancer support group
☐ 2. a referral to the social worker
☐ 3. how to contact a home health care agency
☐ 4. when to contact a plastic surgeon

33. A client is to have radiation therapy after a modified radical mastectomy. What instruction should the nurse give the client about caring for the skin at the site of the radiation therapy?
☐ 1. Wash the area with water.
☐ 2. Expose the area to dry heat.
☐ 3. Apply an ointment to the area.
☐ 4. Use talcum powder on the area.

34. A client is to have radiation therapy following a mastectomy. What should the nurse tell the client to expect as a normal local tissue response to radiation?
☐ 1. atrophy of the skin
☐ 2. scattered pustule formation
☐ 3. redness of the surface tissue
☐ 4. sloughing of two layers of skin

35. The nurse is providing discharge instructions about preventing infection to a client who had a modified radical mastectomy and will be pruning flowers when they return to work. To prevent infection, what should the nurse instruct the client to do?
☐ 1. Wear protective gloves when gardening.
☐ 2. Avoid crowded areas.
☐ 3. Keep cuticles cut.
☐ 4. Remove underarm hair with a sharp razor.

36. **STEP 1**

The nurse is caring for a 53-year-old female client with breast cancer who is at the infusion center for cycle 3 of neoadjuvant chemotherapy.

> **Nurse's Notes**
>
> **1000:**
> At this visit to the infusion center, the client reports feeling tired and becoming short of breath when walking. The client reports bruises on their arms and bleeding from their gums. The client has been nauseated and does not feel like eating. The client's hair is beginning to fall out.
> Vital signs are temperature 99.9°F (37.3°C); pulse 78 bpm; respiration rate 18 breaths/min; and blood pressure 110/80 mm Hg.

➤ Which findings are most concerning? Answer choices have been underlined.

> **Nurse's Notes**
>
> **1000:**
> At this visit to the infusion center, the client reports feeling tired and becoming <u>short of breath</u> when walking. The client reports <u>bruises on their arms</u> and <u>bleeding from their gums</u>. The client has been <u>nauseated</u> and does not feel like eating. The client's <u>hair is beginning to fall out</u>.
> Vital signs are temperature <u>99.9°F (37.3°C)</u>; pulse 78 bpm; respiration rate 18 breaths/min; and blood pressure 110/80 mm Hg.

37. STEP 2

The nurse is caring for a 53-year-old female client with breast cancer who is at the infusion center for cycle 3 of neoadjuvant chemotherapy.

Nurse's Notes

1000:
At this visit to the infusion center, the client reports feeling tired and becoming short of breath when walking. The client reports bruises on their arms and bleeding from their gums. The client has been nauseated and does not feel like eating. The client's hair is beginning to fall out.

Vital signs are temperature 99.9°F (37.3°C); pulse 78 bpm; respiration rate 18 breaths/min; and blood pressure 110/80 mm Hg.

1015:
Laboratory results available.

Laboratory Results

Diagnostic	Finding	Normal Range	Date
Sodium	138 mEq/L (138 mmol/L)	Adults: 135–145 mEq/L (135–145 mmol/L)	September 15
Potassium	3.7 mEq/L (3.7 mmol/L)	Adults: 3.5–5.2 mEq/L (3.5–5.2 mmol/L)	September 15
Chlorine	100 mEq/L (100 mmol/L)	Adults: 96–106 mEq/L (96–106 mmol/L)	September 15
Blood urea nitrogen	20 mg/dL (7.1 mmol/L)	8–20 mg/dL (2.9–7.5 mmol/L)	September 15
Creatinine	0.9 mg/dL (68.6 μmol/L)	Women: 0.6–1.1 mg/dL (53–97 μmol/L)	September 15
White blood cell (WBC) count	4.0×10^3 cells/mm³ (4.0×10^9/L)	$4.5–10.5 \times 10^3$ cells/mm³ ($4.5–10.5 \times 10^9$/L)	September 15
Red blood cell count	3.6 million/μL (3.6×10^{12}/L)	Women: 3.6–5 million/μL ($3.6–5 \times 10^{12}$/L)	September 15
Hemoglobin	10.8 g/dL (108 g/L)	Women: 12–16 g/dL (120–160 g/L)	September 15
Hematocrit	32% (0.32 proportion of 1.0)	Women: 36%–48% (0.36–0.48 proportion of 1.0)	September 15
Platelet count	100,000/μL (100×10^9/L)	Adults: 140,000–400,000/μL ($140–400 \times 10^9$/L)	September 15

The nurse reviews the client's laboratory results.

➢ For each finding below, click to specify if the finding is consistent with the client's WBC count, platelet count, or hemoglobin. Each finding may support more than one lab value.

Finding	WBC Count	Platelet Count	Hemoglobin
Fatigue	☐	☐	☐
Bruising	☐	☐	☐
Exertional dyspnea	☐	☐	☐
Nausea	☐	☐	☐
Gingival bleeding	☐	☐	☐
Anorexia	☐	☐	☐
Alopecia	☐	☐	☐
Temperature of 99.9°F (37.3°C)	☐	☐	☐

38. STEP 3

The nurse is caring for a client with breast cancer who is at the infusion center for cycle 3 of neoadjuvant chemotherapy.

Nurse's Notes

1000:
At this visit to the infusion center, the client reports feeling tired and becoming short of breath when walking. The client reports bruises on their arms and bleeding from their gums. The client has been nauseated and does not feel like eating. The client's hair is beginning to fall out.

Vital signs are temperature 99.9°F (37.3°C); pulse 78 bpm; respiration rate 18 breaths/min; and blood pressure 110/80 mm Hg.

1015:
Laboratory results available.

1020:
The client notes, "My hair is beginning to fall out and I haven't been eating much because my mouth is so sore. I have lost 5 pounds." On inspection of the mouth, the client has 3 open lesions.

The right upper chest port site is without redness, swelling, or drainage. The port is accessed with a 21-gauge Huber needle. The port has good blood return and flushes easily.

Infusion prepared.

Laboratory Results

Diagnostic	Finding	Normal Range	Date
Sodium	138 mEq/L (138 mmol/L)	Adults: 135–145 mEq/L (135–145 mmol/L)	September 15
Potassium	3.7 mEq/L (3.7 mmol/L)	Adults: 3.5–5.2 mEq/L (3.5–5.2 mmol/L)	September 15
Chlorine	100 mEq/L (100 mmol/L)	Adults: 96–106 mEq/L (96–106 mmol/L)	September 15
Blood urea nitrogen	20 mg/dL (7.1 mmol/L)	8–20 mg/dL (2.9–7.5 mmol/L)	September 15
Creatinine	0.9 mg/dL (68.6 µmol/L)	Women: 0.6–1.1 mg/dL (53–97 µmol/L)	September 15
White blood cell (WBC) count	4.0×10^3 cells/mm^3 (4.0×10^9/L)	4.5–10.5×10^3 cells/mm^3 (4.5–10.5×10^9/L)	September 15
Red blood cell count	3.6 million/µL (3.6×10^{12}/L)	Women: 3.6–5 million/µL (3.6–5×10^{12}/L)	September 15
Hemoglobin	10.8 g/dL (108 g/L)	Women: 12–16 g/dL (120–160 g/L)	September 15
Hematocrit	32% (0.32 proportion of 1.0)	Women: 36%–48% (0.36–0.48 proportion of 1.0)	September 15
Platelet count	100,000/µL (100×10^9/L)	Adults: 140,000–400,000/µL (140–400×10^9/L)	September 15

➤ Complete the following sentence by choosing from the list of options.

The client is most likely concerned about [altered body image / sores in mouth / ineffective coping / severe anxiety]

as evidenced by the client's [weight loss. / feelings about hair loss. / negative past experiences with cancer.]

39. STEP 4

The nurse is caring for a client with breast cancer who is at the infusion center for cycle 3 of neoadjuvant chemotherapy.

Nurse's Notes

1000:
At this visit to the infusion center, the client reports feeling tired and becoming short of breath when walking. The client reports bruises on their arms and bleeding from their gums. The client has been nauseated and does not feel like eating. The client's hair is beginning to fall out.
Vital signs are temperature 99.9°F (37.3°C); pulse 78 bpm; respiration rate 18 breaths/min; and blood pressure 110/80 mm Hg.

1015:
Laboratory results available.

1020:
The client notes, "My hair is beginning to fall out and I haven't been eating much because my mouth is so sore. I have lost 5 pounds." On inspection of the mouth, the client has 3 open lesions.
　The right upper chest port site is without redness, swelling, or drainage. The port is accessed with a 21-gauge Huber needle. The port has good blood return and flushes easily.
　Infusion prepared.

Laboratory Results

Diagnostic	Finding	Normal Range	Date
Sodium	138 mEq/L (138 mmol/L)	Adults: 135–145 mEq/L (135–145 mmol/L)	September 15
Potassium	3.7 mEq/L (3.7 mmol/L)	Adults: 3.5–5.2 mEq/L (3.5–5.2 mmol/L)	September 15
Chlorine	100 mEq/L (100 mmol/L)	Adults: 96–106 mEq/L (96–106 mmol/L)	September 15
Blood urea nitrogen	20 mg/dL (7.1 mmol/L)	8–20 mg/dL (2.9–7.5 mmol/L)	September 15
Creatinine	0.9 mg/dL (68.6 μmol/L)	Women: 0.6–1.1 mg/dL (53–97 μmol/L)	September 15
White blood cell (WBC) count	4.0×10^3 cells/mm³ (4.0×10^9/L)	$4.5–10.5 \times 10^3$ cells/mm³ ($4.5–10.5 \times 10^9$/L)	September 15
Red blood cell count	3.6 million/μL (3.6×10^{12}/L)	Women: 3.6–5 million/μL ($3.6–5 \times 10^{12}$/L)	September 15
Hemoglobin	10.8 g/dL (108 g/L)	Women: 12–16 g/dL (120–160 g/L)	September 15
Hematocrit	32% (0.32 proportion of 1.0)	Women: 36%–48% (0.36–0.48 proportion of 1.0)	September 15
Platelet count	100,000/μL (100×10^9/L)	Adults: 140,000–400,000/μL ($140–400 \times 10^9$/L)	September 15

➤ The nurse is preparing to begin the infusion of the chemotherapeutic agents. Which nursing action(s) would be indicated? Select all that apply.

- ☐ 1. Calculate the drip rate to infuse the medications by gravity.
- ☐ 2. Administer corticosteroids after the infusions are complete.
- ☐ 3. Monitor the client for rash or flushing during the infusion.
- ☐ 4. Wear appropriate personal protective equipment.
- ☐ 5. Monitor the client's respiratory status.
- ☐ 6. Review the client's cholesterol and triglyceride levels.
- ☐ 7. Verify the five rights of medication administration with a second registered nurse (RN).
- ☐ 8. Administer the prescribed antiemetic before starting the infusion.

40. STEP 5

The nurse is caring for a client with breast cancer who is at the infusion center for cycle 3 of neoadjuvant chemotherapy.

Nurse's Notes

1000:
At this visit to the infusion center, the client reports feeling tired and becoming short of breath when walking. The client reports bruises on their arms and bleeding from their gums. The client has been nauseated and does not feel like eating. The client's hair is beginning to fall out.

Vital signs are temperature 99.9°F (37.3°C); pulse 78 bpm; respiration rate 18 breaths/min; and blood pressure 110/80 mm Hg.

1015:
Laboratory results available.

1020:
The client notes, "My hair is beginning to fall out and I haven't been eating much because my mouth is so sore. I have lost 5 pounds" On inspection of the mouth, the client has 3 open lesions. The right upper chest port site is without redness, swelling, or drainage.

The port is accessed with a 21-gauge Huber needle. The port has good blood return and flushes easily. Infusion prepared.

Laboratory Results

Diagnostic	Finding	Normal Range	Date
Sodium	138 mEq/L (138 mmol/L)	Adults: 135–145 mEq/L (135–145 mmol/L)	September 15
Potassium	3.7 mEq/L (3.7 mmol/L)	Adults: 3.5–5.2 mEq/L (3.5–5.2 mmol/L)	September 15
Chlorine	100 mEq/L (100 mmol/L)	Adults: 96–106 mEq/L (96–106 mmol/L)	September 15
Blood urea nitrogen	20 mg/dL (7.1 mmol/L)	8–20 mg/dL (2.9–7.5 mmol/L)	September 15
Creatinine	0.9 mg/dL (68.6 μmol/L)	Women: 0.6–1.1 mg/dL (53–97 μmol/L)	September 15
White blood cell (WBC) count	4.0×10^3 cells/mm³ (4.0×10^9/L)	$4.5–10.5 \times 10^3$ cells/mm³ ($4.5–10.5 \times 10^9$/L)	September 15
Red blood cell count	3.6 million/μL (3.6×10^{12}/L)	Women: 3.6–5 million/μL ($3.6–5 \times 10^{12}$/L)	September 15
Hemoglobin	10.8 g/dL (108 g/L)	Women: 12–16 g/dL (120–160 g/L)	September 15
Hematocrit	32% (0.32 proportion of 1.0)	Women: 36%–48% (0.36–0.48 proportion of 1.0)	September 15
Platelet count	100,000/μL (100×10^9/L)	Adults: 140,000–400,000/μL ($140–400 \times 10^9$/L)	September 15

The nurse implements a teaching plan in response to the client's reported sores in their mouth.

➢ For each nursing action, click to specify if the action is indicated or contraindicated.

Nursing Action	Indicated	Contraindicated
Assess the client's food and drink preferences	○	○
Recommend spicy or highly seasoned foods	○	○
Propose snack ideas that have a crunchy texture	○	○
Suggest protein sources such as eggs, cheese, or yogurt	○	○
Advise the client to use alcohol-based mouthwash	○	○
Remind the client to use a soft-bristled toothbrush	○	○
Encourage gentle oral care before and after meals	○	○

41. STEP 6

The nurse is caring for a client with breast cancer who is at the infusion center for cycle 3 of neoadjuvant chemotherapy.

Nurse's Notes

1000:
At this visit to the infusion center, the client reports feeling tired and becoming short of breath when walking. The client reports bruises on their arms and bleeding from their gums. The client has been nauseated and does not feel like eating. The client's hair is beginning to fall out.
Vital signs are temperature 99.9°F (37.3°C); pulse 78 bpm; respiration rate 18 breaths/min; and blood pressure 110/80 mm Hg.

1015:
Laboratory results available.

1020:
The client notes, "My hair is beginning to fall out and I haven't been eating much because my mouth is so sore. I have lost 5 pounds" On inspection of the mouth, the client has 3 open lesions. The right upper chest port site is without redness, swelling, or drainage. The port is accessed with a 21-gauge Huber needle. The port has good blood return and flushes easily. Infusion prepared.

Laboratory Results

Diagnostic	Finding	Normal Range	Date
Sodium	138 mEq/L (138 mmol/L)	Adults: 135–145 mEq/L (135–145 mmol/L)	September 15
Potassium	3.7 mEq/L (3.7 mmol/L)	Adults: 3.5–5.2 mEq/L (3.5–5.2 mmol/L)	September 15
Chlorine	100 mEq/L (100 mmol/L)	Adults: 96–106 mEq/L (96–106 mmol/L)	September 15
Blood urea nitrogen	20 mg/dL (7.1 mmol/L)	8–20 mg/dL (2.9–7.5 mmol/L)	September 15
Creatinine	0.9 mg/dL (68.6 µmol/L)	Women: 0.6–1.1 mg/dL (53–97 µmol/L)	September 15
White blood cell (WBC) count	4.0×10^3 cells/mm^3 (4.0×10^9/L)	$4.5–10.5 \times 10^3$ cells/mm^3 ($4.5–10.5 \times 10^9$/L)	September 15
Red blood cell count	3.6 million/µL (3.6×10^{12}/L)	Women: 3.6–5 million/µL ($3.6–5 \times 10^{12}$/L)	September 15
Hemoglobin	10.8 g/dL (108 g/L)	Women: 12–16 g/dL (120–160 g/L)	September 15
Hematocrit	32% (0.32 proportion of 1.0)	Women: 36%–48% (0.36–0.48 proportion of 1.0)	September 15
Platelet count	100,000/µL (100×10^9/L)	Adults: 140,000–400,000/µL ($140–400 \times 10^9$/L)	September 15

After reviewing current laboratory results and instructing the client about self-care during the chemotherapy infusion, the nurse evaluates the effectiveness of the teaching.

> Which client statement(s) would indicate the effectiveness of the teaching based on the laboratory results? Select all that apply.

- [ ] 1. "I will avoid crowds of people."
- [ ] 2. "I will eat cooked greens, enriched bread, beans, and lean meats."
- [ ] 3. "I will space out activities with periods of rest."
- [ ] 4. "I will take aspirin as needed for pain."
- [ ] 5. "I will stay 6 feet from housemates."
- [ ] 6. "I will go to the dentist to have my teeth cleaned next week."
- [ ] 7. "I will wash my hands often."
- [ ] 8. "I should get the MMR (measles-mumps-rubella) booster vaccine soon."

The Adult with Benign Prostatic Hypertrophy

42. An adult male client has been unable to void for the past 12 hours. What is the **best** method for the nurse to use when assessing for bladder distention in a male client?
☐ 1. Palpate for a rounded swelling above the pubis.
☐ 2. Percuss dullness in the lower left quadrant.
☐ 3. Determine rebound tenderness below the symphysis.
☐ 4. Inspect the urethral meatus for urine discharge.

43. The nurse is inserting a catheter for a client with a distended bladder following surgery for benign prostatic hypertrophy. The nurse should allow the urine to drain from the bladder slowly to prevent which complication?
☐ 1. renal failure
☐ 2. abdominal cramping
☐ 3. possible shock
☐ 4. atrophy of bladder musculature

44. The nurse has inserted an indwelling catheter in a male client. Which problem is prevented if the nurse tapes the catheter laterally to the thigh?
☐ 1. pressure at the penoscrotal angle
☐ 2. catheter kinking in the urethra
☐ 3. accidental catheter removal
☐ 4. obstructing urine flow when the client turns

45. The nurse is providing preoperative instructions to a client who is having a transurethral resection of the prostate (TURP). What should the nurse tell the client?
☐ 1. "You will have a central venous access inserted just before the procedure."
☐ 2. "Plan on being in the hospital anywhere from 5 to 7 days following the procedure."
☐ 3. "You will be taught care of the incision and suture line before your discharge home."
☐ 4. "Expect blood in your urine in the first couple of days following the procedure."

46. The nurse is teaching a client about continuous bladder irrigation (CBI) following prostate surgery. What should the nurse tell the client?
☐ 1. "The catheter is disconnected from the drainage tubing one time per shift to enable manual irrigation of the bladder."
☐ 2. "The purpose of the irrigation is to keep bladder drainage clear and to prevent the formation of blood clots in the bladder."
☐ 3. "The fluid drips into the bladder at a slow rate to prevent the effects of overhydration and hyponatremia."
☐ 4. "The catheter is clamped off approximately 4 hours after you return to the nursing unit."

47. The nurse is planning care for a client with a history of benign prostatic hypertrophy (BPH). What action(s) should the nurse plan to take? Select all that apply.
☐ 1. Provide privacy and time for the client to void.
☐ 2. Monitor intake and output.
☐ 3. Catheterize the client for postvoid residual urine.
☐ 4. Ask the client if they have urinary retention.
☐ 5. Test the urine for hematuria.

48. A client has prostatic hypertrophy. When conducting a focused assessment of the client's ability to urinate, the nurse should expect which finding?
☐ 1. voiding at less frequent intervals
☐ 2. difficulty starting the flow of urine
☐ 3. painful urination
☐ 4. increased force of the urine stream

49. A client is scheduled to undergo transurethral resection of the prostate. The procedure is to be done under spinal anesthesia. What should the nurse assess the client for after surgery?
☐ 1. seizures
☐ 2. cardiac arrest
☐ 3. renal shutdown
☐ 4. respiratory paralysis

50. A client with benign prostatic hypertrophy (BPH) is being treated with terazosin 2 mg at bedtime. What should the nurse tell the client to monitor regularly?
☐ 1. glucosuria glucose
☐ 2. restlessness
☐ 3. blood pressure
☐ 4. pulse

51. A client who had a transurethral resection of the prostate (TURP) has a three-way indwelling urinary catheter with continuous bladder irrigation. In which circumstance should the nurse increase the flow rate of the continuous bladder irrigation?
Increase it when drainage:
☐ 1. is continuous but slow.
☐ 2. appears cloudy and dark yellow.
☐ 3. becomes bright red.
☐ 4. of urine and irrigating solution stops.

52. A client is to receive belladonna and opium suppositories, as needed, postoperatively after transurethral resection of the prostate (TURP). The nurse should give the client these drugs when they demonstrate signs of which symptom?
☐ 1. a urinary tract infection
☐ 2. urine retention
☐ 3. frequent urination
☐ 4. pain from bladder spasms

53. An unlicensed assistive personnel (UAP) tells the nurse, "I think the client is confused. They keep telling me they have to void, but that's not possible because they have a catheter in place that is draining well." What should the nurse tell the UAP?
☐ 1. "The catheter is probably plugged. I will irrigate it."
☐ 2. "That is a common problem after prostate surgery. The client only imagines the urge to void."
☐ 3. "The urge to void is usually created by the large catheter, and they may be having some bladder spasms."
☐ 4. "I think the client may be somewhat confused."

54. A health care provider (HCP) has prescribed amoxicillin 100 mg orally (PO) two times a day. What should the nurse instruct the client to do? Select all that apply.
☐ 1. Drink 300 to 500 mL of fluids daily.
☐ 2. Void frequently, at least every 2 to 3 hours.
☐ 3. Take time to empty the bladder completely.
☐ 4. Take the last dose of the antibiotic for the day at bedtime.
☐ 5. Take the antibiotic with or without food.

55. The nurse is planning for home care with a client after transurethral resection of the prostate (TURP). What should the nurse tell the client about dribbling of urine after this surgery? Dribbling of urine:
☐ 1. can be a chronic problem.
☐ 2. can persist for several months.
☐ 3. is an abnormal sign that requires intervention.
☐ 4. is a sign of healing within the prostate.

56. A client is being discharged home 3 days after undergoing transurethral resection of the prostate (TURP). What should the nurse instruct the client to do? Select all that apply.
☐ 1. Drink at least 12 cups (about 1 L) of water per day.
☐ 2. Increase calorie intake by eating six small meals a day.
☐ 3. Report bright red bleeding to the health care provider.
☐ 4. Take deep breaths and cough every 2 hours.
☐ 5. Report a temperature over 99°F (37.2°C).

57. A client with benign prostatic hypertrophy has an elevated prostate-specific antigen (PSA) level. What should the nurse do **next**?
☐ 1. Instruct the client to request a colonoscopy before coming to conclusions about the PSA results.
☐ 2. Instruct the client that a urologist will monitor the PSA level biannually when elevated.
☐ 3. Determine if the prostatic palpation was done before or after the blood sample was drawn.
☐ 4. Ask the client if they emptied their bladder before the blood sample was obtained.

The Adult with a Sexually Transmitted Disease

58. The nurse is developing a teaching plan with a client diagnosed with genital herpes. What is the **most** important information for the nurse to include in the teaching plan?
☐ 1. Use condoms at all times during sexual intercourse.
☐ 2. A urologist should be seen only when lesions occur.
☐ 3. Oral sex is permissible without a barrier.
☐ 4. Determine if your partner has received a vaccine against herpes.

59. A sexually active client asks the nurse about using preexposure prophylaxis (PrEP) for HIV. The nurse should tell the client the drug, a combination of 300 mg tenofovir disoproxil fumarate and 200 mg emtricitabine (TDF/FTC) can be used for which group of people who are at risk for becoming infected with human immunodeficiency virus (HIV)?
☐ 1. anyone who is in an ongoing sexual relationship with an HIV-infected partner
☐ 2. people who do not use condoms when in a sexual relationship
☐ 3. persons with a sexually transmitted disease that is not being treated
☐ 4. anyone with a compromised immune system

60. A client who is in a sexual relationship with a partner who has human immunodeficiency virus (HIV) has a prescription for preexposure prophylaxis (PrEP) using a combination of 300 mg tenofovir disoproxil fumarate and 200 mg emtricitabine (TDF/FTC). What should the nurse instruct the client about taking this drug?
☐ 1. Renew your prescription every year.
☐ 2. Take the medication daily.
☐ 3. It is not necessary to use condoms when using the medication.
☐ 4. The drug is 100% effective.

61. A client with human immunodeficiency virus (HIV) infection is taking zidovudine (AZT). What is the expected outcome of AZT for this client?
☐ 1. Destroy the virus.
☐ 2. Enhance the body's antibody production.
☐ 3. Enable slow replication of the virus.
☐ 4. Neutralize toxins produced by the virus.

62. The nurse is teaching a 20-year-old client about the importance of being vaccinated for human papillomavirus (HPV). The nurse should emphasize that the client is at risk for which health problem?
☐ 1. sterility
☐ 2. cervical cancer
☐ 3. uterine fibroid tumors
☐ 4. irregular menses

63. The nurse is teaching a client about controlling the spread of human immunodeficiency virus (HIV). Which strategy is the **most** effective way to control the spread of HIV infection?
☐ 1. premarital serologic screening
☐ 2. prophylactic treatment of exposed people
☐ 3. laboratory screening of pregnant women
☐ 4. ongoing sex education about preventive behaviors

64. A male client with human immunodeficiency virus (HIV) infection becomes depressed and tells the nurse: "I have nothing worth living for now." Which statement would be the **best** response by the nurse?
☐ 1. "You're a young person and have a great deal to live for."
☐ 2. "You shouldn't be too depressed; we're close to finding a cure for acquired immunodeficiency syndrome (AIDS)."
☐ 3. "You're right; it's very depressing to have HIV."
☐ 4. "Tell me more about how you're feeling about being HIV positive."

65. The nurse is obtaining a health history from a client with a sexually transmitted disease. Which description from the client indicates the likelihood of syphilis?
"In my genital area I have:
☐ 1. tender pimples."
☐ 2. a wart."
☐ 3. a moist ulcer."
☐ 4. itching."

66. The nurse is interviewing a client with newly diagnosed syphilis. To prevent the spread of the disease, the nurse should focus the interview on which approach?
☐ 1. motivating the client to undergo treatment
☐ 2. obtaining a list of the client's sexual contacts
☐ 3. increasing the client's knowledge of the disease
☐ 4. reassuring the client that medical records are confidential

67. The health care provider has prescribed benzathine penicillin G, 2.4 million units intramuscularly (IM) to treat an adult with primary syphilis. In which muscle should the nurse administer the injection?
☐ 1. deltoid
☐ 2. ventrogluteal
☐ 3. quadriceps lateralis
☐ 4. dorsogluteal

68. An 18-year-old female client is to have a pelvic examination. Which response by the nurse would be **best** when the client says that they are nervous about the upcoming pelvic examination?
☐ 1. "Can you tell me more about how you're feeling?"
☐ 2. "You're not alone. Most clients feel uncomfortable about this examination."
☐ 3. "Don't worry about Dr. Smith. The provider is a specialist in female problems."
☐ 4. "We will do everything we can to avoid embarrassing you."

69. When educating a female client with gonorrhea, the nurse should emphasize which information? In women, gonorrhea:
☐ 1. is often marked by symptoms of dysuria or vaginal bleeding.
☐ 2. does not lead to serious complications.
☐ 3. can be treated but not cured.
☐ 4. may not cause symptoms until serious complications occur.

70. The nurse is planning an education program about the incidence of sexually transmitted diseases. Which age group has experienced the **greatest** rise in the incidence of sexually transmitted diseases (STDs) over the past two decades?
☐ 1. teenagers and young adults
☐ 2. people who have divorced and remarried
☐ 3. young married couples
☐ 4. single older adults

71. A sexually active male client has burning on urination and a milky discharge from the urethral meatus. What documentation should be included in the client's medical record? Select all that apply.
☐ 1. history of unprotected sex (sex without a condom)
☐ 2. length of time since symptoms presented
☐ 3. history of fever or chills
☐ 4. presence of any enlarged lymph nodes on examination
☐ 5. names and phone numbers of all sexual contacts
☐ 6. allergies to any medications

72. The health care provider (HCP) has prescribed 50 mg of doxycycline twice a day for a client who has been diagnosed with a chlamydial infection. The most cost-effective form of the medication is a 100-mg scored tablet. How should the nurse instruct the client to take this drug?
_____ tablet(s) each dose.

73. A female client with gonorrhea informs the nurse that they had sexual intercourse with their male partner and asks the nurse, "Would they have any symptoms?" The nurse can tell the client which symptoms of gonorrhea occur in men?
    ☐ 1. impotence
    ☐ 2. scrotal swelling
    ☐ 3. urine retention
    ☐ 4. dysuria

74. The nurse is assessing the mouth and oral cavity of a client with human immunodeficiency virus (HIV) infection. Opportunistic infections in clients with HIV initially present with which symptom?
    ☐ 1. herpes simplex virus (HSV) lesions on the lips
    ☐ 2. oral candidiasis
    ☐ 3. cytomegalovirus (CMV) infection
    ☐ 4. aphthae on the gingiva

75. The nurse is administering didanosine to a client with human immunodeficiency virus (HIV). Before administering this medication, the nurse should check which lab test result(s)? Select all that apply.
    ☐ 1. elevated serum creatinine
    ☐ 2. elevated blood urea nitrogen (BUN)
    ☐ 3. elevated aspartate aminotransferase (AST)
    ☐ 4. elevated alanine aminotransferase (ALT)
    ☐ 5. elevated serum amylase

76. The nurse is caring for a client from Southeast Asia who has human immunodeficiency virus (HIV)/ acquired immunodeficiency syndrome (AIDS). The client does not speak or comprehend the English language. What should the nurse do?
    ☐ 1. Contact the hospital's chaplain.
    ☐ 2. Do an internet search for the Joint United Nations Programme on HIV/AIDS.
    ☐ 3. Utilize language-appropriate interpreters.
    ☐ 4. Ask a family member to obtain informed consent.

The Adult with Cancer of the Cervix

77. The nurse is preparing a 45-year-old female client for a vaginal examination. The nurse should place the client in which position?
    ☐ 1. lateral recumbent position
    ☐ 2. lithotomy position
    ☐ 3. genupectoral position
    ☐ 4. dorsal recumbent position

78. The nurse is teaching a middle-age woman about risk factors for cervical cancer. Which is a likely risk factor for this client?
    ☐ 1. having frequent sex with one partner
    ☐ 2. observing a sedentary lifestyle
    ☐ 3. being overweight
    ☐ 4. having had a human papillomavirus infection

79. A woman tells the nurse, "There has been a lot of cancer in my family." The nurse should instruct the client to report which possible sign of cervical cancer?
    ☐ 1. pain
    ☐ 2. leg edema
    ☐ 3. urinary and rectal symptoms
    ☐ 4. light bleeding or watery vaginal discharge

80. A young woman will receive 6 months of chemotherapy for cervical cancer. They are a single parent of two young children and can no longer work. The nurse contacts a social worker to help plan continuing care. The client states, "I feel overwhelmed. How can the social worker help me?" Which response(s) by the nurse about the role of the social worker would be appropriate? Select all that apply.
    ☐ 1. "The social worker is a part of a multidisciplinary team that provides care for clients with cancer."
    ☐ 2. "The social worker can assist in locating resources and programs to assist you during your treatment."
    ☐ 3. "Based on your financial situation and need to care for your children, the social worker can help you identify needed resources at this time."
    ☐ 4. "Your entire family will be included in the treatment plan. Your needs and those of your children will be assessed and determined so that referrals can be made to appropriate resources."
    ☐ 5. "The social worker can authorize temporary funds to help you with childcare and pay your bills while you are sick."

81. The spouse of a client with cervical cancer says to the nurse, "The doctor told my spouse that their cancer is curable. Is the doctor just trying to make us feel better?" Which would be the nurse's **most** accurate response?
    ☐ 1. "When cervical cancer is detected early and treated aggressively, the cure rate is almost 100%."
    ☐ 2. "The 5-year survival rate is about 75%, which makes the odds pretty good."
    ☐ 3. "Saying a cancer is curable means that 50% of all women with the cancer survive at least 5 years."
    ☐ 4. "Cancers of the female reproductive tract tend to be slow growing and respond well to treatment."

82. A client with suspected cervical cancer had a colposcopy with conization. What information should the nurse give the client about their menstrual periods after this surgery?
☐ 1. Their period will return to normal after 6 months.
☐ 2. Their next two or three periods may be heavier and more prolonged than usual.
☐ 3. Their next two or three periods will be lighter than normal.
☐ 4. They may skip their next two periods.

83. A client with cervical cancer is undergoing internal radium implant therapy. A lead-lined container and a pair of long forceps have been placed in the client's hospital room. What should the nurse tell the client about how these will be used?
The forceps and container will be used for:
☐ 1. disposal of emesis or other bodily secretions.
☐ 2. handling of a dislodged radiation source.
☐ 3. disposal of the client's eating utensils.
☐ 4. storage of the radiation dose.

84. The mother of a client who has a radium implant asks why so many nurses are involved in their daughter's care. They state, "The doctor said I can be in the room for up to 2 hours each day, but the nurses say they are restricted to being here for 30 minutes." What should the nurse explain to the client?
Nurses:
☐ 1. touch the client, which increases their radiation exposure.
☐ 2. work with many clients and could carry infection to a client receiving radiation therapy if exposure is prolonged.
☐ 3. work with radiation on an ongoing basis, while visitors have infrequent exposure to radiation.
☐ 4. are at greater risk from the radiation because they are younger than the mother.

85. A client with human papillomavirus (HPV) infection is being treated by a colposcopy. The client asks the nurse if this procedure is really necessary. The nurse can tell the client that if the HPV infection is not treated which health problem is likely to occur?
☐ 1. infertility
☐ 2. cervical cancer
☐ 3. pelvic inflammatory disease
☐ 4. rectal cancer

86. The nurse is planning care for a client with cervical cancer who has an internal radium implant in place, Which action should be included in the nursing care plan?
☐ 1. Offer the bed pan every 2 hours.
☐ 2. Provide perineal care twice daily.
☐ 3. Check the position of the applicator hourly.
☐ 4. Offer a low-residue diet.

87. A client is being treated with internal radium implants. The nurse should assess the client for which adverse effect associated with radiation therapy to the cervix?
☐ 1. severe vaginal itching
☐ 2. confusion
☐ 3. high fever in the afternoon or evening
☐ 4. nausea and a foul vaginal discharge

The Adult with Cancer of the Ovaries

88. The nurse is teaching a client about ovarian cancer. Which information should the nurse include in the teaching plan? Select all that apply.
☐ 1. details about the prognosis
☐ 2. staging and grading of ovarian cancer
☐ 3. need for routine colonoscopy beginning at age 30
☐ 4. procedures for diagnosis if there is a pelvic mass
☐ 5. symptoms occurring early in the disease process

89. Interprofessional management of ovarian cancer includes which measure(s)? Select all that apply.
☐ 1. combination chemotherapy to cure the cancer
☐ 2. bilateral salpingo-oophorectomy to remove diseased organs
☐ 3. radiation therapy to eliminate all cancer cells
☐ 4. referral to social services for supportive care
☐ 5. nutrition therapy for parenteral lipids

90. A client with ovarian cancer asks the nurse, "What is the cause of this cancer?" Which is the **most** accurate response by the nurse?
☐ 1. Use of oral contraceptives increases the risk for ovarian cancer.
☐ 2. Women who have had at least two live births are protected from ovarian cancer.
☐ 3. There is less chance of developing ovarian cancer when one lives in an industrialized country.
☐ 4. The risk for developing ovarian cancer is related to environmental, endocrine, and genetic factors.

91. The nurse is planning a presentation about ovarian cancer to a group of women. Which topic should receive **priority** attention in the lesson plan?
☐ 1. Ovarian cancer signs and symptoms are often vague until late in development.
☐ 2. Ovarian cancer should be considered in any woman older than 30 years of age.
☐ 3. A rigid, boardlike abdomen is the most common sign.
☐ 4. Methods for early detection have made a dramatic reduction in the mortality rate of ovarian cancer.

The Adult with Testicular Disease

92. A 28-year-old client is diagnosed with acute epididymitis. What should the nurse assess the client for when conducting a focused assessment?
☐ 1. burning and pain during urination
☐ 2. severe tenderness and swelling in the scrotum
☐ 3. foul-smelling ejaculate
☐ 4. foul-smelling urine

93. A 30-year-old client is being treated for epididymitis. What information should the nurse include in the teaching plan about the likely cause of epididymitis?
☐ 1. virus
☐ 2. parasite
☐ 3. sexually transmitted infection
☐ 4. protozoon

94. The nurse is teaching a client about the best time to perform testicular self-examination. What should the nurse tell the client?
Perform testicular self-examination:
☐ 1. after intercourse.
☐ 2. at the end of the day.
☐ 3. after a warm bath or shower.
☐ 4. after exercise.

95. The nurse is assessing a client's testes. Which finding indicates the testes are normal?
☐ 1. soft
☐ 2. egg-shaped
☐ 3. spongy
☐ 4. lumpy

96. The nurse is obtaining a health history from a middle-age male client. Which is a risk factor for testicular cancer for this client?
☐ 1. undescended testes
☐ 2. sexual relations at an early age
☐ 3. seminal vesiculitis
☐ 4. epididymitis

97. A client with a testicular malignancy undergoes a radical orchiectomy. What should the nurse assess the client for during the **immediate** postoperative period?
☐ 1. bladder spasms
☐ 2. urine output
☐ 3. pain
☐ 4. nausea

98. A right orchiectomy is performed on a client with a testicular malignancy. The client expresses concerns regarding their sexuality. What information should the nurse give the client to address their concerns?
The client:
☐ 1. is not a candidate for sperm banking.
☐ 2. should retain normal sexual drive and function.
☐ 3. will be impotent.
☐ 4. will have a change in secondary sexual characteristics.

99. A client diagnosed with seminomatous testicular cancer expresses fear and questions the nurse about their prognosis. Which information should the nurse give the client about the prognosis for testicular cancer?
☐ 1. Testicular cancer can be cured.
☐ 2. Testicular cancer has a cure rate of 90% when diagnosed early.
☐ 3. Surgery is the treatment of choice for testicular cancer.
☐ 4. Testicular cancer has a 50% cure rate when diagnosed early.

The Adult with Cancer of the Prostate

100. The nurse is developing an educational program about prostate cancer. The nurse should provide information about which topic?
☐ 1. The prostate-specific antigen (PSA) test is reliable for detecting the presence of prostate cancer.
☐ 2. For all men, age 50 and older, the American Cancer Society and the Canadian Cancer Society recommend an annual rectal examination.
☐ 3. Men over 50 should have a colonoscopy.
☐ 4. Regular sexual activity promotes the health of the prostate gland, which prevents cancer.

101. The nurse is caring for a client who will have a bilateral orchiectomy. The client asks what is involved with this procedure. Which statement is the nurse's **most** appropriate response?
"The surgery:
☐ 1. removes the entire prostate gland, prostatic capsule, and seminal vesicles."
☐ 2. tends to cause urinary incontinence and impotence."
☐ 3. freezes prostate tissue, killing cells."
☐ 4. results in a reduction of the major circulating androgen, testosterone."

102. The nurse is teaching a client about prostate cancer. Which point(s) should be included in the instruction? Select all that apply.
☐ 1. Prostate cancer is usually multifocal and slow growing.
☐ 2. Most prostate cancers are adenocarcinoma.
☐ 3. The incidence of prostate cancer is higher in men of African descent, and the onset is earlier.
☐ 4. A prostate-specific antigen (PSA) lab test result higher than 4 ng/mg will require another test and further monitoring.
☐ 5. Cancer cells are detectable in the urine.

103. The nurse is developing a care plan for a client who is receiving hormone replacement for prostate cancer. Which action(s) should the nurse take? Select all that apply.
☐ 1. Inform the client that increased libido is expected with hormone therapy.
☐ 2. Reassure the client that erectile dysfunction will not occur as a consequence of hormone therapy.
☐ 3. Provide the client the opportunity to communicate concerns and needs.
☐ 4. Utilize communication strategies that enable the client to gain some feeling of control.
☐ 5. Suggest that an appointment be made to see a psychiatrist.

104. A client asks the nurse why a prostate-specific antigen (PSA) level is determined before a digital rectal examination. What should the nurse tell the client?
☐ 1. "It is easier for the client."
☐ 2. "A prostate examination can possibly decrease the PSA."
☐ 3. "A prostate examination can possibly increase the PSA."
☐ 4. "If the PSA is normal, the client will not have to undergo the rectal examination."

105. A client is undergoing a total prostatectomy for prostate cancer. The client asks questions about their sexual function. What should the nurse tell the client?
"Loss of the prostate gland means that you will:
☐ 1. be impotent."
☐ 2. be infertile and there will be no ejaculation."
☐ 3. have no loss of sexual function and drive."
☐ 4. have erectile capability immediately after surgery."

106. STEP 1

The nurse is caring for a 63-year-old male client with prostate cancer who had a robotic-assisted radical prostatectomy 12 hours ago.

Nurse's Notes

1900:
A 63-year-old client had a robotic-assisted radical prostatectomy this morning. The client has slept since arriving on the unit at 1500 but arouses when their name is called, is oriented to person and place, follows commands, and moves all extremities equally. The client has five 2½-cm (1-inch) abdominal incisions and one smaller one in the umbilicus. The client has one left abdominal drain attached to bulb suction with 20 mL of serosanguinous drainage. Adhesive closures are intact. Lung sounds are diminished in both bases, and bowel sounds are absent. Oxygen saturation is 91% on 3 L via nasal cannula. An 18Fr three-way urinary catheter is draining pink-tinged urine with very small clots. Intravenous (IV) fluids of 5% dextrose and 0.45% sodium chloride (D_5 0.45 NaCl) are infusing at 150 mL per hour in the left forearm. The client has consumed 100 mL of ice chips over the last 2 hours.

1915:
The client states, "I'm suddenly in terrible pain. It's at least a 9 out of 10. It's cramping so bad. It feels like my bladder is going to burst. It feels wet around that tube going into my bladder. I really need to pee right now."

The client is restless, agitated, and shifting in bed. The abdomen is distended, and there is bruising around the incisions. Pink-tinged urine is leaking from the catheter insertion site.

Vital Signs

Day of Surgery	1600	1915
Heart rate (HR)	80 bpm	104 bpm
Blood pressure (BP) systolic	122 mm Hg	162 mm Hg
BP diastolic	74 mm Hg	86 mm Hg
Respiratory rate	16 breaths/min	22 breaths/min
Oxygen saturation	96% on 4 L	92% on 3 L
Temperature	98.6°F (37°C)	99.9°F (37.7°C)
Pain rating on a 0-to-10 scale	2	9

➢ For each client finding below, click to specify if the finding is expected or unexpected.

Symptom	Expected	Unexpected
HR 104 bpm	○	○
Incisional discomfort rated as 2 on a 0-to-10 scale	○	○
Cramping pelvic pain rated as 9 on a 0-to-10 scale	○	○
Restless and agitated	○	○
Bruising around incisions	○	○
Abdominal distention	○	○
Temperature of 99.9°F (37.7°C)	○	○

107. STEP 2

The nurse is caring for a 63-year-old male client with prostate cancer who had a robotic-assisted radical prostatectomy 12 hours ago.

Nurse's Notes

1900:
A 63-year-old client had a robotic-assisted radical prostatectomy this morning. The client has slept since arriving on the unit at 1500 but arouses when their name is called, is oriented to person and place, follows commands, and moves all extremities equally. The client has five 2½-cm (1-inch) abdominal incisions and a smaller one in the umbilicus. The client has one left abdominal drain attached to bulb suction with 20 mL of serosanguinous drainage. Adhesive closures are intact. Lung sounds are diminished in both bases, and bowel sounds are absent. Oxygen saturation is 91% on 3 L via nasal cannula. An 18Fr three-way urinary catheter is draining pink-tinged urine with very small clots. Intravenous (IV) fluids of 5% dextrose and 0.45% sodium chloride (D_5 0.45 NaCl) are infusing at 150 mL per hour in the left forearm. The client has consumed 100 mL of ice chips over the last 2 hours.

1915:
The client states, "I'm suddenly in terrible pain. It's at least a 9 out of 10. It's cramping so bad. It feels like my bladder is going to burst. It feels wet around that tube going into my bladder. I really need to pee right now."

The client is restless, agitated, and shifting in bed. The abdomen is distended, and there is bruising around the incisions. Pink-tinged urine is leaking from the catheter insertion site.

Vital Signs

Day of Surgery	1600	1915
Heart rate (HR)	80 bpm	104 bpm
Blood pressure (BP) Systolic	122 mm Hg	162 mm Hg
BP diastolic	74 mm Hg	86 mm Hg
Respiratory rate	16 breaths/min	22 breaths/min
Oxygen saturation	96% on 4 L	92% on 3 L
Temperature	98.6°F (37°C)	99.9°F (37.7°C)
Pain rating on a 0-to-10 scale	2	9

Following surgery, the nurse is analyzing the client's findings.

➢ For each client finding below, click to specify if the finding is consistent with bladder spasm or atelectasis.

Finding	Bladder Spasm	Atelectasis
Diminished breath sounds	○	○
Cramping pelvic pain	○	○
Sense of urgency to urinate	○	○
Temperature of 99.9°F (37.7°C)	○	○
Urine leakage around the catheter	○	○
Oxygen saturation 92% per pulse oximetry on 2 L via nasal cannula	○	○

108. STEP 3

The nurse is caring for a 63-year-old male client with prostate cancer who had a robotic-assisted radical prostatectomy 12 hours ago.

Nurse's Notes

1900:
A 63-year-old client had a robotic-assisted radical prostatectomy this morning. The client has slept since arriving on the unit at 1500 but arouses when their name is called, is oriented to person and place, follows commands, and moves all extremities equally. The client has five 2½-cm (1-inch) abdominal incisions and a smaller one in the umbilicus. The client has one left abdominal drain attached to bulb suction with 20 mL of serosanguinous drainage. Adhesive closures are intact. Lung sounds are diminished in both bases, and bowel sounds are absent. Oxygen saturation is 91% on 3 L via nasal cannula. An 18Fr three-way urinary catheter is draining pink-tinged urine with very small clots. Intravenous (IV) fluids of 5% dextrose and 0.45% sodium chloride (D_5 0.45 NaCl) are infusing at 150 mL per hour in the left forearm. The client has consumed 100 mL of ice chips over the last 2 hours.

1915:
The client states, "I'm suddenly in terrible pain. It's at least a 9 out of 10. It's cramping so bad. It feels like my bladder is going to burst. It feels wet around that tube going into my bladder. I really need to pee right now."

The client is restless, agitated, and shifting in bed. The abdomen is distended, and there is bruising around the incisions. Pink-tinged urine is leaking from the catheter insertion site.

Vital Signs

Day of Surgery	1600	1915
Heart rate (HR)	80 bpm	104 bpm
Blood pressure (BP) systolic	122 mm Hg	162 mm Hg
BP diastolic	74 mm Hg	86 mm Hg
Respiratory rate	16 breaths/min	22 breaths/min
Oxygen saturation	96% on 4 L	92% on 3 L
Temperature	98.6°F (37°C)	99.9°F (37.7°C)
Pain rating on a 0-to-10 scale	2	9

➤ Which finding requires the **most** immediate nursing action? Complete the following sentence by choosing from the list of options.

The client's
- blood pressure
- pulse
- lung sounds
- urine output

warrants an assessment of the
- rate of the intravenous infusion.
- pupillary reaction to light.
- patency of the bladder catheter.
- strength of dorsalis pedis pulses.

109. STEP 4

The nurse is caring for a 63-year-old male client with prostate cancer who had a robotic-assisted radical prostatectomy 12 hours ago.

Nurse's Notes

1900:
A 63-year-old client had a robotic-assisted radical prostatectomy this morning. The client has slept since arriving on the unit at 1500 but arouses when their name is called, is oriented to person and place, follows commands, and moves all extremities equally. The client has five 2½-cm (1-inch) abdominal incisions and a smaller one in the umbilicus. The client has one left abdominal drain attached to bulb suction with 20 mL of serosanguineous drainage. Adhesive closures are intact. Lung sounds are diminished in both bases, and bowel sounds are absent. Oxygen saturation is 91% on 3 L via nasal cannula. An 18Fr three-way urinary catheter is draining pink-tinged urine with very small clots. Intravenous (IV) fluids of 5% dextrose and 0.45% sodium chloride (D_5 0.45 NaCl) are infusing at 150 mL per hour in the left forearm. The client has consumed 100 mL of ice chips over the last 2 hours.

1915:
The client states, "I'm suddenly in terrible pain. It's at least a 9 out of 10. It's cramping so bad. It feels like my bladder is going to burst. It feels wet around that tube going into my bladder. I really need to pee right now."

The client is restless, agitated, and shifting in bed. The abdomen is distended, and there is bruising around the incisions. Pink-tinged urine is leaking from the catheter insertion site.

Vital Signs

Day of Surgery	1600	1915
Heart rate (HR)	80 bpm	104 bpm
Blood pressure (BP) systolic	122 mm Hg	162 mm Hg
BP diastolic	74 mm Hg	86 mm Hg
Respiratory rate	16 breaths/min	22 breaths/min
Oxygen saturation	96% on 4 L	92% on 3 L
Temperature	98.6°F (37°C)	99.9°F (37.7°C)
Pain rating on a 0-to-10 scale	2	9

The nurse is developing a postoperative care plan.

➤ An unlicensed assistive personnel (UAP) is assigned to care for the client with the registered nurse (RN). Which element(s) of the care plan could the nurse delegate to the UAP? Select all that apply.

☐	1. Assist with position changes.
☐	2. Bathe as needed.
☐	3. Assess lung sounds.
☐	4. Take vital signs.
☐	5. Teach the client to use an incentive spirometer.
☐	6. Empty the catheter bag.
☐	7. Evaluate pain relief.

110. STEP 5

The nurse is caring for a client with prostate cancer who had a robotic-assisted radical prostatectomy 2 days ago.

Nurse's Notes

1900:
A 63-year-old client had a robotic-assisted radical prostatectomy this morning. The client has slept since arriving on the unit at 1500 but arouses when their name is called, is oriented to person and place, follows commands, and moves all extremities equally. The client has five 2½-cm (1-inch) abdominal incisions and a smaller one in the umbilicus. The client has one left abdominal drain attached to bulb suction with 20 mL of serosanguinous drainage. Adhesive closures are intact. Lung sounds are diminished in both bases, and bowel sounds are absent. Oxygen saturation is 91% on 3 L via nasal cannula. An 18Fr three-way urinary catheter is draining pink-tinged urine with very small clots. Intravenous (IV) fluids of 5% dextrose and 0.45% sodium chloride (D_5 0.45 NaCl) are infusing at 150 mL per hour in the left forearm. The client has consumed 100 mL of ice chips over the last 2 hours.

1915:
The client states, "I'm suddenly in terrible pain. It's at least a 9 out of 10. It's cramping so bad. It feels like my bladder is going to burst. It feels wet around that tube going into my bladder. I really need to pee right now." The client is restless, agitated, and shifting in bed. The abdomen is distended, and there is bruising around the incisions. Pink-tinged urine is leaking from the catheter insertion site.

Day 2, 0800:
A client underwent a robotic-assisted radical prostatectomy 2 days ago. The client is alert and oriented to person, place, and time. The client also follows commands and moves all extremities equally. The client has five 2½-cm (1-inch) abdominal incisions and a smaller one in the umbilicus. Adhesive closures are intact. Lung sounds are clear in both bases, and bowel sounds are normally active in all four quadrants. Oxygen saturation is 95% on room air. An 18Fr three-way urinary catheter is draining clear yellow urine with a few red flecks. A saline lock is present in the left forearm. The surgeon discontinued the Jackson-Pratt drain and wrote orders to discharge the client home with a catheter in place. The client will see the surgeon in 1 week to discontinue the catheter.

Vital Signs

Day of Surgery	1600	1915
Heart rate (HR)	80 bpm	104 bpm
Blood pressure (BP) systolic	122 mm Hg	162 mm Hg
BP diastolic	74 mm Hg	86 mm Hg
Respiratory rate	16 breaths/min	22 breaths/min
Oxygen saturation	96% on 4 L	92% on 3 L
Temperature	98.6°F (37°C)	99.9°F (37.7°C)
Pain rating on a 0-to-10 scale	2	9

The nurse is preparing a teaching plan for the client who will be going home with a catheter in place for 1 week.

➤ For each possible topic in a discharge teaching plan, click to specify if it is essential, nonessential, or inappropriate.

Possible Topic	Essential	Nonessential	Inappropriate
Demonstrate cleaning the urethral meatus	○	○	○
Illustrate how the catheter lumens differ			
Explain why the urine collection bag must be kept lower than the bladder	○	○	○
Emphasize why the catheter tubing should be secured to the ankle	○	○	○
Show the client how to change to a leg bag during the day	○	○	○
Explain the French sizing system for urinary catheters	○	○	○
Teach the client how to remove the catheter in 1 week	○	○	○

111. STEP 6

The nurse is caring for a client with prostate cancer who had a robotic-assisted radical prostatectomy 2 days ago and has orders to discharge to home with a catheter in place for 1 week.

Nurse's Notes

1900:
A 63-year-old client had a robotic-assisted radical prostatectomy this morning. The client has slept since arriving on the unit at 1500 but arouses when their name is called, is oriented to person and place, follows commands, and moves all extremities equally. The client has five 2½-cm (1-inch) abdominal incisions and a smaller one in the umbilicus. The client has one left abdominal drain attached to bulb suction with 20 mL of serosanguinous drainage. Adhesive closures are intact. Lung sounds are diminished in both bases, and bowel sounds are absent. Oxygen saturation is 91% on 3 L via nasal cannula. An 18Fr three-way urinary catheter is draining pink-tinged urine with very small clots. Intravenous (IV) fluids of 5% dextrose and 0.45% sodium chloride (D_5 0.45 NaCl) are infusing at 150 mL per hour in the left forearm. The client has consumed 100 mL of ice chips over the last 2 hours.

1915:
The client states, "I'm suddenly in terrible pain. It's at least a 9 out of 10. It's cramping so bad. It feels like my bladder is going to burst. It feels wet around that tube going into my bladder. I really need to pee right now."

The client is restless, agitated, and shifting in bed. The abdomen is distended, and there is bruising around the incisions. Pink-tinged urine is leaking from the catheter insertion site.

Day 2, 0800:
A client underwent a robotic-assisted radical prostatectomy 2 days ago. The client is alert and oriented to person, place, and time. The client also follows commands and moves all extremities equally. The client has five 2½-cm (1-inch) abdominal incisions and a smaller one in the umbilicus. Adhesive closures are intact. Lung sounds are clear in both bases, and bowel sounds are normally active in all four quadrants. Oxygen saturation is 95% on room air. An 18Fr three-way urinary catheter is draining clear yellow urine with a few red flecks. A saline lock is present in the left forearm. The surgeon discontinued the Jackson-Pratt drain and wrote orders to discharge the client home with a catheter in place. The client will see the surgeon in 1 week to discontinue the catheter.

0900:
The client also follows commands and moves all extremities equally. The client has five 2½-cm (1-inch) abdominal incisions and a smaller one in the umbilicus. Adhesive closures are intact. Lung sounds are clear in both bases, and bowel sounds are normally active in all four quadrants. Oxygen saturation is 95% on room air. An 18Fr three-way urinary catheter is draining clear yellow urine with a few red flecks. A saline lock is present in the left forearm. The surgeon discontinued the Jackson-Pratt drain and wrote orders to discharge the client home with a catheter in place. The client will see the surgeon in 1 week to discontinue the catheter.

Vital Signs

Day of Surgery	1600	1915
Heart rate (HR)	80 bpm	104 bpm
Blood pressure (BP) Systolic	122 mm Hg	162 mm Hg
BP diastolic	74 mm Hg	86 mm Hg
Respiratory rate	16 breaths/min	22 breaths/min
Oxygen saturation	96% on 4 L	92% on 3 L
Temperature	98.6°F (37°C)	99.9°F (37.7°C)
Pain rating on a 0-to-10 scale	2	9

➤ In response to the client's questions, the nurse has instructed the client about incontinence management. Which client statement(s) would indicate the nurse's teaching has been effective? Select all that apply.

- ☐ 1. "I should remember to urinate every 2 hours."
- ☐ 2. "I will remember to drink fluids before bedtime."
- ☐ 3. "I will tighten and relax my pelvic muscles 50 times daily after my catheter is out."
- ☐ 4. "I should limit fluids to about 2 cups (about ½ L) per day."
- ☐ 5. "I can use disposable undergarments or pads."
- ☐ 6. "I will set a goal of losing 20 lb (9.1 kg) this year."

---

112. A 65-year-old client has been told by the health care provider that their prostate cancer was graded at stage IIB. The client inquires if this means they are going to die soon. What is the **best** response by the nurse?
"Prostate cancer at this stage:
- ☐ 1. is very slow growing."
- ☐ 2. is very fast growing."
- ☐ 3. has spread to the bone."
- ☐ 4. is difficult to predict."

113. A client with prostate cancer is treated with a luteinizing hormone-releasing hormone agonist and antagonist goserelin. What symptom should the nurse instruct the client to expect while receiving this treatment?
- ☐ 1. tenderness of the scrotum
- ☐ 2. flushing
- ☐ 3. loss of pubic hair
- ☐ 4. decreased blood pressure

The Adult with Erectile Dysfunction

114. The client is taking sildenafil orally for erectile dysfunction. What instruction should the nurse give the client?
☐ 1. Sildenafil may be taken more than one time per day.
☐ 2. The health care provider (HCP) should be notified promptly if the client experiences sudden or diminished vision.
☐ 3. Sildenafil offers protection against some sexually transmitted diseases (STDs).
☐ 4. Sildenafil does not require sexual stimulation to work.

115. A male client reports having impotence. The nurse should teach the client that which medication is a contributing factor to impotence?
☐ 1. aspirin
☐ 2. antihypertensives
☐ 3. nonsteroidal antiinflammatory drugs
☐ 4. anticoagulants

116. A 65-year-old male client with erectile dysfunction (ED) asks the nurse, "Is all this just in my head? Am I crazy?" What should the nurse tell the client?
☐ 1. "ED is believed to be psychogenic in most cases."
☐ 2. "More than 50% of the cases are attributed to organic causes."
☐ 3. "Evaluation of nocturnal erections does not help differentiate psychogenic or organic causes."
☐ 4. "ED is an uncommon problem among men older than age 65."

117. The nurse is teaching a client with erectile dysfunction (ED) to alter their lifestyle. Which change should the nurse recommend?
☐ 1. avoiding alcohol
☐ 2. following a low-salt diet
☐ 3. stopping smoking
☐ 4. increasing attempts at sexual intercourse

Managing Care, Quality, and Safety of Adults with Reproductive Health Problems

118. The nurse is assigning tasks to the unlicensed assistive personnel (UAP) for a client with an abdominal hysterectomy on the first postoperative day. Which task **cannot** be delegated to the UAP?
☐ 1. taking vital signs
☐ 2. recording intake and output
☐ 3. giving perineal care
☐ 4. assessing the incision site

119. The nurse-manager on a gynecologic surgical unit is addressing reports from clients that they have to wait too long on the night shift for their pain medication. Which course of action should the nurse-manager take **first**?
☐ 1. Change the staffing schedule on nights to include a medication nurse.
☐ 2. Consult the nursing supervisor.
☐ 3. Consult the nurses on the evening shift about their evaluation of the night nurses regarding these reports from the clients.
☐ 4. Complete a quality improvement study with the night nurses to document the waiting times for pain medication and other data, including staffing and client acuity.

120. A nurse is reviewing the health care provider's (HCP's) admitting prescriptions for a postmenopausal woman scheduled for a dilatation and curettage. The nurse is unable to decipher the handwriting but thinks the medication prescription reads either *metoprolol* or *topiramate*. What should the nurse do **next**?
☐ 1. Ask the client if they have hypertension.
☐ 2. Ask the client if they have migraines.
☐ 3. Call the HCP to clarify the prescription.
☐ 4. Ask the pharmacist to interpret the prescription.

121. The unlicensed assistive personnel (UAP) reports to the nurse that the client with an abdominal hysterectomy who returned from the recovery room 1 hour earlier has saturated the blue pad with bright red blood. What should the nurse do?
☐ 1. Call the surgeon to report the bleeding.
☐ 2. Ask the UAP to obtain vital signs while the nurse calls the surgeon.
☐ 3. Ask the UAP to increase the flow of intravenous (IV) fluids to prevent shock.
☐ 4. Assess the client again in 15 minutes before the nurse takes any further action.

Answers, Rationales, and Test-Taking Strategies

The answers and rationales for each question follow below, along with keys (🔑) to the client need (CN) and cognitive level (CL) for each question. In addition, questions that measure clinical judgment will be coded (CJ). As you check your answers, use the **Content Mastery and Test-Taking Skill Self-Analysis** worksheet (tear-out worksheet in the back of the book) to identify the reason(s) for not answering the questions correctly. For additional information about test-taking skills and strategies for answering questions, refer to pages 12–51 in Part 1 of this book.

The Adult with a Vaginal Infection

1. **1, 3, 4.** The client's discharge may be a symptom of bacterial vaginosis, a clinical syndrome resulting from the replacement of the normal vaginal *Lactobacillus* species with the overgrowth of anaerobic bacteria that cause a cluster of symptoms. Often the discharge disappears, but the nurse should instruct the client to seek care from their HCP if the discharge has a fishy odor, there is abdominal pain, or the client has an elevated temperature. The client's menstrual cycles will continue as normal. A decreased appetite is not a sign of a vaginal infection.

   🔑 CN: Health promotion and maintenance; CL: Analyze

2. **3.** Douching may disrupt the normal flora of the vaginal lactobacilli and change the pH, which could result in overgrowth of other bacteria. Coffee, intercourse during menses, and tampons are not related to changes in vaginal pH or the incidence of bacterial vaginosis.

   🔑 CN: Health promotion and maintenance; CL: Apply

3. **4.** Metronidazole interacts with alcohol and can cause a serious disulfiram-type reaction, with severe, prolonged vomiting. The client should not douche unless following a medical prescription, but douching does not interact with metronidazole. Sexual intercourse and hot tub baths are not known to affect the incidence or treatment of bacterial vaginosis.

   🔑 CN: Pharmacological and parenteral therapies; CL: Analyze

4. **1, 2, 3.** Women with underlying medical conditions, such as uncontrolled diabetes and HIV infection or cancer-causing immunosuppression, correlate with an increasing severity of candidiasis. Hypertension and asthma are not related to immunosuppression or complicated candidiasis.

   🔑 CN: Health promotion and maintenance; CL: Analyze

5. **1.** Antibiotics may decrease the effectiveness of oral contraceptives. The client should be instructed to continue the contraceptives and use a barrier method as a backup method of birth control until the next menstrual cycle. The client should not stop taking their oral contraceptives, and there is no indication for or benefit to taking the antibiotic 2 hours after the contraceptive. There is no incidence of the adverse effects of increased hunger and fluid retention with the interaction of antibiotic therapy and oral contraceptives.

   🔑 CN: Pharmacological and parenteral therapies; CL: Create

6. **4.** Due to an increased risk for pelvic inflammatory disease, candidates for the IUD should be in a monogamous relationship. Smoking and hypertension are not contraindications for an IUD. The frequency of sexual relations will not affect IUD use.

   🔑 CN: Pharmacological and parenteral therapies; CL: Analyze

The Adult with Uterine Fibroids

7. **2.** The best approach for a client who is fearful about having surgery is to allow the client opportunities to express their fears. Open-ended questions should elicit the client's individual and specific fears. This then allows the nurse to provide clarification, information, and support and possibly to offer other resources. The other actions are not supportive and deny the client the opportunity to express their feelings.

   🔑 CN: Psychosocial adaptation; CL: Analyze

8. **1, 2.** A woman with uterine fibroids and dysmenorrhea is at risk for iron deficiency anemia. The hemoglobin and hematocrit indicate the likelihood that the fibroids causing heavy menstrual blood loss have resulted in anemia. A hemoglobin level of less than 12 g/dL (120 g/L) in women is considered low. The white blood cell count and potassium levels are within normal parameters, and normocytic red blood cells are normal.

   🔑 CN: Management of care; CL: Analyze

9. 2. It is a priority that the client knows they will not be able to eat or drink for 8 hours before admission. A client who consumes food and fluid before receiving a general anesthetic is at risk for aspiration, which can lead to aspiration pneumonia, respiratory arrest, and even death. The clothing they should wear to the hospital and the type of medication they will receive are important, but they are not the priority. Information on exercise and resumption of normal activities can be included in the discharge teaching.

🔑 CN: Reduction of risk potential; CL: Analyze

10. 2. The client needs to understand that with the removal of the uterus, they will no longer be able to bear children or have menstrual periods. The surgical procedure should not change the client's libido or sexual functioning. Research does not support the idea that hysterectomy contributes to depression or weight gain. Research demonstrates that women who have managed health problems for some time before the hysterectomy may actually have a more positive effect, with less worry about their health condition, contraception, or pregnancy.

🔑 CN: Management of care; CL: Apply

11. 4, 1, 3, 2. After gathering appropriate supplies, the nurse should prepare a sterile field. After lubricating the catheter adequately with a water-soluble lubricant to minimize trauma to the urethra, the nurse should insert the catheter far enough into the bladder so the retention balloon does not traumatize urethral tissues. Ensuring a free flow of urine prevents infection; improper drainage occurs when tubing is kinked or twisted.

🔑 CN: Management of care; CL: Apply

12. 4. The discomfort associated with gas pains is likely to be relieved when the client ambulates. The gas will be more easily expelled with exercise. The anesthesia, analgesics, and immobility have altered normal peristalsis. Peristalsis will be stimulated by exercise. Offering a hot beverage, providing extra warmth, and applying an abdominal binder are not recommended and could aggravate the discomfort of postoperative gas pains.

🔑 CN: Physiological adaptation; CL: Analyze

13. 3. An elevated temperature on the second postoperative day is suggestive of a respiratory tract infection. Respiratory infections most often occur during the first 48 hours after surgery. The nurse should encourage the client to take deep breaths frequently. The nurse should also monitor the client's vital signs and report significant changes to the surgeon. Signs of infection, if present in the wound or urinary tract, are likely to occur later in the postoperative period. There is no indication that the IV catheter is the source of infection.

🔑 CN: Physiological adaptation; CL: Analyze

14. 3. When a dressing sticks to a wound, it is best to moisten the dressing with sterile normal saline solution and then remove it carefully. Trying to remove a dry dressing is likely to irritate the skin and wound. This may contribute to tension or tearing along the suture line.

🔑 CN: Reduction of risk potential; CL: Apply

15. 2. The social worker will be able to coordinate respite care for the son and other community resources for this family. Home health care would provide care for the client, but respite care for the son is the priority need for this family. Pastoral care provides spiritual care. The volunteer department would not be responsible for the coordination of care at the client's home.

🔑 CN: Management of care; CL: Apply

16. 2. Assessment is the first step in planning client education. Assessing social support resources is a key aspect of discharge planning that begins when the client is admitted to the hospital. It is imperative to know what assistance and support the client has at home. Assessment includes obtaining data about any family or home responsibilities the client is concerned with during the recovery period. It is within the scope of nursing practice to provide discharge instructions. A social worker is not needed at this time. The nurse should assess the client's needs before determining whether using a video or reading instructions to the client is appropriate.

🔑 CN: Health promotion and maintenance; CL: Create

17. 2. The nurse's first action is to notify the surgeon as the amount of bleeding on the perineal pad is not normal. Excessive bleeding is also indicated by elevated heart rate and decreased blood pressure. Urinary catheters are not removed until the second or third postoperative day. The surgeon may prescribe an increase in the rate of IV fluids. The nurse changes the perineal pad and offers comfort measures once the client is stable.

🔑 CN: Physiological adaptation; CL: Analyze

18. 3. The client should be prepared for what to expect after surgery. The client should not drive until they can use the brake pedal without abdominal pain. The nurse should teach the client to avoid activities that may increase pelvic congestion, such as dancing or brisk walking, for several months, whereas activities, such as swimming and leisurely walking, may be both physically and mentally helpful. Heavy lifting should be avoided for 2 months, but the client can lift up to 10 lb (4.5 kg) as long as there is no tension on the abdomen or abdominal pain.

🗝 CN: Physiological adaptation; CL: Analyze

19. 1. The nurse must first assess the intensity of the client's pain before selecting the correct analgesia. A high score would necessitate administering morphine. If the intensity rating is low, an oral analgesic would be appropriate. If acetaminophen is given without assessing the intensity of the client's pain, the nurse must wait 4 hours before administering another analgesic.

🗝 CN: Pharmacological and parenteral therapies; CL: Analyze

20. 3. The nurse should withhold administering docusate sodium, a stool softener, and document that the woman has had loose stools. The nurse is responsible for assessing contraindications and adverse effects of medications, and administering the medication when the client already has loose stools is unsafe. The assessment should also include auscultation of bowel sounds and inquiry about gas pains, but the stool softener should still be withheld.

🗝 CN: Pharmacological and parenteral therapies; CL: Analyze

21. ➖➕ 1, 4. The average age of menopause is 50 to 52 years, although some variation exists. Vaginal infections do not necessarily increase during menopause. Hot flashes occur in about 80% of women; they can range from mild to very debilitating with disruption of sleep patterns. Depression is not usual during menopause; if symptoms of depression do occur, the nurse should refer the client to their health care provider. Contraception should be used until menses has ceased for a full year.

🗝 CN: Physiological adaptation; CL: Create

The Adult with Breast Cancer

22. 3. The upper outer quadrant is the area of the breast in which most breast tumors are found. This area should be palpated thoroughly. Although breast tumors can be found in any area of the breast, including the nipple, they are most often found in the upper outer quadrant.

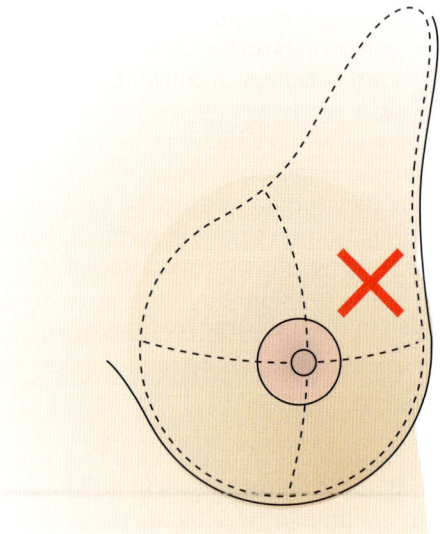

🗝 CN: Health promotion and maintenance; CL: Apply

23. 2. The breasts may vary in size before menstruation because of breast engorgement caused by hormonal changes. A client may then note that their bra fits more tightly than usual. Benign cysts do not cause variation in breast size. A change in breast size that does not follow hormonal changes could warrant further assessment. The breasts normally are about the same size, though some women have one breast slightly larger than the other.

🗝 CN: Health promotion and maintenance; CL: Apply

24. 2. The nurse should explain that the incidence of breast cancer increases with age and current guidelines recommend women have a mammogram every 2 years until age 74. While mammograms are less painful as breast tissue becomes softer, the nurse should advise the woman to have the mammogram. Family history is important, but only about 5% of breast cancers are genetic. Several breast cancer screening guidelines recommend against breast self-examinations for women.

🗝 CN: Health promotion and maintenance; CL: Analyze

25. 1. An important nursing responsibility is preoperative teaching, and the most frequently recommended guide for teaching is to tell the client as much as they want to know and can understand. Delaying discussion of issues about which the client has concerns is likely to aggravate the situation and cause the client to feel distrust. As a general guide, the client would not ask the question if they were not ready to discuss their

The Adult with Reproductive Health Problems 615

situation. The nurse is available to answer the client's questions and concerns and should not delay discussing these with the client.

 CN: Psychosocial adaptation; CL: Analyze

26. **1.** The nurse documents serosanguineous drainage of 100 to 200 mL because this is normal during the first 24 hours after surgery. The nurse notifies the surgeon only if there is excessive or very bloody drainage. The surgeon removes the drain within 24 to 48 hours. The client is instructed to keep their arm on the affected side and supported in an adducted position.

 CN: Physiological adaptation; CL: Analyze

27. **4.** Atropine sulfate, a cholinergic blocking agent, is given preoperatively to reduce secretions in the mouth and respiratory tract, which assists in maintaining the integrity of the respiratory system during general anesthesia. Atropine is not used to promote muscle relaxation, decrease nausea and vomiting, or decrease pulse and respiratory rates. It causes the pulse to increase.

 CN: Pharmacological and parenteral therapies; CL: Evaluate

28. **3.** The nurse should respond with an open-ended statement that elicits further exploration of the client's feelings. Women with cancer may feel guilt or shame. Previous life decisions, sexuality, and religious beliefs may influence a client's adjustment to a diagnosis of cancer. The nurse should not contradict the client's feelings of punishment or offer advice such as confiding in the husband. A social worker referral may be beneficial in the future, but it is not the first response needed to elicit exploration of the client's feelings.

 CN: Psychosocial adaptation; CL: Analyze

29. **4.** Lymph nodes can be removed from the axillary area when a modified radical mastectomy is done and each of the nodes is biopsied. To facilitate drainage from the arm on the affected side, the client's arm should be elevated on pillows with their hand higher than their elbow and their elbow higher than their shoulder. A sentinel node biopsy procedure is associated with a decreased risk for lymphedema because fewer nodes are excised.

 CN: Physiological adaptation; CL: Analyze

30. **1, 3, 5, 6.** Blood pressures or blood draws in the affected arm, sun exposure, trauma with a sharp razor, and immobilization increase the risk for lymphedema. Elevation of the arm and hand pump exercises promote lymph flow and reduce edema.

 CN: Health promotion and maintenance; CL: Create

31. **2.** Tamoxifen is an antiestrogen drug that is effective against metastatic breast cancer and can improve the survival rate. The drug causes hot flashes as an adverse effect.

 CN: Pharmacological and parenteral therapies; CL: Analyze

32. **1.** Giving the client a list of community resources that could provide support and guidance assists the client in maintaining their self-image and independence. The support group will include other clients who have undergone similar therapies and can offer suggestions for breast products and wigs. Because the client is asking about specific resources, they do not need a referral to a social worker, home health agency, or plastic surgeon.

 CN: Management of care; CL: Analyze

33. **1.** A client receiving radiation therapy should avoid lotions, ointments, and anything that may irritate the skin, such as exposure to sunlight, heat, or talcum powder. The area may safely be washed with water if it is done gently and care is taken not to injure the skin.

 CN: Reduction of risk potential; CL: Analyze

34. **3.** The most common reaction of the skin to radiation therapy is redness of the surface tissues. Dryness, tanning, and capillary dilation are also common. Atrophy of the skin, pustules, and sloughing of two layers would not be expected and should be reported to the radiologist.

 CN: Reduction of risk potential; CL: Apply

35. **1.** This client is at risk for lymphedema and infection. Precautions to avoid creating an entry site for infection in the affected arm include wearing protective gloves, using cuticle cream, not cutting cuticles, using an electric razor, using a thimble when sewing, and avoiding having injections or blood drawn from that arm. They do not need to avoid crowds; the client is not at high risk for respiratory infection.

 CN: Reduction of risk potential; CL: Analyze

36.

STEP 1

Nurse's Notes

At this visit to the infusion center, the client reports feeling tired and becoming short of breath when walking. The client reports bruises on their arms and bleeding from their gums. The client has been nauseated and does not feel like eating. The client's hair is beginning to fall out.
Vital signs are temperature 99.9°F (37.3°C); pulse 78 bpm; respiration rate 18 breaths/min; and blood pressure 110/80 mm Hg.

This is the client's third visit to the infusion center, and they are beginning to show side effects of the chemotherapy. It is concerning that the client is short of breath, has bruising on their arms and bleeding from their gums. Also of concern is that the client is nauseated and does not feel like eating and has a temperature. Other vital signs are within normal limits.

CJ: Case study; Step 1: Recognize cues; CL: Understand

37.

STEP 2

Finding	WBC Count	Platelet Count	Hemoglobin
1. Fatigue			X
2. Bruising		X	
3. Exertional dyspnea			X
4. Nausea			
5. Gingival bleeding		X	
6. Anorexia			
7. Alopecia			
8. Temperature of 99.9°F (37.3°C)	X		

The client has an elevated WBC count, which is why the client has an elevated temperature. The findings related to the platelet count include bruising and gingival bleeding; the findings related to the hemoglobin value include fatigue and exertional dyspnea. The findings from the laboratory report—nausea, anorexia, and alopecia—are not related to the complete blood count (CBC) results.

Myelosuppression is a common effect of chemotherapy. The CBC reveals leukopenia, thrombocytopenia, and anemia. The recent slight temperature elevation could be an indicator of an infection. Although it has resolved and did not exceed 101.4°F (38.6°C), the nurse should monitor clients receiving chemotherapy for the presence of a fever. Clients with leukopenia, especially neutropenia, can develop life-threatening infections and sepsis. The client may experience abnormal hemostasis due to the low platelet count, which puts the client at risk for prolonged bleeding from minor trauma. Fatigue and exertional dyspnea may occur because anemia decreases the oxygen-carrying capacity of the blood. Nausea and anorexia are likely not due to myelosuppression but may occur because the cells of the gastrointestinal tract are highly proliferative and sensitive to chemotherapy. The chemotherapeutic agents used in the client's protocol damage the hair follicles, which results in hair loss during treatment.

CJ: Case study; Step 2: Analyze cues; CL: Analyze

38.

STEP 3

0/1 The client is most concerned about **sores in the mouth** as evidenced by the client's **concern about weight loss.**

The chemotherapeutic regimen destroys mucous membranes and can cause open sores in the mouth. The client has difficulty eating and is losing weight. Although the client is beginning to experience hair loss, they do not express concerns about that or being unable to cope or being anxious. The nurse should be alert to cues about changes clients experience as they undergo chemotherapy.

CJ: Case study; Step 3: Prioritize hypothesis; CL: Analyze

39.

STEP 4

−/+ 3, 4, 5, 7, 8. Chemotherapeutic agents are high-risk medications; therefore, an infusion pump must be used, and two nurses should verify the correct medication, calculation method, dose, route, time, and client with at least two identifiers. In compliance with chemotherapy administration safety standards, the nurse should don personal protective equipment that is appropriate for use when handling hazardous drugs such as chemotherapy-tested gloves and gowns. The nurse should assess the client's respiratory status and the presence of a rash because hypersensitivity reactions can occur with chemotherapeutic agents. The lipid panel is not relevant in this situation. It is most important for the nurse to review the client's CBC and metabolic panel before starting the infusion. Corticosteroids and antiemetic medications should both be administered as prescribed before the infusion to prevent nausea and vomiting and hypersensitivity reactions.

CJ: Case study; Step 4: Generate solutions; CL: Create

40.

STEP 5

Nursing Action	Indicated	Contraindicated
1. Assess the client's food and drink preferences	X	
2. Recommend spicy or highly seasoned foods		X
3. Propose snack ideas that have a crunchy texture		X
4. Suggest protein sources such as eggs, cheese, or yogurt	X	
5. Advise the client to use an alcohol-based mouthwash		X
6. Remind the client to use a soft-bristled toothbrush	X	
7. Encourage gentle oral care before and after meals	X	

Because the client has several sores in their mouth, the nurse should consider nursing actions, such as assessing the client's food and drink preferences, suggesting increasing the protein in the diet, reminding the client to use a soft-bristled toothbrush, and encouraging oral care before and after meals. Nursing actions that are contraindicated include eating spicy or highly seasoned foods or foods with a crunchy texture and using an alcohol-based mouthwash.

Rapid cellular destruction by chemotherapeutic agents can cause inflammation or ulceration of the mucosa of the highly proliferative cells of the gastrointestinal mucosa. Assessing the client's preferences is an important first step in maintaining adequate nutrition to prevent dehydration and weight loss. Spicy, highly seasoned, or hard, crunchy foods can cause further irritation and discomfort with eating. Sources of protein that are smooth and bland in texture include foods such as eggs, cheese, cottage cheese, yogurt, and milkshakes. Alcohol-based mouthwashes can further dry irritated oral mucosa. The client should be encouraged to perform gentle oral care frequently with a soft-bristled toothbrush, saline rinses, or non–alcohol-based mouthwash to keep the mouth moist, clean, and free of debris.

🗝️ CJ: Case study; Step 5: Take action; CL: Apply

41.

STEP 6

–/+ **1, 2, 3, 7.** The CBC reveals leukopenia, thrombocytopenia, and anemia, and the client is experiencing mucositis and fatigue. The nurse should instruct the client about self-care to decrease the client's risk for infection, bleeding, and activity intolerance. Avoiding crowds and diligent handwashing will decrease the risk for infection; however, the client only needs to physically distance themself from family members who are febrile or who have been exposed to or have symptoms of an infection. Immunocompromised clients should not receive vaccines that contain live virus. Aspirin inhibits platelet cyclooxygenase, which can further increase bleeding risk. If possible, a dental cleaning should be performed before the client begins the first cycle of chemotherapy. Excessive bleeding could occur during a dental cleaning at this point in the client's treatment. The food selections listed are high in iron and protein, which are needed for red blood cell production. Alternating periods of activity and rest will help conserve the energy of the client with anemia.

🗝️ CJ: Case study; Step 6: Evaluate outcomes; CL: Evaluate

The Adult with Benign Prostatic Hypertrophy

42. 1. The best way to assess for a distended bladder in either a male or female client is to check for a rounded swelling above the pubis. This swelling represents the distended bladder rising above the pubis into the abdominal cavity. Dullness does not indicate a distended bladder. The client might experience tenderness or pressure above the symphysis. No urine discharge is expected; the urine flow is blocked by the enlarged prostate.

🗝️ CN: Reduction of risk potential; CL: Analyze

43. 3. Rapid emptying of an overdistended bladder may cause hypotension and shock due to the sudden change of pressure within the abdominal viscera. The nurse should empty the bladder slowly. Removal of urine from the bladder does not cause renal failure. The client may experience cramping, but the primary concern is the potential for shock. Bladder muscles will not atrophy because of catheterization.

🗝️ CN: Reduction of risk potential; CL: Apply

44. 1. The primary reason for taping an indwelling catheter to the lateral aspect of the thigh of a male client is so that the penis is held in a lateral position to prevent pressure at the penoscrotal angle. Prolonged pressure at the penoscrotal angle can cause a ureterocutaneous fistula. This position of the catheter does not prevent kinking in the urethra, accidental removal, or obstruction of the urine flow if the client turns.

🗝️ CN: Reduction of risk potential; CL: Apply

45. 4. TURP is a common surgical procedure used to treat male clients with benign prostate enlargement. The surgery commonly results in blood from the surgery in the urine for the first few days, and the client should not be concerned; the urine will become clear within 2 to 3 days. Central venous access is not expected for this type of surgery. Peripheral intravenous access can be expected. Clients are instructed to anticipate hospitalization for 1 to 3 days. Because the procedure is performed transurethrally (via the urethra), there is no outward incision.

🗝️ CN: Physiological adaptation; CL: Analyze

46. 2. CBI is performed when urinary surgery (typically prostate surgery) results in hematuria. It is accomplished using an indwelling Foley catheter with three lumens. One port is for the balloon, a second port allows irrigant inflow, and a third port enables outflow. The purpose of the irrigation is to achieve and maintain clear outflow and to prevent clot formation within the bladder. Manual irrigation is used as an intermittent type of bladder irrigation and is not the same as CBI. CBI involves irrigation of the bladder; it is not an intravascular infusion. The rate is often initially fast to achieve a clear outflow. Stopping and clamping the irrigant inflow is done only under a health care provider's direction and is typically not expected until at least 1 day after the procedure.

🗝️ CN: Physiological adaptation; CL: Analyze

47. –/+ **1, 2, 4, 5.** Because of the history of BPH, the nurse should provide privacy and time for the client to void. The nurse should also monitor intake and output, assess the client for urinary retention, and test the urine for hematuria. It is not necessary to catheterize the client.

🗝️ CN: Physiological adaptation; CL: Analyze

48. 2. Signs and symptoms of prostatic hypertrophy include difficulty starting the flow of urine, urinary frequency and hesitancy, decreased force of the urine stream, interruptions in the urine stream when voiding, and nocturia. The prostate gland surrounds the urethra, and these symptoms are all attributed to obstruction of the urethra resulting from prostatic hypertrophy. Nocturia from incomplete emptying of the bladder is common. Straining and urine retention are usually the symptoms that prompt the client to seek care. Painful urination is generally not a symptom of prostatic hypertrophy.

 CN: Physiological adaptation; CL: Analyze

49. 4. If paralysis of vasomotor nerves in the upper spinal cord occurs when spinal anesthesia is used, the client is likely to develop respiratory paralysis. Artificial ventilation is required until the effects of the anesthesia subside. Seizures, cardiac arrest, and renal shutdown are not likely results of spinal anesthesia.

 CN: Physiological adaptation; CL: Analyze

50. 3. Terazosin is an antihypertensive drug that is also used in the treatment of BPH. The client should monitor their blood pressure to ensure they do not develop hypotension, syncope, or orthostatic hypotension. The client should be instructed to change positions slowly. Terazosin does not cause glycosuria, restlessness, or changes in the heart rate.

 CN: Pharmacological and parenteral therapies; CL: Analyze

51. 3. The decision by the surgeon to insert a catheter after TURP or prostatectomy depends on the amount of bleeding that is expected after the procedure. During continuous bladder irrigation after a TURP or prostatectomy, the rate at which the solution enters the bladder should be increased when the drainage becomes brighter red. The color indicates the presence of blood. Increasing the flow of irrigating solution helps flush the catheter well so that clots do not plug it. There would be no reason to increase the flow rate when the return is continuous or when the return appears cloudy and dark yellow. Increasing the flow would be contraindicated when there is no return of urine and irrigating solution.

 CN: Pharmacological and parenteral therapies; CL: Analyze

52. 4. Belladonna and opium suppositories are prescribed and administered to reduce bladder spasms that cause pain after TURP. Bladder spasms frequently accompany urologic procedures. Antispasmodics offer relief by eliminating or reducing spasms. Antimicrobial drugs are used to treat an infection. Belladonna and opium do not relieve urine retention or urinary frequency.

 CN: Pharmacological and parenteral therapies; CL: Analyze

53. 3. The indwelling urinary catheter creates the urge to void and can also cause bladder spasms. The nurse should ensure adequate bladder emptying by monitoring urine output and characteristics. Urine output should be at least 30 to 50 mL per hour. A plugged catheter, imagining the urge to void, and confusion are less likely reasons for the client's problem.

 CN: Reduction of risk potential; CL: Analyze

54. 2, 3, 4, 5. Amoxicillin may be given with or without food, but the nurse should instruct the client to obtain an adequate fluid intake of 10½ to 12½ cups (2½ to 3 L) to promote urinary output and flush out bacteria from the urinary tract. The nurse should also encourage the client to void frequently (every 2 to 3 hours) and empty the bladder completely. Taking the antibiotic at bedtime, after emptying the bladder, helps ensure an adequate concentration of the drug during the overnight period.

 CN: Physiological adaptation; CL: Analyze

55. 2. Dribbling of urine can occur for several months after TURP. The client should be informed that this is expected and is not an abnormal sign. The nurse should teach the client perineal exercises to strengthen sphincter tone. The client may need to use pads for temporary incontinence. The client should be reassured that continence will return in a few months and will not be a chronic problem. Dribbling is not a sign of healing but is related to the trauma of surgery.

 CN: Basic care and comfort; CL: Analyze

56. 1, 3, 5. The nurse should instruct the client to drink a large amount of fluids (12 cups [about 1 L]) to keep the urine clear. The urine should be almost without color. About 2 weeks after TURP, when desiccated tissue is sloughed out, a secondary hemorrhage could occur. The client should be instructed to call the surgeon or go to the emergency department if at any time the urine turns bright red. The nurse should also instruct the client to report signs of infection such as a temperature over 99°F (37.2°C). The client is not specifically at risk for nutritional problems after TURP and can resume a diet as tolerated. The client is not specifically at risk for airway problems because the procedure is done under spinal anesthesia and the client does not need to take deep breaths and cough.

 CN: Physiological integrity; CL: Analyze

57. 3. Rectal and prostate examinations can increase serum PSA levels. The prostatic palpation should be done after the blood sample is drawn. The PSA level must be monitored more often than biannually when it is elevated. Having a colonoscopy is not related to the findings of the PSA test. It is not necessary to void before having PSA blood levels tested.

🗝️ CN: Health promotion and maintenance; CL: Analyze

The Adult with a Sexually Transmitted Disease

58. 1. The client should be taught to abstain from sexual intercourse while lesions are present. Condoms should be used at all times as the virus can be shed without lesions present. Multiple partners would promote the spread of genital herpes. There is no vaccine available to prevent genital herpes. Although periodic examinations should be advised, a urologist does not necessarily need to be seen when lesions occur.

🗝️ CN: Physiological adaptation; CL: Analyze

59. 1. PrEP is primarily available to anyone who is in an ongoing sexual relationship with an HIV-infected partner. Others at risk, such as those who are having sex with partners who are at risk for HIV such as drug users or who are themselves sharing equipment with people who are at risk for HIV, may also receive PrEP. The drug is not used for people who do not use condoms, have untreated sexually transmitted diseases, or have a compromised immune system.

🗝️ CN: Pharmacological and parenteral therapies; CL: Application

60. 2. It is imperative that the client take the medication daily; the client should also use condoms. The client should have HIV testing every 3 months, and prescriptions are written for renewal every 3 months. The drug is about 92% effective, but its effectiveness increases when condoms are used.

🗝️ CN: Pharmacological and parenteral therapies; CL: Application

61. 3. AZT interferes with the replication of HIV and thereby slows the progression of HIV infection to acquired immunodeficiency syndrome (AIDS). There is no known cure for HIV infection. Today, clients are not treated with monotherapy but are usually on triple therapy due to a much-improved clinical response. Decreased viral loads with the drug combinations have improved the longevity and quality of life in clients with HIV/AIDS. AZT does not destroy the virus, enhance the body's antibody production, or neutralize toxins produced by the virus.

🗝️ CN: Pharmacological and parenteral therapies; CL: Evaluate

62. 2. Women who have HPV are much more likely to develop cervical cancer than women who have never had the disease. Cervical cancer is now considered a sexually transmitted disease. Regular examinations, including Papanicolaou tests, are recommended to detect and treat cervical cancer at an early stage. Girls and women as well as boys and men (around ages 9 to 26 depending on the vaccine) should receive a vaccine to prevent HPV. HPV does not cause sterility, uterine fibroid tumors, or irregular menses.

🗝️ CN: Health promotion and maintenance; CL: Analyze

63. 4. Education to prevent behaviors that cause HIV transmission is the primary method of controlling HIV infection. Behaviors that place people at risk for HIV infection include unprotected sexual intercourse and sharing of needles for intravenous drug injection. Educating clients about using condoms during sexual relations is a priority in controlling HIV transmission.

🗝️ CN: Safety and infection control; CL: Apply

64. 4. The nurse should respond with a statement that allows the client to express their thoughts and feelings. After sharing feelings about their diagnosis, clients will need information, support, and community resources. Statements of encouragement or agreement do not provide an opportunity for the client to express themself.

🗝️ CN: Psychosocial adaptation; CL: Analyze

65. 3. The chancre of syphilis is characteristically a painless, moist ulcer. The serous discharge is very infectious. Because the chancre is usually painless and disappears, the client may not be aware of it or may not seek care. The chancre does not appear as pimples or warts and does not itch, thus making diagnosis difficult.

🗝️ CN: Physiological adaptation; CL: Analyze

66. 2. An important aspect of controlling the spread of sexually transmitted diseases (STDs) is obtaining a list of the sexual contacts of an infected client. These contacts, in turn, should be encouraged to obtain immediate care. Many people with STDs are reluctant to reveal their sexual contacts, which makes controlling STDs difficult. Increasing clients' knowledge of the disease and reassuring clients that their records are confidential can motivate them to seek treatment, which helps control the spread of the disease, but it is not as critical as information about the client's sexual contacts.

🗝️ CN: Health promotion and maintenance; CL: Analyze

67. 2. Because of the large dose, the upper ventrogluteal is the recommended site. The deltoid, dorsogluteal, and quadriceps lateralis muscles are not large enough for the recommended dose.

🗝️ CN: Pharmacological and parenteral therapies; CL: Apply

68. 1. Asking the client to describe their nervousness gives them the opportunity to express their concerns. It also allows the nurse to understand the client better and gives the nurse a base to respond to the client's stated fears, questions, or need for further information. Responses that make assumptions about the source of the concern or offer reinforcement are not supportive and block successful communication.

🗝️ CN: Psychosocial adaptation; CL: Analyze

69. 4. Many women do not seek treatment because they are unaware that they have gonorrhea. They may be symptom-free or have only very mild symptoms until the disease progresses to pelvic inflammatory disease. Dysuria and vaginal bleeding are not present in gonorrhea. Gonorrhea can lead to very serious complications. It can be cured with the proper treatment.

🗝️ CN: Physiological adaptation; CL: Analyze

70. 1. Statistics reveal that the incidence of STDs is rising more rapidly among people 15 to 24 (teenagers and young adults) than among any other age group. Many reasons have been given for this trend, including a change in societal mores and increasing sexual activity among teenagers. During this developmental stage, teenagers and young adults may engage in high-risk sexual behaviors because they often are living in the present and believe it will not happen to them.

🗝️ CN: Health promotion and maintenance; CL: Apply

71. ⊟ 1, 2, 3, 4, 6. The client is suspected of having a sexually transmitted infection. Therefore, the client's sexual history, assessment, and examination must be documented, including symptoms (such as fever, chills, and enlarged glands) and their onset and duration. Allergies are critical to document for every client but are especially noteworthy in this case because antibiotics will be prescribed. If a sexually transmitted infection is confirmed, sexual contacts need to be treated. To protect privacy, the names and phone numbers should never be placed in the medical record. The public health department will also assist in obtaining information and treating known sexual contacts.

🗝️ CN: Safety and infection control; CL: Analyze

72. one half tablet per dose. The nurse should instruct the client to cut the 100-mg tablet in two and take one half of a tablet for each of the two doses a day that the HCP has prescribed.

🗝️ CN: Pharmacological and parenteral therapies; CL: Apply

73. 4. Dysuria and a mucopurulent urethral discharge characterize gonorrhea in men. Gonococcal symptoms are so painful and bothersome for men that they usually seek treatment with the onset of symptoms. Impotence, scrotal swelling, and urine retention are not associated with gonorrhea.

🗝️ CN: Physiological adaptation; CL: Apply

74. 2. The most common opportunistic infection in HIV infection initially presents as oral candidiasis, or thrush. The client with HIV should always have an oral assessment. HSV and CMV are opportunistic infections that present later in acquired immunodeficiency syndrome. Aphthous stomatitis, or recurrent canker sores, is not an opportunistic infection, though the sores are thought to occur more often when the client is under stress.

🗝️ CN: Health promotion and maintenance; CL: Apply

75. ⊟ 3, 4, 5. The nurse should withhold the medication and notify the health care provider immediately if the client develops manifestations of pancreatitis or hepatic failure, including nausea and vomiting, severe abdominal pain, elevated bilirubin, or elevated serum enzymes (e.g., amylase, AST, ALT). If both BUN and creatinine are elevated, the client may have kidney disease.

🗝️ CN: Pharmacological and parenteral therapies; CL: Analyze

76. 3. Interpreters are essential in enabling the nurses' communications to be understood accurately. The chaplain may not know the client's language. The Joint United Nations Programme on HIV/AIDS has the number of reported cases of AIDS. It is not necessary for the family member to obtain informed consent.

🗝️ CN: Management of care; CL: Analyze

The Adult with Cancer of the Cervix

77. 2. Although other positions may be used, the preferred position for a vaginal examination is the lithotomy position. This position offers the best visualization. If the client is an older adult and frail, staff members may need to support the client's flexed legs while the examiner conducts the examination and performs the Papanicolaou test. Positioning the client in the other positions will make visualization more difficult and may not be as comfortable for the client.

 CN: Health promotion and maintenance; CL: Apply

78. 4. A primary cause of cervical cancer is a history of sexually transmitted disease, particularly human papillomavirus infection. Other risk factors include young age at first pregnancy, a family history of the disease, sexual experience with multiple partners, and having human immunodeficiency virus. Sexual relations with one partner, sedentary lifestyle, and obesity are not risk factors for cervical cancer.

 CN: Health promotion and maintenance; CL: Apply

79. 4. In its early stages, cancer of the cervix is usually asymptomatic, which underscores the importance of regular Papanicolaou tests. A light bleeding or serosanguineous discharge may be apparent as the first noticeable symptom. Pain, leg edema, urinary and rectal symptoms, and weight loss are late signs of cervical cancer.

 CN: Physiological adaptation; CL: Apply

80. 1, 2, 3, 4. The social worker is part of the comprehensive, holistic health care team. Because the client is now unemployed and is a single parent, the social worker can provide information about sources of financial support. The needs of the client and the family members are included in the treatment plan. The social worker cannot authorize temporary funds.

 CN: Management of care; CL: Apply

81. 1. When cervical cancer is detected early and treated aggressively, the cure rate approaches 100%. The incidence of cervical cancer has increased among women of African descent, Native American and Aboriginal women, and Latinas, and these women often have a poorer prognosis because the cancer is not identified early. Papanicolaou tests and colposcopy have the potential to decrease mortality from invasive carcinoma when these screening and treatment programs are utilized by women.

 CN: Physiological adaptation; CL: Analyze

82. 2. The client should be informed that their next two or three periods could be heavy and prolonged. The client is instructed to report any excessive bleeding. The nurse should reinforce the necessity for the follow-up check and the review of the biopsy results with the client. The client's periods will not be normal for 2 to 3 months.

 CN: Reduction of risk potential; CL: Analyze

83. 2. Dislodged radioactive materials should not be touched with bare or gloved hands. Forceps are used to place the material in the lead-lined container, which shields the radiation. Exposure to radiation can occur only by direct exposure to the encased radioactive substance; it cannot result from contact with emesis or urine or from touching the client. Disposal of eating utensils cannot lead to radiation exposure. Radioactive dose materials are kept only in the radiation department.

 CN: Safety and infection control; CL: Apply

84. 3. The three factors related to radiation safety are time, distance, and shielding. Nurses on radiation oncology units work with radiation frequently and so must limit their contact. Nurses are physically closer to clients than are visitors, who are often asked to sit 6 feet (182.9 cm) away from the client. Touching the client does not increase the amount of radiation exposure. Aseptic technique and isolation prevent the spread of infection. Age is a risk factor for people in their reproductive years.

 CN: Safety and infection control; CL: Apply

85. 2. HPV infection, or genital warts, can lead to dysplastic changes of the cervix, referred to as *cervical intraepithelial neoplasia*. The development of cervical cancer remains the largest threat of all condyloma-associated neoplasias. Infertility, pelvic inflammatory disease, and rectal cancer are not complications of genital warts.

 CN: Health promotion and maintenance; CL: Apply

86. 4. Bowel movements can be difficult with the radium applicator in place. The purpose of the low-residue diet is to decrease bowel movements. The bowel is cleaned before therapy, and the woman is maintained on a low-residue diet during treatment to prevent bowel distention and defecation. To prevent dislodgment of the applicator, the client is maintained on strict bed rest and allowed only to turn from side to side. Perineal care is omitted during radium implant therapy, though any vaginal discharge should be reported to the health care provider. It is rare for the applicator to extrude, so this does not need to be checked every hour.

 CN: Basic care and comfort; CL: Analyze

87. 4. Nausea, vomiting, and a foul vaginal discharge are common adverse effects of internal radiation therapy for cervical cancer. A foul-smelling discharge may develop from the destruction and sloughing of cells. Vaginal discharge may persist for some time. General signs and symptoms of radiation syndrome include nausea, vomiting, anorexia, and malaise. Vaginal itching, confusion, and high fever are not typical adverse effects of radiation therapy for cervical cancer.

CN: Safety and infection control; CL: Apply

The Adult with Cancer of the Ovaries

88. 2, 4. Client teaching emphasizes the importance of regular gynecologic examinations. If a pelvic mass is found, the nurse should completely explain the procedures for diagnosis, presurgical and postsurgical instructions, and the terminology particular to staging and grading of cancer, when appropriate. The nurse should refer all questions about the prognosis to the health care provider. Routine colonoscopies are typically begun at age 50 unless family history warrants otherwise. Ovarian tumors are commonly occult until symptoms of advanced disease are present.

CN: Health promotion and maintenance; CL: Create

89. 2, 4. Ovarian cancer is a malignant tumor of the ovary. Ovarian cancer is the fourth most common gynecologic cancer, and it is the most lethal. It is usually found in advanced stages because clients are often without symptoms in the early stages of the disease. Interdisciplinary management may involve chemotherapy, radiation therapy, surgery, and supportive services. Chemotherapy may be used to achieve remission of the disease; it is not, however, curative. Surgery is the treatment of choice, usually involving total hysterectomy with bilateral salpingo-oophorectomy and removal of the omentum. Radiation therapy may be performed for palliative purposes only. The nurse should provide a referral to home health services, financial assistance, psychological counseling, clergy, and other social services, as appropriate. Nutrition therapy for parenteral lipids is not part of the management of ovarian cancer.

CN: Management of care; CL: Create

90. 4. A definitive cause of carcinoma of the ovary is unknown, and the disease is multifactorial. The risk for developing ovarian cancer is related to environmental, endocrine, and genetic factors. The highest incidence is in industrialized Western countries. Endocrine risk factors for ovarian cancer include women who are nulliparous. The use of oral contraceptives does not increase the risk for developing ovarian cancer, and it may actually be protective.

CN: Health promotion and maintenance; CL: Apply

91. 1. Ovarian cancer is rarely diagnosed early. Methods for mass screening and early detection have not been successful. Signs and symptoms are often vague until late in development. Ovarian cancer should be considered in any woman older than 40 years of age who has vague abdominal or pelvic discomfort or enlargement, a sense of bloating, or flatulence. Enlargement of the abdomen due to the accumulation of fluid is the most common sign.

CN: Health promotion and maintenance; CL: Analyze

The Adult with Testicular Disease

92. 2. Epididymitis causes acute tenderness and pronounced swelling of the scrotum. Gradual onset of unilateral scrotal pain, urethral discharge, and fever are other key signs. Epididymitis is occasionally, but not routinely, associated with urinary tract infection. Burning and pain on urination and foul-smelling ejaculate or urine are not classic symptoms of epididymitis.

CN: Physiological adaptation; CL: Analyze

93. 3. Among men younger than age 35, epididymitis is most frequently caused by a sexually transmitted infection. Causative organisms are usually chlamydia or *Neisseria gonorrhoeae*. The other major form of epididymitis is bacterial, caused by the *Escherichia coli* or *Pseudomonas* organisms. The nurse should always include safe-sex teaching for a client with epididymitis. The client should also be advised against anogenital intercourse because this is a mode of transmission of gram-negative rods to the epididymis.

CN: Health promotion and maintenance; CL: Apply

94. 3. After a warm bath or shower, the testes hang lower and are both relaxed and in the ideal position for manual evaluation and palpation. The testes are not relaxed or in the best position after intercourse, at the end of the day, or after exercise.

CN: Health promotion and maintenance; CL: Apply

95. **2.** Normal testes feel smooth, egg-shaped, and firm to the touch, without lumps. The surface should feel smooth and rubbery. The testes should not be soft or spongy to the touch. Testicular malignancies are usually nontender, nonpainful hard lumps. Lumps, swelling, nodules, or signs of inflammation should be reported to the health care provider.

CN: Health promotion and maintenance; CL: Analyze

96. **1.** Cryptorchidism (undescended testes) carries a greatly increased risk for testicular cancer. Undescended testes occur in about 3% of male infants, with an increased incidence in premature infants. Other possible causes of malignancy include chemical carcinogens, trauma, orchitis, and environmental factors. Testicular cancer is not associated with early sexual relations in men, even though cervical cancer is associated with early sexual relations in women. Testicular cancer is not associated with seminal vesiculitis or epididymitis.

CN: Health promotion and maintenance; CL: Apply

97. **3.** Because of the location of the incision in the high inguinal area, pain is a major problem during the immediate postoperative period. The incisional area and discomfort caused by movement contribute to increased pain. Bladder spasms and elimination problems are more commonly associated with prostate surgery. Nausea is not a priority problem.

CN: Physiological adaptation; CL: Analyze

98. **2.** Unilateral orchiectomy alone does not result in impotence if the other testis is normal. The other testis should produce enough testosterone to maintain normal sexual drive, functioning, and characteristics. Sperm banking before treatment is commonly recommended because radiation or chemotherapy can affect fertility.

CN: Psychosocial adaptation; CL: Analyze

99. **2.** When diagnosed early and treated aggressively, testicular cancer has a cure rate of about 90%. Treatment of testicular cancer is based on tumor type, and seminoma cancer has the best prognosis. Modes of treatment include combinations of orchiectomy, radiation therapy, and chemotherapy. The chemotherapeutic regimen used currently is responsible for the successful treatment of testicular cancer. The nurse should not indicate to the client that the cancer will be cured, even though cure rates are high.

CN: Physiological adaptation; CL: Apply

The Adult with Cancer of the Prostate

100. **2.** Most cases of prostate cancer are adenocarcinomas. An adenocarcinoma is palpable on rectal examination because it arises from the posterior portion of the gland. Although the PSA is not a perfect screening test, the American Cancer Society and the Canadian Cancer Society recommend an annual rectal examination and blood PSA level for all men age 50 years and older, or starting at age 40 years if the client is of African descent, or if there is a family history of prostate cancer. A colonoscopy is performed to diagnose colon cancer, not prostate cancer. Regular sexual activity does not prevent cancer of the prostate.

CN: Health promotion and maintenance; CL: Analyze

101. **4.** Bilateral orchiectomy (removal of testes) results in a reduction of the major circulating androgen, testosterone, as a palliative measure to reduce symptoms and progression of prostate cancer. A radical prostatectomy (removal of the entire prostate gland, prostatic capsule, and seminal vesicles) may include pelvic lymphadenectomy. Complications include urinary incontinence, impotence, and rectal injury with the radical prostatectomy. Cryosurgery freezes prostate tissue, killing tumor cells without prostatectomy.

CN: Reduction of risk potential; CL: Apply

102. **1, 2, 3, 4.** Cancer of the prostate gland is the second leading cause of cancer death among American and Canadian men and is the most common carcinoma in men older than age 65. The incidence of prostate cancer is higher in men of African descent, and the onset is earlier. Most prostate cancers are adenocarcinoma. Prostate cancer is usually multifocal and slow growing and can spread by local extension, by lymphatics, or through the bloodstream. If the client has a PSA test result higher than 4 ng/mg, the health care provider will recommend a repeat test and further monitoring. Additional examinations may include a skeletal x-ray, a bone scan, and computed tomography or magnetic resonance imaging to detect local extension and bone and lymph node involvement. Urine does not have prostate cancer cells.

CN: Health promotion and maintenance; CL: Create

103. **3, 4.** Hormone manipulation deprives tumor cells of androgens or their by-products and, thereby, alleviates symptoms and retards disease progression. Complications of hormonal manipulation include hot flashes, nausea and vomiting, gynecomastia, and sexual dysfunction. As part of supportive care, the nurse should provide explanations of diagnostic tests and treatment options and help the client gain some feeling of control over their disease and decisions related to it. To help achieve optimal sexual function, the nurse should give the client the opportunity to communicate concerns and sexual needs. The nurse should also inform the client that decreased libido is expected after hormonal manipulation therapy and that impotence may result from some surgical procedures and radiation. A psychiatrist is not needed.

CN: Psychosocial adaptation; CL: Analyze

104. 3. Manipulation of the prostate during a digital rectal examination may falsely increase PSA levels. The PSA determination and the digital rectal examination are no longer recommended as screening tools for prostate cancer. Prostate cancer is the most common cancer in men and the second leading cause of death from cancer among men in the United States and Canada. Its incidence increases sharply with age, and the disease is predominant in men in their 60s and 70s.

CN: Health promotion and maintenance; CL: Apply

105. 2. Loss of the prostate gland interrupts the flow of semen, so there will be no ejaculation fluid. The sensations of orgasm remain intact. The client needs to be advised that the return of erectile capability is often disrupted after surgery, but within 1 year, 95% of men have returned to normal erectile function with sexual intercourse.

CN: Physiological adaptation; CL: Analyze

106.

STEP 1

Symptom	Expected	Unexpected
HR 104 bpm		X
Incisional discomfort rated as 2 on a 0-to-10 scale	X	
Cramping pelvic pain rated as 9 on a 0-to-10 scale		X
Restless and agitated		X
Bruising around incisions	X	
Abdominal distention	X	
Temperature of 99.9°F (37.7°C)	X	

Expected findings for clients who have undergone a radical prostatectomy via the robotic-assisted laparoscopic approach include less pain than those who have the traditional surgical approach. Incisional discomfort rated 2 to 3, bruising around the port access incisions, abdominal distention, and a low-grade fever also are expected findings. Unexpected, abnormal findings include severe cramping pelvic pain associated with tachycardia and restlessness, and the nurse should further assess the client and report these findings to the surgeon.

CJ: Case study; Step 1: Recognize cues; CL: Understand

107.

STEP 2

Finding	Bladder Spasm	Atelectasis
Diminished breath sounds		X
Cramping pelvic pain	X	
Sense of urgency to urinate	X	
Temperature of 99.9°F (37.7°C)		X
Urine leakage around the catheter	X	
Oxygen saturation 92% per pulse oximetry on 2 L via nasal cannula		X

Following prostate surgery, clients often have bladder spasms that can occur when a urinary catheter is in place. Clients who have undergone a radical prostatectomy may be at risk for bladder spasms for 1 to 2 weeks because the prostate lies directly below the bladder wall. The client may also experience a sense of urgency to urinate and have urine leakage around the catheter. The nurse should assess the client for these symptoms and reassure the client that they are expected.

After surgery, clients may have postoperative atelectasis as a result of general anesthesia, retained secretions, and obesity, which may decrease respiratory excursion. The nurse should assess the client for signs of atelectasis, such as decreased breath sounds, increased temperature, and decreased oxygen saturation. The nurse should also initiate deep-breathing exercises and request an order for incentive spirometry if it has not already been ordered.

CJ: Case study; Step 2: Analyze cues; CL: Analyze

108.

STEP 3

The client's **urine output** warrants an assessment of the **patency of the bladder catheter**.

The client has IV fluids infusing at 150 mL per hour and has started taking ice chips. Urine output has exceeded intake until the last hour when urine output dropped to 40 mL; urine is leaking around the catheter, and the client feels bladder discomfort and the urge to void. The nurse's top priority at this time is to assess the patency of the urinary catheter. The client is experiencing severe pain, which can increase the heart rate and blood pressure above baseline. Assessing the infusion rate, pupillary reaction, and dorsalis pedis pulses would be a lower priority for this client problem.

🗝️ CJ: Case study; Step 3: Prioritize hypothesis; CL: Analyze

109.
STEP 4

–/+ **1, 2, 4, 6.** The RN can delegate vital signs; bathing; dressing; assisting with position changes and ambulation; and emptying, measuring, and documenting the urine in the catheter bag. Assessing lung sounds, teaching the client to use an incentive spirometer, and evaluating pain relief are within the scope of practice of the RN and cannot be delegated to UAP.

🗝️ CJ: Case study; Step 4: Generate solutions; CL: Create

110.
STEP 5

Possible Topic	Essential	Nonessential	Inappropriate
Demonstrate cleaning the urethral meatus	X		
Illustrate how the catheter lumens differ		X	
Explain why the urine collection bag must be kept lower than the bladder	X		
Emphasize why the catheter tubing should be secured to the ankle			X
Show the client how to change to a leg bag during the day	X		
Explain the French sizing system for urinary catheters		X	
Teach the client how to remove the catheter in 1 week			X

It is <u>essential</u> for the nurse to teach the client how to clean the urethral meatus to prevent infection. The nurse should keep the collection bag lower than the bladder to avoid backflow into the bladder. To facilitate ambulation and decrease the risk for dislodging the catheter during activity, the nurse can use a smaller collection bag attached to the thigh. To minimize infection risk, the nurse should demonstrate proper technique. It is <u>not essential</u> for the nurse to explain the details about the parts and size of the catheter unless the client specifically asks. The nurse should focus on what the client needs for safe self-care. Securing the tubing to the ankle would increase the risk for dislodgement during walking or a fall. It is <u>inappropriate</u> for the nurse to teach the client how to remove the catheter because approximately 1 week after surgery, a qualified health care provider will remove the urinary catheter.

🗝️ CJ: Case study; Step 5: Take action; CL: Apply

111.
STEP 6

1, 3, 5. The client understands how to manage care at home when they state that they will plan to void on a fixed schedule at least every 2 hours while awake to begin to develop urinary control and continence. The client also understands the importance of doing pelvic floor muscle (Kegel) exercises to strengthen the muscles and improve bladder support provided by strong pelvic floor muscles. These exercises can be started after the surgeon removes the catheter. Incontinence may improve over time; however, wearing incontinence pads or undergarments can limit embarrassing odor and enhance confidence in resuming social activities. Losing excess weight will decrease pressure on the bladder, which will improve incontinence, and the client understands that they should lose 20 lb (9.1 kg) over the next year. Limiting fluids to 2 cups (about ½ L) per day is overly restrictive and could cause dehydration. Drinking fluids before bedtime may worsen nocturnal incontinence.

🗝️ CJ: Case study; Step 6: Evaluate outcomes; CL: Evaluate

112. 1. Clients who have stage IA or IIB prostate cancer have an excellent survival rate. Prostate cancer is usually slow growing, and many men who have prostate cancer do not die from it. A stage I or II tumor is confined to the prostate gland and has not spread to the extrapelvic region or bone.

🗝️ CN: Physiological adaptation; CL: Analyze

113. 2. Goserelin is used to decrease testosterone production in men to slow or stop the production of cancer cells. A common side effect is flushing or hot flashes. Changes in blood pressure, tenderness of the scrotum, and dramatic changes in secondary sexual characteristics should not occur.

🗝️ CN: Pharmacological and parenteral therapies; CL: Apply

The Adult with Erectile Dysfunction

114. 2. The client should notify their HCP promptly if they experience sudden or decreased vision loss in one or both eyes. Sildenafil should not be taken more than once per day. Sildenafil offers no protection against STDs. Sildenafil has no effect in the absence of sexual stimulation.

🗝️ CN: Pharmacological and parenteral therapies; CL: Analyze

115. 2. Antihypertensives, especially beta-blockers such as propranolol, can cause impotence. When a male client has impotence, the nurse should always examine their medication regimen as a potential contributing factor. Aspirin, nonsteroidal antiinflammatory drugs, and anticoagulants do not cause erectile dysfunction.

🔑 CN: Pharmacological and parenteral therapies; CL: Analyze

116. 2. ED is multifactorial in origin, and more than 50% of the cases can be attributed to organic causes, which include alteration in vascular supply, hormonal changes, neurologic dysfunction, medications, and associated systemic diseases, such as diabetes mellitus or alcoholism. The presence of nocturnal erections is the first evaluation to differentiate between organic and psychogenic causes. ED is a common problem among men older than age 65.

🔑 CN: Physiological adaptation; CL: Apply

117. 1. Avoidance of alcohol can improve the outcome of therapy. Alcohol and smoking can affect a man's ability to have and maintain an erection. The client should be encouraged to follow a healthy diet, but no specific diet is associated with improvement of sexual function. The client should cease smoking, not just decrease smoking. Increasing attempts at intercourse without treatment will not facilitate improvement. The client should be reassured that ED is a common problem and that help is available.

🔑 CN: Reduction of risk potential; CL: Analyze

Managing Care, Quality, and Safety of Adults with Reproductive Health Problems

118. 4. The registered nurse (RN) is responsible for monitoring the surgical site for the condition of the dressing, the status of the incision, and signs and symptoms of complications. UAP who have been trained to report abnormalities to the RN supervising the care may take vital signs, record intake and output, and give perineal care.

🔑 CN: Management of care; CL: Analyze

119. 4. To determine the cause of this problem, a quality improvement study should be conducted. Before implementing solutions to a problem, the precise issues in the hospital system must be observed and documented. Consulting with the evening nurses may result in biased observations because the evening nurses are not conducting care under the same environment as the night nurses. Including a medication nurse is not the first step in understanding the problem and may be an unrealistic or expensive solution. The supervisor is not directly involved with the problem and should only be consulted if the problem cannot be solved by those involved.

🔑 CN: Management of care; CL: Analyze

120. 3. The nurse must clarify this prescription with the admitting HCP to ensure medication accuracy and client safety. In health care settings without computerized medical records or computer prescribing, misinterpretation of handwriting remains a leading cause of medication errors. It is not safe practice to question the client regarding a diagnosis and assume the medication is correctly prescribed. The pharmacist will need clarification of the prescription as well. It is not the role of the pharmacist to interpret the prescription.

🔑 CN: Pharmacological and parenteral therapies; CL: Analyze

121. 2. The surgeon should be notified when a client who has had an abdominal hysterectomy develops vaginal bleeding that saturates a blue pad in 1 hour, and care should be managed so that other personnel can obtain vital signs while the nurse contacts the surgeon. The client may need to have IV fluids increased, but the surgeon needs to be notified first. Waiting 15 minutes while the client is having bright red bleeding is an unsafe nursing action; the client may lose a large amount of blood.

🔑 CN: Management of care; CL: Analyze

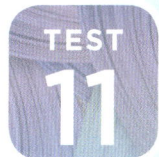

TEST 11: The Adult with Neurologic Health Problems

- The Adult with a Head Injury
- The Adult with Seizures
- The Adult with a Stroke
- The Adult with Parkinson's Disease
- The Adult with Multiple Sclerosis
- The Adult with Myasthenia Gravis
- The Unconscious Adult
- The Adult in Pain
- Managing Care, Quality, and Safety of Adults with Neurologic Health Problems
- Answers, Rationales, and Test-Taking Strategies

The Adult with a Head Injury

1. The nurse has established a goal to maintain intracranial pressure (ICP) within the normal range for a client who had a craniotomy 12 hours ago. What action(s) should the nurse take? Select all that apply.
   ☐ 1. Encourage the client to cough to expectorate secretions.
   ☐ 2. Elevate the head of the bed 30 degrees.
   ☐ 3. Contact the health care provider (HCP) if the ICP is higher than 28 mm Hg.
   ☐ 4. Monitor neurologic status using the Glasgow Coma Scale.
   ☐ 5. Stimulate the client with active range-of-motion exercises.

2. The nurse is monitoring a client with increased intracranial pressure (ICP). What indicator(s) would be the **most** critical for the nurse to monitor? Select all that apply.
   ☐ 1. systolic blood pressure
   ☐ 2. urine output
   ☐ 3. breath sounds
   ☐ 4. cerebral perfusion pressure (CPP)
   ☐ 5. level of pain

3. A nurse is assessing a client with increasing intracranial pressure. What is a client's mean arterial pressure (MAP) in mm Hg when blood pressure (BP) is 120/60 mm Hg?
   _____ mm Hg.

4. A client with a contusion has been admitted for observation following a motor vehicle collision when they were driving their pregnant spouse to the hospital. The next morning, instead of asking about their spouse and baby, the client asked to see the football game on television that they think is starting in 5 minutes. The client is agitated because the nurse will not turn on the television. What should the nurse do **next**? Select all that apply.
   ☐ 1. Find a television so the client can view the football game.
   ☐ 2. Determine if the client's pupils are equal and react to light.
   ☐ 3. Ask the client if they have a headache.
   ☐ 4. Arrange for the client to be with their spouse and baby.
   ☐ 5. Administer a sedative.

5. The nurse is assessing the level of consciousness in a client with a head injury who has been unresponsive for the last 8 hours. Using the Glasgow Coma Scale, the nurse notes that the client opens their eyes only as a response to pain, responds with sounds that are not understandable, and has an abnormal extension of their extremities. What should the nurse do?

Glasgow Coma Scale

Parameter	Finding	Score
Eye opening	Spontaneously	4
	To speech	3
	To pain	2
	Do not open	1
Best verbal responses	Oriented	5
	Confused	4
	Inappropriate speech	3
	Incomprehensible sounds	2
	No verbalization	1
Best motor response	Obeys command	6
	Localizes pain	5
	Withdraws from pain	4
	Abnormal flexion	3
	Abnormal extension	2
	No motor response	1

Interpretation: Best score = 15; worst score = 3; 7 or less general indicates coma; changes from baseline are most important.

☐ 1. Attempt to arouse the client.
☐ 2. Reposition the client with the extremities in normal alignment.
☐ 3. Chart the client's level of consciousness as coma.
☐ 4. Notify the health care provider (HCP).

6. An unconscious client with multiple injuries to the head and neck arrives in the emergency department. What should the nurse do **first**?
☐ 1. Establish an airway.
☐ 2. Determine the identity of the client.
☐ 3. Stop bleeding from open wounds.
☐ 4. Check for a neck fracture.

7. A client has delirium following a head injury. The client is agitated and has managed to lower the side rail at the upper right side of the bed. In which order from first to last should the nurse initiate care for this client? All options must be used.

| 1. Request a prescription for haloperidol. |
| 2. Maintain a quiet environment. |
| 3. Raise the side rail. |
| 4. Speak to the client using short sentences. |
| |
| |
| |

8. A client is at risk for increased intracranial pressure (ICP). Which finding is the **priority** for the nurse to monitor?
☐ 1. unequal pupil size
☐ 2. decreasing systolic blood pressure
☐ 3. tachycardia
☐ 4. decreasing body temperature

9. The nurse is planning care for a client with a head injury. What should the nurse do **first** when the client begins to have clear drainage from the nose?
☐ 1. Compress the nares.
☐ 2. Tilt the head back.
☐ 3. Collect the drainage.
☐ 4. Administer an antihistamine for postnasal drip.

10. The nurse is assessing the respiratory pattern of a client with a head injury. Which respiratory pattern indicates increasing intracranial pressure in the brain stem?
☐ 1. slow, irregular respirations
☐ 2. rapid, shallow respirations
☐ 3. asymmetric chest excursion
☐ 4. nasal flaring

11. A client with a head injury has an intracranial pressure (ICP) of 20 mm Hg. What should the nurse do **next**?
☐ 1. Give the client a warming blanket.
☐ 2. Administer low-dose barbiturates.
☐ 3. Encourage the client to take deep breaths to hyperventilate.
☐ 4. Restrict fluids.

12. The nurse is assessing a client with increasing intracranial pressure (ICP). The nurse should notify the health care provider (HCP) about which early change in the client's condition?
    ☐ 1. widening pulse pressure
    ☐ 2. decrease in the pulse rate
    ☐ 3. dilated, fixed pupils
    ☐ 4. decrease in the level of consciousness (LOC)

13. A client with a head injury has a sustained increased intracranial pressure (ICP) of 20 mm Hg. Which position is **most** appropriate?
    ☐ 1. the head of the bed elevated 15 to 20 degrees
    ☐ 2. Trendelenburg position
    ☐ 3. lateral recumbent position
    ☐ 4. the head elevated on two pillows

14. The nurse administers mannitol to the client with increased intracranial pressure (ICP). Which parameter requires close monitoring?
    ☐ 1. muscle relaxation
    ☐ 2. intake and output
    ☐ 3. widening of the pulse pressure
    ☐ 4. pupil dilation

15. The nurse is assessing a client for movement after halo traction placement for a C8 fracture. What should the nurse do to test the client's ability to move?
    Ask the client to:
    ☐ 1. shrug their shoulders against downward resistance.
    ☐ 2. pull their arm up from a resting position against resistance.
    ☐ 3. straighten their arm from a flexed position against resistance.
    ☐ 4. grasp the nurse's hands with both hands and squeeze.

16. A client who is regaining consciousness after a craniotomy becomes restless and attempts to pull out the intravenous (IV) line. The nurse contacts the health care provider (HCP) and explains the situation and background. What type of restraint should the nurse recommend the HCP order?
    ☐ 1. a jacket restraint
    ☐ 2. soft "mitten" restraints
    ☐ 3. placing the client's arms under the sheet and securing the sheet
    ☐ 4. a wrist restraint on each arm

17. The nurse is planning care for a client with a head injury who is at risk for increased intracranial pressure (ICP). Which activity should the nurse instruct the client to avoid?
    ☐ 1. deep-breathing exercises
    ☐ 2. turning
    ☐ 3. vigorous coughing
    ☐ 4. passive range-of-motion (ROM) exercises

18. A client who had a serious head injury with increased intracranial pressure and short-term memory loss is to be discharged to a rehabilitation facility. Which outcome of rehabilitation during the first 3 days is realistic for the client?
    The client will:
    ☐ 1. exhibit no further episodes of short-term memory loss.
    ☐ 2. be able to return to a construction job in 3 weeks.
    ☐ 3. actively participate in the rehabilitation process.
    ☐ 4. be emotionally stable and display preinjury personality traits.

19. Four hours after supratentorial surgery, the client is receiving intravenous (IV) fluid at 80 mL per hour, and the nurse is monitoring the client's neurologic status using the Glasgow Coma Scale. At 1015, the client has turned to the left side and is lying flat. At 1030, the nurse notes changes in the client's status (see chart). What should the nurse do next?

Glasgow Coma Scale	1000	1015	1030
Eye opening	4	4	3
Verbal response	5	5	4
Motor response	6	6	6
Total score	15	15	13

    ☐ 1. Note the changes, and continue to assess the client every 15 minutes.
    ☐ 2. Notify the surgeon of these findings.
    ☐ 3. Position the client supine with the head of the bed elevated at 30 degrees.
    ☐ 4. Slow the rate of the intravenous (IV) fluid to 60 mL per hour.

20. The nurse is assessing a client's motor response after brain surgery. The nurse pinches the client's skin to elicit a response and observes the client's arms and legs moving straight out and the feet and toes bending downward. How should the nurse document this response?
    ☐ 1. flaccid paralysis
    ☐ 2. flexion posturing
    ☐ 3. chronic spastic paralysis
    ☐ 4. extension posturing

21. A client receiving continuous mandatory ventilation begins to experience cluster breathing after recent intracranial occipital bleeding. What should the nurse do?
    ☐ 1. Count the rate to be sure that ventilations are deep enough to be sufficient.
    ☐ 2. Notify the health care provider (HCP) of the client's breathing pattern.
    ☐ 3. Increase the rate of ventilations.
    ☐ 4. Increase the tidal volume on the ventilator.

22. The nurse is planning the care for a client who has had a posterior fossa (infratentorial) craniotomy. What should the nurse **avoid** when positioning the client?
    - ☐ 1. keeping the client flat on one side or the other
    - ☐ 2. elevating the head of the bed to 30 degrees
    - ☐ 3. logrolling or turning as a unit when turning
    - ☐ 4. keeping the neck in a neutral position

23. A young adult is admitted to the hospital with a head injury and possible temporal skull fracture sustained in a motorcycle accident. On admission, the client was conscious but lethargic; vital signs included a temperature of 99°F (37°C), pulse of 100 bpm, respiration rate of 18 breaths/min, and blood pressure of 140/70 mm Hg. The nurse should report which change(s) to the health care provider (HCP)? Select all that apply.
    - ☐ 1. decreasing urinary output
    - ☐ 2. decreasing systolic blood pressure
    - ☐ 3. bradycardia
    - ☐ 4. widening pulse pressure
    - ☐ 5. tachycardia
    - ☐ 6. increasing diastolic blood pressure

24. A client with a head injury regains consciousness after several days. When the client **first** awakes, what should the nurse say to the client?
    - ☐ 1. "I'll get your family."
    - ☐ 2. "Can you tell me your name and where you live?"
    - ☐ 3. "I'll bet you are a little confused right now."
    - ☐ 4. "You're in the hospital. You were in an accident and unconscious."

The Adult with Seizures

25. The nurse sees a client walking in the hallway who begins to have a seizure. What should the nurse do in order of priority from first to last? All options must be used.

1. Maintain a patent airway.
2. Record the seizure activity observed.
3. Ease the client to the floor.
4. Obtain vital signs.

26. A client is in the ictal phase of a generalized tonic-clonic seizure. Which finding is expected?
    - ☐ 1. jerking in one extremity that spreads gradually to adjacent areas
    - ☐ 2. vacant staring and abruptly ceasing all activity
    - ☐ 3. facial grimaces, patting motions, and lip smacking
    - ☐ 4. loss of consciousness, body stiffening, and violent muscle contractions

27. It is the night before a client is to have a computed tomography (CT) scan of the head without contrast. What should the nurse tell the client to do to prepare for this test?
    - ☐ 1. "You must shampoo your hair tonight to remove all oil and dirt."
    - ☐ 2. "You may drink fluids until midnight, but after that, drink nothing until the scan is completed."
    - ☐ 3. "You will have some hair shaved to attach the small electrode to your scalp."
    - ☐ 4. "You will need to hold your head very still during the examination."

28. The client will have an electroencephalogram (EEG) in the morning. Which instruction should the nurse give to the client about dietary preparation the morning of the test?
    - ☐ 1. Do not have any food or drink.
    - ☐ 2. Have only coffee or tea.
    - ☐ 3. Eat a full breakfast as desired, but no coffee, tea, or energy drinks
    - ☐ 4. Observe a liquid diet such as fruit juice, oatmeal, or smoothie

29. The client is scheduled to receive phenytoin through a nasogastric (NG) tube and has a tube-feeding supplement running continuously. The head of the bed is elevated to 30 degrees. Before administering the medication, the nurse should take which action?
    - ☐ 1. Elevate the head of the bed to 60 degrees.
    - ☐ 2. Draw blood to determine the phenytoin level after giving the morning dose to determine if the client has a toxic blood level.
    - ☐ 3. Stop the tube feeding 1 hour before giving phenytoin, and hold the tube feeding for 1 hour after giving the medication.
    - ☐ 4. Flush the NG tube with 150 mL of water before and after giving the phenytoin.

30. The nurse is developing a teaching plan with a client with seizures who is going home with a prescription for gabapentin. What information should the nurse give the client about taking gabapentin?
    - ☐ 1. Take all the medication until it is gone.
    - ☐ 2. Notify the health care provider (HCP) if vision changes occur.
    - ☐ 3. Store gabapentin in the refrigerator.
    - ☐ 4. Take gabapentin with an antacid to protect against ulcers.

31. The nurse is planning care for a client in the postictal phase of a seizure. What action should the nurse take **first**?
☐ 1. Reorient the client to time, person, and place.
☐ 2. Determine the client's level of sleepiness.
☐ 3. Assess the client's breathing pattern.
☐ 4. Position the client comfortably.

32. The nurse is planning to minimize the risk for seizure activity in a client who is undergoing diagnostic studies after having experienced several episodes of seizures. What action should the nurse take?
☐ 1. Maintain the client on bed rest.
☐ 2. Administer a sedative as prescribed.
☐ 3. Close the door to the room to minimize stimulation.
☐ 4. Administer oral carbamazepine 200 mg twice daily.

33. The nurse is assessing a client who is in the beginning of the ictal phase of a seizure. What information about the seizure should the nurse document? Select all that apply.
☐ 1. time of onset
☐ 2. level of consciousness
☐ 3. blood pressure
☐ 4. oxygen saturation per pulse oximeter
☐ 5. movement of the head
☐ 6. pupil size
☐ 7. muscle rigidity
☐ 8. time of the last dose of anticonvulsant medication

34. The nurse is assessing a client in the postictal phase of a generalized tonic-clonic seizure. The nurse would expect that the client will have which symptom following the seizure?
☐ 1. drowsiness
☐ 2. inability to move
☐ 3. paresthesia
☐ 4. hypotension

35. The health care provider has prescribed phenytoin sodium therapy for a client with seizures. What should the nurse explain to the client about stopping the drug suddenly?
☐ 1. Physical dependency develops over time.
☐ 2. Status epilepticus may occur.
☐ 3. A hypoglycemic reaction is likely.
☐ 4. Heart block can happen.

36. The nurse is teaching a client with seizures to recognize an aura. What should the nurse instruct the client to notice as indicating the onset of an aura?
☐ 1. a postictal state of amnesia
☐ 2. a hallucination that occurs during a seizure
☐ 3. a symptom that occurs just before a seizure
☐ 4. a feeling of relaxation as the seizure begins to subside

37. The nurse is teaching a client with a seizure disorder how to take topiramate. Which statement indicates the client has understood the nurse's instruction about this drug? "I will:
☐ 1. take the medicine before going to bed."
☐ 2. drink six to eight glasses of water a day."
☐ 3. eat plenty of fresh fruits."
☐ 4. take the medicine with a meal or snack."

38. The nurse is assessing a client with a seizure disorder who has been taking phenytoin sodium for 2 years. Which is an expected outcome of long-term phenytoin sodium therapy?
☐ 1. weight gain
☐ 2. insomnia
☐ 3. excessive growth of gum tissue
☐ 4. deteriorating eyesight

39. A 21-year-old female client takes clonazepam. What should the nurse ask this client about? Select all that apply.
☐ 1. seizure activity
☐ 2. pregnancy status
☐ 3. alcohol use
☐ 4. cigarette smoking
☐ 5. intake of caffeine and sugary drinks

The Adult with a Stroke

40. Which outcome(s) would indicate effective management of a conscious client who is being treated with recombinant tissue plasminogen therapy during the initial phase of an ischemic cerebral vascular accident (CVA)? Select all that apply.
☐ 1. headache reduced
☐ 2. dysphagia improved
☐ 3. visual disturbances improved
☐ 4. responds to comfort measures
☐ 5. no signs or symptoms of bleeding

41. A client admitted with possible ischemic stroke has been aphasic for 3 hours and has a blood pressure (BP) of 220/120 mm Hg. Which prescription by the health care provider should the nurse question?
☐ 1. labetalol infusion to keep the BP lower than 120/80 mm Hg
☐ 2. tissue plasminogen activator (t-PA) per protocol
☐ 3. normal saline intravenously at 75 mL per hour
☐ 4. bed elevated 30 degrees

42. Following a stroke, a client has dysphagia and left-sided facial paralysis. Which feeding technique will be **most** helpful at this time?
☐ 1. Have the client sip liquids from a straw.
☐ 2. Position the client with the bed at a 30-degree angle.
☐ 3. Offer thickened or solid foods from the unaffected side of the mouth.
☐ 4. Feed the client a soft diet from a spoon into the cheek on the left side of the mouth.

43. A client is being monitored for transient ischemic attacks. The client is oriented, can open the eyes spontaneously, and follows commands. What is the Glasgow Coma Scale score?

Glasgow Coma Scale		
Parameter	Finding	Score
Eye opening	Spontaneously	4
	To speech	3
	To pain	2
	Do not open	1
Best verbal responses	Oriented	5
	Confused	4
	Inappropriate speech	3
	Incomprehensible sounds	2
	No verbalization	1
Best motor response	Obeys command	6
	Localizes pain	5
	Withdraws from pain	4
	Abnormal flexion	3
	Abnormal extension	2
	No motor response	1
Interpretation: Best score = 15; worst score = 3; 7 or less general indicates coma; changes from baseline are most important.		

_____ points.

44. The nurse is teaching a client about taking prophylactic warfarin sodium. Which statement(s) would indicate that the client understands how to take the drug? Select all that apply.
☐ 1. "The drug's action peaks in 2 hours."
☐ 2. "Maximum dosage is not achieved until 3 to 4 days after starting the medication."
☐ 3. "Effects of the drug continue for 4 to 5 days after discontinuing the medication."
☐ 4. "Protamine sulfate is the antidote for warfarin."
☐ 5. "I should have my blood levels tested periodically."

45. The nurse is observing the unlicensed assistive personnel (UAP) give mouth care to a client who has had a stroke and is unconscious. The nurse should intervene if the UAP does which?
☐ 1. positions the client on the back with a small pillow under the head
☐ 2. keeps portable suctioning equipment at the bedside
☐ 3. opens the client's mouth with a padded tongue blade
☐ 4. cleans the client's mouth and teeth with a toothbrush

46. A client arrives in the emergency department with an ischemic stroke. What should the nurse do before the client receives tissue plasminogen activator (t-PA)?
☐ 1. Ask what medications the client is taking.
☐ 2. Complete a history and health assessment.
☐ 3. Identify the time of onset of the stroke.
☐ 4. Determine if the client is scheduled for any surgical procedures.

47. A client has received thrombolytic treatment for an ischemic stroke. The nurse should notify the health care provider (HCP) if there is a rapid increase in which vital sign?
☐ 1. pulse
☐ 2. respirations
☐ 3. blood pressure
☐ 4. temperature

48. STEP 1

The nurse is caring for a 50-year-old male client in the emergency department (ED).

Nurse's Notes

Today: 0800
A client presented to the ED with a headache, slurred speech, and right-sided arm weakness. The client was brought to the ED by a family member, who states they were at lunch when the client began to show symptoms about 30 minutes ago.
   The client is alert and oriented to person, place, time, and situation. Vital signs are temperature 97.7°F (36.5°C); heart rate 89 bpm; respiration rate 22 breaths/min; blood pressure 170/89 mm Hg; and oxygen saturation 96% on room air. PERRLA assessment reveals a 4-mm pupil size. The client reports a headache pain of 8 on a scale of 0 to 10. The client has a medical history of high blood pressure, diabetes, and high cholesterol.

➤ Which four findings require **immediate** follow-up?

- [ ] 1. Right-sided arm weakness
- [ ] 2. Slurred speech
- [ ] 3. Heart rate of 89 bpm
- [ ] 4. Headache
- [ ] 5. Confusion
- [ ] 6. Respiration rate of 22 breaths/min

49. STEP 2

The nurse is caring for a 50-year-old male client in the emergency department (ED).

Nurse's Notes

Today: 0800
A client presented to the ED with a headache, slurred speech, and right-sided arm weakness. The client was brought to the ED by a family member, who states they were at lunch when the client began to show symptoms about 30 minutes ago.
   The client is alert and oriented to person, place, time, and situation. Vital signs are temperature 97.7°F (36.5°C); heart rate 89 bpm; respiration rate 22 breaths/min; blood pressure 170/89 mm Hg; and oxygen saturation 96% on room air. PERRLA assessment reveals a 4-mm pupil size. The client reports a headache pain of 8 on a scale of 0 to 10. The client has a medical history of high blood pressure, diabetes, and high cholesterol.

The nurse is caring for a 50-year-old male client in the emergency department (ED).

➤ Complete the following sentence by using the list of drop-down options.

The nurse determines that the client is at risk for [cranial hemorrhaging / clotting / paralysis] if the client were to be administered tissue plasminogen activator (t-PA) when experiencing a(n) [ischemic / hemorrhagic / transient] stroke because the blood vessels of the brain have already [ruptured. / clotted. / narrowed.]

50. STEP 3

The nurse is caring for a 50-year-old male client in the emergency department (ED).

Nurse's Notes

Today: 0800
A client presented to the ED with a headache, slurred speech, and right-sided arm weakness. The client was brought to the ED by a family member, who states they were at lunch when the client began to show symptoms about 30 minutes ago.

The client is alert and oriented to person, place, time, and situation. Vital signs are temperature 97.7°F (36.5°C); heart rate 89 bpm; respiration rate 22 breaths/min; blood pressure 170/89 mm Hg; and oxygen saturation 96% on room air. A PERRLA assessment reveals a 4-mm pupil size. The client reports a headache pain of 8 on a scale of 0 to 10. The client has a medical history of high blood pressure, diabetes, and high cholesterol.

Orders

Date	Time	
08/13	0845	Computed tomography (CT) scan stat
08/13	0845	Cranial x-ray
08/13	0845	Enoxaparin sodium 150 mEq
08/13	0845	Neurologic assessment every 15 minutes
08/13	0845	Blood glucose stat
08/13	0845	Intravenous (IV) placement
08/13	0845	t-PA stat

The nurse has received orders from the health care provider.

➢ Which three orders should the nurse perform **right away**?

- ☐ 1. CT scan stat
- ☐ 2. Cranial x-ray
- ☐ 3. Enoxaparin sodium 150 mEq
- ☐ 4. Neurologic assessment every 15 minutes
- ☐ 5. Blood glucose stat
- ☐ 6. t-PA stat

51. STEP 4

The nurse is caring for a 50-year-old male client in the emergency department (ED).

Nurse's Notes

Today: 0800
A client presented to the ED with a headache, slurred speech, and right-sided arm weakness. The client was brought to the ED by a family member, who states they were at lunch when the client began to show symptoms about 30 minutes ago.
 The client is alert and oriented to person, place, time, and situation. Vital signs are temperature 97.7°F (36.5°C); heart rate 89 bpm; respiration rate 22 breaths/min; blood pressure 170/89 mm Hg; and oxygen saturation 96% on room air. PERRLA assessment reveals a 4-mm pupil size. The client reports a headache pain of 8 on a scale of 0 to 10. The client has a medical history of high blood pressure, diabetes, and high cholesterol.

Today: 0915
The health care provider has ordered t-PA to be administered at 0.9 mg/kg over 60 minutes. The client's blood glucose level is 109 mg/dL (6.05 mmol/L); CT scan results indicate that no hemorrhagic stroke was evident. The client verbalizes consent for treatment.

Orders

Date	Time	
08/13	0845	Computed tomography (CT) scan stat
08/13	0845	Cranial x-ray
08/13	0845	Enoxaparin sodium 150 mEq
08/13	0845	Neurologic assessment every 15 minutes
08/13	0845	Blood glucose stat
08/13	0845	Intravenous (IV) placement
08/13	0845	Tissue plasminogen activator stat

The nurse is determining if the client has any contraindications to receiving t-PA medication.

➤ Which finding(s) would be a contraindication to the administration of t-PA? Select all that apply.

☐	1. The symptoms began less than 3 hours ago.
☐	2. The client is experiencing disabling stroke symptoms.
☐	3. The blood pressure is lower than 185/110 mm Hg.
☐	4. The client currently uses anticoagulant medications.
☐	5. The client had a gastrointestinal bleed 2 weeks ago.
☐	6. The client is younger than 85 years of age.
☐	7. The client takes metformin for diabetes.

52. STEP 5

The nurse is caring for a client who has been diagnosed with an ischemic stroke and transferred to the medical-surgical unit.

Nurse's Notes

Today: 0800
A client presented to the ED with a headache, slurred speech, and right-sided arm weakness. The client was brought to the ED by a family member, who states they were at lunch when the client began to show symptoms about 30 minutes ago.

The client is alert and oriented to person, place, time, and situation. Vital signs are temperature 97.7°F (36.5°C); heart rate 89 bpm; respiration rate 22 breaths/min; blood pressure 170/89 mm Hg; and oxygen saturation 96% on room air. PERRLA assessment reveals a 4-mm pupil size. The client reports a headache pain of 8 on a scale of 0 to 10. The client has a medical history of high blood pressure, diabetes, and high cholesterol.

Today: 0915
The health care provider has ordered t-PA to be administered at 0.9 mg/kg over 60 minutes. The client's blood glucose level is 109 mg/dL (6.05 mmol/L); CT scan results indicate that no hemorrhagic stroke was evident. The client verbalizes consent for treatment.

Today: 1300
The client is transferred to the medical-surgical floor after receiving t-PA while in the emergency department.

The client was found to have an ischemic stroke with associated signs and symptoms of right-sided arm weakness, headache, and slurred speech. The client is alert and oriented to person, place, time, and situation. The client relates headache pain is now rated as a 1 on a scale of 0 to 10. The client continues to state that their right arm feels weak with unequal grips. The client is noted to have regained some resistance to gravity with the right upper extremity; however, they continue to exhibit some slurred speech with slight drooling.

The client will be admitted to the medical-surgical unit for continued observation and initiation of physical therapy and occupational therapy.

Orders

Date	Time	
08/13	0845	Computed tomography (CT) scan stat
08/13	0845	Cranial x-ray
08/13	0845	Enoxaparin sodium 150 mEq
08/13	0845	Neurologic assessment every 15 minutes
08/13	0845	Blood glucose stat
08/13	0845	Intravenous (IV) placement
08/13	0845	Tissue plasminogen activator stat

The nurse is developing a plan of care to prevent the client from aspirating.

➤ Which step(s) can the nurse take to prevent aspiration? Select all that apply.

- ☐ 1. Raise the head of the bed above 90 degrees.
- ☐ 2. Complete a dysphagia screening before providing the client with solids or fluids.
- ☐ 3. Liquify solid foods.
- ☐ 4. Introduce foods on the unaffected side when the client first takes food.
- ☐ 5. Request a consultation with occupational therapy.
- ☐ 6. Teach the client to tuck their chin before swallowing.

53. STEP 6

The nurse is caring for a client who has been diagnosed with an ischemic stroke and has been transferred to the medical-surgical unit.

Nurse's Notes

Today: 0800
A client presented to the ED with a headache, slurred speech, and right-sided arm weakness. The client was brought to the ED by a family member, who states they were at lunch when the client began to show symptoms about 30 minutes ago.
The client is alert and oriented to person, place, time, and situation. Vital signs are temperature 97.7°F (36.5°C); heart rate 89 bpm; respiration rate 22 breaths/min; blood pressure 170/89 mm Hg; and oxygen saturation 96% on room air. PERRLA assessment reveals a 4-mm pupil size. The client reports a headache pain of 8 on a scale of 0 to 10. The client has a medical history of high blood pressure, diabetes, and high cholesterol.

Today: 0915
The health care provider has ordered t-PA to be administered at 0.9 mg/kg over 60 minutes. The client's blood glucose level is 109 mg/dL (6.05 mmol/L); CT scan results indicate that no hemorrhagic stroke was evident. The client verbalizes consent for treatment.

Today: 1300
The client is transferred to the medical-surgical floor after receiving t-PA while in the emergency department.
The client was found to have an ischemic stroke with associated signs and symptoms of right-sided arm weakness, headache, and slurred speech. The client is alert and oriented to person, place, time, and situation. The client relates headache pain is now rated as a 1 on a scale from 0 to 10. The client continues to state that their right arm feels weak with unequal grips. The client is noted to have regained some resistance to gravity with the right upper extremity; however, the client continues to exhibit some slurred speech with slight drooling.
The client will be admitted to the medical-surgical unit for continued observation and initiation of physical therapy and occupational therapy.

Today: 2000
The client is on the medical-surgical floor after receiving t-PA while in the emergency department. The client was found to have an ischemic stroke with associated signs and symptoms of right-sided arm weakness, headache, and slurred speech. The client is alert and oriented to person, place, time, and situation. Pupils are equal and respond to light and accommodation (PERRLA). The client relates their headache pain is now rated as a 1 on a scale of 0 to 10. The client's vital signs are temperature 98.1°F (36.7°C); heart rate 99 bpm and normal sinus rhythm on the monitor; respirations 18 breaths/min; and blood pressure 135/76 mm Hg. The blood glucose level is 105 mg/dL (5.83 mmol/L). Lung sounds are clear and equal, and bowel sounds are normoactive. The client continues to state that the right arm feels weak with unequal grips, with slight weakness observed in the right hand. The client is noted to have regained resistance to gravity with the right upper extremity but continues to exhibit some slurred speech.

Orders

Date	Time	
08/13	0845	Computed tomography (CT) scan stat
08/13	0845	Cranial x-ray
08/13	0845	Enoxaparin sodium 150 mEq
08/13	0845	Neurologic assessment every 15 minutes
08/13	0845	Blood glucose stat
08/13	0845	Intravenous (IV) placement
08/13	0845	Tissue plasminogen activator stat

The nurse is evaluating the client after receiving t-PA 12 hours ago.

➤ Which findings indicate that the t-PA has been effective? Select all that apply.

- ☐ 1. Headache pain rated as 1 on a scale of 0 to 10
- ☐ 2. Slightly slurred speech
- ☐ 3. Blood glucose 105 mg/dL (5.83 mmol/L)
- ☐ 4. Client exhibiting resistance to gravity
- ☐ 5. Pupils are equal and respond to light and accommodation (PERRLA)
- ☐ 6. Temperature 98.1°F (36.7°C)

54. The nurse is planning care for a client in the **first** 24 hours after admission for a thrombotic stroke. Which assessment is a **priority** for the nurse to make during this time?
☐ 1. cholesterol level
☐ 2. pupil size and response
☐ 3. bowel sounds
☐ 4. echocardiogram

55. A client with a hemorrhagic stroke is slightly agitated and has a heart rate of 118 bpm and a respiration rate of 22 breaths/min. Bilateral rhonchi are auscultated, SpO$_2$ is 94%, blood pressure is 144/88 mm Hg, and the client has copious amounts of oral secretions. In which order, from first to last, should the nurse suction the client's mouth and airway to prevent increased intracranial pressure (ICP)? All options must be used.

| 1. Suction the airway. |
| 2. Hyperoxygenate. |
| 3. Suction the mouth. |
| 4. Explain the procedure. |
| |
| |
| |
| |

56. The nurse is developing a care plan for a client who has had a stroke. The nurse asks about the client's functional status before the stroke. How will the nurse incorporate this information into the care plan?

The client's functional status before the stroke will:
☐ 1. guide the rehabilitation plan.
☐ 2. help predict outcomes.
☐ 3. help the client recognize physical limitations.
☐ 4. determine if the client can be expected to regain most functional status.

57. The nurse is positioning a client who has hemiparalysis. Which technique is **most** effective when there is only one person to assist the client to move from the left side to the right side?
☐ 1. rolling the client onto the side
☐ 2. sliding the client to move up in bed
☐ 3. lifting the client when moving the client up in bed
☐ 4. having the client help lift off the bed using a trapeze

58. The nurse is caring for a client who has paraplegia as the result of a stroke. At home, the client uses a wheelchair for mobility and can transfer independently. The client is now being treated with intravenous (IV) antibiotics for a sacral wound via a peripherally inserted central catheter. The client is alert and oriented and has no previous history of falling. Using the Morse Fall Scale (see exhibit), what is this client's total score?

Morse Fall Risk/Scale

Item	Scale	Scoring
1. History of falling; immediate or within 3 months	No 0 Yes 25	
2. Secondary diagnosis	No 0 Yes 15	

3. Ambulatory aid
  Bed rest/nurse assist
  Crutches/cane/walker
  Furniture
	
	0
	15
	30	

4. IV/Heparin Lock	No 0 Yes 20	

5. Gait/Transferring
  Normal/bedrest/immobile
  Weak
  Impaired
	
	0
	10
	20	

6. Mental status
  Oriented to own ability
  Forget limitations
	
	0
	15	

_____ fall risk score.

59. The nurse is planning care for a client who has had a stroke. Which is the **most** effective means of preventing plantar flexion in a client who has had a stroke with residual paralysis?
☐ 1. Place the client's feet against a firm footboard.
☐ 2. Reposition the client every 2 hours.
☐ 3. Have the client wear ankle-high tennis shoes at intervals throughout the day.
☐ 4. Massage the client's feet and ankles regularly.

60. The nurse is planning the care of a client with hemiplegia to prevent joint deformities of the arm and hand. Which position(s) would be appropriate? Select all that apply.
☐ 1. placing a pillow in the axilla so the arm is away from the body
☐ 2. inserting a pillow under the slightly flexed arm so the hand is higher than the elbow
☐ 3. immobilizing the extremity in a sling
☐ 4. positioning a hand cone in the hand so the fingers are barely flexed
☐ 5. keeping the arm at the side using a pillow

61. The nurse is planning care for a client who is experiencing expressive aphasia. Which nursing action is **most** helpful in promoting communication?
☐ 1. speaking loudly and slowly
☐ 2. using a "picture board" for the client to point to pictures
☐ 3. writing directions so the client can read them
☐ 4. speaking in short sentences

62. The nurse is teaching the family of a client with dysphagia about decreasing the risk for aspiration while eating. Which measure(s) should the nurse include in the teaching plan? Select all that apply.
☐ 1. maintaining an upright position while eating
☐ 2. restricting the diet to liquids until swallowing improves
☐ 3. introducing foods on the unaffected side of the mouth
☐ 4. keeping distractions to a minimum
☐ 5. cutting food into large pieces of finger food

63. The nurse is assisting a client with a stroke who has homonymous hemianopia. The nurse should understand that the client will do what when eating?

The client will:
☐ 1. have a preference for foods high in salt.
☐ 2. eat food on only half of the plate.
☐ 3. forget the names of foods.
☐ 4. be unable to swallow liquids.

64. A nurse is teaching a client who had a stroke about ways to adapt to a visual disability. What does the nurse identify as the **primary** safety precaution to use?
☐ 1. Wear a patch over one eye.
☐ 2. Place personal items on the sighted side.
☐ 3. Lie in bed with the unaffected side toward the door.
☐ 4. Turn the head from side to side when walking.

65. A client is experiencing mood swings after a stroke and often has episodes of tearfulness that are distressing to the family. Which is the **best** technique for the nurse to instruct family members to try when the client experiences a crying episode?
☐ 1. Sit quietly with the client until the episode is over.
☐ 2. Ignore the behavior.
☐ 3. Attempt to divert the client's attention.
☐ 4. Tell the client that this behavior is unacceptable.

66. The nurse is developing a care plan to help a client with expressive aphasia communicate. Which action(s) would be helpful? Select all that apply.
☐ 1. Present one thought at a time.
☐ 2. Avoid writing messages.
☐ 3. Speak at a normal volume.
☐ 4. Make use of gestures.
☐ 5. Encourage pointing to the needed object.

67. The nurse is administering a thrombolytic drug to a client who has had a stroke. What is the expected outcome of this drug?
☐ 1. increased vascular permeability
☐ 2. vasoconstriction
☐ 3. dissolved blood clot
☐ 4. prevention of hemorrhage

The Adult with Parkinson's Disease

68. The nurse is planning care for a client with Parkinson's disease who is experiencing freezing of gait with difficulty initiating movement. Which action should the nurse take?
☐ 1. Pull the client forward to initiate walking.
☐ 2. Instruct the client to use a wheelchair.
☐ 3. Have the client remain still.
☐ 4. Tell the client to march in place.

69. A health care provider (HCP) has prescribed carbidopa-levodopa four times per day for a client with Parkinson's disease. The client wants "to end it all now that the Parkinson's disease has progressed." What should the nurse do? Select all that apply.
☐ 1. Explain that the new prescription for carbidopa-levodopa will treat the depression.
☐ 2. Encourage the client to discuss feelings as the carbidopa-levodopa is being administered.
☐ 3. Contact the HCP before administering the carbidopa-levodopa.
☐ 4. Determine if the client is on antidepressants or monoamine oxidase (MAO) inhibitors.
☐ 5. Determine if the client is at risk for suicide.

70. The nurse is assessing a client with Parkinson's disease. Which is an initial sign of Parkinson's disease?
☐ 1. rigidity
☐ 2. tremor
☐ 3. bradykinesia
☐ 4. akinesia

71. The nurse develops a teaching plan for a client newly diagnosed with Parkinson's disease. Which topic is **most** important to include in the plan?
☐ 1. maintaining a balanced nutritional diet
☐ 2. enhancing the immune system
☐ 3. maintaining a safe environment
☐ 4. engaging in diversional activity

72. The nurse observes that when a client with Parkinson's disease unbuttons their shirt, the upper arm tremors disappear. Which statement **best** guides the nurse's analysis of this observation about the client's tremors?
    ☐ 1. The tremors are probably psychological and can be controlled at will.
    ☐ 2. The tremors sometimes disappear with purposeful and voluntary movements.
    ☐ 3. The tremors disappear when the client's attention is diverted by some activity.
    ☐ 4. There is no explanation for the observation; it is a chance occurrence.

73. The nurse is teaching a client with Parkinson's disease about managing hyperkinesia. At what time of day should the nurse encourage the client to schedule the **most** demanding physical activities to minimize the effects of hypokinesia?
    ☐ 1. early in the morning, when the client's energy level is high
    ☐ 2. when the peak action of drug therapy occurs
    ☐ 3. immediately after a rest period
    ☐ 4. when family members will be available

74. The nurse is working with an interprofessional team to plan care for a client with Parkinson's disease. Which goal is **best** collaboratively established by the client with Parkinson's disease, the nurse, and the physical therapist?
    ☐ 1. maintaining joint flexibility
    ☐ 2. building muscle strength
    ☐ 3. improving muscle endurance
    ☐ 4. reducing ataxia

75. A client is being switched from levodopa (L-dopa) to carbidopa-levodopa. The nurse should monitor for which possible complication during medication changes and dosage adjustments?
    ☐ 1. euphoria
    ☐ 2. jaundice
    ☐ 3. vital sign fluctuation
    ☐ 4. signs and symptoms of diabetes

76. A client with Parkinson's disease needs a long time to complete morning care but becomes annoyed when the nurse offers assistance and refuses all help. Which action should the nurse take?
    ☐ 1. Tell the client firmly that they need assistance and help with the morning care.
    ☐ 2. Praise the client for the desire to be independent, and give extra time and encouragement.
    ☐ 3. Tell the client that they are being unrealistic about their abilities and must accept the fact that they need help.
    ☐ 4. Ask the client to at least modify the morning care routine if they insist on self-care.

The Adult with Multiple Sclerosis

77. The nurse is assessing a client with multiple sclerosis for potential complications of the disease. Which symptom(s) would indicate the development of a complication? Select all that apply.
    ☐ 1. dehydration
    ☐ 2. falls
    ☐ 3. seizures
    ☐ 4. skin breakdown
    ☐ 5. fatigue

78. The nurse is teaching a client with bladder dysfunction from multiple sclerosis (MS) about bladder training at home. Which instruction(s) should the nurse include in the teaching plan? Select all that apply.
    ☐ 1. Restrict fluids to about 4 cups (1 L) every 24 hours.
    ☐ 2. Drink 1½ to 2 cups (400 to 500 mL) of fluids with each meal.
    ☐ 3. Drink fluids midmorning, midafternoon, and late afternoon.
    ☐ 4. Attempt to void at least every 2 hours.
    ☐ 5. Use intermittent catheterization as needed.

79. The nurse is assessing a client with multiple sclerosis (MS). Which clinical manifestation(s) of multiple sclerosis would the nurse expect to observe in the client? Select all that apply.
    ☐ 1. hypertension
    ☐ 2. euphoria
    ☐ 3. double vision
    ☐ 4. loss of muscle tone
    ☐ 5. muscle tremors
    ☐ 6. sudden bursts of energy

80. A client with multiple sclerosis (MS) is receiving baclofen. The nurse determines that the drug is effective when it produces which outcome?
    ☐ 1. induces sleep
    ☐ 2. stimulates the client's appetite
    ☐ 3. relieves muscular spasticity
    ☐ 4. reduces the urine bacterial count

81. A client has had multiple sclerosis (MS) for 15 years and has received various drug therapies. What is the **primary** reason the nurse has found it difficult to evaluate the effectiveness of the drugs that the client has used?

    The client:
    ☐ 1. exhibits intolerance to many drugs.
    ☐ 2. experiences spontaneous remissions from time to time.
    ☐ 3. requires multiple drugs simultaneously.
    ☐ 4. endures long periods of exacerbation before the illness responds to a particular drug.

82. The nurse is teaching a client with multiple sclerosis (MS) who has slurred speech how to improve verbal communication. Which is the **most** effective strategy for the nurse to suggest to the client?
    ☐ 1. Speak slowly.
    ☐ 2. Write long words on a whiteboard.
    ☐ 3. Repeat indistinguishable words.
    ☐ 4. Speak louder.

83. The right hand of a client with multiple sclerosis trembles severely whenever they attempt a voluntary action. The client spills their coffee twice at lunch and cannot get their dress fastened securely. Which is the **best** legal documentation in the nurse's notes of the medical record for this client assessment?
    ☐ 1. "The client has an intention tremor of the right hand."
    ☐ 2. "The client's right-hand tremor worsens with purposeful acts."
    ☐ 3. "The client needs assistance with dressing and eating due to severe trembling and clumsiness."
    ☐ 4. "The client's slight shaking of the right hand increases to a severe tremor when the client tries to button their clothes or drink from a cup."

84. A client with multiple sclerosis (MS) is experiencing bowel incontinence and is starting a bowel retraining program. What information should the nurse include in the teaching plan for this client?
    ☐ 1. eating a diet low in fiber
    ☐ 2. setting a regular time for elimination
    ☐ 3. using a stool softener daily
    ☐ 4. limiting fluid intake to about 4 cups (1 L) a day

85. The nurse is assisting a client with multiple sclerosis (MS) set long-term goals. Which goal is realistic?
    ☐ 1. greater joint flexibility
    ☐ 2. improved muscle strength
    ☐ 3. clearer thinking
    ☐ 4. fewer mood swings

86. The nurse is preparing a client with multiple sclerosis (MS) for discharge from the hospital to home. What information should the nurse include in the teaching plan?
    ☐ 1. "You'll need to accept the necessity of a quiet and inactive lifestyle."
    ☐ 2. "Keep active, use stress-reduction strategies, and avoid fatigue."
    ☐ 3. "Follow good health habits to change the course of the disease."
    ☐ 4. "Practice using the mechanical aids that you'll need when future disabilities arise."

87. The nurse is developing a discharge teaching plan with a client with multiple sclerosis who has an impaired peripheral sensation. Which information should the nurse include in the discharge teaching plan? Select all that apply.
    ☐ 1. Carefully test the temperature of bath water.
    ☐ 2. Avoid kitchen activities because of the risk for injury.
    ☐ 3. Avoid hot water bottles and heating pads.
    ☐ 4. Inspect the skin daily for injury or pressure points.
    ☐ 5. Wear warm clothing when outside in cold temperatures.

88. A client with multiple sclerosis has urinary incontinence. Which intervention should the nurse suggest to help the client avoid episodes of urinary incontinence?
    ☐ 1. Limit fluid intake to about 4 cups (1 L) a day.
    ☐ 2. Insert an indwelling urinary catheter.
    ☐ 3. Establish a regular voiding schedule.
    ☐ 4. Administer prophylactic antibiotics as prescribed.

89. A client with multiple sclerosis (MS) lives with their daughter and 3-year-old granddaughter. The daughter asks the nurse what they can do at home to help the client. Which measure would be **most** beneficial?
    ☐ 1. psychotherapy
    ☐ 2. regular exercise
    ☐ 3. daycare for the granddaughter
    ☐ 4. weekly visits by another person with MS

The Adult with Myasthenia Gravis

90. The nurse is developing a teaching plan with a client with myasthenia gravis. The nurse should include information about the risk for which health problem?
    ☐ 1. aspiration
    ☐ 2. bladder dysfunction
    ☐ 3. hypertension
    ☐ 4. sensory loss

91. The nurse is discussing discharge instructions with a client with myasthenia gravis who is taking pyridostigmine. What should the nurse instruct the client to do?
    ☐ 1. Administer artificial tears.
    ☐ 2. Avoid contact with crowds.
    ☐ 3. Take pyridostigmine in the afternoon.
    ☐ 4. Decrease protein in the diet.

92. After teaching a client about myasthenia gravis, the nurse would judge that the client has formed a realistic concept of the disease and the treatment plan when the client makes which statement?
    ☐ 1. "I'll live longer, but ultimately the disease will cause death."
    ☐ 2. "My symptoms will be controlled, and eventually I will be cured."
    ☐ 3. "I'll be able to control the disease and enjoy a healthy lifestyle."
    ☐ 4. "I won't be so tired, but I can expect occasional periods of muscle weakness."

The Unconscious Adult

93. A client is brought to the emergency department unconscious. An empty bottle of aspirin was found in the car, and a drug overdose is suspected. Which medication should the nurse have available for further emergency treatment?
    ☐ 1. vitamin K
    ☐ 2. dextrose 50%
    ☐ 3. activated charcoal powder
    ☐ 4. sodium thiosulfate

94. The nurse is assessing a client diagnosed with an overdose of a cholinergic agent. Which clinical manifestation(s) should the nurse assess? Select all that apply.
    ☐ 1. dry mucous membranes
    ☐ 2. urinary incontinence
    ☐ 3. central nervous system (CNS) depression
    ☐ 4. seizures
    ☐ 5. skin rash

95. The nurse is caring for a client who is unconscious following an attempted suicide by drug overdose. When speaking with the client's distraught spouse, what should the nurse do **first**?
    ☐ 1. Explain that because the client was found on hospital property, they were probably asking for help and did not intentionally overdose.
    ☐ 2. Ask the spouse if they would like to speak to a member of the clergy.
    ☐ 3. Encourage the spouse to express their feelings and concerns, and listen carefully.
    ☐ 4. Allow the spouse to help care for the client by rubbing their back when the client is turned.

96. The nurse is caring for an unconscious intubated client with normal intracranial pressure. What should the nurse include in the care plan?
    ☐ 1. Monitor the oral temperature, keep the room temperature at 70°F (21.1°C), and place the client on a cooling blanket if the client's temperature is higher than 101°F (38.3°C).
    ☐ 2. Clean the mouth carefully, apply a thin coat of a lubricant, and move the endotracheal tube to the opposite side daily.
    ☐ 3. Position the client in the supine position with the head to the side and slightly elevated on two pillows.
    ☐ 4. Turn the client with a draw-sheet, and place a pillow behind the back and one between the legs.

97. An unconscious client is to be placed in a right side-lying position. The nurse should intervene when observing the client in which position?
    ☐ 1. The head is placed on a small pillow.
    ☐ 2. The right leg is extended without pillow support.
    ☐ 3. The left arm is rested on the mattress with the elbow flexed.
    ☐ 4. The left leg is supported on a pillow with the knee flexed.

98. The nurse and physical therapist have planned for an unconscious client to receive passive range-of-motion (ROM) exercises. What indicates these exercises are having their intended outcome?
    ☐ 1. preservation of muscle mass
    ☐ 2. prevention of bone demineralization
    ☐ 3. increase in muscle tone
    ☐ 4. maintenance of joint mobility

99. The nurse observes that the right eye of an unconscious client does not close completely. Which nursing intervention is **most** appropriate?
    ☐ 1. Have the client wear eyeglasses at all times.
    ☐ 2. Lightly tape the eyelid shut.
    ☐ 3. Instill artificial tears once every shift.
    ☐ 4. Clean the eyelid with a washcloth every shift.

100. The nurse is administering intermittent enteral feeding via a percutaneous enterostomy tube to an unconscious client. What action should the nurse take?
    ☐ 1. Heat the formula in a microwave.
    ☐ 2. Place the client in a semi-Fowler position.
    ☐ 3. Obtain a sterile gavage bag and tubing.
    ☐ 4. Weigh the client before administering the feeding.

101. An unconscious client is to receive 200 mL of tube feeding every 4 hours. The nurse checks for the client's gastric residual before administering the next scheduled feeding and obtains 40 mL of gastric residual. What should the nurse do **next**?
☐ 1. Withhold the tube feeding, and notify the health care provider (HCP).
☐ 2. Dispose of the residual, and continue with the feeding.
☐ 3. Delay feeding the client for 1 hour, and then recheck the residual.
☐ 4. Readminister the residual to the client, and continue with the feeding.

The Adult in Pain

102. The health care provider (HCP) prescribes morphine sulfate 2 to 4 mg intravenous (IV) push every 2 hours as needed (PRN) for a client who has postoperative pain following abdominal surgery. Before performing an abdominal dressing change with packing at 1000, the nurse assesses the client's pain level as 1 on a scale of 0 to 10, with 0 being no pain and 10 being the worst pain. The client is awake and oriented, and their vital signs are within normal limits. The nurse reviews the pain medication record (see chart). What action should the nurse take?

Medication Record

Time	Pain Level	Intervention
0700	8	Morphine 4 mg IV
0900	4	Morphine 2 mg IV
1000	1	

☐ 1. Perform the dressing change.
☐ 2. Administer morphine 2 mg IV before the dressing change.
☐ 3. Administer morphine 4 mg IV after the dressing change.
☐ 4. Call the HCP for a new medication prescription.

103. A client is arousing from a coma and keeps saying, "Just stop the pain." The nurse responds based on the knowledge that the client's **first** response to pain will be to do what?
☐ 1. Tolerate the pain.
☐ 2. Decrease the perception of pain.
☐ 3. Escape the source of pain.
☐ 4. Divert attention from the source of pain.

104. Ergotamine tartrate is prescribed for a client's migraine headaches. What is an expected outcome of the use of this drug?
☐ 1. prevention of the migraine
☐ 2. aborting the developing migraine
☐ 3. relief from the sleeplessness experienced in the past after a migraine
☐ 4. relief from the vision problems experienced in the past after a migraine

105. A client is using biofeedback to manage pain. The nurse can explain to the client that biofeedback will enable the client to exert control over physiologic processes by which mechanism?
☐ 1. regulating the body processes through electrical control
☐ 2. shocking the client when an undesirable response is elicited
☐ 3. monitoring the body processes for the therapist to interpret
☐ 4. translating the signals of body processes into observable forms

106. A client is receiving massage therapy to relieve pain. Which statement explains why massage is an effective way to relieve pain?
Massage therapy:
☐ 1. blocks pain impulses from the spinal cord to the brain.
☐ 2. blocks pain impulses from the brain to the spinal cord.
☐ 3. stimulates the release of endorphins.
☐ 4. distracts the client's focus on the source of the pain.

107. A client is using patient-controlled analgesia (PCA) to manage postoperative pain. What should the nurse do when assisting the client with the PCA?
☐ 1. Reassure the client that pain will be relieved.
☐ 2. Document the client's response to pain medication.
☐ 3. Instruct the client to continue pressing the system's button whenever pain occurs.
☐ 4. Titrate pain medication until the client is free from pain.

108. A client has a patient-controlled analgesia (PCA) infusion to manage postoperative pain. Despite receiving a dose of pain medication, the client rates the pain at 8 on a 0 to 10 pain scale. What should the nurse do **first**?
☐ 1. Check the PCA pump function.
☐ 2. Inspect the infusion site.
☐ 3. Assess vital signs.
☐ 4. Notify the health care provider (HCP).

109. A client is using healing touch therapy to manage pain. What should the nurse tell the client about how healing touch can be effective in pain management?
Healing touch involves:
☐ 1. directing the flow of energy fields.
☐ 2. lightly touching the client's skin.
☐ 3. massaging the client's muscles.
☐ 4. increasing endorphin production.

110. The nurse is assessing a client for pain. Which finding is **most** significant?
The client:
☐ 1. protects a specific area of the body.
☐ 2. tells the nurse about experiencing pain.
☐ 3. has a change in vital signs.
☐ 4. appears to be uncomfortable.

111. A client who is 89 years of age is in traction for a broken hip. At 1100 on March 26, the client is experiencing pain. Prescriptions include morphine sulfate 2 to 4 mg intravenous (IV) push every 2 to 4 hours for pain. The client rates the pain as an 8 on the visual analog scale (0 to 10). Before intervening to manage the pain, the nurse reviews the progress notes (see exhibit).

Nurse's Notes

Date	Time	Progress Notes
3/26	0900	Client is alert and oriented. Vital signs: pulse 80, respirations 14, BP 100/80 mm Hg, and oxygen saturation by pulse oximeter 9.2%. Received morphine sulfate 2 mg by intravenous push (IVP).
3/26	1000	Client has pain of 4 on the Visual Analog Scale (0–10). Respirations are 10.

At 1100 on March 26, what should the nurse do?
☐ 1. Reposition the client for comfort, and administer pain medication in another 2 hours.
☐ 2. Administer 2 mg morphine sulfate IV push now, and reassess in 10 to 15 minutes.
☐ 3. Call the health care provider for supplemental medication to relax the client and promote sedation.
☐ 4. Administer 2 mg morphine sulfate IV push in 2 hours if the respirations are above 12 breaths/min.

Managing Care, Quality, and Safety of Adults with Neurologic Health Problems

112. The nurse is planning care for a client with Guillain-Barré syndrome. Which activity can the nurse delegate to the unlicensed assistive personnel (UAP)?
☐ 1. Assess weakness with range-of-motion exercises.
☐ 2. Reposition the client every 2 hours.
☐ 3. Suction the endotracheal tube.
☐ 4. Show the client how to do deep-breathing exercises.

113. An unlicensed assistive personnel (UAP) is providing care to a client with left-sided paralysis. Which action by the UAP indicates that the nurse should provide further instruction?
☐ 1. providing passive range-of-motion exercises to the left extremities during the bed bath
☐ 2. elevating the foot of the bed to reduce edema
☐ 3. pulling up the client under the left shoulder when getting the client out of bed to a chair
☐ 4. putting high-top tennis shoes on the client after bathing

114. The nurse notices that a client with Parkinson's disease is coughing frequently when eating. Which action should the nurse take?
☐ 1. Have the client hyperextend the neck when swallowing.
☐ 2. Tell the client to place the chin firmly against the chest when eating.
☐ 3. Thicken all liquids before offering them to the client.
☐ 4. Place the client on a clear liquid diet.

115. The nurse is assigned to four clients. After receiving a change-of-shift report at 0700, the nurse should assess which client **first**?
☐ 1. a 23-year-old with a migraine headache who has severe nausea associated with retching
☐ 2. a 45-year-old who is scheduled for a craniotomy in 30 minutes and needs preoperative teaching
☐ 3. a 59-year-old with Parkinson's disease who will need a swallowing assessment before breakfast
☐ 4. a 63-year-old with multiple sclerosis who has an oral temperature of 101.8°F (38.8°C) and flank pain

116. The nurse has asked the unlicensed assistive personnel (UAP) to ambulate a client with Parkinson's disease. The nurse observes the UAP pulling on the client's arms to get the client to walk forward. What should the nurse do?
☐ 1. Have the UAP keep a steady pull on the client to promote forward ambulation.
☐ 2. Explain how to overcome a freezing gait by telling the client to march in place.
☐ 3. Assist the UAP with getting the client back in bed.
☐ 4. Give the client a muscle relaxant.

117. The nurse is assessing an unconscious client. Which pressure point area(s) should the nurse monitor for this client when positioned on the right side (see figure). Select all that apply.

☐ 1. ankles
☐ 2. ear
☐ 3. greater trochanter
☐ 4. heels
☐ 5. shoulder

118. The nurse ascertains that there is a discrepancy in the records of the use of a controlled substance for a client who is taking large doses of narcotic pain medication. What should the nurse do **next**?
☐ 1. Notify the police.
☐ 2. Contact the hospital's administration or legal department.
☐ 3. Notify the pharmacy technician who delivered the controlled substance.
☐ 4. Notify the nursing supervisor of the clinical unit.

119. The nurse is caring for a client who continues to be confused about time and place. The client has intravenous fluid infusing. The nurse attempts to reorient the client, but the client remains unable to understand. To maintain client safety, the nurse should do what **first**?
☐ 1. Ask the family to stay with the client.
☐ 2. Contact the health care provider, and request a prescription for soft wrist restraints.
☐ 3. Increase the frequency of client observation.
☐ 4. Administer a sedative.

120. The nurse finds a confused client with soft wrist restraints in place (see figure). What should the nurse do **first**?

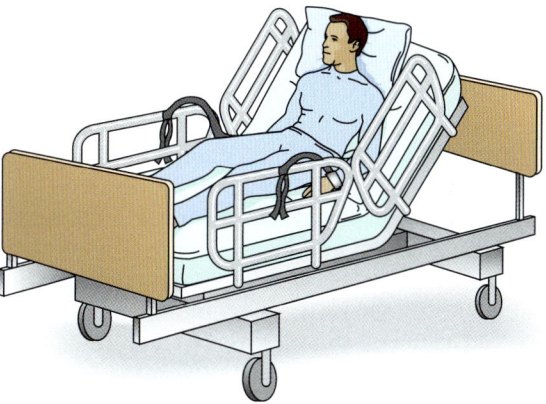

☐ 1. Assess and document the condition of the client's skin beneath the restraint.
☐ 2. Untie the restraint, and resecure it to the bed frame using a quick-release knot.
☐ 3. Release the restraint, and perform passive range-of-motion exercises.
☐ 4. Ask if the client needs to use the restroom.

Answers, Rationales, and Test-Taking Strategies

The answers and rationales for each question follow below, along with keys (🔑) to the client need (CN) and cognitive level (CL) for each question. In addition, questions that measure clinical judgment will be coded (CJ). As you check your answers, use the **Content Mastery and Test-Taking Skill Self-Analysis** worksheet (tear-out worksheet in the back of the book) to identify the reason(s) for not answering the questions correctly. For additional information about test-taking skills and strategies for answering questions, refer to pages 12–51 in Part 1 of this book.

The Adult with a Head Injury

1. **2, 3, 4.** The nurse should maintain ICP by elevating the head of the bed 30 degrees and monitoring neurologic status. An ICP of 28 mm Hg with 20 to 25 mm Hg as the upper limit of normal indicates increased ICP, and the nurse should notify the HCP. Coughing and range-of-motion exercises will increase ICP and should be avoided in the early postoperative stage.

    🔑 CN: Physiological adaptation; CL: Analyze

2. **1, 4.** The nurse must monitor the systolic and diastolic blood pressure to obtain the mean arterial pressure (MAP), which represents the pressure needed for each cardiac cycle to perfuse the brain. The nurse must also monitor the CPP, which is obtained from the ICP and the MAP. The nurse should also monitor urine output, respirations, and pain; however, crucial measurements needed to maintain CPP are ICP and MAP. When ICP equals MAP, there is no CPP.

    🔑 CN: Management of care; CL: Analyze

3. **80 mm Hg**

    To obtain the MAP, use this formula:

    $\text{MAP} = [\text{systolic BP} + (2 \times \text{diastolic BP})] \div 3$

    $\text{MAP} = [120 + (2 \times 60)] \div 3$

    $\text{MAP} = 240 \div 3 = 80$.

    🔑 CN: Management of care; CL: Apply

4. **2, 3.** The nurse should determine if the client's pupils are equal and react to light and ask the client if they have a headache. Confusion, agitation, and restlessness are subtle clinical manifestations of increased intracranial pressure (ICP). At this time, it is not appropriate for the nurse to find a television or arrange for the client to see their spouse and baby. Administering a sedative at this time will obscure the assessment of increased ICP.

    🔑 CN: Management of care; CL: Analyze

5. **3.** The client has a score of 6 (eye opening to pain = 2; verbal response, incomprehensible sounds = 2; best motor response, abnormal extension = 2); a score lower than 7 is indicative of coma. Although the nurse should continue to speak to the client, at this time, the client will not be able to be aroused. The nurse should continue to provide skin care and appropriate alignment, but the client will continue to have a motor response of limb extension. It is not necessary to notify the HCP as this assessment does not represent a significant change in neurologic status.

    🔑 CN: Physiological adaptation; CL: Analyze

6. **1.** The highest priority for a client with multiple head and neck injuries is to establish an open airway for effective ventilation and oxygenation. Unless the client has a patent airway, other care measures will be futile. Determining the client's identity and the amount of blood lost, stopping bleeding from open wounds, and checking for a neck fracture are important nursing interventions to be completed after the airway and ventilation are established.

    🔑 CN: Safety and infection control; CL: Analyze

7. **4, 3, 2, 1.** The first step in providing care for a client with delirium is to ensure the client's safety by raising the side rail. The nurse should speak calmly to the client using short sentences when explaining the care given. The nurse should maintain a quiet environment to prevent overstimulation by removing extraneous noises, dimming the lights, and limiting visitors. When the underlying problems related to the head injury are resolved, the delirium likely will improve.

    🔑 CN: Physiological adaptation; CL: Analyze

8. **1.** Increasing ICP causes unequal pupils as a result of pressure on the third cranial nerve. Increasing ICP causes an increase in the systolic pressure, which reflects the additional pressure needed to perfuse the brain. It increases the pressure on the vagus nerve, which produces bradycardia, and it causes an increase in body temperature from hypothalamic damage.

    🔑 CN: Reduction of risk potential; CL: Analyze

9. **3.** The clear drainage must be analyzed to determine whether it is nasal drainage or cerebrospinal fluid (CSF). The nurse should not give the client tissues because it is important to

know how much leakage of CSF is occurring. Compressing the nares will obstruct the drainage flow. It is inappropriate to tilt the head back, which would allow the fluid to drain down the throat and not be collected for a sample. It is inappropriate to administer an antihistamine because the drainage may not be from postnasal drip.

🗝 CN: Reduction of risk potential; CL: Analyze

10. **1.** Neural control of respiration takes place in the brain stem. Deterioration and pressure produce slow and irregular respirations. Rapid and shallow respirations, asymmetric chest movements, and nasal flaring are more characteristic of respiratory distress or hypoxia.

🗝 CN: Physiological adaptation; CL: Apply

11. **3.** Normal ICP is 15 mm Hg or less for 15 to 30 seconds or longer. Hyperventilation causes vasoconstriction, which reduces cerebrospinal fluid and blood volume, two important factors for reducing a sustained ICP of 20 mm Hg. A cooling blanket is used to control the elevation of temperature because a fever increases the metabolic rate, which in turn increases ICP. High doses of barbiturates may be used to reduce the increased cellular metabolic demands. Fluid volume and inotropic drugs are used to maintain cerebral perfusion by supporting the cardiac output and keeping the cerebral perfusion pressure higher than 80 mm Hg.

🗝 CN: Physiological adaptation; CL: Analyze

12. **4.** A decrease in the client's LOC is an early indicator of the deterioration of the client's neurologic status. Changes in LOC, such as restlessness and irritability, may be subtle. Widening of the pulse pressure, a decrease in the pulse rate, and dilated, fixed pupils occur later if the increased ICP is not treated.

🗝 CN: Physiological adaptation; CL: Analyze

13. **1.** The client's ICP is elevated, and the client should be positioned to avoid extreme neck flexion or extension. The head of the bed is usually elevated 15 to 20 degrees to drain the venous sinuses and thus decrease the ICP. Trendelenburg's position places the client's head lower than the body, which would increase ICP. Lateral recumbent position and elevating the head on two pillows may extend or flex the neck, which increases ICP.

🗝 CN: Reduction of risk potential; CL: Analyze

14. **2.** After administering mannitol, the nurse closely monitors intake and output because mannitol promotes diuresis and is given primarily to pull water from the extracellular fluid of the edematous brain. Mannitol can cause hypokalemia and may lead to muscle contractions, not muscle relaxation. Signs and symptoms, such as widening pulse pressure and pupil dilation, should not occur because mannitol serves to decrease ICP.

🗝 CN: Pharmacological and parenteral therapies; CL: Analyze

15. **4.** The correct motor function test for C8 is a hand-grasp check. The motor function check for C4 to C5 is shoulders shrugging against the downward pressure of the examiner's hands. The motor function check for C5 to C6 is an arm pulling up from a resting position against resistance. The motor function check for C7 is an arm straightening out from a flexed position against resistance.

🗝 CN: Management of care; CL: Analyze

16. **2.** It is best for the client to wear mitts, which help prevent the client from pulling on the IV without causing additional agitation. Using a jacket or wrist restraint or tucking the client's arms and hands under the sheet restricts movement and adds to feelings of being confined, all of which would add to the agitation and increase the client's intracranial pressure.

🗝 CN: Physiological adaptation; CL: Analyze

17. **3.** Vigorous coughing is contraindicated for a client at risk for increased ICP because coughing increases ICP. If the client has a cough, the nurse can consider requesting a prescription for a cough suppressant. The client can continue deep-breathing exercises. Turning and passive ROM exercises can be continued with care not to extend or flex the neck.

🗝 CN: Reduction of risk potential; CL: Analyze

18. **3.** Recovery from a serious head injury is a long-term process that may continue for months or years. Depending on the extent of the injury, clients who are transferred to rehabilitation facilities most likely will continue to exhibit cognitive and mobility impairments as well as behavior and personality changes. The client would be expected to participate in the rehabilitation efforts to the extent they are capable. Family members and significant others will need long-term support to help them cope with the changes that have occurred in the client.

🗝 CN: Physiological adaptation; CL: Evaluate

19. **3.** The Glasgow Coma Scale is used to determine the extent of neurologic changes, which can include increased intracranial pressure (ICP).

The decreases in this score are an early indicator of increasing ICP. The nurse should first position the client in the supine position with the head of the bed elevated at 30 degrees. A side-lying position or having the head of the bed elevated beyond 30 degrees can decrease cerebral perfusion. Continued assessment and a more in-depth neurologic examination will help determine this. If repositioning the client improves the Glasgow Coma Scale score, the nurse does not need to contact the surgeon and should continue to monitor the client for changes. The nurse should determine the total amount of fluid intake before considering adjusting the fluid rate.

CN: Physiological adaptation; CL: Synthesis

20. 4. The client is exhibiting extension posturing indicating severe brain stem or midbrain damage, which may be a sign of irreversible damage. Flaccid paralysis occurs when there is no resistance to passive range of motion or voluntary movement. Flexion posturing is a sign of brain damage and communication with nerves in the spinal cord and is not as dangerous a sign as extension posturing. Chronic spastic paralysis results from damage to the voluntary movement system between the brain and the muscles.

CN: Physiological Adaptation; CL: Analysis

21. 2. Cluster breathing consists of clusters of irregular breaths followed by periods of apnea on an irregular basis. A lesion in the upper medulla or lower pons is usually the cause of cluster breathing. Because the client had a bleed in the occipital lobe, which is just superior and posterior to the pons and medulla, clinical manifestations that indicate a new lesion are monitored very closely in case another bleed ensues. The nurse should notify the HCP immediately so that treatment can begin before respirations cease. The client is not obtaining sufficient oxygen, and the depth of breathing is assisted by the ventilator. The HCP will determine changes in the ventilator settings.

CN: Physiological adaptation; CL: Analyze

22. 2. Elevating the head of the bed to 30 degrees is contraindicated for infratentorial craniotomies because it could cause herniation of the brain down onto the brain stem and spinal cord, resulting in sudden death. Elevation of the head of the bed to 30 degrees with the head turned to the side opposite the incision, if not contraindicated by the increased intracranial pressure, is used for supratentorial craniotomies.

CN: Physiological adaptation; CL: Analyze

23. 3, 4. The nurse should immediately report changes that indicate increasing intracranial pressure (ICP): bradycardia, increasing systolic pressure, and widening pulse pressure. As ICP increases and the brain becomes more compressed, respirations become rapid, blood pressure decreases, and the pulse slows further; these are very ominous signs. Decreased arterial blood pressure and tachycardia can indicate bleeding elsewhere in the body. Decreasing urinary output indicates decreased tissue perfusion. The nurse monitors changes and notifies the HCP if trends continue.

CN: Physiological adaptation; CL: Analyze

24. 4. It is important to first explain where a client is to orient them to time, person, and place. Offering to get the family and asking questions to determine orientation are important, but the first comments should let the client know where they are and what has happened. It is useful to be empathetic to the client, but making a comment such as "I'll bet you are a little confused" is not helpful and may cause anxiety.

CN: Psychosocial adaptation; CL: Analyze

The Adult with Seizures

25. 3, 1, 4, 2. To protect the client from falling, the nurse first should ease the client to the floor. It is important to protect the head and maintain a patent airway since altered breathing and excessive salivation can occur. The assessment of the postictal period should include the level of consciousness and vital signs. The nurse should record details of the seizure once the client is stable. The events preceding the seizure, timing with descriptions of each phase, body parts affected and sequence of involvement, and autonomic signs should be recorded.

CN: Safety and infection control; CL: Analyze

26. 4. A generalized tonic-clonic seizure involves both a tonic phase and a clonic phase. The tonic phase consists of loss of consciousness, dilated pupils, and muscular stiffening or contraction, which lasts about 20 to 30 seconds. The clonic phase involves repetitive movements. The seizure ends with confusion, drowsiness, and resumption of respiration. A partial seizure starts in one region of the cortex and may stay focused or spread (e.g., jerking in the extremity that spreads to other areas of the body). An absence seizure usually occurs in children and involves a vacant stare with a brief loss of consciousness that often goes unnoticed. A complex partial seizure involves facial grimacing with patting and smacking.

CN: Physiological adaptation; CL: Analyze

27. 4. The client will be asked to hold their head very still during the examination, which lasts about 30 to 60 minutes. In some instances, food and fluids may be withheld for 4 to 6 hours before the procedure if a contrast medium is used because the radiopaque substance sometimes causes nausea. There is no special preparation for a CT scan, so a shampoo the night before is not required. The client may drink fluids until 4 hours before the scan is scheduled. Electrodes are not used for a CT scan, nor is the head shaved.

🔑 CN: Physiological adaptation; CL: Analyze

28. 3. Beverages containing caffeine, such as coffee, tea, cola, and energy drinks, are withheld before an EEG because of the stimulating effects of the caffeine on the brain waves. A meal should not be omitted before an EEG because low blood sugar could alter brain wave patterns; the client can have the entire meal except for the coffee. The client does not need to be on a liquid diet or NPO.

🔑 CN: Physiological adaptation; CL: Analyze

29. 3. For phenytoin to be properly absorbed and provide maximum benefit to the client, nutritional supplements must be stopped before and after delivery. The head of the bed is elevated 30 degrees since this client has a tube feeding infusing; it is not necessary to elevate the bed any further. Blood levels are usually drawn before giving a dose of phenytoin, not after. It is not necessary to flush with such a large amount of water (150 mL) before and after administering phenytoin.

🔑 CN: Pharmacological and parenteral therapies; CL: Analyze

30. 2. Gabapentin may impair vision. Changes in vision, concentration, or coordination should be reported to the HCP. Gabapentin should not be stopped abruptly because of the potential for status epilepticus; this is a medication that must be tapered off. Gabapentin is to be stored at room temperature and out of direct light. It should not be taken with antacids.

🔑 CN: Pharmacological and parenteral therapies; CL: Analyze

31. 3. A priority for the client in the postictal phase (after a seizure) is to assess the client's breathing pattern for effective rate, rhythm, and depth. The nurse should apply oxygen and ventilation to the client as appropriate. Other interventions, to be completed after the airway has been established, include reorientation of the client to time, person, and place. Determining the client's level of sleepiness is useful, but it is not a priority. Positioning the client comfortably promotes rest but is of less importance than ascertaining that the airway is patent.

🔑 CN: Reduction of risk potential; CL: Analyze

32. 4. Carbamazepine is an anticonvulsant that helps prevent further seizures and is the most effective intervention for preventing seizure risk while the client is undergoing diagnostic tests for seizures. Bed rest, sedation, and providing privacy do not minimize the risk for seizures.

🔑 CN: Pharmacological and parenteral therapies; CL: Analyze

33. -/+ **1, 2, 4, 5, 6, 7.** During a seizure, the nurse should note the time of onset of the seizure; the level of consciousness; the movement of the client's head and eyes; the pupil size; and muscle rigidity, especially when the seizure first begins. This information helps locate the trigger focus in the brain. It is typically not possible to assess the client's heart rate, blood pressure, or oxygen saturation during a tonic-clonic seizure because the muscle contractions make assessment difficult. The nurse can obtain information about when the last dose of anticonvulsant medication was administered once the client has recovered from the seizure.

🔑 CN: Physiological adaptation; CL: Analyze

34. 1. The nurse should expect a client in the postictal phase to experience drowsiness to somnolence because exhaustion results from the abnormal spontaneous neuron firing and tonic-clonic motor response. An inability to move a muscle part is not expected after a tonic-clonic seizure because a lack of motor function would be related to a complication, such as a lesion, tumor, or stroke, in the correlating brain tissue. A change in sensation would not be expected because this would indicate a complication such as an injury to the peripheral nerve pathway to the corresponding part of the central nervous system. Hypotension is not typically a problem after a seizure.

🔑 CN: Physiological adaptation; CL: Analyze

35. 2. Anticonvulsant drug therapy should never be stopped suddenly; doing so can lead to life-threatening status epilepticus. Phenytoin sodium does not carry a risk for physical dependency or lead to hypoglycemia. Phenytoin has antiarrhythmic properties, and discontinuation does not cause heart block.

🔑 CN: Pharmacological and parenteral therapies; CL: Apply

36. 3. An aura is a premonition of an impending seizure. Auras usually are of a sensory nature (e.g., an olfactory, visual, gustatory, or auditory sensation); some may be of a psychic nature. Evaluating an aura may help identify the area of the brain from which the seizure originates. Auras occur before a seizure, not during or after (postictal). They are not similar to hallucinations or amnesia or related to relaxation.

CN: Physiological adaptation; CL: Analyze

37. 2. Toxic effects of topiramate include nephrolithiasis, and clients are encouraged to drink six to eight glasses of water a day to dilute the urine and flush the renal tubules to avoid stone formation. Topiramate is taken in divided doses because it produces drowsiness. Although eating fresh fruits is desirable from a nutritional standpoint, this is not related to the topiramate. The drug does not have to be taken with meals.

CN: Pharmacological and parenteral therapies; CL: Evaluate

38. 3. A common adverse effect of long-term phenytoin therapy is an overgrowth of gingival tissues. Problems may be minimized with good oral hygiene, but in some cases, overgrown tissues must be removed surgically. Phenytoin does not cause weight gain, insomnia, or deteriorating eyesight.

CN: Pharmacological and parenteral therapies; CL: Evaluate

39. −/+ **1, 2, 3.** The nurse should assess the number and type of seizures the client has experienced since starting clonazepam monotherapy for seizure control. The nurse should also determine if the client might be pregnant because clonazepam crosses the placental barrier. The nurse should also ask about the client's use of alcohol because alcohol potentiates the action of clonazepam. Although the nurse may want to check on the client's diet or use of cigarettes for health maintenance and promotion, such information is not specifically related to clonazepam therapy.

CN: Pharmacological and parenteral therapies; CL: Evaluate

The Adult with a Stroke

40. −/+ **1, 4, 5.** A headache (which is treated with analgesics) is commonly associated with an ischemic CVA. A conscious client responds to comfort measures. Bleeding is a side effect of recombinant tissue plasminogen (t-PA) therapy to dissolve the clots; the absence of bleeding is a desired outcome. The reduction of dysphagia and visual disturbances is unpredictable and less likely to occur during this phase.

CN: Pharmacological and parenteral therapies; CL: Evaluate

41. 1. The nurse should question the prescription to administer labetalol to decrease the BP to less than 20/80 mm Hg. It is not recommended that diastolic blood pressure is less than 90 mm Hg. Mean arterial pressure (MAP) should be kept between 80 and 110 mm Hg. The client's presenting BP is 220/120 mm Hg, which would indicate a MAP of 146 mm Hg. When a client has a stroke, autoregulation is a protective mechanism used to protect the brain. Elevated blood pressure helps increase cerebral perfusion. The standard of care is to administer t-PA within 4.5 hours of signs and symptoms of a stroke. Normal saline is an isotonic solution recommended for a client experiencing an ischemic stroke. Keeping the head of the bed at 30 degrees helps decrease intracranial pressure.

CN: Safe and effective care environment; CL: Analysis

42. 3. Following a stroke, it is easiest for clients with dysphagia (difficulty swallowing) to swallow solid foods; the nurse should introduce foods on the unaffected side and verify that the client has swallowed the food and is not retaining it in the cheek. Liquid foods are difficult to swallow, and the nurse can instruct the client and family to offer thickened liquids. The client with facial paralysis will have difficulty sipping using a straw. The nurse can raise the head of the bed to 90 degrees, or instruct the client to sit up, if possible, while eating to prevent choking and aspiration.

CN: Physiological adaptation; CL: Apply

43. 15 points

The Glasgow Coma Scale provides three objective neurologic assessments: spontaneity of eye opening, best motor response, and best verbal response on a scale of 3 to 15. The client who scores the best on all three assessments scores 15 points.

CN: Reduction of risk potential; CL: Apply

44. −/+ **2, 3, 5.** The maximum dosage of warfarin sodium is not achieved until 3 to 4 days after starting the medication, and the effects of the drug continue for 4 to 5 days after discontinuing the medication. The client should have blood levels tested periodically to make sure that the desired level is maintained. Warfarin has a peak action of 9 hours. Vitamin K is the antidote for warfarin; protamine sulfate is the antidote for heparin.

CN: Pharmacological and parenteral therapies; CL: Evaluate

The Adult with Neurologic Health Problems **651**

45. 1. The UAP should position an unconscious client on the side, not on the back, with the head flat. A lateral position helps secretions escape from the throat and mouth, minimizing the risk for aspiration. It may be necessary to suction the client if they aspirate. Suction equipment should be nearby. It is safe to use a padded tongue blade, and the client should receive oral care, including brushing with a toothbrush.

🗝️ CN: Reduction of risk potential; CL: Analyze

46. 3. Studies show that clients who receive recombinant t-PA treatment within 3 hours after the onset of a stroke have better outcomes. The time from the onset of a stroke to t-PA treatment is critical. A complete health assessment and history are not possible when a client is receiving emergency care. Upcoming surgical procedures may need to be delayed because of the administration of t-PA, which is a priority in the immediate treatment of the current stroke. While the nurse should identify which medications the client is taking, it is more important to know the time of the onset of the stroke to determine the course of action for administering t-PA.

🗝️ CN: Pharmacological and parenteral therapies; CL: Analyze

47. 3. Control of blood pressure is critical during the first 24 hours after treatment because an intracerebral hemorrhage is the major adverse effect of thrombolytic therapy. Vital signs are monitored, and blood pressure is maintained as identified by the HCP and specific to the client's ischemic tissue needs and risk for bleeding from treatment. The other vital signs are important, but the priority is to monitor blood pressure.

🗝️ CN: Reduction of risk potential; CL: Analyze

48.
STEP 1

0/1 1, 2, 4, 5. The client has right-sided arm weakness, headache, and notable slurred speech, which are findings that indicate the client may be having a stroke. The heart rate and the respiration rate are within normal limits.

🗝️ CJ: Case study; Step 1: Recognize cues; CL: Understand

49.
STEP 2

0/1 The nurse determines that the client is at risk for cranial **hemorrhaging** if the client were to be administered tissue plasminogen activator (t-PA) when experiencing a(n) **hemorrhagic** stroke because the blood vessels of the brain have already **ruptured**.

In an ischemic stroke or transient ischemic attach, the client is experiencing a blood clot that has fully or partially blocked off blood flow to the brain. The client can be administered t-PA to dissolve the clot and return blood flow. If a client were to be given t-PA with a hemorrhagic stroke, the bleeding of the blood vessels would be made significantly worse.

🗝️ CJ: Case study; Step 2: Analyze cues; CL: Analyze

50.
STEP 3

0/1 1, 4, 5. The client needs a CT scan as soon as possible to determine if they are experiencing a stroke and the type of stroke. The nurse should perform neurologic assessments every 15 minutes, and a blood glucose check should be obtained to ensure the client is not exhibiting signs and symptoms of hypoglycemia, which could mimic a stroke. An x-ray is not needed at this time because the CT scan allows more views of the anatomy being scanned. Potassium is not needed until a laboratory report indicates a low potassium level. t-PA may be required, but it should not be administered before determining the type of stroke because of the risk for hemorrhage.

🗝️ CJ: Case study; Step 3: Prioritize hypothesis; CL: Analyze

51.
STEP 4

−/+ 4, 5. If the client is currently taking anticoagulant medications with elevated clotting times, t-PA should not be administered. Additionally, if the client has had gastrointestinal bleeding within the past 3 weeks, t-PA should not be administered. It is appropriate to administer the medication if the client's symptoms began less than 4 hours ago, if the client is experiencing disabling stroke symptoms, and if the client is younger than 85 years. Metformin is not a contraindication to receiving t-PA.

🗝️ CJ: Case study; Step 4: Generate solutions; CL: Create

52.
STEP 5

−/+ 2, 4, 5. 6. The nurse should obtain a dysphagia screening before introducing any solids or liquids to prevent aspiration. If it is safe for the client to be presented with solids and liquids, the nurse should introduce the foods on the unaffected side. The nurse can contact occupational therapy to request they work with the client to improve their swallowing technique. The nurse can teach the client to tuck their chin (chin tuck) to improve swallowing. The client does not need to sit up above 90 degrees; the head of the bed should be raised above 30 degrees. A client with dysphagia commonly has more difficulty swallowing fluids than solids; liquids should be thickened to avoid aspiration.

🗝️ CJ: Case study; Step 5: Take action; CL: Apply

53.

STEP 6

-/+ 1, 2, 4. The client's headache pain is significantly less, indicating that blood flow has returned in the brain and that the blood pressure has lowered. The client's slurred speech is found to be improving, also indicating that the medication is having the intended action. The client is now exhibiting resistance against gravity with the right upper extremity, indicating the medication is improving blood flow in the brain. Pupillary response is critical to monitor for changes in the cranial nerves caused by the stroke; however, the client's pupils were not found to be affected by the client's ischemic stroke. If the client began to experience any signs of cerebral edema, having a valid assessment of the pupil size and pupillary response could help detect these changes. The glucose level is important to monitor after medication administration because the levels may become erratic as a response to a stroke, but the blood glucose levels were both within normal limits. The client's temperature has not changed significantly, but the nurse should continue to monitor the temperature to determine if the increase is becoming a trend.

CJ: Case study; Step 6: Evaluate outcomes; CL: Analyze

54. 2. It is crucial to monitor the pupil size and pupillary response to indicate changes around the cranial nerves. The cholesterol level is not a priority assessment, though it may be an assessment to be addressed for long-term healthy lifestyle rehabilitation. Bowel sounds need to be assessed because an ileus or constipation can develop, but this is not a priority in the first 24 hours when the primary concerns are cerebral hemorrhage and increased intracranial pressure. An echocardiogram is not needed for a client with a thrombotic stroke without heart problems.

CN: Physiological adaptation; CL: Analyze

55. 4, 2, 1, 3. Increased agitation with suctioning will increase ICP, and the nurse should explain the procedure and calm the patient first. The nurse should then hyperoxygenate the client before and after suctioning to prevent hypoxia since hypoxia causes vasodilation of the cerebral vessels and increases ICP. The airway should then be suctioned for no more than 10 seconds. The mouth can be suctioned once the airway is clear to remove oral secretions. Once the mouth is suctioned, the suction catheter should be discarded.

CN: Physiological adaptation; CL: Analyze

56. 1. The primary reason for the nursing assessment of a client's functional status before the stroke is to guide the rehabilitation plan. The assessment does not help predict how far the rehabilitation team can help the client recover from the residual effects of the stroke, only what plans can help a client who has moved from one functional level to another. The nursing assessment of the client's functional status does not help the client recognize limitations.

CN: Physiological adaptation; CL: Apply

57. 1. Rolling the client with hemiparalysis is the most effective method to use when there is only one person to help the client change positions from one side to another. The nurse must keep the client in anatomically neutral positions and ensure that the limbs are properly supported. Sliding a client on a sheet causes friction and is to be avoided. Friction injures the skin and predisposes to pressure ulcer formation. The client may be lifted as long as the nurse has assistance and uses proper body mechanics to avoid injury. Before asking the client to use a trapeze to use the bedpan, the nurse should assess the client's strength and ability to assist.

CN: Reduction of risk potential; CL: Analyze

58. 35. This client has a fall risk score of 35 and is at medium fall risk due to the client's secondary diagnosis (15) and IV access (20). Although the client has paraplegia, this does not affect the client's fall risk assessment as the client will be either in bed or in a wheelchair; therefore, the client is not assessed points on the fall risk for "ambulatory aid" or "gait."

CN: Safety and infection control; CL: Evaluate

59. 3. The use of ankle-high tennis shoes is most effective in preventing plantar flexion (footdrop) because they add support to the foot and keep it in the correct anatomic position. Footboards stimulate spasms and are not routinely recommended. Regular repositioning and range-of-motion exercises are important interventions, but the client's foot needs to be in the correct anatomic position to prevent overextension of the muscle and tendon. Massaging does not prevent plantar flexion and, if rigorous, could release emboli.

CN: Reduction of risk potential; CL: Analyze

60. -/+ 1, 2, 4. Placing a pillow in the axilla so the arm is away from the body keeps the arm abducted and prevents skin from touching skin to avoid skin breakdown. Placing a pillow under the slightly flexed arm so the hand is higher than the elbow prevents dependent edema. Positioning a hand cone (not a rolled washcloth) in the hand prevents hand contractures. Immobilization of the extremity may cause a painful shoulder-hand syndrome. Flexion contractures of the hand, wrist, and elbow can result from immobility of the weak or paralyzed extremity. It is better to extend the arms to prevent contractures.

🔑 CN: Reduction of risk potential; CL: Analyze

61. 2. Expressive aphasia is a condition in which the client understands what is heard or written but cannot say what they want to say. A communication or picture board helps the client communicate with others in that the client can point to objects or activities that they desire. Receptive aphasia is a condition in which the client does not comprehend what is being said. For this client, it is helpful to speak clearly, using short sentences or writing out directions.

🔑 CN: Physiological adaptation; CL: Analyze

62. -/+ 1, 3, 4. A client with dysphagia (difficulty swallowing) commonly has the most difficulty ingesting thin liquids, which are easily aspirated. Liquids should be thickened to avoid aspiration. Maintaining an upright position while eating is appropriate because it minimizes the risk for aspiration. Introducing foods on the unaffected side allows the client to have better control over the food bolus. The client should concentrate on chewing and swallowing; therefore, distractions should be avoided. Large pieces of food could cause choking; the food should be cut into bite-sized pieces.

🔑 CN: Safety and infection control; CL: Analyze

63. 2. Homonymous hemianopia is blindness in half of the visual field; therefore, the client would see only half of the plate. Eating only the food on half of the plate results from an inability to coordinate visual images and spatial relationships. There may be an increased preference for foods high in salt after a stroke, but this would not be related to homonymous hemianopia. Forgetting the names of foods is a sign of aphasia, which involves a cerebral cortex lesion. Being unable to swallow liquids is dysphagia, which involves motor pathways of cranial nerves IX and X, including the lower brain stem.

🔑 CN: Physiological adaptation; CL: Analyze

64. 4. To expand the visual field, the partially sighted client should be taught to turn the head from side to side when walking. Neglecting to do so may result in accidents. This technique helps maximize the use of remaining sight. Covering an eye with a patch will limit the field of vision. Personal items can be placed within sight and reach, but most accidents occur from tripping over items that cannot be seen. It may help the client to see the door, but walking presents the primary safety hazard.

🔑 CN: Reduction of risk potential; CL: Analyze

65. 3. A client who has brain damage may be emotionally labile and may cry or laugh for no explainable reason. Crying is best dealt with by attempting to divert the client's attention. Ignoring the behavior will not affect the mood swing or the crying and may increase the client's sense of isolation. Telling the client to stop is inappropriate.

🔑 CN: Psychosocial adaptation; CL: Analyze

66. -/+ 1, 3, 4, 5. The goal of communicating with a client with aphasia is to minimize frustration and exhaustion. The nurse should encourage the client to write messages or use alternative forms of communication to avoid frustration. Presenting one thought at a time decreases stimuli that may distract the client, as does speaking in a normal volume and tone. The nurse should ask the client to point to objects and encourage the use of gestures to assist in communicating.

🔑 CN: Psychosocial adaptation; CL: Analyze

67. 3. Thrombolytic enzyme agents are used for clients with a thrombotic stroke to dissolve emboli, thus reestablishing cerebral perfusion. They do not increase vascular permeability, cause vasoconstriction, or prevent further hemorrhage.

🔑 CN: Pharmacological and parenteral therapies; CL: Evaluate

The Adult with Parkinson's Disease

68. 4. When a freezing gait occurs, having the client march in place or step over actual lines, imaginary lines, or objects on the floor can promote walking. Instructing the client to take one step backward and two steps forward may also stimulate walking. Pulling the client forward can cause imbalance. The nurse does not instruct the client to use a wheelchair. The client obtains much exercise as possible; having the client remain still does not help the client obtain the momentum needed to walk.

🔑 CN: Health promotion and maintenance; CL: Apply

69. -/+ 3, 4, 5. The nurse should contact the HCP before administering carbidopa-levodopa because this medication can cause further symptoms of depression. Suicide threats in clients with a chronic illness should be taken seriously. The nurse should also determine if the client is on an MAO inhibitor because concurrent use with carbidopa-levodopa can cause a hypertensive crisis. Carbidopa-levodopa is not a treatment for depression. Having the client discuss feelings is appropriate when the prescription is finalized.

🔑 CN: Pharmacological and parenteral therapies; CL: Analyze

70. **2.** The first sign of Parkinson's disease is usually tremors. The client commonly is the first to notice this sign because the tremors may be minimal at first. Rigidity is the second sign, and bradykinesia is the third sign. Akinesia is a later stage of bradykinesia.

CN: Physiological adaptation; CL: Analyze

71. **3.** The primary focus is on maintaining a safe environment because the client with Parkinson's disease usually has a propulsive gait, characterized by a tendency to take increasingly quicker steps while walking. This type of gait commonly causes the client to fall or have trouble stopping. The client should maintain a balanced diet, enhance the immune system, and enjoy diversional activities; however, safety is the primary concern.

CN: Reduction of risk potential; CL: Create

72. **2.** Voluntary and purposeful movements often temporarily decrease or stop the tremors associated with Parkinson's disease. In some clients, however, tremors may increase with voluntary effort. Tremors associated with Parkinson's disease are not psychogenic but are related to an imbalance between dopamine and acetylcholine. Tremors cannot be reduced by distracting the client.

CN: Physiological adaptation; CL: Analyze

73. **2.** Demanding physical activity should be performed during the peak action of drug therapy. Clients should be encouraged to maintain independence in self-care activities to the greatest extent possible. Although some clients may have more energy in the morning or after rest, tremors are managed with drug therapy.

CN: Physiological adaptation; CL: Analyze

74. **1.** The primary goal of physical therapy and nursing interventions is maintaining joint flexibility and muscle strength. Parkinson's disease involves a degeneration of dopamine-producing neurons; therefore, it would be an unrealistic goal to attempt to build muscles or increase endurance. The decrease in dopamine neurotransmitters results in ataxia secondary to extrapyramidal motor system effects. Attempts to reduce ataxia through physical therapy would not be effective.

CN: Physiological adaptation; CL: Analyze

75. **3.** Vital signs should be monitored, especially during periods of adjustment. Changes, such as orthostatic hypotension, cardiac irregularities, palpitations, and light-headedness, should be reported immediately. The client may experience suicidal or paranoid ideation instead of euphoria. The nurse should monitor the client for elevated liver enzyme levels, such as lactate dehydrogenase, aspartate aminotransferase, alanine aminotransferase, blood urea nitrogen, and alkaline phosphatase, but the client should not be jaundiced. The client should not experience signs and symptoms of diabetes or a low serum glucose level, but the nurse should check the hemoglobin and hematocrit levels.

CN: Pharmacological and parenteral therapies; CL: Analyze

76. **2.** Ongoing self-care is a major focus for clients with Parkinson's disease. The client should be given additional time as needed and praised for efforts to remain independent. Firmly telling the client that they need assistance will undermine self-esteem and defeat efforts to be independent. Telling the client that their perception of the situation is unrealistic does not foster hope in their ability to perform self-care measures. Suggesting that the client modify their morning routine seems to put the hospital or the nurse's schedule before the client's needs. This will only decrease the client's self-esteem and desire to try to continue self-care, which is obviously important to the client.

CN: Psychosocial adaptation; CL: Analyze

The Adult with Multiple Sclerosis

77. **-/+** **2, 4, 5.** The client with multiple sclerosis is at risk for falls due to muscle weakness, skin breakdown due to bowel and bladder incontinence, and fatigue. The client is not at risk for dehydration; seizures are not associated with myelin destruction.

CN: Physiological integrity; CL: Analyze

78. **-/+** **2, 3, 4, 5.** Maintaining urinary function in a client with neurogenic bladder dysfunction from MS is an important goal. The client should ideally drink 1½ to 2 cups (about 400 to 500 mL) of fluids with each meal; drink about a cup (200 mL) of fluid midmorning, midafternoon, and late afternoon; and attempt to void at least every 2 hours to prevent infection and stone formation. The client may need to self-catheterize to drain residual urine in the bladder. Restricting fluids during the day will not produce sufficient urine. However, in bladder training for nighttime continence, the client may restrict fluids for 1 to 2 hours before going to bed. The client should drink at least 8 cups (about 2000 mL) of fluids every 24 hours.

CN: Physiological adaptation; CL: Create

79. ☐ **2, 3, 4, 5.** Clients with MS may have euphoria, visual disturbances such as double vision, weakness in the extremities, and loss of muscle tone and tremors. Sudden bursts of energy are not likely due to muscle weakness, and hypertension is not a direct symptom of MS.

🔑 CN: Physiological adaptation; CL: Analyze

80. 3. Baclofen is a centrally acting skeletal muscle relaxant that helps relieve the muscle spasms common in MS. Drowsiness is an adverse effect, and driving should be avoided if the medication produces a sedative effect. Baclofen does not stimulate the appetite or reduce bacteria in the urine.

🔑 CN: Pharmacological and parenteral therapies; CL: Evaluate

81. 2. Evaluating drug effectiveness is difficult because a high percentage of clients with MS exhibit unpredictable episodes of remission, exacerbation, and steady progress without apparent cause. Clients with MS do not necessarily have increased intolerance to drugs, nor do they endure long periods of exacerbation before the illness responds to a particular drug. Multiple drug use is not what makes evaluation of drug effectiveness difficult.

🔑 CN: Pharmacological and parenteral therapies; CL: Analyze

82. 1. To help the client with MS communicate effectively, the nurse can suggest that the client speak slowly and distinctly. It is not necessary for the client to use a whiteboard or to repeat words unless necessary. Speaking louder will not improve communication and may require unnecessary energy.

🔑 CN: Psychosocial adaptation; CL: Analyze

83. 4. The nurse's notes should be concise, objective, clearly stated, and relevant. This client trembles when they attempt voluntary actions, such as drinking a beverage or fastening clothing. This activity should be described exactly as it occurs so that others reading the note will not doubt the nurse's observation of the client's behavior. Identifying the "intentional" activity of daily living will help the interdisciplinary team individualize the client's plan of care. Clarifying what is meant by "worsening" with a purposeful act will facilitate the interrater reliability of the team. It is better to state what the client did than to give vague nursing orders in the nurse's notes.

🔑 CN: Management of care; CL: Apply

84. 2. The nurse can teach the client with MS who is in a bowel retraining program to set a regular time each day for elimination. A diet with adequate amounts of fiber facilitates having a bowel movement. It is not necessary to use a stool softer if bowel training, fluid intake, and the diet are having the intended outcomes. Limiting fluid intake is likely to aggravate rather than relieve symptoms when a bowel retraining program is being implemented. Furthermore, water imbalance, as well as electrolyte imbalance, tends to aggravate the signs and symptoms of MS.

🔑 CN: Physiological adaptation; CL: Analyze

85. 2. MS is a progressive, chronic neurologic disease characterized by patchy demyelination throughout the central nervous system. This interferes with the transmission of electrical impulses from one nerve cell to the next. Care for the client with MS is directed toward maintaining muscle strength, preventing deformities, preventing and treating depression, and providing client motivation. MS affects speech, coordination, and vision, but not cognition.

🔑 CN: Reduction of risk potential; CL: Analyze

86. 2. The nurse's most positive approach is to encourage a client with MS to keep active, use stress-reduction strategies, and avoid fatigue because it is important to support the immune system while remaining active. A quiet, inactive lifestyle is not necessarily indicated. Good health habits are not likely to alter the course of the disease, though they may help minimize complications. Practicing using aids that will be needed for future disabilities may be helpful but also can be discouraging.

🔑 CN: Physiological adaptation; CL: Analyze

87. ☐ **1, 3, 4, 5.** A client with impaired peripheral sensation does not feel pain as readily as does someone whose sensation is unimpaired; therefore, water temperatures should be tested carefully. The client should be advised to avoid using hot water bottles or heating pads and to protect against cold temperatures. Because the client cannot rely on minor pain as an indicator of damaged skin or sore spots, the client should carefully inspect the skin daily to visualize any injuries that they cannot feel. The client should not be instructed to avoid kitchen activities out of fear of injury; independence and self-care are also important. However, the client should meet with an occupational therapist to learn about assistive devices and techniques that can reduce injuries, such as burns and cuts that are common in kitchen activities.

🔑 CN: Reduction of risk potential; CL: Create

88. **3.** Maintaining a regular voiding pattern is the most appropriate measure to help the client avoid urinary incontinence. Fluid intake is not related to incontinence. Incontinence is related to the strength of the detrusor and urethral sphincter muscles. Inserting an indwelling catheter would be a treatment of last resort because of the increased risk for infection. If catheterization is required, intermittent self-catheterization is preferred because of its lower risk for infection. Antibiotics do not influence urinary incontinence.

   CN: Physiological adaptation; CL: Analyze

89. **2.** An individualized regular exercise program helps the client relieve muscle spasms. The client can be trained to use unaffected muscles to promote coordination because MS is a progressive, debilitating condition. The data do not indicate that the client needs psychotherapy, daycare for the granddaughter, or visits from other clients.

   CN: Physiological adaptation; CL: Analyze

The Adult with Myasthenia Gravis

90. **1.** Loss of motor function to the face and throat can cause dysphagia and places the client at risk for aspiration. Bladder dysfunction and hypertension are not associated with myasthenia gravis. Myasthenia affects nerve impulses at the neuromuscular junction, causing loss of motor function; there is no sensory deficit.

   CN: Reduction of risk potential; CL: Analyze

91. **1.** The nurse instructs the client regarding the use of artificial tears because eyelid and extraocular muscles are frequently affected by myasthenia gravis and there is a risk for corneal abrasion if the eyelids do not close completely. The client is encouraged to maintain social contacts and prevent social isolation by staying at home. Medication is taken in the morning, before activities, so the client can complete them. A nutritious diet is encouraged, and there is no indication to limit protein.

   CN: Reduction of risk potential; CL: Analyze

92. **3.** With a well-managed regimen, a client with myasthenia gravis should be able to control symptoms, maintain a normal lifestyle, and achieve a normal life expectancy. Myasthenia gravis can be controlled and need not be a fatal disease. Myasthenia gravis can be controlled, not cured. Episodes of increased muscle weakness should not occur if treatment is well managed.

   CN: Physiological adaptation; CL: Evaluate

The Unconscious Adult

93. **3.** Activated charcoal powder is administered to absorb remaining particles of salicylate. Vitamin K is an antidote for warfarin sodium. Dextrose 50% is used to treat hypoglycemia. Sodium thiosulfate is an antidote for cyanide.

   CN: Pharmacological and parenteral therapies; CL: Analyze

94. **2, 3, 4.** An excess of cholinergic agents produces urinary and fecal incontinence, increased salivation, diarrhea, and diaphoresis. In a severe overdose, CNS depression; seizures and muscle fasciculations; bradycardia or tachycardia; weakness; and respiratory arrest due to respiratory muscle paralysis occur. Anticholinergics produce dry mucous membranes. Skin rash is not a sign of overdose with a cholinergic agent.

   CN: Pharmacological and parenteral therapies; CL: Analyze

95. **3.** The spouse's initial response to this crisis is high anxiety. Anxiety must dissipate before a person can deal with the actual situation. Allowing the spouse to express their feelings can help diffuse their anxiety. The reasons for the client's actions are unknown; assumptions must be validated before they become facts. The nurse should first listen to the spouse's needs before recommending meeting with clergy. Asking the spouse to help with the client's care is appropriate at a later time.

   CN: Psychosocial adaptation; CL: Analyze

96. **2.** The nurse must clean the unconscious client's mouth carefully, apply a thin coat of a lubricant, and move the endotracheal tube to the opposite side daily to prevent dryness, crusting, inflammation, and parotiditis. The unconscious client's temperature should be monitored by a route other than oral (e.g., rectal, tympanic) because oral temperatures will be inaccurate. The client should be positioned in a lateral or semiprone position, not a supine position, to allow for drainage of secretions and for the jaw and tongue to fall forward. The client should not be dragged when turned, as may happen when a drawsheet is used. Care should be taken to lift the client's heels, buttocks, arms, and head off of the sheets when turning. Trochanter rolls, splints, foam boot aids, specialty beds, and so on—not just two pillows—should be used to keep the client in the correct body position and to decrease pressure on bony prominences.

   CN: Reduction of risk potential; CL: Analyze

97. **3.** The client is not in proper body alignment if when in the right side-lying position, the client's left arm rests on the mattress with the elbow flexed. This positioning of the arm pulls the left shoulder out of good alignment, restricting respiratory movements. The arm should be supported on a pillow. The client's head also should be placed on a small pillow to keep it in alignment with the body. The right leg should be extended on the mattress without a pillow to avoid hyperrotation of the hip. A pillow should be placed between the left and right legs with the left knee flexed so that on no parts of the legs is skin touching skin.

CN: Physiological adaptation; CL: Analyze

98. **4.** The goal of performing passive ROM exercises is to maintain joint mobility. Active exercise is needed to preserve bone and muscle mass. Passive ROM movements do not prevent bone demineralization or have a positive effect on the client's muscle tone.

CN: Physiological adaptation; CL: Evaluate

99. **2.** When the blink reflex is absent or the eyes do not close completely, the cornea may become dry and irritated. Corneal abrasion can occur. Taping the eye closed will prevent injury. Having the client wear eyeglasses or cleaning the eyelid will not protect the cornea from dryness or irritation. Artificial tears instilled once per shift are not frequent enough to prevent dryness.

CN: Reduction of risk potential; CL: Analyze

100. **2.** The client should be placed in a semi-Fowler position to reduce the risk for aspiration. The formula should be at room temperature, not heated. Administering enteral tube feedings is a clean procedure, not a sterile one; therefore, sterile supplies are not required. Clients receiving enteral feedings should be weighed regularly but not necessarily before each feeding.

CN: Reduction of risk potential; CL: Analyze

101. **4.** Gastric residuals are checked before administration of enteral feedings to determine whether gastric emptying is delayed. A residual of less than 50% of the previous feeding volume is usually considered acceptable. In this case, the amount is not excessive, and the nurse should reinstill the aspirate through the tube and then administer the feeding. If the amount of gastric residual is excessive, the nurse should notify the HCP and withhold the feeding. Disposing of the residual can cause electrolyte and fluid losses.

CN: Reduction of risk potential; CL: Analyze

The Adult in Pain

102. **2.** Morphine 2 mg was given 1 hour ago, and the client can have up to 4 mg every 2 hours. Although the pain level is at 1, the nurse should give medication before the dressing change with packing that is likely to cause discomfort. A 4-mg dose of morphine would exceed the 2-hour limit and, if given after the dressing change, would not manage pain during the procedure. The client has been responding to the pain medication dosing, and a new prescription is not required at this time.

CN: Pharmacological and parenteral therapies; CL: Analyze

103. **3.** The client's innate responses to pain are directed initially toward escaping from the source of pain. Variations in tolerance and perception of pain are apparent only in conscious clients, and only conscious clients can employ distraction to help relieve pain.

CN: Physiological adaptation; CL: Apply

104. **2.** Ergotamine tartrate is used to help abort a migraine attack. It should be taken as soon as prodromal symptoms appear. Reduced migraine severity and relief from sleeplessness and vision problems address symptoms that occur after the migraine has occurred and are not effects of ergotamine.

CN: Pharmacological and parenteral therapies; CL: Evaluate

105. **4.** Biofeedback translates body processes into observable signs so that the client can develop some control over certain body processes. Biofeedback does not involve electrical stimulation. The use of unpleasant stimuli such as electrical shock is a form of aversion therapy. Biofeedback does not involve monitoring body processes for the therapist to interpret; rather, it is a self-directed, self-care activity that reinforces learning because the client can see the results of their actions.

CN: Physiological adaptation; CL: Apply

106. **1.** A back rub stimulates the large-diameter cutaneous fibers, which block the transmission of pain impulses from the spinal cord to the brain. It does not block the transmission of pain impulses or stimulate the release of endorphins. A back rub may distract the client, but the physiologic process of fiber stimulation is the main reason a back rub is used as therapy for pain relief.

CN: Basic care and comfort; CL: Apply

107. 2. It is essential that the nurse document the client's response to pain medication on a routine, systematic basis. Reassuring the client that pain will be relieved is often not realistic. A client who continually presses the PCA button may not be getting adequate pain relief, but through careful assessment and documentation, the effectiveness of pain relief interventions can be evaluated and modified. Pain medication is not titrated until the client is free from pain but rather until an acceptable level of pain management is reached.

CN: Pharmacological and parenteral therapies; CL: Analyze

108. 2. The nurse should first check the infusion site to be sure the site has not been infiltrated. Next, the nurse should check the PCA pump to determine if it is functioning properly. Assessing vital signs would be important to provide additional data about the possible cause of pain, but this is not the first action at this time. It is not necessary to notify the HCP unless the infusion site or pump is malfunctioning and other methods of managing the pain are required.

CN: Pharmacological and parenteral therapies; CL: Analyze

109. 1. The nurse using healing touch affects a client's pain primarily through assessing and directing the flow of energy fields. Healing touch removes energy congestion so energy channels can facilitate integration of the body, mind, and soul to promote healing. Healing touch can involve touching, but it does not have to involve body contact. Massage is not involved with healing touch. The goal of healing touch is not to increase the production of endorphins.

CN: Basic care and comfort; CL: Apply

110. 2. Pain is whatever the client perceives it is; using a pain scale is the best way to have the client quantify the amount of pain. The fact that the client is protecting an area of the body, the client's vital signs, and the client's appearance of discomfort are objective rather than subjective findings; the nurse should confirm the meaning of these changes before assuming the client has pain.

CN: Basic care and comfort; CL: Analyze

111. 2. The nurse administers between 2 and 4 mg of morphine sulfate IV push every 2 to 4 hours according to the prescription for pain management. Even though the client received pain medication 2 hours ago, the client is still experiencing pain of the intensity of 8 on a scale of 0 to 10. Older adult clients may have slowed pain perception but not diminished pain intensity. The nurse starts conservatively, administering 2 mg of morphine sulfate IV push and reassessing in 15 minutes to determine the effectiveness of pain management and respiratory effort. If pain is still not relieved, the titration of morphine sulfate upward to 4 mg is optional. The single provision of nonpharmacologic interventions such as repositioning is not sufficient pain management when a client rates pain at 8 on a scale of 0 to 10. Requesting a prescription for sedation only causes the client to be unable to express their pain and does not treat the pain. Although the nurse continues to monitor the client's respirations, the respirations are not dangerously depressed, and waiting another 2 hours to administer pain medication does not address the client's need for pain relief.

CN: Pharmacological parenteral therapies; CL: Analyze

Managing Care, Quality, and Safety of Adults with Neurologic Health Problems

112. 2. Assessments, teaching, and suctioning are roles of the nurse. Basic care with frequent positioning is the most appropriate to delegate to the UAP.

CN: Management of care; CL: Apply

113. 3. Pulling the client up under the arm can cause shoulder displacement. A belt around the waist should be used to move the client. Passive range-of-motion exercises prevent contractures and atrophy. Raising the foot of the bed assists in venous return to reduce edema. High-top tennis shoes are used to prevent foot drop.

CN: Management of care; CL: Analyze

114. 3. Clients with Parkinson's disease can experience dysphagia. Thickening liquids assists with swallowing, preventing aspiration. Hyperextending the neck opens the airway and can increase the risk for aspiration. Pressing the chin firmly on the chest makes swallowing more difficult. The chin should be slightly tucked to promote swallowing. The nurse should suggest a speech therapy consult for evaluation of the client's ability to swallow.

CN: Health promotion and maintenance; CL: Analyze

115. 4. Urinary tract infections are a frequent complication in clients with multiple sclerosis because of the effect on bladder function; therefore, that client should be seen first by the nurse. The elevated temperature and flank pain suggest that this client may have pyelonephritis. The client should be notified immediately so that antibiotic therapy can be started quickly. The other clients should be assessed soon but do not have needs as urgent as this client.

CN: Management of care; CL: Analyze

116. 2. Clients with Parkinson's disease may experience a freezing gait when they are unable to move forward. Instructing the client to march in place, step over lines in the flooring, or visualize stepping over a log allows them to move forward. It is important to ambulate the client and not keep them on bed rest. A muscle relaxant is not indicated.

CN: Management of care; CL: Analyze

117. -/+ 1, 2, 3, 5. Pressure points in the side-lying position include the ears, shoulders, ribs, greater trochanter, medial or lateral condyles, and ankles. The sacrum, occiput, and heels are pressure point areas affected in the supine position.

CN: Safety and infection control; CL: Analyze

118. 4. All health care facilities in which controlled medications are stored for dispensing or administrating to clients are required to follow procedures for the proper maintenance of narcotic inventory. Narcotic inventory maintenance includes, but is not limited to, thorough and appropriate documentation of any discrepancy with accompanying reasons (i.e., tablet, ampule, or vial breakage and additional medication volume), timely resolution of inventory discrepancies, and timely notification of persons in oversight areas (i.e., pharmacy, security, nursing house supervisor). In the event of a significant incident, the proper external authorities will be notified by the quality and risk management/legal department.

CN: Pharmacological and parenteral therapies; CL: Analyze

119. 3. The first intervention for a confused client is to increase the frequency of observation, by moving the client closer to the nurses' station if possible and delegating the unlicensed assistive personnel (UAP) to check on the client more frequently. If the family can stay with the client, that is an option, but it is the nurse's responsibility, not the family's, to keep the client safe. Wrist restraints are not used simply because a client is confused; there is no mention of this client pulling at intravenous lines, which is one of the main reasons to use wrist restraints. Administering a sedative simply because a client is confused is not appropriate nursing care and may potentiate the problem.

CN: Safety and infection control; CL: Analyze

120. 2. To ensure the client's safety when using restraints, the restraint must be secured to the bed frame (not the side rail) using a quick-release slip knot (not a square knot). Assessing and documenting skin should be done regularly when restraints are in use, but safety is the priority. Regularly releasing restraints and performing range-of-motion exercises are essential but not the priority in this case. Providing for the client's basic needs while in restraints (i.e., toileting) is important but not the priority.

CN: Safety and infection control; CL: Analyze

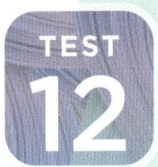

TEST 12 — The Adult with Musculoskeletal Health Problems

- The Adult with Rheumatoid Arthritis
- The Adult with Osteoarthritis
- The Adult with a Hip Fracture
- The Adult Having Hip Replacement Surgery
- The Adult Having Knee Replacement Surgery
- The Adult with a Herniated Disk
- The Adult with an Amputation due to Peripheral Vascular Disease
- The Adult with Fractures
- The Adult with a Femoral Fracture
- The Adult with a Spinal Cord Injury
- Managing Care, Quality, and Safety of Adults with Musculoskeletal Health Problems
- Answers, Rationales, and Test-Taking Strategies

The Adult with Rheumatoid Arthritis

1. During a visit to the clinic, a client reports the onset of early symptoms of rheumatoid arthritis. The nurse should conduct a focused assessment for which symptom?
   - ☐ 1. limited motion of joints
   - ☐ 2. deformed joints of the hands
   - ☐ 3. early morning stiffness
   - ☐ 4. rheumatoid nodules

2. A client with rheumatoid arthritis states, "I can't do my household chores without becoming tired. My knees hurt whenever I walk." Which goal for this client should take **priority**?
   - ☐ 1. Conserve energy.
   - ☐ 2. Adapt self-care skills.
   - ☐ 3. Develop coping skills.
   - ☐ 4. Employ a housekeeping service.

3. The nurse is planning an education program for a group of clients. Which person(s) would be at risk for developing rheumatoid arthritis (RA)? Select all that apply.
   - ☐ 1. a client between the age of 20 and 50 years
   - ☐ 2. a client with the Epstein-Barr virus
   - ☐ 3. a male client
   - ☐ 4. a client with the genetic link HLA-DR4
   - ☐ 5. a client with osteoarthritis

4. A client is in the acute phase of rheumatoid arthritis. In which order of priority from first to last should the nurse establish the goals? All options must be used.

1. Relieve pain.
2. Preserve joint function.
3. Maintain the usual ways of accomplishing tasks.
4. Prevent joint deformity.

5. The nurse teaches a client about heat and cold treatments to manage arthritis pain. Which statement indicates that the client still has a knowledge deficit?
   ☐ 1. "I can use heat and cold as often as I want."
   ☐ 2. "With heat, I should apply it for no longer than 20 minutes at a time."
   ☐ 3. "Heat-producing liniments can be used with other heat devices."
   ☐ 4. "Ten to 15 minutes per application is the maximum time for cold applications."

6. The client with rheumatoid arthritis tells the nurse, "I have a friend who took gold shots and had a wonderful response. Why didn't my health care provider (HCP) let me try that?" Which response by the nurse would be **most** appropriate?
   ☐ 1. "It's the HCP's prerogative to decide how to treat you. They have chosen what is best for your situation."
   ☐ 2. "Tell me more about your friend's arthritic condition. Maybe I can answer that question for you."
   ☐ 3. "That drug is used for cases that are more advanced than yours. You're not eligible for this treatment now."
   ☐ 4. "Every person is different. What works for one client may not always be effective for another."

7. The teaching plan for a client with rheumatoid arthritis includes rest promotion. What position of the involved joints should the nurse tell the client to **avoid** when at rest?
   ☐ 1. keeping all joints aligned
   ☐ 2. elevating the affected joints
   ☐ 3. lying in a prone position
   ☐ 4. maintaining the joints in a flexed position

8. The nurse is teaching a client with rheumatoid arthritis about measures to conserve energy in activities of daily living involving the small joints. Which activity, if observed by the nurse, indicates the need for additional teaching?
   ☐ 1. pushing with palms when rising from a chair
   ☐ 2. holding packages close to the body
   ☐ 3. sliding objects
   ☐ 4. carrying a laundry basket with clenched fingers and fists

9. The nurse is teaching the client with severe rheumatoid arthritis how to take methotrexate. Which statement indicates the need for further teaching?
   ☐ 1. "I'll take my vitamins while I'm on this drug."
   ☐ 2. "I must not drink any alcohol while I'm taking this drug."
   ☐ 3. "I should brush my teeth after every meal."
   ☐ 4. "I'll continue taking my birth control pills."

10. A 25-year-old client taking hydroxychloroquine for rheumatoid arthritis reports difficulty seeing out of their left eye. What does this finding indicate?
    ☐ 1. development of a cataract
    ☐ 2. possible retinal degeneration
    ☐ 3. part of the disease process
    ☐ 4. a coincidental occurrence

11. A client with rheumatoid arthritis is taking high doses of nonsteroidal anti-inflammatory medications. What should the nurse teach the client about taking these medications?
    ☐ 1. "Take prescribed medication with food to lessen the likelihood of an upset stomach."
    ☐ 2. "Do not stop taking the medication suddenly; the dose needs to be decreased gradually."
    ☐ 3. "Use mouthwash to rinse the mouth after taking this medication."
    ☐ 4. "Do not drive or use heavy machinery if dizziness occurs."

12. A client with rheumatoid arthritis tells the nurse, "I know it's important to exercise my joints so I won't lose mobility, but my joints are so stiff and painful that exercising is difficult." Which response by the nurse would be **most** appropriate?
    ☐ 1. "You're probably exercising too much. Decrease your exercise to every other day."
    ☐ 2. "Tell the health care provider about your symptoms. Maybe your analgesic medication can be increased."
    ☐ 3. "Stiffness and pain are part of the disease. Learn to cope by focusing on activities you enjoy."
    ☐ 4. "Take a warm tub bath or shower before exercising. This may help with your discomfort."

13. The nurse is preparing a client for an arthrocentesis. Which information should the nurse include in the teaching plan? Select all that apply.
    ☐ 1. "A local anesthetic agent may be injected into the joint site for your comfort."
    ☐ 2. "A syringe and needle will be used to withdraw fluid from your joint."
    ☐ 3. "The procedure, although not painful, will provide immediate relief."
    ☐ 4. "We will want you to keep your joint active after the procedure to increase blood flow."
    ☐ 5. "You will need to wear a compression bandage for several days after the procedure."

The Adult with Osteoarthritis

14. A client with osteoarthritis will undergo arthrocentesis on a painful, edematous knee. What information should be included in the nursing plan of care? Select all that apply.
☐ 1. Explain the procedure.
☐ 2. Administer preoperative medication 1 hour before surgery.
☐ 3. Instruct the client to immobilize the knee for 2 days after the surgery.
☐ 4. Assess the site for bleeding.
☐ 5. Offer pain medication.

15. A postmenopausal client is scheduled for a bone density scan. What should the nurse instruct the client to do?
☐ 1. Remove all metal objects on the day of the scan.
☐ 2. Consume foods and beverages with a high content of calcium for 2 days before the test.
☐ 3. Ingest 600 mg of calcium gluconate by mouth for 2 weeks before the test.
☐ 4. Report any significant pain to the health care provider at least 2 days before the test.

16. A health care provider (HCP) prescribes a lengthy x-ray examination for a client with osteoarthritis with severe pain. Which action by the nurse would demonstrate client advocacy?
☐ 1. Contact the x-ray technician to see if the lengthy session can be divided into shorter sessions.
☐ 2. Contact the HCP to determine if an alternative examination could be scheduled.
☐ 3. Request a prescription for acetaminophen before the examination.
☐ 4. Request padding and careful positioning for the hard x-ray table.

17. The nurse is completing the history and physical examination of a client diagnosed with osteoarthritis. The nurse should obtain information about which condition?
☐ 1. anemia
☐ 2. osteoporosis
☐ 3. weight loss
☐ 4. local joint pain

18. The nurse is developing a teaching plan with a client with osteoporosis. Which information should be included in the plan? Select all that apply.
☐ 1. Maintain a diet with adequate amounts of vitamin D.
☐ 2. Choose calcium-rich foods.
☐ 3. Use alcohol in moderation.
☐ 4. Swim to maintain bone mass.
☐ 5. Avoid high-fat foods.

19. The nurse has explained to a client with osteoarthritis how to use capsaicin cream. Which statement indicates the client has understood the nurse's explanation?
☐ 1. "I always wash my hands right after I apply the cream."
☐ 2. "After I apply the cream, I wrap my knee with an elastic bandage."
☐ 3. "I keep the cream in the cabinet above the stove in the kitchen."
☐ 4. "I also use the same cream when I get a cut or a burn."

20. The nurse is teaching a client with osteoarthritis when to take ibuprofen to minimize gastric mucosal irritation. What time is **best**?
☐ 1. at bedtime
☐ 2. on arising
☐ 3. immediately after a meal
☐ 4. on an empty stomach

21. A client diagnosed with osteoarthritis tells the nurse, "My friend takes steroid pills for their rheumatoid arthritis. Should I be taking steroids, too?" What should the nurse tell the client?
☐ 1. Intra-articular corticosteroid injections are used to treat osteoarthritis.
☐ 2. Oral corticosteroids can be used in osteoarthritis.
☐ 3. A systemic effect is needed in osteoarthritis.
☐ 4. Rheumatoid arthritis and osteoarthritis are two similar diseases.

22. The nurse is teaching a client with osteoarthritis about the importance of regular exercise. Which statement indicates the client has understood the teaching?
☐ 1. "Performing range-of-motion exercises will increase my joint mobility."
☐ 2. "Exercise helps drive synovial fluid through the cartilage."
☐ 3. "Joint swelling should determine when to stop exercising."
☐ 4. "Exercising in the outdoors year-round promotes joint relaxation."

The Adult with a Hip Fracture

23. A client in a double-hip spica cast is constipated. The surgeon cuts a window into the front of the cast. Which outcome is intended?
The window in the cast will allow:
☐ 1. the nurse to palpate the superior mesenteric artery.
☐ 2. the surgeon to manipulate the fracture site.
☐ 3. the nurse to reposition the client.
☐ 4. relief from pressure due to abdominal distention.

24. A client has an intracapsular hip fracture. The nurse should conduct a focused assessment to detect which change near the fracture?
☐ 1. internal rotation
☐ 2. muscle flaccidity
☐ 3. shortening of the affected leg
☐ 4. absence of pain in the area

25. A client with an extracapsular hip fracture is scheduled for surgical internal fixation with the insertion of a pin. What can the nurse tell the client about the reason for this type of treatment for the fracture?
☐ 1. Hemorrhage at the fracture site is prevented.
☐ 2. Neurovascular impairment risk is decreased.
☐ 3. The risk for infection at the site is lessened.
☐ 4. The client can be mobilized sooner.

26. A client with an extracapsular hip fracture returns to the nursing unit after internal fixation and pin insertion with a drainage tube at the incision site. The client's spouse asks, "Why do they have this tube inserted in their hip?" Which response would be **best**?
☐ 1. "The tube helps us detect a wound infection."
☐ 2. "This way we will not have to irrigate the wound."
☐ 3. "Fluid will drain and not accumulate at the site."
☐ 4. "We have a way to administer antibiotics into the wound."

27. A client with a hip fracture has undergone surgery for the insertion of a femoral head prosthesis. Which activity should the nurse instruct the client to avoid?
☐ 1. crossing the legs while sitting down
☐ 2. sitting on a raised commode seat
☐ 3. using an abductor splint while lying on the side
☐ 4. rising straight from a chair to a standing position

28. The nurse is caring for an older adult male client who had an open reduction internal fixation of the right hip 24 hours ago. The client is now experiencing shortness of breath and reports having "tightness in my chest." The nurse reviews the recent lab test results. The nurse should report which lab test result to the health care provider?
☐ 1. hematocrit: 40% (0.4 proportion of 1.0)
☐ 2. serum glucose: 120 mg/dL (6.7 mmol/L)
☐ 3. troponin: 1.4 mcg/L (1.4 µg/L)
☐ 4. erythrocyte sedimentation rate (ESR): 22 mm per hour

29. The nurse is advising a client who underwent femoral head prosthesis placement on the type of chair to sit in during the first 6 to 8 weeks after surgery. Which chair would be the correct type to recommend?
☐ 1. a desk-type swivel chair
☐ 2. a padded upholstered chair
☐ 3. a high-backed chair with armrests
☐ 4. a recliner with an attached footrest

30. The nurse is to apply a sequential compression device (intermittent pneumatic compression). Identify the area of the compression device that is placed on the client's calf.

31. The nurse is assessing the home environment of an older adult client who is using crutches during the postoperative recovery phase after hip pinning. Which finding poses the **greatest** hazard to the client as a risk for falling at home?
☐ 1. a 4-year-old cocker spaniel
☐ 2. scatter rugs
☐ 3. snack tables
☐ 4. rocking chairs

The Adult Having Hip Replacement Surgery

32. An older adult with a hip fracture is to use an alternating air pressure mattress at home to prevent pressure ulcers while recovering from surgery. The nurse is showing the client's family how to place the mattress (see below). What should the nurse instruct the family to do?

☐ 1. Turn the mattress over so the air cells face the mattress of the bed, and cover the mattress with a bedsheet.
☐ 2. Put a thick pad over the pressure mattress to prevent soiling, and place the bedsheet on top of the pad.
☐ 3. Make the bed with the bedsheet on top of the pressure mattress.
☐ 4. Place the sheet on the bed, and then remove the pillow to allow full use of the mattress on the neck.

33. A client had a posterolateral total hip replacement 2 days ago. What information should the nurse include in the client's plan of care? Select all that apply.
    ☐ 1. When using a walker, encourage the client to keep the toes pointing inward.
    ☐ 2. Position a pillow between the legs to maintain abduction.
    ☐ 3. Allow the client to be in the supine position or in the lateral position on the unoperated side.
    ☐ 4. Do not allow the client to bend down to tie or slip on shoes.
    ☐ 5. Place ice on the incision after physical therapy.

34. The nurse is developing a teaching plan for a client who had an anterolateral approach for a total hip replacement and is being discharged home. Which information should the nurse include in the discharge plan? Select all that apply.
    ☐ 1. Avoid turning the toes or knee outward.
    ☐ 2. Use an abduction pillow between the legs when in bed.
    ☐ 3. Use an elevated toilet seat and shower chair.
    ☐ 4. Do not extend the operative leg backward.
    ☐ 5. Restrict motion for 2 weeks after surgery.

35. The nurse is assessing a client for neurologic impairment after a total hip replacement. Which finding indicates impairment in the affected extremity?
    ☐ 1. decreased distal pulse
    ☐ 2. inability to move
    ☐ 3. diminished capillary refill
    ☐ 4. coolness to the touch

36. The nurse is instructing a client who will have a total hip replacement tomorrow. Which information is **most** important to include in the teaching plan at this time?
    ☐ 1. Teach how to prevent hip flexion.
    ☐ 2. Demonstrate coughing and deep-breathing techniques.
    ☐ 3. Show the client what an actual hip prosthesis looks like.
    ☐ 4. Assess the client's fears about the procedure.

37. After surgery and insertion of a total hip prosthesis, a client develops severe sudden pain and an inability to move the extremity. What do these findings indicate?

    The client:
    ☐ 1. is developing an infection.
    ☐ 2. is bleeding in the operative site.
    ☐ 3. has a joint dislocation.
    ☐ 4. has glue seepage into soft tissue.

38. The nurse is assessing a client who had a total hip replacement 2 days ago. The client has profuse diaphoresis. Vital signs are temperature 101°F (38.3°C); pulse 90 bpm; and respiration rate 20 breaths/min. The intravenous (IV) line is infusing at 31 drops per minute. The client received morphine 1 hour ago and reports a pain level of 2 on a 0 to 10 scale. The client had eggs, toast, and orange juice for breakfast. The dressing is dry. The nurse reviews the client's prescriptions. Which action(s) should the nurse take to prevent the client from becoming dehydrated? Select all that apply.

    Prescriptions

    1. Diet as tolerated
    2. Physical therapy to ambulate the client two times a day
    3. Acetaminophen 325 mg, 2 tablets every 4 hours for a temperature over 100°F (37.7°C)
    4. Morphine 10 mg, IV push every 4 hours
    5. 10,000 mL dextrose 5% in water (D5W) every 8 hours

    ☐ 1. Encourage the client to drink 500 mL of fluids each shift.
    ☐ 2. Teach the client how to inspect the incision site for bleeding.
    ☐ 3. Have the client maintain bed rest.
    ☐ 4. Administer morphine.
    ☐ 5. Administer acetaminophen.
    ☐ 6. Ask the health care provider to increase the amount of IV fluids.

39. A client had a total hip replacement today. How should the nurse position the client when the client is transferred from the transport cart to the bed?
    ☐ 1. Place weights alongside the affected extremity to keep the extremity from rotating.
    ☐ 2. Elevate both feet on two pillows.
    ☐ 3. Keep the lower extremities adducted by placing an immobilization device around both legs.
    ☐ 4. Maintain the affected extremity in slight abduction by using an abduction splint or placing pillows between the thighs.

40. The nurse is instructing an unlicensed assistive personnel (UAP) on how to move and position a client who had a total hip replacement yesterday. What should the nurse tell the UAP to do? Select all that apply.
    ☐ 1. With the aid of a coworker, turn the client from the supine to the prone position every 2 hours.
    ☐ 2. Encourage the client to use the overhead trapeze to assist with position changes.
    ☐ 3. For meals, elevate the head of the bed to 90 degrees.
    ☐ 4. Use a fracture bedpan when needed by the client.
    ☐ 5. When the client is in bed, prevent thromboembolism by encouraging the client to do toe-pointing exercises.

41. A client is to have a total hip replacement. What nursing action(s) should the preoperative plan include? Select all that apply.
   ☐ 1. Administer antibiotics as prescribed to ensure therapeutic blood levels.
   ☐ 2. Apply a leg compression device.
   ☐ 3. Request a trapeze be added to the bed.
   ☐ 4. Teach isometric exercises for the quadriceps and gluteal muscles.
   ☐ 5. Demonstrate crutch walking with a three-point gait.
   ☐ 6. Place Buck's traction on the bed.

42. The nurse is teaching a client to administer enoxaparin after a total hip replacement. What should the nurse instruct the client to do? Select all that apply.
   ☐ 1. Report promptly any difficulty breathing, rash, or itching.
   ☐ 2. Notify the health care provider (HCP) of unusual bruising.
   ☐ 3. Avoid all aspirin-containing medications.
   ☐ 4. Wear or carry medical identification.
   ☐ 5. Expel the air bubble from the syringe before the injection.
   ☐ 6. Remove the needle immediately after the medication is injected.

43. A client who had a total hip replacement 4 days ago is worried about dislocation of the prosthesis. How should the nurse respond to the client's concern?
   ☐ 1. "Don't worry. Your new hip is very strong."
   ☐ 2. "Using a cushioned toilet seat helps prevent dislocation."
   ☐ 3. "Activities that tend to cause adduction of the hip tend to cause dislocation, so try to avoid them."
   ☐ 4. "Decreasing use of the abductor pillow will strengthen the muscles to prevent dislocation."

44. The nurse is assessing a client who had a left hip replacement 36 hours ago. Which finding(s) would indicate the prosthesis is dislocated? Select all that apply.
   ☐ 1. The client reported a "popping" sensation in the hip.
   ☐ 2. The left leg is shorter than the right leg.
   ☐ 3. The client has sharp pain in the groin.
   ☐ 4. The client cannot move the right leg.
   ☐ 5. The client cannot wiggle the toes on the left leg.

45. A client who has had a total hip replacement has a dislocated hip prosthesis. What should the nurse do **first**?
   ☐ 1. Stabilize the leg with Buck's traction.
   ☐ 2. Apply an ice pack to the affected hip.
   ☐ 3. Position the client toward the opposite side of the hip.
   ☐ 4. Notify the orthopedic surgeon.

46. The nurse has established a goal with a client to improve mobility following hip replacement. Which outcome is realistic at the time of discharge from the surgical unit?

The client can:
   ☐ 1. walk throughout the nursing unit with a walker.
   ☐ 2. walk the length of a hospital hallway with minimal pain.
   ☐ 3. be more independent when transferring from bed to chair.
   ☐ 4. raise the affected leg 6 inches (15.2 cm) with assistance.

47. The nurse is assessing a client who had a total hip replacement yesterday for potential complications. Which complication has the **greatest** likelihood of occurring?
   ☐ 1. deep vein thrombosis (DVT)
   ☐ 2. polyuria
   ☐ 3. displacement of the new joint
   ☐ 4. wound evisceration

The Adult Having Knee Replacement Surgery

48. In preparation for total knee surgery, a 200-lb (90.7-kg) client with osteoarthritis must lose weight. Which exercise should the nurse recommend as **best** if the client has no contraindications?
   ☐ 1. weight lifting
   ☐ 2. walking
   ☐ 3. aquatic exercise
   ☐ 4. tai chi exercise

49. The client has just had a total knee replacement. When assessing the client, the nurse understands that which finding indicates possible nerve damage?
   ☐ 1. numbness
   ☐ 2. bleeding
   ☐ 3. dislocation
   ☐ 4. pinkness

50. After knee arthroplasty, the client has a sequential compression device (SCD). What should the nurse do?
   ☐ 1. Elevate the SCD on two pillows.
   ☐ 2. Change the settings on the SCD to make the client more comfortable.
   ☐ 3. Stop the SCD to remove dressings, and bathe the leg.
   ☐ 4. Discontinue the SCD when the client is ambulatory.

51. A client returns from the first session of scheduled physical therapy following total knee replacement surgery. The nurse assesses that the client's knee is swollen, slightly erythematous, and painful. The client rates the pain as a 7 on a scale of 0 to 10 and has not had any scheduled or as-needed (PRN) pain medication today. What should the nurse do? Select all that apply.
    ☐ 1. Gently massage the area to increase circulation to reduce pain.
    ☐ 2. Administer pain medication as prescribed.
    ☐ 3. Elevate the leg and apply a cold pack.
    ☐ 4. Notify the health care provider (HCP).
    ☐ 5. Call the physical therapy team to cancel the next treatment.

52. The nurse is preparing a client who underwent a knee replacement with a metal joint to go home. What should the nurse instruct the client to do? Select all that apply.
    ☐ 1. Notify the health care provider (HCP) about the joint before undergoing invasive procedures.
    ☐ 2. Inform the HCP before having magnetic resonance imaging (MRI) scans.
    ☐ 3. Notify airport security that the joint may set off alarms on metal detectors.
    ☐ 4. Refrain from carrying items weighing more than 5 lb (2.3 kg).
    ☐ 5. Eat a low-fat, low-carbohydrate diet.

53. The laboratory notifies the nurse that a client who had a total knee replacement 3 days ago and is receiving heparin has an activated partial thromboplastin time (aPTT) of 95 seconds. After verifying the values, the nurse calls the health care provider (HCP). What prescription for the client should the nurse recommend the HCP consider?
    ☐ 1. protamine sulfate
    ☐ 2. vitamin K
    ☐ 3. warfarin
    ☐ 4. packed red blood cells

54. The nurse is assessing a client's left leg for neurovascular changes following a total left knee replacement. Which finding(s) would be expected as normal? Select all that apply.
    ☐ 1. moderate edema of the left knee
    ☐ 2. skin warm to touch
    ☐ 3. capillary refill response of less than 3 seconds
    ☐ 4. moves toes
    ☐ 5. pain absent
    ☐ 6. pulse on the left leg weaker than the right leg

55. On the evening of surgery for a total knee replacement, a client wants to get out of bed. What should the nurse do to safely assist the client?
    ☐ 1. Encourage the client to apply full weight bearing.
    ☐ 2. Ask the health care provider (HCP) to prescribe a walker for the client.
    ☐ 3. Place a straight-backed chair at the foot of the bed.
    ☐ 4. Apply a knee immobilizer.

56. The nurse is preparing a client for discharge from the hospital after a total knee replacement. Which information should the nurse include in the discharge plan? Select all that apply.
    ☐ 1. Report signs of infection to the health care provider (HCP).
    ☐ 2. Keep the affected leg and foot on the floor when sitting in a chair.
    ☐ 3. Remove antiembolism stockings when sleeping.
    ☐ 4. Understand that the physical therapist will encourage progressive ambulation with the use of assistive devices.
    ☐ 5. Change the dressing daily.

The Adult with a Herniated Disk

57. The nurse is observing a client who is recovering from back strain as they lift a box as shown below. What should the nurse do?

    ☐ 1. Praise the client for using correct body mechanics.
    ☐ 2. Suggest that the client put both knees on the floor before attempting to lift the box.
    ☐ 3. Advise the client to bend from the waist rather than stretch the back in this position.
    ☐ 4. Instruct the client to keep the back straight by squatting with both knees parallel.

58. A client has low back pain. What should the nurse instruct the client to **avoid** doing?
    ☐ 1. keeping light objects below the level of the elbows when lifting
    ☐ 2. leaning forward while bending the knees
    ☐ 3. exceeding the prescribed exercise program
    ☐ 4. sleeping on the side with legs flexed

59. A client is discharged with the following prescription for severe back pain from a herniated intravertebral disc: hydrocodone 5 mg, acetaminophen 500 mg, one-half to one tablet by mouth each, every 8 to 12 hours as needed. How should the nurse instruct the client to follow this prescription?
☐ 1. Start with a half tablet of each tablet, and take one every 12 hours.
☐ 2. Start with a half tablet of each tablet, and take one every 8 hours.
☐ 3. Start with one tablet of each tablet, and take one every 8 hours.
☐ 4. Start with one tablet of each tablet, and take one every 12 hours.

60. A client attempting to get out of bed stops midway because of low back pain radiating down to the right heel and lateral foot. What should the nurse do in order of priority from first to last? All options must be used.

1. Apply a warm compress to the client's back.
2. Notify the health care provider (HCP).
3. Assist the client to lie down.
4. Administer the prescribed celecoxib.

61. A client with a ruptured intervertebral disc at L4–L5 stands with a flattened spine slightly tilted forward and slightly flexed to the affected side. How should the nurse interpret this finding?

The client has:
☐ 1. motor changes.
☐ 2. postural deformity.
☐ 3. alteration of reflexes.
☐ 4. sensory changes.

62. The nurse is positioning a client with a ruptured disc at L5–S1 right. In which position will the client be **most** comfortable?
☐ 1. prone
☐ 2. supine with the legs flexed
☐ 3. high Fowler's
☐ 4. right semiprone position

63. A client tells the nurse about having numbness from the back of their left buttock to the dorsum of their foot and big toe. The client is scheduled to undergo a laminectomy, and the operative consent form states "a left lumbar laminectomy of L3–L4." What should the nurse do **next**?
☐ 1. Have the client sign the consent form.
☐ 2. Call the surgeon.
☐ 3. Change the consent form.
☐ 4. Review the client's history.

64. Immediately after a lumbar laminectomy, the nurse administers ondansetron hydrochloride to the client as prescribed. The nurse determines that the drug is effective when which sign is controlled?
☐ 1. muscle spasms
☐ 2. nausea
☐ 3. shivering
☐ 4. dry mouth

65. After a laminectomy, the client states, "The doctor said that I can do anything I want to." Which activity that the client intends to do indicates the need for further teaching?
☐ 1. drying the dishes
☐ 2. sitting outside on firm cushions
☐ 3. making the bed by walking from one side of the bed to the other
☐ 4. sweeping the front porch

66. The nurse is developing a discharge teaching plan for a client after a lumbar laminectomy of L4–L5. What action should the nurse encourage the client to **avoid** when returning to work in 6 weeks?
☐ 1. placing one foot on a step stool during prolonged standing
☐ 2. sleeping on the back with support under the knees
☐ 3. maintaining average body weight for height
☐ 4. sitting whenever possible

67. A male client underwent a lumbar spinal fusion yesterday. Which nursing assessment should alert the nurse to the development of a possible complication?
☐ 1. lateral rotation of the head and neck
☐ 2. clear yellowish fluid on the dressing
☐ 3. use of the standing position to void
☐ 4. nonproductive cough

68. The nurse is teaching a client about wearing a back brace after a spinal fusion. Which statement indicates the client understands how to wear the back brace?
☐ 1. "I will apply lotion before putting on the brace."
☐ 2. "I will be sure to pad the area around my iliac crest."
☐ 3. "I can use baby powder under the brace to absorb perspiration."
☐ 4. "I should wear a thin cotton undershirt under the brace."

69. The nurse develops a teaching plan for a client scheduled for a spinal fusion. What should the nurse tell the client?
☐ 1. The client will typically experience more pain at the donor site than at the fusion site.
☐ 2. The surgeon will apply a simple gauze dressing to the donor site.
☐ 3. Neurovascular checks are unnecessary if the fibula is the donor site.
☐ 4. The client's level of activity restriction is determined by the amount of pain.

70. A client who has had a lumbar laminectomy with a spinal fusion is sitting in a chair. Which is the correct position for this client?
☐ 1. with the feet flat on the floor
☐ 2. on a low footstool
☐ 3. in any comfortable position with legs uncrossed
☐ 4. on a high footstool so the feet are level with the chair seat

71. The nurse develops a plan of care for a client in the initial postoperative period following a lumbar laminectomy. Which activity is **contraindicated**?
☐ 1. assisting with daily hygiene activities
☐ 2. lying flat in bed
☐ 3. walking in the hall
☐ 4. sitting all afternoon in their room

72. The nurse is following up with the physical therapist's exercise plan for a client who had a lumbar laminectomy. Which exercises should the nurse remind the client are helpful to continue to do at home? Select all that apply.
☐ 1. knee-to-chest lifts
☐ 2. hip tilts
☐ 3. sit-ups
☐ 4. pelvic tilts

The Adult with an Amputation due to Peripheral Vascular Disease

73. The nurse is assessing the risk for a client who is to have an amputation of the foot because of peripheral vascular disease (PVD). Which factor(s) would place this client at risk? Select all that apply.
☐ 1. uncontrolled diabetes mellitus for 15 years
☐ 2. a 20-pack-year history of cigarette smoking
☐ 3. a hemoglobin level of 14.2 g/dL (142 g/L)
☐ 4. a serum cholesterol concentration of 275 mg/dL (15.3 mmol/L)
☐ 5. work that requires prolonged standing
☐ 6. oxygen saturation of 94% on pulse oximetry

74. A client has severe arterial occlusive disease and gangrene of the left great toe. Which finding is expected?
☐ 1. edema around the ankle
☐ 2. loss of hair on the lower leg
☐ 3. thin, soft toenails
☐ 4. warmth in the foot

75. A client with absent peripheral pulses and pain at rest is scheduled for an arterial Doppler study of the affected extremity. When preparing the client for this test, the nurse should take which action?
☐ 1. Have the client sign an informed consent form for the procedure.
☐ 2. Administer a pretest sedative as appropriate.
☐ 3. Keep the client tobacco free for 30 minutes before the test.
☐ 4. Wrap the client's affected foot with a blanket.

76. The nurse is teaching a client with peripheral arterial disease about how to promote circulation. Which instruction will be **most** helpful?
☐ 1. resting with the legs elevated above the level of the heart
☐ 2. walking slowly but steadily for 30 minutes twice a day
☐ 3. minimizing activity as much and as often as possible
☐ 4. wearing antiembolism stockings at all times when out of bed

77. The nurse is developing a teaching plan with a client with arterial insufficiency to the feet. What information should be included in the plan?
☐ 1. Lubricate the feet daily.
☐ 2. Soak the feet in warm water.
☐ 3. Apply antiembolism stockings.
☐ 4. Wear firm, supportive leather shoes.

78. A client says, "I hate the idea of being an invalid after they cut off my leg." Which response by the nurse would be the **most** therapeutic?
☐ 1. "At least you'll still have one good leg to use."
☐ 2. "Tell me more about how you're feeling."
☐ 3. "Let's finish the preoperative teaching."
☐ 4. "You're lucky to have a spouse to care for you."

79. The client asks the nurse, "Why won't the health care provider tell me exactly how much of my leg they are going to take off? Don't you think I should know that?" On which information should the nurse base the response?
☐ 1. the need to remove as much of the leg as possible
☐ 2. the adequacy of the blood supply to the tissues
☐ 3. the ease with which a prosthesis can be fitted
☐ 4. the client's ability to walk with a prosthesis

80. A client who has had an above-the-knee amputation develops a dime-sized bright red spot on the dressing after 45 minutes in the postanesthesia recovery unit. What should the nurse do **first**?
☐ 1. Elevate the stump.
☐ 2. Reinforce the dressing.
☐ 3. Call the surgeon.
☐ 4. Draw a mark around the site.

81. A client in the postanesthesia care unit with a left below-the-knee amputation has pain in the left big toe. What should the nurse do **first**?
☐ 1. Tell the client it is impossible to feel the pain.
☐ 2. Show the client that the toes are not there.
☐ 3. Explain to the client that the pain is real.
☐ 4. Give the client the prescribed opioid analgesic.

82. The client with an above-the-knee amputation is to use crutches while the prosthesis is being adjusted. Which exercises will **best** prepare the client for using crutches?
☐ 1. abdominal exercises
☐ 2. isometric shoulder exercises
☐ 3. quadriceps setting exercises
☐ 4. triceps strengthening exercises

83. The nurse is teaching a client about using crutches. On which part of the body should the nurse instruct the client to support the body weight?
☐ 1. axillae
☐ 2. elbows
☐ 3. upper arms
☐ 4. hands

84. The client is to be discharged on a low-fat, low-cholesterol, low-sodium diet. When teaching the client about the diet, the nurse should take which action **first**?
☐ 1. Determine the client's knowledge level about cholesterol.
☐ 2. Ask the client to name foods that are high in fat, cholesterol, and salt.
☐ 3. Explain the importance of complying with the diet.
☐ 4. Assess the client's and family's typical food preferences.

The Adult with Fractures

85. A client has a leg immobilized in traction. Which observation by the nurse indicates that the client understands actions to take to prevent muscle atrophy?

The client:
☐ 1. adducts the affected leg every 2 hours.
☐ 2. rolls the affected leg away from the body's midline twice per day.
☐ 3. performs isometric exercises to the affected extremity three times per day.
☐ 4. asks the nurse to add a 5-lb (2.3-kg) weight to the traction for 30 minutes a day.

86. A client with a fractured tibia has an external fixation. The health care provider has prescribed a solution of ½ normal saline and ½ hydrogen peroxide to clean the pin site twice a day. In which order should the nurse cleanse the pin from first to last? All options must be used.

1. Inspect the site for redness, swelling, or discharge.
2. Clean the pin with a cotton swab dipped in the prescribed solution, wiping from the insertion site to the tip of the pin.
3. Clean the pin insertion site with a cotton swab dipped in the prescribed solution, removing the crust and wiping away from the site.
4. Clean the area around the pin insertion site with cotton swabs, dipped in the prescribed solution.

87. A client with a fractured tibia has been taking methocarbamol. Which finding indicates that the drug is having the intended effect?
☐ 1. lack of infection
☐ 2. reduction in itching
☐ 3. relief of muscle spasms
☐ 4. decrease in nervousness

88. The nurse is developing a teaching plan for a client who is prescribed acetaminophen for muscle pain. Which information should the nurse include in the teaching plan? Select all that apply.
☐ 1. The drug can be used if the person is allergic to aspirin.
☐ 2. Acetaminophen does not affect platelet aggregation.
☐ 3. This drug causes little or no gastric distress.
☐ 4. Acetaminophen exerts a strong anti-inflammatory effect.
☐ 5. The client should have the international normalized ratio (INR) checked regularly.

89. A client who has been taking hydrocodone with acetaminophen at home for 6 weeks following a fractured tibia is admitted with a blood pressure of 80/50 mm Hg, a pulse rate of 115 bpm, and respirations of 8 breaths/min and shallow. What do these findings indicate?
    ☐ 1. expected common adverse effects of the hydrocodone
    ☐ 2. hypersensitivity reaction to the acetaminophen
    ☐ 3. possible habituation effect of long-term drug use
    ☐ 4. hemorrhage from gastrointestinal irritation associated with the pain medication

90. The nurse is caring for a client who is 30 years of age with a fracture of the right femur and left tibia. Both legs have casts. The nurse assesses that the client's respiration rate is 30 breaths/min and respirations are rapid and shallow; there is the presence of a faint expiratory wheeze; and coughing produces thin pink sputum. The client is yelling at the nurse and wants to be released from the hospital; this is behavior unlike that previously reported. The last pain medication was administered 3 hours ago. What should the nurse do **first**?
    ☐ 1. Cut slits in the top of the casts.
    ☐ 2. Administer pain medication.
    ☐ 3. Notify the health care provider (HCP).
    ☐ 4. Obtain a chest x-ray.

91. A client is being discharged following an open reduction and internal fixation of the left ankle and is to wear a non–weight-bearing cast for 2 weeks. What should the nurse teach the client to do when using crutches?
    ☐ 1. Use a four-point gait.
    ☐ 2. Maintain two to three finger widths between the axillary fold and underarm piece grip.
    ☐ 3. Keep the leg dependent when sitting.
    ☐ 4. Maintain balance by supporting the body's weight on the axillae.

92. The nurse is caring for an adult with a grade III compound fracture of the right femur; the client has been placed in skeletal traction. What is the intended outcome of the traction?
    ☐ 1. Prevent skin breakdown.
    ☐ 2. Prevent movement in the bed.
    ☐ 3. Preserve the normal length of the leg.
    ☐ 4. Reduce and immobilize the fracture.

93. An older adult is admitted with a fracture of the femur. What should the nurse assess **first** about this client?
    ☐ 1. ability to change positions
    ☐ 2. type of pain
    ☐ 3. mechanism of injury
    ☐ 4. extent of anxiety

94. The nurse is admitting a client with a fractured tibia. Which area should the nurse assess **first**?
    ☐ 1. area proximal to the fracture
    ☐ 2. actual fracture site
    ☐ 3. area distal to the fracture
    ☐ 4. opposite extremity for baseline comparison

95. The nurse is teaching a client about cast care. Which statement indicates the nurse should provide additional information to the client?
    ☐ 1. "I will elevate the cast above my heart initially."
    ☐ 2. "I will exercise my joints above and below the cast."
    ☐ 3. "I can pull out cast padding to scratch inside the cast."
    ☐ 4. "I will apply ice for 10 minutes to control edema for the first 24 hours."

96. The nurse is planning care for a client who is in a double-hip spica cast. Which nursing action(s) should be included in the care plan? Select all that apply.
    ☐ 1. encouraging the intake of cranberry juice
    ☐ 2. advising the client to eat large amounts of cheese
    ☐ 3. establishing regular times for elimination
    ☐ 4. having the client dangle at the bedside
    ☐ 5. wiping the cast with a damp cloth when the cast is dirty
    ☐ 6. placing a protective cloth around the cast when eating.

97. The nurse is preparing a teaching plan for a client about crutch walking using a two-point gait pattern. What information should the nurse include?
    ☐ 1. Advance a crutch on one side, and then advance the opposite foot; repeat on the opposite side.
    ☐ 2. Advance a crutch on one side, and simultaneously advance and bear weight on the opposite foot; repeat on the opposite side.
    ☐ 3. Advance both crutches together, and then follow by lifting both lower extremities to the level of the crutches.
    ☐ 4. Advance both crutches together, and then follow by lifting both lower extremities past the level of the crutches.

98. A client returned from surgery with a debrided open tibial fracture and has a three-way drainage system. The client's vital signs are within normal limits. What should the nurse do **next**?
    ☐ 1. Review the results of culture and sensitivity testing of the wound.
    ☐ 2. Change the dressing at the surgery site.
    ☐ 3. Determine if the client has increased pain from exposed nerve endings.
    ☐ 4. Check laboratory results for electrolyte imbalances.

99. A client has a left tibial fracture that required casting. Approximately 5 hours later, the client has increasing pain distal to the fracture despite the morphine injection administered 30 minutes ago. Which area should be the nurse's **next** assessment?
☐ 1. distal pulses
☐ 2. pain with a pain rating scale
☐ 3. vital sign changes
☐ 4. potential for drug tolerance

100. A client with a fracture develops compartment syndrome. Which sign should alert the nurse to impending organ failure?
☐ 1. crackles
☐ 2. jaundice
☐ 3. generalized edema
☐ 4. dark, scanty urine

The Adult with a Femoral Fracture

101. The nurse is planning care for a client with a femoral fracture who is in balanced suspension traction. Which nursing care can be included in the plan of care?
☐ 1. using a fracture bedpan when the client uses the trapeze to raise the hips
☐ 2. turning the client from side to side to give back care
☐ 3. raising the head of the bed to 90 degrees to sit the client up
☐ 4. giving the client a complete bed bath

102. A client in balanced suspension traction is transported to surgery for closed reduction and internal fixation of a fractured femur. What should the nurse do when transporting the client to the operating room?
☐ 1. Transfer the client to a cart with manually suspended traction.
☐ 2. Call the surgeon to request a prescription to temporarily remove the traction.
☐ 3. Send the client on the bed with extra help to stabilize the traction.
☐ 4. Remove the traction, and send the client on a cart.

103. A client is in balanced suspension traction to maintain alignment of a fractured tibia. Which activities are safe for the client?
☐ 1. Eat while lying flat.
☐ 2. Raise the hips using a trapeze.
☐ 3. Rotate from side to side.
☐ 4. Flex and extend the ankle on the affected side.

104. A client has a Pearson attachment on the traction setup. What is the purpose of this attachment?
☐ 1. to support the lower portion of the leg
☐ 2. to support the thigh and upper leg
☐ 3. to allow attachment of the skeletal pin
☐ 4. to prevent flexion deformities in the ankle and foot

105. The nurse is assessing a client with a fracture of the right femur for signs of complications. Which finding indicates the client may be developing a fat embolus?
☐ 1. acute respiratory distress syndrome
☐ 2. migraine-like headaches
☐ 3. numbness in the right leg
☐ 4. muscle spasms in the right thigh

106. A client in traction for a fractured femur is having difficulty managing self-care activities. Which outcome indicates successful completion of a goal of promoting independence for this client?
The client:
☐ 1. assists as much as possible in care, demonstrating increased participation over time.
☐ 2. allows the nurse to complete care in an efficient manner without interfering.
☐ 3. allows the spouse to assume total responsibility for care.
☐ 4. accepts that self-care is not possible while in traction.

107. A client with an open femoral fracture was discharged to home and reports having a fever, night sweats, chills, restlessness, and restrictive movement of the fractured leg. The nurse should interpret these findings as the client may be experiencing which complication?
☐ 1. pulmonary embolus
☐ 2. osteomyelitis
☐ 3. fat embolus
☐ 4. urinary tract infection

108. The nurse is planning care for a client with osteomyelitis. The client is taking an antibiotic, but the infection has not resolved. What should the nurse advise the client to do?
☐ 1. Use herbal supplements.
☐ 2. Eat a diet high in protein and vitamins C and D.
☐ 3. Ask the health care provider for a change of antibiotics.
☐ 4. Encourage frequent passive range of motion to the affected extremity.

The Adult with a Spinal Cord Injury

109. The nurse is directing the care team as they plan to move a person with a possible spinal cord injury. The nurse should direct the team to move the client using which procedure?
  ☐ 1. Limit movement of the arms by wrapping them next to the body.
  ☐ 2. Move the person gently to help reduce pain.
  ☐ 3. Immobilize the head and neck to prevent further injury.
  ☐ 4. Cushion the back with pillows to ensure comfort.

110. The nurse is caring for a client with a spinal cord injury. The client is experiencing blurred vision and has a blood pressure of 204/102 mm Hg. What should the nurse do **first**?
  ☐ 1. Position the client on the left side.
  ☐ 2. Control the environment by turning the lights off and decreasing stimulation for the client.
  ☐ 3. Check the client's bladder for distention.
  ☐ 4. Administer pain medications.

111. The nurse is taking care of a client with a spinal cord injury. The extent of the client's injury is shown below. Which finding is expected when assessing this client?

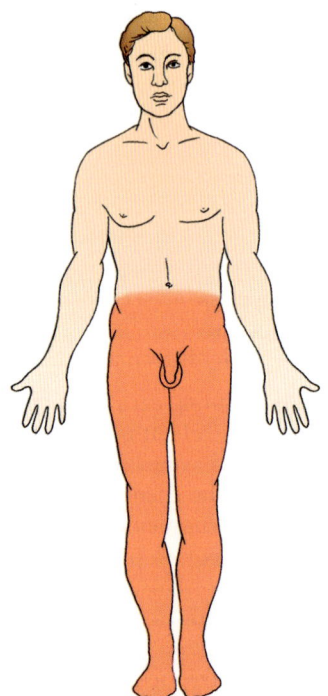

  ☐ 1. inability to move the arms
  ☐ 2. loss of sensation in the hands and fingers
  ☐ 3. dysfunction of bowel and bladder
  ☐ 4. difficulty breathing

112. The nurse is assessing a client with a cord transection above T5 for possible complications. For which complication(s) should the nurse assess the client? Select all that apply.
  ☐ 1. diarrhea
  ☐ 2. paralytic ileus
  ☐ 3. lack of movement in arms
  ☐ 4. stress ulcers
  ☐ 5. intra-abdominal bleeding

113. The nurse is assessing a client with a spinal cord injury for the development of deep vein thrombosis. Which is the **most** effective way to determine deep vein thrombosis in this client?
  ☐ 1. Detect a positive Homans' sign.
  ☐ 2. Rate the amount of pain.
  ☐ 3. Assess for tenderness.
  ☐ 4. Measure leg girth.

114. A client with a spinal cord injury has spinal shock. What should the nurse expect the client's bladder function to be at this time?
  ☐ 1. spastic
  ☐ 2. normal
  ☐ 3. atonic
  ☐ 4. uncontrolled

115. After 1 month of therapy, a client in spinal shock begins to experience muscle spasms in the legs and calls the nurse in excitement to report the leg movement. Which response by the nurse would be the **most** accurate?
  ☐ 1. "These movements indicate that the damaged nerves are healing."
  ☐ 2. "This is a good sign. Keep trying to move all the affected muscles."
  ☐ 3. "The return of movement means that eventually you should be able to walk again."
  ☐ 4. "The movements occur from muscle reflexes that cannot be initiated or controlled by the brain."

116. A client with a spinal cord injury asks the nurse why the dietitian has recommended decreasing the total daily intake of calcium. Which response by the nurse would provide the **most** accurate information?
  ☐ 1. "Excessive intake of dairy products makes constipation more common."
  ☐ 2. "Immobility increases calcium absorption from the intestine."
  ☐ 3. "Lack of weight bearing causes demineralization of the long bones."
  ☐ 4. "Dairy products likely will contribute to weight gain."

117. As a first step in teaching a female client with a spinal cord injury and quadriplegia about their sexual health, the nurse assesses the client's understanding of their current sexual functioning. Which statement by the client indicates they understand their current ability?
☐ 1. "I won't be able to have sexual intercourse until the urinary catheter is removed."
☐ 2. "I can participate in sexual activity but might not experience orgasm."
☐ 3. "I can't have sexual intercourse because it causes hypertension, but other sexual activity is okay."
☐ 4. "I should be able to participate in sexual activity, but I'll be infertile."

118. A client with a spinal cord injury who has been active in sports and outdoor activities talks almost obsessively about past activities. In tears, one day they ask the nurse, "Why can't I stop talking about these things? I know those days are gone forever." Which response by the nurse conveys the **best** understanding of the client's behavior?
☐ 1. "Be patient. It takes time to adjust to such a massive loss."
☐ 2. "Talking about the past is a form of denial. We have to help you focus on today."
☐ 3. "Reviewing your losses is a way to help you work through your grief and loss."
☐ 4. "It's a simple escape mechanism to go back and live again in happier times."

Managing Care, Quality, and Safety of Adults with Musculoskeletal Health Problems

119. The nurse is ensuring that all clients who are at risk for falls are wearing red slipper socks that identify clients who are at risk for falling. Which client(s) should receive red slipper socks? Select all that apply.
a client who is:
☐ 1. 45 years of age, in hospice with terminal cancer, and receiving morphine every 2 hours
☐ 2. 70 years of age, hospitalized for a lung biopsy, and receiving no medications
☐ 3. 62 years of age, recovering from breast biopsy in outpatient surgery, and has a fear of falling
☐ 4. 80 years of age and in a locked facility for clients with cognitive impairment
☐ 5. 75 years of age and recovering at home from hip replacement surgery on the left hip

120. Four days after surgery for internal fixation of a C3–C4 fracture, a nurse is moving a client from the bed to the wheelchair. The nurse is checking the wheelchair for correct features for this client. Which feature(s) of the wheelchair would be appropriate for the needs of this client? Select all that apply.
☐ 1. back at the level of the client's scapula
☐ 2. back and head that are high
☐ 3. seat that is lower than normal
☐ 4. seat with firm cushions
☐ 5. chair controlled by the client's breath

121. The nurse is planning care for a group of clients who have had a total hip replacement. Of the clients listed below, who is at the **highest** risk for infection and should be assessed **first**?
☐ 1. a 55-year-old client who is 6 feet (180 cm) tall and weighs 180 lb (81.7 kg)
☐ 2. a 90-year-old who lives alone
☐ 3. a 74-year-old who has periodontal disease with periodontitis
☐ 4. a 75-year-old who has asthma and uses an inhaler

122. The nurse is documenting the care of a client who is restrained in bed with bilateral wrist restraints. Following assessment of the restraints, what should the nurse's documentation include? Select all that apply.
☐ 1. nutrition and hydration needs
☐ 2. capillary refill
☐ 3. continued need for restraints
☐ 4. need for medication
☐ 5. skin integrity

123. The nurse is instituting a falls prevention program. Which personnel should be involved in the program? Select all that apply.
☐ 1. registered nurses
☐ 2. insurance providers
☐ 3. unlicensed assistive personnel
☐ 4. housekeeping services
☐ 5. family members
☐ 6. client

124. The nurse unit manager is making rounds on a team of clients and notices a client with a color-coded armband that indicates the client is at risk for falling while walking down the hall unassisted. The client is at the end of the hallway and far from their room, but they are not tired. What should the nurse do **first**?
☐ 1. Obtain a wheelchair, and take the client back to the room.
☐ 2. Walk with the client back to the room, and assist the client to get in bed or a chair.
☐ 3. Locate an unlicensed nursing personnel (UAP) to walk with the client back to the room.
☐ 4. Instruct the client to walk only in the room at this time.

125. The health care provider has prescribed 5 mg of warfarin given orally for a hospitalized client. In planning care for this client, the nurse understands that which service(s) would be contacted? Check all that apply.
☐ 1. pharmacy
☐ 2. dietary
☐ 3. laboratory
☐ 4. discharge planning
☐ 5. risk management

126. Unlicensed assistive personnel (UAP) are helping a client who had knee surgery 2 days ago get into bed. As the nurse makes rounds, which information requires the nurse to intervene?
☐ 1. The call light is pinned to the head of the bed in the client's reach.
☐ 2. The night light is dimmed, giving low-level lighting to the room.
☐ 3. There is a clear path to the bathroom.
☐ 4. The side rails on the head and foot of the bed are in the up position.

127. The nurse is going to lunch and is conducting a "hand-off of care" to the charge nurse. Which information should the nurse communicate to the charge nurse during the hand-off of care communication?
☐ 1. Tell the charge nurse that the nurse is going to lunch.
☐ 2. Verify that the charge nurse has assigned someone else to take care of the client.
☐ 3. Give the charge nurse information about what care should be given while the nurse is at lunch.
☐ 4. Remind the charge nurse about the client's history and current medications.

128. The client has been diagnosed with septic arthritis in a hip joint. Which outcome(s) would be desired from a client-focused teaching plan? Select all that apply.
☐ 1. Report pain that is severe enough to limit activities.
☐ 2. Discuss how to take prescribed medications.
☐ 3. Describe how the application of a heating pad set on "high" readily resolves edema.
☐ 4. Describe the septic arthritis physiologic process.
☐ 5. Explain the importance of supporting the affected joint.
☐ 6. Describe how to use ambulatory aids and assistive devices.

129. The nurse is identifying clients who should receive passive range-of-motion (PROM) exercises when the unlicensed assistive personnel (UAP) are providing care. For which client(s) should the nurse instruct the UAPs to perform PROM exercises? Select all that apply.
a client who:
☐ 1. has septic joints
☐ 2. has a temporary loss of sensation
☐ 3. is unconscious
☐ 4. has plantar flexion of the foot
☐ 5. has supination of the hand

130. A client is at moderate risk for falling according to a fall risk assessment scale. What should the nurse instruct the unlicensed assistive personnel (UAP) to do?
☐ 1. Remain with the client during toileting.
☐ 2. Reorient the client to time and place every hour.
☐ 3. Activate the bed and chair alarms.
☐ 4. Apply a protective chest restraint.

131. The nurse is planning care for a client who is at low risk for falling. What information would be included in the care plan? Select all that apply.
☐ 1. Place the call bell within easy reach.
☐ 2. Secure locks on beds, stretchers, and wheelchairs.
☐ 3. Remain with the client during toileting.
☐ 4. Keep the bed in the lowest position when possible.
☐ 5. Place a commode next to the bed for easy access.
☐ 6. Employ a seat belt whenever a wheelchair is in use.

Answers, Rationales, and Test-Taking Strategies

The answers and rationales for each question follow below, along with keys (🔑) to the client need (CN) and cognitive level (CL) for each question. In addition, questions that measure clinical judgment will be coded (CJ). As you check your answers, use the **Content Mastery and Test-Taking Skill Self-Analysis** *worksheet (tear-out worksheet in the back of the book) to identify the reason(s) for not answering the questions correctly. For additional information about test-taking skills and strategies for answering questions, refer to pages 12–51 in part 1 of this book.*

The Adult with Rheumatoid Arthritis

1. **3.** Initially, most clients with early symptoms of rheumatoid arthritis report early morning stiffness or stiffness after sitting still for a while. Later symptoms of rheumatoid arthritis include limited joint range of motion; deformed joints, especially of the hand; and rheumatoid nodules.

    🔑 CN: Physiological adaptation; CL: Analyze

2. **1.** Based on the information from the client, the nurse should develop a plan with the client that will conserve energy and decrease episodes of fatigue. Although the client may develop a self-care deficit related to increased joint pain, they are voicing concerns about household chores and difficulty around the house and yard, not self-care issues. Over time, the client may have difficulty coping, but that is not the current concern. Employing cleaning services may not be within the client's budget, and they should first try a plan that balances rest and activity.

    🔑 CN: Basic care and comfort; CL: Analyze

3. –/+ **1, 2, 4.** RA affects women three times more often than men between the ages of 20 and 55 years. Research has determined that RA occurs in clients who have had an infectious disease, such as the Epstein-Barr virus. A genetic link, specifically HLA-DR4, has been found in 65% of clients with RA. People with osteoarthritis are not necessarily at risk for developing RA.

    🔑 CN: Reduction of risk potential; CL: Analyze

4. **1, 2, 4, 3.** Pain relief is the highest priority during the acute phase because pain is typically severe and interferes with the client's ability to function. Preserving joint function is the next goal to set, followed by preventing joint deformity during the acute phase to promote an optimal level of functioning and reduce the risk for contractures. Maintaining the usual ways of accomplishing tasks is the goal with the lowest priority during the acute phase. Rather, the focus is on developing less stressful ways of accomplishing routine tasks.

    🔑 CN: Health promotion and maintenance; CL: Analyze

5. **3.** Heat-producing liniment can produce a burn if used with other heat devices that could intensify the response to the heat. Heat and cold can be used as often as the client desires. However, each application of heat should not exceed 20 minutes, and each application of cold should not exceed 10 to 15 minutes. Application for longer periods results in the opposite of the intended effect: vasoconstriction instead of vasodilation with heat and vasodilation instead of vasoconstriction with cold.

    🔑 CN: Reduction of risk potential; CL: Evaluate

6. **4.** The nurse's most appropriate response is one that is therapeutic. The basic principle of therapeutic communication and a therapeutic relationship is honesty. Therefore, the nurse needs to explain truthfully that each client is different and that there are various forms of arthritis and arthritis treatment. To state that it is the HCP's prerogative to decide how to treat the client implies that the client is not a member of their own health care team and is not a participant in their care. The statement also is defensive, which serves to block any further communication or questions. Asking the client to tell more about the friend presumes that the client knows correct and complete information, which is not a valid assumption to make. The nurse does not know about the client's friend and should not make statements about another client's condition. Stating that the drug is for advanced disease demonstrates that the nurse is making assumptions that are not necessarily valid or appropriate. Also, telling the client that they are not eligible for the drug now is not within the scope of the nurse's practice.

    🔑 CN: Psychosocial adaptation; CL: Analyze

7. **4.** Positions of flexion should be avoided to prevent loss of functional ability of affected joints. Proper body alignment during rest periods is encouraged to maintain correct muscle and joint placement. Lying in the prone position is encouraged to avoid further curvature of the spine and internal rotation of the shoulders.

    🔑 CN: Physiological adaptation; CL: Analyze

8. **4.** Carrying a laundry basket with clenched fingers and fists is not an example of conserving energy of small joints. The laundry basket should be held with both hands opened as wide as possible and with outstretched arms so that pressure is not placed on the small joints of the fingers. When rising from a chair, the palms should be used instead of the fingers so as to distribute weight over the larger area of the palms. Holding packages close to the body provides greater support to the shoulder, elbow, and wrist joints because the muscles of the arms and hands are used to stabilize the weight against the body. This decreases the stress and weight or pull on small joints, such as the fingers. Objects can be slid with the palm of the hand, which distributes weight over the larger area of the palms instead of stressing the small joints of the fingers to pick up the weight of the object to move it to another place.

    CN: Basic care and comfort; CL: Evaluate

9. **1.** Because some over-the-counter vitamin supplements contain folic acid, the client should avoid self-medication with vitamins while taking methotrexate, a folic acid antagonist. Because methotrexate is hepatotoxic, the client should avoid the intake of alcohol, which could increase the risk for hepatotoxicity. Methotrexate can cause bone marrow depression, placing the client at risk for infection. Therefore, meticulous mouth care is essential to minimize the risk for infection. Contraception should be used during methotrexate therapy and for 8 weeks after the therapy has been discontinued because of its effect on mitosis. Methotrexate is considered teratogenic.

    CN: Pharmacological and parenteral therapies; CL: Evaluate

10. **2.** Difficulty seeing out of one eye, when evaluated in conjunction with the client's medication therapy regimen, leads to the suspicion of possible retinal degeneration. The possibility of an irreversible retinal degeneration caused by deposits of hydroxychloroquine in the layers of the retina requires an ophthalmologic examination before therapy is begun and at 6-month intervals. Although cataracts may develop in young adults, they are less likely, and damage from the hydroxychloroquine is the most obvious at-risk factor. Eyesight is not affected by the disease process of rheumatoid arthritis.

    CN: Pharmacological and parenteral therapies; CL: Analyze

11. **1.** Gastric upset is a side effect of nonsteroidal anti-inflammatory medications; taking medication with food minimizes this effect. Corticosteroids affect adrenal gland function and are discontinued by lowering the dose gradually, but this is not true of nonsteroidal anti-inflammatory medications. It is not necessary to rinse the mouth, as stomatitis is not a usual side effect. Dizziness is not an effect of this drug.

    CN: Pharmacological and parenteral therapies; CL: Analyze

12. **4.** Superficial heat applications, such as tub baths, showers, and warm compresses, can be helpful in relieving pain and stiffness. Exercises can be performed more comfortably and more effectively after heat applications. A client with rheumatoid arthritis must balance rest with exercise every day, not every other day. Typically, large doses of analgesics, which can lead to hepatotoxic effects, are not necessary. Learning to cope with the pain by refocusing is inappropriate.

    CN: Basic care and comfort; CL: Analyze

13. **1, 2, 5.** An arthrocentesis is performed to aspirate excess synovial fluid, pus, or blood from a joint cavity to relieve pain or to diagnose inflammatory diseases such as rheumatoid arthritis. A local agent may be used to decrease the pain of the needle insertion through the skin and into the joint cavity. Aspiration of the fluid into the syringe can be very painful because of the size and inflammation of the joint. Usually, a steroid medication is injected locally to alleviate the inflammation; a compression bandage is applied to help decrease swelling; and the client is asked to rest the joint for up to 24 hours afterward to help relieve the pain and promote rest to the inflamed joint. The client may experience pain during this time until the inflammation begins to resolve and swelling decreases.

    CN: Reduction of risk potential; CL: Create

The Adult with Osteoarthritis

14. **1, 4, 5.** To prepare a client for arthrocentesis, the nurse should tell the client that a local anesthetic administered by the health care provider will decrease discomfort. There may be bleeding after the procedure, so the nurse should check the dressing. The client may experience pain. The nurse should offer pain medication and evaluate outcomes for pain relief. Because a local anesthetic is used, the client will not require preoperative medication. The client will rest the knee for 24 hours and then should begin range-of-motion and muscle-strengthening exercises.

    CN: Safety and infection control; CL: Create

The Adult with Musculoskeletal Health Problems 677

15. 1. Metal will interfere with the test. Metallic objects within the examination field, such as jewelry, earrings, and dental amalgams, may inhibit organ visualization and can produce unclear images. Ingesting foods and beverages days before the test will not affect bone mineral status. Short-term calcium gluconate intake will also not influence bone mineral status. The client may already have had chronic pain as a result of a bone fracture or osteoporosis.

🔑 CN: Management of care; CL: Analyze

16. 1. Shorter sessions will allow the client to rest between the sessions. Changing the HCP's prescription to a different examination will not provide the information needed for this client's treatment. Acetaminophen is a nonopioid analgesic and an antipyretic, not an anti-inflammatory agent; thus, it would not help this client avoid the adverse effects of a lengthy x-ray examination. Although the x-ray table is hard, it is not possible to provide padding and obtain the needed diagnostic x-rays.

🔑 CN: Management of care; CL: Analyze

17. 4. Osteoarthritis is a degenerative joint disease with local manifestations such as local joint pain. Rheumatoid arthritis has systemic manifestations such as anemia and osteoporosis. Weight loss occurs in rheumatoid arthritis, whereas most clients with osteoarthritis are overweight.

🔑 CN: Physiological adaptation; CL: Analyze

18. −/+ **1, 2, 3.** A diet with adequate amounts of vitamin D aids in the regulation, absorption, and subsequent utilization of calcium and phosphorus, which are necessary for the normal calcification of bone. Figs, broccoli, and almonds are very good sources of calcium. A moderate intake of alcohol has no known negative effects on bone density, but excessive alcohol intake does reduce bone density. Swimming, biking, and other non–weight-bearing exercises do not maintain bone mass. Walking and running, which are weight-bearing exercises, do maintain bone mass. The client should eat a balanced diet but does not need to avoid high-fat foods.

🔑 CN: Health promotion and maintenance; CL: Create

19. 1. Capsaicin cream, which produces analgesia by preventing the reaccumulation of substance P in the peripheral sensory neurons, is made from the active ingredients of hot peppers. Therefore, clients should wash their hands immediately after applying capsaicin cream, if they do not wear gloves, to avoid possible contact between the cream and mucous membranes. Clients are instructed to avoid wearing tight bandages over areas where capsaicin cream has been applied because swelling may occur from inflammation of arthritis in the joint and lead to constriction on the peripheral neurovascular system. Capsaicin cream should be stored at a temperature between 59°F and 86°F (15°C and 30°C). The cabinet over the stove in the kitchen would be too warm. Capsaicin cream should not come in contact with irritated and broken skin, mucous membranes, or eyes. Therefore, it should not be used on cuts or burns.

🔑 CN: Pharmacological and parenteral therapies; CL: Evaluate

20. 3. Drugs that cause gastric irritation, such as ibuprofen, are best taken after or with a meal, when stomach contents help minimize the local irritation. Taking the medication on an empty stomach at any time during the day will lead to gastric irritation. Taking the drug at bedtime with food may cause the client to gain weight, possibly aggravating osteoarthritis. When the client arises, they are stiff from immobility and should use warmth and stretching until they get food in the stomach.

🔑 CN: Pharmacological and parenteral therapies; CL: Analyze

21. 1. Corticosteroids are used for clients with osteoarthritis to obtain a local effect. Therefore, they are given only via intra-articular injection. Oral corticosteroids are avoided because they can cause an acceleration of osteoarthritis. Rheumatoid arthritis and osteoarthritis are two different diseases.

🔑 CN: Pharmacological and parenteral therapies; CL: Analyze

22. 2. Weight-bearing exercise plays a very important role in stimulating the regeneration of cartilage, which lacks blood vessels, by driving synovial fluid through the joint cartilage. Joint mobility is increased by weight-bearing exercises, not range-of-motion exercises, because surrounding muscles, ligaments, and tendons are strengthened. Pain is an early sign of degenerative joint bone problems. Swelling may not occur for some time after pain, if at all. Osteoarthritic pain is worsened in cold, damp weather; therefore, exercising outdoors is not recommended year-round in all settings.

🔑 CN: Health promotion and maintenance; CL: Evaluate

The Adult with a Hip Fracture

23. 4. The hip spica cast is used for the treatment of femoral fractures; it immobilizes the affected extremity and the trunk securely. A double-hip spica cast extends from above the nipple line to the base of the foot of both extremities. Constipation, possibly caused by lack of mobility, can cause abdominal distention or bloating. When the spica cast becomes too tight because of distention, the cast will compress the superior mesenteric artery against the duodenum. The compression produces abdominal pain, abdominal pressure, nausea, and vomiting. To relieve the compression, the surgeon can cut a "window" in the cast. The nurse should assess the abdomen for decreased bowel sounds, not the superior mesenteric artery. The surgeon cannot manipulate a fracture through a small window in a double-hip spica cast. The nurse cannot use the window to aid in repositioning because the window opening can break and negate the effect of the cast.

CN: Reduction of risk potential; CL: Evaluate

24. 3. With an intracapsular hip fracture, the affected leg is shorter than the unaffected leg because of muscle spasms and external rotation. The client also experiences severe pain in the region of the fracture.

CN: Physiological adaptation; CL: Analyze

25. 4. The insertion of a pin for the internal fixation of an extracapsular fractured hip provides good fixation of the fracture. The fracture site is stabilized, and fractured bone ends are well approximated. As a result, the client is able to be mobilized sooner, thus reducing the risks of complications related to immobility. Internal fixation with a pin insertion does not prevent hemorrhage or decrease the risk for neurovascular impairment, which are potential complications associated with any joint or bone surgery. It does not lessen the client's risk for infection at the site.

CN: Reduction of risk potential; CL: Apply

26. 3. The primary purpose of the drainage tube is to prevent fluid accumulation in the wound. Fluid, when it accumulates, creates dead space. Elimination of the dead space by keeping the wound free of fluid greatly enhances wound healing and helps prevent abscess formation. Although the characteristics of the drainage from the tube, such as a change in color or appearance, may suggest a possible infection, this is not the tube's primary purpose. The drainage tube does not eliminate the need for wound irrigation or provide a way to instill antibiotics into the wound.

CN: Reduction of risk potential; CL: Apply

27. 1. Any activity or position that causes flexion, adduction, or internal rotation of more than 90 degrees should be avoided until the soft tissue surrounding the prosthesis has stabilized, at approximately 6 weeks. Crossing the legs while sitting down causes internal rotation and can lead to dislocation of the femoral head from the hip socket. Sitting on a raised commode seat prevents hip flexion and adduction. Using an abductor splint while side-lying keeps the hip joint in abduction, thus preventing adduction and possible dislocation. Rising straight from a chair to a standing position is acceptable for this client because this action avoids hip flexion, adduction, and internal rotation of more than 90 degrees.

CN: Reduction of risk potential; CL: Analyze

28. 3. Troponin is a cardiac biomarker and is normally almost undetectable in the blood. A level of 1.4 mcg/L (1.4 µg/L) means there has likely been some damage to the heart muscle. Although the serum glucose level (normal is 60 to 100 mg/dL [3.3 to 5.5 mmol/L]) and the ESR (normal is less than 20 mm per hour for men older than 50 years) are slightly elevated, this could be explained by normal stress and an inflammatory response to surgery. The hematocrit level is low (normal is 40% to 45% [0.4 to 0.5 proportion of 1.0] for men), but it is also not unexpected for a client following surgery.

CN: Physiological adaption; CL: Analyze

29. 3. A high-backed straight chair with armrests is recommended to help keep the client in the best possible alignment after surgery for femoral head prosthesis placement. Using this type of chair helps prevent dislocation of the prosthesis from the socket. A desk-type swivel chair, a padded upholstered chair, or a recliner should be avoided because they do not provide good body alignment and can cause the overly flexed femoral head to dislocate.

CN: Reduction of risk potential; CL: Analyze

30. The air cell should be centered on the back of the client's calf.

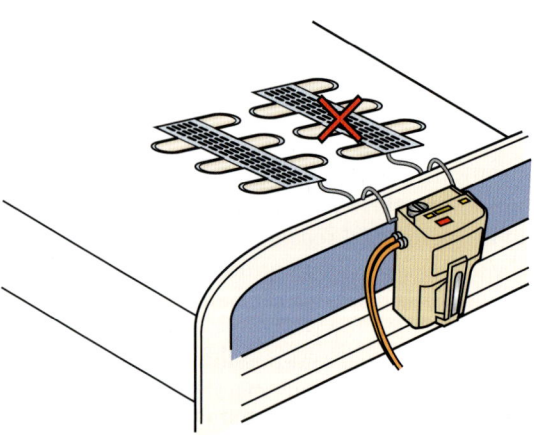

CN: Safety and infection control; CL: Apply

31. **2.** Although pets and furniture, such as snack tables and rocking chairs, may pose a problem, scatter rugs are the single greatest hazard in the home, especially for older adults who are unsure and unsteady with walking. Falls have been found to account for almost half the accidental deaths that occur in the home. The risk for falls is further compounded by the client's need for crutches.

CN: Safety and infection control; CL: Analyze

The Adult Having Hip Replacement Surgery

32. **3.** To obtain the best results, one sheet should be used to cover the mattress. The air cells should be facing up as shown. Thick pads should not be used; if the client is incontinent, a "breathable" incontinent pad can be added. The client can use a pillow as needed.

CN: Basic Care and Comfort; CL: Apply

33. **2, 3, 4, 5.** A client who has had a posterolateral total hip replacement should not adduct the hip joint, which would lead to dislocation of the ball out of the socket; therefore, the client should be encouraged to keep the toes pointed slightly outward when using a walker. An abduction pillow should be kept between the legs to keep the hip joint in an abducted position. The client should rotate between lying supine and lateral on the unoperated side, but not on the operated side. Ice is used to reduce swelling on the operative side. The client should not flex the operated hip beyond a 90-degree angle, such as when bending down to tie or slip on shoes. Doing so could lead to joint dislocation.

CN: Reduction of risk potential; CL: Create

34. **1, 3, 4.** A client who has had a total hip replacement via an anterolateral approach has almost the opposite precautions as those for a client who has had a total hip replacement through the posterolateral approach. The hip joint should not be actively abducted. The client should avoid turning the toes or knee outward. The client should keep the legs side by side without a pillow or wedge. The client should use an elevated toilet seat and shower chair and should not extend the operative leg backward. The client should perform range-of-motion exercises as directed by the physical therapist.

CN: Reduction of risk potential; CL: Create

35. **2.** Being unable to move the affected leg suggests neurologic impairment. A decrease in the distal pulse, diminished capillary refill, and coolness to touch of the affected extremity suggest vascular compromise.

CN: Reduction of risk potential; CL: Analyze

36. **4.** The nurse should first identify and discuss the client's fears about the procedure. Only then can the client begin to hear what the nurse has to share about the individualized teaching plan designed to meet the client's needs. In the preoperative period, the client needs to learn how to correctly prevent hip flexion and demonstrate coughing and deep breathing. However, this teaching can be effective only after the client's fears have been assessed and addressed. Although the client may appreciate seeing what a hip prosthesis looks like, so as to understand the new body part, this is not a necessity.

CN: Psychosocial adaptation; CL: Analyze

37. **3.** The joint has dislocated when the client with a total joint prosthesis develops severe sudden pain and an inability to move the extremity. Clinical manifestations of an infection would include inflammation, redness, erythema, and possibly drainage and separation of the wound. Bleeding could be external (e.g., blood visible from the wound or on the dressing) or internal and manifested by signs of shock (e.g., pallor, coolness, hypotension, tachycardia). The seepage of glue into soft tissue would have occurred in the operating room, when the glue is still in liquid form. The glue dries into a hard, fixed form before the wound is closed.

CN: Reduction of risk potential; CL: Analyze

38. **1, 5.** To prevent the client from becoming dehydrated, the nurse should encourage the client to increase their oral fluid intake and administer the acetaminophen to lower the temperature to minimize the fluid loss from diaphoresis. The client is receiving adequate IV fluids, and it is not necessary to request additional fluids at this time. The client is not in severe pain and cannot have another dose of morphine for another 3 hours. The nurse, not the client, should inspect the incision for bleeding. The client does not need to be on bed rest but rather should get out of bed with assistance to promote lung expansion and maintain strength.

CN: Physiological adaptation CL: Analyze

39. **4.** After total hip replacement, proper positioning by the nurse prevents dislocation of the prosthesis. The nurse should place the client in a supine position and keep the affected extremity in slight abduction using an abduction splint or pillows or Buck's extension traction. The client must not abduct or flex the operated hip because this may produce dislocation.

CN: Reduction of risk potential; CL: Analyze

40. 2, 4, 5. Following total hip replacement, the client should use the overhead trapeze to assist with position changes. The head of the bed should not be elevated more than 45 degrees; any height higher than 45 degrees puts a strain on the hip joint and may cause dislocation. To use a fracture bedpan, instruct the client to flex the unoperated hip and knee to lift the buttocks onto the pan. Toe-pointing exercises stimulate circulation in the lower extremities to prevent the formation of thrombi and potential emboli. The prone position is avoided shortly after a total hip replacement.

🔑 CN: Heath promotion and maintenance; CL: Analyze

41. 1, 3, 4. Administration of antibiotics as prescribed will aid in the acquisition of therapeutic blood levels during and immediately after surgery to prevent osteomyelitis. The nurse can request that a trapeze be added to the bed so the client can assist with lifting and turning. The nurse should also demonstrate and have the client practice isometric exercises (muscle setting) of quadriceps and gluteal muscles. The client will not use crutches after surgery; a physical therapy assistant will initially assist the client with walking by using a walker. The client will not use Buck's traction. The client will require antiembolism stockings and the use of a leg compression device to minimize the risk for thrombus formation and potential emboli; the leg compression device is applied during surgery and maintained per prescription.

🔑 CN: Reduction of risk potential; CL: Create

42. 1, 2, 3, 4. Client/family teaching should include advising the client to report any symptoms of unusual bleeding or bruising, dizziness, itching, rash, fever, swelling, or difficulty breathing to the HCP immediately. The nurse should instruct the client to avoid taking aspirin or nonsteroidal anti-inflammatory drugs without consulting the HCP while on therapy. Low-molecular-weight heparin is considered to be a high-risk medication, and the client should wear or carry medical identification. The air bubble should not be expelled from the syringe because the bubble ensures the client receives the full dose of the medication. The client should allow 5 seconds to pass before withdrawing the needle to prevent seepage of the medication out of the site.

🔑 CN: Pharmacological and parenteral therapies; CL: Create

43. 3. Dislocation precautions include avoiding extremes of internal rotation, adduction, and 90-degree flexion of the affected hip for at least 4 to 6 weeks after the procedure. Using an abduction pillow prevents adduction. Decreasing use of the abductor pillow does not strengthen the muscles to prevent dislocation. Informing a client to "not worry" is not therapeutic. A cushioned toilet seat does not prevent hip dislocation.

🔑 CN: Reduction of risk potential; CL: Analyze

44. 1, 2, 3. Dislocation of a hip prosthesis may occur with positioning that exceeds the limits of the prosthesis. The nurse must recognize dislocation of the prosthesis. Signs of prosthesis dislocation include acute groin pain in the affected hip, shortening of the affected leg, restricted ability or inability to move the affected leg, and reported "popping" sensation in the hip. Toe wiggling is not a test for potential hip dislocation.

🔑 CN: Reduction of risk potential; CL: Analyze

45. 4. If a prosthesis becomes dislocated, the nurse should immediately notify the surgeon. This is done so the hip can be reduced and stabilized promptly to prevent nerve damage and maintain circulation. After closed reduction, the hip may be stabilized with Buck's traction or a brace to prevent recurrent dislocation. If prescribed by the surgeon, an ice pack may be applied after reduction to limit edema, though caution must be used because of the potential for muscle spasms. Some orthopedic surgeons may prescribe the client be turned toward the side of the reduced hip, but that is not the nurse's first response.

🔑 CN: Reduction of risk potential; CL: Analyze

46. 3. Expected outcomes for the client at the time of discharge from the surgical unit after a hip replacement include increased independence in transfers, participation in progressive ambulation without pain or assistance, and the ability to raise the affected leg without assistance. The client will not be able to walk throughout the hospital, walk for a distance without some postoperative pain, or raise the affected leg more than several inches. The client may be referred to a rehabilitation unit to achieve additional independence, strength, and pain relief.

🔑 CN: Physiological adaptation; CL: Evaluate

47. 1. DVT is a complication of total joint replacement and may occur during hospitalization or develop later when the client is home. Clients who are obese or have previous a history of a DVT or pulmonary embolism are at high risk. Immobility produces venous stasis, increasing the client's chance to develop a venous thromboembolism. Signs of DVT include unilateral calf tenderness, warmth, redness, and edema (increased calf circumference). Findings should be reported promptly to the health care provider for definitive evaluation and therapy. Polyuria may be indicative of diabetes mellitus. Displacement of the new joint is unlikely. Wound evisceration is more likely to occur after abdominal surgeries.

 CN: Reduction of risk potential; CL: Analyze

The Adult Having Knee Replacement Surgery

48. 3. When combined with a weight loss program, aquatic exercise would be best because it cushions the joints and allows the client to burn off calories. Aquatic exercise promotes circulation, muscle toning, and lung expansion, which promote healthy preoperative conditioning. Weight lifting and walking are too stressful to the joints, possibly exacerbating the client's osteoarthritis. Although tai chi exercise is designed for stretching and coordination, it would not be the best exercise for this client to help with weight loss.

 CN: Health promotion and maintenance; CL: Analyze

49. 1. The nurse should suspect nerve damage if numbness is present. However, whether the damage is short term and related to edema or long term and related to permanent nerve damage would not be clear at this point. The nurse needs to continue to assess the client's neurovascular status, including pain, pallor, pulselessness, paresthesia, and paralysis (the five Ps). Bleeding would suggest vascular damage or hemorrhage. Dislocation would suggest malalignment. A pink color would suggest adequate circulation to the area. Numbness would suggest neurologic damage.

 CN: Reduction of risk potential; CL: Analyze

50. 4. After knee arthroplasty, the knee will be extended and immobilized with a firm compression dressing and an adjustable soft extension splint in place. An SCD will be applied. The SCD can be discontinued when the client is ambulatory, but while the client is in bed, the SCD needs to be maintained to prevent thromboembolism. The SCD should be positioned on the bed, but not on two pillows. Settings for the SCD are prescribed by the orthopedic surgeon. Initial dressing changes are completed by the orthopedic surgeon and changed as needed per prescription.

 CN: Reduction of risk potential; CL: Analyze

51. -/+ 2, 3. It is anticipated that there might be some swelling, redness, and discomfort immediately after activity, including physical therapy. Ideally, pain medication could be offered or given before therapy to reduce posttreatment pain, but it should also be administered now. Elevation and cold packs can also reduce swelling and decrease pain. It is not appropriate to notify the HCP as pain and swelling are normal after therapy. It is also not appropriate to massage the area. This will increase circulation and therefore increase swelling and pain.

 CN: Management of care; CL: Analyze

52. -/+ 1, 2, 3. The nurse should instruct the client to notify the dentist or other HCPs about the joint so the HCP can prescribe prophylactic antibiotics before the client undergoes any invasive procedure (e.g., tooth extraction) because of the potential for bacteremia. The nurse should also advise the client that the metal components of the joint may set off the metal detector alarms in airports. The client should also report having the metal joint before having MRI studies because, depending on the type of joint replacement, the implanted metal components could be pulled toward the large magnet core of the MRI. Any weight bearing that is permitted is prescribed by the orthopedic surgeon and is usually not limited to 5 lb (2.3 kg). After surgery, the client can resume a normal diet with regular fluid intake.

 CN: Health promotion and maintenance; CL: Create

53. 1. The aPTT is at a critical value, and the client should receive protamine sulfate as the antidote for heparin. Vitamin K is the antidote for warfarin. Packed red blood cells are administered to increase the hematocrit.

 CN: Pharmacological and parenteral therapies; CL: Apply

54. -/+ 1, 2, 3, 4. Postoperatively, the knee in a total knee replacement is dressed with a compression bandage, and ice may be applied to control edema and bleeding. Recurrent assessment by the nurse for neurovascular changes can prevent loss of limb. Normal neurovascular findings include color normal, extremity warm, capillary refill less than 3 seconds, moderate edema, tissue not palpably tense, pain controllable, normal sensations, no paresthesia, normal motor abilities, no paresis or paralysis, and pulses strong and equal.

 CN: Reduction of risk potential; CL: Analyze

55. 4. The knee is usually protected with a knee immobilizer (splint, cast, or brace) and is elevated when the client sits in a chair. Before and after surgery, the HCP prescribes weight-bearing limits and the use of assistive devices for progressive ambulation. Positioning a straight-backed chair at the foot of the bed is not an activity conducive to getting the client out of bed on the evening before surgery for a total knee replacement.

 CN: Reduction of risk potential; CL: Analyze

56. -/+ 1, 4. After a total knee replacement, efforts are directed at preventing complications, such as thromboembolism, infection, limited range of motion, and peroneal nerve palsy. The nurse should instruct the client to report signs of infection, such as an increased temperature. To prevent edema, the affected leg must remain elevated when the client sits in a chair. The client will wear antiembolism stockings at all times, including when sleeping. After discharge, the client may undergo physical therapy on an outpatient basis per HCP prescription. The client should leave the dressing in place until the follow-up visit with the surgeon.

 CN: Reduction of risk potential; CL: Create

The Adult with a Herniated Disk

57. 1. The client is using correct body mechanics for lifting because they are keeping their back as straight as possible and holding the box close to their body. The client is using their large leg muscles to lift the box. The client is using a broad base of support by placing their feet as wide apart as possible. The other suggestions would cause the client to put a strain on their back.

 CN: Reduction of risk potential; CL: Analyze

58. 3. A client with low back pain should not exceed the prescribed exercises even though the client may think, "If this will make me well, double will make me well quicker." When exceeding prescribed exercise programs, the client's muscles may be unconditioned and easily tired, leading to injury and increased pain. To use proper body mechanics when lifting light objects, the client should bring the item close to the center of gravity, which occurs when the object is kept below the level of the elbows. Leaning forward while bending the knees allows for the muscles of the thigh to be used instead of those of the lower back. Sleeping on the side with the legs flexed is appropriate because the spine is kept in a neutral position without twisting or pulling on muscles.

 CN: Reduction of risk potential; CL: Analyze

59. 1. The nurse instructs the client to start the prescription by taking the least amount of the medication. The client is advised to monitor their pain level and adjust the dosage according to the amount of pain relief.

 CN: Pharmacological and parenteral therapies; CL: Analyze

60. 3, 4, 1, 2. When the client is not entirely able to get out of bed, the nurse should first assist the client to lie down for comfort and safety before administering the prescribed celecoxib. Applying a warm compress will further promote relaxation of skeletal muscles. The HCP should be kept informed of the client's status and nursing actions already taken.

 CN: Basic care and comfort; CL: Analyze

61. 2. Standing with a flattened spine slightly tilted forward and slightly flexed to the affected side indicates a postural deformity. Motor changes would include findings such as hypotonia or muscle weakness. Absent or diminished reflexes related to the level of herniation would indicate an alteration in reflexes. Sensory changes would include findings such as paresthesia and numbness related to the specific tract of the herniation.

 CN: Physiological adaptation; CL: Analyze

62. 2. A supine position with the client's legs flexed is the most comfortable position because it allows for the disc to recess off of the nerve, thus alleviating pressure and pain. The prone position causes hyperextension of the spine and increased pressure of the disc on the nerve root on the right. A ruptured disc at L5–S1 right identifies a ruptured disc compressing the right nerve root exiting the L5–S1 spinous process; terms such as this are commonly used in the analysis of a magnetic resonance image, myelogram, or history and physical examination. If the ruptured area of the disc were in the central area of the spinous process, the prone position and hyperextension might relieve the disc pressure on the nerve. A high Fowler's or sitting position increases the pressure of the disc on the nerve root because of gravity, as does a right semiprone position.

 CN: Physiological adaptation; CL: Analyze

63. 2. Based on the client's comments, the nurse should call the surgeon to verify the location of the surgery. The client's comments indicate radiculopathy of L4–L5, but the informed consent form states L3–L4. Radiculopathy of L3–L4 involves pain radiating from the back to the buttocks to the posterior thigh to the inner calf. The nurse must act as a client advocate and not ask the client to sign the consent until the correct procedure is identified and confirmed on the consent. The nurse has no legal authority or

responsibility to change the consent. The history is a source of information, but when the client is coherent and the history is contradictory, the health care provider should be contacted to clarify the situation. Ultimately, it is the surgeon's responsibility to identify the site of surgery specified on the surgical consent form.

CN: Management of care; CL: Analyze

64. 2. Ondansetron hydrochloride is a selective serotonin receptor antagonist that acts centrally to control the client's nausea in the postoperative phase. It does not control muscle spasms, shivering, or dry mouth.

CN: Pharmacological and parenteral therapies; CL: Evaluate

65. 4. Sweeping causes a twisting motion, which should be avoided because twisting can cause undue stress on the recently ruptured disc site, muscle spasms, and a potential recurrent disc rupture. Although the client should not bend at the waist, such as when washing dishes at the sink, the client can dry dishes because no bending is necessary. The client can sit in a firm chair that keeps the back anatomically aligned. The client should not twist and pull, so when making the bed, the client should pull the covers up on one side and then walk around to the other side before trying to pull the covers up there.

CN: Physiological adaptation; CL: Evaluate

66. 4. After a lumbar laminectomy of L4–L5, a client who is returning to work should avoid sitting whenever possible. If the client must sit, they should sit only in chairs that allow the knees to be higher than the hips and support the arms to maintain correct body alignment and reduce undue stress on the spine. Maintaining good body posture is most important after a lumbar laminectomy of L4–L5. By 6 weeks after the surgery, the client should have regained stamina. To maintain correct body posture, the client should also place one foot on a step stool during prolonged standing. Sleeping on the back with a support under the knees is effective in maintaining correct body posture. Maintaining an average weight for height is important in maintaining a healthy back because carrying extra weight causes undue stress on back muscles.

CN: Physiological adaptation; CL: Analyze

67. 2. Clear yellowish fluid on the dressing may be cerebrospinal fluid (CSF). This fluid must be tested for glucose to determine whether it is CSF. If so, the client is at great risk for an infection of the central nervous system, which has a high mortality rate. The client should be able to laterally rotate the head and neck, which is above the surgical site in the spinal column. During the nursing postoperative neuromuscular-vascular assessment of movement of the head and neck, the nurse should find results consistent with the preoperative baseline status. Using the standing position to void is normal for a male client. Coughing is the body's defense mechanism to help clear the lungs of the anesthetic agents and to ventilate the lungs in response to a sustained deep inspiration for ventilation of the lower lobes of the lungs. A frequent cough could place a strain on the incision site and should be avoided. Also, a productive cough of thick, yellow sputum would indicate the complication of a respiratory infection.

CN: Reduction of risk potential; CL: Analyze

68. 4. The client should wear a thin cotton undershirt under the brace to prevent the brace from abrading directly against the skin. The cotton material also aids in absorbing any moisture, such as perspiration, that could lead to skin irritation and breakdown. Applying lotion is not recommended before applying the brace because further skin breakdown can result (related to the collection of moisture where microorganisms can grow). Applying extra padding (e.g., to the iliac crests) is not recommended because the padding can become wrinkled, producing more pressure sites and skin breakdown. Use of baby or talcum powder and lotion is not recommended because they can cause irritation and skin breakdown.

CN: Reduction of risk potential; CL: Evaluate

69. 1. Typically, the donor site causes more pain than the fused site does because inflammation, swelling, and venous oozing around the nerve endings in the donor site, where the subcutaneous tissue was removed, occur during the first 24 to 48 hours postoperatively. After surgery, the surgeon applies a pressure dressing to the donor site to compress the veins that were transected for the removal of subcutaneous tissue but that did not stop oozing blood after surgical cauterization. Pressure on a transected vein, which is low pressure, stops the oozing and loss of blood from the venous site. When the donor site is the fibula, neurovascular checks must be performed every hour to ensure adequate neurologic function and circulation to the area. The surgeon, not the degree or amount of pain, specifies activity restrictions.

CN: Physiological adaptation; CL: Analyze

70. 1. A client who has had back surgery should place their feet flat on the floor to avoid strain on the incision. Placing the feet on a low or high footstool or in any other position of comfort with the legs uncrossed increases the pressure on the suture line and increases the inflammation around the involved nerve root, thereby increasing the risk for possible rerupture of the disc site.

CN: Reduction of risk potential; CL: Evaluate

71. 4. After a lumbar laminectomy, a client should not sit for prolonged periods in a chair because of the increased pressure against the nerve root and incision site. Assisting with daily hygiene is an appropriate activity during the initial postoperative period because, as with any surgical procedure, the client needs to return to an optimal level of functioning as soon as possible. There is no limitation on the client's participation in daily hygiene activities except for individual responses of pain, nausea, vomiting, or weakness. Lying flat in bed is appropriate because it does not cause stress on the spinal column where the laminectomy was performed and the disc tissue was removed. Positions that should be avoided are those that would cause twisting and flexion of the spine. Walking in the hall is an acceptable activity. It promotes good postoperative ventilation, circulation, and return of peristalsis, which are needed for all surgical clients. In addition, walking provides the postoperative lumbar laminectomy client an opportunity to build up endurance and muscle strength and to promote circulation to the operative and incision sites for healing without twisting or stressing them.

CN: Physiological adaptation; CL: Analyze

72. 1, 2, 4. The nurse can instruct a client who has had a lumbar laminectomy to do knee-to-chest lifts, hip tilts, and pelvic tilt exercises to strengthen back and abdominal muscles. Sit-ups are not recommended because these exercises place too great a stress on the back.

CN: Reduction of risk potential; CL: Analyze

The Adult with an Amputation due to Peripheral Vascular Disease

73. 1, 2, 4. Uncontrolled diabetes mellitus is considered a risk factor for PVD because of the macroangiopathic and microangiopathic changes that result from poor blood glucose control. Cigarette smoking is a known risk factor for peripheral vascular disease; nicotine is a potent vasoconstrictor. A serum cholesterol level higher than 200 mg/dL (11.1 mmol/L) is considered a risk factor for PVD. The hemoglobin level is within normal range and is not a risk for PVD. Prolonged standing is a risk factor for venous stasis and varicose veins. The oxygen saturation level is within normal limits.

CN: Reduction of risk potential; CL: Analyze

74. 2. The client with severe arterial occlusive disease and gangrene of the left great toe would have lost the hair on the leg due to decreased circulation to the skin. Edema around the ankle and lower leg would indicate venous insufficiency of the lower extremity. Thin, soft toenails (i.e., not thickened and brittle) are a normal finding. Warmth in the foot indicates adequate circulation to the extremity. Typically, the foot would be cool to cold if a severe arterial occlusion were present.

CN: Physiological adaptation; CL: Analyze

75. 3. The client should be tobacco free for 30 minutes before the test to avoid false readings related to the vasoconstrictive effects of smoking on the arteries. Because this test is noninvasive, the client does not need to sign an informed consent form. The client should receive an opioid analgesic, not a sedative, to control the pain as the blood pressure cuffs are inflated during the Doppler studies to determine the ankle-to-brachial pressure index. The client's ankle should not be covered with a blanket because the weight of the blanket on the ischemic foot will cause pain. A bed cradle should be used to keep even the weight of a sheet off the affected foot.

CN: Reduction of risk potential; CL: Analyze

76. 2. Slow, steady walking is a recommended activity for the client with peripheral arterial disease because it stimulates the development of collateral circulation needed to ensure adequate tissue oxygenation. A client with peripheral arterial disease should not minimize activity. Activity is necessary to foster the development of collateral circulation. Elevating the legs above the heart is an appropriate strategy for reducing venous congestion. Wearing antiembolism stockings promotes the return of venous circulation, which is important for clients with venous insufficiency. However, their use in clients with peripheral arterial disease may cause the disease to worsen.

CN: Physiological adaptation; CL: Evaluate

77. 1. Daily lubrication, inspection, cleaning, and patting dry of the feet should be performed to prevent cracking of the skin and possible infection. Soaking the feet in warm water should be avoided because soaking can lead to maceration and subsequent skin breakdown. Additionally, the client with arterial insufficiency typically experiences sensory changes, so the client may be unable to detect water that is too warm, thus placing the client at risk for burns. Antiembolism stockings, appropriate for clients with venous insufficiency, are inappropriate for clients with arterial insufficiency and could lead to a worsening of the condition. Footwear should be roomy, soft, and protective and allow air to circulate. Therefore, firm, supportive leather shoes would be inappropriate.

CN: Reduction of risk potential; CL: Analyze

78. **2.** Encouraging the client who will be undergoing amputation to verbalize their feelings is the most therapeutic response. Asking the client to tell more about how they are feeling helps elicit information, providing insight into their view of the situation and also providing the nurse with ideas to help them cope. The nurse should avoid value-laden responses, such as "At least you will still have one good leg to use," that may make the client feel guilty or hostile, thereby blocking further communication. Furthermore, stating that the client still has one good leg ignores their expressed concerns. The client has verbalized feelings of helplessness by using the term "invalid." The nurse needs to focus on this concern and not try to complete the teaching first before discussing what is on the client's mind. The client's needs, not the nurse's needs, must be met first. It is inappropriate for the nurse to assume to know the relationship between the client and their spouse or the roles they now must assume as dependent client and caregiver. Additionally, the response about the client's spouse caring for them may reinforce the client's feelings of helplessness as an invalid.

CN: Psychosocial adaptation; CL: Analyze

79. **2.** The level of amputation often cannot be accurately determined until during surgery, when the surgeon can directly assess the adequacy of the circulation of the residual limb. From a moral, ethical, and legal viewpoint, the surgeon attempts to remove as little of the leg as possible. Although a longer residual limb facilitates prosthesis fitting, unless the stump is receiving a good blood supply, the prosthesis will not function properly because tissue necrosis will occur. Although the client's ability to walk with a prosthesis is important, it is not a determining factor in the decision about the level of amputation required. Blood supply to the tissue is the primary determinant.

CN: Physiological adaptation; CL: Analyze

80. **4.** The priority action is to draw a mark around the site of bleeding to determine the rate of bleeding. Once the area is marked, the nurse can determine whether the bleeding is increasing or decreasing by the size of the area marked. Because the spot is bright red, the bleeding is most likely arterial in origin. Once the rate and source of bleeding are identified, the surgeon should be notified. The stump is not elevated because adhesions may occur, interfering with the ability to fit a prosthesis. The dressing would be reinforced if the bleeding is determined to be of venous origin, characterized by slow oozing of darker blood that ceases with the application of a pressure dressing. Typically, operative dressings are not changed for 24 hours. Therefore, the dressing is reinforced to prevent organisms from penetrating through the blood-soaked areas of the initial postoperative dressing.

CN: Physiological adaptation; CL: Analyze

81. **4.** The nurse's first action should be to administer the prescribed opioid analgesic to the client because this phenomenon is a phantom sensation and interventions should be provided to relieve it. Pain relief is the priority. Phantom sensation is a real sensation. It is incorrect and inappropriate to tell a client that it is impossible to feel the pain. Although it does relieve the client's apprehensions to be told that phantom sensations are a real phenomenon, the client needs prompt treatment to relieve the pain sensation. Usually, phantom sensation will go away. However, showing the client that the toes are not there does nothing to provide the client with relief.

CN: Physiological adaptation; CL: Analyze

82. **4.** The use of crutches requires significant strength from the triceps muscles. Therefore, efforts are focused on strengthening these muscles in anticipation of crutch walking. Bed and wheelchair push-ups are excellent exercises targeted at the triceps muscles. Abdominal exercises, range-of-motion and isometric exercises of the shoulders, and quadriceps and gluteal setting exercises are not helpful in preparing for crutch walking.

CN: Reduction of risk potential; CL: Analyze

83. **4.** When using crutches, the client is taught to support weight primarily on the hands. Supporting body weight on the axillae, elbows, or upper arms must be avoided to prevent nerve damage from excessive pressure.

CN: Reduction of risk potential; CL: Analyze

84. **4.** Before beginning dietary instructions and interventions, the nurse must first assess the client's and family's food preferences, such as pattern of food intake, lifestyle, food

preferences, and ethnic, cultural, and financial influences. Once this information is obtained, the nurse can begin teaching based on the client's current knowledge level and then build on this knowledge base.

🔑 CN: Health promotion and maintenance; CL: Analyze

The Adult with Fractures

85. **3.** Isometric contractions increase the tension within a muscle but do not produce movement. Repeated isometric contractions make muscles grow larger and stronger. Adduction of the leg puts work onto the hip joint and alters the pull of traction. Rolling the leg, or *external rotation*, alters the pull of traction. Additional weight should not be added to traction unless prescribed by the health care provider; it will not prevent muscle atrophy.

🔑 CN: Reduction of risk potential; CL: Evaluate

86. **4, 3, 1, 2.** The nurse should first clean the area around the pin insertion site, wiping in one direction around the pin and discarding the swabs as they are used. The nurse should then remove any crust that may have formed around the pin. Next, the nurse should inspect the area for infection. Last, the nurse should clean the pin.

🔑 CN: Safety and infection control; CL: Apply

87. **3.** Methocarbamol is a muscle relaxant that acts primarily to relieve muscle spasms. It has no effect on microorganisms or on nervousness, and it does not reduce itching.

🔑 CN: Pharmacological and parenteral therapies; CL: Evaluate

88. -/+ **1, 2, 3.** Acetaminophen is an alternative for a client who is allergic to aspirin. It does not affect platelet aggregation, and the client does not need to have coagulation studies (such as INR). Acetaminophen causes little or no gastric distress. Acetaminophen exerts no anti-inflammatory effects.

🔑 CN: Pharmacological and parenteral therapies; CL: Create

89. **3.** Hypotension and depressed respirations are signs of high levels of ingestion of hydrocodone, and the client may be developing a habit of taking this drug for a prolonged period. Expected common adverse effects of hydrocodone and acetaminophen would include drowsiness, confusion, blurred vision, and constipation. Hemorrhage from gastrointestinal irritation is not associated with this drug. Hypersensitivity reactions would be manifested by pruritus and rashes.

🔑 CN: Pharmacological and parenteral therapies; CL: Evaluate

90. **3.** The nurse's first action is to notify the HCP because the client is likely experiencing a fat embolus. Fat emboli are associated with embolization of marrow or tissue fat or platelets and free fatty acids to the pulmonary capillaries, producing rapid onset of symptoms. Multiple fractures and fractures of the long bones or pelvis increase a client's risk for developing a fat embolus; in addition, young adults between 20 and 30 years of age are at a higher risk for fat emboli with fractures. When fat emboli do occur, hypoxia results; therefore, it is most important for the nurse to assess changes in the client's level of consciousness and observe changes in behavior, such as restlessness and irritability. The nurse does not cut the cast; there is no indication that the casts are obstructing circulation. Arterial blood gas tests are used to confirm the diagnosis, not a chest x-ray. The client's behavior is a result of hypoxemia, not pain.

🔑 CN: Reduction of risk potential; CL: Analyze

91. **2.** The nurse instructs the client to maintain two finger widths between the axillary fold and the underarm piece grip of the crutches to prevent pressure on the brachial plexus. The client is advised to use the three-point gait; in the four-point and two-point gait, there is partial weight bearing of both feet. The client is also advised to keep the affected leg elevated when sitting to prevent swelling and to use the arms, not the axillae, to maintain balance and support.

🔑 CN: Reduction of risk potential; CL: Apply

92. **4.** Skeletal traction is often used to regain normal length of the bone, but in this situation, the main purpose of the traction is to reduce and immobilize the fracture. This type of traction allows the client to move in bed without dislocating the fracture. This client has an open fracture, but skeletal traction will not prevent further skin breakdown.

🔑 CN: Physiological adaptation; CL: Evaluate

93. **3.** The nurse first assesses the mechanism of injury to help determine related injuries, tests needed, and potential treatment options. The next step is to assess the location, type, quality, and intensity of the pain. Neurovascular stasis of the injured site is assessed after pain; therefore, the nurse checks for functional ability or changing positions. Although the nurse can also determine the extent of anxiety while assessing the injury and can use communication strategies to minimize anxiety, it is not the first priority for assessing this client.

🗝️ CN: Physiological adaptation; CL: Analyze

94. 3. The nursing assessment is first focused on the region distal to the fracture for neurovascular injury or compromise. When a nerve or blood vessel is severed or obstructed at the actual fracture site, innervation to the nerve or blood flow to the vessel is disrupted below the site; therefore, the area distal to the fracture site is the area of compromised neurologic input or vascular flow and return, not the area above the fracture site or the fracture site itself. The nurse may assess the opposite extremity at the area proximal to the fracture site for a baseline comparison of pulse quality, color, temperature, size, and so on, but the comparison would be made after the initial neurovascular assessment.

🗝️ CN: Reduction of risk potential; CL: Analyze

95. 3. Clients should not pull out cast padding to scratch inside the cast because of the hazard of skin breakdown and subsequent potential for infection. Clients are encouraged to elevate the casted extremity above the level of the heart to reduce edema and to exercise or move the joints above and below the cast to promote and maintain flexibility and muscle strength. Applying ice for 10 minutes during the first 24 hours helps reduce edema.

🗝️ CN: Reduction of risk potential; CL: Evaluate

96. -/+ 1, 3, 4, 5, 6. To prevent constipation, the nurse should encourage the client in a hip spica cast to eat fresh fruits and vegetables; cheese can cause constipation. The nurse should also instruct the client to increase fluid intake to at least 2500 mL a day. The nurse can also encourage the client to drink cranberry juice, which helps keep urine acidic, thereby avoiding the development of renal calculi. The nurse should instruct the client to establish regular times for elimination to promote regularity in bowel and bladder habits. To prevent orthostatic hypotension, the nurse should teach the client to do dangling and standing exercises. The nurse can also advise the client to use a protective cloth around the cast when eating to prevent food from getting inside the cast. If the cast does become soiled, the client can wash the cast with a damp cloth.

🗝️ CN: Physiological adaptation; CL: Analyze

97. 2. A two-point gait involves partial weight bearing on each foot, with each crutch advancing simultaneously with the opposing leg. Advancing a crutch on one side and then advancing the opposite foot, and repeating on the opposite side, illustrates the four-point gait. When the client advances both crutches together and follows by lifting both lower extremities to the same level as the crutches, the gait is called a "swing-to" gait. When the client advances both crutches together and follows by lifting both lower extremities past the level of the crutches, the gait is called a "swing-through" gait. The swing-through gait is often used by clients with paraplegia because it allows them to place weight on their legs while the crutches are moved one stride ahead.

🗝️ CN: Reduction of risk potential; CL: Analyze

98. 1. The wound has a three-way drainage system in place to irrigate the debrided wound with normal saline or an antibiotic. Before the debridement, a sample of the wound would be taken for culture and sensitivity testing so that an organism-specific antibiotic could be administered to prevent possible serious sequelae of osteomyelitis. Therefore, the nurse should review the results of the culture and sensitivity report before initiating care. A dressing would not be applied to an open wound. Rather, a wet-to-dry dressing most likely would be used, and the health care provider would write the exact prescription. There should not be increased pain related to the exposure of nerve endings in the subcutaneous tissue of the wound that was left open to the environment. The first priority is to determine if there is an infection as this is the biggest risk to the client; the nurse can check other lab values later.

🗝️ CN: Physiological adaptation; CL: Analyze

99. 1. The nurse should assess the client's ability to move the toes and for the presence of distal pulses, including a neurovascular assessment of the area below the cast. Increasing pain unrelieved by usual analgesics and occurring 4 to 12 hours after the onset of casting or trauma may be the first sign of compartment syndrome, which can lead to permanent damage to nerves and muscles. Although the nurse can use a pain rating scale or assess for changes in vital signs to objectively assess the client's pain, the client's comments suggest early and important signs of compartment syndrome requiring immediate intervention. The nurse should not confuse these signs with the potential for drug tolerance. This assessment might be appropriate once the suspicion of compartment syndrome has been ruled out.

🗝️ CN: Physiological adaptation; CL: Analyze

100. 4. A client with compartment syndrome may release myoglobin from damaged muscle cells into the circulation. This becomes trapped in the renal tubules, resulting in dark, scanty urine, possibly leading to acute renal failure. Crackles may suggest respiratory complications; jaundice suggests liver failure; and generalized edema may suggest heart failure. However, these are not associated with compartment syndrome.

CN: Reduction of risk potential; CL: Analyze

The Adult with a Femoral Fracture

101. 1. A client with a femoral fracture in balanced suspension traction can raise the hips using a trapeze to use the fracture bedpan while maintaining the line of the traction. The client should not turn side to side as it will disrupt the line of traction. The nurse can give back care when the client raises the body using the trapeze. The client should not be given a complete bed bath. Rather, the client is encouraged to participate in self-care and movement in bed, such as with a trapeze. The client should be positioned so that the feet do not press against the footboard. Therefore, elevating the head of the bed no more than 25 degrees is recommended to keep the client from moving down in the bed.

CN: Reduction of risk potential; CL: Analyze

102. 3. The nurse should send the client to the operating room on the bed with extra help to keep the traction from moving to maintain the femur in the proper alignment before surgery. Transferring the client to a cart with manually suspended traction is inappropriate because doing so places the client at risk for additional trauma to the surrounding neurovascular and soft tissues, as would removing the traction. The surgeon need not be called because the decision about transferring the client is an independent nursing action.

CN: Safety and infection control; CL: Analyze

103. 2. The client in balanced suspension traction can raise the hips using a trapeze. The client can then use the bedpan. The client can be in a sitting position to eat. The client should not move from side to side but can turn toward the affected side. The client should not flex or extend the ankle on the affected side.

CN: Basic care and comfort; CL: Analyze

104. 1. The Pearson attachment supports the lower leg and provides increased stability in the overall traction setup. It also makes it easier to maintain correct alignment. It does not support the thigh and upper leg or prevent flexion deformities in the ankle and foot. It is not attached to the skeletal pin.

CN: Reduction of risk potential; CL: Apply

105. 1. Fat emboli usually result in symptoms of acute respiratory distress syndrome, such as apprehension, chest pain, cyanosis, dyspnea, tachypnea, tachycardia, and decreased partial pressure of arterial oxygen resulting from poor oxygen exchange. Migraine-like headaches are not a symptom of a fat embolism, but mental confusion, memory loss, and a headache from poor oxygen exchange may be seen with central nervous system involvement. Numbness in the right leg is a peripheral neurovascular response that most likely is related to the femoral fracture. Muscle spasms in the right thigh are a symptom of a neuromuscular response affecting the local muscle around the femoral fracture site.

CN: Reduction of risk potential; CL: Analyze

106. 1. The client's assistance in self-care and increased participation over time indicate that the client has accomplished self-care by gaining a sense of control. If the client lets the nurse complete the care without interfering, the behavior would indicate passivity, possibly from denial or depression. If the client allows the spouse to assume total responsibility, a successful outcome has not been reached. The client is able to accomplish self-care activities within the limits of immobilization from the traction.

CN: Basic care and comfort; CL: Evaluate

107. 2. Fever, night sweats, chills, restlessness, and restrictive movement of the fractured leg are clinical manifestations of osteomyelitis, which is a pyogenic bone infection caused by bacteria (usually staphylococci), a virus, or a fungus. The bone is inaccessible to macrophages and antibodies for protection against infections, so an infection in this site can become serious quickly. The client with a pulmonary or fat embolus would develop symptoms of pulmonary compromise, such as shortness of breath, chest pain, angina, and mental confusion. Signs and symptoms of urinary tract infection would include pain over the suprapubic, groin, or back region with fever and chills, with no restrictive movement of the leg.

CN: Reduction of risk potential; CL: Analyze

108. 2. The goal of care for this client is healing and tissue growth while the client continues on long-term antibiotic therapy to clear the infection. A diet high in protein and vitamins C and D promotes healing. Herbal supplements may potentiate bleeding (e.g., ginkgo, ginger, turmeric, chamomile, kelp, horse chestnut, garlic, dong quai) and have not been proven through research to promote healing. Frequent passive motion will increase circulation but may also aggravate localized bone pain. It is not appropriate to advise the client to change antibiotics as treatment may take time.

🗝️ CN: Physiological adaptation; CL: Analyze

The Adult with a Spinal Cord Injury

109. 3. The priority concern is to immobilize the head and neck to prevent further trauma when a fractured vertebra is unstable and easily displaced. Although wrapping and supporting the extremities is important, it does not take priority over immobilizing the head and neck. Pain usually is not a significant consideration with this type of injury. Cushioning is contraindicated. The neck should be kept in a neutral position and immobilized. Flexion of the neck is avoided.

🗝️ CN: Safety and infection control; CL: Analyze

110. 3. The client is experiencing autonomic dysreflexia, which is a medical emergency. The nurse should immediately evaluate the client for bladder distention and be prepared to catheterize the client. Positioning the client on the left side, reducing environmental stimuli, and administering pain medications are not used to treat autonomic hyperreflexia.

🗝️ CN: Physiological adaptation; CL: Analyze

111. 3. This client has a spinal cord injury of the sacral region of the spinal cord and will have bladder and bowel dysfunction as well as loss of sensation and muscle control below the injury. The other options are true for a client who has quadriplegia.

🗝️ CN: Physiological adaptation; CL: Analyze

112. -/+ 2, 4, 5. The nurse should assess a client with a spinal cord transection above T5 for a risk for complications. The client may have constipation due to atonia and is at risk for the development of a paralytic ileus because the sympathetic nerve innervation to the vagus nerve, which dominates all the vessels and organs below T5 (e.g., the intestinal tract), has been disrupted and therefore the client has no movement or peristalsis. The client is at risk for the development of stress ulcers because the sympathetic nerve innervation to the stomach has been disrupted, which results in an excessive release of hydrochloric acid in the stomach, allowing contact of hydrochloric acid with the stomach mucosa. The client does not feel subjective signs of stress ulcers (e.g., pain, guarding, tenderness) and therefore is at increased risk for bleeding because complications of an ulcer can develop before early diagnosis. The client can move their arms. The client is not likely to develop diarrhea but may become constipated.

🗝️ CN: Reduction of risk potential; CL: Analyze

113. 4. Measuring the leg girth is the most appropriate method because the usual signs, such as a positive Homans' sign, pain, and tenderness, are not present. Other means of assessing for deep vein thrombosis in a client with a spinal cord injury are through a Doppler examination and impedance plethysmography.

🗝️ CN: Reduction of risk potential; CL: Analyze

114. 3. During the period of spinal shock, the bladder is completely atonic and will continue to fill passively unless the client is catheterized. The bladder will not go into spasms or cause uncontrolled urination. Bladder function will not be normal during the period of spinal shock.

🗝️ CN: Reduction of risk potential; CL: Analyze

115. 4. The movements occur from muscle reflexes and cannot be initiated or controlled by the brain. After the period of spinal shock, the muscles gradually become spastic owing to an increased sensitivity of the lower motor neurons. It is an expected occurrence and does not indicate that healing is taking place or that the client will walk again. The movement is not voluntary and cannot be brought under voluntary control.

🗝️ CN: Physiological adaptation; CL: Analyze

116. 3. Long-bone demineralization is a serious consequence of the loss of weight bearing. An excessive calcium load is brought to the kidneys, and precipitation may occur, predisposing to stone formation. Excessive intake of dairy products may promote constipation. However, this is not the most accurate reason for decreasing calcium intake. Immobility does not increase calcium absorption from the intestine. Dairy products do not necessarily contribute to weight gain.

🗝️ CN: Basic care and comfort; CL: Analyze

117. 2. A woman with a spinal cord injury can participate in sexual activity but might not experience orgasm. Cessation in the nerve pathway may occur in spinal cord injury, but this does not negate the client's mental and emotional needs to creatively participate with their partner in a sexual relationship and to reach orgasm. An indwelling urinary catheter may be left in place during intercourse and need not be removed because the indwelling urinary catheter is placed in the urethra, which is not the channel used for sexual intercourse. There are no contraindications, such as hypertension, to sexual activity in a woman with spinal cord injury. Sexual intercourse is allowed, and hypertension should be manageable. Because a spinal cord injury does not affect fertility, the client should have access to family planning information so that an unplanned pregnancy can be avoided.

CN: Basic care and comfort; CL: Evaluate

118. 3. Spinal cord injury represents a physical loss; grief is the normal response to this loss. Working through grief entails reviewing memories and eventually letting go of them. The process may take as long as 2 years. Telling the client to be patient and that adjustment takes time is a clichéd type of response, one that is not empathetic or responsive to the client's needs. Telling the client to focus on today does not allow time for the grief process, which is necessary for the client to work through and adjust to the loss. The client is not escaping but is reminiscing on what is lost, to work through the grieving process.

CN: Psychosocial adaptation; CL: Analyze

Managing Care, Quality, and Safety of Adults with Musculoskeletal Health Problems

119. **-/+** **1, 3, 4, 5.** Clients who are at risk for falling include the client taking narcotics, the client with a known fear of falling, the client with cognitive impairment, and the client with gait problems. Age and setting are not necessarily risks for fallings.

CN: Management of care; CL: Analyze

120. **-/+** **2, 3, 5.** The client with a C3–C4 fracture has neck control but may tire easily using sore muscles around the incision area to hold up the head. Therefore, the head and neck of the wheelchair should be high. The seat of the wheelchair should be lower than normal to facilitate transfer from the bed to the wheelchair. When a client can use the hands and arms to move the wheelchair, the placement of the back to the client's scapula is necessary. This client cannot use their arms and will need an electric chair with breath, chin, or voice control to manipulate the movement of the chair. A firm or hard cushion adds pressure to bony prominences; the cushion should instead be padded to reduce the risk for pressure ulcers.

CN: Basic care and comfort; CL: Analyze

121. 3. Infection is a serious complication of total hip replacement and may necessitate removal of the implant. Clients who are obese, poorly nourished, or older adults and those who have poorly controlled diabetes, rheumatoid arthritis, or concurrent infections (e.g., dental, urinary tract) are at high risk for infection. Clients who are of normal weight and have well-controlled chronic diseases are not at risk for infection. Living alone is not a risk factor for infection.

CN: Reduction of risk potential; CL: Analyze

122. **-/+** **1, 2, 3, 5.** A restraint is a method of involuntary physical restriction of a client's freedom of movement, physical activity, or normal access to their body. The nurse must monitor and provide care to optimize the physical and psychological well-being of the client including, but not limited to, respiratory and circulatory status, skin integrity, and vital signs. With each assessment, the nurse needs to ascertain that restraints are still required for client safety. The least restrictive intervention based on an individualized assessment of the client's medical or behavioral status or condition is needed.

CN: Safety and infection control; CL: Analyze

123. **-/+** **1, 3, 4, 5, 6.** Client safety is a priority for the client, the client's family, and all of the personnel working on this unit. All of these persons must be engaged in using strategies to prevent falls. The insurance provider does not need to be involved in developing a falls program.

CN: Safety and infection control; CL: Create

124. 2. The client is identified as being at risk for falling, and a staff member or family member should accompany the client when they are walking. The nurse should first accompany the client back to the room. Because the client is not fatigued, they do not need a wheelchair but must have assistance. The nurse can delegate the task of ambulating the client to the UAP, but it may take a while to locate a UAP that is available at this time. Walking only in the room will not provide an opportunity for the client to gain strength and improve ambulation, but the nurse should remind the client to have assistance.

CN: Reduction of risk potential; CL: Analyze

125. 1, 2, 3. To assure client safety when using anticoagulants, the nurse should coordinate care with the pharmacist, dietitian, and laboratory at this time. The pharmacist will collaborate in teaching the client about using the drug;

dietary services will plan a diet that limits foods that have high amounts of vitamin K (spinach, cabbage, blueberries) that will interfere with anticoagulation; and the laboratory will draw daily international normalized ratio (INR) levels to assure accurate dosing. Although the nurse coordinates discharge planning at the time of admission to the hospital, at this point it is too soon for discharge planning services to be involved because it is not known if the client will continue to take the warfarin when discharged. There is no indication that there has been an actual or potential error, and risk management is not needed at this time.

CN: Management of care; CL: Analyze

126. 4. Side rails are considered restraints and are not used at both the head and foot of the bed. Using side rails at the head of the bed will aid the client in sitting up and are safe, but using side rails at both the head and the foot of the bed presents risks for a client who might become wedged between the rail and the bed or attempt to climb over them. The nurse discusses side rail use with the UAP and lowers the side rail at the foot of the bed. The nurse assures the bed is placed in a low position. The accessible call light, dim lighting, and clear path to the bathroom are factors that contribute to fall prevention.

CN: Management of care: CL: Analyze

127. 3. Hand-off of care communication is an interactive communication allowing the opportunity for questioning between the giver and receiver of client information, including up-to-date information regarding the client's care, treatment, and services, as well as the client's current condition and any recent or anticipated changes. Hand-off communication occurs when a nurse is leaving the nursing unit, but the purpose is not to let the charge nurse know that the nurse is going to lunch or to have someone else assigned to care for the client. Hand-off communication focuses on current information, not the client's history.

CN: Management of care; CL: Analyze

128. 1, 2, 4, 5, 6. The nurse should determine that a client with rheumatoid arthritis can describe the septic arthritis physiologic process and knows how to relieve pain using pharmacologic and nonpharmacologic interventions. Prolonged immobility and limited activity may promote the formation of deep vein thrombosis and possibly subsequent pulmonary emboli. The client should also understand the importance of supporting the affected joint and weight-bearing and activity restrictions and how to use ambulatory aids and assistive devices safely to promote recovery of normal function. The local application of heat and cold to an injured body part can provide therapeutic benefits; however, "high" heat may cause a thermal injury and further promote edema formation. The client should inform the health care provider about pain that is not relieved by the current management plan.

CN: Management of care; CL: Evaluate

129. 2, 3. PROM exercises are used to move the client's joints through as full a range of motion as possible. PROM exercises improve or maintain joint mobility and help prevent contractures. These exercises are indicated for the client with temporary or permanent loss of mobility, sensation, or consciousness. Exercises help with joint mobility, strength, and endurance. Plantar flexion of the foot and supination of the hand may be normal joint movements if the client can do active range of motion. Septic joints have infection that may be spread either hematogenously or through trauma.

CN: Reduction of risk potential; CL: Apply

130. 3. The client has a moderate fall risk, and the nurse should direct the UAP to activate the bed and chair alarms. The UAP does not need to remain with the client during toileting unless the client's risk for falling is high. There is no evidence the client is confused, and hourly reorientation could disrupt sleep. Protective devices to restrain clients are used for clients at high risk for a fall and require a prescription from a health care provider.

CN: Management of care; CL: Analyze

131. 1, 2, 4. Since the client is at low risk for falling, it is not necessary to remain during toileting or to place a commode at the client's bedside as the client is able to use the toilet. A wheelchair seat belt is used for clients with a moderate fall risk. The nurse should always make sure the call bell is within easy reach, that all locks are engaged when needed, and that the bed is in the lowest position.

CN: Safety and infection control; CL: Analyze

TEST 13: The Adult with Cancer

- The Adult at Risk for Cancer
- The Adult with Pain
- The Adult Who Is Receiving Chemotherapy
- The Adult Who Is Receiving Radiation Therapy
- The Adult Who Requires Symptom Management
- The Adult Who Is Coping with Loss, Grief, Bereavement, and Spiritual Distress
- The Adult Who Is Experiencing Problems with Sexuality
- Ethical and Legal Issues Related to Adults with Cancer
- End-of-Life Care
- Managing Care, Quality, and Safety of Adults with Cancer
- Answers, Rationales, and Test-Taking Strategies

The Adult at Risk for Cancer

1. The nurse is teaching a wellness class. Which person is at **highest** risk for colorectal cancer?

   The client:
   - ☐ 1. who smoked one pack of cigarettes a day for 30 years.
   - ☐ 2. who follows a vegetarian diet.
   - ☐ 3. who has been treated for Crohn's disease for 20 years.
   - ☐ 4. with a family history of lung cancer.

2. A nurse is conducting a cancer risk screening program. Which client is at **greatest** risk for basal cell cancer?
   - ☐ 1. Women who use indoor tanning booths.
   - ☐ 2. Dark-skinned males.
   - ☐ 3. Teenagers who are on sports teams.
   - ☐ 4. Older adults who have scars from burns.

3. A client diagnosed with testicular cancer expresses concerns about fertility. The client and their spouse desire to eventually have a family, and the nurse discusses the option of sperm banking. What should the nurse tell the couple about the **best** time to donate the sperm?
   - ☐ 1. before treatment is started
   - ☐ 2. once the client is tolerating the treatment
   - ☐ 3. upon completion of treatment
   - ☐ 4. when tumor markers drop to normal levels

4. A nurse is providing education in a community setting about general measures to avoid excessive sun exposure. Which recommendation is appropriate?
   - ☐ 1. Use sunscreen only after going into the water.
   - ☐ 2. Avoid peak exposure hours from 0900 to 1300.
   - ☐ 3. Wear loosely woven clothing for added ventilation.
   - ☐ 4. Apply sunscreen with a sun protection factor (SPF) of 15 or more before sun exposure.

5. A 29-year-old client is concerned about their personal risk factors for malignant melanoma. They are upset because their 49-year-old sibling was recently diagnosed with the disease. After gathering information about the client's history of sun exposure, the nurse should tell the client which information?
   - ☐ 1. Some melanomas have a familial component, and the client should seek medical advice.
   - ☐ 2. The client's personal risk is low because most melanomas occur at age 60 or later.
   - ☐ 3. The client's personal risk is low because melanoma does not have a familial component.
   - ☐ 4. The client should not worry because they did not experience severe sunburn as a child.

6. A client with a family history of cancer asks the nurse what the single **most** important risk factor is for cancer. Which risk factor should the nurse discuss?
   ☐ 1. family history
   ☐ 2. lifestyle choices
   ☐ 3. age
   ☐ 4. hormonal changes

7. A client who is a highway construction worker is concerned about their cancer risks. The client has been married for 18 years, has two children, smokes one pack of cigarettes per day, and occasionally drinks one to two beers. They are 30 lb (13.6 kg) overweight, eat fried fast food often, and rarely eat fresh fruits and vegetables. The client's parent was diagnosed with breast cancer 2 years ago. The client's other parent and an aunt both died of lung cancer. The client had a basal cell carcinoma removed from their cheek 3 years ago. What behavioral change(s) should the nurse coach this client to make to decrease their risk for cancer? Select all that apply.
   ☐ 1. Improve nutrition.
   ☐ 2. Decrease alcohol consumption.
   ☐ 3. Use sunscreen.
   ☐ 4. Stop smoking.
   ☐ 5. Lose weight.
   ☐ 6. Change their job to work inside.

8. The nurse is assessing a client who has hoarseness and a chronic sore throat. What should the nurse determine while conducting a health history with this client? Select all that apply.
   ☐ 1. use of acetaminophen
   ☐ 2. exposure to the sun
   ☐ 3. consumption of a high-fat diet
   ☐ 4. extent of tobacco use
   ☐ 5. amount of alcohol consumption

9. A client is interested in making dietary changes to reduce the risk for colon cancer. What dietary selections should the nurse suggest?
   ☐ 1. croissant, granola and peanut butter squares, and whole milk
   ☐ 2. bran muffin, skim milk, and stir-fried broccoli
   ☐ 3. granola, bagel with cream cheese, and cauliflower salad
   ☐ 4. oatmeal raisin cookies, baked potato with sour cream, and a turkey sandwich

10. The nurse is conducting a cancer risk assessment for a middle-age client. Which risk factor would the nurse focus on when engaging in motivational interviewing as an approach to risk reduction?
    ☐ 1. sex assigned at birth
    ☐ 2. nutrition
    ☐ 3. family history
    ☐ 4. age

11. A client at risk for lung cancer asks about the reason for having a computed tomography (CT) scan as part of the initial examination. What is the nurse's **best** response?
    "A CT scan is:
    ☐ 1. far superior to magnetic resonance imaging for evaluating lymph node metastasis."
    ☐ 2. noninvasive and readily available."
    ☐ 3. useful for distinguishing small differences in tissue density and detecting nodal involvement."
    ☐ 4. used to distinguish a malignant from a nonmalignant adenopathy."

12. The nurse is planning a culturally sensitive health education program. Which action should the nurse take?
    ☐ 1. Locate the program at a facility that will not charge for use.
    ☐ 2. Integrate folk beliefs and traditions of the target population into the content.
    ☐ 3. Prepare materials in the primary language of the program sponsor.
    ☐ 4. Exclude community leaders from the dominant culture from initial planning efforts.

The Adult with Pain

13. A client in a hospice program has increasing pain, and the nurse is collaborating with the client to make a pain management plan. Which plan will be **most** effective for the client?
    ☐ 1. administering doses of analgesic medication when pain is a 5 on a scale of 0 to 10
    ☐ 2. providing enough analgesic medication to keep the client semi-somnolent
    ☐ 3. allowing an analgesic medication–free period so the client can carry out daily hygienic activities
    ☐ 4. administering pain medications over a 24-hour period

14. A client with pancreatic cancer has been receiving morphine via a subcutaneous pump for 2 weeks. The client is requiring an increased dose of morphine to manage their pain. How should the nurse document this finding?
    ☐ 1. tolerating the medication well
    ☐ 2. showing addiction to morphine
    ☐ 3. developing a tolerance for the medication
    ☐ 4. experiencing physical dependence

15. A client had a craniotomy for the removal of a malignant brain tumor in the occipital region. The nurse should question a prescription for which drug?
☐ 1. ibuprofen
☐ 2. naproxen
☐ 3. morphine sulfate
☐ 4. acetaminophen

16. The nurse is conducting a health history with a client taking a nonsteroidal antiinflammatory drug (NSAID) for pain management. The nurse should include specific questions regarding which body system?
☐ 1. gastrointestinal
☐ 2. renal
☐ 3. pulmonary
☐ 4. cardiac

17. A client with lung cancer is being cared for by their spouse at home. The client's pain is increasing in severity. The nurse recognizes that teaching has been effective when the spouse uses which pain relief strategy? Select all that apply.
☐ 1. gives the client a long-acting or sustained-release oral pain medication regularly around the clock
☐ 2. uses an immediate-release medication (oxycodone) for breakthrough pain
☐ 3. avoids long-acting opioids because of the client's concern about addiction
☐ 4. uses music for distraction as well as heat or cold in combination with medications
☐ 5. substitutes acetaminophen to avoid tolerance to the medications
☐ 6. has the client use a pain rating scale to measure the effectiveness of reaching their individual pain goal

18. A client was discharged from the hospital for cancer-related pain. While the client was in the hospital, the pain was well controlled on patient-controlled administration (PCA) of intravenous (IV) morphine, and on discharge 2 days ago, the client was taking oral morphine. The client now reports pain as an 8 on a 10-point scale and is asking the nurse about using PCA for the morphine at home. Which explanation is the **most** likely for the client's reports of inadequate pain control?

The client is:
☐ 1. addicted to the IV morphine.
☐ 2. going through withdrawal from the IV opioid.
☐ 3. physically dependent on the IV morphine.
☐ 4. undermedicated on the oral opioid.

19. A nurse is assessing a client with bone cancer pain. Which part of a thorough pain assessment is **most** significant for this client?
☐ 1. intensity
☐ 2. cause
☐ 3. aggravating factors
☐ 4. location

20. A client with chronic cancer pain has been receiving opiates for 4 months. The client rated the pain as an 8 on a 10-point scale before starting the opioid medication. A thorough examination reveals no new evidence of increased disease, yet the pain is close to 8 again. What is the **most** likely explanation for the increasing pain?
☐ 1. development of an addiction to the opioids
☐ 2. tolerance to the opioid
☐ 3. withdrawal from the opioid
☐ 4. placebo effect has decreased

21. The nurse teaches a client with chronic cancer pain about optimal pain control. Which recommendation is **most** effective for pain control?
☐ 1. Take pain medication as soon as the pain level is a 2 on a 10-point scale.
☐ 2. Take prescribed analgesic medications on an around-the-clock schedule to prevent recurrent pain.
☐ 3. Take analgesic medications only when the pain returns.
☐ 4. Take enough analgesic medications around the clock to be able to sleep 12 to 16 hours a day to block the pain.

The Adult Who Is Receiving Chemotherapy

22. The nurse is preparing to administer a chemotherapeutic agent to a client. Which is the appropriate technique to use when administering chemotherapeutic agents?
☐ 1. Wear two pairs of gloves.
☐ 2. Dispose of chemotherapy wastes in the client's bedside trash.
☐ 3. Use gloves, goggles, and disposable long-sleeved gowns when handling agents.
☐ 4. Administer only prepackaged agents from the manufacturer.

23. A client who is receiving chemotherapy develops stomatitis. What should the nurse instruct the client to do?
☐ 1. Rinse their mouth with hydrogen peroxide every 4 hours.
☐ 2. Use a soft-bristled toothbrush after each meal.
☐ 3. Drink hot tea with honey to soothe the painful oral mucosa.
☐ 4. Avoid using dental floss until the stomatitis is resolved.

24. A client is taking doxorubicin and is distressed about hair loss. What should the nurse do?
  ☐ 1. Have the client wash and massage their scalp daily to stimulate hair growth.
  ☐ 2. Explain that hair loss is temporary and will quickly grow back to its original appearance.
  ☐ 3. Provide resources for a wig selection before hair loss begins.
  ☐ 4. Recommend that the client limit social contacts until hair regrows.

25. A client is receiving chemotherapy for a diagnosis of brain cancer. When teaching the client about contamination from excretion of the chemotherapy drugs within 48 hours, the nurse should tell the client which information?
  ☐ 1. A bathroom can be shared with an adult who is not pregnant.
  ☐ 2. Urinary and bowel excretions are not considered contaminated.
  ☐ 3. Disposable plates and plastic utensils must be used during the entire course of chemotherapy.
  ☐ 4. Any contaminated linens should be washed separately and then washed a second time if necessary.

26. A client is receiving vincristine. What should the nurse instruct the client to do when taking this drug?
  ☐ 1. Use loperamide for diarrhea.
  ☐ 2. Restrict fluids to 6 cups (about 1½ L) a day.
  ☐ 3. Follow a low-fiber, bland diet.
  ☐ 4. Take a stool softener daily.

27. A client who is receiving chemotherapy is not eating well but otherwise feels healthy. What should the nurse suggest the client eat?
  ☐ 1. cereal with milk and strawberries
  ☐ 2. milkshake made with blueberries, bananas, and ice cream
  ☐ 3. broiled chicken, green beans, and cottage cheese
  ☐ 4. steak and French fries

28. A nurse is assessing a client who is receiving the second administration of chemotherapy for breast cancer. When obtaining this client's health history, the nurse should ask the client which question?
  ☐ 1. "Has your hair been falling out in clumps?"
  ☐ 2. "Have you had nausea or vomiting?"
  ☐ 3. "Have you been sleeping at night?"
  ☐ 4. "Do you have your usual energy level?"

29. A client is receiving monthly doses of chemotherapy for the treatment of stage III colon cancer. Which laboratory result(s) should the nurse report to the oncologist before the **next** dose of chemotherapy is administered? Select all that apply.
  ☐ 1. hemoglobin of 14.5 g/dL (145 g/L)
  ☐ 2. platelet count of 40,000/mm^3 (40 × 10^9/L)
  ☐ 3. blood urea nitrogen (BUN) level of 12 mg/dL (4.3 mmol/L)
  ☐ 4. white blood cell count of 2300/mm^3 (2.3 × 10^9/L)
  ☐ 5. temperature of 101.2°F (38.4°C)
  ☐ 6. urine specific gravity of 1.020

30. A client is struggling with the decision of whether or not to continue chemotherapy. The client tells the nurse, "It's making me so sick and ruining whatever time I have with my family." What is the nurse's role when caring for this client?
  ☐ 1. Share stories about how others made this decision.
  ☐ 2. Listen to the client's concerns.
  ☐ 3. Advocate for the client with the health care provider.
  ☐ 4. Teach the client how to logically approach the situation.

31. A client has a saline-only peripherally inserted central catheter (PICC). What should the nurse do to maintain the catheter?
  ☐ 1. Flush the port using 3 mL of saline after each use.
  ☐ 2. Avoid flushing any ports unless they appear blocked.
  ☐ 3. Utilize a 10-mL saline flush to maintain line patency.
  ☐ 4. Add 10 units of heparin to each saline flush to prevent clotting.

32. The nurse is instructing a client with cancer who is receiving chemotherapy about reporting signs of infection. Which is the **most** reliable early indicator of infection in a client who is neutropenic?
  ☐ 1. fever
  ☐ 2. chills
  ☐ 3. tachycardia
  ☐ 4. dyspnea

33. A nurse is caring for a client who is undergoing chemotherapy. Current laboratory values are noted on the medical record. Which action would be **most** appropriate for the nurse to implement?

Laboratory Results

Test	Result	Normal Range
Hemoglobin	12.0 g/dL (120 g/L)	Men: 14–17.4 g/dL (140–174 g/L) Women: 12–16 g/dL (120–160 g/L)
Platelet count	108,000/mm^3 (108 × 10^9/L)	Adults: 140,000–400,000/mm^3 (140–400 × 10^9/L).
White blood cell (WBC) count	1600/mm^3 (1.6 × 10^9/L)	4.5–10.5 × 10^3 cells/mm^3 (4.5–10.5 × 10^9/L)
Absolute neutrophil count (ANC)	Less than 1000/mm^3 (1 × 10^9/L)	3000–7000/mm^3 or 3–7 × 10^9/L

☐ 1. wearing a protective gown and particulate respirator mask when completing treatments
☐ 2. washing hands before and after entering the room
☐ 3. restricting visitors
☐ 4. contacting the health care provider (HCP) for a prescription for hematopoietic factors such as erythropoietin

34. A client is receiving chemotherapy and tells the nurse about also taking herbal therapy. What should the nurse do **next**?
☐ 1. Determine what substances the client is using, and make sure that the health care provider (HCP) is aware of all therapies the client is using.
☐ 2. Guide the client in the decision-making process to select either Western or alternative medicine.
☐ 3. Encourage the client to seek alternative modalities that do not require the ingestion of substances.
☐ 4. Recommend that the client stop using the alternative medicines immediately.

35. A client diagnosed with cancer is receiving chemotherapy. The nurses should assess which diagnostic value while the client is receiving chemotherapy?
☐ 1. bone marrow cells
☐ 2. liver tissues
☐ 3. heart tissues
☐ 4. pancreatic enzymes

36. A client is to start chemotherapy to treat lung cancer. A venous access device has been placed to permit the administration of chemotherapeutic medications. Three days later at the scheduled appointment to receive chemotherapy, the nurse assesses that the client is dyspneic and their skin is warm and pale. The vital signs are blood pressure 80/30 mm Hg, pulse 132 bpm, respirations 28 breaths/min, temperature 103°F (39.4°C), and oxygen saturation 84%. The central line insertion site is inflamed. After the nurse calls the rapid response team, what should the nurse do **next**?
☐ 1. Place cold, wet compresses on the client's head.
☐ 2. Obtain a portable electrocardiogram monitor.
☐ 3. Administer a prescribed antipyretic medication.
☐ 4. Insert a peripheral intravenous fluid line and infuse normal saline.

37. A client receiving chemotherapy for cancer has an elevated serum creatinine level. What should the nurse do **next**?
☐ 1. Cancel the next scheduled chemotherapy.
☐ 2. Administer the scheduled dose of chemotherapy.
☐ 3. Notify the health care provider (HCP).
☐ 4. Obtain a urine specimen.

The Adult Who Is Receiving Radiation Therapy

38. The nurse is instructing a client about skin care while receiving radiation therapy to the chest. What should the nurse instruct the client to do?
☐ 1. Apply lotion if the skin becomes dry.
☐ 2. Shave the chest to prevent contamination from chest hair.
☐ 3. Wash the area with tepid water and mild soap.
☐ 4. Keep the area covered with a nonadherent dressing between treatments.

39. A client with cancer is receiving radiation therapy and develops thrombocytopenia. What is the **priority** nursing goal to prevent which effect of thrombocytopenia for this client?
☐ 1. pain related to spontaneous bleeding episodes
☐ 2. altered nutrition related to anemia
☐ 3. injury related to the decreased platelet count
☐ 4. skin breakdown related to decreased tissue perfusion

40. A client is beginning external beam radiation therapy to the right axilla after a lumpectomy for breast cancer. Which information should the nurse include in client teaching?
☐ 1. Use a heating pad under the right arm.
☐ 2. Immobilize the right arm.
☐ 3. Place ice on the area after each treatment.
☐ 4. Apply deodorant only under the left arm.

41. A client receiving radiation therapy for lung cancer is having difficulty sleeping. What should the nurse do **first** when teaching the client about promoting sleep?
☐ 1. Tell the client to stop watching television before bed.
☐ 2. Ask the client about usual sleep patterns.
☐ 3. Instruct the client to sleep in a darkened room.
☐ 4. Suggest the client stop drinking coffee until the therapy is completed.

42. A female client is currently receiving radiation therapy to the chest wall for recurrent breast cancer. They have pain while swallowing and burning and tightness in their chest. The nurse should further assess the client for indications of which health problem?
☐ 1. hiatal hernia
☐ 2. stomatitis
☐ 3. radiation enteritis
☐ 4. esophagitis

43. A 36-year-old female client is scheduled to receive external radiation therapy and a cesium implant for cancer of the cervix and is asking about the effects of the radiation on sexual relations during and after the radiation therapy. What should the nurse tell the client regarding a potential effect of radiation therapy on sexuality?
☐ 1. "You will be able to have sexual intercourse while the implant is in place."
☐ 2. "You will have vaginal dryness after treatment is completed."
☐ 3. "You will experience vaginal relaxation after treatment is completed."
☐ 4. "You will continue to have normal menstrual periods during treatment."

44. The nurse is caring for a client who is receiving external beam radiation therapy for the treatment of lung cancer. What should the nurse assess the client for while they are receiving radiation therapy?
☐ 1. diarrhea
☐ 2. improved energy level
☐ 3. dysphagia
☐ 4. normal white blood cell count

The Adult Who Requires Symptom Management

45. A client receiving radiation to the head and neck is experiencing stomatitis. What can the nurse recommend to relieve this symptom?
☐ 1. evaluation by a dentist
☐ 2. alcohol-based mouthwash rinses
☐ 3. artificial saliva
☐ 4. vigorous brushing of teeth after each meal

46. A client undergoing chemotherapy has a white blood cell count of 2300/mm^3 (2.3×10^9/L), a hemoglobin level of 9.8 g/dL (98 g/L), a platelet count of 80,000/mm^3 (80×10^9/L), and a potassium level of 3.8 mEq/L (3.8 mmol/L). Which finding should take **priority**?
☐ 1. blood pressure 136/88 mm Hg
☐ 2. emesis of 90 mL
☐ 3. temperature 101°F (38.3°C)
☐ 4. urine output 40 mL per hour

47. A nurse is caring for a client 24 hours after an abdominal-perineal resection for a bowel tumor. The client's spouse asks if they can bring some of the client's favorite home-cooked Italian minestrone soup. What should the nurse tell the spouse?
☐ 1. Auscultate for bowel sounds.
☐ 2. Ask the client if they feel hunger or gas pains.
☐ 3. Consult the dietician.
☐ 4. Encourage the spouse to bring the soup when the client is able to tolerate solid foods.

48. A client with metastatic lung cancer is having difficulty breathing. Which action should the nurse take to help the client breathe more effectively?
☐ 1. Teach the client diaphragmatic breathing techniques.
☐ 2. Administer cough suppressants as prescribed.
☐ 3. Encourage pursed-lip breathing.
☐ 4. Place the client in a low semi-Fowler position.

49. A client with cancer has thrombocytopenia. Which information should the nurse include in the teaching plan? Select all that apply.
☐ 1. Use an electric razor.
☐ 2. Use a soft-bristle toothbrush.
☐ 3. Avoid frequent flossing for oral care.
☐ 4. Include an over-the-counter nonsteroidal antiinflammatory (NSAID) daily for pain control.
☐ 5. Monitor temperature daily.
☐ 6. Report bleeding, such as nosebleed, petechiae, or melena, to the health care provider (HCP).

50. A client with cancer is afraid of experiencing a febrile reaction associated with blood transfusions. What should the nurse tell the client about febrile transfusion reactions?

"Febrile reactions:
☐ 1. are caused when antibodies on the surface of blood cells in the transfusion are directed against antigens of the recipient."
☐ 2. can usually be prevented by administering antipyretics and antihistamines before the start of the transfusion."
☐ 3. are rarely immune-mediated reactions and can be a sign of hemolytic transfusion."
☐ 4. usually occur within 15 minutes after initiation of the transfusion."

51. A client had a right pneumonectomy for lung cancer yesterday and now has dyspnea. What position in bed will be **best** for this client?
☐ 1. lying on the left side
☐ 2. positioned for postural drainage
☐ 3. head of the bed elevated
☐ 4. flat in bed on full bed rest

52. A client undergoing chemotherapy tells the nurse, "I don't want to get out of bed in the morning because I'm so tired." What action should the nurse take **first**?
☐ 1. Ask the physical therapist to plan an exercise program.
☐ 2. Review current laboratory reports for an underlying cause.
☐ 3. Suggest the client set an alarm clock and get out of bed at the same time each day.
☐ 4. Instruct the client to remain on bed rest until chemotherapy is completed.

53. A nurse is reviewing the health record of an adult male with cancer. The health care provider (HCP) has prescribed filgrastim 400 mcg, subcutaneously once daily. When the nurse reviews the laboratory report, which result indicates the treatment has been effective?

Laboratory Results

Laboratory Results	2/1	2/7	Normal Range
Hemoglobin	15 g/dL (150 g/L)	16 g/dL (160/g/L)	Men: 14–17.4 g/dL (140–174 g/L)
Neutrophil count	1200 mcL	3000 mcL	2500–6000 mcL
Platelet count	200,000/mm³ (200 × 10⁹/L)	200,000/mm³ (200 × 10⁹/L)	Adults: 140,000–400,000/µL (140–400 × 10⁹/L)
Red blood cell (RBC) count	4.0 million/mm³ (4.0 × 10¹²/L)	4.3 million/mm³ (4.3 × 10¹²/L)	4.2–5.4 million/µL (4.2–5.4 × 10¹²/L)

☐ 1. Hemoglobin is 16 g/dL (160 g/L)
☐ 2. Neutrophil count is 3,000/mcl
☐ 3. Platelet count is 200,000/mm3 (200 × 109/L)
☐ 4. RBC count is 4.3 million/mm3 (4.3 × 1012/L)

54. The nurse is teaching a client who is receiving chemotherapy and the client's family how to manage possible nausea and vomiting at home. What information should the nurse include in the teaching plan?
☐ 1. Eat frequent, small meals.
☐ 2. Include soft foods in the diet.
☐ 3. Drink a milkshake made with fruit every day.
☐ 4. Limit the amount of fluid intake.

55. A terminally ill client in hospice care is experiencing nausea and vomiting because of a partial bowel obstruction. To respect the client's wishes for palliative care, the nurse can recommend that the client use which measure?
☐ 1. a nasogastric (NG) suction tube
☐ 2. intravenous (IV) antiemetics
☐ 3. osmotic laxatives
☐ 4. a clear liquid diet

56. A client with brown hair is concerned about losing hair as a result of chemotherapy. What should the nurse tell the client?
☐ 1. "The new growth of hair will be gray."
☐ 2. "The hair loss is temporary."
☐ 3. "New hair growth will be the same texture and color as it was before chemotherapy."
☐ 4. "Avoid the use of wigs when possible."

57. An adult with a history of chronic obstructive pulmonary disease (COPD) and metastatic carcinoma of the lung has not responded to radiation therapy and is being admitted to the hospice program. The nurse should conduct a focused assessment for which symptom?
☐ 1. abdominal distension
☐ 2. pleural friction rub
☐ 3. dyspnea
☐ 4. peripheral edema

58. The nurse is planning with a client who has cancer to improve the client's independence in activities of daily living after radiation therapy. What should the nurse do?
☐ 1. Refer the client to a community support group after discharge from the rehabilitation unit.
☐ 2. Make certain that a family member is present for the rehabilitation sessions.
☐ 3. Provide positive reinforcement for skills achieved.
☐ 4. Inform the client of rehabilitation plans made by the rehabilitation team.

59. When teaching about prevention of infection to a client with a long-term venous catheter, the nurse determines that the client has understood discharge instructions when the client makes which statement?
☐ 1. "I won't remove the dressing until I return to the clinic next week."
☐ 2. "My spouse will change the dressing three times a week, using sterile technique."
☐ 3. "I will monitor my temperature every other day."
☐ 4. "I know it's very important to wash my hands after irrigating the catheter."

60. The nurse is caring for a client with a central venous line. Which nursing action(s) should be implemented in the plan of care for chemotherapy administration? Select all that apply.
☐ 1. Verify patency of the line by the presence of a blood return at regular intervals.
☐ 2. Inspect the insertion site for swelling, erythema, or drainage.
☐ 3. Administer a cytotoxic agent to keep the regimen on schedule even if blood return is not present.
☐ 4. Reposition the client if unable to aspirate blood, and encourage the client to cough.
☐ 5. Contact the health care provider about verifying placement if the status is questionable.

61. The nurse is explaining to the client where the distal tip of a central line will be placed. Indicate on the illustration where the central line will be placed.

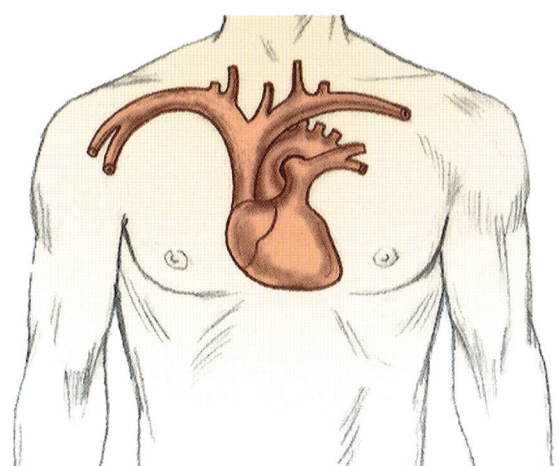

62. A client with pancreatic cancer who has been bedbound for 3 weeks has just returned from having a left subclavian, long-term, tunneled catheter inserted for the administration of analgesic medication. The nurse has not yet received the radiographic results for confirmation of placement. The client becomes restless and dyspneic and has chest pain radiating to the middle of the back. A physical assessment reveals tachycardia and absent breath sounds in the left lung. What complication should the nurse further assess for?
☐ 1. air embolus
☐ 2. pneumothorax
☐ 3. pulmonary embolus
☐ 4. myocardial infarction

63. A client with advanced liver cancer has not been eating a well-balanced diet and has lost weight. Which is a desired outcome for the client?

The client will:
☐ 1. have normalized albumin levels.
☐ 2. return to their ideal body weight.
☐ 3. gain 1 lb (0.5 kg) every 2 weeks.
☐ 4. maintain their current weight.

64. The nurse administers a bolus tube feeding to a client with cancer. To decrease the risk for aspiration, the nurse should take which action?
☐ 1. Place the client on bed rest with the head of the bed elevated to 60 degrees for 2 hours.
☐ 2. Turn the client on their left side with the head of the bed at 45 degrees for 15 minutes.
☐ 3. Assist the client out of bed to sit upright in a chair for 1 hour.
☐ 4. Ask the client to rest in bed with the head of the bed elevated to 30 degrees for 20 minutes.

65. A client with colon cancer had a left hemicolectomy 3 weeks ago. The client is still having difficulty maintaining an adequate oral intake to meet their metabolic needs for optimal healing. The nurse should recommend to the health care provider which nutritional support to maintain the nutritional needs of the client?
☐ 1. total parenteral nutrition through a central catheter
☐ 2. intravenous (IV) infusion of dextrose
☐ 3. nasogastric feeding tube with a protein supplement
☐ 4. jejunostomy for high-caloric feedings

66. A client with colon cancer undergoes surgical removal of a segment of colon and creation of a sigmoid colostomy. What assessment(s) by the nurse would indicate the client is developing complications within the first 24 hours? Select all that apply.
☐ 1. coarse breath sounds auscultated bilaterally at the bases
☐ 2. dusky appearance of the stoma
☐ 3. no drainage in the ostomy appliance
☐ 4. temperature higher than 101.2°F (38.4°C)
☐ 5. decreased bowel sounds

67. A client receiving chemotherapy for metastatic colon cancer is admitted to the hospital because of prolonged vomiting. Assessment findings include an irregular pulse of 120 bpm; blood pressure of 88/48 mm Hg; respiratory rate of 14 breaths/min; serum potassium level of 2.9 mEq/L (2.9 mmol/L); and arterial blood gas test results of pH 7.46, PaCO₂ 45 mm Hg (6.0 kPa), PaO₂ 95 mm Hg (12.6 kPa), and bicarbonate level 29 mEq/L (29 mmol/L). Which prescription should the nurse implement **first**?
☐ 1. oxygen at 4 L per nasal cannula
☐ 2. repeat lab work in 4 hours
☐ 3. 5% dextrose in 0.45% normal saline with potassium chloride (KCl) 40 mEq/L at 125 mL per hour
☐ 4. 12-lead electrocardiogram (ECG)

68. The nurse is making a follow-up telephone call to a client with lung cancer. The client now has a low-grade fever (100.6°F [38.1°C]), a nonproductive cough, and increasing fatigue. The client completed the radiation therapy to the mass in the right lung and mediastinum 10 weeks ago and has a follow-up appointment to see the health care provider (HCP) in 2 weeks. What should the nurse advise the client to do?
☐ 1. Take two acetaminophen tablets every 4 to 6 hours for 2 days, and call the health care provider (HCP) if the temperature increases to 101°F (38.3°C) or greater.
☐ 2. Understand these are expected side effects of the radiation therapy, keep the follow-up appointment in 2 weeks.
☐ 3. Contact the HCP for an appointment today.
☐ 4. Go to the nearest emergency department.

69. A client with malignant pleural effusions has dyspnea and chest pain. In which order of priority from first to last should the nurse manage the client's care? All options must be used.

| 1. Administer morphine sulfate 2 mg IV. |
| 2. Apply oxygen at 2 L via nasal cannula. |
| 3. Educate the client in anticipation of a thoracentesis. |
| 4. Coach the client on deep-breathing exercises. |
| |
| |
| |
| |

70. A client who had a right-side modified radical mastectomy has developed cellulitis in their right arm. What should the nurse tell the client to do to manage the cellulitis?
☐ 1. Take all of the antibiotics as prescribed.
☐ 2. Perform arm exercises as demonstrated by the physical therapist.
☐ 3. Apply ice packs to the affected area for 20-minute periods twice a day.
☐ 4. Keep the right arm lower than the shoulder.

71. An adult client has just had a sclerosing agent instilled after chest tube drainage of a pleural effusion. What should the nurse instruct the client to do?
☐ 1. Lie still to prevent a pneumothorax.
☐ 2. Sit upright with their arms on an overhead table to promote lung expansion.
☐ 3. Change position frequently to distribute the agent.
☐ 4. Lie on the side where the thoracentesis was done to hold pressure on the chest tube site.

72. After surgery for head and neck cancer, a client has a permanent tracheostomy. Which is the **most** important point for the nurse to include in the teaching plan for the client and family?
☐ 1. providing tracheostomy site care
☐ 2. addressing the psychosocial issues related to tracheostomy
☐ 3. observing for early signs and symptoms of skin breakdown around the tracheostomy site
☐ 4. using humidifiers to prevent thick, tenacious secretions

73. A client has a malignant pleural effusion. The nurse should conduct a focused assessment to determine if the client has which sign(s) or symptom(s)? Select all that apply.
☐ 1. hiccups
☐ 2. weight gain
☐ 3. peripheral edema
☐ 4. chest pain
☐ 5. dyspnea

74. A client with suspected lung cancer is undergoing a thoracentesis. Which outcome(s) of the procedure would be expected? Select all that apply.
☐ 1. treatment of a recurrent malignant effusion
☐ 2. diagnosis of underlying disease
☐ 3. palliation of symptoms
☐ 4. relief of acute respiratory distress
☐ 5. removal of the cancer cells

75. The nurse is assessing a client with anemia. To plan nursing care, the nurse should focus the assessment on which sign or symptom?
☐ 1. decreased salivation
☐ 2. bradycardia
☐ 3. cold intolerance
☐ 4. nausea

76. A nurse is assessing an adult who has been receiving chemotherapy. The client has a platelet count of 22,000 cells/mm³ (22 × 10⁹/L) and has petechiae on their lower extremities. What should the nurse instruct the client to do?
☐ 1. Increase the amount of iron in their diet.
☐ 2. Apply lotion to their lower extremities.
☐ 3. Elevate their legs.
☐ 4. Consult the health care provider.

77. A middle-age female client with a history of breast-conserving surgery, axillary node dissection, and radiation therapy reports that their arm is red, warm to touch, and slightly swollen. Which action should the nurse suggest?
☐ 1. Apply warm compresses to the affected arm.
☐ 2. Elevate the arm on two pillows.
☐ 3. Contact the health care provider immediately.
☐ 4. Apply an ice pack to the area of the swelling.

78. The nurse is assessing a middle-age client with cancer who has lost 1 lb (0.5 kg) in 4 weeks. The client is taking ondansetron for nausea and now has a temperature of 101°F (38.3°C). The nurse judges that the fever is a sign of what?
☐ 1. inadequate nutrition
☐ 2. new resistance to current antiemetic therapy
☐ 3. expected response to chemotherapy treatment
☐ 4. infection

79. A nurse is assessing a client with lymphoma who reports distress 9 days after chemotherapy. Because of the risk for septic shock, the nurse should assess the client for which cluster of symptoms?
☐ 1. flushing, decreased oxygen saturation, and mild hypotension
☐ 2. low-grade fever, chills, and tachycardia
☐ 3. elevated temperature, oliguria, and hypotension
☐ 4. high-grade fever, normal blood pressure, and increased respirations

80. A client receiving radiation therapy has fatigue. What should the nurse include in the teaching plan?
☐ 1. increase fluid intake
☐ 2. minimize naps or periods of rest during the day
☐ 3. conserve energy by prioritizing activities
☐ 4. limit dietary intake of high-fiber foods

81. A client receiving chemotherapy has pruritus. To develop a care plan, the nurse should ask the client about which measure?
☐ 1. wearing clothes made from 100% cotton
☐ 2. sleeping in a cool, humidified room
☐ 3. increasing fluid intake to at least 12 cups (about 3 L) a day
☐ 4. taking daily baths with deodorant soap

82. The nurse is developing a long-term care plan with a client who is a cancer survivor concerned about their future quality of life. Which factor should the nurse assess when helping this client focus on plans for the future?
☐ 1. occupation and employability
☐ 2. functional status
☐ 3. evidence of disease
☐ 4. individual values and beliefs

83. A client with breast cancer has abdominal bloating and cramping with no bowel movement for 5 days. The client says they usually have a bowel movement every day after their morning coffee. Bowel sounds are present in all four quadrants. The client received 80 mg of doxorubicin hydrochloride 10 days ago. The nurse should contact the health care provider to request which prescription?
☐ 1. ready-to-use enema to stimulate peristalsis
☐ 2. soapsuds enema until clear
☐ 3. oral cathartic until the client has a bowel movement
☐ 4. mild opioid for abdominal discomfort

84. A client with cancer has diarrhea and inflamed areas of skin around the rectum. What action(s) should the nurse take? Select all that apply.
    ☐ 1. Use sitz baths.
    ☐ 2. Apply zinc oxide ointment to the rectal area after each bowel movement.
    ☐ 3. Apply a skin barrier dressing daily to the rectal area.
    ☐ 4. Clean the rectal area with unscented soap and water after each bowel movement, rinse well, and pat dry.
    ☐ 5. Increase fluid intake.

85. The nurse is explaining the long-term toxic effects of cancer treatments on the immune system to a client who is receiving chemotherapy and radiation therapy for colon cancer. What should the nurse tell the client?
    ☐ 1. Clients with persistent immunologic abnormalities after treatment are at a much greater risk for infection than clients with a history of splenectomy.
    ☐ 2. The use of radiation and combination chemotherapy can result in more frequent and more severe immune system impairment.
    ☐ 3. Long-term immunologic effects have been studied only in clients with breast and lung cancer.
    ☐ 4. The helper T cells recover more rapidly than do the suppressor T cells, which results in a positive helper cell balance that can last 5 years.

The Adult Who Is Coping with Loss, Grief, Bereavement, and Spiritual Distress

86. A client is newly diagnosed with cancer and is beginning a treatment plan. Which action by the nurse will be **most** effective in helping the client cope?
    ☐ 1. Assume decision-making for the client until treatment is completed.
    ☐ 2. Encourage the client to observe strict compliance with all treatment regimens.
    ☐ 3. Inform the client of all possible adverse treatment effects.
    ☐ 4. Identify available resources for the client and family.

87. A client is being treated for breast cancer. The client's adult child is concerned that the client is in denial because when they discuss the diagnosis of breast cancer, the client says that breast cancer is not that serious and then changes the subject. The nurse can tell the client's child that denial can be a healthy defense mechanism if it is used when?
    ☐ 1. to permit the client to seek unconventional treatments
    ☐ 2. when making decisions about the client's care
    ☐ 3. alone and not in combination with other defense mechanisms
    ☐ 4. to allow the client to continue in their role as a parent

88. A client who is a single parent of three teenage children has metastatic breast cancer, and the health care provider has recommended another high-dose chemotherapy. The client's older adult parents live a 10-hour drive away and have only been able to visit twice since the initial diagnosis 14 months ago. The client is concerned about their children's welfare during the treatment. Which potential problem should the nurse help the client solve **first**?
    ☐ 1. using denial as a primary coping mechanism
    ☐ 2. finding support systems
    ☐ 3. making realistic decisions
    ☐ 4. arranging care for the client's children

89. The nurse is helping the spouse of a middle-age client in hospice care for end-stage pancreatic cancer prepare for the client's death. Which factor will **most** adversely impact the spouse's bereavement outcomes?

    The spouse:
    ☐ 1. is preparing for the client's death.
    ☐ 2. has a high socioeconomic status.
    ☐ 3. has strong family support.
    ☐ 4. blames themself for the client's cancer.

90. The nurse is counseling the family of an older adult who died today. Which factor facilitates attainment of a positive bereavement outcome?
    ☐ 1. being a teenager
    ☐ 2. having a history of anxiety
    ☐ 3. being a spouse
    ☐ 4. possessing adequate financial resources

91. A client with end-stage colon cancer is experiencing powerlessness. Which nursing action will be **most** effective when caring for this client?
    ☐ 1. Make certain that all staff members focus only on the client's capabilities.
    ☐ 2. Encourage family members to become more responsible for the client's care.
    ☐ 3. Request a referral to a psychologist.
    ☐ 4. Include the client in decision-making whenever possible.

92. A client has just been diagnosed with cancer. During the initial stage of adaptation to the diagnosis and its treatment, the nurse can facilitate the client's adaptation by using which strategy?
☐ 1. encouraging the client to maintain their usual role
☐ 2. facilitating family-related disagreements and conflicts
☐ 3. supporting the client in their use of denial as a coping strategy
☐ 4. arranging transportation and childcare on treatment days

93. The family of a client is considering end-of-life care for their parent. When explaining hospice care, the nurse should give the family which information?

"Hospice care:
☐ 1. is available 1 month before treatment is no longer curative."
☐ 2. offers end-of-life care that includes palliative care and focuses on the client's physical, emotional, and spiritual needs."
☐ 3. is coordinated by your health care provider."
☐ 4. helps clients die at home."

94. A client's spouse expresses concern that the dying client keeps saying, "I have to go to the store." Which statement by the nurse will be **most** effective in assisting the spouse to understand the dying process?
☐ 1. "Many dying clients are restless and can be treated with sedatives."
☐ 2. "The client may be fighting death, and you should leave them alone."
☐ 3. "Comments related to going somewhere or leaving on a trip are common in dying clients."
☐ 4. "You can tell your spouse that you will take them to the store."

95. The spouse of a terminally ill client asks the nurse, "Why is my spouse having frequent bowel movements if they are not eating?" What should the nurse tell the spouse?
☐ 1. "I know he's having frequent loose stools and it's distressing for you, but that's just the way it is."
☐ 2. "I don't know when the bowels will shut down, but they will eventually."
☐ 3. "The pain medication will eventually help low the process of bowel function."
☐ 4. "The intestines still produce some waste products even when a person is not eating."

96. The client who is in the end stages of cancer is requesting spiritual support. What should the nurse do **next**?
☐ 1. Review the client's medical record to determine the client's religion.
☐ 2. Call a chaplain, and set up an appointment for spiritual guidance.
☐ 3. Request that the family notify the client's spiritual advisor.
☐ 4. Ask the client what spiritual activities would be most helpful.

97. An older adult with end-stage cancer needs assistance with arranging the finances for end-of-life home care. The nurse should refer the client to which person?
☐ 1. business manager of the health care agency
☐ 2. discharge planning coordinator
☐ 3. health care provider (HCP)
☐ 4. executor of the client's will

98. The family members of a client who is near death from colon cancer ask the nurse what to expect if the client becomes dehydrated. What should the nurse tell them?
☐ 1. The health care provider (HCP) will make the decision regarding hydration therapy.
☐ 2. Dehydration may prolong the dying process.
☐ 3. Hydration is used only in extreme situations of dehydration.
☐ 4. Dehydration is expected during the dying process.

99. A client who is at the end of life tells the nurse about experiencing "spiritual distress." What should the nurse do **first**?
☐ 1. Make a referral to a member of the clergy.
☐ 2. Refer the client to a bereavement support group.
☐ 3. Ask if the client would like to pray.
☐ 4. Determine what spiritual distress means to the client.

100. A nurse is caring for a client who is receiving hospice care at home. The client's neighbors have been calling the nurse to inquire about the client's condition. What should the nurse tell the neighbors?
☐ 1. "Please call the oncologist."
☐ 2. "The client is in a coma now."
☐ 3. "Please call the client's sibling."
☐ 4. "The client is not expected to live much longer."

101. A client with breast cancer is concerned that their spouse is depressed by their diagnosis. Which change in their spouse's behavior may confirm their fears?
☐ 1. increased decisiveness
☐ 2. problem-focused coping style
☐ 3. increase in social interactions
☐ 4. disturbance in sleep patterns

102. The nurse is teaching the health care staff about ways to improve communication with clients from a variety of cultures. Which strategy will be **most** effective in improving transcultural communications with clients with cancer and their families?
☐ 1. Use touch to show concern and care for the client.
☐ 2. Focus attention on verbal communication skills only.
☐ 3. Establish a rapport, and listen to their concerns.
☐ 4. Maintain eye contact at all times.

103. The nurse is planning to refer a client with cancer to a cancer support group. Which outcome is expected of the client participating in a cancer support group?
The client can:
☐ 1. choose the best treatment options.
☐ 2. find financial help.
☐ 3. obtain home health care.
☐ 4. cope with cancer.

104. A cancer survivor feels guilty when attending a cancer support group meeting. The nurse can help the client manage feelings of guilt by giving the client which information?
☐ 1. These are feelings of anger at the terminally ill clients in the group.
☐ 2. It is an unexpected response to volatile emotions.
☐ 3. This is a spiritual response to the client's own illness.
☐ 4. This is a normal reaction when surviving a life-threatening experience.

105. A client's only adult child lives too far away to visit often. For which reason is the client at higher risk for psychosocial distress?
The client:
☐ 1. has been successful in dealing with stress throughout life.
☐ 2. does not have to deal with other stressors right now.
☐ 3. is able to use denial as a coping mechanism.
☐ 4. perceives having minimal social support.

106. A client with a diagnosis of cancer is frequently disruptive and challenges the nurse. This behavior may be caused by which factor?
☐ 1. uncertainty and an underlying fear of recurrence
☐ 2. the usual trajectory of a short-term illness
☐ 3. a history of a behavioral illness
☐ 4. the one-time crisis from learning of the diagnosis

107. A parent of a 7-year-old child and a 10-year-old child is concerned about what they should tell their children regarding their spouse's impending death from aggressive breast cancer. How should the nurse respond to the client's spouse?
☐ 1. Refer the family to pastoral care services.
☐ 2. Encourage the client's spouse to come to terms with their own grief.
☐ 3. Suggest that the health care provider (HCP) tell the children about the seriousness of their parent's illness.
☐ 4. Begin education about strategies for communication with their children.

108. While talking to their spouse who is caring for their children, a middle-age female client with stage 4 breast cancer slams the phone down. The client begins to cry and states that they feel guilty for being hospitalized. Which nursing action will **best** support the client emotionally?
☐ 1. Ask the client if they would like to speak with a grief counselor.
☐ 2. Call the health care provider, and request an antidepressant.
☐ 3. Sit with the client, and help them acknowledge and discuss their feelings.
☐ 4. Suggest the client call their spouse when they are calmer.

109. A middle-age client who is receiving radiation therapy tells the nurse that they feel inadequate as a spouse and parent because they can no longer carry out their usual duties with the same energy as before. What recommendations should the nurse make to help the client cope with this situation?
☐ 1. Suggest they reassign all household chores to other members of the family.
☐ 2. Suggest prioritizing activities and asking for help from friends and family.
☐ 3. Ignore the household chores during the crisis period.
☐ 4. Avoid worrying so much because it is normal to be tired during this phase of the therapy.

110. An older adult client who is usually meticulous about their appearance and dress arrives today for their 23rd day of radiation therapy. The client appears disheveled and emotionally labile, and their responses to the usual questions are a little inappropriate. The client's heart rate is 124 bpm, respirations are 32 breaths/min, and their skin is cold and clammy. Based on these findings, the nurse should further assess the client for which condition?
☐ 1. schizophrenia
☐ 2. panic disorder
☐ 3. depression
☐ 4. delirium

111. The nurse is planning future care with a middle-age client who has undergone surgical resection for lung cancer. Which plan will **best** promote adaptation and rehabilitation?
☐ 1. arranging a visit from a client who has recovered from a similar surgery
☐ 2. planning a progressive activity regimen
☐ 3. teaching about dressing care
☐ 4. requesting house-cleaning services for 3 months

112. The nurse is evaluating a client with cancer who has lost all of the hair on their head. Which finding indicates the client is adapting well to body image changes?
The client:
☐ 1. names a relative to call if experiencing suicidal ideation.
☐ 2. continuously looks at their bald head.
☐ 3. discusses a date to return to work.
☐ 4. serves as a volunteer in a client-to-client visitation program.

The Adult Who Is Experiencing Problems with Sexuality

113. A female client has increased vaginal dryness during sexual intercourse. The client has received chemotherapy in the past and has menopausal symptoms due to ovarian suppression. The nurse should instruct the client on the use of which solution for vaginal dryness?
☐ 1. vaginal dilators
☐ 2. douching with a soothing solution
☐ 3. water-soluble vaginal lubricants
☐ 4. relaxation techniques

114. A client with cancer of the larynx has a permanent tracheostomy tube. The client confides to the nurse that they are beginning to avoid sexual activity because of the increased tracheostomy secretions. Which statement by the nurse will be **most** helpful to the client?
☐ 1. "Use a scopolamine patch to decrease secretions."
☐ 2. "Avoid fluid intake 2 hours before sexual activity."
☐ 3. "Place a thin piece of gauze over the tracheostomy."
☐ 4. "Wash the tracheostomy area with deodorizing antibacterial soap before sexual activity."

115. A client is scheduled for a total abdominal hysterectomy for cervical cancer. When discussing the potential impact of this procedure on the client's sexuality, the nurse should offer which response to the client?
☐ 1. "All women experience sexual problems with this surgical procedure. Do you have any questions?"
☐ 2. "When can I schedule an appointment with you and your partner to discuss any issues either of you may have regarding sexuality?"
☐ 3. "Do you anticipate any problems with sex related to your scheduled hysterectomy?"
☐ 4. "Most women have concerns about their sexuality after this type of surgery. Do you have any concerns or questions?"

116. A young male client with early-stage testicular cancer is scheduled for a unilateral orchiectomy. The client confides to the nurse that they are concerned about what effects the surgery will have on their sexual performance. Which response by the nurse provides accurate information about sexual performance after an orchiectomy?
☐ 1. "Most impotence resolves in a couple of months."
☐ 2. "You could have early ejaculation with this type of surgery."
☐ 3. "We will refer you to a sex therapist because you will probably notice erectile dysfunction."
☐ 4. "Because your surgery does not involve other organs or tissues, you will likely not notice much change in your sexual performance."

117. A young female client is receiving chemotherapy and mentions to the nurse that they and their spouse are using a diaphragm for birth control. Which information is **most** important for the nurse to discuss?
☐ 1. inconvenience of the diaphragm
☐ 2. transmission of sexually transmitted infections
☐ 3. body changes related to hormones
☐ 4. infection control

118. The nurse is teaching a client who had a lobectomy for lung cancer and the client's partner how to promote comfort and optimal respiratory expansion during sexual intimacy. What can the nurse suggest the couple do?
☐ 1. Use a nasal decongestant inhaler.
☐ 2. Raise the affected partner's head and upper torso on pillows.
☐ 3. Have the affected partner assume a dependent position.
☐ 4. Limit the duration of the sexual activity.

Ethical and Legal Issues Related to Adults with Cancer

119. A hospitalized client with end-stage pancreatic cancer does not want to be resuscitated. The health care provider (HCP) has written the do-not-resuscitate (DNR) prescription on the client's record. The client has a cardiac arrest, and the spouse tells the nurse they want the client to be resuscitated and asks the nurse to "do something." What should the nurse do?
☐ 1. Begin cardiopulmonary resuscitation (CPR).
☐ 2. Call a "code."
☐ 3. Page the HCP.
☐ 4. Discuss the DNR prescription with the spouse.

120. A registered nurse (RN) is assigning care on the oncology unit and assigns a client with Kaposi's sarcoma and human immunodeficiency virus (HIV) infection to the unlicensed assistive personnel (UAP). The UAP does not want to care for this client. How should the nurse respond?
☐ 1. "I will assign this client to another nurse."
☐ 2. "I will help you take care of this client so you are confident with the care."
☐ 3. "You seem worried about this assignment."
☐ 4. "I will review blood and body fluid precautions with you."

121. A person who is employed full-time wants to request a leave of absence to care for their parent who is being treated for colon cancer 300 miles (480 km) away. What should the nurse advise the person to do **first**?
☐ 1. Contact their employee resources department about policies guiding leaves of absence.
☐ 2. Make a plan to see how long they can be out of work without financial concerns.
☐ 3. Find someone to do their work while they are away.
☐ 4. Ask the parent if they can afford a caregiver.

122. The nurse is developing a care plan for a client with cancer receiving hospice home care. Which would be the **most** appropriate action for managing the client's chronic pain?
☐ 1. Administer analgesic medication regularly and as needed for breakthrough pain.
☐ 2. Sedate the client with tranquilizers.
☐ 3. Avoid intravenous pain medication until the client is terminally ill.
☐ 4. Administer analgesic medication when vital signs indicate increased pain severity.

123. A client and nurse have established a goal for the client to be more autonomous in decision-making. Which situation indicates that the goal has been met?
☐ 1. The health care provider (HCP) directs the client's care.
☐ 2. The nurse provides the client with the facts and then allows the client to make an independent decision.
☐ 3. The nurse respects a client's choice not to know particular information.
☐ 4. The health care team makes health and treatment decisions.

End-of-Life Care

124. A client who is near death is receiving hospice care to manage severe pain. The client is receiving a narcotic pain medication intravenously per a patient-controlled analgesia (PCA) pump. The client is lethargic, is sleeping much of the time, and has not rated their pain recently. What information should the nurse use to make decisions about the care plan? The client:
☐ 1. received too much medication through an overdose of medication administered through the PCA pump.
☐ 2. may be nearing death as specific dosages and time intervals for self-administration of the analgesic are programmed into the PCA pump to prevent overdose.
☐ 3. has obtained sufficient pain relief because they have not had pain in the last 12 hours.
☐ 4. has an IV that has infiltrated, and the analgesic medication has been injected into the subcutaneous tissues and has been absorbed faster than prescribed.

125. The family of a hospitalized client demonstrates understanding of the teaching about legal documents related to end-of-life care such as "advance directive" and "power of attorney" when they make which statement(s)? Select all that apply.
☐ 1. "Advance directives give instructions about future medical care and treatment."
☐ 2. "If people are not capable of communicating their wishes, health care providers and family together can agree on measures or actions that will be taken."
☐ 3. "Ethics experts agree that the family is the sole deciding factor when the client is competent."
☐ 4. "Medical power of attorney gives primarily financial access to the designee."
☐ 5. "Medical power of attorney or durable power of attorney for health care is a document that lists who can make health care decisions if a person is unable to make an informed decision for themself."
☐ 6. "Advance directives give details about the client's medical history."

126. The nurse can be an important advocate for a client who is considering an alternative method of cancer treatment. Which statement **best** demonstrates the nurse as a client advocate? The nurse will:
☐ 1. provide information about standard therapies.
☐ 2. monitor blood tests as indicated by the alternative therapy.
☐ 3. document the client's desire to try an alternative therapy.
☐ 4. allow the client to make health care choices but will assist in ensuring the client is fully informed when making those decisions.

127. After completing the nursing assessment for a client and family entering the palliative care program. Which nursing goal(s) would be appropriate at this time? Select all that apply.
☐ 1. Modify the family's usual coping strategies.
☐ 2. Achieve a dignified and respectful death.
☐ 3. Maximize the client's quality of life.
☐ 4. Provide comfort during the dying process.
☐ 5. Offer support for the client's family.
☐ 6. Prolong life.

128. A client and their family have just received an initial diagnosis of colon cancer. In which way can the nurse act as an advocate?
☐ 1. helping them maintain a sense of optimism and hopefulness
☐ 2. determining their understanding of the results of the diagnostic testing
☐ 3. listening carefully to their perceptions of what their needs are
☐ 4. providing them with written materials about the cancer site and its treatment

129. A client who is dying of acquired immunodeficiency syndrome (AIDS) is admitted to the inpatient psychiatric unit because they attempted suicide. The client's close friend recently died of AIDS. The client begins to talk about their feelings related to the illness and the loss of their friend. The client begins to cry. Which response by the nurse would be **most** appropriate?
☐ 1. Give the client some tissues, and tell them it is okay to cry.
☐ 2. Tell the client to stop crying and that everything will be okay.
☐ 3. Sort the client's mail to distract the client.
☐ 4. Change the subject.

130. The spouse of an older adult who has been admitted to the hospital with kidney failure tells the nurse, "I know they don't want to die in a hospital, but it's so hard for me to take care of them at home. They say they don't want any more treatment, but I'm not ready to let them go. We have so many arrangements to decide before they die." Which statement(s) by the nurse to the client's spouse would be **most** appropriate? Select all that apply.
☐ 1. "Your spouse is not going to die that soon judging by their current symptoms."
☐ 2. "What are your fears about your spouse dying?"
☐ 3. "I can imagine that it's hard for you to care for your spouse at home."
☐ 4. "What do you and your spouse know about advance directives?"
☐ 5. "We can discuss types of hospice and home care available."
☐ 6. "What kind of arrangements do you think need to be made before they die?"

131. A terminally ill client's spouse tells the nurse, "I wish we had taken that trip to Europe last year. We just kept putting it off, and now I'm upset that we didn't go." The nurse interprets the spouse's statement as indicating which stage of adaptation to dying?
☐ 1. anger
☐ 2. denial
☐ 3. bargaining
☐ 4. depression

132. A client who is in the end stages of cancer is increasingly upset about receiving chemotherapy. Which approach by the nurse would likely be **most** helpful in gaining the client's cooperation?
☐ 1. Tell the client how the treatment can be expected to help.
☐ 2. Describe the probable effect that missing a treatment would have.
☐ 3. Explain that being upset makes the treatment more difficult.
☐ 4. Suggest having a massage during the treatment.

133. A client suspects the end of life is near. However, others talk about only pleasant matters and maintain a persistently cheerful façade. The nurse plans care for this client by recognizing that these behaviors will **most** likely cause the client to experience which feeling?
☐ 1. relief
☐ 2. isolation
☐ 3. hope
☐ 4. independence

134. The young sibling of a young adult client with leukemia asks, "Can you check my blood? When my sibling got pneumonia, so did I. And I think I have this, too." How should the nurse respond? Select all that apply.
☐ 1. Ask the client's health care provider to take a sample of the sibling's blood.
☐ 2. Explain to the sibling that leukemia is not a communicable disease.
☐ 3. Discuss the sibling's concern with their parents.
☐ 4. Tell the parents about a group for siblings of clients with terminal illness.
☐ 5. Ask the sibling about their concerns.

135. When talking with the nurse, the sibling of a client with leukemia says, "We used to play pretty rough games together. Maybe some of the bruises they got when I tackled them caused this." Which statement is the nurse's **best** response?
☐ 1. "Don't feel guilty. You didn't cause this illness."
☐ 2. "I can see you're worried. Let's talk about how people get leukemia."
☐ 3. "Here's some information about leukemia for you to read."
☐ 4. "Lots of people worry about things like this. It's not your fault."

Managing Care, Quality, and Safety of Adults with Cancer

136. A nurse is making follow-up phone calls to clients being treated for cancer. In which order of priority from first to last should the nurse return the calls? All options must be used.
The client:

| 1. receiving chemotherapy who has a loss of appetite |
| 2. who underwent a mastectomy 2 weeks ago who called for information on the Reach for Recovery program |
| 3. receiving spinal radiation for bone cancer metastases who has urinary incontinence |
| 4. with colon cancer who has questions about a high-fiber diet |
| |
| |
| |

137. The nurse is making client rounds following the shift report. Which client should the nurse assess **first**?
☐ 1. 38-year-old client receiving internal radiation therapy for cervical cancer
☐ 2. 27-year-old client with leukemia hospitalized for induction of high-dose chemotherapy
☐ 3. 75-year-old client with metastatic prostate cancer with a pathologic fracture of the femur who is in pain
☐ 4. 23-year-old client undergoing surgery for placement of a central venous catheter

138. The nurse is administering intravenous chemotherapy to a client with cancer. Which precaution(s) would be necessary when administering chemotherapy? Select all that apply.
☐ 1. taping all intravenous (IV) tubing connections
☐ 2. wearing gloves when handling the client's urine
☐ 3. disposing of chemotherapy waste as hazardous material
☐ 4. wearing a long-sleeved gown when administering chemotherapy
☐ 5. disposing of sharps in a specifically labeled container

139. During the intravenous (IV) administration of a chemotherapeutic vesicant drug, the nurse observes that there is a lack of blood return from the IV catheter. What should the nurse do **first**?
☐ 1. Stop the administration of the drug.
☐ 2. Reposition the client's arm, and continue with administration of the drug.
☐ 3. Irrigate the catheter with normal saline.
☐ 4. Continue to administer the drug, and assess for edema at the IV site.

140. The nurse is caring for a client with end-stage cancer whose health status is declining. A prescription is written by the attending health care provider (HCP) to withhold all fluid, but the health care team cannot locate a family member or guardian. The nurse requests an ethics consultation. Which information is true of an ethics consultation? Select all that apply.
☐ 1. Persons requesting an ethics consultation may do so without intimidation or fear of reprisal.
☐ 2. Ethics consultations may prevent poor outcomes in cases involving ethical problems.
☐ 3. The recommendations of ethics consultants are advisory only.
☐ 4. Requests for ethics consultations may only be made by the HCP or nurse.
☐ 5. An ethics consultation is intended to provide legal advice on client care.

141. The nurse-manager on the oncology unit wants to improve documentation of the effectiveness of analgesic medication within 30 minutes after administration. What should the nurse-manager do **first**?
☐ 1. Change the policy of documentation to 45 minutes.
☐ 2. Consult the pharmacist.
☐ 3. Consult the nurses on the evening shift where documentation of analgesia is the greatest problem.
☐ 4. Complete a brief quality improvement study and chart audit to document the rate of adherence to the policy and the pattern of documentation over shifts.

142. A registered nurse (RN) instructs an unlicensed assistive personnel (UAP) to check the urine intake and output (I&O) of clients on the oncology unit at the end of the 8-hour shift. It is important for the nurse to instruct the UAP to do what?
☐ 1. Ask the clients if they are thirsty when calculating the I&O.
☐ 2. Report back to the nurse immediately if any client has an output less than 240 mL.
☐ 3. Document the I&O results on the medical records.
☐ 4. Write the I&O results down for the nurse to give a report to the next shift.

143. An alert and oriented older adult client with metastatic lung cancer is admitted to the medical-surgical unit for treatment of heart failure. The client was given 80 mg of furosemide in the emergency department. The nurse is instructing the unlicensed assistive personnel (UAP) to implement a nursing plan to manage potential incontinence. Which instruction will be **most** effective for this client?
☐ 1. prescribing incontinence briefs for the client so they will not have to worry about incontinence
☐ 2. requesting an indwelling urinary catheter to avoid incontinence
☐ 3. padding the bed with extra absorbent linens
☐ 4. placing a commode at the bedside and instructing the client in its use

144. The nursing team on an oncology unit consists of a registered nurse (RN), a licensed practical/vocational nurse (LPN/VN), and one unlicensed assistive personnel (UAP). Which client should be assigned to the RN?
☐ 1. 52-year-old client with lung cancer admitted for acute dyspnea
☐ 2. 45-year-old client receiving tube feedings
☐ 3. 28-year-old client being evaluated for a bone marrow transplant
☐ 4. 65-year-old client diagnosed with endometrial cancer who underwent an abdominal hysterectomy 3 days ago

145. The nurse is to wear personal protective equipment (PPE) to administer a chemotherapeutic agent to a client. What guideline(s) should the nurse follow for PPE use and care? Select all that apply.
☐ 1. Understand the proper use and limitations of PPE.
☐ 2. Use care in removing all items to reduce contamination.
☐ 3. Ensure that PPE is made of materials that allow for air ventilation.
☐ 4. Sanitize the hands with an alcohol-based solution before putting gloves on and after removing gloves.
☐ 5. Discard the PPE in containers for contaminated waste.

146. A client is to receive intravascular chemotherapy for 10 days. Which equipment should the nurse use for this procedure?
☐ 1. short peripheral catheter
☐ 2. central venous access in the femoral vein
☐ 3. intravenous catheter insertion device
☐ 4. peripherally inserted central catheter (PICC)

Answers, Rationales, and Test-Taking Strategies

*The answers and rationales for each question follow below, along with keys (🗝) to the client need (CN) and cognitive level (CL) for each question. In addition, questions that measure clinical judgment will be coded (CJ). As you check your answers, use the **Content Mastery and Test-Taking Skill Self-Analysis** worksheet (tear-out worksheet in the back of the book) to identify the reason(s) for not answering the questions correctly. For additional information about test-taking skills and strategies for answering questions, refer to pages 12–51 in part 1 of this book.*

The Adult at Risk for Cancer

1. **3.** Clients over age 50 who have a history of inflammatory bowel disease are at risk for colon cancer. The client who smokes is at high risk for lung cancer. Although the exact cause is not always known, other risk factors for colon cancer are a diet high in animal fats, including a large amount of red meat and fatty foods with low fiber, and the presence of colon cancer in a first-generation relative.
   🗝 CN: Reduction of risk potential; CL: Analyze

2. **1.** Basal cell carcinoma occurs most commonly in sun-exposed areas of the body. The highest risk for basal cell carcinoma is for those who have had frequent exposure to ultraviolet (UV) radiation from the sun and indoor tanning; fair skinned people; people over 50 years; males and people with a history of other types of skin cancers.
   🗝 CN: Health promotion and maintenance; CL: Analyze

3. **1.** Because of the high risk for infertility with chemotherapy, pelvic irradiation, and retroperitoneal lymph node dissection that may follow an orchiectomy, cryopreservation of sperm is completed before treatment is started and should be discussed with the client.
   🗝 CN: Physiological adaptation; CL: Apply

4. **4.** A sunscreen with an SPF of 15 or higher should be worn on all sun-exposed skin surfaces. It should be applied before sun exposure and reapplied after being in the water. Peak sun exposure usually occurs from 0010 to 1400. Tightly woven clothing, protective hats, and sunglasses are recommended to decrease sun exposure. Sun tanning parlors should be avoided.
   🗝 CN: Health promotion and maintenance; CL: Analyze

5. **1.** Malignant melanoma may have a familial basis, especially in families with dysplastic nevi syndrome. First-degree relatives should be monitored closely. Malignant melanoma occurs most often in the 20- to 45-year-old age group. Severe sunburn as a child does increase the risk; however, this client is at increased risk because of their family history.
   🗝 CN: Health promotion and maintenance; CL: Apply

6. **3.** Because more than 50% of cancers occur in people who are older than age 65, the single most important factor in determining risk would be age. Life-style choices are increasingly thought to contribute to cancer, and hormonal changes are a factor, but age continues to be the most important risk factor.
   🗝 CN: Health promotion and maintenance; CL: Apply

7. **-/+ 1, 3, 4, 5.** The client is at increased risk for the development of lung, skin, or breast cancer. Consequently, the client should improve nutrition (e.g., eating food with lower animal fat content, increasing fiber, adding fruits and vegetables to their diet), stop smoking, use sunscreen, and lose weight. The client's alcohol consumption is not excessive and not a risk. It is not necessary and would be difficult for the client to change jobs to work inside as long as the client uses protection from the sun.
   🗝 CN: Health promotion and maintenance; CL: Analyze

8. **-/+ 4, 5.** Hoarseness and chronic sore throat are indicative of head and neck cancers, particularly cancer of the pharynx. Tobacco use and heavy consumption of alcohol are risk factors for these cancers and may have a synergistic effect. Heavy use of acetaminophen is not a risk factor for head and neck cancer, but it is related to liver failure. Exposure to the sun increases the risk for skin cancers but not cancers of the head and neck. Consuming a high-fat diet is not related to head and neck cancer, but it may be a risk factor for other cancers and heart disease. Exposure to wood dust and other inhaled particles is associated with lung cancer.
   🗝 CN: Health promotion and maintenance; CL: Analyze

9. 2. High-fiber, low-fat diets are recommended to reduce the risk for colon cancer. Stir-frying, poaching, steaming, and broiling are all low-fat methods to prepare foods. Croissants are made of refined flour. They are also high in fat, as are peanut butter squares and whole milk, granola, cream cheese, and sour cream.

CN: Health promotion and maintenance; CL: Apply

10. 2. Motivational interviewing is a technique used to guide clients to make changes in their behavior. A client's diet and nutritional status can be changed. Sex, family history of cancer, and age are risk factors that cannot be changed.

CN: Health promotion and maintenance; CL: Apply

11. 3. CT scanning is the standard noninvasive method used in a workup for lung cancer because it can distinguish small differences in tissue density and can detect nodal involvement. CT is comparable to magnetic resonance imaging in evaluating lymph node metastasis. CT is noninvasive and usually available, but these are not the main reasons for its use. CT can distinguish malignancy in some situations but not all.

CN: Physiological adaptation; CL: Analyze

12. 2. Strategies to reach clients in all cultures should include incorporating the folk beliefs and traditions of the target population into the program. Identification of a centrally located building with available access by the target population, use of materials in the native or primary language of the target population, and involvement by all community leaders will also help the program succeed.

CN: Health promotion and maintenance; CL: Analyze

The Adult with Pain

13. 4. The desired outcome for management of pain is that the client's or family's subjective report of pain is acceptable and documented using a pain scale; the goal is that behavioral and physiologic indicators of pain are absent around the clock. The nurse, client, and the client's family should develop a systematic approach to pain management using information gathered from the client's history and a hierarchy of pain measurement. Pain should be assessed at frequent intervals. The client should not wait to receive medication until the pain is midpoint on the pain scale, nor should the client receive so much pain medication that they are not alert. Continuous pain relief is the goal, not just during particular periods during the day.

CN: Basic care and comfort; CL: Analyze

14. 3. Tolerance develops from taking opioids over an extended period. It is characterized by the need for an increased dose to achieve the same degree of analgesia. Addiction is characterized by a drive to take the medication for the psychological effect rather than the therapeutic effect. Physical dependence is a response to ongoing exposure to a medication manifested by withdrawal symptoms when discontinued abruptly.

CN: Pharmacological and parenteral therapies; CL: Analyze

15. 3. Administration of morphine sulfate is contraindicated because morphine causes respiratory depression. It may also increase intracranial pressure if the client is not ventilating properly, which could result in an accumulation of carbon dioxide, a potent vasodilator. Ibuprofen, naproxen, and acetaminophen are not likely to mask symptoms of increased intracranial pressure or impact respiratory status.

CN: Pharmacological and parenteral therapies; CL: Analyze

16. 1. The most common toxicities from NSAIDs are gastrointestinal disorders (nausea, epigastric pain, ulcers, bleeding, diarrhea, constipation). Renal dysfunction, pulmonary complications, and cardiovascular complications from NSAIDs are much less common.

CN: Pharmacological and parenteral therapies; CL: Analyze

17. 1, 2, 4, 6. The scheduled use of long-acting opioids and around-the-clock dosing are necessary to achieve a steady level of analgesia. Whatever the route or frequency, a prescription should be available for breakthrough pain medication to be administered in addition to the regularly scheduled medication. Oral drug administration is the route of choice for economy, safety, and ease of use. Even severe pain requiring high doses of opioids can be managed orally as long as the client can swallow medication and has a functioning gastrointestinal system. Tolerance occurs because of the need for increasing doses to achieve the same pain relief and will not be avoided with the use of acetaminophen. Addiction is a complex condition in which the drug is used for psychological effect and not analgesia. Nurses need to educate families about the appropriate use of opioids and assure them that addiction is not a concern when managing cancer pain. Nonpharmacologic methods are useful as an adjunct to assist in pain control.

Self-report is the best assessment of pain and is an individual response.

    CN: Pharmacological and parenteral therapies; CL: Evaluate

18. 4. Most clients with cancer who are experiencing inadequate pain control while taking an oral opioid after being switched from IV administration have been undermedicated. Equianalgesic conversions should be made to provide estimates of the equivalent dose needed for the same level of relief as provided by the IV dose. There is research to suggest that clients with cancer do not become addicted to opioids when dosed adequately. There is no evidence to suggest that the client is physically addicted or is having withdrawal symptoms.

    CN: Pharmacological and parenteral therapies; CL: Analyze

19. 1. Intensity is indicative of the severity of pain and is important for evaluating the efficacy of pain management. The cause and location of the pain cannot be managed, but the intensity of the pain can be controlled. The nurse and client can collaborate to reduce aggravating factors; however, the goal will ultimately be to reduce the intensity of the pain.

    CN: Basic care and comfort; CL: Analyze

20. 2. Tolerance to an opioid occurs when a larger dose of the analgesic medication is needed to provide the same level of pain control. The risk for addiction is low with opioids used to treat cancer pain. There are no data to support that this client is experiencing withdrawal. Although the client may have experienced a placebo effect at one time, placebo effects tend to diminish over time, especially in regard to chronic cancer pain.

    CN: Pharmacological and parenteral therapies; CL: Analyze

21. 2. The regular administration of medications provides a consistent serum level of medication, which can help prevent breakthrough pain. Therefore, the nurse should instruct the client to take the pain medication on a regular schedule to manage chronic cancer-related pain. The client should not wait for the intensity of the pain to increase but rather take the medication on a regular basis. There is little risk for the client with cancer-related pain to become addicted. Sleeping 12 to 16 hours a day would not allow the client to participate in usual daily activities or preferred activities.

    CN: Pharmacological and parenteral therapies; CL: Analyze

The Adult Who Is Receiving Chemotherapy

22. 3. Chemotherapeutic agents are very toxic; therefore, precautions are taken, such as the use of safety goggles, gloves, and long-sleeved gowns when handling agents to prevent incidental contact with skin or splashes to the eyes. It is not sufficient to wear only double gloves when administering chemotherapy. The nurse should dispose of articles in contact with chemotherapeutic drugs in biohazard containers according to institution policy. Prepackaged agents can still be hazardous if not handled properly.

    CN: Pharmacological and parenteral therapies; CL: Analyze

23. 2. Stomatitis is an inflammation of the mucous membranes of the mouth resulting from chemotherapy. Using a soft-bristled toothbrush prevents further bleeding and irritation to the already irritated gums and mucous membranes. Hydrogen peroxide can further irritate the mouth. Fluids need to be lukewarm instead of hot; dental floss can be used if it is done gently.

    CN: Basic care and comfort; CL: Analyze

24. 3. Resources should be provided for acquiring a wig since it is easier to match hairstyle and color before hair loss begins. The client has expressed negative feelings of self-image with hair loss. Excessive shampooing and manipulation of hair will increase hair loss. Hair usually grows back in 3 to 4 weeks after the chemotherapy is finished; however, new hair may have a new color or texture. A wig, hairpiece, hat, scarf, or turban can be used to conceal hair loss. Social isolation should be avoided, and the client should be encouraged to socialize with others.

    CN: Pharmacological and parenteral therapies; CL: Analyze

25. 4. The client may excrete the chemotherapeutic agent for 48 hours or more after administration. Blood, emesis, and excretions may be considered contaminated during this time, and the client should not share a bathroom with children or pregnant women. Any contaminated linens or clothing should be washed separately and then washed a second time if necessary. All contaminated disposable items should be sealed in plastic bags and disposed of as hazardous waste.

    CN: Physiological integrity; CL: Analyze

26. 4. A side effect of vincristine is constipation, and the nurse should encourage the client to include high fiber in the diet and drink 10½ to 12 cups (about 2½ to 3 L) of fluids each day. The nurse can instruct the client to take a stool softener as needed and before receiving a dose of vincristine. Loperamide is used to treat diarrhea, and it is not appropriate unless the client has diarrhea.

🔑 CN: Pharmacological and parenteral therapies; CL: Analyze

27. 3. A client receiving chemotherapy may experience loss of appetite along with nausea and vomiting but also requires a diet that includes protein, carbohydrates, and a small amount of fat. Carbohydrates are the first substance used by the body for energy. Proteins are needed to maintain muscle mass, repair tissue, and maintain osmotic pressure in the vascular system. Fats, in a small amount, are needed for energy production. Chicken, green beans, and cottage cheese are the best selection to provide a nutritionally well-balanced diet of carbohydrate, protein, and a small amount of fat. Cereal with milk and strawberries and the milkshake made with fruit and ice cream contain a large number of carbohydrates and not enough protein. Steak and French fries provide some carbohydrates and a good deal of protein; however, they also provide a large amount of fat.

🔑 CN: Health promotion and maintenance; CL: Analyze

28. 2. Chemotherapy agents typically cause nausea and vomiting when not controlled by antiemetic drugs. Antineoplastic drugs attack rapidly growing normal cells, such as in the gastrointestinal tract. These drugs also stimulate the vomiting center in the brain. Hair loss, loss of energy, and sleep are important aspects of the health history, but they are not as critical as the potential for dehydration and electrolyte imbalance caused by nausea and vomiting.

🔑 CN: Pharmacological and parenteral therapies; CL: Analyze

29. -/+ 2, 4, 5. Chemotherapy causes bone marrow suppression and risk for infection. A platelet count of 40,000/mm³ (40 × 10⁹/L) and a white blood cell count of 2300/mm³ (2.3 × 10⁹/L) are low. A temperature of 101.2°F (38.4°C) is high and could indicate an infection. Further assessment and examination should be performed to rule out infection. The BUN, hemoglobin, and specific gravity values are normal.

🔑 CN: Reduction of risk potential; CL: Analyze

30. -/+ 2. The nurse's role while the client is making a decision is to support the client by listening to concerns, asking clarifying questions to help the client think things through, and providing unbiased information. The nurse should not lead the client to what the nurse thinks is best but rather allow the client to make their own decision. Although the nurse may help the client think through the decision, the nurse would not teach the client how to make a decision because this could bias the client toward the nurse's opinion (a subtle form of coercion). There is no need for the nurse to advocate for the client until the client makes a decision.

🔑 CN: Management of care; CL: Synthesis

31. 3. The nurse should use a large syringe for flushing this device because a syringe of smaller size requires an increase in force to instill the fluid, and this force leads to increased pressure that can damage the catheter and even blood vessels. Most manufacturers recommend a 10-mL syringe for this purpose. The 3-mL syringe will lead to high pressure and possible damage to the device. The ports must be flushed on a regular basis per institutional policy. Although heparin is added in a flush in some devices, the correct dosage is 10 units per mL.

🔑 CN: Pharmacological and parenteral therapies; CL: Evaluation

32. 1. Fever is an early sign requiring clinical intervention to identify potential causes. Chills and dyspnea may or may not be observed. Tachycardia can be an indicator in a variety of clinical situations when associated with infection; it usually occurs in response to an elevated temperature or change in cardiac function.

🔑 CN: Reduction of risk potential; CL: Analyze

33. 2. Chemotherapy causes myelosuppression with a decrease in red blood cells (RBCs), WBCs, and platelets. This client's data demonstrate neutropenia, placing the client at risk for infection. An ANC of 500 to 1000/mm³ (0.5 to 1 × 10⁹/L) indicates a moderate risk for infection; an ANC of less than 500/mm³ (0.5 × 10⁹/L) indicates severe neutropenia and a high risk for infection. When the WBC count is low and immature WBCs are present, normal phagocytosis is impaired. Precautions to protect the client from life-threatening infections may be instituted when the ANC is less than 1000/mm³ (1 × 10⁹/L). Handwashing is the best way to avoid the spread of infection. It is not necessary to wear a gown and mask to take care of this client. It is also not necessary to restrict visitors; however, visitors should be screened to avoid exposing the client to possible infections. Erythropoietin is used for stimulating RBCs, not WBCs. Granulocyte colony-stimulating factors or granulocyte-macrophage colony-stimulating factors are useful for treating neutropenia.

CN: Safety and infection control; CL: Analyze

34. 1. The role of the nurse is to assess what substances or medications the client is using and to document and inform other members of the health care team. To avoid adverse interactions, it is very important to encourage the client to keep the HCP informed of all the therapeutic agents, medications, and supplements they are using. It is not appropriate for the nurse to suggest that the client choose either Western or alternative therapies or to discourage the client's use of alternative therapies. The nurse should remain objective about the client's treatment choices and respect the client's autonomy.

CN: Reduction of risk potential; CL: Analyze

35. 1. The fast-growing, normal cells most likely to be affected by certain cancer treatments are blood-forming cells in the bone marrow, as well as cells in the digestive tract, reproductive system, and hair follicles. Fortunately, most normal cells recover quickly when treatment is over. Bone marrow suppression (a decreased ability of the bone marrow to manufacture blood cells) is a common side effect of chemotherapy. A low white blood cell count (neutropenia) increases the risk for infection during chemotherapy, but other blood cells made in the bone marrow can be affected as well. Most cancer agents do not affect tissues and organs, such as the heart, liver, and pancreas.

CN: Physiologic adaptation; CL: Apply

36. 4. The client is experiencing severe sepsis, and it is essential to increase circulating fluid volume to restore the blood pressure and cardiac output. Placing wet compresses, administering antipyretic medication, and monitoring the client's cardiac status may be beneficial for this client but are not the highest priority action at this time. These three interventions may require the nurse to leave the client, which is not advisable.

CN: Physiological adaptation; CL: Analyze

37. 3. Nephrotoxicity caused by chemotherapy is assessed by monitoring the serum creatinine level. Creatinine is the most sensitive indicator of proper kidney function. In this case, the client is experiencing decreased kidney function, most likely due to the chemotherapy. The nurse consults the HCP for guidance. Administering the next dose of chemotherapy could potentially cause further kidney damage. It is inappropriate to cancel the chemotherapy without checking with the HCP or to tell the client that the cancer is spreading. A urine specimen will not provide other helpful information.

CN: Pharmacological and parenteral therapies; CL: Analyze

The Adult Who Is Receiving Radiation Therapy

38. 3. Clients receiving radiation experience dryness or redness in the area of the radiation. The nurse instructs the client to wash the area with soap and water and keep the area dry. The client does not apply lotion, shave, or cover the area.

CN: Basic care and comfort; CL: Apply

39. 3. This client is at high risk for bleeding because of the decreased platelet count. The priority nursing goal is to prevent injury to this client by preventing bleeding occurrences. Spontaneous bleeding may cause pain, but it is not the priority. The client has a low platelet count, not a low hemoglobin count such as exists in anemia. Skin integrity is a risk but not a priority.

CN: Reduction of risk potential; CL: Analyze

40. 4. The nurse should instruct the client to avoid applying chemicals (such as a deodorant) or heat or cold (such as with a heating pad or ice pack) to the area being treated. The client should be encouraged to use the extremity to prevent muscle atrophy and contractures.

CN: Health promotion and maintenance; CL: Analyze

41. 2. Since sleeplessness is often an adverse effect of radiation therapy, the nurse should first assess the client's usual sleep patterns, hours of sleep required before treatment, and usual bedtime routine. Refraining from watching television before bedtime and avoiding caffeine intake may be helpful, depending first on the client's needs. It is also helpful to sleep in a darkened room if the client is not already doing so. Sleeplessness is not always an effect of radiation therapy, and the nurse should develop the care plan according to the client's needs.

CN: Health promotion and maintenance; CL: Analyze

42. 4. Difficulty in swallowing, pain, and tightness in the chest are signs of esophagitis, which is a common complication of radiation therapy on the chest wall. Hiatal hernia is a herniation of a portion of the stomach into the esophagus. The client could experience burning and tightness in the chest secondary to a hiatal hernia, but not pain when swallowing. Also, a hiatal hernia is not a complication of radiation therapy. Stomatitis is an inflammation of the oral cavity characterized by pain, burning, and ulcerations. The client with stomatitis may experience pain with swallowing but not burning and tightness in the chest. Radiation enteritis is a disorder of the large and small bowel that occurs during or after radiation therapy to the abdomen, pelvis, or rectum. Nausea, vomiting, abdominal cramping, the frequent urge to have a bowel movement, and watery diarrhea are the signs and symptoms of radiation enteritis.

CN: Physiological adaptation; CL: Analyze

43. **2.** Radiation fields that include the ovaries usually result in premature menopause. Vaginal dryness will occur without estrogen replacement. There should be no sexual intercourse while the implant is in place. Cesium is a radioactive isotope used for therapeutic irradiation of cancerous tissue. There is no documentation to support vaginal relaxation after treatment. Because the client will have premature menopause, they will not have normal menstrual periods.

CN: Physiological adaptation; CL: Analyze

44. **3.** Radiation-induced esophagitis with dysphagia is particularly common in clients who receive radiation to the chest. The anatomic location of the esophagus is posterior to the mediastinum and is within the field of primary treatment. Diarrhea may occur with radiation to the abdomen. A decreased energy level and a decreased white blood cell count are potential complications of radiation therapy.

CN: Reduction of risk potential; CL: Analyze

The Adult Who Requires Symptom Management

45. **3.** Head and neck radiation can cause the complication of stomatitis and decreased salivary flow. A saliva substitute will assist with dryness, moistening food, and swallowing. Meticulous mouth care is needed; however, alcohol and vigorous brushing will increase irritation. Evaluation by a dentist to perform necessary dental work is done before the initiation of therapy.

CN: Physiological adaptation; CL: Analyze

46. **3.** The client has a low white blood cell count from the chemotherapy and has an elevated temperature. Signs and symptoms of infection may be diminished in a client receiving chemotherapy; therefore, the temperature elevation is significant. Early detection of the source of infection facilitates early intervention. Surveillance for bleeding is important with the low hemoglobin and platelet count; however, high blood pressure does not indicate bleeding. Vomiting is a side effect of chemotherapy and should be treated. The urine output and potassium level are within normal limits.

CN: Physiological adaptation; CL: Analyze

47. **4.** The nurse should tell the spouse that when the client is able to tolerate foods, and there are no dietary restrictions, it will be possible to bring foods the client likes. Clients who undergo gastrointestinal surgery may have decreased peristalsis for several days after surgery. The nurse should perform a thorough assessment of the abdomen and auscultate for bowel sounds in all four quadrants. The nurse should check the abdomen for distention and check with the client and the medical record regarding the passage of flatus or stool. Consulting a dietician at this time would be inappropriate because the client must be kept on nothing-by-mouth status until bowel sounds are present.

CN: Reduction of risk potential; CL: Analyze

48. **3.** For clients with obstructive versus restrictive disorders, extending exhalation through pursed-lip breathing will make the respiratory effort more efficient. The usual position of choice for this client is the upright position, leaning slightly forward to allow greater lung expansion. Teaching diaphragmatic breathing techniques will be more helpful to the client with a restrictive disorder. Administering cough suppressants will not help respiratory effort. A low semi-Fowler position does not encourage lung expansion. Lung expansion is enhanced in the upright position.

CN: Basic care and comfort; CL: Analyze

49. **1, 2, 3, 6.** Thrombocytopenia places the client at risk for bleeding. Therefore, electric razors will reduce the potential for skin nicks and bleeding. Oral hygiene should be provided with a soft toothbrush and with minimal friction to gently clean without trauma. Clients should be instructed to read labels on all over-the-counter medications and avoid medications such as aspirin or NSAIDs because of their effect on platelet adhesiveness. Clients should evaluate mucous membranes, skin, stools, and other sites of potential bleeding.

Monitoring temperature may be an important part of assessment but is focused on neutropenia instead of the problem of thrombocytopenia.

CN: Reduction of risk potential; CL: Create

50. 2. The administration of antipyretic and antihistamine drugs before the initiation of a transfusion in a client who frequently undergoes transfusions can decrease the incidence of febrile reactions. Febrile reactions are immune mediated and are caused by antibodies in the recipient that are directed against antigens present on the granulocytes, platelets, and lymphocytes in the transfused component. They are the most common transfusion reactions and may occur with onset, during transfusion, or hours after transfusion is completed.

CN: Pharmacological and parenteral therapies; CL: Analyze

51. 3. The client will be most comfortable and have the best lung expansion with the head of the bed elevated. When in a side-lying position, the client should lie on their right side to permit expansion of the unaffected lung. Postural drainage positioning will lower the head of the bed and increase dyspnea. Lying flat will increase dyspnea; the client should be encouraged to be out of bed as tolerated.

CN: Physiological adaptation; CL: Analyze

52. 2. Many clients who are receiving chemotherapy experience fatigue. The nurse should review the client's complete blood count report to determine if there is an underlying cause for the fatigue, such as a low hemoglobin or hematocrit level. The client is not ready to plan an exercise program or get out of bed at a fixed time. Bed rest causes muscle atrophy, which adds to fatigue and can contribute to deep vein thrombosis; the nurse should encourage the client to be up out of bed.

CN: Health promotion and maintenance; CL: Analyze

53. 1. Chemotherapy may cause suppression of the immune system, resulting in a reduction in the neutrophil count and placing the client at risk for infection. This client has a normal neutrophil count, indicating that the filgrastim has been effective. A decreased hemoglobin level indicates anemia. The hemoglobin level is within normal limits for a man. A decreased platelet count would indicate thrombocytopenia, and platelets would be prescribed. The platelet count is within normal limits for an adult.

CN: Pharmacologic and parenteral therapy; CL: Evaluate

54. 1. To reduce the adverse effects of chemotherapy such as nausea and vomiting, the nurse can suggest that the client eat small meals more frequently, which will be better tolerated while maintaining adequate nutrition. It is not necessary to eat soft food or milkshakes blended with fruit. Fluid intake should be encouraged to avoid dehydration.

CN: Basic care and comfort; CL: Analyze

55. 4. The use of diet modification is a conservative approach to treating terminally ill clients or clients in hospice who have nausea and vomiting related to bowel obstruction. Osmotic laxatives would be harder for the client to tolerate. An NG tube is more aggressive and invasive. IV antiemetics are also invasive. The hospice philosophy involves comfort and palliative care for terminally ill clients.

CN: Basic care and comfort; CL: Analyze

56. 2. Alopecia from chemotherapy is temporary. The new hair will not be necessarily gray, but the texture and color of new hair growth may be different. Clients who will be receiving chemotherapy should be encouraged to purchase a wig while they still have hair so they can match the color and texture of their hair. Loss of hair, or *alopecia*, is a serious threat to self-esteem and should be addressed quickly before treatment.

CN: Pharmacological and parenteral therapies; CL: Apply

57. 3. Abdominal distension is a distressing symptom in clients with advanced cancer, including metastatic carcinoma of the lung, previous radiation therapy, and coexisting COPD. Abdominal distension occurs in clients with metastatic carcinoma; however, in a client with COPD and lung cancer, dyspnea is a more common finding. A pleural friction rub is usually associated with pneumonia, pleurisy, or pulmonary infarct.

CN: Physiological adaptation; CL: Analyze

58. 3. Positive reinforcement builds confidence and facilitates the achievement of rehabilitation goals. Community support may or may not be applicable after discharge. Although family support is an important component of rehabilitation, reinforcing the skills the client has acquired is of greater importance when they are regaining independence. Rehabilitation plans should include the client, family, or both.

CN: Basic care and comfort; CL: Analyze

59. 2. The most important intervention for infection control is to continue meticulous catheter site care. Dressings are to be changed two to three times per week, depending on institutional policies. Temperature should be monitored at least once a day in someone with a vascular access device. Handwashing before and after irrigation or any manipulation of the site is a must for infection prevention.

🔑 CN: Safety and infection control; CL: Evaluate

60. ➖➕ **1, 2, 4, 5.** A major concern with intravenous (IV) administration of cytotoxic agents is vessel irritation or extravasation. The Oncology Nursing Society and hospital guidelines require frequent reevaluation of blood return when administering vesicant or nonvesicant chemotherapy because of the risk for extravasation. These guidelines apply to peripheral and central venous lines. The nurse should also assess the insertion site for signs of infiltration, such as swelling and redness. In addition, central venous lines may be long-term venous access devices. Thus, difficulty drawing or aspirating blood may indicate the line is against the vessel wall or may indicate the line has occlusion. Having the client cough or move position may change the status of the line if it is temporarily against a vessel wall. Occlusion warrants a more thorough evaluation via an x-ray study to verify placement if the status is questionable and may require a declotting regimen. The nurse should not administer any drug if the IV line is not open or does not have an adequate blood return.

🔑 CN: Pharmacological and parenteral therapies; CL: Create

61. The distal tip of a central line should be placed in the subclavian vein.

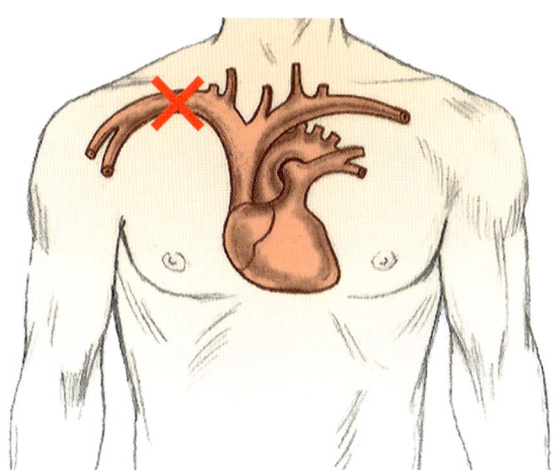

🔑 CN: Pharmacological and parenteral therapies; CL: Apply

62. **2.** The client is exhibiting signs and symptoms of a pneumothorax from the insertion of the subclavian venous catheter. Although it is possible that the client experienced an air embolus during the procedure and the client is at risk for pulmonary emboli because of their immobility, absent breath sounds immediately after insertion of a subclavian line are strongly suggestive of a pneumothorax. Unilateral absent breath sounds are not associated with a myocardial infarction.

🔑 CN: Physiological adaptation; CL: Analyze

63. **4.** An appropriate and realistic outcome would be for the client to maintain their current weight or not lose weight. It is unrealistic to expect that the client with advanced liver cancer will have normal albumin levels or will be able to gain weight.

🔑 CN: Basic care and comfort; CL: Analyze

64. **3.** As long as the client is able to get out of bed, the preferred position and time frame for preventing aspiration after a bolus tube feeding is sitting upright out of bed in a chair for 30 to 60 minutes. The client should have the head of the bed elevated more than 60 degrees; it is not necessary to remain in an upright position for more than an hour after the feeding. Placing the client on their right side, not their left, may facilitate gastric emptying, but this is not the preferred position. Elevating the bed 30 degrees decreases the risk for aspiration, but this elevation must be maintained for at least 45 to 60 minutes.

🔑 CN: Basic care and comfort; CL: Analyze

65. **1.** Total parenteral nutrition solutions supply the body with sufficient amounts of dextrose, amino acids, fats, vitamins, and minerals to meet metabolic needs. Clients who are unable to tolerate adequate quantities of foods and fluids and those who have had extensive bowel surgery may not be candidates for enteral feedings. The nurse would anticipate total parenteral nutrition via a central catheter to promote wound healing. IV dextrose does not supply all the nutrients required to promote wound healing.

🔑 CN: Pharmacological and parenteral therapies; CL: Analyze

66. ➖➕ **1, 2, 4.** An elevated temperature in the first 24 hours along with coarse breath sounds may indicate a respiratory complication or the result of general anesthesia. The use of incentive spirometry and increasing activity would be key interventions. A healthy stoma will be beefy red. A dusky appearance of the stoma indicates decreased blood supply and is of concern. It is not uncommon to have decreased bowel sounds initially after gastrointestinal surgery. In addition, it usually will take time for the ostomy to function.

🗝 CN: Reduction of risk potential; CL: Analyze

67. 3. The vital signs suggest that the client is dehydrated from vomiting, and the nurse should first infuse the intravenous fluids with the addition of potassium chloride. There is no indication that the client needs oxygen at this time because the PaO_2 is 95 mm Hg (12.6 kPa). Although the client has a rapid and irregular pulse, the infusion of fluids may cause the heart rate to return to normal, and the 12-lead ECG can be prescribed after starting the intravenous fluids.

🗝 CN: Physiological adaptation; CL: Analyze

68. 3. The client is exhibiting early symptoms of pulmonary toxicity as a result of the radiation therapy. These are not expected adverse effects of radiation. The client should be examined to differentiate between an infection and radiation pneumonitis. Suggesting that the client take acetaminophen and call back in 2 days is inappropriate. These signs and symptoms are not indicative of a true emergency, but the client should be seen by an HCP before the next appointment.

🗝 CN: Reduction of risk potential; CL: Analyze

69. 2, 1, 4, 3. The client is short of breath. The head of the bed should be elevated to enable breathing, and oxygen should be applied. Morphine should be administered for pain before initiating deep-breathing exercises. Deep-breathing exercises improve lung expansion and decrease dyspnea. Education can be provided on the thoracentesis that is anticipated once the symptoms are managed.

🗝 CN: Physiological adaptation; CL: Analyze

70. 1. Treatment for cellulitis includes administration of oral or intravenous antibiotics for 1 to 2 weeks, elevation of the affected extremity, and application of warm, moist packs to the site. Arm exercises help reduce swelling, but they do not treat the infection.

🗝 CN: Physiological adaptation; CL: Analyze

71. 3. Changing positions frequently aids in distributing the agent to the pleura for sealing. The majority of the pleural fluid is drained, and the lung should already be reexpanded before instillation of the sclerosing agent. A pressure dressing is applied to the chest tube exit site, and it is not necessary to lie on that side to hold pressure on the area.

🗝 CN: Reduction of risk potential; CL: Analyze

72. 4. Providing adequate humidification for the client with a tracheostomy is essential. The client no longer has the functions of the nose for warming, moistening, or filtering the air when breathing through the tracheostomy site. Providing tracheostomy site care, addressing psychosocial issues, and observing for early signs and symptoms of skin breakdown around the tracheostomy site are also important; however, using humidifiers to prevent thick, tenacious secretions is the most important recommendation for long-term management and the prevention of pulmonary infection.

🗝 CN: Physiological adaptation; CL: Analyze

73. -/+ 4, 5. A malignant pleural effusion is an accumulation of excessive fluid within the pleural space that occurs when cancer cells irritate the pleural membrane. Dyspnea can result from increased pressure, which may contribute to increased anxiety and fear of suffocation. Pain is caused by pleural irritation. Hiccups are usually associated with pericardial effusions. Weight gain and peripheral edema may occur with peritoneal effusion.

🗝 CN: Physiological adaptation; CL: Analyze

74. -/+ 2, 3, 4. Thoracentesis is usually successful for the diagnosis of underlying disease, palliation of symptoms, and treatment of acute respiratory distress; alleviation of symptoms and distress is usually short term. Thoracentesis is not used as a treatment for recurrent pleural effusion because the fluid accumulates rapidly. Thoracentesis does not remove cancer cells.

🗝 CN: Reduction of risk potential; CL: Evaluate

75. 3. Cold intolerance may be associated with anemia because of the diminished oxygen supply to the peripheral circulation. Decreased salivation is not associated with anemia. Tachycardia may be expected in severe anemia. Clients with anemia are usually not nauseated.

🗝 CN: Physiological adaptation; CL: Analyze

76. 4. Petechiae are tiny, purplish, hemorrhagic spots visible under the skin. Petechiae usually appear when platelets are depleted. Bleeding gums or oozing of blood may accompany the petechiae, and the client should seek medical assistance immediately. Increasing iron in the diet will not improve the platelet count. Lotion will not treat the petechiae. Elevating the legs will not cause the petechiae to disappear.

🔑 CN: Physiological adaptation; CL: Analyze

77. **3.** Redness, warmth, and swelling are all signs of infection, and the nurse should tell the client to contact the health care provider. Treatment with antibiotics is usually indicated. Infection usually increases fluid accumulation and could worsen lymphedema. Warm compresses could also increase fluid accumulation. Elevating the arm will not treat the infection, nor will applying an ice pack. It is critical that the client not delay treatment.

🔑 CN: Reduction of risk potential; CL: Analyze

78. **4.** Fever is most commonly related to infection. In a client with neutropenia, fever frequently occurs in the absence of the usual clinical signs and symptoms of infection. Inadequate nutrition or antiemetic therapy resistance would not result in fever. Fever is not usually expected with most chemotherapy drugs.

🔑 CN: Physiological adaptation; CL: Analyze

79. **2.** Nine days after chemotherapy, it is expected for the client to be immunocompromised. The clinical signs and symptoms of shock reflect changes in cardiac function, vascular resistance, cellular metabolism, and capillary permeability. Low-grade fever, tachycardia, and chills may be early signs of shock. A client with signs and symptoms of impending septic shock may not have decreased oxygen saturation levels. Oliguria and hypotension are late signs of shock. Urine output can be initially normal or increased.

🔑 CN: Pharmacological and parenteral therapies; CL: Analyze

80. **3.** Prioritizing physical activities helps conserve energy, which promotes adaptation to fatigue. The client should learn to take short naps or short rest periods during the day for additional energy conversation. Increased fluid intake is important but may interrupt rest periods by causing frequent urination. Limiting intake of high-fiber foods can add to constipation, which may be a problem because of inactivity in fatigued clients.

🔑 CN: Basic care and comfort; CL: Analyze

81. **4.** The use of deodorant or fragrant soaps is drying to the skin. Cotton clothing gives the least irritation to the skin. A cool, humidified environment adds to the client's comfort and provides hydration for skin comfort. A fluid intake of 12 cups (about 3 L) a day is recommended for adequate hydration.

🔑 CN: Basic care and comfort; CL: Analyze

82. **4.** Individuals with cancer have various cultural values and beliefs that help them cope with the cancer experience. Quality of life cannot be evaluated solely by quantifiable factors such as employability, functional status, or evidence of disease. The nurse can help cancer survivors identify their own needs within the context of their subjective and individual values and beliefs.

🔑 CN: Psychosocial integrity; CL: Analyze

83. **3.** Constipation lasting 3 days or longer is unusual in this client and warrants immediate action. However, because the client had chemotherapy with doxorubicin 10 days ago, they are susceptible to infection and should avoid rectal medications and treatments. Abdominal discomfort secondary to constipation will be relieved after the client has a bowel movement; an opioid would contribute to constipation.

🔑 CN: Pharmacological and parenteral therapies; CL: Analyze

84. **1, 4, 5.** The rectal area needs to be cleaned and gently dried after each bowel movement to prevent skin breakdown and inhibit the growth of bacteria. Sitz baths are appropriate because they promote comfort. The client should increase fluid consumption to prevent dehydration. Zinc oxide ointment does form a protective skin barrier, but it makes it difficult to thoroughly clean the perirectal area of feces and increases the risk for infection, as do skin barrier dressings.

🔑 CN: Safety and infection control; CL: Analyze

85. **2.** Studies of long-term immunologic effects in clients treated for leukemia, Hodgkin's disease, and breast cancer reveal that combination treatments of chemotherapy and radiation can cause overall bone marrow suppression, decreased leukocyte counts, and profound immunosuppression. Persistent and severe immunologic impairment may follow radiation and chemotherapy (especially multiagent therapy). There is no evidence of a greater risk for infection in clients with persistent immunologic abnormalities. Suppressor T cells recover more rapidly than helper T cells.

🔑 CN: Pharmacological and parenteral therapies; CL: Apply

The Adult Who Is Coping with Loss, Grief, Bereavement, and Spiritual Distress

86. 4. Identifying available resources for the client and family represents a respectful effort to make options available and encourages the client to become involved in treatment decisions. Assuming decision-making for the client may foster dependence. Encouraging strict compliance with all treatment regimens may increase anxiety and limit the client's options and treatment choices. Informing the client of all possible adverse treatment effects may increase anxiety and fear by focusing on adverse outcomes too soon.

🔑 CN: Psychosocial integrity; CL: Analyze

87. 4. Denial is a defense mechanism used to shut out a situation that is too frightening or threatening to tolerate. In this case, denial allows the client to vacillate between acceptance of the illness and its treatment and denial of the actual or potential seriousness of the disease. This may allow the client more psychological freedom to maintain their current roles in the family and elsewhere. Denial can be harmful if the client ignores standard medical therapies in favor of unconventional treatments. Denial is not helpful when it interferes with a client's willingness to seek treatment or make decisions about care. Using any one defense mechanism exclusively usually reflects maladaptive coping. Other defense mechanisms that may be used include regression, humor, and sublimation.

🔑 CN: Psychosocial integrity; CL: Apply

88. 2. The nurse should first assist the client in assessing their resources for coping with their emotional and practical needs and the needs of their family because usual coping strategies and support systems are often inadequate in especially stressful situations. The nurse may be concerned with the client's use of denial, decision-making abilities, and ability to care for their children; however, helping the client obtain support systems will be of more importance in this situation.

🔑 CN: Psychosocial integrity; CL: Analyze

89. 4. Variables that are most predictive of negative bereavement outcomes include anger and self-reproach, low socioeconomic status, lack of preparation for death, and lack of family support. Making preparations suggests that the client is coping with the client's approaching death.

🔑 CN: Psychosocial integrity; CL: Analyze

90. 4. Having adequate financial resources facilitates bereavement. Younger people are at higher risk for negative bereavement outcomes. Having a history of depressive illness or anxiety is a risk factor for negative bereavement outcomes. Being a spouse does not make grieving easier.

🔑 CN: Psychosocial integrity; CL: Analyze

91. 4. Focusing on the client's physical capabilities is important, but powerlessness reflects a perceived lack of control over the current situation and the belief that one's actions will not affect the outcome. Participation in decision-making is key to getting the client involved and feeling more in control of their own care. Apathy and dependence on others are characteristics of powerlessness. Encouraging others to take responsibility for the client's care will increase the client's feelings of powerlessness. A referral to a psychologist is not necessarily indicated. The nurse should implement strategies to involve the client in decisions about the client's care and evaluate the response to this intervention before suggesting a referral.

🔑 CN: Psychosocial integrity; CL: Analyze

92. 1. Maintaining role function has been found to be a supportive source of normalcy and positive self-esteem for clients and their families during the cancer experience. Facilitating family-related disagreements and conflicts is not the nurse's role. Supporting the client in the use of denial as a coping strategy will not help facilitate the client's adaptation to the diagnosis. Arranging transportation and childcare on treatment days may be helpful but does not necessarily facilitate adaptation to the diagnosis.

🔑 CN: Psychosocial integrity; CL: Analyze

93. 2. Hospice care services provide palliative care and also address the client's physical, emotional, and spiritual needs. The focus of the care is on the care of the client and family. Hospice care services can begin 6 months before the illness is terminal and can be renewed, depending on the course of the disease. Hospice care collaborates with the client's HCP, but the HCP does not direct the care. Not all hospice clients want to die at home, nor is it a requirement to be at home to receive hospice care.

🔑 CN: Basic care and comfort; CL: Apply

94. 3. Mental changes and decreased level of consciousness are common in the dying process, and the client may talk about travel, trips, or going somewhere. Suggesting that the client be sedated ignores the spouse's question about what the client is experiencing. Suggesting that the client is fighting death and that the spouse should leave them alone is inappropriate and denies the spouse time to spend with the client. The spouse should not make misleading statements to the client.

🔑 CN: Psychosocial integrity; CL: Analyze

95. 4. It is important to give factual information to answer a loved one's questions and concerns. Stating "That's just the way it is" is unprofessional and uncaring. Saying "I don't know when the bowels will shut down, but they will eventually" projects an uncaring attitude and does not address the spouse's concern for the client or their need for information. Although it may be true that the pain medication will slow bowel function, this does not provide the spouse with the information they are seeking.

🔑 CN: Psychosocial integrity; CL: Apply

96. 4. It is important to allow the client to choose their own form of spiritual support, and the nurse can begin by asking the client what would be most supportive now. It is not necessary to know the client's religion before finding out what is important to the client. The client must be consulted before a referral to a chaplain is made. It is not appropriate for the nurse to ask the family to contact a spiritual advisor; once the nurse understands the client's needs, the nurse and client can make a plan about how to meet them.

🔑 CN: Psychosocial integrity; CL: Analyze

97. 2. The discharge planning coordinator, social services, or a social worker can provide information for supportive services and can help the client determine which resources are necessary at this time. The business office of the health care agency does not provide advice about managing finances. The HCP will be part of the team but will focus on managing the client's health and end-of-life care. The client may or may not have a will; it is not the role of an executor to make financial decisions about health care.

🔑 CN: Psychosocial integrity; CL: Analyze

98. 4. Dehydration is an expected event within the dying process. Hydration may be used in any situation of dehydration as long as it is within the client and family's wishes. Rehydrating the client may actually prolong the dying process. Decisions about treatment are made with the family.

🔑 CN: Basic care and comfort; CL: Apply

99. 4. The nurse must first allow the client to clarify the meaning of spiritual distress and explore their own beliefs and values before making referrals to clergy or a support group. The nurse should allow the client to indicate if praying would be helpful after helping the client clarify the meaning of spiritual distress.

🔑 CN: Psychosocial integrity; CL: Analyze

100. 3. The family is in the best position to give the information they elect to disclose to friends and community members. The hospice nurse and the oncologist must maintain client confidentiality and follow privacy guidelines for the release of confidential information. Therefore, disclosing any information about the client's condition would be inappropriate.

🔑 CN: Management of care; CL: Analyze

101. 4. Depression can be a mixture of affective responses (feelings of worthlessness, hopelessness, sadness), behavioral responses (appetite changes, withdrawal, sleep disturbances, lethargy), and cognitive responses (decreased ability to concentrate, indecisiveness, suicidal ideation). Increased decisiveness, problem-solving ability, and increased social interactions are reflective of adaptive coping.

🔑 CN: Psychosocial integrity; CL: Analyze

102. 3. It is important to establish rapport with the client and family by listening to verbal and nonverbal concerns and showing respect for cultural differences. The use of touch or eye contact is culture-specific and cannot be generalized as an intervention for all individuals with cancer. Miscommunication between individuals of different cultures is often caused by language differences, rules of communication, age, and gender.

🔑 CN: Psychosocial integrity; CL: Analyze

103. 4. Support groups are designed to educate clients and their families experiencing cancer about the disease and methods of coping positively with it. These are self-help and support groups monitored by professionals and cancer survivors who have undergone a training course that helps them facilitate small groups.

🔑 CN: Psychosocial integrity; CL: Apply

104. 4. Many cancer survivors question why they are doing so well and others are not. Often, they express feeling guilty when they hear that others are not doing well. Suggesting that the client does not know how to describe the client's own emotions is inappropriate and may discourage the client from expressing feelings. Although the client may be experiencing volatile emotions, this is not the likely source of feelings of guilt. Guilt about doing well after cancer treatment is not a spiritual response to illness.

CN: Psychosocial integrity; CL: Analyze

105. 4. The person who has minimal social support, has not been successful in dealing with stressors, and has multiple other stressors is at greater risk for psychosocial distress. Being successful in dealing with stress throughout life would decrease the client's risk for psychosocial distress. Not having to deal with other stressors would be helpful in managing the current stressful situation. The denial coping mechanism, if used for short periods, can decrease the risk for psychosocial distress.

CN: Psychosocial integrity; CL: Analyze

106. 1. Clients with cancer report that the lifelong fear of recurrence is one of the most disruptive aspects of the disease. The trajectory of the disease is unpredictable and can be intertwined with many short- and long-term illnesses related to cancer and the treatment modalities. A diagnosis of cancer challenges the individual and the family with a series of crises rather than a time-limited episode. There are no data to indicate that the client has an underlying behavioral disorder.

CN: Psychosocial integrity; CL: Analyze

107. 4. Without clear, consistent communication, the parent-child relationship may become strained during the illness and subsequent death of a parent. A great number of parents do not know how to communicate with their children, especially about difficult emotional topics at a time when they are also under great emotional stress. The nurse should begin by providing information and developmentally appropriate books about the grieving process for children. Referral to pastoral care services may be appropriate; however, the nurse's direct intervention of beginning education about strategies for communication will be of immediate and long-term benefit. The grieving process cannot be rushed for the spouse, nor should an opportunity for the parent and children to communicate and grieve together be delayed. Excluding children from participating in the grieving ritual does not shield them from sorrow and sadness, and having the HCP tell the children does not promote healthy communication between the parent and the children.

CN: Psychosocial integrity; CL: Analyze

108. 3. Acknowledgment and discussion of the client's feelings begin the establishment of a therapeutic relationship between nurse and client. It also acknowledges the seriousness of the current situation and validates the client's feelings. Grief counseling and antidepressant medication may be options if the depression is severe and prolonged. The client is not ready at this point to continue the conversation with their spouse.

CN: Psychosocial integrity; CL: Analyze

109. 2. Individuals who are experiencing fatigue need to prioritize their activities and ask for assistance from others. It is best not to take away all of the client's activities because their role as spouse and parent is obviously important to the client and to their sense of self-worth. Suggesting that they ignore the household chores or telling them not to worry because everyone gets tired disregards the client's feelings and is not appropriate.

CN: Basic care and comfort; CL: Analyze

110. 4. Tachycardia, tachypnea, moist or clammy skin, and disorientation are classic symptoms of delirium. Clients with panic disorder do not exhibit disorientation. Clients with depression exhibit a flat affect, apathy, and sleep disturbances. Clients with schizophrenia have thought disorders such as hallucinations or delusions.

CN: Physiological adaptation; CL: Analyze

111. 2. A progressive activity regimen may be prescribed to increase pulmonary function after surgical lung resection. Rehabilitation should include walking and some stair climbing as tolerated. It is not necessary at this point for the client to speak with someone who has had similar surgery. Depending on the surgeon's preference, there may not be a dressing to change. There is no indication that the client would not be able to manage cleaning the house as their energy increases.

CN: Health promotion and maintenance; CL: Analyze

112. 4. When a client with cancer serves as a volunteer in a client-to-client program, this behavior indicates a higher level of adaptation than attention to self, and the nurse judges that the client is adapting to changes in body image. Discussing suicide is an indication the client is not adapting to the changes in health status. Continuing to look at the site of hair loss indicates the client has not accepted changes in body image. Although looking forward to returning to work is a positive sign, being able to help others demonstrates an integration of the experience into the client's life.

CN: Psychosocial integrity; CL: Evaluate

The Adult Who Is Experiencing Problems with Sexuality

113. **3.** Water-soluble lubricants used during sexual intercourse can augment reduced natural vaginal lubrication caused by ovarian dysfunction and decreased circulating estrogen related to chemotherapy. The use of vaginal dilators, relaxation techniques, or nightly douches would not increase vaginal lubrication. Frequent douching can disrupt the normal vaginal environment.

CN: Health promotion and maintenance; CL: Analyze

114. **3.** Placing a thin piece of gauze over the tracheostomy during sexual activity will help contain the secretions and yet allow ventilation. Although a scopolamine patch may depress the salivary and bronchial secretions, it is not recommended for long-term use and would not be indicated in this situation. Avoiding fluids before sexual activity is not recommended to decrease secretions. Washing the tracheostomy area with any deodorizing soap may cause skin irritation and place the client at risk for infection.

CN: Health promotion and maintenance; CL: Analyze

115. **4.** This question introduces some basic information and allows for support for the client who may be experiencing some sexuality concerns. Not all women experience sexual problems after undergoing a hysterectomy. Assuming that the client will want to schedule an appointment with their partner is inappropriate and may embarrass the client. Simply asking the client whether they expect to have problems with sex is too abrupt and does not provide any information.

CN: Psychosocial integrity; CL: Analyze

116. **4.** Although there may not be a big change in sexual function with a unilateral orchiectomy, the loss of a gonad and testosterone may result in decreased libido and sterility. Sperm banking may be an option worth exploring if the number and motility of the sperm are adequate. The population most affected by testicular cancer is generally young men between the ages of 15 and 34, and in this crucial stage of life, sexual anxieties may be a large concern. Since there will likely not be a big change in sexual function, it is not appropriate to tell the client they will experience impotence, have early ejaculation, or require a referral to a sex therapist.

CN: Psychosocial integrity; CL: Analyze

117. **4.** The risk for becoming neutropenic during chemotherapy is very high. Therefore, an inserted foreign object such as a diaphragm may be a nidus for infection. Although the nurse may wish to inform the client about the ease with which various contraceptive modalities may be used, the focus of this discussion should be on preventing an infection, which can be fatal for the neutropenic client. There are no data to suggest the client is at risk for acquiring a sexually transmitted disease. The client will not be experiencing body changes directly related to hormonal changes.

CN: Safety and infection control; CL: Analyze

118. **2.** Raising the upper torso for the affected partner facilitates respiratory function. The client should not use inhalers that are not a part of the treatment plan, and if the client's health is well managed, it is not necessary to take additional medications to improve respiratory function. A dependent position may compromise respiratory expansion, even though energy may be conserved. Duration of sexual activity is not necessarily related to exertion.

CN: Health promotion and maintenance; CL: Analyze

Ethical and Legal Issues Related to Adults with Cancer

119. **4.** The nurse must respect the wishes of the client who has indicated that they do not wish to be resuscitated and not to initiate CPR. Nurses who resuscitate clients who have directed otherwise may be considered to be battering the client. In this situation, the HCP has written the DNR prescription, and it is not necessary for the nurse to page the HCP. The nurse can be most helpful by explaining the client's decision to the spouse and helping them manage to understand the client's wishes and manage their own grief.

CN: Management of care; CL: Analyze

120. **3.** The RN assigning care should first give the UAP the opportunity to explore concerns and fears about caring for a client with HIV infection. Reassigning care for this client, assisting with care, and reviewing precautions do not address the present concern or create an environment that will generate useful knowledge regarding future assignments for client care.

CN: Management of care; CL: Analyze

121. 1. The nurse should advise the person to check with their employer to determine the policies and legislation followed there regarding leaves of absence. Although the client can consider the other options, the first step is to obtain information from their employer.

 CN: Management of care; CL: Apply

122. 1. Maintaining a steady blood level of analgesic medication is beneficial for the client with chronic cancer pain. Administering analgesic medication regularly helps control pain more efficiently. Additional doses of medication may be necessary as needed for breakthrough pain. Keeping the client overly sedated may not help control pain. Intravenous analgesic medications are more effective than oral medications at controlling pain because their distribution is more predictable. Vital signs are not a reliable indicator of how much pain the client is experiencing.

 CN: Management of care; CL: Apply

123. 3. The goal of client autonomy is to respect the client's choice not to know particular information. The client's best interests should be determined by the client after they receive all the necessary information and in conjunction with other people of the client's choice, including family, the HCP, and other health care personnel. The client's best interests are not totally directed by the HCP or the health care team.

 CN: Management of care; CL: Evaluate

End-of-Life Care

124. 2. The client is likely becoming more comatose and is not self-administering the pain medication. The client is not receiving too much medication because the PCA pump has controls to prevent overdose. The client is likely having pain but is not able to recognize it. There is no indication that the IV has infiltrated.

 CN: Pharmacological and parenteral therapies; CL: Analyze

125. 1, 2, 5. Advance directives are written statements of a person's wishes related to health care if they are unable to decide for themselves. Power of attorney is a written authorization to represent or act on another's behalf in private affairs, business, or some other legal matter. These documents relate to current or future health care and not medical history. Competent adults are responsible for their own health care decisions and their own right to accept or refuse treatment. Advance directives are used when the person cannot make the decision. *Medical power of attorney* is a term used to describe the person who makes health care decisions if someone is unable to make informed decisions for themself. The focus is not primarily on financial access.

 CN: Management of care; CL: Evaluate

126. 4. The advocacy role of the nurse implies that the nurse will ensure that the client's wishes are being respected and the client is making informed decisions. Therefore, the nurse will assist in ensuring that the client is fully informed. The other interventions are appropriate for the nurse but are not related to client advocacy. The client may not understand or have all the necessary information for standard therapy. A client who is taking an alternative therapy should be monitored for adverse effects. If a client is taking an alternative therapy, it is essential for the health care provider to know so that the therapy can be incorporated into the client's treatment plan and to ensure that there are no incompatibilities with other therapies or medications.

 CN: Management of care; CL: Evaluate

127. 2, 3, 4, 5. Palliative care is health care aimed at symptom management rather than curative treatment for diseases. Nursing care goals include providing comfort and support for the client and family and maximizing the client's quality of life. Grief counseling is a component, and efforts would be to enhance the coping of all involved, but the family's usual coping methods would not be altered. Palliative care does not involve advocating to prolong the client's life.

 CN: Management of care; CL: Create

128. 3. The best nursing advocacy intervention is listening carefully to the client's and family's perceptions of their needs. Studies have demonstrated that these needs are not necessarily what the nurse thinks they are. Intervening without listening carefully may result in a lack of responsiveness to the real needs. Helping the client and family maintain a sense of optimism and hopefulness is appropriate but is not necessarily advocacy. Determining the client's and family's understanding of the results of the diagnostic testing and providing written materials about the cancer site and its treatment are examples of the nurse's role as educator.

 CN: Psychosocial integrity; CL: Analyze

129. 1. The nurse would give the client a tissue and indicate that it is okay to cry to convey acceptance and empathy. The client needs to know that it is natural to have tremendous feelings of loss and sadness. Telling the client to stop crying, busying oneself in the client's room, and changing the subject are not helpful to the client because they ignore the client's needs and inhibit the expression of emotion.

CN: Psychosocial integrity; CL: Analyze

130. -/+ 2, 3, 4, 5, 6. With serious, chronic, and terminal illnesses, it is important to help clients and families address fears, difficulties with home care, advance directives, hospice and home care options, and final arrangements. Predicting the length of life for this client is not appropriate at admission.

CN: Psychosocial integrity; CL: Analyze

131. 1. The client's spouse is experiencing anger, much of which stems from feelings of guilt about not taking the trip. During the stage of denial, the spouse is more likely to deny the client's diagnosis and prognosis. During the stage of bargaining, the spouse would offer to do certain things in exchange for more time before the client dies. In the stage of depression, the spouse is likely to make few or no comments and to act dejected.

CN: Psychosocial integrity; CL: Analyze

132. 1. The best course of action when the client has outbursts concerning treatments is to explain how the treatment is expected to help. Describing the effect if the client misses a treatment is a negative approach and may be threatening to the client. Explaining the effects of being upset does not deal with the client's feelings. Offering to arrange for a massage during the chemotherapy may be helpful, but it does not deal with the client's immediate feelings.

CN: Psychosocial integrity; CL: Analyze

133. 2. Clients tend to experience isolation and loneliness when those around them are trying to hide or mask the truth. They are then left to face the realities of death alone. Clients do not experience relief or hopefulness when others are falsely cheerful. Independence is promoted by offering realistic choices about care at the end of life.

CN: Psychosocial integrity; CL: Analyze

134. -/+ 3, 4, 5. Taking a blood sample is an unnecessary, invasive procedure that would not directly address the sibling's fear. Leukemia is not considered a communicable disease. The nurse should first determine the sibling's concerns, and then alert the parents to the sibling's concerns. the nurse should also tell the parents about resources that are available to assist siblings in coping with a terminal illness in the family.

CN: Psychosocial integrity; CL: Analyze

135. 2. A response that acknowledges the sibling's concern and provides them with information is most helpful. Therefore, telling the sibling that the nurse sees that they are worried and then following this up with a discussion about leukemia is most appropriate. Providing reassurance or information without acknowledging the expressed concern is not as helpful as acknowledging the concern and providing the information. Although acknowledging the sibling's worry is appropriate, it is more important that the sibling receives factual information about the disease.

CN: Psychosocial integrity; CL: Analyze

Managing Care, Quality, and Safety of Adults with Cancer

136. 3, 1, 4, 2. Using the Maslow hierarchy of needs to set priorities, the nurse should first call the client with bone cancer metastases to the spine because this client is at risk for compression, damage, or severing of the spinal cord. The nurse should evaluate the client immediately for urinary incontinence, paralysis, difficulty ambulating, and possible weakness or loss of motor function. The nurse should next call the client with loss of appetite to assess weight loss and suggest ways to increase the appetite. The client with colon cancer requires assistance with diet planning, also a physiologic need, but this client is not at high risk for weight loss. Lastly, the nurse should obtain information on Reach to Recovery and return the call to the client with a mastectomy. The needs of this client are the least urgent.

CN: Reduction of risk potential; CL: Analyze

137. 3. The nurse should first assess the 75-year-old client with prostate cancer because of the client's age, need for pain management, extended bed rest, and potential for preexisting nutritional deficits. The nurse should plan to spend a focused but short time with the client receiving internal radiation. The client who will receive chemotherapy will require more observation after receiving the medication. The nurse can assess the client who will have a central venous catheter after assuring the older client is comfortable.

CN: Management of care; CL: Analyze

138. -/+ 2, 3, 4, 5. Nurses preparing and administering chemotherapy wear gloves and a disposable, long-sleeved gown. Antineoplastic agents are disposed of as hazardous material, and gloves are always worn when handling the excretions of clients who have received chemotherapy. Sharps must be disposed of in a sharps container labeled "chemotherapy items." It is not appropriate to tape IV tubing connections; antineoplastic agents are administered using LuerLok fittings on all intravenous tubing to minimize the risk for exposure from a needlestick injury.

🔑 CN: Pharmacological and parenteral therapies; CL: Analyze

139. **1.** An IV catheter with no blood return is most likely occluded and not patent. A chemotherapeutic vesicant drug extravasates into the surrounding skin tissue and causes tissue necrosis. The nurse stops administration of the drug immediately. Repositioning the arm does not improve patency. Irrigating the catheter may cause the medication to enter tissue. It is inappropriate to wait and see if the arm becomes edematous because of the vesicant action of the drug.

🔑 CN: Pharmacological and parenteral therapies; CL: Analyze

140. -/+ **1, 2, 3.** An ethics consultation seeks to facilitate communication and shared decision-making in client care. Ethics consultations also tend to increase knowledge of clinical ethics, improve client care, and prevent poor outcomes in cases involving ethical problems. Requests for ethics consultations can be made by any member of the health care team and by clients, family members, guardians, students, or others with a legitimate interest in the client. The recommendations of ethics consultants are advisory only; the ethics consultation process is intended to supplement and support existing departmental and institutional mechanisms for making decisions and resolving conflict in clinical practice. Clinicians are encouraged to seek an ethics consultation when the client is incapacitated and when no family members or guardians exist or can be found or when the client's family members disagree about the ethically appropriate action to be taken. An ethics consultation is not intended or authorized to provide legal advice on client care. Persons requesting an ethics consultation may do so without intimidation or fear of reprisal.

🔑 CN: Management of care; CL: Analyze

141. **4.** To determine the cause of this problem, a quality improvement study should be conducted along with a chart audit. Before implementing solutions to a problem, the precise issues in the hospital system must be observed and documented. Changing the time to chart from 30 minutes to 45 minutes does not solve the problem. It is not the pharmacist's role to provide consultation about the documentation of drugs administered by nurses. Consulting the evening nurses may be helpful, but this is a systems issue for the entire unit and involves every registered nurse administering analgesic medication.

🔑 CN: Management of care; CL: Create

142. **2.** The RN is responsible for describing to the UAP when to report to the RN a result that indicates a potential client problem with dehydration. The RN must assess and interpret results but must also give concrete feedback to the UAP on what is an expected situation or a specific result to report back to the RN. Urine output should be at least 30 mL per hour or 240 mL over the 8-hour shift. Dehydrated clients may be thirsty, and the UAP can ask if the client is thirsty and offer water if permitted. However, because urine output is the critical indicator of dehydration, the UAP should document I&O and give results outside the normal range to the nurse. The nurse is specifically assessing dehydration and should request to receive this information from the UAP before it is charted and reported to the next shift.

🔑 CN: Management of care; CL: Analyze

143. **4.** A bedside commode should be near the client for easy, safe access. Measurement of urine output is also important in a client with heart failure. Putting diapers on an alert and oriented individual would be demeaning and inappropriate. Indwelling catheters are associated with an increased risk for infection and are not a solution to possible incontinence. There is no reason to think that the client would not be able to use the bedside commode.

🔑 CN: Safety and infection control; CL: Analyze

144. **1.** Ongoing assessment by the RN is required to evaluate the client with dyspnea to monitor for potential deterioration of the respiratory status. If the RN is the care provider, the RN will have greater interaction with the individual client. The RN is responsible for the assessment of all the clients. The other clients would not be considered unstable, and maintaining a patent airway is always the priority in providing care. Care for the other clients could be assigned safely, according to the abilities of the LPN/VN and UAP.

🔑 CN: Management of care; CL: Analyze

145. -/+ **1, 2, 5.** Employers should provide appropriate PPE to protect workers who handle hazardous drugs in the workplace. The following general guidelines apply to PPE use and care: select specific respirators and protective clothing based on an assessment of the potential exposure to hazardous drugs; understand the proper use and limitations of any selected PPE to ensure that it functions properly; and use care when donning and removing all items to prevent damage to PPE and to reduce the spread of contamination. The PPE must be constructed of materials that are appropriate for hazardous drug exposure. Hands must be thoroughly washed with soap and water both before donning and after removing gloves. Consider all PPE worn when handling hazardous drugs as being contaminated; contain and dispose of such PPE as contaminated waste.

⚿ CN: Safety and infection control; CL: Analyze

146. 4. When the duration of intravascular therapy is likely to be more than 6 days, a midline catheter or a PICC is preferred to a short peripheral catheter. In adult clients, use of the femoral vein for central venous access should be avoided. Steel needles should be avoided when administering fluids and medications that might cause tissue necrosis if extravasation occurs.

⚿ CN: Reduction of risk potential; CL: Apply

TEST 14: The Adult Having Surgery

- The Adult Who Is Preparing for Surgery
- The Adult Who Is Receiving or Recovering from Anesthesia
- The Adult Who Has Had Surgery
- Legal and Ethical Issues Associated with Surgery
- Managing Care, Quality, and Safety of Adults Having Surgery
- Answers, Rationales, and Test-Taking Strategies

The Adult Who Is Preparing for Surgery

1. A client tells the nurse on admission that they are uneasy about having to leave their children with a relative while being in the hospital for surgery. What should the nurse do?
   ☐ 1. Reassure the client that their children will be fine and they should stop worrying.
   ☐ 2. Contact the relative to determine their capacity to be an adequate care provider.
   ☐ 3. Encourage the client to call the children to make sure they are doing well.
   ☐ 4. Gather more information about the client's feelings about the childcare arrangements.

2. A client has a latex allergy. What should the nurse teach the client to do before having surgery? Select all that apply.
   ☐ 1. Determine that there will be a latex-safe environment for surgery.
   ☐ 2. Report symptoms experienced with the latex allergy (e.g., rhinitis, conjunctivitis, flushing).
   ☐ 3. Notify the health care providers (HCPs) at the surgery center.
   ☐ 4. Wear a stainless steel medical alert bracelet into the surgical suite.
   ☐ 5. Ask to have the surgery at a hospital.

3. When the nurse asks the client who is having abdominal surgery today if the client understands the procedure, the client replies, "No, not really; I talked about several different things with my surgeon, and I'm just not sure." What should the nurse do **next**?
   ☐ 1. Teach the client all the details of the planned procedure.
   ☐ 2. Utilize a second witness when the client signs for consent.
   ☐ 3. Notify the surgeon of the client's expressed lack of understanding.
   ☐ 4. Administer the prescribed preoperative narcotics or sedatives.

4. When the nurse is removing personal protective covering, what action should this nurse (see figure) take to avoid spreading nosocomial infections?

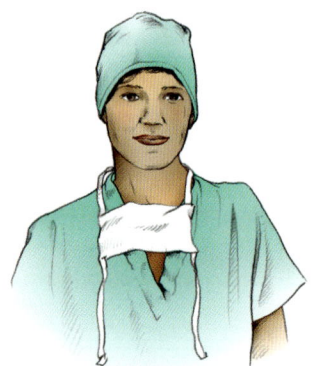

   ☐ 1. Remove the face mask.
   ☐ 2. Place the face mask over the mouth and nose before removing the hair covering.
   ☐ 3. Wash hands before tying the strings on the mask.
   ☐ 4. Tie the dangling strings of the mask around the neck.

5. The client is to have surgery on the fourth metatarsal. Identify the place on the illustration below where the client should confirm the operative site to the health care provider.

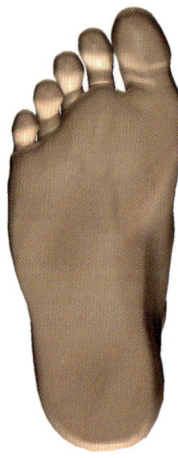

6. The nurse is reviewing the medical record of a client who is scheduled for a lumbar laminectomy. The nurse should report which finding to the surgeon?
- ☐ 1. pimple on the lower back
- ☐ 2. abnormal electrocardiogram (ECG)
- ☐ 3. hearing aid
- ☐ 4. allergy to iodine

7. Prior to going to surgery, the client tells the nurse that it is not possible to hear without a hearing aid and asks to wear it to surgery and recovery. What is the nurse's **best** response?
- ☐ 1. Explain to the client that it is policy not to take personal items to surgery because they may be lost or broken.
- ☐ 2. Tell the client that a nurse will bring the hearing aid to the postanesthesia care unit as soon as the client wakes up.
- ☐ 3. Explain to the client that the premedication will cause sleepiness and it will not be necessary to hear anything.
- ☐ 4. Call the surgery unit to explain the client's concern, and ask if the client can wear the hearing aid to surgery.

8. The adult daughters of an older adult client inform the nurse that they fully expect their parent to be combative after surgery. Preoperatively, they request that the nurse put all four side rails up and use restraints to keep their parent safe. What should the nurse tell the daughters?
- ☐ 1. "Certainly; we will want to be sure to keep your parent safe too."
- ☐ 2. "We will call the health care provider to get a prescription right away."
- ☐ 3. "We will first try to keep them safe without restraint."
- ☐ 4. "Restraint use is prohibited at our hospital at all times."

9. Before surgery, the client is to take nothing by mouth after 0400. Which statement indicates the client did not follow the preoperative directions? The client:
- ☐ 1. ate a gelatin dessert at 0330.
- ☐ 2. brushed their teeth at 0400 but did not swallow.
- ☐ 3. held a cold washcloth against their lips.
- ☐ 4. smoked a cigarette at 0600.

10. The surgeon prescribes cefazolin 1 g to be given intravenously (IV) at 0730 when the client's surgery is scheduled at 0800. What is the **primary** reason to start the antibiotic exactly at 0730?
- ☐ 1. Legally, the medication has to be given at the prescribed time.
- ☐ 2. The antibiotic is most effective in preventing infection if it is given 30 to 60 minutes before the operative incision is made.
- ☐ 3. The postoperative dose of cefazolin needs to be started exactly 8 hours after the preoperative dose of cefazolin.
- ☐ 4. The peak and titer levels are needed for antibiotic therapy.

11. A client who is to receive general anesthesia has a serum potassium level of 5.8 mEq/L (5.8 mmol/L). What action should the nurse take **first**?
- ☐ 1. Call the operating room to cancel the surgery.
- ☐ 2. Send the client to surgery.
- ☐ 3. Make a note on the client's record.
- ☐ 4. Notify the anesthesiologist.

12. Before being transported to the surgery suite, the nurse asks the client whether the client has any allergies. The client responds, "Does anyone communicate with anyone? I've been asked that question over and over!" What is the nurse's **best** response?
- ☐ 1. "I'm sorry! I just have to ask that question for the record."
- ☐ 2. "It's an important question, and we just have to check."
- ☐ 3. "You will hear it again and again as you go through surgery."
- ☐ 4. "This question is asked for verification and safety with each new phase of treatment."

13. On the day of surgery, a client with diabetes who takes insulin on a sliding scale is to have nothing by mouth and all medications withheld. The client's 0600 glucose level is 300 mg/dL (16.7 mmol/L). What should the nurse do?
- ☐ 1. Withhold all medications.
- ☐ 2. Administer the insulin dose dictated by the sliding scale.
- ☐ 3. Call the health care provider (HCP) for specific prescriptions based on the glucose level.
- ☐ 4. Notify the surgery department.

14. The nurse is preparing a preoperative teaching plan for a client who is undergoing a bilateral breast reduction. Which aspect of the plan is the **priority**?
- ☐ 1. reduction of risk potential
- ☐ 2. physiologic adaptation
- ☐ 3. psychosocial integrity
- ☐ 4. health promotion and maintenance

15. A client is scheduled to have an elective mandibular osteotomy to correct a mandibular fracture sustained in an accident 6 months earlier. Which statement by the client indicates to the nurse that the client is having difficulty coping?
- ☐ 1. "I'll be glad to have my jaw fixed because my spouse thinks I don't look like myself."
- ☐ 2. "I'm somewhat afraid to have the surgery, but I feel okay about it."
- ☐ 3. "My spouse will help me, but I don't think I'll need that much help."
- ☐ 4. "I'm ready to get this over with."

16. The nurse is assessing a client's nutritional status before surgery. Which observation would indicate poor nutrition in a 5-foot 7-inch (170-cm) female client who is 21 years of age?
☐ 1. poor posture
☐ 2. brittle nails
☐ 3. dull expression
☐ 4. weight of 128 lb (58.1 kg)

17. An older adult is being discharged following a repair of an inguinal hernia. The client is independent and lives alone, but the client's family lives 60 miles from the client's house. When at home, the client is to cleanse and inspect the incision for signs of infection. The client and family are able to read and understand written instructions. When giving discharge instructions, the nurse should perform which action(s)? Select all that apply.
☐ 1. Explain the instructions to the client.
☐ 2. Ask the client to demonstrate the procedure.
☐ 3. Explain the instructions to a family member.
☐ 4. Provide written instructions for the client.
☐ 5. Give the family a link to a video showing the procedure.

18. A client is admitted for an arthroscopy of the right shoulder through same-day surgery. Which nurse is responsible for starting the client's discharge planning?
☐ 1. preadmission nurse
☐ 2. preoperative nurse
☐ 3. intraoperative nurse
☐ 4. postoperative nurse

19. The nurse is preparing to administer a preoperative medication that includes a sedative to a client who is having abdominal surgery. What should the nurse do **first**?
☐ 1. Have the family present.
☐ 2. Ensure that the operative area has been shaved.
☐ 3. Have the client empty the bladder.
☐ 4. Make sure the client is covered with a warm blanket.

20. Before surgery, a client expresses a fear of surgery because 10 years ago the client's sibling died in surgery related to complications of anesthesia. What action should the nurse take?
☐ 1. Reassure the client that technology has changed over the last 10 years.
☐ 2. Encourage the client to further express concerns.
☐ 3. Explain to the client that it is normal to be afraid.
☐ 4. Ask the client if any family members had trouble when they had surgery.

21. The nurse is preparing to start an intravenous (IV) infusion and has raised the head of the client's bed. After the nurse applies gloves to insert an IV catheter, the client begins to rub the eyes and wipe away nasal drainage. What should the nurse do **first**?
☐ 1. Distract the client's attention.
☐ 2. Assess the client for pain.
☐ 3. Remove the gloves, and assess the client's vital signs.
☐ 4. Lower the head of the client's bed.

22. When attempting to check the pupils of a client scheduled to receive general anesthesia, the nurse notices that the client has trouble tilting their head back. What is the **primary** concern related to this finding?
☐ 1. The client has limited movement of the neck.
☐ 2. The client may have postoperative neck pain.
☐ 3. The client is at risk for difficult intubation.
☐ 4. The ability to assess the client's pupils is limited.

23. A client is to have a below-the-knee amputation. Before the surgery, what should the circulating nurse in the operating room do?
☐ 1. Insert a Foley catheter.
☐ 2. Start an intravenous (IV) infusion.
☐ 3. Initiate a time-out.
☐ 4. Verify that the surgeon possesses the degree of expertise needed.

24. The nurse is developing a plan to teach a client deep-breathing exercises to expand collapsed alveoli and prevent postoperative atelectasis and pneumonia. What information should be included in the plan? Select all that apply.
☐ 1. Splint or support the incision to promote maximal comfort.
☐ 2. Inhale slowly through the nostrils; exhale through pursed lips.
☐ 3. Hold the breath for about 5 seconds to expand the alveoli.
☐ 4. Repeat this breathing method 5 to 10 times hourly.
☐ 5. Close one nostril while inhaling.

25. The nurse receives the preoperative blood work report for a client who is scheduled to undergo surgery. Which laboratory finding should the nurse report to the surgeon and anesthesiologist?
☐ 1. red blood cells, 4.5 million/mm^3 (4.5×10^{12}/L)
☐ 2. creatinine, 2.6 mg/dL (198 µmol/L)
☐ 3. hemoglobin, 12.2 g/dL (122 g/L)
☐ 4. blood urea nitrogen, 15 mg/dL (5.4 mmol/L)

26. A client will receive intravenous midazolam hydrochloride during surgery. Which finding indicates a therapeutic effect?
☐ 1. amnesia
☐ 2. nausea
☐ 3. mild agitation
☐ 4. blurred vision

27. The nurse is administering intravenous midazolam hydrochloride to a client. What action should the nurse take?
☐ 1. Assess the blood pressure.
☐ 2. Monitor the pulse oximeter.
☐ 3. Have the client take deep breaths.
☐ 4. Help the client relax.

28. When the nurse administers intravenous midazolam hydrochloride, the client demonstrates signs of an overdose. What should the nurse do **next**?
☐ 1. Ventilate with an oxygenated bag valve mask.
☐ 2. Prepare electrocardiogram paddles in case the client has a cardiac arrest.
☐ 3. Administer 0.5 mL of 1:1000 epinephrine.
☐ 4. Titrate flumazenil to reverse the effects of the midazolam hydrochloride.

29. Metoclopramide is prescribed as a premedication for a client about to undergo a gastroduodenoscopy. What expected therapeutic effect of this drug should the nurse assess in this client?
☐ 1. increased gastric pH
☐ 2. increased gastric emptying
☐ 3. reduced anxiety
☐ 4. inhibited respiratory secretions

30. The nurse has administered glycopyrrolate to a client who is going to surgery. Which outcome is expected?
☐ 1. increased heart rate
☐ 2. increased respiratory rate
☐ 3. decreased secretions
☐ 4. decreased amnesia

31. The nurse is administering enoxaparin to a client 6 hours before the scheduled time of laparoscopically assisted vaginal hysterectomy. Which is the intended therapeutic action of the enoxaparin?
☐ 1. increase in red blood cell production
☐ 2. reduction of postoperative thrombi
☐ 3. decrease in postoperative bleeding
☐ 4. promotion of tissue healing

32. During the preoperative interview, the nurse obtains information about the client's medication history. Which information is necessary to record about the client? Select all that apply.
☐ 1. current use of medications, herbs, and vitamins
☐ 2. over-the-counter medication use in the last 6 weeks
☐ 3. steroid use in the last year
☐ 4. all drugs taken in the last 18 months
☐ 5. which medications to take after surgery.

33. When the nurse is conducting a preoperative interview with a client who is having a vaginal hysterectomy, the client states that they forgot to tell the surgeon that they had a total hip replacement 3 years ago. Why should the nurse communicate this information to the perioperative nurse?
☐ 1. The prosthesis may cause a problem with the electrosurgical unit used to control bleeding.
☐ 2. The client should not have their hip externally rotated when they are positioned for the procedure.
☐ 3. The perioperative nurse can inform the rest of the team about the total hip replacement.
☐ 4. There is not enough time to notify the surgeon and note this finding on the history and physical information before the procedure.

34. The nurse learns that a client who is scheduled for a tonsillectomy has been taking 40 mg of oral prednisone daily for the last week for poison ivy on the leg. What should the nurse do **first**?
☐ 1. Document the prednisone with current medications.
☐ 2. Notify the surgeon of the poison ivy.
☐ 3. Notify the anesthesiologist of the prednisone administration.
☐ 4. Withhold all preoperative medications.

35. A client who is scheduled for an open cholecystectomy has been smoking a pack of cigarettes a day for 20 years. For which postoperative complication is the client **most** at risk?
☐ 1. deep vein thrombosis
☐ 2. atelectasis
☐ 3. delayed wound healing
☐ 4. intolerance to fatty foods

36. The nurse explains to a family that they cannot go with the client past the doors that separate the public from the restricted area of the operating room suite. What is the purpose of this restriction?
☐ 1. protection of the privacy of clients
☐ 2. prevention of electrical sparks that could ignite the anesthetic gases
☐ 3. separation of the family from the surgical team during the operation
☐ 4. maintenance of an aseptic environment to prevent infection

37. The nurse teaches a client who had a cystoscopy about the urge to void when the procedure is over. What other information should the nurse tell the client to expect to do?
    ☐ 1. Ignore the urge to void.
    ☐ 2. Increase intake of fluids.
    ☐ 3. Ask for the bedpan.
    ☐ 4. Ring for assistance to go to the bathroom.

38. The nurse is developing a care plan for a client who had abdominal surgery today. Which nursing action will be **most** important in preventing postoperative complications?
    ☐ 1. progressive diet planning
    ☐ 2. pain management
    ☐ 3. bowel and elimination monitoring
    ☐ 4. early ambulation

39. The nurse is preparing a teaching plan for a client about general anesthesia induction. Which explanation would be **most** appropriate?
    ☐ 1. "Your premedication will put you to sleep."
    ☐ 2. "You will breathe in an inhalant anesthetic mixed with oxygen through a facial mask and receive intravenous medication to make you sleepy."
    ☐ 3. "You will receive intravenous (IV) medication to make you sleepy."
    ☐ 4. "You will breathe in medication through a facial mask to make you sleepy."

The Adult Who Is Receiving or Recovering from Anesthesia

40. A client who had a gastrectomy has been in the postanesthesia recovery room for 30 minutes when the vital signs suddenly change. The nurse checks the recovery room record (see chart). In addition to notifying the health care provider, the nurse should take what other action **immediately**?

Vital Signs			
Date	06/30	06/30	06/30
Time	1345	1400	1415
Pulse	70	82	90
Respiration	12	14	20
Blood pressure	100/60 mm Hg	110/70 mm Hg	140/90 mm Hg
Temperature	98°F (36.7°C)	99°F (37.2°C)	102°F (38.9°C)

    ☐ 1. Administer dantrolene.
    ☐ 2. Elevate the head of the bed 30 degrees.
    ☐ 3. Administer a bolus of intravenous (IV) fluids.
    ☐ 4. Insert an indwelling urinary catheter.

41. A female client is worried about being placed in the lithotomy position for surgery. What action should the nurse take?
    ☐ 1. Explain in detail what will occur in the operating room.
    ☐ 2. Determine what the client is concerned about.
    ☐ 3. Pad the stirrups for comfort.
    ☐ 4. Reassure the client that an all-female surgical team will be present.

42. A client is to receive medication by a continuous nerve block route. Prior to insertion of the catheter by the anesthesiologist, what information must the nurse document? Select all that apply.
    ☐ 1. vital signs
    ☐ 2. weakness/numbness
    ☐ 3. location of pain
    ☐ 4. results of laboratory tests
    ☐ 5. allergies

43. A client who is having surgery will have an epidural/intrathecal catheter placed. What should the nurse instruct the client to do while the catheter is in place? Select all that apply.
    ☐ 1. Take showers instead of baths.
    ☐ 2. Tell the nurse about having nausea or vomiting.
    ☐ 3. Call for assistance with turning or repositioning while in bed.
    ☐ 4. Inform the nurse of numbness or weakness in the legs.
    ☐ 5. Take shallow breaths to prevent dislodging the catheter.
    ☐ 6. Call the nurse if the catheter becomes dislodged.

44. A client arrives from surgery to the postanesthesia care unit. Which respiratory assessment should the nurse complete **first**?
    ☐ 1. oxygen saturation
    ☐ 2. respiratory rate
    ☐ 3. breath sounds
    ☐ 4. airway flow

45. The nurse is assessing a client who had epidural anesthesia 4 hours ago. What should the nurse assess **first**?
    ☐ 1. bladder distention
    ☐ 2. headache
    ☐ 3. postoperative pain
    ☐ 4. ability to move the legs

46. The nurse is assessing a client who has had spinal anesthesia. Which finding is expected?
    ☐ 1. The client feels pain before moving their legs.
    ☐ 2. The client's blood pressure is significantly increased.
    ☐ 3. Sensation returns to the toes first and then progresses to the perineal area.
    ☐ 4. The client has a headache while in the lying position.

47. The nurse in the postanesthesia care unit notes that one of the client's pupils is larger than the other. What should the nurse do **next**?
☐ 1. Rate the client on the Glasgow Coma Scale.
☐ 2. Administer oxygen.
☐ 3. Check the client's baseline data.
☐ 4. Call the surgeon.

48. A client is admitted to the postanesthesia care unit following a left hip replacement. The initial nursing assessment is temperature 96.6°F (35.9°C); pulse 90 bpm; respiration rate 14 breaths/min; and blood pressure 128/80 mm Hg. The client only responds with moaning when spoken to. What should the nurse do **first**?
☐ 1. Observe the surgical dressing.
☐ 2. Position the client on the right side.
☐ 3. Remove the oral airway remaining from surgery.
☐ 4. Administer a sedation reversal agent such as flumazenil.

49. The surgical floor receives a client from the postanesthesia care unit. Ten minutes ago, the final assessment in the postanesthesia care unit indicated that the client had a patent airway and stable vital signs. The client's pain level was 2. What should the nurse do **next**?
☐ 1. Check the dressing for signs of bleeding.
☐ 2. Empty any peri-incisional drains.
☐ 3. Reassess the client's pain level.
☐ 4. Determine if the client has a full bladder.

50. A client with impaired cardiac functioning is having abdominal surgery. Sodium thiopental is being used during anesthesia induction. What should the nurse monitor the client for during the surgery?
☐ 1. bradycardia
☐ 2. complete muscle relaxation
☐ 3. hypotension
☐ 4. tachypnea

51. A client received propofol as the induction and maintenance agent for general anesthesia. What outcome of this drug should the nurse expect?
☐ 1. minimal nausea and vomiting
☐ 2. hypertension
☐ 3. slow induction of anesthesia
☐ 4. small tremors of the skeletal muscles

52. A 250-lb (113-kg) male client is recovering from general anesthesia. The client's vital signs are tympanic temperature 99.8°F (37.7°C); pulse 150 bpm; respiratory rate 28 breaths/min; and blood pressure 90/50 mm Hg. The client has rigid muscles. How should the nurse interpret these findings?
☐ 1. The client is recovering as expected from the anesthesia; the nurse should continue monitoring them.
☐ 2. The client is exhibiting the effects of excessive blood loss experienced in the operating room; the nurse should increase the rate of the intravenous infusion.
☐ 3. The client is in the early stages of malignant hyperthermia; the nurse should obtain emergency medications and notify the anesthesiologist.
☐ 4. The client is in pain; the nurse should offer the client pain medication.

53. The nurse is assessing a client recovering from anesthesia. Which finding is an early indicator of hypoxemia?
☐ 1. somnolence
☐ 2. restlessness
☐ 3. chills
☐ 4. urgency

54. The nurse is administering flumazenil intravenously to a client who is recovering from anesthesia for reversal of sedation. What action(s) should the nurse take? Select all that apply.
☐ 1. Administer the medication as a 2-mg bolus.
☐ 2. Give the medication undiluted in incremental doses.
☐ 3. Be alert for shivering and hypotension.
☐ 4. Use only a free-flowing intravenous (IV) line in a large vein.
☐ 5. Monitor the client's level of consciousness.

55. An older adult client had spinal anesthesia for a transurethral resection of the prostate and received 4000 mL of room-temperature isotonic bladder irrigation. The client now has continuous irrigation through a three-way indwelling urinary catheter. Which postoperative nursing intervention is **most** important to include in the plan of care?
☐ 1. Empty the catheter drainage bag.
☐ 2. Cover the client with warm blankets.
☐ 3. Hang new bags of irrigation.
☐ 4. Turn the client.

56. Before having a broken arm casted, a client received an intravenous regional nerve block. After surgery, the casted arm is elevated on a pillow. What action should the nurse encourage the client to avoid until sensation returns?
    ☐ 1. holding the operated arm close to the face
    ☐ 2. holding the operated arm with the unoperated arm
    ☐ 3. using the unoperated arm
    ☐ 4. using pain medication

57. The health care provider prescribed intravenous naloxone to reverse the respiratory depression from morphine administration. After administration of the naloxone, what should the nurse do?
    ☐ 1. Check respirations in 5 minutes because naloxone is immediately effective in relieving respiratory depression.
    ☐ 2. Check respirations in 30 minutes because the effects of morphine will have worn off by then.
    ☐ 3. Monitor respirations frequently for 4 to 6 hours because the client may need repeated doses of naloxone.
    ☐ 4. Monitor respirations each time the client receives morphine sulfate 10 mg intramuscularly.

58. The nurse is administering naloxone to a client who is recovering from anesthesia. The nurse should monitor the surgical client closely for which clinical manifestation?
    ☐ 1. restlessness
    ☐ 2. dizziness
    ☐ 3. bleeding
    ☐ 4. urine retention

59. The nurse is to administer midazolam 2.5 mg. The medication is available in a 5-mg/mL vial. How many milliliters should the nurse administer? Record your answer using one decimal point.
    _____ mL.

The Adult Who Has Had Surgery

60. On the first day after abdominal surgery, the nurse auscultates a client's abdomen for bowel sounds; there are none. What should the nurse do **next**?
    ☐ 1. Notify the health care provider (HCP).
    ☐ 2. Ask another nurse to validate the absence of bowel sounds.
    ☐ 3. Encourage the client to take more ice chips.
    ☐ 4. Document assessment findings in the client's medical record.

61. Three days after a cholecystectomy, a client states, "I feel like my stomach is going to burst." The client is taking a regular diet. After determining that vital signs are stable, in which order of priority from first to last does the nurse assist the client? All options must be used.

| 1. Position the client on the right side. |
| 2. Offer 120 mL of hot liquids. |
| 3. Auscultate for bowel sounds. |
| 4. Encourage ambulation. |
| |
| |
| |
| |

62. The nurse assesses that a client is restless and becoming agitated in the immediate postoperative period. The client's oxygen saturation is 91%. What should the nurse do **next**?
    ☐ 1. Administer a sedative.
    ☐ 2. Offer ice chips.
    ☐ 3. Administer oxygen.
    ☐ 4. Apply wrist restraints.

63. A client requests a narcotic analgesic shortly after the oncoming nurse receives the change-of-shift report. The nurse who is leaving reported that the client had received morphine 10 mg intramuscularly 2 hours ago. In what order from first to last should the oncoming registered nurse (RN) perform the actions? All options must be used.

   1. Take the client's vital signs.

   2. Assess the client for pain using a pain scale.

   3. Review the prescription for dose and frequency of administration.

   4. Determine the client's sedation level using the Opioid-induced Sedation Scale.

64. A client is prescribed morphine sulfate intramuscularly (IM). Which is true regarding the administration of this controlled substance?
    ☐ 1. Morphine may only be administered by a registered nurse.
    ☐ 2. Another nurse must observe the disposal of unused medication.
    ☐ 3. Another nurse must validate the administration of the medication.
    ☐ 4. A registered nurse must observe the licensed practical/vocational nurse administer the medication.

65. A client who is a Jehovah's Witness consented to surgery only and **not** to receiving any blood products, including autotransfusion. During surgery, the client lost blood, the blood pressure dropped, and two units of blood were administered. Following surgery and during handover, the nurse was informed that the blood had been administered. In which order, from first to last should the nurse complete these tasks?
    ☐ 1. Complete an incident report.
    ☐ 2. Initiate an ethics consultation.
    ☐ 3. Notify the unit manager.
    ☐ 4. Inform the next oncoming nurse during the hand-off-of-care report.

66. On the day of surgery, a client has been breathing room air. Their vital signs are normal, and their oxygen saturation is 89%. What should the nurse do **first**?
    ☐ 1. Turn the client to one side.
    ☐ 2. Notify the health care provider (HCP).
    ☐ 3. Assist the client to take several deep breaths and cough.
    ☐ 4. Administer oxygen by nasal cannula as prescribed at 2 L per minute.

67. A client has been unable to void since having abdominal surgery 7 hours ago. What should the nurse do **first**?
    ☐ 1. Encourage the client to increase their oral fluid intake.
    ☐ 2. Insert an intermittent urinary catheter.
    ☐ 3. Use an ultrasound bladder scanner to determine urine volume in the bladder.
    ☐ 4. Assist the client up to the toilet to attempt to void.

68. Following abdominal surgery, a client refuses to deep breathe and cough every 2 hours as prescribed. What should the nurse do **first**?
    ☐ 1. Ask the client's wife to insist that the client take deep breaths every 2 hours.
    ☐ 2. Respect the client's wishes, and turn the client from side to side more frequently.
    ☐ 3. Suggest that the client increase the daily fluid intake to at least 10½ cups (about 2½ L).
    ☐ 4. Explain the risks of not expanding the lungs and why the exercise is important.

69. Eight hours after laparoscopic abdominal surgery, a client has a distended bladder and is unable to void in bed using a urinal. The client can be out of bed as tolerated but has not done so yet. What should the nurse do **next**?
    ☐ 1. Assist the client to stand at the bedside to use the urinal.
    ☐ 2. Pour running water over the perineum to stimulate emptying of the bladder.
    ☐ 3. Encourage the client to ambulate to prevent further bladder distention.
    ☐ 4. Notify the health care provider to request a prescription for catheterization.

70. The nurse is assessing the level of consciousness of a client who just had open heart surgery. When asked, the client can give their name but is not sure about where they are or the time of day. What should the nurse do **next**?
    ☐ 1. Notify the surgeon.
    ☐ 2. Rub the client's sternum to arouse the client.
    ☐ 3. Encourage the client's wife to orient the client.
    ☐ 4. Tell the client where they are and the time of day.

71. Following surgery, a client is receiving 1000 mL of normal saline intravenously (IV) with 40 mEq (40 mmol/L) of potassium chloride (KCl), which has been prescribed to be infused at 125 mL per hour. The client states, "My IV hurts." What should the nurse do **first**?
☐ 1. Contact the client's health care provider (HCP) for a different IV prescription.
☐ 2. Slow down the infusion to a keep-open rate (20 to 50 mL per hour).
☐ 3. Assess the IV site for signs of phlebitis, extravasation, or IV-related infection.
☐ 4. Check the hanging parenteral fluid and administration set for documentation as to when they were last changed.

72. A nurse is assessing a client when they return from same-day surgery for a dilatation and curettage. The nurse checks preoperative vital signs at 0830 to compare them with the current vital signs at 2230 (see chart). What should the nurse do **first**?

Vital Signs	0830	2230
Pulse	80	90
Respirations	16	20
Blood pressure	90/60 mm Hg	100/80 mm Hg
Temperature	99.5°F (37.5°C)	97°F (36.1°C)

☐ 1. Call the health care provider for pain medication.
☐ 2. Cover the client with warmed blankets.
☐ 3. Administer oxygen at 4 L per minute.
☐ 4. Increase the intravenous (IV) fluid rate.

73. The nurse is caring for a client receiving morphine in an intravenous infusion using a patient-controlled anesthesia pump (PCA) for relief of postoperative pain. On assessment, the client's vital signs are: heart rate 84 bpm; respiration rate 8 breaths/min; blood pressure 104/56 mm Hg; and oxygen saturation 88% on room air. What should the nurse do **first**?
☐ 1. Contact the health care provider (HCP) to request a prescription for naloxone.
☐ 2. Stop the infusion of morphine.
☐ 3. Assist the client to sit and stimulate coughing and deep breathing.
☐ 4. Call the rapid response team.

74. A client had a colectomy 8½ hours ago and received 1500 mL of dextrose 5% in water with normal saline solution. The client has just used a patient-controlled analgesia pump to administer morphine for pain, has been repositioned for comfort, and has a stable pulse rate, respiration rate, and blood pressure. What should the nurse do **next**?
☐ 1. Check that the family is comfortable.
☐ 2. Assess vital signs following the use of morphine.
☐ 3. Dim the lights in the room.
☐ 4. Increase nasal oxygen from 2 L to 3 L.

75. A client who underwent esophageal hernia repair 4 hours ago has a temperature of 100.4°F (38°C); pulse of 90 bpm; respiration rate of 16 breaths/min; blood pressure of 130/80 mm Hg; and pulse oximeter reading of 91% on room air. What should the nurse do **first**?
☐ 1. Obtain a culture of the incision.
☐ 2. Notify the surgeon to obtain an antibiotic prescription.
☐ 3. Offer pain medication.
☐ 4. Assist the client to a sitting position to take deep breaths.

76. The nurse is teaching the client how to use the patient-controlled analgesia (PCA) pump. The nurse determines that the client understands the use of the PCA pump when the client makes which statement?
☐ 1. "It's okay for my family to press the button for me if I'm too tired to do it myself."
☐ 2. "I should wait until the pain is really bad before I push the button to get more pain medicine."
☐ 3. "The machine will only give me the prescribed amount of pain medication even if I push the button too soon."
☐ 4. "I have to be careful about pushing the button too many times or I will overdose myself."

77. A client had a total abdominal hysterectomy and bilateral oophorectomy for ovarian carcinoma yesterday. They received 2 mg of morphine sulfate intravenously by patient-controlled analgesia (PCA) 10 minutes ago. The nurse was assisting the client from the bed to a chair when the client felt dizzy and fell into the chair. What should the nurse do **next**?
☐ 1. Discontinue the PCA pump.
☐ 2. Administer oxygen.
☐ 3. Take the client's blood pressure.
☐ 4. Assist the client back to bed.

78. Immediately following pelvic surgery, a client has an indwelling urinary catheter. Which nursing action would be **most** helpful to prevent a catheter-related urinary tract infection?
- ☐ 1. Provide catheter and perineal care twice daily.
- ☐ 2. Monitor the color, clarity, and amount of urine output.
- ☐ 3. Advocate for limited use of and duration of indwelling urinary catheters.
- ☐ 4. Palpate for lower abdominal distension once per shift.

79. A nurse is instructing a client who had abdominal surgery that day to do deep-breathing exercises. In which order from first to last should the nurse teach the client to perform diaphragmatic breathing and coughing? All options must be used.

1. Inhale through the nose.
2. Cough deeply from the lungs.
3. Exhale through pursed lips.
4. Splint the incisional site.

80. The postoperative nursing assessment of a client's ability to swallow fluids before providing oral fluids is based on the type of anesthesia given. Which client would **not** have delayed fluid restrictions?
the client who had:
- ☐ 1. a bronchoscopy under local anesthesia
- ☐ 2. a transurethral resection of a bladder tumor under general anesthesia
- ☐ 3. a repair of carpal tunnel syndrome under local anesthesia
- ☐ 4. an inguinal herniorrhaphy with spinal and intravenous conscious sedation

81. A client has just returned to bed following the first ambulation since abdominal surgery. The client's heart rate and blood pressure are slightly elevated; oxygen saturation is 91% on room air. The client reports being "a little short of breath" but does not have dizziness or pain. What should the nurse do **next**?
- ☐ 1. Obtain a 12-lead electrocardiogram (ECG).
- ☐ 2. Administer pain medication.
- ☐ 3. Allow the client to rest for a few minutes, then reassess.
- ☐ 4. Request new activity prescriptions from the health care provider.

82. Eight hours after bowel surgery, the nurse observes that the client's urine output has decreased from 50 to 20 mL per hour. The nurse should assess the client further for which condition?
- ☐ 1. bowel obstruction
- ☐ 2. adverse effects of opioid analgesics
- ☐ 3. hemorrhage
- ☐ 4. hypertension

83. A client who had a left thoracoscopy sustained an injury secondary to the surgery position. The nurse should assess the client for which sign?
- ☐ 1. foot drop
- ☐ 2. knee swelling and pain
- ☐ 3. tingling in the arm
- ☐ 4. absence of the Achilles reflex

84. The nurse is evaluating a client who is using a flow incentive spirometer (see figure) following abdominal surgery 1 day ago. The client is performing the procedure correctly when the client does what? Select all that apply.

- ☐ 1. inhales before using the spirometer
- ☐ 2. inhales for 3 seconds following fully expanding the lungs
- ☐ 3. coughs after using the spirometer
- ☐ 4. uses the spirometer once every 8 hours
- ☐ 5. exhales passively before using the spirometer
- ☐ 6. sits upright

85. The nurse is teaching a client how to take care of an incision at home. What should the nurse tell the client?
    ☐ 1. "Don't touch your incision before your next appointment."
    ☐ 2. "Clean your incision three times a day with hydrogen peroxide and water."
    ☐ 3. "Don't be concerned about uneven lumps under the suture lines."
    ☐ 4. "If the staples don't come out by themselves before your next appointment, the surgeon will remove them."

86. The nurse is removing the client's staples from an abdominal incision when the client sneezes and the incision splits open, exposing the intestines. What should the nurse do **first**?
    ☐ 1. Press the emergency alarm to call the resuscitation team.
    ☐ 2. Cover the abdominal organs with sterile dressings moistened with sterile normal saline.
    ☐ 3. Have all visitors and family leave the room.
    ☐ 4. Call the surgeon to come to the client's room immediately.

87. On the fourth day after surgery, a client's incision is red and inflamed. There is moderate drainage from the incision. The client has a temperature of 102°F (38.9°C). The total white blood cell (WBC) count is 10,000/mm³ (10 × 10⁹/L). What should the nurse do **first**?
    ☐ 1. Encourage the client to increase their fluid intake.
    ☐ 2. Cleanse the incision site with soap and water.
    ☐ 3. Place an absorbent dressing over the incision.
    ☐ 4. Notify the health care provider (HCP).

88. The nurse is making rounds and observes a client receiving oxygen (see figure). What should the nurse do **next**?

    ☐ 1. Position the mask lower on the client's nose.
    ☐ 2. Verify that the reservoir bag remains deflated.
    ☐ 3. Confirm that the flow rate is set to deliver oxygen at 6 to 10 L per minute.
    ☐ 4. Loosen the elastic band on the client's face.

89. The nurse is changing a wet-to-dry dressing covering a surgical wound. Which is the appropriate procedure for changing this type of dressing?
    ☐ 1. Place a dry dressing in the wound.
    ☐ 2. Use an aqueous solution of aluminum acetate (Burow's solution) to wet the dressing.
    ☐ 3. Pack the wet dressing tightly into the wound.
    ☐ 4. Cover the wet packing with a dry sterile dressing.

90. Two days following abdominal surgery, a client is refusing to take narcotic pain medication, even though their pain rating is an 8 on a 0-to-10 scale. The client tells the nurse, "I don't want to get dependent on that stuff." Which response from the nurse is the **most** appropriate?
    ☐ 1. "You will recover more quickly and more effectively if you take pain medication now."
    ☐ 2. "Newer pain medications don't cause dependence or addiction."
    ☐ 3. "It's your right to not take pain medication."
    ☐ 4. "You don't need to worry about becoming addicted so soon."

91. The nurse empties a Jackson-Pratt drainage bulb. Which nursing action ensures correct functioning of the drain?
    ☐ 1. irrigating it with normal saline
    ☐ 2. connecting it to low intermittent suction
    ☐ 3. compressing it and then plugging it to establish suction
    ☐ 4. connecting it to a drainage bag and clamping it off

92. The nurse is planning care for a client who had abdominal surgery. To prevent pulmonary emboli in this client, the nurse should take which action?
    ☐ 1. Have the client perform leg exercises every hour while awake.
    ☐ 2. Encourage the client to cough and deep breathe.
    ☐ 3. Massage the client's calves.
    ☐ 4. Have the client wear antiembolism stockings when out of bed.

93. The nurse assesses a client who has just received morphine sulfate. The client's pulse is 58 bpm; the respiration rate is 4 breaths/min; and the blood pressure is 90/50 mm Hg. What should the nurse do **first**?
    ☐ 1. Call the rapid response team.
    ☐ 2. Administer naloxone hydrochloride.
    ☐ 3. Start oxygen at 2 L per minute via nasal cannula.
    ☐ 4. Begin rescue breathing.

94. The nurse observes the client with an intermittent compression device in place after abdominal surgery (see figure). What should the nurse do **next**?

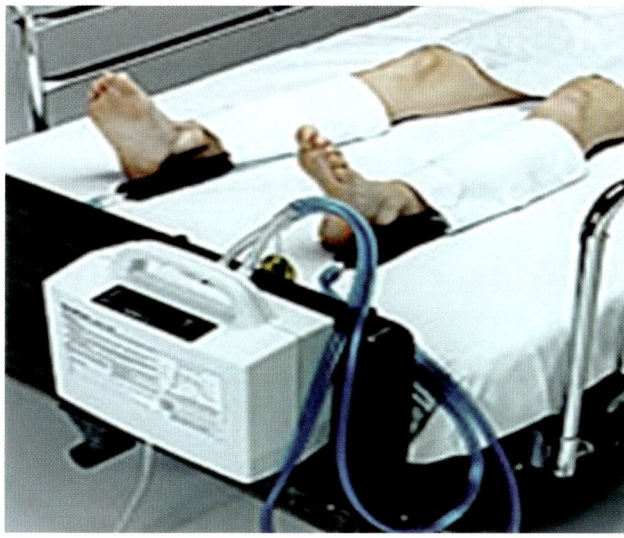

☐ 1. Elevate the client's legs.
☐ 2. Apply thromboembolic stockings to be worn under the device.
☐ 3. Instruct the client not to move while the device is inflated.
☐ 4. Make sure the client is comfortable.

95. A client is being discharged from same-day surgery. Which statement indicates that the client does not understand postoperative instructions about transportation home?
☐ 1. "My husband is taking the day off from work to drive me home."
☐ 2. "I can drive myself home after surgery."
☐ 3. "I am taking a taxi home, and my daughter will meet me at home."
☐ 4. "My son will be here at noon to take me home."

96. The initial postoperative assessment is completed on a client who had an arthroscopy of the knee. Which information is **not** necessary to obtain every 15 minutes during the first postoperative hour?
☐ 1. vital signs including pulse oximeter
☐ 2. pain rating of the operative site
☐ 3. urine output
☐ 4. neurovascular check distal to the operative site

97. After surgery, a client was treated for postoperative nausea and vomiting and now is experiencing hypotension and tachycardia. The nurse should review the medication record to determine if the client has received which medication?
☐ 1. ondansetron hydrochloride
☐ 2. droperidol
☐ 3. prochlorperazine
☐ 4. promethazine

98. A client has an epidural catheter for postoperative pain management. What action should the nurse take when managing the catheter?
☐ 1. Assess but not disturb the epidural dressing.
☐ 2. Change the epidural dressing daily.
☐ 3. Change the epidural dressing daily only if it is wet.
☐ 4. Use strict aseptic technique when handling the epidural catheter.

99. After surgery, the client is receiving epidural pain management. The client wants to get out of bed and walk to the bathroom. The nurse should base the decision to ambulate on which information?
☐ 1. The analgesia is periodically administered through the epidural catheter.
☐ 2. A low concentration of analgesia is used with the catheter.
☐ 3. The analgesia from the epidural catheter bathes the spinal fluid.
☐ 4. The epidural medication affects sympathetic and motor function.

100. The nurse is caring for a client who is using a portable wound suction unit (see figure). Six hours after surgery, the drainage unit is full. What should the nurse do **first**?

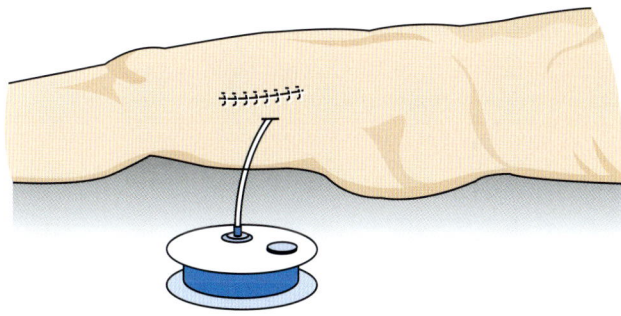

☐ 1. Remove the drain from the incision.
☐ 2. Notify the surgeon.
☐ 3. Empty the drainage.
☐ 4. Record the amount in the unit as output on the client's medical record.

101. Three days after surgery, a client continues to take hydrocodone 7.5 mg and acetaminophen 500 mg for postoperative pain. What should the nurse ask the client before administering the pain medication?
☐ 1. "When did you last have a bowel movement?"
☐ 2. "Have you emptied your bladder?"
☐ 3. "How long has it been since your last dose?"
☐ 4. "Is your pain better than before you had surgery?"

102. Upon waking up in the postanesthesia care unit and seeing a drain with bright red fluid in it exiting from their total hip incision, a client asks the nurse, "Is this the way it's supposed to be?" What should the nurse tell the client?
☐ 1. "The drainage is blood and fluid that must be drained out for healing."
☐ 2. "Don't worry about it. I'll explain it when you are more awake."
☐ 3. "This blood is being kept sterile and will be given back to you."
☐ 4. "I'll give you something to make you sleep so you won't worry."

103. A client has a Jackson-Pratt drainage tube in place the first day after surgical repair of a ruptured diverticulum. The client asks the nurse the purpose of the drain. What should the nurse tell the client? "The drainage tube is used to prevent:
☐ 1. infection in the peritoneal cavity."
☐ 2. bleeding into the peritoneal cavity."
☐ 3. pressure on the bladder."
☐ 4. pressure on the gallbladder."

104. A client who had a cholecystectomy has a biliary drainage tube in place. What color of the drainage is expected?
☐ 1. pinkish red
☐ 2. dark yellow-orange
☐ 3. clear
☐ 4. green

105. A client is to be discharged from same-day surgery 7 hours after inguinal hernia repair. Which nursing observation indicates this client is ready to be discharged?
The client:
☐ 1. voids 500 mL of urine.
☐ 2. tolerates eating a hamburger.
☐ 3. is pain free.
☐ 4. walks in the hallway unassisted.

106. A client has requested to have patient-controlled analgesia (PCA) after surgery. When is it appropriate for a client to receive PCA?
☐ 1. A family member is able to assist with self-dosing.
☐ 2. There are advanced directives in place.
☐ 3. The client has the ability to self-administer.
☐ 4. There is a nurse to assist with self-administration.

107. A nurse is assessing a client's blood pressure 8 hours after surgery. The client's blood pressure before surgery was 120/80 mm Hg, and on admission to the postsurgical nursing unit it was 110/80 mm Hg. The client's blood pressure is now 90/70 mm Hg. After determining that other vital signs are normal, what should the nurse do **first**?
☐ 1. Notify the health care provider (HCP).
☐ 2. Elevate the head of the bed.
☐ 3. Administer pain medication.
☐ 4. Call the rapid response team.

108. A client has been positioned in the lithotomy position under general anesthesia for a pelvic procedure. In which anatomic area may the client expect to experience postoperative discomfort?
☐ 1. shoulders
☐ 2. thighs
☐ 3. legs
☐ 4. feet

109. The nurse has established a goal for a client who had abdominal surgery to prevent atelectasis. Which measure(s) should the nurse include in the care plan? Select all that apply.
☐ 1. offering pain relief before having the client cough
☐ 2. providing a minimum of 4 cups (about 1 L) of fluid per day
☐ 3. using an incentive spirometer every 2 to 4 hours
☐ 4. assisting with early ambulation
☐ 5. turning the client to a prone position every 8 hours

110. The nurse is teaching the client about deep-breathing techniques. Which statement from the client indicates the need for additional education?
☐ 1. "I will use my incentive spirometer every hour while I am awake."
☐ 2. "I should place my hands lightly over my lower ribs and upper abdomen."
☐ 3. "I should get into a comfortable position before doing my breathing exercises."
☐ 4. "I should take four deep breaths and then cough deeply from the lungs."

111. A client has had a nasogastric tube connected to low intermittent suction. What is the client at risk for?
☐ 1. confusion
☐ 2. muscle cramping
☐ 3. edema
☐ 4. tremors

Legal and Ethical Issues Associated with Surgery

112. On admission to same-day surgery, the nurse reviews the medical record to verify the client's identification documentation. Which information is **most** important?
☐ 1. admitting record
☐ 2. preprinted labels
☐ 3. identification bracelet
☐ 4. location of family

113. A 12-year-old client needs lifesaving emergency surgery, but the relatives live an hour away from the hospital and cannot sign the consent form. What is the nurse's **best** response?
  ☐ 1. Send the client to surgery without the consent.
  ☐ 2. Call the family for a consent over the telephone, and have another nurse listen as a witness.
  ☐ 3. No action is necessary in this case because consent is not needed.
  ☐ 4. Have the family sign the consent form as soon as they arrive.

114. A client who has type 1 diabetes is being prepared to have a craniotomy. The nurse is evaluating the client's understanding of the informed consent before witnessing the client's signature on the operative consent form. Which statement from the client indicates that the nurse needs to contact the surgeon for further communication with the client?
  ☐ 1. "We talked about the effect of my diabetes on healing."
  ☐ 2. "The surgeon explained how the craniotomy was done."
  ☐ 3. "There are no major risks from this surgery."
  ☐ 4. "I will die if the tumor is not removed from my brain."

115. The nurse is helping to prepare a client for nonemergency surgery. What should the nurse do?
  ☐ 1. Obtain informed consent from the client.
  ☐ 2. Explain the surgical procedure in detail.
  ☐ 3. Verify that the client understands the informed consent form.
  ☐ 4. Inform the client about the risks of the surgery to be performed.

116. The nurse is helping a client sign an informed consent for surgery. The client cannot read or write but understands what the nurse is explaining about the surgery. What action should the nurse take after reading the consent in the presence of two witnesses?
  ☐ 1. Have the client's next of kin sign the informed consent.
  ☐ 2. Have the client put an "X" on the signature line.
  ☐ 3. Have a court appoint a guardian for the client.
  ☐ 4. Have a hospital quality management coordinator sign for the client.

Managing Care, Quality, and Safety of Adults Having Surgery

117. The nurse is verifying that all clients who are going to surgery today have had blood glucose levels drawn. The nurse should review the glucose level of which client(s) going to surgery today? Select all that apply.
  ☐ 1. a client with diabetes mellitus controlled by diet
  ☐ 2. a client with a high stress response to surgery
  ☐ 3. a client receiving corticosteroids for the past 3 months
  ☐ 4. a client with a family history of diabetes receiving dextrose 5% in lactated Ringer's solution (D_5LR) intravenous (IV) fluids
  ☐ 5. a client who consumes a high-carbohydrate diet

118. The nurse is assessing clients who are going to surgery today to determine if any client has a possible latex allergy. Which client has the **greatest** risk for latex allergies?
  ☐ 1. a woman who is admitted for their seventh surgery
  ☐ 2. a man who works as a sales clerk
  ☐ 3. a man with well-controlled type 2 diabetes
  ☐ 4. a woman who is having laser surgery

119. A client is admitted on the day of surgery for arthroscopy of the left knee. Which nursing action(s) should be completed prior to administering anesthesia to the client to avoid wrong-site surgery? Select all that apply.
  ☐ 1. Verify that the surgeon has marked with a permanent marker the correct knee for the surgical site.
  ☐ 2. Ask the client to state their name, surgical site, and procedure.
  ☐ 3. Verify the correct client with the correct operative site from medical records and diagnostic reports.
  ☐ 4. Call a "time-out" in the operating room to have the surgeon verify the correct knee before making the incision.
  ☐ 5. Show the client an anatomic model of the surgery site.

120. The nurse is planning care for a client with severe postoperative pain. There is a prescription for morphine written as "10 mg MSO_4" on the medical record. What should the nurse do **first**?
  ☐ 1. Obtain an intravenous (IV) infusion system.
  ☐ 2. Prepare the medication for administration.
  ☐ 3. Contact the pharmacy department.
  ☐ 4. Contact the health care provider (HCP) who prescribed the medication.

121. The client has returned to the surgery unit from the postanesthesia care unit (PACU). The client's respirations are rapid and shallow, their pulse is 120 bpm, and their blood pressure is 88/52 mm Hg. The client's level of consciousness is declining. What should the nurse do **first**?
☐ 1. Call the PACU.
☐ 2. Call the health care provider (HCP).
☐ 3. Call the respiratory therapist.
☐ 4. Call the rapid response team (RRT)/medical emergency team.

122. When completing the preoperative checklist on the nursing unit, the nurse discovers an allergy that the client has not reported. What should the nurse do **first**?
☐ 1. Withhold the prescribed preanesthetic medication.
☐ 2. Note this new allergy prominently on the medical record.
☐ 3. Contact the scrub nurse in the operating room.
☐ 4. Inform the anesthesiologist.

123. The nurse is making a staffing plan. Which task(s) should the nurse assign to the unlicensed assistive personnel (UAP) to assist in the care of postoperative clients? Select all that apply.
☐ 1. Empty and measure indwelling urinary catheter collection bags.
☐ 2. Reposition clients for pain relief.
☐ 3. Teach clients the proper use of the incentive spirometer.
☐ 4. Tell the nurse if clients report they are having pain.
☐ 5. Assess intravenous (IV) insertion sites for redness.

124. The client's identification armband was cut and removed to start an IV line as a part of the preoperative preparation. The transport team has arrived to transport the client to the operating room. The nurse notices that the client's identification band is not on either wrist. What should the nurse do?
☐ 1. Send the removed armband with the medical record and the client to the operating room.
☐ 2. Place a new identification armband on the client's wrist before transport.
☐ 3. Tape the cut armband back onto the client's wrist.
☐ 4. Send the client without an armband because the client is alert and can respond to questions about their identity.

125. At 0800, the nurse reviews the nurse's notes for an older adult who had surgery yesterday.

> **Nurse's Notes**
>
> **0700:**
> Heart rate is 98 bpm; respiration rate is 32 breaths/min; blood pressure is 148/92 mm Hg; and oxygen saturation is 88% on 4 L per minute via nasal cannula. Breath sounds are coarse and wet bilaterally with a loose, productive cough. The client voided 100 mL of very dark, concentrated urine during the last 4 hours. There is bilateral pitting pedal edema.
> After verifying the client's vital signs and breath sounds, using the SBAR (Situation-Background-Assessment-Recommendation) method to notify the health care provider of current assessment findings, the nurse should recommend which prescription?

☐ 1. antihypertensive medication
☐ 2. additional fluid intake
☐ 3. diuretic medication
☐ 4. increased oxygen liter flow rate

126. The nurse has just received the morning change-of-shift report on four clients. In what order from first to last should the nurse perform the actions? All options must be used.

1. Discuss the plan for the day with the unlicensed assistive personnel (UAP), delegating duties as appropriate.
2. Assess the client who has been vomiting according to the report from the night nurse.
3. Begin discharge paperwork for a client who is eager to go home.
4. Notify the health care provider (HCP) about a client who has a serum potassium level of 6.2 mEq/L (6.2 mmol/L).

127. While making rounds, the nurse observes that a client's primary bag of intravenous (IV) solution is light yellow. The label on the IV bag says the solution is dextrose 5% in water (D_5W). What should the nurse do **first**?
☐ 1. Continue to monitor the bag of IV solution.
☐ 2. Ask another nurse to look at the solution.
☐ 3. Notify the health care provider (HCP).
☐ 4. Hang a new bag of D_5W, and complete an incident report.

128. A client informs the nurse that the venipuncture site "hurts." The nurse should assess the site for which finding(s)? Select all that apply.
☐ 1. redness
☐ 2. pain
☐ 3. coolness
☐ 4. blanching
☐ 5. firmness
☐ 6. edema

129. A client has accidentally received twice the normal dose of a medication that was administered on the previous shift. What should the nurse who discovers the error do **first**?
☐ 1. Call the person who made the error, and request that an incident report be completed.
☐ 2. Assess the client, and note any changes in condition.
☐ 3. Call the health care provider (HCP) to obtain a prescription for additional intravenous (IV) fluids to dilute the drug.
☐ 4. Administer a drug antidote per standing prescription.

130. A client is in the operating room having surgery to replace a hip. Before the surgery, there is confusion about the view of the hip on the x-ray. The surgical team requests a "time-out" and stops the surgery. When can surgery continue? Select all that apply.
☐ 1. The surgeon verifies the correct procedure.
☐ 2. The surgeon verifies the correct surgical site.
☐ 3. The nurse reestablishes the sterile field.
☐ 4. The surgical team identifies the client using two sources of identification.
☐ 5. Another x-ray is obtained.

131. A client is being transferred from the recovery room to the medical-surgical nursing unit. The nurse from the recovery room should report which information to the nurse in the medical-surgical unit? Select all that apply.
☐ 1. type of surgery
☐ 2. current vital signs
☐ 3. names of all surgeons participating in the surgery
☐ 4. amount of blood loss
☐ 5. fluids infusing including rate and type of fluid

132. A client with a history of myocardial infarction 3 years ago was admitted at 0700 for a cholecystectomy scheduled at 0900. The client has been nothing by mouth (NPO) since midnight. At 0830, the client reports having chest pains. At 0700, the client's vital signs were pulse, 80 bpm; respiration rate, 14 breaths/min; and blood pressure, 110/70 mm Hg. At 0830 the nurse takes the vital signs again: pulse is 110 bpm; respiration rate is 20 breaths/min; and blood pressure is 90/60 mm Hg. The nurse calls the surgeon and, using the SBAR (Situation-Background-Assessment-Recommendation) communication protocol, should discuss which information with the surgeon? Select all that apply.
☐ 1. that the client has remained NPO
☐ 2. history of myocardial infarction and current report of chest pains
☐ 3. the change in vital signs
☐ 4. the type of surgery scheduled
☐ 5. request for an electrocardiogram (ECG)
☐ 6. request to administer nitroglycerin

133. When taking a client's vital signs on the first postoperative day, the unlicensed assistive personnel (UAP) reports to the nurse that the oral temperature is 100°F (37.8°C). After encouraging the client to use the incentive spirometer, the nurse should delegate which activity to the UAP?
☐ 1. Apply an ice cap to a client's forehead.
☐ 2. Bathe the client with cool water.
☐ 3. Place a hyperthermia blanket on the client's bed.
☐ 4. Continue to monitor the client's temperature.

134. A nurse is working with an unlicensed assistive personnel (UAP). Which client(s) should the nurse assign to the UAP? Select all that apply.
☐ 1. adult client newly diagnosed with diabetes who is learning to administer insulin
☐ 2. older adult client who had hip replacement surgery and needs to walk in the hall with a walker
☐ 3. adult client who had abdominal surgery yesterday and requires a dressing change
☐ 4. young adult client who requires tube feedings
☐ 5. adult client who had a hysterectomy 3 days ago and requires vital sign checks every 4 hours

135. A nurse is caring for a postsurgical client with two types of drains. Which task(s) can the nurse delegate to the unlicensed assistive personnel (UAP)? Select all that apply.
  ☐ 1. Assess the drainage of an open drainage system, such as a Penrose drain.
  ☐ 2. Document the drain site and surrounding tissue status.
  ☐ 3. Stabilize an open drainage system, such as a Penrose drain.
  ☐ 4. Empty a closed drainage system, such as a Jackson-Pratt drain or Hemovac drain.
  ☐ 5. Record the output from a closed-drainage system, such as a Jackson-Pratt drain or Hemovac drain.

136. The nurse is teaching a client with limited English language skills how to change a dressing on an abdominal incision. Which action should the nurse take to be sure the client can change the dressing at home?
  ☐ 1. Read written instructions to the client, and have an interpreter translate.
  ☐ 2. Show the client a video on the client's phone so the client can review it again at home.
  ☐ 3. Demonstrate how to change the dressing, and have the client return the demonstration.
  ☐ 4. Give the client a handout with the steps of the procedure illustrated.

137. A client who does not speak English is to be discharged from the hospital following outpatient surgery. Using an interpreter, the nurse reviewed all postoperative instructions, including the need to come in for the follow-up appointment in 2 weeks. The nurse also explained the reconciled medication list, including when to resume taking each medication and the signs and symptoms that would require a call to the health care provider. To ensure the client will continue ongoing care management, the nurse should do what **next**?

  ☐ 1. Schedule follow-up visits, and inform the client of dates and times.
  ☐ 2. Provide the reconciled client medication list.
  ☐ 3. Obtain the client's signature following receipt of discharge materials.
  ☐ 4. Provide a copy of the discharge materials to the interpreter.

138. A nurse is caring for a group of clients. After receiving the shift report, the nurse should make rounds on the clients in which order? Place in order of the highest to lowest priority. All options must be used.

| 1. female client who is 34 years of age and just returning from the recovery room following an abdominal hysterectomy; intravenous (IV) line is running at 50 drops per minute with 100 mL remaining |

| 2. client who is 50 years of age and diagnosed with diabetes mellitus 3 days ago who is learning to administer insulin |

| 3. client who is 75 years of age with a fractured hip of 4 days who needs to be turned frequently |

| 4. client who is 79 years of age, who has had a tracheotomy for 4 years, and who had surgery for removal of cancer of the colon 2 days ago |

| |

| |

| |

| |

139. A client scheduled for surgery is confused and shows signs of dementia. The nurse should ask which person to sign the consent for the client?
  ☐ 1. minister
  ☐ 2. nursing supervisor
  ☐ 3. attorney
  ☐ 4. spouse

140. A client who has an abdominal dressing has asked to use the urinal. A nurse drops a clean glove on the floor while attempting to don gloves. In which order, from first to last, should the nurse proceed?
  ☐ 1. Apply new, clean gloves.
  ☐ 2. Assess the client's surgical dressing.
  ☐ 3. Dispose of the glove on the floor.
  ☐ 4. Reposition the client's urinal.

Answers, Rationales, and Test-Taking Strategies

*The answers and rationales for each question follow below, along with keys (🔑) to the client need (CN) and cognitive level (CL) for each question. In addition, questions that measure clinical judgment will be coded (CJ). As you check your answers, use the **Content Mastery and Test-Taking Skill Self-Analysis** worksheet (tear-out worksheet in the back of the book) to identify the reason(s) for not answering the questions correctly. For additional information about test-taking skills and strategies for answering questions, refer to pages 12–51 in part 1 of this book.*

The Adult Who Is Preparing for Surgery

1. **4.** The health history is conducted to ascertain a client's state of wellness or illness. A personal dialogue between a client and a nurse is conducted to obtain information. To achieve a relationship of mutual trust and respect, the nurse must have the ability to communicate a sincere interest in the client. The therapeutic communication must be adapted to the responses, problems, and needs of the client. Reassurance and the remaining options do not demonstrate that the nurse is genuinely interested in the client's needs.

   🔑 CN: Psychosocial integrity; CL: Analyze

2. **-/+ 1, 2, 3.** Treatment and diagnostic evaluation must be done in a latex-safe environment. Signs and symptoms of latex allergy may range from mild to anaphylaxis. Clients with a latex allergy are advised to notify their HCPs and to wear medical identification; however, all metal and jewelry must be removed before surgery as they could conduct an electrical current. The surgery can be safely performed at a free-standing surgery center as long as latex precautions are observed.

   🔑 CN: Safety and infection control; CL: Create

3. **3.** It is the surgeon's responsibility to discuss the planned procedure and review the risks, benefits, and alternatives to the planned procedure. If the client verbalizes that they do not understand the procedure that is planned, it is the nurse's responsibility to notify the surgeon of this lack of understanding right away, before any additional nursing actions. In this case, when the client verbalizes a lack of understanding, the nurse should not teach about the procedure; the surgeon needs to do this. The nurse cannot assist the client to sign for consent and should not administer narcotics or sedatives until the client understands and agrees to the procedure.

   🔑 CN: Management of care; CL: Analyze

4. **1.** The nurse should remove the face mask. The face mask contains nasal and oral droplets, which are easily transmitted to the hands as the mask dangles when left hanging around the neck. When a face mask is not worn over the mouth and nose, it should be completely removed.

   🔑 CN: Safety and infection control; CL: Analyze

5. This is the correct surgical site.

   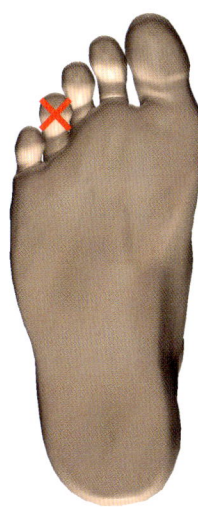

   🔑 CN: Physiological adaptation; CL: Apply

6. **1.** A pimple close to the incision site may be a reason for the surgeon to cancel the surgical procedure because it increases the risk for infection. If the client had an abnormal ECG, the nurse would notify the anesthesiologist who will be administering the anesthesia. The anesthesiologist is the decision-maker regarding the implications of the anesthesia on the cardiac system. The surgical team should be notified of the client's hearing disability, but the surgeon, who has already met the client, does not need to be notified. The surgical team should be notified of the client's allergy to iodine, and it should be documented in all the appropriate places, but the surgeon would not need to be notified in advance of the surgical procedure.

   🔑 CN: Safety and infection control; CL: Analyze

7. **4.** The nurse serves as a client advocate when helping in addressing a client's concern. The nurse should call the operating room and inform the intraoperative nurse about the client's request. A

special container with correct identification can be prepared so that when the client is anesthetized and their hearing aid is removed, it will not be lost or broken. It is usual policy not to send personal belongings to surgery because they are easily broken or lost in the transfer of an anesthetized client with higher priority needs, but special needs do exist. In some instances, the nurse does bring a client's personal belongings to the postanesthesia care unit, but in this case, the item involves the client's ability to communicate. Because the trend is to use little premedication, clients are more alert and may want to talk with their surgical team before going to sleep. Decreasing the client's anxieties preoperatively affects the amount of medication used to induce the client and their overall psychological and physiologic status. Telling the client that they will not need to hear is insensitive.

CN: Basic care and comfort; CL: Analyze

8. **3.** A least-restraint environment should always be provided as much as possible. Nursing staff are required to attempt lesser restrictive alternatives (e.g., use of family or sitter, reorientation, distraction, toileting schedule) before notifying the provider of the need for restraints. Nursing staff are also required to document clinical conditions requiring restraint, lesser restrictive alternatives attempted, and the client and family education provided regarding restraint use. Provider prescriptions for restraints must be time limited and specific regarding the type of restraint. Additionally, if restraints are implemented, nursing staff must monitor clients for safety (including skin checks and range of motion) and provide frequent food, fluids, and toileting.

CN: Safety and infection control; CL: Analyze

9. **4.** The client has deficient knowledge if they smoked a cigarette after 0400 because, even though they did not have anything to eat or drink, smoking has increased the production of gastric hydrochloric acid, which can increase the risk for aspiration in an anesthetized client. The client consumed the gelatin dessert prior to the 0400 restriction for being NPO. Comfort measures, such as brushing the teeth without swallowing or holding a cold washcloth against the lips, are acceptable for a client who is to have nothing by mouth.

CN: Reduction of risk potential; CL: Evaluate

10. **2.** The antibiotic is most effective in preventing infection, according to research, if it is given 30 to 60 minutes before the operative incision is made. When the surgeon prescribes the antibiotic to be given at a specific time related to the scheduled time of the surgical procedure, it is imperative that the antibiotic is given on time. Legally, the nurse considers 30 minutes on either side of the scheduled time to be acceptable for administering medications; however, in this situation, giving the antibiotic 30 minutes too soon can make the prophylactic antibiotic ineffective. The postoperative dose of the antibiotic is not timed according to the preoperative dose. Peak and titer levels are measured for some antibiotics, but in this case, the primary reason is to have the antibiotic infused before the time of the incision.

CN: Reduction of risk potential; CL: Apply

11. **4.** The nurse should notify the anesthesiologist because a serum potassium level of 5.8 mEq/L (5.8 mmol/L) places the client at risk for arrhythmias when under general anesthesia. It is not the role of the nurse to cancel surgery. The nurse should not automatically send a client with abnormal laboratory findings to surgery because the procedure may be canceled. Once the client is inside the operating room and sterile supplies have been opened up for the procedure, the client is usually charged. The nurse should call ahead of time to communicate the abnormal laboratory result instead of noting the finding on the client's record. The information on the record should not be reviewed until after the client has been transported to the operating room and the supplies have been opened.

CN: Reduction of risk potential; CL: Analyze

12. **4.** Clients should be made aware that some questions are asked for verification and safety with each new phase of treatment. Indicating that the nurse is sorry, or needs to check several times, or telling the client that the question will be asked again does not tell the client why it is necessary to continue to verify information essential to the client's safety.

CN: Psychosocial integrity; CL: Analyze

13. **3.** The nurse should notify the HCP directly for specific prescriptions based on the client's glucose level. The nurse cannot ignore the elevated glucose level. The surgical experience is stressful, and the client needs specific insulin coverage during the perioperative period. The nurse should not administer the insulin without checking with the surgeon because there are specific prescriptions to withhold all medications. It is not necessary to notify the surgery department unless the HCP cancels the surgery.

CN: Pharmacological and parenteral therapies; CL: Analyze

14. **3.** Psychosocial integrity issues, including coping mechanisms, situational role changes, and body image changes, are more common in a client who undergoes elective cosmetic surgical procedures. Reduction of risk potential, physiologic adaptation, and health promotion and maintenance are greater needs for clients who are undergoing surgical correction of functional, anatomic, or physiologic defects in nonelective surgical procedures.

CN: Psychosocial integrity; CL: Analyze

15. **1.** A client should not elect surgery to meet someone else's needs. The nurse should encourage the client to share their feelings and their perception of the deformity and to clarify their reasons for electing to have the surgery. It is normal to be somewhat afraid, and it is good if a client says they feel "okay" about the surgery. The fact that a client believes that their spouse will help them after surgery and that they will also be relatively independent reflects appropriate adaptation. It is a common feeling among preoperative clients that they are ready to "get this over with," indicating that the waiting period is stressful.

CN: Psychosocial integrity; CL: Evaluate

16. **2.** Brittle nails indicate poor nutrition. Poor posture indicates that the client does not stand up straight and use their muscles to support themself. A dull expression reflects the client's affect and emotional status. The client's weight of 128 lb (58.1 kg) is within normal range.

CN: Health promotion and maintenance; CL: Analyze

17. **1, 2, 4.** The nurse should explain and demonstrate the discharge instructions and then ask the client to give a return demonstration. The Joint Commission and Health Canada require that discharge instructions be written for the postoperative client. Clients need to be given discharge instructions orally and in written form because of stress, medications, and the volume of material to be learned. Explaining all the instructions to a family member and giving them a link to a video is important but does not replace the need for written instructions. Since the family does not live nearby, the nurse must be certain the client can manage the instructions by themself.

CN: Health promotion and maintenance; CL: Analyze

18. **1.** The preadmission nurse, the first person in contact with the client, starts the discharge planning for the client undergoing surgery. All nurses involved with the client, from preadmission through postoperative recovery, should continue to reinforce the discharge plan.

CN: Health promotion and maintenance; CL: Apply

19. **3.** The nurse should have the client empty the bladder before the premedication is administered. This will be more comfortable and safer for the client. The purpose of the premedication is to decrease anxiety and promote a relaxed state. The client must have an empty bladder before being transferred to the operating room, where the client will be immobilized and receive intravenous fluids. The family does not have to be present, but it is usually desired. Shaving the operative area is not generally recommended because it can cause small nicks that harbor bacteria. If the client must be shaved, it is usually done in the operating room holding area. The client should be comfortable at all times and offered a warm blanket before or after the premedication.

CN: Basic care and comfort; CL: Analyze

20. **4.** The nurse should immediately think of the congenital metabolic tendency for malignant hyperthermia, which occurs in the presence of certain kinds of anesthetics. Whenever a preoperative client states that a family member has had problems with anesthesia or surgery, the nurse should inquire about the nature of the problems and whether other family members have had similar problems. Reassuring the client that technology has changed will do little to affect their fears and misses the opportunity to evaluate the risk for malignant hyperthermia. Encouraging the client to further express their concerns and reassuring them that their feelings are normal are important, but missing a familial tendency of malignant hyperthermia could be fatal.

CN: Reduction of risk potential; CL: Analyze

21. **3.** Although most clinical agencies use latex-free materials, the nurse should assess the vital signs of the client who exhibits urticaria, rhinitis, and conjunctivitis a few seconds after coming in contact with rubber gloves, a plastic catheter, plastic IV tubing, or a plastic IV solution bag. The nurse should recognize that these symptoms indicate that a type I allergic reaction is occurring. Although many health care agencies now use latex-free materials, it is possible that the products contain latex or other materials that might be precipitating the client's allergic response. The client does not need to be distracted or assessed for pain. It is not necessary to lower the head of the bed.

CN: Safety and infection control; CL: Analyze

22. 3. The client is at risk for a difficult intubation because the neck must be hyperextended to pass the endotracheal tube. Assessment of the pupils should not be limited. If the client is positioned appropriately during surgery, there is no risk for postoperative neck pain or limited neck movement.

🗝 CN: Reduction of risk potential; CL: Analyze

23. 3. The Universal Protocol is used to prevent wrong-site, wrong-procedure, and wrong-person surgery. The actions included in the protocol are: conduct a preprocedure verification process; mark the procedure site; and perform a time-out. Exceptions to the Universal Protocol are routine or "minor" procedures, such as venipuncture, peripheral IV line placement, insertion of oral/nasal drainage or feeding tubes, or Foley catheter insertion. Prior to closure, the surgeon or circulating nurse will initiate a time-out to verbally confirm a review of informed consent and procedures completed; all specimens are identified, accounted for, and accurately labeled; and all foreign bodies have been removed. The chief of surgery and medical director are the ones who will verify the surgeons' levels of expertise.

🗝 CN: Safety and infection control; CL: Apply

24. -/+ **1, 2, 3, 4.** Splinting the incision is important to avoid stress on the surgical site and to promote comfort so that the client will adhere to the plan of care. Inhaling through the nostrils and exhaling through pursed lips are important to bring in adequate oxygen and clear out carbon dioxide; however, closing one nostril when inhaling would be inappropriate and ineffective. The most important step is asking the client to hold the inhaled breath for about 5 seconds, which keeps the alveoli expanded. This step should be stressed the most. Repeating the exercise 5 to 10 times hourly is the second most important point to emphasize in this teaching plan.

🗝 CN: Reduction of risk potential; CL: Create

25. 2. The nurse should call the surgeon for a serum creatinine level of 2.6 mg/dL (198 μmol/L), which is higher than the normal range of 0.1 to 0.4 mg/dL (8 to 31 μmol/L). An elevated serum creatinine value indicates that the kidneys are not filtering effectively and has important implications for the surgical client because many anesthesia and analgesia medications need to be filtered out through the renal system. The red blood cell count, hemoglobin level, and blood urea nitrogen level are within normal limits and do not need to be reported to the surgeon.

🗝 CN: Reduction of risk potential; CL: Analyze

26. 1. Midazolam hydrochloride causes antegrade amnesia or decreased ability to remember events that occurred around the time of sedation. Nausea, mild agitation, and blurred vision are adverse effects of midazolam.

🗝 CN: Pharmacological and parenteral therapies; CL: Evaluate

27. 3. The client should be encouraged to take slow, deep breaths because midazolam hydrochloride is a respiratory depressant. The nurse should assess the client's blood pressure, monitor the pulse oximeter, and keep the client calm and relaxed, but the client will slip into very shallow, ineffective breathing if not encouraged to deep breathe.

🗝 CN: Pharmacological and parenteral therapies; CL: Analyze

28. 1. The nurse should have a bag valve mask in the client's room because midazolam hydrochloride can lead to respiratory arrest if it is administered too quickly. The client does not need to be shocked back into a normal rhythm or receive epinephrine unless cardiac compromise develops after the respiratory arrest. The client would receive titrated dosing of flumazenil to reverse the midazolam, but first, the nurse should ventilate the client.

🗝 CN: Pharmacological and parenteral therapies; CL: Analyze

29. 2. Metoclopramide is an antiemetic given because of its gastric emptying ability, which is necessary in gastrointestinal procedures. It does not increase gastric pH, reduce anxiety, or inhibit respiratory secretions.

🗝 CN: Pharmacological and parenteral therapies; CL: Evaluate

30. 3. Glycopyrrolate is an anticholinergic agent given for its ability to reduce oral and respiratory secretions before general anesthesia. An increased heart rate or respiratory rate would be an adverse effect of the drug. Amnesia should not be an effect of the drug.

🗝 CN: Pharmacological and parenteral therapies; CL: Apply

31. 2. Research findings have shown that enoxaparin and low-dose heparin given 6 to 12 hours preoperatively reduce the incidence of deep vein thrombosis and pulmonary emboli by 60% in clients who are at risk for deep vein thrombosis, such as those who are placed in the lithotomy position. Enoxaparin has no effect on red blood cell production, postoperative bleeding, or tissue healing.

🗝 CN: Pharmacological and parenteral therapies; CL: Evaluate

32. -/+ **1, 2, 3, 4.** The nurse should record all drugs the client is currently taking, including herbs and vitamins, over-the-counter medications such as aspirin taken in the past 6 weeks, the amount of alcohol consumed, and the use of illegal drugs, because these can interfere with anesthetic and analgesic agents. Steroid use is of concern because it can suppress the adrenal cortex for up to 1 year, and supplemental steroids may need to be administered in times of stress such as surgery. The nurse does not need to ask about all drugs used in the last 18 months if the client is not currently taking them as these drugs will not affect the use of anesthesia. The nurse should not discuss with the client what medications will be used after surgery, as that information is not known at this time.

CN: Reduction of risk potential; CL: Apply

33. 2. The nurse should notify the surgery department and document the past surgery in the medical record in the preoperative notes so that the client's hip is not externally rotated and the hip dislocated while they are in the lithotomy position. The prosthesis should not be a problem as long as the perioperative nurse places the return electrode away from the prosthesis site. The perioperative nurse will inform the rest of the team, but the primary reason to inform the perioperative nurse is related to the safe positioning of the client. The surgeon should enter this information on the client's medical record at this time.

CN: Reduction of risk potential; CL: Apply

34. 3. The nurse should notify the anesthesiologist because supplemental prednisone suppresses the adrenal cortex's natural ability to produce increased corticosteroids in times of stress such as surgery. The anesthesiologist may need to prescribe supplemental steroid coverage during the perioperative period. The nurse should document the prednisone with current medications, but it is a priority to inform the anesthesiologist. Because the poison ivy is not in the surgical field, the surgeon does not need to be called regarding the skin disruption. It is not the nurse's responsibility to decide to withhold the preoperative medications.

CN: Pharmacological and parenteral therapies; CL: Analyze

35. 2. The client who has a significant cigarette smoking history and an operative manipulation close to the diaphragm (the gallbladder is against the liver) is at increased risk for atelectasis and pneumonia. Postoperatively, this client will be reluctant to deep breathe because of pain, in addition to having residual lung damage from smoking. Therefore, the client is at greater-than-average risk for pulmonary complications. The client does not have an increased risk for intolerance to fatty foods (the client will follow a diet as tolerated), deep vein thrombosis (as long as the client performs leg exercises), or delayed wound healing (as long as the client maintains appropriate nutrition).

CN: Reduction of risk potential; CL: Analyze

36. 4. The purpose of separating the public from the restricted-attire area of the operating room is to provide an aseptic environment and prevent contamination of the environment by organisms. The client's privacy is protected, but the main purpose is infection control. Anesthetics currently in use do not pose a risk for being ignited.

CN: Safety and infection control; CL: Apply

37. 2. After a scope or catheter has been inserted into the urethra, the mucosal membrane is irritated, and the client feels the need to void even though the bladder may not be full. The nurse should encourage the client to force fluids to make the urine dilute. The client should not ignore the urge to void. The client should be encouraged to use the bathroom; there is no need to use the bedpan. The client does not need assistance to the bathroom because this procedure does not require any anesthesia except a topical anesthetic for the male client.

CN: Basic care and comfort; CL: Analyze

38. 4. Early ambulation is the most significant general nursing measure to prevent postoperative complications and has been advocated for more than 40 years. Walking the client increases vital capacity and maintains normal respiratory functioning, stimulates circulation, prevents venous stasis, improves gastrointestinal and genitourinary function, increases muscle tone, and increases wound healing. The client should maintain a healthy diet, manage pain, and have regular bowel movements. However, early ambulation is the most important intervention.

CN: Reduction of risk potential; CL: Analyze

39. 2. Adult clients are induced for general anesthesia by breathing in an inhalant anesthetic mixed with oxygen through a facial mask and receiving IV medication to make them sleepy. Clients are not induced with the premedication. Clients usually are not induced with the IV infusion or the mask alone.

CN: Reduction of risk potential; CL: Analyze

The Adult Who Is Receiving or Recovering from Anesthesia

40. 1. The client is demonstrating signs of malignant hyperthermia. Unless the body is cooled and the influx of calcium into the muscle cells is reversed, lethal cardiac arrhythmia and hypermetabolism occur. The client's body temperature can rise as high as 109°F (42.8°C) as body muscles contract. Dantrolene, an IV skeletal muscle relaxant, is used to reverse muscle rigidity. Elevating the head of the bed will not reverse the hyperthermia. Adding fluids and inserting an indwelling urinary catheter are not immediately beneficial steps in reversing the progression of malignant hyperthermia.

CN: Management of care; CL: Analyze

41. 2. The nurse should first attempt to find out what the client's concerns are and address them. Providing too much information with details can increase the client's anxiety and does not address specific concerns. Padding the stirrups will provide comfort, but this does not address concerns. Having an all-female team may or may not be the source of the client's concerns and probably is not possible.

CN: Psychosocial integrity; CL: Analyze

42. 1, 2, 3, 5. Prior to the catheter insertion, the nurse must document the location of pain and the pain rating, the level of consciousness (LOC), vital signs, and weakness or numbness, especially in the legs. The nurse should also ask if the client has allergies before medication administration. It is not the nurse's responsibility to chart laboratory results; the results will be documented on the client's health record.

CN: Safety and infection control; CL: Analyze

43. 2, 3, 4, 6. Complications may develop when a client is receiving medication via epidural, intrathecal, or continuous nerve block routes. The nurse should inform the health care provider (HCP) if there is a dislodged catheter, disconnected tubing, or an occluded line. The nurse must also notify the HCP if the client has nausea or vomiting as the movement involved could dislodge the catheter. Numbness or weakness in the legs could also indicate a dislodged catheter, and the nurse must assess the client for these signs and report them if they occur. The client should call for assistance when getting out of bed or ambulating. The client should not take a shower or a bath while the catheter is in place. The client does not need to take shallow breaths, and the nurse should encourage the client to breathe normally and take deep breaths regularly.

CN: Safety and infection control; CL: Analyze

44. 4. Airway flow is always the first assessment. Once the nurse establishes that the client has a patent airway, the pulse oximeter is applied to measure the oxygen saturation, the respiratory rate is counted, and the breath sounds are auscultated bilaterally.

CN: Physiological adaptation; CL: Analyze

45. 1. The last area to regain sensation is the perineal area, and the nurse should check the client for a distended bladder. The client has received a large volume of intravenous fluids since the epidural was inserted, and the client may not feel the urge to void or may be unable to void. In that case, the nurse should obtain a prescription to catheterize the client before the bladder becomes so distended as to cause bladder spasms. The nurse should assess for a spinal headache, postoperative pain, and the client's ability to move after determining whether the bladder is distended.

CN: Reduction of risk potential; CL: Analyze

46. 3. Spinal anesthesia is an extensive conduction nerve block that is produced when a local anesthetic is introduced into the subarachnoid space at the lumbar level. A few minutes after induction of a spinal anesthetic, anesthesia and paralysis affect the toes and perineum and then, gradually, the legs and abdomen. When the autonomic nervous system is blocked, vasodilation and hypotension occur. The client will feel sensation in the toes before the perineal area. A spinal headache due to loss of fluid is a severe headache that occurs while in the upright position but is relieved in the lying position.

CN: Physiological adaptation; CL: Analyze

47. 3. The nurse should check the client's baseline data to ascertain whether the client's pupil has always been enlarged or if this is a new finding. The preoperative assessment is valuable as the baseline for comparison of all subsequent assessments made throughout the perioperative period. The nurse may determine that a more involved neurologic examination is indicated or may choose to assess other signs using the Glasgow Coma Scale, administer oxygen, or call the surgeon, but the nurse still needs to know the baseline data before proceeding.

CN: Physiological adaptation; CL: Analyze

48. 2. During the immediate postanesthesia period, the unconscious client should be positioned on the side to maintain an open airway and promote drainage of secretions; because of the type of surgery, the client should be positioned on the right side. Removing the oral airway and observing the surgical dressing are appropriate, but other actions should be implemented before these. Respiratory depression can occur in a client after a procedure requiring sedation. If the client cannot be aroused, the sedation drugs can be reversed by administering a sedation reversal agent, but this client's respiratory rate is 14 breaths/min, and the client is moaning, indicating expected recovery from anesthetics.

🔑 CN: Physiological adaptation; CL: Analyze

49. 1. The nurse should check the dressing for signs of bleeding to establish a baseline for future assessments of the dressing and to verify that there is no obvious sign of hemorrhage. The nurse does not need to empty peri-incisional drains at this time. All drains should have been emptied and reconstituted by the postanesthesia care nurse before the client was transferred to the surgical floor. Assessing the client's pain level and assessing the bladder are important; however, it is more important to assess the surgical site for bleeding because hemorrhage is a life-threatening complication of any surgical procedure.

🔑 CN: Physiological adaptation; CL: Analyze

50. 3. Sodium pentothal, a short-acting barbiturate, can cause hypotension, which may be especially problematic for the client with impaired cardiac functioning. Sodium pentothal does not cause bradycardia, complete muscle relaxation, hypertension, or tachypnea.

🔑 CN: Pharmacological and parenteral therapies; CL: Apply

51. 1. Propofol, a nonbarbiturate anesthetic agent, causes less nausea and vomiting than other induction agents because of a direct antiemetic action. It does not cause hypertension or skeletal muscle movement, and it does not act slowly.

🔑 CN: Pharmacological and parenteral therapies; CL: Analyze

52. 3. A heart rate of 150 bpm or greater, hypotension, and muscle rigidity are early signs of malignant hyperthermia. The nurse should quickly assemble emergency supplies and personnel because malignant hyperthermia is potentially and rapidly fatal in more than 50% of cases. A rapid, extreme rise in temperature is a late sign. Another factor influencing the analysis is that the client has a large body frame, and having large, bulky muscles is a risk factor for malignant hyperthermia. The client's vital signs are well out of the range of normal; analysis of the data and swift intervention are indicated. Excessive blood loss is unlikely, and the data do not support this conclusion. Although clients have changes in vital signs when in acute pain, the nurse would expect the client to be hypertensive, not hypotensive.

🔑 CN: Physiological adaptation; CL: Analyze

53. 2. One of the earliest signs of hypoxia is restlessness and agitation. Decreased level of consciousness and somnolence are later signs of hypoxia. Chills can be related to the anesthetic agent used but are not indicative of hypoxia. Urgency is not related to hypoxia.

🔑 CN: Physiological adaptation; CL: Analyze

54. 2, 3, 4, 5. Flumazenil should be administered in small quantities such as 0.2 mg over 15 to 30 seconds but never as a bolus. Flumazenil may be given undiluted in incremental doses. Adverse effects of flumazenil may include shivering and hypotension. The nurse should monitor the client's level of consciousness while recovering from sedation. Flumazenil should be administered through a free-flowing IV line in a large vein because extravasation causes local irritation.

🔑 CN: Pharmacological and parenteral therapies; CL: Analyze

55. 2. It is important for the nurse to cover this client with warm blankets because they are at high risk for hypothermia secondary to age, spinal anesthesia, placement in a lithotomy position in the cool operating room for 1½ hours, instillation of 4000 mL of room-temperature bladder irrigation, and ongoing bladder irrigation. Spinal anesthesia causes vasodilation, which results in heat loss from the core to the periphery. The nurse will empty the catheter drainage bag and hang new bags of irrigation as needed, but the client's potential for hypothermia should be addressed first. The client will not be turned at this time.

🔑 CN: Reduction of risk potential; CL: Analyze

56. 1. The nurse should encourage the client to avoid holding the operated arm, the arm with the intravenous regional nerve block (Bier block), close to the face because the client does not have motor control over it. With the cast in place, the client could hit the eye, nose, or mouth and cause soft tissue damage. It is acceptable for the client to hold the operated arm with the unoperated arm or to use the unoperated arm. The nurse should administer the analgesic before the intravenous regional anesthetic completely wears off so that the pain does not peak before pain medication is administered.

🔑 CN: Reduction of risk potential; CL: Analyze

57. 3. The nurse should monitor the client's respirations closely for 4 to 6 hours because naloxone has a shorter duration of action than opioids. The client may need repeated doses of naloxone to prevent or treat a recurrence of respiratory depression. Naloxone is usually effective in a few minutes; however, its effects last only 1 to 2 hours, and ongoing monitoring of the client's respiratory rate will be necessary. The client's dosage of morphine will be decreased or a new drug will be prescribed to prevent another instance of respiratory depression.

CN: Pharmacological and parenteral therapies; CL: Analyze

58. 1. The nurse should monitor the client who has received naloxone for reversal of opioid overdose or anesthesia recovery for side effects such as restlessness, agitation, and potential cardiac arrhythmias. Bleeding, dizziness, and urine retention are not typical side effects of naloxone.

CN: Pharmacological and parenteral therapies; CL: Analyze

59. 0.5 mL. To obtain the answer, treat the volume to be administered as X.

$$\frac{2.5 \text{ mg}}{X \text{ mL}} = \frac{5 \text{ mg}}{1 \text{ mL}}$$

$$5X = 2.5$$

$$X = \frac{2.5}{5} = 0.5$$

CN: Pharmacological and parenteral therapies; CL: Apply

The Adult Who Has Hvad Surgery

60. 4. Bowel sounds are not present until the third or fourth postoperative day; the nurse should document the assessment findings. Since this is an expected finding, it is not necessary to notify the HCP or have another nurse validate the findings. Too many ice chips may promote abdominal distention, especially if the client is not ambulating in the intermediate postoperative period.

CN: Physiological adaptation; CL: Analyze

61. 3, 2, 1, 4. The nurse first auscultates the abdomen for bowel sounds to determine if peristalsis has resumed and is present. The nurse then administers hot liquids to stimulate peristalsis and promote expulsion of the gas that is causing the client to be uncomfortable. Positioning the client on the right side permits gas to rise along the transverse colon and facilitates its release. Abdominal distention may be minimized by early and frequent ambulation, which stimulates intestinal motility. The nurse also assists the client to ambulate.

CN: Physiological adaptation; CL: Analyze

62. 3. Restlessness in the immediate postoperative period may be a sign of cerebral hypoxia as a result of depression on the central nervous from anesthetic agents and sedatives. Administering sedatives would depress the central nervous system further. A client may aspirate ice chips when they are restless. Wrist restraints may increase agitation and cannot be used without justification.

CN: Physiological adaptation; CL: Analyze

63. 2, 1, 4, 3. The oncoming nurse should first assess the client for pain using a pain scale. Next, the nurse should check the client's vital signs and then check the client's level of sedation using a scale that assesses levels of sedation for clients receiving opioids such as the Opioid-induced Sedation Scale. Last, the nurse should review the prescription to see how often and at what dose the client can receive the pain medication.

CN: Pharmacological and parenteral therapies; CL: Analyze

64. 2. Morphine sulfate and other narcotics are carefully controlled by state and federal guidelines, including observation and documentation of any unused ("wasted") medication. While administering morphine intravenously is not within the scope of practice of a licensed nurse, IM morphine may be given by a registered or licensed nurse without observation or validation by another nurse.

CN: Pharmacological and parenteral therapies; CL: Analyze

65. 2, 3, 1, 4. Anyone (client, family, nurse) can initiate an ethics consultation for guidance in the event an ethical or legal concern arises. As a requirement for accreditation, ethics teams are available for consultation at all times, and the nurse could initiate a request for this consultation. The nurse manager would be notified shortly after the ethics consultation request. The nurse manager will consult with corporate legal and risk management related to the next steps. An incident report would be completed, and all parties would be notified, including the surgeon and client. During the shift hand-off-of-care report, the oncoming nurse would be informed of the incident and the actions completed.

CN: Management of care; CL: Analyze

66. **3.** The nurse should instruct the client to first take deep breaths and cough to increase lung expansion and prevent the accumulation of secretions in postoperative clients. Oxygen saturation of 89% is not an unexpected or emergency finding immediately following surgery. Frequent coughing and deep breathing will likely quickly remedy an oxygen saturation of 89% and will also effectively help prevent atelectasis and pneumonia in the remainder of the postoperative period. It is not necessary to notify the HCP prior to intervening with coughing and deep breathing, and it is not appropriate to turn the client to the side because this would make it more difficult for the client to take deep breaths. Oxygen may be necessary, but the nurse should assist the client to cough and deep breathe first to attempt to improve the client's oxygenation and saturation.

CN: Physiological integrity; CL: Analyze

67. **4.** Urinary retention is common following abdominal surgery. The nurse should first assist the client to an anatomically comfortable position to void before resorting to other strategies such as cauterization. If the client is unable to void, the nurse can use a bladder scanner to determine the volume of retained urine, and then, if necessary, use an intermittent urinary catheter. While increasing fluid intake is important, it will not help the client void now.

CN: Basic care and comfort; CL: Analyze

68. **4.** Following surgery, clients are at risk for respiratory complications and should take the necessary actions to prevent these. The nurse should first be sure that the client understands how to do the exercises and the potential complications if they are not done. It is not the spouse's responsibility to make the client do the exercise, but they can help. Increasing fluid intake and frequent turning are appropriate, but these measures are not sufficient for aerating the lungs.

CN: Health promotion and maintenance; CL: Analyze

69. **1.** The nurse should first try to facilitate the client's ability to void by having the client stand at the bedside and use the urinal. Pouring running water over the perineum is a strategy that could be used if the client cannot void in a standing position. Ambulation will not help the client void. If such conservative methods fail, the nurse should obtain a prescription to catheterize the client, but an indwelling urinary catheter increases the risk for urinary tract infection because microbes ascend the catheter and travel to the bladder.

CN: Reduction of risk potential; CL: Analyze

70. **4.** The first cognitive response that returns after anesthesia is orientation to person. The nurse assesses this by asking the client his name. Orientation to place and time usually occurs after orientation by the nurse because of confusion from anesthesia and waking in an unfamiliar place. The nurse can then continue to assess and document the client's cognitive ability to remember information. The nurse does not need to notify the surgeon. The client's cognitive response is normal. It is not necessary to ask the spouse to reorient the client; however, the spouse can continue to talk to the client and help them regain consciousness.

CN: Physiological adaptation; CL: Analyze

71. **3.** Potassium in an IV solution may be irritating to a vein. The nurse should assess the IV site before taking any of the other actions listed. The infusion may have to be slowed or stopped and the HCP contacted. An outdated parenteral fluid setup does not cause pain, but it may be a source of infection.

CN: Pharmacological and parenteral therapies; CL: Analyze

72. **2.** The client's body temperature dropped 2.5°F (1.4°C) from the preoperative to postoperative phase. The client lost heat during the preoperative period. The client has not had time to regain the heat they lost and should not be discharged postoperatively until their postoperative vital signs, which include body temperature, are closer to their preoperative vital signs. The client's pulse rate, respiratory rate, and blood pressure have compensated according to the client's hypothermic state and will reflect changes as the client warms up. There are no indications that the client needs more pain medication, oxygen, or IV fluids.

CN: Physiological adaptation; CL: Analyze

73. **3.** The client still has a respiratory rate of 8 breaths/min; the nurse should first assist the client to sit and stimulate the client to take deep breaths and cough. This action will also help the nurse to determine what the client's level of sedation is; if the client is too sedated to cooperate with coughing and deep breathing, it will be important to slow or stop the infusion of narcotics and to consider contacting the HCP for a prescription for naloxone. The client is still breathing, so it is not necessary to call the rapid response team.

CN: Physiologic adaptation; CL: Analyze

74. **3.** The nurse is helping the client manage pain and comfort level. The nurse has completed the assessment of the client and should now dim the lights and create a quiet environment. Such nonpharmacologic measures as adjusting the light level in the room facilitate pain management.

Decreasing stimulation from the environment, such as brightness to the optic nerve, promotes the client's ability to relax skeletal muscles and fall asleep. It is too soon to reassess vital signs. Checking that the family is comfortable is important, but it is not the next thing to do for this client. Increasing the oxygen flow rate is not indicated and, if needed, should have been done before repositioning the client.

🔑 CN: Management of care; CL: Analyze

75. **4.** When a client has a temperature of 100°F (37.8°C) or higher in the first 24 hours after surgery, the temperature elevation is usually related to atelectasis. Because this client had upper abdominal surgery with manipulation around the diaphragm, the client is more prone to guarding the operative site and shallow breathing. Encouraging the client to take deep breaths is an appropriate measure to prevent atelectasis and pulmonary infection. Changing the client's position from lying to sitting for deep breathing will expand the alveoli in the lower posterior lobes. There is no indication that a surgical wound infection is occurring. An antibiotic is not indicated at this time. Pain medication will decrease respirations, and the client is not indicating pain at the moment.

🔑 CN: Physiological adaptation; CL: Analyze

76. **3.** The client must be able to verbalize understanding about receiving no more pain medication than is prescribed no matter how many times the button is pushed. Only the client should press the button for the PCA. The client should administer the pain medication when the pain is first noticed, well before the pain is out of control. One of the advantages of the PCA is that the amount of pain medication is controlled; therefore, overdosing is not a client concern when using a PCA.

🔑 CN: Pharmacological and parenteral therapies; CL: Evaluate

77. **3.** The nurse should take the client's blood pressure. The client is likely experiencing orthostatic hypotension. The PCA pump does not need to be discontinued because as soon as the blood pressure stabilizes the pain medication can be resumed. Administering oxygen is not necessary unless the oxygen saturation also drops. The client should sit in the chair until the blood pressure stabilizes.

🔑 CN: Pharmacological and parenteral therapies; CL: Analyze

78. **3.** Urinary catheters should be limited in use and duration only as needed for client care. The guideline also specifies that if used, the catheter should be inserted using aseptic technique, secured to provide unobstructed flow and drainage, and maintained in a way that protects the sterility of the catheter and the drainage system. It is not necessary to provide catheter care or cleanse the meatus as these can be a source of introducing an infection; it is not necessary to check for bladder distention if the catheter is draining correctly.

🔑 CN: Safety and infection control; CL: Analyze

79. **4, 1, 3, 2.** The client must first splint the incision to avoid increased pain, so the client can take deep breaths. The next step is to inhale oxygen to expand the alveoli for a few seconds and then exhale carbon dioxide in successive steps 5 to 10 times. The client should try to cough at the end of the exhalation to remove retained secretions from the larger airways.

🔑 CN: Reduction of risk potential; CL: Analyze

80. **3.** The client who had a repair of carpal tunnel syndrome under local anesthesia has not had the gag reflex anesthetized because the area being anesthetized was the tissue in the wrist. Therefore, this client would not have delayed fluid restrictions. The client who had a bronchoscopy received a local anesthetic on the vocal cords, and the nurse should check the gag reflex or ability to swallow before administering fluids. Clients who had general anesthesia or intravenous conscious sedation received medication for central nervous system sedation, and the nurse should assess the level of consciousness and ability to swallow before administering fluids.

🔑 CN: Reduction of risk potential; CL: Analyze

81. **3.** The client is experiencing activity intolerance, which is common following the first ambulation following surgery. The nurse should allow the client to rest and continue to monitor vital signs. Since the client is not dizzy or in pain, the nurse should wait to see if the client recovers from ambulating and reports having pain before administering pain medication. There is no need to request different activity prescriptions; it will still be important for the client to ambulate. The client is not having chest pain; it is not necessary to obtain a 12-lead ECG.

🔑 CN: Basic care and comfort; CL: Analyze

82. **3.** When the urine output is less than 30 mL per hour, the nurse should assess for potential causes such as hypovolemia or hemorrhage. The nurse should assess and evaluate the client's vital signs, intake and output, dressing, and available laboratory values and notify the health care provider. Bowel obstruction, though possible after surgery, is characterized most notably by abdominal distention and absent bowel sounds, not decreased urine output. The nurse would not expect the client to have hypertension, but rather hypotension.

🔑 CN: Physiological adaptation; CL: Analyze

83. **3.** A client who had a left thoracoscopy is placed in the lateral position, in which the most common injury is an injury to the brachial plexus. Numbness and tingling in the arm suggest a brachial plexus injury. There is no undue pressure on the ankles or knees during thoracic surgery.

🔑 CN: Physiological adaptation; CL: Analyze

84. **2, 3, 5, 6.** The client should be in an upright position when using the spirometer. The client should exhale fully prior to using the spirometer and then inhale to expand the lungs and continue inhaling for 3 more seconds. The client should relax and exhale before inhaling for the next use of the spirometer. The client should cough and clear retained secretions following the use of the spirometer. The client should use the spirometer every 2 hours during the immediate postoperative period.

🔑 CN: Physiological adaptation; CL: Evaluate

85. **3.** The nurse should inform the client that as the incision heals, uneven lumps might appear under the incision line because the collagen is growing new tissue at different rates. Eventually, the lumps will even out, and the tissue will be smooth. The client can touch the incision with clean hands as needed to perform incisional care. The client should not clean the incision with hydrogen peroxide because it may dry out the natural skin oils. The surgeon will remove the staples for the client.

🔑 CN: Reduction of risk potential; CL: Analyze

86. **2.** When a wound eviscerates (abdominal organs protruding through the opened incision), the nurse should cover the open area with a sterile dressing moistened with sterile normal saline and then cover it with a dry dressing. The surgeon should then be notified to take the client back to the operating room to close the incision under general anesthesia. The nurse should not press the emergency alarm because this is not a cardiac or respiratory arrest. The nurse should have the visitors and family leave the room to decrease the chance of airborne contamination, but the primary focus should be on covering the wound with a moist, sterile covering.

🔑 CN: Safety and infection control; CL: Analyze

87. **4.** The findings (WBC count above normal; inflammation and drainage at the incision site; and an elevated temperature) indicate that the client has an infection. The nurse should first notify the HCP. Encouraging fluids will be helpful, but it is not the first action. The nurse should not cleanse the site or place a dressing over the incision until the HCP writes a prescription to do so.

🔑 CN: Physiological adaptation; CL: Analyze

88. **3.** The client is receiving oxygen using a partial rebreathing mask, which is positioned correctly. The correct flow rate for this type of oxygen mask is 6 to 10 L of oxygen per minute. To be effective, the mask must cover the client's face. The elastic band must be tight enough to secure the mask. When used correctly, the reservoir bag should inflate during the inspiratory phase.

🔑 CN: Physiological adaptation; CL: Analyze

89. **4.** A wet-to-dry dressing should be able to dry out between dressing changes. Thus, the dressing should be moist, not dry, when applied. As the moist dressing dries, the wound will be debrided of necrotic tissue and exudate. Normal saline is most commonly used to moisten the sponge; Burow's solution will irritate the wound. The sponge should not be packed into the wound tightly because the circulation to the site could be impaired. The moist sponge should be placed so that all surfaces of the wound are in contact with the dressing. Then the sponge is covered and protected by a dry sterile dressing to prevent contamination from the external environment.

🔑 CN: Safety and infection control; CL: Analyze

90. **1.** Common client misconceptions regarding pain and pain medication administration include a concern that taking pain medication regularly will lead to addiction. However, this misconception overstates the risk for addiction and greatly understates the risk for immobility due to poor pain control, including atelectasis, decubitus formation, and delayed healing. The nurse should assist the client to understand the importance of adequate pain medication to support and promote client mobilization following surgery and client/family satisfaction with care. There is a potential for dependence and addiction with all narcotic drugs, though this is not likely during the postoperative period.

🔑 CN: Basic care and comfort; CL: Analyze

91. **3.** After emptying a Jackson-Pratt drainage bulb, the nurse should compress the bulb, plug it to establish suction, and then document the amount and type of drainage emptied. Irrigating a Jackson-Pratt drain is inappropriate because it could contaminate the wound. The Jackson-Pratt drain is not usually connected to wall suction. The purpose of the Jackson-Pratt drain is to remove bloody drainage from the deep tissues of the incision; clamping the drain would be counterproductive.

  CN: Safety and infection control; CL: Analyze

92. 1. Performing leg exercises, including ankle pumping, ankle rotation, and quadriceps setting exercises, will help prevent stasis of blood in the lower extremities, which can lead to blood clot formation. Encouraging the client to cough and deep breathe is an important postoperative intervention; however, it is directed at preventing pneumonia, not pulmonary emboli. The nurse should not massage the calves because a deep vein thrombus could dislodge and travel to the pulmonary vasculature. Antiembolism stockings should be worn continuously during the postoperative period.

  CN: Physiological adaptation; CL: Analyze

93. 2. The nurse should first administer naloxone hydrochloride, which is the antidote for morphine sulfate. The signs of overdose on morphine sulfate are a respiration rate of 2 to 4 breaths/min, bradycardia, and hypotension. If the client does not respond, the nurse can call the rapid response team. The client's respirations should improve after receiving the naloxone. If it becomes necessary for the nurse to call the rapid response team, they can determine if the client requires rescue breaths or CPR.

  CN: Pharmacological and parenteral therapies; CL: Analyze

94. 4. The device is applied correctly, and the nurse should ensure the client's comfort. The client's legs should remain extended as shown while using the device; the legs may be elevated, but it is not necessary to elevate the client's legs. The device should be placed directly on the client's legs; it is not necessary to apply antiembolic stockings under them. The client may move in bed as needed; active and isometric movement is encouraged to promote blood flow.

  CN: Health promotion and maintenance; CL: Analyze

95. 2. The client admitted for same-day surgery should not drive home after the surgical procedure because it is unsafe. Even without an anesthetic, the surgical event can be more stressful than anticipated. It is acceptable to have someone arrive after the surgery has started to take the client home. A taxi is permissible but not desirable.

  CN: Safety and infection control; CL: Evaluate

96. 3. The urine output does not have to be checked every 15 minutes for a client who has had an arthroscopy because this client probably does not have a catheter in place. If the client voids, the output would be recorded. Assessments every 15 minutes during the first hour would include vital signs, pulse oximeter values, and pain to monitor the client's comfort level and check for compartment syndrome. Neurovascular checks distal to the operative site are especially vital because a tourniquet was used proximal to the operative site during the surgical procedure and because edema may develop during the postoperative period.

  CN: Reduction of risk potential; CL: Analyze

97. 2. Hypotension and tachycardia are common adverse effects of droperidol and should be monitored closely by the nurse. Hypotension and tachycardia are not common adverse effects of ondansetron hydrochloride, prochlorperazine, or promethazine.

  CN: Pharmacological and parenteral therapies; CL: Analyze

98. 1. The nurse should assess but not disturb the epidural dressing because the catheter can be easily dislodged and organisms can easily be transmitted into the central nervous system. The nurse should not have to change the dressing at all if a waterproof dressing is applied over the epidural site. Even with strict aseptic technique, a drain into a sterile cavity is a direct route for transmission of organisms and places a client at increased risk for infection, and the nurse should not handle the dressing or the catheter.

  CN: Pharmacological and parenteral therapies; CL: Apply

99. 2. The client who has epidural pain management postoperatively can ambulate because a low concentration of local analgesia causes sensory blockage only. The catheter is placed so that constant pain management plus patient-controlled administration of an analgesic dose can block sensory innervation. Motor function should not be affected since the catheter is placed above the dura lining the spinal fluid. If the catheter would move through the dura sac, spinal analgesia would occur, affecting motor function as well as sympathetic nervous system function.

  CN: Pharmacological and parenteral therapies; CL: Apply

100. 3. Portable wound suction units can be emptied and drained. The nurse should compress the unit after emptying to create suction before reinserting the plug. It is normal for the suction unit to be full

6 hours after surgery, and the nurse does not need to notify the surgeon. The drainage unit should be emptied when full or every 8 hours. The drain in the incision should remain in place until the surgeon removes it. While all drainage should be noted as output on the medical record, recording the amount without emptying the drainage unit is not accurate, nor is it safe practice.

🗝️ CN: Safety and infection control; CL: Analyze

101. 1. The nurse should ask the client about having a bowel movement because acetaminophen with hydrocodone is an opioid, which can be constipating. By the third day, many clients become constipated and are feeling distended, with sharp, cramping pain due to gas, which is treated with ambulation, not more opioids. The client's emptying the bladder should not affect the pain level. The nurse should look at the client's medical record to determine when the client's last dose of pain medication was administered, rather than asking the client. The client's statement regarding the pain level before the surgery is not relevant to whether the nurse should administer the acetaminophen and hydrocodone.

🗝️ CN: Physiological adaptation; CL: Analyze

102. 1. Blood and serous fluid is drained from the operative site to prevent hematoma formation or a collection of fluid that could become a site for infection. This also minimizes postoperative swelling, which can be painful. A simple explanation such as this is appropriate because the client is just waking up from surgery. Blood from the operative site can be collected through an autotransfusion system so that it can be transfused to the client during or immediately after surgery. However, strict guidelines about the volume of blood lost, how quickly the device fills, and how long the blood has been out of the client's body govern whether the blood can be transfused. Therefore, although it is possible that the drainage system to which the client refers is an autotransfusion system, it is more likely that the client has a simple Hemovac drain. It is incorrect to tell a client not to worry about something even if they are in the drowsy state of awakening from anesthesia. It is inappropriate to ignore the client and give the client something to make them drowsy instead of addressing their concerns.

🗝️ CN: Psychosocial integrity; CL: Analyze

103. 1. The purpose of the Jackson-Pratt drainage tube is to drain off the purulent drainage from the sterile peritoneal cavity and prevent peritonitis. A Jackson-Pratt drain cannot prevent bleeding. The Jackson-Pratt drain has no effect on pressure on the bladder. There is no reason to be concerned about pressure on the gallbladder.

🗝️ CN: Reduction of risk potential; CL: Apply

104. 2. Biliary drainage tubes (T-tubes) are placed in the common bile duct and drain bile, which is dark yellow-orange. Serosanguineous drainage is thin and pinkish red. Bile is not clear and is not green unless it comes in contact with gastric fluid.

🗝️ CN: Reduction of risk potential; CL: Analyze

105. 1. Urinary elimination in the first 8 hours postoperatively is a requirement before the client who has had an inguinal hernia repair can be discharged from same-day surgery. Ingestion of fluids without nausea and vomiting is important, but eating solid foods is not a requirement for discharge from same-day surgery. Being completely pain free is an unrealistic expectation for the time frame and is not a requirement for leaving same-day surgery. However, the client should be comfortable, and their pain should be controlled. It is not a requirement for the client to ambulate in the hallway, but the client should be able to sit up and go to the bathroom without assistance.

🗝️ CN: Reduction of risk potential; CL: Analyze

106. 3. The ability to self-administer the drug is a requirement for the client to use PCA. Having a family member or advance directives is not a requirement for initiating PCA. The nurse teaches the client about how to use PCA and monitors the effectiveness of the pain medication; however, it is not necessary for the nurse to assist with the administration of the drug.

🗝️ CN: Pharmacological and parenteral therapies; CL: Evaluate

107. 1. The client's systolic blood pressure is dropping, and the pulse pressure is narrowing, indicating impending shock. The nurse should immediately notify the HCP. Elevating the head of the bed will not increase blood pressure. Administering pain medication could cause the blood pressure to drop further. It is not necessary to activate the rapid response team unless the client's vital signs change before the HCP evaluates the client.

🗝️ CN: Reduction of risk potential; CL: Analyze

108. 1. The client who has been positioned in the lithotomy position under general anesthesia may experience discomfort in the shoulders postoperatively because the client is placed in the

Trendelenburg position to expose the perineal area. The client's weight is then shifted toward the shoulders, and the client experiences muscle soreness postoperatively. Although there may be pressure on the nerves in the thighs, legs, or feet from pressure from the stirrups, there should be no discomfort if the stirrups are well padded.

CN: Basic care and comfort; CL: Apply

109. -/+ **1, 3, 4.** After surgery, the nurse should administer pain medication before assisting the client to take deep breaths and expectorate retained secretions. The client should use the incentive spirometer every 2 to 4 hours. The nurse should monitor the client's breath sounds and temperature to detect early signs of infection. The nurse should assist with early ambulation. The client should drink a minimum of 10 cups (about 1 L) of fluid per day (not 4 cups [1 L]) to keep secretions liquefied and easier to cough up and eliminate from the upper respiratory tract. Placing this client in a prone position will limit the ability to expand the chest when breathing.

CN: Reduction of risk potential; CL: Analyze

110. 3. The client should sit in an upright position when doing breathing exercises to allow for full chest expansion of both lungs and all fields and bases. Using an incentive spirometer every hour while awake is appropriate and allows the client visual feedback. Placing their hands lightly over the lower ribs and upper abdomen allows the client to see muscles of inspiration and expiration and is appropriate. Coughing deeply from the lungs after four deep breaths allows the client to effectively cough up secretions.

CN: Reduction of risk potential; CL: Evaluate

111. 2. Muscle cramping is a sign of hypokalemia. Potassium is an electrolyte lost with nasogastric suctioning. Confusion is seen with hypercalcemia. Edema is seen with protein deficit or fluid volume overload. Tremors are seen with hypomagnesemia.

CN: Reduction of risk potential; CL: Analyze

Legal and Ethical Issues Associated with Surgery

112. 3. The most critical piece of information is the client identification bracelet. Misidentification of clients can result in serious harm to the client. The nurse also needs the admitting records and any preprinted labels as part of verifying the client's identification. The location of the family is not included in verifying identification.

CN: Reduction of risk potential; CL: Analyze

113. 2. While laws in states and provinces may vary, generally, when the client cannot sign the operative consent and it is a true lifesaving emergency, consent may be obtained over the telephone from the client's next of kin or guardian. The surgeon must obtain the telephone consent, but if it is a true lifesaving emergency, the surgeon often is already in surgery, so the nurse makes the telephone call, and another nurse witnesses the call. Some institutions have a special consent form for emergency surgery. Consent can be waived in situations in which no family is available; however, if the family can be reached by telephone before surgery, verbal consent is legally required.

CN: Management of care; CL: Analyze

114. 3. There are risks with both the surgical procedure and the general anesthesia required for a craniotomy. The risks involved in the procedure are a part of the informed consent. Other information that is part of an informed consent includes potential complications, expected benefits, the inability of the surgeon to predict results, the irreversibility of the procedure (if applicable), and other available treatments. Talking about the effects of diabetes on healing, explaining how the craniotomy is performed, and explaining the consequences of declining treatment (e.g., death if the tumor is not removed) represent appropriate actions to provide information to the client.

CN: Management of care; CL: Evaluate

115. 3. The surgeon is responsible for explaining the surgical procedure to be performed and the risks of the procedure, as well as for obtaining informed consent from the client. A nurse may be responsible for obtaining and witnessing a client's signature on the consent form. The nurse is the client's advocate, verifying that a client (or family member) understands the consent form and its implications and that consent for the surgery is truly voluntary.

CN: Reduction of risk potential; CL: Apply

116. 2. When the client cannot read or write, the consent can be read to the client, and the client can sign in the presence of two witnesses. The client (not the next of kin) should always sign for self unless they are a minor or not of sound mind. The court does not appoint a guardian for a person of sound mind just because they cannot read or write. Hospital personnel would not and could not sign a consent form for a client.

 CN: Management of care; CL: Apply

Managing Care, Quality, and Safety of Adults Having Surgery

117. 1, 2, 3. Clients who have diabetes mellitus controlled by diet, those with a high stress response to surgery, or those who have been on steroid treatment for the last 3 months should have their serum glucose level assessed. A client with a family history of diabetes receiving D_5LR IV fluids does not need to have the serum glucose level checked unless other clinical manifestations are present. The client who has a high-carbohydrate diet should be able to metabolize the glucose unless there are other health problems.

 CN: Reduction of risk potential; CL: Analyze

118. 1. Clients who have had long-term multiple exposures to latex products, such as would occur with six previous surgeries and recoveries, are at increased risk for latex allergies. The nurse should explore what types of surgeries these were, how involved the client's recoveries were, and whether signs of latex allergies have occurred in the past. Working as a sales clerk, having type 2 diabetes, and undergoing laser surgery do not expose a client to latex or increase the risk for latex allergy.

 CN: Safety and infection control; CL: Analyze

119. 1, 2, 3, 4. The root cause of wrong-site surgery involves a breakdown in communication between the client and family and the health care team. Information retrieved from the client in the preoperative assessment, such as the client's name, surgical site, and procedure, should be verbally assessed and verified with medical records and radiographic diagnostic reports. This information should be compiled in a checklist that the intraoperative team can recheck, thus avoiding unnecessary distraction and delay in the operating room. The nurse in the operating room is responsible for calling a time-out so that every surgical team member can double-check the correct site of surgery, verify the site using the operative consent form, and verify that the surgeon has marked the operative site on the client. Showing the client an anatomic model will assist the client in understanding the location of the surgery, but it will not prevent anyone from identifying the wrong site on the client.

 CN: Safety and infection control; CL: Apply

120. 4. The nurse should first contact the HCP because the prescription for the morphine is not complete. The Joint Commission of the United States and the Institute for Safe Medication Practices Canada recommend not to use MSO_4 because it can apply to morphine as well as to magnesium sulfate. There is no mention of an IV system being needed. The morphine should not be in the medication cabinet because the prescription is not complete. Although the pharmacy staff may offer a suggestion as to what the medication prescribed is, the best means to confirm the intent of the prescription is to contact the HCP who wrote the prescription.

 CN: Safety and infection control; CL: Analyze

121. 4. The nurse should first call the RRT or the medical emergency team that provides a team approach to evaluate and treat immediately clients with alterations in vital signs or neurologic deterioration. The client's vital signs have changed since the client was in the PACU, and immediate action is required to manage the changes; the staff in PACU are not responsible for managing care once the client is transferred to the surgical unit. The respiratory therapist may be a part of the RRT but should not be called first.

 CN: Safety and infection control; CL: Analyze

122. 4. The anesthesiologist who administers the anesthetic agent and monitors the client's physical status throughout the surgery must have knowledge of all known allergies for client safety. The completed record (with the preoperative checklist) must be available to all members of the surgical team, and any unusual last-minute observations that may have a bearing on anesthesia or surgery are noted prominently at the front of the medical record. The nurse should first notify the anesthesiologist of the allergy; it is not the nurse's responsibility to withhold the preoperative medications unless the anesthesiologist rewrites the preoperative orders. The nurse in the scrub role provides sterile instruments and supplies to the surgeon during the procedure and does not determine if the client's allergy will cause the surgery to be canceled.

 CN: Safety and infection control; CL: Analyze

123. 1, 2, 4. Nurses can delegate to the UAP the tasks of observing clients and promoting their comfort following surgery as well as emptying and measuring urinary catheter drainage bags. UAPs cannot teach clients; that is the responsibility of the registered nurse (RN) or respiratory therapist. UAPs cannot assess IV insertion sites, which is the responsibility of an RN.

🔑 CN: Management of care; CL: Analyze

124. **2.** The client must have an identification bracelet properly secured on the wrist before being transported to the operating room to ensure correct identification. It is incorrect to send the client without a properly secured identification bracelet. The perioperative nurse must verify the client's identification by checking for the same name on the medical record, armband, and schedule and by the client's statement. The preoperative nurse may be asked to physically identify the client and obtain a new armband.

🔑 CN: Management of care; CL: Analyze

125. **3.** The client is experiencing a fluid overload and has vital signs that are outside of normal limits. The provider must be notified of the client's current status. It would be appropriate to recommend the provider administer a diuretic to correct the fluid overload. It is not appropriate to administer an antihypertensive medication or administer more fluids. It may be appropriate to administer additional oxygen, but because of the fluid volume excess the client exhibits, diuretic administration is most important.

🔑 CN: Physiologic adaptation; CL: Analyze

126. **4, 2, 1, 3.** The nurse should first notify the HCP of the high serum potassium level. A normal serum potassium level is 3.5 to 5.0 mEq/L; a level of 6.2 mEq/L must be called to the HCP immediately because hyperkalemia may cause serious cardiac arrhythmias, potentially leading to death if left untreated. The nurse should next assess the client who has been vomiting and if necessary contact the HCP for a prescription for an antiemetic if none has been prescribed. After assessing all clients, the nurse should discuss the plan for the day, with the UAP delegating duties as appropriate. Though the client is eager to go home, the discharge paperwork must wait until all clients have been assessed and immediate needs met.

🔑 CN: Reduction of risk potential; CL: Analyze

127. **4.** Maintenance of IV sites and systems includes regular assessment and rotation of the site and periodic changes of the dressing, solution, and tubing; these measures help prevent complications. The nurse should also observe the solution for discoloration, turbidity, and particulates. An IV solution is changed every 24 hours or as needed, and because the nurse noted an abnormal color, the nurse should change the bag of D_5W and note this on an incident report. It is not necessary to verify this action with another nurse. Paging the HCP is not necessary; maintaining the IV and using the correct solutions is a nursing responsibility. Although the first action is to hang a new bag, hospital policy should be followed if there is a question as to whether there could have been an unknown substance in the bag that caused it to change color.

🔑 CN: Safety and infection control; CL: Analyze

128. -/+ **1, 2, 3, 4, 5, 6.** The venipuncture site must be assessed for signs of infection (redness and pain at the puncture site), infiltration (coolness, blanching, and edema at the site), and thrombophlebitis (redness, firmness, pain along the path of the vein, and edema).

🔑 CN: Pharmacological and parenteral therapies; CL: Analyze

129. **2.** In any situation that involves a medication error, the nurse first assesses the client immediately to determine any changes in condition and the need for urgent interventions. Calling the HCP or administering an antidote is not done until the client is assessed and the necessary data are gathered. The nurse finding the error can complete an incident report after the client's safety is established and any emergency treatments are completed.

🔑 CN: Management of care; CL: Analyze

130. -/+ **1, 2, 4.** When a time-out is called prior to surgery, the surgical team must read back all prescriptions, verify the correct site, identify the client again, and double-check the echocardiogram. The sterile field has not been disrupted and does not need to be set up again. It is not necessary to obtain another x-ray as long as the confusion is clarified and the surgical team is satisfied that all are ready to begin the surgery.

🔑 CN: Management of care; CL: Apply

131. -/+ **1, 2, 4, 5.** Transfer reports must include information about the client's surgery; all current treatments and medications; vital signs, including pain level; fluid status, including blood loss; and current intravenous infusions. It is not necessary to identify the surgeons who were present during the surgery.

🔑 CN: Management of care; CL: Apply

132. -/+ **2, 3, 5, 6.** Using SBAR, the nurse informs the surgeon of the current situation (chest pains), the background (history of myocardial infarction), and assessment (chest pains, vital signs changes, likelihood of having a myocardial infarction). The nurse should also discuss recommendations and suggestions for prescriptions such as the ECG and nitroglycerin. The nurse is focusing on the chest pain and change in vital signs and communicating recommendations for managing the chest pain; it is not necessary to report at this time that the client has been NPO or the type of surgery the client will have.

CN: Management of care; CL: Analyze

133. **4.** Temperature variation in the postoperative period provides valuable information about a client's status. Fever may occur at any time during the postoperative period. A mild elevation (up to 100.4°F [38°C]) during the first 48 hours usually reflects the surgical stress response. After the first 48 hours, a moderate to marked elevation (higher than 99.9°F [37°C]) is usually caused by infection. It is not appropriate to do any of the other options to lower a client's temperature at this time.

CN: Management of care; CL: Analyze

134. **2, 5.** The UAP can assist clients with ambulation and take vital signs. It is within the registered nurse's scope of practice to teach the client to administer insulin, change dressings, and administer tube feedings.

CN: Management of care; CL: Analyze

135. **4, 5.** The nurse may delegate to the UAP emptying the closed drainage system and recording the output to the unlicensed assistive personnel. A closed drainage system, such as a Jackson-Pratt drain or Hemovac drain, is anchored to the skin with one or more sutures. However, open-drainage systems, such as the Penrose drain, are not anchored to the skin. For this type of drain, it is important for the nurse to care for the drain so as to prevent inadvertent dislodgment. Assessing and documenting the drain site is a nursing responsibility.

CN: Management of Care; CL: Analyze

136. **3.** The most effective way for the nurse to teach the client how to change the dressing and determine that the client has understood the directions for changing the dressing is to use a "teach-back" approach. Demonstrating the procedure and then asking the client to do the procedure ensures that the client will be able to do the procedure at home. Asking an interpreter to translate verbal instructions does not offer the opportunity for the client to perform the procedure and for the nurse to give feedback. Although showing a video on the client's phone or using an illustrated handout will provide a helpful review for the client, the nurse needs to verify that the client can perform the procedure.

CN: Health promotion and maintenance; CL: Analyze

137. **1.** Making appointments and navigating the health care system is a major obstacle for non–English-speaking clients. To support ongoing care management, the nurse can help the client by making the appointment for the follow-up visit, and providing dates and times. Providing the reconciled medication list and obtaining the client's signature are part of the discharge process. Providing a copy of the discharge materials to the interpreter is not part of the discharge process and would be a violation of the Health Insurance Portability and Accountability Act (HIPAA).

CN: Reduction of risk; CL: Analyze

138. **1, 4, 3, 2.** The nurse establishes priorities based on airway, breathing, circulation, and disability as well as the immediacy of client needs. The client who is just returning from surgery needs to be assessed; the nurse will also need to check the IV. The client with cancer of the colon also needs to have vital signs, pain, and dressings checked; the tracheotomy is established, and in the report, there was no mention of distress. The client with the fractured hip is at risk for pressure ulcers and should be seen next. The nurse should then make rounds on the client with diabetes and schedule a time to continue teaching injection techniques at that time.

CN: Management of care; CL: Analyze

139. **4.** Although practices for signing informed consent documents may vary across practice jurisdictions, generally, the spouse or another responsible family member may sign the consent form for a client with dementia. The minister, supervisor, and attorney cannot provide legal consent for surgery for this client.

CN: Management of care; CL: Analyze

140. **1, 2, 4, 3.** The nurse should always work from the least contaminated to the most contaminated area. If the nurse picks up and disposes of the glove on the floor, the hands are contaminated, and the nurse will need to repeat hand hygiene before caring for the client. The nurse should first put on a new pair of clean gloves and then assess the client's surgical dressing. The nurse can next assist the client with using the urinal, and last, the nurse can pick up and dispose of the glove on the floor. It is more time efficient to dispose of fallen objects when all client care is complete unless the fallen object is required to proceed with client care.

CN: Safety and infection control; CL: Analyze

TEST 15: The Adult with Health Problems of the Eyes, Ears, Nose, and Throat

- The Adult with Cataracts
- The Adult with Retinal Detachment
- The Adult with Glaucoma
- The Adult with Adult Macular Degeneration
- The Adult Undergoing Nasal Surgery
- The Adult with a Hearing Disorder
- The Adult with Ménière's Disease
- The Adult with Cancer of the Larynx
- Managing Care, Quality, and Safety of Adults with Health Problems of the Eyes, Ears, Nose, and Throat
- Answers, Rationales, and Test-Taking Strategies

The Adult with Cataracts

1. The nurse is observing a spouse administer eye drops, as shown in the figure. What should the nurse instruct the spouse to do?

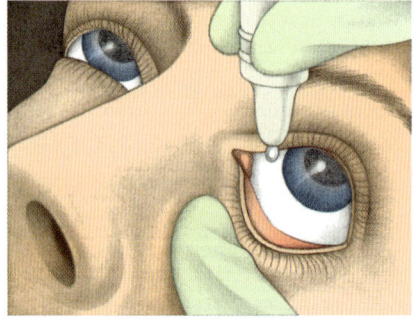

   ☐ 1. Move the dropper to the inner canthus.
   ☐ 2. Have the client raise their eyebrows.
   ☐ 3. Administer the drops in the center of the lower lid.
   ☐ 4. Have the client squeeze both eyes after administering the drops.

2. One day after cataract surgery, the client is having discomfort from bright light. What should the nurse advise the client to do?
   ☐ 1. Dim lights in the house, and stay inside for 1 week.
   ☐ 2. Attach sun shields to existing eyeglasses when in direct sunlight.
   ☐ 3. Use sunglasses that wrap around the side of the face when in bright light.
   ☐ 4. Patch the affected eye when in bright light.

3. The nurse is discharging a client who just had cataract removal and intraocular lens implantation. What statement(s) would indicate that the client understands discharge instructions? Select all that apply.
   ☐ 1. "I understand the schedule for my eye drops and will use the medications."
   ☐ 2. "I feel good and am ready to drive home now."
   ☐ 3. "I will call in the morning if I cannot see clearly."
   ☐ 4. "I will wear the eye shield at night to protect my eye."
   ☐ 5. "I will avoid lifting or pulling anything over 15 lb (6.8 kg)."
   ☐ 6. "I will call if I still have eye pain after taking acetaminophen."

4. A client is having a cataract removed and will use eyeglasses after the surgery. What information should the nurse include in the teaching plan? Select all that apply.
   ☐ 1. Images will appear one-third larger.
   ☐ 2. Look through the center of the glasses.
   ☐ 3. The changes will be immediate.
   ☐ 4. Use handrails when climbing stairs.
   ☐ 5. Stay out of the sun for 2 weeks.

5. The client has had a cataract removed. When explaining discharge instructions, the nurse should tell the client to perform which action?
   ☐ 1. Keep the head aligned straight.
   ☐ 2. Utilize bright lights in the home.
   ☐ 3. Use an eye shield at night.
   ☐ 4. Change the eye patch as needed.

6. A client with a cataract tells the nurse about being afraid of being awake during eye surgery. Which response by the nurse would be the **most** appropriate?
☐ 1. "Have you ever had any reactions to local anesthetics in the past?"
☐ 2. "What is it that disturbs you about the idea of being awake?"
☐ 3. "By using a local anesthetic, you will not have nausea and vomiting after the surgery."
☐ 4. "There is really nothing to fear about being awake. You will be given a medication that will help you relax."

7. A client tells the nurse that their vision is blurred and hazy throughout the entire day. What should the nurse recommend that the client do?
☐ 1. Purchase a pair of magnifying glasses.
☐ 2. Wear glasses with tinted lenses.
☐ 3. Schedule an appointment with an optician.
☐ 4. Schedule an appointment with an ophthalmologist.

8. The nurse is to instill drops of phenylephrine hydrochloride into the client's eye before cataract surgery. Which is the expected outcome?
☐ 1. dilation of the pupil and blood vessels
☐ 2. dilation of the pupil and constriction of blood vessels
☐ 3. constriction of the pupil and constriction of blood vessels
☐ 4. constriction of the pupil and dilation of blood vessels

9. A short time after cataract surgery, a client has nausea. What should the nurse do **first**?
☐ 1. Instruct the client to take a few deep breaths until the nausea subsides.
☐ 2. Explain that this is a common feeling that will pass quickly.
☐ 3. Tell the client to call the nurse promptly if vomiting occurs.
☐ 4. Medicate the client with an antiemetic, as prescribed.

10. The nurse is instructing a client about postoperative care following cataract removal. What position should the nurse teach the client to use?
☐ 1. Remain in a semi-Fowler position.
☐ 2. Position the feet higher than the body.
☐ 3. Lie on the operative side.
☐ 4. Place the head in a dependent position.

11. After returning home, a client who has had cataract surgery will need to continue to instill eye drops in the affected eye. The client is instructed to apply slight pressure against the nose at the inner canthus of the eye after instilling the eye drops. What is the expected outcome of applying pressure?
Pressure:
☐ 1. prevents the medication from entering the tear duct.
☐ 2. keeps the drug from running down the client's face.
☐ 3. allows the sensitive cornea to adjust to the medication.
☐ 4. facilitates the distribution of the medication over the eye surface.

12. The nurse is teaching a client who has had cataract surgery how to decrease intraocular pressure. What should the nurse instruct the client to avoid?
☐ 1. lying supine
☐ 2. coughing
☐ 3. deep breathing
☐ 4. ambulation

13. After cataract-removal surgery on the left eye, the client sits up and reports having sharp pain in the operative eye. What should the nurse do **next**?
☐ 1. Cover the eye with a moist sterile sponge.
☐ 2. Administer eye drops for pain.
☐ 3. Have the client lie on the right side.
☐ 4. Contact the health care provider (HCP).

The Adult with Retinal Detachment

14. The client is diagnosed with a detached retina in the right eye. What should the nurse do **first**?
☐ 1. Apply compresses to the eye.
☐ 2. Instruct the client to lie prone.
☐ 3. Remove all bed pillows.
☐ 4. Promote measures that limit mobility.

15. The nurse is placing patches on both eyes of a client with detachment of the retina. What is the expected outcome of patching?
☐ 1. reduced rapid eye movements
☐ 2. decreased irritation caused by light entering the damaged eye
☐ 3. protection of the injured eye from infection
☐ 4. minimized eye strain on the uninvolved eye

16. The client with retinal detachment in the right eye is extremely apprehensive and tells the nurse, "I am afraid of going blind. It would be so hard to live that way." What factor should the nurse consider before responding to this statement?
- ☐ 1. Repeat surgery is impossible, so if this procedure fails, vision loss is inevitable.
- ☐ 2. The surgery will only delay blindness in the right eye, but vision is preserved in the left eye.
- ☐ 3. More and more services are available to help newly blind people adapt to daily living.
- ☐ 4. Optimism is justified because surgical treatment has a 90% to 95% success rate.

17. The nurse is teaching the client who has had laser surgery for retinal detachment. What should the nurse tell the client about activity while recovering from surgery?
The activity level is:
- ☐ 1. increased gradually; the client can resume usual activities in 5 to 6 weeks.
- ☐ 2. determined by the client's tolerance; clients can be as active as they wish.
- ☐ 3. restricted for about 2 months; the client should plan on being sedentary.
- ☐ 4. not restricted; clients can resume usual activities.

18. The nurse is planning care with a client who has undergone surgery for retinal detachment. Which goal is a **priority**?
- ☐ 1. Control pain.
- ☐ 2. Prevent an increase in intraocular pressure.
- ☐ 3. Cleanse the eye with soap and water.
- ☐ 4. Maintain a darkened environment.

The Adult with Glaucoma

19. A client with glaucoma is to receive 3 gtt of acetazolamide in the left eye. What should the nurse do?
- ☐ 1. Ask the client to close the right eye while administering the drug in the left eye.
- ☐ 2. Have the client look up while the nurse administers the eye drops.
- ☐ 3. Have the client lift the eyebrows while the nurse positions the hand with the dropper on the client's forehead.
- ☐ 4. Wipe the eyes with a tissue following administration of the drops.

20. A client who has been treated for chronic open-angle glaucoma (COAG) for 5 years asks the nurse, "How does glaucoma damage my eyesight?" What should the nurse tell the client?
"Your glaucoma:
- ☐ 1. results from chronic eye inflammation."
- ☐ 2. causes increased intraocular pressure."
- ☐ 3. leads to detachment of the retina."
- ☐ 4. is caused by decreased blood flow to the retina."

21. A client has chronic open-angle glaucoma (COAG). What should the nurse ask the client about when conducting a focused assessment?
- ☐ 1. eye pain
- ☐ 2. excessive lacrimation
- ☐ 3. colored light flashes
- ☐ 4. decreasing peripheral vision

22. A client is having an eye examination that will include tonometry. What information should the nurse provide when preparing the client for tonometry?
- ☐ 1. Oral pain medication will be given before the procedure.
- ☐ 2. It is a painless procedure with no adverse effects.
- ☐ 3. Blurred or double vision may occur after the procedure.
- ☐ 4. Medication will be given to dilate the pupils before the procedure.

23. A client uses timolol maleate eye drops. What is the expected outcome of this drug?
- ☐ 1. constricting the pupils
- ☐ 2. dilating the canals of Schlemm
- ☐ 3. reducing aqueous humor formation
- ☐ 4. improving the ability of the ciliary muscle to contract

24. The nurse observes the client instill eye drops. The client says, "I just try to hit the middle of my eyeball so the drops do not run out of my eye." What should the nurse tell the client about this method of instilling eye drops?
This method may cause:
- ☐ 1. scleral staining.
- ☐ 2. corneal injury.
- ☐ 3. excessive lacrimation.
- ☐ 4. systemic drug absorption.

25. The nurse is assessing a client who has acute angle-closure glaucoma. The nurse should determine if the client has experienced which symptom?
- ☐ 1. gradual loss of central vision
- ☐ 2. acute light sensitivity
- ☐ 3. loss of color vision
- ☐ 4. sudden eye pain

26. A client has been diagnosed with an acute episode of angle-closure glaucoma. The client asks the nurse what will be done. What should the nurse tell the client about this health problem?
Acute angle-closure glaucoma:
- ☐ 1. frequently resolves without treatment.
- ☐ 2. is typically treated with sustained bed rest.
- ☐ 3. is a medical emergency that can rapidly lead to blindness.
- ☐ 4. is most commonly treated with steroid therapy.

The Adult with Adult Macular Degeneration

27. The nurse is assessing a client with macular degeneration. The nurse should determine if the client is experiencing which symptom?
☐ 1. loss of central vision
☐ 2. loss of peripheral vision
☐ 3. total blindness
☐ 4. blurring of vision

28. A client has a history of macular degeneration. What is the **priority** nursing goal while the client is in the hospital?
☐ 1. Provide education regarding community services for clients with adult macular degeneration (AMD).
☐ 2. Provide health care related to monitoring the eye condition.
☐ 3. Promote a safe, effective care environment.
☐ 4. Improve vision.

29. The nurse is teaching a client with adult macular degeneration (AMD) about safety precautions. Which information should the nurse include in the teaching plan?
☐ 1. Wear a patch over one eye.
☐ 2. Place personal items on the sighted side.
☐ 3. Lie in bed with the unaffected side toward the door.
☐ 4. Turn the head from side to side when walking.

30. The nurse is assessing a client with macular degeneration. Identify the illustration that **best** depicts what clients with this disorder typically see.

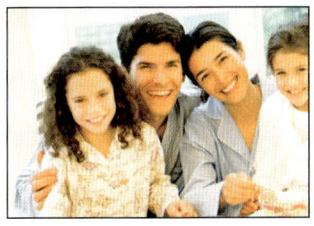 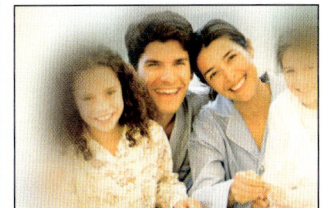
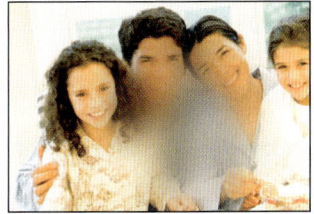 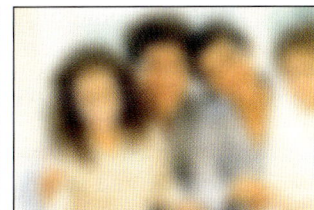

31. The nurse is assisting a client who has new-onset vision loss to transition to home from the hospital. The client can see shadows and light in the right eye only. When at home, what is the client's **greatest** risk?
☐ 1. loss of sensory perception
☐ 2. injury from falls
☐ 3. denial of changes in vision
☐ 4. isolation from social activities

The Adult Undergoing Nasal Surgery

32. A young adult is admitted for elective nasal surgery for a deviated septum. Which sign would be an important indicator of bleeding even if the nasal drip pad remained dry and intact?
☐ 1. presence of nausea
☐ 2. repeated swallowing
☐ 3. rapid respiratory rate
☐ 4. feelings of anxiety

33. A client is ready for discharge after surgery for a deviated septum. Which instruction would be appropriate?
☐ 1. Avoid activities that elicit the Valsalva maneuver.
☐ 2. Take aspirin to control nasal discomfort.
☐ 3. Avoid brushing the teeth until the nasal packing is removed.
☐ 4. Apply heat to the nasal area to control swelling.

34. The nurse is teaching a client who had a repair of the nasal septum about postoperative care at home. Which statement indicates that the client has understood the discharge instructions?
☐ 1. "I shouldn't shower until my packing is removed."
☐ 2. "I will take stool softeners and modify my diet to prevent constipation."
☐ 3. "Coughing every 2 hours is important to prevent respiratory complications."
☐ 4. "It's important to blow my nose each day to remove the dried secretions."

The Adult with a Hearing Disorder

35. The nurse is entering the room of a client who is deaf. What should the nurse do **first**?
☐ 1. Knock on the room's door loudly.
☐ 2. Close and open the vertical blinds rapidly.
☐ 3. Talk while walking into the room.
☐ 4. Get the client's attention.

36. A 75-year-old client who has been taking furosemide regularly for 4 months tells the nurse about having trouble hearing. What should the nurse do?
☐ 1. Tell the client that at age 75 years, it is inevitable that there will be hearing loss.
☐ 2. Report the hearing loss to the health care provider.
☐ 3. Schedule the client for audiometric testing and a hearing aid.
☐ 4. Tell the client that the hearing loss is only temporary; when the body adjusts to the furosemide, hearing will improve.

37. The nurse is providing preoperative instructions to a client who is deaf. Which strategy is **most** effective in assuring that the client understands the information?
☐ 1. Stand in front of the client, and slowly explain the instructions.
☐ 2. Provide instructions to the spouse, and have the spouse explain them to the client.
☐ 3. Give the client written material to read, and follow up with time for questions.
☐ 4. Show the client a video with instructions.

38. A client who is prescribed by the health care provider (HCP) to take aspirin daily to prevent thrombus formation reports having ringing in their ears. The nurse advises the client to take which measure?
☐ 1. Increase fluid intake.
☐ 2. Stop taking the aspirin.
☐ 3. Use acetaminophen instead.
☐ 4. Contact the HCP.

39. The adult child of an older adult reports that their parent just "stares off into space" more and more in the last several months but then eagerly smiles and nods once the son can get their attention. What additional assessment should the nurse make to better understand the client's behavior?
☐ 1. dementia
☐ 2. hearing loss
☐ 3. frustration
☐ 4. depression

40. The nurse has been assigned to a client who is hearing impaired and reads speech. Which care measure(s) should the nurse incorporate when communicating with the client? Select all that apply.
☐ 1. Avoid being silhouetted against strong light.
☐ 2. Do not block out the person's view of the speaker's mouth.
☐ 3. Face the client when talking.
☐ 4. Have bright light behind so the individual can see.
☐ 5. Ensure the client is familiar with the subject material before discussing it.
☐ 6. Talk to the client while doing other nursing procedures.

41. The nurse is to instill ear drops in the client's left ear to soften cerumen. Which action(s) should the nurse take to instill the ear drops? Select all that apply.
☐ 1. Have the client lie in bed on the client's left side.
☐ 2. Place a pillow under the head.
☐ 3. Pull the ear up and back.
☐ 4. Warm the ear drops to body temperature by holding the bottle in the hand.
☐ 5. Allow the ear drops to remain in the ear for 2 to 5 minutes.

42. What should the nurse instruct a client who has cerumen buildup in the ear to do? Select all that apply.
☐ 1. Wash the external ear with a washcloth.
☐ 2. Instill cerumenolytic drops in the ear canal.
☐ 3. Use cotton-tipped applicators to remove the wax from the ear canal.
☐ 4. Use small forceps to extract the wax.
☐ 5. Irrigate the ear with sterile water after softening the wax with a cerumenolytic solution.

43. A client is about to have a tympanoplasty and asks the nurse what the surgical procedure involves. What should the nurse do **first** when answering the question?
☐ 1. Assess the client's understanding of what the health care provider has explained.
☐ 2. Describe the surgical procedure.
☐ 3. Tell the client that the procedure will close the perforation and prevent recurrent infection.
☐ 4. Explain that the procedure will improve hearing.

44. An older adult takes two 81-mg aspirin tablets daily to prevent a heart attack. The client reports having a constant "ringing" in both ears. How should the nurse respond to the client's comment?
☐ 1. Tell the client that ringing in the ears is associated with the aging process.
☐ 2. Refer the client to have a Weber test.
☐ 3. Schedule the client for audiometric testing.
☐ 4. Explain to the client that the ringing may be related to the aspirin.

The Adult with Ménière's Disease

45. An older adult has vertigo accompanied by tinnitus as the result of Ménière's disease. The nurse should instruct the client to restrict which dietary element?
☐ 1. protein
☐ 2. potassium
☐ 3. fluids
☐ 4. sodium

46. A client has vertigo. Which goal(s) would be **most** appropriate to prevent injury related to altered immobility and gait disturbances? Select all that apply.
The client:
☐ 1. assumes a safe position when dizzy.
☐ 2. experiences no falls.
☐ 3. performs vestibular/balance exercises.
☐ 4. demonstrates family involvement.
☐ 5. keeps the head still when dizzy.

47. A client with Ménière's disease is instructed to modify their diet. The nurse should explain that what is the **most** frequently recommended diet modification for Ménière's disease?
☐ 1. low sodium
☐ 2. high protein
☐ 3. low carbohydrate
☐ 4. low fat

48. A client has asked the nurse about the expected course of Ménière's disease. The nurse should give the client which information?
☐ 1. "The disease process will gradually extend to the eyes."
☐ 2. "Control of the episodes is usually possible, but a cure is not yet available."
☐ 3. "Continued medication therapy will cure the disease."
☐ 4. "Bilateral deafness is an inevitable outcome of the disease."

49. The risk for injury during an attack of Ménière's disease is high. The nurse should instruct the client to take which **immediate** action when experiencing vertigo?
☐ 1. "Place your head between your knees."
☐ 2. "Concentrate on rhythmic deep breathing."
☐ 3. "Close your eyes tightly."
☐ 4. "Assume a reclining or flat position."

The Adult with Cancer of the Larynx

50. Following a laryngectomy, the nurse notices that the client has saliva collecting beneath the skin flaps. What should the nurse do **next**?
☐ 1. Place an absorbent dressing over the area.
☐ 2. Circle the area, and monitor it for increased accumulation of saliva.
☐ 3. Ask the client to expectorate the saliva into an emesis basin.
☐ 4. Notify the health care provider (HCP).

51. The nurse is developing a care plan with a client who had a laryngectomy 3 days ago. What step(s) should the nurse take to assure adequate client nutrition? Select all that apply.
☐ 1. Weigh weekly and report weight loss.
☐ 2. When eating, sit and lean slightly forward.
☐ 3. Have the serum albumin level checked regularly.
☐ 4. Receive enteral tube feedings as prescribed.
☐ 5. Manipulate the nasogastric tube daily.

52. The client with a laryngectomy is being discharged. The nurse should determine that the client understands the need for which self-care measure(s)? Select all that apply.
☐ 1. Provide humidification in the home.
☐ 2. Use a protective shield over the stoma for bathing.
☐ 3. Consume a liberal intake of fluids (8 to 12 cups [about 2 to 3 L] a day).
☐ 4. Limit spicy seasonings on food.
☐ 5. Follow a low-fiber diet.

53. After a total laryngectomy, a client has a feeding tube. What is the purpose of the feeding tube? The feeding tube:
☐ 1. provides nutrition.
☐ 2. minimizes aspiration.
☐ 3. prevents fistula formation.
☐ 4. maintains an open airway.

54. The nurse is planning care with a client who 2 days earlier had a total laryngectomy with creation of a new tracheostomy. Which is a **priority** goal for the client?
☐ 1. Decrease secretions.
☐ 2. Learn to care for the tracheostomy.
☐ 3. Relieve anxiety related to the tracheostomy.
☐ 4. Maintain a patent airway.

Managing Care, Quality, and Safety of Adults with Health Problems of the Eyes, Ears, Nose, and Throat

55. A client with glaucoma is scheduled for a hip replacement. Which prescription would require clarification before the nurse carries it out?
☐ 1. Administer morphine sulfate.
☐ 2. Administer atropine sulfate.
☐ 3. Teach deep-breathing exercises.
☐ 4. Teach leg lifts and muscle-setting exercises.

56. The nurse is planning care for a hospitalized client who is blind. What should the nurse do to ensure safety for this client?
☐ 1. Require that the client has a sitter for each shift.
☐ 2. Request that the client stays in bed until the nurse can assist them.
☐ 3. Orient the client to the room environment.
☐ 4. Keep the side rails up when the client is alone.

57. The nurse is taking care of a client who had a laryngectomy yesterday. To assure client safety, the nurse should give hand-off reports at which time(s)? Select all that apply.
☐ 1. change of shift
☐ 2. change of nurses
☐ 3. when the nurse goes to lunch
☐ 4. when the unit clerk goes to a staff meeting
☐ 5. when new medication prescriptions are written

58. The nurse is admitting a client with glaucoma. The client brings prescribed eye drops from home and insists on using them in the hospital. What should the nurse do?
☐ 1. Allow the client to keep the eye drops at the bedside and use them as prescribed on the bottle.
☐ 2. Place the eye drops in the hospital medication drawer, and administer them as labeled on the bottle.
☐ 3. Explain to the client that the health care provider (HCP) will write a prescription for the eye drops to be used at the hospital.
☐ 4. Ask the client's spouse to assist the client in administering the eye drops while the client is in the hospital.

59. The nurse is assigned to care for a client with an ocular prosthesis who is having surgery under a local anesthetic. What should the nurse do before the surgery?
☐ 1. Maintain surgical asepsis when caring for the prosthesis.
☐ 2. Leave the prosthesis in place.
☐ 3. Cleanse the ocular prosthesis with full-strength hydrogen peroxide.
☐ 4. Instruct the client to cleanse the prosthesis daily.

60. A client has been diagnosed with insulin-requiring diabetes. The nurse should instruct the client about which factor(s) that can contribute to the risk for diabetic retinopathy? Select all that apply.
☐ 1. poor control of blood sugar
☐ 2. nearsightedness
☐ 3. length of time of being diagnosed with diabetes
☐ 4. hypertension
☐ 5. elevated cholesterol

Answers, Rationales, and Test-Taking Strategies

*The answers and rationales for each question follow below, along with keys (🔑) to the client need (CN) and cognitive level (CL) for each question. In addition, questions that measure clinical judgment will be coded (CJ). As you check your answers, use the **Content Mastery and Test-Taking Skill Self-Analysis** worksheet (tear-out worksheet in the back of the book) to identify the reason(s) for not answering the questions correctly. For additional information about test-taking skills and strategies for answering questions, refer to pages 12–51 in Part 1 of this book.*

The Adult with Cataracts

1. 3. The spouse has positioned the dropper and the client correctly to prevent injury to the client's eye. The spouse should administer the drops in the center of the lower lid. Following administration of the eye drops, the client should blink the eyes to distribute the medication; squeezing or rubbing the eyes might cause the medication to drip out of the eye.

🔑 CN: Pharmacological and parenteral therapies; CL: Apply

2. 3. To prevent discomfort from bright light, the client should wear sunglasses that cover the front and side of the face, thus minimizing light that comes into the eye from any direction. It is not necessary to remain in dim light or inside. Attaching sun shields or sunglasses to existing glasses will not cover the eye sufficiently, and bright light will come in on the side of the face. It is not necessary to patch the affected eye.

🔑 CN: Basic care and comfort; CL: Analyze

3. ➕ **1, 4, 5, 6.** To promote the success of lens implantation without complication (infection, inflammation, hemorrhage), it is important for the client to instill eye drops as prescribed, protect the eye, and avoid placing any stress on the eye by lifting, pulling, or pushing objects that weigh more than 15 lb (6.8 kg). Pain should be minimal and relieved with acetaminophen; if not, the client should notify the health care provider (HCP). Clients should not expect to drive or see clearly immediately following lens implantation; it may take several days for vision to clear, and limitations will be discussed at the follow-up appointment.

🔑 CN: Reduction of risk potential; CL: Evaluate

4. ⊟ **1, 2, 4.** The use of glasses following cataract surgery does not totally restore binocular vision. Glasses will cause images to appear larger, and peripheral vision will be distorted; the client should look through the center of the glasses and turn their head to view objects in the periphery. The client should also use caution when walking or climbing stairs until they have adjusted to the change in vision. Changes in vision following cataract surgery are not immediate, and the nurse can instruct the client to be patient while adjusting to the changes. The client does not need to stay out of the sun but should wear dark glasses to prevent discomfort from photophobia.

🗝 CN: Reduction of risk potential; CL: Create

5. 3. Using an eye shield at night prevents rubbing the eye. The head should be turned to the side to scan the entire visual field to compensate for impaired peripheral vision. Eye medications may initially cause sensitivity to bright light. The surgeon changes the eye patch on the second postoperative day.

🗝 CN: Reduction of risk potential; CL: Analyze

6. 2. The nurse should give a client who seems fearful of surgery an opportunity to express their feelings. Only after identifying the client's concerns can the nurse intervene appropriately. Asking the client about previous reactions to local anesthetics may be warranted, but it does not address the client's concerns in this instance. Telling the client that they will not have nausea or vomiting ignores the client's feelings of fear and does not provide any data about the client's feelings. More data would help the nurse plan care. Telling the client that there is nothing to be afraid of minimizes the client's feelings and does not address their concerns. Premature explanations and clichés do not provide the needed assessment data and ignore the client's feelings.

🗝 CN: Psychosocial integrity; CL: Analyze

7. 4. An ophthalmologist is a health care provider who specializes in the treatment of disorders of the eye, and the nurse should advise the client to see an ophthalmologist. An optician makes glasses, and it is not known at this point what the best treatment for the client is. Magnifying glasses, or glasses with tinted lenses, do not correct hazy or blurred vision. If glasses are needed to correct refractive errors, they should be prescription glasses.

🗝 CN: Health promotion and maintenance; CL: Analyze

8. 2. Instilled in the eye, phenylephrine hydrochloride acts as a mydriatic, causing the pupil to dilate. It also constricts small blood vessels in the eye.

🗝 CN: Pharmacological and parenteral therapies; CL: Evaluate

9. 4. A prescribed antiemetic should be administered as soon as the client has nausea following cataract extraction. Vomiting can increase intraocular pressure, which should be avoided after eye surgery because it can cause complications. Deep breathing is unlikely to relieve nausea. Postoperative nausea may be common; however, it does not necessarily pass quickly and can lead to vomiting. Telling the client to call only if vomiting occurs ignores the client's need for comfort and intervention to prevent complications.

🗝 CN: Pharmacological and parenteral therapies; CL: Analyze

10. 1. The nurse should instruct the client to remain in a semi-Fowler position or on the nonoperative side. Positioning the feet higher than the body does not affect the operative eye; placing the head in a dependent position could increase pressure within the eyes.

🗝 CN: Reduction of risk potential; CL: Analyze

11. 1. Applying pressure against the nose at the inner canthus of the closed eye after administering eye drops prevents the medication from entering the lacrimal (tear) duct. If the medication enters the tear duct, it can enter the nose and pharynx, where it may be absorbed and cause toxic symptoms. Eye drops should be placed in the eye's lower conjunctival sac. Applying pressure will not prevent the drug from running down the face as long as the drops are instilled in the eye. Pressure does not affect the cornea or facilitate distribution of the medication over the eye surface.

🗝 CN: Pharmacological and parenteral therapies; CL: Apply

12. 2. Coughing is contraindicated after cataract extraction because it increases intraocular pressure. Other activities that are contraindicated because they increase intraocular pressure include turning to the operative side, sneezing, crying, and straining. Lying supine, ambulating, and deep breathing do not affect intraocular pressure.

🗝 CN: Physiological adaptation; CL: Analyze

13. 4. Sudden, sharp pain after eye surgery may indicate that the client has intraocular hemorrhage. The nurse should immediately contact the HCP. Covering the eye will not manage intraocular hemorrhage. Pain medication will not be effective to manage hemorrhage. The nurse should help the client return to a recumbent position.

🗝 CN: Physiological adaptation; CL: Analyze

The Adult with Retinal Detachment

14. 4. Promoting measures that limit mobility may prevent further injury. Following surgical repair of a detached retina, cool or warm compresses are applied to edematous eyelids, if prescribed. The client should avoid lying face down, stooping, or bending preoperatively. It is not necessary to remove all pillows.

🗝 CN: Safety and infection control; CL: Analyze

15. 1. Patching the eyes helps decrease random eye movements that could enlarge and worsen retinal detachment. Although clients with eye injuries frequently are light sensitive, and preventing infection is important, the specific goal is to reduce rapid eye movements. Using the uninvolved eye would not cause eye strain, but random movements of one eye will involve the other eye.

🗝 CN: Safety and infection control; CL: Evaluate

16. 4. Untreated retinal detachment results in increasing detachment and eventual blindness, but 90% to 95% of clients can be successfully treated with surgery. If necessary, the surgical procedure can be repeated about 10 to 14 days after the first procedure. Many more services are available for newly blind people, but ideally, this client will not need them. Surgery does not delay blindness.

🗝 CN: Physiological adaptation; CL: Analyze

17. 1. After laser surgery, the retinal tear needs time to heal completely. This may take up to 2 months. Therefore, resumption of activity should be gradual; typically, the client may resume usual activities in 5 to 6 weeks. Successful healing should allow the client to return to a previous level of functioning.

🗝 CN: Basic care and comfort; CL: Analyze

18. 2. After surgery to correct a detached retina, prevention of increased intraocular pressure is the priority goal. Control of pain with analgesics is a secondary goal. The client should avoid getting soap and water in the eye when bathing. Maintaining a darkened environment is not necessary for this client.

🗝 CN: Physiological adaptation; CL: Analyze

The Adult with Glaucoma

19. 2. The client should look up while the nurse instills the eye drops. The client will need to keep both eyes open while the nurse administers the drug. If the client raises the eyebrows while the nurse's hand is positioned on the eyebrows, the movement of the forehead may cause the dropper to move and injure the eye. The client should gently blink the eyes after the eye drops have been instilled. Using a tissue to wipe the eyes could remove some of the medication; excess fluid can be removed with a cotton ball.

🗝 CN: Pharmacological and parenteral therapies; CL: Apply

20. 2. In COAG, there is an obstruction to the outflow of aqueous humor, leading to increased intraocular pressure. The increased intraocular pressure eventually causes destruction of the retina's nerve fibers. This nerve destruction causes painless vision loss. The exact cause of glaucoma is unknown. Glaucoma does not lead to retinal detachment.

🗝 CN: Physiological adaptation; CL: Analyze

21. 4. Although COAG is usually asymptomatic in the early stages, peripheral vision gradually decreases as the disorder progresses. Eye pain is not a feature of COAG but is common in clients with angle-closure glaucoma. Excessive lacrimation is not a symptom of COAG; it may indicate a blocked tear duct. Flashes of light are a common symptom of retinal detachment.

🗝 CN: Physiological adaptation; CL: Analyze

22. 2. Tonometry, which measures intraocular pressure, is a simple, noninvasive, and painless procedure that requires no particular preparation or postprocedure care and carries no adverse effects. It is not necessary to dilate the pupils for tonometry.

🗝 CN: Reduction of risk potential; CL: Analyze

23. 3. Timolol maleate is commonly administered to control glaucoma. The drug's action is not completely understood, but it is believed to reduce aqueous humor formation, thereby reducing intraocular pressure. Timolol does not constrict the pupils; miotics are used for pupillary constriction and contraction of the ciliary muscle. Timolol does not dilate the canal of Schlemm.

🗝 CN: Pharmacological and parenteral therapies; CL: Evaluate

24. 2. The cornea is sensitive and can be injured by eye drops falling onto it. Therefore, eye drops should be instilled into the lower conjunctival sac of the eye to avoid the risk for corneal damage. The drops do not cause scleral staining or excessive lacrimation. Systemic absorption occurs when eye drops enter the tear ducts.

CN: Pharmacological and parenteral therapies; CL: Evaluate

25. 4. Acute angle-closure glaucoma produces abrupt changes in the angle of the iris. Clinical manifestations include severe eye pain, colored halos around lights, and rapid vision loss. Gradual loss of central vision is associated with macular degeneration. The loss of color vision, or achromatopsia, is a rare symptom that occurs when a stroke damages the fusiform gyrus. It most often affects only half of the visual field.

CN: Physiological adaptation; CL: Analyze

26. 3. Acute angle-closure glaucoma is a medical emergency that rapidly leads to blindness if left untreated. Treatment typically involves miotic drugs and surgery, usually iridectomy or laser therapy. Both procedures create a hole in the periphery of the iris, which allows the aqueous humor to flow into the anterior chamber. Bed rest does not affect the progression of acute angle-closure glaucoma. Steroids are not a treatment for acute angle-closure glaucoma; in fact, they are associated with the development of glaucoma.

CN: Physiological adaptation; CL: Apply

The Adult with Adult Macular Degeneration

27. 1. Macular degeneration generally involves loss of central vision. Gradual blurring of vision can occur as the disease progresses and may result in blindness; however, loss of central vision is the most common finding. Tiny yellowish spots, known as drusen, develop beneath the retina. Loss of peripheral vision is characteristic of glaucoma.

CN: Physiological adaptation; CL: Analyze

28. 3. AMD generally affects central vision. Confusion may result because of the changes in the client's environment and the client's inability to see the environment clearly. Therefore, providing safety is the priority goal in the care of this client. Educating the client regarding community resources or monitoring their AMD may have been done at an earlier date or can be done after assessing their knowledge base and experience with the disease process. Improving the client's vision may not be possible.

CN: Safety and infection control; CL: Analyze

29. 4. To expand the visual field, the partially sighted client should be taught to turn the head from side to side when walking. Neglecting to do so may result in accidents. This technique helps maximize the use of remaining sight. A patch does not address the problem of hemianopsia. Appropriate client positioning and placement of personal items will increase the client's ability to cope with the problem but will not affect safety.

CN: Health promotion and maintenance; CL: Analyze

30. In macular degeneration, the center vision is blackened out, and only the outer visual fields are clear.

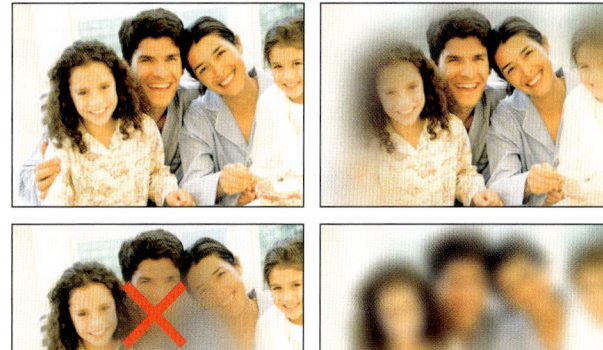

CN: Physiological adaptation; CL: Analyze

31. 2. Because of the client's recent vision loss, the client is at high risk for injury. Sensory alterations often affect other areas of functional ability, including leaving clients with sensory deficits at risk for injuries as a result. Disturbed sensory perception, denial of and difficulty adjusting to vision loss, and social isolation may also be of concern and may accompany changes in sensory function, but they are not a higher priority than the risk for injury.

CN: Management of care; CL: Analyze

The Adult Undergoing Nasal Surgery

32. 2. Because of the dense packing, it is relatively unusual for bleeding to be apparent through the nasal drip pad. Instead, the blood runs down the throat, causing the client to swallow frequently. The back of the throat can be assessed with a flashlight. An accumulation of blood in the stomach may cause nausea and vomiting, but it is not an initial sign of bleeding. Increased respiratory rate occurs in shock and is not an early sign of bleeding in the client after nasal surgery. Feelings of anxiety are not indicative of nasal bleeding.

CN: Physiological adaptation; CL: Analyze

33. **1.** The client should be instructed to avoid any activities that cause the Valsalva maneuver (e.g., straining at stool, vigorous coughing, exercise) to reduce stress on suture lines and bleeding. The client should not take aspirin because of its antiplatelet properties, which may cause bleeding. Oral hygiene is important to rid the mouth of old dried blood and to enhance the client's appetite. Cool compresses, not heat, should be applied to decrease swelling and control discoloration of the area.

    CN: Reduction of risk potential; CL: Analyze

34. **2.** Constipation can cause straining during defecation, which can induce bleeding. Showering is not contraindicated. The client should take measures to prevent coughing. The client should avoid blowing their nose for 48 hours after the packing is removed. Thereafter, the client should blow their nose gently using the open-mouth technique to minimize bleeding in the surgical area.

    CN: Health promotion and maintenance; CL: Evaluate

The Adult with a Hearing Disorder

35. **4.** The nurse should avoid startling the client who is deaf and should obtain the attention of the client before speaking. The client who is deaf cannot hear knocking on the door or talking. Opening the blinds is not a helpful way to get the client's attention.

    CN: Psychosocial integrity; CL: Analyze

36. **2.** Furosemide may cause ototoxicity. The nurse should tell the client to promptly report the hearing loss, dizziness, or tinnitus to help prevent permanent ear damage. Hearing loss is not inevitable, and it is inappropriate to make assumptions about the cause of symptoms without a thorough evaluation. The client's system will not "adjust," and hearing loss will not resolve.

    CN: Pharmacological and parenteral therapies; CL: Analyze

37. **3.** A client who is deaf benefits most from reading information and then having an opportunity to ask questions and follow up. Verbal communication, while appropriate, may not be sufficient. The spouse can be included in the teaching, but the nurse is responsible for ensuring that the client understands the instructions. Videos may be helpful, but unless they have closed captioning, key points may be missed in the audio portion.

    CN: Reduction of risk potential; CL: Analyze

38. **4.** Because aspirin is ototoxic, the ringing in the client's ears is likely caused by long-term aspirin use. The nurse advises the client to contact the HCP; if the aspirin is to be discontinued, other drugs may be prescribed. The client is not instructed to stop taking the drug without discussing the change with the HCP. Acetaminophen does not have the same antithrombotic properties as aspirin. Increasing fluid intake will not stop the ringing in the client's ears.

    CN: Physiological adaptation; CL: Analyze

39. **2.** Blank looks, decreased attention span, positioning of the head toward sound, and smiling/nodding in agreement once attention is gained are all behaviors that indicate hearing loss in adults. It is common to confuse sensory deficits for a change in cognitive status such as dementia. The nurse should focus assessments of sensory function on considering any pathophysiology of existing or new-onset deficits and consider all client factors that might contribute to deficits. The blank looks do not indicate that this client is frustrated or depressed.

    CN: Basic care and comfort; CL: Analyze

40. **-/+ 1, 2, 3, 5.** When working with a client who is hearing impaired and reads speech, the presenter must face the person directly and devote full attention to the communication process. In addition, it will be useful for the client that the speaker is not too silhouetted against strong light, that the speaker's mouth is not blocked from the client's view, and that there are no objects in the mouth of the speaker. Finally, it is recommended that the presenter provide the client with the needed information to study before reviewing. This will provide the client with the ability to use contextual clues in speech reading.

    CN: Basic care and comfort; CL: Analyze

41. **-/+ 3, 4, 5.** To instill ear drops in an adult, the nurse places a towel on the bed and has the client lie in bed on the side *opposite* the affected ear. To straighten the adult client's ear canal, the nurse pulls the auricle of the ear up and back. Ear drops should be administered at body temperature. The drops should remain in the ear for 2 to 5 minutes.

    CN: Pharmacological and parenteral therapies; CL: Apply

42. **-/+ 1, 2, 5.** The nurse can advise the client with cerumen that is impacted in the ear to use a washcloth to clean the exterior part of the ear. The client can also instill cerumenolytic drops to soften the earwax. The client can then irrigate the ear

canal with sterile water using a small bulb syringe. The client should not use cotton-tipped applicators as they often push the cerumen further into the ear canal. The client should never put forceps in the ear.

CN: Pharmacological and parenteral therapies; CL: Analyze

43. 1. The nurse should first assess the client's knowledge base. Working within the framework of the client's knowledge and educational level, the nurse then can describe the procedure and its benefits.

CN: Reduction of risk potential; CL: Analyze

44. 4. Tinnitus (ringing in the ears) is an adverse effect of aspirin. Aspirin contains salicylate, which is an ototoxic drug that can induce reversible hearing loss and tinnitus. The nurse should explain this to the client and then encourage the client to inform the health care provider of the symptom. Tinnitus is not a function of aging. The Weber test and audiometric testing are useful for determining hearing loss but are not necessarily helpful in the management or diagnosis of drug-induced tinnitus.

CN: Pharmacological and parenteral therapies; CL: Analyze

The Adult with Ménière's Disease

45. 4. Ménière's disease is commonly seen in older women; the disorder is caused by pressure within the labyrinth of the inner ear as a result of excess endolymph resulting in swelling in the cochlea. Therefore, the nurse should instruct the client on dietary restrictions of sodium to reduce fluid retention. Pharmacologic treatment includes drugs to treat vertigo and diuretics. If the client is prescribed a diuretic, fluid and electrolytes are monitored. The amount of protein does not have a direct influence on this disease process.

CN: Physiological adaptation; CL: Analyze

46. 1, 2, 3, 5. Assessment of vertigo, including history, onset, description of attacks, duration, frequency, and associated ear symptoms, is important. Vestibular/balance therapy or exercises should be taught and practiced. The client needs to be instructed to sit down when dizzy and decrease the amount of head movement. The client will benefit from recognizing whether they experience an "aura" before an attack so appropriate action can be taken. Finally, it is recommended that the client keep the eyes open and look straight ahead when lying down. These expected outcomes will prevent the problem of injury. Family involvement is essential when dealing with a client experiencing vertigo, but it is not essential for this client who must manage vertigo with or without family involvement.

CN: Reduction of risk potential; CL: Analyze

47. 1. A low-sodium diet is frequently an effective mechanism for reducing the frequency and severity of the disease episodes. About three-quarters of clients with Ménière's disease respond to treatment with a low-salt diet. A diuretic may also be prescribed. Other dietary changes, such as high protein, low carbohydrate, and low fat, do not have an effect on Ménière's disease.

CN: Basic care and comfort; CL: Apply

48. 2. There is no cure for Ménière's disease, but the wide range of medical and surgical treatments allows for adequate control in many clients. The disease often worsens, but it does not spread to the eyes. The hearing loss is usually unilateral.

CN: Physiological adaptation; CL: Evaluate

49. 4. The client needs to assume a safe and comfortable position during an attack, which may last several hours. The client's location when the attack occurs may dictate the most reasonable position. Ideally, the client should lie down immediately in a reclining or flat position to control the vertigo. The danger of a serious fall is real. Placing the head between the knees will not help prevent a fall and is not practical because the attack may last several hours. Concentrating on breathing may be a useful distraction, but it will not help prevent a fall. Closing the eyes does not help prevent a fall.

CN: Safety and infection control; CL: Analyze

The Adult with Cancer of the Larynx

50. 4. The nurse should next notify the HCP. A salivary fistula is suspected when there is saliva collecting beneath skin flaps or leaking through the suture line or drain site. Salivary fistula or skin necrosis usually precedes carotid artery rupture. Using a dressing, observing for increased drainage, or having the client expectorate the saliva are not appropriate actions until the HCP has determined the presence and extent of a fistula.

CN: Reduction of risk potential; CL: Analyze

51. −/+ **1, 2, 3, 4.** The nurse should monitor nutritional status through frequent weighing and checking the serum albumin level. The nurse also should administer enteral tube feedings until there is sufficient healing of the pharynx and the client can consume sufficient oral feedings to meet body needs. The nurse should avoid manipulation of the nasogastric tube during this time so it does not disrupt the suture line. The nurse should place the client in a sitting position, leaning slightly forward, which allows the larynx to move forward and the hypopharynx to partially open; the epiglottis normally prevents fluid and food from entering the larynx during swallowing.

CN: Physiological adaptation; CL: Create

52. −/+ **1, 2, 3.** The nurse should advise the client to provide humidification at home. Instruct the client to use a protective shield for bathing, showering, shampooing, or cutting hair to prevent aspiration. The nurse can also encourage the client to drink 8 to 12 cups (about 2 to 3 L) of fluids daily to help liquefy secretions. To counteract any loss of smell and impairment of taste sensation, the client can add additional seasoning to food. The client should follow a high-fiber diet and use stool softeners because they may not be able to hold their breath and bear down for bowel movements.

CN: Health promotion and maintenance; CL: Evaluate

53. 1. The goal of postoperative care is to maintain physiologic integrity. Therefore, inserting a feeding tube is a strategy to ensure that the fluid and nutritional needs of the client are met as the surgical site is healing. The feeding tube helps prevent aspiration by preventing ingested fluid from leaking through the wound into the trachea before healing occurs; however, the primary rationale is to meet the client's nutritional and fluid needs. A tracheoesophageal fistula is a rare complication of total laryngectomy and may occur if radiation therapy has compromised wound healing. A feeding tube does not help maintain an open airway.

CN: Reduction of risk potential; CL: Evaluate

54. 4. The main goal for a client with a new tracheostomy is to maintain a patent airway. A fresh tracheostomy frequently causes bleeding and excess secretions, and clients may require frequent suctioning to maintain patency. Decreasing secretions may be a component of a client's care after laryngectomy and tracheostomy, and relieving anxiety is always an important goal; however, the primary goal is to maintain a patent airway. Instruction on how to care for a tracheostomy is a priority later in the client's recovery.

CN: Physiological adaptation; CL: Analyze

Managing Care, Quality, and Safety of Adults with Health Problems of the Eyes, Ears, Nose, and Throat

55. 2. Atropine sulfate causes pupil dilation. This action is contraindicated for the client with glaucoma because it increases intraocular pressure. The drug does not have this effect on intraocular pressure in people who do not have glaucoma. Morphine causes pupil constriction. Deep-breathing exercises will not affect glaucoma. The client should resume taking all medications for glaucoma immediately after surgery.

CN: Pharmacological and parenteral therapies; CL: Analyze

56. 3. The priority goal of care for a client who is blind is safety and preventing injury. The initial action is to orient the client to a new environment. Taking time to identify the objects and where they are located in the room can achieve this goal. It is unrealistic to have someone stay with the client at all times or for the client to stay in bed until the nurse can assist. Using side rails creates unnecessary barriers and may be a safety hazard.

CN: Safety and infection control; CL: Analyze

57. −/+ **1, 2, 3.** Effective communication is essential when managing client safety and preventing errors. "Hand-off reports" should be made at shift change, when there is a change of nurses or when the nurse leaves the unit, and when the client is discharged or transferred to another unit. There does not need to be a hand-off report when the unit clerk leaves the unit or when new medication prescriptions are written.

CN: Management of care; CL: Apply

58. 3. To prevent medication errors, clients may not use medications they bring from home; the HCP will prescribe the eye drops as required. It is not safe to place the eye drops in the client's medication box or permit the client to use them at the bedside. The nurse should ask the spouse to take the eye drops home.

CN: Safety and infection control; CL: Analyze

59. 2. The nurse should maintain medical asepsis to care for an ocular prosthesis. Because the client will have a local anesthetic, the nurse should leave the prosthesis in place. Daily removal and cleansing are not necessary and may be irritating to the socket; removal for cleansing once or twice a month is sufficient. The nurse should never use anything stronger than liquid soap and water to cleanse an ocular prosthesis.

 CN: Reduction of risk potential; CL: Apply

60. 1, 3, 4, 5. The risk for diabetic retinopathy increases for clients with diabetes who have poorly controlled blood sugar and for clients with other health problems such as hypertension and hypercholesterolemia. The risk for diabetic retinopathy also corresponds with the length of time the client has had the disease. Being nearsighted is not a risk factor. The nurse should include information about risk factors and how to prevent or minimize them when developing a teaching plan for all clients with diabetes.

 CN: Health promotion and maintenance; CL: Analyze

TEST 16: The Adult with Health Problems of the Integumentary System

- The Adult with Burns
- The Older Adult with General Problems of the Integumentary System
- The Adult with Shingles
- The Adult with a Pressure Injury
- The Adult with Skin Cancer
- Managing Care, Quality, and Safety of Adults with Health Problems of the Integumentary System
- Answers, Rationales, and Test-Taking Strategies

The Adult with Burns

1. There has been a fire in an apartment building. All residents have been evacuated, but many are burned. Which client(s) should be transported **immediately** to a burn center for treatment? Select all that apply.
  - ☐ 1. 8-year-old client with third-degree burns over 10% of the body surface area (BSA)
  - ☐ 2. 20-year-old client who inhaled the smoke of the fire
  - ☐ 3. 50-year-old client with diabetes who has first- and second-degree burns on their left forearm (about 5% of the body surface area [BSA])
  - ☐ 4. 30-year-old client with second-degree burns on the back of their left leg (about 9% of body surface area [BSA])
  - ☐ 5. 40-year-old client with second-degree burns on the right arm (about 10% of BSA)

2. The nurse is assessing an 80-year-old client who has scald burns on their hands and both forearms (first- and second-degree burns on 10% of their body surface area). What should the nurse do **first**?
  - ☐ 1. Clean the wounds with warm water.
  - ☐ 2. Apply antibiotic cream.
  - ☐ 3. Refer the client to a burn center.
  - ☐ 4. Cover the burns with a sterile dressing.

3. During the emergency (resuscitative) phase of burn injury, which finding indicates that the client requires additional volume with fluid resuscitation?
  - ☐ 1. serum creatinine level of 2.5 mg/dL (221 μmol/L)
  - ☐ 2. little fluctuation in daily weight
  - ☐ 3. hourly urine output of 60 mL
  - ☐ 4. serum albumin level of 3.8 mg/dL (38 g/L)

4. A client is admitted to the hospital after sustaining burns to the front of their body. The burned areas include the front of the chest and abdomen as well as the skin on the front of the right arm and right leg, as shown in the shaded areas in the illustration. Using the "rule of nines," estimate what percentage of the client's body surface has been burned.

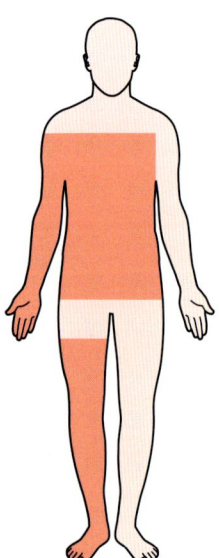

  - ☐ 1. 18%
  - ☐ 2. 27%
  - ☐ 3. 45%
  - ☐ 4. 64%

5. The nurse is caring for a client with severe burns who is receiving fluid resuscitation. Which finding indicates that the client is responding to the fluid resuscitation?
  ☐ 1. pulse rate of 112 bpm
  ☐ 2. blood pressure of 94/64 mm Hg
  ☐ 3. urine output of 30 mL per hour
  ☐ 4. serum sodium level of 136 mEq/L (136 mmol/L)

6. A client is admitted with a 45% partial-thickness and full-thickness burn. Which finding would alert the nurse that the client has a deficiency in fluid volume during the first 24 hours?
  ☐ 1. serum creatinine of 1.1 mg/dL (97.2 μmol/L)
  ☐ 2. serum potassium level of 3.7 mEq/L
  ☐ 3. oxygen saturation of 94%
  ☐ 4. urine output of less than 30 mL per hour

7. A client with burns is to have a whirlpool bath and dressing change. What should the nurse do 30 minutes before the bath?
  ☐ 1. Soak the dressing.
  ☐ 2. Remove the dressing.
  ☐ 3. Administer an analgesic agent.
  ☐ 4. Slit the dressing with blunt scissors.

8. A client with a major burn injury receives total parenteral nutrition (TPN). What is the expected outcome of TPN?
  ☐ 1. Correct water and electrolyte imbalances.
  ☐ 2. Allow the gastrointestinal tract to rest.
  ☐ 3. Provide supplemental vitamins and minerals.
  ☐ 4. Ensure adequate caloric and protein intake.

9. A client is to receive biologic burn grafts. What should the nurse tell the client's family is the advantage of using biologic burn grafts such as porcine (pigskin) grafts?

Porcine grafts:
  ☐ 1. encourage the formation of tough skin.
  ☐ 2. promote the growth of epithelial tissue.
  ☐ 3. provide for permanent wound closure.
  ☐ 4. facilitate the development of subcutaneous tissue.

10. The health care team is developing a care plan for a client who has burns on 30% of their body. When should the team initiate rehabilitation plans for this client?
  ☐ 1. immediately after the burn has occurred
  ☐ 2. after the client's circulatory status has been stabilized
  ☐ 3. after grafting of the burn wounds has occurred
  ☐ 4. after the client's pain has been eliminated

11. The nurse is reviewing the lab reports for a client who has burns on 40% of their body. Lab values indicating which problem are of **greatest** concern during the first 3 days of burn care?
  ☐ 1. hypernatremia
  ☐ 2. hyponatremia
  ☐ 3. metabolic alkalosis
  ☐ 4. hyperkalemia

12. The nurse is planning care for a group of clients who have been burned. Which client will **most** likely require an endotracheal or tracheostomy tube?
a client who has:
  ☐ 1. electrical burns on the hands and arms causing arrhythmias
  ☐ 2. thermal burns to the head, face, and airway resulting in hypoxia
  ☐ 3. chemical burns on the chest and abdomen
  ☐ 4. secondhand smoke inhalation

13. A client is receiving fluid replacement with lactated Ringer's solution after 40% of the body was burned 10 hours ago. The assessment reveals a temperature of 97.1°F (36.2°C), heart rate of 122 bpm, blood pressure of 84/42 mm Hg, central venous pressure (CVP) of 2 mm Hg, and urine output of 25 mL for the last 2 hours. The intravenous (IV) rate is currently at 375 mL per hour. Using the SBAR (Situation-Background-Assessment-Recommendation) technique for communication, the nurse should request which prescription from the health care provider?
  ☐ 1. furosemide
  ☐ 2. fresh frozen plasma
  ☐ 3. IV rate increase
  ☐ 4. dextrose 5%

14. The nurse is planning care for a client with a burn after the initial phase of the burn injury. Which goal should the nurse establish with the client?
  ☐ 1. developing a positive self-concept
  ☐ 2. promoting hygiene
  ☐ 3. preventing infection
  ☐ 4. managing care of the skin grafts

15. A client has burns on both hands and upper arms. Which nursing action(s) will be **most** helpful in preventing contractures? Select all that apply.
  ☐ 1. Keep the hands elevated.
  ☐ 2. Administer narcotic pain medications every 3 hours.
  ☐ 3. Wash the fingers, hands, and upper arms with cool water.
  ☐ 4. Apply moisturizer to the hands and fingers.
  ☐ 5. Apply splints as prescribed.
  ☐ 6. Collaborate with the physical therapist.

16. The nurse is assessing a client with a burn injury for indications of disruptions of the gastrointestinal system. The nurse should assess the client for which potential problem?
☐ 1. paralytic ileus
☐ 2. gastric distention
☐ 3. hiatal hernia
☐ 4. Curling ulcer

17. A client in the acute phase of burn injury rates their pain as 9 on a scale of 0 to 10. Which pain medication would be **most** effective to decrease the client's perception of the pain?
☐ 1. oral analgesic medications
☐ 2. intravenous opioids
☐ 3. intramuscular opioids
☐ 4. oral antianxiety agents

The Older Adult with General Problems of the Integumentary System

18. The nurse is assessing an older adult's skin. The assessment will involve inspecting the skin for color, pigmentation, and vascularity. What should the nurse assess?
☐ 1. similarities from one side to the other
☐ 2. changes from the normally expected findings
☐ 3. appearance of age-related wrinkles
☐ 4. skin turgor

19. The nurse is assessing the skin of an older adult. Which are signs of normal skin changes in an older adult? Select all that apply.
☐ 1. diminished hair on the scalp and pubic areas
☐ 2. dusky rubor of the left lower extremity
☐ 3. solar lentigo
☐ 4. wrinkles
☐ 5. xerosis
☐ 6. yellow pigmentation

20. An older adult is having abdominal surgery. The nurse should assess the client for which postoperative concern related to normal changes in the integumentary system of an older adult?
☐ 1. increased scarring
☐ 2. decreased melanin and melanocytes
☐ 3. decreased healing
☐ 4. increased immunocompetence

21. The nurse is instructing an older adult about ways to promote skin integrity. Which health maintenance behavior by the client is **most** helpful?
☐ 1. drinks 6 cups (about 1½ L) of fluids per day
☐ 2. consumes a balanced diet of 1200 calories a day
☐ 3. walks briskly for 10 minutes three times per week
☐ 4. sleeps at least 8 hours each night

22. The nurse is developing a care plan for a client who will have abdominal surgery tomorrow. Which factor puts an older adult at the **greatest** risk for impaired wound healing after abdominal surgery?
☐ 1. age over 75 years
☐ 2. poorly controlled diabetes
☐ 3. history of one myocardial infarction
☐ 4. chronic peripheral vascular disease

23. An older adult has several areas of ecchymosis on the left arm. What should the nurse further assess? Select all that apply.
☐ 1. elder abuse
☐ 2. self-inflicted injury
☐ 3. increased capillary fragility and permeability
☐ 4. increased blood supply to the skin
☐ 5. shingles

24. An older adult reports being cold in the room even though the thermostat is set at 75°F (24°C). The nurse can tell the client that older adults may feel cold for which reason?

Older adults have:
☐ 1. increased cellular cohesion.
☐ 2. increased moisture content of the stratum corneum.
☐ 3. slower cellular renewal time.
☐ 4. decreased ability to thermoregulate.

25. A client has tinea capitis. What should the nurse instruct the client with tinea capitis to do? Select all that apply.
☐ 1. Place a dressing saturated with vinegar and water on the area.
☐ 2. Apply topical antibacterial ointment to the area.
☐ 3. Shampoo hair two or three times with selenium sulfide shampoo.
☐ 4. Use antibacterial soap for bathing.
☐ 5. Take antifungal medication as prescribed.

26. An older adult has pruritus on the arms and legs and is scratching the affected areas. Which is the **priority** nursing care for this client?
☐ 1. preventing infection
☐ 2. instructing the client not to scratch
☐ 3. increasing fluid intake
☐ 4. avoiding social isolation

27. The nurse is applying a hand mitt restraint for a client with pruritus (see figure). What should the nurse do **first**?

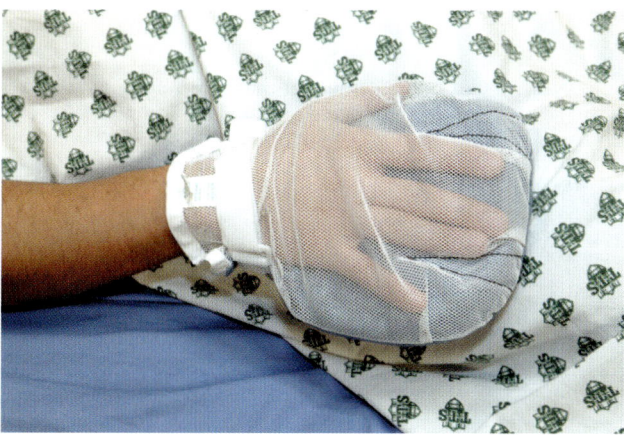

☐ 1. Verify the prescription to use the restraint.
☐ 2. Secure the mitt with ties around the wrist tied to the bed frame.
☐ 3. Place a folded pillow under the wrist.
☐ 4. Place the mitt on top of the hand.

28. An older adult client in stage 2 of Parkinson disease is being discharged with cellulitis of the right lower extremity. The nurse should base the discharge plan on which information? Select all that apply.
The client has:
☐ 1. decreased tissue perfusion.
☐ 2. risk for skin breakdown.
☐ 3. potential for falls.
☐ 4. difficulty communicating.
☐ 5. limited activity.

29. The nurse is discharging an older adult to home after hospitalization for cellulitis of the right foot, followed by an infection. After reviewing discharge instructions, what statement by the client indicates the need for further teaching by the nurse? "I will:
☐ 1. eat lots of fruit and vegetables and take vitamin C to help this heal."
☐ 2. be sure to wear shoes to protect my feet when I go out to get the mail."
☐ 3. manage my pain by putting this foot up on a pillow when it hurts."
☐ 4. take the antibiotics until the redness goes away and my foot feels better."

30. The nurse is assessing a group of older adults. Which client is at the **greatest** risk for skin breakdown?
a person who has:
☐ 1. altered balance
☐ 2. reduced sensation of pressure
☐ 3. impaired hearing ability
☐ 4. impaired visual acuity

The Adult with Shingles

31. A client has been diagnosed with herpes zoster (shingles). The nurse should include which information in a teaching plan? Select all that apply.
☐ 1. Instruct the client about taking antiviral agents as prescribed.
☐ 2. Demonstrate how to apply wet-to-dry dressings.
☐ 3. Explain how to follow proper hand hygiene techniques.
☐ 4. Assure the client that the pain from herpes zoster will be gone within 7 days.
☐ 5. Tell the client to remain in isolation in a bedroom until the lesions have healed.

32. A client is asking the nurse about receiving the current shingles vaccine (Shingrix). Which factor indicates the client should receive the vaccine? The client:
☐ 1. has never had chickenpox.
☐ 2. is at risk for genital herpes.
☐ 3. is over 50 years of age.
☐ 4. has a compromised immune system.

33. A 65-year-old client received the Zostavax vaccine for shingles 5 years ago. The client asks the nurse if the vaccine is still effective. What should the nurse tell the client?
☐ 1. "Your vaccine is still up to date."
☐ 2. "This vaccine is no longer effective."
☐ 3. "You should be revaccinated with a newer vaccine."
☐ 4. "You can have the new vaccine when you are 70."

34. A nurse is caring for an older adult with shingles. The client is experiencing considerable pain related to open blisters on the client's abdomen and back. The client is taking acyclovir and low-dose prednisone. The nurse has several prescriptions available. What additional medication(s) or nursing care measure(s) to promote comfort may be helpful? Select all that apply.
☐ 1. diphenhydramine 25 mg by mouth every 6 hours as needed (PRN)
☐ 2. calamine lotion applied to the affected areas
☐ 3. cool, wet compresses to the affected areas
☐ 4. acetaminophen 325 mg by mouth every 6 hours PRN
☐ 5. ondansetron 4 mg by mouth every 4 hours PRN
☐ 6. diversionary activities to prevent client scratching

The Adult with a Pressure Injury

35. The nurse is assessing a client with dark skin for the presence of a stage I pressure injury. Which is the **best** approach to making this assessment?
    ☐ 1. Use a fluorescent light source to assess the skin.
    ☐ 2. Inspect the skin only when the Braden score is above 12.
    ☐ 3. Look for skin color that is darker than the surrounding tissue.
    ☐ 4. Avoid touching the skin during the inspection.

36. The nurse is assessing a client who is immobile and notes that an area of sacral skin is reddened but not broken. The reddened area continues to blanch and refill with fingertip pressure. What should the nurse do **next**?
    ☐ 1. Apply a wet to moist dressing, being careful to pack just the wound bed.
    ☐ 2. Consult with a wound-ostomy-continence nurse specialist.
    ☐ 3. Reposition the client off of the reddened skin, and reassess in a few hours.
    ☐ 4. Complete and document a Braden skin breakdown risk score for the client.

37. A nurse utilizes an interpreter to teach a non–English-speaking client how to change a dressing. After explaining the procedure through the interpreter and giving the client an education document with pictures of the procedure, the nurse asks if the client understands the information. The client nods yes. What should the nurse do **next**? Select all that apply.
    ☐ 1. Ask the interpreter to repeat the question to confirm the response.
    ☐ 2. Request the client demonstrate the dressing change.
    ☐ 3. Have the client sign the education document to confirm understanding.
    ☐ 4. Review the educational instruction with the client a second time.
    ☐ 5. Ask a question that does not involve a yes or no response.

38. The nurse is assessing a hospitalized older client for the presence of pressure injuries. The nurse notes that the client has a 1- × 1-inch (3- × 3-cm) area on the sacrum in which there is skin breakdown as far as the dermis. What should the nurse note on the medical record?
    ☐ 1. stage I pressure injury
    ☐ 2. stage II pressure injury
    ☐ 3. stage III pressure injury
    ☐ 4. stage IV pressure injury

39. The nurse is assessing a client with a pressure injury. Which finding indicates the client has a stage II pressure injury?
    ☐ 1. redness in the involved area
    ☐ 2. muscle spasms in the involved area
    ☐ 3. pain in the involved area
    ☐ 4. tissue necrosis in the involved area

40. The nurse is using home telehealth monitoring to manage care for an 80-year-old client who is homebound. The client spends most of the day in bed. Two months ago, the nurse detected sacral redness from friction and shearing force of being in bed. Last month, the client had increased sacral redness, and the area was classified as a stage I pressure injury. During this visit, the nurse is assessing the sacral area using a video camera. The nurse compares the site from a visit made 1 month ago (see figure part **A**) with the assessment made at this visit (see figure part **B**). Upon comparing the change of the pressure injury from this visit with the previous visit, the nurse should do what **next**?

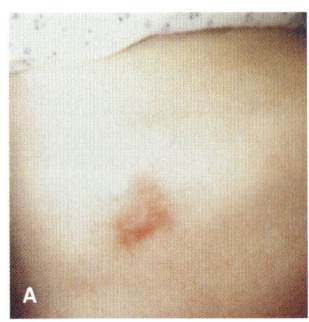 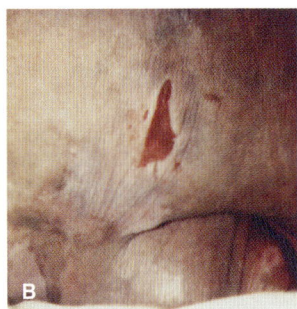

   ☐ 1. Instruct the home health aide to reposition the client every 2 hours while the client is awake.
   ☐ 2. Ask the client's adult child to take pictures of the area and send them to the nurse.
   ☐ 3. Contact the health care provider to request a hydrocolloid dressing.
   ☐ 4. Make a home visit to verify the changes in the ulcer.

41. STEP 1

[stem] The nurse is caring for a 68-year-old male client who had an above-the-knee amputation 1 week ago and has a stage II pressure injury. The client is being transferred to a long-term care facility.

Nurse's Notes

1300:
A client was admitted from the hospital after an above-the-knee amputation of a gangrenous left foot 1 week ago. The client has very limited mobility and sensation in both legs. The client is well nourished but obese and has diabetes, hypertension, end-stage renal disease requiring hemodialysis three times a week, dementia, and depression. The client's health care proxy is their adult child. The client is alert and oriented to person only. Occasionally, the client yells out, "I want to see my child." The client receives 10 mg of morphine orally every 4 hours for pain, and the last dose was at 1100. Vital signs are within normal limits. A stage II pressure injury in the coccyx measures 1 × 1 × 0.1 cm, is red, and does not blanche to touch; the client receives wet-to-dry dressings daily. The client is up ad lib to a chair using a ceiling lift and is on a regular diet. The client is incontinent of urine.

➤ Identify the **four** assessment findings that require follow-up.

☐	1. Vital signs
☐	2. Wants to see son
☐	3. Infection risk
☐	4. Client mental status
☐	5. Nutritional status
☐	6. Pain control
☐	7. Respiratory status
☐	8. Skin breakdown

42. STEP 2

The nurse is caring for a 68-year-old male client who had an above-the-knee amputation 1 week ago and has a stage II pressure injury. The client is being transferred to a long-term care facility.

Nurse's Notes

1300:
A client was admitted from the hospital after an above-the-knee amputation of a gangrenous left foot 1 week ago. The client has very limited mobility and sensation in both legs. The client is well nourished but obese and has diabetes, hypertension, end-stage renal disease requiring hemodialysis three times a week, dementia, and depression. The client's health care proxy is their adult child. The client is alert and oriented to person only. Occasionally, the client yells out, "I want to see my child." The client receives 10 mg of morphine orally every 4 hours for pain, and the last dose was at 1100. Vital signs are within normal limits. A stage II pressure injury in the coccyx measures 1 × 1 × 0.1 cm, is red, and does not blanche to touch; the client receives wet-to-dry dressings daily. The client is up ad lib to a chair using a ceiling lift and is on a regular diet. The client is incontinent of urine.

➤ Using the Braden Scale, highlight the client's risk for pressure injury.

Braden Scale for Pressure Injury Risk					
Sensory Perception	1. Completely limited	2. Very limited	3. Slightly limited	4. No impairment	
Moisture	1. Constantly moist	2. Very moist	3. Occasionally moist	4. Rarely moist	
Activity	1. Bedfast	2. Chairfast	3. Walks occasionally	4. Walks frequently	
Mobility	1. Completely immobile	2. Very limited	3. Slightly limited	4. No limitations	
Nutrition	1. Very poor	2. Probably inadequate	3. Adequate	4. Excellent	
Friction and Shear	1. Problem	2. Potential problem	3. No apparent problem		
Total Score					
If the score is less than 19, the client is at risk for developing pressure injuries.					

43. STEP 3

The nurse is caring for a 68-year-old male client who had an above-the-knee amputation 1 week ago and has a stage II pressure injury. The client is being transferred to a long-term care facility.

Nurse's Notes

1300:
A client was admitted from the hospital after an above-the-knee amputation of a gangrenous left foot 1 week ago. The client has very limited mobility and sensation in both legs. The client is well nourished but obese and has diabetes, hypertension, end-stage renal disease requiring hemodialysis three times a week, dementia, and depression. The client's health care proxy is their adult child. The client is alert and oriented to person only. Occasionally, the client yells out, "I want to see my child." The client receives 10 mg of morphine orally every 4 hours for pain, and the last dose was at 1100. Vital signs are within normal limits. A stage II pressure injury in the coccyx measures 1 × 1 × 0.1 cm, is red, and does not blanche to touch; the client receives wet-to-dry dressings daily. The client is up ad lib to a chair using a ceiling lift and is on a regular diet. The client is incontinent of urine.

➤ Identify the top four findings that **most** likely contribute to the client's risk for pressure injury.

☐	1. Dementia
☐	2. Immobility
☐	3. Poor circulation
☐	4. Diabetes
☐	5. Incontinence
☐	6. Adequate nutrition
☐	7. Friction and shear

44. STEP 4

The nurse is caring for a 68-year-old male client who had an above-the-knee amputation 1 week ago and has a stage II pressure injury. The client is being transferred to a long-term care facility.

Nurse's Notes

1300:
A client was admitted from the hospital after an above-the-knee amputation of a gangrenous left foot 1 week ago. The client has very limited mobility and sensation in both legs. The client is well nourished but obese and has diabetes, hypertension, end-stage renal disease requiring hemodialysis three times a week, dementia, and depression. The client's health care proxy is their adult child. The client is alert and oriented to person only. Occasionally, the client yells out, "I want to see my child." The client receives 10 mg of morphine orally every 4 hours for pain, and the last dose was at 1100. Vital signs are within normal limits. A stage II pressure injury in the coccyx measures 1 × 1 × 0.1 cm, is red, and does not blanche to touch; the client receives wet-to-dry dressings daily. The client is up ad lib to a chair using a ceiling lift and is on a regular diet. The client is incontinent of urine.

Orders

- Record calorie counts.
- Change wet-to-dry dressings daily.
- Insert an indwelling urinary catheter.
- Order a pressure-relief mattress.
- Administer 500 mL 0.9% sodium chloride intravenously (IV) once.
- Administer 10 mg morphine orally every 4 hours as needed for pain.

The nurse has received orders from the health care provider.

➤ For each order, click to specify if it is indicated, not indicated, or contraindicated.

Intervention	Indicated	Not Indicated	Contraindicated
Record calorie counts	○	○	○
Change wet-to-dry dressings daily	○	○	○
Insert an indwelling urinary catheter	○	○	○
Order a pressure-relief mattress	○	○	○
Administer 500 mL 0.9% sodium chloride IV once	○	○	○
Administer 10 mg morphine orally every 4 hours as needed	○	○	○

45. STEP 5

The nurse is caring for a 68-year-old male client who had an above-the-knee amputation 1 week ago and has a stage II pressure injury. The client is being transferred to a long-term care facility.

Nurse's Notes

1300:
A client was admitted from the hospital after an above-the-knee amputation of a gangrenous left foot 1 week ago. The client has very limited mobility and sensation in both legs. The client is well nourished but obese and has diabetes, hypertension, end-stage renal disease requiring hemodialysis three times a week, dementia, and depression. The client's health care proxy is their adult child. The client is alert and oriented to person only. Occasionally, the client yells out, "I want to see my child." The client receives 10 mg of morphine orally every 4 hours for pain, and the last dose was at 1100. Vital signs are within normal limits. A stage II pressure injury in the coccyx measures 1 × 1 × 0.1 cm, is red, and does not blanche to touch; the client receives wet-to-dry dressings daily. The client is up ad lib to a chair using a ceiling lift and is on a regular diet. The client is incontinent of urine.

Orders

- Record calorie counts.
- Change wet-to-dry dressings daily.
- Insert an indwelling urinary catheter.
- Order a pressure-relief mattress.
- Administer 500 mL 0.9% sodium chloride intravenously (IV) once.
- Administer 10 mg morphine orally every 4 hours as needed for pain.

➤ The nurse has developed a plan of care for this client. Which task(s) can the nurse delegate to the unlicensed assistive personnel (UAP)? Select all that apply.

- ☐ 1. Administer pain medication.
- ☐ 2. Change the wound dressing.
- ☐ 3. Empty and record urine output.
- ☐ 4. Evaluate for new skin breakdown.
- ☐ 5. Flush the peripheral IV with saline.
- ☐ 6. Order lunch for the client.
- ☐ 7. Record food intake.
- ☐ 8. Teach the client about prevention.
- ☐ 9. Turn and reposition the client.

46. STEP 6

The nurse is caring for a 68-year-old male client who had an above-the-knee amputation 1 week ago and has a stage II pressure injury. The client is being transferred to a long-term care facility.

Nurse's Notes

1300:
A client was admitted from the hospital after an above-the-knee amputation of a gangrenous left foot 1 week ago. The client has very limited mobility and sensation in both legs. The client is well nourished but obese and has diabetes, hypertension, end-stage renal disease requiring hemodialysis three times a week, dementia, and depression. The client's health care proxy is their adult child. The client is alert and oriented to person only. Occasionally, the client yells out, "I want to see my child." The client receives 10 mg of morphine orally every 4 hours for pain, and the last dose was at 1100. Vital signs are within normal limits. A stage II pressure injury in the coccyx measures 1 × 1 × 0.1 cm, is red, and does not blanche to touch; the client receives wet-to-dry dressings daily. The client is up ad lib to a chair using a ceiling lift and is on a regular diet. The client is incontinent of urine.

Orders

- Record calorie counts.
- Change wet-to-dry dressings daily.
- Insert an indwelling urinary catheter.
- Order a pressure-relief mattress.
- Administer 500 mL 0.9% sodium chloride intravenously (IV) once.
- Administer 10 mg morphine orally every 4 hours as needed for pain.

The nurse is reassessing the pressure injury.

➤ Identify the top **four** findings that indicate the pressure injury is healing.

- ☐ 1. The area of injury is 20% smaller.
- ☐ 2. The injury shows signs of cellulitis.
- ☐ 3. Skin blanches to touch.
- ☐ 4. The injury needs debridement.
- ☐ 5. The client is in less pain.
- ☐ 6. The skin in the injury area appears red.
- ☐ 7. A fatty area in the injury is exposed.

The Adult with Skin Cancer

47. The nurse is teaching a wellness class to a group of adults. The nurse should tell the group that which factor places a person at the **greatest** risk for skin cancer?
☐ 1. fair skin and history of chronic sun exposure
☐ 2. fair skin and history of hypertension
☐ 3. dark skin and family history of skin cancer
☐ 4. dark skin and history of hypertension

48. A nurse is teaching a client about skin cancer. Which risk factor(s) for skin cancer should the nurse explain? Select all that apply.
☐ 1. increasing age
☐ 2. exposure to chemical pollutants
☐ 3. long-term exposure to the sun
☐ 4. increased pigmentation
☐ 5. genetics
☐ 6. immunosuppression

49. The nurse is in the recovery room caring for a 55-year-old male client who had a gastrectomy.

Nurse's Notes

1345:
The client was admitted to the postanesthesia recovery room. The client is sedated and not responding to voice. An intravenous (IV) line of dextrose 5% in water (D_5W) is running at 125 gtt/min. Vital signs are recorded.

1415:
The client is having muscle spasms in their arms and legs, and their body is warm. Their temperature has risen 4°F (2.2°C).

Vital Signs

Date	06/30	06/30	06/30
Time	1345	1400	1415
Pulse	70 bpm	82 bpm	90 bpm
Respiration rate	12 breaths/min	14 breaths/min	20 breaths/min
Blood pressure	100/60 mm Hg	110/70 mm Hg	140/90 mm Hg
Temperature	98°F (36.7°C)	99°F (37.2°C)	102°F (38.9°C)

The nurse is reviewing the record of the vital signs.

➤ Which action(s) should the nurse take? Select all that apply.
☐ 1. Administer dantrolene as ordered.
☐ 2. Elevate the head of the bed 30 degrees.
☐ 3. Administer a bolus of IV fluids.
☐ 4. Insert an indwelling urinary catheter.
☐ 5. Notify the surgeon.
☐ 6. Place a warming blanket over the client.

50. The nurse is developing a program about skin cancer prevention for a community group. Which information should be included in the program? Select all that apply.
☐ 1. Purchase sunscreen containing benzophenones to block ultraviolet (UV) A and UVB rays.
☐ 2. Use sunscreen with a minimum of 30 sun protection factor (SPF).
☐ 3. Obtain genetic screening to identify the risk for melanoma.
☐ 4. Apply sunscreen only on sunny days, especially between 1000 and 1400.
☐ 5. Have a pigmented lesion biopsied by shaving if it looks suspicious.

51. A client with malignant melanoma asks the nurse about their prognosis. The nurse should tell the client that their prognosis depends on which factor?
☐ 1. amount of ulceration of the lesion
☐ 2. age of the client
☐ 3. location of the lesion on the body
☐ 4. thickness of the lesion

Managing Care, Quality, and Safety of Adults with Health Problems of the Integumentary System

52. The nurse finds an unlicensed assistive personnel (UAP) massaging the reddened bony prominences of a client on bed rest. What should the nurse do?
☐ 1. Reinforce the UAP's use of this intervention over the bony prominences.
☐ 2. Explain that massage is effective because it improves blood flow to the area.
☐ 3. Inform the UAP that massage is even more effective when combined with lotion during the massage.
☐ 4. Instruct the UAP that massage is contraindicated because it decreases blood flow to the area.

53. The nurse manager on the orthopedic unit is reviewing a report that indicates that in the last month, five clients were diagnosed with pressure ulcers. What should the nurse manager do?
☐ 1. Use benchmarking procedures to compare the findings with other nursing units in the hospital.
☐ 2. Ask the staff education department to conduct an educational session about preventing pressure ulcers.
☐ 3. Institute a quality improvement plan that identifies contributing factors, proposes solutions, and sets improvement outcomes.
☐ 4. Conduct a chart audit to determine which nurses on which shifts were giving nursing care to the clients with pressure ulcers.

54. A client has been admitted to the hospital with draining foot lesions. What should the nurse do? Select all that apply.
☐ 1. Place the client in a room with negative air pressure.
☐ 2. Admit the client to a semiprivate room.
☐ 3. Admit the client to a private room.
☐ 4. Post a "contact isolation" sign on the door.
☐ 5. Wear a protective gown when in the client's room.
☐ 6. Wear gloves when providing direct care.

55. The nurse is to administer an antibiotic to a client with burns, but there is no medication in the client's medication box. What should the nurse do **first**?
☐ 1. Inform the unit's shift coordinator.
☐ 2. Contact the client's health care provider (HCP).
☐ 3. Call the pharmacy department.
☐ 4. Borrow the medication from another client.

56. A client has a wound on the ankle that is not healing. The nurse should assess the client for which risk factor(s) for delayed wound healing? Select all that apply.
☐ 1. atrial fibrillation
☐ 2. advancing age
☐ 3. type 2 diabetes mellitus
☐ 4. hypertension
☐ 5. smoking

57. The nurse is assessing the left lower extremity of a client with type 2 insulin-requiring diabetes and cellulitis. What should the nurse do?
☐ 1. Instruct the client to elevate the left leg when sitting in the chair.
☐ 2. Encourage the client to ambulate in the halls on the unit.
☐ 3. Massage the left leg with alcohol to stimulate circulation.
☐ 4. Cleanse the left lower leg with perfumed liquid soap.

58. A client is admitted with pneumonia and shingles with draining lesions over the right anterior and posterior chest wall. Of the nurses scheduled for the shift, which nurse(s) may be assigned to care for this client? Select all that apply.
☐ 1. 43-year-old nurse who had a preexposure varicella vaccination
☐ 2. 48-year-old nurse who had shingles 1 year ago
☐ 3. 32-year-old nurse who is in the first trimester of pregnancy
☐ 4. 24-year-old nurse who has never had the pneumococcal vaccine
☐ 5. 36-year-old nurse taking steroids for an autoimmune disease

Answers, Rationales, and Test-Taking Strategies

*The answers and rationales for each question follow below, along with keys to the client need (CN) and cognitive level (CL) for each question. In addition, questions that measure clinical judgment will be coded (CJ). As you check your answers, use the **Content Mastery and Test-Taking Skill Self-Analysis** worksheet (tear-out worksheet in the back of the book) to identify the reason(s) for not answering the questions correctly. For additional information about test-taking skills and strategies for answering questions, refer to pages 12–51 in part 1 of this book.*

The Adult with Burns

1. **1, 2, 3.** Clients who should be transferred to a burn center include children under age 10 or adults over age 50 with second- and third-degree burns on 10% or greater of their BSA, clients between ages 11 and 49 with second- and third-degree burns over 20% of their BSA, clients of any age with third-degree burns on more than 5% of their BSA, clients with smoke inhalation, and clients with chronic diseases, such as diabetes and heart or kidney disease.
   CN: Management of care; CL: Analyze

2. **3.** The nurse should have the client transported to a burn center. The client's age and the extent of the burns require care by a burn team, and the client meets triage criteria for referral to a burn center. Because of the age of the client and the extent of the burns, the nurse should not treat the burn.

Scald burns are not at high risk for infection and do not need to be cleaned, covered, or treated with antibiotic cream at this time.

🔑 CN: Physiological adaptation; CL: Analyze

3. 1. Fluid shifting into the interstitial space causes intravascular volume depletion and decreased perfusion to the kidneys. This would increase the serum creatinine level. Urine output should be frequently monitored and adequately maintained with intravenous fluid resuscitation that would be increased when a drop in urine output occurs. Urine output should be at least 30 mL per hour. Fluid replacement is based on the Parkland or Brooke formula and also the client's response by monitoring urine output, vital signs, and central venous pressure readings. Daily weight is important to monitor for fluid status. Little fluctuation in weight suggests that there is no fluid retention and the intake is equal to output. Exudative loss of albumin occurs in burns, causing a decrease in colloid osmotic pressure. The normal serum albumin is 3.5 to 5 g/dL (35 to 50 g/L).

🔑 CN: Physiological adaptation; CL: Analyze

4. 3. According to the rule of nines, this client, as shown in the figure, has sustained burns on about 45% of their body surface. The right arm is calculated as being 9%, the right leg is 18%, and the anterior trunk is 18%, for a total of 45%.

🔑 CN: Reduction of risk potential; CL: Apply

5. 3. Ensuring a urine output of 30 to 50 mL per hour is the best measure of adequate fluid resuscitation. The heart rate is elevated, but this is not an indicator of adequate fluid balance. The blood pressure is low, likely related to the hypovolemia, but the urinary output is the more accurate indicator of fluid balance and kidney function. The sodium level is within normal limits.

🔑 CN: Physiologic adaptation; CL: Evaluate

6. 4. It is critical that the nurse monitor the client's vital signs, hemodynamics, and urine output during the emergency and resuscitative phase of the burn injury. A urine output of less than 30 mL per hour is an indication of hypovolemia in this client. The serum creatinine, serum potassium, and oxygen saturation levels are all within acceptable limits.

🔑 CN: Physiological adaptation; CL: Analyze

7. 3. Removing dressings from severe burns exposes sensitive nerve endings to the air, which is painful. The client should be given a prescribed analgesic agent about one-half hour before the dressing change to promote comfort. The other activities are done as part of the whirlpool and dressing change process and not one-half hour beforehand.

🔑 CN: Reduction of risk potential; CL: Analyze

8. 4. Nutritional support with sufficient calories and protein is extremely important for a client with severe burns because of the loss of plasma protein through injured capillaries and an increased metabolic rate. Gastric dilation and paralytic ileus commonly occur in clients with severe burns, making oral fluids and foods contraindicated. Water and electrolyte imbalances can be corrected by the administration of intravenous fluids with electrolyte additives, though TPN typically includes all necessary electrolytes. Resting the gastrointestinal tract may help prevent paralytic ileus, and TPN provides vitamins and minerals; however, the primary reason for starting TPN is to provide the protein necessary for tissue healing.

🔑 CN: Pharmacological and parenteral therapies; CL: Evaluate

9. 2. Biologic dressings such as porcine grafts serve many purposes for a client with severe burns. They enhance the growth of epithelial tissues, minimize the overgrowth of granulation tissue, prevent loss of water and protein, decrease pain, increase mobility, and help prevent infection. They do not encourage the growth of tougher skin, provide for permanent wound closure, or facilitate the growth of subcutaneous tissue.

🔑 CN: Physiological adaptation; CL: Apply

10. 2. Rehabilitation efforts are implemented as soon as the client's condition is stabilized. Early emphasis on rehabilitation is important to decrease complications and to help ensure that the client will be able to make the adjustments necessary to return to an optimal state of health and independence. It is not possible to eliminate the client's pain; pain control is a major challenge in burn care.

🔑 CN: Basic care and comfort; CL: Analyze

11. 4. Immediately after a burn, excessive potassium from cell destruction is released into the extracellular fluid. Hyponatremia is a common electrolyte imbalance in a client with burns that occurs within the first week after being burned. Metabolic acidosis usually occurs as a result of the loss of sodium bicarbonate.

🔑 CN: Reduction of risk potential; CL: Analyze

12. **2.** Airway management is the priority in caring for a burn client. Tracheostomy or endotracheal intubation is anticipated when significant thermal and smoke inhalation burns occur. Clients who have experienced burns to the face and neck usually will be compromised within 1 to 2 hours. Electrical burns on the hands and arms, even with cardiac arrhythmias, or a chemical burn on the chest and abdomen is not likely to result in the need for intubation. Secondhand smoke inhalation influences an individual's respiratory status, but it does not require intubation unless the individual has an allergic reaction to the smoke.

CN: Physiological adaptation; CL: Analyze

13. **3.** The decreased urine output, low blood pressure, low CVP, and high heart rate indicate hypovolemia and the need to increase fluid volume replacement. Furosemide is a diuretic that should not be given due to the existing fluid volume deficit. Fresh frozen plasma is not indicated. It is given for clients with deficient clotting factors who are bleeding. Fluid replacement used for burns is lactated Ringer's solution, normal saline, or albumin.

CN: Management of care; CL: Analyze

14. **3.** The inflammatory response begins when a burn is sustained. As a result of the burn, the immune system becomes impaired. There is a decrease in immunoglobulins, changes in white blood cells, alterations of lymphocytes, and decreased levels of interleukin. The human body's protective barrier, the skin, has been damaged. As a result, the burn client becomes vulnerable to infections. Education and interventions to maintain a positive self-concept would be appropriate during the rehabilitation phase. Promoting hygiene helps the client feel comfortable; however, the primary focus is on reducing the risk for infection.

CN: Safety and infection control; CL: Analyze

15. **1, 5, 6.** The most helpful strategies to prevent and manage contractures when a client has burns on the hands are to keep the hands elevated, use hand splints, and engage in physical therapy. The nurse should collaborate with the entire burn team to prevent contractures. The nurse should administer pain medication and provide hygiene measures as prescribed, but these do not directly prevent contractures. The nurse should check with the health care provider before applying moisturizer or other substances to the burned area.

CN: Health promotion and maintenance; CL: Analyze

16. **4.** A Curling ulcer, or gastrointestinal ulceration, occurs in about half of clients with a burn injury. The incidence of ulceration appears proportional to the extent of the burns, and the ulceration is believed to be caused by hypersecretion of gastric acid and compromised gastrointestinal perfusion. Paralytic ileus and gastric distention do not result from hypersecretion of gastric acid and stress and thus are not expected findings at this time. Hiatal hernia is not necessarily a potential complication of a burn injury.

CN: Physiological adaptation; CL: Analyze

17. **2.** The severe pain experienced by burn clients requires opioid analgesic medications. In addition, opioids such as morphine sedate and alleviate apprehension. Oral analgesic medications such as ibuprofen or acetaminophen are unlikely to be strong enough to effectively manage the intense pain experienced by the client who is severely burned. Because of the altered tissue perfusion from the burn injury, intravenous medications are preferred. Antianxiety agents are not effective against pain.

CN: Pharmacological and parenteral therapies; CL: Analyze

The Older Adult with General Problems of the Integumentary System

18. **2.** Noting changes from the normally expected findings is the most important component when assessing an older client's integumentary system. Comparing one extremity with the contralateral extremity (i.e., comparing one side with the other) is an important assessment step; however, the most important component is noting changes from an expected normal baseline. Noting wrinkles related to age is not of much consequence unless the client is admitted for cosmetic surgery to reduce the appearance of age-related wrinkling. Noting skin turgor is an assessment of fluid status, not an assessment of the integumentary system.

CN: Health promotion and maintenance; CL: Analyze

19. **1, 3, 4, 5.** Skin changes associated with aging include diminished hair on the scalp and pubic areas, solar lentigo (liver spots), wrinkles, and xerosis (dryness). Dusky rubor of the left lower extremity may indicate the client has a venous stasis problem in the affected extremity and is generally associated with "unsuccessful aging." Yellow pigmentation of the skin that may be associated with liver inflammation is generally known as jaundice.

CN: Health promotion and maintenance; CL: Analyze

20. **3.** Normal aging consists of a decreased proliferative capacity of the skin. Decreased collagen slows capillary growth, impairs phagocytosis among older clients, and results in slow healing. Increased scarring is not a result of age-related skin changes. Both melanin and melanocytes give color to the skin and hair but are increased with aging. There is a decrease in the immunocompetence of the aging client.

CN: Health promotion and maintenance; CL: Analyze

21. **1.** Drinking at least 6 cups (about 1½ L) of fluid per day helps the client stay well hydrated. Maintaining optimal fluid balance is important for all body systems, particularly the skin. Caloric intake varies according to an individual's size and activity level. An intake of 1200 calories a day may be insufficient for some older clients. Walking 10 minutes a day is useful, but an otherwise healthy older client should try to walk 20 to 30 minutes a day three or more times a week. It is important to get adequate rest; however, the amount of sleep needed varies with the individual.

CN: Health promotion and maintenance; CL: Evaluate

22. **2.** Poorly controlled diabetes is a serious risk factor for postoperative wound infection. Other factors that delay wound healing include nutritional deficiencies (vitamin C, protein, zinc), use of corticosteroids, infection, mechanical friction on the wound, obesity, anemia, and poor general health. A previous myocardial infarction is not a risk factor for wound infection. Peripheral vascular disease is not as much of a risk factor for infection of an abdominal wound as it might be for more distal parts of the body. Being frail is not a specific risk factor for wound infection.

CN: Reduction of risk potential; CL: Analyze

23. **1, 2, 3.** The nurse should always assess an older adult who has signs of bruising (ecchymosis) for signs of abuse, self-inflicted injuries, or injuries that might have occurred from falls. Also, the aging process involves increased capillary fragility and permeability, and because older adults have a decreased amount of subcutaneous fat, it is also likely that there is an increased incidence of bruise-like lesions caused by a collection of extravascular blood in the loosely structured dermis. In addition, older clients do not always realize that injury has occurred because of a diminished awareness of pain, touch, and peripheral vibration. Blood supply to the skin decreases with aging and thus is not a cause of ecchymosis. Shingles presents as a red rash and fluid-filled blisters.

CN: Health promotion and maintenance; CL: Analyze

24. **4.** Older clients have a decreased thermoregulation that is related to decreased blood supply and reabsorption of body fat. As a result, older adults are at risk for hypothermia. Cellular cohesion and moisture content diminish with age, and cellular renewal time is slowed; however, these do not result in impaired thermoregulation.

CN: Health promotion and maintenance; CL: Analyze

25. **3, 5.** Tinea capitis is a contagious fungal infection of the hair shaft. The hair should be shampooed two or three times with selenium sulfide shampoo. An oral medication will typically be prescribed as well since the shampoo alone will not cure tinea capitis. Vinegar and water may be used to treat tinea pedis. The most common fungal skin infection is tinea (also called *ringworm* because of its characteristic appearance of a ring or rounded tunnel under the skin). Tinea infections affect the head, body, groin, feet, and nails. Antibacterial ointment and soap are not effective for treating fungal infections.

CN: Physiological adaptation; CL: Create

26. **1.** The client is at risk for infection because of the pruritus, and the nurse should institute measures to help the client control the scratching such as cutting fingernails, using protective gloves or mitts, and, if necessary, using antianxiety medications. More information is required regarding the knowledge level of the client, but learning cannot take place when an individual's attention is distracted by pruritus. Increasing fluid intake is not a priority at this time. There are no data to indicate the client is experiencing social isolation.

CN: Reduction of risk potential; CL: Analyze

27. **1.** Before using any restraints, the nurse must verify that a health care provider has prescribed the restraint. The mitt does not need to be secured with ties. The client can move the hand as needed. It is not necessary to place a pillow under the wrist. The nurse should place the mitt on the palmar surface of the hand.

CN: Safety and infection control; CL: Analyze

28. **2, 3.** Usual aging is associated with dry skin; however, seborrhea (oily skin and dandruff) is one result of the biochemical changes associated with Parkinson disease. The client with Parkinson disease has a higher risk for skin breakdown because of the moist and oily skin. To maintain skin integrity, a client with Parkinson disease needs frequent skin care and aeration of the skin. Gait instability in a client with Parkinson disease is a result of muscle rigidity, change in the center of gravity, and gait shuffling. Because of these changes in gait and balance, the client is at higher risk for injuries in the environment, such as hitting furniture or obstacles in the client's path. As a result, the environment should be evaluated for potential injury or falls. Tissue perfusion and verbal communication are not problems typically associated with Parkinson disease. The client should not experience activity intolerance from the cellulitis or Parkinson disease.

CN: Health promotion and maintenance; CL: Analyze

29. **4.** It is important for the client to understand the need to complete the entire course of oral antibiotics as prescribed to prevent recurrence or worsening of cellulitis. If the pain and redness continue despite antibiotics, the client should follow up with the health care provider. Extra vitamin C, protective footwear, and elevating the foot are strategies to promote healing.

CN: Management of care; CL: Analyze

30. **2.** Pressure ulcers usually occur over bony prominences. An alteration in the protective pressure sensation results from a decline in the number of Meissner and Pacinian corpuscles. Older adults have altered balance that may result in falls, but not skin breakdown. Impaired hearing and vision do not contribute to pressure ulcers.

CN: Reduction of risk potential; CL: Analyze

The Adult with Shingles

31. **1, 2, 3.** The nurse should instruct the client and family members about the importance of taking antiviral agents as prescribed. The client must be taught how to apply wet dressings or medication to the lesions and to follow proper hand hygiene techniques to avoid spreading the virus. The healing time varies from 7 to 26 days. The most common complication is postherpetic neuralgia, which may last longer than 6 months. It is not necessary for the client to remain in isolation.

CN: Health promotion and maintenance; CL: Create

32. **3.** People older than 50 years should receive the shingles vaccine to prevent the disease. The vaccine is not effective for genital herpes. The vaccine can be given to persons who have or have not had chickenpox. The vaccine is not advised for persons with a compromised immune system, for example, those receiving chemotherapy or radiation therapy.

CN: Health promotion and maintenance; CL: Apply

33. **3.** A newer vaccine, Shingrix, is available and offers greater protection against the shingles virus. The vaccine is administered in two doses 2 to 6 months apart. Even though the client has been vaccinated with Zostavax, the client should be revaccinated with the newer vaccine. The vaccine with Zostavax is not considered up to date, but it is effective; however, it does not offer the same protection as being revaccinated. Clients over the age of 50 should receive the newer vaccine or be revaccinated as needed.

CN: Health promotion and maintenance; CL: Analyze

34. **1, 2, 3, 4, 6.** Diphenhydramine is an antihistamine that reduces allergic reactions, calamine lotion is a topical antipruritic, and acetaminophen is an analgesic medication. These medications may help increase client comfort by reducing pain, inflammation, and itching, which, in turn, may reduce client scratching and potentially spreading the virus. Cool wet compresses also relieve itching and pain. Ondansetron is an antiemetic and would not be helpful for this client's discomfort.

CN: Physiological integrity; CL: Analyze

The Adult with a Pressure Ulcer

35. **3.** When assessing a client with dark skin for the presence of a pressure ulcer, the nurse should observe for skin that is darker, brownish, purplish, or bluish compared to surrounding skin. Fluorescent light casts a blue light, making skin assessment difficult; natural or halogen light sources help the nurse accurately assess the skin. Risk assessment using the Braden Scale should be performed on all clients. A Braden score of 12 indicates a high risk for pressure ulcer, and the lower the Braden score, the higher the risk (no risk: 19 to 23; at risk: 15 to 18; moderate risk: 13 to 14; high risk: 10 to 12, and very high risk: 9 or below). The nurse should touch the skin to assess consistency and temperature differences.

CN: Physiological adaptation; CL: Analyze

36. **3.** A stage I ulcer presents as an area of intact, nonblanchable redness, usually over a bony prominence, caused by pressure. If a reddened area blanches and refills with fingertip pressure, it indicates that there is still some blood flow to the injured area, and the redness may be reversible. It may be appropriate to complete and document a Braden score or consult a wound nurse specialist, but it is imperative to reposition the client off the reddened skin area first. Since there is no break in the skin, it is not appropriate to apply a wet to moist dressing.

    CN: Basic care and comfort; CL: Analyze

37. **2, 5.** Clients from some cultures highly respect educated professionals and will nod "yes" in response to questions out of respect. Clients may also nod their heads to avoid loss of face if they do not understand the information. Having the interpreter repeat the question to confirm the response will result in the same response and uncertainty related to understanding. Having the client sign the patient education document to confirm understanding would not confirm the client's understanding. Unless the nurse tries a different approach to instructing the client, the client may continue to not understand how to change the dressing; observing the client change the dressing or having the client explain the procedure are effective ways to evaluate the client's understanding of the procedure.

    CN: Reduction of risk potential; CL: Analyze

38. **2.** Stage I pressure ulcers appear as nonblanching macules that are red in color. Stage II ulcers have breakdown of the dermis. Stage III ulcers have full-thickness skin breakdown. In stage IV ulcers, the bone, muscle, and supporting tissue are involved. The nurse should immediately initiate plans to relieve the pressure, ensure good nutrition, and protect the area from abrasion.

    CN: Reduction of risk potential; CL: Analyze

39. **3.** A stage II skin breakdown involves epidermal sloughing and pain. Redness without blanching is noted in stage I. Stage III involves tissue necrosis with subcutaneous involvement. Stage IV involves muscle or bone destruction. Muscle spasm is not a criterion used in the staging process.

    CN: Physiological adaptation; CL: Analyze

40. **3.** The pressure ulcer has changed from stage I to stage II and requires the use of a protective dressing. Repositioning and use of foam mattresses are appropriate interventions for stage I pressure ulcers. While the daughter can take pictures and send them to the nurse, it is the nurse's responsibility to make decisions about needed care. Telehealth monitoring equipment is providing sufficient visualization of the skin changes; the nurse does not need to make a home visit at this time.

    CN: Reduction of risk potential; CL: Analyze

41.

STEP 1

0/1 **3, 4, 6, 8.** The immediate concerns of the nurse are the client's risk for infection with a stage II pressure injury and risk for new or further skin breakdown, especially since the client is incontinent and now requires complete care. The client has postoperative pain and is currently receiving morphine, and the nurse should plan pain management strategies with the client. Also, the nurse should monitor the client's mental status at this time as they are only oriented to person and have diagnoses of dementia and depression. The vital signs are within normal limits. After the nurse follows up with immediate needs, they can follow up on the client's request to see their adult child, who is the client's health care proxy. The client's nutritional status is important for wound healing and establishing a weight control plan, but it does not require immediate follow-up.

CJ: Case study; Step 1: Recognize cues; CL: Analyze

42.

STEP 2

Braden Scale for Pressure Injury Risk				
Sensory Perception	1. Completely limited	2. Very limited	3. Slightly limited	4. No impairment
Moisture	1. Constantly moist	2. Very moist	3. Occasionally moist	4. Rarely moist
Activity	1. Bedfast	2. Chairfast	3. Walks occasionally	4. Walks frequently
Mobility	1. Completely immobile	2. Very limited	3. Slightly limited	4. No limitations
Nutrition	1. Very poor	2. Probably inadequate	3. Adequate	4. Excellent
Friction and Shear	1. Problem	2. Potential problem	3. No apparent problem	
Total Score				

If the score is less than 19, the client is at risk for developing pressure injuries.

The client has <u>very limited</u> sensory perception as the client has limited sensation in both legs. The client is incontinent of urine, so this risk would be rated as <u>occasionally moist</u>. The client is <u>chairfast</u> as they cannot get out of bed independently and are not ambulatory; the client's <u>mobility is very limited</u> since the client moves from the bed to the chair using a ceiling lift, which contributes to the client's comorbidities. The nurse rates the client's nutrition as <u>excellent</u> as the client has a good appetite and is eating most of their meals. The nurse rates the client as having a <u>problem with friction and shear</u> since the client already has a pressure ulcer and spends most time in bed or in a chair, which puts pressure on the coccyx.

🗝️ CJ: Case study; Step 2: Analyze cues; CL: Analyze

43.

STEP 3

0/1 **2, 3, 5, 7.** The nurse should prevent the client's risk for further development of the pressure injury. Decreased mobility due to amputation, friction and shear caused by limited mobility, bed rest and position in a chair, poor circulation due to lack of activity and diabetes, and incontinence that leads to moist skin are findings that increase the client's risk for further development of the pressure injury. The client's dementia does not directly contribute to the risk for pressure injury. Having adequate nutrition promotes wound healing and is not a contributing factor to the risk for pressure injury.

🗝️ CJ: Case study; Step 3: Prioritize hypothesis; CL: Analyze

44.

STEP 4

Intervention	Indicated	Not Indicated	Contraindicated
Record calorie counts	X		
Change wet-to-dry dressings daily	X		
Insert an indwelling urinary catheter			X
Order a pressure-relief mattress	X		
Administer 500 mL 0.9% sodium chloride IV once		X	
Administer 10 mg morphine orally every 4 hours as needed	X		

The nurse should record calorie counts, change wet-to-dry dressings daily, and order a pressure-relief mattress to promote circulation and healing and prevent further skin breakdown. The nurse should also administer pain medication as needed for a client with a recent amputation and a pressure injury. Inserting an indwelling urinary catheter is contraindicated since it creates a portal for infection; the nurse should try other measures first, such as using incontinence pads or bladder training. The client's vital signs are stable, and the client is taking oral foods and fluids; there is no indication that there is a need to administer the one-time dose of 500 mL of 0.9% sodium chloride.

🗝️ CJ: Case study; Step 4: Generate solutions; CL: Apply

45.

STEP 5

−/+ **3, 6, 7, 9.** The UAP can empty and record the urine output, order lunch, record food intake, and turn and reposition the client. The nurse's role is to supervise the UAP, who is responsible for performing basic supportive care, such as ambulating, turning and repositioning, bathing, recording intake and output, toileting, feeding, obtaining vital signs, and weighing the client. The nurse should not delegate a task to the UAP if the task requires *t*eaching, *a*ssessing, *p*lanning, and *ev*aluating (*Remember: TAPE).

🗝️ CJ: Case study; Step 5: Take action; CL: Apply

46.

STEP 6

0/1 **1, 3, 5, 6.** The client was admitted with a stage II pressure injury that was 8 cm, red, and did not blanche. Signs of healing include the area decreases in size, the skin blanches to touch, the tissue is red in color, and the client has less pain in the area. Cellulitis is a sign of infection and may require debridement. The ability to visualize a fatty layer indicates the pressure ulcer is increasing in size and depth.

🗝️ CJ: Case study; Step 6: Evaluate outcomes; CL: Evaluate

0/1

The Adult with Skin Cancer

47. **1.** People who have fair skin and high exposure to ultraviolet light are at increased risk for malignant neoplasms of the skin. The other risk factors include exposure to tar and arsenicals and family history. A history of hypertension is a coronary artery disease risk factor. Clients with dark skin have increased melanin and are not as prone to skin cancer.

🗝️ CN: Health promotion and maintenance; CL: Analyze

48. **−/+** **1, 2, 3, 5, 6.** Risk factors associated with skin cancer include age, exposure to chemical pollutants, exposure to the sun, genetics, and immunosuppression. As individuals age, the risk for developing skin cancer increases. Longtime exposure to the sun and exposure to chemical pollutants (nitrates, coal, tar, etc.) increase the risk for skin cancer. Individuals who have less skin pigmentation (e.g., fair, blue-eyed people) have a higher risk for skin cancer because they tend to incur sunburns rather than tan. Family history plays a role in cancer. Regardless, immunosuppressed individuals are at a higher risk for the development of any type of cancer, as the body's defenses are not functioning properly.

◦— CN: Health promotion and maintenance; CL: Apply

49. -/+ **1, 5.** The client is experiencing malignant hyperthermia, a reaction to anesthesia. Signs include elevated body temperature, muscle rigidity, and increased heart rate. Unless the body is cooled and the influx of calcium into the muscle cells is reversed, lethal cardiac arrhythmia and hypermetabolism occur. The client's body temperature can rise as high as 109°F (42.8°C) as body muscles contract. The nurse should administer dantrolene, an IV skeletal muscle relaxant used to reverse muscle rigidity. The nurse should also notify the surgeon. Elevating the head of the bed will not reverse hyperthermia. Adding fluids and inserting an indwelling urinary catheter are not immediately beneficial steps in reversing the progression of malignant hyperthermia. Ice packs are used to lower body temperature, not a heated blanket.

◦— CJ: Standalone trend; CL: Analyze

50. -/+ **1, 2.** Sunscreen should be applied 20 to 30 minutes before going outside, even in cloudy weather. Sunscreen with a minimum of 30 SPF should be used. Sunscreen containing benzophenones blocks both UVA and UVB rays. The rays of the sun are most dangerous between 1000 and 1400. Genetic screening is not indicated, though a mutated gene has been identified in some families with a high incidence of melanoma. A prior diagnosis of melanoma and having a first-degree relative diagnosed with melanoma increase a person's risk. Lesions should not be shave biopsied; an excisional biopsy technique is used.

◦— CN: Health promotion and maintenance; CL: Create

51. **4.** Tumor or lesion thickness is the predictive factor for survival. Cutaneous melanoma that is confined to the epidermis has a high cure rate. Asymmetry, border, color, and diameter are known as the "ABCDs" of melanoma. Thus, the amount of ulceration, age, and location are not clearly associated with the prognosis.

◦— CN: Health promotion and maintenance; CL: Analyze

Managing Care, Quality, and Safety of Adults with Health Problems of the Integumentary System

52. **4.** Massaging areas that are reddened due to pressure is contraindicated because it further reduces blood flow to the area. The UAP should not massage the bony prominences or use lotion on the area. Massage improves circulation and blood flow to muscle areas; however, because the area is reddened, the client is at risk for further skin breakdown.

◦— CN: Management of care; CL: Analyze

53. **3.** The problem of pressure ulcers in hospitalized clients is best addressed by using quality improvement techniques to identify the problem, determining strategies for improvement, and setting goals for outcomes. Benchmarking for comparison will indicate where this nursing unit compares with other units, but it does not address the problem for this unit; having clients with pressure ulcers on any unit is not acceptable. Educational programs are more effective after there is an understanding of the problem. Chart audits and blaming do not solve the problem or address quality improvement measures.

◦— CN: Management of care; CL: Analyze

54. -/+ **3, 4, 5, 6.** Infection control policies must be followed to prevent the spread of infection. Until the pathogens are identified, the client must be isolated in a private room. Utilizing contact isolation and wearing a protective isolation gown and clean gloves, in addition to following isolation protocol to exit the room, may aid in preventing the spread of infectious agents to others. A draining foot lesion does not require a negative air pressure room, which is primarily reserved for preventing the spread of tuberculosis.

◦— CN: Safety and infection control; CL: Analyze

55. **3.** By contacting the pharmacy to report the absence of the medication, the pharmacy can bring the medication to the client's medication box. From there on, the pharmacy can make sure the correct medications are present. Contacting the shift coordinator or the client's HCP will not correct the original cause of the variance. It is never appropriate to "borrow" a medication from another client.

◦— CN: Management of care; CL: Analyze

56. -/+ **2, 3, 5.** Advancing age, type 2 diabetes mellitus, and smoking are risk factors for delayed healing. Advanced age slows collagen because of a decrease in fibroblasts, impairs circulation, and requires a longer time for epithelialization of the skin. Type 2 diabetes mellitus reduces the supply of oxygen and nutrients secondary to vascular complications. Nicotine is a potent vasoconstrictor and impedes blood flow, which reduces the supply of oxygen and nutrients necessary for healing. Atrial fibrillation causes venous stasis in the atria, but it

does not affect wound healing. Hypertension does not affect healing.

 CN: Reduction of risk potential;
CL: Analyze

57. 1. The client has cellulitis and should elevate the affected area above heart level. Ambulation stimulates circulation and promotes the deposition of pathogens in other areas of the body. Alcohol and perfumed soaps are drying to the skin. Massaging the lower extremities could dislodge a clot.

 CN: Reduction of risk potential;
CL: Analyze

58. 1, 2, 4. While the 43-year-old nurse has not had chickenpox, they have been vaccinated against the disease. A person can have shingles twice, but there is nothing in the 48-year-old nurse's history that precludes them from caring for this client. Having or not having the pneumococcal vaccine does not preclude a health care worker from caring for someone with pneumonia or shingles. Anyone who is immunocompromised or pregnant is at an increased risk for contracting varicella and should not be assigned to care for a client with shingles. All health care workers should have evidence of immunity to varicella, and if not, they should receive two doses of the vaccine at the recommended intervals at the time of employment. However, in this scenario, the immunity status of the pregnant nurse is not given, and risk reduction is warranted.

 CN: Management of care; CL: Analyze

TEST 17
Responding to Emergencies, Mass Casualties, and Disasters

- Emergencies
- Mass Casualties
- Disasters
- Managing Care, Quality, and Safety of Adults
- Answers, Rationales, and Test-Taking Strategies

Emergencies

1. A client is admitted to the emergency department with a headache, weakness, and slight confusion. The health care provider diagnoses carbon monoxide poisoning. After starting an intravenous infusion, the nurse should take which action **next**?
   - ☐ 1. Initiate gastric lavage.
   - ☐ 2. Maintain body temperature.
   - ☐ 3. Administer 100% oxygen by mask.
   - ☐ 4. Determine if the client was suicidal.

2. Three hours ago, an adult was thrown from a car into a ditch. The client is now in the emergency department in stable condition. Vital signs are within normal limits. The client has an open fracture of the right tibia. For which sign should the nurse be especially alert?
   - ☐ 1. hemorrhage
   - ☐ 2. infection
   - ☐ 3. deformity
   - ☐ 4. shock

3. A client admitted to the emergency department with atrial fibrillation has a heart rate of 160 bpm. The nurse should implement which prescription **first**?
   - ☐ 1. Administer a heparin bolus.
   - ☐ 2. Administer a beta-blocker.
   - ☐ 3. Administer oxygen via nasal cannula.
   - ☐ 4. Prepare the client for an immediate cardioversion.

4. A client is admitted to the emergency department with atrial fibrillation and does not recall how long the rapid pulse and irregular heart rate have been occurring. The nurse should include which goal(s) of care at this time? Select all that apply.
   - ☐ 1. Convert the heart rate to sinus rhythm.
   - ☐ 2. Decrease cardiac output and workload.
   - ☐ 3. Maintain bed rest.
   - ☐ 4. Maintain a ventricular response below 100 bpm.
   - ☐ 5. Prevent an embolic stroke.

5. The nurse is discharging a client who had a fish hook embedded in their eye. The fish hook was removed surgically in the emergency department, but the client currently has no vision in that eye. The surgeon has informed the client that a corneal transplant may restore some vision but the surgery cannot be performed for 6 to 8 weeks and only if no infection occurs. What information should the nurse include in the discharge teaching plan?
   - ☐ 1. resting to reduce strain on the eye and promote healing after surgery
   - ☐ 2. washing hands carefully to keep the area clean and decrease the risk for infection
   - ☐ 3. verbalizing feelings regarding vision loss
   - ☐ 4. eating a healthy diet to promote healing and prevent constipation

6. A client with a laceration to their finger is in the triage area of the emergency department, waiting to be seen by a health care provider. The client has a runny nose and is sneezing and coughing. To prevent the spread of infection to others in the area, the nurse should take which action? Select all that apply.
   - ☐ 1. Place the client in an isolation room.
   - ☐ 2. Seat the client 6 feet away from others.
   - ☐ 3. Give the client a surgical mask to wear.
   - ☐ 4. Give the client sanitizing wipes to wash their hands.
   - ☐ 5. Instruct the client to dispose of any tissues or wipes in a no-touch receptacle.

7. There has been a car collision involving four vehicles. The nearest emergency department is 30 minutes away. Which client should be transported by helicopter rather than an ambulance to the nearest hospital?
   ☐ 1. a 10-year-old client with a simple fracture of the femur who is crying and looking for their parents
   ☐ 2. a middle-age client with cold, clammy skin and a heart rate of 120 bpm who is unconscious
   ☐ 3. a middle-age client with severe asthma and a heart rate of 120 bpm who is having difficulty breathing
   ☐ 4. an older adult client with a severe headache who is conscious

8. The nurse notices a fire in a wastebasket in a client's room. In which order of priority from first to last should the nurse perform the actions? All options must be used.

1. Confine the fire by closing the door to the client's room.
2. Extinguish the fire.
3. Remove the client from the room.
4. Pull the fire alarm at the alarm pull station.

9. A client is admitted to the emergency department with a full-thickness burn to the right arm. Upon assessment, the arm is edematous, the fingers are mottled, and the radial pulse is now absent. The client rates the pain as 8 on a scale of 0 to 10. What should the nurse do **next**?
   ☐ 1. Administer morphine sulfate intravenous (IV) push for the severe pain.
   ☐ 2. Call the health care provider (HCP) to report the loss of the radial pulse.
   ☐ 3. Continue to assess the arm every hour for any additional changes.
   ☐ 4. Instruct the client to exercise the fingers and wrist.

10. A client is brought to the emergency department with abdominal trauma following an automobile crash. The vital signs are temperature 97.0°F (36.1°C); heart rate 132 bpm; respiration rate 28 breaths/min; blood pressure 84/58 mm Hg; and oxygen saturation 89% on room air. Which prescription should the nurse implement **first**?
    ☐ 1. Administer 1 L 0.9% normal saline intravenously.
    ☐ 2. Draw a complete blood count with hematocrit and hemoglobin.
    ☐ 3. Obtain an abdominal x-ray.
    ☐ 4. Insert an indwelling urinary catheter.

11. A middle-age client collapses in the emergency department waiting room. What should the nurse do **first**?
    ☐ 1. Shake the client and shout their name.
    ☐ 2. Perform the head tilt/chin lift to open the client's airway.
    ☐ 3. Feel for any air movement from the client's nose or mouth.
    ☐ 4. Watch the client's chest for respirations.

12. A client is experiencing an allergic response. The nurse should perform the actions in which order from first to last? All options must be used.

1. Assess for urticaria.
2. Assess the airway and breathing pattern.
3. Notify the health care provider (HCP).
4. Activate the rapid response team.

13. A visitor to the hospital has a cardiac arrest. When determining to use an automated external defibrillator (AED), the nurse should consider that AEDs are used in cardiac arrest in which circumstances?
    ☐ 1. early defibrillation in cases of atrial fibrillation
    ☐ 2. cardioversion in cases of atrial fibrillation
    ☐ 3. pacemaker placement
    ☐ 4. early defibrillation in cases of ventricular fibrillation

14. A person in the hospital waiting room has collapsed and does not have a pulse. The nurse obtains the automatic external defibrillator. Indicate on the illustration where the nurse should place the other electrode of the automated external defibrillator.

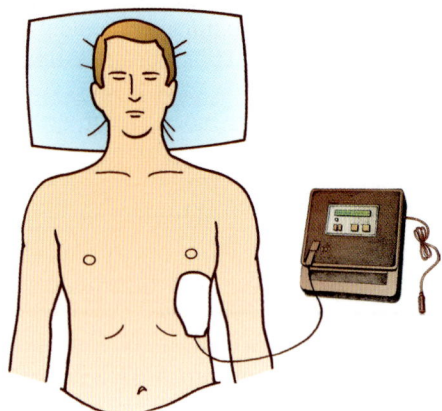

15. An adult has been admitted to the emergency department and diagnosed with food poisoning following an outdoor picnic. What should the nurse do? Select all that apply.
    ☐ 1. Tell the family to discard contaminated food.
    ☐ 2. Collect specimens for laboratory examination.
    ☐ 3. Assess vital signs.
    ☐ 4. Initiate support for the respiratory system.
    ☐ 5. Monitor fluid and electrolyte status.
    ☐ 6. Provide antiemetics, as prescribed.

16. The nurse in the emergency department reports there is a possibility of having had direct contact with the blood of a client who is suspected of having human immunodeficiency virus (HIV)/acquired immunodeficiency syndrome (AIDS). The nurse requests that the client have a blood test. Which circumstance(s) would indicate that the client does not need to give consent for HIV testing? Select all that apply.
    ☐ 1. An emergency medical provider has been exposed to the client's blood or body fluids.
    ☐ 2. Testing is prescribed by a health care provider (HCP) under emergency circumstances.
    ☐ 3. Testing is prescribed by a court, based on evidence that the client poses a threat to others.
    ☐ 4. Testing is done on blood collected anonymously in an epidemiologic survey.
    ☐ 5. An HCP who is taking care of a client suspected of having HIV/AIDS requests a blood test.

Mass Casualties

17. Thirty people are injured in a train derailment. Which client should be transported to the hospital **first**?
    ☐ 1. 20-year-old who is unresponsive and has a high injury to their spinal cord
    ☐ 2. 80-year-old who has a compound fracture of the arm
    ☐ 3. 10-year-old with a laceration on their leg
    ☐ 4. 25-year-old with a sucking chest wound

18. An explosion at a chemical plant produces flames and smoke. More than 20 persons, all adults, have burn injuries. Which client(s) should be transported to a burn center? Select all that apply. the client who has:
    ☐ 1. chemical spills on both arms
    ☐ 2. third-degree burns on both legs
    ☐ 3. first-degree burns on both hands
    ☐ 4. respiratory distress
    ☐ 5. inhaled smoke

19. An apartment fire spreads to seven apartment units. Clients experience burns, minor injuries, and broken bones from jumping from windows. Which client should be transported **first**?
    a client:
    ☐ 1. who is 5 months pregnant with no apparent injuries
    ☐ 2. with no injuries who has rapid respirations and coughs
    ☐ 3. with a simple fracture of the humerus who is in severe pain
    ☐ 4. with first-degree burns on their hands and forearms

20. There is a shooting in a shopping mall. Three clients with gunshot wounds are brought to the emergency department. What should the nurse do to preserve forensic evidence? Select all that apply.
    ☐ 1. Remove clothing without destroying evidence.
    ☐ 2. Place each item of clothing in a separate paper bag.
    ☐ 3. Hang wet clothing to dry.
    ☐ 4. Refrain from documenting client statements.
    ☐ 5. Place bullets in a sterile container.

21. An airplane crash results in mass casualties. The nurse is directing personnel to tag all clients. Which information should be placed on the tag? Select all that apply.
    ☐ 1. triage priority
    ☐ 2. identifying information when possible (such as name and age)
    ☐ 3. medications and treatments administered
    ☐ 4. presence of jewelry
    ☐ 5. next of kin

22. Four people who have been injured in a car crash are admitted to the emergency department. According to the emergency severity index (ESI), in which order from first to last should the clients be seen by a health care provider (HCP)? All options must be used.

1. an adult with bleeding through a pressure dressing from a laceration in the leg

2. a child with lacerations on the arms and legs

3. an adult with a history of asthma and respirations of 22 breaths/min

4. an older adult with normal vital signs, but is confused

23. A small airplane crashes in a neighborhood of 10 houses. One of the clients appears to have a cervical spine injury. What should first aid for this client include? Select all that apply.
☐ 1. Establish an airway, if needed, using the jaw-thrust maneuver.
☐ 2. Immobilize the spine by keeping the client flat.
☐ 3. Logroll the client to a side-lying position.
☐ 4. Elevate the feet 6 inches (15.2 cm).
☐ 5. Place a cervical collar around the neck.

24. Thirty-two children are brought to the emergency department after a school bus crash. Two children were killed along with the three people in the car who caused the crash. Before the clients arrive, in addition to ensuring that the hospital staff is prepared for the emergency, the nurse should anticipate carrying out which step?
☐ 1. calling the nearest crisis response team
☐ 2. alerting the news media
☐ 3. notifying the hospital volunteer office
☐ 4. calling the school to inform teachers of the crash

25. The nurse in the emergency department is triaging clients of an airplane crash. Prioritize the clients in the order in which they should be treated from first to last. All options must be used.

1. a 75-year-old client with a 2-inch (5.1-cm) laceration to their left forearm

2. a 22-year-old client with a 2-inch (5.1-cm) laceration to their left temple who is slightly confused

3. a 14-year-old client with a 2-inch (5.1-cm) laceration to the chin, a history of asthma, a respiration rate of 26 breaths/min, and audible wheezing

4. a 22-year-old client who is 36 weeks pregnant and experiencing contractions every 10 to 15 minutes

Disasters

26. A suspected outbreak of anthrax has been transmitted by skin exposure. A client is admitted to the emergency department with lesions on the hands. The health care provider prescribes antibiotics and sends the client home. What should the nurse instruct the client to do? Select all that apply.
☐ 1. Take the prescribed antibiotics for 60 days.
☐ 2. Avoid contact with other members of the family during the treatment period.
☐ 3. Wear a mask for 60 days.
☐ 4. Expect the skin lesions to clear up within 1 to 2 weeks.
☐ 5. Wash hands frequently.

27. An epidemic of severe acute respiratory syndrome (SARS) is occurring in a community of 10,000 people. Three people are being admitted to the emergency department. Two people are vomiting. Which type of precautions should the nurse institute?
☐ 1. enteric precautions
☐ 2. handwashing precautions
☐ 3. reverse isolation precautions
☐ 4. airborne precautions

28. Several clients who work in the same building are brought to the emergency department. They all have fever, headache, a rash over the entire body, and abdominal pain with vomiting and diarrhea. Upon initial assessment, the nurse finds that each client has low blood pressure and has developed petechiae in the area where the blood pressure cuff was inflated. Which isolation precautions should the nurse initiate?
    - ☐ 1. contact isolation with double gloving and shoe covers
    - ☐ 2. respiratory isolation with positive pressure rooms
    - ☐ 3. enteric precautions
    - ☐ 4. reverse isolation

29. Eight farm workers are admitted to the emergency department after they were splashed with "a couple of chemicals" at work 30 minutes ago. They have watery and itchy eyes, a slight cough, diaphoresis, and constricted pupils, and they are conscious and oriented. Their clothes are wet. What action should the nurse do **first**?
    - ☐ 1. Apply oxygen at 3 L per nasal cannula.
    - ☐ 2. Remove their clothing.
    - ☐ 3. Begin a decontamination shower.
    - ☐ 4. Isolate the clients.

30. The nurse is triaging clients who were removed from a building following its collapse from an earthquake. Which clients should be classified as red? Select all that apply.
    - ☐ 1. a 10-year-old client with a crushing chest wound and tachypnea with labored breathing who is unconscious and has an impaled object in their forehead
    - ☐ 2. a 49-year-old client with crushing chest pain radiating to the jaw who is diaphoretic and nauseated and has an open fracture of the left wrist
    - ☐ 3. a 75-year-old awake and alert client with an obvious fracture of the femur; absent pedal pulses on the affected side; a heart rate of 110 bpm; a respiration rate of 34 breaths/min; and diaphoretic skin who rates their pain as 10 on a scale of 0 to 10
    - ☐ 4. a 32-year-old client who is unconscious with a 3-inch (7.6-cm) laceration to their forehead; ecchymosis behind the ears; shallow respirations of 10 breaths/min; a weak, thready, rapid radial pulse; and no breath sounds on the right side

Managing Care, Quality, and Safety of Adults

31. A client who sustained a gunshot wound was treated in the emergency department and died. What can the nurse direct the unlicensed assistive personnel (UAP) to do during postmortem care? Select all that apply.
    - ☐ 1. Remove all tubes and intravenous (IV) lines.
    - ☐ 2. Cover the body with a sheet.
    - ☐ 3. Notify the family.
    - ☐ 4. Transport the body to the morgue.
    - ☐ 5. Notify the chaplain.

32. The nurse in the emergency department is administering a prescription for 20 mg intravenous furosemide, which is to be given immediately. The nurse scans the client's identification band and the medication barcode. The medication administration system does not verify that furosemide is prescribed for this client; however, the furosemide is prepared in the accurate unit dose for an intravenous infusion. What should the nurse do **next**?
    - ☐ 1. Contact the pharmacist immediately to check the prescription and the barcode label for accuracy.
    - ☐ 2. Administer the medication now, knowing the medication is labeled and the client is identified.
    - ☐ 3. Report the problem to the information technology team to have the barcode system recalibrated.
    - ☐ 4. Ask another nurse to verify the medication and the client so the medication can be given now.

33. The nurse notices a pair of nervous-acting individuals entering the emergency department. When reporting suspicious activity, the nurse should include which information in the report? Select all that apply.
    - ☐ 1. description of their vehicle or vehicles
    - ☐ 2. current location of the parties involved
    - ☐ 3. names and phone numbers of the parties involved
    - ☐ 4. relationship to the hospitalized client
    - ☐ 5. tone of voice of each party involved

34. There has been an increase in medication errors and errors in prescribing laboratory studies in the emergency department. The nurse manager is conducting a staff education session on when to use "read-back" procedures. Read-back procedures should be performed in which situation(s)? Select all that apply.
- ☐ 1. when a medication prescription or critical laboratory result is received verbally or over the telephone
- ☐ 2. when any verbal or phone prescription is received
- ☐ 3. whenever a written prescription or printed critical test result is received
- ☐ 4. when the unit secretary takes a phone prescription
- ☐ 5. when the agency uses computerized health care records

35. Several clients are in the emergency department. Which client should the nurse see **first**?
a client:
- ☐ 1. experiencing a "ripping" sensation in their chest
- ☐ 2. with a blood pressure of 170/95 mm Hg
- ☐ 3. with a urine output of 240 mL in 12 hours
- ☐ 4. taking anticoagulants with bloody stool

Answers, Rationales, and Test-Taking Strategies

*The answers and rationales for each question follow below, along with keys (🔑) to the client need (CN) and cognitive level (CL) for each question. In addition, questions that measure clinical judgment will be coded (CJ). As you check your answers, use the **Content Mastery and Test-Taking Skill Self-Analysis** worksheet (tear-out worksheet in the back of the book) to identify the reason(s) for not answering the questions correctly. For additional information about test-taking skills and strategies for answering questions, refer to pages 12–51 in part 1 of this book.*

Emergencies

1. 3. Carbon monoxide poisoning develops when carbon monoxide combines with hemoglobin. Because carbon monoxide combines more readily with hemoglobin than oxygen does, tissue anoxia results. The nurse should administer 100% oxygen by mask to reduce the half-life of carboxyhemoglobin. Gastric lavage is used for ingested poisons. With tissue anoxia, metabolism is diminished, with a subsequent lowering of the body's temperature; thus, steps to increase body temperature would be required. Once the effects of the carbon monoxide poisoning have been managed, the nurse can complete a history and physical examination and determine the possible cause of the poisoning.

🔑 CN: Physiological adaptation; CL: Analyze

2. 2. Because of the degree of contamination of the open fracture and the time that has passed since the crash, the risk for infection is very high. Therefore, the nurse should be especially alert for signs and symptoms of possible existing infection or early signs of infections, such as debris in the wound site, temperature abnormalities, results of laboratory studies (such as complete blood cell count and wound culture and sensitivities), or heat or redness around or in the wound. Because the client's vital signs and cardiovascular status are stable at this time, hemorrhage is not the primary concern. The client is talking coherently at this point, which does not suggest shock. However, the nurse should continue to assess the client for signs and symptoms of hemorrhage and shock. The fracture would be corrected by surgery as soon as possible, thereby minimizing the risk for deformity.

🔑 CN: Physiological adaptation; CL: Analyze

3. 3. The nurse should first administer oxygen; in atrial fibrillation, the workload of the heart is increased, and as a result, myocardial oxygen demands are also increased. A heparin bolus may be prescribed; it is not clear how long the client has been in atrial fibrillation, and it is critical to determine this before treatment is initiated. Beta-blockers and cardioversion are not primary interventions, and it is important first to determine if the client is hemodynamically stable and the length of time the client has had atrial fibrillation.

🔑 CN: Physiological integrity; CL: Analyze

4. ➖/➕ **3, 4, 5.** Clients who experience atrial fibrillation for more than 48 hours are at an increased risk for developing blood clots due to stasis of blood in the atria. Initially, it will be important to maintain a ventricular heart rate of less than 100 bpm and prevent complications related to clot formation, including an embolic stroke. It is not necessary to limit activities; the client can resume normal activities and slowly increase exercise tolerance. Treating the atrial fibrillation and decreasing the heart rate will help increase exercise tolerance. Atrial fibrillation causes a decrease in cardiac output, and a goal of therapy would be to increase cardiac output. It is imperative to determine the length of time a client has been in atrial fibrillation before performing a cardioversion. If a client has been in atrial fibrillation longer than 48 hours and a cardioversion is performed, a clot may be dislodged and become lodged in vessels of the brain, lungs, or coronary arteries.

🔑 CN: Physiological integrity; CL: Analyze

5. 2. Infection prevention is the immediate priority for this client to promote healing and a successful corneal transplant with the potential restoration of vision. Rest and a diet rich in nutrients and fiber to prevent straining due to constipation are important considerations as well as allowing the client to discuss feelings regarding vision loss. However, these are currently lower priority than infection prevention.

🔑 CN: Reduction of risk potential; CL: Analyze

6. -/+ **2, 3, 4, 5.** To prevent infections in hospitals, the nurse institutes measures to contain respiratory secretions in symptomatic clients. The nurse should ask the client to sit 6 feet away from others and give the client a mask to wear. The nurse can give the client sanitizing wipes to wash their hands and instruct the client to dispose of used wipes and tissues in a no-touch receptacle. It is not necessary to place the client in isolation unless the client also has a fever.

🔑 CN: Safety and infection control; CL: Analyze

7. 2. The middle-age woman is likely in shock; this client is classified as a triage level 1 and requires immediate care. The child with moderate trauma is classified as triage level 3, urgent, and can be treated within 30 minutes. The man with asthma and the man with the severe headache are classified as emergencies, triage level 2, and can be transported by ambulance and reach the hospital within 15 minutes.

🔑 CN: Management of care; CL: Analyze

8. 3, 4, 1, 2. The nurse uses the RACE procedure to manage a fire: Rescue, Alarm, Confine, Extinguish.

🔑 CN: Safety and infection control; CL: Apply

9. 2. Circulation can be impaired by circumferential burns and edema, causing compartment syndrome. Early recognition and treatment of impaired blood supply are key. The HCP should be informed since an escharotomy (incision through full-thickness eschar) is frequently performed to restore circulation. Pain management is important for clients with burns, but restoration of circulation is the priority. Assessments should be performed every 15 minutes while the radial pulse is absent. Exercise will not restore the obstructed circulation.

🔑 CN: Reduction of risk potential; CL: Analyze

10. -/+ **1.** The client is demonstrating vital signs consistent with fluid volume deficit, likely due to bleeding or hypovolemic shock as a result of the automobile crash. The client will need intravenous fluid volume replacement using an isotonic fluid (e.g., 0.9% normal saline) to expand or replace blood volume and normalize vital signs. The other prescriptions can be implemented once the intravenous fluids have been initiated.

🔑 CN: Physiologic adaptation; CL: Analyze

11. 1. Calling the client's name and gently shaking them is used to establish unresponsiveness. The head-tilt, chin-lift maneuver is used to open the client's airway. Feeling for any air movement from the client's nose or mouth indicates whether they are breathing on their own. The rescuer can watch the client's chest for respirations to see if they are breathing.

🔑 CN: Physiological adaptation; CL: Analyze

12. 2, 1, 4, 3. If a client is experiencing an allergic response, the nurse's initial action is to assess the client for signs and symptoms of anaphylaxis, first checking the airway, breathing pattern, and vital signs, with particular attention to signs of increasing edema and respiratory distress. The nurse should then assess for other indications of anaphylaxis, such as urticaria, feelings of impending doom or fright, weakness, sweating (because a severe systemic response to an allergen can result in massive vasodilation), increased capillary permeability, decreased perfusion, decreased venous return, and subsequent decreased cardiac output. The nurse should call the rapid response team and then notify the HCP.

🔑 CN: Reduction of risk potential; CL: Analyze

13. 4. AEDs are used for early defibrillation in cases of ventricular fibrillation. The American Heart Association and the Canadian Heart and Stroke Foundation place major emphasis on early defibrillation for ventricular fibrillation and the use of the AED as a tool to increase sudden cardiac arrest survival rates.

🔑 CN: Safety and infection control; CL: Apply

14. One electrode is placed to the right of the upper sternum just below the right clavicle. The other is placed, as shown, over the fifth or sixth intercostal space at the left anterior axillary line.

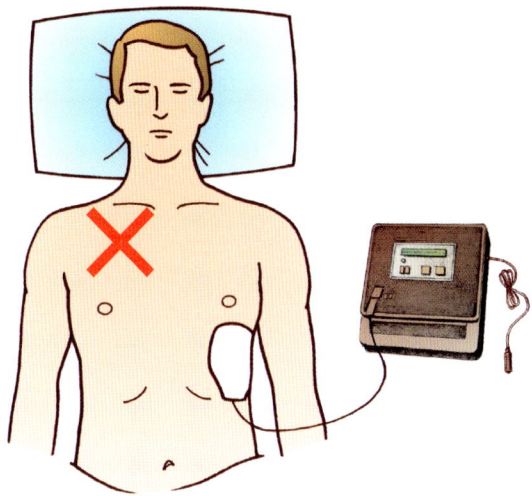

🔑 CN: Safety and infection control; CL: Apply

15. 🔢 2, 3, 4, 5, 6. Food poisoning is a sudden illness that occurs after ingestion of contaminated food or drink. The nurse should first assess vital signs and then ensure that the client is not in respiratory distress because death from respiratory paralysis can occur with botulism, fish poisoning, and other food poisonings. Measures to control nausea are important to prevent vomiting, which could exacerbate fluid and electrolyte imbalance. Because large volumes of electrolytes and water are lost by vomiting and diarrhea, fluid and electrolyte status needs to be continuously monitored. The key to treatment is determining the source and type of food poisoning. If possible, rather than discarding the food, the suspected food should be brought to the medical facility and a history obtained from the client or family.

🔑 CN: Physiological adaptation; CL: Analyze

16. 🔢 1, 2, 3, 4. Upon an HCP's written prescription requesting an HIV test for a client, consent for HIV testing must be obtained. Consent exceptions include the following: testing is prescribed by an HCP under emergency circumstances, and the test is medically necessary to diagnose or treat the client's condition; testing is prescribed by a court, based on clear and convincing evidence of a serious and present health threat to others posed by an individual; testing is done on blood collected or tested anonymously as part of an epidemiologic survey; or an emergency medical provider has been exposed to the client's blood or body fluids.

🔑 CN: Safety and infection control; CL: Apply

Mass Casualties

17. 4. During a disaster, the nurse must make difficult decisions about which persons to treat first. The guidelines for triage offer general priorities for immediate, delayed, minimal, and expectant care. The client with a sucking chest wound needs immediate attention and will likely survive. The 80-year-old is classified as delayed; emergency response personnel can immobilize the fracture and cover the wound. The 10-year-old has minimal injuries and can wait to be treated. The client with a spinal cord injury is not likely to survive and should not be among the first to be transported to the health care facility.

🔑 CN: Management of care; CL: Analyze

18. 🔢 1, 2, 4, 5. Clients with chemical burns, second- and third-degree burns over more than 20% of their body surface area, and those with inhalation injuries should be transported to a burn center. The client with first-degree burns on their hands can be treated with first aid on the scene and referred to a health care facility.

🔑 CN: Management of care; CL: Analyze

19. 2. The client with respiratory distress and coughing should be transported first because they are probably experiencing smoke inhalation. The pregnant client is not in imminent danger or likely to have a precipitous birth. The 10-year-old client is not at risk for infection and could be treated in an outpatient facility. First-degree burns are considered less urgent.

🔑 CN: Management of care; CL: Analyze

20. 🔢 2, 3. Preserving forensic evidence is essential for investigative purposes following injuries that may be caused by criminal intent. The nurse should put each item of clothing in a separate paper bag and label it; wet clothing should be hung to dry. The nurse should not cut or otherwise unnecessarily handle clothing, particularly clothing with such evidence as blood or body fluids. The nurse should document carefully the client's description of the incident and use quotes around the client's exact words where possible. The documentation will become a part of the client's record and can be subpoenaed for subsequent investigation. The nurse should not handle bullets from the client because they are an important piece of forensic evidence.

🔑 CN: Management of care; CL: Apply

21. 🔢 1, 2, 3. Tracking clients who experience disasters is important for casualty planning and management. All clients should receive a tag, securely attached, that indicates the triage priority, any available identifying information, and what

care, if any, has been given along with the time and date. Tag information should be recorded in a disaster log and used to track clients and inform families. It is not necessary to document the presence of jewelry or next of kin.

🗝️ CN: Management of care; CL: Apply

22. 1, 3, 2, 4. Using the ESI, the nurse should triage the clients to be seen by an HCP as follows: the adult with severe bleeding through a pressure dressing is categorized as level 1, life-threatening and should be seen first; the adult with asthma and increased respirations is in the emergency category and should be seen next; the child with lacerations is categorized as less urgent and can be seen next; and the older adult has vital signs within normal range and is assessed as being nonurgent and can be seen last.

🗝️ CN: Management of care; CL: Analyze

23. -/+ 1, 2. The client with a neck injury should be immobilized and moved as little as possible. It is also important to ensure an open airway; this can be accomplished with the jaw-thrust maneuver, which does not require tilting the head. The client should not be rolled to a side-lying position nor have the feet elevated. Both actions can cause additional injury to the spinal cord. Placing a cervical collar causes movement of the spinal column and should not be done as a first-aid measure.

🗝️ CN: Management of care; CL: Analyze

24. 1. The children and their families are at risk for experiencing a crisis. Disaster teams are available for crisis intervention in such emergencies. Usually, the news media monitors emergency radio frequencies and most likely are aware of the crash already. Although volunteers may help in some ways, they are not responsible for crisis intervention. Calling the school might be done, but the emergency issues take precedence.

🗝️ CN: Psychosocial integrity; CL: Analyze

25. 3, 2, 4, 1. The 14-year-old client with asthma needs immediate, lifesaving interventions for the wheezing and should be seen first. The 22-year-old client who is confused should be seen next to assess for head injury; the location of the laceration could indicate a significant blunt force traumatic injury. The pregnant client requires assessment but is not urgent unless other symptoms appear. The 75-year-old client is nonurgent and can wait safely for several hours.

🗝️ CN: Management of care; CL: Evaluate

Disasters

26. -/+ 1, 4. Anthrax is treated with antibiotics, and the client must continue the prescription for 60 days, even if symptoms do not persist. The client may have skin lesions at the point of contact, with macula or papule formation; the eschar will fall off in 1 to 2 weeks. Clients with anthrax are not contagious; the client does not need to follow isolation procedures at home. Anthrax from skin exposure is not transmitted by respiratory contact, and the client does not need to wear a mask.

🗝️ CN: Safety and infection control; CL: Analyze

27. 4. Transmission of SARS or other diseases such as Covid-19 that are transmitted by a respiratory route can be contained by full airborne precautions that include an isolation room with negative pressure, use of an N95 respirator, and use of personal protective equipment. The disease is spread by the respiratory, not enteric, route. Handwashing alone is not sufficient to prevent transmission. Reverse isolation (protection of the client) is not sufficient to prevent transmission.

🗝️ CN: Safety and infection control; CL: Analyze

28. 1. The nurse should institute treatment for hemorrhagic fever viruses, including contact isolation with double gloving and shoe covers, strict hand hygiene, and protective eyewear. The nurse should start respiratory isolation with negative pressure rooms, not positive pressure rooms. Enteric precautions are not needed because the virus is spread by droplets and contact. Reverse isolation protects the client; in this situation, the health care team also needs protection.

🗝️ CN: Safety and infection control; CL: Analyze

29. 4. The safety of the staff and others is the first priority. Isolating reduces the chance of contaminating others (secondary contamination). Vital signs can be obtained when it is safe—after protecting staff, clients, and visitors from secondary contamination. Oxygen is not indicated for any of the listed symptoms. Removing clothing is important to prevent further exposure to the client, but it must be done safely to prevent secondary contamination to others. The clients can remove their own clothes and place them in plastic bags. After the safety of the staff and others is addressed, the facility is prepared, and properly trained staff is ready, the clients can be given a decontamination shower. If the staff is not trained, 911 may be the most appropriate response. Finding out which chemicals were involved is important but does not take priority over preventing secondary contamination.

🗝️ CN: Management of care; CL: Analyze

30. -/+ **2, 3.** The client with crushing chest pain has an acute cardiac condition and can have a successful outcome if immediate interventions are initiated. The client with the open fracture could be stabilized and is not a significant factor in triage in a mass casualty incident. The client with a displaced femur fracture can also be classified as immediate because the fracture can impair circulation. There are also signs of shock and severe pain. All conditions can improve with interventions. In a mass casualty incident, the goal is to do the greatest good for the greatest number—which sometimes means that limited resources are not allocated to the very critically injured who have a very low probability of survival. The other two clients are categorized as expectant or may have a black tag because of their critical injuries and the unavailability of advanced trauma care.

🗝️ CN: Management of care; CL: Analyze

Managing Care, Quality, and Safety of Adults

31. -/+ **2, 4.** The UAP can cover the body and transport it to the morgue. Deaths by gunshot wound are considered reportable deaths. All evidence in a reportable death, including tubes and IV lines, should remain intact until the coroner has been contacted. The health care provider should be the one to notify the family. The nurse should be the one to notify the chaplain.

🗝️ CN: Management of care; CL: Analyze

32. 1. The nurse should contact the pharmacist first to be sure the medication is labeled for administration to this client. The nurse should not administer the drug until all safety precautions have been observed; the nurse should also not ask another nurse to verify the medication or client. Later, if the problem cannot be resolved by relabeling the medication, the nurse or pharmacist can contact the information technology team to check the barcode system.

🗝️ CN: Safety and infection control; CL: Analyze

33. -/+ **1, 2.** All suspicious individuals or activities should be reported as soon as possible to the security department. When reporting an incident, nurses/employees should provide the following information: (a) type of incident, (b) persons involved/physical description, (c) vehicles involved and description, (d) date and time the incident occurred, (e) location where the incident occurred, (f) weapons involved, and (g) current location of parties involved. All reports of threats, actual episodes of violence, or suspicious individuals or activities must be investigated.

🗝️ CN: Safety and infection control; CL: Analyze

34. -/+ **1, 2.** A goal of client safety is to improve the effectiveness of communication among caregivers. For verbal or telephone prescriptions or telephone reporting of critical test results, one must verify the complete prescription or test result by having the individual receiving the information read back the complete prescription or test result. The unit secretary is not a licensed health care professional who has a scope of practice or the authority to receive prescriptions or results. The type of charting system used by the health care agency is not a factor in using read-back prescriptions.

🗝️ CN: Management of care; CL: Analyze

35. 1. A "ripping" sensation in the chest is indicative of a ruptured thoracic aneurysm and warrants immediate intervention. While a blood pressure of 170/95 mm Hg is high, there is not enough information that suggests that this client is a higher priority than the others. A urine output of 240 mL in 12 hours is less than 30 mL per hour; however, this is this client's only problem now, and the nurse can investigate the cause next. A client experiencing bloody stools will need to be seen; however, no other information is present that would warrant this client being seen first.

🗝️ CN: Management of care; CL: Analyze

The Nursing Care of Clients with Psychiatric Disorders and Mental Health Problems

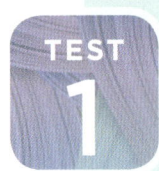

Mood Disorders

- The Client with Major Depression
- The Client with Bipolar Disorder, Manic Phase
- The Client with Suicidal Ideation and Suicide Attempt
- The Client with Psychosexual Disorders
- Managing Care, Quality, and Safety of Clients with Mood Disorders
- Answers, Rationales, and Test-Taking Strategies

The Client with Major Depression

1. The nurse is planning care with a Latino client who is diagnosed with a depressive disorder. The client uses treatment by a root healer. Which intervention is **most** indicated?
   ☐ 1. Avoid talking to the client about the root healer.
   ☐ 2. Explain to the client that Western medicine has a scientific, not mystical, basis.
   ☐ 3. Explain that such beliefs are superstitious and should be forgotten.
   ☐ 4. Involve the root healer in a consultation with the client, health care provider, and nurse.

2. After a period of unsuccessful treatment with amitriptyline, a client diagnosed with depression is switched to tranylcypromine. Which statement by the client indicates the client understands the side effects of tranylcypromine?
   ☐ 1. "I need to increase my intake of sodium."
   ☐ 2. "I must refrain from strenuous exercise."
   ☐ 3. "I must refrain from eating aged cheese or yeast products."
   ☐ 4. "I should decrease my intake of foods containing sugar."

3. A client visits the mental health clinic and reports being lethargic, experiencing pain in the back, having difficulty concentrating, and feeling depressed. The nurse observes patches of hair loss on the client's scalp. Which referral should the nurse make **first**?
   ☐ 1. occupational therapist
   ☐ 2. physical therapist
   ☐ 3. psychologist
   ☐ 4. health care provider

4. A client has been taking 30 mg of duloxetine twice daily for 2 months because of depression and vague aches and pains. While interacting with the nurse, the client discloses a pattern of drinking a six-pack of beer daily for the past 10 years to help with sleep. What should the nurse do **first**?
   ☐ 1. Refer the client to the concurrent disorders program at the clinic.
   ☐ 2. Share the information at the next interdisciplinary treatment conference.
   ☐ 3. Report the client's beer consumption to the health care provider (HCP).
   ☐ 4. Teach the client relaxation exercises to perform before bedtime.

5. A client was admitted to the inpatient unit 3 days ago with a flat affect, psychomotor deficits, anorexia, hopelessness, and suicidal ideation. The health care provider prescribed 75 mg of venlafaxine extended release to be given every morning. The client interacted minimally with the staff and spent most of the day in their room. At the beginning of the shift, the nurse observes that the client is smiling and cheerful and appears to be relaxed. What should the nurse interpret as the **most** likely cause of the client's behavior?
   - ☐ 1. The venlafaxine is helping the client's symptoms of depression significantly.
   - ☐ 2. The client's sudden improvement calls for close observation by the staff.
   - ☐ 3. The staff can decrease their observation of the client.
   - ☐ 4. The client is nearing discharge due to the improvement of symptoms.

6. A 16-year-old client is prescribed 10 mg of paroxetine at bedtime for major depression. The nurse should instruct the client and parents to monitor the client closely for which adverse effect?
   - ☐ 1. headache
   - ☐ 2. nausea
   - ☐ 3. fatigue
   - ☐ 4. agitation

7. A client diagnosed with major depression spends most of the day lying in bed with the sheet pulled over the head. Which approach by the nurse is **most** therapeutic?
   - ☐ 1. Wait for the client to begin the conversation.
   - ☐ 2. Initiate contact with the client frequently.
   - ☐ 3. Sit outside the client's room.
   - ☐ 4. Question the client until the client responds.

8. A client exhibits a flat affect, psychomotor deficits, and depressed mood. The nurse attempts to engage the client in an interaction, but the client does not respond to the nurse. Which response by the nurse is **most** appropriate?
   - ☐ 1. "I'll sit here with you for 15 minutes."
   - ☐ 2. "I'll come back a little bit later to talk."
   - ☐ 3. "I'll find someone else for you to talk with."
   - ☐ 4. "I'll get you something to read."

9. After a few minutes of conversation, a client who is depressed wearily asks the nurse, "Why pick me to talk to? Go talk to someone else." Which reply by the nurse is **best**?
   - ☐ 1. "I'm assigned to care for you today, if you'll let me."
   - ☐ 2. "You have a lot of potential, and I'd like to help you."
   - ☐ 3. "I'll talk to someone else later."
   - ☐ 4. "I'm interested in you and want to help you."

10. The health care provider prescribes fluoxetine orally every morning for a 72-year-old client with depression. Which transient adverse effect of this drug requires **immediate** action by the nurse?
    - ☐ 1. nausea
    - ☐ 2. dizziness
    - ☐ 3. sedation
    - ☐ 4. dry mouth

11. A client is taking trazodone as prescribed by the health care provider. Which statement by the client indicates to the nurse that further teaching about the medication is needed?
    - ☐ 1. "I'll continue to take my medication after a light snack."
    - ☐ 2. "Taking trazodone at night will help me to sleep."
    - ☐ 3. "My depression will be gone in about 5 to 7 days."
    - ☐ 4. "I will not drink alcohol while taking trazodone."

12. A middle-age client with severe depression and psychotic symptoms is scheduled for electroconvulsive therapy (ECT) tomorrow morning. The client's adult child asks the nurse, "How painful will the treatment be for my parent?" The nurse should respond with which statement?
    - ☐ 1. "Your parent will be given something for pain before the treatment."
    - ☐ 2. "The health care provider (HCP) will make sure your parent does not suffer needlessly."
    - ☐ 3. "Your parent will be asleep during the treatment and will not be in pain."
    - ☐ 4. "Your parent will be able to talk to us and tell us if they are in pain."

13. During a group session, a client who is depressed tells the group, "I just lost my job." Which response by the nurse is **best**?
    - ☐ 1. "It must have been very upsetting for you."
    - ☐ 2. "Would you tell us about your job?"
    - ☐ 3. "You'll find another job when you're better."
    - ☐ 4. "You were probably too depressed to work."

14. A client who is very depressed exhibits psychomotor deficits, a flat affect, and apathy. The nurse observes that the client needs grooming and hygiene. Which nursing action is **most** appropriate?
    - ☐ 1. explaining the importance of hygiene to the client
    - ☐ 2. asking the client if they are ready to shower
    - ☐ 3. waiting until the client's family can participate in the client's care
    - ☐ 4. stating to the client that it is time for them to take a shower

15. A client is to receive electroconvulsive therapy (ECT). Which intervention(s) should the nurse include in the plan of care to prepare a client for ECT? Select all that apply.
    ☐ 1. Maintain nothing-by-mouth (NPO) status.
    ☐ 2. Verify if consent is signed.
    ☐ 3. Orient the client to place and time.
    ☐ 4. Remove dentures.
    ☐ 5. Request the client to void.
    ☐ 6. Assess the client's vital signs every 30 minutes.

16. A teaches the client about the prescribed medication sertraline. Which comment indicates that a client understands the nurse's teaching?
    ☐ 1. "Sertraline will probably cause me to gain weight."
    ☐ 2. "This medicine can cause delayed ejaculation."
    ☐ 3. "Dry mouth is a permanent side effect of sertraline."
    ☐ 4. "I can take my medicine with St. John's wort."

17. The client with recurring depression will be discharged from the psychiatric unit. What instructions for the family are **most** important to include in the plan of care?
    ☐ 1. Discourage visitors while the client is at home.
    ☐ 2. Provide a schedule of activities outside the home.
    ☐ 3. Involve the client in usual at-home activities.
    ☐ 4. Encourage the client to sleep as much as possible.

18. A client with major depression and psychotic features is admitted involuntarily to the hospital. The client will not eat because "my bowels have turned to jelly," which the client states is punishment for wickedness. The client requests to leave the hospital. The nurse denies the request because commitment papers have been initiated by the health care provider. The nurse understands this client is legally committable based on which criterion?
    ☐ 1. evidence of psychosis
    ☐ 2. being gravely disabled
    ☐ 3. risk for harm to self or others
    ☐ 4. diagnosis of mental illness

19. The client states to the nurse, "I take citalopram 40 mg every day as my health care provider prescribed. I have also been taking St. John's wort 750 mg daily for the past 2 weeks." Which findings would indicate that the client is developing serotonin syndrome? Select all that apply.
    ☐ 1. confusion
    ☐ 2. restlessness
    ☐ 3. constipation
    ☐ 4. diaphoresis
    ☐ 5. ataxia

20. A client is prescribed phenelzine. Which food should the nurse tell the client to avoid while taking the medication?
    ☐ 1. roasted chicken
    ☐ 2. salami
    ☐ 3. fresh fish
    ☐ 4. hamburger

21. A client is taking phenelzine 15 mg orally three times a day. The nurse is about to administer the next dose when the client tells the nurse about having a throbbing headache. Which action should the nurse do **first**?
    ☐ 1. Give the client an analgesic medication prescribed as needed.
    ☐ 2. Call the health care provider (HCP) to report the symptom.
    ☐ 3. Administer the client's next dose of phenelzine.
    ☐ 4. Obtain the client's vital signs.

22. The nurse is caring for a severely depressed client. Which statement by the nurse is **best** when talking to the client on the patient care unit?
    ☐ 1. "Everybody feels down once in a while."
    ☐ 2. "Things will get better."
    ☐ 3. "You're wearing a new shirt today."
    ☐ 4. "I like the shoes you wore yesterday."

23. The nurse assesses a client with depressive disorder for discharge readiness. Which behavior would lead the nurse to determine that the client is ready for discharge?
    ☐ 1. interactions with staff and peers
    ☐ 2. sleeping for 4 hours at a time
    ☐ 3. verbalization of feeling in control of self and situations
    ☐ 4. statements of dissatisfaction over not being able to perform at work

24. The client with major depression and suicidal ideation has been taking bupropion 100 mg orally three times daily for 5 days. Assessment reveals the client is somewhat less withdrawn, able to perform activities of daily living with minimal assistance, and eating 50% of each meal. At this time, the nurse should monitor the client specifically for which behavior?
    ☐ 1. seizure activity
    ☐ 2. suicide attempt
    ☐ 3. visual disturbances
    ☐ 4. increased libido

25. A client exhibits psychomotor deficits, withdrawal, minimal eye contact, and unresponsiveness to the nurse's questions. Which outcome should the nurse include in the initial plan of care?
    The client will:
    ☐ 1. initiate interactions with peers.
    ☐ 2. participate in milieu activities.
    ☐ 3. discuss adaptive coping techniques.
    ☐ 4. interact with the nurse.

26. The nurse prepares a teaching plan for a client about imipramine. Which substance should the nurse tell the client to avoid while taking the medication?
☐ 1. caffeinated coffee
☐ 2. sunscreen
☐ 3. alcohol
☐ 4. artificial tears

27. The client with depression who is taking imipramine states to the nurse, "My psychiatrist wants me to have an electrocardiogram (ECG) in 2 weeks, but my heart is fine." Which response by the nurse is **most** appropriate?
☐ 1. "It's routine practice to have an ECG periodically because there is a slight chance that the drug may affect the heart."
☐ 2. "It's probably a precautionary measure because I'm not aware that you have a cardiac condition."
☐ 3. "Try not to worry too much about this. Your health care provider (HCP) is just being very thorough in monitoring your condition."
☐ 4. "You had an ECG before you were prescribed imipramine, and the procedure will be the same."

28. The nurse assesses a client who is receiving tricyclic antidepressant therapy. The nurse should be alert for which finding that could suggest the client is experiencing anticholinergic effects?
☐ 1. tremors and cardiac arrhythmias
☐ 2. sedation and delirium
☐ 3. respiratory depression and convulsions
☐ 4. urine retention and blurred vision

29. The health care provider (HCP) prescribes mirtazapine 30 mg orally at bedtime for a client diagnosed with depression. Which nursing action is indicated?
☐ 1. Give the medication as prescribed.
☐ 2. Question the HCP's prescription.
☐ 3. Request to give the medication in the morning.
☐ 4. Give the medication in three divided doses.

30. The nurse develops a teaching plan for a client about the medications prescribed for depression. Which component is **most** important for the nurse to include?
☐ 1. pharmacokinetics of the medication
☐ 2. current research related to the medication
☐ 3. management of common adverse effects
☐ 4. dosage regulation and adjustment

31. A client diagnosed with severe major depression has been taking escitalopram 10 mg daily for the past 2 weeks. Which parameter should the nurse monitor **most** closely at this time?
☐ 1. suicidal ideation
☐ 2. sleep
☐ 3. appetite
☐ 4. energy level

32. A client taking paroxetine 40 mg orally every morning tells the nurse, "My mouth feels like cotton." Which statement by the client necessitates further assessment by the nurse?
☐ 1. "I'm sucking on ice chips."
☐ 2. "I'm using sugarless gum."
☐ 3. "I'm sucking on sugarless candy."
☐ 4. "I'm drinking a glass of water every hour."

33. A client with a depressive disorder has been consistent with taking 12.5 mg of paroxetine extended release daily. The nurse judges the client to be benefiting from this drug therapy when the client demonstrates which behavior(s)? Select all that apply.
☐ 1. takes 2-hour evening naps daily
☐ 2. completes homework assignments
☐ 3. decreases pacing
☐ 4. increases somatization
☐ 5. verbalizes feelings

34. A client with a major depressive disorder comes to the mental health clinic for a follow-up visit. The client has been taking escitalopram for 3 months and reports feeling "like my old self again." Now the client wants to stop taking medication. "I don't want to be dependent on meds like my parent." What is the nurse's **best** initial response?
☐ 1. "After another 3 months of stability, it might be safe for you to go off the escitalopram."
☐ 2. "After two significant episodes, you'll need to take an antidepressant indefinitely."
☐ 3. "Research indicates that individuals who have had two major depressive episodes have a 70% chance of having a third episode."
☐ 4. "It's likely that you can learn to manage your depression with a regular exercise regime and a healthy diet."

35. An adolescent has just begun taking an antidepressant. Which client statement would indicate the need for further teaching?
☐ 1. "Now that I've been taking my antidepressant for a week, I'm going to feel better about myself."
☐ 2. "A week ago when I started my antidepressant, I didn't care about eating, but now I want to eat a bit more."
☐ 3. "After a week of taking my antidepressant, I can sleep a little better—6 hours or so each night."
☐ 4. "Now that I've had a week of my antidepressant, it's a little easier to get up in the morning."

The Client with Bipolar Disorder, Manic Phase

36. A client is taking 50 mg of lamotrigine daily for bipolar disorder. The client shows the nurse a rash on their arm. What should the nurse do?
- ☐ 1. Report the rash to the health care provider (HCP).
- ☐ 2. Explain that the rash is a temporary adverse effect.
- ☐ 3. Give the client an ice pack for the arm.
- ☐ 4. Question the client about recent sun exposure.

37. In a predischarge program to educate clients with bipolar disorder and their family members, the nurse emphasizes that which symptom is the **most** significant indicator for the onset of relapse?
- ☐ 1. a sense of pleasure and motivation for new endeavors
- ☐ 2. decreased need for sleep and racing thoughts
- ☐ 3. self-concern about an increase in energy
- ☐ 4. leaving a good job to start a new business

38. A client is prescribed lithium. Which statement by a client **most** indicates a need for more teaching?
- ☐ 1. "I don't have to worry about my levels because my last level was normal."
- ☐ 2. "I've been getting a lot of good exercise playing on a local soccer team."
- ☐ 3. "I'm trying hard to watch my diet and eat healthy."
- ☐ 4. "I've learned to take my lithium even when I have the stomach flu."

39. A young woman comes to the mental health clinic for their routine medication follow-up. The client has been married for 2 years and reports that they and their spouse are ready to start a family. The client has a diagnosis of bipolar disorder and has been well managed on divalproex for at least 3 years. What is the **most** essential counsel for the nurse to give the client?
- ☐ 1. "Schedule an appointment for a complete gynecological examination if you haven't had one in the past year."
- ☐ 2. "Pay careful attention to eating healthy from this point on to maximize the health of both birth parent and baby."
- ☐ 3. "Check with your health care provider as divalproex carries an increased risk for birth defects."
- ☐ 4. "Learning to reduce stress now is important to reduce your chances of developing postpartum depression."

40. A health care provider (HCP) has prescribed valproic acid for a client with bipolar disorder who has achieved limited success with lithium carbonate. Which information should the nurse teach the client about taking valproic acid?
- ☐ 1. Follow-up blood tests are necessary while on this medication.
- ☐ 2. The extended-release tablet can be crushed if necessary for ease of swallowing.
- ☐ 3. Tachycardia and upset stomach are common side effects.
- ☐ 4. Consumption of a moderate amount of alcohol is safe if the medication is taken in the morning.

41. A young adult client diagnosed with bipolar disorder has been managing the disorder effectively with medication and treatment for several years. The client suddenly becomes manic. The nurse reviews the client's medication record. Which new medication may have contributed to the development of their manic state?

Medication Record
• Amitriptyline 50 mg orally (PO) daily at bedtime
• Prednisone 20 mg PO three times a day
• Buspirone HCl 5 mg PO three times a day
• Gabapentin 300 mg PO three times a day

- ☐ 1. amitriptyline
- ☐ 2. prednisone
- ☐ 3. buspirone
- ☐ 4. gabapentin

42. A client with acute mania has been admitted to the inpatient unit voluntarily. The nurse approaches the client with medication to be taken orally as prescribed by the health care provider. The client states, "I don't need that stuff." Which response by the nurse is **best**?
- ☐ 1. "You can't refuse to take this medication."
- ☐ 2. "If you don't take it orally, I'll give you a shot."
- ☐ 3. "The medication will help you feel calmer."
- ☐ 4. "I'll get you some written information about the medication."

43. A nurse observes a client who is hyperactive and intrusive sitting very close to another client with their arm around the other client's shoulders. The nurse hears the client tell a sexually explicit joke. The nurse approaches the client and asks them to walk down the hallway. Which statement by the nurse should benefit the client?
- ☐ 1. "They won't want to be around you with that kind of talk."
- ☐ 2. "Telling sexual jokes and touching others is not permitted here."
- ☐ 3. "You need to be careful about what you say to other people."
- ☐ 4. "I think a time-out in your room would be appropriate now."

44. The nurse is preparing to administer a controlled substance to a client who was admitted to an inpatient unit after being injured during a manic episode. The single-dose vial contains more than is needed for the prescribed dose. Which nursing action is appropriate?
  ☐ 1. Document wasting of the excess medication with a second witness.
  ☐ 2. Document the excess, and return excess medication to the pharmacy.
  ☐ 3. Document the excess, and return it to the excess medication drawer for future use.
  ☐ 4. Document the prescribed dose, and notify the charge nurse of the waste.

45. A client with mania is irritable and insulting to an unlicensed assistive personnel (UAP). The UAP states, "I can't believe this client is so rude. I thought people with mania were overly happy." Which response by the nurse should help the UAP understand the client's behavior?
  ☐ 1. "It's our responsibility to listen to clients even though we might not like what they are saying."
  ☐ 2. "We must reprimand the client for doing that because there's no reason to behave like that."
  ☐ 3. "I'll go and speak to the client about this behavior and emphasize the need to control what they are saying."
  ☐ 4. "I know it's difficult, but being irritable is a symptom of the client's mania."

46. A client has acute mania. Which milieu activity should the nurse recommend? Select all that apply.
  ☐ 1. resting during scheduled periods
  ☐ 2. performing relaxation exercises
  ☐ 3. listening to soft music
  ☐ 4. watching television
  ☐ 5. taking a walk

47. A nurse is assessing a client with a history of mania who wants to stop taking mood-stabilizing medication because the client is "feeling good," has a high energy level, and reports being productive at work. Which response by the nurse is **most** appropriate?
  ☐ 1. "Are you thinking about hurting yourself?"
  ☐ 2. "If you stop your medication, your behavior will quickly spiral out of control."
  ☐ 3. "I believe you were hospitalized the last time you stopped your medication."
  ☐ 4. "Why don't you cut your medication dosage in half for a while and see how you respond?"

48. A client with acute mania is prescribed 600 mg of lithium orally (PO) three times per day. The health care provider (HCP) also prescribes 5 mg of haloperidol PO at bedtime. Which action should the nurse take?
  ☐ 1. Administer the medication as prescribed.
  ☐ 2. Question the HCP about the prescription.
  ☐ 3. Administer the haloperidol but not the lithium.
  ☐ 4. Consult with the nursing supervisor before administering the medications.

49. The client with a diagnosis of bipolar disorder, manic phase, states to the nurse, "I am the Queen of England. Bow before me." The nurse interprets this statement as important to document in which area of the mental status examination?
  ☐ 1. psychomotor behavior
  ☐ 2. mood and affect
  ☐ 3. attitude toward the nurse
  ☐ 4. thought content

50. The client is laughing and telling jokes to a group of clients. Suddenly, the client is crying and talking about a death in the family. A moment later, the client is laughing and joking again. What should the nurse do?
  ☐ 1. Call the health care provider (HCP) for a prescription for lorazepam as needed.
  ☐ 2. Place the client in seclusion and call the HCP for a prescription for the seclusion.
  ☐ 3. Ignore the client's behavior to avoid giving the client too much attention.
  ☐ 4. Ask the client to come to a quiet area to talk to the nurse individually.

51. A client with acute mania exhibits euphoria, pressured speech, and flight of ideas. The client has been talking to the nurse nonstop for 5 minutes, and lunch has arrived on the unit. What should the nurse do **next**?
  ☐ 1. Excuse oneself while telling the client to come to the dining room for lunch.
  ☐ 2. Tell the client to stop talking because it is time to eat lunch.
  ☐ 3. Do not interrupt the client, but wait for the client to finish talking.
  ☐ 4. Walk away, and approach the client in a few minutes before the food gets cold.

52. A client with acute mania brings six suitcases and three shopping bags of personal belongings on admission to the unit. When informed that some of the suitcases and bags need to be returned home because of a lack of storage space, the client begins to use profanity against the nurse. Which response by the nurse is **most** therapeutic?
  ☐ 1. "You're acting inappropriately."
  ☐ 2. "I won't tolerate your talking to me like that."
  ☐ 3. "Swearing and profanity are unacceptable here."
  ☐ 4. "We don't want to put you in seclusion yet."

53. The spouse of a client who is experiencing acute mania and swearing and using profanity apologizes to the nurse for the client's behavior. Which reply by the nurse is **most** therapeutic?
    ☐ 1. "This must be difficult for you."
    ☐ 2. "It's okay. We've heard worse."
    ☐ 3. "How long has your partner been like this?"
    ☐ 4. "Your partner needs some medication."

54. The nurse is caring for a client with acute mania who is euphoric and flirtatious. The nurse overhears the client describing a sexual exploit with a group of clients seated at a table. What **immediate** action should the nurse take?
    ☐ 1. Continue walking down the hall, ignoring the conversation.
    ☐ 2. Speak to the client later in private while saying nothing at this time.
    ☐ 3. Tell the client others may not want to hear about sex, and invite the client to play a game of ping-pong.
    ☐ 4. Inform the client that continuing to talk about sex will alienate others.

55. A client with acute mania states to the nurse, "I am the prince of peace and can save the world. Those against me will find me and take me to another world. They will come. I know it." The client is beginning to scan the room and starts to repeat their delusion. Which response by the nurse is **most** therapeutic?
    ☐ 1. "Describe the people who will come."
    ☐ 2. "The staff and I will protect you."
    ☐ 3. "You're not the prince of peace. Your name is Joe."
    ☐ 4. "Let us walk around the unit for a while."

56. A client with bipolar disorder, manic phase, is scheduled for a chest x-ray. What should the nurse do before taking the client to the radiology department?
    ☐ 1. Give a thorough explanation of the procedure.
    ☐ 2. Explain the procedure in simple terms.
    ☐ 3. Call security to be on standby for possible problems.
    ☐ 4. Cancel the appointment until the client can go unescorted.

57. A client with bipolar disorder, manic phase, appears at the nurse's station wearing a transparent shirt, miniskirt, high heels, 10 bracelets, and 8 necklaces. The client's makeup is overdone, and they are not wearing underwear. What should the nurse do?
    ☐ 1. Tell the client to dress appropriately while out of their room.
    ☐ 2. Ask the client to put on hospital pajamas until they can dress appropriately.
    ☐ 3. Instruct the client to go to their room and change clothes.
    ☐ 4. Escort the client to their room, and assist with choosing appropriate attire.

58. A client diagnosed with bipolar disorder and experiencing acute mania states to the nurse, "Where is my son? I love Lucy. Rain, rain go away. Dogs eat dirt." Another client approaches the nurse and says, "Man, are they ever nuts! They are driving me crazy with all their weird talk." Which response by the nurse to the second client is **most** appropriate?
    ☐ 1. "I agree. They're a little hard to take sometimes."
    ☐ 2. "Just walk away and leave the other client alone. There's nothing else you can do."
    ☐ 3. "I realize their behavior bothers you, but they can't control it right now."
    ☐ 4. "I really cannot discuss other clients with you."

59. A client with mania is skipping up and down the hallway, nearly running into other clients. The nurse should include which activity in the client's plan of care?
    ☐ 1. leading a group activity
    ☐ 2. watching television
    ☐ 3. reading the newspaper
    ☐ 4. cleaning the dayroom tables

60. A client admitted to the nursing unit with bipolar disorder, manic phase, is accompanied by the client's partner. The partner states that the client has been overly energetic and happy, talking constantly, purchasing many unneeded items, and sleeping about 4 hours a night for the past 5 days. When completing the client's daily assessment, the nurse should be especially alert for which finding?
    ☐ 1. exhaustion
    ☐ 2. vertigo
    ☐ 3. gastritis
    ☐ 4. bradycardia

61. The partner of a client with bipolar disorder, manic phase, states to the nurse, "My partner is acting so crazy. What did they do to get this way?" The nurse bases the response on which understanding of this disorder?
    Bipolar disorder is:
    ☐ 1. caused by underlying psychological difficulties.
    ☐ 2. caused by disturbed family dynamics in the client's early life.
    ☐ 3. the result of an imbalance of chemicals in the brain.
    ☐ 4. the result of a genetic inheritance from someone in the family.

62. A client diagnosed with bipolar disorder asks the nurse why it is necessary to have a serum lithium level drawn every 3 to 4 months. The nurse's response should be based on which factor?
    ☐ 1. to monitor compliance with the medication
    ☐ 2. to prevent toxicity related to the drug's therapeutic range
    ☐ 3. to monitor the client's white blood cell count
    ☐ 4. to comply with governmental safety requirements

63. The health care provider (HCP) prescribes a serum lithium level tomorrow for a client with bipolar disorder, manic phase, who has been receiving lithium 300 mg orally three times daily for the past 5 days. At what time should the nurse plan to have the blood specimen obtained?
☐ 1. before bedtime
☐ 2. after lunch
☐ 3. before breakfast
☐ 4. during the afternoon

64. A client will be discharged on lithium carbonate 600 mg three times daily. When teaching the client and the family about lithium therapy, the nurse determines that teaching has been effective if the client and family state that they will notify the prescribing health care provider (HCP) **immediately** with which symptoms? Select all that apply.
☐ 1. nausea
☐ 2. muscle weakness
☐ 3. vertigo
☐ 4. fine hand tremor
☐ 5. vomiting

65. The nurse teaches a client with bipolar disorder about lithium therapy. Which client statement indicates the need for additional teaching?
☐ 1. "It's important to keep using a regular amount of salt in my diet."
☐ 2. "It's okay to double my next dose of lithium if I forget a dose."
☐ 3. "I should drink about 8 to 10 cups (about 2 to 2½ L) of water each day."
☐ 4. "I need to take my medicine at the same time each day."

66. A client with acute mania is to receive lithium carbonate 600 mg orally (PO) three times daily and 2 mg of haloperidol PO at bedtime. Which action should the nurse take?
☐ 1. Refuse to give the medications as prescribed.
☐ 2. Give the lithium only.
☐ 3. Request a decreased dosage of lithium.
☐ 4. Give the medications as prescribed.

67. A client with bipolar disorder, manic phase, has a subtherapeutic valproic acid level. Which client behaviors should the nurse judge to be due to this level of valproic acid? Select all that apply.
☐ 1. irritability
☐ 2. grandiosity
☐ 3. anhedonia
☐ 4. hypersomnia
☐ 5. flight of ideas

68. A client with rapid-cycling bipolar disorder who is about to receive the 1700 hours dose of carbamazepine reports a sore throat and chills. What should the nurse do **next**?
☐ 1. Administer the prescribed dose of carbamazepine.
☐ 2. Give the client acetaminophen as prescribed PRN.
☐ 3. Report the symptoms to the health care provider (HCP) in the morning.
☐ 4. Call the HCP immediately to report changes.

69. A client's spouse states, "I don't know what to do sometimes. It's so hard being married to someone with a mental illness like bipolar disorder." After the nurse talks with the client's spouse about their feelings and difficulties, which action is **most** appropriate?
☐ 1. Suggest that the spouse see their own health care provider (HCP).
☐ 2. Give the spouse information about a support group.
☐ 3. Recommend that the spouse talk with a close friend.
☐ 4. Have the spouse share feelings with the client.

70. A client with bipolar disorder is approaching discharge after being hospitalized with a first episode of acute mania. The client's spouse asks the nurse what to do to help them. What recommendation for the spouse should the nurse anticipate including in the teaching plan?
☐ 1. Help the client to be free from worry and anxiety.
☐ 2. Communicate openly and offer support.
☐ 3. Relieve the client of all responsibilities.
☐ 4. Remind the client to control their symptoms.

71. A client experiencing a manic episode has been talking loudly, pacing the unit, and trying to draw other clients into debates about the value of self-determination. Arrange in order the steps a nurse should take to help calm this client. All options must be used.

1. Use oral medication to decrease anxiety and increase appropriate social interaction.

2. Talk with the client about the anxiety and stress the client is feeling.

3. Take the client to a quiet area, such as their room, to decrease stimuli.

4. Teach the client coping strategies to deal with stressors.

72. A client with bipolar disorder, manic phase, states to the nurse, "You're looking good. I'm taking you out to dinner." What reply by the nurse is **most** therapeutic?
- ☐ 1. "I don't want to go out to dinner."
- ☐ 2. "I can't go out to dinner with you."
- ☐ 3. "It doesn't matter how I look; the answer is no."
- ☐ 4. "I'm Chris Smith, a nurse working on this unit."

73. The nurse administers an antipsychotic drug to a client with acute mania. The client still refuses to lie down on the bed, pushes other clients in the hallways, and screams threatening remarks to the staff. What should the nurse do **next**?
- ☐ 1. Follow the client, and ask the client to calm down.
- ☐ 2. Tell the client to lie down on the sofa in the community room.
- ☐ 3. Seclude the client, and use restraints if necessary.
- ☐ 4. Tell the staff to ignore the client's remarks.

74. As the nurse is turning off the television, a client with bipolar disorder, manic phase, says, "I want the television on so I can watch the late show. I'm not tired, and you can't tell me what to do. I want it on!" What should the nurse tell the client?
- ☐ 1. "I'll let you watch television just this once, but you have to turn the sound off."
- ☐ 2. "I'll turn the television off when you get sleepy. Don't ask me to do this again."
- ☐ 3. "Television hours are from 1900 hours to 2200 hours. It's 2200, and the television goes off so everyone can sleep."
- ☐ 4. "The television goes off at 2200 hours. I've been telling you this for the past three evenings."

The Client with Suicidal Ideation and Suicide Attempt

75. The nurse reviews discharge protocols. Which strategies would be helpful in preventing suicide for clients about to be discharged from a psychiatric inpatient unit? Select all that apply.
- ☐ 1. At discharge, give all depressed clients a card containing the crisis phone line number for their area.
- ☐ 2. Have all clients who have expressed suicidal ideation just prior to or during hospitalization make a written personal suicide prevention plan.
- ☐ 3. Require that all clients who have had previous suicidal ideation, plans, or attempts refill all prescriptions every 2 weeks rather than monthly.
- ☐ 4. Educate family and friends of previously suicidal clients in ways to help clients remain safe after discharge.
- ☐ 5. Suggest that family and friends of previously suicidal clients know the client's whereabouts at all times.

76. The nurse manager in the emergency department (ED) conducts an in-service for the nursing staff about screening clients for suicide. One of the nurses states, "Questioning adolescents about suicide will only increase their thinking about self-harm, and they wouldn't admit it to me anyhow." How should the nurse manager respond? Select all that apply.
- ☐ 1. "Suicide is a leading cause of death in adolescents."
- ☐ 2. "We'll limit the assessment to adolescents with psychiatric diagnoses."
- ☐ 3. "It's a myth that talking about suicide leads to suicide attempts.
- ☐ 4. "If you think the adolescent isn't telling you the truth, you can question the parents."
- ☐ 5. "Adolescents will disclose suicidal thoughts when asked directly."

77. The nurse assesses a client for their risk for suicide. Which method of suicide, if identified by the client, should the nurse identify as **most** lethal?
☐ 1. overdosing on aspirin
☐ 2. poisoning with carbon monoxide
☐ 3. jumping off an 8-foot bridge
☐ 4. slashing both wrists

78. The nurse manager overhears two staff members talking in the snack room. One of the staff members states, "Those superficial cuts are just a means of getting our attention. That client never should have been admitted. I hope they are out of here soon." Which response by the nurse manager is **most** appropriate?
☐ 1. "It's our job to help clients no matter how we feel about them or what they did. This client will be discharged soon."
☐ 2. "I won't tolerate that kind of discussion from my staff. Now, it's time for you to go back to work."
☐ 3. "I know it's hard to understand, but we need to do the best we can even though this client will be back."
☐ 4. "No matter what the intent, all suicidal behavior is serious and deserves our serious consideration."

79. The history of a client who has just been admitted to the unit and is very depressed reveals a weight loss of 10 lb (4.5 kg) in 2 weeks, sleeping 3 hours a night, and poor hygiene. The client states, "I'm no good to anyone. Everyone would be better off without me." Which question should the nurse ask **first**?
☐ 1. "What do you mean?"
☐ 2. "Are you thinking about hurting yourself?"
☐ 3. "Does your family not care about you?"
☐ 4. "What happened to make you think that?"

80. The unlicensed assistive personnel (UAP) states to the nurse, "My client talks about how awful and useless they are. Sometimes, they sound angry for no reason. I'm tired of listening to them." Which response by the nurse is **most** appropriate?
☐ 1. "I'll switch your assignment to someone who is less depressed and less tiring."
☐ 2. "It's important for you to listen because they need to verbalize how they are feeling."
☐ 3. "Don't worry about it. I know you haven't done anything to make them angry."
☐ 4. "Clients with depression are hard to deal with, but don't take what they say seriously."

81. A client who was recently discharged from the psychiatric unit telephones the unit to speak to the nurse. The client reports taking their children to the neighbors' house and has turned on the gas to attempt suicide. Which action should the nurse take **next**?
☐ 1. Refer the caller to a 24-hour suicide hotline.
☐ 2. Tell the caller that another nurse will telephone the police.
☐ 3. Ask whether the caller telephoned their health care provider (HCP).
☐ 4. Instruct the caller to telephone their family for help.

82. A client walks into the clinic and tells the nurse they want to die because their partner broke up with them. The client states, "I'll show them. They'll be sorry." The nurse notes which underlying theme and method to deal with the client?
☐ 1. Sadness—ask the client to reveal how long they have felt this way.
☐ 2. Escape—ask the client to indicate what they want to escape.
☐ 3. Loneliness—ask the client to state who they believe to be their friends.
☐ 4. Retaliation—ask the client about their specific plans to harm themself or their partner.

83. A client has been hospitalized for major depression and suicidal ideation. Which statement indicates to the nurse that the client is improving?
☐ 1. "I couldn't kill myself because I don't want to go to hell."
☐ 2. "I don't think about killing myself as much as I used to."
☐ 3. "I'm of no use to anyone anymore."
☐ 4. "I know my kids don't need me anymore since they're grown."

84. A client states to the nurse at the outpatient clinic, "I don't feel ready to go back to work. It's only been a week since I left the hospital." Assessment reveals a flat affect, disheveled appearance, poor posture, and minimal eye contact during interaction. The nurse asks if they are thinking about self-harm. The client reports having a loaded revolver at home and says, "I will probably use it." What should the nurse do **next**?
☐ 1. Tell the client to go and remove the gun from the home.
☐ 2. Ask the client to call the nurse every hour after returning home.
☐ 3. Ask the client to promise not to attempt harm.
☐ 4. Initiate plans for hospitalization immediately.

85. The spouse of a client who successfully completed suicide tearfully says, "I feel guilty because I'm so angry at them for committing suicide. It must have been what they wanted." After assisting the spouse with dealing with their feelings, which intervention is **most** helpful?
☐ 1. Refer the spouse to a group for survivors of suicide.
☐ 2. Encourage the spouse to receive counseling from a chaplain.
☐ 3. Provide the spouse with the local suicide hotline number.
☐ 4. Suggest the spouse receive individual therapy by the nurse.

86. A client with depression is exhibiting a brighter affect and an ability to attend to hygiene and grooming tasks and is beginning to participate in group activities. The nurse asks the client to identify three personal strengths. After much hesitation and thinking, the client identifies being a nice person, a good cook, and a hard worker. What should the nurse do **next**?
☐ 1. Ask the client to identify additional three strengths.
☐ 2. Volunteer the client to lead the cooking group later in the day.
☐ 3. Educate the client about the importance of medication.
☐ 4. Reinforce the client for identifying and sharing strengths.

87. The friend of a client with depression and suicidal ideation asks the nurse, "How should I act around them?" What should the nurse tell the friend? Select all that apply.
☐ 1. "Try to cheer them up."
☐ 2. "Be caring and genuine."
☐ 3. "Remind them that suicide would hurt their family."
☐ 4. "Avoid asking how they are feeling."
☐ 5. "Listen and let them tell their story."

88. The nurse is completing an assessment in the outpatient clinic on a client with depression who has been talking about how "it would be better if I wasn't here anymore." What questions are important for the nurse to ask the client? Select all that apply.
☐ 1. "Do you want to hurt yourself?"
☐ 2. "How long do you think it would take you to feel different?"
☐ 3. "Do you have a gun at your home?"
☐ 4. "How many of your medication, imipramine, tablets do you have at home?"
☐ 5. "Do you live alone?"

89. A client is escorted to the psychiatric unit from the emergency department (ED) by staff and a security officer. The client's shoulder is bandaged, and their arm is in a sling because of a self-inflicted gunshot wound to the shoulder. Later, the client's spouse follows with a bag of the client's belongings. Which nursing action is **most** appropriate at this time?
☐ 1. Tell the spouse to take the items home because the client is suicidal.
☐ 2. Instruct the spouse to unpack the bag and put the client's things in the dresser.
☐ 3. Ask the spouse whether the bag contains anything dangerous.
☐ 4. Inspect the bag and its contents in the presence of the client and spouse.

90. A suicidal client is placed in the seclusion room and given lorazepam because they tried to harm themself by banging their head against the wall. After 10 minutes, the client starts to bang their head against the wall in the seclusion room. Which action should the nurse take **next**?
☐ 1. Call hospital security for assistance.
☐ 2. Place the client in restraints.
☐ 3. Call the health care provider (HCP) for additional medication prescriptions.
☐ 4. Instruct a staff member to sit in the room with the client.

91. A client lives in a group home and visits the community mental health center regularly. During one visit with the nurse, the client states, "The voices are telling me to hurt myself again." Which question by the nurse is **most** important to ask?
☐ 1. "When do you hear the voices?"
☐ 2. "Are you going to hurt yourself?"
☐ 3. "How long have you heard the voices?"
☐ 4. "Why are the voices starting again?"

92. A 20-year-old client diagnosed with paranoid schizophrenia is recovering from the first psychotic break. Before discharge from the hospital, the client becomes depressed and states, "I don't want this illness. I'm about to begin my junior year in college." Which issue would be **most** important for the nurse to address at this time?
☐ 1. disturbed thought process
☐ 2. disturbed sensory perceptions
☐ 3. communication problems
☐ 4. potential for medication noncompliance

93. The nurse is teaching two unlicensed assistive personnel who are new to the inpatient unit about caring for a client who is suicidal. The nurse determines that additional teaching is needed when which statement is made?
☐ 1. "I need to check the client precisely at 15-minute intervals."
☐ 2. "Documenting suicide checks is absolutely necessary."
☐ 3. "Clients on one-to-one suicide precautions can never be left alone."
☐ 4. "All clients using razors must be supervised by staff."

94. The nurse cares for a client with suicide ideation on an inpatient unit. Which activity should the nurse recommend when the client has thoughts of suicide?
☐ 1. keeping track of feelings in a journal
☐ 2. engaging in physical activity
☐ 3. talking with the nurse
☐ 4. playing a card game with other clients

95. A client is receiving outpatient treatment for depression and suicidal ideation. What is the correct amount of imipramine to have at one time?
☐ 1. 30-day supply
☐ 2. 21-day supply
☐ 3. 14-day supply
☐ 4. 7-day supply

96. Which statement by the nurse reflects the **best** understanding of suicide in an individual with depression?
☐ 1. "The more severe the depression, the greater the probability for suicidal behavior."
☐ 2. "The person who talks about suicide is less likely to try it."
☐ 3. "Every client with depression is potentially suicidal."
☐ 4. "Suicide is less likely when the individual is receiving antidepressant therapy."

The Client with Psychosexual Disorders

97. A couple informs the nurse that they have been having some "problems in the bedroom." What is the **most** appropriate response by the nurse?
☐ 1. "I can refer you to a therapist."
☐ 2. "I need to obtain your admission history first."
☐ 3. "I'd like to hear your concerns."
☐ 4. "Let me refer you to a marriage counselor."

98. A client who is admitted to the adult unit of a mental health care facility with depression tells the nurse that they have pedophilia. What should the nurse do?
☐ 1. Be aware of personal opinions and views.
☐ 2. Recognize that because the client is depressed, the client will not be able to discuss the pedophilia.
☐ 3. Ensure that the client is never alone with other clients on the unit.
☐ 4. Refer the client to group therapy.

99. A client and their partner come to the clinic stating they have been unable to have sexual intercourse. The female client states they have pain and their "vagina is too tight." The client was raped at age 15 years of age. Which nursing problem is **most** appropriate for this client?
☐ 1. dysfunctional grieving related to loss of self-esteem because of lack of sexual intimacy
☐ 2. risk for trauma related to fear of vaginal penetration
☐ 3. vaginismus related to vaginal constriction
☐ 4. sexual dysfunction related to sexual trauma

100. A client with erectile disorder is taking sildenafil. What instructions should the nurse give the client?
☐ 1. Take the medication 8 hours before having intercourse.
☐ 2. Use nitroglycerin if chest pains occur during intercourse.
☐ 3. Take up to three tablets within 24 hours.
☐ 4. Expect an erection that may last up to 4 hours.

Managing Care, Quality, and Safety of Clients with Mood Disorders

101. The nurse is caring for a client with bipolar disorder who was recently admitted to an inpatient unit and is experiencing a manic episode. What is a **priority** nursing intervention for this client?
☐ 1. Prescribe and administer all medications in a liquid form.
☐ 2. Base permission for family visits on the client's attendance at therapy groups.
☐ 3. Closely monitor the client's eating and sleeping habits.
☐ 4. Encourage the client to keep a journal about feelings and emotions.

102. A client receives the diagnosis they are HIV positive. Which reaction to the diagnosis would put the client in **greatest** need of intervention by the nurse?
☐ 1. a client who is angry, hostile, and alienated from their family
☐ 2. a client who is obsessed with cleanliness and showers many times a day
☐ 3. a client who is unable to make decisions and is helpless and tearful
☐ 4. a client who says, "I've found a solution for this mess"

103. The nurse reviews nursing protocols for an inpatient psychiatric unit. Which actions would represent an ethical breach regarding the rights of clients in psychiatric care situations?
☐ 1. The nurse discusses the client's care with out-of-town family members who the client has formally indicated are allowed to know about the client's hospital care.
☐ 2. The nurse discusses the client's history and hospital course of treatment with a consulting health care provider (HCP).
☐ 3. The nurse discusses with the HCP content overheard in a client's phone call to their family.
☐ 4. The nurse discusses the client's care with the admission coordinator of a retirement home that the client plans to enter after discharge from the hospital.

104. The nurse is part of a team charged with making recommendations to create a healthy work environment. What workplace measure(s) would **most** likely support the health and well-being of workers? Select all that apply.
☐ 1. workshops for workers nearing retirement
☐ 2. counseling for workers exposed to traumatic events
☐ 3. interventions for workers with substance-related problems
☐ 4. standard work hours that include scheduled rest periods
☐ 5. education for workers regarding customary workplace practices

105. The nurse develops appropriate assignments for the staff. Which client should the nurse judge to be at **highest** risk for suicide completion?
☐ 1. 85-year-old White man who lives alone after their spouse's death
☐ 2. 34-year-old single Latino woman who has recently been diagnosed with cancer
☐ 3. 15-year-old girl of African descent whose partner broke up with them
☐ 4. 52-year-old man of Asian descent who was terminated from their job because of downsizing

106. An adolescent client tells the nurse that the reason they are depressed and suicidal is that they are being bullied at school. While discussing the circumstances of the bullying, the client indicates that they are gay, which they think contributes to the bullying. The client tells the nurse their sexual orientation in confidence, stating that their parents do not know and that the client does not want that information revealed to them. Which action(s) should the nurse take? Select all that apply.
☐ 1. Give the client the crisis phone line number.
☐ 2. Provide contact information for a support group for gay teens.
☐ 3. Question the client about the bullying.
☐ 4. Assess the client's current status regarding suicidal thoughts or plans.
☐ 5. Help the client develop a safety plan regarding suicidal thoughts or plans.
☐ 6. Notify the school about the bullying without identifying the specific student.

107. A spouse brings a client to the emergency department with a bleeding gunshot wound to the leg. The spouse tells the nurse that the client was trying to commit suicide. In what order should the nurse perform the actions from first to last? All options must be used.

1. Assess current suicide risk.
2. Assign constant observation.
3. Check the area for potentially harmful objects.
4. Assess the severity of the bleeding.

108. The nurse is caring for a client prescribed phenelzine for depression who has not responded to other medications. When reviewing the dietary restrictions associated with this medication, the client reports that most of their favorite foods are now going to be restricted. Which collaborative action would **best** meet the needs of the client?
☐ 1. Review the diet restrictions with the client, and make a schedule of when the preferred foods can be eaten.
☐ 2. Identify the primary meal preparer in the family, and review a meal plan with that person to decrease client stress.
☐ 3. Discuss the client's noncompliance with the health care provider so the medication can be adjusted to a previous prescription.
☐ 4. Schedule a case conference with the health care team to review medication options.
☐ 5. Collaborate with the dietitian to counsel the client on additional foods or preparation methods that are acceptable with the medication.

109. The nurse is caring for a 40-year-old female client who was admitted to the inpatient unit 3 days ago for a manic episode.

Nurse's Notes

1430:
The client has been taking lithium and olanzapine with good effect and has been out of their room with limited participation in unit activities. The client's appetite has increased.

1440:
The unlicensed assistive personnel reported attempting to take the client's vital signs in the dayroom but found them stiff and unable to move their arms. The client was diaphoretic and unable to respond coherently, and their skin was hot to touch. Vital signs are temperature 102.4°F (39.1°C); pulse 110 bpm, respiration rate 18 breaths/min; and blood pressure 136/90 mm Hg.

➤ Complete the diagram by specifying what condition the client is most likely experiencing, two actions the nurse should take to address that condition, and two parameters the nurse should monitor to assess the client's progress.

Action to Take — Condition Most Likely Experiencing — Parameter to Monitor

Action to Take — Parameter to Monitor

Actions to Take	Potential Conditions	Parameters to Monitor
Give antibiotics	Anaphylaxis	Urine output
Apply a cooling blanket	Meningitis	Breath sounds
Administer epinephrine	Neuroleptic malignant syndrome	Vital signs
Start intravenous (IV) fluids	Lithium toxicity	Deep tendon reflexes
Administer a neuroleptic agent		Intracranial pressure

Answers, Rationales, and Test-Taking Strategies

The answers and rationales for each question follow below, along with keys (🗝) to the client need (CN) and cognitive level (CL) for each question. In addition, questions that measure clinical judgment will be coded (CJ). As you check your answers, use the **Content Mastery and Test-Taking Skill Self-Analysis** *worksheet (tear-out worksheet in the back of the book) to identify the reason(s) for not answering the questions correctly. For additional information about test-taking skills and strategies for answering questions, refer to pages 12–51 in Part 1 of this book.*

The Client with Major Depression

1. 4. Including the root healer gives credibility and respect to the client's cultural beliefs. Avoiding talking about the healer demonstrates either ignorance or disregard for the client's cultural values. A negative comparison of root healing with Western medicine not only denigrates the client's beliefs but also is likely to alienate the client and cause them to end treatment.

🗝 CN: Psychosocial integrity; CL: Analyze

2. 3. Cheese and yeast products contain tyramine, which the client should avoid to prevent a negative interaction with tranylcypromine, a monoamine oxidase (MAO) inhibitor. Sodium will not interact with tranylcypromine, and neither exercise nor sugar needs to be limited.

🗝 CN: Pharmacological and parenteral therapies; CL: Evaluate

3. 4. The client is exhibiting signs of hypothyroidism, which includes hair loss, pain, fatigue, and increased sensitivity to cold. Hypothyroidism may be impacting the client's mood, ability to concentrate, physical sensations, and energy levels. Resolving potential biological causes of symptoms takes priority over rehabilitation strategies or psychological approaches.

🗝 CN: Management of care; CL: Analyze

4. 3. The nurse should report the client's beer consumption to the HCP. Duloxetine should not be administered to a client with renal or hepatic insufficiency because the medication can elevate liver enzymes and, together with substantial alcohol use, can cause liver injury. Referring the client to the concurrent diagnosis program, sharing information at the next interdisciplinary treatment conference, and teaching the client relaxation exercises are helpful interventions for the nurse to implement. However, reporting the findings to the HCP is most important.

🗝 CN: Pharmacological and parenteral therapies; CL: Analyze

5. 2. The client's sudden improvement and decrease in anxiety most likely indicate that the client is relieved because the client has made the decision to kill themself and may now have the energy to complete the suicide. Symptoms of severe depression do not suddenly abate because most antidepressants work slowly and take 2 to 4 weeks to provide a maximum benefit. The client will improve slowly due to the medication. The sudden improvement in symptoms does not mean the client is nearing discharge, and decreasing observation of the client compromises the client's safety.

🗝 CN: Psychosocial adaptation; CL: Analyze

6. 4. The nurse closely monitors the client taking paroxetine for the development of agitation, which could lead to self-harm in the form of a suicide attempt. Headache, nausea, and fatigue are transient adverse effects of paroxetine.

🗝 CN: Pharmacological and parenteral therapies; CL: Analyze

7. 2. The nurse should initiate brief, frequent contacts throughout the day to let the client know that they are important to the nurse. This will positively affect the client's self-esteem. The nurse's action conveys acceptance of the client as a worthwhile person and provides some structure to the seemingly monotonous day. Waiting for the client to begin the conversation with the nurse is not helpful because the depressed client resists interaction and involvement with others. Sitting outside of the client's room is not productive and not necessary in this situation. If the client were actively suicidal, then a one-on-one client-to-staff assignment would be necessary. Questioning the client until they respond would overwhelm them because they could not meet the nurse's expectations to interact.

🗝 CN: Psychosocial integrity; CL: Analyze

8. 1. The most appropriate action is for the nurse to remain with the client even if the client does not engage in conversation with the nurse. A client with severe depression may be unable to engage in an interaction with the nurse because the client feels worthless and lacks the necessary energy to do so. However, the nurse's presence conveys acceptance and caring, thus helping to increase the client's self-worth. Telling the client that the nurse will come back later, stating that the nurse will find someone else for the client to talk with, or telling the client that the nurse will get something to read conveys that the client is not important, reinforcing the client's negative view of self. Additionally, such statements interfere with the client's development of a sense of security and trust in the nurse.

🗝 CN: Psychosocial integrity; CL: Analyze

9. 4. The nurse tells the client that the nurse is interested in the client to increase the sense of importance, worth, and self-esteem. Also, stating that the nurse wants to help conveys to the client a message of being worthwhile and important. Saying that the nurse is assigned to care for the client is impersonal and implies that the client is being uncooperative. Telling the client that the nurse is there because the client has potential for improvement will not help a client with low self-esteem because most people develop a sense of self-worth through accomplishment. Simply saying that the client has a lot of potential will not convince the client of being worthwhile. Telling the client that the nurse will talk to someone else later is not client focused and does not address the client's question or concern.

🗝 CN: Psychosocial integrity; CL: Analyze

10. 2. The presence of dizziness could indicate orthostatic hypotension, which may cause injury to the client from falling. Nausea, sedation, and dry mouth do not require immediate intervention by the nurse.

🗝 CN: Pharmacological and parenteral therapies; CL: Analyze

11. 3. Symptom relief can occur during the first week of therapy, with optimal effects possible within 2 weeks. For some clients, 2 to 4 weeks is needed for optimal effects. The client's statement that the depression will be gone in 5 to 7 days indicates to the nurse that clarification and further teaching are needed. Trazodone should be taken after a meal or light snack to enhance its absorption. Trazodone can cause drowsiness, and therefore the major portion of the drug should be taken at bedtime. The depressant effects of central nervous system depressants and alcohol may be potentiated by this drug.

🗝 CN: Pharmacological and parenteral therapies; CL: Evaluate

12. 3. The nurse should explain that ECT is a safe treatment and that the client is given an ultrashort-acting anesthetic to induce sleep before ECT and a muscle relaxant to prevent musculoskeletal complications during the convulsion, which typically lasts 30 to 60 seconds to be therapeutic. Atropine is given before ECT to inhibit salivation and respiratory tract secretions and thereby minimize the risk for aspiration. Medication for pain is not necessary and is not given before or during the treatment. Some clients experience a headache after the treatment and may request and be given an analgesic such as acetaminophen. Telling the client's child that the HCP will ensure that the client does not suffer needlessly would not provide accurate information about ECT. This statement also implies that the client will have pain during the treatment, which is untrue.

CN: Reduction of risk potential; CL: Analyze

13. 1. By stating "It must have been very upsetting for you," the nurse conveys empathy to the client by recognizing the underlying meaning of a painful occurrence. The nurse's statement invites the client to verbalize feelings and thoughts and lets the client know that the nurse is listening to and respects the client. Telling the client to talk about the job disregards the client's feelings and is nontherapeutic for the depressed client because of underlying feelings of worthlessness and guilt that are commonly present. Telling the client that they will find another job when they are better or that they were probably too depressed to work is inappropriate because it disregards the client's feelings and may promote additional feelings of failure and inadequacy in the client.

CN: Psychosocial integrity; CL: Analyze

14. 4. The client with depression is preoccupied, has decreased energy, and cannot make decisions, even simple ones. Therefore, the nurse presents the situation, "It's time for a shower," and assists the client with personal hygiene to preserve dignity and self-esteem. Explaining the importance of good hygiene to the client is inappropriate because the client may know the benefits of hygiene but is too fatigued and preoccupied to pay attention to self-care. Asking if the client is ready for a shower is not helpful because the client with depression commonly cannot make even simple decisions. This action also reinforces the client's feeling about not caring about showering. Waiting for the family to visit to help with the client's hygiene is inappropriate and irresponsible on the part of the nurse. The nurse is responsible for making basic decisions for the client until the client can make decisions for themself.

CN: Psychosocial integrity; CL: Analyze

15. 1, 2, 4, 5. NPO status, a signed consent, removal of dentures, and preprocedure voiding are all preparations prior to a procedure involving anesthesia, such as ECT. Orientation and frequent assessment of vital signs occur after the procedure.

CN: Reduction of risk potential; CL: Analyze

16. 2. Sertraline, like other selective serotonin reuptake inhibitors (SSRIs), can cause decreased libido and sexual dysfunction such as delayed ejaculation in men and an inability to achieve orgasm in women. SSRIs do not typically cause weight gain but may cause loss of appetite and weight loss. Dry mouth is a possible side effect, but it is temporary. The client should be told to take sips of water, suck on ice chips, or use sugarless gum or candy. St. John's wort should not be taken with SSRIs because a severe reaction could occur.

CN: Pharmacological and parenteral therapies; CL: Evaluate

17. 3. It is best to involve the client in usual at-home activities as much as the client can tolerate them. Discouraging visitors may not be in the client's best interest because visits with supportive significant others will help reinforce supportive relationships, which are important to the client's self-worth and self-esteem. A schedule of activities outside the home may be overwhelming for the client initially. Involving the client in planning for outside activities would be appropriate. Encouraging the client to sleep as much as possible is nontherapeutic and promotes withdrawal from others.

CN: Management of care; CL: Analyze

18. 2. Criteria for commitment include being gravely disabled and posing harm to self or others. This client is not threatening to commit self-harm in the form of suicide or to harm others. The client is gravely disabled because of an inability to care for self—namely, not eating because of the delusion. Evidence of psychosis or psychotic symptoms or diagnosis of a mental illness alone does not make the client legally eligible for commitment.

CN: Management of care; CL: Apply

19. 1, 2, 4, 5. Serotonin syndrome can occur if a selective serotonin reuptake inhibitor is combined with a monoamine oxidase inhibitor, a tryptophan-serotonin precursor, or St. John's wort. Signs and symptoms of serotonin syndrome include mental status changes (such as confusion, restlessness, or agitation), headache, diaphoresis, ataxia, myoclonus, shivering, tremor, diarrhea, nausea, abdominal cramps, and hyperreflexia. Constipation is not associated with serotonin syndrome.

CN: Pharmacological and parenteral therapies; CL: Analyze

20. 2. Phenelzine is a monoamine oxidase inhibitor (MAOI). MAOIs block the enzyme monoamine oxidase, which is involved in the decomposition and inactivation of norepinephrine, serotonin, dopamine, and tyramine (a precursor to the previously stated neurotransmitters). Foods high in tyramine—those that are fermented, pickled, aged, or smoked—must be avoided because when they are ingested in combination with MAOIs a hypertensive crisis occurs. Some examples include salami, bologna, dried fish, sour cream, yogurt, aged cheese, bananas, pickled herring, caffeinated beverages, chocolate, licorice, beer, red wine, and alcohol-free beer.

🗝️ CN: Pharmacological and parenteral therapies; CL: Apply

21. 4. The nurse should first take the client's vital signs because the client could be experiencing a hypertensive crisis, which requires prompt intervention. Signs and symptoms of a hypertensive crisis include occipital headache, a stiff or sore neck, nausea, vomiting, sweating, dilated pupils and photophobia, nosebleed, tachycardia, bradycardia, and constricting chest pain. Giving this client an analgesic medication without taking vital signs first is inappropriate. After the client's vital signs have been obtained, the nurse would call the HCP to report the client's problems and vital signs. Administering the client's next dose of phenelzine before taking vital signs could result in a dangerous situation if the client is experiencing a hypertensive crisis.

🗝️ CN: Pharmacological and parenteral therapies; CL: Analyze

22. 3. Pointing out facts of the present day draws the client into reality. Offering inane platitudes such as "everybody feels down once in a while" or "things will get better" minimizes the client's feelings and may increase their feelings of worthlessness. Informing the client that the nurse liked something the client wore yesterday could make the client feel the nurse did not like other things they wore and requires the client to remember what that item was—often difficult with severe depression.

🗝️ CN: Psychosocial integrity; CL: Apply

23. 3. A client who verbalizes feeling in control of self and situations no longer feels powerless to affect an outcome but realizes that one's actions can have an impact on self and situations. It is common for a client with depression to feel powerless to affect an outcome and to feel a lack of control over a situation. Although interacting with staff and peers is a positive action, the client could be conversing in a negative or nontherapeutic manner. Sleeping only 4 hours at a time is evidence of symptomatology and does not indicate improvement or recovery. Verbalizing dissatisfaction over not being able to perform at work indicates that the client is most likely focusing on shortcomings and powerlessness.

🗝️ CN: Psychosocial integrity; CL: Analyze

24. 2. The nurse must monitor the client for a suicide attempt at this time when the client is starting to feel better because the depressed client may now have enough energy to carry out an attempt. Bupropion inhibits dopamine reuptake; it is an activating antidepressant and could cause agitation. Although bupropion lowers the seizure threshold, especially at doses higher than 450 mg a day, and visual disturbances and increased libido are possible adverse effects, the nurse must closely monitor the client for a suicide attempt. As the client with major depression begins to feel better, the client may have enough energy to carry out an attempt.

🗝️ CN: Psychosocial integrity; CL: Analyze

25. 4. In the initial plan of care, the most appropriate outcome would be that the client will interact with the nurse. First, the client would begin interacting with one individual, the nurse. The nurse would gradually assist the client to engage in interactions with other clients in one-on-one contact, progressing toward informal group gatherings and eventually taking part in structured group activities. The client needs to experience success according to the client's level of tolerance. Initiating interactions with peers occurs when the client can gain a measure of confidence and self-esteem instead of feeling intimidated or unduly anxious. Discussing adaptive coping techniques is an outcome the client may be able to reach when symptoms are not as severe and the client can concentrate on improving coping skills.

🗝️ CN: Psychosocial integrity; CL: Analyze

26. 3. Imipramine, a tricyclic antidepressant, in combination with alcohol will produce additive central nervous system depression. Although caffeinated coffee is safe to use when the client is taking imipramine, it is not recommended for a client with depression who may be experiencing sleep disturbances. Imipramine may cause photosensitivity, so the client would be instructed to use sunscreen and protective clothing when exposed to the sun. Reduced lacrimation may occur as a side effect of imipramine. Therefore, the use of artificial tears may be recommended.

🗝️ CN: Pharmacological and parenteral therapies; CL: Analyze

27. 1. Telling the client that ECGs are done routinely for all clients taking imipramine, a tricyclic antidepressant, is an honest and direct response. Additionally, it provides some reassurance for the client. Commonly, a client with depression will ruminate, leading to needless increased anxiety. Tricyclic antidepressants may cause tachycardia, ECG changes, and cardiotoxicity. Telling the client that it is probably a precautionary measure because the nurse is not aware of a cardiac condition instills doubt and may cause undue anxiety for the client. Telling the client not to worry because the HCP is very thorough dismisses the client's concern and does not give the client adequate information. Explaining that the client had an ECG before initiating therapy with imipramine and that the procedure will be the same does not answer the client's question.

🔑 CN: Pharmacological and parenteral therapies; CL: Analyze

28. **4.** Anticholinergic effects, which result from blockage of the parasympathetic nervous system, include urine retention, blurred vision, dry mouth, and constipation. Tremors, cardiac arrhythmias, and sexual dysfunction are possible side effects, but they are caused by increased norepinephrine availability. Sedation and delirium are not anticholinergic effects. Sedation may be a therapeutic effect because many clients with depression experience agitation and insomnia. Delirium, typically not a side effect, would indicate toxicity, especially in older adult clients. Respiratory depression, convulsions, ataxia, agitation, stupor, and coma indicate tricyclic antidepressant toxicity.

🔑 CN: Pharmacological and parenteral therapies; CL: Analyze

29. **1.** The nurse should give the medication as prescribed. Mirtazapine is given once daily, preferably at bedtime to minimize the risk for injury resulting from postural hypotension and sedative effects. The usual dosage ranges from 15 to 45 mg. There is no reason to question the HCP's prescriptions. The nurse should administer the medication as prescribed. Requesting to give the medication in three divided doses is inappropriate and demonstrates the nurse's lack of knowledge about the drug.

🔑 CN: Pharmacological and parenteral therapies; CL: Analyze

30. **3.** Compliance with medication therapy is crucial for the client with depression. Medication noncompliance is the primary cause of relapse among psychiatric clients. Therefore, the nurse needs to teach the client about managing common adverse effects to promote compliance with medication. Teaching the client about the medication's pharmacokinetics may help the client to understand the reason for the drug. However, teaching about how to manage common adverse effects to promote compliance is crucial. Current research about the medication is more important to the nurse than to the client. Teaching about dosage regulation and adjustment of medication may be helpful, but typically, the HCP, not the client, is the person in charge of this aspect.

🔑 CN: Pharmacological and parenteral therapies; CL: Analyze

31. **1.** After about 2 weeks of medication therapy, the nurse should expect improvements in sleep, appetite, and energy, though mood may not have improved significantly yet. The increased energy related to better sleep and food intake gives the client the ability to act on thoughts to harm themselves (suicide) since the depressed mood has not completely lifted.

🔑 CN: Pharmacological and parenteral therapies; CL: Analyze

32. **4.** Dry mouth is a common, temporary side effect of paroxetine. The nurse needs to further assess the client's water intake when the client reports drinking lots of water. Excessive intake of water could be harmful to the client and could lead to electrolyte imbalance. Dry mouth is caused by the medication, and drinking a lot of water will not eliminate it. Sucking on ice chips or using sugarless gum or candy is appropriate to ease the discomfort of dry mouth associated with paroxetine.

🔑 CN: Pharmacological and parenteral therapies; CL: Evaluate

33. **2, 3, 5.** Symptoms of depression include depressed mood, anhedonia, appetite disturbance, sleep disturbance, psychomotor disturbance, fatigue, feelings of worthlessness, excessive or inappropriate guilt, decreased concentration, and recurrent thoughts of death or suicide. Paroxetine is a selective serotonin reuptake inhibitor antidepressant that also can be used to treat anxiety. Improved concentration, verbalization of feelings, and decreased agitation or pacing are signs of improvement. Taking 2-hour evening naps daily is still a sign of fatigue or lack of energy, and the increased use of somatization (bodily problems) could be a sign of continued symptoms of depression.

🔑 CN: Pharmacological and parenteral therapies; CL: Evaluate

34. **3.** After two episodes of a major depressive disorder, the likelihood of a third episode increases to 70%. This information would be useful to convey prior to discussing the importance of continuing the medication. This client also has a family history of depression. A healthy diet and exercise are very significant adjuncts to the therapeutic plan but may not be sufficient as stand-alone therapy.

🔑 CN: Physiological integrity; CL: Analyze

35. 1. In the first week or so of taking an antidepressant, the vegetative symptoms of depression (poor sleep, appetite, and energy level) improve. However, it takes 3 to 4 weeks for improvement in self-concept and self-esteem to take place.

    CN: Pharmacological and parenteral therapies; CL: Evaluate

The Client with Bipolar Disorder, Manic Phase

36. 1. The nurse should immediately report the rash to the HCP because lamotrigine can cause Stevens-Johnson syndrome, a toxic epidermal necrolysis. The rash is not a temporary adverse effect. Giving the client an ice pack and questioning the client about recent sun exposure are irresponsible nursing actions because of the possible seriousness of the rash.

    CN: Pharmacological and parenteral therapies; CL: Analyze

37. 2. Decreased need for sleep and racing thoughts are the most prominent hallmarks of mania. Feelings of pleasure, motivation, and increased energy, within reason, are desired experiences. Also, leaving a job to start a new business is not, in itself, a sign of impending illness.

    CN: Psychosocial integrity; CL: Apply

38. 4. The therapeutic serum level for lithium ranges from 0.6 to 1.2 mEq/L (0.6 to 1.2 mmol/L), but levels do fluctuate with fluid intake and output. Therefore, the most urgent matter for teaching is the client's comment about taking the lithium during an excessive loss of fluids during an episode of "stomach flu" with diarrhea. Exercising is only concerning if the client becomes dehydrated. A healthy diet is indicated while taking lithium.

    CN: Pharmacological and parenteral therapies; CL: Analyze

39. 3. All of these options need to be addressed. However, it is vital that this young woman receive counseling about the serious birth defects that have an increased incidence with the taking of divalproex during the first trimester of pregnancy. These problems include craniofacial abnormalities (cleft palate), organ malformations (holes in the heart and urinary tract problems), limb deficiencies, and developmental delays. The chances of preeclampsia and premature labor are also increased.

    CN: Reduction of risk potential; CL: Analyze

40. 1. Valproic acid can cause hepatotoxicity, so regular liver function tests are needed. Other side effects include nausea and drowsiness. Extended-release tablets should not be split or crushed; doing so changes their absorption. Alcohol should never be mixed with this medication. There will be medication in the client's body at all times. Nausea and tachycardia are not common side effects of valproic acid.

    CN: Pharmacological and parenteral therapies; CL: Analyze

41. 2. The use of prednisone or other steroids can initiate a manic state in a bipolar client even if the client is well controlled on medication. The other medications would decrease the client's depression, mood swings, and anxiety, making them calmer rather than more agitated.

    CN: Pharmacological and parenteral therapies; CL: Analyze

42. 3. The nurse should first attempt a collaborative approach to increasing adherence to the prescribed medication regimen. Giving written medication information to a client with acute mania is poor nursing judgment because a client with acute mania cannot benefit from written information as a result of impaired ability to focus and concentrate. The client was a voluntary admission and has the right to refuse any medication. Giving the medication as an injection against the client's consent constitutes battery.

    CN: Management of care; CL: Analyze

43. 2. The nurse clearly informs the client about behavior that is unacceptable on the unit, such as voicing jokes with sexual content and touching others. Setting limits on behavior provides safety and security to the client and conveys to the client that they are worthy of help. Saying "They will not want to be around you with that kind of talk" and "You need to be careful about what you say to others" does not clearly inform the client about behaviors that are unacceptable and implies that the client can control behaviors if they choose. A time-out in the client's room does not inform the client about the inappropriateness of their behavior and could be interpreted by the client as punitive as well as diminishing their self-esteem.

    CN: Psychosocial integrity; CL: Analyze

44. 1. Wasting controlled substances requires an independent witness and documentation; at least one, but preferably both, of the witnesses should be licensed. For single-dose vials, the excess is not returned to the pharmacy or saved for a future dose of medication. The waste is witnessed and

documented per agency protocols. It is unnecessary to inform the charge nurse about wasted medication when agency protocols for wasting controlled substances have been followed.

🔑 CN: Pharmacological and parenteral therapies; CL: Evaluate

45. 4. The nurse should help the UAP understand the client's behavior by stating that the irritable mood is a symptom of mania. Not all clients with mania are euphoric or have an expansive mood. Saying "It is our responsibility to listen to clients even though we might not like what they are saying" does not help the UAP understand a client with mania. Reprimanding the client for the behavior and asking the client to control the behavior are inappropriate actions and show poor nursing judgment and a lack of understanding of the manic client.

🔑 CN: Psychosocial integrity; CL: Analyze

46. −/+ 1, 2, 3, 5. Scheduled rest periods, relaxation exercises, and listening to soft music are activities that reduce environmental stimuli for the client who is hyperactive, talkative, easily distracted, irritable, and angry. Walking is also beneficial to discharge some of the client's need to be active. Watching television is not therapeutic because it would stimulate a client with acute mania.

🔑 CN: Psychosocial integrity; CL: Apply

47. 3. Reminding the client of past consequences of stopping the medication may help the client realize the risks of stopping the medication again. While increases in energy may precipitate suicide attempts, the priority here is to reinforce the need for maintenance medications. Encouraging the client to reduce the medication dose reinforces the client's misperception of needing medication only when feeling depressed or manic rather than recognizing that the mood stabilizer can prevent experiencing those extreme highs and lows. Saying the client will "spiral out of control" if the client stops the medication is not as specific as identifying the need for hospitalization.

🔑 CN: Pharmacological and parenteral therapies; CL: Analyze

48. 1. The nurse should administer the medication as prescribed. Lithium has a clinical response lag time of 1 to 2 weeks. Haloperidol is prescribed temporarily to produce a neuroleptic effect until the lithium starts to produce a clinical response. Haloperidol is usually discontinued when the lithium starts to take effect. There is no need to contact the HCP or supervisor as the prescription is appropriate.

🔑 CN: Pharmacological and parenteral therapies; CL: Analyze

49. 4. The client's statement "I am the Queen of England. Bow before me" is an example of a grandiose delusion and refers to thought content in the mental status examination. Examples of psychomotor behavior to be documented would include excited, typically exaggerated, and repetitive physical movements, and excessive talking and gesturing. Mood is a subjective state, and affect is an observable expression of emotion. Mood is what a client tells you they are feeling, and affect is what you see the client feeling. For example, the client may state that they feel sad or happy in reference to mood. Affect refers to the display of physical emotion, commonly described as "appropriate" or "flat." Attitude toward the nurse refers to the client's behavior in the presence of the nurse during the mental status examination (pleasant, cooperative, irritable, and guarded).

🔑 CN: Psychosocial integrity; CL: Analyze

50. 4. Decreasing external stimuli is the intervention most likely to decrease the emotional lability and minimize its effect on other clients. While the client is displaying emotional lability, this behavior has not reached the level where involuntary isolation (seclusion) or physical restraint is needed. The client is not totally out of control or threatening others. However, ignoring the behavior will not result in a decrease in lability. Lorazepam can be used, but benzodiazepines can lead to dependence and should not be used before other measures have been tried.

🔑 CN: Psychosocial integrity; CL: Analyze

51. 1. The nurse would request to be excused, showing respect and regard for the client, while telling the client to come to the dining room for lunch. Acutely manic clients need clear, concise comments and directions. Telling the client to stop talking because it is lunchtime is disrespectful and does not give the client directions for what the client needs to do. Using the familiar skill of waiting without interrupting until the person pauses would not be effective with the very talkative, manic client. Walking away and approaching the client after a few minutes before the food gets cold is not helpful because the client would probably continue talking.

🔑 CN: Psychosocial integrity; CL: Analyze

52. 3. By stating to the client "Swearing and profanity is unacceptable here," the nurse is setting limits in a nonpunitive manner for behavior that is inappropriate or threatening to other clients and staff. Setting limits helps the client regain self-control, prevents alienation from others, and preserves self-esteem. It is common for the irritable manic client to misperceive the nurse's and others' statements and intentions, feel threatened, and respond in a manner that is out of character for the client when not in a manic phase. Stating that the client is acting very inappropriately or that the nurse will not tolerate the client's swearing and profanity or threatening to put the client in seclusion is threatening and punitive and thus nontherapeutic.

☞ CN: Psychosocial integrity; CL: Analyze

53. 1. Stating that this must be difficult for the spouse conveys empathy and understanding and offers the opportunity to voice feelings to the nurse. Telling the spouse that it is okay and that the nurse has heard worse is inappropriate and minimizes the impact of the client's illness on the spouse. Asking about the length of the client's illness or telling the spouse that the client needs some medication ignores the spouse's feelings, thereby minimizing self-respect.

☞ CN: Psychosocial integrity; CL: Analyze

54. 3. Telling the client that others may not want to hear about sex and inviting the client to play a game of ping-pong with the nurse informs the client that even though the behavior is unacceptable, the nurse considers the client worthy of help. The client's thoughts and actions are out of control, and directing the client to an activity with the nurse is an appropriate way of regaining control. The nurse is responsible for providing safety and security to this client and others on the unit. Continuing to walk down the hall while ignoring the conversation does nothing to meet the needs of this or other clients. Doing so also diminishes trust in the nurse. Speaking to the client later in private while saying nothing at the time allows the client to continue the provocative behavior instead of focusing energy on productive activity. Informing the client that continuing to talk about sex will alienate others is not helpful because the behavior is a symptom of the illness, and the statement diminishes self-worth.

☞ CN: Psychosocial integrity; CL: Analyze

55. 4. The nurse suggests an activity such as walking around the unit to distract the client from the paranoid grandiose delusion that could result in loss of control. This action interrupts the client's anxious state and helps the client redirect energy and focus on an activity based in reality. The focus must be on the underlying need or feeling of the delusion and not on the content. Asking the client to describe the people who will come challenges the client and forces them to cling to the delusion. Stating that the nurse and staff will protect the client conveys agreement with the client's belief system, reinforcing their delusion. Telling the client that they are not the prince of peace and repeating their name challenges the client and their present belief system. Doing so may lead to decreased trust in the nurse and an aggressive response, or it may force the client to defend their beliefs.

☞ CN: Psychosocial integrity; CL: Analyze

56. 2. The nurse needs to explain the procedure in simple terms because the client in a manic phase has difficulty concentrating, is easily distracted, and can misinterpret what the nurse states. Giving a thorough explanation of the procedure is not helpful and can confuse the client. Calling security to be on standby is inappropriate. If the nurse judges that the client might elope or become agitated, the nurse should schedule the appointment for another time. Canceling the appointment until the client can go unescorted is impractical and may not follow unit or hospital policy and the client's treatment plan.

☞ CN: Psychosocial integrity; CL: Analyze

57. 4. The nurse escorts the client to their room and assists with choosing appropriate attire to preserve the client's dignity and self-esteem and prevent ridicule from others on the unit. It is common for a client with bipolar disorder, manic phase, to exhibit poor judgment, provocative behavior, and hyperactivity. The client in the manic phase commonly dresses inappropriately and changes clothes many times throughout the day. The nurse needs to assist the client with hygiene, grooming, and proper attire until their judgment improves. Telling the client to dress appropriately while out of their room may be perceived by the client as an attack. Additionally, the client may be incapable of making that decision. Asking the client to put on hospital pajamas until they can dress appropriately is punitive and demeaning. Because of the client's cognitive difficulties, the client may not understand the instructions to go to their room to change clothes. Additionally, the client may become distracted by stimuli on the unit and may not reach their room.

☞ CN: Psychosocial integrity; CL: Analyze

58. 3. Although the client who is psychotic can upset other clients, the nurse must respond to the second client with both empathy for the client's feelings and a general explanation that the behavior is out of the psychotic client's control. Agreeing with the second client or telling them that they cannot discuss other clients does not help the upset client gain empathy for the peer and only temporarily deals with the problem.

☞ CN: Psychosocial integrity; CL: Analyze

59. 4. The client with mania is very active and needs to have this energy channeled into a constructive task, such as cleaning or tidying the dayroom. Because the client is distracted easily and can concentrate only for short periods, the successful completion of a helpful task would give the nurse the opportunity to thank the client for the help, thereby enhancing the client's self-esteem. Leading a group activity is too stimulating for the client. Participating in this type of activity also may cause the client to be disruptive. Watching television or reading the newspaper would be inappropriate for a client who cannot sit for a period of time.

   CN: Psychosocial integrity; CL: Analyze

60. 1. The client in the manic phase experiences insomnia, as evidenced by sleeping only for about 4 hours a night for the past 5 days. The client experiencing an acute manic episode is not capable of judging the need for sleep. Therefore, the nurse should assess the amount of rest the client is receiving daily to prevent exhaustion. The development of vertigo, gastritis, or bradycardia typically does not result from acute mania.

   CN: Psychosocial integrity; CL: Analyze

61. 3. Bipolar disorder is a biochemical disorder caused by an imbalance of neurotransmitters in the brain. Manic episodes seem to be related to excessive levels of norepinephrine, serotonin, and dopamine. Psychopharmacologic therapy aims to restore the balance of neurotransmitters. In the past, it was thought that bipolar disorder may have been caused by early psychodynamics or disturbed families, but the current view emphasizes the role of biology. Bipolar disorder could be genetic or inherited from someone in the family, but it is best for the client and family to understand the disease concept related to neurotransmitter imbalance. This understanding also helps them to refrain from placing blame on anyone. Siblings and close relatives have a higher incidence of bipolar disorder and mood disorders in general when compared with the general population.

   CN: Psychosocial integrity; CL: Apply

62. 2. The serum lithium level has nothing to do with the client's white blood cell count, and there are no government safety regulations for blood testing. Although obtaining a periodic serum lithium level could help monitor whether or not a client was taking the prescribed medication, the most important reason for the blood test is to periodically assess the client's lithium level and prevent even mild toxicity on an ongoing basis.

   CN: Pharmacological and parenteral therapies; CL: Apply

63. 3. Because lithium reaches peak blood levels in 1 to 3 hours, blood specimens for serum lithium concentration determinations are usually drawn before the first dose of lithium in the morning (which is usually 8 to 12 hours after the previous dose) or before breakfast. Stat lithium levels can be drawn at any time, usually when toxicity is suspected.

   CN: Pharmacological and parenteral therapies; CL: Apply

64. 2, 3, 5. Serious side effects that may indicate lithium toxicity include muscle weakness, vertigo, vomiting, extreme hand tremor, and sedation. The prescribing HCP should be notified immediately when these symptoms occur. When lithium is initiated, mild or transient side effects can occur, such as nausea, fine hand tremor, anorexia, increased thirst and urination, and diarrhea or constipation.

   CN: Pharmacological and parenteral therapies; CL: Evaluate

65. 2. The therapeutic and toxic range of lithium is very narrow. If the client forgets to take a scheduled dose of lithium, they need to wait until the next scheduled time to take it because taking twice the amount of lithium can cause lithium toxicity. The client needs to maintain a regular diet and regular salt intake. Lithium and sodium are eliminated from the body through the kidneys. An increase in salt intake leads to decreased plasma lithium levels because lithium is excreted more rapidly. A decrease in salt intake leads to increased plasma lithium levels. The client needs to drink 8 to 10 cups (about 2 to 2½ L) of water daily to maintain fluid balance and decrease thirst. Decreased water intake can lead to an increase in the lithium level and consequently a risk for toxicity. Lithium must be taken on a regular basis at the same time each day to ensure the maximum therapeutic effect.

   CN: Pharmacological and parenteral therapies; CL: Evaluate

66. 4. Lithium commonly is combined with an antipsychotic agent, such as haloperidol, or a benzodiazepine such as lorazepam. Antipsychotic agents, such as haloperidol, are prescribed to produce a neuroleptic effect until the lithium produces a clinical response. After a clinical response is achieved, the antipsychotic agent usually is discontinued. Additionally, the dosages of each drug listed are appropriate. Therefore, the nurse would administer the drugs as prescribed.

   CN: Pharmacological and parenteral therapies; CL: Analyze

67. 1, 2, 5. The therapeutic level of valproic acid is 50 to 100 mg/mL (347 to 693 mmol/L). Clients with subtherapeutic valproic acid levels most likely would be manifesting symptoms of mania. Irritability, euphoria, grandiosity, pressured speech, flight of ideas, distractibility, and a decreased need for sleep are some characteristics of a manic episode. Anhedonia and hypersomnia are related to a depressive illness and not mania.

🔑 CN: Pharmacological and parenteral therapies; CL: Analyze

68. 4. The nurse should call the HCP to report symptoms of a sore throat, fever, and chills because these symptoms may be signs of serious adverse effects of the medication, including potentially fatal hematologic, cardiovascular, and hepatic complications. Giving the dose of carbamazepine is contraindicated in this situation. Giving the acetaminophen would be inappropriate and potentially detrimental to the client's health. Waiting until the morning to report the client's symptoms is a serious error in judgment.

🔑 CN: Pharmacological and parenteral therapies; CL: Analyze

69. 2. The nurse's most appropriate action is to give the spouse information about a support group in the area. Family members need and want education and support. Suggesting that the spouse see an HCP is not necessary in this situation. The spouse needs support and education. Recommending talking with a close friend may be helpful if the spouse so chooses. However, this is not as helpful as attending a support group. Here, the spouse can learn, share, obtain support from, and provide support to others with similar situations. Having the spouse share feelings with the client may or may not be appropriate or helpful to either individual. The client may be unable to help the spouse with adaptive coping, and therefore the client's self-esteem could be diminished.

🔑 CN: Psychosocial integrity; CL: Analyze

70. 2. The nurse should encourage the spouse to support and communicate openly with the client to maintain effective family-client interactions. During any illness, open communication and support help the relationship between partners. It is unrealistic for any individual to be free from anxiety or worry and impossible for the spouse to be able to control what the client may think or feel. Relieving the client of all responsibilities is unrealistic and not helpful. The client needs to resume activities as soon as they can manage them. Reminding the client to control symptoms is not appropriate and indicates that the spouse needs further teaching about this condition.

🔑 CN: Psychosocial integrity; CL: Apply

71. 3, 1, 2, 4. None of the other interventions will be successful unless the stimuli that fuel the client's mania are removed or decreased. Once the client is in a quieter setting, oral medication will help calm the client so they can be calmer. Once the medication has taken effect, the nurse can help the client explore the client's feelings and problems. Finally, teaching coping techniques can be effective in addressing client problems after they have become calmer.

🔑 CN: Psychosocial integrity; CL: Analyze

72. 4. The nurse should state their name and purpose on the unit to clarify their identity and to counteract other beliefs the client may have. Stating that the nurse does not want to or cannot go out to dinner is not therapeutic because it fails to clarify the client's misperceptions or erroneous beliefs, as is the statement, "It doesn't matter how I look; the answer is no."

🔑 CN: Psychosocial integrity; CL: Analyze

73. 3. The client is visibly out of control, and other measures have not helped. Therefore, the nurse needs to seclude the client and use restraints if necessary to protect the client and others from harm. Following the client and asking the client to calm down or telling the client to lie down on the sofa is not helpful; the client's level of anxiety is too high for the client to attempt to calm down without help, and the client cannot control the behavior. Telling the staff to ignore the client's remarks is not helpful because the client needs external means of control to protect the client, other clients on the unit, and the staff. Safety is the priority.

🔑 CN: Safety and infection control; CL: Analyze

74. 3. When the client in a manic state attempts to manipulate the nurse or demands privileges, the nurse must restate the unit rules in a calm and matter-of-fact manner. "The television hours are from 1900 hours to 2200 hours. It's 2200, and the television goes off so everyone can sleep" is the most therapeutic response because it restates the rules and is nonthreatening. During a manic phase, the client is impulsive and has difficulty concentrating. The client needs consistency and structure from the staff. The statement "I'll let you watch television just this once" allows the client to manipulate the nurse, as does "I'll turn the television off when you get sleepy. Don't ask me to do this again." In addition, the last portion of the statement is a threat. The statement, "The television goes off at 2200 hours; I've been telling you this for the past three evenings," is inappropriate because it is authoritative and demeaning to the client.

🔑 CN: Psychosocial integrity; CL: Analyze

The Client with Suicidal Ideation and Suicide Attempt

75. **1, 2, 4.** Having resources such as a crisis phone line number and a specific prevention plan helps clients know what to do if they begin to feel they want to harm themselves. Likewise, having support people educated about how to help the client stay safe also improves the client's safety. Not all medications are lethal enough that access to a month's supply of medication should be limited. Further, such a limitation is likely to increase costs for the clients, which may increase the client's stress. It is unrealistic and potentially distressing to the client and family/friends to have the client under constant surveillance.

CN: Safety and infection control; CL: Apply

76. **1, 3, 5.** Suicide is a leading cause of death in adolescents. Therefore, it is important to assess clients in the ED for suicide risk so that those with the potential can receive help before discharge. Many visitors to the ED have no other source for health care. It is a myth that talking about suicide will cause young people to think about suicide, and evidence exists that they will talk about suicide if asked directly. Limiting the assessment of suicide risk only to adolescents with psychiatric diagnoses falsely assumes that other young people are not at risk for suicide. Questioning the parents about their adolescent's suicide risk may be an unreliable method because the parents may not be aware that suicide risk is present.

CN: Psychosocial integrity; CL: Analyze

77. **2.** A crucial factor in determining the lethality of a method is the amount of time that occurs between initiating the method and the delivery of the lethal impact of the method. Lethal methods of suicide include using a gun, jumping from a high place, hanging, drowning, poisoning with carbon monoxide, and overdosing on certain drugs, such as central nervous system depressants, alcohol, and barbiturates. The more detailed the suicide plan, the more lethal and accessible the method, and the more effort exerted to block rescue, the greater the chance is for the suicide to be completed. Impulsive attempts at suicide even with rescuers in sight may be lethal depending on the method. Less lethal methods may include overdosing on aspirin and wrist cutting. Jumping off an 8-foot bridge may cause injury, but it is not likely to be lethal.

CN: Psychosocial integrity; CL: Apply

78. **4.** The statement "No matter what the intent, all suicidal behavior is serious and deserves our serious consideration" is most appropriate because it provides accurate information for the staff. Superficial cuts may be termed *suicide gestures*. Nevertheless, these gestures are a cry for help and may indicate ambivalence about dying. Clients have accidentally and unintentionally killed themselves because previous attempts were not taken seriously, they acted on impulse, or rescue attempts were foiled. Stating "It's our job to help clients no matter how we feel about them or what they did. This client will be discharged soon" is inappropriate because it does not provide the staff members with accurate information. Stating "I won't tolerate that kind of discussion from my staff; now it's time for you to go back to work" is authoritarian and punitive. Additionally, it does not help the staff members gain insight. Stating "I know it's hard to understand, but we need to do the best we can even though this client will back" voices agreement with the staff's bias and lack of knowledge. As such, this statement is inappropriate.

CN: Management of care; CL: Analyze

79. **2.** On hearing the client's statement, the nurse must ask the client directly whether they intend to attempt suicide. It is erroneous to think that talking to the client about suicide will drive the client to it. Asking directly about suicidal intent is absolutely necessary. Commonly, doing so provides the client with a sense of relief. In addition, the nurse conveys concern for and a sense of worth to the client, thus enabling appropriate planning for care. Asking "What do you mean?" is an indirect method of inquiry that provides the client with the opportunity to evade the nurse's intent. Asking "Does your family not care about you?" shows poor judgment on the nurse's part and is demeaning to the client. Asking "What happened to make you think that?" conveys a lack of knowledge of psychopathology.

CN: Psychosocial integrity; CL: Analyze

80. **2.** The nurse's best response is to teach the UAP about the appropriate intervention and why it is important for the client. Staff members need to be client focused and understand why a specific intervention is important and appropriate. Telling the UAP that the assignment will be switched or not to worry about it is not appropriate because it does not teach the UAP about the client's illness and appropriate client care. The statement "Clients who are depressed are hard to deal with, but do not take what they say seriously" does not help the staff member understand why listening is important and may jeopardize the client's safety.

CN: Management of care; CL: Analyze

81. **2.** The immediate priority is to save the caller's life. Therefore, the nurse should tell the caller that another nurse will telephone the police. The immediate goal is to rescue the caller because the suicide attempt has begun. Referring the caller to a 24-hour suicide hotline or instructing the caller to telephone family for help may be appropriate as part of discharge planning. Asking whether the caller has telephoned their own HCP is not appropriate. The nurse is responsible for notifying the HCP.

CN: Psychosocial integrity; CL: Analyze

82. **4.** The statement refers to the suicidal client's wish to use their own death to retaliate or get even with their partner. If a client wishes to retaliate, discovering their specific plans would be important to maintain their safety as well as possibly their partner's. Although sadness, escape, and loneliness can all be themes expressed by a suicidal client, they do not apply to the comment made by this client.

CN: Psychosocial integrity; CL: Analyze

83. **2.** The statement "I don't think about killing myself as much as I used to" indicates a lessening of suicidal ideation and improvement in the client's condition. The statement "I couldn't kill myself because I don't want to go to hell" indicates that the client will not attempt suicide but could still be thinking about death. The statements "I'm of no use to anyone anymore" and "I know my kids don't need me anymore since they're grown" indicate that the client feels worthless and may be experiencing suicidal ideation.

CN: Psychosocial integrity; CL: Evaluate

84. **4.** Based on the client's statement, the nurse must initiate plans for hospitalization immediately because the client has suicidal ideation with a definite plan, lethal method, and immediate access to the method. Telling the client to remove the gun, call the nurse, or promise not to hurt themselves does not sufficiently reduce the risk for suicide.

CN: Psychosocial integrity; CL: Analyze

85. **1.** The survivor of suicide, in this situation, would be referred to a group for survivors of suicide to help them with their feelings and to work through the grief reaction. This group provides support and understanding of what the individual is experiencing by members who are experiencing similar reactions, including anger and guilt. Depression and unresolved grief can occur when the survivor does not receive appropriate help. Counseling by a chaplain or individual therapy by the nurse may be appropriate in addition to referral to the group. Giving the survivor the suicide hotline number would be appropriate if the survivor was thinking about suicide.

CN: Psychosocial integrity; CL: Analyze

86. **4.** After the client identifies and shares personal strengths, the nurse reinforces the client for the ability to evaluate themselves in a positive manner. Doing so promotes self-esteem and offers hope for improvement. Asking the client to identify three additional strengths or volunteering the client to lead the cooking group could be too overwhelming for the client at this time and may increase anxiety and feelings of worthlessness. Although educating the client about the importance of medication is important, doing so at another time would be more appropriate.

CN: Psychosocial integrity; CL: Analyze

87. **-/+ 2, 5.** The nurse should advise the visitor to be caring and genuine to the client as a friend normally would. Family and friends are commonly afraid or at a loss about how to act or what to say to someone with a mental illness or to someone who may voice thoughts of self-harm. The nurse should also advise the friend to listen when the client talks without being judgmental or trying to offer ways to fix the problems. The statement "Try to cheer them up" is inappropriate because the client may feel overwhelmed and thus become more despondent when unable to meet or match the cheerful demeanor. Telling the client that their suicide would hurt others is a form of arguing that is not helpful in addressing the client's underlying depressed feelings. The statement "Avoid asking how they are feeling" is inappropriate because it conveys a lack of interest in and concern for the client.

CN: Psychosocial integrity; CL: Analyze

88. **-/+ 1, 3, 4, 5.** The question "Do you want to harm yourself?" is straightforward and asks the question regarding suicidal plans. A gun in the home as well as more than a week's worth of imipramine are lethal suicidal methods. Living alone allows the client to carry out suicidal plans more easily than if the client lives with another person or persons. Asking how long it could take to feel different does not address the plan or the lethality of suicide.

CN: Psychosocial integrity; CL: Apply

89. **4.** The nurse inspects the bag and its contents in the presence of the client and the spouse so that they know what is allowed on the unit and what should be returned home and why. The nurse is responsible for the client's safety and that of the other clients and staff. Telling the spouse to take the client's things home because the client is suicidal diminishes the client's self-worth and is inaccurate. Instructing the spouse to unpack the bag and put the client's things away is inappropriate because it is the nurse's responsibility to manage safety issues pertaining to the client and the unit. Asking the spouse whether the bag contains anything dangerous would be poor judgment on the part of the nurse because the spouse would not be knowledgeable about the safety factors.

CN: Safety and infection control; CL: Analyze

90. **2.** The nurse and staff should place the client in restraints to protect the client from further self-harm. The client's behavior is out of control and necessitates external controls for safety. The health care team is trained to deal with this type of behavior, so there is no reason to call hospital security at this time. Calling the HCP for additional medication prescriptions is not appropriate because the lorazepam given by the nurse may take effect if the client remains still. The nurse is responsible for judging whether additional medication is needed later. Instructing a staff member to sit in the room with the client is unsafe for the client and the staff member.

CN: Safety and infection control; CL: Analyze

91. **2.** The nurse needs to ask whether the client is going to attempt self-harm to determine the client's ability to cope with the voices and to assess the client's impulse control. The nurse's assessment will then determine the course of action to take regarding the client's safety. Asking when the client hears the voices and how long the client has heard them is important but not as important as determining whether the client will act on what the voices are saying. Asking "Why are the voices starting again?" would be inappropriate because the client may not know why and may not be able to answer the nurse.

CN: Safety and infection control; CL: Analyze

92. **4.** Though disturbed thoughts and sensory perceptions would be a concern to the nurse, as would communication issues, the primary issue for this client in terms of the comments would be the potential for medication noncompliance and relapse. Most college students want to be like their peers and perceive themselves as capable and well. These beliefs can lead a young client with schizophrenia to stop taking medication, which leads to relapse.

CN: Psychosocial integrity; CL: Analyze

93. **1.** Clients on 15-minute suicide checks must be observed by a staff member every 15 minutes. However, the staff member must stagger the timing of the check so that the client cannot predict the precise time. The staff member could check the client at 10 minutes and then at 8 minutes, and so on, to protect the client from self-harm. The nurse would further explain the necessity of this procedure to help the staff understand its importance. Documenting that suicide checks have been done is absolutely necessary. Clients on one-to-one suicide precautions can never be left alone. All clients using razors must be supervised by staff.

CN: Management of care; CL: Evaluate

94. **3.** Talking with a staff member when suicidal thoughts occur is an important part of contracting for safety. The nurse or another staff member can then assess whether the client will act on the thoughts and assist the client with methods of coping when suicidal ideation occurs. Writing in a journal, engaging in physical activity, or playing games with others does not allow the client to verbalize suicidal thoughts to the nurse.

CN: Safety and infection control; CL: Analyze

95. **4.** Because the client has a history of recurring depression and suicidal ideation, the nurse would give the client a 7-day supply of imipramine to prevent possible overdose. Giving the client a 14-, 21-, or 30-day supply of medication would provide the client with enough medication to complete a suicide attempt. Tricyclic antidepressants are associated with a higher rate of death than selective serotonin reuptake inhibitors.

CN: Pharmacological and parenteral therapies; CL: Apply

96. **3.** Statistics do not apply when focusing on one individual, and every depressed client is potentially suicidal. During the most severe symptom period, the individual often does not have the energy to act on their suicidal ideation. Most people who complete suicide have talked about it or left clues to their intention. During the initial treatment period, the risk for suicide may be higher due to the delay of therapeutic onset.

CN: Psychosocial integrity; CL: Analyze

The Client with Psychosexual Disorders

97. **3.** Telling the couple that the nurse would like to hear about their concerns invites open communication. Telling the clients that admission history is needed first gives the client the impression that the issue is not important; the couple may not want to bring the subject up in the future. Referring the client to a therapist or marriage counselor is appropriate only after determining the nature of the problem.

🗝️ CN: Psychosocial integrity; CL: Apply

98. 1. The nurse must be aware of personal opinions and views when caring for clients with psychosexual disorders. The care plan for the client will be developed to manage both the depression and the pedophilia. It is not necessary to restrict the client's interactions with others on this adult mental health unit. The health care provider will determine the type of therapy that will be most appropriate for this client.

🗝️ CN: Management of care; CL: Apply

99. 4. Sexual dysfunction is the problem that is the most appropriate. Dysfunctional grieving because of lack of intimacy is not correct as the couple may have emotional intimacy. The trauma occurred when the female client was 15 years of age and thus is not an acute problem. Vaginismus is a medical diagnosis.

🗝️ CN: Psychosocial integrity; CL: Apply

100. 4. An expected outcome of taking sildenafil is an erection that can last up to 4 hours. The nurse instructs the client to take the medication 1 hour before having intercourse as an erection will occur within 1 hour and to take only one tablet in 24 hours. The nurse advises the client to avoid taking the drug if they take nitrate therapy, such as nitroglycerin, to avoid unsafe decreases in blood pressure.

🗝️ CN: Pharmacological and parenteral therapies; CL: Apply

Managing Care, Quality, and Safety of Clients with Mood Disorders

101. 3. Distraction and disorganization may prevent clients from eating or sleeping. Monitoring for needed intervention can prevent exhaustion and malnutrition. Liquid medications are indicated only if the client cannot or will not swallow tablets. Manic clients tend to disrupt group therapy, so this treatment usually is not for them. Family visits should not be tied to compliance with treatment. The client is unlikely to be able to concentrate and complete a journal at this time.

🗝️ CN: Psychological integrity; CL: Analyze

102. 4. The statement by the person who says "I have found a solution for this mess" contains suicidal ideation, and that person is more of a safety risk than the angry, alienated client or the obsessed or helpless one. The other clients may need intervention as well, but the potentially suicidal client has the greatest need for nursing intervention.

🗝️ CN: Management of care; CL: Analyze

103. 3. Hospitalized clients retain the right to privacy when they engage in personal communications with friends and family. Nurses commit an ethical breach when they share information overheard in a private phone call. The exception to the rule would be if the conversation included information that indicated the client was at risk for self-harm or harm to others. The nurse communicates with consulting HCPs and referral agencies as part of the client's continuity of care to which the client consented when admitted to the unit. The communication with the family also has the client's consent.

🗝️ CN: Management of care; CL: Apply

104. -/+ 1, 2, 3. Strategies that assist and support the needs of specific workers or groups of workers most effectively promote and protect health and well-being. Standard hours of work and customary workplace practices do not support or address individual worker needs.

🗝️ CN: Management of care; CL: Analyze

105. 1. High-risk factors that have been related to suicide include hopelessness, White race, male gender, advanced age, living alone, previous suicide attempts, family history of suicide attempts, family history of substance abuse, general medical illnesses, psychosis, and substance abuse. The highest suicide rate is among people over the age of 65, particularly White males age 85 and over. Psychiatric diagnosis is considered to be the most reliable factor for suicide, especially for those with depression, schizophrenia, and substance disorders. Therefore, an 85-year-old White man who lives alone after their spouse's death is at high risk for suicide completion.

🗝️ CN: Management of care; CL: Analyze

106. -/+ 1, 2, 3, 4, 5. The priority is for the nurse to provide for the student's safety. The nurse should immediately assess the client's suicide risk and help the client develop a safety plan, which may include using a crisis intervention hotline. After addressing the suicide risk, the nurse would explore the bullying and provide sexual orientation support resources. The nurse would not notify the school about the bullying as the conversation was shared in confidence.

🗝️ CN: Management of care; CL: Apply

107. 4, 3, 2, 1. The nurse first assesses and treats the bleeding gunshot wound. Next, the nurse removes any objects the client could use to attempt self-harm and ensures that the client will have constant observation. The nurse then assesses the client's immediate risk for suicide and bases subsequent decisions on the level of risk. Once the client is safe and the wound is treated, the nurse contacts the crisis intervention team.

⚭ CN: Safety and infection control; CL: Analyze

108. 4. Nurses rely on the expertise of other disciplines to assist in meeting client needs. Collaborating with the dietician to identify foods agreeable to the client provides client-centered care for the therapeutic plan. "Scheduling" the intake of restricted foods puts the client at risk for adverse reactions. Bypassing the client in making meal plans undermines trust and may create problems between the client and the meal preparer. The client has not responded to other medications, so a health care meeting about medication options is less likely to lead to an outcome that improves the depression.

⚭ CN: Management of care; CL: Analyze

109.

0/1	Apply a cooling blanket	Neuroleptic malignant syndrome	Urine output
	Start intravenous (IV) fluids		Vital signs

The client's symptoms indicate that they are experiencing neuroleptic malignant syndrome (NMS), a life-threatening condition that can develop in reaction to antipsychotic drugs such as olanzapine. Primary symptoms of NMS include mental status changes, severe muscle rigidity, and autonomic changes such as increased temperature, heart rate, and blood pressure. Immediate treatment includes holding all antipsychotic/neuroleptic medications and providing supportive treatment to treat dehydration and hyperthermia. A cooling blanket and IV fluids are most needed. The nurse would monitor the vital signs closely, especially the temperature. The nurse must monitor urine output closely because renal damage can occur as the kidneys filter by-products of muscle tissue breakdown. Lithium toxicity would have a gradual onset with early signs of muscle weakness, tremors, and gastrointestinal disturbances. Fever is associated with anaphylaxis, but the client does not have respiratory symptoms or a rash. Fever is also associated with meningitis, but the nurse would expect the client to have a headache. Monitoring breath sound changes are most needed with anaphylaxis. Monitoring intracranial pressure is most needed with meningitis. Deep tendon reflexes are not accurate assessments in clients with rigidity.

⚭ CJ: Standalone bowtie; CL: Create

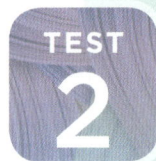

TEST 2: Schizophrenia, Other Psychoses, and Cognitive Disorders

- The Client with Schizophrenia or a Psychotic Disorder
- Clients and Families Affected by Chronic Mental Illnesses
- The Client with Cognitive Disorders
- The Client with Delirium
- The Client with Dementia
- The Client with Alzheimer's Disease
- Managing Care, Quality, and Safety of Clients with Schizophrenia, Other Psychoses, and Cognitive Disorders
- Answers, Rationales, and Test-Taking Strategies

The Client with Schizophrenia or a Psychotic Disorder

1. A newly admitted client describes their mission in life as one of saving their child by eliminating the "provocative sluts" of the world. There are several attractive young people on the unit. What action should the nurse take **first**?
   ☐ 1. Ask the client for their definition of "provocative sluts."
   ☐ 2. Discuss the dress code with all clients at the next group meeting.
   ☐ 3. Have the client discuss their concerns in the next group session.
   ☐ 4. Ask the client to inform the staff if they have negative thoughts about other clients.

2. A young client diagnosed with paranoid schizophrenia is talking with the nurse and says, "You know, when I thought everyone was out to get me, I was staying in my apartment all the time. Now, I would like to get out and do things again." What is the **best** initial response by the nurse?
   ☐ 1. "With whom do you want to do things?"
   ☐ 2. "What activities did you enjoy in the past?"
   ☐ 3. "What kind of transportation do you use?"
   ☐ 4. "How much money can you spend?"

3. The nurse recognizes the client in the emergency department from a picture in the local paper. The client has recently received a major scholarship for high academic achievement. The client tells the nurse that they hear voices that tell them they are worthless. The client has tried to kill themself. What statement is the most appropriate for the nurse to use **first** when attempting to establish a therapeutic relationship?
   ☐ 1. "You have a lot to live for."
   ☐ 2. "The voices are not real."
   ☐ 3. "I'm sorry this is happening to you."
   ☐ 4. "Would you like me to call your parents?"

4. A client who is neatly dressed and clutching a leather briefcase tightly in their arms scans the adult inpatient unit on their arrival at the hospital and backs away from the window. The client requests that the nurse move away from the window. The nurse recognizes that doing as the client requested is contraindicated for which reason?
   ☐ 1. The action will make the client feel that the nurse is humoring them.
   ☐ 2. The action indicates nonverbal agreement with the client's false ideas.
   ☐ 3. The client will then think that they will have their way when they wish.
   ☐ 4. The nurse will be demonstrating a lack of composure over the situation.

5. A client reports having thoughts of being followed by foreign agents who are after their secret papers. Which response by the nurse is **most** appropriate when responding to the client's disturbed thought process?
   ☐ 1. "I don't see any foreign agents."
   ☐ 2. "I think these thoughts are frightening to you."
   ☐ 3. "I don't know what you mean."
   ☐ 4. "I would like you to come to group with me right now."

6. A client who has been stabilized on medications for several months is at the clinic for a medication check. During a conversation with the nurse, the client suddenly jumps up, begins pacing, and wrings their hands. In what order should the nurse do the following interventions from first to last? All options must be used.

   | 1. Walk with the client to help decrease their anxiety. |
   | 2. Discuss productive ways to solve the problems causing anxiety. |
   | 3. Share observations about their anxiety-related behaviors. |
   | 4. Ask the client about the sources of their anxiety. |
   | |
   | |
   | |
   | |

7. A client on haloperidol has stiff muscles, restlessness, and internal jumpiness. The client has all of the following medications prescribed as needed. Which one would be **most** appropriate for the nurse to administer to decrease the client's symptoms?
   ☐ 1. lorazepam
   ☐ 2. benztropine
   ☐ 3. trazodone
   ☐ 4. olanzapine

8. The parents of a 20-year-old client diagnosed with paranoid schizophrenia admitted 4 days ago are attending a family psychoeducation group in the hospital. Which statement by the parent indicates that they understand the client's illness and management?
   ☐ 1. "I know that I'll have to do everything for my child when they come home."
   ☐ 2. "Tasks as simple as getting out of bed and showering in the morning may be difficult for them."
   ☐ 3. "I know that visits from their friends at home should be discouraged for a while."
   ☐ 4. "They won't experience a relapse as long as they take their prescribed medication."

9. During a home visit for a client diagnosed with paranoid schizophrenia and discharged 1 week ago, the client's parent tearfully states, "I can hardly sleep because I'm so worried about my child. I'm afraid to leave them alone in the house. What if something happens while I'm gone?" Which caregiver problem would be the **most** inclusive one for the nurse to incorporate into the client's plan of care?
   ☐ 1. caregiver role strain
   ☐ 2. anxiety
   ☐ 3. fear
   ☐ 4. disturbed sleep pattern

10. When conducting a mental status examination with a newly admitted client who has a diagnosis of paranoid schizophrenia, the client states, "I'm being followed; it's not safe. They are monitoring my every move." In which area of the mental status examination should the nurse document this information?
    ☐ 1. thought content
    ☐ 2. quality of speech
    ☐ 3. insight
    ☐ 4. judgment

11. The spouse of a client admitted for treatment of newly diagnosed paranoid schizophrenia visits 2 days after the client's admission and states to the nurse, "Why aren't they eating? They're still talking about their food being poisoned." Which appraisal by the nurse is **most** accurate?
    ☐ 1. The spouse's inquiry is reasonable.
    ☐ 2. Education about the client's medications is needed.
    ☐ 3. The spouse's expectations of the client are realistic.
    ☐ 4. An increase in the client's medication is indicated.

12. A client states that they hear God's voice telling them that they have sinned and they need to be punished. Which response by the nurse is **most** important?
    ☐ 1. "How do you think you'll be punished?"
    ☐ 2. "Do you think you need to punish yourself now?"
    ☐ 3. "What exactly do you think you've done to be punished?"
    ☐ 4. "Let's talk about your strengths."

13. The nurse develops the plan of care for a client who is staying in their room because they perceive that staff want to harm them. Which outcome of care planning is **most** realistic?
    ☐ 1. Within 2 days, the client will complete activities of daily living.
    ☐ 2. Within 3 days, the client will participate in recreation with other clients.
    ☐ 3. Within 4 days, the client will demonstrate an absence of verbal aggression.
    ☐ 4. Within 5 days, the client will seek out staff to talk about feelings.

14. A client diagnosed with paranoid schizophrenia is still withdrawn, unkempt, and unmotivated to get out of bed. An unlicensed assistive personnel (UAP) asks the nurse why the client is behaving this way after being on fluphenazine 10 mg for 7 days. What should the nurse tell the UAP?
    ☐ 1. "Fluphenazine is most effective with the positive symptoms of schizophrenia."
    ☐ 2. "The client will be less withdrawn and unmotivated when the fluphenazine takes effect."
    ☐ 3. "The client's fluphenazine dose probably needs to be increased again."
    ☐ 4. "Lack of motivation is a common side effect of fluphenazine."

15. A pregnant client in their third trimester is started on chlorpromazine 25 mg 4 times daily. Which instructions are **most** important for the nurse to include in the client's teaching plan?
    ☐ 1. "Don't drive because there is a possibility of seizures occurring."
    ☐ 2. "Avoid going out in the sun without sunscreen with a sun protection factor of at least 30."
    ☐ 3. "Stop the medication immediately if constipation occurs."
    ☐ 4. "Tell your health care provider if you experience an increase in blood pressure."

16. A client reports that people in blue clothes keep looking in their window and talking about them. Which response by the nurse is **most** appropriate?
    ☐ 1. "Those people are groundskeepers. They are talking about their work, not you."
    ☐ 2. "Don't take things so personally. Not everyone who is talking is talking about you."
    ☐ 3. "Let's not pay attention to them. Let's play cards instead."
    ☐ 4. "I'll close the drapes so you can't see them."

17. The nurse prepares a teaching plan for a client who is to start clozapine. Which information is **crucial** to include?
    ☐ 1. description of akathisia and drug-induced parkinsonism
    ☐ 2. measures to relieve episodes of diarrhea
    ☐ 3. the importance of reporting insomnia
    ☐ 4. an emphasis on the need for weekly blood tests

18. A client is sitting in the corner of the dayroom cocking their head to one side as if they hear something, but no one is nearby. The nurse suspects the client is having auditory hallucinations. Which question should the nurse ask **first**?
    ☐ 1. "Are you seeing someone other than me?"
    ☐ 2. "What are you hearing right now?"
    ☐ 3. "What is going on with you right now?"
    ☐ 4. "Do you want to go to the recreation room?"

19. A client who is newly diagnosed with paranoid schizophrenia tells the nurse, "The aliens are telling me that I am defective and need to be eliminated." Which response by the nurse is **most** appropriate initially?
    ☐ 1. "I know those voices are real to you, but I don't hear them."
    ☐ 2. "You're having hallucinations as a result of your illness."
    ☐ 3. "I want you to agree to tell staff when you hear these voices."
    ☐ 4. "Your medications will help control these voices you are hearing."

20. An outpatient client who has a history of paranoid schizophrenia and chronic alcohol dependency has been taking risperidone for several months. The client reports that they stopped drinking 4 days ago. The client is very frightened by the tactile hallucinations of bugs crawling under their skin. Which factor should the nurse incorporate into the plan of care when explaining the tactile hallucinations?
    ☐ 1. alcohol intoxication
    ☐ 2. ineffectiveness of risperidone
    ☐ 3. alcohol withdrawal
    ☐ 4. interaction of alcohol and risperidone

21. A newly admitted client diagnosed with paranoid schizophrenia is pacing rapidly and wringing their hands. They state that another client is out to get them. Then they say, "Protect me, select me, reject me." What action should the nurse take **next**?
    ☐ 1. Administer oral lorazepam and haloperidol as needed.
    ☐ 2. Place the client in temporary seclusion.
    ☐ 3. Call the health care provider (HCP) for a prescription for restraints.
    ☐ 4. Ask the other clients to leave the immediate area.

22. A new nurse is leading a family education group for those who have relatives with paranoid schizophrenia. Which statement by the new nurse indicates the need for further teaching about symptom management?
    ☐ 1. "When the clients get overwhelmed, it's best if they spend some time in their room."
    ☐ 2. "The more we push the clients to spend time with friends, the more their voices decrease."
    ☐ 3. "Until we get the clients up and going, they seem to have no motivation to do anything."
    ☐ 4. "We still have to remind the clients that we do not hear the voices they do."

23. A client is being successfully treated with clozapine. Which statement by the client reflects a need for further teaching about managing the drug's adverse effects?
☐ 1. "If I eat too many fruits, I'll get constipated."
☐ 2. "I need to take the medicine with food to avoid nausea."
☐ 3. "I have to get up slowly so I don't get dizzy."
☐ 4. "Sometimes I have to push myself because I'm sleepy."

24. The client has been newly diagnosed with paranoid schizophrenia. Which client statement indicates increased insight about being stabilized on medications?
☐ 1. "Now that the voices are gone, I can decrease my medicines."
☐ 2. "I'd feel better if I knew there wasn't poison in my food."
☐ 3. "Since I feel better, I know I can restart school next week."
☐ 4. "The voices go away when I tell them to, except if I'm really nervous."

25. A client who is suspicious of others, including the staff, is brought to the hospital wearing a wrinkled dress with stains on the front. The assessment also reveals a flat affect, confusion, and slow movements. Which goal should the nurse identify as the **initial priority** when planning this client's care?
☐ 1. helping the client feel safe and accepted
☐ 2. introducing the client to other clients
☐ 3. giving the client information about the program
☐ 4. providing the client with clean, comfortable clothes

26. The parent of a young adult client diagnosed with paranoid schizophrenia is asking questions about their child's antipsychotic medication, ziprasidone. Which statement by the parent reflects a need for further teaching?
☐ 1. "If they experience restlessness or muscle stiffness, they should tell their health care provider (HCP)."
☐ 2. "I should give them benztropine to help prevent constipation from the ziprasidone."
☐ 3. "If they become dizzy, I'll make sure they don't drive."
☐ 4. "The ziprasidone should help them be more motivated and less withdrawn."

27. The nurse cares for a 23-year-old male client with schizophrenia in the outpatient clinic.

Flow Sheet			
Weights	June 10 140 lb (63.5 kg)	September 5 159 lb (72.1 kg)	December 1 188 lb (85.2 kg)
Nurse's Notes	6/10. The client was started on olanzapine 10 mg orally (PO) per day for treatment of schizophrenia with auditory hallucinations. 9/5. The client is occasionally hearing voices. Olanzapine was increased to 15 mg PO per day. 12/1. Symptoms are controlled, but the client wants to stop treatment because of weight gain. The client's prescription was changed to ziprasidone 20 mg PO twice a day.		

After a prescription change from olanzapine to ziprasidone, the client tells the nurse, "I don't want to take this ziprasidone either. I don't like the side effects, and I can't gain any more weight."

➤ Which response(s) by the nurse are appropriate for this client? Select all that apply.
☐ 1. "Ziprasidone causes less weight gain than do the other atypical antipsychotics."
☐ 2. "We can give it to you as an injection rather than in capsule form."
☐ 3. "Abnormal movements are not as common with ziprasidone."
☐ 4. "You can take it just before bedtime, so you won't need a snack."
☐ 5. "I can request a referral for dietary counseling to help you manage the weight gain risk."

28. As hospital-based care has become more oriented to crisis intervention, criteria for admission to the hospital have also changed. Which client(s) would have **priority** for admission to an acute care facility? Select all that apply.
Clients who:
☐ 1. live alone
☐ 2. are acutely psychotic
☐ 3. are acutely depressed
☐ 4. are dangerous to self or others
☐ 5. are not sleeping and have a lack of appetite
☐ 6. are not complying with medication regimens

29. An older adult client is brought to the outpatient clinic by their caregiver for a routine medication evaluation. The caregiver reports that the client is quite stable and has no adverse effects from the risperidone they are taking. Then, the caregiver says, "I just think the client could be even better if they were on a larger dosage. My son takes 1 mg of risperidone every day and the client is only on 0.5 mg." What is the **most** helpful response by the nurse?
☐ 1. "Maybe your son is sicker than the client."
☐ 2. "We could increase the client's dosage if you want."
☐ 3. "Older clients generally need lesser doses than do younger people."
☐ 4. "I am not seeing any symptoms of illness in the client. Let us wait until the next visit."

30. At an outpatient visit 3 months after discharge from the hospital, a client says they have stopped their olanzapine even though it controls their symptoms of schizophrenia better than other medications. "I've gained 20 lb (9.1 kg) already. I can't stand it anymore." Which response by the nurse is **most** appropriate?
    ☐ 1. "I don't think you look fat; why do you think so?"
    ☐ 2. "I can help you with a diet and exercise plan to keep your weight down."
    ☐ 3. "You can be switched to another medicine."
    ☐ 4. "Your weight gain will level off if you stay on the medication for 3 more months."

31. A client diagnosed with schizophrenia is being switched to risperidone long-acting injection. The client is told that they will remain on an oral dose of risperidone daily for approximately 1 month. The client says, "I didn't have to take pills when I was on fluphenazine shots in the past." What should the nurse tell the client?
    ☐ 1. "Taking fluphenazine orally and by injection would not be as effective as the injection alone."
    ☐ 2. "Risperidone is less potent than fluphenazine."
    ☐ 3. "Your health care provider did not believe you would take both the pills and fluphenazine injections."
    ☐ 4. "Risperidone initially takes a little longer to reach the ideal blood level."

32. The nurse is instructing the client who has a prescription for lurasidone HCL for schizoaffective disorder. Which nursing instruction is the **most** appropriate?
    "Take the dose:
    ☐ 1. in the morning with a full breakfast of eggs, toast, juice, and coffee."
    ☐ 2. in the evening with a sandwich and a glass of milk."
    ☐ 3. at noon with an apple and celery."
    ☐ 4. in the midafternoon with water."

33. A client perceives that their roommate's stuffed animal is their own dog at home. The nurse determines that this misperception of reality (illusion) is improving when the client makes which statement?
    ☐ 1. "Jan's stuffed dog looks somewhat like my dog."
    ☐ 2. "Jan's dog and my dog could be twins."
    ☐ 3. "I wish Jan had not had my dog stuffed."
    ☐ 4. "I guess Jan needs a dog as much as I do."

34. When asked about their stresses before admission, an anxious client stares blankly at the nurse and mutters unintelligibly. Which description of the client's behaviors should the nurse document in the client's medical record?
    "The client:
    ☐ 1. cannot answer any questions asked at this time."
    ☐ 2. is uncooperative during the admission procedure, refusing to answer any questions."
    ☐ 3. responded to questions with a blank look and incomprehensible mumble."
    ☐ 4. stared at the wall when asked questions and was disoriented and incoherent."

35. The nurse plans care for a client with schizophrenia who lacks the motivation to shower and dress. Which outcome should the nurse expect the client to achieve by the end of 4 days?
    ☐ 1. Verbalize the need to shower and dress.
    ☐ 2. Recognize the need to shower and dress.
    ☐ 3. Explain reasons for showering and dressing.
    ☐ 4. Perform showering and dressing.

36. A client diagnosed with schizophrenia is brought to the hospital from a group home where they became agitated, threw a chair at another client, and have been refusing medication for 8 weeks. The client exhibits a flat affect, is not caring for their hygiene, and has become increasingly withdrawn and asocial. The health care provider prescribes treatment with risperidone to improve the client's negative and positive symptoms of schizophrenia. When evaluating the drug's effectiveness on the client's negative symptoms, the nurse should expect improvement in which symptom?
    ☐ 1. apathy, affect, social isolation
    ☐ 2. agitation, delusions, hallucinations
    ☐ 3. hostility, ideas of reference, tangential speech
    ☐ 4. aggression, bizarre behavior, illusions

37. A 77-year-old client is brought to the emergency department by their caregiver. The client has a severe headache and lack of sleep because "I am so worried about everything." The caregiver says that the client has heart failure and schizophrenia. "In addition to all of their heart medicines, they're on aripiprazole, which was increased to 30 mg by their health care provider (HCP) 3 days ago." In addition to documenting all of the client's medications and exact dosages, the nurse should **particularly** investigate which factor(s)? Select all that apply.
    ☐ 1. the qualifications of the client's HCP
    ☐ 2. the client's symptoms of schizophrenia
    ☐ 3. the dose of aripiprazole
    ☐ 4. the client's symptoms of heart failure
    ☐ 5. the client's relationship with their caregiver

38. A client with schizophrenia comes to the outpatient mental health clinic 5 days after being discharged from the hospital. The client was given a 1-week supply of clozapine. The client tells the nurse that they have too much saliva and frequently need to spit. The nurse interprets the client's statement as being consistent with which factor?
☐ 1. delusion, requiring further assessment
☐ 2. unusual reaction to clozapine
☐ 3. expected adverse effect of clozapine
☐ 4. unresolved symptom of schizophrenia

39. A client's nursing care plan includes the following prescription: "Assess for auditory hallucinations." What behavior would suggest to the nurse the client may be experiencing auditory hallucinations?
☐ 1. inflated sense of power, knowledge, or identity
☐ 2. elevated mood, hyperactivity, distractibility
☐ 3. poor eye contact, tilted head, mumbling to self
☐ 4. distrust, fear, suspicion

40. The nurse hands the medication cup to a client who is psychotic and exhibiting concrete thinking and tells the client to take their medicine. The client takes the cup, holds it in their hand, and stares at it. What action should the nurse take **next**?
☐ 1. Tell the client to put the medicine in their mouth and swallow it with some water.
☐ 2. Instruct the client to sit in the dayroom and wait for the nurse to assist them.
☐ 3. Ask another staff member to stay with the client until the client takes the medication.
☐ 4. Say nothing, and wait for the client to put the medication in their mouth and swallow it.

41. The nurse cares for a client who is delusional. Which action by the nurse is **most** likely to increase the anxiety and suspiciousness of the client? Select all that apply.
☐ 1. informing the client of schedule changes
☐ 2. whispering with others where the client can observe
☐ 3. telling the client gently that the nurse does not share the client's view
☐ 4. inviting the client to join in leisure activities
☐ 5. maintaining personal space during interactions

42. A client with schizophrenia tells the nurse that they do not go out much because they do not have anywhere to go, and they do not know anyone in the apartment building where they are staying. Which action is **most** beneficial for the client at this time?
☐ 1. encouraging them to call their family to visit more often
☐ 2. making an appointment for the client to see the nurse daily for 2 weeks
☐ 3. thinking about the need for rehospitalization for the client
☐ 4. arranging for the client to attend day treatment at the clinic

43. The plan of care for an outpatient client with schizophrenia includes risperidone therapy. The nurse prepares to administer this drug based on the understanding of which factor?
☐ 1. The positive symptoms of schizophrenia are usually more prominent than the negative symptoms.
☐ 2. Agranulocytosis is less of a risk with risperidone therapy than with clozapine.
☐ 3. Typical antipsychotics help with negative symptoms, but not as well as risperidone does.
☐ 4. Risperidone is less expensive than traditional antipsychotics.

44. A client diagnosed with schizophrenia is being discharged on aripiprazole 5 mg every night. When developing the teaching plan about the most common adverse effects, the nurse should include which information? Select all that apply.
☐ 1. headaches
☐ 2. transient mild anxiety
☐ 3. insomnia
☐ 4. torticollis
☐ 5. pill-rolling movements

45. A newly admitted client with an acute exacerbation of psychotic symptoms of schizophrenia is having trouble deciding whether to live in a group home or a supervised apartment. Based on the client's current cognitive functioning, which activity is **most** appropriate for the nurse to ask the client to do initially?
☐ 1. List the pros and cons of each housing option.
☐ 2. Choose between apple and orange juice for breakfast.
☐ 3. Identify why the client cannot live in an unsupervised apartment.
☐ 4. Decide which staff member the client would like to have today.

46. An outpatient client who has been receiving haloperidol for 2 days develops muscular rigidity, altered consciousness, a temperature of 103°F (39.4°C), and trouble breathing on day 3. The nurse interprets these findings as indicating which complication?
☐ 1. neuroleptic malignant syndrome
☐ 2. tardive dyskinesia
☐ 3. extrapyramidal adverse effects
☐ 4. drug-induced parkinsonism

47. A client with schizophrenia reports doing very little all day except sleeping and eating. Which intervention should the nurse use with this client?
☐ 1. Suggest exercise periods three times a day.
☐ 2. Ask a relative to call the client several times a day.
☐ 3. Help the client set up a daily activity schedule.
☐ 4. Arrange for the client to attend structured group activities.

48. The nurse notes that a client sitting in a chair has not gotten up in 1 hour. The client does not respond to verbal directions, and their arm has been extended over the armrest for 30 minutes. What action should the nurse take **next**?
☐ 1. Help the client out of the chair and lead them back to bed.
☐ 2. Give prescribed doses of haloperidol and lorazepam as needed (PRN).
☐ 3. Ask the client to describe what they are experiencing right now.
☐ 4. Sit quietly with the client until they begin to respond.

49. An outpatient client with schizophrenia has been withdrawn from friends and family for 3 weeks. What is the **most** appropriate long-term goal for the client?
☐ 1. calling the client's parent once a day
☐ 2. attending day therapy three times a week
☐ 3. allowing two friends to visit every day
☐ 4. remaining out of bed for 10 hours a day

50. A client has catatonic behaviors. Which outcome would indicate a medication has been **most** effective in improving long-term behavior? The client:
☐ 1. can move all extremities occasionally.
☐ 2. walks with the nurse to the client's room.
☐ 3. responds to verbal directions to eat.
☐ 4. initiates simple activities without directions.

51. The parent of a client with schizophrenia calls the visiting nurse in the outpatient clinic to report that their child has not answered the phone in 10 days. "They were doing so well for months. I don't know what's wrong. I'm worried." Which response by the nurse is **most** appropriate?
☐ 1. "Maybe they're just mad at you. Did you have an argument?"
☐ 2. "They may have stopped taking their medications. I'll check on them."
☐ 3. "Don't worry about this. It happens sometimes."
☐ 4. "Go over to their apartment and see what's going on."

52. During a home visit, the nurse discovers that the client is less verbal, less active, less responsive to directions, severely anxious, and more dazed. The nurse interprets these findings to indicate that the client needs which intervention?
☐ 1. stress management
☐ 2. clinic appointment
☐ 3. increase in medication
☐ 4. immediate medical evaluation

53. A client admitted with a diagnosis of schizoaffective disorder, manic phase, who is currently taking fluoxetine, valproic acid, and olanzapine as prescribed, has had an increase in manic symptoms in the past week. The health care provider prescribes a valproic acid blood level to be drawn at once. What does the nurse understand is the rationale for this prescription?
☐ 1. All clients taking valproic acid need periodic valproic acid levels drawn.
☐ 2. Fluoxetine can decrease the effectiveness of valproic acid.
☐ 3. A decrease in the level of valproic acid could explain the increase in manic symptoms.
☐ 4. The valproic acid level is needed before a short course of lorazepam for agitation can be prescribed.

54. A 22-year-old client is being admitted with a diagnosis of brief psychotic disorder. Which finding would the nurse expect to find during the admission interview that is consistent with the client's diagnosis?
☐ 1. current treatment for pneumonia
☐ 2. regular use of alcohol or marijuana
☐ 3. evidence of delusions or hallucinations
☐ 4. a history of chronic depression

55. A client brought to the clinic after being arrested for harassing and stalking their ex-spouse denies any other symptoms or problems except anger about being arrested. The ex-spouse reports to the police, "They're fine except for this irrational belief that we'll remarry." When collaborating with the health care provider about a plan of care, which intervention would be **most** effective for the client at this time?
☐ 1. prescription for olanzapine 10 mg daily
☐ 2. joint session with the client and their ex-spouse
☐ 3. prescription for fluoxetine 20 mg every morning
☐ 4. referral to an outpatient counselor

Clients and Families Affected by Chronic Mental Illnesses

56. A nurse working at an outpatient mental health center primarily with chronically mentally ill clients receives a telephone call from the parent of a client who lives at home. The parent reports that the client has not been taking their medication and now is refusing to go to the work center where they have worked for the past year. What action should the nurse take **first**?
- ☐ 1. Call the director of the work center for information about the client.
- ☐ 2. Reserve an inpatient bed in preparation for the client's admission.
- ☐ 3. Ask to speak to the client directly on the phone.
- ☐ 4. Make an appointment for the client to see the health care provider (HCP).

57. A nurse is teaching the families of clients with chronic mental illnesses about causes of relapse and rehospitalization. What should the nurse include as the **primary** cause?
- ☐ 1. loss of family support
- ☐ 2. noncompliance with medications
- ☐ 3. sudden changes in medications
- ☐ 4. nonattendance at treatment programs

58. The director of an outpatient rehab program tells the nurse that a client with schizophrenia had done well for 6 months until last week when a new person started the program. This new person worked faster than the client did and took their place as leader of the group. Based on this information, which intervention is **most** appropriate?
- ☐ 1. Make a home visit and tell the client that if they do not return to the program, they will lose their place there.
- ☐ 2. Ask the director to assign the client to another group when they return to the program.
- ☐ 3. Make an appointment to meet the client at the mental health center and ask them about the situation.
- ☐ 4. Arrange for the placement of the client in a skill training program.

59. A 25-year-old client diagnosed with schizophrenia states, "I stopped my medications a week ago. I was just tired of not being able to drink with my friends. Besides, I feel fine without them." Which response by the nurse is **most** appropriate?
- ☐ 1. "It's important for you to go back on your medicines."
- ☐ 2. "I hear how difficult it must be to live with the changes caused by your illness."
- ☐ 3. "You'll have to talk to your health care provider (HCP) about stopping your medications."
- ☐ 4. "Your buddies will understand that you can't drink anymore."

60. A 23-year-old client diagnosed with schizophrenia cheerfully announces, "My parents and I are so excited that I'm pregnant. They're willing to help us take care of the baby too." Which reason should cause the nurse to be concerned about this situation?
- ☐ 1. The client did not say that the parent of the baby was excited about this.
- ☐ 2. The client's parents are not likely to provide enough help for what the client needs.
- ☐ 3. Symptom management will be difficult in early pregnancy without medications.
- ☐ 4. The client will have difficulty financially supporting the baby.

61. The nurse is reviewing the laboratory values of a client receiving clozapine. Which laboratory value does the nurse **immediately** report to the health care provider (HCP)?
- ☐ 1. white blood cell (WBC) count of 3500/μL (3.5×10^9/L)
- ☐ 2. hemoglobin of 11.9 g/dL (119 g/L)
- ☐ 3. sodium level of 136 mEq/L (136 mmol/L)
- ☐ 4. hyaline casts in the urinalysis

62. A client is being discharged before complete stabilization of symptoms. When developing a discharge plan for this client, the nurse should ensure that the client will have which factor in place?
- ☐ 1. more medical consultations after discharge
- ☐ 2. monthly outpatient visits
- ☐ 3. many coordinated services
- ☐ 4. a caring and supportive family

63. The nurse works with a team developing a community-based service program for clients with chronic mental illness. Which facility would the nurse rank as the lowest **priority** to expand?
- ☐ 1. partial hospitalization programs
- ☐ 2. psychiatric home care
- ☐ 3. residential services
- ☐ 4. long-term hospitals

64. Crisis intervention plays a major role in the management of care for clients with chronic mental illnesses. Although the safety of the client and others is always a priority, these clients typically need crisis intervention in which situations? Select all that apply.
- ☐ 1. inability to keep outpatient appointments
- ☐ 2. signs of relapse and decompensation
- ☐ 3. threat of eviction from housing
- ☐ 4. unpaid bills and lack of food
- ☐ 5. occasionally missing a dose of medication

65. The most common reason given by mentally ill clients for noncompliance with medications is their uncomfortable adverse effects. When teaching families, the nurse should identify which need as the **greatest**?
☐ 1. alternative ways to manage the adverse effects
☐ 2. home visits to set up a week's supply of medications
☐ 3. family monitoring of the administration of medication
☐ 4. outpatient monitoring of medication compliance

66. The stigma related to having a mental illness, especially a chronic illness, persists despite improvements in the management of illnesses and an increase in public education. Which view **most** perpetuates the stigma?
☐ 1. Mental illness is hereditary.
☐ 2. Mental illnesses have biochemical bases.
☐ 3. Clients cannot prevent mental illness if they want to do so.
☐ 4. Clients can recover from mental illness if they have willpower.

The Client with Cognitive Disorders

67. An older adult experiences short-term memory problems and occasional disorientation a few weeks after their spouse's death. The client also is not sleeping, has urinary frequency and burning, and sees rats in the kitchen. The home care nurse calls the client's health care provider to discuss the client's situation and background, assess, and give recommendations. The nurse concludes that the client most likely has which problem?
☐ 1. the onset of Alzheimer's disease
☐ 2. trouble adjusting to living alone without their spouse
☐ 3. delayed grieving related to their Alzheimer's disease
☐ 4. delirium and a urinary tract infection (UTI)

68. An older adult client was prescribed lorazepam 1 mg three times a day to help calm anxiety after their spouse's death. The next day, the client calls their adult child asking when they are picking them up to go to the graveside. The client says they have been walking up and down the driveway for the past hour waiting for their child. Noting the client's agitation, hyperactivity, and insistence, the adult child calls the nurse to report the client's behavior. Which finding would the nurse suspect as the cause of the client's behavior, and what action would the nurse suggest? The client is:
☐ 1. manic and may need a sleeping pill.
☐ 2. experiencing a medication interaction and should go to the emergency department.
☐ 3. experiencing a paradoxical reaction to the lorazepam and should stop the new medication immediately.
☐ 4. overcome by grief and probably needs an antidepressant.

69. The adult child of an older adult client who has cognitive impairments approaches the nurse and says, "I'm so upset. The health care provider says I have 4 days to decide on where my parent is going to live." The nurse responds to the concerns, gives the adult child a list of types of living arrangements, and discusses the needs, abilities, and limitations of the client. The nurse should intervene further if the family member makes which comment?
☐ 1. "Boy, I have a lot to think about before I see the social worker tomorrow."
☐ 2. "I think I can handle most of their needs with the help of some home health care."
☐ 3. "I'm so afraid of making the wrong decision, but I can move them later if I need to."
☐ 4. "I want the social worker to make this decision so my parent won't blame me."

70. A client has been transferred to the hospital's psychiatric unit from a nursing home for increasing confusion. The client's behavior is found to be the result of cerebral arteriosclerosis. Which nursing staff action(s) should positively influence the client's behavior? Select all that apply.
☐ 1. limiting the client's choices
☐ 2. accepting the client as they are
☐ 3. allowing the client to do as they wish
☐ 4. acting nonchalantly
☐ 5. explaining to the client what they need to do step by step

71. The nurse observes a client in a group who is reminiscing about their past. Which effect should the nurse expect reminiscing to have on the client's functioning in the hospital?
☐ 1. Increase the client's confusion and disorientation.
☐ 2. Cause the client to become sad.
☐ 3. Decrease the client's feelings of isolation and loneliness.
☐ 4. Keep the client from participating in therapeutic activities.

The Client with Delirium

72. An older adult client is admitted and diagnosed with delirium. Later in the day, they try to get out of the locked unit. They yell, "Unlock this door. I've got to go see my doctor. I just can't miss my monthly Friday appointment." Which of the following responses by the nurse is **most** appropriate?
☐ 1. "Please come away from the door. I'll show you your room."
☐ 2. "It's 5 o'clock Tuesday, and you're in the hospital. I'm Taylor, a nurse."
☐ 3. "The door is locked to keep you from getting lost."
☐ 4. "I want you to eat your lunch before you go for your appointment."

73. An older adult client is admitted to the unit after being examined in the emergency department (ED) and diagnosed with delirium. After the admission interviews with the client and their grandchild, the nurse explains that there will be more laboratory tests and x-rays done that day. The grandchild says, "They've already been stuck several times and had a brain scan or something. Just give them some medicine and let them rest." What should the nurse tell the grandchild? Select all that apply.
☐ 1. "I agree they need to rest, but there's no one specific medicine for your grandparent's condition."
☐ 2. "The health care provider will look at the results of those tests in the ED and decide what other tests are needed."
☐ 3. "Delirium commonly results from underlying medical causes that we need to identify and correct."
☐ 4. "Tell me about your grandparent's behaviors, and maybe I could figure out what medicine they need."
☐ 5. "I'll ask the health care provider to postpone more tests until tomorrow."

74. The nurse attempts to draw blood from a client with a diagnosis of delirium who was admitted last evening. The client yells out, "Stop! Leave me alone! What are you trying to do to me? What's happening to me?" Which response by the nurse is **most** appropriate?
☐ 1. "The tests of your blood will help us figure out what's happening to you."
☐ 2. "Please hold still so I don't have to stick you a second time."
☐ 3. "After I get your blood, I'll get some medicine to help you calm down."
☐ 4. "I'll tell you everything after I get your blood tests to the laboratory."

75. An older adult client diagnosed with major depression is suddenly experiencing sleep disturbances, inability to focus, poor recent memory, altered perceptions, and disorientation to time and place. Lab test results indicate the client has a urinary tract infection (UTI) and dehydration. After explaining the situation and giving the background and assessment data, the nurse should make which recommendation to the client's health care provider?
☐ 1. prescription to place the client in restraints
☐ 2. reevaluation of the client's mental status
☐ 3. transfer of the client to a medical unit
☐ 4. transfer of the client to a nursing home

76. The nurse cares for the client diagnosed with delirium. The nurse should investigate which condition as the **most** important?
☐ 1. cancer of any kind
☐ 2. impaired hearing
☐ 3. prescription drug intoxication
☐ 4. heart failure

77. The nurse cares for a client with changes in cognition. Which characteristic would make the nurse suspect that a client has delirium?
☐ 1. disturbances in cognition and consciousness that fluctuate during the day
☐ 2. the failure to identify objects despite intact sensory functions
☐ 3. significant impairment in social or occupational functioning over time
☐ 4. memory impairment to the degree of being called amnesia

78. The nurse cares for a client experiencing delirium. What intervention is **essential** to include in the plan of care?
☐ 1. controlling behavioral symptoms with low-dose psychotropics
☐ 2. identifying the underlying causative condition or illness
☐ 3. manipulating the environment to increase orientation
☐ 4. decreasing or discontinuing all previously prescribed medications

79. The nurse creates a plan of care for a client with delirium. What is a realistic short-term goal to be accomplished in 2 to 3 days?
☐ 1. Explain the experience of having delirium.
☐ 2. Resume a normal sleep-wake cycle.
☐ 3. Regain orientation to time and place.
☐ 4. Establish normal bowel and bladder function.

80. The nurse integrates an understanding of the disturbances in orientation in the plan of care for a client with delirium. What should the nurse expect to include as a **priority** for the client?
☐ 1. identifying self and making sure that the nurse has the client's attention
☐ 2. eliminating the client's napping in the daytime as much as possible
☐ 3. engaging the client in reminiscing with relatives or visitors
☐ 4. avoiding arguing with a suspicious client about their perceptions of reality

81. A client has been in the critical care unit for 3 days following a severe myocardial infarction. Although they are medically stable, they have begun to have fluctuating episodes of consciousness, illogical thinking, and anxiety. They are picking at the air to "catch these baby angels flying around my head." While the client waiting for medical and psychiatric consults, which need(s) would have the **highest priority**? Select all that apply.
☐ 1. decreasing as many abnormal stimuli as possible
☐ 2. avoiding challenging the client's perceptions about "baby angels"
☐ 3. orienting the client about their medical condition
☐ 4. gently presenting reality as needed
☐ 5. calling the client's family to report the onset of dementia

The Client with Dementia

82. The nurse is assessing an older adult for signs of dementia. The nurse gives the client three words to remember: "cat," "crackers," and "toys." After having the client perform a short task, the nurse asks the client to repeat the words. The client says "toys," "boys," and "joys." What action should the nurse take **next**?
    ☐ 1. Ask the client to repeat the original words one more time.
    ☐ 2. Note on the medical record that the client has echolalia.
    ☐ 3. Refer the client to a health care provider for further follow-up.
    ☐ 4. Repeat the test when a family member is present.

83. The nurse is caring for a hospitalized client who has a disorder of the amygdala. Which symptom can the nurse anticipate that the client will have?
    ☐ 1. impulsive acts of aggression
    ☐ 2. sleep disturbance
    ☐ 3. unable to recognize objects by touch
    ☐ 4. difficulties with speech

84. A client has been admitted to the emergency department. The client's family tells the nurse that the client has suddenly become lethargic and is "not making sense." The client has not had anything to eat or drink for the last 8 hours. The nurse further assesses the client using the Confusion Assessment Method (CAM). The client's responses to questions are rambling, and the client is not able to focus clearly to answer the nurse's questions. Based on these findings, the nurse should report that the client has which problem?
    ☐ 1. dementia
    ☐ 2. depression
    ☐ 3. delirium
    ☐ 4. dehydration

85. A nurse on the geropsychiatric unit receives a call from the caregiver of a recently discharged client. The caregiver reports that the client just got a prescription for memantine to take "on top of their donepezil." The caregiver then asks, "Why do they have to take extra medicines?" What should the nurse tell the son?
    ☐ 1. "Maybe the donepezil alone is not improving their dementia fast enough or well enough."
    ☐ 2. "Memantine and donepezil are commonly used together to slow the progression of dementia."
    ☐ 3. "Memantine is more effective than donepezil. Your parent will be tapered off the donepezil."
    ☐ 4. "Donepezil has a short half-life, and memantine has a long half-life. They work well together."

86. An older adult diagnosed with dementia wanders the halls of the locked nursing unit during the day. To ensure the client's safety while walking in the halls, what action should the nurse take?
    ☐ 1. Administer PRN haloperidol.
    ☐ 2. Assess the client's gait for steadiness.
    ☐ 3. Restrain the client in a geriatric chair.
    ☐ 4. Administer PRN lorazepam.

87. A client with dementia who prefers to stay in their room has been brought to the dayroom. After 10 minutes, the client becomes agitated and retreats to their room again. The nurse decides to assess the conditions in the dayroom. Which is the **most likely** occurrence that is disturbing to this client?
    ☐ 1. There is only one other client in the dayroom; the rest are in a group session in another room.
    ☐ 2. There are three staff members and one health care provider (HCP) in the nurse's station working on charting.
    ☐ 3. A relaxation tape is playing in one corner of the room, and a television airing a special on crime is playing in the opposite corner.
    ☐ 4. A housekeeping staff member is washing off the countertops in the kitchen, which is on the far side of the dayroom.

88. During a home visit to an older adult with mild dementia, the client's adult child reports that they have one major problem with their parent. The child says, "They sleep most of the day and are up most of the night. I can't get a decent night's sleep anymore." Which suggestion(s) should the nurse make to the client's child? Select all that apply.
    ☐ 1. Ask the client's health care provider for a strong sleep medicine.
    ☐ 2. Establish a set routine for rising, hygiene, meals, short rest periods, and bedtime.
    ☐ 3. Engage the client in simple, brief exercises or a short walk when they get drowsy during the day.
    ☐ 4. Promote relaxation before bedtime with a warm bath or relaxing music.
    ☐ 5. Have the client's child encourage the use of caffeinated beverages during the day to keep the client awake.

89. A client with early dementia exhibits disturbances in mental awareness and orientation to reality. The nurse should expect to assess a loss of ability in what other areas?
    ☐ 1. speech
    ☐ 2. judgment
    ☐ 3. endurance
    ☐ 4. balance

90. A client with dementia states to the nurse, "I know you. You're the kid who lives down the street from me." Which response by the nurse is **most** therapeutic?
    ☐ 1. "Mrs. Jones, I'm Shaun, a nurse here at the hospital."
    ☐ 2. "Now Mrs. Jones, you know who I am."
    ☐ 3. "Mrs. Jones, I told you already, I'm Shaun, and I don't live down the street."
    ☐ 4. "I think you forgot that I'm Shaun, Mrs. Jones."

91. While assessing a client diagnosed with dementia, the nurse notes that the client's spouse is concerned about what they should do when the client uses vulgar language with them. What should the nurse tell the spouse?
    ☐ 1. Tell the client that they are very rude.
    ☐ 2. Ignore the vulgarity and distract the client.
    ☐ 3. Tell the client to stop swearing immediately.
    ☐ 4. Say nothing and leave the room.

92. A client has severe dementia and motor apraxia. The nurse understands that the client may be able to perform which action?
    ☐ 1. Balance a checkbook accurately.
    ☐ 2. Brush the teeth when handed a toothbrush.
    ☐ 3. Use confabulation when telling a story.
    ☐ 4. Find misplaced car keys.

93. The nurse communicates with the client who is experiencing dementia and exhibiting decreased attention and increased confusion. Which intervention should the nurse employ as the **first** step?
    ☐ 1. using gentle touch to convey empathy
    ☐ 2. rephrasing questions the client does not understand
    ☐ 3. eliminating distracting stimuli such as turning off the television
    ☐ 4. asking the client to go for a walk while talking

94. During family teaching, the caregiver of a client with dementia mentions to the nurse that the client distorts things. The nurse understands that the caregiver needs further teaching about dementia when they make which statement?
    ☐ 1. "I tell them reality, such as 'That noise is the wind in the trees.'"
    ☐ 2. "I understand the misperceptions are part of the disease."
    ☐ 3. "I turn off the radio when we're in another room."
    ☐ 4. "I tell them they're wrong, and then I tell them what's right."

The Client with Alzheimer's Disease

95. The nurse discusses the possibility of a client's attending day treatment for clients with early Alzheimer's disease. What is the **best** rationale for encouraging day treatment?
    ☐ 1. The client would have more structure to their day.
    ☐ 2. The staff are excellent in the treatment they offer clients.
    ☐ 3. The client would benefit from increased social interaction.
    ☐ 4. The family would have more time to engage in their daily activities.

96. The nurse is planning care for a client admitted for vascular dementia. Which action is **most** appropriate in assisting the client with activities of daily living?
    ☐ 1. Perform activities for the client during hospitalization.
    ☐ 2. Document all activities the nurse expects the client to complete during the shift.
    ☐ 3. Inform the client that if morning care is not completed by 0830 hours, the unlicensed assistive personnel (UAP) will complete it.
    ☐ 4. Encourage the client to complete as many activities as possible and provide ample time to complete them.

97. The family of a client diagnosed with Alzheimer's disease wants to keep the client at home. They say that they have the most difficulty in managing the client's wandering. What should the nurse instruct the family to do? Select all that apply.
    ☐ 1. Ask the health care provider for sleeping medication.
    ☐ 2. Install motion and sound detectors.
    ☐ 3. Have a relative sit with the client all night.
    ☐ 4. Have the client wear a medical alert bracelet.
    ☐ 5. Install door alarms and high door locks.

98. A client with Alzheimer's disease is experiencing difficulty processing and completing complex tasks. What is a **priority** to include in the plan of care?
    ☐ 1. repeating the directions until the client follows them
    ☐ 2. asking the client to do one step of the task at a time
    ☐ 3. demonstrating to the client how to do the task
    ☐ 4. maintaining routine and structure for the client

99. The nurse helps the families of clients with Alzheimer's disease cope with vulgar or sexual behaviors. Which suggestion is **most** helpful?
    ☐ 1. Ignore the behaviors, but try to identify the underlying need for the behaviors.
    ☐ 2. Give feedback on the inappropriateness of the behaviors.
    ☐ 3. Employ anger management strategies.
    ☐ 4. Administer the prescribed risperidone.

100. The nurse provides family education to the family of a client with Alzheimer's disease. The nurse determines that a family member needs further education about the disease when they make which statement?
☐ 1. "I didn't realize the deterioration would be so incapacitating."
☐ 2. "The Alzheimer's support group has so much good information."
☐ 3. "I get tired of the same old stories, but I know it's important for them."
☐ 4. "I woke up this morning expecting that my old parent would be back."

101. The spouse of a client who was diagnosed 6 years ago with Alzheimer's disease approaches the nurse and says, "I'm so excited that my spouse is starting to use donepezil for their illness." What should the nurse tell the spouse?
☐ 1. The medication is effective mostly in the early stages of the illness.
☐ 2. The adverse effects of the drug are numerous.
☐ 3. The client will attain a functional level equal to that of 6 years ago.
☐ 4. Effectiveness in the terminal phase of the illness is scientifically proven.

102. The health care provider prescribes risperidone for a client with Alzheimer's disease. The nurse anticipates administering this medication to help decrease which behavior?
☐ 1. sleep disturbances
☐ 2. concomitant depression
☐ 3. agitation and aggression
☐ 4. confusion and withdrawal

103. The nurse makes a home visit to a client diagnosed with Alzheimer's disease. The client is recently started on lorazepam due to increased anxiety. The nurse is cautioning the family about the use of lorazepam. The nurse should instruct the family to report which significant side effect to the health care provider?
☐ 1. paradoxical excitement
☐ 2. headache
☐ 3. slowing of reflexes
☐ 4. fatigue

104. The nurse provides family education for those who have a relative with Alzheimer's disease about minimizing stress. Which suggestion is **most** relevant?
☐ 1. Allow the client to go to bed four to five times during the day.
☐ 2. Test the cognitive functioning of the client several times a day.
☐ 3. Provide reality orientation even if the memory loss is severe.
☐ 4. Maintain consistency in environment, routine, and caregivers.

Managing Care, Quality, and Safety of Clients with Schizophrenia, Other Psychoses, and Cognitive Disorders

105. An older adult client who has been diagnosed with delusional disorder for many years is exhibiting early symptoms of dementia. The client's adult child lives with them to help the client manage daily activities. The client attends a daycare program for seniors during the week while the caregiver works. A nurse at the daycare center hears the client say, "If my neighbor puts up a fence, I'll blow them away with my shotgun. They've never respected my property line, and I've had it!" Which action should the nurse take?
☐ 1. Observe the client more closely, but do not report the threat since the client will likely not be able to follow through with it because of dementia.
☐ 2. Report the comment to the caregiver so they can observe the client more closely, but refrain from telling the neighbor due to privacy regulations.
☐ 3. Report the comment to the neighbor, the intended victim, but refrain from telling the caregiver since they will worry about the actions of their parent they cannot control.
☐ 4. Report the comment to the neighbor, the caregiver, and the police since there is the potential for a criminal act.

106. A client reports having blurred vision after 4 days of taking haloperidol 1 mg twice a day and benztropine 2 mg twice a day. The nurse contacts the health care provider to explain the situation, background, and assessment and make a recommendation. Which information reported to the HCP is the assessment of the situation?
☐ 1. "The client is taking 1 mg of haloperidol twice a day and benztropine 2 mg twice a day."
☐ 2. "I think the client might need a lower dose of benztropine."
☐ 3. "The client reports having blurred vision since this morning."
☐ 4. "The higher dose of benztropine could be causing the client's blurred vision."

107. The nurse cares for a client who has an involuntary commitment or formal admission status. What should be charted by the nurse?
☐ 1. Nothing should be charted. The forms are in the chart; there is no need to duplicate them.
☐ 2. The client's receipt of information about status and rights should be charted.
☐ 3. The client's willingness to cooperate with seclusion should be charted.
☐ 4. The name of the health care provider (HCP) officially signing the certificates should be charted.

108. The nurse assesses an aggressive client. Which behavior warrants the nurse's prompt reporting and use of safety precautions?
☐ 1. crying when talking about their divorce
☐ 2. starting a petition to delay bedtime
☐ 3. declining attendance at a daily group therapy session
☐ 4. naming another client as their adversary

109. A nurse plans care for an older adult client with cognitive impairment who is still living at home. Which action should the nurse identify as a **priority** for safety in planning care for this client?
☐ 1. having two people accompany the client whenever the client is up and about
☐ 2. ensuring the removal of objects in the client's path that may cause them to trip
☐ 3. putting the client's favorite belongings in a safe place so they will not lose them
☐ 4. giving the client their medications in liquid form to make certain that they swallow the medication

110. The nurse manager of a psychiatric unit notices that one of the nurses commonly avoids a 75-year-old client's company. Which factor should the nurse manager identify as being the **most** likely cause of this nurse's discomfort with older clients?
☐ 1. fear and conflict about aging
☐ 2. dislike of physical contact with older people
☐ 3. a desire to be surrounded by beauty and youth
☐ 4. recent experiences with their parent's older adult friends

Answers, Rationales, and Test-Taking Strategies

*The answers and rationales for each question follow below, along with keys (🔑) to the client need (CN) and cognitive level (CL) for each question. In addition, questions that measure clinical judgment will be coded (CJ). As you check your answers, use the **Content Mastery and Test-Taking Skill Self-Analysis** worksheet (tear-out worksheet in the back of the book) to identify the reason(s) for not answering the questions correctly. For additional information about test-taking skills and strategies for answering questions, refer to pages 12–51 in part 1 of this book.*

The Client with Schizophrenia or a Psychotic Disorder

1. **4.** It is critical for the nurse to ensure the safety of others by knowing who the client might think needs elimination. Asking the client to explain what they mean and discussing their concerns at the group session are possible interventions for later in the client's hospital stay. Wearing appropriate clothing while hospitalized is generally a unit expectation for all clients.

    🔑 CN: Psychosocial integrity; CL: Analyze

2. **2.** Knowing the client's interests is the best place to begin to help the client resocialize. Knowing with whom the client wishes to socialize, what transportation they have, or how much spending money they have may be relevant questions, but these questions should be asked after the question concerning what activities the client enjoyed in the past.

    🔑 CN: Psychosocial integrity; CL: Analyze

3. **3.** Demonstrating empathy is an effective means of beginning an effective therapeutic relationship. Challenging the client's beliefs or thoughts is not the most effective in establishing a trusting relationship. Determining what supports are needed is done after an initial assessment.

    🔑 CN: Management of care; CL: Apply

4. **2.** The nurse's nonverbal behavior, moving away from the window as the client requests, indicates agreement with the client's false ideas. The client's behavior is likely to be reinforced if the nurse takes steps to agree with the false ideas the client holds.

    🔑 CN: Psychosocial integrity; CL: Analyze

5. 2. The client's disturbed thought process likely reflects this client's paranoid delusions. The nurse should acknowledge that the thoughts are frightening the client. Telling the client the nurse does not see any foreign agents is an appropriate nursing response if the client is having disturbed visual sensory perception and is having visual hallucinations. Telling the client the nurse does not understand what the client means is an appropriate response if the client has impaired verbal communication. Suggesting that a client participate in group activities would be appropriate if the client had a nursing diagnosis of social isolation and was staying in their room.

CN: Psychosocial integrity; CL: Analyze

6. 1, 3, 4, 2. The nurse should first walk with the client to reduce their anxiety because the client must be at a mild level of anxiety before learning can occur. Sharing observations with the client conveys a sense of caring. Later, the nurse can help the client connect the anxiety-related behaviors to their feelings of anxiety. Once the client can identify the source of their anxiety, they can talk about solutions.

CN: Management of care; CL: Analyze

7. 2. The reported symptoms are signs of extrapyramidal side effects. The medication of choice is benztropine, an antiparkinson medicine. Lorazepam is an antianxiety agent. Trazodone is an antidepressant used to enhance sleep. Olanzapine is an antipsychotic medication that could aggravate the extrapyramidal side effects.

CN: Pharmacological and parental therapies; CL: Analyze

8. 2. Clients with paranoid schizophrenia experience alterations in thought resulting in introspection, confusion, and distraction from external reality. Simple tasks that require concentration and effort, including activities involving self-care, may be difficult for the client, especially during the acute phase of the illness. However, the parent should not need to do everything for their child. Rather, the parent should encourage the child to do things for themself with guidance. Visits from friends should be discussed with the client, and the client should be encouraged to visit with friends to minimize the risk for social isolation. Although relapse typically occurs with medication noncompliance, vulnerability to stress, a low threshold for stress, the number of stresses, and the client's lack of adaptive coping behaviors contribute to relapse.

CN: Safety and infection control; CL: Evaluate

9. 1. The nurse recognizes the parent's feelings of being overwhelmed with the issues concerning the management of their child at home as caregiver role strain. Anxiety, fear, and sleep disturbances all contribute to caregiver role strain. The nurse should help the parent elicit the support of other family members or friends, continue with psychoeducation, and help the family connect with a support group.

CN: Psychosocial integrity; CL: Analyze

10. 1. The client is voicing paranoid delusions of being followed and monitored. The presence of delusions is described in the area of thought content in the mental status examination. The speech section would typically include documentation of disturbances in speech or pressured speech. In the insight section, the nurse would document information reflecting a lack of insight—for example, statements such as "I don't have a problem." In the judgment section, the nurse would document information reflecting a lack of judgment—for example, poor choices such as buying a gun for self-protection.

CN: Psychosocial integrity; CL: Analyze

11. 2. For the client with paranoid schizophrenia, 2 days on medication is too short a time for improvement to be seen. Therefore, the nurse evaluates the client's spouse as needing education or knowledge about paranoid schizophrenia, the course of the illness, and medications. Expecting an absence of delusions by the end of the client's second day of hospitalization is unrealistic. Rather, the nurse would reasonably expect delusions to decrease, disappearing by 5 to 9 days of hospitalization. The spouse's inquiry is not reasonable because not enough time has elapsed to evaluate the effectiveness of treatment. An increase in the client's medication would be unreasonable because not enough time has elapsed to evaluate the effectiveness of the medication. Generally, a time frame of 5 to 7 days is needed before the effectiveness of medications can be determined.

CN: Pharmacological and parenteral therapies; CL: Analyze

12. 2. The client is at risk for harming themself because of the command auditory hallucinations. It is most important for the staff to know if the client currently thinks they need to punish themself. Then it is important to know how they think they might punish themself. Knowing what they think they have done is relevant for changing negative thinking. Focusing on strengths would help improve the client's self-esteem.

CN: Psychosocial integrity; CL: Analyze

13. 4. The client is exhibiting suspiciousness of and a lack of trust in the staff, not aggression. Seeking out staff indicates the development of trust and decreased suspiciousness. Although completing activities of daily living and participating in recreation with other clients are important, the major problem presented is related to the client's isolation and perception of being harmed—not, for example, showering, hygiene, or other clients.

CN: Psychosocial integrity; CL: Analyze

14. 1. Fluphenazine is most effective with the positive symptoms of schizophrenia. The client's symptoms reflect the negative symptoms. Fluphenazine generally is effective in 3 to 7 days for the positive symptoms. An increased dose or longer time on fluphenazine will not help the negative symptoms of being withdrawn and unmotivated.

CN: Pharmacological and parental therapies; CL: Apply

15. 2. Chlorpromazine is a low-potency antipsychotic that is likely to cause sun-sensitive skin. Therefore, the client needs instructions about using sunscreen with a sun protection factor of 30 or higher. Typically, chlorpromazine is not associated with an increased risk for seizures. Although constipation is a common adverse effect of this drug, it can be managed with diet, fluids, and exercise. The drug does not need to be discontinued. Chlorpromazine is associated with postural hypotension, not hypertension. Additionally, if postural hypotension occurs, safety measures, such as changing positions slowly and dangling the feet before arising, not stopping the drug, are instituted.

CN: Pharmacological and parenteral therapies; CL: Analyze

16. 1. The nurse needs to present the reality of the situation. By explaining that the people are groundskeepers and probably talking about work, the nurse is reinforcing reality to counter the client's illusion (misinterpretation of reality). Additionally, this response voices doubt about the client's paranoid interpretation. Telling the client not to take things personally is flippant and judgmental. Telling the client to not pay attention to the people fails to address the client's misinterpretations and misperceptions. Closing the drapes so that the client does not see the people ignores the client's misperceptions and misinterpretation.

CN: Psychosocial integrity; CL: Analyze

17. 4. Clozapine is associated with agranulocytosis. Therefore, the nurse must instruct the client about the need for weekly blood tests to monitor for this adverse effect. Akathisia and drug-induced parkinsonism are associated with high-potency antipsychotics. These effects are not common with this atypical antipsychotic agent. Constipation and sedation may occur with this drug.

CN: Pharmacological and parenteral therapies; CL: Analyze

18. 2. Before intervening with the client experiencing hallucinations, the nurse must validate what the client is experiencing. Asking the client what they hear right now accomplishes this. Asking about seeing someone near the client would be appropriate to validate visual hallucinations. Asking the client about what is going on may be helpful. However, the question is too general to validate that the client is experiencing auditory hallucinations. Asking the client if they want to go to the recreation room might be appropriate after the nurse has validated what the client is experiencing.

CN: Psychosocial integrity; CL: Analyze

19. 3. The client may act on command hallucinations and harm himself or others. Therefore, the staff needs to know when the client is hearing such commands, to ensure safety first. Telling the client that the voices are real but that the nurse does not hear them would be an appropriate response later in the client's hospitalization when the client's safety is no longer an issue because antipsychotics are beginning to take effect. Telling the client that the hallucinations are part of the illness or that medications will help control the voices would be appropriate once the client has developed some insight into the symptoms of the illness.

CN: Safety and infection control; CL: Analyze

20. 3. Tactile hallucinations are more common in alcohol withdrawal than in schizophrenia. Therefore, the nurse should explain that these hallucinations are the result of withdrawal from alcohol. Because the client stopped drinking 4 days ago, the client is not intoxicated. Risperidone has little effect on symptoms of alcohol withdrawal. It is prescribed for symptoms of schizophrenia. Alcohol and risperidone have an additive effect but do not cause hallucinations.

CN: Physiological adaptation; CL: Analyze

21. 1. The client's anxiety as reflected in rapid pacing and clang associations is rising as a result of their paranoid delusions. Administering the lorazepam and haloperidol will help the anxiety and delusions. The client is not threatening others at this point, so seclusion, restraints, and asking clients to leave the area are not necessary.

CN: Pharmacological and parenteral therapies; CL: Apply

22. 2. Pushing a suspicious client into social situations is likely to increase anxiety, which increases, not decreases, the hallucinations. The statement about spending some time alone if the client is overwhelmed indicates awareness and understanding of how to intervene when the client is exposed to stress. The statement about lack of motivation indicates awareness and understanding of avolition. The statement about reminding the client that the family does not hear the voices indicates awareness and understanding of the client's hallucinations.

CN: Psychosocial integrity; CL: Evaluate

23. 1. Clozapine is the one atypical antipsychotic associated with severe anticholinergic adverse effects such as constipation. Consuming fruits would not be the cause of the client's constipation. The client should take clozapine with food to avoid nausea. Getting up slowly indicates that the client understands that postural hypotension may occur with clozapine. The statement about sleepiness indicates that the client understands that sedation may occur with this drug.

CN: Pharmacological and parenteral therapies; CL: Evaluate

24. 4. The statement about the voices occurring if the client is nervous reflects an awareness that stress and anxiety can increase the positive symptoms of schizophrenia. Decreasing the medications because the voices are gone reveals a lack of awareness about the need for the medications to control the client's symptoms. Stating that there is still poison in their food demonstrates a lack of insight into the client's delusions. Restarting school in a week reflects an unrealistic expectation for a client who is newly diagnosed and being stabilized on medications.

CN: Psychosocial integrity; CL: Evaluate

25. 1. The initial priority for this client is to help them overcome their suspiciousness of others, including staff, and thereby feel safe and accepted. Introducing the client to others, giving the client information about the program, and providing clean clothes are important, but these are of lower priority than helping the client feel safe and accepted.

CN: Psychosocial integrity; CL: Apply

26. 2. Constipation caused by medication is best managed by diet, fluids, and exercise. Benztropine can increase constipation. However, it may be prescribed for restlessness and stiffness. Restlessness and stiffness should be reported to the HCP. Drowsiness and dizziness are adverse effects of ziprasidone. Clients should not drive if they are experiencing dizziness. Ziprasidone does help improve the negative symptoms of schizophrenia such as avolition.

CN: Pharmacological and parenteral therapies; CL: Evaluate

27. 1, 5. Most clients experience less weight gain when taking ziprasidone. Dietary counseling, exercise programs, and cognitive and behavioral strategies prevention and intervention strategies have been shown to have modest effects on weight. Although ziprasidone can be administered intramuscularly, it can be used only on an as-needed basis by this route. Ziprasidone has fewer extrapyramidal side effects, but that is not this client's major concern. Ziprasidone is better absorbed when taken with food, so a bedtime snack is needed.

CJ: Standalone trend; CL: Analyze

28. 2, 4. Safety issues, including protection of the client and others, are the priorities for admission. Acute psychosis commonly involves issues of safety. Living alone is not a sufficient reason to be admitted to a health care facility. Depression, insomnia, lack of appetite, and noncompliance are important issues but not sufficient for admission unless combined with one of the other criteria.

CN: Management of care; CL: Analyze

29. 3. Older adult clients are typically on lower dosages of antipsychotic medications because of the metabolic changes of aging. Comparing dosages is not relevant. Each client is unique in metabolizing medications. Changing medication dosages is based on an assessment of illness symptoms and the adverse effect profile, not on family preferences. Urging the client's child to wait discounts their concerns and gives no rationale for waiting.

CN: Pharmacological and parenteral therapies; CL: Analyze

30. 2. Helping the client control their weight is the most appropriate approach. The nurse's contradiction of the client's statement is inappropriate. Most atypical antipsychotics cause weight gain and are not a solution to the weight gain. There is little evidence that weight gain from taking olanzapine decreases with time.

CN: Pharmacological and parenteral therapies; CL: Analyze

31. 4. Achieving a therapeutic blood level is a slower process with risperidone long-acting injection. Oral fluphenazine does not decrease the effectiveness of the intramuscular version and might increase the incidence of adverse effects. There is no evidence that the potency of the two medications is significantly different. Blaming the client for noncompliance with these two medications is inappropriate.

🗝 CN: Pharmacological and parenteral therapies; CL: Apply

32. 2. Lurasidone HCL should be taken in the later hours of the day with a total of 350 calories. A sandwich and a glass of milk will provide this number of calories. Another effect of lurasidone is drowsiness after administration, so taking it in the evening is preferred by many clients. Taking the medication in the morning with a large breakfast provides too many calories and allows the drowsiness to manifest. Taking with an apple and celery or just water also is not enough calories. Clients report abdominal discomfort.

🗝 CN: Pharmacological and parental therapies; CN: Apply

33. 1. Recognition by the client that there is a difference between the stuffed animal and their live dog indicates that the client perceives the reality of the situation. Stating that the stuffed animal and the client's dog could be twins reflects the client's continued misperception of reality, thinking that the stuffed animal and their dog are one and the same. Stating that they wish their dog had not been stuffed reflects their continued misperception of reality. Stating that the roommate needs a dog as much as they do is unrelated to the client's perception or misperception of reality.

🗝 CN: Psychosocial integrity; CL: Evaluate

34. 3. The nurse must be objective in documenting the client's behavior, recording exactly what the client did or did not say or do in a particular situation. Recording that the client could not answer any questions, was uncooperative and refused to answer questions, or was disoriented and incoherent is not described and is a subjective interpretation on the nurse's part.

🗝 CN: Management of care; CL: Apply

35. 4. By the end of 4 days, the client should be able to perform showering and dressing for themselves. The client with schizophrenia commonly appears to be apathetic and lack initiative. Therefore, demonstrating the ability to complete the tasks indicates improvement. Although the client may be able to recognize, verbalize, or explain the need to shower and dress, they may be unable to do so because of the ambivalence associated with schizophrenia that impedes the client's ability to initiate and complete self-care. Therefore, evidence of improvement would be lacking.

🗝 CN: Management of care; CL: Analyze

36. 1. When determining the effectiveness of risperidone, the nurse would expect improvement in the client's negative symptoms of apathy, flat affect, and social withdrawal. Delusions, hallucinations, illusions, and ideas of reference are positive symptoms of schizophrenia. Agitation, hostility, and aggression are also the result of the positive symptoms.

🗝 CN: Pharmacological and parenteral therapies; CL: Evaluate

37. -/+ 2, 3, 4. The client's symptoms are likely to be adverse effects of aripiprazole, especially at the reported dose. The normal adult dose is 5 to 10 mg. The older adult client commonly needs a lower dose compared with other adults. The anxiety and sleep disturbance could be symptoms of schizophrenia or medication adverse effects. A holistic approach would include assessing the client's heart failure. Questioning the qualifications of the family's HCP is unproductive. There are no indications of problems in the client's relationship with their child.

🗝 CN: Pharmacological and parenteral therapies; CL: Analyze

38. 3. Excessive salivation, or sialorrhea, is commonly associated with clozapine therapy. The client can use a washcloth to wipe the saliva instead of spitting. It is an expected adverse effect of the drug, not a delusion, an unusual reaction, or an unresolved symptom of schizophrenia.

🗝 CN: Pharmacological and parenteral therapies; CL: Analyze

39. 3. Cues that the client is experiencing auditory hallucinations include eyes looking around the room as though looking for a speaker, tilting the head to one side as though listening, and mumbling or talking aloud as though responding to someone. An inflated sense of power, knowledge, or identity is associated with delusions. Elevated mood and hyperactivity are features of a manic episode. Distrust and suspicion are prevalent in paranoia.

🗝 CN: Psychosocial integrity; CL: Evaluate

40. 1. The nurse instructs the client clearly and directly to put the medication in their mouth and then to swallow it with some water. Clear, step-by-step directions assist the client to process what the nurse is saying. Telling the client to sit in the dayroom and wait, asking another staff member to stay with the client, or saying nothing is not helpful.

🗝 CN: Pharmacological and parenteral therapies; CL: Apply

41. -/+ 2. Whispering and laughing with another person where the client can see or observe the nurse but not hear the conversation increases the client's anxiety and suspiciousness. Therefore, this action should be avoided. Informing the client of schedule changes, telling the client gently that the nurse does not share the client's interpretation of an event, and inviting the client to participate in leisure activities help the client to decrease anxiety and suspiciousness and to focus on actual or realistic events. Invading the personal space of a client experiencing delusions is likely to cause agitation.

🗝️ CN: Psychosocial integrity; CL: Analyze

42. 4. Because the client can live in an apartment setting, further development of independent functioning and the skills to gain as much independence as they are capable of need to be fostered, including getting out and developing new friendships. Arranging for participation in day treatment is most beneficial at this time. Family visits and daily nursing visits do not encourage the client to do this. Making an appointment for 2 weeks later puts the client's needs off. A lack of social relationships is not a sufficient reason for rehospitalization.

🗝️ CN: Psychosocial integrity; CL: Analyze

43. 2. One advantage of using risperidone is that it is not associated with agranulocytosis like clozapine and does not require the same lab monitoring. In schizophrenia, negative symptoms are more prominent than positive. Negative symptoms do not respond to typical antipsychotics such as haloperidol. Agranulocytosis is commonly associated with clozapine. Because it is a newer drug, risperidone usually is more expensive than typical antipsychotics.

🗝️ CN: Pharmacological and parenteral therapies; CL: Apply

44. -/+ 1, 2, 3. Headaches, transient anxiety, and insomnia are the most common adverse effects of aripiprazole. Torticollis and pill rolling are more common with older antipsychotics.

🗝️ CN: Pharmacological and parenteral therapies; CL: Apply

45. 2. The client is in an acute psychotic state and cannot process complex decisions or explain complex situations. Therefore, the nurse would focus on decision-making involving simple choices. Listing the pros and cons of each housing option and identifying why the client cannot live in an unsupervised apartment involve complex decision-making skills. Deciding which staff member to have today is a difficult and threatening decision for a client who is psychotic.

🗝️ CN: Management of care; CL: Analyze

46. 1. The client is exhibiting hallmark signs and symptoms of life-threatening neuroleptic malignant syndrome induced by the haloperidol. Tardive dyskinesia usually occurs later in treatment, typically months to years later. Extrapyramidal adverse effects (dystonia, akathisia) and drug-induced parkinsonism, though common, are not life-threatening.

🗝️ CN: Reduction of risk potential; CL: Analyze

47. 3. The client with schizophrenia needs more structure every day to improve functioning. Therefore, helping the client to set up a daily activity schedule is most appropriate. Suggesting the client exercise three times a day and arranging group activities does not take into account the client's preferences. Asking a relative to call the client several times per day is unrealistic given the typical daily responsibilities of a healthy relative.

🗝️ CN: Psychosocial integrity; CL: Apply

48. 2. The client is exhibiting catatonic behavior, an acutely serious result of severe anxiety and psychosis. In this situation, the nurse needs to administer the PRN prescribed doses of haloperidol and lorazepam; they can be given together safely. Assisting the client out of the chair to go back to bed or sitting quietly until the client responds ignores the seriousness of the client's condition. It is unlikely that the client can describe what is being experienced.

🗝️ CN: Psychosocial integrity; CL: Apply

49. 2. Attending day therapy three times per week is a long-term goal that will show the most progress in overcoming withdrawal. The client's calling their parent is a first step in getting out of a severe withdrawal. Allowing two friends to visit every day would be appropriate if the client is successful with calling their parent once a day. Insufficient information is presented in the scenario to indicate that excessive sleep is a problem.

🗝️ CN: Psychosocial integrity; CL: Analyze

50. 4. Although all the actions indicate improvement, the ability to initiate simple activities without directions indicates the most improvement in the catatonic behaviors. Moving all extremities occasionally, walking with the nurse to the client's room, and responding to verbal directions to eat represent single steps toward the client initiating the client's own actions.

🗝️ CN: Pharmacological and parenteral therapies; CL: Evaluate

51. **2.** Noncompliance with medications is common in a client with schizophrenia. The nurse has the responsibility to assess this situation. Asking the parent if they have argued or if the client is mad at the parent or telling the parent to go over to the apartment and see what is going on places the blame and responsibility on the parent and therefore is inappropriate. Telling the parent not to worry ignores the seriousness of the client's symptoms.

 CN: Management of care; CL: Analyze

52. **4.** The client is exhibiting symptoms of becoming catatonic and unable to care for themself and needs immediate evaluation and possible hospitalization. Stress management is not sufficient to treat this client. The client's worsening condition dictates action without waiting for a clinic appointment. An increase in medication may be indicated, but hospitalization is required first for safety.

 CN: Management of care; CL: Analyze

53. **3.** Valproic acid is commonly used to treat manic symptoms. Therefore, a decrease in the valproic acid level could explain the increase in manic symptoms. Periodic determinations of the valproic acid level are necessary to determine the effectiveness of the drug. However, the stat nature of the specimen to be drawn indicates an immediate problem. Fluoxetine is not known to decrease the effectiveness of valproic acid. The valproic acid level is not needed before beginning a short course of therapy with lorazepam.

 CN: Pharmacological and parenteral therapies; CL: Apply

54. **3.** A diagnosis of brief psychotic disorder is made when the client exhibits delusions, hallucinations, and disorganized speech or behaviors in the absence of a mood disorder, substance-induced disorder, or general medical condition.

 CN: Reduction of risk potential; CL: Analyze

55. **4.** Follow-up counseling is appropriate because of the client's anger and inappropriate behaviors. The goal is to help the client deal with the end of their marriage. A joint session might have been useful before the divorce and arrest, but not after. The client is exhibiting no signs or symptoms of schizophrenia or psychosis, so olanzapine is not indicated. The client is not exhibiting signs of depression, so fluoxetine is not indicated.

 CN: Management of care; CL: Analyze

Clients and Families Affected by Chronic Mental Illnesses

56. **3.** The first thing that the nurse should do is to speak with the client on the phone and question them about perceptions or reasons that are interfering with them going to the sheltered workshop. This conveys that the nurse is interested and willing to help the client. The nurse should call the director of the work center for information only if the nurse receives the client's permission. Making preparations for the client's admission is inappropriate and would not be done until the client's needs have been assessed and it is determined that the client requires hospitalization. Making an appointment with the HCP is inappropriate until the nurse has assessed the client's needs.

 CN: Management of care; CL: Analyze

57. **2.** Noncompliance with medications is documented as the primary cause of relapse. Although loss of family support, sudden changes in medications, and nonattendance at treatment programs may contribute to relapse, these factors are not as significant as medication noncompliance as causes of relapse.

 CN: Psychosocial integrity; CL: Analyze

58. **3.** The most therapeutic action at this time is for the nurse to make an appointment with the client at the mental health center to explore their feelings and behavior. Doing so acknowledges the client's importance and makes them a partner in resolving the problem. The nurse needs to determine what is going on in the situation first and then plan accordingly. Threatening the client with loss of the position, asking for a new assignment for the client, or arranging for the placement of the client in a skill training program is inappropriate and premature.

 CN: Management of care; CL: Analyze

59. **2.** By acknowledging the difficulties of living with the illness, the nurse conveys empathy for the client's feelings and opens up the lines of communication. Although it is important for the client to maintain compliance with medication therapy, telling the client that it is important to start taking them again or to talk with the HCP about stopping the medications ignores the underlying feelings of the client's initial statements. Stating that the client's buddies will understand may or may not be true. Additionally, this statement ignores the underlying feelings.

 CN: Psychosocial integrity; CL: Analyze

60. 3. Because antipsychotic agents cross the placental barrier and can be teratogenic, they are to be avoided during pregnancy, especially during the first trimester. Later in the pregnancy, low doses of medications may be given if necessary. Although the degree of excitement by the other parent, the pregnant parent's ability to provide help, and the client's financial situation may or may not be of concern, the priority in this situation is the safety of the fetus and the risks associated with the need for antipsychotic therapy.

CN: Reduction of risk potential; CL: Analyze

61. 1. A side effect of clozapine is leukopenia. A WBC count is drawn every week, and if it starts to drop, the HCP is notified. Slightly low hemoglobin levels or a normal sodium level is not significant. Hyaline casts occur because of protein in the urine, and a small amount is normally found in the urine, especially after exercise.

CN: Reduction of risk potential; CL: Analyze

62. 3. Many coordinated services are needed, including medication management, more frequent outpatient visits, day treatment, or some combination of these, to decrease the risk for relapse, which is common among chronically ill clients. Medical consultations (if needed) would be included in the coordinated services provided. Chronically mentally ill clients, who are discharged early before becoming truly stable, typically require more than monthly outpatient visits because of the high risk for relapse. A caring and supportive family is ideal for all clients but not always available.

CN: Management of care; CL: Analyze

63. 4. For a community-based program, the need for long-term hospitalization is least needed if the other services, such as partial hospitalization programs, psychiatric home care, and residential services, are available and accessible.

CN: Management of care; CL: Apply

64. 2, 3, 4. Although all of the situations require immediate attention, the inability to keep outpatient appointments is less critical than signs of relapse and decompensation, threat of eviction, unpaid bills, and lack of food. Occasionally missing a dose of medication usually will not precipitate a crisis for a client.

CN: Psychosocial integrity; CL: Analyze

65. 1. Providing ways to decrease or manage adverse effects without additional medications is crucial. Although home visits, family monitoring, and outpatient monitoring may help, if the adverse effects are not controlled, the client is less likely to take the drug, which would interfere with its effectiveness.

CN: Pharmacological and parenteral therapies; CL: Analyze

66. 4. Many still believe that recovery from mental illness is a matter of willpower—for example, "pull yourself up by your bootstraps" or "just get over it." This belief persists despite awareness that mental illness can be hereditary and has a biochemical basis. Mental illness can be prevented only if there is early intervention. Clients cannot prevent it just by the desire to do so.

CN: Psychosocial integrity; CL: Evaluate

The Client with Cognitive Disorders

67. 4. Delirium is commonly due to a medical condition such as a UTI in the older adult. Delirium often involves memory problems, disorientation, and hallucinations. It develops rather quickly. There are not enough data to suggest Alzheimer's disease, especially given the quick onset of symptoms. Delayed grieving and adjusting to being alone are unlikely to cause hallucinations.

CN: Reduction of risk potential; CL: Analyze

68. 3. Paradoxical responses to benzodiazepines are more common in children and older adults than in other age groups and generally occur at the beginning of treatment. Grief and depression in the older adult are more likely to result in fatigue and withdrawal than hyperactivity and agitation. Treatment with a sleeping medication chemically related to the benzodiazepines is likely to result in an increase rather than decrease in agitation symptoms in older adult clients. A medication interaction is possible, but it is less likely because most pharmacies screen for drug interactions when filling prescriptions.

CN: Pharmacological and parenteral therapies; CL: Analyze

69. 4. Expecting the social worker to make the decision indicates that the adult child is avoiding participating in decisions about the client. The other responses convey that the son understands the importance of a careful decision, the availability of resources, and the ability to make new plans if needed.

CN: Management of care; CL: Analyze

70. 1, 2, 5. Confused clients need fewer choices, acceptance as a person, and step-by-step directions. Allowing the client to do as they wish can lead to substandard care and the risk for harm. Acting nonchalantly conveys a lack of caring.

CN: Psychosocial integrity; CL: Analyze

Schizophrenia, Other Psychoses, and Cognitive Disorders 853

71. 3. Reminiscing can help reduce depression in an older adult client and lessen feelings of isolation and loneliness. Reminiscing encourages a focus on positive memories and accomplishments as well as shared memories with other clients. An increase in confusion and disorientation is most likely the result of other cognitive and situational factors, such as loss of short-term memory, not reminiscing. The client will not likely become sad because reminiscing helps the client connect with positive memories. Keeping the client from participating in therapeutic activities is less likely with reminiscing.

CN: Psychosocial integrity; CL: Evaluate

The Client with Delirium

72. 2. Loss of orientation, especially for time and place, is common in delirium. The nurse should orient the client by telling the client the time, date, place, and who the client is with. Taking the client to their room and telling them why the door is locked do not address their disorientation. Telling the client to eat before going to their medical appointment reinforces their disorientation.

CN: Psychosocial integrity; CL: Analyze

73. 1, 2, 3. The client does need rest, and it is true that there is no specific medicine for delirium, but it is crucial to identify and treat the underlying causes of delirium. Other tests will be based on the results of already completed tests. Although some medications may be prescribed to help the client with their behaviors, this is not the primary basis for medication prescriptions. Because the underlying medical causes of delirium could be fatal, treatment must be initiated as soon as possible. It is not the nurse's role to determine medications for this client. Postponing tests until the next day is inappropriate.

CN: Psychosocial integrity; CL: Apply

74. 1. Explaining why blood is being taken responds to the client's concerns or fears about what is happening. Threatening more pain or promising to explain later ignores or postpones meeting the client's need for information. The client's statements do not reflect a loss of self-control requiring medication intervention.

CN: Psychosocial integrity; CL: Analyze

75. 3. The client is showing symptoms of delirium, a common outcome of UTI in older adults. The nurse can request a transfer to a medical unit for acute medical intervention. The client's symptoms are not just due to a worsening of the depression. There are no indications that the client needs restraints or a transfer to a nursing home at this point.

CN: Management of care; CL: Apply

76. 3. Polypharmacy is much more common in the older adult. Drug interactions increase the incidence of intoxication from prescribed medications, especially with combinations of digoxin and analgesic, diuretic, and anticholinergic medications. With drug intoxication, the onset of delirium typically is quick. Although cancer, impaired hearing, and heart failure could lead to delirium in the older adult, the onset would be more gradual.

CN: Reduction of risk potential; CL: Analyze

77. 1. In addition to developing over a period of hours or days, fluctuating symptoms are characteristic of delirium. The failure to identify objects despite intact sensory functions, significant impairment in social or occupational functioning over time, and memory impairment to the degree of being called amnesia all indicate dementia.

CN: Physiological adaptation; CL: Analyze

78. 2. The most critical aspect of caring for a client with delirium is to institute measures to correct the underlying causative condition or illness. Controlling behavioral symptoms with low-dose psychotropics, manipulating the environment, and decreasing or discontinuing all medications may be dangerous to the client's health.

CN: Reduction of risk potential; CL: Apply

79. 3. In approximately 2 to 3 days, the client should be able to regain orientation and thus become oriented to time and place. Being able to explain the experience of having delirium is something that the client is expected to achieve later in the course of the illness, but ultimately before discharge. Resuming a normal sleep-wake cycle and establishing normal bowel and bladder function probably will take longer, depending on how long it takes to resolve the underlying condition.

CN: Psychosocial integrity; CL: Analyze

80. 1. Identifying oneself and making sure that the nurse has the client's attention address the difficulties with focusing, orientation, and maintaining attention. Eliminating daytime napping is unrealistic until the cause of the delirium is determined and the client's ability to focus and maintain attention improves. Engaging the client in reminiscing and avoiding arguing are also unrealistic at this time.

CN: Psychosocial integrity; CL: Apply

81. -/+ 1, 2, 4. The abnormal stimuli of the critical care unit can aggravate the symptoms of delirium. Arguing with hallucinations is inappropriate. When a client has illogical thinking, gently presenting reality is appropriate, but orienting the client to their condition is unlikely to be helpful. Dementia is not the likely cause of the client's symptoms. The client is experiencing delirium, not dementia.

 CN: Psychosocial integrity; CL: Analyze

The Client with Dementia

82. 3. That the client is not able to recall the three words is a likely indicator of dementia; the nurse should make a referral for further testing. It is recommended not to repeat the test a second time if the client is not able to recall the words. Although the client repeated rhyming words, echolalia refers to the repetition of the same word. It is not necessary to have a family member present when conducting the test, but the nurse should communicate the findings to the family and encourage them to seek follow-up assessment.

 CN: Reduction of risk potential; CL: Analyze

83. 1. Impulsive acts of aggression and violence have been linked to dysregulation of the amygdala. The hypothalamus regulates basic human activities such as sleep-rest patterns. The parietal lobe contains the primary somatosensory area. The temporal lobes contain the primary auditory areas.

 CN: Management of care; CL: Analyze

84. 3. Based on CAM's assessment tool, the client has an acute onset of behaviors, is inattentive, has disorganized thinking, and is lethargic (decreased level of consciousness). This cluster of behaviors constitutes delirium. Dementia has a slow onset, the client's level of consciousness is usually normal, and the client can focus attention. Clients who are depressed are alert and oriented and able to focus attention, though they may be easily distracted. Further assessment is needed to determine if the client also is dehydrated.

 CN: Reduction of risk potential; CL: Analyze

85. 2. Memantine and donepezil are commonly given together. Neither medicine will improve dementia, but they may slow the progression. Neither medicine is more effective than the other; they act differently in the brain. Both medicines have a half-life of 60 or more hours.

 CN: Pharmacological and parenteral therapies; CL: Apply

86. 2. Older adult clients with dementia have an increased risk for falls due to balance problems, medication use, and decreased eyesight. Haloperidol may cause extrapyramidal side effects, which increase the risk for falls. The client is not agitated, so restraints are not indicated. Lorazepam may increase fall risk and cause paradoxical excitement.

 CN: Reduction of risk potential; CL: Apply

87. 3. The tape and television are competing, even conflicting, stimuli. Crime events portrayed on television could be misperceived as a real threat to the client. A low number of clients and the presence of a few staff members quietly working are less intense stimuli for the client and not likely to be disturbing.

 CN: Management of care; CL: Analyze

88. -/+ 2, 3, 4. A set routine and brief exercises help decrease daytime sleeping. Decreasing caffeine and fluids and promoting relaxation at bedtime promote nighttime sleeping. A strong sleep medicine for an older adult client is contraindicated due to changes in metabolism, increased adverse effects, and the risk for falls. Using caffeinated beverages may stimulate metabolism but can also have long-lasting adverse effects and may prevent sleep at bedtime.

 CN: Management of care; CL: Apply

89. 2. Clients with chronic cognitive disorders experience defects in memory orientation and intellectual functions, such as judgment and discrimination. Loss of other abilities, such as speech, endurance, and balance, is less typical.

 CN: Psychosocial integrity; CL: Analyze

90. 1. Because of the client's short-term memory impairment, the nurse gently corrects the client by stating their name and who they are. This approach decreases anxiety, embarrassment, and shame and maintains the client's self-esteem. Telling the client that they know who the nurse is or that they forgot can elicit feelings of embarrassment and shame. Saying "I told you already" sounds condescending, as if blaming the client for not remembering.

 CN: Psychosocial integrity; CL: Analyze

91. 2. Vulgar language is common in clients with dementia when they are having trouble communicating about a topic. Ignoring the vulgarity and distracting them is appropriate. Telling the client they are rude or to stop swearing will have no lasting effect and may cause agitation. Just leaving the room is abandonment that the client will not understand.

 CN: Psychosocial integrity; CL: Apply

92. 2. Highly conditioned motor skills, such as brushing teeth, may be retained by the client who has dementia and motor apraxia. Balancing a checkbook involves calculations, a complex skill that is lost with severe dementia. Confabulation is fabrication of details to fill a memory gap. This is more common when the client is aware of a memory problem, not when dementia is severe. Finding keys is a memory factor, not a motor function.

CN: Psychosocial integrity; CL: Analyze

93. 3. Competing and excessive stimuli lead to sensory overload and confusion. Therefore, the nurse should first eliminate any distracting stimuli. After this is accomplished, using touch and rephrasing questions are appropriate. Going for a walk while talking has little benefit on attention and confusion.

CN: Psychosocial integrity; CL: Analyze

94. 4. Telling the client that they are wrong and then telling them what is right is argumentative and challenging. Arguing with or challenging distortions is least effective because it increases defensiveness. Telling the client about reality indicates an awareness of the issues and is appropriate. Acknowledging that misperceptions are part of the disease indicates an understanding of the disease and an awareness of the issues. Turning off the radio helps to limit environmental stimuli and indicates an awareness of the issues.

CN: Psychosocial integrity; CL: Evaluate

The Client with Alzheimer's Disease

95. 3. The best rationale for day treatment for the client with Alzheimer's disease is the enhancement of social interactions. More daily structure, excellent staff, and allowing caregivers more time for themselves are all positive aspects, but they are less focused on the client's needs.

CN: Psychosocial integrity; CL: Apply

96. 4. By fostering independence and providing as much time as possible, the nurse is helping the client continue to complete as many tasks as possible. Performing activities for the client is counterproductive. A list may cause the client to become frustrated if the list is not completed or if it becomes lost. Informing the client that the UAP will complete activities may be perceived as a threat.

CN: Basic care and comfort; CL: Apply

97. 2, 4, 5. Motion and sound detectors, a medical alert bracelet, and door alarms and locks are all appropriate interventions for wandering. Sleep medications do not prevent wandering before and after the client is asleep and may have negative effects. Having a relative sit with the client is usually an unrealistic burden.

CN: Psychosocial integrity; CL: Apply

98. 2. Because the client is experiencing difficulty processing and completing complex tasks, the priority is to provide the client with only one step at a time, thereby breaking the task up into simple steps, ones that the client can process. Repeating the directions until the client follows them or demonstrating how to do the task is still too overwhelming to the client because of the multiple steps involved. Although maintaining structure and routine is important, it is unrelated to task completion.

CN: Psychosocial integrity; CL: Analyze

99. 1. The vulgar or sexual behaviors are commonly expressions of anger or more sensual needs that can be addressed directly. Therefore, the families should be encouraged to ignore the behaviors but attempt to identify their purpose. Then the purpose can be addressed, possibly leading to a decrease in the behaviors. Because of impaired cognitive function, the client is not likely to be able to process the inappropriateness of the behaviors if given feedback. Likewise, anger management strategies would be ineffective because the client would probably be unable to process the inappropriateness of the behaviors. Risperidone may decrease agitation, but it does not improve social behaviors.

CN: Psychosocial integrity; CL: Apply

100. 4. The statement about expecting that the old parent would be back conveys a lack of acceptance of the irreversible nature of the disease. The statement about not realizing that the deterioration would be so incapacitating is based in reality. The statement about the Alzheimer's group is based in reality and demonstrates the family member's involvement with managing the disease. Stating that reminiscing is important reflects a realistic interpretation on the son's part.

CN: Psychosocial integrity; CL: Evaluate

101. 1. When compared with other similar medications, donepezil has fewer adverse effects. Donepezil is effective primarily in the early stages of the disease. The drug helps to slow the progression of the disease if started in the early stages. After the client has been diagnosed for 6 years, improvement to the level seen 6 years ago is highly unlikely. Data are not available to support the drug's effectiveness for clients in the terminal phase of the disease.

🔑 CN: Pharmacological and parenteral therapies; CL: Apply

102. 3. Antipsychotics are most effective with agitation and aggression. Antipsychotics have little effect on sleep disturbances, concomitant depression, or confusion and withdrawal.

🔑 CN: Pharmacological and parenteral therapies; CL: Apply

103. 1. Although all of the side effects listed are possible with lorazepam, paradoxical excitement is cause for immediate discontinuation of the medication. (Paradoxical excitement is the opposite reaction to lorazepam than is expected.) The other side effects tend to be minor and usually are transient.

🔑 CN: Pharmacology and parental therapies; CL: Apply

104. 4. Change increases stress. Therefore, the most important and relevant suggestion is to maintain consistency in the client's environment, routine, and caregivers. Although rest periods are important, going to bed interferes with the sleep-wake cycle. Rest in a recliner chair is more useful. Testing cognitive functioning and reality orientation are not likely to be successful and may increase stress if memory loss is severe.

🔑 CN: Psychosocial integrity; CL: Apply

Managing Care, Quality, and Safety of Clients with Schizophrenia, Other Psychoses, and Cognitive Disorders

105. 4. The neighbor could be harmed as well as the caregiver if they should try to stop the client from using the gun, so both should be notified. Any use of firearms against another person requires the involvement of the police. The nurse has a legal/ethical responsibility to warn potential victims and other involved parties as well as law enforcement authorities when one person makes a threat against another person. This duty supersedes confidentiality statutes. Failure to do so and to document it can result in civil penalties. The client's early dementia would likely not prevent them from carrying through the threat.

🔑 CN: Management of care; CL: Analyze

106. 4. Benztropine has a common side effect of blurred vision. After evaluating the relative doses of haloperidol and benztropine, the *assessment* would be that the higher dose of benztropine compared with the dose of haloperidol is responsible for the blurred vision. (High doses of haloperidol can cause blurred vision at times.) Reporting that the client has blurred vision is the *situation*. Listing the medications and doses is describing the *background*. The *recommendation* would be a lower dose of benztropine.

🔑 CN: Management of care; CL: Analyze

107. 2. Nurses are required to document that clients have been given information about their status and rights. Seclusion is not related to people becoming involuntary or certified clients. Including details contained within the certificates, such as an HCP signing the certificates, is not required.

🔑 CN: Management of care; CL: Apply

108. 4. The client exhibits aggression against a perceived adversary when they name another client as their adversary. The staff will need to watch the client carefully for signs of impending violent behavior that may injure others. Crying about a divorce would be appropriate, not pathologic, behavior demonstrating grief over a loss. A petition to delay bedtime would be a positive, direct action aimed at a bothersome situation. Although declining to attend group therapy needs follow-up, there may be any number of unknown reasons for this action.

🔑 CN: Safety and infection control; CL: Analyze

109. 2. When caring for a client with cognitive impairment, the priority is to ensure that all objects in the client's path are removed to prevent the client from falling. Additional measures, such as having two people accompany the client when they ambulate, placing their favorite things in safekeeping, and giving medications in a liquid form to be sure they swallow them, are less crucial.

🔑 CN: Safety and infection control; CL: Analyze

110. 1. The most common reason for the nurse's discomfort with older adult clients is that the nurse has not examined their own fears and conflicts about aging. Until nurses resolve their fears, it is unlikely that they will feel comfortable with older adult clients. A dislike of physical contact with older people, a desire to be surrounded by beauty and youth, and recent experiences with a parent's older adult friends are possible explanations, but not common or likely.

🔑 CN: Management of care; CL: Analyze

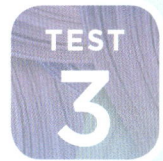

TEST 3: Personality Disorders, Substance-Related Disorders, Anxiety Disorders, and Anxiety-Related Disorders

- The Client with a Personality Disorder
- The Client with an Alcohol-Related Disorder
- The Client with Disorders Related to Other Addictive Substances
- The Client with Anxiety Disorders and Anxiety-Related Disorders
- The Client with a Somatoform Disorder
- Managing Care, Quality, and Safety of Clients with Personality Disorders, Substance-Related Disorders, Anxiety Disorders, and Anxiety-Related Disorders
- Answers, Rationales, and Test-Taking Strategies

The Client with a Personality Disorder

1. A client has been diagnosed with avoidant personality disorder. The client reports loneliness but has fears about making friends. The client also reports anxiety about being rejected by others. In a long-term treatment plan, in what order, from first to last, should the nurse list interventions for the client? All options must be used.

| 1. Teach the client anxiety management and social skills. |
| 2. Ask the client to join in a chosen activity with the nurse and two other clients. |
| 3. Talk with the client about self-esteem and fears. |
| 4. Help the client make a list of small group activities at the center that the client would find interesting. |
| |
| |
| |
| |

2. A client diagnosed with borderline personality disorder has self-inflicted cuts on the arms. The nurse is assessing the client for the risk of suicide. What should the nurse ask the client **first**?
- ☐ 1. about medications the client has taken recently
- ☐ 2. if the client is taking antidepressants
- ☐ 3. if the client has a suicide plan
- ☐ 4. why the client self-inflicted the cuts

3. The nurse develops the plan of care for a client diagnosed with a personality disorder. The nurse plans to assist the client **primarily** with what factor?
- ☐ 1. specific dysfunctional behaviors
- ☐ 2. psychopharmacologic compliance
- ☐ 3. examination of developmental conflicts
- ☐ 4. manipulation of the environment

4. A client diagnosed with paranoid personality disorder is hospitalized for physically threatening their spouse because they suspect the spouse of having an affair with a coworker. What approach should the nurse employ with this client?
- ☐ 1. authoritarian
- ☐ 2. parental
- ☐ 3. matter of fact
- ☐ 4. controlling

5. The nurse plans care for a client diagnosed with schizotypal personality disorder. Which intervention helps the client become involved with others?
- ☐ 1. participating solely in group activities
- ☐ 2. being involved with primarily one-to-one activities
- ☐ 3. leading a sing-along in the afternoon
- ☐ 4. attending an activity with the nurse

6. A client is reporting to other clients about not being allowed by staff to keep food in their room. What action should the nurse take?
   ☐ 1. Ignore the client's behavior.
   ☐ 2. Set limits on the behavior.
   ☐ 3. Reprimand the client.
   ☐ 4. Allow snacks to be kept in the client's room.

7. A client with a diagnosis of antisocial personality disorder has a potential for violence and aggressive behavior. Which short-term client outcome is **most** appropriate for the nurse to include in the plan of care?
   ☐ 1. Use humor when expressing anger.
   ☐ 2. Discuss feelings of anger with staff.
   ☐ 3. Ask the nurse for medication when upset.
   ☐ 4. Use indirect behaviors to express anger.

8. A new client on the psychiatric unit has been diagnosed with depression and obsessive-compulsive personality disorder (OCPD). During visiting hours, the client's spouse states to the nurse that they do not understand this OCPD and what can be done about it. What information should the nurse share with the client and their spouse? Select all that apply.
   ☐ 1. "Perfectionism and overemphasis on tasks usually interfere with friendships and leisure time."
   ☐ 2. "It will help to interrupt the client with tasks and tell them you are going out for the evening."
   ☐ 3. "There are medicines, such as clomipramine or fluoxetine, that may help."
   ☐ 4. "Remind your spouse that it is "OK" to be human and make mistakes."
   ☐ 5. "Reinforce with the client that they are not allowed to expect the whole family to be perfect too."
   ☐ 6. "This disorder typically involves inflexibility and a need to be in control."

9. A young client with a diagnosis of major depression and dependent personality disorder has been living at home with very supportive parents. The client is thinking about independent living on the recommendation of the treatment team. The client states to the nurse, "I don't know if I can make it in an apartment without my parents." How should the nurse respond to the client?
   ☐ 1. "You're an adult now, so you should rely on the health care team for help."
   ☐ 2. "Your parents will not be around forever. After all, they're getting older."
   ☐ 3. "Your parents need a break, and you need a break from them."
   ☐ 4. "Your parents have been supportive and will continue to be even if you live apart."

10. A client moves in with their family after their roommate of 4 weeks told the client to leave. The client is admitted to the subacute unit after reporting feeling empty and lonely, being unable to sleep, and eating very little for the last week. The client's arms are scarred from frequent self-mutilation. What should the nurse do in order of priority from first to last? All options must be used.

    | 1. Monitor for suicide and self-mutilation. |
    | 2. Discuss the issues of loneliness and emptiness. |
    | 3. Monitor sleeping and eating behaviors. |
    | 4. Discuss options for housing after discharge. |
    | |
    | |
    | |
    | |

11. A client approaches various staff with numerous requests and needs to the point of disrupting the staff's work with other clients. The nurse meets with the staff to decide on a consistent, therapeutic approach for this client. Which approach will be **most** effective?
    ☐ 1. telling the client to stay in the client's room until staff approach
    ☐ 2. limiting the client to the dayroom and dining area
    ☐ 3. giving the client a list of permissible requests
    ☐ 4. having the client discuss needs with the staff person assigned

12. A client with diagnosed borderline personality disorder tells the nurse, "You're the best nurse here. I can talk to you and you listen. You're the only one here that can help me." Which response by the nurse is **most** therapeutic?
    ☐ 1. "Thank you; you're a good person."
    ☐ 2. "All of the nurses here provide good care."
    ☐ 3. "Other clients have told me that too."
    ☐ 4. "Mary and Sam are good nurses too."

13. The nurse assesses a client to be at risk for self-mutilation and implements a safety contract with the client. Which client behavior(s) would indicate that the contract is working? Select all that apply. The client:
    ☐ 1. withdraws to the client's room when feeling overwhelmed.
    ☐ 2. notifies staff when anxiety is increasing.
    ☐ 3. suppresses feelings when angry.
    ☐ 4. displaces feelings onto the health care provider (HCP).
    ☐ 5. identifies the triggers that have led to self-mutilation in the past.

14. A client diagnosed with borderline personality disorder who is to be discharged soon threatens to "do something" to themself if discharged. What action should the nurse take **first**?
☐ 1. Request that the client's discharge be canceled.
☐ 2. Ignore the client's statement because it is a sign of manipulation.
☐ 3. Ask a family member to stay with the client at home temporarily.
☐ 4. Discuss the meaning of the client's statement with them.

15. A young adult client is admitted to a psychiatric unit with a diagnosis of alcohol use disorder and personality disorder. The client's parent states, "They're always in trouble, just like when they were little. Now they're just a bigger prankster and out of control." In view of the client's history, which intervention is **most** important initially?
☐ 1. letting the client know the staff has the authority to subdue them if they get unruly
☐ 2. keeping the client isolated from other clients until they are better known by the staff
☐ 3. emphasizing to the client that they will have to pay for any damage they cause
☐ 4. closely observing the client's behavior to establish a baseline pattern of functioning

16. A client tells the nurse at the outpatient clinic that they do not need to attend groups because they are "not a regular like these other people here." How should the nurse respond to the client?
☐ 1. "Because you're not a regular client, sit in the hall when the others are in group."
☐ 2. "Your family wants you to attend, and they'll be very disappointed if you don't."
☐ 3. "I'll have to mark you absent from the clinic today and speak to the health care provider about it."
☐ 4. "You say you're not a regular here, but you're experiencing what others are experiencing."

17. A client who has a history of angry outbursts when frustrated begins to curse at the nurse during an appointment after being informed that they will have to wait to have their medication refilled. Which response by the nurse is **most** appropriate?
☐ 1. "You are upsetting the other clients."
☐ 2. "I'm sorry if you can't wait."
☐ 3. "I won't continue to talk with you if you curse."
☐ 4. "Come back tomorrow, and your medication will be ready."

18. Which behavior indicates to the nurse that a client diagnosed with avoidant personality disorder is improving?
☐ 1. interacting with two other clients
☐ 2. listening to music with headphones
☐ 3. sitting at a table and painting
☐ 4. talking on the telephone

19. One evening, a client takes the nurse aside and whispers, "Don't tell anybody, but I'm going to call in a bomb threat to this hospital tonight." Which action is the **priority**?
☐ 1. warning the client that their telephone privileges will be taken away if they abuse them
☐ 2. assessing the details of the client's plan to determine if the threat is real.
☐ 3. notifying the proper authorities after saying nothing until the client has actually completed the call
☐ 4. explaining to the client that this information will have to be shared immediately with the staff and the health care provider (HCP)

20. The nurse orients an unlicensed assistive personnel (UAP) new to the mental health unit about the principles for the care of a client diagnosed with a personality disorder. What information should the nurse include?
☐ 1. The clients are accepted, though their behavior may not be.
☐ 2. The clients need limits on their behavior.
☐ 3. The staff members are the primary ones left to care about these clients.
☐ 4. The staff should use minimal humor when working with these clients.

21. The nurse is talking with a client who has been diagnosed with antisocial personality disorder about how to socialize during activities without being seductive. The nurse should focus the discussion on which area?
☐ 1. explaining the negative reactions of others toward their behavior
☐ 2. suggesting they apologize to others for their behavior
☐ 3. asking them to explain the reasons for their seductive behavior
☐ 4. discussing the client's relationship with their parent

22. The nurse cares for a client with narcissistic personality disorder. Which approach is **most** appropriate to use when discrepancies exist between what the client states and what actually exists?
☐ 1. limit setting
☐ 2. supportive confrontation
☐ 3. consistency
☐ 4. rationalization

23. A client with histrionic personality disorder is melodramatic and responds to others and situations in an exaggerated manner. The nurse should recommend which activity for this client?
☐ 1. party planning
☐ 2. music group
☐ 3. cooking class
☐ 4. role-playing

The Client with an Alcohol-Related Disorder

24. A client has been diagnosed with dementia related to chronic and heavy alcohol consumption. In a family meeting with the client, discharge plans are being discussed. Which point(s) should the nurse share with the family and client? Select all that apply.
☐ 1. Even after all alcohol has been removed from the home, clients frequently find ways to get more.
☐ 2. Without continued alcohol intake, the client will gradually get better.
☐ 3. With the memory loss, answer the client's question once, and then ignore that question when asked again.
☐ 4. Safety alarms on the doors will help keep the client from wandering off.
☐ 5. As the need for supervision increases, it may be necessary for the client to be placed in an extended care facility.

25. In an outpatient addiction group, a recovering client said that before treatment, their spouse drank on social occasions. "Now they drink at home, from the time they come home from work and to until they go to bed. They say that they don't like me anymore and that I expect them to do more work on the house and yard. I used to ignore that stuff. I don't know what to do." In which order of priority from first to last would the nurse make the comments? All options must be used.

1. "What do you think you could do to have your spouse come in for an evaluation?"
2. "I hear how confused and frustrated you are."
3. "It can happen that as one person sobers up, the spouse deteriorates."
4. "What have you tried to do about your spouse's behaviors?"

26. A client is having difficulty falling asleep at night because of withdrawal symptoms from alcohol, which are abating. Which nursing intervention is likely to be **most** effective?
☐ 1. inviting the client to play a board game with the nurse
☐ 2. allowing the client to sit in the community room until the client feels sleepy
☐ 3. advising the client to take multiple short naps during the day until symptoms improve
☐ 4. teaching the client relaxation exercises to use before bedtime

27. The nurse assesses a client experiencing alcohol withdrawal. Which symptom(s) would indicate that a client has alcohol withdrawal delirium? Select all that apply.
☐ 1. tachycardia
☐ 2. tachypnea
☐ 3. dry, flushed skin
☐ 4. thirst
☐ 5. hypertension
☐ 6. abdominal cramping

28. A client has been admitted to the emergency department with alcohol withdrawal delirium.

Progress Note				
Vital Signs	10/24 2100	10/25 0100	10/25 0500	10/25 0900
	Temperature (T) 99°F (37.2°C) Pulse (P) 110 bpm Respiration rate (RR) 18 breaths/min Blood pressure (BP) 140/90 mm Hg Arterial oxygen saturation (SaO₂) 97	T 99.2°F (37.3°C) P 90 bpm RR 14 breaths/min BP 130/80 mm Hg SaO₂ 98	T 99°F (37.2°C) P 70 bpm RR 14 breaths/min BP 126/80 mm Hg SaO₂ 97	T 99°F (37.2°C) P 50 bpm RR 10 breaths/min BP 100/60 mm Hg SaO₂ 95
Nurse's Notes				
10/24 2100	An IV of dextrose 5% in water was started at 60 mL/h in the left hand. Diazepam was administered. Oriented to person, place, and time.			
10/25 0100	The client is resting quietly.			
10/25 0500	The client is oriented to person, place, and time.			
10/25 0900	The client is confused.			

The nurse compares these findings with the nurse's progress notes from admission 24 hours ago. What action should the nurse take **first**?
☐ Contact the health care provider (HCP).
☐ Increase the rate of the IV infusion.
☐ Attempt to arouse the client.
☐ Administer magnesium sulfate.

29. An intoxicated client is admitted to the hospital for alcohol withdrawal. What should the nurse do to help the client become sober?
☐ 1. Give the client black coffee to drink.
☐ 2. Walk the client around the unit.
☐ 3. Have the client take a cold shower.
☐ 4. Provide the client with a quiet room to sleep in.

30. A client is admitted to the hospital for alcohol detoxification. Which intervention(s) should the nurse use? Select all that apply.
☐ 1. taking vital signs
☐ 2. monitoring intake and output
☐ 3. placing the client in restraints as a safety measure
☐ 4. reinforcing reality if the client is disoriented or hallucinating
☐ 5. explaining to the client that the symptoms of withdrawal are temporary

31. The nurse is assessing a client who has fallen twice in the last 2 days. The client has been diagnosed with delirium tremens (DTs) following withdrawal from alcohol use. The nurse should further evaluate the client for which complication(s)? Select all that apply.
☐ 1. disorientation
☐ 2. paralysis
☐ 3. elevated temperature
☐ 4. diaphoresis
☐ 5. visual or auditory hallucinations

32. A client was discharged from an alcohol rehabilitation program on clonazepam 0.5 mg three times a day. Several months later, the client reports having insomnia, shakiness, sweating, and one seizure. The nurse should **first** assess the client for which possible symptoms cause?
☐ 1. drinking alcohol with the clonazepam
☐ 2. developing tolerance to the clonazepam
☐ 3. stopping the clonazepam suddenly
☐ 4. increasing the clonazepam dose independently

33. A client is entering the chemical dependency unit for treatment of alcohol dependency and treatment with disulfiram. Which possession(s) belonging to the client should the nurse remove from the area? Select all that apply.
☐ 1. toothpaste
☐ 2. aftershave
☐ 3. dental floss
☐ 4. shaving cream
☐ 5. antiseptic mouthwash
☐ 6. facial astringents

34. A client is entering rehabilitation for alcohol dependency as an alternative to going to jail for multiple arrests for driving under the influence. While obtaining the client's history, the nurse asks about the amount of alcohol the client consumes daily. The client responds, "I just have a few drinks with my friends after work." Which response by the nurse is **most** therapeutic?
☐ 1. "That's what all the clients here say at first."
☐ 2. "Then you should have had a designated driver for yourself."
☐ 3. "I guess you just can't handle a few drinks."
☐ 4. "You say you have a few drinks, but you have multiple arrests."

35. While admitting a client to the alcohol treatment program, the nurse asks the client how long they have been drinking, how much they have been drinking, and when they had their last drink. The client replies that they have been drinking about a liter of vodka a day for the past week and their last drink was about an hour ago. This information helps the nurse to determine which factor?
☐ 1. severity of the disease
☐ 2. severity of withdrawal symptoms
☐ 3. possibility of alcoholic hallucinosis
☐ 4. occurrence of delirium tremens

36. A client who is experiencing alcohol withdrawal exhibits tremors, diaphoresis, and hyperactivity. Blood pressure is 190/87 mm Hg, and pulse is 92 bpm. Which medication should the nurse expect to administer?
☐ 1. haloperidol
☐ 2. lorazepam
☐ 3. benztropine
☐ 4. naloxone

37. The health care provider prescribes a medication to help treat alcohol withdrawal in a client. Which assessment provides the **best** information about the client's physiologic response and the effectiveness of the medication?
☐ 1. nutritional status
☐ 2. evidence of tremors
☐ 3. vital signs
☐ 4. sleep pattern

38. A client who had been drinking heavily over the weekend could not remember specific events of where the client had been or what the client had done. The nurse interprets this information as indicating that the client experienced which condition?
☐ 1. blackout
☐ 2. hangover
☐ 3. tolerance
☐ 4. delirium tremens

39. A client is entering the alcohol treatment program for the fourth time in 5 years. Which statement by the nurse will be **most** helpful to the client?
- ☐ 1. "I hope you're serious about maintaining your sobriety this time."
- ☐ 2. "I don't know you from past attempts, but you'll get it right this time."
- ☐ 3. "I know someone who was successful after the fifth program."
- ☐ 4. "I'm a nurse in the program. The staff and I will help you through the program."

40. The spouse of a client with alcohol dependency tells the nurse, "I'm tired of making excuses to their boss and coworkers when they can't make it into work. I believe them every time they say they're going to quit." The nurse recognizes the spouse's statement as indicating which behavior?
- ☐ 1. helpfulness
- ☐ 2. self-defeat
- ☐ 3. enabling
- ☐ 4. masochism

41. The nurse is participating in a group confrontation with a coworker. Which statement is **most** helpful in reducing the coworker's denial about alcohol being a problem?
- ☐ 1. "Your behavior is unprofessional."
- ☐ 2. "As a nurse, you should have sought help earlier."
- ☐ 3. "Nurses are the worst when it comes to asking for help."
- ☐ 4. "You have alcohol on your breath."

42. A nurse working in an alcohol rehabilitation program is teaching staff how to give clients constructive feedback. Which statement given as an example illustrates that the staff member understands the nurse's teaching regarding the use of constructive feedback?
- ☐ 1. "I think you're a real con artist."
- ☐ 2. "You're dominating the conversation."
- ☐ 3. "You interrupted twice in 4 minutes."
- ☐ 4. "You don't give anyone a chance to finish talking."

43. A client ashamedly tells the nurse that they hit their spouse while intoxicated and asks the nurse if the spouse will ever forgive them. What is the nurse's **most** appropriate response?
- ☐ 1. "Perhaps you could ask your spouse and find out."
- ☐ 2. "That is something you can explore in family therapy."
- ☐ 3. "It would depend on how much they really care for you."
- ☐ 4. "You seem to have some feelings about hitting your spouse."

44. A client is admitted to the emergency department with an elevated blood alcohol level. The authorities state the client was driving on the wrong side of the road. The client is transferred to the acute care unit where they awaken the next morning. Vital signs are stable, and the client has a headache. What action should the nurse take **first** when caring for this client?
- ☐ 1. Work through personal feelings related to substance use disorder.
- ☐ 2. Be persistent with the client regarding the substance use disorder.
- ☐ 3. Help to make abstinence and sobriety worthwhile for the client.
- ☐ 4. Suggest a treatment program within the client's home area.

45. The nurse cares for a client experiencing severe symptoms of alcohol withdrawal. Which nursing action is contraindicated?
- ☐ 1. helping the client walk
- ☐ 2. monitoring intake and output
- ☐ 3. assessing vital signs
- ☐ 4. using short, concrete statements

46. The nurse performs medication teaching for a client prescribed disulfiram. Which client statement indicates to the nurse that the client needs further teaching about disulfiram?
- ☐ 1. "I can drink one or two beers and not get sick while on disulfiram."
- ☐ 2. "I can take disulfiram at bedtime if it makes me sleepy."
- ☐ 3. "A metallic or garlic taste in my mouth is normal when starting on disulfiram."
- ☐ 4. "I'll read the labels on cough syrup and mouthwash for possible alcohol content."

47. While receiving disulfiram therapy, a client becomes nauseated and vomits severely. Which question should the nurse ask **first**?
- ☐ 1. "How long have you been taking disulfiram?"
- ☐ 2. "Do you feel like you have the flu?"
- ☐ 3. "How much alcohol did you drink today?"
- ☐ 4. "Have you eaten any foods cooked in wine?"

48. A client being treated for alcohol addiction is receiving thiamine. What is the expected outcome for using thiamine with this client?
- ☐ 1. Prevent the development of Wernicke encephalopathy.
- ☐ 2. Decrease the client's withdrawal symptoms.
- ☐ 3. Aid the client in regaining strength sooner.
- ☐ 4. Promote the elimination of alcohol from the body faster.

49. The nurse teaches a client about preventing alcohol relapse. Which client statement indicates an understanding of the risk of alcohol relapse?
☐ 1. "I know I can stay dry if my spouse keeps alcohol out of the house."
☐ 2. "Stopping support groups and not expressing feelings can lead to relapse."
☐ 3. "I'll have my support group sponsor keep the list of symptoms for me."
☐ 4. "If someone tells me I'm about to relapse, I'll be sure to do something about it."

50. A client sees no connection between their liver disorder and their alcohol intake. The client believes that they drink very little and that their family is making something out of nothing. The nurse interprets these behaviors as indicative of the client's use of which defense mechanisms?
☐ 1. denial
☐ 2. displacement
☐ 3. rationalization
☐ 4. reaction formation

51. The nurse plans care for a client experiencing alcohol withdrawal. Which food should the nurse eliminate from the client's diet?
☐ 1. milk
☐ 2. regular coffee
☐ 3. orange juice
☐ 4. eggs

52. A client with alcohol dependency has peripheral neuropathy. The nurse should develop a teaching plan that emphasizes which action?
☐ 1. washing and drying the feet daily
☐ 2. massaging the feet with lotion
☐ 3. trimming the toenails carefully
☐ 4. avoiding use of an electric blanket

53. A client experiencing alcohol withdrawal wakes up and screams, "There is something crawling under my skin! Help me!" What should the nurse do in order of priority from first to last? All options must be used.

1. Remind the client that this is a withdrawal symptom and that these symptoms will be treated.
2. Administer a dose of lorazepam depending on the severity of the withdrawal symptoms.
3. Assess the client for other withdrawal symptoms.
4. Take the client's vital signs.

54. The nurse cares for a client with alcohol withdrawal delirium. Which measure should the nurse include in the plan of care?
☐ 1. using restraints continuously
☐ 2. touching the client before saying anything
☐ 3. remaining with the client when the client is confused or disoriented
☐ 4. informing the client about alcohol treatment programs

55. A client is to be discharged from an alcohol rehabilitation program. What should the nurse emphasize in the discharge plan as a **priority**?
☐ 1. supportive friends
☐ 2. a list of goals
☐ 3. returning to work
☐ 4. follow-up care

56. A client is to be discharged from the hospital after a safe, medically supervised withdrawal from alcohol. Which outcome(s) would indicate client readiness for an outpatient alcohol treatment program? Select all that apply.
The client:
☐ 1. states the need to cut down on alcohol intake.
☐ 2. verbalizes the damaging effects of alcohol on the body.
☐ 3. plans to attend support group meetings.
☐ 4. takes naltrexone daily.
☐ 5. expresses a desire to get back to a normal routine.

57. A client diagnosed with major depression and substance use disorder is being admitted to the concurrent disorder treatment unit. In explaining the focus of this program, the nurse should tell what information to the client?
☐ 1. The addiction will be treated first, then the depression.
☐ 2. The depression will be treated first, then the addiction.
☐ 3. There will be simultaneous treatment of the addiction and depression.
☐ 4. As the addiction is treated, the depression will clear up on its own.

58. The nurse cares for a client who has bipolar disorder and alcohol use disorder. Which area is the **priority** for daily assessment?
☐ 1. sleep pattern
☐ 2. mental status
☐ 3. eating habits
☐ 4. self-care ability

59. The nurse cares for a client admitted to the emergency department after being found lying on the bathroom floor with several empty pill bottles around them. While waiting for a psychiatric consult, the nurse discovers that the client's partner has recently broken up with them. Which response is **most** likely to build and maintain a therapeutic relationship within the emergency department?
☐ 1. "I know what it is like to go through a bad breakup."
☐ 2. "I know that this hurts."
☐ 3. "Why did you try to kill yourself?"
☐ 4. "What can I do to help while you are here?"

The Client with Disorders Related to Other Addictive Substances

60. A client is admitted to the hospital following an inadvertent overdose of oxycodone. The client reveals that they have chronic back pain that resulted from an injury on a construction site. The client states, "I know I took too much oxycodone at once, but I can't live with this pain without them. You can't take them away from me." Which response by the nurse is **most** appropriate?
☐ 1. "Once you're tapered off the oxycodone, you will find that nonaddictive pain medicines will be enough to control your pain."
☐ 2. "You're going to be switched from the oxycodone to methadone for long-term pain management."
☐ 3. "The oxycodone will be stopped tomorrow, but you'll have lorazepam to help you with the withdrawal symptoms."
☐ 4. "Your pain will be controlled by tapering doses of oxycodone and with other pain management strategies and medicines."

61. A school nurse is planning a program for parents on "Drugs Commonly Abused by Teenagers." Which information should be included about inhalants? Select all that apply.
☐ 1. Monitor for paper bags and rags that may have been used for breathing inhalants.
☐ 2. Brain damage is unlikely with the use of inhalants.
☐ 3. Use of inhalants by teens is on the decline.
☐ 4. Deaths from inhalants occur from asphyxiation, suffocation, and aspiration of vomit.
☐ 5. Inhalants usually cause depression of the central nervous system.
☐ 6. The basic groups of inhalants are hydrocarbon solvents such as glue, aerosol propellants from spray cans, and anesthetics and gases.

62. A client is brought to the emergency department by a friend who states, "They were using a lot of heroin until they ran out of money about 2 days ago." The nurse judges the client to be in opioid withdrawal if they exhibit which sign(s) or symptom(s)? Select all that apply.
☐ 1. rhinorrhea
☐ 2. diaphoresis
☐ 3. piloerection
☐ 4. synesthesia
☐ 5. formication

63. The nurse assesses a client with a history of heroin use. Which finding should the nurse expect to assess for a client who is exhibiting late signs of heroin withdrawal?
☐ 1. vomiting and diarrhea
☐ 2. yawning and diaphoresis
☐ 3. lacrimation and rhinorrhea
☐ 4. restlessness and irritability

64. The nurse teaches a client about methadone therapy for opioid addiction. The nurse should instruct the client that methadone is useful primarily for what reason?
☐ 1. It is not an addictive substance.
☐ 2. A maintenance dose is taken twice a day.
☐ 3. The client will no longer be addicted to opioids.
☐ 4. The client may work and live normally.

65. A client recovering from narcotic addiction states to the nurse, "I'm not going anymore to support group meetings. I felt out of place there." Which response by the nurse is **best**?
☐ 1. "Try attending a meeting at a different location; you may feel more comfortable there."
☐ 2. "Maybe it just wasn't a good day for you. Everybody has bad days now and then."
☐ 3. "Perhaps you weren't paying close enough attention to what they were saying."
☐ 4. "Sometimes the meetings can seem like a waste of time, but you need to attend to stay clean."

66. A client is recovering from narcotic addiction. Which outcome should the nurse use as the **best** measure to determine a client's progress in rehabilitation?
☐ 1. the kinds of friends the client makes
☐ 2. the number of drug-free days the client has
☐ 3. the way the client gets along with their parents
☐ 4. the amount of responsibility the client's job entails

67. The nurse assesses a client with a history of substance use disorder. Which finding would lead the nurse to suspect that a client is addicted to heroin?
☐ 1. hilarity
☐ 2. aggression
☐ 3. labile mood
☐ 4. hypoactivity

68. A client brought by ambulance to the emergency department after taking an overdose of barbiturates is comatose. The nurse should assess the client for which complication?
☐ 1. kidney failure
☐ 2. cerebrovascular accident
☐ 3. status epilepticus
☐ 4. respiratory failure

69. A client's spouse reports that the client has been taking about 800 mg of secobarbital daily, besides drinking more alcohol than usual. The spouse asks anxiously, "Do you think they will live?" Which response by the nurse is **most** appropriate?
☐ 1. "We can only wait and see. It's too soon to tell."
☐ 2. "This must be quite a shock. How long have you been married?"
☐ 3. "The client is very ill and may not live. Some do not pull through."
☐ 4. "The client's condition is serious. You sound very worried about them."

70. Before hospitalization, a client needed increasingly larger doses of barbiturates to achieve the same euphoric effect the client initially realized from their use. From this information, the nurse develops a plan of care that considers that the client is likely experiencing what problem?
☐ 1. drug tolerance
☐ 2. drug addiction
☐ 3. substance abuse
☐ 4. drug dependence

71. A client with a barbiturate overdose awakens in a confused state and exhibits stable vital signs. Which statement by the nurse is **most** appropriate?
☐ 1. "I'm here to help you beat your drug habit. But it's you who will need to work hard."
☐ 2. "It's time to get straight and stay clean and put an end to your torture."
☐ 3. "I'm glad you pulled through; it was touch and go with you for a while."
☐ 4. "You're in the hospital because of a drug problem; I'm one of the nurses who will help you."

72. A client states that their "life has gone down the tubes" since their divorce 6 months ago. Then, after they lost their job and apartment, they took an overdose of barbiturates so they "could go to sleep and never wake up." Which statement by the nurse should be made **first**?
☐ 1. "It seems as if your self-esteem has been affected by all your losses."
☐ 2. "I know you took an overdose of barbiturates. Are you thinking of suicide now?"
☐ 3. "Helplessness is common after losing a job. Are you having trouble making decisions?"
☐ 4. "You sound hopeless about the future since your divorce."

73. A client who has experienced the loss of their spouse through divorce, the loss of their job and apartment, and the development of drug dependency is experiencing situational low self-esteem. Which outcome is **most** appropriate initially?
The client will:
☐ 1. discuss their feelings related to their losses.
☐ 2. identify two positive qualities.
☐ 3. explore their strengths.
☐ 4. prioritize problems.

74. The nurse notices that a client recovering from a barbiturate overdose spends most of their time with other young adults who have substance-related problems. This group of clients is a dominant force on the unit, keeping the nondrug users entertained with stories of their "highs." Which method is **best** to use when dealing with this problem?
☐ 1. providing additional recreation
☐ 2. breaking up drug-oriented discussions
☐ 3. speaking with the clients individually about their behavior
☐ 4. discussing the behavior at the daily community meeting

75. A client recovering from a drug overdose is interacting with the nurse and recounting their exploits at numerous parties they attended. Which action is **most** therapeutic?
☐ 1. allowing the client to continue with their stories
☐ 2. telling the client you have heard the stories before
☐ 3. questioning the client further about their exploits
☐ 4. directing the conversation to realistic concerns

76.

The nurse cares for a 92-year-old female client who was admitted to the medical-surgical unit from home with a urinary tract infection.

Admission Note

The client is accompanied by their caregiver who found the client this morning disoriented, lying in a pool of urine, and unable to get out of bed. Before today, the client's caregiver reports that the client was living independently, though their memory was starting to fade, and that the client cries frequently since their spouse died 6 months ago. The client is incontinent of urine and oriented to person only. The client answers questions only by saying yes or no indiscriminately. The client is very agitated and appears to be swatting at objects in the air. Vital signs are temperature 102.2°F (39°C); pulse 100 bpm; respiration rate 20 breaths/min; blood pressure 92/60 mm Hg; and oxygen saturation 98% on room air.

The nurse reviews the client's admission data to begin the plan of care.

➢ Complete the diagram by specifying what condition the client is most likely experiencing, two actions the nurse should take to address that condition, and two parameters the nurse should monitor to assess the client's progress.

Action to Take — Condition Most Likely Experiencing — Parameter to Monitor
Action to Take — Parameter to Monitor

Action to Take	Potential Conditions	Parameters to Monitor
Administer antibiotics	Delirium	Short-term memory
Administer antidepressants	Dementia	Agitation
Administer lithium	Depression	Self-concept
Administer benzodiazepines	Psychosis	Orientation
Administer antipsychotics		Mood

77. A young client is being admitted to the psychiatric unit after their obstetrician's staff suspected they were experiencing postpartum psychosis. The client's spouse said they were doing fine for 2 weeks after the birth of the baby, except for pain from a cesarean birth and trouble sleeping. These symptoms subsided over the next 4 weeks. Three days ago, however, the client started having anxiety, irritability, vomiting, diarrhea, and delirium, resulting in their inability to care for the baby. The spouse says, "I saw that my bottles of alprazolam and oxycodone were empty even though I have not been taking them." What action should the nurse take **first**?
- ☐ 1. Call the health care provider for prescriptions for appropriate treatment for opiate and benzodiazepine withdrawal.
- ☐ 2. Immediately place the client on withdrawal precautions.
- ☐ 3. Confirm with the client that they have in fact been using their spouse's medications.
- ☐ 4. Assess the client for prior and current use of any other substances.

78. A 68-year-old client is admitted to the addiction unit after treatment in the emergency department for an overdose of oxycodone. The client's adult child calls the unit and expresses intense anger that their parent is being treated as a "common street addict." The child says the client has severe back pain and was given that prescription by their health care provider. "My parent just accidentally took a few too many pills last night." Which reply by the nurse is **most** therapeutic?
- ☐ 1. "I understand that your parent may not have intentionally taken too many pills. This medication can cause one to forget how many have been taken."
- ☐ 2. "It may be appropriate for your parent to be referred to a pain management program."
- ☐ 3. "Unfortunately, it's fairly common for clients with pain to increase their use of pain pills over time."
- ☐ 4. "I can hear how upset you are. You sound very concerned about your parent."

79. A client is admitted to the addiction unit for a confirmed and long-term addiction to alprazolam. The client continues to strongly deny their addiction, stating they were prescribed the alprazolam to control their "panic attacks." Which procedure(s) would be the **most** important during the admission process? Select all that apply.
☐ 1. Assess the client for suicide, escape, and aggression risks.
☐ 2. Perform a search for contraband and restricted items.
☐ 3. Initiate withdrawal precautions.
☐ 4. Explain the unit routine and types of groups.
☐ 5. Obtain a urine specimen for a urine drug screen.

80.

The nurse cares for a 24-year-old female client in the emergency department with a suspected overdose.

Nurse's Notes

2200:
The client was brought to the emergency department by a friend who became worried about their behavior at a party. The friend reports that the client became very talkative and stated that the client had been talking with aliens. The friend did not know what the client might have taken. The client's pupils are dilated, and they appear diaphoretic and agitated. Vital signs are temperature 100.9°F (38.3°C); pulse 108 bpm; respiration rate 22 breaths/min; blood pressure 150/104 mm Hg; and oxygen saturation 96% on room air. IV access is obtained.

➤ Complete the diagram by specifying what condition the client is most likely experiencing, two actions the nurse should take to address that condition, and two parameters the nurse should monitor to assess the client's progress.

Action to Take — Condition Most Likely Experiencing — Parameter to Monitor
Action to Take — Parameter to Monitor

Action to Take	Potential Conditions	Parameters to Monitor
Administer naloxone	Alcohol overdose	Blood alcohol levels
Give fluid bolus	Inhalant overdose	Urine output
Perform gastric lavage	Opioid overdose	Neuro-checks
Administer lorazepam	Stimulant overdose	Vital signs
Implement seizure precautions		Serum electrolytes

81. A client walks into the clinic and tells the nurse they have run out of money for crack and have crashed and they want something to help them feel better. Which factor is **most** important for the nurse to assess?
☐ 1. suspiciousness
☐ 2. loss of appetite
☐ 3. drug craving
☐ 4. suicidal ideation

82. A client is fidgeting and has trouble sitting still. They have difficulty concentrating and are erratic. Which intervention(s) should help decrease this client's level of anxiety? Select all that apply.
☐ 1. refocusing attention
☐ 2. allowing ventilation
☐ 3. suggesting a time-out
☐ 4. giving intramuscular medication
☐ 5. assisting with problem-solving

83. The nurse cares for a client who has overdosed on phencyclidine (PCP). The nurse should be especially cautious about which client behavior?
☐ 1. visual hallucinations
☐ 2. violent behavior
☐ 3. bizarre behavior
☐ 4. loud screaming

84. The nurse cares for a client who is intoxicated on phencyclidine (PCP). Which liquid should the nurse administer to hasten excretion of the chemical?
☐ 1. water
☐ 2. milk
☐ 3. cranberry juice
☐ 4. grape juice

85. The nurse assesses a client with possible alcohol poisoning. The nurse should investigate the client's use of which substance while drinking alcohol?
☐ 1. marijuana
☐ 2. lysergic acid diethylamide
☐ 3. peyote
☐ 4. psilocybin

86. A client with a cocaine dependency is irritable, anxious, highly sensitive to stimuli, and overreacting to clients and staff on the unit. Which action is **most** therapeutic for this client?
☐ 1. secluding and restraining the client as needed
☐ 2. telling the client to stay in their room until they can control themself
☐ 3. providing the client with frequent "time-outs"
☐ 4. confronting the client about their behaviors

87. A client with symptoms of amphetamine psychosis that are improving is anxious and still experiencing some delusions. When developing the client's plan of care, which measure should the nurse include?
☐ 1. Assign the client to a group meeting about the physiologic effects of drugs.
☐ 2. Advise the client to watch television.
☐ 3. Wait for the client to approach the nurse.
☐ 4. Invite the client to play a game of ping-pong with the nurse.

88. In consultation with their outpatient psychiatrist, a client is admitted for detoxification from methadone. The client states, "I got addicted to morphine for my chronic knee pain. Methadone worked for a long time. Since I had my knee replacement surgery 3 months ago and physical therapy, I don't think I need methadone anymore." It is important to discuss which information with this client? Select all that apply.
☐ 1. "Detoxification will likely occur with slowly decreasing doses of methadone."
☐ 2. "Oxycodone will be available if needed for breakthrough pain."
☐ 3. "You will be monitored closely for withdrawal symptoms and treated as needed (PRN)."
☐ 4. "Physical therapy and nonchemical pain management techniques can be prescribed if needed."
☐ 5. "If you have knee stiffness or pain, it is likely to be managed by nonnarcotic pain medicines."

89. A client approaches the medication nurse and states, "I can't believe you are NOT helping me with my cravings for my fentanyl patches! When I got off alcohol 2 years ago, they gave me naltrexone for my cravings, and it really helped. I can't stand the cravings and back pain anymore, and I'm getting angry." Which response(s) by the nurse would be helpful for this client? Select all that apply.
☐ 1. "Naltrexone can interfere with opiate cravings in some clients."
☐ 2. "Cravings are hard to deal with, especially when you are in pain too."
☐ 3. "I hear your frustration about how your detoxification is going."
☐ 4. "I'm positive naltrexone can help with your cravings for fentanyl."
☐ 5. "I can ask your health care provider (HCP) if they think naltrexone might help you."

The Client with Anxiety Disorders and Anxiety-Related Disorders

90. An adolescent client who has been treated for an anxiety disorder since middle school with behavioral treatment and as-needed (PRN) anxiety medication is preparing to go to college. The parents are concerned that their child will experience an exacerbation of symptoms attending college out of town and want their child to attend the local community college and live at home. The client believes they can handle the challenge of leaving home for college. How should the nurse in the outpatient clinic respond to the family's concerns? Select all that apply.
☐ 1. "Your parents have a point; transitions have been hard for you in the past."
☐ 2. "There are many pros and cons here that we all need to discuss together."
☐ 3. "Every high school graduate deserves the chance to take on new challenges."
☐ 4. "It may be premature for you to think of college at this point in time."
☐ 5. "Let's discuss the things that you would need to know to manage your health if you left home."

91. An adolescent client who is academically gifted is about to graduate from high school early since they have completed all courses needed to earn a diploma. Within the last 3 months, the client has begun to experience panic attacks that have forced them to leave classes early and occasionally miss a day of school. The client is concerned that these attacks may hinder their ability to pursue a college degree. What would be the **best** response by the school nurse who has been helping them deal with panic attacks?
☐ 1. "It's natural to be worried about going into a new environment. I'm sure with your abilities you'll do well once you get settled."
☐ 2. "You're putting too much pressure on yourself. You just need to relax more, and things will be alright."
☐ 3. "It might be best for you to postpone going to college. You need to get these panic attacks controlled first."
☐ 4. "It sounds like you have real concern about transitioning to college. I can refer you to a health care provider (HCP) for assessment and treatment."

92. A client takes diazepam while establishing a therapeutic dose of antidepressants for generalized anxiety disorder. Which instruction(s) should the nurse give this client? Select all that apply.
☐ 1. Consult with their health care provider before they stop taking the drug.
☐ 2. Avoid eating cheese and other tyramine-rich foods.
☐ 3. Take the medication on an empty stomach.
☐ 4. Avoid the use of alcohol while taking the drug.
☐ 5. Stop taking the drug if they experience swelling of the lips and face and difficulty breathing.

93. An adult client diagnosed with anxiety disorder becomes anxious when they touch fruits and vegetables. What action should the nurse take?
☐ 1. Instruct the client to avoid touching these foods.
☐ 2. Ask the client why they become anxious in these situations.
☐ 3. Assist the client to make a plan for their family to do the food shopping and preparation.
☐ 4. Teach the client to use cognitive-behavioral approaches to manage their anxiety.

94. A client who is pacing and wringing their hands states "I just need to walk" when questioned by the nurse about what they are feeling. Which response by the nurse is **most** therapeutic?
☐ 1. "You need to sit down and relax."
☐ 2. "Are you feeling anxious?"
☐ 3. "Is something bothering you?"
☐ 4. "You must be experiencing a problem now."

95. A client brought to the emergency department is perspiring profusely, breathing rapidly, and having dizziness and palpitations. Problems of a cardiovascular nature are ruled out, and the client's diagnosis is tentatively listed as a panic attack. After the symptoms pass, the client states, "I thought I was going to die." Which is the nurse's **best** response?
☐ 1. "It was very frightening for you."
☐ 2. "We would not have let you die."
☐ 3. "I would have felt the same way."
☐ 4. "But you are okay now."

96. A client commonly jumps when spoken to and reports feeling uneasy. The client says, "It's as though something bad is going to happen." In which order, from first to last, should the nursing actions be done? All options must be used.

1. Teach problem-solving strategies.
2. Ask the client to deep breathe for 2 minutes.
3. Discuss the client's feelings in more depth.
4. Reduce environmental stimuli.

97. A client with panic disorder is taking alprazolam 1 mg orally three times daily. The nurse understands that this medication is effective in blocking the symptoms of panic because of its specific action on which neurotransmitters?
☐ 1. gamma-aminobutyrate
☐ 2. serotonin
☐ 3. dopamine
☐ 4. norepinephrine

98. A client is diagnosed with generalized anxiety disorder (GAD) and given a prescription for venlafaxine. Which information should the nurse include in a teaching plan for this client? Select all that apply.
☐ 1. various strategies for reducing anxiety
☐ 2. the benefits and mechanisms of actions of venlafaxine in treating GAD
☐ 3. how venlafaxine will eliminate their anxiety at home and work
☐ 4. the management of the common side effects of venlafaxine
☐ 5. substituting adaptive coping strategies for maladaptive ones
☐ 6. the positive effects of venlafaxine being evident in 4 to 5 days

99. A client has been prescribed alprazolam. Which food should the nurse instruct the client to avoid?
☐ 1. coffee
☐ 2. cheese
☐ 3. alcohol
☐ 4. shellfish

100. A client has been taking buspirone as prescribed for 2 days. Which client statement indicates the need for further teaching?
☐ 1. "This medication will help my tight, aching muscles."
☐ 2. "I may not feel better for 7 to 10 days."
☐ 3. "The drug does not cause physical dependence."
☐ 4. "I can take the medication with food."

101. A week ago, a tornado destroyed a client's home and seriously injured their spouse. The client has been walking around the hospital in a daze without any outward display of emotions. The client tells the nurse that they feel like they are going crazy. Which intervention should the nurse use **first**?
☐ 1. Explain the effects of stress on the mind and body.
☐ 2. Reassure the client that their feelings are typical reactions to serious trauma.
☐ 3. Reassure the client that their symptoms are temporary.
☐ 4. Acknowledge the unfairness of the client's situation.

102. After being discharged from the hospital with acute stress disorder, a client is referred to the outpatient clinic for follow-up. What is **most** important for the client to use for continued alleviation of anxiety?
☐ 1. recognizing when they are feeling anxious
☐ 2. understanding reasons for their anxiety
☐ 3. using adaptive and palliative methods to reduce anxiety
☐ 4. describing the situations preceding their feelings of anxiety

103. A client with acute stress disorder states to the nurse, "I keep having horrible nightmares about the car accident that killed my child. I should not have taken them with me to the store." Which response by the nurse is **most** therapeutic?
☐ 1. "Don't keep torturing yourself with such horrible thoughts."
☐ 2. "Stop blaming yourself. It's only hurting you."
☐ 3. "Let's talk about something that's a bit more pleasant."
☐ 4. "The accident just happened and couldn't have been predicted."

104. A client who is a veteran with posttraumatic stress disorder tells the nurse about the horror and mass destruction of war. The client states, "I killed all of those people for nothing." Which response by the nurse is appropriate?
☐ 1. "You did what you had to do at that time."
☐ 2. "Maybe you didn't kill as many people as you think."
☐ 3. "How many people did you kill?"
☐ 4. "War is a terrible thing."

105. A client with acute stress disorder has avoided feelings of anger toward their rapist and cannot verbally express them. The nurse suggests which action(s) to assist the client with expressing their feelings? Select all apply.
☐ 1. working on a puzzle
☐ 2. writing in a journal
☐ 3. engaging in art therapy
☐ 4. meditating
☐ 5. listening to music

106. The nurse develops the plan of care for a client with acute stress disorder who lost their sibling in a boating accident. Which intervention should the nurse initiate?
☐ 1. helping the client to evaluate their sibling's behavior
☐ 2. telling the client to avoid details of the accident
☐ 3. facilitating a progressive review of the accident and its consequences
☐ 4. postponing discussion of the accident until the client brings it up

107. A soldier on their second tour of duty was notified of the date that they will be redeployed. As this date approaches, the client is showing signs of excessive anxiety and irritability and inability to sleep at night because of nightmares of explosive device tragedies, all leading to poor work performance. The client's commanding officer refers them to the base hospital for an evaluation. What should the nurse do in order of priority from first to last? All options must be used.

1. Remind the client that any feelings and problems they are having are typical in their current situation.

2. Ask them to talk about their upsetting experiences.

3. Remove any weapons and dangerous items they have in their possession.

4. Acknowledge any injustices or unfairness related to their experiences, and offer empathy and support.

108. A newly admitted young adult client diagnosed with posttraumatic stress disorder (PTSD) reluctantly reveals that they were the victim of human trafficking 2 years ago. The client says, "Nobody will ever believe the horrible things people did to me, and no one never stopped them." Which response is appropriate for the nurse to make?
  ☐ 1. "I'll believe anything you tell me. You can trust me."
  ☐ 2. "I understand that you do not want to keep reliving the pain. I won't ask you questions."
  ☐ 3. "Tell me what they did to you. It's important that I understand the details."
  ☐ 4. "It must be difficult to talk about what happened. I'm willing to listen."

109. An adolescent client diagnosed with posttraumatic stress disorder (PTSD) is admitted to the unit after slicing both arms with a razor blade. The client says, "Maybe my parent will listen to me now. They tell me I'm just crazy when I say I'm screwed up because my stepparent had sex with me for years." What should the nurse ask **first**?
Ask the client:
  ☐ 1. about the stepparent possibly abusing younger children in the family.
  ☐ 2. to be specific about what they mean by "screwed up."
  ☐ 3. to state what they will do if they feel the urge to hurt themself.
  ☐ 4. to talk about appropriate ways to express anger toward their parent.

110. A client diagnosed with posttraumatic stress disorder is readmitted for suicidal thoughts and continued trouble sleeping. They report that when they close their eyes, they have vivid memories of being awakened at night, stating, "My parent would be on top of me trying to have sex with me. I couldn't breathe." Which suggestion(s) would be appropriate for the nurse to make for the insomnia? Select all that apply.
  ☐ 1. trying relaxation techniques to help decrease anxiety before bedtime
  ☐ 2. taking the quetiapine 25 mg as needed as prescribed by the health care provider
  ☐ 3. staying in the dayroom and trying to sleep in the recliner chair near staff
  ☐ 4. listening to calming music as the client tries to fall asleep
  ☐ 5. processing the content of their flashbacks no less than an hour before bedtime
  ☐ 6. leaving their door slightly open to decrease noise during the nightly checks

111. A client with posttraumatic stress disorder needs to find new housing and wants to wait for a month before setting another appointment to see the nurse. How should the nurse interpret this action?
  ☐ 1. method of avoidance
  ☐ 2. detriment to progress
  ☐ 3. burnout going to therapy
  ☐ 4. necessary break in treatment

112. The nurse teaches a client who is taking a benzodiazepine about possible medication interactions. Which medication should the nurse warn the client to avoid?
  ☐ 1. antacids
  ☐ 2. acetaminophen
  ☐ 3. vitamins
  ☐ 4. aspirin

113. The nurse evaluates a client's understanding of benzodiazepines. Which client statement indicates the need for additional teaching about benzodiazepines?
☐ 1. "I can't drink alcohol while taking diazepam."
☐ 2. "I can stop taking the diazepam anytime I want."
☐ 3. "Diazepam can make me drowsy, so I shouldn't drive for a while."
☐ 4. "Diazepam will help my tight muscles feel better."

114. A client is diagnosed with agoraphobia without panic disorder. Which type of therapy would **most** the nurse expect to see included in the plan of care?
☐ 1. insight therapy
☐ 2. group therapy
☐ 3. behavior therapy
☐ 4. psychoanalysis

115. A client diagnosed with a fear of eating in public places or in front of other people has finished eating lunch in the dining area in the nurse's presence. Which statement by the nurse should reinforce the client's positive action?
☐ 1. "It wasn't so hard, now was it?"
☐ 2. "At supper, I hope to see you eat with a group of people."
☐ 3. "You must have been hungry today."
☐ 4. "It's progress for you to eat in the dining room with me."

116. A client diagnosed with agoraphobia refuses to walk down the hall to the group room. Which response by the nurse is **most** appropriate?
☐ 1. "I know you can do it."
☐ 2. "Try holding onto the wall as you walk."
☐ 3. "You can miss group this one time."
☐ 4. "I will walk with you."

117. A client diagnosed with obsessive-compulsive disorder has been taking sertraline but would like to have more energy every day. At their monthly checkup, the client reports that their massage therapist recommended they take St. John's wort to help with depression. What should the nurse tell the client?
☐ 1. "St. John's wort is a harmless herb that might be helpful in this instance."
☐ 2. "Combining St. John's wort with the sertraline can cause a serious reaction called *serotonin syndrome*."
☐ 3. "If you take St. John's wort, we will have to decrease the dose of your sertraline."
☐ 4. "St. John's wort is not consistently effective for treating depression, but we can increase your sertraline dose."

118. A client diagnosed with obsessive-compulsive disorder arrives late for an appointment with the nurse at the outpatient clinic. During the interview, the client fidgets restlessly, has trouble remembering what topic is being discussed, and says they think they are going crazy. Which statement by the nurse is **best**?
☐ 1. "What do you mean when you say you think you're going crazy?"
☐ 2. "Most people feel that way occasionally."
☐ 3. "I don't know you well enough to judge your mental state."
☐ 4. "I haven't heard you make a crazy statement."

119. A client with obsessive-compulsive disorder reveals that they were late for their appointment "because of my dumb habit. I have to take off my socks and put them back on 41 times! I can't stop until I do it just right." The nurse interprets the client's behavior as **most** likely representing which factor?
☐ 1. relief from anxiety
☐ 2. control of their thoughts
☐ 3. attention from others
☐ 4. safe expression of hostility

120. A client with obsessive-compulsive disorder, who was admitted early yesterday morning, must make their bed 22 times before they can have breakfast. Because of this behavior, the client missed having breakfast yesterday with the other clients. Which action should the nurse institute to help the client be on time for breakfast?
☐ 1. Tell the client to make their bed one time only.
☐ 2. Wake the client an hour earlier to perform their ritual.
☐ 3. Insist that the client stop their activity when it is time for breakfast.
☐ 4. Advise the client to have breakfast first before making the bed.

121. The nurse notices that a client diagnosed with major depression and social phobia must get up and move to another area when someone sits next to them. Which action by the nurse is appropriate?
☐ 1. Ignore the client's behavior.
☐ 2. Question the client about their avoidance of others.
☐ 3. Convey awareness of the client's anxiety about being around others.
☐ 4. Have nursing staff follow the client as they move away.

122. The nurse is developing a long-term care plan for an outpatient client diagnosed with dissociative identity disorder. Which intervention(s) should be included in this plan? Select all that apply.
☐ 1. learning how to manage feelings, especially anger and rage
☐ 2. joining several outpatient support groups that are process oriented
☐ 3. identifying resources to call when there is a risk of suicide or self-mutilation
☐ 4. selecting a method for alter personalities to communicate with each other, such as journaling
☐ 5. trying different medicines to find one that eliminates the dissociative process

123. A client with a long history of experiencing dissociative identity disorder is admitted to the unit after the cuts on their legs were sutured in the emergency department. During the admission interview, the client tearfully states that they do not know what happened to their legs. Then, a stronger, alter personality states that the client is useless, weak, and needs to be eliminated completely. The nurse should do which action **first**?
☐ 1. Explore the alter personalities' attitudes toward the client more thoroughly.
☐ 2. Place the client in restraints when the alter personality emerges.
☐ 3. Contract with the alter personality to tell the nurse when they have the urge to harm the client and the body they both share.
☐ 4. Keep the client in a stress-free environment so that the stronger alter personality does not get a chance to emerge.

The Client with a Somatoform Disorder

124. At 1000 hours, a client with a diagnosis of pain disorder demands that the nurse call the health care provider (HCP) for more pain medication because they are still in pain after the 0900 analgesic medication. What action should the nurse take **next**?
☐ 1. Call the HCP as the client requests.
☐ 2. Suggest the client lie down while waiting for their next dose.
☐ 3. Tell the client that the HCP will be in later to talk to them about it.
☐ 4. Inform the client that the nurse cannot give their additional medication at this time.

125. The unlicensed assistive personnel (UAP) tells the nurse that the client with a somatoform disorder is sick and is not coming to the dining room for lunch. The nurse should direct the UAP to do which intervention?
☐ 1. Take the client a lunch tray, and let them eat in their room.
☐ 2. Tell the client they will need to wait until supper to eat if they miss lunch.
☐ 3. Invite the client to lunch and accompany them to the dining room.
☐ 4. Inform the client that they have 10 minutes to get to the dining room for lunch.

126. A client diagnosed with conversion disorder has a paralyzed arm. A staff member states, "I would just tell the client their arm is paralyzed because they had an affair and neglected their baby's care to the point where the baby had to be hospitalized for dehydration." Which response by the nurse is **best**?
☐ 1. "Ignore the client's behaviors and treat them with respect."
☐ 2. "Pushing insight will increase the client's anxiety and the need for physical symptoms."
☐ 3. "Pushing awareness will be helpful and further the client's recovery."
☐ 4. "We will meet with the client and confront them about their behavior."

127. The health care provider (HCP) refers a client diagnosed with somatization disorder to the outpatient clinic because of problems with nausea. The client's past symptoms involved back pain, chest pain, and problems with urination. The client tells the nurse that the nausea began when their spouse asked them for a divorce. Which intervention is **most** appropriate?
☐ 1. asking the client to describe their problem with nausea
☐ 2. directing the client to describe their feelings about their impending divorce
☐ 3. allowing the client to talk about the HCPs they have seen and the medications they have taken
☐ 4. informing the client about a different medication for their nausea

128. A client diagnosed with pain disorder has a history of ruminating on pain in their arm. The client is talking with the nurse about fishing when they suddenly revert to talking about the pain in the arm. What action should the nurse take **next**?
☐ 1. Allow the client to talk about the pain.
☐ 2. Ask the client if they need more pain medication.
☐ 3. Suggest the client practice relaxation techniques.
☐ 4. Redirect the interaction back to fishing.

129. The nurse evaluates the progress of a client being treated for somatoform disorder. Which statement indicates to the nurse that the client is progressing toward recovery from a somatoform disorder?
☐ 1. "I understand my pain will feel worse when I am worried about my divorce."
☐ 2. "My stomach pain will go away once I get properly diagnosed."
☐ 3. "My headache feels better when I time my medication dose."
☐ 4. "I need to find a health care provider (HCP) who understands what my pain is like."

Managing Care, Quality, and Safety of Clients with Personality Disorders, Substance-Related Disorders, Anxiety Disorders, and Anxiety-Related Disorders

130. A client is brought to the emergency department (ED) by a friend who states that the client recently ran out of their lorazepam and has been having a grand mal seizure for the last 10 minutes. The nurse observes that the client is still seizing. What should the nurse do in order of priority from first to last? All options must be used.

| 1. Place seizure pads on the cart rails. |
| 2. Record the time, duration, and nature of the seizures. |
| 3. Obtain a stat prescription for diazepam. |
| 4. Ask the friend about the client's medical history and current medications. |
| |
| |
| |

131. A client is in the emergency department with their partner. The client is just recovering from a temporary drug-induced psychosis from lysergic acid diethylamide (LSD). The client is still frightened and a little suspicious. Which nursing action is **most** appropriate?
☐ 1. having an unlicensed assistive personnel (UAP) stay with the client to decrease the client's fear
☐ 2. placing the client next to the nursing desk
☐ 3. leaving the client alone until the "trip" is over
☐ 4. having the partner check on the client frequently

132. The nurse is teaching unlicensed staff about caring for the client with alcohol dependency. Which statement by the staff indicates the need for additional teaching?
☐ 1. "Alcohol dependency affects the entire family."
☐ 2. "The client is a weak individual and could stop if they desire."
☐ 3. "Alcohol is a problem when it interferes with the client's daily life."
☐ 4. "The client who cannot stop drinking, even though they want to, is alcohol dependent."

133. The nurse is serving on the hospital ethics committee that is considering the ethics of a proposal for the nursing staff to search the room of a client diagnosed with substance use disorder while the client is off the unit and without their knowledge. What should be considered concerning the relationship between ethical and legal standards of behavior?
Ethical standards:
☐ 1. are generally higher than those required by law.
☐ 2. are equal to those required by law.
☐ 3. bear no relationship to legal standards for behavior.
☐ 4. are irrelevant when the health of a client is at risk.

Personality Disorders, Substance-Related Disorders, Anxiety Disorders, and Anxiety-Related Disorders 875

134. A client with a history of cocaine use disorder is receiving intravenous therapy and exits the hospital "to visit a friend." The client returns to the nursing unit 1 hour later, agitated, aggressive, combative, and reporting "chest pain." Place the nurse's actions in priority order from first to last. All options must be used.

   1. Contact the security department.
   2. Obtain an electrocardiogram (ECG).
   3. Initiate a referral to obtain drug rehabilitation counseling.
   4. Obtain a urine sample.

135. During a unit meeting attended by clients and staff, several clients are criticizing their primary nurses. These clients have also been intimidating two other clients who have recently been admitted to the unit, and now the new clients have stopped sharing their opinions during the meeting. What is the **first** action for the nurse to take?
   ☐ 1. Help the new clients express the reasons they have stopped sharing their ideas.
   ☐ 2. Ask the clients criticizing their nurses to suggest some possible solutions for the practices they are criticizing.
   ☐ 3. Give the clients who are publicly criticizing the nurses a verbal warning that this behavior is not acceptable.
   ☐ 4. Use the next unit meeting to discuss respect and the importance of collaboration with the treatment team.

136. Two nurses disagree on what is the **most** important information for a client with addictions to have during a discharge teaching session. How should the nurse assigned to provide the discharge teaching proceed?
   ☐ 1. Share all the information that both nurses thought was important.
   ☐ 2. Review the policies related to required discharge teaching.
   ☐ 3. Be aware of different interpretations and personal biases held by nurses.
   ☐ 4. Ask the client what is most important to them as they prepare for discharge.

Answers, Rationales, and Test-Taking Strategies

*The answers and rationales for each question follow below, along with keys (🔑) to the client need (CN) and cognitive level (CL) for each question. In addition, questions that measure clinical judgment will be coded (CJ). As you check your answers, use the **Content Mastery and Test-Taking Skill Self-Analysis** worksheet (tear-out worksheet in the back of the book) to identify the reason(s) for not answering the questions correctly. For additional information about test-taking skills and strategies for answering questions, refer to pages 12–51 in Part 1 of this book.*

The Client with a Personality Disorder

1. **3, 1, 4, 2.** The client needs a stepwise plan for developing a social life. The client needs to first work on self-esteem and reduce fears of rejection before talking about how to decrease anxiety and learn new social skills. Helping the client choose interesting activities is important before suggesting an activity. Then, the client will be ready to try a structured activity with the nurse present for support and role modeling.
   🔑 CN: Psychosocial integrity; CL: Analyze

2. **3.** The client is at risk for suicide, and the nurse should determine how serious the client is, including if the client has a plan and the means to implement the plan. While medication history may be important, the nurse should first attempt to determine suicide risk. Asking why the client made the self-inflicted cuts will likely cause the client to respond with insufficient information to determine suicide risk.
   🔑 CN: Reduction of risk potential; CL: Analyze

3. **1.** The nurse should plan to assist the client who has a personality disorder primarily with specific dysfunctional behaviors that are distressing to the client or others. The client with a personality disorder has lifelong, inflexible, and dysfunctional patterns of relating and behaving. The client commonly does not view the behavior as distressful. The client becomes distressed because of others' reactions and behaviors toward the client, which causes the client emotional pain and discomfort. Psychopharmacologic compliance is not a primary need because medication does not cure a personality disorder. Medication is prescribed if the client has a severe symptom that

interferes with functioning, such as severe anxiety or depression. Examination of developmental conflicts usually is not helpful because of the ingrained dysfunctional ways of thinking and behaving. It is more useful to help the client with changing dysfunctional behaviors. Although milieu management is a component of care, the client usually is proficient enough in the manipulation of the environment to meet personal needs.

🔑 CN: Psychosocial integrity; CL: Analyze

4. 3. For this client, the nurse needs to use a calm, matter-of-fact approach to create a nonthreatening and secure environment because the client is experiencing problems with suspiciousness and trust. The use of "I" statements and responses would be therapeutic to reduce the client's suspiciousness and increase their trust in the staff and the environment. An authoritarian approach is nontherapeutic and inappropriate because the client may perceive this approach as an attack, subsequently responding with anger and threatening behavior. A parental or controlling approach may be perceived as authoritarian, and the client may become defensive and angry.

🔑 CN: Safety and infection control; CL: Apply

5. 4. Attending an activity with the nurse helps the client to become involved with others slowly. The client with a schizotypal personality disorder needs support, kindness, and gentle suggestion to improve social skills and interpersonal relationships. The client commonly has problems in thinking, perceiving, and communicating and appears similar to clients with schizophrenia except that psychotic episodes are infrequent and less severe. Participation solely in group activities or leading a sing-along would be too overwhelming for the client, subsequently increasing the client's anxiety and withdrawal. Engaging primarily in one-to-one activities would not be helpful because of the client's difficulty with social skills and interpersonal relationships. However, activities with the nurse could be used to establish trust. Then, the client could proceed to activities with others.

🔑 CN: Psychosocial integrity; CL: Analyze

6. 2. The nurse needs to set limits on the client's manipulative behavior to help the client control dysfunctional behavior. The manipulative client bends rules to have needs met without regard for rules or the needs or rights of others. A consistent approach by the staff is necessary to decrease manipulation. Ignoring the client's behavior reinforces or promotes the continuation of the client's manipulative behavior. Reprimanding the client may be perceived as a threat, resulting in aggressive behavior. Allowing the client to keep a snack in the client's room reinforces the dysfunctional behavior.

🔑 CN: Psychosocial integrity; CL: Apply

7. 2. The nurse assists the client with identifying and putting feelings into words during one-to-one interactions. This helps the client express their feelings in a nonthreatening setting and avoid directing anger toward other clients. A client with an antisocial personality disorder needs to understand how others feel and react to their behaviors and why they react the way they do. The client also needs to understand the consequences of their behaviors. Using humor or indirect behaviors to express anger is a passive-aggressive method that will not help the client learn how to express their anger appropriately. Asking the nurse for medication when upset is a way to avoid dealing with feelings and is not helpful. However, medication may be necessary if talking, and engaging in physical activity has not been effective in lowering anxiety or if the client is about to lose control of their behavior.

🔑 CN: Psychosocial integrity; CL: Analyze

8. -/+ **1, 3, 4, 6.** Inflexibility, need to be in control, perfectionism, overemphasis on work or tasks, and a fear of making mistakes are common symptoms of OCPD. Clomipramine and fluoxetine may help with the obsessive symptoms. Interrupting the client's tasks is likely to increase their anxiety even more. Telling the client that they cannot expect the family to be perfect is likely to create a power struggle.

🔑 CN: Psychosocial integrity; CL: Apply

9. 4. Some characteristics of a client with a dependent personality are an inability to make daily decisions without advice and reassurance and the preoccupation with fear of being alone to care for oneself. The client needs others to be responsible for important areas of the client's life. The nurse should respond, "Your parents have been supportive of you and will continue to be supportive even if you live apart" to gently challenge the client's fears and suggest that they may be unwarranted. The client can be encouraged to look to both parents and the health care team for support. Stating, "You're an adult now, not a child who needs to be cared for" or "Your parents need a break, and you need a break from them" is reprimanding and would diminish the client's self-worth. Stating, "Your parents will not be around forever; after all, they're getting older" may be true, but it is an insensitive response that may increase the client's anxiety.

🔑 CN: Psychosocial integrity; CL: Apply

10. **1, 3, 2, 4.** Safety is the priority concern, and then eating and sleeping patterns need to be reestablished. After the nurse intervenes to meet basic needs, delving into the loneliness and emptiness are important for determining underlying issues that need to be followed up in outpatient counseling. Although the client is living with their family currently, other options might be appropriate for them to consider.

   CN: Safety and infection control; CL: Analyze

11. **4.** For the client with attention-seeking behaviors, the nurse would institute a behavioral contract with the client to help decrease dysfunctional behaviors and promote self-sufficiency. Having the client approach only the assigned staff person sets limits on the attention-seeking behavior. Telling the client to stay in the client's room until staff approach, limiting the client to a certain area, or giving the client a list of permissible requests is punitive and does nothing to help the client gain control over the dysfunctional behavior.

   CN: Management of care; CL: Analyze

12. **2.** The most therapeutic response is "All of the nurses here provide good care." This statement corrects the client's unrealistic and exaggerated perception. "Splitting," defined as the inability to integrate good and bad aspects of an individual and the self, is a hallmark behavior of a client with borderline personality disorder. The client sees themself and others as all good or all bad. Components of "splitting" include behaviors that idealize and devalue others. It is a defense that allows the client to avoid pain and feelings associated with past abuse or a current situation involving the threat of rejection or abandonment. The other statements promote the client's idealistic view and do nothing to help correct the client's distortion.

   CN: Psychosocial integrity; CL: Apply

13. **2, 5.** For the client who is at risk for self-mutilation, the nurse develops a contract to assist the client with assuming responsibility for their behavior and helping the client develop adaptive methods of coping with feelings. Self-mutilation is usually an expression of intense anxiety, anger, helplessness, or guilt or a means to block psychological pain by inducing physical pain. The contract would also describe the triggers that have led to self-mutilation so the client can anticipate using coping strategies. A typical contract helpful to the client would have the client notify staff when anxiety is increasing. Withdrawing to their room when feeling overwhelmed, suppressing feelings when angry, or displacing feelings onto the HCP is not an adaptive method to help the client deal with feelings and could still result in self-mutilation.

   CN: Safety and infection control; CL: Evaluate

14. **4.** Any suicidal statement must be assessed by the nurse. The nurse should discuss the client's statement with them to determine its meaning in terms of suicide, overwhelming feelings of anxiety, abandonment, or other needs that the client cannot express appropriately. It is not uncommon for a client with borderline personality disorder to make threatening comments before discharge. Extending the hospital stay is inappropriate because it would encourage dependency and manipulation. Ignoring the client's statement on the assumption that it is a sign of manipulation is an error in judgment. Asking a family member to stay with the client temporarily at home is not appropriate and places the responsibility for the client on the family instead of the client.

   CN: Psychosocial integrity; CL: Analyze

15. **4.** The best initial course of action when admitting a client is to observe them to establish baseline information. This assessment provides valuable information about the client's behavior and forms the basis for the plan of care. Telling the client that the staff has the authority to subdue them if they get unruly or that they will have to pay for any damage they cause is threatening and may incite or provoke trouble. Isolating a client is not recommended unless there is a very good reason for it, such as a very active, combative client who is dangerous to themself and others.

   CN: Psychosocial integrity; CL: Analyze

16. **4.** The best response is "You say you're not a regular here, but you're experiencing what others are experiencing." This statement helps the client to identify factors that precipitate denial by helping them confront that which inhibits compliance. Denial is used to help a client feel better and more secure when a situation provokes a high level of anxiety and is threatening to the client. The statement "Because you are not a regular client, sit in the hall when the others are in group" agrees with and promotes denial in the client and interferes with treatment. The statement "Your family wants you to attend and they will be disappointed if you do not" causes the client to feel guilty and decreases their self-esteem. The statement "I'll have to mark you absent from the clinic today and speak to the health care provider about it" is punitive and threatening to the client, subsequently decreasing their self-esteem.

   CN: Psychosocial integrity; CL: Analyze

17. 3. Stating "I won't continue to talk with you if you curse" sets limits on the client's behavior and points out the negative effects of their behavior. Therefore, this response is most appropriate and therapeutic. The statement "you are upsetting the other clients" reprimands the client without putting limits on the behavior. The statement "I'm sorry if you can't wait" fails to provide feedback to the client about their behavior. The statement "Come back tomorrow, and your medication will be ready" ignores the client's behavior, failing to provide feedback to the client about the behavior. It also shows poor nursing judgment because the client may need their medication before tomorrow or may not return to the clinic the following day.

CN: Psychosocial integrity; CL: Analyze

18. 1. The client with avoidant personality disorder is showing signs of improvement when interacting with two other clients. A client with avoidant personality disorder is timid, socially uncomfortable, withdrawn, and hypersensitive to criticism. Social contact with others decreases isolation and withdrawal. Listening to music with headphones, sitting at a table and painting, and talking on the telephone are solitary activities and therefore do not indicate improvement, which is evidenced by social contact.

CN: Psychosocial integrity; CL: Analyze

19. 4. The priority is to explain to the client that this information has to be shared immediately with the staff and the HCP because of its serious nature. Safety of all is crucial regardless of whether the client follows through on their plan. It is possible that the client is asking to be stopped and that they are indirectly pleading for help in a dysfunctional manner. Determining the viability of a bombing plan should be assessed by other professionals. Bargaining with the client, such as warning them that their telephone privileges will be taken away if they abuse them, or offering to disregard the plan if the client does not go through with it is inappropriate. Saying nothing to anyone until the client has actually completed the call and then notifying the proper authorities would represent serious negligence on the part of the nurse.

CN: Safety and infection control; CL: Analyze

20. 1. The most basic and important idea to convey to a client is that, as a person, they are accepted, though their behavior may not be. Empathy is conveyed for emotional pain regardless of the client's behavior. Although some clients need limits placed on their behavior, not all clients require limit setting. That the staff members are the primary ones left to care about these clients is not necessarily true, nor is it true that the staff should use very little humor with these clients. Clients who are rigid and perfectionists and who have a restricted affect may need help with displaying humor.

CN: Management of care; CL: Apply

21. 1. The nurse should explain the negative reactions of others toward the client's behaviors to make them aware of the impact of their seductive behaviors on others. Suggesting that the client apologize to others for poor behavior is futile because the client cannot feel remorse for wrongdoing. Asking the client to explain their reasons for their seductive behavior is not helpful because this client is skillful at using projection and rationalization. Discussing the client's relationship with their parent is not helpful because the focus should be oriented to the present situation and managing their behavior at the present time.

CN: Psychosocial integrity; CL: Analyze

22. 2. The nurse would specifically use supportive confrontation with the client to point out discrepancies between what the client states and what actually exists to increase the client's responsibility for themselves. Although limit setting and consistency also may be used to help the client control unacceptable behavior and reduce the frequency of negative behaviors, these approaches do not entail pointing out discrepancies. Rationalization is typically used by the client, not the nurse, to blame others, make excuses, and provide alibis for self-centered behaviors.

CN: Psychosocial integrity; CL: Analyze

23. 4. The nurse should use role-playing to teach the client appropriate responses to others in various situations. This client dramatizes events, draws attention to self, and is unaware of and does not deal with feelings. The nurse works to help the client clarify true feelings and learn to express them appropriately. Party planning, music group, and cooking class are therapeutic activities, but they will not help the client specifically learn how to respond appropriately to others.

CN: Psychosocial integrity; CL: Analyze

The Client with an Alcohol-Related Disorder

24. 1, 4, 5. As with any dementia, there is a need to protect the client from wandering off and risking harm to self. Dementia is progressive and eventually requires 24-hour supervision. The client

Personality Disorders, Substance-Related Disorders, Anxiety Disorders, and Anxiety-Related Disorders 879

will find a way to get more alcohol if quitting is not a personal goal. Not answering the client's question will generally increase the client's anger. Once the dementia is evident, a lack of alcohol intake will not reverse the condition.

 CN: Psychosocial integrity; CL: Analyze

25. **2, 3, 4, 1.** The client's feelings and concerns need to be validated so they can open up more. The client should know that the changes in their spouse are not unusual. It helps to know the client has tried with their spouse to determine if they are appropriate or not. Then, there can be a discussion about getting help for their spouse so that their efforts to stay sober are not compromised.

 CN: Reduction of risk potential; CL: Analyze

26. **4.** The best action by the nurse to help a client who has difficulty falling asleep would be to teach the client relaxation exercises to use before bedtime to reduce anxiety and promote relaxation. This activity will also be useful for the client when out of the hospital. Inviting the client to play a board game is inappropriate because this activity can be competitive and thus stimulate the client. Allowing the client to sit in the community room until feeling sleepy is inappropriate because it does nothing to help the client relax. Taking frequent naps can worsen the ability to fall asleep at night.

 CN: Basic care and comfort; CL: Analyze

27. **1, 2, 5.** When a client is developing impending alcohol withdrawal delirium, the initial symptoms are a fast pulse and respiratory rate and an elevated blood pressure. Red, flushed, dry skin and reports of thirst occur with diabetic ketoacidosis. Abdominal cramping and severe diarrhea are symptoms of opiate withdrawal.

 CN: Reduction of risk potential; CL: Analyze

28. **1.** The nurse should first contact the HCP. The client's vital signs and level of consciousness are deteriorating, indicating complications of withdrawal, which can be life-threatening. Increasing the rate of the infusion may cause fluid overload and has not been prescribed by the HCP. Arousing the client will not address the underlying problems. Magnesium sulfate is used to treat seizures precipitated by alcohol withdrawal, but the client is not demonstrating signs of actual or impending seizures.

 CN: Safety and infection control; CL: Analyze

29. **4.** The nurse should provide the client with a quiet room to sleep in. Alcohol is destroyed and oxidized in the body at a slow, steady rate. The rate of alcohol metabolism is not influenced by drinking black coffee, walking around the unit, or taking a cold shower. Therefore, it is best to have the client sleep off the effects of the alcohol.

 CN: Reduction of risk potential; CL: Apply

30. **1, 2, 4, 5.** For the client experiencing symptoms of alcohol withdrawal, the nurse monitors vital signs and intake and output; reinforces reality for the client who is confused, disoriented, or hallucinating; explains that the symptoms of withdrawal are temporary; reduces stimulation; and stays with the client if they are confused or agitated. The nurse administers medications to prevent the progression of symptoms, such as seizures and delirium tremens, and to ensure the client's safety. Restraints are not used as a precautionary measure. Restraints are used only as a least restrictive measure to protect the client and others when the client is a danger to themself or others.

 CN: Psychosocial integrity; CL: Apply

31. **1, 3, 4, 5.** Two or three days after cessation of alcohol, clients may experience DTs, as evidenced by disorientation, nightmares, abdominal pain, nausea, and diaphoresis, as well as elevated temperature, pulse, and blood pressure, and visual and auditory hallucinations. If the client had a traumatic brain injury after falling, the client might have paralysis, but there is no association of paralysis from DTs.

 CN: Physiologic adaptation; CL: Analyze

32. **3.** The nurse should first confirm that the client has stopped taking the clonazepam because the client is reporting symptoms of benzodiazepine withdrawal from stopping the clonazepam abruptly. The client would report symptoms of being sedated if the client took alcohol with the clonazepam. Tolerance symptoms would be increased anxiety, not these physical symptoms. The client's symptoms are consistent with clonazepam withdrawal, not excess; thus, asking about increased use is not relevant.

 CN: Pharmacological and parenteral therapies; CL: Analyze

33. **2, 5, 6.** Disulfiram produces very unpleasant side effects when combined with alcohol in the body. Disulfiram reactions most commonly happen when alcohol is ingested, but they may also occur with topical applications of alcohol. Antiseptic mouthwash commonly contains alcohol and should be kept in a locked area

unless labeling clearly indicates that the product does not contain alcohol. A client with an intense craving for alcohol may drink mouthwash that contains alcohol. Aftershaves, perfumes, and skin astringents also often contain enough alcohol to cause a reaction. Personal care items, such as toothpaste, dental floss, and shaving cream, do not contain alcohol, and the client would be allowed to keep them in the room.

🗝 CN: Safety and infection control; CL: Analyze

34. 4. The best way to intervene with a client's minimization or denial of alcohol problems is to point out the consequences of the drinking—the multiple arrests. The other responses are superficial and discount the seriousness of the client's problem.

🗝 CN: Psychosocial integrity; CL: Analyze

35. 2. The client's response helps the nurse determine the severity of withdrawal symptoms because the length and extent of drinking alcohol have an effect on the severity of symptoms the client experiences during withdrawal. Decreased use of alcohol can also result in withdrawal symptoms in the client who has developed a high tolerance to alcohol and is physically dependent. The severity of the disease, the possibility of hallucinations, and the occurrence of delirium tremens are not determined by the information given. The diagnosis of alcohol dependency is just that—it is not classified as mild, moderate, or severe. Alcoholic hallucinosis is a state of auditory hallucinations that develops about 48 hours after the client has stopped drinking. The client hears voices or noises within the context of a clear sensorium, meaning that the auditory hallucination is the only symptom the client experiences. Severe withdrawal symptoms that are not managed medically can progress to delirium tremens or severe abstinence syndrome. Delirium tremens occurs about 3 to 5 days after a client's last drink and is characterized by confusion, agitation, severe psychomotor activity, hallucinations, sleeplessness, tachycardia, elevated blood pressure, elevated temperature, and possibly seizures.

🗝 CN: Reduction of risk potential; CL: Analyze

36. 2. The nurse would most likely administer a benzodiazepine, such as lorazepam, to the client who is experiencing symptoms of alcohol withdrawal. The benzodiazepine substitutes for the alcohol to suppress withdrawal symptoms. The client experiences symptoms of withdrawal because of the "rebound phenomenon" when sedation of the central nervous system (CNS) from alcohol begins to decrease. Haloperidol is an antipsychotic and is not indicated for alcohol withdrawal symptoms. Benztropine is used to treat extrapyramidal symptoms associated with antipsychotic therapy. Naloxone is used in opioid overdose to reverse the CNS depression caused by the opioid.

🗝 CN: Pharmacological and parenteral therapies; CL: Apply

37. 3. Monitoring vital signs provides the best information about the client's overall physiologic status during alcohol withdrawal and the physiologic response to the medication used. Vital signs reflect the degree of central nervous system irritability and indicate the effectiveness of the medication in easing withdrawal symptoms. Although assessment of nutritional status and sleep pattern and assessment for evidence of tremors are important, they provide only indirect information about single aspects of the client's physiologic status.

🗝 CN: Reduction of risk potential; CL: Analyze

38. 1. A client is experiencing a blackout when the client cannot recall what they did while under the influence of alcohol. A hangover refers to symptoms experienced the day after a bout of heavy drinking. Common symptoms include headaches and gastrointestinal distress, typically after heavy alcohol consumption. Tolerance refers to the need to increase the amount of the substance or to ingest the substance more often to achieve the same effects. Delirium tremens refers to severe alcohol withdrawal or abstinence syndrome with confusion, psychomotor agitation, sleeplessness, hallucinations, and elevated vital signs.

🗝 CN: Physiological adaptation; CL: Analyze

39. 4. Stating "I'm a nurse in the program; the staff and I will help you" is a nonjudgmental, caring approach that promotes trust and a therapeutic relationship. The statement "I hope you're serious about maintaining your sobriety this time" blames the client, subsequently decreasing the client's self-worth. Saying "You'll get it right this time" is threatening to the client, possibly leading to decreased self-worth by reinforcing the client's past failures at maintaining sobriety. The statement "I know someone who was successful after the fifth program" is impersonal and irrelevant to the client's situation.

🗝 CN: Psychosocial integrity; CL: Analyze

40. 3. The spouse of the client with alcohol dependency is exhibiting enabling behavior when they make excuses for the client's absenteeism.

Enabling behavior is not helpful to the client but rescues them from adverse consequences in relation to employment. Self-defeating behavior would be evidenced by putting oneself in a position that will lead to failure. Masochistic behavior would be evidenced by the need to experience emotional or physical pain to become sexually aroused.

CN: Psychosocial integrity; CL: Analyze

41. 4. To be most helpful, the nurse should calmly and objectively present facts by saying "You have alcohol on your breath" to help the coworker overcome denial and resistance. This statement also helps reinforce the coworker's awareness of the problem. The other statements blame the coworker and may reinforce denial. Blaming, nagging, and yelling diminish self-esteem in the individual with a substance use disorder who has low frustration tolerance.

CN: Psychosocial integrity; CL: Analyze

42. 3. The statement "You interrupted twice in 4 minutes" indicates an understanding of the use of constructive feedback by describing specifically what was seen and heard in an objective manner. The other statements are judgmental and blame the client without specifying what the objectionable behavior is.

CN: Psychosocial integrity; CL: Evaluate

43. 4. The client is feeling remorse about hitting their spouse. It is best to make a comment that will help them focus on their feelings and express them. Reflecting what the client has said is a good technique to accomplish these goals. Suggesting the client ask their spouse or explore the issue in family therapy is inappropriate because it gives advice and ignores the client's underlying feelings. Saying "It would depend on how much they really care for you" is inappropriate because it ignores the client's feelings and reinforces the negative aspects such as the shamefulness of the behavior.

CN: Psychosocial integrity; CL: Analyze

44. 1. The nurse must work through personal feelings related to substance use. Negative feelings towards individuals with substance use problems may make the nurse prejudiced against this client. Being persistent with the client regarding the substance use disorder, helping to make abstinence and sobriety worthwhile for the client, and suggesting a treatment program near the client's home all are interventions that the nurse can accomplish after the initial approach to the client.

CN: Psychosocial integrity; CL: Analyze

45. 1. Having the client who is experiencing severe symptoms of alcohol withdrawal walk is contraindicated because increased activity and stimulation may confuse the client and promote hallucinations. The client may also sustain an injury if the client has a seizure as part of the alcohol withdrawal process. The nurse should monitor intake and output to ensure fluid and electrolyte balance and hydration. The nurse should assess vital signs to assess the physiologic status of the client and the response to medications. The nurse should use short, concrete statements to decrease confusion and ambiguity.

CN: Reduction of risk potential; CL: Apply

46. 1. Any amount of alcohol consumed while taking disulfiram can cause an alcohol-disulfiram reaction. The reaction experienced is in proportion to the amount of alcohol ingested. The alcohol-disulfiram reaction can begin 5 to 10 minutes after alcohol is ingested. Symptoms can be mild, as in flushing, throbbing in the head and neck, nausea, and diaphoresis. Other symptoms include vomiting, respiratory difficulty, hypotension, vertigo, syncope, and confusion. Severe reactions involve respiratory depression, convulsions, coma, and even death. Disulfiram can be taken at bedtime if the client feels sleepy from the medication. Some clients experience a metallic or garlic taste when initiating disulfiram treatment. Anything containing alcohol, such as cough medicine, aftershave lotion, and mouthwash, can cause a reaction. Therefore, the client needs to check the labels of these items for their alcohol content.

CN: Pharmacological and parenteral therapies; CL: Evaluate

47. 3. The first question should be to ask the client how much alcohol they had today because nausea with severe vomiting is a sign of an alcohol-disulfiram reaction. Asking whether the client feels flu symptoms is important after inquiring about alcohol intake. Foods cooked in an alcoholic beverage, such as wine, could also cause a reaction, but the reaction would be less severe because the alcohol dissipates with cooking. Asking how long the client has been taking disulfiram would be least important at this time.

CN: Pharmacological and parenteral therapies; CL: Analyze

48. 1. Thiamine specifically prevents the development of Wernicke encephalopathy, a reversible amnestic disorder caused by a diet deficient in thiamine secondary to poor nutritional intake that commonly accompanies chronic alcoholism. It is characterized by nystagmus, ataxia, and mental status changes. Because the client would rather drink alcohol than eat, the client is depleted of vitamins and nutrients. Alcohol also is an irritant that causes a "malabsorption syndrome" in which vitamins and nutrients are not absorbed properly in the gastrointestinal tract. Thiamine is not associated with decreasing withdrawal symptoms, helping clients regain their strength, or promoting elimination of alcohol from the body.

🔑 CN: Pharmacological and parenteral therapies; CL: Apply

49. 2. The statement "Stopping support groups and not expressing feelings can lead to relapse" indicates the client's understanding of the risk of relapse. The client is responsible for sobriety and must understand the risk and signs of relapse. Other antecedents to relapse include severe craving, being around users, and severe emotional crises. The other statements place the responsibility for the client's sobriety on someone else.

🔑 CN: Reduction of risk potential; CL: Evaluate

50. 1. The client is using denial, an unconscious defense mechanism, when they refuse to acknowledge that they have a problem with alcohol. This is further evidenced by the client's inability to connect the liver disorder with alcohol ingestion. Displacement involves transfer of a feeling to someone else or to an object. Rationalization involves an attempt to make or prove that one's feeling or behavior is justifiable. Reaction formation is a conscious behavior that is the exact opposite of an unconscious feeling.

🔑 CN: Psychosocial integrity; CL: Analyze

51. 2. Regular coffee contains caffeine, which acts as a psychomotor stimulant and leads to feelings of anxiety and agitation. Serving coffee to the client may add to tremors and wakefulness. Milk, orange juice, and eggs are part of a well-balanced, high-protein diet needed by the client in alcohol withdrawal, who is nutritionally depleted.

🔑 CN: Reduction of risk potential; CL: Apply

52. 4. The nurse should teach the client with peripheral neuropathy to avoid using an electric blanket because the client is likely to have decreased sensitivity in the extremities owing to the damaging effects of alcohol on the nerve endings. It is particularly important to guard against burns because the client may not be able to discern the appropriate degree of heat on the feet. Daily washing and drying, massaging with lotion, and trimming the toenails are appropriate foot care measures for any client.

🔑 CN: Reduction of risk potential; CL: Analyze

53. 1, 4, 3, 2. After the nurse reminds the client about this withdrawal symptom, the nurse should take the client's vital signs and then assess for other symptoms, such as visual and auditory disturbances, tremors, anxiety, nausea, and excess perspiration. The elevation of the vital signs also helps determine the amount of lorazepam needed to control the withdrawal symptoms.

🔑 CN: Physiological adaptation; CL: Analyze

54. 3. The client with alcohol withdrawal delirium should not be left unattended when confused, disoriented, or hallucinating. Injury or unintentional suicide is a possibility when the client attempts to get away from hallucinations. Restraints are used only when the client loses control and is a danger to themself or others. Touching the client before saying anything is an additional stimulus that would most likely add to the client's agitation. Informing the client about the alcohol treatment program while the client is delirious is inappropriate and shows poor nursing judgment. The client should be given information about alcohol treatment when the withdrawal symptoms are lessening and the client can comprehend the information.

🔑 CN: Safety and infection control; CL: Analyze

55. 4. Follow-up care is essential to prevent relapse. Recovery has just begun when the treatment program ends. The first few months after program completion can be difficult and dangerous for the chemically dependent client. The nurse is responsible for discharge plans that include arrangements for counseling, self-help group meetings, and other forms of aftercare. Supportive friends, a list of goals, and returning to work may be important and helpful to the client, but follow-up care is essential.

🔑 CN: Management of care; CL: Analyze

56. -/+ **2, 3, 4.** The client who plans to attend support group meetings, verbalizes the damaging effects of alcohol on the body, and takes naltrexone daily may be ready for alcohol rehabilitation. Other key outcomes include admitting that a problem with alcohol exists and realizing the negative effects of alcohol on their life. Stating that they only need to cut down on alcohol intake is a sign of denial of an alcohol problem. Desiring to get back to a normal routine may indicate they want to resume previous lifestyle patterns that included alcohol.

🔑 CN: Management of care; CL: Evaluate

Personality Disorders, Substance-Related Disorders, Anxiety Disorders, and Anxiety-Related Disorders   883

57. 3. The best approach is to treat both illnesses simultaneously. Treating one and not the other is ineffective. The depression will not clear just by becoming sober or clean.

   CN: Management of care; CL: Analyze

58. 2. The nurse should assess the client's mental status daily to note changes that could occur from exacerbation of the mental illness or withdrawal from alcohol. Changes in mental status are important for treatment issues such as medication and participation in groups. Assessment of mental status takes priority because mental status affects the client's ability to sleep, eat, and care for themself. Flexibility is necessary on the part of nurses and staff members who are working with a heterogeneous client population.

   CN: Management of care; CL: Analyze

59. 4. Using a client-centered approach to care will most effectively establish a therapeutic relationship. Stating "I know what it is like to go through a bad breakup" shifts the focus away from the client's experience to the nurse. Minimizing the pain the client experiences because of the breakup does not acknowledge that at the present time the client is in significant distress. Asking "why" suggests that the nurse is judging the appropriateness of the actions and does not demonstrate empathy.

   CN: Psychosocial integrity; CL: Apply

The Client with Disorders Related to Other Addictive Substances

60. 4. Tapering doses of oxycodone, pain management strategies, and other pain control medicines are found to be the most helpful with opiate addictions resulting from chronic pain. Nonaddictive (over-the-counter) medicines alone are generally insufficient for chronic pain management. Methadone is an addictive opioid that involves substituting one addiction with another, so now clients are being detoxed off methadone as well. Lorazepam may help with anxiety during withdrawal from opiates, but it does not control the other symptoms of opiate withdrawal.

   CN: Pharmacological and parenteral therapies; CL: Analyze

61. 1, 4, 5, 6. The nurse should instruct the parents to monitor their children for use of paper bags or rags. The nurse should present information about brain damage from inhalants, including damage to the frontal lobe, cerebellum, and hippocampus, and that death is possible. Rather than use being on the decline, teenagers are experimenting even more with many types of inhalants, such as Freon, ground-up candy disks, and spray cleaners for computer and TV screens.

   CN: Health promotion and maintenance; CL: Apply

62. 1, 2, 3. Symptoms of opioid withdrawal include yawning, rhinorrhea, sweating, chills, piloerection (goose bumps), tremors, restlessness, irritability, leg spasms, bone pain, diarrhea, and vomiting. Symptoms of withdrawal occur within 36 to 72 hours of usage and subside within a week. Withdrawal from heroin is seldom fatal and usually does not necessitate medical intervention. Synesthesia (a blending of senses) is associated with lysergic acid diethylamide use, and formication (feeling of bugs crawling beneath the skin) is associated with cocaine use.

   CN: Physiological adaptation; CL: Analyze

63. 1. Vomiting and diarrhea are usually late signs of heroin withdrawal, along with muscle spasm, fever, nausea, repetitive sneezing, abdominal cramps, and backache. Early signs of heroin withdrawal include yawning, tearing (lacrimation), rhinorrhea, and sweating. Intermediate signs of heroin withdrawal are flushing, piloerection, tachycardia, tremor, restlessness, and irritability.

   CN: Reduction of risk potential; CL: Analyze

64. 4. The client takes methadone primarily to be able to work, live normally, and function productively without the mental and physical deterioration caused by opioid addiction. Methadone lessens physiologic dependence on opioids and is used to prevent withdrawal symptoms. Methadone, a substance similar to morphine, is an addictive substance; the client is still considered addicted to opioids. Because methadone has a long half-life of 15 to 30 hours, it can be taken once a day on an outpatient basis.

   CN: Psychosocial integrity; CL: Apply

65. 1. Suggesting that the client try attending a meeting at a different location is a supportive, positive response and encourages the client to continue participating in treatment. Saying "Maybe it just wasn't a good day for you" or "Perhaps you weren't paying close enough attention" places blame on the client and is not helpful. The statement "Sometimes the meetings can seem like a waste of time, but you need to attend to stay clean" diminishes the importance of the self-help group and offers little support to the client.

   CN: Management of care; CL: Analyze

66. 2. The best measure to determine a client's progress in rehabilitation is the number of drug-free days the client has. The longer the client abstains, the better the prognosis is. Although the kinds of friends the client makes, the way the client gets along with their parents, and the degree of responsibility the client's job requires could influence the client's decision to stay clean, the number of drug-free days is the best indicator of progress.

CN: Management of care; CL: Evaluate

67. 4. The client who is addicted to heroin is most likely to exhibit hypoactivity. Initially, the client feels euphoric. This is followed by drowsiness, hypoactivity, anorexia, and a decreased sex drive. Hilarity, aggression, and a labile mood usually are not associated with heroin addiction.

CN: Psychosocial integrity; CL: Analyze

68. 4. Because barbiturates are central nervous system depressants, the nurse should be especially alert for the possibility of respiratory failure. Respiratory failure is the most likely cause of death from barbiturate overdose. Kidney failure, cerebrovascular accident, and status epilepticus are not associated with barbiturate overdose.

CN: Reduction of risk potential; CL: Analyze

69. 4. When a spouse asks whether a seriously ill client will live, it is best for the nurse to respond by explaining the seriousness of the client's condition and acknowledging the spouse's concern. This type of comment does not offer false hope. Telling the spouse to wait and see and that it is too soon to tell is a stereotypical statement that offers no support. Asking the spouse to describe the length of their relationship with the client ignores the spouse's concern and does not focus on the problem. Simply saying that the client is very ill and may not live and that some do not pull through is harsh and not supportive.

CN: Psychosocial integrity; CL: Analyze

70. 1. Tolerance for a drug occurs when a client requires increasingly larger doses to obtain the desired effect. Therefore, the plan of care would address the client's state of tolerance. The term *addiction* refers to psychological and physiologic symptoms indicating that an individual cannot control their use of psychoactive substances. This term has been replaced with the term *dependence*. *Substance abuse* refers to the excessive use of a substance that differs from societal norms. Drug dependence occurs when the client must take a usual or increasing amount of the drug to prevent the onset of abstinence symptoms, cannot keep drug intake under control, and continues to use even though physical, social, and emotional processes are compromised.

CN: Physiological adaptation; CL: Analyze

71. 4. For a client who is confused when awakening after taking a large dose of barbiturates, the nurse should speak in concrete terms using simple statements in a calm, nonjudgmental, gentle manner to assist the client with cognitive-perceptual impairment, enhance understanding, and decrease anxiety. The other statements contain abstract information and some slang terms that may further confuse the client and thus increase the client's anxiety.

CN: Psychosocial integrity; CL: Analyze

72. 2. The highest priority is assessing for suicide risk. When the client is safe, then the self-esteem, helplessness, and hopelessness issues can be addressed.

CN: Psychosocial integrity; CL: Analyze

73. 1. The most appropriate initial outcome for the client is to discuss thoughts and feelings related to their losses. The nurse should help the client identify and verbalize their feelings so that they can externalize their thoughts and emotions and begin to deal with them. This prevents the client from internalizing feelings, which leads to depression and self-harm. The ability to identify two positive qualities, explore strengths, and prioritize problems would be appropriate after the client has explored their thoughts and feelings, gained awareness of the issues, and then can participate in the treatment plan.

CN: Psychosocial integrity; CL: Evaluate

74. 4. The best method to deal with the problem is to discuss observations with clients at the daily community meeting because the problem involves all of the clients, and this provides them with the opportunity to offer their views. Peer pressure is valuable in confronting self-defeating and destructive behaviors. Providing additional recreation avoids or ignores the problem and is damaging to all clients because it decreases trust in the nurse. Breaking up drug-oriented discussions would not be sufficient to stop the behavior. Speaking with the clients individually about their behavior is not as effective as dealing with the problem openly and directly with everyone.

CN: Psychosocial integrity; CL: Analyze

75. 4. The nurse directs the conversation to realistic concerns or issues to decrease denial and focus on rebuilding a substance-free life. Allowing the client to continue with the stories or questioning the client further about their exploits reinforces the denial. Telling the client you have heard the stories before is nondirective. Additionally, these actions do nothing to help the client focus on rebuilding a substance-free life.

🔑 CN: Psychosocial integrity; CL: Analyze

76.

Administer antibiotics	Delirium	Agitation
Administer antipsychotics		Orientation

The client is exhibiting symptoms of delirium, which is a sudden change in attention, orientation, and cognition that cannot be accounted for by a preexisting neurocognitive disorder. Visual hallucinations and disorientation are common with delirium. Dementia is a chronic progressive loss of intellectual functioning that typically evolves over time. Psychosis typically evolves more slowly, involves auditory hallucinations, and does not involve severe disorientation. The client's primary symptoms are cognitive, not mood, changes that would signal depression. Management of delirium includes identifying and treating the underlying medical condition causing the change and managing the symptoms. The fever and incontinence suggest the cause is most likely a urinary tract infection and needs to be treated with antibiotics. An antipsychotic may be needed to treat psychomotor agitation, which could present a safety issue. Benzodiazepines should be avoided as they can worsen the delirium. The client is not showing signs of a depressive disorder to warrant lithium or antidepressants. The client is presenting with disorientation and agitation; thus, it is most important for the nurse to monitor for those parameters to return to baseline. Monitoring short-term memory, self-concept, and mood are secondary assessments.

🔑 CJ: Standalone bowtie; CL: Create

77. 3. It is crucial to confirm that the client was taking their spouse's opiates and benzodiazepines and that their symptoms are due to the sudden withdrawal from these medications. After that information is obtained, the nurse should assess whether the client has been using other substances (such as alcohol) that may cause other withdrawal symptoms. Even before calling for prescriptions, the nurse can initiate withdrawal precautions for client safety.

🔑 CN: Safety and infection control; CL: Apply

78. 4. Acknowledging the client's son's feelings is the most therapeutic intervention because they are not likely to hear the nurse's information until anger and other feelings are addressed and subside. Then, it is important to acknowledge that oxycodone, especially in older clients, can interfere with remembering how many pills were taken. It is common for clients with chronic pain to inadvertently overuse or become addicted to pain medications. Pain management programs help clients to withdraw from the medication and start on a multifaceted system for controlling the pain.

🔑 CN: Psychosocial integrity; CL: Analyze

79. 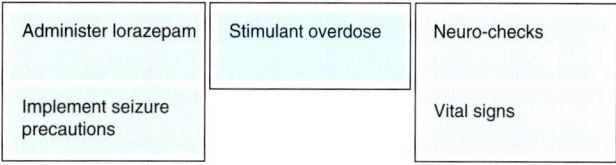 **1, 2, 3, 5.** Clients who deny an addiction and the need for treatment can be at risk for a suicide attempt, efforts to escape the unit, and aggression directed at staff. A contraband search is a safety measure to look for concealed drugs and dangerous items. Depending on the last use of the substance, withdrawal symptoms can begin quickly. A urine drug screen is crucial to determine what other substances the client may be using that may cause other withdrawal symptoms. Explaining the unit routines and groups can wait until the client is calmer and more receptive.

🔑 CN: Safety and infection control; CL: Analyze

80.

Administer lorazepam	Stimulant overdose	Neuro-checks
Implement seizure precautions		Vital signs

The client is presenting with symptoms of a stimulant (amphetamine or cocaine) overdose. Stimulants cause central nervous system irritation that can manifest as euphoria, talkativeness, agitation, grandiosity, or hallucinations. Physiologic changes with stimulant overdose can include tachycardia, elevated blood pressure, respiratory distress, and fever. The client may be diaphoretic and have dilated pupils. Alcohol, opioid, and inhalant overdoses would be expected to manifest with respiratory depression. Clients who have overdosed on stimulants are at the greatest risk for seizures. The nurse would implement seizure precautions and give medications to decrease central nervous system irritation, such as lorazepam. Antipsychotics may also be used. A fluid bolus is not indicated with an elevated blood pressure. Gastric lavage may be indicated to treat alcohol overdose. Naloxone is used to treat opioid overdose. Treatment for inhalant overdose is supportive. The nurse would monitor vital signs and the client's neurologic status to determine the success of treatment.

🔑 CJ: Standalone bowtie; CL: Create

81. 4. The nurse assesses the client for feelings of depression and suicidal ideation. After the client experiences an instantaneous high from crack, a crash immediately follows, and the client has an intense craving for more crack. A crash commonly leads to a cocaine-induced depression when additional crack is unavailable. At times, the depression is so severe that users attempt suicide. Although suspiciousness, loss of appetite, and drug craving are also associated with cocaine use, they are less of a priority than suicidal ideation.

CN: Psychosocial integrity; CL: Analyze

82. 1, 2, 5. The client is exhibiting symptoms of moderate anxiety. At this level of anxiety, the nurse should help the client decrease anxiety by allowing ventilation, crying, exercise, and relaxation techniques. The nurse would further assist the client by refocusing their attention, relating behaviors and feelings to anxiety, and then assisting with problem-solving. Oral medication may be needed if the client's anxiety is prolonged or does not decrease with the nurse's interventions. Suggesting a time-out and giving intramuscular medication are possible interventions for a client whose anxiety level is severe.

CN: Psychosocial integrity; CL: Analyze

83. 2. The nurse must be especially cautious when providing care to a client who has taken PCP because of unpredictable, violent behavior. The client can appear to be in a calm state or even in a coma, then become violent, and then return to a calm or comatose state. Visual hallucinations, bizarre behavior, and loud screaming are associated with PCP-intoxicated clients. However, the unpredictable, violent behavior presents a major issue of safety for clients and staff.

CN: Safety and infection control; CL: Analyze

84. 3. An acid environment aids in the excretion of PCP. Therefore, the nurse should give the client with PCP intoxication cranberry juice to acidify the urine to a pH of 5.5 and accelerate excretion. Water, milk, or grape juice will not acidify the urine.

CN: Reduction of risk potential; CL: Analyze

85. 1. Smoking marijuana while using alcohol can lead to alcohol poisoning because marijuana masks the nausea and vomiting associated with excessive alcohol consumption. Marijuana contains tetrahydrocannabinol (THC), which is responsible for suppressing nausea. With dangerous levels of alcohol in the body, respiratory depression, coma, and death can occur. Lysergic acid diethylamide, peyote, and psilocybin do not contain THC.

CN: Reduction of risk potential; CL: Analyze

86. 3. Providing frequent "time-outs" when the client is highly anxious, sensitive, irritable, and overreactive is needed to calm the client and reduce the possibility of escalating behaviors and violence. Secluding and restraining the client are not appropriate actions and would only be used if the client was threatening others and other alternative actions had been unsuccessful. Telling the client to stay in their room until they can control themself is unrealistic and futile because the client cannot eliminate behaviors induced by chemicals. Confronting the client about their behaviors would most likely lead to aggression and possibly violent behavior.

CN: Safety and infection control; CL: Analyze

87. 4. The nurse should invite the client who is anxious to participate in an activity that involves gross motor movements. Doing so helps direct energy toward a therapeutic activity. Appropriate activities include walking, riding a stationary bicycle, or playing volleyball. Assigning the client to an educational group is not helpful because the anxious client would be unable to sit in a group setting and concentrate on what was occurring in the group. Watching television may be too stimulating for the client, possibly increasing anxiety. Additionally, the client may be too anxious to sit and focus. Waiting for the client to approach the nurse is not helpful or appropriate. The nurse is responsible for initiating contact with the client.

CN: Psychosocial integrity; CL: Analyze

88. 1, 3, 4, 5. Since methadone is an addictive medication, the client will be gradually tapered off of it while being monitored for withdrawal symptoms. Any residual pain is likely to be controlled with other pain management techniques and nonnarcotic pain medication. It is very unlikely that oxycodone would be prescribed PRN since it is a very addictive medication.

CN: Reduction of risk potential; CL: Apply

89. 1, 2, 3, 5. Acknowledgment of the client's frustration, pain, and cravings is important to decrease the client's anger. Naltrexone can help with detoxification from alcohol and opiates. Asking the HCP about the possibility of adding naltrexone is appropriate. The nurse can never promise that a medication will help this client since naltrexone is effective in only 20% to 30% of clients with opiate cravings.

CN: Pharmacological and parental therapies; CL: Analyze

The Client with Anxiety Disorders and Anxiety-Related Disorders

90. ⬛ **2, 5.** The nurse cannot appear to take the side of either the student or their parents, so discussing the situation together where all points of view can be presented and evaluated is important. Young adults often rely on their parents to manage their health needs. The nurse should begin the discussion of preparing for a transition to adult care so both parties understand where the teen is in the readiness process. To avoid college altogether is likely to only escalate both parties' anxiety.

🔑 CN: Psychosocial integrity; CL: Apply

91. 4. The client's concerns are real and serious enough to warrant assessment by an HCP rather than being dismissed as trivial. Although the client is very intelligent, their intelligence cannot overcome their anxiety, and in fact, the anxiety is likely to interfere with the client's ability to perform in college if no assessment and treatment are received. Just postponing college is likely to increase the client's anxiety rather than lower it since it does not address the panic they are experiencing.

🔑 CN: Psychosocial integrity; CL: Analyze

92. ⬛ **1, 4, 5.** The nurse should instruct the client who is taking diazepam to take the medication as prescribed; stopping the medication suddenly can cause withdrawal symptoms. This medication is used for a short time only. The drug dose can be potentiated by alcohol, and the client should not drink alcoholic beverages while taking this drug. Swelling of the lips and face and difficulty breathing are signs and symptoms of an allergic reaction. The client should stop taking the drug and seek medical assistance immediately. The client does not need to avoid eating foods containing tyramine because it interacts with monoamine oxidase inhibitors, not benzodiazepines. The client can take the medication with food.

🔑 CN: Health promotion and maintenance; CL: Analyze

93. 4. Cognitive-behavioral therapy is effective in treating anxiety disorders. The nurse can assist the client in identifying the onset of the fears that cause the anxiety and develop strategies to modify the behavior associated with the fears. Avoiding touching foods, asking about reasons for the anxiety, and providing ways to work around touching the foods do not deal with the anxiety and are not interventions that will help this client.

🔑 CN: Psychosocial integrity; CL: Analyze

94. 2. Asking, "Are you feeling anxious?" helps the client label the feeling as anxiety so they can begin to understand and manage it. Some clients need assistance with identifying what they are feeling so they can recognize what is happening to them. Stating "You need to sit down and relax" is not appropriate because the client needs to continue their pacing to feel better. Asking if something is bothering the client or saying that they must be experiencing a problem is vague and does not help the client identify their feelings as anxiety.

🔑 CN: Psychosocial integrity; CL: Analyze

95. 1. The nurse responds with the statement "It was very frightening for you" to express empathy, thus acknowledging the client's discomfort and accepting their feelings. The nurse conveys respect and validates the client's self-worth. The other statements do not focus on the client's underlying feelings, convey active listening, or promote trust.

🔑 CN: Psychosocial integrity; CL: Analyze

96. 4, 2, 3, 1. Immediate anxiety-reducing strategies are decreasing stimuli and performing deep breathing. Once the anxiety is lessened, the client's feelings can be explored for triggers and underlying issues. Then, problem-solving strategies can be discussed to handle the triggers and issues appropriately.

🔑 CN: Psychosocial integrity; CL: Analyze

97. 1. Alprazolam, a benzodiazepine used on a short-term or temporary basis to treat symptoms of anxiety, increases gamma-aminobutyrate (GABA), a major inhibitory neurotransmitter. Because GABA is increased and the reticular activating system is depressed, incoming stimuli are muted, and the effects of anxiety are blocked. Alprazolam does not directly target serotonin, dopamine, or norepinephrine.

🔑 CN: Pharmacological and parenteral therapies; CL: Apply

98. ⬛ **1, 2, 4, 5.** It is appropriate to provide education on medication mechanisms, benefits, and managing side effects. No medication will eliminate all anxiety, so teaching about anxiety reduction and adaptive coping is needed. Venlafaxine is a serotonin-norepinephrine reuptake inhibitor antidepressant, and it will take 2 to 4 weeks to feel the effects.

🔑 CN: Pharmacological and parenteral therapies; CL: Apply

99. 3. Using alcohol or any central nervous system depressant while taking a benzodiazepine, such as alprazolam, is contraindicated because of additive depressant effects. Ingestion of cheese or shellfish is not problematic. Coffee in large amounts works against the desired effects of alprazolam but may be consumed in moderation.

  CN: Pharmacological and parenteral therapies; CL: Apply

100. 1. Buspirone, a nonbenzodiazepine anxiolytic, is particularly effective in treating the cognitive symptoms of anxiety, such as worry, apprehension, difficulty with concentration, and irritability. Buspirone is not effective for the somatic symptoms of anxiety (muscle tension). Therapeutic effects may be experienced in 7 to 10 days, with full effects occurring in 3 to 4 weeks. This drug is not known to cause physical or psychological dependence. It can be taken with food or small meals to reduce gastrointestinal upset.

  CN: Pharmacological and parenteral therapies; CL: Evaluate

101. 2. The nurse initially reassures the client that their feelings and behaviors are typical reactions to serious trauma to help decrease anxiety and maintain self-esteem. Explaining the effects of stress on the body may be helpful later. Telling the client that their symptoms are temporary is less helpful. Acknowledging the unfairness of the client's situation does not address the client's needs at this time.

  CN: Psychosocial integrity; CL: Analyze

102. 3. The client with anxiety may be able to learn to recognize when they are feeling anxious, understand the reasons for their anxiety, and be able to describe situations that preceded their feelings of anxiety. However, the client is likely to continue to experience symptoms unless they have also learned to use adaptive and palliative methods to reduce anxiety.

  CN: Psychosocial integrity; CL: Analyze

103. 4. Saying "The accident just happened and couldn't have been predicted" provides the client with an objective perception of the event instead of the client's perceived role. This type of statement reflects active listening and helps reduce feelings of blame and guilt. Saying "Don't keep torturing yourself" or "Stop blaming yourself" is inappropriate because it tells the client what to do, subsequently delaying the therapeutic process. The statement "Let's talk about something that's a bit more pleasant" ignores the client's feelings and changes the subject. The client needs to verbalize feelings and decrease feelings of isolation.

  CN: Psychosocial integrity; CL: Analyze

104. 1. The nurse states "You did what you had to do at that time" to help the client evaluate past behavior in the context of the trauma. Clients commonly feel guilty about past behaviors when viewing them in the context of current values. The other statements are inappropriate because they do not help the client evaluate past behavior in the context of the trauma.

  CN: Psychosocial integrity; CL: Analyze

105. 2, 5. Writing in a journal can help the client safely express feelings, particularly anger, when the client cannot verbalize them. Art therapy can also help clients heal by helping reveal deep thoughts and feelings. Listening to music, meditating, and working on a puzzle may be relaxing, but these actions will not help the client express their feelings. Safely externalizing anger by writing in a journal helps the client maintain control over their feelings.

  CN: Psychosocial integrity; CL: Analyze

106. 3. The nurse should facilitate a progressive review of the accident and its consequences to help the client integrate feelings and memories and begin the grieving process. Helping the client evaluate the sibling's behavior, telling the client to avoid details of the accident, or postponing the discussion of the accident until the client brings it up is not therapeutic and does not facilitate the development of trust in the nurse. Such actions do not facilitate a review of the accident, which is necessary to help the client integrate feelings and memories and begin the grieving process.

  CN: Management of care; CL: Apply

107. 3, 1, 4, 2. Safety is the first priority in clients experiencing acute stress disorder (ASD). ASD symptoms are typical reactions to an abnormal situation that are not being handled effectively. When the client believes they are "normal," being accepted, understood, and supported, they will be able to discuss their thoughts and feelings related to the traumas of the war.

  CN: Safety and infection control; CL: Analyze

108. 4. Survivors of trauma or torture have a lot of difficulty with trust and do not readily talk about the horrible events they experienced. Therefore, empathy and a willingness to listen without pressuring the client are crucial. Telling the client "I understand that you do not want to keep reliving the pain" shows empathy, but saying "I won't ask you questions" does not open the door for the client to talk about what they are ready to share. Knowing the details is not necessary to provide care and puts pressure on the client to relive painful memories. Believing everything may or may not be possible and does not convey empathy.

   CN: Psychosocial integrity; CL: Analyze

109. 3. The nurse should first assure the client's safety after the client's self-mutilation by assessing the client's intentions for self-harm. Then the nurse can address whether the stepparent possibly may be abusing younger children. If so, a police report may need to be filed. It is important to follow up on what the client means exactly by "screwed up" to identify other emotions and behaviors that need attention. It is very common for survivors of childhood sexual abuse to have intense anger at those who did not stop or prevent the abuse, and once the other steps have been taken, the nurse can begin to help the client manage their anger.

   CN: Reduction of risk potential; CL: Analyze

110. 1, 2, 4, 6. Relaxation techniques and listening to calming music decrease anxiety and promote sleep. Quetiapine is often effective in decreasing nightmares and flashbacks and has a beneficial side effect of drowsiness. Leaving the client's door slightly open will decrease the noise of making 15-minute checks at night. Staying in the dayroom in a recliner with all the noise and lights is not likely to help. Processing memories an hour or two before bedtime does not allow enough time to calm down before sleep.

   CN: Psychosocial integrity; CL: Analyze

111. 4. The nurse judges the client's request for an interruption in treatment as a necessary break in treatment. A "time-out" is common and necessary to enable the client to focus on pressing problems and solutions. It is not necessarily an indication of burnout, a method of avoidance, or a detriment to progress. A problem like housing can be very stressful and require all of the client's energy and attention, with none left for the emotional stress of treatment.

   CN: Management of care; CL: Analyze

112. 1. Combining a benzodiazepine with an antacid impairs the absorption rate of the benzodiazepine. Acetaminophen, vitamins, and aspirin are safe to take with a benzodiazepine because no major drug interactions occur.

   CN: Pharmacological and parenteral therapies; CL: Analyze

113. 2. Diazepam, like any benzodiazepine, cannot be stopped abruptly. The client must be slowly tapered off of the medication to decrease withdrawal symptoms, which would be similar to withdrawal from alcohol. Alcohol in combination with a benzodiazepine produces an increased central nervous system depressant effect and therefore should be avoided. Diazepam can cause drowsiness, and the client should be warned about driving until tolerance develops. Diazepam has muscle relaxant properties and will help tight, tense muscles feel better.

   CN: Pharmacological and parenteral therapies; CL: Evaluate

114. 3. The nurse should suggest behavior therapy, which is most successful for clients with phobias. Systematic desensitization, flooding, exposure, and self-exposure treatments are most therapeutic for clients with phobias. Self-exposure treatment is being increasingly used to avoid frequent therapy sessions. Insight therapy, exploration of the dynamics of the client's personality, is not helpful because the process of anxiety underlies the disorder. Group therapy or psychoanalysis, which deals with repressed, intrapsychic conflicts, is not helpful for the client with phobias because it does not help manage the underlying anxiety or disorder.

   CN: Psychosocial integrity; CL: Apply

115. 4. Saying "It's progress to eat in the dining area with me" conveys positive reinforcement and gives the client hope and confidence, thus reinforcing the adaptive behavior. Stating "It wasn't so hard, now was it" decreases the client's self-worth and minimizes their accomplishment. Stating "At supper, I hope to see you eat with a group of people" will overwhelm the client and increase anxiety. Stating "You must have been hungry today" ignores the client's positive behavior and shows the nurse's lack of understanding of the dynamics of the disorder.

   CN: Psychosocial integrity; CL: Analyze

116. 4. The nurse should walk with the client to activate adaptive coping for the client experiencing high anxiety and decreased motivation and energy. Stating "I know you can do it," "Try holding on to the wall," or "You can miss group this one time" maintains the client's avoidance, thus reinforcing the client's behavior, and does not help the client begin to cope with the problem.

   CN: Psychosocial integrity; CL: Analyze

117. 2. The effectiveness of St. John's wort with depression is unconfirmed. The critical issue is that the combination of St. John's wort and sertraline (a selective serotonin reuptake inhibitor [SSRI] antidepressant) can produce serotonin syndrome, which can be fatal. The client should not take the St. John's wort while taking sertraline.

   CN: Pharmacological and parenteral therapies; CL: Apply

118. 1. When the client says they think they are "going crazy," it is best for the nurse to ask them what "crazy" means. The nurse must have a clear idea of what the client means by their words and actions. Using an open-ended question facilitates client description to help the nurse assess their meaning. The other statements minimize and dismiss the client's concern and do not give them the opportunity to openly discuss their feelings, possibly leading to increased anxiety.

CN: Psychosocial integrity; CL: Analyze

119. 1. A client who is exhibiting compulsive behavior is attempting to control their anxiety. The compulsive behavior is performed to relieve discomfort and to bind or neutralize anxiety. The client must perform the ritual to avoid an extreme increase in tension or anxiety even though the client is aware that the actions are absurd. The repetitive behavior is not an attempt to control thoughts; the obsession or thinking component cannot be controlled. It is not an attention-seeking mechanism or an attempt to express hostility.

CN: Psychosocial integrity; CL: Analyze

120. 2. The nurse should wake the client an hour earlier to perform their ritual so that they can be on time for breakfast with the other clients. The nurse provides the client with the time needed to perform rituals because the client needs to keep their anxiety in check. The nurse should never take away a ritual because panic will ensue. The nurse should work with the client later to slowly set limits on the frequency of the action.

CN: Pharmacological and parenteral therapies; CL: Analyze

121. 3. The nurse conveys empathy and awareness of the client's need to reduce anxiety by showing acceptance and understanding to the client, thereby promoting trust. Ignoring the behavior, questioning the client about their avoidance of others, or telling other clients to follow them when they move is not therapeutic or appropriate.

CN: Psychosocial integrity; CL: Analyze

122. 1, 3, 4. Managing suicidal thoughts, urges to self-mutilate, and the intense anger are critical safety issues. Then, the focus can switch to communication methods for each alter and the integration issues. Process groups can be overwhelming when too much is revealed or when child alters are unable to understand the group content. There are no known medicines to stop the process of dissociating.

CN: Management of care; CL: Apply

123. 3. The no-harm contract with any destructive alters is essential along with the reminder that the alters share the same body. Later, the alter's attitudes toward the client can be explored in more depth. When alter personalities emerge, their behaviors are not predictable. Restraints could not be placed on the client soon enough. There are no behaviors to justify restraints at this point. Creating a stress-free environment is not possible.

CN: Safety and infection control; CL: Analyze

The Client with a Somatoform Disorder

124. 4. The nurse sets limits by informing the client in a matter-of-fact manner that the nurse cannot give them additional pain medication at this time. The nurse can then invite the client to participate in another activity, such as a card game, to decrease rumination about pain by directing the client's attention to an activity. By telling the client the nurse will call the HCP as requested, the nurse is manipulated to do what the client demands. Suggesting that the client lie down because they have to wait for the next dosage or telling the client that the HCP will be in later ignores the client and their needs and is not helpful in decreasing rumination about their pain.

CN: Psychosocial integrity; CL: Analyze

125. 3. The nurse instructs the UAP to invite the client to lunch and accompany them to the dining room to decrease manipulation, secondary gain, dependency, and reinforcement of negative behavior while maintaining the client's self-worth. Taking the client a lunch tray and allowing them to eat in their room reinforces negative behaviors and secondary gain. Telling the client they will need to wait until supper to eat if they miss lunch or informing the client that they have 10 minutes to get to the dining room challenges the client and may increase feelings of anger and the need for physical concerns.

CN: Management of care; CL: Analyze

126. 2. Pushing insight or awareness into conflicts or problems increases anxiety and the need for physical symptoms to handle or take care of the anxiety. Awareness or insight must be developed slowly as the client's need for symptoms diminishes. Saying "Ignore the client's behavior and treat them with respect" is not helpful to the staff member or the client. This statement fails to educate the staff member about the client's disorder and simply dismisses the needs of both. It is not true that pushing awareness will be helpful and further the client's recovery; this is the opposite of what is needed. Meeting with the client to confront their behavior is not therapeutic and will greatly increase the client's anxiety and the need for the conversion symptoms.

🗝 CN: Management of care; CL: Analyze

127. 2. The nurse helps the client to focus on their feelings about an impending divorce to decrease the client's anxiety and decrease focus on physical ailments. The client with a somatoform disorder typically has problems with identifying, describing, and dealing with feelings. Internalizing feelings leads to increased anxiety and the need for protective mechanisms. Asking the client to describe their problem with nausea, allowing the client to talk about the many HCPs they have seen and the medications they have taken, and informing the client about a different medication for nausea are counterproductive toward recovery because they reinforce the focus on the symptoms.

🗝 CN: Psychosocial integrity; CL: Analyze

128. 4. The nurse should redirect the interaction back to fishing or another focus whenever the client begins to ruminate about physical symptoms or impairment. Doing so helps the client talk about topics that are more therapeutic and beneficial to recovery. Allowing the client to talk about their pain or asking if they need additional pain medication is not therapeutic because it reinforces the client's need for the symptom. Recommending relaxation techniques can be tried next if the nurse is unable to redirect the client to the previous conversation.

🗝 CN: Psychosocial integrity; CL: Analyze

129. 1. The client who states "I understand my pain will feel worse when I am worried about my divorce" recognizes the connection between their pain and the divorce and indicates developing insight into their problem. The nurse should then be able to assist the client with developing adaptive coping strategies. The other statements indicate a lack of insight into the disorder and a lack of progress toward recovery. The client is still searching for the "right" diagnosis, medication, and HCP.

🗝 CN: Psychosocial integrity; CL: Evaluate

Managing Care, Quality, and Safety of Clients with Personality Disorders, Substance-Related Disorders, Anxiety Disorders, and Anxiety-Related Disorders

130. 3, 1, 2, 4. The nurse should first obtain a stat prescription for diazepam and administer it to stop the status epilepticus. The nurse should next prevent injury by using seizure pads. Recording the time, duration, and nature of the seizures will be important for ongoing treatment. Finally, the nurse can attempt to obtain information about medication use and abuse history from the friend until the client is able to do so for themself.

🗝 CN: Safety and infection control; CL: Analyze

131. 1. Having a UAP stay with the client provides reassurance and safety. Being next to the nursing desk will increase stimuli and confusion. Being alone will increase the client's fears and anxiety. It is inappropriate to ask the partner to provide client supervision for the nurse.

🗝 CN: Safety and infection control; CL: Analyze

132. 2. The statement "The client is a weak individual and could stop if they desire" is false and indicates a lack of understanding regarding alcohol dependency. Criteria for substance dependency include the inability to stop using even when wanting to do so. The client cannot stop or control the amount used when dependent on a substance. Alcohol dependency affects individuals from every culture and socioeconomic background and has nothing to do with being a "weak" individual. The devastating effects of alcohol dependency are felt by every member of the family and not just the individual with the alcohol problem. Family members need education about the physical, physiologic, and psychological effects of alcohol and referrals to self-help groups for support. They have felt and lived with the devastating effects of the disease. A simple and commonly held view of alcoholism is that alcohol is a problem when it interferes with life or disrupts family, work, or social relationships.

🗝 CN: Management of care; CL: Evaluate

133. 1. Some behavior that is legally allowed might not be considered ethically appropriate. Legal and ethical standards are often linked, such as in the commandment "Thou shalt not kill." Ethical standards are never irrelevant, though a client's safety or the safety of others may pose an ethical dilemma for health care personnel. Searching a client's room when they are not there is a violation of privacy. Room searches can be done with a health care provider's prescription and generally are done with the client present.

🗝️ CN: Management of care; CL: Apply

134. **1, 2, 4, 3.** The nurse should first provide for the safety of the client and the staff by requesting assistance from the security department. Next, the nurse should obtain an ECG because the client reports having chest pain. The nurse should then obtain a urine sample to identify if the client has been using illegal drugs. When the client is stabilized, the nurse can develop a care plan that includes treatment goals to support the respiratory and cardiovascular functions and enhance clearance of the agent and initiate a referral for treatment where access to the drug is eliminated and drug rehabilitation is provided as part of therapeutic management of clients with substance use disorder or a drug overdose.

🗝️ CN: Reduction of risk potential; CL: Analyze

135. **2.** Recognizing that the clients are part of the solution to the issues they are presenting demonstrates a client-centered approach to care. Having the new clients challenge the behaviors of other clients does not facilitate the development of a therapeutic milieu. Warning clients that behaviors are unacceptable reinforces a sense of client powerlessness and does not build a therapeutic relationship. Discussing respect and collaboration would happen after the criticisms have been acknowledged and the clients have been asked for their opinions.

🗝️ CN: Management of care; CL: Analyze

136. **4.** The discharge teaching session will be most effective if the nurse uses a client-centered approach to better assess what the client needs and, therefore, what information to share. Sharing all the information does not respect the knowledge that the client already has. Reviewing the policies is one area to help identify important areas for teaching, but to ensure that client needs are met, further assessment is required. Awareness of personal biases should not be used to determine what is important for the client.

🗝️ CN: Management of care; CL: Analyze

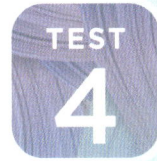

TEST 4

Stress, Crisis, Anger, and Violence

- The Client Managing Stress
- The Client Coping with Physical Illness
- The Client in Crisis
- The Client with Problems Expressing Anger
- The Client with Interpersonal Violence
- Managing Care, Quality, and Safety of Clients with Stress, Crisis, Anger, and Violence
- Answers, Rationales, and Test-Taking Strategies

The Client Managing Stress

1. The nurse cares for a middle-age client with a below-the-knee amputation. Which statement indicates the need for further assessment of the client's body image?
   - ☐ 1. "When I get my prosthesis, I want to learn to walk so I can participate in walkathons."
   - ☐ 2. "I hope to get skilled enough at using my prosthesis to help others like me adjust."
   - ☐ 3. "Whenever I start to feel sorry for myself, I remember that my buddy died in that accident."
   - ☐ 4. "I hope I can handle having a prosthesis, but I'm really wondering what my spouse will think."

2. A 75-year-old client is newly diagnosed with diabetes. The nurse is instructing them about blood glucose testing. After the session, the client states, "I can't be expected to remember all this stuff." The nurse should recognize this response as **most** likely related to which factor?
   - ☐ 1. moderate to severe anxiety
   - ☐ 2. disinterest in the illness
   - ☐ 3. early-onset dementia
   - ☐ 4. normal reaction to learning a new skill

3. Anxiety occurs in degrees, from a level that stimulates productive problem solving to a level that is severely debilitating. At a mild, productive level of anxiety, the nurse should expect to see what cognitive characteristic of mild anxiety?
   - ☐ 1. slight muscle tension
   - ☐ 2. occasional irritability
   - ☐ 3. accurate perceptions
   - ☐ 4. loss of contact with reality

4. Nursing interventions with an anxious client change as the anxiety level increases. At a low level of anxiety, what is the **primary** focus of intervention?
   - ☐ 1. taking control of the situation for the client
   - ☐ 2. learning and problem solving
   - ☐ 3. reducing stimuli and pressure
   - ☐ 4. using tension-reduction activities

5. A client's coping has become dysfunctional enough to require admission to the hospital. The nurse expects that the client would be exhibiting what behaviors?
   - ☐ 1. objective and rational problem solving
   - ☐ 2. tension-reduction activities and then problem solving
   - ☐ 3. anger management strategies with no problem solving
   - ☐ 4. minimal functioning with new problems developing

6. A client has severe anxiety after hearing about a death in the immediate family. The client is not able to focus on the questions asked of them. They will not eat, drink any fluids, or attend to personal care. The client keeps asking what they could have done differently for the deceased individual. Which instruction by the nurse is **best**?
   - ☐ 1. "You've got to take care of yourself."
   - ☐ 2. "Here, drink this glass of milk."
   - ☐ 3. "They wouldn't want to see you like this."
   - ☐ 4. "When do you think you can take care of yourself?"

7. A client is experiencing a relationship problem. Which client statement indicates that the client has coped effectively with the problem?
   ☐ 1. "My spouse will be happy to know that I can spend less time at work now."
   ☐ 2. "My spouse and I are talking about our likes and dislikes in activities."
   ☐ 3. "I can understand how my spouse and I see things differently."
   ☐ 4. "We are really listening to each other about our different views on issues."

8. The nurse cares for a client with stress. In an ongoing assessment, the nurse should identify the client's thoughts and feelings about a situation in addition to what other factor?
   ☐ 1. whether the client's behavior is appropriate in the context of the current situation
   ☐ 2. whether the client is motivated to decrease dysfunctional behaviors
   ☐ 3. which of the client's problems has the highest priority
   ☐ 4. which of the client's behaviors necessitates a safety plan

9. A client is hospitalized with a stress-related disorder. What short-term goal for the client is **most** realistic?

   The client will:
   ☐ 1. demonstrate a positive self-image.
   ☐ 2. describe plans for how to get back into school.
   ☐ 3. write a list of strengths and needs.
   ☐ 4. practice assertiveness skills in confronting their parent.

10. The nurse is counseling a client with cancer who is experiencing anxiety. Which goal will provide the **best** long-term client outcome?
    ☐ 1. Keep follow-up appointments with mental health providers.
    ☐ 2. Understand medication effects and adverse effects.
    ☐ 3. Take medication as prescribed.
    ☐ 4. Solve problems independently.

11. The nurse is planning care for a client experiencing stress. What area should the nurse focus on when integrating the concepts underlying the cognitive-behavioral model into the client's plan of care?
    ☐ 1. substitution of rational beliefs for self-defeating thinking and behaving
    ☐ 2. insight into unconscious conflicts and processes
    ☐ 3. analysis of fears and barriers to growth
    ☐ 4. reduction of bodily tensions and stress management

12. The nurse assesses the progress of a client who has behavioral manifestations of stress. Which client statement indicates that the client has gained insight into the use of the defense mechanism of displacement?
    ☐ 1. "I can't think about the weekend right now. I've got to study for the examination."
    ☐ 2. "I know I'm not good in sports, but I feel good about my grades."
    ☐ 3. "Now when I am mad at my spouse, I talk to them instead of taking it out on the kids."
    ☐ 4. "For years I couldn't remember being molested; now I know I have to face it."

13. The nurse educates staff on common legal issues. In which situation does the nurse teach the staff that a client's confidentiality can legally be breached?
    ☐ 1. to answer a request from a client's spouse about the client's medication
    ☐ 2. in a student nurse's clinical paper about a client
    ☐ 3. when a client near discharge is threatening to harm an ex-partner
    ☐ 4. when a client's employer requests the client's diagnosis to initiate medical claims

14. The nurse is helping a client deal with personal issues and painful feelings. What does the nurse identify as a **crucial** goal of therapeutic communication?
    ☐ 1. communicating empathy through gentle touch
    ☐ 2. conveying client respect and acceptance even if not all of the client's behaviors are tolerated
    ☐ 3. mutual sharing of information, spontaneity, emotions, and intimacy
    ☐ 4. guaranteeing total confidentiality and anonymity for the client

15. An 18-year-old pregnant college student presented at the prenatal clinic for an initial visit at 14 weeks' gestation. The client's history revealed that they have taken fluoxetine 20 mg orally daily for posttraumatic stress disorder (PTSD) and depression. Their medication was recently increased to 40 mg daily because of reports of increased stress and suicide ideation. Which side effect of fluoxetine would the nurse judge to be the **greatest** risk for the client and their developing fetus at this stage in the pregnancy?
    ☐ 1. insomnia
    ☐ 2. nausea/anorexia
    ☐ 3. headache
    ☐ 4. decreased libido

16. The nurse encourages client evaluation of their own behavior. Which probe should the nurse use?
☐ 1. "I can hear that it's still hard for you to talk about this."
☐ 2. "So what does this all mean to you now?"
☐ 3. "What did you do differently with your coworker this time?"
☐ 4. "What will it take to carry out your new plans?"

17. Even when a client understands problems and is motivated to change, the client may have fears about failing. Which intervention is **most** likely to facilitate change?
☐ 1. performing reality testing about the need for change
☐ 2. asking the client about fears that need to be overcome
☐ 3. teaching new communication skills
☐ 4. having the client practice new behaviors

The Client Coping with Physical Illness

18. A mastectomy is recommended for a 68-year-old client diagnosed with breast cancer a week ago. When approached about giving consent for the mastectomy, the client says, "What's the use in trying to get rid of the cancer? It will just come back! I can't handle another thing—having diabetes is enough. Besides, I'm getting old. It would be different if I were younger and had more energy." What action should the nurse take?
☐ 1. Accept the client's decision because it is their right to choose to obtain treatment or not.
☐ 2. Give the client information about the survival rates for clients who underwent mastectomies.
☐ 3. Notify the health care provider about the client's hopeless attitude about the future.
☐ 4. Explore with the client their feelings about their health problems and proposed surgery.

19. An 18-year-old client is recently diagnosed with leukemia. What is the **most** appropriate short-term goal for the nurse and client to establish?
☐ 1. accepting the client's death as imminent
☐ 2. expressing the client's angry feelings to the nurse
☐ 3. decreasing interaction with peers to conserve energy
☐ 4. gaining an intellectual understanding of the illness

20. The nurse has been asked to develop a medication education program for clients with chronic mental illness in the rehabilitation program. When the nurse is developing the course outline, which topic is **most** important to include?
☐ 1. a categorization of many psychotropic drugs
☐ 2. interventions for common side effects of psychotropic drugs
☐ 3. how to use medication reminders
☐ 4. effects of combining common street drugs with psychotropic medication

21. The health care provider (HCP) recommends that a client have a partial bowel resection and an ileostomy. Later, the client says to the nurse, "That doctor of mine surely likes to play big. I will bet the more the doctor can cut, the better they like it." Which reply by the nurse is **most** therapeutic?
☐ 1. "I can tell you more about the surgery if you like."
☐ 2. "What do you mean by that statement?"
☐ 3. "Why don't you think about getting a second opinion?"
☐ 4. "Does that remark have something to do with the operation the doctor wants you to have?"

22. A client becomes increasingly irritable after being diagnosed with cancer. The client is rude to visitors and pushes nurses away when they attempt to give medications and treatments. What should the nurse do when the client has a hostile outburst? Select all that apply.
☐ 1. Offer the client positive reinforcement each time the client cooperates.
☐ 2. Encourage the client to discuss immediate concerns and feelings.
☐ 3. Continue with the assigned tasks and duties as though nothing has happened.
☐ 4. Limit visitation until the client is less irritable.
☐ 5. Maintain appropriate personal space.

23. Arrangements are made for a member of the colostomy support group to meet with a client before bowel surgery. What is accomplished by having a representative from the group meet the client preoperatively?
☐ 1. letting the client know that there are resources in the community that can help
☐ 2. providing support for the health care provider's (HCP's) plan of therapy for the client
☐ 3. providing the client with support and realistic information on the colostomy
☐ 4. explaining that the surgery will not be disfiguring and that the client can lead a full life

24. A nurse is working in the emergency department when a visitor comes in reporting that they were notified that their spouse was just admitted following an accident. The visitor is pacing and tearful, and their attention span seems poor. The nurse recognizes that the visitor is having moderate anxiety. What should be the nurse's **first** response?
    - ☐ 1. "I'm really glad you are here. I work on this unit and was here when your spouse came in."
    - ☐ 2. "Your spouse is awake and stable right now. I'll take you to their room."
    - ☐ 3. "Your spouse had an x-ray and might have a fractured femur. Their hemoglobin and hematocrit are stable. They are diaphoretic. They have had an analgesic while awaiting an orthopedic consultation."
    - ☐ 4. "You seem really nervous about all of this. Maybe you should complete the admission paperwork before seeing your spouse."

25. The nurse teaches a client with acute cardiac illness about lifestyle changes. Which statement would lead the nurse to determine that a client lacks understanding or the ability to make lifestyle changes?
    - ☐ 1. "I already have my airline ticket, so I won't miss my meeting tomorrow."
    - ☐ 2. "These relaxation tapes sound okay; I'll see if they help me."
    - ☐ 3. "No more working 10 hours a day for me unless it's an emergency."
    - ☐ 4. "I talked with my spouse yesterday about working on a new budget together."

26. A client has been rehospitalized with a severe exacerbation of lupus. The client's spouse approaches the nurse and says, "My spouse is scaring me, saying they don't want to live with this illness anymore. Our kids are grown, and they feel useless as a parent and a spouse." Which statement(s) would be the **most** appropriate response(s) to the client's spouse? Select all that apply.
    - ☐ 1. "I'll have a talk with your spouse to see if they are suicidal."
    - ☐ 2. "You need to be strong and optimistic when you are with them."
    - ☐ 3. "I'm glad you shared this with me. I can imagine that this is scary for you."
    - ☐ 4. "I'm sure your spouse will feel differently when we get this episode under control."
    - ☐ 5. "We can talk about what you can say to your spouse that may help."

27. A client with kidney stones refuses to eat lunch and rudely tells the nurse to get out of their room. Which response by the nurse is **most** appropriate?
    - ☐ 1. "I'll leave, but you need to eat."
    - ☐ 2. "I'll get you something for your pain."
    - ☐ 3. "Your anger doesn't bother me. I'll be back later."
    - ☐ 4. "You sound angry. What's upsetting you?"

28. A client diagnosed with ulcerative colitis also experiences obsessive-compulsive anxiety disorder (OCD). In helping the client understand their illness, the nurse should respond with which statement?
    - ☐ 1. "Your ulcerative colitis has made you perfectionistic, and it has caused your OCD."
    - ☐ 2. "There is no relationship at all between your colitis and your OCD. They are separate disorders."
    - ☐ 3. "The perfectionism and anxiety related to your obsessions and compulsions have led to your colitis."
    - ☐ 4. "It's possible that your desire to have everything be perfect has caused stress that may have worsened your colitis, but there is no proof that either disorder caused the other."

29. A client receiving dialysis directs profanities at the nurse and then abruptly hangs their head and pleads, "Please forgive me. Something just came over me. Why do I say those things?" The nurse interprets this as which finding?
    - ☐ 1. neologism
    - ☐ 2. confabulation
    - ☐ 3. flight of ideas
    - ☐ 4. emotional lability

30. On an oncology unit, the nurse hears noises coming from a client's room. The client is found throwing objects at the walls and has just picked up the phone and is screaming, "How can God do this to me? It's the third type of cancer I've had. I've gone through all the treatment for nothing." In what order of priority from first to last should the nurse make the interventions? All options must be used.

1. "Tell me what you are feeling right now."
2. "Please put the telephone down so we can talk."
3. "I can hear how upset you are about the cancer."
4. "I wonder if you would like to talk to a member of the hospital clergy."

31. A client who has had acquired immune deficiency syndrome (AIDS) for years is being treated for a serious episode of pneumonia. A psychiatric nurse consult was arranged after the client stated, "I'm tired of being in and out of the hospital. I'm not coming in here anymore. I have other options." The nurse would evaluate the psychiatric nurse consult as helpful if the client makes which statement?
  ☐ 1. "Nobody wants me to commit suicide."
  ☐ 2. "If I talk about suicide, I'll be transferred to the psychiatric unit."
  ☐ 3. "I realize that I really do have more time to enjoy my family and friends."
  ☐ 4. "I would probably screw up suicide anyway."

The Client in Crisis

32. The nurse assists a client in responding to a loss. What is the **best** approach for the nurse to use with this client?
  ☐ 1. Make sure the client progresses through all of the stages of the grief process.
  ☐ 2. Encourage the client to work to resolve lingering family conflicts.
  ☐ 3. Assist the client to engage in the work associated with the normal grieving process.
  ☐ 4. Allow the client to express anger.

33. The nurse is assessing a client who has just experienced a crisis. The nurse should **first** assess this client for which behavior?
  ☐ 1. effective problem solving
  ☐ 2. level of anxiety
  ☐ 3. attention span
  ☐ 4. help seeking

34. The nurse is working with a family in crisis. What should the nurse do **first**?
  ☐ 1. Make a plan for managing the crisis.
  ☐ 2. Develop strategies to reduce symptoms.
  ☐ 3. Assess the family's resources.
  ☐ 4. Identify the family member in crisis.

35. An anxious young adult is brought to the interviewing room of a crisis shelter, sobbing and saying that they think they are pregnant but do not know what to do. Which nursing intervention is **most** appropriate at this time?
  ☐ 1. Ask the client about the type of things that they have thought of doing.
  ☐ 2. Give the client some ideas about what to expect to happen next.
  ☐ 3. Recommend a pregnancy test after acknowledging the client's distress.
  ☐ 4. Question the client about their feelings and possible parental reactions.

36. A client who had been sexually assaulted as an adolescent saw their assailant after 5 years. The client cut their wrists and was brought into the emergency department by a family member who discovered the client hiding on a closet floor. Which question(s) should the nurse ask to assess the client's perception of this event? Select all that apply.
  ☐ 1. "Has anything upsetting happened to you within the past few days or weeks?"
  ☐ 2. "Who can you talk to when you feel overwhelmed?"
  ☐ 3. "What was happening in your life before you started to feel like hurting yourself?"
  ☐ 4. "Describe how you are feeling now."
  ☐ 5. "Who is available to help you?"

37. A 40-year-old client who is quite anxious says that they would "rather die than be pregnant." Which response by the nurse is **most** helpful?
  ☐ 1. "Try not to worry until after the pregnancy test."
  ☐ 2. "You know, pregnancy is a normal event."
  ☐ 3. "You're only 40 years old and not too old to have a baby."
  ☐ 4. "I see you're upset. Take some deep breaths to relax a little."

38. On a crisis shelter hotline, the nurse talks to two 11-year-old children who think a friend abuses inhalants. They say the friend's breath sometimes smells like glue and they act drunk. They say they are afraid to tell their parents about the friend. When the nurse is formulating a reply, what is the **most** important factor for the nurse to consider?
  ☐ 1. The callers probably fear punishment.
  ☐ 2. Inhalant abuse is illegal.
  ☐ 3. The callers' observations could be wrong.
  ☐ 4. Inhalant abuse is a minor form of substance abuse.

39. While the nurse is teaching a group of volunteers for a crisis hotline, a volunteer asks, "What if I'm not sure why someone is calling?" Which statement by the nurse is **most** helpful?
  ☐ 1. "Ask the caller to tell you why they are calling you today."
  ☐ 2. "Tell the caller to make an appointment at the walk-in crisis clinic."
  ☐ 3. "Instruct the caller to go to the nearest emergency department."
  ☐ 4. "Tell the caller to let you speak to anyone else in the house."

40. After teaching a group of students who are volunteering for a local crisis hotline, the nurse judges that further education about crisis and intervention is needed when a student makes which statement?
- ☐ 1. "Callers to a crisis line use this service when they are overwhelmed and exhausted."
- ☐ 2. "People use crisis hotlines when they are in the most pain and nothing is working for them."
- ☐ 3. "Most people in crisis will be calling the line once every day for at least a year."
- ☐ 4. "One benefit is that a person will know how to handle stressful situations better in the future."

41. A true crisis state, involving a period of severe disorganization, is difficult to endure emotionally and physically. The nurse recognizes that a client will only be able to tolerate being in crisis for how long?
- ☐ 1. 1 to 2 weeks
- ☐ 2. 4 to 6 weeks
- ☐ 3. 12 to 14 weeks
- ☐ 4. 24 to 26 weeks

42. The nurse incorporates the underlying premise of crisis intervention into the plan of care. What is the initial goal of providing "the right kind of help at the right time?"
- ☐ 1. regaining emotional security and equilibrium
- ☐ 2. resolving underlying emotional problems
- ☐ 3. developing insight and personal growth
- ☐ 4. formulating more effective support systems

43. The nurse understands that with the right help at the right time, a client can successfully resolve a crisis and function better than before the crisis. Which factor supports improved functioning?
- ☐ 1. relinquishment of dysfunctional coping
- ☐ 2. reestablishment of lost support systems
- ☐ 3. acquisition of new coping skills
- ☐ 4. gain of crisis prevention knowledge

44. A distraught parent is waiting for their child to come out of surgery. The parent accidentally backed the car into the child, causing multiple fractures and a serious head injury. Which statement by the parent would **most** alert the nurse to the need for a psychiatric consultation?
- ☐ 1. "My child will be fine, but I may be charged with reckless driving."
- ☐ 2. "This accident will probably cost me my marriage."
- ☐ 3. "I just did not see them run behind the car."
- ☐ 4. "If my child dies, there will be nothing for me to do but join them."

45. An adult grandchild calls the crisis center expressing concern about their grandparent, who lost their spouse a month ago. The family member states, "They've been in bed for a week and are not eating or showering. My grandparent told me that they didn't want to kill themself, but it's not like them to lay in bed and not shower. They won't even talk to me when I visit." The nurse encourages the grandchild to bring their grandparent to the center for evaluation based on which reason?
- ☐ 1. The behaviors may reflect passive suicidal thoughts.
- ☐ 2. The behaviors reflect altered role performance.
- ☐ 3. Seeing the grandchild and grandparent together will be helpful.
- ☐ 4. Refusing to talk to the grandchild alone indicates a major problem.

46. An adolescent client who is being seen by the crisis nurse after making several superficial cuts on their wrist states that all their friends are siding with their ex-partner and will not talk to the client anymore. The client says that although they know the relationship is over, "If I can't have my ex, no one else will." Which client problem takes the **highest priority**?
- ☐ 1. situational low self-esteem
- ☐ 2. risk for other-directed violence
- ☐ 3. risk for suicide
- ☐ 4. risk-prone health behavior

47. A client who comes to the crisis center in a very distressed state tells the nurse, "I just can't get over being fired last week. I've asked for help. I've talked to friends. I've tried everything to get through this, but nothing is working. Help me!" Which initial crisis intervention strategy should the nurse use?
- ☐ 1. referral for counseling
- ☐ 2. support system assessment
- ☐ 3. emotion management
- ☐ 4. unemployment assistance

48. A major role in crisis intervention is getting a client's family and friends involved in helping with the immediate crisis as soon as possible. The nurse should determine that the support persons are prepared to help when they verbalize what information?
- ☐ 1. the name and phone number of the client's health care provider
- ☐ 2. emergency resources and when to use them
- ☐ 3. the coping strategies they are using
- ☐ 4. long-term solutions they plan to tell the client to use

The Client with Problems Expressing Anger

49. A client was experiencing marital discord with a spouse of 4 years. When the spouse walked out, the client became angry and began to throw things and break dishes. A friend talked the client into seeking help at the local mental health center. Which of these questions should the nurse ask **initially** to begin to assess this client's **immediate** problem?
- ☐ 1. "Do you feel in control of yourself at this time?"
- ☐ 2. "What did you do to cause your spouse to leave?"
- ☐ 3. "In hindsight, how might you have managed this situation differently?"
- ☐ 4. "What led you to come in for help today?"

50. A client is being admitted to a psychiatric outpatient program for counseling for ongoing emotional symptoms. Asked to rate the severity of the depression, anxiety, and anger that the client is feeling, the client states, "I don't have any anger anymore. I lost my temper once and nearly hurt my spouse. I never got angry again." In which order of priority from first to last should the principles related to anger be shared with this client? All options must be used.

1. "You can learn effective ways to discuss anger with others and still maintain control."

2. "Anger is a natural emotion occurring in all human relationships."

3. "Holding your anger inside contributes to your depression."

4. "Unexpressed anger has a negative effect on the human body and mind."

51. The parent of a soldier who was killed 2 days ago is admitted after a serious suicide attempt. The client is medically stable, and a safety plan is in place. During a talk with the nurse, the client says, "Terrorism and war are holding me and the whole world hostage. It's so unfair. I would rather be dead than live alone in constant fear." Which nursing intervention(s) would be important in the **next** few days? Select all that apply.
- ☐ 1. discussing effective ways to express justifiable anger
- ☐ 2. teaching stress management and relaxation techniques
- ☐ 3. identifying community groups for relatives of military personnel
- ☐ 4. recommending an antiwar advocacy group
- ☐ 5. strategizing about ways to increase a personal sense of security

52. In developing a plan of care for a client who has had previous episodes of angry verbal outbursts, the nurse plans to take an educational approach to the problem. Arrange the steps the nurse should take from first to last. All options must be used.

1. Assist the client to recognize the early cues of anger.

2. Help the client identify triggers for anger.

3. Practice with the client appropriate ways to express anger.

4. Identify alternate ways to express anger.

53. The treatment team recommends that a client take an assertiveness training class offered in the hospital. Which behavior indicates that the client is becoming more assertive?
- ☐ 1. The client arrives late for unit activities, and when asked about the lateness, the client says, "Because I feel like it!"
- ☐ 2. The client asks the nurse to call the client's employer about obtaining insurance.
- ☐ 3. The client asks a roommate to put away dirty clothes because the untidiness bothers the client.
- ☐ 4. The client follows the nurse's advice of asking the health care provider (HCP) about being passive aggressive.

54. The nurse assesses a client for physiologic responses to stress. Which finding would suggest to the nurse that the client is not experiencing anger?
    ☐ 1. increased respiratory rate
    ☐ 2. decreased blood pressure
    ☐ 3. increased muscle tension
    ☐ 4. decreased peristalsis

55. When planning the care of a client experiencing aggression, the nurse incorporates the principle of "least restrictive alternative," meaning that less restrictive interventions must be tried before more restrictive measures are employed. What measure should the nurse consider to be the **most** restrictive?
    ☐ 1. tension-reduction strategies
    ☐ 2. haloperidol given orally
    ☐ 3. voluntary seclusion or time-out
    ☐ 4. haloperidol given intramuscularly

56. An angry client becomes more agitated while talking about problems. The nurse decides to ask for staff assistance in taking control of the situation when the client demonstrates which behavior?
    ☐ 1. swearing about a spouse's behaviors when discussing marital problems
    ☐ 2. picking up a pool cue stick and telling the nurse to get out of the way
    ☐ 3. making a fist and pounding loudly on the table
    ☐ 4. coming out of the room instead of staying in time-out

57. When a client is about to lose control, the extra staff who come to help commonly stay at a distance from the client unless asked to move closer by the nurse who is talking to the client. What statement **best** explains the primary rationale for staying at a distance initially?
    ☐ 1. The client is more likely to act out if there is an audience, even additional staff.
    ☐ 2. The nurse talking to the client makes the decisions about other staff actions.
    ☐ 3. The client is likely to perceive others as being closer than they are and feel threatened.
    ☐ 4. When the extra staff is visible, the client is less likely to regain self-control.

58. When preparing to use seclusion as an alternative to restraint for a client who has not yet lost control, the nurse expects to use a room with limited furniture and no access to dangerous articles. What should the nurse also consider as critical for the safety of the client?
    ☐ 1. a security window in the door or a room camera
    ☐ 2. lights that can be dimmed from outside the room
    ☐ 3. a staff member to stay in the room with the client
    ☐ 4. a prescription for the seclusion before it is initiated

59. The nurse is required initially to restrain all four of a client's extremities. For what reason would the nurse anticipate the need to add a full-length restraint blanket?
    ☐ 1. The client states that restraints are tight and uncomfortable.
    ☐ 2. There is a medical need to maintain body alignment.
    ☐ 3. The client is at risk for injury from fighting the restraints.
    ☐ 4. Staff assessment reveals that the client will feel more secure under the blanket.

60. A client who has lost control has been put into restraints. Which nursing intervention is the **highest priority** when a client is placed in restraints?
    ☐ 1. monitoring the client every 15 minutes
    ☐ 2. assisting with nutrition and elimination
    ☐ 3. performing range-of-motion exercises for each limb, one at a time
    ☐ 4. changing the client's position every 2 hours

61. According to hospital protocol, after a client is restrained, the staff meet and discuss the restraint situation. In addition to sharing feelings and offering support, the nurse should identify which long-term goal for the debriefing?
    ☐ 1. providing feedback to each other on how procedures were handled
    ☐ 2. comparing the perceptions of the various staff members
    ☐ 3. deciding when to release the client from restraints
    ☐ 4. improving the staff's use of restraint procedures

The Client with Interpersonal Violence

62. A client has a history of violence toward others and an inability to cope with anger. What should the nurse use as the **most** important indicator of goal achievement before discharge?
    ☐ 1. acknowledgment of the client's angry feelings
    ☐ 2. ability to describe situations that provoke angry feelings
    ☐ 3. development of a list of how anger has been handled in the past
    ☐ 4. verbalization of feelings in an appropriate manner

63. A client is admitted to the psychiatric hospital for evaluation after numerous incidents of threatening others, angry outbursts, and two episodes of hitting a coworker at the client's place of employment. The client is very anxious and tells the nurse, "I didn't mean to hit them. They made me so mad that I just couldn't help it. I hope I don't hit anyone here." To ensure a safe environment, what should the nurse do **first**?
☐ 1. Let other clients know that the client has a history of hitting others so that they will not provoke the client.
☐ 2. Put the client in a private room, and limit the client's time out of the room to when staff can be with the client.
☐ 3. Tell the client that hitting others is unacceptable behavior and ask the client to tell a staff member when feeling angry.
☐ 4. Obtain a prescription for a medication to be administered to decrease the client's anxiety and threatening behavior.

64. A client loses control and throws two chairs toward another client. What should the nurse do **next**?
☐ 1. Ask the client to go to the quiet area, and talk about the behavior.
☐ 2. Administer an oral as-needed (PRN) tranquilizer, and prepare for a show of determination.
☐ 3. Process the incident with the client, and discuss alternative behaviors.
☐ 4. Call for assistance to restrain the client, and administer a PRN intramuscular tranquilizer.

65. A female client who was raped in their home was brought to the emergency department by their spouse. After being interviewed by the police, the spouse talks to the nurse. "I don't know why they didn't keep the doors locked like I said. I can't believe they had sex with another person now." How should the nurse respond?
☐ 1. "Let's talk about how you feel. Maybe it would help to talk to other people who have been through this."
☐ 2. "Maybe the doors were locked, but the rapist broke in anyway."
☐ 3. "Your spouse needs your support right now, not your criticism."
☐ 4. "It wasn't consensual sex. Let's see if your spouse was physically injured."

66. A 75-year-old female client was brought to the crisis center by their spouse. The spouse reports that the client has been in shock and anxious since their purse was stolen outside of their home. The client blames themself for being robbed, is worried about their stolen wallet and credit cards, and is afraid to go home. What nursing action(s) would be indicated? Select all that apply.
☐ 1. Request a prescription for lorazepam to decrease the client's anxiety.
☐ 2. Encourage the client to talk about the robbery and their feelings.
☐ 3. Discuss what changes at home would help them feel safe.
☐ 4. Investigate if the client has physical injuries from the robbery.
☐ 5. Ask the client what they think they could have done to prevent the robbery.

67. A 35-year-old has been killed as a result of a terrorist attack. What should the nurse advise the friends and relatives of the victim to do during the early stages of the recovery process? Select all that apply.
☐ 1. Keep in contact with other family and friends.
☐ 2. Attend memorial or religious services.
☐ 3. Use relaxation techniques and physical activities.
☐ 4. Speak out publicly about the impact of the loss.
☐ 5. Attend community meetings with others who have lost loved ones.

Managing Care, Quality, and Safety of Clients with Stress, Crisis, Anger, and Violence

68. STEP 1

The nurse cares for a 55-year-old male client brought to the hospital on 48-hour emergency detention.

Nurse's Notes

1800:
A court order for 48-hour emergency detention and psychiatric evaluation was obtained after reports that the client had not left their car for three nights. The client appears badly disheveled and dehydrated. The client states, "My spouse kicked me out and is divorcing me. It wasn't my fault I was fired from work. My spouse and boss are plotting against me because I'm smarter than they are." The client refused to cooperate and became very agitated when it was attempted to take vital signs. The client pounded their fists on the table and stated, "I'm not staying here, and you can't stop me."

➢ What are the top **four** findings that require immediate follow-up?

- ☐ 1. Disheveled appearance
- ☐ 2. Living in car
- ☐ 3. Impending divorce
- ☐ 4. Dehydration
- ☐ 5. Recent job loss
- ☐ 6. Threats to leave
- ☐ 7. Agitation
- ☐ 8. Refusal of vital signs

69. STEP 2

The nurse cares for a 55-year-old male client brought to the hospital on 48-hour emergency detention.

Nurse's Notes

1800:
A court order for 48-hour emergency detention and psychiatric evaluation was obtained after reports that the client had not left their car for three nights. The client appears badly disheveled and dehydrated. The client states, "My spouse kicked me out and is divorcing me. It wasn't my fault I was fired from work. My spouse and boss are plotting against me because I'm smarter than they are." The client refused to cooperate and became very agitated when it was attempted to take vital signs. The client pounded their fists on the table and stated, "I'm not staying here, and you can't stop me."

The nurse obtains additional admission assessment data.

➢ Which assessment(s) would be essential for the nurse to obtain? Select all that apply.

- ☐ 1. Self-harm or violent urges
- ☐ 2. Feelings of depression, desperation, or rage
- ☐ 3. Normalcy of sensory and thought processes
- ☐ 4. Presence of medical issues, medications, or allergies
- ☐ 5. Contact information for the spouse
- ☐ 6. Recent eating and sleep patterns
- ☐ 7. Health-related goals
- ☐ 8. Use of alcohol, street drugs, or tobacco

70. STEP 3

The nurse cares for a 55-year-old male client brought to the hospital on 48-hour emergency detention.

Nurse's Notes

1800:
A court order for 48-hour emergency detention and psychiatric evaluation was obtained after reports that the client had not left their car for three nights. The client appears badly disheveled and dehydrated. The client states, "My spouse kicked me out and is divorcing me. It wasn't my fault I was fired from work. My spouse and boss are plotting against me because I'm smarter than they are." The client refused to cooperate and became very agitated when it was attempted to take vital signs. The client pounded their fists on the table and stated, "I'm not staying here, and you can't stop me."

1830:
The client denies any significant medical history or substance use. When it was attempted to collect admission information, the client began pacing, hyperventilating, and pounding their fists into each other. The client had difficulty focusing to answer admission questions.

➢ Complete the following sentences from the list of drop-down options.

The client is most likely manifesting signs of [anxiety. / delirium. / mania.]

The nurse should prioritize [using de-escalation strategies. / managing the confusion. / administering antipsychotics.]

71. STEP 4

The nurse cares for a 55-year-old male client brought to the hospital on 48-hour emergency detention.

Nurse's Notes

1800:
A court order for 48-hour emergency detention and psychiatric evaluation was obtained after reports that the client had not left their car for three nights. The client appears badly disheveled and dehydrated. The client states, "My spouse kicked me out and is divorcing me. It wasn't my fault I was fired from work. My spouse and boss are plotting against me because I'm smarter than they are." The client refused to cooperate and became very agitated when it was attempted to take vital signs. The client pounded their fists on the table and stated, "I'm not staying here, and you can't stop me."

1830:
The client denies any significant medical history or substance use. When it was attempted to collect admission information, the client began pacing, hyperventilating, and pounding their fists into each other. The client had difficulty focusing to answer admission questions.

The nurse begins to create the plan of care.

➢ What intervention(s) should be included in the client's **immediate** plan of care? Select all that apply.

- ☐ 1. obtaining collateral information from the spouse and boss
- ☐ 2. anxiety and anger management
- ☐ 3. appropriate housing
- ☐ 4. divorce counseling
- ☐ 5. assault and escape precautions
- ☐ 6. suspiciousness and grandiosity issues

72. STEP 5

The nurse cares for a 55-year-old male client brought to the hospital on 48-hour emergency detention.

Nurse's Notes

1800:
A court order for 48-hour emergency detention and psychiatric evaluation was obtained after reports that the client had not left their car for three nights. The client appears badly disheveled and dehydrated. The client states, "My spouse kicked me out and is divorcing me. It wasn't my fault I was fired from work. My spouse and boss are plotting against me because I'm smarter than they are." The client refused to cooperate and became very agitated when it was attempted to take vital signs. The client pounded their fists on the table and stated, "I'm not staying here, and you can't stop me."

1830:
The client denies any significant medical history or substance use. When it was attempted to collect admission information, the client began pacing, hyperventilating, and pounding their fists into each other. The client had difficulty focusing to answer admission questions.

Orders

1. Admit to a locked mental health unit on 48-hour emergency detention.
2. Follow routine unit orders.
3. Obtain a psychiatric consult.

After reviewing the orders, the nurse educates the client about their rights during their admission to the mental health unit.

➢ What right(s) would the nurse tell the client they retain? Select all that apply.

- ☐ 1. to have reasonable access to a telephone to make and receive confidential calls
- ☐ 2. to refuse medical treatment or treatment with medications except in an emergency
- ☐ 3. to leave the hospital against medical advice
- ☐ 4. to have or not have other persons notified if they are hospitalized
- ☐ 5. to decline to take part in any research project or medical experiment

73. STEP 6

The nurse cares for a 55-year-old male client brought to the hospital on 48-hour emergency detention.

Nurse's Notes

1800:
A court order for 48-hour emergency detention and psychiatric evaluation was obtained after reports that the client had not left their car for three nights. The client appears badly disheveled and dehydrated. The client states, "My spouse kicked me out and is divorcing me. It wasn't my fault I was fired from work. My spouse and boss are plotting against me because I'm smarter than they are." The client refused to cooperate and became very agitated when it was attempted to take vital signs. The client pounded their fists on the table and stated, "I'm not staying here, and you can't stop me."

1830:
The client denies any significant medical history or substance use. When it was attempted to collect admission information, the client began pacing, hyperventilating, and pounding their fists into each other. The client had difficulty focusing to answer admission questions.

Day 3, 0900:
The client is alert and oriented and denies any urges to harm self or others. The client is showering without being told. The client is eating 75% of their meals and slept 4 hours last night. The client states that they are ready for discharge. They report that they have the names and phone numbers of two divorce lawyers. They also have a list of support persons and community resources.

Orders
1. Admit to a locked mental health unit on 48-hour emergency detention.
2. Follow routine unit orders.
3. Obtain a psychiatric consult.

The client received the diagnosis of acute stress disorder after the psychiatric evaluation. The nurse is evaluating the client's readiness to be discharged to outpatient treatment.

➤ Highlight findings that suggest the client is ready for discharge. Answer choices have been underlined.

Nurse's Notes

Day 3, 0900:
The <u>client is alert and oriented</u> and <u>denies any urges to harm self or others</u>. The client is <u>showering without being told</u>. The client is <u>eating 75% of their meals</u> and <u>slept 4 hours last night</u>. The <u>client states that they are ready for discharge</u>. They <u>report that they have the names and phone numbers of two divorce lawyers</u>. They also <u>have a list of support persons and community resources</u>.

---

74. The nurse manager on a psychiatric unit is reviewing the outcomes of staff participation in an aggression management program. What indicator would the nurse use to evaluate the effectiveness of such a program?
☐ 1. fewer client injuries during restraint procedures
☐ 2. a reduction of complaints by clients' relatives
☐ 3. fewer staff injuries during restraint procedures
☐ 4. a reduction in the total number of restraint procedures

75. A young female client has been stalked and then beaten by an ex-partner. Treatment of injuries is complete, and the client is ready for discharge. What should the nurse do to ensure the client's safety and security prior to discharge? Select all that apply.
☐ 1. Determine if the client knows the location of the ex-partner.
☐ 2. Ask if the client plans to see the ex-partner again.
☐ 3. Provide information on resources and a safety plan.
☐ 4. Ensure that the client has a safe place to stay after discharge.
☐ 5. Obtain consent to send emergency department records to the client's family health care provider.

76. The nurse is planning care for a group of clients. Which client should the nurse identify as needing the **most** assistance in accepting being ill?
☐ 1. 8-year-old male client who alternately cries for their parent and is angry with the nurse about being hospitalized after a bike accident
☐ 2. 32-year-old female client diagnosed with depression related to lupus erythematosus who discusses their medication's adverse effects with the nurse
☐ 3. 45-year-old male client who recently experienced a severe myocardial infarction and talks to the nurse about concerns regarding resuming sexual relations with their spouse
☐ 4. 60-year-old female client diagnosed with chronic obstructive pulmonary disease who refuses to wear an oxygen mask even though poor oxygenation makes them confused

77. The nurse is managing the care of a client in a disaster shelter who broke a femur and has lost their family home in a hurricane. What measure(s) should the nurse take? Select all that apply.
☐ 1. Supervise the care provided to the client during the crisis.
☐ 2. Obtain a prescription for antipsychotic medications for the client.
☐ 3. Act as a client advocate for the client in crisis.
☐ 4. Discuss with the interdisciplinary team available community resources for the client.
☐ 5. Obtain accurate identification, including name, age, address, contact information, and names of relatives.

78. During a meeting with nurse managers from the crisis intake unit, acute mental health unit, and mental health long-term care unit, the hospital risk manager says, "Approximately 57% of our client safety problems can be directly attributed to poor handoffs." What solution might the nurse managers implement to improve these statistics?
☐ 1. All shift handoff reports should be face to face instead of being tape-recorded.
☐ 2. Nursing staff should complete a checklist to take more care in interpreting primary health care provider prescriptions.
☐ 3. Nursing staff should complete and document admission history and physicals within 1 hour of arrival on a unit.
☐ 4. Initiate a template of transfer information to be communicated when a client is transferred from one care setting to another.

79. The nurse teaches a client about the benefits of participation in self-help groups. What information does the nurse include in the teaching plan? Select all that apply.
☐ 1. It increases knowledge about mental illness.
☐ 2. It develops stronger social networks and support.
☐ 3. It is more cost-effective than hospitalization.
☐ 4. It increases the client's sense of well-being.
☐ 5. It facilitates the development of advocacy skills.

80. During a unit meeting attended by clients and staff, several clients are criticizing their primary nurses. These clients have also been intimidating two other clients who have recently been admitted to the unit, and now the new clients have stopped sharing their opinions during the meeting. What is the **first** action for the nurse to take?
☐ 1. Help the new clients express the reasons they have stopped sharing their ideas.
☐ 2. Ask the clients criticizing their nurses to suggest some possible solutions for the practices they are criticizing.
☐ 3. Give the clients who are publicly criticizing the nurses a verbal warning that this behavior is not acceptable.
☐ 4. Use the next unit meeting to discuss respect and the importance of collaboration with the treatment team.

81. Two nurses disagree on what is the most important information for a client with a stress-related illness to have during a discharge teaching session. How should the nurse assigned to provide the discharge teaching proceed?
☐ 1. Share all the information that both nurses thought was important.
☐ 2. Review the policies related to required discharge teaching.
☐ 3. Be aware of different interpretations and personal biases held by nurses.
☐ 4. Ask the client what is most important for them as they prepare for discharge.

82. Despite education and role-play practice of restraint procedures, a staff member is injured when actually restraining a client. When helping the uninjured staff deal with the incident, the nurse should address which factor?
☐ 1. The emotional responses may be similar to those of other crime victims.
☐ 2. The member is likely to resign after experiencing such an injury.
☐ 3. Legal action against the client will take time and energy.
☐ 4. The member must debrief with the assaultive client before returning.

83. A nurse calls the unit manager to report that their purse has been stolen from the locked break room. The nurse says they think they know which staff stole the purse. Which action(s) by the nurse manager would be appropriate? Select all that apply.
  ☐ 1. Confront the person the nurse suspects stole the purse.
  ☐ 2. Call hospital security to initiate an investigation.
  ☐ 3. Ask the nurse to document all the facts related to the stolen purse.
  ☐ 4. Alert nursing administration that a staff's purse has been stolen.
  ☐ 5. Ask other staff to report any suspicious activity they may have observed.

84. A nurse's ex-partner enters the unit and states, "If I can't have them, no one will." Hospital security escorts the ex out of the building and warns them not to return. The unit manager holds a staff meeting to confirm that which workplace violence policy or procedure will be implemented? Select all that apply.
  ☐ 1. Give a quick overview of the hospital's workplace violence policies and procedures.
  ☐ 2. Offer counseling for the nurse and any other staff threatened by their ex-partner.
  ☐ 3. Work with security and the nurse to initiate workplace precautions related to the ex-partner.
  ☐ 4. Ask security to help the nurse understand how to initiate a protective order against the nurse's ex-partner.
  ☐ 5. Ask the nurse to take a leave of absence until their ex-partner is notified of the protective order.

Answers, Rationales, and Test-Taking Strategies

*The answers and rationales for each question follow below, along with keys (🔑) to the client need (CN) and cognitive level (CL) for each question. In addition, questions that measure clinical judgment will be coded (CJ). As you check your answers, use the **Content Mastery and Test-Taking Skill Self-Analysis** worksheet (tear-out worksheet in the back of the book) to identify the reason(s) for not answering the questions correctly. For additional information about test-taking skills and strategies for answering questions, refer to pages 12–51 in Part 1 of this book.*

The Client Managing Stress

1. 4. The client expressing doubts about their spouse's response to their amputation, as well as possible doubt on the client's part, is still struggling with body image issues. Looking forward to participating in walkathons and helping others indicate plans for the future that imply an acceptance of their amputee status. Remembering that their friend died in the accident that caused their amputation indicates that the client is aware that there was a worse end result to the accident than their amputation.

🔑 CN: Psychosocial integrity; CL: Evaluate

2. 1. Anxiety, especially at higher levels, interferes with learning and memory retention. After the client's anxiety lessens, it will be easier for the client to learn the steps of blood glucose monitoring. Because the client's illness is a chronic, lifelong illness that severely changes lifestyle, it is unlikely that the client is uninterested in the illness or how to treat it. It is also unlikely that dementia would be the cause of the client's frustration and lack of memory. The client's response indicates anxiety. Client responses that would indicate lessening anxiety would be questions to the nurse or requests to repeat part of the instruction.

🔑 CN: Psychosocial integrity; CL: Analyze

3. 3. With mild anxiety, perceptions are accurate. Slight muscle tension reflects a motor response. Occasional irritability is an emotional response. Loss of contact with reality is a cognitive characteristic of severe anxiety.

🔑 CN: Psychosocial integrity; CL: Analyze

4. **2.** Mild anxiety motivates the client to focus on issues and resolve them. Therefore, learning and problem solving can occur at a mild level of anxiety. Taking control of the client is reserved for a near-panic level of anxiety. Severe anxiety interferes with reasoning and functioning. Therefore, reducing stimuli and pressure is crucial at a severe level. Tension reduction is appropriate at a moderate level to help the client think more clearly and engage in problem solving.

CN: Psychosocial integrity; CL: Analyze

5. **4.** Minimal functioning, which can cause new problems to develop, is a reflection of dysfunctional coping. The ability to objectively and rationally solve problems demonstrates adaptive coping. Tension-reduction activities demonstrate palliative coping. However, such activities alone do not solve problems; they must be followed by problem solving. Anger management alone may prevent new problems, such as violence toward oneself or others, but it does not solve problems directly. It is considered maladaptive coping.

CN: Psychosocial integrity; CL: Analyze

6. **2.** When a client is experiencing severe anxiety, the nurse should use firm, short, and simple statements. Telling the client to drink milk is firm, short, and simple and provides the client with some protein. The statement, "You've got to take care of yourself" suggests that the client can solve the problem. Telling the client that the deceased person would not like to see the client like this puts blame on the anxious client. Asking the client, "When do you think you can take care of yourself?" implies that the client can make that decision. Clients with severe anxiety cannot make decisions, so providing an answer as to when they can perform self-care would not be possible at this time.

CN: Psychosocial integrity; CN: Apply

7. **4.** The client's statement that both the client and their spouse listen to each other reflects improved efforts at communicating about issues. The other statements provide some insight into the need for better communication; however, they are but steps along the way to coping effectively with the problem.

CN: Psychosocial integrity; CL: Evaluate

8. **1.** Assessment examines the client's thoughts, feelings, and behaviors within a context. Whether the client's behavior is appropriate for the situation is important assessment data. Setting priorities is part of making nursing diagnoses and planning; motivation to change and identifying the need for a safety plan are part of the planning stage.

CN: Psychosocial integrity; CL: Analyze

9. **3.** Writing a list of strengths and needs is short term, achievable, and measurable. Achieving positive self-esteem would occur over the long term. Going to school involves complex future steps to a long-term goal. Using skills is likely to be stressful and is best attempted after the client has done a self-assessment.

CN: Psychosocial integrity; CL: Analyze

10. **4.** The ultimate outcome is to have clients solve problems by themselves, collaborating in their own care. Client follow-up with mental health providers, while desirable, does not ensure that the client will fully comply with treatment or medication. Knowledge of the medication's effects and adverse effects and compliance can help the client, but it will not ensure success unless the client knows how to address and solve problems independently.

CN: Health promotion and maintenance; CL: Analyze

11. **1.** Substituting rational beliefs is a major goal when using cognitive-behavioral models, which focus more on thinking and behaviors than feelings. Unconscious processes are the focus of psychoanalytic models. Analysis of fears and barriers to growth is the focus of developmental models. Tension and stress are targets of the stress models.

CN: Psychosocial integrity; CL: Apply

12. **3.** Displacement refers to a defense mechanism that involves taking feelings out on a less-threatening object or person instead of tackling the issue or problem directly. Talking to their spouse directly reflects insight into the client's use of the defense mechanism and their ability to overcome it. Not thinking about the weekend is suppression. Here, the client is focusing on the issue with the highest priority. Focusing on academic rather than athletic achievement is compensation, highlighting one's strengths instead of weaknesses. Not remembering the molestation is repression.

CN: Psychosocial integrity; CL: Evaluate

13. **3.** Legally, there is a duty to warn a potential victim of a client's intent to harm. Staff can be held accountable if the client injures the ex-partner and the staff failed to warn that person. The client's permission is needed to share information with a spouse. Student papers should not contain identifying information. The release of information is made directly to the client's insurance company, not to the employer.

CN: Management of care; CL: Apply

14. **2.** The nurse is required to set limits on inappropriate behavior while conveying respect and acceptance of that person. Doing so conveys that the client is worthy without posing any harm or embarrassment to the client. Touch is a complex issue that must be used cautiously. Touch may be misinterpreted or misperceived by a client who has been abused or who has perceptual or thought disturbances. Mutual sharing reflects a social friendship, not a therapeutic one. Total confidentiality is not desirable. For example, treatment team members and insurance companies need selected information to ensure quality services.

CN: Psychosocial integrity; CL: Apply

15. 2. Growth of the fetus is important, so nausea and anorexia that would interfere with the client's nutrition would cause the most harm to the developing fetus. It could also lead to electrolyte imbalance if the client did not take in enough fluid. While insomnia could cause problems long term, this side effect could be mitigated through adjustment of the dosing time (earlier in the day), by decreasing the dosage to their former 20 mg daily, or by changing to every other day dosing of 40 mg since fluoxetine has a long half-life. Headaches are uncomfortable but can be treated with mild analgesic medication or other treatments, such as cold cloths, that would not harm the fetus. Decreased libido, while not enjoyable for the client or their sexual partner, does not pose any risks for the fetus.

CN: Pharmacological and parenteral therapy; CL: Analyze

16. 3. Asking for descriptions of changes in behavior (what the client did differently) encourages evaluation. Conveying empathy, such as stating that it is still hard for the client to talk about it, encourages data collection. Asking for meaning helps with the nursing diagnosis. Asking the client about what it will take to follow out a plan is part of planning.

CN: Psychosocial integrity; CL: Apply

17. 4. Practicing new behaviors builds confidence and reinforces appropriate behaviors. Reality testing, asking about fears, and teaching new communication skills are some of the many steps when trying out new behaviors.

CN: Psychosocial integrity; CL: Apply

The Client Coping with Physical Illness

18. 4. While the client does have a right to accept or reject treatment, the client has not explored their feelings, their possible mastectomy, or the future. The nurse should assist the client in exploring their feelings and moving toward a fuller understanding of their options. Giving the client survival rates indicates that the nurse feels they should have the surgery and negates their fears and concerns. The health care provider would need to be notified if the client decided not to have treatment or there were concerns that a mental health referral was needed, but this step should be done after the client has explored their feelings.

CN: Management of care; CL: Apply

19. 2. Diagnosis of a serious illness would be a shock to anyone but particularly a young person. Feelings of anger are normal and should be expressed. Gaining an intellectual understanding of their illness would also be necessary, but such learning will not take place if the client's feelings have not been addressed. There is no indication that the client needs to conserve energy because of the client's condition, nor is it clear that death is imminent. Neither situation is likely at the point of first diagnosis unless the disease is well advanced, which is not indicated here.

CN: Management of care; CL: Apply

20. 2. The psychotropic drugs used to treat chronic mental illnesses have side effects that can lead to noncompliance. Therefore, teaching the clients measures to deal with the common side effects would be most important. Teaching should be focused on the need for compliance and the specific interests of the target audience. Teaching should concentrate on the medications commonly used to treat chronic mental illness, not on many psychotropic drugs or those used in acute illness. Such topics as the role of medication in the treatment of chronic mental illness and the effects of using common street drugs with psychotropic medication should be discussed after the issue of compliance is addressed. Using medication reminders can be helpful, but choosing not to take medication because of side effects is a more common compliance problem that should be addressed first.

CN: Health promotion and maintenance; CL: Analyze

21. 2. When a client seems to be questioning the HCP's goals, it is best for the nurse to present an open statement and ask what the client means. This technique helps the client express feelings. Telling the client about the surgery is less therapeutic when the client is upset. While it is the client's right to get a second opinion, this suggestion does not address the client's feelings. Making assumptions can also interfere with communication, especially if the assumption is incorrect.

CN: Psychosocial integrity; CL: Analyze

22. **-/+ 2, 5.** When a client has hostile outbursts, it is best for the nurse to help the client express feelings. This serves as a release valve for the client. Keeping appropriate personal space helps the client from feeling overwhelmed or threatened while also protecting the nurse. Offering positive reinforcement for cooperation does not help the client express feelings appropriately. Continuing with assigned tasks ignores the client's feelings and may lead to further escalation. Limiting visitation reduces the client's support systems and does not address the underlying problem.

CN: Psychosocial integrity; CL: Apply

23. **3.** Preoperative visits and talks with others who have made successful adjustments to colostomies are helpful and tend to make the client less fearful of the operation and its consequences. Knowing about resources in the community will be helpful as the client approaches discharge. Supporting the HCP is less important than supporting the client and giving the client information. The client will have a change in body image, with disfigurement due to the creation of a colostomy. However, the client should be able to lead a full life.

CN: Management of care; CL: Apply

24. **2.** When people are experiencing moderate anxiety, their attention span is limited, and they are only able to focus on immediate concerns, so being brief and concise with communication initially is best. Giving the client too many detail or using medical terms prior to their knowing the immediate condition of their spouse, will just increase their anxiety. At this point, the client is also unable to focus on details such as paperwork as their immediate concern is the spouse.

CN: Psychosocial integrity; CL: Apply

25. **1.** Leaving the hospital and immediately flying to a meeting indicate poor judgment by the client and little understanding of what lifestyle changes the client needs to make. The other statements show that the client understands some of the changes that need to be made to decrease stress and lead a healthier lifestyle.

CN: Psychosocial integrity; CL: Evaluate

26. **-/+ 1, 3, 5.** Suicide is a risk with chronic illnesses. The spouse needs validation of their feelings and support as well as suggestions for helping the client with their concerns. Telling the client to be strong and optimistic ignores the client's needs. It is false to assume that the client will no longer be suicidal when the lupus is under control.

CN: Safety and infection control; CL: Analyze

27. **4.** The nurse's best response is one that directly expresses the nurse's observations to the client and offers the client the opportunity to talk about feelings or concerns to decrease somatization (the need to express feelings through physical symptoms). Leaving, offering to provide pain medication, and stating that anger does not bother the nurse are actions that ignore the client's needs.

CN: Psychosocial integrity; CL: Synthesize

28. **4.** Although ulcerative colitis and OCD have some features in common and stress can make both illnesses worse, there is no definitive cause-effect relationship between ulcerative colitis and OCD. Therefore, the only appropriate nursing response would be to acknowledge the effect of stress on both illnesses and indicate there is no proof that either illness causes the other.

CN: Physiological adaptation; CL: Analyze

29. **4.** This type of behavior illustrates *emotional lability*, which is a readily changeable or unstable emotional affect. *Neologism* is using a word when it can have two or more meanings, or a play on words. *Confabulation* involves replacing memory loss with fantasy to hide confusion; it is unconscious behavior. *Flight of ideas* refers to a rapid succession of verbal expressions that jump from one topic to another and are only superficially related.

CN: Psychosocial integrity; CL: Analyze

30. **2, 3, 1, 4.** The first priority is a safe environment so the client and nurse are not hurt by the phone. Then, it is important to acknowledge the client's anger to help diffuse it. As the client calms down, the nurse can explore the client's feelings in more depth. Since the client implies anger at God, a clergy consult may be appropriate.

CN: Safety and infection control; CL: Analyze

31. **3.** Focusing on enjoying time with family and friends conveys a renewal of hope for the future and a decreased risk for suicide. Simply saying that no one wants the client to commit suicide does not say the client does not want to do it. Avoiding a transfer to a psychiatric unit does not mean the client is no longer suicidal. Fear of not being successful with suicide usually is not a deterrent.

CN: Reduction of risk potential; CL: Evaluate

The Client in Crisis

32. 3. Individuals progress through the stages of loss at their own pace. Not everyone experiences each phase, and no one can be forced to advance to the next stage until ready. The best approach for helping the client to work through the pain of loss is to assist the client in processing and engaging in the pain of loss. This process may involve working on family conflicts or anger issues, but it is not the primary goal.

CN: Health promotion and maintenance; CL: Analyze

33. 2. During the first phase of crisis, the client exhibits elevated anxiety. A client who can use problem-solving capabilities is not in crisis. A shortened attention span is characteristic of the fourth phase of crisis. Reaching out to others for help is indicative of the third phase of crisis.

CN: Management of care; CL: Apply

34. 4. The nurse must first identify which member is exhibiting crisis symptoms. Next, the nurse would identify strategies to reduce the most severe symptoms. The nurse then assesses the family's resources. The family member in crisis may have such overwhelming feelings that they are unable to identify or describe the feelings.

CN: Psychosocial integrity; CL: Apply

35. 3. Before any interventions can occur, knowing whether the client is pregnant is crucial in formulating a plan of care. Asking the client about what things they had thought about doing, giving the client some ideas about what to expect next, and questioning the client about their feelings and possible parental reactions would be appropriate after it is determined that the client is pregnant.

CN: Psychosocial integrity; CL: Analyze

36. 1, 3, 4. To clearly define the problem, the nurse needs to assess the client's perception of the precipitating events. The question of whether anything upsetting happened to them within the past few days or weeks, what was happening in their life before they started to feel like hurting themselves, and requesting the client to describe how they are feeling all reflect how the client is perceiving the problem now. The questions about who can the client talk to when feeling overwhelmed or who is available to help them are situational support assessment questions.

CN: Psychosocial integrity; CL: Apply

37. 4. Because people in an emotional crisis find it difficult to focus their thinking, the goal is to return the client to noncrisis functioning. Pointing out and decreasing the client's level of anxiety is the first step in attaining this goal. Telling an obviously distressed person not to worry is ineffective because it ignores the client's distress and concerns. Although pregnancy is a normal event, and 40 years of age may not be too old for pregnancy, these responses also ignore the client's distress and feelings.

CN: Psychosocial integrity; CL: Analyze

38. 1. Telephoning the crisis shelter indicates that the children are alarmed but are reluctant to talk with their parents. They may fear that their parents will assume that they have been abusing inhalants and punish them. The nurse should focus on helping the children talk with their parents. The legality of using inhalants varies, but crisis hotlines are geared at providing supportive services. To prove that the observations are incorrect requires an intervention beginning with the children's parents. Inhalant abuse is a very dangerous, not minor, form of substance abuse.

CN: Management of care; CL: Analyze

39. 1. The crisis worker needs to use active focusing techniques to determine the crisis-precipitating event or the immediate problem. Asking the caller, "Why are you calling today?" or "What is the immediate problem?" will assist the caller to focus on the specific need or event. Telling the client to make an appointment is inappropriate because the problem might be life-threatening. Telling the caller to go to the nearest emergency department is precipitous and may be unnecessary. Asking to speak to someone else in the home may be futile because the caller might be alone. This action also ignores the caller and their feelings.

CN: Management of care; CL: Analyze

40. 3. The concern that someone may call the crisis hotline every day for a year indicates that further understanding of crisis and crisis intervention is needed. A crisis situation is time limited, typically resolving in 4 to 6 weeks if handled effectively. If a person calls the line daily for a year, that person has not been properly dealt with or is probably in a highly disorganized state requiring an alternative intervention. The nurse needs to further review and clarify the material presented. Callers are typically in pain, overwhelmed, and exhausted when they call. A crisis can help an individual cope better in the future if the individual learns to handle the situation.

CN: Management of care; CL: Evaluate

41. 2. Generally, 4 to 6 weeks is viewed as the length of time a client can tolerate the severe level of disturbance of a true crisis. In the first week or two, the client usually is still trying to use normal coping skills and support systems. After 6 weeks of continuous crisis, a client is probably becoming so physically and emotionally drained that the client has sought or has been brought by others for medical or psychiatric care.

🔑 CN: Management of care; CL: Apply

42. 1. The initial goal in crisis intervention is helping the client regain emotional security and equilibrium. Resolving the underlying emotional problems, developing insight and personal growth, and formulating more effective support systems are goals to address as the crisis subsides.

🔑 CN: Psychosocial integrity; CL: Apply

43. 3. Learning new coping skills is the major factor necessary for higher functioning. Better coping is likely to lead to regaining support systems, giving up dysfunctional coping, and awareness of how to prevent future crises.

🔑 CN: Psychosocial integrity; CL: Apply

44. 4. The statement about joining the child if they die indicates potential for self-harm and subsequent suicide, always a risk during crisis. Although the parent may be charged with reckless driving, this is not an indication for a psychiatric consultation. Verbalizing that the accident may lead to divorce may or may not be a real risk; however, this situation is not urgent. The statement about not seeing the child run behind the car illustrates the parent's attempts at trying to process the situation.

🔑 CN: Psychosocial integrity; CL: Evaluate

45. 1. Passive suicidal thoughts, such as a wish to die or giving up on self-care, can be as much of a risk as active suicidal ideation (the idea of killing oneself directly), especially for older clients because they commonly lack the means, energy, and motivation for an active suicide attempt. Seeing the grandson and grandmother together may help later. Not talking to the grandchild and experiencing altered role performance may be real issues, but these are not as critical as the risk for indirect (passive) suicide.

🔑 CN: Psychosocial integrity; CL: Analyze

46. 2. The threat toward the ex-partner is the most immediate concern now, as the client turns their anger toward their ex-partner instead of themselves. Although situational low self-esteem, risk for suicide, and risk-prone health behavior are evident, these problems are less of a concern at this time.

🔑 CN: Safety and infection control; CL: Analyze

47. 3. Letting the client express feelings (emotion management) is essential before trying to solve the problem or deciding what kind of referral is appropriate. A referral for counseling, assessment of the client's support system, and unemployment assistance may be appropriate after the client's anxiety is reduced.

🔑 CN: Psychosocial integrity; CL: Apply

48. 2. During a crisis, support persons demonstrate preparedness to help the client by verbalizing the emergency resources available and knowing when to use them. Follow-up medical care may be helpful as the crisis subsides. The coping strategies used by the support persons may or may not be relevant to the client's needs and situation. Long-term solutions and advice may or may not be appropriate. The focus needs to be on the client's immediate needs and situation.

🔑 CN: Psychosocial integrity; CL: Analyze

The Client with Problems Expressing Anger

49. 4. Beginning with an open-ended question that brings out the client's view of their situation and reasons for seeking treatment is the most neutral beginning and helps to gain the client's perception of events. Blaming the client for problems is accusatory and nonproductive. A time for reviewing what could have been done differently will come later.

🔑 CN: Psychosocial integrity; CL: Apply

50. 2, 4, 3, 1. Clients need to understand that anger is a normal emotion and if it is not expressed, it can have negative effects on the body and mind. Then, the nurse should begin to focus on the client's personal situation and help the client understand that holding in anger can aggravate depressive symptoms as well. One focus of outpatient counseling will be learning safe, effective ways to express anger.

🔑 CN: Reduction of risk potential; CL: Analyze

51. -/+ **1, 2, 3, 5.** Dealing with anger, stress, and anxiety; identifying resources and support groups; and increasing a sense of safety and security are appropriate interventions at this time. However, recommending an antiwar advocacy group may or may not be appropriate, even much later in the client's recovery.

🔑 CN: Psychosocial integrity; CL: Analyze

52. **2, 1, 4, 3.** Angry clients may not realize what makes them angry and the cues that their behavior is becoming out of control. The nurse should first help the client identify what triggered the anger. Once the cause of the anger and cues to the loss of control are discovered, the nurse should assist the client in identifying safe and appropriate alternative expressions of anger and then practice those techniques prior to facing a real anger-producing situation.

  CN: Psychosocial integrity; CL: Analyze

53. **3.** By requesting that the roommate respect the client's rights (asking the roommate to put the dirty clothes on the floor away after telling them that this bothers the client), the client is asserting themself. Arriving late is commonly passive resistance and thus not an indicator that the client is becoming assertive. Asking the nurse to call is dependent behavior. Although asking the HCP about being passive aggressive is more assertive, the client is relying on the nurse's direction to do so.

  CN: Psychosocial integrity; CL: Analyze

54. **2.** Blood pressure, as well as respiratory rate and muscle tension, increases during anger because of the autonomic nervous system's response to epinephrine secretion. Peristalsis decreases.

  CN: Physiological adaptation; CL: Apply

55. **4.** When given intramuscularly, haloperidol is considered most restrictive because it is intrusive and a client usually does not receive the drug voluntarily. Oral haloperidol is considered less restrictive because the client usually accepts the pill voluntarily. Tension-reduction strategies and voluntary seclusion are considered less restrictive because they are not intrusive and the client usually **consents** to their use.

  CN: Safety and infection control; CL: Apply

56. **2.** Asking the staff for assistance is appropriate when the client demonstrates behaviors that involve the direct threat of violence. Holding a stick and telling the nurse to move is the most direct threat of violence. Swearing and pounding on a table may be disturbing, but these actions are less of a threat. The client coming out of their room may indicate noncompliance with directions. However, further assessment is needed to determine whether this behavior was a direct threat of violence.

  CN: Management of care; CL: Analyze

57. **3.** A client who is about to lose control is experiencing a high degree of anxiety or agitation, which alters the client's ability to perceive reality. Initially, the client may feel threatened by the presence of others. A client who is out of control is not thinking about having an audience. Although the nurse with the client who is about to lose control is generally the one giving directions, this is not a rationale for staying at a distance. When seeing extra staff, the client may or may not be able to gain self-control.

  CN: Safety and infection control; CL: Apply

58. **1.** When using seclusion, the nurse understands that the safety of the client is paramount. Therefore, staff must be able to see the client in seclusion at all times, such as through a security window in the door or with a room camera. Although outside access for dimming the lights to decrease stimuli may be appropriate, it is not critical for the client's safety. Having one staff member stay in a room alone with a potentially violent client is unsafe. A prescription for seclusion can be obtained before or after it is initiated.

  CN: Safety and infection control; CL: Synthesize

59. **3.** A full-length restraint blanket is added when the client is at risk for injury from fighting the restraints. The increased degree of restriction is justified only when the risk for client injury increases and should not be used to treat other medical problems like alignment More. Client statements that restraints are tight and uncomfortable require the nurse to assess the situation and adjust the restraints if necessary to ensure adequate circulation. Four-way restraints already provide adequate protection for the staff.

  CN: Safety and infection control; CL: Apply

60. **1.** Safety of the client and staff is the utmost priority. Therefore, the client must be monitored closely and frequently, such as every 15 minutes, to ensure that the client is safe and free from injury. Assisting with nutrition and elimination, performing range-of-motion exercises on each limb, and changing the client's position every 2 hours are important after the safety of the client and staff is ensured by close, frequent monitoring.

  CN: Safety and infection control; CL: Analyze

61. **4.** The long-term goal of the debriefing after restraining a client is to improve aggression management procedures so that prevention of aggression improves and the frequency of restraint use decreases. Providing feedback and comparing perceptions are single aspects that would eventually lead to the ultimate goal of improving

The Client with Interpersonal Violence

62. 4. Verbalizing feelings, especially feelings of anger, in an appropriate manner is an adaptive method of coping that reduces the chance that the client will act out these feelings toward others. The client's ability to verbalize feelings indicates a change in behavior, a crucial indicator of goal achievement. Although acknowledging feelings of anger and describing situations that precipitate angry feelings are important in helping the client reach their goal, they are not appropriate indicators that behavior has changed. Asking the client to list how anger has been handled in the past is helpful if the nurse discusses coping methods with the client. However, based on this client's history, this would not be helpful because the nurse and client are already aware of the client's aggression toward others.

CN: Safety and infection control; CL: Evaluate

63. 3. The nurse must clearly address behavioral expectations, such as telling the client that hitting is unacceptable, and also provide alternatives for the client, such as letting staff members know when the client begins to feel angry. Making others responsible for the client's behavior or isolating the client in a room is inappropriate because it does not include the client in managing the behavior. Although medication may be helpful, this action does not give the client responsibility for the behavior and is not warranted at this time.

CN: Safety and infection control; CL: Apply

64. 4. The client is in the crisis phase of the assault cycle. Therefore, the nurse must act immediately, using restraints and an intramuscular tranquilizer to prevent injury to others or further property damage. It is too late to ask the client to go to a quiet area to talk because the client's behavior is past the triggering phase. Giving the client an oral tranquilizer and preparing for a show of determination are nursing interventions used in the escalation phase. Processing the incident with the client and discussing alternative behaviors are interventions used in the postcrisis phase.

CN: Safety and infection control; CL: Apply

65. 1. The nurse should respond to the spouse's needs and concerns and should offer support. Protecting or defending the client against criticism ignores the spouse's needs.

CN: Psychosocial integrity; CL: Apply

66. 2, 3, 4. After the impact of a crime, the client's most important needs are physical safety and emotional security. There is no indication that the client has a severe level of anxiety; therefore, lorazepam is not indicated. Asking the client how they could have prevented the robbery implies that they could be at fault.

CN: Psychosocial integrity; CL: Analyze

67. 1, 2, 3, 5. Receiving support from family, friends, other survivors, and community services is generally helpful after such events. Relaxation and participation in activities help manage stress reactions. Speaking out publicly may or may not be helpful later in the recovery process but may actually hinder recovery in the early stages.

CN: Psychosocial integrity; CL: Apply

Managing Care, Quality, and Safety of Clients with Stress, Crisis, Anger, and Violence

68.

STEP 1

1, 4, 6, 7. A client may be hospitalized against their will if there is reason to believe that they are a danger to themself or others or if they are perceived to be gravely disabled and unable to care for themselves. The most important things for the nurse to follow up on are immediate safety issues and the client's physical health. Agitation and threats to leave can easily progress to aggression and violence. Evidence of dehydration and extreme disheveled appearance indicate self-neglect, which may or may not be purposeful. Addressing possible homelessness, job loss, and impending divorce are issues that can be addressed after safety and physiological needs are met.

CJ: Case study; Step 1: Recognize cues; CL: Analyze

69.

STEP 2

1, 2, 3, 4, 6, 8. The client has been admitted against their will, so the nurse should focus on the most critical aspects of admission assessment necessary to keep the client safe. Self-harm urges, depression, desperation, and rage all are safety concerns. The nurse needs to assess if the client is oriented and in contact with reality. It is important to know if the client has any significant history, including the use of medications or allergies. The nurse should try to determine how the client has been sleeping and eating, especially as sleep deprivation can lead to psychosis. Finally, the nurse should determine the client's substance use patterns to help determine if withdrawal might occur. The client does not have to provide contact information for the spouse. The client is unlikely to share health-related goals since the hospitalization was not voluntary.

CJ: Case study; Step 2: Analyze cues; CL: Analyze

70.

STEP 3

0/1 *The client is most likely manifesting signs of* **anxiety**. *The nurse should prioritize using* **de-escalation strategies**.

The pacing, pounding fists, hyperventilating, and decreased attention suggest that the client is acutely experiencing a high level of anxiety. The nurse should implement de-escalation strategies to help prevent a panic attack. The client is not displaying high levels of energy, rapid speech, or flight of ideas to indicate experiencing a manic episode. Although the client is having difficulty focusing to answer questions, there is little evidence to suggest delirium, which is an acute state of confusion that is typically precipitated by a medical illness or injury.

🗝️ CJ: Case study; Step 3: Prioritize hypothesis; CL: Analyze

71.

STEP 4

−/+ 2, 5. The client is showing increased anxiety and anger as well as refusing to stay in the hospital, which are immediate and crucial concerns at admission. The client is not likely to give permission to talk to the spouse and boss at this point. Housing issues and divorce counseling may be relevant before discharge, but not initially. Suspiciousness and grandiosity may be relevant after the client's anxiety and anger are under control.

🗝️ CJ: Case study; Step 4: Generate solutions; CL: Apply

72.

STEP 5

−/+ 1, 2, 4, 5. When a client is committed involuntarily, the right to leave against medical advice is forfeited. All the other rights are preserved unless there is further court action or a case of imminent danger to self or others (hitting staff, cutting self). The client may refuse treatment, including medications, unless the situation is an emergency or a court judge has determined that the client is incapable of making their own decisions. Clients may make confidential phone calls and have the right to determine who or who will not be notified of their hospitalizations. The exception is if there is reason to believe that a person is at risk for harm. Then the duty to notify applies. Clients retain the right to decline to participate in research studies.

🗝️ CJ: Case study; Step 5: Take action; CL: Apply

73.

STEP 6

−/+ | **Nurse's Notes**

> **Day 3, 0900:**
> The client is alert and oriented and denies any urges to harm self or others. The client is showering without being told. The client is eating 75% of their meals and slept 4 hours last night. The client states that they are ready for discharge. They report that they have the names and phone numbers of two divorce lawyers. They also have a list of support persons and community resources.

The reasons for the hospitalization were to assess the client's safety risk and their ability to care for their basic needs. Being alert and oriented, denying urges to harm self or others, eating most of their meals, and taking care of basic hygiene needs indicate that the client has functional abilities. The risk for relapse persists for months after a crisis has abated. Therefore, it is important for the client to be able to verbalize information about appropriate support persons and community resources and to have this information readily available. Sleeping 4 only hours a night remains a risk factor. Although the client may state feeling ready to be discharged, this is not the most reliable indicator as the client did not want to be admitted. Having a divorce lawyer may or may not be appropriate at this point but does factor into determining if the client is ready for discharge.

🗝️ CJ: Case study; Step 6: Evaluate outcomes; CL: Evaluate

74. 4. The primary goal of an aggression management program is to prevent violence. This goal is evidenced by a reduction in the total number of restraint procedures used or needed. Although fewer client and staff injuries are important, these goals are secondary to prevention. Reduction in the number of complaints by clients' relatives is affected by more variables than just restraint procedures.

🗝️ CN: Management of care; CL: Evaluate

75. −/+ 1, 2, 3, 4. The crucial interventions involve safety and support. Asking for consent is a health privacy issue, not a safety issue, and is not essential to the discharge process.

🗝️ CN: Safety and infection control; CL: Apply

76. **4.** The 60-year-old female client is acting in a way that worsens their physical and mental condition because they do not want to be sick. The 8-year-old child is acting normally for someone their age who is unexpectedly hospitalized. The cooperation demonstrated by the client with lupus and the client who had a myocardial infarction indicates a level of acceptance of their illnesses and of their role as being ill.

CN: Management of care; CL: Analyze

77. **1, 3, 4, 5.** The nurse who is managing the care of the client in a disaster shelter provides for the management of care by supervising the care for the client in crisis. In a disaster, the nurse also must be sure that the client is identified and contact information about the client is documented. The nurse also acts as a client advocate for the client in crisis and discusses available community resources for the client with the interdisciplinary team assigned to this client. There are no data to indicate that antipsychotic medications are needed for this client at this time.

CN: Management of care; CL: Apply

78. **4.** Handoffs occur when a client is transferred from one care setting to another, or from one caregiver to another. The use of a template to standardize the information communicated at the time of transfer can address safety concerns. Giving a report face-to-face does not guarantee all critical information is included. Handoffs are not associated with admission history and physicals, though clinical guidelines often play a part in initiating care. Health care provider checklists may impact safety but are not part of the hand-off process.

CN: Management of care; CL: Analyze

79. **1, 2, 4.** Participation in self-help groups has been shown to increase knowledge, coping skills, self-esteem, confidence, sense of well-being, and a sense of being in control. Improving social and support networks is also a common outcome of client engagement in self-help groups. If symptoms are severe or life-threatening, hospitalization may be the most appropriate action and as a result potentially more cost-effective. The development of personal advocacy skills is not a primary outcome of client participation in self-help groups.

CN: Management of care; CL: Apply

80. **2.** Recognizing that the clients are part of the solution to the issues they are presenting demonstrates a client-centered approach to care. Having the new clients challenge the behaviors of other clients does not facilitate the development of a therapeutic milieu. Warning clients that behaviors are unacceptable reinforces a sense of client powerlessness and does not build a therapeutic relationship. Discussing respect and collaboration would happen after the criticisms have been acknowledged and the clients have been asked for their opinions.

CN: Management of care; CL: Apply

81. **4.** The discharge teaching session will be most effective if the nurse uses a client-centered approach to better assess what the client needs and, therefore, what information to share. Sharing all the information does not respect the knowledge that the client already has. Reviewing the policies is one area to help identify important areas for teaching, but to ensure that client needs are met, further assessment is required. Awareness of personal biases should not be used to determine what is important for the client.

CN: Management of care; CL: Apply

82. **1.** Being injured by a client can result in emotional responses similar to those of other crime victims. A resignation after being injured is relatively rare. Legal action against the client is sometimes discussed but rarely initiated. Debriefing with the client may be inappropriate or unnecessary to resolve the situation.

CN: Management of care; CL: Analyze

83. **2, 3, 4, 5.** It is appropriate for the nurse manager to initiate a security investigation and ask the nurse to document all the facts about the missing purse. Alerting nursing administration is required. Seeking information from other staff will help with the investigation. It is inappropriate to confront any possible suspects while the investigation is ongoing.

CN: Management of care; CL: Analyze

84. **1, 2, 3, 4.** National guidelines exist for managing workplace violence. Unit staff, hospital administration, and hospital security personnel develop and enforce the resulting policies. These include training all staff about workplace violence, processes for reporting such violence, and counseling for the staff victim. Protecting staff and clients may include posting the ex-partner's picture at employee entrances and a protective order initiated by the nurse. With these policies and procedures in place, it is counterproductive to ask the nurse to take a leave of absence.

CN: Management of care; CL: Analyze

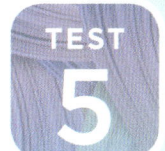

TEST 5: Abuse and Mental Health Problems of Children, Adolescents, and Families

- The Client Experiencing Abuse
- The Adolescent with Eating Disorders
- Children and Adolescents with Behavioral Problems
- The Child and Adolescent with Adjustment Disorders
- Children and Adolescents with Autism
- Managing Care, Quality, and Safety of Clients with Abuse and Mental Health Problems
- Answers, Rationales, and Test-Taking Strategies

The Client Experiencing Abuse

1. A married female client has been referred to the mental health center because they are depressed. The nurse notices bruises on their upper arms and asks about them. After denying any problems, the client starts to cry and says, "My spouse did not really mean to hurt me, but I hate for the kids to see this. I'm so worried about them." What is the **most** crucial information for the nurse to determine?
- ☐ 1. type and extent of abuse occurring in the family
- ☐ 2. potential of immediate danger to the client and their children
- ☐ 3. resources available to the client
- ☐ 4. whether the client wants to allow the spouse in the clinic

2. A client with suspected abuse describes their spouse as a good person who works hard and provides well for their family. The client does not work outside the home and states that they are proud to be a spouse and parent just like their own parent. The nurse interprets the family pattern described by the client as **best** illustrating which characteristic of abusive families?
- ☐ 1. tight, impermeable boundaries
- ☐ 2. unbalanced power ratio
- ☐ 3. role stereotyping
- ☐ 4. learned helplessness

3. The nurse plans the care for a client who is being abused. Which measure is **most** important to include?
- ☐ 1. being compassionate and empathetic
- ☐ 2. teaching the client about abuse and the cycle of violence
- ☐ 3. explaining to the client about the client's personal and legal rights
- ☐ 4. helping the client develop a safety plan

4. A nurse is assessing a client who is being abused. The nurse should assess the client for which characteristic(s)? Select all that apply.
- ☐ 1. assertiveness
- ☐ 2. self-blame
- ☐ 3. alcohol abuse
- ☐ 4. suicidal thoughts
- ☐ 5. guilt

5. After months of counseling, a client abused by their spouse tells the nurse that they have decided to stop treatment. There has been no abuse during this time, and they feel better able to cope with the needs of their spouse and children. How should the nurse begin the discussion of the decision with the client?
- ☐ 1. Tell the client that this is a bad decision that they will regret in the future.
- ☐ 2. Find out more about the client's rationale for their decision to stop treatment.
- ☐ 3. Warn the client that abuse commonly stops when one partner is in treatment, only to begin again later.
- ☐ 4. Remind the client of their duty to protect their children by continuing treatment.

6. A school-age child is referred to the mental health clinic by the school nurse because they are fearful, anxious, and socially isolated. After meeting with the client, the nurse talks with their parent, who says, "It's that school nurse again. They have done nothing but try to make trouble for our family since my child started school. And now you're in on it." What is the nurse's **most** appropriate response?
   ☐ 1. "The school nurse is concerned about your child and is only doing their job."
   ☐ 2. "You don't need to feel singled out. We see a number of children who go to your child's school."
   ☐ 3. "You sound pretty angry with the school nurse. Tell me what's happened."
   ☐ 4. "Let me tell you why your child was referred, and then you can tell me about your concerns."

7. The parent of a school-age child tells the nurse, "For most of the past year, my husband was unemployed, and I worked a second job. Twice during the year, I spanked my child repeatedly when they refused to obey. It hasn't happened again. Our family is back to normal." After assessing the family, the nurse decides that the child is still at risk for abuse. Which observation **best** supports this conclusion?
   ☐ 1. The parents say they are taking away privileges when their child refuses to obey.
   ☐ 2. The child has talked about family activities with the nurse.
   ☐ 3. The parents are less negative toward the nurse.
   ☐ 4. The child wears long-sleeved shirts and long pants, even in warm weather.

8. When caring for a client who was a victim of a crime, the nurse is aware that recovery from any crime can be a long and difficult process depending on the meaning it has for the client. Arrange the goals, in order from first to last, that the nurse expects the client to achieve as the client reconstructs their life. All options must be used.

   | 1. getting through the shock and confusion |
   | 2. carrying out home and work routines |
   | 3. resolving grief over any losses |
   | 4. regaining a sense of security and safety |
   | |
   | |
   | |

9. A client tells the nurse that they have been raped but have not reported it to the police. After determining whether the client was injured, whether it is still possible to collect evidence, and whether the client wants to file a report, the nurse's **next priority** is to offer which intervention to the client?
   ☐ 1. legal assistance
   ☐ 2. crisis intervention
   ☐ 3. rape support group
   ☐ 4. medication for disturbed sleep

10. The nurse cares for a client who was raped. Which intervention is **most** important for the nurse to implement?
    ☐ 1. continuing to encourage the client to report the rape to the legal authorities
    ☐ 2. recommending that the client resume sexual relations with their partner as soon as possible
    ☐ 3. periodically reminding the client that they did not deserve and did not cause the rape
    ☐ 4. telling the client that the rapist will eventually be caught, put on trial, and jailed

11. In the process of dealing with intense feelings about being raped, victims commonly verbalize that they were afraid they would be killed during the rape and wish that they had been. The nurse should decide that further counseling is needed if the client makes which statement?
    ☐ 1. "I didn't fight them, but I guess I did the right thing because I'm alive."
    ☐ 2. "Suicide would be an easy escape from all this pain, but I couldn't do it to myself."
    ☐ 3. "I wish they gave the death penalty to all rapists and other sexual predators."
    ☐ 4. "I get so angry at times that I have to have a couple of drinks before I sleep."

12. One of the myths about sexual abuse of young children is that it usually involves physically violent acts. Which behavior is more likely to be used by the abusers?
    ☐ 1. tying the child down
    ☐ 2. offers of payment with money
    ☐ 3. coercion as a result of the trusting relationship
    ☐ 4. bribery with expensive gifts

13. A preadolescent child is suspected of being sexually abused because they demonstrate the self-destructive behaviors of self-mutilation and attempted suicide. Which common behavior should the nurse also expect to assess?
    ☐ 1. inability to play
    ☐ 2. truancy and running away
    ☐ 3. head banging
    ☐ 4. overcontrol of anger

14. Adolescents and adults who were sexually abused as children commonly mutilate themselves. How does the nurse interpret this behavior? Select all that apply.
☐ 1. the need to make themselves less sexually attractive
☐ 2. an alternative to binging and purging
☐ 3. use of physical pain to avoid dealing with emotional pain
☐ 4. an alternative to getting high on drugs
☐ 5. an inability to express how they are feeling

15. A young child who has been sexually abused has difficulty putting feelings into words. Which approach should the nurse employ with the child?
☐ 1. engaging in play therapy
☐ 2. role-playing
☐ 3. giving the child's drawings to the abuser
☐ 4. reporting the abuse to a prosecutor

16. A client who has been sexually assaulted is admitted to the emergency department (ED). Which is the most important initial statement by the nurse?
☐ 1. "Did you know the person who did this to you?"
☐ 2. "I'll get the emergency rape kit."
☐ 3. "I'll stay with you while you're here."
☐ 4. "Don't worry, security guards protect this area."

17. A client reveals a history of childhood sexual abuse. What question should the nurse ask **first**?
☐ 1. "What other forms of abuse did you experience?"
☐ 2. "How long did the abuse go on?"
☐ 3. "Was there a time when you did not remember the abuse?"
☐ 4. "Does your abuser still have contact with young children?"

18. The nurse obtains a history from parents who are suspected of abusing their child. Which characteristic about the parents should the nurse **particularly** assess?
☐ 1. attentiveness to the child's needs
☐ 2. self-blame for the injury to the child
☐ 3. ability to relate the child's developmental achievements
☐ 4. difficulty with controlling aggression

19. A preschool-age child with a history of being abused has blood drawn. The child lies very still and makes no sound during the procedure. Which comment by the nurse would be **most** appropriate?
☐ 1. "It's okay to cry when something hurts."
☐ 2. "That really didn't hurt, did it?"
☐ 3. "We must seem mean to hurt you that way."
☐ 4. "You were very good not to cry with the needle."

20. The nurse interviews a preschool-age girl who has been sexually abused about the event. Which approach would be **most** effective?
☐ 1. Describe what happened during the abusive act.
☐ 2. Draw a picture, and explain what it means.
☐ 3. "Play out" the event using anatomically correct dolls.
☐ 4. Name the perpetrator.

21. The nurse performs a health assessment on a 15-month-old toddler. Which observation by the nurse suggests the toddler has been abused?

The child:
☐ 1. appears happy when personnel work with them.
☐ 2. plays alongside others contentedly.
☐ 3. is underdeveloped for their age.
☐ 4. sucks their thumb.

22. The nurse plans interventions for parents who are abusive. The nurse should incorporate knowledge of which factor as a common parental indicator?
☐ 1. lower socioeconomic group
☐ 2. unemployment
☐ 3. low self-esteem
☐ 4. loss of emotional family attachments

The Adolescent with Eating Disorders

23. An adolescent client is being admitted with an eating disorder. Which initial assessment finding is of **greatest** concern for the nurse?
☐ 1. systolic blood pressure of 86 mm Hg
☐ 2. weight loss of 10% over 6 months
☐ 3. potassium level of 2.5 mEq/L (2.5 mmol/L)
☐ 4. heart rate of 57 bpm

24. A hospitalized adolescent diagnosed with anorexia nervosa refuses to comply with their daily before-breakfast weigh-in. The client states that they just drank a glass of water, which they feel will unfairly increase their weight. What is the nurse's **best** response to the client?
☐ 1. "You're here to gain weight, so that will work in your favor."
☐ 2. "Don't drink or eat for 2 hours, and then I'll weigh you."
☐ 3. "You must weigh in every day at this time. Please step on the scale."
☐ 4. "If you don't get on the scale, I'll be forced to call your health care provider."

25. The nurse discovers that an adolescent client with anorexia nervosa is taking diet pills rather than complying with the diet. What should the nurse do **first**?
☐ 1. Explain to the client how diet pills can jeopardize health.
☐ 2. Listen to the client discuss fears of losing control of eating while being treated.
☐ 3. Talk with the client about how weight loss worries the health care provider (HCP).
☐ 4. Inquire about concerns of the client's family regarding the client's health.

26. The nurse teaches a group of adolescents about anorexia nervosa. The nurse should describe this disorder as being characterized by which factors?
☐ 1. excessive fear of becoming obese, near-normal weight, and a self-critical body image
☐ 2. obsession with the weight of others, chronic dieting, and an altered body image
☐ 3. extreme concern about dieting, calorie counting, and an unrealistic body image
☐ 4. intense fear of becoming obese, emaciation, and a disturbed body image

27. The nurse reviews laboratory work for a female client who is admitted to the acute psychiatric unit for an eating disorder.

Laboratory Results		
Test	Results	Normal Range
Albumin level	2.8 g/dL (28 g/L)	Adults: 3.5–5 g/dL (35–50 g/L)
Sodium level	145 mEq/L (145 mmol/L)	Adults: 135–145 mEq/L (135–145 mmol/L)
Hemoglobin level	10.8 g/dL (108 g/L)	Women: 12–16 g/dL (120–160 g/L)
Potassium level	2.7 mEq/L (2.7 mmol/L)	Adults: 3.5–5.2 mEq/L (3.5–5.2 mmol/L)
Hematocrit level	37% (0.37 proportion of 1.0)	Women: 36%–48% (0.36–0.48 proportion of 1.0)

Which finding(s) would the nurse report to the health care provider? Select all that apply.
☐ 1. albumin level
☐ 2. sodium level
☐ 3. hemoglobin level
☐ 4. potassium level
☐ 5. hematocrit level

28. The parents of an adolescent client newly diagnosed with anorexia nervosa are meeting with the nurse during the admission process. Which remark should the nurse interpret as typical for parents of a client with anorexia nervosa?
☐ 1. "We've given them everything, and look how they repay us!"
☐ 2. "They've had behavior problems for the past year both at home and at school."
☐ 3. "They've been a model child. We've never had any problems with them."
☐ 4. "We have five children, all normal kids with some problems at times."

29. A young adult client is brought to the emergency department by their roommate to seek treatment for gastrointestinal problems. The client reveals that they attend college and work at a coffee shop each evening. A diet history indicates that the client has unhealthy eating habits, commonly eating large amounts of carbohydrates and junk food with few fruits and vegetables. "Their stomach is upset a lot," the roommate says. The roommate further reports that the client is "in the bathroom all the time." Which referral is **most** important for the nurse to make for the client?
☐ 1. mental health clinic
☐ 2. weight-loss program
☐ 3. overeating support group
☐ 4. client's health care provider (HCP)

30. A nurse is working with a client with bulimia. Which goal(s) should be included in the care plan? Select all that apply.
The client will:
☐ 1. maintain a normal weight.
☐ 2. comply with medication therapy.
☐ 3. achieve a positive self-concept.
☐ 4. acknowledge the disorder.
☐ 5. never have the desire to purge again.

31. A nurse works with a client diagnosed with bulimia. What is the **most** appropriate long-term client goal for this client?
☐ 1. Eat meals at home without binging or purging.
☐ 2. Be able to eat out without binging or purging.
☐ 3. Manage stresses in life without binging or purging.
☐ 4. Be able to attend college without binging or purging.

32. A client newly diagnosed with bulimia is attending the nurse-led group at the mental health center. The client tells the group that they only came because their spouse said they would divorce the client if the client did not get help. Which response by the nurse is appropriate?
- ☐ 1. "You sound angry with your spouse. Is that correct?"
- ☐ 2. "You'll find that you like coming to group. These people are a lot of fun."
- ☐ 3. "Tell me more about why you're here and how you feel about that."
- ☐ 4. "Tell me something about what has caused you to be bulimic."

33. A client diagnosed with bulimia tells the nurse that they only eat excessively when upset with their best friend and then they vomit to avoid gaining a lot of weight. What should the nurse do **next**?
- ☐ 1. Schedule daily family therapy sessions.
- ☐ 2. Enroll the client in a coping skills group.
- ☐ 3. Work with the client to limit purging.
- ☐ 4. Obtain an as-needed (PRN) prescription for lorazepam.

34. A community health nurse working with a group of fifth-grade girls is planning primary prevention to help the girls avoid developing eating disorders during their teen years. The nurse should focus on which factor(s)? Select all that apply.
- ☐ 1. working with the school nurse to closely monitor the girls' weight during middle school
- ☐ 2. discussing ways to build positive self-esteem
- ☐ 3. limiting the girls' access to media images of very thin models and celebrities
- ☐ 4. telling the girls' parents to monitor their daughter's weight and media access
- ☐ 5. helping the girls accept and appreciate their bodies

Children and Adolescents with Behavioral Problems

35. An adolescent client who has been taking an antidepressant for 6 weeks has returned to the clinic for a medication check. When the nurse talks with the client and their parent, the parent reports that they have to remind the client to take their antidepressant every day. The client says, "Yeah, I'm pretty bad about remembering to take my meds, but I never miss a dose because my parent always bugs me about taking it." Which response would be effective for the nurse to make to the client?
- ☐ 1. "It's a good thing your parent takes care of you by reminding you to take your meds."
- ☐ 2. "It seems there are some difficulties with being responsible for your medications that we need to address."
- ☐ 3. "You'll never be able to handle your medication administration at college next year if you are so dependent on your parent."
- ☐ 4. "I'm surprised your parent allows you to be so irresponsible."

36. The nurse assesses a school-age client who excessively cleans and categorizes. The parents report that the client has always been orderly, but since the client's sibling died of cancer 6 months ago, the cleaning and categorizing have escalated. In school, the client reads instead of playing with other children. These behaviors are now interfering with homework and leisure activities. To bolster the client's self-esteem, the nurse should encourage the child to engage in which activity?
- ☐ 1. Serve as a library helper.
- ☐ 2. Volunteer to organize a party for the class.
- ☐ 3. Lead a group project with four peers.
- ☐ 4. Be a member of the kickball team.

37. An adolescent is a heavy user of marijuana and alcohol. When the nurse confronts the client about their drug and alcohol use, they admit previous heavy use to feel more comfortable around peers and achieve social acceptance. They say they have been trying to stay clean since their parents found out and had them seek treatment. When the nurse develops a plan of care with the client, what should be the **highest priority** to help them maintain sobriety?
- ☐ 1. peer recognition that does not involve substance use
- ☐ 2. support and guidance from their parents
- ☐ 3. a strict no-drug policy at their high school
- ☐ 4. the threat of legal charges if caught drinking or smoking marijuana

38. An adolescent client is admitted to a psychiatric day treatment program due to severe lower back pain since their parent's death 3 years ago. Medical examinations have not discovered a physical cause for the pain. The client cares for four younger siblings after school and on weekends because of their other parent's long work hours. Which predischarge statement indicates that treatment for their condition has been successful?
☐ 1. "I understand now why my father spends so much time away from home."
☐ 2. "My back pain is worse on weekends with more responsibility and homework."
☐ 3. "I don't want to talk about my family. It's my back that's hurting."
☐ 4. "I just need more rest and relaxation, and then my back will feel fine."

39. When collaborating with the health care provider to develop the plan of care for a child diagnosed with attention deficit hyperactivity disorder (ADHD), the treatment plan will likely include which treatment?
☐ 1. antianxiety medications, such as buspirone, and homeschooling
☐ 2. antidepressant medications, such as imipramine, and family therapy
☐ 3. anticonvulsant medications, such as carbamazepine, and monthly blood levels
☐ 4. psychostimulant medications, such as methylphenidate, and behavior modification

40. The nurse meets with the parent of a child diagnosed with attention deficit hyperactivity disorder. The parent states, "I feel so guilty that they have this disease, like I did something wrong. I feel like I need to be with my child constantly for them to get better. But still, sometimes I feel like I'm going to lose control and hurt them." The nurse should suggest which intervention to the parent?
☐ 1. arranging for respite care to watch the child and give the parent a regular break
☐ 2. taking a job to allow the parent to feel some success because their child will not ever improve
☐ 3. arranging to have coffee with friends daily as a way to begin a support group
☐ 4. considering foster care if they feel that they cannot handle their child's problems

41. The nurse is with the parents of an adolescent client who recently attempted suicide. The nurse cautions the parents to be especially alert for which changes in their child?
☐ 1. expression of a desire to date
☐ 2. decision to try out for an extracurricular activity
☐ 3. giving away valued personal items
☐ 4. desire to spend more time with friends
☐ 5. engaging in more risk-taking or reckless behaviors

42. An adolescent client has struggled academically throughout high school and realizes during their last semester in school that they are not going to graduate with their class, which will delay admission to college. In the past, the client has intermittently used drugs and alcohol to deal with anxiety, but now their involvement with substances escalates to daily use. In what order of priority from first to last should the nurse, who has become aware of the problem, take the actions? All options must be used.
Refer the client to:
☐ 1. the school authorities to address academic issues so they can graduate next semester.
☐ 2. a program at the local community college to improve their readiness for college and decrease anxiety.
☐ 3. an outpatient program that treats clients with chemical dependency issues.
☐ 4. a psychiatric clinic so they can get an appropriate diagnosis and medication for their anxiety.

43. A parent states to the nurse in the health care provider's (HCP's) office that they are frustrated regarding their school-age child's nightly enuresis for the past 3 years. The client says they have limited evening fluids, eliminated all caffeine and soft drinks from their diet, and have had them wash their own sheets, but their child still wets the bed almost every night. The spouse has told the parent that they were a bed wetter as a child. The spouse thinks the child will "get over it." The parent is worried that it could negatively affect the child's peer relationships as they grow older. Which action should the nurse take?
☐ 1. Reinforce that the parent should be patient since their spouse's enuresis stopped without intervention.
☐ 2. Suggest asking the HCP about medication treatment to deal with the enuresis.
☐ 3. Discuss a behavioral treatment plan to improve the child's social skills.
☐ 4. Suggest the parent ask the HCP about a complete renal workup.

44.

Medical Record			
Weights	October 10 56.9 lb (25.8 kg)	November 10 55.1 lb (25 kg)	December 10 51.8 lb (23.5 kg)
Nurse's Notes	10/10 – An 8-year-old otherwise healthy child begins methylphenidate extended release for a diagnosis of attention deficit hyperactivity disorder (ADHD). 11/10 – The parents state school performance has improved, but it is difficult to get the client up and ready for school in the morning unless they are given the medication as soon as they awaken. 12/12 – The client continues to do well at school, but the parents report the child does not eat breakfast or very much of their lunch at school; the child eats dinner, but only an average amount of food.		

Which action should the nurse suggest the parent do **first**?
- ☐ 1. Have the child eat a breakfast bar, banana, and a glass of milk at their bedside at the same time they take their medication every morning.
- ☐ 2. Monitor the child's weight closely for a month since they are likely to stop losing weight when the school year ends in 2 weeks.
- ☐ 3. Request a change of medication to a nonstimulant drug that will treat the client's ADHD without causing their appetite to decrease.
- ☐ 4. Supplement that the parent supplement the child's dinner with a high-protein drink or other food that will increase their caloric intake.

45. An adolescent is brought to the emergency department (ED) after accidentally taking an overdose of heroin. The adolescent is semiconscious, unable to respond appropriately to questions, slurs words, and has constricted pupils; the client's vital signs are blood pressure 60/50 mm Hg, pulse 50 bpm, and respirations 8 breaths/min. Naloxone is administered to temporarily reverse the effects of the heroin. Which finding would **first** indicate that the naloxone administration has been effective?
- ☐ 1. The client's blood opiate level drops to a nontoxic level.
- ☐ 2. The client becomes talkative and physically active.
- ☐ 3. The client's memory and attention become normal.
- ☐ 4. The client's respirations improve to 12 breaths/min.

46. The nurse caring for pediatric clients performs a suicide risk assessment. What information does the nurse need to know about suicide risk in children and adolescents?
- ☐ 1. Children rarely commit suicide unless one of their parents has already committed suicide, especially in the past year.
- ☐ 2. The risk for suicide increases during adolescence, with those who have recently experienced a loss, abuse, or family discord being most at risk.
- ☐ 3. Children do have a suicidal risk that coincides with some significant event such as a recent gun purchase in the family.
- ☐ 4. Adolescents typically do not choose suicide unless they live in certain geographical regions of the United States and Canada.

47. A child is being seen at the clinic for an attention deficit hyperactivity disorder (ADHD) assessment. What symptom(s) would the nurse expect to find? Select all that apply.
- ☐ 1. excessive climbing and running
- ☐ 2. excessive fidgeting
- ☐ 3. pouting behaviors
- ☐ 4. cannot wait to take turns
- ☐ 5. easily distracted

48. A school-age girl whose maternal parent and a female relative have been diagnosed as having bipolar disorder and whose paternal parent is diagnosed with depression is brought to the clinic because of problems with behavior and attention in school and inability to sleep at night. The child says, "My brain does not turn off at night." The child is diagnosed as experiencing attention deficit hyperactivity disorder (ADHD) with a possibility of bipolar disorder as well. What should the nurse say to the parent to explain what the provider said? Select all that apply.
- ☐ 1. "Your child was diagnosed as having ADHD because of their attention and behavior problems at school."
- ☐ 2. "ADHD involves difficulty with attention, impulse control, and hyperactivity at school, home, or in both settings."
- ☐ 3. "Your provider does not know how to diagnose your child's illness since they have symptoms of both bipolar disorder and ADHD."
- ☐ 4. "The child's description of their inability to sleep is irrelevant to diagnosing their condition since they stay up late."
- ☐ 5. "Your provider is considering a bipolar diagnosis because of your child's family history of bipolar disorder and their sleep issues."

49. At the admission interview, the parent of a 4-year-old male client with attention deficit hyperactivity disorder (ADHD) says to the nurse, "I know that my spouse or I must have caused this disease." What is the nurse's **best** response?
☐ 1. "ADHD is more common within families, but there is no evidence that problems with parenting cause this disorder."
☐ 2. "What do you think you might have done that could have led to causing this disorder to develop in your child?"
☐ 3. "Many parents feel this way, but I doubt there's anything that you did that caused ADHD to develop in your child."
☐ 4. "Let's not focus on the cause but rather on what needs to be done to help your child get better. I know that you and your spouse are very interested in helping them to improve their behavior."

50. A member of a nurse-led group for depressed adolescents tells the group that they are not coming back because they are taking medication and no longer need to talk about their problems. Which response by the nurse is **most** appropriate?
☐ 1. "I'm glad that you're taking your medication, but how can we know that you will continue to take it? After all, you haven't been on it for very long, and you might decide to stop taking it."
☐ 2. "I think that it's important to let everyone respond to what you said, so let's go around the group and let everyone give their thoughts about what you've decided."
☐ 3. "The purpose of the group is to provide each of you with a place to discuss the problems of being a teenager with depression with others who also are experiencing a similar situation."
☐ 4. "You don't have to stay in the group if you don't want to, but if you choose to leave, then you won't be able to change your mind later and return to the group."

51. The nurse assesses a 17-year-old client with depression for suicide risk. Which question is **most** appropriate to use?
☐ 1. "What movies about death have you watched lately?"
☐ 2. "Can you tell me what you think about suicide?"
☐ 3. "Has anyone in your family ever committed suicide?"
☐ 4. "Are you thinking about killing yourself?"

52. A teacher is talking to the nurse about a child in their classroom who has a tic disorder. The teacher mentions that the student frequently trips other children, though no one has ever been hurt. The teacher then further states that they ignore the student when that happens because it is part of their disorder. What should the nurse tell the teacher?
☐ 1. "Tripping other children is not a tic, so you can respond to that as you would in any other child."
☐ 2. "I can't believe that you actually allow the student to get away with that!"
☐ 3. "I think that's the best choice unless some parents of the other children start to protest about it."
☐ 4. "If no one else is getting hurt, then it seems harmless and might prevent the development of a worse behavior."

53. A 15-year-old boy client successfully treated for Tourette's syndrome tells the nurse, "I'm not going to take this medication anymore. Anyone who is really my friend will accept me as I am, tics and all!" What is the nurse's **best** response?
☐ 1. "You and your family came to the clinic for treatment, so you can terminate it whenever you wish."
☐ 2. "Will your lack of medication cause more tics and make you less attractive to other people?"
☐ 3. "Let's talk about what brought you into treatment and why you now want to stop taking medication."
☐ 4. "I think that's a very unwise decision, but you're entitled to do whatever you wish."

54. An adolescent client is sent to the school clinic with dizziness and nausea. While assessing the student, who denies any health problems, the nurse smells alcohol on their breath. Which response by the nurse is **most** appropriate?
☐ 1. "Your breath tells me that have been drinking alcohol this morning!"
☐ 2. "What is the real reason that you are feeling sick this morning?"
☐ 3. "Tell me everything that you have had to eat and drink yesterday and today."
☐ 4. "I know that high school is stressful, but drinking alcohol is not the best way to handle it."

55. A school-age child was recently hospitalized at a child psychiatric unit for inattention and acting out behavior at school and home. The client's provider prescribed the methylphenidate patch to control their attention deficit hyperactivity disorder symptoms, and inpatient unit staff worked with them on behavioral control measures. During the child's first office visit after discharge from the hospital, the office nurse discovers that the child has been taking off their patch during the day, which is causing problems at school and at home. In which order of priority from first to last should the nurse take the actions? All options must be used.

1. Explain to the family, in terms the child can understand, the benefits of their medication in dealing with school and home problems they are experiencing.

2. Explore the parents' attitudes about medication administration in general and their child's medication in particular.

3. Explore the child's reasons for removing the patch during the day rather than at the end of the day.

4. Have the provider discuss with the child and parents a trial of a different medication.

56. A school-age client is diagnosed with conduct disorder. After admission, the nurse identifies the client's problematic behaviors as cruelty to animals, stealing, truancy, aggression with peers, lying, and explosive angry outbursts resulting in destruction of property. The nurse is now talking with the client about their behavioral contract. What crucial component(s) should the contract include? Select all that apply.
☐ 1. taking prescribed medications
☐ 2. acceptable methods for expressing anger
☐ 3. consequences for unacceptable behaviors
☐ 4. rules for interacting with staff and other clients
☐ 5. personal possessions allowed on the unit

57. The nurse is meeting weekly with an adolescent recently diagnosed with depression to monitor progress with therapy and antidepressant medication. The nurse should be **most** concerned when the client reports what information?
☐ 1. An acquaintance hanged themself 2 days ago.
☐ 2. The client is experiencing intermittent headaches as a side effect of taking the antidepressant.
☐ 3. The client received a low score on their last history test.
☐ 4. The client's younger sibling has been starting fights with them for the last week.

The Child and Adolescent with Adjustment Disorders

58. A 19-year-old client with cystic fibrosis (CF) is hospitalized for a serious lung infection and needs a lung transplant. However, the client has a rare blood type that complicates the process of obtaining a donor organ. The client has also been diagnosed with bipolar disorder and treated successfully since mid-adolescence with medication and therapy. The client requests to see a chaplain to help them make plans for a funeral. The client would also like to donate their body to science after death. How should the nurse interpret the client's request?
It is a signal of:
☐ 1. the depressive side of the client's bipolar disorder, and they should be checked for suicidal thoughts/plans.
☐ 2. an exacerbation of the client's CF and warrants further assessment by their lung specialist.
☐ 3. the client's awareness they are likely to have a shortened life span and should be supported by unit staff.
☐ 4. delirium as a result of the many medications they are taking and requires further assessment by the pharmacist or health care provider.

59. A 6-year-old client has experienced the death of one parent in the last 3 months. The client and their other parent are involved in a grief support program that has sessions for all ages. A nurse is educating the parents in the group about the normal grief reactions of children to help them distinguish normal behavior from behavior that is unusual and possibly indicative of depression or other psychological issues. Which represents normal grief behavior for this young child after the death of a parent? Select all that apply.
☐ 1. talking to their deceased parent as if they were present in the room
☐ 2. crying followed in a few minutes by laughing
☐ 3. playing with a rope, saying they are going to be with their deceased parent
☐ 4. yelling and being angry at their deceased parent for leaving them
☐ 5. playing with a friend right after saying they miss their deceased parent

60. The nurse counsels a 5-year-old child who recently experienced the loss of a parent. Which statement reflects the typical understanding of death at this age?
☐ 1. "My mommy died last week, but I'm going to see them again."
☐ 2. "My daddy said mommy went to heaven, and I'm glad God took them there."
☐ 3. "My dog died and now we got another one."
☐ 4. "I think Mommy went to heaven and I will get to see them someday when I die."

61. A shy 12-year-old child who must change school systems just before they begin junior high school begins cutting their arms to relieve the stress that they feel about leaving long-standing friends, having to develop new friendships, and meeting high academic standards in their new school. After the client has been cutting for a few weeks, a parent discovers the injuries and takes the child to a mental health provider who prescribes a therapeutic group at the local mental health center and medication to help decrease anxiety. Which finding(s) would indicate that the child had made appropriate progress toward recovery? Select all that apply.
☐ 1. The child indicated that they have joined three clubs at school and agreed to be an officer in one of them.
☐ 2. The child says they have developed a friendship with a student in class and one in their therapy group.
☐ 3. The child wears short-sleeved or sleeveless tops when the weather is warm.
☐ 4. The child's grades are good, and hours of study are not excessive.
☐ 5. The child begins saying they must study hard to get into a good university.

Children and Adolescents with Autism

62. The parents of a preschool-age child diagnosed with autism must take their child on a plane flight and are concerned about how they can make the experience less stressful for their child and fellow travelers. The nurse suggests a dry run to the airport in which they simulate going through security and boarding a plane. In addition, the nurse suggests taking items to help the child be calm during the flight. Which item should the nurse suggest **first** to help modify stressors?
☐ 1. DVD player with headphones and favorite program
☐ 2. favorite stuffed toy animal or other soft toy
☐ 3. favorite nonelectronic game
☐ 4. medication that can be given as needed to calm the child

63. A nurse is conducting a group session for parents of toddlers recently diagnosed with autism. Which parent statement indicates a need for additional teaching?

"Children with autism may:
☐ 1. develop normally until 18 to 24 months old."
☐ 2. have poor coordination of the large muscles."
☐ 3. be extremely sensitive to sounds and smells."
☐ 4. be overwhelmed by rules and structure."

64. The nurse cares for a school-age child with autism who has been admitted to the hospital. Which intervention(s) should the nurse include in the plan of care? Select all that apply.
☐ 1. Allow a family member in the room 24 hours a day.
☐ 2. Encourage the child to alert the nurse whenever they are in pain.
☐ 3. Dim lights and keep noise levels low.
☐ 4. Show medical equipment to the child before procedures.
☐ 5. Bring in possessions from home.

65. A parent brings their adolescent with autism to the emergency department with a bleeding forehead laceration resulting from head banging. In what order should the nurse perform the actions from first to last? All options must be used.
☐ 1. Ensure constant observation.
☐ 2. Assess the head laceration.
☐ 3. Provide education on self-harming behavior.
☐ 4. Recommend a head computed tomography scan.

66. The nurse is assessing a 7-month-old infant. Which assessment finding(s) would require further evaluation for autism? Select all that apply.
☐ 1. poor eye contact
☐ 2. only responds to name when spoken by a parent
☐ 3. absence of social play
☐ 4. no social smile
☐ 5. fixation on objects

67. The parent of a school-age child with autism asks the nurse how they should tell their child that they have autism. Which response by the nurse is **most** therapeutic?
☐ 1. "Explain to your child that they have a developmental disorder that makes them different from other children their age."
☐ 2. "Schedule a case conference where the health care team can tell your child about their diagnosis of autism."
☐ 3. "Tell your child that they are different from other kids their age and that you will always be there to support them."
☐ 4. "Explain the definition of autism and emphasize your child's strengths as well as their areas of challenge."

68. A 5-year-old child with autism has been diagnosed with the eating disorder pica. When educating the family about pica, the nurse should include which information?
☐ 1. Pica will improve as the child gets older.
☐ 2. The child will require periodic lead screening.
☐ 3. Avoid feeding the child foods high in zinc.
☐ 4. The child will require periodic abdominal x-rays.

69. The parent of a child with autism tells the nurse that their child is only sleeping 2 to 3 hours per night. When educating the parent about treatment for the child's sleep disturbance, the nurse should include what information?
☐ 1. Behavioral interventions including sleep-hygiene measures are often effective in treating sleep disturbance.
☐ 2. Exercising before bed will tire the child and promote quality sleep.
☐ 3. Complete elimination of caffeine from the child's diet will effectively treat the sleep disturbance.
☐ 4. Zolpidem given each night 1 hour before bed will help promote quality sleep.

70. The parent of an autistic child visits the clinic and tells the nurse that their child has been acting out in school, particularly in the cafeteria and during gym class. Understanding that the child may be having difficulty with sensory processing, the nurse should suggest that the health care provider refer the child to which professional?
☐ 1. physical therapist
☐ 2. mental health provider
☐ 3. occupational therapist
☐ 4. speech-language pathologist

71. A 6-year-old child with autism has been prescribed risperidone to treat aggression and self-injury behaviors. When educating the family about risperidone, the nurse should include which information?
☐ 1. Notify the child's health care provider if a dose of risperidone is missed.
☐ 2. Notify the child's health care provider if the child is exhibiting lip-smacking behaviors.
☐ 3. The child may experience weight loss after beginning risperidone.
☐ 4. The child will have improved behavior about 1 week after starting risperidone.

Managing Care, Quality, and Safety of Clients with Abuse and Mental Health Problems

72. The nurse assesses a group of pediatric clients for mental health risk factors. Which child would the nurse identify as being **most** at risk for an episode of major depression?
☐ 1. 16-year-old male who has been struggling in school, earning only Cs and Ds
☐ 2. 13-year-old female who was upset over not being chosen as a cheerleader
☐ 3. 10-year-old male who has never liked school and has few friends
☐ 4. 14-year-old female who recently moved to a new school after their parents' divorce

73. A nurse on the mental health unit tells the nurse manager, "Kids with conduct disorders might as well be jailed because they all end up as adults with antisocial personality disorder anyway." What is the **best** reply by the nurse manager?
☐ 1. "You really sound burned out. Do you have a vacation coming up soon?"
☐ 2. "These children are more likely to have problems with depression and anxiety disorder as adults."
☐ 3. "You sound really frustrated. Let's talk about the meaning of their behavior."
☐ 4. "My experience hasn't been that negative. Let's see what the other staff members think; maybe I'm wrong."

74. The nurse performs wellness checks in the pediatric clinic. Which child would the nurse assess as demonstrating behaviors that need further evaluation?
☐ 1. 2-year-old who refuses to be toilet trained and talks to themself
☐ 2. 6-year-old who sucks their thumb when tired and has never spent the night with a friend
☐ 3. 10-year-old who frequently tells their parent that they are going to run away whenever they argue
☐ 4. 2-year-old who is indifferent to other children and adults and is mute

75. A nurse has been caring for an adolescent client in a residential facility. The child has been through a series of foster placements since infancy with no success in any placement until the age of 7 when placed with a middle-age single woman. The client thrived there until the foster parent was killed in a car accident. The client attempted suicide after their foster parent died in response to the loss, and the child was placed in the residential facility. The nurse has become close to this client and wants to help them address their issues and move on with their life. Which comment to the manager demonstrates that the nurse understands the client's issues and is able to respond appropriately to the client's needs?
☐ 1. "It's difficult for the client to love and trust again after their losses. In this facility, they can learn to deal with their loss in a less emotionally charged environment than a foster home."
☐ 2. "The client just needs someone who will love them and give them the things they have missed out on in life. An adoptive family needs to be found for them as soon as possible."
☐ 3. "I'm not sure they are going to be able to get past all the loss and rejection they have experienced. I don't think adoption will ever be a viable option."
☐ 4. "I know the client well and am familiar with their issues. I think the best chance for success for them would be if they were adopted into my family."

76. The nurse screens adolescent clients for high-risk health behaviors. Which client would the nurse determine needs further evaluation?
☐ 1. young adolescent girl whose mood changes when upset with their parents, though they have been in trouble in school or the community
☐ 2. young adolescent boy who coughs for 5 minutes after trying their first marijuana cigarette and declares they do not want to do it again
☐ 3. young adolescent boy who restricts their food and fluid intake to be able to box in a lower weight class
☐ 4. young adolescent girl who reads "dark" novels and questions why God allows innocent people to be harmed

77. A new client has just been admitted to an adolescent psychiatric inpatient unit. The charge nurse and an unlicensed assistive personnel (UAP) are discussing the client's needs. The UAP says, "They're just showing off to try and get our sympathy. There is no need for the client to cut themself. Why would adolescents want to do such a thing to themselves?" What response by the charge nurse is **most** indicated?
☐ 1. "They're not doing the cutting for attention since they always wear clothing that covers up their injuries, and further, they're not willing to talk about it."
☐ 2. "It's hard to see a young person harm themself as they do, but they have serious family issues and don't know better ways to handle them, so we have to help them with that."
☐ 3. "You don't understand their problems and don't take them seriously, so you shouldn't be allowed to work with them during their hospitalization."
☐ 4. "Working with adolescents can be extremely difficult at times. Would you prefer that I change your assignment?

78. A teenage client is admitted to the psychiatric unit with both bulimia nervosa and anorexia nervosa. Which initial intervention(s) would be appropriate for this client? Select all that apply.
☐ 1. Assign a staff member to accompany the client when using the bathroom.
☐ 2. Have the client keep a self-monitoring journal as a coping strategy.
☐ 3. Weigh the client in the same amount of clothing and facing away from the scale at daily scheduled intervals.
☐ 4. Inform the client that parenteral nutrition will be necessary if the client does not gain weight.
☐ 5. Assign a staff member to sit with the client during meals and for 1½ hours after meals.
☐ 6. Provide liquid protein supplements when the client is unable to eat meals.

79. A young adult who was admitted to the psychiatric hospital 2 months ago with an eating disorder is being discharged. Which action indicates the client understands discharge instructions?

The client:
☐ 1. returns to the same living situation as they had prior to hospitalization.
☐ 2. attends a social club at their local church.
☐ 3. returns to the lab for routine lab tests.
☐ 4. enrolls in a health club.

80. STEP 1

The nurse is caring for a 19-year-old female client admitted to the emergency department after a fainting episode.

Nurse's Notes

1230:
A female college student was transported by ambulance after fainting during class. The client is drowsy but oriented to person, place, and time. Their affect is blunted. They offer no spontaneous information, and eye contact is poor. Their skin is dry, lips are cracked, and body is covered with fine hair. The client is a freshman majoring in biology and a member of the cross-country track team. They were accompanied by a roommate who states that the client has fainted at least two other times in the past few weeks. Vital signs are temperature (T) 97.6°F (36.4°C); pulse (P) 40 bpm; respiration rate (RR) 16 breaths/min; blood pressure (BP) 80/48 mm Hg; and oxygen saturation 97% on room air. The client weighs 87 lb (39.6 kg) and has a body mass index (BMI) of 15 kg/m². A complete metabolic panel was drawn.

➢ Select the three findings that require **immediate** follow-up.

☐ 1. BMI
☐ 2. Client affect
☐ 3. Recent exercise
☐ 4. Previous fainting episodes
☐ 5. Skin characteristics
☐ 6. Vital signs

81. STEP 2

The nurse is caring for a 19-year-old female client admitted to the emergency department after a fainting episode.

Nurse's Notes

1230:
A female college student was transported by ambulance after fainting during class. The client is drowsy but oriented to person, place, and time. Their affect is blunted. They offer no spontaneous information, and eye contact is poor. Their skin is dry, lips are cracked, and body is covered with fine hair. The client is a freshman majoring in biology and a member of the cross-country track team. They were accompanied by a roommate who states that the client has fainted at least two other times in the past few weeks. Vital signs are temperature (T) 97.6°F (36.4°C); pulse (P) 40 bpm; respiration rate (RR) 16 breaths/min; blood pressure (BP) 80/48 mm Hg; and oxygen saturation 97% on room air. The client weighs 87 lb (39.6 kg) and has a body mass index (BMI) of 15 kg/m². A complete metabolic panel was drawn.

1315:
The client is lying on the stretcher with their eyes closed. They are unable to provide a urine sample and are vague regarding when they last ate or drank anything. The client thinks their last menstrual period was 3 months ago. Dentition appears normal. The client became agitated when asked additional questions, stating, "Does any of this really matter? I'd be better off if I died."

➤ For each possible finding, specify if the finding is consistent with anorexia nervosa or bulimia nervosa. Each finding may support one or both conditions.

Finding	Anorexia Nervosa	Bulimia Nervosa
Amenorrhea	☐	☐
Dehydration	☐	☐
Bradycardia	☐	☐
Normal dentition	☐	☐
Lanugo	☐	☐
BMI less than 85% of normal	☐	☐
Suicide ideation	☐	☐

Note: Each column must have at least one response option selected.

82. STEP 3

The nurse is caring for a 19-year-old female client admitted to the emergency department after a fainting episode.

Nurse's Notes

1230:
A female college student was transported by ambulance after fainting during class. The client is drowsy but oriented to person, place, and time. Their affect is blunted. They offer no spontaneous information, and eye contact is poor. Their skin is dry, lips are cracked, and body is covered with fine hair. The client is a freshman majoring in biology and a member of the cross-country track team. They were accompanied by a roommate who states that the client has fainted at least two other times in the past few weeks. Vital signs are temperature (T) 97.6°F (36.4°C); pulse (P) 40 bpm; respiration rate (RR) 16 breaths/min; blood pressure (BP) 80/48 mm Hg; and oxygen saturation 97% on room air. The client weighs 87 lb (39.6 kg) and has a body mass index (BMI) of 15 kg/m². A complete metabolic panel was drawn.

1315:
The client is lying on the stretcher with their eyes closed. They are unable to provide a urine sample and are vague regarding when they last ate or drank anything. The client thinks their last menstrual period was 3 months ago. Dentition appears normal. The client became agitated when asked additional questions, stating, "Does any of this really matter? I'd be better off if I died."

Laboratory Results

Lab	Value	Normal range
Sodium	138 mEq/L (138 mmol/L)	Adults: 135–145 mEq/L (135–145 mmol/L)
Potassium	2.9 mEq/L (2.9 mmol/L)	Adults: 3.5–5.2 mEq/L (3.5–5.2 mmol/L)
Hemoglobin	11 g/dL (110 g/L)	Women: 12–16 g/dL (120–160 g/L)
Hematocrit	35% (0.35 proportion of 1)	Women: 36%–48% (0.36–0.48 proportion of 1.0)

The nurse reviews the client's lab test results and prioritizes care.

➤ Complete the sentence from the list of drop-down options.

The nurse should prioritize treating the [dehydration / bradycardia / malnutrition]

and the [anemia. / hypokalemia. / suicide risk.]

83. STEP 4

The nurse is caring for a 19-year-old female client admitted to the emergency department after a fainting episode.

Nurse's Notes

1230:
A female college student was transported by ambulance after fainting during class. The client is drowsy but oriented to person, place, and time. Their affect is blunted. They offer no spontaneous information, and eye contact is poor. Their skin is dry, lips are cracked, and body is covered with fine hair. The client is a freshman majoring in biology and a member of the cross-country track team. They were accompanied by a roommate who states that the client has fainted at least two other times in the past few weeks. Vital signs are temperature (T) 97.6°F (36.4°C); pulse (P) 40 bpm; respiration rate (RR) 16 breaths/min; blood pressure (BP) 80/48 mm Hg; and oxygen saturation 97% on room air. The client weighs 87 lb (39.6 kg) and has a body mass index (BMI) of 15 kg/m^2. A complete metabolic panel was drawn.

1315:
The client is lying on the stretcher with their eyes closed. They are unable to provide a urine sample and are vague regarding when they last ate or drank anything. The client thinks their last menstrual period was 3 months ago. Dentition appears normal. The client became agitated when asked additional questions, stating, "Does any of this really matter? I'd be better off if I died."

Laboratory Results

Lab	Value	Normal range
Sodium	138 mEq/L (138 mmol/L)	Adults: 135–145 mEq/L (135–145 mmol/L)
Potassium	2.9 mEq/L (2.9 mmol/L)	Adults: 3.5–5.2 mEq/L (3.5–5.2 mmol/L)
Hemoglobin	11 g/dL (110 g/L)	Women: 12–16 g/dL (120–160 g/L)
Hematocrit	35% (0.35 proportion of 1)	Women: 36%–48% (0.36–0.48 proportion of 1.0)

The health care provider diagnoses the client with anorexia nervosa (restricting type) and orders inpatient psychiatric hospitalization for safety.

➤ Select the anticipated provider orders from each of the following categories. Each category must have at least one option selected.

Category	Possible Order
Nursing	☐ 1. Activity ad lib
	☐ 2. Intake and output
	☐ 3. Daily weights
Consults	☐ 1. Dietary
	☐ 2. Psychiatry
	☐ 3. Cardiology
Medications	☐ 1. IV Dextrose 5% in 0.45% normal saline
	☐ 2. Total parenteral therapy
	☐ 3. Potassium supplements

84. STEP 5

The nurse is caring for a 19-year-old female client admitted to the emergency department after a fainting episode.

Nurse's Notes

1230:
A female college student was transported by ambulance after fainting during class. The client is drowsy but oriented to person, place, and time. Their affect is blunted. They offer no spontaneous information, and eye contact is poor. Their skin is dry, lips are cracked, and body is covered with fine hair. The client is a freshman majoring in biology and a member of the cross-country track team. They were accompanied by a roommate who states that the client has fainted at least two other times in the past few weeks. Vital signs are temperature (T) 97.6°F (36.4°C); pulse (P) 40 bpm; respiration rate (RR) 16 breaths/min; blood pressure (BP) 80/48 mm Hg; and oxygen saturation 97% on room air. The client weighs 87 lb (39.6 kg) and has a body mass index (BMI) of 15 kg/m^2. A complete metabolic panel was drawn.

1315:
The client is lying on the stretcher with their eyes closed. They are unable to provide a urine sample and are vague regarding when they last ate or drank anything. The client thinks their last menstrual period was 3 months ago. Dentition appears normal. The client became agitated when asked additional questions, stating, "Does any of this really matter? I'd be better off if I died."

Laboratory Results

Lab	Value	Normal range
Sodium	138 mEq/L (138 mmol/L)	Adults: 135–145 mEq/L (135–145 mmol/L)
Potassium	2.9 mEq/L (2.9 mmol/L)	Adults: 3.5–5.2 mEq/L (3.5–5.2 mmol/L)
Hemoglobin	11 g/dL (110 g/L)	Women: 12–16 g/dL (120–160 g/L)
Hematocrit	35% (0.35 proportion of 1)	Women: 36%–48% (0.36–0.48 proportion of 1.0)

Orders

- Suicide precautions
- Give 1000 mL IV Dextrose 5% in 0.45% normal saline.
- Begin potassium 20 mEq orally twice daily after the client urinates.
- Obtain an electrocardiogram.
- Psychiatric consult
- Cardiology consult
- Dietary consult
- Daily weights
- Intake and output
- Refeeding protocol

The nurse transfers the client with anorexia nervosa from the emergency department to the inpatient psychiatric unit. The nurse reviews the initial admission orders.

➢ What does the nurse teach the client about the plan of care? Select all that apply.

- ☐ 1. "You must eat within view of a staff member."
- ☐ 2. "You may not go to the bathroom for one-half hour after eating."
- ☐ 3. "We will increase your calories gradually."
- ☐ 4. "You will likely tolerate liquid foods best when beginning treatment."
- ☐ 5. "You may not discuss food with other clients in treatment."
- ☐ 6. "You will be on restricted activity until you are able to gain 1 lb (0.5 kg)."
- ☐ 7. "You will remain on suicide precautions until you are discharged."

85. STEP 6

The nurse is caring for a 19-year-old female client admitted to the emergency department after a fainting episode.

Nurse's Notes

1230:
A female college student was transported by ambulance after fainting during class. The client is drowsy but oriented to person, place, and time. Their affect is blunted. They offer no spontaneous information, and eye contact is poor. Their skin is dry, lips are cracked, and body is covered with fine hair. The client is a freshman majoring in biology and a member of the cross-country track team. They were accompanied by a roommate who states that the client has fainted at least two other times in the past few weeks. Vital signs are temperature (T) 97.6°F (36.4°C); pulse (P) 40 bpm; respiration rate (RR) 16 breaths/min; blood pressure (BP) 80/48 mm Hg; and oxygen saturation 97% on room air. The client weighs 87 lb (39.6 kg) and has a body mass index (BMI) of 15 kg/m^2. A complete metabolic panel was drawn.

1315:
The client is lying on the stretcher with their eyes closed. They are unable to provide a urine sample and are vague regarding when they last ate or drank anything. The client thinks their last menstrual period was 3 months ago. Dentition appears normal. The client became agitated when asked additional questions, stating, "Does any of this really matter? I'd be better off if I died."

Day 2: 1100:
The client slept 5 hours last night. They have eaten a total of 2 spoons of scrambled eggs and drank 250 mL of coffee. Vital signs are T 98.0°F (36.7°C); P 52 bpm and regular; RR 16 breaths/min; and BP 82/50 mm Hg. The client's morning weight is 89 lb (40.1 kg), which is up 1.1 lb (0.5 kg) from their admission weight. Potassium this morning is 3.3 mEq/L (3.3 mmol/L). The client insists that they are fine and need to be discharged because they need to practice for a track meet. The client has spent most of the day in their room, refusing to participate in group.

Laboratory Results

Lab	Value	Normal range
Sodium	138 mEq/L (138 mmol/L)	Adults: 135–145 mEq/L (135–145 mmol/L)
Potassium	2.9 mEq/L (2.9 mmol/L)	Adults: 3.5–5.2 mEq/L (3.5–5.2 mmol/L)
Hemoglobin	11 g/dL (110 g/L)	Women: 12–16 g/dL (120–160 g/L)
Hematocrit	35% (0.35 proportion of 1)	Women: 36%–48% (0.36–0.48 proportion of 1.0)

Orders

- Suicide precautions
- Give 1000 mL IV Dextrose 5% in 0.45% normal saline.
- Begin potassium 20 mEq orally twice daily after the client urinates.
- Obtain an electrocardiogram.
- Psychiatric consult
- Cardiology consult
- Dietary consult
- Daily weights
- Intake and output
- Refeeding protocol

The nurse evaluates the client's progress on day 2.

➤ Highlight the findings that indicate the client's status is improving. Answer choices have been underlined.

Nurse's Notes

Day 2: 1100:
The client <u>slept 5 hours last night</u>. They have <u>eaten a total of 2 spoons of scrambled eggs and drank 250 mL of coffee</u>. Vital signs are T 98.0°F (36.7°C); <u>P 52 bpm and regular</u>; <u>RR 16 breaths/min</u>; and <u>BP 82/50 mm Hg</u>. The client's <u>morning weight is 89 lb (40.1 kg), which is up 1.1 lb (0.5 kg) from their admission weight</u>. <u>Potassium this morning is 3.3 mEq/L (3.3 mmol/L)</u>. The client <u>insists that they are fine and need to be discharged because they need to practice for a track meet</u>. The client has spent most of the day in their room, refusing to participate in group.

Answers, Rationales, and Test-Taking Strategies

The answers and rationales for each question follow below, along with keys (🔑) to the client need (CN) and cognitive level (CL) for each question. In addition, questions that measure clinical judgment will be coded (CJ). As you check your answers, use the **Content Mastery and Test-Taking Skill Self-Analysis** *worksheet (tear-out worksheet in the back of the book) to identify the reason(s) for not answering the questions correctly. For additional information about test-taking skills and strategies for answering questions, refer to pages 12–51 in Part 1 of this book.*

The Client Experiencing Abuse

1. **2.** The safety of the client and their children is the most immediate concern. If there is immediate danger, action must be taken to protect them. The other options can be discussed after the client's safety is assured.

    🔑 CN: Psychosocial integrity; CL: Analyze

2. **3.** The traditional and rigid gender roles described by the client are examples of role stereotyping. Impermeable boundaries, unbalanced power ratio, and learned helplessness are also common in abusive families.

    🔑 CN: Safety and infection control; CL: Analyze

3. **4.** The client's safety, including the need to stay alive, is crucial. Therefore, helping the client develop a safety plan is most important to include in the plan of care. Being empathetic, teaching about abuse, and explaining the person's rights are also important after safety is ensured.

    🔑 CN: Psychosocial integrity; CL: Analyze

4. -/+ **2, 3, 4, 5.** A person who experiences abuse is usually compliant with the spouse and feels guilt, shame, and some responsibility for the battering. Self-blame, substance abuse, and suicidal thoughts and attempts are possible dysfunctional coping methods used by abuse victims. A person who is abused is not likely to demonstrate assertiveness.

    🔑 CN: Psychosocial integrity; CL: Analyze

5. **2.** The nurse needs more information about the client's decision before deciding what intervention is most appropriate. Judgmental responses could make it difficult for the client to return for treatment should they want to do so. Telling the client that this is a bad decision that they will regret is inappropriate because the nurse is making an assumption. Warning the client that abuse commonly stops when one partner is involved in treatment may be true for some clients. However, until the nurse determines the basis for the client's decision, this type of response is an assumption and therefore inappropriate. Reminding the client about their duty to protect the children would be appropriate if the client had talked about episodes of current abuse by their partner and the fear that their children might be hurt by them, but the scenario offers no evidence that the other spouse has threatened the children.

    🔑 CN: Psychosocial integrity; CL: Apply

6. **3.** The parent's feelings are the priority here. Addressing the parent's feelings and asking for their view of the situation is most important in building a relationship with the family. Ignoring the parent's feelings will hinder the relationship. Defending the school nurse and the school puts the client's parent on the defensive and stifles communication.

    🔑 CN: Psychosocial integrity; CL: Analyze

7. **4.** Parental use of nonviolent discipline, the child's talk about what the family is doing, and the easing of the parent's negativity toward the school nurse are all signs of progress. Avoidance and wearing clothes inappropriate for the weather imply that the child has something to hide, likely signs of physical abuse.

    🔑 CN: Psychosocial integrity; CL: Analyze

8. **1, 2, 3, 4.** Ultimately, a victim of a crime needs to move from being a victim to being a survivor. The client must first get through the initial shock. Next, the client would be expected to begin to carry out home and work routines. The nurse would then expect the client to resolve grief over any losses. The goal that would be expected to take the longest to achieve is gaining a reasonable sense of safety and security.

    🔑 CN: Psychosocial integrity; CL: Analyze

9. **2.** The experience of rape is a crisis. Crisis intervention services, especially with a rape crisis nurse, are essential to help the client begin dealing with the aftermath of a rape. Legal assistance may be recommended if the client decides to report the rape and only after crisis intervention services have been provided. A rape support group can be helpful later in the recovery process. Medications for sleep disturbance, especially benzodiazepines, should be avoided if possible. Benzodiazepines are potentially addictive and can be used in suicide attempts, especially when consumed with alcohol.

    🔑 CN: Psychosocial integrity; CL: Analyze

10. **3.** Guilt and self-blame are common feelings that need to be addressed directly and frequently. The client needs to be reminded periodically that they did not deserve and did not cause the rape. Continually encouraging the client to report the rape pressures the client and is not helpful. In most cases, resuming sexual relations is a difficult process that is not likely to occur quickly. It is not necessarily true that the rapist will be caught, tried, and jailed. Most rapists are not caught or convicted.

CN: Psychosocial integrity; CL: Apply

11. **4.** Use of alcohol reflects unhealthy coping mechanisms. The client's report of needing alcohol to calm down needs to be addressed. Survival is the most important goal during a rape. The client's acknowledging this indicates that they are aware that they made the right choice. Although suicidal thoughts are common, the statement that suicide is an easy escape but the client would be unable to do it indicates low risk. Fantasies of revenge, such as giving the death penalty to all rapists, are natural reactions and are a problem only if the client intends to carry them out directly.

CN: Psychosocial integrity; CL: Evaluate

12. **3.** Coercion is the most common strategy used because the child commonly trusts the abuser. Tying the child down usually is not necessary. Typically, the abusive person can control the child by their size and weight alone. Bribery and expensive gifts usually are not necessary because the child wants love and affection from the abusive person, not money.

CN: Psychosocial integrity; CL: Apply

13. **2.** Truancy and running away are common symptoms for young children and adolescents. The stress of the abuse interferes with school success, leading to the avoidance of school. Running away is an effort to escape the abuse or lack of support at home. Rather than an inability to play or a lack of play, play is likely to be aggressive with sexual overtones. Children tend to act out anger rather than control it. Head banging is a behavior typically seen with very young children who are abused.

CN: Psychosocial integrity; CL: Analyze

14. **3, 5.** Dealing with the physical pain associated with mutilation is viewed as easier than dealing with the intense anger and emotional pain. The client often does not know how to express their emotions or fears an aggressive outburst when anger and emotional pain increase. Self-mutilation seems easier and safer. Additionally, self-mutilation may occur if the client feels unreal or numb or is dissociating. Here, the mutilation proves to the client that they are alive and capable of feeling. The client may want to be less sexually attractive, but this aspect usually is not related to self-mutilation. Binging and purging are commonly done in addition to, not instead of, self-mutilation. Although a few clients report an occasional high with self-mutilation, usually the experience is just relief from anger and rage.

CN: Psychosocial integrity; CL: Analyze

15. **1.** The dolls and toys in a play therapy room are useful props to help the child remember situations and reexperience the feelings, acting out the experience with the toys rather than putting the feelings into words. Role-playing without props commonly is more difficult for a child. Although drawing itself can be therapeutic, having the abuser see the pictures is usually threatening to the child. Reporting abuse to authorities is mandatory but does not help the child express feelings.

CN: Psychosocial integrity; CL: Apply

16. **3.** The priority of care for the client is safety. Staying with the client at all times is a priority. The perpetrator most likely threatened the victim that if they informed anyone about the incident, the rapist will severely harm or kill the victim. Staying with the client also supports the development of trust in the nurse by the client. The question regarding the identity of the perpetrator is within the realm of the authorities—not the nurse. Leaving the ED to obtain the rape kit is not the safety priority; this action can be delegated to another individual. Telling an individual to "not worry" is nontherapeutic communication and will not allay the fears of a client who has undergone the trauma of a physical sexual assault.

CN: Safety and infection control; CL: Apply

17. **4.** The safety of other children is a primary concern. It is critical to know whether other children are at risk for being sexually abused by the same perpetrator. Asking about other forms of abuse, how long the abuse went on, and if the victim did not remember the abuse are important questions after the safety of other children is determined.

CN: Psychosocial integrity; CL: Analyze

18. **4.** Parents of an abused child have difficulty controlling their aggressive behaviors. They may blame the child or others for the injury, may not ask questions about treatment, and may not know developmental information.

CN: Psychosocial integrity; CL: Analyze

19. 1. It is not normal for a preschooler to be totally passive during a painful procedure. Typically, a preschooler reacts to a painful procedure by crying or pulling away because of the fear of pain. However, an abused child may become "immune" to pain and may find that crying can bring on more pain. The child needs to learn that appropriate emotional expression is acceptable. Telling the child that it really did not hurt is inappropriate because it is untrue. Telling the child that nurses are mean does not build a trusting relationship. Praising the child will reinforce the child's response not to cry, even though it is acceptable to do so.

CN: Psychosocial integrity; CL: Analyze

20. 3. A 3-year-old child has limited verbal skills and should not be asked to describe an event, explain a picture, or respond verbally or nonverbally to questions. More appropriately, the child can act out an event using dolls. The child is likely to be too fearful to name the perpetrator or will not be able to do so.

CN: Psychosocial integrity; CL: Analyze

21. 3. An almost universal finding in descriptions of abused children is underdevelopment for age. This may be reflected in small physical size or in poor psychosocial development. The child should be evaluated further until a plausible diagnosis can be established. A child who appears happy when personnel work with them is exhibiting normal behavior. Children who are abused often are suspicious of others, especially adults. A child who plays alongside others is exhibiting normal behavior, that of parallel play. A child who sucks their thumb contentedly is also exhibiting normal behavior.

CN: Psychosocial integrity; CL: Analyze

22. 3. Parents who are abusive often suffer from low self-esteem, commonly because of the way they were parented, including not being able to develop trust in caregivers and not being encouraged or offered emotional support by parents. Therefore, the nurse works to bolster the parents' self-esteem. This can be achieved by praising the parents for appropriate parenting. Employment and socioeconomic status are not indicators of abusive parents. Abusive parents usually are attached to their children and do not want to give them up to foster care. Parents who are abusive usually love their children and feel close to them emotionally.

CN: Psychosocial integrity; CL: Analyze

The Adolescent with Eating Disorders

23. 3. Hypokalemia can result from excessive vomiting or laxative use in clients with eating disorders. Potassium levels of 2.5 mEq/L (2.5 mmol/L) or less are considered life-threatening and in need of urgent attention. A 10% weight loss over 6 months indicates gradual rather than rapid weight loss. Depending on the client's height and exact age, a systolic blood pressure of 86 mm Hg can be near normal limits. Low heart rates are frequently seen in clients with very restricted calorie intakes. While a heart rate of 57 bpm indicates bradycardia, if there are no other signs of poor perfusion, it is not immediately life-threatening.

CN: Reduction of risk potential; CL: Analyze

24. 3. In responding to the client, the nurse must be nonjudgmental and matter of fact. Telling them that weight gain is in their favor ignores the client's extreme fear of gaining weight. Putting off the weigh-in for 2 hours allows the client to manipulate the nurse and interferes with the need to weigh the client at the same time each day. Threatening to call the care provider is not likely to build rapport or a working relationship with the client.

CN: Psychosocial integrity; CL: Analyze

25. 2. A client with anorexia nervosa commonly has an extreme fear of not being able to control weight. The nurse should address this fear. Explaining the dangers of diet pills or discussing the HCP or family concerns focuses on the effect of the client's weight loss on other people rather than the client. Unless the client is motivated to stop, the client will likely not be successful.

CN: Psychosocial integrity; CL: Apply

26. 4. An intense fear of becoming obese, emaciation, and a disturbed body image all are considered to be characteristics of anorexia nervosa. Near-normal weight is not associated with anorexia. The weight of others is not a primary factor. "Concern about dieting" is not strong enough language to describe the control of food intake in the individual with anorexia nervosa.

CN: Psychosocial integrity; CL: Apply

27. 1, 3, 4. The normal albumin level is 3.5 to 5 g/dL (35 to 50 g/L), the normal hemoglobin level is 12 to 16 g/dL (120 to 160 g/L), and the normal potassium is 3.5 to 5 mEq/L (3.5 to 5 mmol/L). These levels are all low. The client is likely not eating a sufficient amount of protein;

therefore, the albumin and hemoglobin are low. The potassium level would be low if the client was purging. The sodium level is normally 136 to 145 mEq/L (136 to 145 mmol/L), so this is in the normal range; however, it can be high in a client with an eating disorder. The normal hematocrit level is 37% to 47% (0.37 to 0.47 proportion of 1.0) in an adult.

 CN: Reduction of risk potential; CL: Analyze

28. **3.** Parents commonly describe their child as a model child who is a high achiever and compliant. These adolescents are typically well liked by teachers and peers. It is not typical for behavior problems to be reported. The description about having given the child everything and being repaid is more likely to describe an adolescent who is exhibiting behavior problems.

 CN: Psychosocial integrity; CL: Analyze

29. **1.** The large carbohydrate intake and significant time in the bathroom are characteristics of bulimia. To address the problem, the client must obtain an evaluation of their physical and psychological status. Suggesting going to a weight-loss program or overeating support group frames the problem as strictly a weight issue and ignores the psychological etiology of the problem. Seeing the family's HCP does not address the psychological aspect of the client's illness, and the client must make the appointment themself.

 CN: Psychosocial integrity; CL: Apply

30. **1, 2, 3.** Because of the large number of calories ingested in a binge and the fact that a purge does not eliminate all calories consumed, the client with bulimia is of more normal weight but still must have a goal of maintaining that weight. Research has shown that selective serotonin reuptake inhibitors are effective in treating bulimia, and the client is usually amenable to taking the medication. The client with an eating disorder (bulimia and anorexia) has negative self-concepts that fuel their disordered eating, and attaining a positive self-concept is an appropriate goal. The nurse should work with the client with bulimia to help them recognize their eating as disordered. That recognition can make the client more amenable to treatment. It is not realistic to establish a goal that the client with bulimia will never have the desire to purge again.

 CN: Psychosocial integrity; CL: Analyze

31. **3.** A successful outcome for a bulimic client is to avoid using the eating disorder as a coping measure when dealing with stress. Being able to attend college, eat at home, and eat out without binging and purging are important goals, but they do not address the primary problem of stress management and its connection to eating.

 CN: Psychosocial integrity; CL: Analyze

32. **3.** Encouraging the client to talk about why they are here and their feelings may reveal more information about what led the client to come to the group and what led to their diagnosis. It also provides the nurse with valuable information needed to develop an appropriate plan of care. The comment that the client sounds angry presumes what the client is feeling and focuses the talk on their spouse. The focus should be on the client, not the spouse. Telling the client that they will like coming to group imposes the nurse's view onto the client. The statement also focuses on having fun in the group instead of stressing the therapeutic value. Having the client tell the nurse something about the cause of their bulimia ignores the client's original statement. In addition, it requires the client to have insight into the cause of their disease, which may not be possible at this point. Also, it may be too early in the relationship to discuss this disorder.

 CN: Psychosocial integrity; CL: Analyze

33. **2.** Because the client eats excessively when upset, the best treatment would be a group to help them learn alternative coping skills. Trying to limit purging without controlling binging would result in weight gain and likely increase the client's purging. Daily family therapy sessions are not realistic. Taking lorazepam whenever the client feels they need to binge may temporarily calm the client but does not address the cause of the binging and purging and will lead to drug dependence with long-term use.

 CN: Psychosocial integrity; CL: Apply

34. **2, 5.** The goals of a primary prevention program for eating disorders are for the girls to have positive feelings about themselves and their bodies. Monitoring of weight by parents or nurses might note eating disorders early, particularly anorexia, but will not address the cause of the disorder. Limiting the girls' access to media would be impossible and does not prevent distress with one's body image.

 CN: Psychosocial integrity; CL: Analyze

Children and Adolescents with Behavioral Problems

35. **2.** The client and parent need to address the issue of responsibility for medication administration. Reinforcing the parent's overinvolvement in medication taking or making negative comments

36. **1.** This child is demonstrating signs of anxiety and withdrawal. Being a library helper enables the client to use an interest (reading) when interacting with others and gain pride in helping others. Most interactions will be one-to-one and with adults, which is likely to be more comfortable for them in their state of anxiety. Organizing a class party, working on a group project with their peers, and being a member of a kickball team involve multiple peer interactions, which are likely to be difficult for the client at this time. Also, there is no mention of the child liking sports, so kickball would not be an appropriate activity.

🗝 CN: Psychosocial integrity; CL: Analyze

37. **1.** Peer acceptance and recognition is a very powerful force in the lives of adolescents, leading to positive or negative behavior depending on the child's peers. Although the influence of parents remains strong, peer acceptance combined with the adolescent's desire for independence can lead to disobeying the parents. The sanctions provided at school and in the community by law enforcement will support those teens that have other support in their lives but are generally not sufficient to prevent substance use in adolescents lacking support at home and with peers.

🗝 CN: Psychosocial integrity; CL: Analyze

38. **2.** This statement indicates insight into possible emotional causes for their pain. After insight is achieved, the client can make behavior changes to effectively cope with their anxiety-related disorder. Saying that they understand why their parent is away so often demonstrates insight into their parent's actions rather than their own. Wanting to discuss their pain and not their family indicates denial of any connection between their pain and stress, which perpetuates the current situation. Although rest may help their back, the client's statement does not address psychological issues related to the back pain.

🗝 CN: Psychosocial integrity; CL: Evaluate

39. **4.** ADHD is typically managed by psychostimulant medications, such as methylphenidate and pemoline, along with behavior modification. Antianxiety medications, such as buspirone, are not appropriate for treating ADHD. Homeschooling commonly is not a possibility because both parents work outside the home. Antidepressants, such as imipramine, are indicated for major depressive disorders and must be used with extreme caution in children because they carry the risk for suicidal thinking. Family therapy may be a part of the treatment. Anticonvulsant medications, such as carbamazepine, are not appropriate for ADHD. Also, carbamazepine levels are obtained weekly early during therapy to avoid toxicity and ascertain therapeutic levels.

🗝 CN: Pharmacological and parenteral therapies; CL: Apply

40. **1.** Suggesting that the parent arrange for respite care so that they can have a regular break would help to alleviate some of the stress that they feel when they are with their child constantly. The parent also could use family and friends to provide some care, thereby helping provide a break. The child may improve, so suggesting that the parent take a job to provide a feeling of success would be inappropriate. Having coffee daily with friends may provide some opportunities for socialization. However, friends may not be able to provide the verbal support that the parent needs. Rather, attending a support group of other parents with children with attention deficit hyperactivity disorder might be helpful. Placing the child in foster care is an extreme measure that may damage the therapeutic relationship with the nurse and dramatically and negatively affect the relationship between the parent and child.

🗝 CN: Psychosocial integrity; CL: Apply

41. **3. 5.** Giving away personal items has consistently been shown to be an indicator of suicide plans in a depressed and suicidal individual. Increased risk-taking or reckless behavior is associated with increased thoughts of suicide, especially when the risk-taking behaviors include illicit drug use. Expression of a desire to date, trying out for an extracurricular activity, or the desire to spend more time with friends indicates a return of interest in normal adolescent activities.

🗝 CN: Psychosocial integrity; CL: Analyze

42. **4, 3, 1, 2.** The client's anxiety seems to fuel their substance abuse, so treatment for their anxiety is paramount, followed by treatment for substance abuse. Those two interventions should increase their readiness to profit from academic aid offered by the school. Referral to a community college program would help them get ready for college, which will likely decrease anxiety.

🗝 CN: Psychosocial integrity; CL: Analyze

43. **2.** The parent's distress and length of time the problem has existed combined with the efforts they have made to address the problem demonstrate that medication treatment should be considered. The absence of any other symptoms makes a renal workup unnecessary at this time. It is unlikely that social skills training alone will change the client's nocturnal enuresis. Just waiting for the behavior to stop is likely to further tax the parent and client.

🔑 CN: Psychosocial integrity; CL: Apply

44. 1. Because weight loss is a common side effect of methylphenidate and because the child's symptoms are controlled with the stimulant, the first action should be to increase the child's oral intake before the medication's side effects begin. Weight should be monitored, but since the child has already lost weight, a remedy is needed as well as monitoring. The weight loss is directly due to the medication's side effects, so the child will continue to lose weight unless an intervention is made whether or not they are enrolled in school or on summer vacation. A high-protein drink could work, but then the child is taking in all their calories in the evening, which is not best nutritionally. A change of medication should be the last resort because methylphenidate is the most effective medication for ADHD and has been successful with this child.

🔑 CN: Pharmacological and parenteral therapies; CL: Analyze

45. 4. Decreased respirations and coma are the two most dangerous effects of a heroin overdose, so an increase in respirations after administration of the naloxone demonstrates initial effectiveness of the medication. Changes in cognition and psychomotor activity will take more time to become apparent. The client's blood opioid level may not drop to a nontoxic level for a few days.

🔑 CN: Pharmacological and parenteral therapies; CL: Evaluate

46. 2. Adolescents are more likely than children to attempt or commit suicide. Loss, abuse, and family discord remain significant risk factors. There is no evidence to support that children rarely commit suicide. Additionally, evidence fails to support the belief that children who have lost a parent to suicide will attempt it themselves. Significant events, such as a recent firearm purchase, have not been linked to suicide attempts in children. No geographical region in the United States or Canada is free from adolescent suicide.

🔑 CN: Psychosocial integrity; CL: Apply

47. −/+ 1, 2, 4, 5. A child with ADHD will manifest excessive climbing and running, excessive fidgeting, inability to take turns, and distractibility. This child does not exhibit pouting or moody behaviors.

🔑 CN: Psychosocial integrity; CL: Analyze

48. −/+ 1, 2, 5. The client's school problems, the presence of first-degree relatives diagnosed with bipolar disorder and depression, and their inability to sleep at night mirror aspects of both ADHD and bipolar disorder, which are difficult to distinguish from each other in children. Health care providers are reluctant to diagnose young children as bipolar at this age. The client may have only one disorder or the other or both. Further monitoring and their response to medication will differentiate whether they have one of the disorders or both. Any comments indicating that the provider does not know what they are doing or that the child's perceptions of their illness are not valid will undermine any trust the parent and child might be developing in their caregiver and so should be avoided.

🔑 CN: Psychosocial integrity; CL: Apply

49. 1. Stating that attention deficit hyperactivity disorder occurs more commonly in families takes the opportunity for teaching while also helping the parent realize that the parent and their spouse are not to blame. Parents who are commonly blamed by society for their child's behavior need help with education. Questioning the parent about what they think they may have done implies that the parents played some role in this disorder, possibly contributing to the parent's guilt. Telling the parent that other parents also feel this way and that the nurse does not think the parents are at fault is premature at this point. Telling the parent that they should focus on what needs to be done, rather than what caused the disorder, minimizes the parent's concerns and feelings.

🔑 CN: Psychosocial integrity; CL: Analyze

50. 3. Focusing on the purpose of the group is the best response. Adolescents are greatly influenced by their peers. Medication alone is not typically the most successful treatment strategy. Questioning whether the client will continue the medication is negative and is not the reason for them to stay in the group. Asking the rest of the group to respond may or may not give the nurse support for the teenager remaining in the group. Groups commonly have rules regarding movement of members in and out of the group, but this does not address the reasons for the client to remain in the group.

🔑 CN: Psychosocial integrity; CL: Analyze

51. 4. Asking whether the client is thinking about killing themselves is the most direct and therefore the best way to assess suicidal risk. Knowing whether the client has watched movies on suicide and death, what the client thinks about suicide, and whether other family members have committed suicide will not tell the nurse whether the client is thinking about committing suicide right now.

🔑 CN: Psychosocial integrity; CL: Analyze

52. **1.** The teacher needs to be informed that this behavior is inappropriate. Therefore, educating the teacher and encouraging them to respond to misbehavior consistently are correct. Telling the teacher that the nurse cannot believe the teacher lets the child get away with the behavior is demeaning and condescending. Allowing the child to continue the misbehavior is counterproductive to discipline and could create other problems.

CN: Psychosocial integrity; CL: Apply

53. **3.** When an adolescent wants to stop treatment with medication, it represents a desire for more control over their life as well as a wish to be free of the disorder with which they have been diagnosed. If the caregiver merely acknowledges the client's right to stop treatment or warns of consequences if the client stops medication, they abdicate the adult role of health care advisor. Before any action is taken, the nurse should explore the client's reasoning to see if anything in the medication regimen could be changed to make it more palatable for the client. The client also needs to know that if their current objections cannot be overcome, they can return later to restart their medication.

CN: Psychosocial integrity; CL: Analyze

54. **3.** Asking the client to report everything that they had to eat and drink yesterday and today is the least judgmental approach and also provides helpful information. Confronting the client about drinking alcohol or asking them to admit the real reason for feeling sick can put the client on the defensive and block further communication. The nurse should avoid putting the client on the defensive to facilitate communication that may eventually enable the nurse to get the truth and identify interventions.

CN: Psychosocial integrity; CL: Analyze

55. **3, 2, 1, 4.** First, the child's reasons for removing the patch need to be explored to determine what needs to be done to solve the problem of inadequate medication administration. Since the child is probably heavily influenced by their parents' attitudes about taking medications, their attitudes need to be addressed next to determine if they openly or subtly oppose the medication or its method of administration. Once the knowledge of the child's and parent's feelings about medication are known, education can be offered to be sure the child understands how the medication can help them cope better in school and at home. If the child continues to take off their patch or demonstrates an allergic response to the patch, or if it is determined that their parents are not supportive of the patch, discussion of a trial of another medication to treat the child's symptoms should occur.

CN: Pharmacological and parenteral therapies; CL: Analyze

56. **1, 2, 3, 4.** The crucial elements of a behavioral contract include compliance with the medication regimen if medication is prescribed, appropriate anger management, consequences for unacceptable behaviors, and rules for interactions with others. Personal possessions may be limited by unit rules but are not part of an individualized behavioral contract.

CN: Psychosocial integrity; CL: Analyze

57. **1.** While all the occurrences could upset the client in the early stage of treatment, the one involving the most risk to safety is the suicide completion of a peer. Adolescents are susceptible to "copycat" suicides. The fact that the client knows the method of the suicide of the acquaintance and is at a critical period in treatment, when their antidepressant may have given them increased energy while still experiencing low self-esteem, can put the client at significant risk for suicide.

CN: Safety and infection control; CL: Analyze

The Child and Adolescent with Adjustment Disorders

58. **3.** A client who has endured serious chronic illness (both psychiatric and medical) would be well aware of their shortened life span, particularly if they are unable to get a lung transplant. It would not be unusual for them to want to plan ahead so their wishes would be honored in the event of their death. In the absence of other physical signs, an exacerbation of CF or delirium is not demonstrated. Likewise, the client's successful bipolar treatment in the absence of any other signs rules depression out as a reason for their behavior. Although it may be difficult to think about a young person in terms of dying, the client's consideration of the future is a rational decision.

CN: Psychosocial integrity; CL: Analyze

59. **1, 2, 4, 5.** Young children cannot be sad all the time after a loss, but that does not mean they grieve less. Their moods change more quickly, and they often work out their issues through play rather than talking. Because young children do not have a full understanding of death's finality, they may talk to a deceased loved one as if they are present. They also may not understand the circumstances of the death and so may think the loved one left voluntarily and be angry at the deceased for leaving them. Play involving a dangerous object such as a rope, coupled with a stated desire to join the deceased parent, would be cause for alarm as the child could harm themself either purposely or accidentally.

🗝️ CN: Psychosocial integrity; CL: Apply

60. 1. Five-year-old children view death as reversible, so talking about seeing their parent again is a normal statement for a child of this age. A child of this age would not usually state that they are glad God took their parent but instead might be afraid that God would also take the life of other family members. The idea of replacing their parent with a new one, as hinted in the statement that they got another dog after the dog died, has not been supported by studies of grieving children. Stating that the parent went to heaven and that the child will see them someday when the child dies is reflective of more advanced abstract thinking than a 5-year-old would demonstrate.

🗝️ CN: Health promotion and maintenance; CL: Analyze

61. -/+ 2, 3, 4. The development of friendships and good grades with moderate amounts of study are positive signs since friends and grades in the new school were sources of stress and anxiety for the child. The ability to wear clothes appropriate to the weather rather than hiding their arms is a sign they are no longer injuring their arms. Joining three clubs and being an officer in one of them is unlikely and would probably be an additional source of stress for the child as would be pushing themself to extraordinary academic achievement to secure a place in college when they have just entered junior high.

🗝️ CN: Psychosocial integrity; CL: Evaluate

Children and Adolescents with Autism

62. 1. Electronic games and stories are favorites of most children but are particularly enjoyed by children on the autism spectrum. The headphones block out some of the noises that might be upsetting to a child on the autism spectrum. If the child cannot be engaged electronically, a favorite nonelectronic toy would be the next choice. Stuffed animals or other soft toys can soothe a child who is starting to become upset. Medication should be a last resort as it can have a paradoxical effect if it is an antianxiety medication or may cause too much sedation during the flight.

🗝️ CN: Psychosocial integrity; CL: Analyze

63. 4. Children with autism spectrum disorder tend to function best with clear rules, routine, and daily structure. Children with autism may develop normally until 18 to 24 months old at which time their development may be stifled or they may regress. Many people with autism have difficulty with muscle tone and coordination, which can affect their ability to reach developmental milestones. Children with autism often have sensory dysfunction and are extremely sensitive to sounds, smells, textures, and tastes.

🗝️ CN: Health promotion; CL: Evaluate

64. -/+ 1, 3, 4, 5. Children with autism prefer routine and familiarity. Having a family member in the room 24 hours a day may decrease the child's anxiety. Dimming lights and keeping noise levels low will reduce sensory stimulation. Introducing autistic children to equipment before a procedure may help reduce their anxiety. Bringing in possessions from home will help with routine and familiarity. People with autism often have a limited ability to communicate. Health care providers need to approach autistic children carefully with minimal touch and clear and concise instructions; their interactions should be brief.

🗝️ CN: Psychosocial integrity; CL: Apply

65. 2, 1, 4, 3. The nurse first assesses and treats the bleeding head laceration. Next, the nurse assures that the parent or a staff member remains with the child to ensure that the child does not engage in additional self-harming behaviors. Next, the nurse makes a recommendation to the provider for a computed tomography scan to determine if there is any additional injury to the brain or skull. Finally, the nurse provides the parent with education on self-harming behaviors.

🗝️ CN: Physiological adaptation; CL: Analyze

66. -/+ 4, 5. Symptoms of autism are often unrecognized during infancy. Autistic behaviors can be recognized as early as 6 months of age and include poor eye contact, lack of a social smile, and fixation on objects rather than people. Children with autism rarely respond to their name regardless of who is attempting to get their attention. All infants lack social play.

🗝️ CN: Management of care; CL: Analyze

67. 4. Using age-appropriate terminology, parents should explain the definition of autism to their child, focusing on the child's individual strengths and challenges. Providing examples of the child's strengths and challenges and comparing them with the strengths and challenges of other children can assist the child in understanding how they are different from others. A 9-year-old will not understand the definition of a developmental disorder. Autistic children prefer familiarity; therefore, it is not advised to have a health care team explain the diagnosis of autism. It is important for parents to let their autistic child know that they will support the child, but they should explain the diagnosis of autism.

🔑 CN: Psychosocial integrity; CL: Apply

68. 2. Children with pica often ingest substances that contain toxic ingredients like lead. Periodic blood lead levels will indicate if the child is at risk for lead poisoning. Pica usually improves as kids get older. However, in children with autism, pica is often an ongoing problem. Providing balanced nutrition and addressing nutritional deficiencies are essential for a child with pica. There is no need to avoid zinc. Children with pica may need an abdominal x-ray if there is a suspected abdominal obstruction, but periodic scheduled x-rays are not necessary.

🔑 CN: Physiological adaptation; CL: Apply

69. 1. Behavioral interventions have been found to be effective in treating sleep disturbances in children with autism. Exercising 20 to 30 minutes a day can aid in promoting health, but children should not exercise within a few hours of going to bed or it may cause additional sleep disturbances. Although restricting caffeine within a few hours of bed may help promote sleep, completely eliminating caffeine from a child's diet may be extremely difficult. Medication is not often recommended to treat sleep disorders in autistic children and can be habit-forming. Zolpidem is a sedative used to treat insomnia, but it is not recommended for children.

🔑 CN: Basic care and comfort; CL: Apply

70. 3. Occupational therapists can help evaluate sensory processing issues and fine motor difficulties. Many occupational therapists are also trained in coping strategies to help individuals feel more comfortable in their surroundings. Physical therapists primarily work on gross motor skills, often working closely with occupational therapy to develop effective exercise programs for autistic clients. A mental health provider will help the child and family manage emotional and mental health concerns. Speech-language pathologists evaluate communication deficits and assist clients in developing functional communication skills.

🔑 CN: Management of care; CL: Analyze

71. 2. Notify the health care provider if the child exhibits lip-smacking behavior as it may be an indication that the child is developing tardive dyskinesia. If the child misses a dose of risperidone, give the missed dose as soon as possible. If it is near the next scheduled dose, skip the missed dose. Weight gain is a common side effect of risperidone. It takes about 3 to 4 weeks of treatment with risperidone to see major changes in behavior.

🔑 CN: Pharmacologic and parental therapies; CL: Apply

Managing Care, Quality, and Safety of Clients with Abuse and Mental Health Problems

72. 4. Children who experience serious losses, especially multiple losses, such as old friends or a parent, are more at risk for depression. Girls also are at greater risk than boys during the adolescent years. While doing poorly in school is a risk factor for depression, it is not as great as having two sudden losses. Being upset over not being selected over being a cheerleader indicates represents a loss, but not multiple or serious losses. Not doing well in school is a risk, but developing new friends shows a positive perspective.

🔑 CN: Health promotion and maintenance; CL: Analyze

73. 3. The nurse manager needs to focus on the frustration that the nurse is expressing. Additionally, the nurse manager needs to correct any misinformation or misinterpretation that the staff nurse has. Saying that the nurse sounds burned out and asking about a vacation do not focus on the nurse's frustration or address the inaccuracy of the nurse's statement. There is no evidence to suggest that children with conduct disorder have more than the average adult's risk for depression or anxiety. Therefore, this response is inaccurate and inappropriate. Anecdotal information from personal experience does not supply the nurse with accurate, reliable information.

🔑 CN: Management of care; CL: Analyze

74. 4. Indifference to other people and mutism may be indicators of autism and would require further investigation. A 2-year-old who talks to themself and refuses to cooperate with toilet training is displaying behaviors typical for this age. Occasional thumb sucking and not having spent the night with a friend would be normal at age 6. Threatening to run away when angry is considered within the range of normal behaviors for a 10-year-old child.

🔑 CN: Health promotion and maintenance; CL: Analyze

75. 1. The severe emotional trauma the child has experienced will likely make it difficult for them to be successful in an adoptive placement at the present time, whether that placement is with someone they know (the nurse) or another adoptive family. Additionally, adoption by the nurse is inappropriate because it blurs the lines between their professional and personal life and is likely to confuse the client. It is clear that the client has many issues and that love alone is not likely to solve all their problems. Treatment at the residential facility will allow the client to work through emotional issues in a more therapeutic environment. Though not currently ready for adoption, the client may be ready for adoption in the future after sufficient treatment.

CN: Management of care; CL: Evaluate

76. 3. Restricting intake to lose weight is a first step toward an eating disorder for males as well as females, so this behavior should be investigated further, especially since males of this age are usually unconcerned about their weight. Quick mood changes are common in young adolescents, particularly girls. Such mood changes should not be considered problematic if the adolescent is not experiencing trouble in major areas of their life. Experimenting with alcohol or other substances is fairly common in the teen years, but one or two uses do not generally lead to addiction. The negative effect of the coughing may be a deterrent to further use. Religious questioning and exploration of "dark" subjects are common among teens and are part of the development of mature thinking. In the absence of other signs of depression, it does not warrant further evaluation.

CN: Management of care; CL: Evaluate

77. 2. The UAP is concerned about the behavior of the client and confused about why it is occurring, so the nurse needs to explain a bit about the issues involved as well as demonstrate empathy for the aide. It is appropriate to explain that the client is not cutting for attention, but the nurse's response does not address the reason for the teen's behavior and is therefore inadequate. It could also appear that the nurse is denigrating the UAP, which will not encourage the aide to listen to what the nurse has to say. The comments that the UAP cannot work with the client are punitive. Asking the UAP if they want their assignment changed does nothing to help the UAP understand self-mutilation and sets a bad precedent that the UAP can pick and choose an assignment.

CN: Management of care; CL: Analyze

78. −/+ **1, 2, 3, 5, 6.** Interventions for the client with both bulimia nervosa and anorexia nervosa involve assigning a staff member to accompany the client to the bathroom; promoting a self-monitoring journal as a nonfood coping strategy; providing daily weight measurement in the same clothing at the same times of the week, while facing the client away from the scale readout; assigning a staff member to sit with the client during meals and stay with the client for 1½ hour after meals; and providing liquid protein supplements when the client is unable to eat meals. Telling the client that parenteral nutrition will be necessary may be perceived as a threat and is not an appropriate initial intervention.

CN: Management of care; CL: Apply

79. 3. The client with an eating disorder is instructed to receive regular lab tests to monitor nutritional compliance. Frequently, the living situation from before hospitalization was dysfunctional, and returning to the situation can result in recurrent health problems. Attending a social club is not a priority for the client, and enrolling in a health club could result in the client exercising excessively.

CN: Management of care; CL: Evaluate

80.

STEP 1

0/1 1, 5, 6. A normal BMI is 18.5 to 25. The client is severely underweight and most likely severely malnourished. The dry skin, cracked lips, and low blood pressure suggest dehydration. The low heart rate suggests the fainting may be cardiac related. Following up on affect can wait until after the client's physiological status has been stabilized. The nurse does not need to fully understand recent exercise patterns and circumstances surrounding previous fainting episodes to begin client treatment.

CJ: Case study; Step 1: Recognize cues; CL: Analyze

81.

STEP 2

−/+

Finding	Anorexia Nervosa	Bulimia Nervosa
Amenorrhea	X	
Dehydration	X	X
Bradycardia	X	
Normal dentition.	X	
Lanugo	X	
BMI less than 85% of normal	X	
Suicidal ideation	X	X

Anorexia nervosa is a life-threatening eating disorder characterized by an intense fear of gaining weight, refusal or inability to maintain a normal body weight, and refusal to acknowledge the seriousness of the problem. Clients with anorexia have a body weight that is 85% or less of the expected weight for age and height. Amenorrhea is common among women with the disorder. Other findings may include fine body hair (lanugo), hypotension, hypothermia, hypovolemia, bradycardia, arrhythmias, electrolyte imbalances, anemia, and liver dysfunction. Anorexia can be of the restricting or purging type. Clients with restricting type often have normal dentition. Bulimia nervosa is characterized by recurrent episodes of binging and an inappropriate compensatory mechanism such as purging, fasting, or exercising excessively. Gastric acid commonly leads to dental damage. Purging can also lead to fluid and electrolyte imbalances and dehydration. Clients with bulimia can have near normal weights and even be slightly overweight. Suicide is a major cause of death in clients with both types of eating disorders.

CJ: Case study; Step 2: Analyze cues; CL: Analyze

82.

STEP 3

0/1 *The nurse should prioritize immediately treating the* **dehydration** *and the* **suicide risk**.

The nurse should prioritize the problems that are immediately life-threatening. The inability to urinate, low blood pressure, and drowsiness are signs of severe dehydration. Because the client has expressed that they might be better off dead, the nurse must immediately assess the suicide risk. A potassium level less than 3 mEq/L (3 mmol/L) can lead to ventricular fibrillation and sudden cardiac death, but potassium cannot be given until the dehydration is corrected and the client voids. The client's underlying problem, malnutrition, will require long-term treatment. The hemoglobin and hematocrit levels suggest anemia, but it is mild and not life-threatening. The bradycardia is a sign of physiologic instability that will need to be addressed, but it is not immediately life-threatening.

CJ: Case study; Step 3: Prioritize hypothesis; CL: Analyze

83.

STEP 4

–/+

Category	Possible Order
Nursing	☐ 1. Activity ad lib
	☒ 2. Intake and output
	☒ 3. Daily weights
Consults	☒ 1. Dietary
	☒ 2. Psychiatry
	☒ 3. Cardiology
Medications	☒ 1. IV Dextrose 5% in 0.45% normal saline
	☐ 2. Total parenteral therapy
	☒ 3. Potassium supplements

The nurse anticipates keeping intake and output records on any client with dehydration. Daily weights are indicated to ensure progress is being made toward weight restoration. A dietary consult is needed to establish a refeeding plan. The nurse anticipates obtaining a psychiatric consult to evaluate suicide ideation and develop a comprehensive treatment. A cardiology consult is needed to evaluate the bradycardia and possible cardiac involvement. IV fluids with dextrose and sodium are needed to treat the hypoglycemia and dehydration. Potassium supplements are anticipated to correct the hypokalemia. The client is expected to have activity restrictions, including limiting exercise and being placed on suicide precautions. Complete parenteral nutrition would not be ordered while electrolyte balances were still being corrected or until after oral nutritional therapy had been judged as unsuccessful.

CJ: Case study; Step 4: Generate solutions; CL: Apply

84.

STEP 5

–/+ **1, 2, 3, 4.** Clients are supervised closely during meals to ensure they do not dispose of food to avoid calories. Use of the bathroom is restricted for 30 minutes to an hour after meals to discourage purging. Before treatment, clients with anorexia may have restricted their own intake to 250 to 500 calories per day. Intake is incrementally increased to avoid abdominal pain and vomiting. Liquid foods are more rapidly absorbed and tend to cause less bloating when first trying to increase intake. The nurse cannot prohibit the client from discussing food. Although the client will likely be on activity restrictions at the beginning of treatment for safety reasons, linking restrictions to weight gain would be a punitive approach to treatment. The length of treatment for anorexia is dependent on the severity and can last months. The client's mental status will be monitored closely. Suicide precautions will remain in effect only while the client is suicidal.

CJ: Case study; Step 5: Take action; CL: Apply

85.

STEP 6

–/+

Nurse's Notes

Day 2: 1100:
The client slept 5 hours last night. They have eaten a total of 2 spoons of scrambled eggs and drank 250 mL of coffee. Vital signs are T 98.0°F (36.7°C); P 52 bpm and regular; RR 16 breaths/min; and BP 82/50 mm Hg. The client's morning weight is 89 lb (40.1 kg), which is up 1.1 lb (0.5 kg) from their admission weight. Potassium this morning is 3.3 mEq/L (3.3 mmol/L). The client insists that they are fine and need to be discharged because they need to practice for a track meet. The client has spent most of the day in their room, refusing to participate in group

A heart rate higher than 50 bpm indicates an improvement in cardiac physiology. Other vital signs are similar to those at admission. The weight being up 1.1 lb (0.5 kg) suggests the dehydration has improved. The potassium is not yet normal but has improved. The amount of sleep is less than desired. The oral intake is insufficient. While solids may have to be reintroduced slowly, the client would be expected to drink nutritional supplements. Insisting they need to practice for a meet and refusing to participate in group therapy show that the client has not accepted the seriousness of the eating disorder.

CJ: Case study; Step 6: Evaluate outcomes; CL: Evaluate

5

The Nursing Care of Clients Receiving Pharmacological and Parenteral Therapies

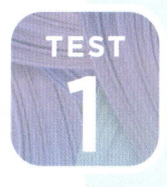

TEST 1 — Managing Care, Quality, and Safety of Clients Receiving Pharmacological and Parenteral Therapies

1. Rho(D) immune globulin is prescribed for a client before they are discharged after a spontaneous abortion. The nurse instructs the client that this drug is used to prevent which condition?
   ☐ 1. development of a future Rh-positive fetus
   ☐ 2. an antibody response to Rh-negative blood
   ☐ 3. a future pregnancy resulting in abortion
   ☐ 4. development of Rh-positive antibodies

2. The primary health care provider prescribes intravenous magnesium sulfate for a primigravid client at 38 weeks' gestation diagnosed with severe preeclampsia. Which medication would be **most** important for the nurse to have readily available?
   ☐ 1. diazepam
   ☐ 2. hydralazine
   ☐ 3. calcium gluconate
   ☐ 4. phenytoin

3. The primary health care provider prescribes whole blood replacement for a multigravid client with abruptio placentae. What should the nurse do **first** before administering the intravenous blood product?
   ☐ 1. Validate client information and the blood product with another nurse.
   ☐ 2. Check the vital signs before transfusing over 5 to 6 hours.
   ☐ 3. Ask the client if they have ever had any allergies.
   ☐ 4. Administer 100 mL of 5% dextrose solution intravenously.

4. The primary health care provider (HCP) prescribes betamethasone for a 34-year-old multigravid client at 32 weeks' gestation who is experiencing preterm labor. Previously, the client experienced one infant death due to preterm birth at 28 weeks' gestation. The nurse explains that this drug is given for which reason?
   ☐ 1. to enhance fetal lung maturity
   ☐ 2. to counter the effects of tocolytic therapy
   ☐ 3. to treat chorioamnionitis
   ☐ 4. to decrease neonatal production of surfactant

5. A multigravid laboring client has an extensive history of drug abuse disorder. The client's last reported usage was 5 hours ago. They are 2 cm dilated with contractions every 3 minutes of moderate intensity. The health care provider prescribes nalbuphine 15 mg slow IV push for pain relief followed by an epidural when the client is 4 cm dilated. Within 10 minutes of receiving the nalbuphine, the client states they think they are going to have their baby now. Of the drugs available at the time of the birth, which should the nurse avoid using with this client in this situation?
   - ☐ 1. lidocaine 1%
   - ☐ 2. naloxone
   - ☐ 3. local anesthetic
   - ☐ 4. pudendal block

6. A full-term client is admitted for induction of labor. When admitted, the client's cervix is effaced 25% but has not dilated. The initial goal is cervical ripening before labor induction. Which drug will prepare the cervix for induction?
   - ☐ 1. nalbuphine
   - ☐ 2. oxytocin
   - ☐ 3. dinoprostone
   - ☐ 4. betamethasone

7. The nurse is explaining the medication options available for pain relief during labor. The nurse realizes the client needs further teaching when the client makes which statement?
   - ☐ 1. "Nalbuphine and promethazine will give relief from pain and nausea during early labor."
   - ☐ 2. "I can have an epidural as soon as I start contracting."
   - ☐ 3. "If I have a cesarean, I can have an epidural."
   - ☐ 4. "If I have an emergency cesarean, I may be put to sleep for the birth."

8. When instilling erythromycin ointment into the eyes of a neonate 1 hour old, the nurse would explain to the parents that the medication is used to prevent which problem?
   - ☐ 1. chorioretinitis from cytomegalovirus
   - ☐ 2. blindness secondary to gonorrhea
   - ☐ 3. cataracts from beta-hemolytic streptococcus
   - ☐ 4. strabismus resulting from neonatal maturation

9. The health care provider prescribes ampicillin 100 mg/kg per dose for a newly admitted neonate. The neonate weighs 1350 g (2.97 lb). How many milligrams should the nurse administer? Record your answer using one decimal place.

   _____ mg

10. The nurse caring for a postterm client scheduled for an induction of labor has completed the necessary assessments. The client has been placed on electronic fetal monitoring, and venous access has been established. After reviewing a titrated prescription for oxytocin (see graphic), the nurse should perform what action **next**?

    Prescriptions
    1. Start an intravenous infusion of oxytocin 30 units/500 mL lactated Ringer's at 2 milliunits per minute.
    2. Increase by 1 to 2 milliunits per minute every 30 minutes until adequate process of labor is established or contractions are every 2 to 3 minutes apart.
    3. Discontinue oxytocin infusion immediately for uterine hyperactivity or fetal distress.

    - ☐ 1. Begin the oxytocin infusion at 2 milliunits per minute.
    - ☐ 2. Contact the health care provider to clarify the prescription.
    - ☐ 3. Ensure that adult resuscitation equipment is in the room.
    - ☐ 4. Implement a two-nurse verification of high-alert medications.

11. The new nurse is initiating intravenous (IV) therapy in a newborn. Which action if taken by the new nurse would the nurse's preceptor question?
    - ☐ 1. Offer oral sucrose during the IV insertion.
    - ☐ 2. Ensure the site is covered with a sterile transparent dressing.
    - ☐ 3. Flush the IV site every 4 hours.
    - ☐ 4. Document the IV status hourly.

12. An infant has been diagnosed with neonatal abstinence syndrome (NAS) and is receiving therapeutic weaning doses of methadone. What measure is **most** needed to ensure client safety when administering methadone?
    - ☐ 1. Document vital signs for drug administration.
    - ☐ 2. Notify the health care provider of the administration of the medication.
    - ☐ 3. Obtain an independent double check of the medication from another nurse.
    - ☐ 4. Wake the infant for an assessment before the administration of the medication.

13.

The clinic nurse is caring for an 8-month-old female client with congenital heart disease in the pediatric clinic.

Nurse's Notes

The parent reports that the infant takes digoxin twice a day and furosemide daily as prescribed for congestive heart failure. The infant also takes ferrous sulfate drops daily. This morning, the infant seemed more tired than usual and had a poor appetite. The client vomited 30 minutes after taking their morning medication. The client has also had four loose stools in the last 24 hours. Vital signs are temperature 97.8°F (36.6°C); pulse 88 bpm; respiration rate 30 breaths/min; blood pressure 80/56 mm Hg; and oxygen saturation 95% on room air. The client's last weight at 6 months was 15 lb 3 oz (6.9 kg), and their weight today is 16 lb 14 oz (7.6 kg). Point-of-care testing shows electrolytes are within normal limits.

The nurse reviews the assessment data to begin the plan of care.

➤ Complete the diagram by dragging from the choices below to specify the condition the client is most likely experiencing, two actions to take, and two parameters to monitor to assess the client's progress.

Action to Take — Condition Most Likely Experiencing — Parameter to Monitor
Action to Take — Parameter to Monitor

Action to Take	Potential Conditions	Parameters to Monitor
Obtain a stool culture	Fluid overload	Heart rate
Obtain a digitalis level	Digitalis toxicity	Breath sounds
Obtain a chest x-ray	Gastroenteritis	Pulse oximetry
Obtain hemoglobin and hematocrit levels	Anemia	Intake and output
Obtain an electrocardiogram		Color

14. The nurse is teaching an adolescent with asthma how to use a metered-dose inhaler. In which order should the nurse instruct the client to follow the steps from first to last? All options must be used.

1. Put the inhaler in your mouth.
2. Breathe out.
3. Depress the top of the inhaler.
4. Begin to slowly breathe in.
5. Hold your breath for 5 to 10 seconds.
6. Shake the inhaler.

15. An adolescent girl is prescribed amoxicillin for an ear infection. The nurse should teach the adolescent about the risks associated with their concurrent use of which medication?
☐ 1. over-the-counter antihistamines
☐ 2. oral contraceptives
☐ 3. multiple vitamins
☐ 4. ibuprofen

16. Nonsteroidal anti-inflammatory drugs are the first choice in treating a child with juvenile idiopathic arthritis. Which adverse effect(s) should the nurse include in the teaching plan for the parents? Select all that apply.
☐ 1. weight gain
☐ 2. abdominal pain
☐ 3. blood in the stool
☐ 4. folic acid deficiency
☐ 5. reduced blood clotting ability

17. An 18-month-old with a congenital heart defect is to receive digoxin twice a day. Which instruction should the nurse give the parents?
☐ 1. Digoxin enables the heart to pump more effectively with a slower and more regular rhythm.
☐ 2. Signs of digoxin toxicity include increased pulse and visual disturbances.
☐ 3. Digoxin is absorbed better if taken with meals.
☐ 4. Repeat the digoxin dosage if the child vomits within 15 minutes of administration.

18. The health care provider prescribes 30 mg of methylphenidate to a child with autism. The methylphenidate is to be given in two divided doses. The concentration is 10 mg/5 mL. How many milliliters of methylphenidate should the nurse give per dose?

_____ mL

19. A child weighing 23 kg (50.7 lb) is admitted to the hospital for a surgical procedure. The nurse reviews the standing intravenous fluid prescription (see exhibit). At what hourly rate should the nurse infuse the maintenance fluid?

Nurse's Notes	
Insert a peripheral IV	
Include dextrose 5% in 0.45% saline per weight protocol:	
Weight	mL/kg per day
First 10 kg (weight kg or less)	100 mL/kg per day
For the next 10 kg (weight 10–20 kg)	50 mL/kg per day
More than 20 kg, a child requires 20 mL/kg per day	20 mL/kg per day

_____ mL per hour

20. The parents of a child on sulfamethoxazole and trimethoprim for a urinary tract infection report that the child has a red, blistery rash. What instruction should the nurse give the parents?
☐ 1. Apply an anti-itch lotion to the affected areas at least twice a day.
☐ 2. Discontinue the medicine, and come for immediate further evaluation.
☐ 3. Use sunblock, and avoid midday sun while on the medication.
☐ 4. Increase the child's fluid intake to at least 2500 mL a day.

21. What should be part of the nurse's teaching plan for a child with epilepsy being discharged on a regimen of phenytoin?
☐ 1. Drink plenty of fluids.
☐ 2. Brush the teeth after each meal.
☐ 3. Have someone be with the child during waking hours.
☐ 4. Report signs of infection.

22. A client's intravenous (IV) site on the left arm is cool, pale, and swollen, and the alarm on the infusion pump is sounding. What should the nurse do **first**?
☐ 1. Reset the alarm on the infusion pump.
☐ 2. Assess the site for infiltration.
☐ 3. Elevate the client's left arm.
☐ 4. Stop the infusion.

23. The health care provider has prescribed a saline lock for a client. In which order from first to last should the nurse implement this prescription? All options must be used.

1. Use the nondominant hand to stabilize the vein by pulling the skin taut.

2. Apply clean gloves, and locate and clean the venipuncture site.

3. Stabilize the catheter, and apply a dressing to secure the saline lock.

4. Insert an over-the-needle catheter, advancing the catheter once flashback is observed.

24. At 0900, the nurse started an infusion of 1 L of 5% dextrose and normal saline (D_5NS) infusing at a keep-vein-open rate. At 0945, the client reports a pounding headache, is dyspneic, is experiencing chills, and has a heart rate of 116 bpm. The nurse notes that the IV bag has 400 mL remaining. The nurse should take which action **first**?
☐ 1. Slow the IV infusion.
☐ 2. Assess the client's blood pressure.
☐ 3. Remove the IV catheter.
☐ 4. Call the health care provider (HCP).

25. A client is receiving a transfusion of two units of packed red blood cells. Thirty minutes after starting the transfusion of the first unit, the nurse determines the client is having a reaction and stops the infusion. What should the nurse do **next**?
☐ 1. Remove the intravenous (IV) line, and obtain a culture of the tip.
☐ 2. Wait 15 minutes, and restart the blood transfusion.
☐ 3. Run normal saline at a keep-vein-open rate.
☐ 4. Call the health care provider (HCP) to report the suspected transfusion reaction.

26. A client had surgery 6 hours ago. The client has a prescription for a narcotic medication for pain every 3 to 4 hours. The last dose was administered at 1500. When the nurse enters the room at 1800, the client is restless and grimacing. What action should the nurse take **first**?
☐ 1. Ask the unlicensed assistive personnel (UAP) to help reposition the client.
☐ 2. Administer the narcotic medication to relieve the pain.
☐ 3. Assess the client to determine the cause of the grimacing.
☐ 4. Turn the lights down to minimize the client's restlessness.

27. A client has a triple lumen central line with lactated Ringer's (LR) currently infusing at 80 mL per hour. The health care provider writes a new prescription for total parenteral nutrition (TPN), 1500 mL to infuse over 24 hours plus lipids to infuse at 250 mL over 12 hours. What is the new infusion rate for LR if the total fluid intake for 24 hours is prescribed to be 125 mL per hour?

_____ mL per hour

28. Upon entering the room, a nurse notes that there is a cap missing on the central venous access device. The client is experiencing shortness of breath, coughing, and chest pain. What would the nurse do **first** after replacing the cap on the open port?
☐ 1. Reassure the client that the symptoms will resolve very quickly.
☐ 2. Place the client in low Fowler position to facilitate easier breathing.
☐ 3. Obtain an electrocardiogram (ECG) to rule out possible myocardial infarction.
☐ 4. Notify the health care provider (HCP) of the incident.

29. When delivering medication through an intermittent peripheral access device, the nurse should take which action **immediately** after cleaning the access port with an antimicrobial swab?
☐ 1. Aspirate to check for a blood return.
☐ 2. Flush the line with a normal saline flush.
☐ 3. Reconfirm the client's identity.
☐ 4. Instill the medication.

30. The nurse is to administer omeprazole to a female client. What information should the nurse obtain from the client before administering the drug?
☐ 1. Does the client have a history of gastrointestinal ulcers?
☐ 2. Is the client sexually active or pregnant?
☐ 3. Does the client have an ulcer induced by *Helicobacter pylori*?
☐ 4. Will the client be able to crush the pill if necessary?

31. Which statement by a client who is taking atorvastatin indicates a need for further teaching?
☐ 1. "I'll increase my activity level to lower my cholesterol."
☐ 2. "My diet should include foods that are low in saturated fat."
☐ 3. "I should always take this medication with grapefruit juice."
☐ 4. "My liver and kidney function will be checked to make sure there is no toxicity."

32. A client is to take rosuvastatin. What information should the nurse determine before administering the drug?
☐ 1. Can the client swallow a pill, or does the client need a liquid form?
☐ 2. Is the client of Asian descent?
☐ 3. Will the client be able to afford the medication?
☐ 4. Does the client have a history of cardiovascular disease?

33. The nurse reviews a client's medication administration record and notes the scheduled medications (see chart). When planning to administer the medications, the nurse must administer which medication within 30 minutes of its scheduled administration time?

> **Prescriptions**
>
> - Lisinopril 20 mg by mouth once daily.
> - Ampicillin 500 mg by mouth every 6 hours.
> - Metoprolol 25 mg by mouth twice daily.
> - Pneumococcal vaccine 0.5 mL intramuscularly today as a one-time occurrence.

☐ 1. lisinopril
☐ 2. ampicillin
☐ 3. metoprolol
☐ 4. pneumococcal vaccine

34. The nurse is to inject an intravenous medication via a locked peripheral intravenous port. The nurse flushes the port with saline, administers the intravenous medication, and again flushes the port with saline. During this process, when should the nurse clean the injection port with an antiseptic swab?
☐ 1. before entering the capped injection port the first time
☐ 2. when administering the intravenous medication
☐ 3. at each entry of the capped injection port
☐ 4. after the first and last entry of the capped injection port

35. A client has several intravenous infusions, each running to a separate location. Which intravenous infusion line does the nurse select to attach secondary tubing to infuse an intravenous piggyback medication over 30 minutes?
☐ 1. 25,000 units of heparin sodium in 250 mL 5% dextrose in water at 10 mL per hour.
☐ 2. 1000 mL normal saline at 50 mL per hour.
☐ 3. 350 mL of packed red blood cells at 100 mL per hour.
☐ 4. parenteral nutrition at 83 mL per hour.

36. When injecting an intravenous push medication into intravenous tubing with a solution infusing, the nurse should select which injection port?
☐ 1. the port adjacent to the drip chamber
☐ 2. the port just above the automated infusion pump
☐ 3. the port just below the automated infusion pump
☐ 4. the port closest to the client

37. When administering an intravenous medication, the nurse should explain which teaching point(s) to the client? Select all that apply.
☐ 1. date the medication will expire
☐ 2. incompatibilities with other medications
☐ 3. name of the medication
☐ 4. purpose of the medication
☐ 5. possible adverse effects
☐ 6. manufacturer of the medication

38. Before administering an opioid prescribed for pain management, the nurse assesses a client using the Pasero Opioid-Induced Sedation Scale (POSS) (see chart). The nurse assigns a score of 3 based on the assessment criteria for the scale. What should the nurse do **next**?

PASERO OPIOID-INDUCED SEDATION SCALE

1 = Awake and alert
2 = Slightly drowsy, easily aroused
3 = Frequently drowsy, arousable, drifts off to sleep during conversation
4 = Somnolent, minimal or no response to verbal and physical stimulation

☐ 1. Continue to administer the medication because the client is well sedated.
☐ 2. Increase the dose if the client becomes restless.
☐ 3. Contact the health care provider (HCP) to request a decreased dose of the medication.
☐ 4. Prepare to administer a reversal agent.

39. In the first 12 hours after starting a patient-controlled analgesia (PCA) infusion to administer an opioid, what should the nurse monitor every 1 to 2 hours? Select all that apply.
☐ 1. arterial blood gas values
☐ 2. level of sedation
☐ 3. muscle strength
☐ 4. oxygen saturation
☐ 5. vital signs

40. The nurse is adding the 8-hour intake for a client with a quadruple lumen central line intravenous access. See the intake-output record below. Based on the documentation, the nurse should document the client's intake as how many milliliters? Record your answer in whole numbers.

Intake and Output Record	
Intake	• 5% dextrose and 0.49% sodium chloride intravenously at 83 mL/h to the proximal lumen • Vancomycin 1 g in 250 mL 5% dextrose in water to the distal lumen • ½ L of intravenous normal saline as a one-time fluid bolus to the distal lumen. ½ cup of ice chips by mouth.
Output	Urine–500 mL

_____ mL

41. A nurse has attempted to insert a peripheral intravenous catheter into the median cubital vein of a client who has one arm amputated above the elbow. The nurse was not successful in inserting the catheter into the vein. In which location does the nurse **next** attempt catheter insertion?
☐ 1. basilic vein of the forearm
☐ 2. cephalic vein of the upper arm
☐ 3. cephalic vein of the wrist
☐ 4. dorsal metacarpal vein

42. A nurse has inserted a peripheral intravenous catheter. Which type of dressing is **most** appropriate to use to cover the insertion site?
☐ 1. transparent
☐ 2. adhesive
☐ 3. hydrocolloid
☐ 4. gauze

43. The client has a peripheral intravenous infusion of 1000 mL 0.9% sodium chloride infusing at 125 mL per hour and received 4 g piperacillin/0.5 g tazobactam in 100 mL of 0.9% sodium chloride as a 4-hour intravenous piggyback infusion. How should the nurse document the client's intravenous intake for an 8-hour shift? Record your answer in whole numbers.

_____ mL

44. A client with a history of smoking and peripheral artery disease reports leg pain. The health care provider has prescribed 400 mg of pentoxifylline by mouth three times a day. What should the nurse instruct the client to do? Select all that apply.
☐ 1. "Avoid driving or operating heavy machinery when first taking this medication."
☐ 2. "Avoid smoking while taking this medication."
☐ 3. "Don't stop taking this medication without the approval of your health care provider."
☐ 4. "Decrease the amount of green leafy vegetables you eat."
☐ 5. "You'll need to have weekly labs drawn with this medication."

45. The nurse is instructing a client about how to take clopidogrel. Which statement(s) by the client would indicate the need for further teaching? Select all that apply.
☐ 1. "I should inform all of my health care providers that I take clopidogrel."
☐ 2. "I understand I may experience a fever while taking clopidogrel."
☐ 3. "I should apply pressure to any injuries that won't stop bleeding."
☐ 4. "I'll take omeprazole to prevent gastrointestinal upset."
☐ 5. "I'll need to have my platelets monitored."

46. A client is receiving warfarin for newly diagnosed atrial fibrillation. Which laboratory result would indicate that the nurse should withhold the medication and contact the health care provider?
☐ 1. international normalized ratio (INR) of 1.8
☐ 2. INR of 4.8
☐ 3. partial thromboplastin time (APTT) of 65 seconds
☐ 4. APTT of 70 seconds

47. Following surgery, a client is receiving morphine 5 mg IV every 2 hours as needed (PRN) for pain. To ensure safe medication administration when administering this drug, the nurse should take which action(s)? Select all that apply.
☐ 1. Assess the client's pain level 45 to 60 minutes after giving the medication.
☐ 2. Check the medication administration record to see when the last dose was administered.
☐ 3. Consult a drug manual to determine whether the amount prescribed is safe.
☐ 4. Document the reason the medication was given in the client's electronic health record.
☐ 5. Use two identifiers to confirm that the medication is given to the correct client.

48. The nurse is teaching a client who has a new prescription for rivaroxaban. The nurse understands that teaching has been effective when the client makes which comment(s)? Select all that apply.
☐ 1. "I'll take this medication with a full glass of water."
☐ 2. "I'll take this medication at the same time each day."
☐ 3. "I'll take a dose if I miss as soon as I remember unless it is 2 hours before I will take the next dose"
☐ 4. "I'll report any bleeding from my gums to my health care provider."
☐ 5. "I'll stop taking this medication if I have an upset stomach."

49. A client reports having crushing chest pain. The electrocardiogram shows ST elevations indicating an anterior myocardial infarction. The client takes captopril twice a day and nitroglycerin sublingual as needed (PRN). The nurse reviews the client's vital signs and blood tests to report to the health care provider. Which information indicates the client has absolute contraindications for receiving fibrinolytic therapy? Select all that apply.
☐ 1. blood urea nitrogen of 20 mg/dL (14.28 mmol/L) and creatinine of 1.1 mg/dL (97.2 μmol/L)
☐ 2. history of intracranial hemorrhage
☐ 3. symptoms or signs suggestive of an aortic dissection active bleeding
☐ 4. hip replacement within the past 3 weeks
☐ 5. systolic blood pressure of 185 mm Hg

50. The nurse is preparing to administer benazepril to a client with hypertension. To help minimize potential adverse effects, the nurse should review which laboratory result(s)? Select all that apply.
☐ 1. alanine transaminase (ALT) and aspartate transaminase (AST)
☐ 2. albumin
☐ 3. blood urea nitrogen (BUN) and creatinine
☐ 4. blood glucose levels
☐ 5. serum electrolytes

51. A client who is 85 kg has a prescription for acyclovir 10 mg/kg in 100 mL sodium chloride to infuse over 1 hour. The client's intravenous infusion infiltrates 8 minutes before the infusion is completed. How much of the acyclovir has the client received? Round to one decimal point.

_____ mg

52. The nurse administers the wrong dose of a medication. Instead of giving furosemide 20 mg orally, the nurse forgets to break the tablet in half and gives furosemide 40 mg orally. The client experienced no harm as a result. What should the nurse do? Select all that apply.
☐ 1. Continue to monitor the client's vital signs and urinary output.
☐ 2. Notify the health care provider, supervisor, and client.
☐ 3. Complete an incident report, outlining the events of the incident.
☐ 4. Document the time and amount of medication given.
☐ 5. Nothing, because no harm came to the client and no further action is needed.

53. The nurse is developing a care plan with a client who is receiving ziprasidone and has stopped taking the drug. Which side effect(s) that may occur and be a reason the client is noncompliant with taking this medication should the nurse discuss? Select all that apply.
☐ 1. drowsiness
☐ 2. weight gain
☐ 3. diarrhea
☐ 4. nausea
☐ 5. headache

54. A client taking risperidone reports stiff muscles, difficulty breathing, and increased perspiration. When the nurse asks the client what day it is, the client answers, "New Year's Eve" when it is late July. Which action should the nurse perform **first**?
☐ 1. Call the client's family member.
☐ 2. Request a prescription for benztropine.
☐ 3. Administer the next dose of risperidone.
☐ 4. Check the client's vital signs.

55. A client with major depressive disorder is receiving phenelzine. The nurse intervenes when the client orders which food for lunch?
☐ 1. pepperoni pizza
☐ 2. yogurt with fruit
☐ 3. Salisbury steak
☐ 4. green beans

56. The nurse is caring for an older adult experiencing depression and chronic pain. The client is requesting a prescription for an opioid pain medication similar to the one prescribed for knee surgery 5 years ago. What education should the nurse provide for the client? Select all that apply.
☐ 1. Physical dependence can develop quickly with opioid medications.
☐ 2. Opioid use is appropriate in chronic pain accompanied by depression.
☐ 3. Opioid use is more appropriate for acute pain than chronic pain.
☐ 4. Opioid use increases the risk for cognitive impairment.
☐ 5. Treatment for depression can improve pain symptoms as well as depression.
☐ 6. Using opioids to control chronic pain will decrease the level of depression.

57. A client with depression is taking a prescribed antidepressant that can cause anticholinergic side effects. The nurse anticipates that this client is at particular risk for developing which anticholinergic side effect?
☐ 1. vomiting
☐ 2. constipation
☐ 3. diarrhea
☐ 4. weight loss

58. The nurse is caring for a client who is taking haloperidol. The client comes to the nurse's station and states that they feel frightened and their muscles hurt. The client is unable to turn their head to look at the nurse, the client's face is stiff, and they cannot move their tongue very well. Which prescribed as-needed (PRN) medication would be appropriate for the nurse to administer?
☐ 1. benztropine
☐ 2. meperidine
☐ 3. diphenhydramine
☐ 4. lorazepam

59. A client recently diagnosed with depression has been prescribed sertraline and is now being discharged. Which statement by the spouse indicates understanding of the medication teaching?
☐ 1. "We should monitor for increased depression if my spouse takes any cold or allergy medication."
☐ 2. "We can expect improvement of my spouse's mood and energy within the next 1 to 2 weeks."
☐ 3. "I can give my spouse the herb St. John's wort as a sleep aid until the depression is better."
☐ 4. "I should encourage my spouse to take the medication in the morning to prevent insomnia."

60. The nurse is caring for a client who has been prescribed a benzodiazepine medication for acute anxiety. What information is **most** important for the nurse to include when teaching the client about the medication?
☐ 1. "Take the medication as prescribed as there is risk for addiction."
☐ 2. "You can only take this medication for a few days due to the side effects."
☐ 3. "This medication may keep you awake, so plan to take it in the morning."
☐ 4. "This medication should be taken with food for best absorption."

61. The client's health care provider prescribes buspirone hydrochloride for increased anxiety. The nurse understands the health care provider's choice of this medication is based on what principle? Buspirone:
☐ 1. is often administered on an as-needed basis.
☐ 2. does not have any drug side effects.
☐ 3. is not habit forming.
☐ 4. is chemically similar to benzodiazepine medications.

62. A nurse overhears the following conversation between coworkers: "Older people have lost many friends and family and also have health problems. Their anxiety and worries can be so severe that they need higher doses of benzodiazepines than most people." What is the **most** appropriate response for the nurse to make to the coworkers?
☐ 1. "You're right. Many older adults have had anxiety for so long that it's more difficult to treat."
☐ 2. "That's not right. Older people need lower doses than most people because of reduced liver and kidney function."
☐ 3. "You're wrong. It's not safe to use benzodiazepines at all in older adults because of the side effects."
☐ 4. "Older people should get the same dose as any other adult. It doesn't make any difference."

63. After administering naloxone, an opioid antagonist, the nurse should monitor the client carefully for which problem?
☐ 1. cerebral edema
☐ 2. kidney failure
☐ 3. seizure activity
☐ 4. respiratory depression

64. A client is taking increased amounts of alprazolam for about 6 months for anxiety. The client asks the nurse how they can "get off the alprazolam." What is the nurse's **best** response?
☐ 1. "There will be an immediate discontinuation of the alprazolam, and haloperidol will be available if needed."
☐ 2. "Instead of alprazolam, you'll take lorazepam in decreasing doses and frequency over a period of 3 to 4 days."
☐ 3. "The alprazolam will be tapered down over a period of 48 hours."
☐ 4. "Alprazolam will be available on an as-needed basis (PRN) for 4 to 5 days."

65. What should the nurse include in the teaching plan for the parents of a child who is receiving methylphenidate?
☐ 1. Give the medication at the same time every evening.
☐ 2. Have the child take two doses at the same time if the last dose was missed.
☐ 3. Give the single-dose form of the medication early in the day.
☐ 4. Allow concurrent use of any over-the-counter medications with this drug.

66. The nurse is reviewing the laboratory report with the client's lithium level before administering the 1700 hours dose. The lithium level is 1.8 mEq/L (1.8 mmol/L). What action should the nurse take?
☐ 1. Administer the 1700 hours dose of lithium.
☐ 2. Hold the 1700 hours dose of lithium.
☐ 3. Give the client 240 mL of water with the lithium.
☐ 4. Give the lithium after the client's supper.

67. A client is receiving paroxetine 20 mg every morning. After taking the first three doses, the client tells the nurse that the medication upsets the stomach. How should the nurse instruct the client to take the paroxetine?
☐ 1. an hour before breakfast
☐ 2. with some food
☐ 3. at bedtime
☐ 4. with 4 oz (120 mL) of orange juice

68. A client who has been taking venlafaxine 25 mg orally three times a day for the past 2 days states, "This medicine isn't doing me any good. I'm still so depressed." Which response by the nurse is **most** appropriate?
☐ 1. "Perhaps we'll need to increase your dose."
☐ 2. "Let's wait a few days and see how you feel."
☐ 3. "It takes about 2 to 4 weeks to receive the full effects."
☐ 4. "It's too soon to tell if your medication will help you."

69. A client taking mirtazapine is disheartened about a 20-lb (9-kg) weight gain over the past 3 months. The client tells the nurse, "I stopped taking my mirtazapine 15 days ago. I don't want to get depressed again, but I feel awful about my weight." Which response by the nurse is **most** appropriate?
  ☐ 1. "Focusing on diet and exercise alone should control your weight."
  ☐ 2. "Your depression is much better now, so your medication is helping you."
  ☐ 3. "Look at all the positive things that have happened to you since you started mirtazapine."
  ☐ 4. "I hear how difficult this is for you and will help you approach your health care provider (HCP) about it."

70. A client comes to the mental health clinic saying that they feel so down and lacking in energy with "loss of interest in everything." The client tells the nurse that they received some samples of a new medication from their health care provider last week to relieve depression. The nurse recalls that this client has a history of bipolar disorder with hospitalization for a significant manic episode. With this knowledge, the nurse would have special concern if the client is taking which category of medication?
  ☐ 1. atypical antipsychotics
  ☐ 2. mood stabilizers/antimanics
  ☐ 3. antianxiety agents/benzodiazepines
  ☐ 4. selective serotonin reuptake inhibitor antidepressants

71. When preparing to insert an intravenous catheter to administer fluids to a client who is going to surgery, the nurse selects the median cubital vein. Identify the location of the median cubital vein on the illustration.

72. The parent of a 28-year-old client who is taking clozapine states, "Something's wrong. My son is drooling like a baby." What response by the nurse would be **most** helpful?
  ☐ 1. "I wonder if they are having an adverse reaction to the medicine."
  ☐ 2. "Excess saliva is common with this drug; here's a paper cup for the client to spit into."
  ☐ 3. "Don't worry about it; this is only a minor inconvenience compared to its benefits."
  ☐ 4. "I've seen this happen to other clients who are taking clozapine."

73. Which medication should the nurse anticipate administering in the event of a heparin overdose?
  ☐ 1. warfarin sodium
  ☐ 2. protamine sulfate
  ☐ 3. aspirin
  ☐ 4. atropine sulfate

74. The nurse has administered aminophylline to a client with emphysema. Which finding indicates the medication has been effective?
  ☐ 1. relief from spasms of the diaphragm
  ☐ 2. relaxation of smooth muscles in the bronchioles
  ☐ 3. efficient pulmonary circulation
  ☐ 4. stimulation of the medullary respiratory center

75. When teaching a client with bipolar disorder who has started to take valproic acid about possible side effects of this medication, the nurse should instruct the client to report which side effect?
  ☐ 1. increased urination
  ☐ 2. slowed thinking
  ☐ 3. sedation
  ☐ 4. weight loss

76. A 36-month-old child weighing 44 lb (20 kg) is to receive ceftriaxone 2 g IV every 12 hours. The recommended dose of ceftriaxone is 50 to 75 mg/kg per day in divided doses. How should the nurse proceed?
  ☐ 1. Administer the medication as prescribed.
  ☐ 2. Administer half the prescribed dose.
  ☐ 3. Call the laboratory to check the therapeutic serum level of ceftriaxone.
  ☐ 4. Withhold administering the ceftriaxone, and notify the health care provider (HCP).

77. The health care provider's (HCP's) prescription for an intravenous (IV) infusion is 3% normal saline to infuse at 125 mL per hour. The client's most recent sodium level is 132 mEq/L (132 mmol/L). What should the nurse do **next**?
  ☐ 1. Hang 0.9% normal saline at 125 mL per hour.
  ☐ 2. Start the IV solution as prescribed.
  ☐ 3. Consult the prescriber about the prescription.
  ☐ 4. Hang the IV solution prescribed at 62 mL per hour.

78. A client is admitted to the emergency department experiencing syncope. The nurse speaks with the family concerning the client's condition and current medications. The client's family states that the client takes several medications and has brought all the client's medications with them. To determine the correct medications required for this client, the nurse performs which step of the required process to ensure safe administration of medications?
☐ 1. verification
☐ 2. clarification
☐ 3. documentation
☐ 4. reconciliation

79. The health care provider prescribes an intramuscular injection of vitamin K for a term neonate. The nurse explains to the parent that this medication is used to prevent which problem?
☐ 1. hypoglycemia
☐ 2. hyperbilirubinemia
☐ 3. hemorrhage
☐ 4. polycythemia

80. A client's peripheral intravenous access does not have a blood return. To determine patency, the nurse should assess for which finding(s)? Select all that apply.
☐ 1. presence of localized swelling
☐ 2. date of intravenous catheter insertion
☐ 3. saline flush is met with resistance
☐ 4. client's report of discomfort with flushing
☐ 5. location of the catheter

Answers, Rationales, and Test-Taking Strategies

*The answers and rationales for each question follow below, along with keys (🔑) to the client need (CN) and cognitive level (CL) for each question. In addition, questions that measure clinical judgment will be coded (CJ). As you check your answers, use the **Content Mastery and Test-Taking Skill Self-Analysis** worksheet (tear-out worksheet in the back of the book) to identify the reason(s) for not answering the questions correctly. For additional information about test-taking skills and strategies for answering questions, refer to pages 12–54 in Part 1 of this book.*

1. 4. Rh sensitization can be prevented by Rho(D) immune globulin, which clears the maternal circulation of Rh-positive cells before sensitization can occur, thereby blocking maternal antibody production to Rh-positive cells. Administration of this drug will not prevent future Rh-positive fetuses, nor will it prevent future abortions. An antibody response will not occur to Rh-negative cells. Rh-negative birth parents do not develop sensitivities if the fetus is also Rh negative.

🔑 CN: Pharmacological and parenteral therapies; CL: Apply

2. 3. The client receiving magnesium sulfate intravenously is at risk for possible toxicity. The antidote for magnesium sulfate toxicity is calcium gluconate, which should be readily available at the client's bedside. Diazepam is used to treat anxiety, and usually it is not given to pregnant women. Hydralazine would be used to treat hypertension, and phenytoin would be used to treat seizures.

🔑 CN: Pharmacological and parenteral therapies; CL: Apply

3. 1. When administering blood replacement therapy, extreme caution is needed. Before administering any blood product, the nurse should validate the client's information and the blood product with another nurse to prevent administration of the wrong blood transfusion. Although baseline vital signs are necessary, the nurse should initiate the infusion of blood slowly for the first 10 to 15 minutes. Then, if there is no evidence of a reaction, the nurse should adjust the rate of infusion to ensure that the blood product is infused over 2 to 4 hours. The nurse can ask the client if they have ever had a reaction to a blood product, but a general question about allergies may not elicit the most complete response about any reactions to blood product administration. Blood transfusions are typically given with intravenous normal saline solution, not dextrose solutions.

🔑 CN: Pharmacological and parenteral therapies; CL: Apply

4. 1. Betamethasone therapy is indicated when the fetal lungs are immature. The fetus must be between 28 and 34 weeks' gestation, and birth must be delayed for 24 to 48 hours for the drug to achieve a therapeutic effect. Antibiotics would be used to treat chorioamnionitis. Betamethasone is not an antagonist for tocolytic therapy. It increases, not decreases, the production of neonatal surfactant.

🔑 CN: Pharmacological and parenteral therapies; CL: Apply

5. 2. Naloxone would not be used in a client who has a history of drug addiction. Naloxone would abruptly withdraw this client from the drug the client is addicted to as well as the nalbuphine. The withdrawal would occur within a few minutes of injection and, if severe enough, could jeopardize the client and fetus. Lidocaine is a local anesthetic and numbs rather than decreases the effects of nalbuphine. The local anesthetic and the pudendal block are both appropriate for this birth but are used to numb the maternal perineum for birth.

🗝️ CN: Pharmacological and parenteral therapies; CL: Analyze

6. 3. Cervical ripening, or creating a cervix that is soft, anterior, and dilated to 2 to 3 cm, must occur before the cervix can efface and dilate with oxytocin. Drugs to accomplish this goal include dinoprostone, misoprostol, and prostaglandin E2. Nalbuphine is a narcotic analgesic medication used in early labor and has no influence on the cervix. Betamethasone is a corticosteroid given to mature fetal lungs.

🗝️ CN: Pharmacological and parenteral therapies; CL: Apply

7. 2. Typically, a client will be able to have an epidural when they are 3 to 4 cm dilated or the active phase of labor has been established. Waiting until the cervix is dilated to this point ensures that the client is in labor and the epidural is less likely to halt labor contractions. Nalbuphine and promethazine are used to provide relief until the client is about 7 cm dilated. If given after this time, narcotic medication may cause neonatal respiratory depression in the neonate. The majority of clients have an epidural or spinal for a cesarean birth. The only time general anesthesia is used is for an emergency cesarean birth.

🗝️ CN: Pharmacological and parenteral therapies; CL: Evaluate

8. 2. The instillation of erythromycin into the neonate's eyes provides prophylaxis for ophthalmia neonatorum, or neonatal blindness caused by gonorrhea in the birth parent. Erythromycin is also effective in the prevention of infection and conjunctivitis from *Chlamydia trachomatis*. The medication may result in redness of the neonate's eyes, but this redness will eventually disappear. Erythromycin ointment is not effective in treating neonatal chorioretinitis from cytomegalovirus. No effective treatment is available for a birth parent with cytomegalovirus. Erythromycin ointment is not effective in preventing cataracts. Additionally, neonatal infection with beta-hemolytic streptococcus results in pneumonia, bacterial meningitis, or death. Cataracts in the neonate may be congenital or may result from maternal exposure to rubella. Erythromycin ointment is also not effective for preventing and treating strabismus (crossed eyes). Infants may exhibit intermittent strabismus until 6 months of age.

🗝️ CN: Pharmacological and parenteral therapies; CL: Apply

9. **135 mg.**

The recommended dose of ampicillin for a neonate is 100 mg/kg per dose. First, determine the neonate's weight in kilograms, and then multiply the kilograms by 100 mg. The nurse should use this formula:

$$1{,}000 \text{ g} = 1 \text{ kg}$$
$$1{,}350 \text{ g} = 1.35 \text{ kg}$$
$$100 \text{ mg} \times 1.35 \text{ kg} = 135 \text{ mg/kg}$$

🗝️ CN: Pharmacological and parenteral therapies; CL: Apply

10. 2. Titration prescriptions must include the medication name, route, starting rate of infusion (dose/min), incremental units the rate can be increased or decreased, frequency for incremental doses (how often the dose [rate] can be increased or decreased), maximum rate (dose) of infusion, and an objective clinical endpoint. This prescription does not contain a maximum rate and therefore must be clarified before administering the medication. The nurse cannot begin the infusion without clarification. Oxytocin infusions are not associated with respiratory or cardiac arrests to require the placement of adult resuscitation equipment in the room. Oxytocin is a high-alert medication that should be verified by two nurses, but only after the prescription is clarified.

🗝️ CN: Pharmacological and parental therapies; CL: Apply

11. 3. Routine flushing is not necessary for IV maintenance. Oral sucrose is an effective measure to reduce procedural pain. A sterile transparent dressing helps reduce infection while making the insertion site visible for continual assessment. Due to the fragility of an infant's blood vessels, hourly assessments for infiltrations are important to prevent tissue or skin damage.

🗝️ CN: Pharmacological and parenteral therapies; CL: Analyze

12. 3. Methadone is a controlled narcotic medication that needs an independent double check before the drug is given to assure the rights of drug administration. Vital signs are not necessary just before the administration of this drug. Infants with NAS will be assessed over a 3- to 6-hour period of time for behaviors; waking the infant for an assessment is not appropriate. The drug was prescribed by the health care provider, who is expecting the nurse to give and document the drug administration. No other notification is necessary unless there are other concerns.

🗝️ CN: Pharmacological and parenteral therapies; CL: Apply

13.

Obtain a digitalis level	Digitalis toxicity	Heart rate
Obtain an electrocardiogram		Intake and output

The infant's bradycardia, lethargy, diarrhea, and vomiting most suggest the infant has digitalis toxicity. The findings of a stable respiratory status and typical 2-month weight gain suggest that the infant does not have fluid overload. The weight, vital signs, and electrolytes do not indicate the infant is dehydrated as would be expected with gastroenteritis. Tachycardia or poor growth would be expected if the infant had anemia. The nurse should obtain a digitalis level and an electrocardiogram to check for arrhythmias. Stool cultures are not needed unless the diarrhea persists. Obtaining hemoglobin and hematocrit levels is not critical because the infant is on iron and gaining weight. A chest x-ray is not needed because the respiratory status is stable. The nurse will monitor the heart rate and hold digitalis for rates less than 90 bpm. The nurse will also monitor intake and output for resolution of the diarrhea. The nurse would continue with routine monitoring of breath sounds, color, and pulse oximetry. Since these parameters are normal, they are not the best indicators of the infant's progress.

CJ: Standalone bowtie; CL: Create

14. 6, 2, 1, 3, 4, 5. When dispensing medication from an inhaler, the client should first shake the inhaler and then breathe out through their mouth before putting the inhaler in their mouth. The client then presses the canister to dispense the medication and inhales slowly. The client should hold their breath for 5 to 10 seconds before exhaling.

CN: Pharmacological and parenteral therapies; CL: Apply

15. 2. When a person is taking amoxicillin as well as an oral contraceptive, it renders the contraceptive less effective. Because pregnancy can occur in such a situation, the nurse should advise the client to use additional means of birth control during the time they are taking the antibiotic. There are no risks associated with the concurrent use of amoxicillin and over-the-counter antihistamines, vitamins, or ibuprofen.

CN: Pharmacological and parenteral therapies; CL: Apply

16. 2, 3, 5. Adverse effects from nonsteroidal anti-inflammatory drugs include abdominal pain, blood in stool, and reduced clotting ability. Weight gain is common with corticosteroids. Folic acid deficiency is associated with methotrexate therapy.

CN: Pharmacological and parenteral therapies; CL: Apply

17. 1. Digoxin's effect is to slow the rate of electrical conduction through the heart and increase the strength of the heart's contraction. Signs of toxicity include anorexia and decreased heart rate, not visual changes or increases in heart rate. Digoxin should be taken 1 hour before meals or 2 hours after meals to obtain better absorption of the drug. If the child vomits within 15 minutes of administration, the dose should not be repeated because it is not known how much of the medication has been absorbed.

CN: Pharmacological and parenteral therapies; CL: Apply

18. 7.5 mL.

$$\frac{mL}{dose} = \frac{5\ mL}{10\ mg} \times \frac{30\ mg}{1\ day} \times \frac{1\ day}{2\ doses} = \frac{7.5\ mL}{dose}$$

CN: Pharmacologic and parental therapies; CL: Apply

19. 65 mL/h.

10 kg × 100 mL = 1,000 mL

10 kg × 50 mL = 500 mL

3 kg × 20 mL = 60 mL

1,000 mL + 500 mL + 60 mL = 1,560 mL/day

$$\frac{1,560\ mL}{24} = 65\ mL/h$$

CN: Pharmacologic and parental therapies; CL: Apply

20. 2. Sulfonamides have been associated with severe adverse reactions. A blistering rash may be a sign of Stevens-Johnson syndrome, a severe allergic reaction that manifests as skin lesions. This reaction is life-threatening and requires immediate attention. Lotion should not be applied to skin with blisters. Sulfamethoxazole and trimethoprim may cause photosensitivity, but this usually appears as a mild red rash, not blisters. Increasing the child's fluid intake may help the urinary tract infection but does not address the rash.

CN: Pharmacological and parenteral therapies; CL: Apply

21. 2. Phenytoin can cause gingival hyperplasia. Children taking phenytoin should brush their teeth after every meal and at bedtime and visit their dentist regularly. Drinking plenty of fluids is not required while taking phenytoin. A child on phenytoin does not need to be observed during waking hours because the seizures should be under control. Infections do not occur with an increased incidence in clients receiving phenytoin.

⚿ CN: Pharmacological and parenteral therapies; CL: Apply

22. 2. Pallor, coolness of the skin, swelling, or discomfort may occur at the insertion site if an IV infiltrates because IV fluid is being deposited in the subcutaneous tissue rather than in the vein. When the pressure in the tissues exceeds the pressure in the tubing, the flow of the IV solution will stop, eventually causing the alarms on the pump to sound. The nurse should first determine the reason for the alarm. Once the nurse has determined that the infusion has infiltrated, the nurse will turn the alarm off and then can elevate the client's arm and stop the infusion.

⚿ CN: Pharmacological and parenteral therapies; CL: Analyze

23. 2, 1, 4, 3. Clean gloves must be donned before any invasive procedure to protect both the client and the nurse from encountering bodily fluids. The vein is stabilized before needle insertion so the vein is less likely to "roll" and the catheter may be more easily threaded into the vein. Flashback signifies that the needle is in the vein, and the catheter is advanced into the vein, using the needle as a guide. Once the catheter is in the vein and connected to the saline lock, it must be stabilized and secured with a transparent dressing so the nurse can monitor the site.

⚿ CN: Pharmacological and parenteral therapies; CL: Create

24. 1. The nurse notes that 600 mL of D5NS has been infused over 45 minutes. The client is showing signs of circulatory overload, and the first action the nurse should take is to slow the IV infusion as the source of the problem. The nurse can then elevate the head of the bed to improve the client's ability to breathe and notify the HCP of the change in condition. The nurse should not remove the IV catheter unless there is infiltration as the open line may be needed for administration of medications.

⚿ CN: Pharmacological and parenteral therapies; CL: Analyze

25. 3. Infusing normal saline at a slow rate will maintain IV access and help maintain the client's intravascular volume. Culturing the catheter tip is not necessary because the catheter should not be removed and the concern is transfusion reaction, not infection. If a transfusion reaction is suspected, the nurse should not restart the blood. The HCP should be notified of the suspected reaction after the nurse has stopped the infusion of blood and started an infusion of normal saline.

⚿ CN: Pharmacological and parenteral therapies; CL: Analyze

26. 3. The nurse should carefully assess the client to determine the reason for the grimacing and restlessness. The nurse should not assume by the client's nonverbal communication that the client is in pain and requires pain medication; the nurse must validate the message rather than make assumptions. The nurse should assess the client first before changing the client's position or turning down the lights.

⚿ CN: Pharmacological and parenteral therapies; CL: Analyze

27. **41 mL per hour.** To determine the prescribed infusion rate, the nurse needs to calculate the drip rate for all drugs:

TPN: 1500 mL divided by 24 hours = 62.5, rounded to 63 mL per hour

Lipids: 250 mL divided by 12 hours = 20.8 rounded to 21 mL per hour

LR: 125 (total fluid intake) − (63 + 21) = 41 mL per hour (decreased from 80 mL per hour)

⚿ CN: Pharmacological and parenteral therapies; CL: Apply

28. 4. The client has signs of an air embolus. An air embolism occurs when a bolus of air enters the client's body through an open access in the venous system. Once the cap has been replaced, no more air will enter. The HCP should be informed immediately. The chest pain will not resolve on its own, and an ECG would be obtained immediately after notifying the HCP. Having the client sit in the low Fowler position will not improve oxygenation.

⚿ CN: Pharmacological and parenteral therapies; CL: Analyze

29. 1. Before the nurse flushes the line and adds the medication, gently aspirating will determine the patency of the device. A return of blood indicates the line is in the vein. After determining the line is patent, the nurse can flush the line with saline. This is not the time to reconfirm that this is the correct client because this has been accomplished before beginning this procedure. The medication can only be administered after the nurse has flushed the line with saline.

⚿ CN: Pharmacological and parenteral therapies; CL: Analyze

The Nursing Care of the Childbearing Family 959

30. 2. Omeprazole has not been approved or determined safe to use during pregnancy as it might harm the fetus. It is highly likely the client has some type of gastrointestinal condition, and this category of drugs is used for ulcers. Omeprazole has been recommended to treat *H. pylori* ulcers in combination with other medications. This medication should never be crushed as it will render the medication ineffective.

CN: Pharmacological and parenteral therapies; CL: Evaluate

31. 3. Grapefruit juice is contraindicated when taking this medication because it slows the metabolism of the drug, which increases the levels of it in the client's system, potentially causing liver damage or rhabdomyolysis. Increasing exercise will be a part of a healthy plan to decrease cardiac disease. Low-fat diets will also help lower the chances of coronary artery disease. Liver and kidney function tests will help determine the client's ability to metabolize and excrete the medication.

CN: Pharmacological and parenteral therapies; CL: Evaluate

32. 2. Rosuvastatin has been shown to reach higher serum levels in persons of Asian descent and should not be used in this group of clients. There is no liquid form for this medication. The cost is always important, but this is not the most significant concern at this point. It is not uncommon to have this drug prescribed to clients with a history of cardiovascular disease as a means of preventing the progression of the disease.

CN: Pharmacological and parenteral therapies; CL: Analyze

33. 2. Time-critical medications are those medications that can cause client harm or subtherapeutic blood levels and should be administered within 30 minutes of the scheduled time. These include antibiotics, anticoagulants, immunosuppressants, insulin, and antiseizure medications. Non–time-critical medications, such as lisinopril, metoprolol, and the pneumococcal vaccine, should generally be administered within 1 to 2 hours of the scheduled time. However, agency policy dictates the window of time to administer non–time-critical medications and may vary by institution.

CN: Pharmacological and parenteral therapies; CL: Analyze

34. 3. The nurse should clean the capped injection port prior to each time it is entered. It is not necessary to clean the injection port at other times, and the other options do not address the importance of cleaning a port before every entry.

CN: Pharmacological and parenteral therapies; CL: Apply

35. 2. The nurse should use the intravenous line with the normal saline. When the intravenous piggyback medication is infusing, the primary line will not infuse. Therefore, the nurse should not interfere with the infusion of heparin, even if compatible, because the partial thromboplastin time may become subtherapeutic. Additionally, no medication line should ever be added to blood or blood products or to parenteral nutrition.

CN: Pharmacological and parenteral therapies; CL: Apply

36. 4. The nurse should inject the medication into the port closest to the client. Administering the medication higher in the tubing makes flushing the tubing difficult and has the potential to interfere with the rate of administration, either of which could alter complete delivery of the medication.

CN: Pharmacological and parenteral therapies; CL: Apply

37. 3, 4, 5. The nurse should always tell the client the name of the medication. The nurse should also tell the client, in lay terms, the purpose of the medication and potential adverse effects that the client may experience and should report to the nurse. The expiration date and incompatibilities with other medications should be noted by the nurse, but they do not need to be communicated to the client. The client does not need to know the manufacturer of the medication.

CN: Pharmacological and parenteral therapies; CL: Apply

38. 3. A standardized sedation scale such as the Pasero Opioid-Induced Sedation Scale (POSS) is used to monitor the client for excessive sedation. A score of 3 on this scale indicates the client is oversedated, and the nurse should contact the HCP to request to administer 25% to 50% less of the medication for this dose. The nurse should not administer the medication or increase the dose. A reversal agent, such as naloxone, is not warranted unless the client has reached a POSS score of 4 or is showing signs of respiratory depression.

CN: Pharmacological and parenteral therapies; CL: Analyze

39. -/+ **2, 4, 5.** When a client is receiving an infusion of self-administered analgesia, the nurse should monitor the level of sedation, oxygen saturation, and vital signs. An oxygen saturation reading may be obtained by oximetry or capnography. The latter is helpful in the identification of respiratory depression secondary to opioid use. Arterial blood gas values will provide oxygenation levels as well, but the invasive nature of arterial blood gases is not necessary for a client beginning patient-controlled analgesia. Muscle strength may be impacted by excessive analgesia, but it is not a routine part of client monitoring with patient-controlled analgesia.

CN: Pharmacological and parenteral therapies; CL: Apply

40. 1474 mL. An intravenous infusion at 83 mL per hour will infuse 664 mL over 8 hours. The vancomycin volume is 250 mL, and the ½ liter of normal saline is 500 mL. Ice melts to one-half of its volume in water. Since a cup is 240 mL, and the client consumed ½ a cup or 120 mL, the client had a total oral intake of 60 mL. This totals 664 mL + 250 mL + 500 mL + 60 mL = 1474 mL.

CN: Pharmacological and parenteral therapies; CN: Apply

41. 1. The nurse should attempt to use insertion sites from most distal to proximal. Therefore, the nurse should next attempt to insert the intravenous catheter in the cephalic vein of the upper arm. The metacarpal vein, the hand, and the wrist and forearm sites are all distal to the median cubital vein.

CN: Pharmacological and parenteral therapies; CL: Analyze

42. 1. A transparent dressing is optimal since it allows assessment of the insertion site. A sterile gauze dressing must be changed every 48 hours or more often if needed according to agency protocol. Adhesive bandages are not occlusive, cover a small surface area, and often irritate the skin. Hydrocolloid and foam dressings are used on pressure ulcers and not peripheral intravenous sites.

CN: Pharmacological and parenteral therapies; CL: Analyze

43. 600 mL. Because the primary infusion does not run when an intravenous piggyback is infusing, the normal saline at 125 mL per hour was off during the 4-hour infusion of the piperacillin and tazobactam. Therefore, the client received 500 mL of the 0.9% sodium chloride infusion and 100 mL of the antibiotic infusion for a total of 600 mL.

CN: Pharmacological and parenteral therapies; CL: Apply

44. -/+ **1, 2, 3.** Pentoxifylline is used to treat pain for clients with peripheral vascular disease. The drug does not have an immediate action, and it is important that this medication is taken until a therapeutic effect has been achieved. Smoking causes vasoconstriction, and pentoxifylline causes vasodilation. Pentoxifylline can also cause dizziness or blurred vision; the nurse should instruct clients taking this medication to avoid driving and operating heavy machinery until they know how it affects them. Pentoxifylline does not require weekly laboratory studies, and clients taking pentoxifylline do not have to restrict the amount of green leafy vegetables they eat.

CN: Pharmacological and parenteral therapies; CL: Apply

45. -/+ **2, 4.** Clopidogrel is an antiplatelet agent. A potential side effect of this medication is neutropenia. The client should report an elevated body temperature as this could indicate neutropenia and should be reported to the primary care provider. Omeprazole is contraindicated in clients taking clopidogrel. Omeprazole utilizes the same CYP2C19 pathway and can interfere with the metabolism of clopidogrel.

CN: Pharmacological and parenteral therapies; CL: Evaluate

46. 2. INR is the diagnostic test used to determine the effectiveness of warfarin. The therapeutic range for clients with atrial fibrillation is 2 to 3. The nurse should contact the health care provider because the client's INR exceeds the normal range. APTT is the diagnostic test for clients receiving heparin.

CN: Pharmacological and parenteral therapies; CL: Apply

47. -/+ **2, 3, 4, 5.** To administer this drug safely and follow the rights of medication administration for this drug, the nurse should verify the medication is the right drug, right dose, right route, right time, right client, and the right documentation. The nurse should use two identifiers before administering any medication. It is also essential to determine when the last dose is given and whether or not the amount prescribed is correct. Documenting the reason for the medication is an important part of the documentation. The nurse should evaluate the client's response to the morphine within 15 to 30 minutes of administering the drug.

CN: Pharmacological and parenteral therapies; CL: Apply

48. -/+ **2, 3, 4.** Rivaroxaban is an anticoagulant, and it should be taken at the same time every day. Rivaroxaban can be taken with or without food; it is not necessary to take the medication with a full glass of water. If a dose is missed, clients should take the medication as soon as they remember and then take the next dose at the regularly scheduled time. A client should not stop taking rivaroxaban abruptly as clotting may occur.

  CN: Pharmacological and parenteral therapies; CL: Evaluate

49. 2, 3. *Absolute* contraindications for a client to receive fibrinolytic medication include a history of any intracranial hemorrhage; symptoms or signs suggestive of aortic dissection; history of ischemic stroke within the preceding 3 months (unless it is an acute ischemic stroke occurring within the last 3 hours, then fibrinolysis is useful!); the presence of a cerebral vascular malformation or a primary or metastatic intracranial malignancy; or significant closed-head or facial trauma within the preceding 3 months. *Relative contradictions* include severe hypertension or uncontrolled hypertension (blood pressure higher than 180 mm Hg systolic or higher than 110 mm Hg diastolic); ischemic stroke more than 3 months ago; major surgery within the last 3 weeks; or internal bleeding within the last 2 to 4 weeks.

  CN: Pharmacological and parenteral therapies; CL: Analyze

50. 3, 5. Benazepril is an angiotensin-converting enzyme (ACE) inhibitor. ACE inhibitors can cause severe renal insufficiency and exacerbate it in other susceptible clients. Therefore, the client should have their BUN and creatinine levels monitored frequently. In addition, ACE inhibitors can cause hyperkalemia because of the inhibition of aldosterone. Clients receiving ACE inhibitors need to have their potassium levels monitored. ACE inhibitors do not affect liver enzymes such as AST or ALT, blood glucose levels, or albumin.

  CN: Pharmacological and parenteral therapies; CL: Analyze

51. 736.7 mg.

$$X \text{ mg} = 85 \text{ kg} \times 10 \text{ mg}/1 \text{ kg} = 850 \text{ mg}/60 \text{ min} \times (60 - 8 \text{ min}) = 736.67 \text{ mg}$$

  CN: Pharmacological and parenteral therapies; CL: Apply

52. 1, 2, 3. The medication given was double the amount prescribed, and it is important to document the amount given and continue to monitor the client. An incident report needs to be completed that outlines the events, provides the client's status, and documents that all parties involved were notified of the events and the client's current status. The incident report is a process used by health care organizations to monitor events that occur. Documenting this information on the client's chart allows a legal team the option to subpoena the document. Doing nothing prevents a health care organization from analyzing the near misses or errors that occur and facilitating identification of system processes that need to be changed.

  CN: Management of care; CL: Apply

53. 1, 2, 4, 5. Ziprasidone can cause drowsiness, weight gain (can be excessive), nausea, and headache; these side effects may preclude noncompliance with this medication. Diarrhea is not a common side effect of ziprasidone.

  CN: Pharmacological and parenteral therapies; CL: Analyze

54. 4. Clients taking risperidone may develop signs and symptoms of neuroleptic malignant syndrome. The client's vital signs may be markedly elevated. The nurse should then contact the health care provider. The nurse would not call the family at this point in the incident. The medication will be held if the client does have neuroleptic malignant syndrome, so administering another dose is not therapeutic. Benztropine is used to treat symptoms of Parkinson disease or involuntary movements, not neuroleptic malignant syndrome.

  CN: Pharmacological and parental therapies; CL: Analyze

55. 1. Clients taking phenelzine, a monoamine oxidase inhibitor, cannot take foods with high tyramine content. Pepperoni is a sausage with a high tyramine content. Yogurt with fruit, Salisbury steak, and green beans have little or no tyramine.

  CN: Pharmacological and parental therapies; CL: Analyze

56. 1, 3, 4, 5. Additional caution and increased monitoring to lessen the increased risk for opioid use disorder are needed among clients with mental health conditions (including depression, anxiety disorders, and posttraumatic stress disorder). When used for acute pain, opioids should be used for fewer than 7 days due to the risk for dependence. Cognitive impairment is a common risk for opioid therapy among older adults. Adequate treatment for depression can have a positive impact on chronic pain levels. There is an increased risk for drug overdose among clients with depression, making opioids more of a risk to use for chronic pain. Opioids are not the best therapeutic option for controlling chronic pain: nonpharmacologic and nonopioid pain medications should be used to manage chronic pain.

  CN: Pharmacological and parenteral therapies; CL: Apply

57. 2. The anticholinergic effects of the client's medication may cause blurry vision, urine retention, constipation, and dry mouth. Gastrointestinal motility may be further compromised by a decreased level of activity associated with depression. Constipation needs to be addressed to prevent additional gastrointestinal problems. Anticholinergic effects do not result in vomiting, diarrhea, or weight loss.

CN: Pharmacological and parental therapies; CL: Analyze

58. 1. The client is experiencing the side effect of dystonia, an extrapyramidal symptom (EPS). Treatment for EPS is with an antiparkinson drug class, which includes benztropine. Lorazepam is prescribed for anxiety, which may be appropriate for fear, but it does not resolve the underlying pathophysiological process. Diphenhydramine is an antihistamine commonly used in allergy reactions and may cause sleepiness. Meperidine is a narcotic pain medication that will not resolve the cause of the client's pain.

CN: Pharmacological and parental therapies; CL: Analyze

59. 4. The client and spouse need to understand the features of taking sertraline hydrochloride, a selective serotonin reuptake inhibitor (SSRI). It should be taken in the morning to counter the expected side effect of insomnia. It takes 4 to 6 weeks for the SSRI to reach therapeutic levels, and St. John's wort should not be taken with any other type of antidepressant medication; it may also interact with multiple medications. Cold or allergy medications do not affect the effectiveness of an SSRI.

CN: Pharmacological and parenteral therapies; CL: Evaluate

60. 1. Benzodiazepines are a central nervous system depressant, and the client should be monitored regularly for increased tolerance and risk for addiction. Although there is a risk for tolerance and addiction, the medication can be safely used with proper monitoring. Drowsiness, not wakefulness, is a common side effect, and food is not needed to increase absorption.

CN: Pharmacological and parenteral therapies; CL: Apply

61. 3. Buspirone is not habit-forming, is administered on a schedule, and does not work immediately. Buspirone may have side effects such as chest pain, dizziness, headache, drowsiness, or nausea. Buspirone hydrochloride is not chemically or pharmacologically related to benzodiazepines or other sedative medications.

CN: Pharmacological and parental therapies; CL: Analyze

62. 2. Reduced liver and kidney function are expected in older adults; benzodiazepines and many other medications should be administered cautiously to them. Older adults are also at increased risk for falls because of oversedation that can occur with benzodiazepines. While benzodiazepines may be prescribed in lower doses, they can still be used in older adults with monitoring for safety.

CN: Pharmacological and parenteral therapies; CL: Analyze

63. 4. After administering naloxone, the nurse should monitor the client's respiratory status carefully because the drug is short acting and respiratory depression may recur after its effects wear off. Cerebral edema, kidney failure, and seizure activity are not directly related to opioid overdose or naloxone therapy.

CN: Pharmacological and parenteral therapies; CL: Analyze

64. 2. Lorazepam, as opposed to alprazolam, is available in dosage ranges that allow more gradual tapering down of doses over 3 to 4 days. Haloperidol is not effective for benzodiazepine withdrawal. Tapering alprazolam in 48 hours is too rapid. Offering alprazolam as a PRN does not deal with the need to gradually reduce the dose and frequency over time.

CN: Pharmacological and parenteral therapies; CL: Analyze

65. 3. The single-dose form of methylphenidate should be taken 10 to 14 hours before bedtime to prevent problems with insomnia, which can occur when the daily or last dose of the medication is taken within 6 hours (for multiple dosing) or 10 to 14 hours (for single dosing) before bedtime. It is recommended that a missed dose be taken as soon as possible; the dose is skipped if it is not remembered until the next dose is due. Any other medication, including over-the-counter medications, should be discussed with the health care provider before use to eliminate the risk for a possible drug interaction.

CN: Pharmacological and parenteral therapies; CL: Apply

66. 2. The nurse should hold the 1700 hours dose of lithium because a level of 1.8 mEq/L (1.8 mmol/L) can cause adverse reactions, including diarrhea, vomiting, drowsiness, muscle weakness, and lack of coordination, which are early signs of lithium toxicity. The nurse should report the lithium level to the health care provider, including any symptoms of toxicity. Administering the 1700 hours dose of lithium, giving the client the lithium with 240 mL of water, or giving it after supper would increase the lithium level, thus increasing the risk for lithium toxicity.

⚷ CN: Pharmacological and parenteral therapies; CL: Apply

67. 2. Nausea and gastrointestinal upset are common, but usually temporary, side effects of paroxetine. Therefore, the nurse would instruct the client to take the medication with food to minimize nausea and stomach upset. Other more common side effects are dry mouth, constipation, headache, dizziness, sweating, loss of appetite, ejaculatory problems in men, and decreased orgasms in women. Taking the medication an hour before breakfast would most likely lead to further gastrointestinal upset. Taking the medication at bedtime is not recommended because paroxetine can cause nervousness and interfere with sleep. Because orange juice is acidic, taking the medication with it, especially on an empty stomach, may lead to nausea or increase the client's gastrointestinal upset.

⚷ CN: Pharmacological and parenteral therapies; CL: Apply

68. 3. The client needs to be informed of the time lag involved with antidepressant therapy. Although improvement in the client's symptoms will occur gradually over 1 to 2 weeks, typically it takes 2 to 4 weeks to get the full effects of the medication. This information will help the client be compliant with medication and will also help decrease any anxiety the client has about not feeling better. The client's dose may not need to be increased; it is too early to determine the full effectiveness of the drug. Additionally, such a statement may increase the client's anxiety and diminish self-worth. Telling the client to wait a few days discounts the client's feelings and is inappropriate. Although it is too soon to tell whether the medication will be effective, telling this to the client may cause the client undue distress. This statement is somewhat negative because it is possible that the medication will not be effective, possibly further compounding the client's anxiety about not feeling better.

⚷ CN: Pharmacological and parenteral therapies; CL: Analyze

69. 4. The nurse should express concern for the client and offer to help the client speak with the HCP, which will lend support to the client's concerns. The client who has stopped the medication must be taken seriously because medication noncompliance could result in a recurrence of symptoms of depression. Telling the client to focus on diet and exercise ignores the client's feelings and subtly implies the weight gain is the client's fault. Pointing out that the medication has helped and that positive things have happened since the depression lifted may be true, but it does not address the client's current feelings or needs.

⚷ CN: Pharmacological and parenteral therapies; CL: Analyze

70. 4. The most urgent consideration for intervention and teaching is the fact that for individuals with a history of bipolar disorder, antidepressants when taken alone can push the person into mania. Antipsychotics are sometimes prescribed for clients with bipolar disorder and would not pose a special concern. Individuals with bipolar disorder are typically treated with mood stabilizers, and benzodiazepines are sometimes used in the short term to give a client relief before the mood stabilizers can take effect.

⚷ CN: Pharmacological and parenteral therapies; CL: Analyze

71. The median cubital vein is located in the approximate center of the antecubital space.

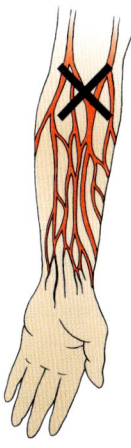

⚷ CN: Pharmacological and parenteral therapies; CL: Apply

72. 2. Telling the parent that excess saliva is a common adverse effect of the drug is most helpful because it gives the parent information about the problem, thereby helping to decrease anxiety about what is occurring with the client. By offering the paper cup, the nurse also demonstrates concern for the client, thereby leading to increased trust. Saying "I wonder if they are having an adverse reaction to the medicine" shows the nurse's lack of knowledge about the drug, decreases confidence in the nurse, and indicates poor judgment. Saying "Don't worry about it, it's only a minor inconvenience compared to its benefits" or telling the parent that the nurse has seen this happening to other clients is insensitive and does not assuage the parent's anxiety.

CN: Pharmacological and parenteral therapies; CL: Analyze

73. 2. Protamine sulfate is a heparin antagonist. It is administered intravenously very slowly (over at least 10 minutes). Warfarin sodium and aspirin have anticoagulant properties and would be contraindicated. Atropine sulfate is an anticholinergic drug and would not be effective in treating a heparin overdose.

CN: Pharmacological and parenteral therapies; CL: Apply

74. 2. Aminophylline, a bronchodilator that relaxes smooth muscles in the bronchioles, is used in the treatment of emphysema to improve ventilation by dilating the bronchioles. Aminophylline does not affect the diaphragm or the medullary respiratory center and does not promote pulmonary circulation.

CN: Pharmacological and parenteral therapies; CL: Evaluate

75. 3. Valproic acid causes sedation as well as nausea, vomiting, and indigestion. Sedation is important because the client needs to be cautioned about driving or operating machinery that could be dangerous while feeling sedated from the medication. Valproic acid does not cause increased urination, slowed thinking, or weight loss. However, some clients may experience weight gain.

CN: Pharmacological and parenteral therapies; CL: Analyze

76. 4. The HCP should be notified because the maximum daily recommended dosage for ceftriaxone for this child's weight would be 1500 g a day, and giving this dose would administer 4 g a day. The nurse cannot administer a different dose than that prescribed. There is no therapeutic serum level of ceftriaxone.

CN: Pharmacological and parenteral therapies; CL: Apply

77. 3. Three percent saline is a hypertonic solution, which will pull fluid from the interstitial and intracellular spaces into the bloodstream. Its use is usually reserved for severe hyponatremia (sodium level of less than 115 mEq/L). If this client were experiencing a fluid volume deficit, this IV solution could worsen the condition. The nurse should consult with the HCP about this prescription. The nurse does not have prescribing rights and cannot change the prescription. The IV rate of 62 mL per hour may still be dangerous for this client, and the rate was prescribed at 125 mL per hour.

CN: Pharmacologic and parenteral therapy; CL: Analyze

78. 2. Clarification is the process of confirming the appropriate medication and doses for any client. Verification is the process of collecting medication history. Reconciliation is the process of documenting medication prescription changes for a client across the continuum of care. Documentation is included as a step in the three steps of a formal medication reconciliation program.

CN: Pharmacological and parenteral therapies; CL: Apply

79. 3. Vitamin K acts as a preventive measure against neonatal hemorrhagic disease. At birth, the neonate does not have the intestinal flora to produce vitamin K, which is necessary for coagulation. Hypoglycemia is prevented and treated by feeding the infant. Hyperbilirubinemia severity can be decreased by early feeding and passage of meconium to excrete the bilirubin. Hyperbilirubinemia is treated with phototherapy. Polycythemia may occur in neonates who are large for gestational age or post term. Clamping of the umbilical cord before pulsations cease reduces the incidence of polycythemia. Generally, polycythemia is not treated unless it is extremely severe.

CN: Pharmacological and parenteral therapies; CL: Apply

80. -/+ 1, 3, 4. Swelling indicates infusion into the soft tissue rather than the vein. While ease of flushing may or may not indicate patency, meeting resistance indicates that the intravenous catheter is not patent. Infiltration may cause client discomfort and is also an indicator of patency. The date of catheter insertion should be noted, as should catheter location, but these are not indicators of catheter patency.

CN: Pharmacological and parenteral therapies; CL: Apply

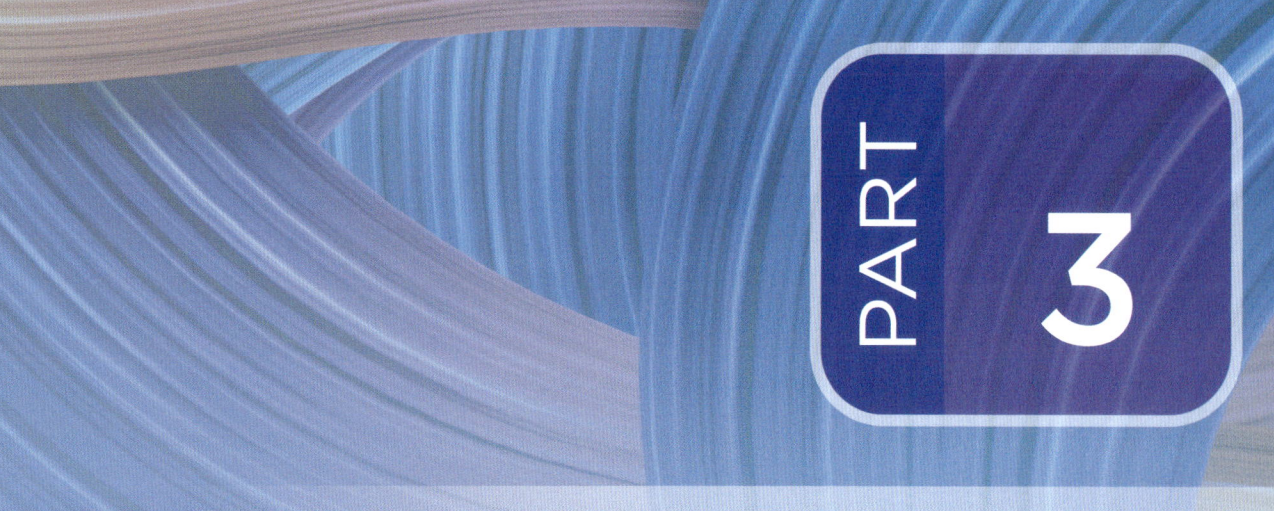

POSTREVIEW TESTS

1

Comprehensive Test

This test has 85 questions. Time yourself as you take the test so you can determine the approximate amount of time it takes to complete this many questions. This test reflects the minimum number of items you might receive on the actual licensing exam.

1. A client with human immunodeficiency virus (HIV) and acquired immunodeficiency syndrome confides that their employer does not know their HIV status. Which response by the nurse is **best**?
   - ☐ 1. "Would you like me to help you tell your employer?"
   - ☐ 2. "The information you confide in me is confidential."
   - ☐ 3. "I must share this information with your family."
   - ☐ 4. "I must share this information with your employer."

2. An older adult client is being admitted to same-day surgery for cataract extraction. The client has several diamond rings. What information should the nurse give the client about how the rings will be secured during surgery?
   - ☐ 1. The rings will be taped on the fingers before the surgery.
   - ☐ 2. The rings will be placed in an envelope, the client will sign the envelope, and the envelope will be placed in a safe.
   - ☐ 3. The rings will be locked in the narcotic box.
   - ☐ 4. The nursing supervisor will hold onto the rings until the client returns from the recovery room.

3. The nurse is conducting a health assessment on an adult client. The nurse may communicate medical information without the client's consent when:
   - ☐ 1. certifying the client's absence from work.
   - ☐ 2. requested by the client's family.
   - ☐ 3. treating the client with a sexually transmitted infection.
   - ☐ 4. prescribed by another health care provider (HCP).

4. A young adult client is brought to the emergency department with their fiancée after being involved in a serious motor vehicle crash. The client's Glasgow Coma Scale score is 7, and they demonstrate evidence of decorticate posturing. Which action is appropriate for obtaining permission to place a catheter for intracranial pressure (ICP) monitoring?
   - ☐ 1. The nurse will obtain a signed consent from the client's fiancée because the fiancée is of legal age and the couple is engaged to be married.
   - ☐ 2. The health care provider (HCP) will get a consultation from another HCP and proceed with the placement of the ICP catheter until the family arrives to sign the consent.
   - ☐ 3. Two nurses will receive verbal consent by telephone from the client's next of kin before inserting the catheter.
   - ☐ 4. The health care provider will document the emergency nature of the client's condition and that an ICP catheter for monitoring was placed without consent.

5. The nurse notices that a cart being used to transport a client has a nonfunctioning clasp on the safety belt. What should the nurse do **next**?
   - ☐ 1. Call the safety/security department to report the problem.
   - ☐ 2. Use a draw sheet to secure the client during transport.
   - ☐ 3. Contact the clinical engineering department to repair the clasp.
   - ☐ 4. Request that the transporter bring a different cart with a functional clasp.

6. The nurse is coaching a client about improving their health. Which strategy is the **most** effective for the nurse to use to help the client take an active role in their health care?
  ☐ 1. Give the client a questionnaire about their health to complete.
  ☐ 2. Provide the client with written instructions about health management.
  ☐ 3. Ask the client about their views of health and health care.
  ☐ 4. Determine if the client has any questions about their health.

7. The nurse is planning care for a client who chews the fingers constantly, leading to broken skin. Before applying mitten restraints, the nurse could try which intervention(s)? Select all that apply.
  ☐ 1. Ask the client to rub lotion over the hands every day after bathing.
  ☐ 2. Encourage physical activity, such as ambulation.
  ☐ 3. Provide frequent contacts for communication and socialization.
  ☐ 4. Educate the family on self-injury prevention strategies.
  ☐ 5. Encourage involvement of family and friends in the plan of care.

8. A client with major depression states, "Life is not worth living anymore. Nothing matters." Which response by the nurse is **best**?
  ☐ 1. "Are you thinking about killing yourself?"
  ☐ 2. "Things will get better, you know."
  ☐ 3. "Why do you think that way?"
  ☐ 4. "You should not feel that way."

9. A client with bipolar disorder has been prescribed olanzapine 5 mg two times a day and lamotrigine 25 mg two times a day. Which adverse effect(s) should the nurse report to the health care provider **immediately**? Select all that apply.
  ☐ 1. rash
  ☐ 2. nausea
  ☐ 3. sedation
  ☐ 4. hyperthermia
  ☐ 5. muscle rigidity

10. The nurse is planning care for an older adult with a pressure ulcer (see figure). What should the nurse do? Select all that apply.

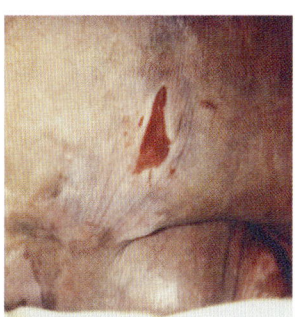

  ☐ 1. Elevate the head of the bed to 50 degrees.
  ☐ 2. Obtain daily cultures.
  ☐ 3. Cover the ulcer with protective dressing.
  ☐ 4. Reposition the client every 2 hours.
  ☐ 5. Request an alternating pressure mattress.

11. A client takes hydrochlorothiazide (HCTZ) for treatment of hypertension. The nurse should instruct the client to report which effect(s)? Select all that apply.
  ☐ 1. muscle twitching
  ☐ 2. abdominal cramping
  ☐ 3. diarrhea
  ☐ 4. confusion
  ☐ 5. lethargy
  ☐ 6. muscle weakness

12. STEP 1

The nurse admits a preschool-age male client with gastroenteritis to the pediatric floor.

Nurse's Notes

0900:
The parent reports that the 4-year-old client has had vomiting and diarrhea for 48 hours. In the last 24 hours, the client had 10 green liquid stools and vomited 8 times. The client is lethargic and refuses fluids. The client last voided before going to bed last night. The last known weight was 37.5 lb (17 kg) at the pediatrician's office 2 months ago. The client is otherwise healthy with some environmental allergies that can cause wheezing. Immunizations are up to date. Weight is 34.8 lb (15.8 kg). Vital signs are oral temperature 100°F (37.8°C); pulse 125 bpm; respiration rate 32 breaths/min; and blood pressure 90/60 mm Hg. Pulse oximetry reading is 96% on room air.

➤ Which vital sign(s) does the nurse recognize as being abnormal for a preschool-age client? Select all that apply.

- ☐ 1. temperature
- ☐ 2. heart rate
- ☐ 3. respiratory rate
- ☐ 4. blood pressure
- ☐ 5. oxygen saturation

13. STEP 2

The nurse admits a preschool-age male client with gastroenteritis to the pediatric floor.

Nurse's Notes

0900:
The parent reports that the 4-year-old client has had vomiting and diarrhea for 48 hours. In the last 24 hours, the client had 10 green liquid stools and vomited 8 times. The client is lethargic and refuses fluids. The client last voided before going to bed last night. The last known weight was 37.5 lb (17 kg) at the pediatrician's office 2 months ago. The client is otherwise healthy with some environmental allergies that can cause wheezing. Immunizations are up to date. Weight is 34.8 lb (15.8 kg). Vital signs are oral temperature 100°F (37.8°C); pulse 125 bpm; respiration rate 32 breaths/min; and blood pressure 90/60 mm Hg. Pulse oximetry reading is 96% on room air.

➤ What additional information does the nurse need to gather **next** to assess the client's hydration status? Select all that apply.

- ☐ 1. bowel sounds
- ☐ 2. capillary refill
- ☐ 3. eyes
- ☐ 4. oral mucosa
- ☐ 5. posturing
- ☐ 6. presence of tears
- ☐ 7. skin temperature
- ☐ 8. skin turgor

14. STEP 3

The nurse admits a preschool-age male client with gastroenteritis to the pediatric floor.

Nurse's Notes

0900:
The parent reports that the 4-year-old client has had vomiting and diarrhea for 48 hours. In the last 24 hours, the client had 10 green liquid stools and vomited 8 times. The client is lethargic and refuses fluids. The client last voided before going to bed last night. The last known weight was 37.5 lb (17 kg) at the pediatrician's office 2 months ago. The client is otherwise healthy with some environmental allergies that can cause wheezing. Immunizations are up to date. Weight is 34.8 lb (15.8 kg). Vital signs are oral temperature 100°F (37.8°C); pulse 125 bpm; respiration rate 32 breaths/min; and blood pressure 90/60 mm Hg. Pulse oximetry reading is 96% on room air.

0915:
The eyes are slightly sunken, the capillary refill is 2 seconds, the skin is cool and moist, the mucous membranes are dry, and tears are absent.

The nurse completes the admission assessment and creates a problem list.

➤ Use words from the choices below to fill in each blank found in the following sentence.

The top priorities for this client are treating the _____ and the _____.

word choices
diarrhea
fever
fluid volume deficit
infection
vomiting

15. STEP 4

The nurse admits a preschool-age male client with gastroenteritis to the pediatric floor.

Nurse's Notes

0900:
The parent reports that the 4-year-old client has had vomiting and diarrhea for 48 hours. In the last 24 hours, the client had 10 green liquid stools and vomited 8 times. The client is lethargic and refuses fluids. The client last voided before going to bed last night. The last known weight was 37.5 lb (17 kg) at the pediatrician's office 2 months ago. The client is otherwise healthy with some environmental allergies that can cause wheezing. Immunizations are up to date. Weight is 34.8 lb (15.8 kg). Vital signs are oral temperature 100°F (37.8°C); pulse 125 bpm; respiration rate 32 breaths/min; and blood pressure 90/60 mm Hg. Pulse oximetry reading is 96% on room air.

0915:
The eyes are slightly sunken, the capillary refill is 2 seconds, the skin is cool and moist, the mucous membranes are dry, and tears are absent.

➤ Select the orders from each of the categories that the nurse anticipates including in the plan of care. Each category may have more than one order.

Category	Anticipated Orders
Nursing	☐ Vital signs every 30 minutes
	☐ Clear liquids and advance diet as tolerated
	☐ Weights every shift
Medications	☐ Ondansetron intravenously (IV) now
	☐ Acetaminophen with codeine orally (PO) every 4 hours as needed (PRN) for fever.
	☐ 250 mL lactated Ringer's IV fluid bolus now
Laboratory	☐ Urine culture
	☐ Stool culture
	☐ Electrolytes

Note: Each category must have at least one response option selected.

16. STEP 5

The nurse admits a preschool-age male client with gastroenteritis to the pediatric floor.

Nurse's Notes

0900:
The parent reports that the 4-year-old client has had vomiting and diarrhea for 48 hours. In the last 24 hours, the client had 10 green liquid stools and vomited 8 times. The client is lethargic and refuses fluids. The client last voided before going to bed last night. The last known weight was 37.5 lb (17 kg) at the pediatrician's office 2 months ago. The client is otherwise healthy with some environmental allergies that can cause wheezing. Immunizations are up to date. Weight is 34.8 lb (15.8 kg). Vital signs are oral temperature 100°F (37.8°C); pulse 125 bpm; respiration rate 32 breaths/min; and blood pressure 90/60 mm Hg. Pulse oximetry reading is 96% on room air.

0915:
The eyes are slightly sunken, the capillary refill is 2 seconds, the skin is cool and moist, the mucous membranes are dry, and tears are absent.

Medications

Home Scheduled Medications

Drug Name	Dose	Route	Frequency	Ordered (Y/N)
Cetirizine over the counter (OTC)	15-mg tablet	PO	Daily	N

Home PRN Medications

Drug Name	Dose	Route	Frequency	Ordered (Y/N)
Loperamide OTC	1 mg/5 mL	PO	Every 8 hours	N

➤ The nurse completes a home medication reconciliation and finds neither home medication is on the prescription list. Which action is needed?

☐ 1. Obtain a prescription to continue the cetirizine.
☐ 2. Request a prescription for loperamide.
☐ 3. Get prescriptions for both cetirizine and loperamide.
☐ 4. Continue implementing the plan of care without requesting cetirizine or loperamide.

17. STEP 6

The nurse admits a preschool-age male client with gastroenteritis to the pediatric floor.

Nurse's Notes

0900:
The parent reports that the 4-year-old client has had vomiting and diarrhea for 48 hours. In the last 24 hours, the client had 10 green liquid stools and vomited 8 times. The client is lethargic and refuses fluids. The client last voided before going to bed last night. The last known weight was 37.5 lb (17 kg) at the pediatrician's office 2 months ago. The client is otherwise healthy with some environmental allergies that can cause wheezing. Immunizations are up to date. Weight is 34.8 lb (15.8 kg). Vital signs are oral temperature 100°F (37.8°C); pulse 125 bpm; respiration rate 32 breaths/min; and blood pressure 90/60 mm Hg. Pulse oximetry reading is 96% on room air.

0915:
The eyes are slightly sunken, the capillary refill is 2 seconds, the skin is cool and moist, the mucous membranes are dry, and tears are absent.

1000:
An IV line is started in the client's right hand. A fluid bolus is started. Ondansetron is given. A stool culture, a urine culture, and electrolytes are sent to the lab.

1100:
A fluid bolus of lactated Ringer's solution is complete. An IV of lactated Ringer's is now infusing in the client's right hand at 60 mL per hour. The client took 60 mL orally and voided 50 mL of dark yellow urine. Capillary refill is 3 seconds. A preliminary stool culture is negative. Vital signs are oral temperature 99.4°F (37.4°C); heart rate 118 bpm; respiration rate 14 breaths/min; blood pressure 90/60 mm Hg; and pulse oximetry 97% on room air.

Medications

Home Scheduled Medications

Drug Name	Dose	Route	Frequency	Ordered (Y/N)
Cetirizine over the counter (OTC)	15-mg tablet	PO	Daily	N

Home PRN Medications

Loperamide OTC	1 mg/5 mL	PO	Every 8 hours	N

The nurse reassesses the client after administering the prescribed fluid bolus and ondansetron.

➤ For each finding, specify whether the finding indicates the interventions were effective, ineffective, or unrelated.

Assessment Findings	Effective	Ineffective	Unrelated
Respiratory rate	○	○	○
Heart rate	○	○	○
Temperature	○	○	○
Urine output	○	○	○
Stool culture	○	○	○
Oral intake	○	○	○
Capillary refill	○	○	○

18. A client has been taking imipramine for depression for 2 days. The client's sibling asks the nurse, "Why is my sibling still so depressed?" Which response by the nurse is **most** appropriate?
- ☐ 1. "They are experiencing a very serious depression."
- ☐ 2. "I will be sure to convey your concern to the health care provider (HCP)."
- ☐ 3. "It takes 2 to 4 weeks for the drug to reach its full effect."
- ☐ 4. "Perhaps we need to change the medication."

19. The nurse plans care for an adolescent with cystic fibrosis (CF). Which finding would require **immediate** intervention?
- ☐ 1. delayed puberty
- ☐ 2. chest pain with dyspnea
- ☐ 3. poor weight gain
- ☐ 4. large, foul-smelling, bulky stools

20. The nurse's assessment of a client starting on lithium reveals dry mouth, nausea, thirst, and mild hand tremor. Based on an analysis of these findings, what should the nurse do **next**?
- ☐ 1. Obtain a stat lithium level.
- ☐ 2. Immediately notify the health care provider (HCP).
- ☐ 3. Reassure the client that these temporary side effects will subside.
- ☐ 4. Assess the client for signs and symptoms of hypernatremia.

21. A client newly diagnosed with hypothyroidism asks the nurse how long it will be necessary to take the prescribed levothyroxine sodium. What should the nurse tell the client?
- ☐ 1. "It will be necessary to take the medication for the rest of your life."
- ☐ 2. "Because the medication is expensive, the health care provider will check your progress, and the dose may be able to be reduced in a few months."
- ☐ 3. "If your thyroid responds to the medication, the medication can be gradually withdrawn in 1 to 2 years."
- ☐ 4. "The medication can be discontinued when your thyroid-stimulating hormone (TSH) level is normal."

22. The nurse teaches a client about bipolar disorder. Which statement indicates that the client has developed insight about the diagnosis?
- ☐ 1. "I enjoy feeling high; I don't need much sleep then and get really creative."
- ☐ 2. "My medicine really helped me. I know I won't need it in about another week."
- ☐ 3. "I'm cured now. I was really wild for a while even though I got into trouble."
- ☐ 4. "I know I'm getting sick when I don't need much sleep and start buying things."

23. A client admitted with a gastric ulcer has been vomiting bright red blood. The hemoglobin level is 5.11 g/dL (51.1 g/L), and the blood pressure is 100/50 mm Hg. The client and family state that their religious beliefs do not support the use of blood products and refuse blood transfusions as a treatment for the bleeding. The nurse should collaborate with the health care provider and family to plan to take which action **next**?
- ☐ 1. Discontinue all measures.
- ☐ 2. Notify the hospital attorney.
- ☐ 3. Attempt to stabilize the client through the use of fluid replacement.
- ☐ 4. Give enough blood to keep the client from dying.

24. The nurse is caring for a 70-year-old woman admitted to the intensive care unit (ICU) with sudden-onset chest pain.

Nurse's Notes

1000:
The client was admitted with sudden-onset chest pain that was rated as a 5 on a 10-point scale. Vital signs are heart rate of 80 bpm; respiration rate of 22 breaths/min; and blood pressure of 140/82 mm Hg. Pulse oximetry reading on room air is 92%. The cardiac rhythm is a normal sinus rhythm on telemetry. An intravenous (IV) line of 1000 mL sodium chloride 9% is running at 75 mL per hour. Lab tests have been ordered. Morphine 2 mg was administered via IV push.

1020:
The client reports severe chest pain rated as a 10 on a 10-point scale and is restless and diaphoretic. Cardiac rhythm on telemetry is 6 premature ventricular contractions per minute.

➤ Complete the diagram by specifying what condition the client is most likely experiencing at 1020, two actions the nurse should take to address that condition, and two parameters the nurse should monitor to assess the client's progress.

Action to Take — Condition Most Likely Experiencing — Parameter to Monitor

Action to Take — Parameter to Monitor

Action to Take	Potential Conditions	Parameters to Monitor
Increase the IV infusion	Hypertension	Cardiac rhythm
Call the rapid response team	Premature ventricular contractions	Vital signs
Administer 5 mg metoprolol IV push as prescribed	Chest pain	Oxygen saturation
Notify the health care provider	Anxiety	Need for defibrillation
Prepare for defibrillation		Chest pain

25. A client is receiving nonsteroidal antiinflammatory drugs (NSAIDs) to manage the pain of rheumatoid arthritis. What information should the nurse give to the client about taking these medications?
☐ 1. Take NSAIDs only when experiencing pain.
☐ 2. Perform joint exercises before taking the next dose of the medication.
☐ 3. Take antacids 1 hour after taking NSAIDs.
☐ 4. Take NSAIDs with food.

26. A client is to receive an intramuscular (IM) injection using the Z-track injection technique. The nurse holds the gauze pledget against an IM injection site while removing the needle from the muscle. What is the intended outcome of this technique?
☐ 1. Seal off the track left by the needle in the tissue.
☐ 2. Speed the spread of the medication in the tissue.
☐ 3. Avoid the discomfort of the needle pulling on the skin.
☐ 4. Prevent organisms from entering the body through the skin puncture.

27. A client in treatment for alcohol dependency begins to talk about not having a problem with alcohol. What is the **best** approach for the nurse to use?
☐ 1. Question the client about how much alcohol the client consumes each day.
☐ 2. Confront the client about being intoxicated 2 days ago.
☐ 3. Point out the consequences of the client's drinking behaviors.
☐ 4. Ask the client about their reasons for not staying sober.

28. The nurse is caring for a toddler in contact isolation for respiratory syncytial virus. In what order from first to last should the nurse remove personal protective equipment (PPE)? All options must be used.

| 1. gloves |
| 2. goggles |
| 3. gown |
| 4. mask |
| |
| |
| |
| |

29. The nurse is teaching a hospitalized client with newly diagnosed type 1 diabetes about using finger-stick glucose monitoring. The client tells the nurse that the finger-stick strip shows a blood glucose level of 48 mg/dL (48 mmol/L). What should the nurse do **first**?
    ☐ 1. Start an intravenous infusion.
    ☐ 2. Have the client repeat the finger stick in 30 minutes.
    ☐ 3. Notify the health care provider (HCP) of the results.
    ☐ 4. Obtain a serum glucose level.

30. A client who has a diagnosis of borderline personality disorder is manipulative and very disruptive on the hospital unit. The client is not dangerous to themselves or others but is clearly not making any therapeutic progress. The client consistently refuses any medications. The nurse realizes that legally this client has which option?
    ☐ 1. Refuse treatment.
    ☐ 2. Receive forced treatment if the nursing team concurs.
    ☐ 3. Be medicated if the client's family signs permission for treatment.
    ☐ 4. Be guided to accept treatment recommendations by threatening loss of privileges.

31. A client who has a prescription to receive nothing by mouth (NPO) is constantly asking for a drink of water. Which nursing action is the **most** appropriate?
    ☐ 1. Explain again why it is not possible to have a drink of water.
    ☐ 2. Offer ice chips every hour to decrease thirst.
    ☐ 3. Offer the client frequent oral hygiene care.
    ☐ 4. Divert the client's attention by turning on the television.

32. An older adult who is to be on bed rest has become incontinent of urine. To prevent pressure ulcers, the nurse should do which task(s)? Select all that apply.
    ☐ 1. Use a sanitary napkin to absorb urine.
    ☐ 2. Institute a turning schedule.
    ☐ 3. Inspect the groin for wetness.
    ☐ 4. Have the client wear incontinence briefs.
    ☐ 5. Anchor a Foley catheter.

33. A nurse is teaching a new parent how to prevent burns in the home. Which statement by the parent indicates more teaching is required?
    ☐ 1. "I will set my hot water heater to 120°F (49°C)."
    ☐ 2. "I will not hold my infant while drinking coffee."
    ☐ 3. "I will heat my infant's formula in the microwave."
    ☐ 4. "I will keep loose appliance cords tied up on the counter."

34. The nurse teaches a primigravid client at 10 weeks' gestation about the recommendations for exercise during pregnancy. Which client statement indicates successful teaching?
    ☐ 1. "While pregnant, I should avoid contact sports."
    ☐ 2. "Even though I'm pregnant, I can learn to ski next month."
    ☐ 3. "While we are on vacation next month, I can continue to scuba dive."
    ☐ 4. "Sitting in a hot tub after exercise will help me to relax."

35. A client with rheumatoid arthritis is receiving antiinflammatory drugs and physical therapy. What is the expected outcome of these actions? The client will be able to:
    ☐ 1. manage joint pain and fatigue to perform activities of daily living.
    ☐ 2. maintain full range of motion in joints.
    ☐ 3. prevent the development of further pain and joint deformity.
    ☐ 4. take antiinflammatory medications as needed for pain.

36. A nurse has been exposed to hepatitis B through a needlestick injury. The nurse received the hepatitis B vaccine 3 years ago. Which actions should be included in the postexposure management plan? Select all that apply.
    ☐ 1. Wash the needlestick site with soap and water.
    ☐ 2. Wipe the site with an antiseptic solution.
    ☐ 3. Obtain a booster dose of hepatitis B vaccine.
    ☐ 4. Request a blood test for the virus.
    ☐ 5. Notify the nurse's supervisor.

37. An older adult who is alert and oriented is admitted to the hospital for treatment of cellulitis of the left shoulder. Which fall prevention strategy is **most** appropriate for this client?
    ☐ 1. Keep all the lights on in the room at all times.
    ☐ 2. Use a nightlight in the bathroom.
    ☐ 3. Keep all four side rails up at all times.
    ☐ 4. Use a medical alert system.

38. STEP 1

The nurse is caring for a 72-year-old female client in the telemetry unit.

Nurse's Notes

Today: 1900
The client was admitted earlier today to the telemetry unit for dehydration. The client states they were gardening yesterday and this morning in the hot sun. They started feeling lightheaded and weak at home; the client's son suggested seeing a health care provider.
The client takes hydrochlorothiazide for hypertension. The client is alert and oriented and denies pain, shortness of breath, or any other problems at this time. Vital signs are temperature 98.9°F (37.2°C); pulse 96 bpm; respirations 14 breaths/min; and blood pressure 118/70 mm Hg. The pulse oximetry reading is 97% on room air. The lungs are clear, bowel sounds are normal in all four quadrants, and heart sounds are normal. A peripheral intravenous (IV) line of 0.9% normal saline at 100 mL per hour is infusing without difficulty.

Today: 1930
The client reports their heart is racing and skipping and that they feel slightly short of breath.

➤ Which assessment(s) should the nurse obtain **immediately**?

- ☐ 1. Pulse
- ☐ 2. Blood pressure
- ☐ 3. Temperature
- ☐ 4. Heart rhythm
- ☐ 5. Skin turgor
- ☐ 6. Intake and output
- ☐ 7. Oxygen saturation

39. STEP 2

The nurse is caring for a 72-year-old female client in the telemetry unit.

Nurse's Notes

Today: 1900
The client was admitted earlier today to the telemetry unit for dehydration. The client states they were gardening yesterday and this morning in the hot sun. They started feeling lightheaded and weak at home; the client's son suggested seeing a health care provider.
The client takes hydrochlorothiazide for hypertension. The client is alert and oriented and denies pain, shortness of breath, or any other problems at this time. Vital signs are temperature 98.9°F (37.2°C); pulse 96 bpm; respirations 14 breaths/min; and blood pressure 118/70 mm Hg. The pulse oximetry reading is 97% on room air. The lungs are clear, bowel sounds are normal in all four quadrants, and heart sounds are normal. A peripheral intravenous (IV) line of 0.9% normal saline at 100 mL per hour is infusing without difficulty.

Today: 1930
The client reports their heart is racing and skipping and that they feel slightly short of breath.

The nurse obtains updated assessment data on the client.

➤ For each client finding below, specify if the finding is consistent with the disease process of dehydration or atrial fibrillation. Each finding may support more than one disease process.

Client Finding	Dehydration	Atrial Fibrillation
1. Increased pulse	☐	☐
2. Increased respirations	☐	☐
3. Decreased skin turgor	☐	☐
4. Decreased pulse oximetry	☐	☐
5. Decreased urine output	☐	☐
6. Decreased blood pressure	☐	☐

40. STEP 3

The nurse is caring for a 72-year-old female client in the telemetry unit.

Nurse's Notes

Today: 1900
The client was admitted earlier today to the telemetry unit for dehydration. The client states they were gardening yesterday and this morning in the hot sun. They started feeling lightheaded and weak at home; the client's son suggested seeing a health care provider.
The client takes hydrochlorothiazide for hypertension. The client is alert and oriented and denies pain, shortness of breath, or any other problems at this time. Vital signs are temperature 98.9°F (37.2°C); pulse 96 bpm; respirations 14 breaths/min; and blood pressure 118/70 mm Hg. The pulse oximetry reading is 97% on room air. The lungs are clear, bowel sounds are normal in all four quadrants, and heart sounds are normal. A peripheral intravenous (IV) line of 0.9% normal saline at 100 mL per hour is infusing without difficulty.

Today: 1930
The client reports their heart is racing and skipping and that they feel slightly short of breath.

Today: 1940
The client's vital signs are temperature 98.8°F (37.1°C); pulse 128 bpm; respiration rate 22 breaths/min; and blood pressure 100/58 mm Hg. The oxygen saturation per pulse oximetry is 92% on room air. Telemetry shows this rhythm:

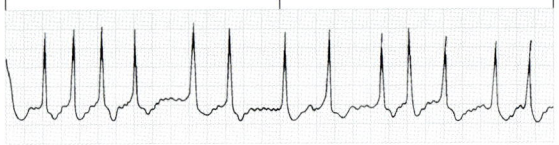

The nurse reviews updated assessment data on the client.

➢ Complete the following sentence by choosing from the lists of options.

The client's [respiratory assessment / cardiac assessment / fluid assessment]

is highly suggestive of the **priority** problem of [dehydration / atrial fibrillation].

41. STEP 4

The nurse is caring for a 72-year-old female client in the telemetry unit.

Nurse's Notes

Today: 1900
The client was admitted earlier today to the telemetry unit for dehydration. The client states they were gardening yesterday and this morning in the hot sun. They started feeling lightheaded and weak at home; the client's son suggested seeing a health care provider.
The client takes hydrochlorothiazide for hypertension. The client is alert and oriented and denies pain, shortness of breath, or any other problems at this time. Vital signs are temperature 98.9°F (37.2°C); pulse 96 bpm; respirations 14 breaths/min; and blood pressure 118/70 mm Hg. The pulse oximetry reading is 97% on room air. The lungs are clear, bowel sounds are normal in all four quadrants, and heart sounds are normal. A peripheral intravenous (IV) line of 0.9% normal saline at 100 mL per hour is infusing without difficulty.

Today: 1930
The client reports their heart is racing and skipping and that they feel slightly short of breath.

Today: 1940
The client's vital signs are temperature 98.8°F (37.1°C); pulse 128 bpm; respiration rate 22 breaths/min; and blood pressure 100/58 mm Hg. The pulse oximetry reading is 92% on room air. Telemetry shows this rhythm:

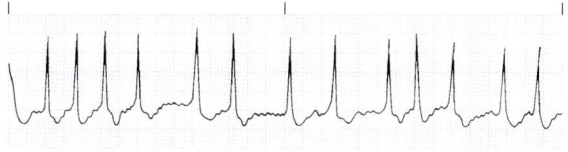

> For each intervention, specify whether the order is indicated, nonessential, or contraindicated.

Potential Intervention	Indicated	Nonessential	Contraindicated
An order for adenosine	○	○	○
An order to decrease the IV fluid to 50 mL/h	○	○	○
An order for an anticoagulant	○	○	○
An order to prepare the client for defibrillation	○	○	○
An order for a calcium channel blocker	○	○	○
An order to initiate oxygen	○	○	○

42. STEP 5

The nurse is caring for a 72-year-old female client in the telemetry unit.

Nurse's Notes

Today: 1900
The client was admitted earlier today to the telemetry unit for dehydration. The client states they were gardening yesterday and this morning in the hot sun. They started feeling lightheaded and weak at home; the client's son suggested seeing a health care provider.
The client takes hydrochlorothiazide for hypertension. The client is alert and oriented and denies pain, shortness of breath, or any other problems at this time. Vital signs are temperature 98.9°F (37.2°C); pulse 96 bpm; respirations 14 breaths/min; and blood pressure 118/70 mm Hg. The pulse oximetry reading is 97% on room air. The lungs are clear, bowel sounds are normal in all four quadrants, and heart sounds are normal. A peripheral intravenous (IV) line of 0.9% normal saline at 100 mL per hour is infusing without difficulty.

Today: 1930
The client reports their heart is racing and skipping and that they feel slightly short of breath.

Today: 1940
The client's vital signs are temperature 98.8°F (37.1°C); pulse 128 bpm; respiration rate 22 breaths/min; and blood pressure 100/58 mm Hg. The pulse oximetry reading is 92% on room air. Telemetry shows this rhythm:

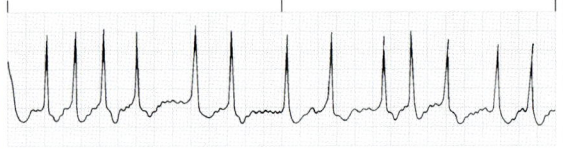

Orders

Today 1945	Obtain a 12-lead electrocardiogram
	Obtain daily international normalized ratio levels
	Give diltiazem 20 mg IV bolus; then start a drip at 5 mg/h
	Draw a basic metabolic panel and complete blood count
	Start warfarin 5 mg orally daily
	Place on oxygen at 2 L via nasal cannula; increase to keep saturations greater than 96%
	Start a second peripheral IV

The nurse calls the health care provider and receives the following orders.

➤ Highlight below the three orders that the nurse should perform **immediately**.

Orders

Today 1945	Obtain a 12-lead electrocardiogram
	Obtain daily international normalized ratio levels
	Give diltiazem 20 mg IV bolus; then start a drip at 5 mg/h
	Draw a basic metabolic panel and complete blood count
	Start warfarin 5 mg orally daily
	Place on oxygen at 2 L via nasal cannula; increase to keep saturations greater than 96%
	Start a second peripheral IV

43. STEP 6

The nurse is caring for a 72-year-old female client in the telemetry unit.

Nurse's Notes

Today: 1900
The client was admitted earlier today to the telemetry unit for dehydration. The client states they were gardening yesterday and this morning in the hot sun. They started feeling lightheaded and weak at home; the client's son suggested seeing a health care provider.
The client takes hydrochlorothiazide for hypertension. The client is alert and oriented and denies pain, shortness of breath, or any other problems at this time. Vital signs are temperature 98.9°F (37.2°C); pulse 96 bpm; respirations 14 breaths/min; and blood pressure 118/70 mm Hg. The pulse oximetry reading is 97% on room air. The lungs are clear, bowel sounds are normal in all four quadrants, and heart sounds are normal. A peripheral intravenous (IV) line of 0.9% normal saline at 100 mL per hour is infusing without difficulty.

Today: 1930
The client reports their heart is racing and skipping and that they feel slightly short of breath.

Today: 1940
The client's vital signs are temperature 98.8°F (37.1°C); pulse 128 bpm; respiration rate 22 breaths/min; and blood pressure 100/58 mm Hg. The pulse oximetry reading is 92% on room air. Telemetry shows this rhythm:

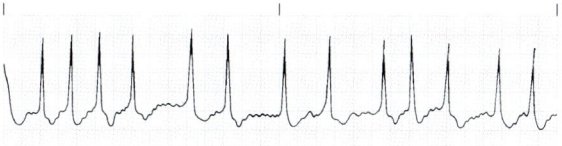

Today: 1945
Telemetry strip shows the client is in normal sinus rhythm. The client's vital signs are pulse 78 bpm; respirations 20 breaths/min, and blood pressure 102/60 mm Hg. Oxygen saturation per pulse oximeter on 2 L of oxygen per nasal cannula is 92%. The client is oriented to time, place, and person and talking about gardening.

Orders

Today 1945	Obtain a 12-lead electrocardiogram
	Obtain daily international normalized ratio levels
	Give diltiazem 20 mg IV bolus; then start a drip at 5 mg/h
	Draw a basic metabolic panel and complete blood count
	Start warfarin 5 mg orally daily
	Place on oxygen at 2 L via nasal cannula; increase to keep oxygen saturation greater than 96%
	Start a second peripheral IV

The nurse is evaluating the outcomes of the interventions.

➢ For each assessment finding, specify if the finding indicates that the client's condition has improved, has not changed, or has declined.

Assessment Finding	Improved	No Change	Declined
Normal sinus rhythm per ECG	○	○	○
Blood pressure 102/60 mm Hg	○	○	○
Heart rate 78 bpm	○	○	○
Oxygen saturation 92% with 2 L nasal oxygen	○	○	○
Conversing with nurse	○	○	○

44.
A client is taking hydrochlorothiazide to treat heart failure. Which adverse effect should the nurse instruct the client to report to the health care provider?
- ☐ 1. urinary retention
- ☐ 2. muscle weakness
- ☐ 3. confusion
- ☐ 4. diaphoresis

45.
The child of a client with Alzheimer's disease excitedly tells the nurse, "My parent was singing a favorite old song. I think they're getting their memory back!" What response by the nurse is **most** appropriate?
- ☐ 1. "Your parent still has long-term memory, but short-term memory will not return."
- ☐ 2. "I'm so happy to hear that. Maybe your parent is getting better."
- ☐ 3. "Don't get your hopes up. This is only a temporary improvement."
- ☐ 4. "I'm glad your parent can sing even if they can't talk to you."

46. A client has the leg immobilized in a long leg cast. Which finding indicates the beginning of circulatory impairment?
☐ 1. inability to move toes
☐ 2. cyanosis of toes
☐ 3. sensation of cast tightness
☐ 4. tingling of toes

47. A multigravid client at 34 weeks' gestation who is leaking amniotic fluid has just been hospitalized with a diagnosis of preterm premature rupture of membranes and preterm labor. The client's contractions are 20 minutes apart, lasting 20 to 30 seconds. The client's cervix is dilated to 2 cm. The nurse reviews prescriptions (see chart). Which prescription should the nurse initiate **first**?

Prescription
• Continuous external fetal and contraction monitoring • IV of D5LR @ 125 mL/h • I&O catheterization for urinalysis and culture and sensitivity • Betamethasone 12 mg IM daily × 2 days

☐ 1. Initiate fetal and contraction monitoring.
☐ 2. Start the intravenous infusion.
☐ 3. Obtain the urine specimen.
☐ 4. Administer betamethasone.

48. The nurse is advising a client with schizophrenia about what to do when beginning to get agitated. The client has been compliant with taking medications and has worked with clinic staff on dealing with the illness and recognizing feelings of agitation. Indicate the order from first to last in which the nurse should suggest the actions be taken. All options must be used.

1. "Take your oral lorazepam."
2. "Take your oral haloperidol."
3. "Go to a quiet place."
4. "Tell trusted people that you are becoming upset."

49. The nurse is collaborating with the client to develop a plan of care to manage the client's ongoing cancer pain. What approach should the nurse use to develop the pain management plan with the client?
☐ 1. Individualize the pain medication regimen for the client.
☐ 2. Select medications that are least likely to lead to addiction.
☐ 3. Plan for the client to administer the medication when the pain is acute.
☐ 4. Change pain medications periodically to avoid drug tolerance.

50. The nurse teaches a multigravid client at 36 weeks' gestation diagnosed with severe hydramnios about the possible complications of this condition. Which client statement(s) indicate the need for further instruction? Select all that apply.
☐ 1. "Because I have hydramnios, I may gain weight."
☐ 2. "Hydramnios has been associated with gastrointestinal disorders in the fetus."
☐ 3. "I should continue to eat high-fiber foods and avoid constipation."
☐ 4. "I can continue to work at my job at the automobile factory until labor starts."
☐ 5. "I will need frequent stress tests until birth."

51. The nurse is instructing a client on how to care for skin that has become dry after radiation therapy. Which statement by the client indicates that they understand the teaching?
☐ 1. "I should take antihistamines to decrease the itching I'm experiencing."
☐ 2. "It's safe to apply a nonperfumed lotion to my skin."
☐ 3. "A heating pad, set on the lowest setting, will help decrease my discomfort."
☐ 4. "I can apply an over-the-counter medicated ointment to relieve the dryness."

52. A nurse is preparing to administer intravenous medication to a client. In addition to the client's name, which additional identifier does the nurse check?
☐ 1. allergies
☐ 2. health care provider's name
☐ 3. birth date
☐ 4. room number

53. The nurse has just removed a client's nasogastric (NG) tube. What should the nurse do **next**?
☐ 1. Provide the client with oral hygiene.
☐ 2. Offer the client liquids to drink.
☐ 3. Encourage the client to cough and deep breathe.
☐ 4. Auscultate the client's bowel sounds.

54. The nurse is making a home visit to an older adult who is living with their child. The client has scald burns on the hands, both forearms, and the neck (10% first- and second-degree burns). What should the nurse do? Select all that apply.
   ☐ 1. Rinse the wounds with cool water.
   ☐ 2. Apply antibiotic cream.
   ☐ 3. Remove clothing near the area.
   ☐ 4. Call for transport to a hospital.
   ☐ 5. Cover the burns with a sterile dressing.
   ☐ 6. Investigate the possibility of older adult abuse.

55. An infant is to receive the diphtheria, tetanus, and acellular pertussis (DTaP) and inactivated polio vaccine (IPV) immunizations. The child is recovering from a cold and is afebrile. The child's sibling has cancer and is receiving chemotherapy. Which action is **most** appropriate?
   ☐ 1. Give the DTaP and withhold the IPV.
   ☐ 2. Administer the DTaP and IPV immunizations.
   ☐ 3. Postpone both immunizations until the sibling is in remission.
   ☐ 4. Withhold both immunizations until the infant is well.

56. A tour bus has overturned on an exit ramp. Many passengers are injured, but there are no fatalities. The injured passengers will be transported to an emergency center. The nurse at the emergency center who will receive the passengers should plan to respond to which situation in addition to treating injuries?
   ☐ 1. The passengers will be experiencing grief and mourning.
   ☐ 2. The passengers may be experiencing feelings of victimization.
   ☐ 3. Someone should be available to coordinate calls from relatives about the passengers.
   ☐ 4. Some of the passengers will need psychiatric hospitalization.

57. The nurse teaches the parents of an infant who has had surgery to correct imperforate anus how to position the infant to prevent tension on the perineum. The nurse determines more teaching is needed when the parents put the infant in which position?
   ☐ 1. abdomen, with legs pulled up under the body
   ☐ 2. back, with legs suspended at a 90-degree angle
   ☐ 3. left side, with hips elevated
   ☐ 4. right side, with hips elevated

58. The nurse develops the plan of care for a 14-year-old client who is bored due to being immobilized in a cast. Which activity is **most** appropriate?
   ☐ 1. playing a card game with a client the same age
   ☐ 2. putting together a puzzle with the client's parent
   ☐ 3. playing video games with a 9-year-old
   ☐ 4. watching a movie with the client's younger sibling

59. After surgery to create a urinary diversion, the client is at risk for a urinary tract infection. What should the nurse do to prevent a urinary tract infection?
   ☐ 1. Clamp the urinary appliance at night.
   ☐ 2. Empty the urinary appliance before it is one-third to one-half full.
   ☐ 3. Limit the client's walking with the appliance.
   ☐ 4. Change the urinary appliance daily.

60. A client with cancer of the throat had a tracheostomy tube inserted 2 days ago. The client has moderate secretions and can take deep breaths without pain. When suctioning a client's tracheostomy tube, the nurse should take which action?
   ☐ 1. Oxygenate the client before suctioning.
   ☐ 2. Insert the suction catheter about 5 cm (2 inches) into the cannula.
   ☐ 3. Use a bolus of sterile water to stimulate coughing.
   ☐ 4. Use clean gloves during the procedure.

61. A 14-month-old child has a severe diaper rash. Which recommendation should the nurse provide to the parents?
   ☐ 1. Continue to use baby wipes.
   ☐ 2. Change the diaper every 4 to 6 hours.
   ☐ 3. Wash the buttocks using mild soap.
   ☐ 4. Apply powder to the diaper area.

62. An adolescent thinks they have infectious mononucleosis. The nurse should assess the client for which symptom(s)? Select all that apply.
   ☐ 1. sore throat
   ☐ 2. malaise
   ☐ 3. weight loss
   ☐ 4. rash
   ☐ 5. swollen lymph glands

63. While assessing the fundus of a multiparous client on the first postpartum day, the nurse performs handwashing and puts on clean gloves. What should the nurse do **next**?
   ☐ 1. Place the nondominant hand above the symphysis pubis and the dominant hand at the umbilicus.
   ☐ 2. Ask the client to assume a side-lying position with the knees flexed.
   ☐ 3. Perform massage vigorously at the level of the umbilicus if the fundus feels boggy.
   ☐ 4. Place the client on a bedpan in case the uterine palpation stimulates the client to void.

64. A nulligravid client in active labor receives an epidural anesthetic. What should be the nurse's **priority** assessment?
☐ 1. level of consciousness
☐ 2. blood pressure
☐ 3. cognitive function
☐ 4. contraction pattern

65. The nurse is reviewing the serum electrolyte levels of a client with heart failure who has been taking digoxin for 6 months. The nurse should report which finding from the lab report to the health care provider?
☐ 1. hyponatremia
☐ 2. hypomagnesemia
☐ 3. hypocalcemia
☐ 4. hypokalemia

66. After abdominal surgery 3 days ago, the client continues to have pain every 4 to 6 hours, ranging from 3 to 7 on a 10-point scale. The client has prescriptions for morphine 10 mg intramuscularly (IM) every 3 to 4 hours and acetaminophen with codeine 30 mg every 3 to 4 hours as needed for pain. The client has been taking the morphine every 4 hours for the past 3 days but tells the nurse that the morphine is no longer lasting 4 hours and wants to receive pain medication every 3 hours. The nurse reviews the progress notes that indicate the client has obtained pain relief for 5 to 6 hours after receiving the morphine. What should the nurse do to help the client manage the pain?
☐ 1. Administer the morphine every 3 hours.
☐ 2. Suggest that the client take the acetaminophen with codeine every 3 hours.
☐ 3. Continue to administer the morphine every 4 hours.
☐ 4. Encourage the client to ambulate more frequently.

67. STEP 1

The nurse is caring for a 43-year-old female client in the clinic.

> Identify the findings that require further follow-up. Answer choices have been underlined.

Nurse's Note

Today: 0900
A 43-year-old client presents to the clinic reporting frequent urination, blurred vision, and a sore on the ankle that is slowly healing.
    The client states the symptoms have been ongoing for the past few weeks. The client denies any medical history and reports they do not take any medications at this time besides ibuprofen for the occasional headache.
    The client weighs 250 lb (113.63 kg). The client's blood pressure is 132/87 mm Hg, and the heart rate is 78 bpm. The respiration rate is 12 breaths/min, and the lungs are clear and equal bilaterally. The skin is warm, dry, and appropriate for ethnicity. A small sore on the ankle was noted with minimal, nonodorous drainage. The client reports having a constantly dry mouth and needs to urinate almost every hour. The client also reports having blurred vision that comes and goes but has noticed it more over the past few months.

Nurse's Note

Today: 0900
A 43-year-old client presents to the clinic reporting <u>frequent urination</u>, <u>blurred vision</u>, and an <u>open sore on the ankle that is slowly healing</u>.
    The client states the symptoms have been ongoing for the past few weeks. The client denies any medical history and reports they do not take any medications at this time besides <u>ibuprofen</u> for the occasional headache.
    The client weighs <u>250 lb (113.4 kg)</u> and has a <u>blood pressure of 132/87 mm Hg</u> and a <u>heart rate of 78 bpm</u>. The <u>respiration rate is 12 breaths/min</u>, and the lungs are clear and equal bilaterally. The skin is appropriate for ethnicity, warm, and dry. A small sore on the ankle was noted with minimal, nonodorous drainage. The client reports having a constantly dry mouth and needs to urinate almost every hour. The client also reports having blurred vision that comes and goes but has noticed it more over the past few months.

68. STEP 2

The nurse is caring for a 43-year-old female client in the clinic.

Nurse's Notes

Today: 0900
A 43-year-old client presents to the clinic reporting frequent urination, blurred vision, and a sore on the ankle that is slowly healing.
 The client states the symptoms have been ongoing for the past few weeks. The client denies any medical history and reports they do not take any medications at this time besides ibuprofen for the occasional headache.
 The client weighs 250 lb (113.63 kg). The client's blood pressure is 132/87 mm Hg, and the heart rate is 78 bpm. The respiration rate is 12 breaths/min, and the lungs are clear and equal bilaterally. The skin is warm, dry, and appropriate for ethnicity. A small sore on the ankle was noted with minimal, nonodorous drainage. The client reports having a constantly dry mouth and needs to urinate almost every hour. The client also reports having blurred vision that comes and goes but has noticed it more over the past few months.

Laboratory Results

Labs	Value	Normal Range	Date	Time
Sodium	140 mg/dL (140 mmol/L)	Adults: 135–145 mEq/L (135–145 mmol/L)	1 week ago	1500
Potassium	3.8 mg/dL (3.8 mmol/L)	Adults: 3.5–5.2 mEq/L (3.5–5.2 mmol/L)	1 week ago	1500
Blood urea nitrogen (BUN)	16 mg/dL (5.71 mmol/L)	8–20 mg/dL (2.9–7.5 mmol/L)	1 week ago	1500
Creatinine	1.1 mg/dL (97.24 µmol/L)	Women: 0.6–1.1 mg/dL (53–97 µmol/L)	1 week ago	1500
Glucose	185 mg/dL (10.27 mmol/L)	Adults: less than or equal to 110 mg/dL (less than or equal to 5.6 mmol/L)	1 week ago	1500
White blood cells	6.8×10^3 cells/mm^3 (6.8×10^9/L)	$4.5–10.5 \times 10^3$ cells/mm^3 ($4.5–10.5 \times 10^9$/L)	1 week ago	1500
Hemoglobin	12.5 g/dL (125 g/L)	Women: 12–16 g/dL (120–160 g/L)	1 week ago	1500
Hematocrit	37.2% (0.37)	Women: 36%–48% (0.36–0.48).	1 week ago	1500
Urinalysis: glucose	More than 1000 mg/dL	Urinalysis: glucose negative	1 week ago	1500
Hemoglobin A1C	8.8% of total hemoglobin (0.09 proportion of total hemoglobin)		1 week ago	1500

The nurse is reviewing the client's laboratory report.

➤ Identify the laboratory value(s) that indicate the client may have type 2 diabetes. Select all that apply.

☐	1. glucose 185 mg/dL (10.27 mmol/L)
☐	2. white blood cell count 6.8×10^3 cells/mm^3 (6.8×10^9/L)
☐	3. hemoglobin 12.5 mg/dL (125 g/L)
☐	4. hemoglobin A1C 8.8% (0.09 proportion of total hemoglobin)
☐	5. sodium 140 mg/dL (140 mmol/L)
☐	6. urinalysis: glucose more than 1000 mg/dL

69. STEP 3

The nurse is caring for a 43-year-old female client in the clinic.

Nurse's Notes

Today: 0900
A 43-year-old client presents to the clinic reporting frequent urination, blurred vision, and a sore on the ankle that is slowly healing.
 The client states the symptoms have been ongoing for the past few weeks. The client denies any medical history and reports they do not take any medications at this time besides ibuprofen for the occasional headache.
 The client weighs 250 lb (113.63 kg). The client's blood pressure is 132/87 mm Hg, and the heart rate is 78 bpm. The respiration rate is 12 breaths/min, and the lungs are clear and equal bilaterally. The skin is warm, dry, and appropriate for ethnicity. A small sore on the ankle was noted with minimal, nonodorous drainage. The client reports having a constantly dry mouth and needs to urinate almost every hour. The client also reports having blurred vision that comes and goes but has noticed it more over the past few months.

Laboratory Results

Labs	Value	Normal Range	Date	Time
Sodium	140 mg/dL (140 mmol/L)	Adults: 135–145 mEq/L (135–145 mmol/L)	1 week ago	1500
Potassium	3.8 mg/dL (3.8 mmol/L)	Adults: 3.5–5.2 mEq/L (3.5–5.2 mmol/L)	1 week ago	1500
Blood urea nitrogen (BUN)	16 mg/dL (5.71 mmol/L)	8–20 mg/dL (2.9–7.5 mmol/L)	1 week ago	1500
Creatinine	1.1 mg/dL (97.24 µmol/L)	Women: 0.6–1.1 mg/dL (53–97 µmol/L)	1 week ago	1500
Glucose	185 mg/dL (10.27 mmol/L)	Adults: less than or equal to 110 mg/dL (less than or equal to 5.6 mmol/L)	1 week ago	1500
White blood cells	6.8×10^3 cells/mm^3 (6.8×10^9/L)	4.5–10.5×10^3 cells/mm^3 (4.5–10.5×10^9/L)	1 week ago	1500
Hemoglobin	12.5 g/dL (125 g/L)	Women: 12–16 g/dL (120–160 g/L)	1 week ago	1500
Hematocrit	37.2% (0.37)	Women: 36%–48% (0.36–0.48).	1 week ago	1500
Urinalysis: glucose	More than 1000 mg/dL	Urinalysis: glucose negative	1 week ago	1500
Hemoglobin A1C	8.8% of total hemoglobin (0.09 proportion of total hemoglobin)		1 week ago	1500

The nurse is interpreting the information obtained from the client's current history and laboratory report.

➤ Identify one condition and one client finding to fill in each blank in the following sentence.

The client is at risk for chronic complications associated with type 2 diabetes such as ▢ peripheral neuropathy / diabetic ketoacidosis / hypoglycemia / oliguria ▢

as evidenced by the client's ▢ sore on the ankle. / weight. / blurred vision. / dry mouth. ▢

70. STEP 4

The nurse is caring for a 43-year-old female client in the clinic.

Nurse's Notes

Today: 0900
A 43-year-old client presents to the clinic reporting frequent urination, blurred vision, and a sore on the ankle that is slowly healing.

The client states the symptoms have been ongoing for the past few weeks. The client denies any medical history and reports they do not take any medications at this time besides ibuprofen for the occasional headache.

The client weighs 250 lb (113.63 kg). The client's blood pressure is 132/87 mm Hg, and the heart rate is 78 bpm. The respiration rate is 12 breaths/min, and the lungs are clear and equal bilaterally. The skin is warm, dry, and appropriate for ethnicity. A small sore on the ankle was noted with minimal, nonodorous drainage. The client reports having a constantly dry mouth and needs to urinate almost every hour. The client also reports having blurred vision that comes and goes but has noticed it more over the past few months.

Laboratory Results

Labs	Value	Normal Range	Date	Time
Sodium	140 mg/dL (140 mmol/L)	Adults: 135–145 mEq/L (135–145 mmol/L)	1 week ago	1500
Potassium	3.8 mg/dL (3.8 mmol/L)	Adults: 3.5–5.2 mEq/L (3.5–5.2 mmol/L)	1 week ago	1500
Blood urea nitrogen (BUN)	16 mg/dL (5.71 mmol/L)	8–20 mg/dL (2.9–7.5 mmol/L)	1 week ago	1500
Creatinine	1.1 mg/dL (97.24 µmol/L)	Women: 0.6–1.1 mg/dL (53–97 µmol/L)	1 week ago	1500
Glucose	185 mg/dL (10.27 mmol/L)	Adults: less than or equal to 110 mg/dL (less than or equal to 5.6 mmol/L)	1 week ago	1500
White blood cells	6.8 x 10^3 cells/mm^3 (6.8 x 10^9/L)	4.5–10.5 x 10^3 cells/mm^3 (4.5–10.5 x 10^9/L)	1 week ago	1500
Hemoglobin	12.5 g/dL (125 g/L)	Women: 12–16 g/dL (120–160 g/L)	1 week ago	1500
Hematocrit	37.2% (0.37)	Women: 36%–48% (0.36–0.48).	1 week ago	1500
Urinalysis: glucose	More than 1000 mg/dL	Urinalysis: glucose negative	1 week ago	1500
Hemoglobin A1C	8.8% of total hemoglobin (0.09 proportion of total hemoglobin)		1 week ago	1500

The nurse is developing a discharge plan.

➢ For each potential nursing intervention, specify whether the intervention is indicated or not essential to include in the discharge plan.

Nursing Intervention	Include in the Discharge Plan	Not Essential to Include in the Discharge Plan
1. Assess that the client is ready for the learning experience.	○	○
2. Assess the client's preferred learning style.	○	○
3. Schedule the client to be seen by an outpatient dietician for diet planning.	○	○
4. Schedule the client to be seen by an outpatient neurologist for blurred vision.	○	○
5. Ask the client to watch a video about type 2 diabetes before being discharged.	○	○
6. Teach the client how to check blood glucose at home.	○	○
7. Provide the client with sufficient time to ask questions during the education.	○	○

71. STEP 5

The nurse is caring for a 43-year-old female client in the clinic.

Nurse's Notes

Today: 0900
A 43-year-old client presents to the clinic reporting frequent urination, blurred vision, and a sore on the ankle that is slowly healing.

The client states the symptoms have been ongoing for the past few weeks. The client denies any medical history and reports they do not take any medications at this time besides ibuprofen for the occasional headache.

The client weighs 250 lb (113.63 kg). The client's blood pressure is 132/87 mm Hg, and the heart rate is 78 bpm. The respiration rate is 12 breaths/min, and the lungs are clear and equal bilaterally. The skin is warm, dry, and appropriate for ethnicity. A small sore on the ankle was noted with minimal, nonodorous drainage. The client reports having a constantly dry mouth and needs to urinate almost every hour. The client also reports having blurred vision that comes and goes but has noticed it more over the past few months.

Today: 0945
The health care provider has reviewed the client's laboratory values and has informed the client that they have type 2 diabetes. The client is to take metformin 500 mg, once in the morning and once at night.

Laboratory Results

Labs	Value	Normal Range	Date	Time
Sodium	140 mg/dL (140 mmol/L)	Adults: 135–145 mEq/L (135–145 mmol/L)	1 week ago	1500
Potassium	3.8 mg/dL (3.8 mmol/L)	Adults: 3.5–5.2 mEq/L (3.5–5.2 mmol/L)	1 week ago	1500
Blood urea nitrogen (BUN)	16 mg/dL (5.71 mmol/L)	8–20 mg/dL (2.9 to 7.5 mmol/L)	1 week ago	1500
Creatinine	1.1 mg/dL (97.24 µmol/L)	Women: 0.6–1.1 mg/dL (53–97 µmol/L)	1 week ago	1500
Glucose	185 mg/dL (10.27 mmol/L)	Adults: less than or equal to 110 mg/dL (less than or equal to 5.6 mmol/L)	1 week ago	1500
White blood cells	6.8 x 10^3 cells/mm^3 (6.8 x 10^9/L)	4.5–10.5 x 10^3 cells/mm^3 (4.5–10.5 x 10^9/L)	1 week ago	1500
Hemoglobin	12.5 g/dL (125 g/L)	Women: 12–16 g/dL (120–160 g/L)	1 week ago	1500
Hematocrit	37.2% (0.37)	Women: 36%–48% (0.36–0.48).	1 week ago	1500
Urinalysis: glucose	More than 1000 mg/dL	Urinalysis: glucose negative	1 week ago	1500
Hemoglobin A1C	8.8% of total hemoglobin (0.09 proportion of total hemoglobin)		1 week ago	1500

The nurse is educating the client about the use of metformin.

➢ Which information should the nurse include in the teaching plan about the use of metformin? Select all that apply.

☐ 1. facilitates the pancreas to produce more insulin
☐ 2. should be held for 48 hours after any imaging procedure using contrast dye
☐ 3. can cause gastrointestinal upset
☐ 4. can cause an increase in lactic acidosis
☐ 5. can cause a disulfiram-like effect with alcohol
☐ 6. can cause frequent episodes of hypoglycemia

72. STEP 6

The nurse is caring for a 43-year-old female client in the clinic.

Nurse's Notes

Today: 0900
A 43-year-old client presents to the clinic reporting frequent urination, blurred vision, and a sore on the ankle that is slowly healing.
The client states the symptoms have been ongoing for the past few weeks. The client denies any medical history and reports they do not take any medications at this time besides ibuprofen for the occasional headache.
The client weighs 250 lb (113.4 kg) and has a blood pressure of 132/87 mm Hg and a heart rate of 78 bpm. The respiration rate is 12 breaths/min, and the lungs are clear and equal bilaterally. The skin is warm, dry, and appropriate for ethnicity. A small sore on the ankle was noted with minimal, nonodorous drainage. The client reports having a constantly dry mouth and needs to urinate almost every hour. The client also reports having blurred vision that comes and goes but has noticed it more over the past few months.

Today: 0945
The health care provider has reviewed the client's laboratory values and has informed the client that they have type 2 diabetes. The client is to take metformin 500 mg, once in the morning and once at night.

Today: 1000
The client has been discharged from the clinic.

Laboratory Results

Labs	Value	Normal Range	Date	Time
Sodium	140 mg/dL (140 mmol/L)	Adults: 135–145 mEq/L (135–145 mmol/L)	1 week ago	1500
Potassium	3.8 mg/dL (3.8 mmol/L)	Adults: 3.5–5.2 mEq/L (3.5–5.2 mmol/L)	1 week ago	1500
Blood urea nitrogen (BUN)	16 mg/dL (5.71 mmol/L)	8–20 mg/dL (2.9–7.5 mmol/L)	1 week ago	1500
Creatinine	1.1 mg/dL (97.24 µmol/L)	Women: 0.6–1.1 mg/dL (53–97 µmol/L)	1 week ago	1500
Glucose	185 mg/dL (10.27 mmol/L)	Adults: less than or equal to 110 mg/dL (less than or equal to 5.6 mmol/L)	1 week ago	1500
White blood cells	6.8 × 10^3 cells/mm^3 (6.8 × 10^9/L)	4.5–10.5 × 10^3 cells/mm^3 (4.5–10.5 × 10^9/L)	1 week ago	1500
Hemoglobin	12.5 g/dL (125 g/L)	Women: 12–16 g/dL (120–160 g/L)	1 week ago	1500
Hematocrit	37.2% (0.37)	Women: 36%–48% (0.36–0.48).	1 week ago	1500
Urinalysis: glucose	More than 1000 mg/dL	Urinalysis: glucose negative	1 week ago	1500
Hemoglobin A1C	8.8% of total hemoglobin (0.09 proportion of total hemoglobin)		1 week ago	1500

The nurse is evaluating the client's understanding of the teaching plan.

➢ Which client comment(s) indicate the client has understood how to manage their care? Select all that apply.

☐	1. "I will begin to follow a healthy diet that is lower in calories and fats."
☐	2. "I will schedule a follow-up appointment with a dietician to facilitate a meal plan."
☐	3. "I can use a phone app to help track my meals."
☐	4. "Minimal exercise should be performed because it may increase insulin resistance."
☐	5. "I will call my doctor if I begin to show signs and symptoms of irregular heartbeat, dizziness, light-headedness, muscle aches, or abdominal pain."
☐	6. "I will check my hemoglobin A1C every day."
☐	7. "I should see an eye doctor and foot doctor every year for regular examinations."

73. The nurse assesses a 7-month-old infant's growth and development. Which behavior would the nurse consider unusual?
☐ 1. drinking from a cup and spilling little of the liquid
☐ 2. raising the chest and upper abdomen off the bed with the hands
☐ 3. imitating sounds that the nurse makes
☐ 4. crying loudly in protest when the parent leaves the room

74. A 13-year-old client is dying of cancer. When providing care for this client, the nurse would incorporate the developmental tasks for this age. According to Erikson's developmental model, the child normally is expected to be working on which psychosocial issue?
☐ 1. lifetime vocation
☐ 2. social conscience
☐ 3. personal values
☐ 4. sense of competence

75. The nurse is performing Leopold maneuvers on a client who is in their eighth month of pregnancy. The nurse is palpating the uterus as shown below. Which maneuver is the nurse performing?

☐ 1. first maneuver
☐ 2. second maneuver
☐ 3. third maneuver
☐ 4. fourth maneuver

76. The nurse is instructing an unlicensed assistive personnel (UAP) on how to help clients prevent postoperative pulmonary complications. Which statement indicates that the UAP has understood the nurse's instructions?
☐ 1. "I will turn the client every 2 hours."
☐ 2. "I will keep the client's head elevated."
☐ 3. "I should suction the client every 2 hours."
☐ 4. "I will have the client take 5 to 10 deep breaths every hour."

77. The nurse observes that the client with multiple sclerosis looks untidy and sad. The client suddenly says, "I can't even find the strength to comb my hair," and bursts into tears. Which response by the nurse is **best**?
☐ 1. "It must be frustrating not to be able to care for yourself."
☐ 2. "How many days have you been unable to comb your hair?"
☐ 3. "Why hasn't your spouse been helping you?"
☐ 4. "Tell me more about how you're feeling."

78. The nurse is planning care for an obese client. The client experiences dribbling urine when they cough, sneeze, or change positions. The nurse should instruct the client to promote urinary health by encouraging which action(s)? Select all that apply.
☐ 1. Increase consumption of fluids such as coffee and tea.
☐ 2. Use an indwelling catheter.
☐ 3. Participate in a weight-loss program.
☐ 4. Perform muscle-strengthening exercises (Kegel exercises).
☐ 5. Use adult diapers as needed.

79. A nurse interviews the parent of a middle-school student who is exhibiting behavioral problems, including substance abuse, after a sibling's suicide. The parent says, "I'm a single parent who has to work hard to support my family, and now I've lost a child, and my other child is acting out and making me crazy! I just can't take all this stress!" Which issue is the **priority**?
☐ 1. the parent's ability to emotionally support the adolescent in this crisis
☐ 2. the potential suicidal thoughts and plans of both family members
☐ 3. the adolescent's anger
☐ 4. the parent's frustration

80. Following surgery, the nurse is to apply a sequential compression device to the client's legs. Before the nurse applies the device, which action should be performed **first**?
☐ 1. Confirm the client's identity using two client identifiers.
☐ 2. Position the client in the bed.
☐ 3. Explain the sequential compression therapy to the client.
☐ 4. Determine the size of sleeve that is needed.

81. The nurse is caring for a previously healthy adult who is alert and oriented and is being admitted to the hospital for unexplained vomiting and abdominal pain. The client has intravenous fluids infusing through a saline lock and has been ambulating in the hallway with a steady gait. Using the Morse Fall Risk Scale (see chart), what is this client's total score, and what is their risk level?

Morse Fall Risk/Scale		
Item	Scale	Scoring
1. History of falling, immediate or within 3 months	No 0 Yes 25	
2. Secondary diagnosis	No 0 Yes 15	

3. Ambulatory aid
    Bed rest/nurse assist
    Crutches/cane/walker
    Furniture
	
	0
	15
	30	

4. IV/heparin lock	No 0 Yes 20	

5. Gait/transferring
    Normal/bed rest/immobile
    Weak
    Impaired
	
	0
	10
	20	

6. Mental status
    Oriented to own ability
    Forgets limitations
	
	0
	15	

☐ a. Score _____ Risk _____.

82. The nurse cares for a pregnant client in the first trimester. Which client statement(s) are consistent with this stage of pregnancy? Select all that apply.
    ☐ 1. "My husband told his friends we'll have to give up the convertible for a minivan."
    ☐ 2. "Oh my, how did this happen? I don't need this now."
    ☐ 3. "I can't wait to see my baby. Do you think it will have my blond hair and blue eyes?"
    ☐ 4. "I used a princess theme for decorating the room."
    ☐ 5. "I wonder how it will feel to buy maternity clothes and be fat."
    ☐ 6. "We went to the mall yesterday to buy a crib and dressing table."

83. A client comes to the emergency department (ED) with abdominal pain. This is the client's third visit to the ED in the past month with the same pain. When the nurse asks the client about taking prescribed medications, the nurse discovers the client has stopped taking the prescribed medication because of the cost. Which action(s) should the nurse take? Select all that apply.
    ☐ 1. Refer the client to a case manager to review insurance and health care benefits.
    ☐ 2. Explain to the client the importance of taking the prescribed medication.
    ☐ 3. Help the client make a budget that will include purchasing medication.
    ☐ 4. Determine if there is a less costly form of the medication.
    ☐ 5. Ask the client about the frequency and duration of pain and if alternative pain management strategies are effective.

84. A client is admitted to the emergency department with crushing chest injuries sustained in a car crash. The nurse is assessing the client's respiratory status. Which sign indicates a possible complication that the nurse should report to the health care provider **immediately**?
    ☐ 1. oxygen saturation of 70% on room air
    ☐ 2. increased fremitus
    ☐ 3. absent breath sounds on the affected side
    ☐ 4. pain on the affected side of 6 on a scale of 1 to 10 when the client breathes

85. A primigravid client at 35 weeks' gestation is scheduled for a biophysical profile. After the nurse instructs the client about the test, which client statement about what the test measures indicates the nurse's teaching has been effective?
    ☐ 1. "A biophysical profile will measure my amniotic fluid volume."
    ☐ 2. "My health care provider can determine placenta placement with a biophysical profile."
    ☐ 3. "Biophysical profiles are useful in determining amniotic fluid color."
    ☐ 4. "The best way to determine fetal gestational age is through a biophysical profile."

Answers, Rationales, and Test-Taking Strategies

*The answers and rationales for each question follow below, along with keys (🔑) to the client need (CN) and cognitive level (CL) for each question. In addition, questions that measure clinical judgment will be coded (CJ). As you check your answers, use the **Content Mastery and Test-Taking Skill Self-Analysis** worksheet (tear-out worksheet in the back of the book) to identify the reason(s) for not answering the questions correctly. For additional information about test-taking skills and strategies for answering questions, refer to pages 12–51 in Part 1 of this book.*

1. **2.** The nurse is responsible for maintaining the confidentiality of this disclosure by the client. The nurse cannot discuss the client's health problems with the family or employer. It is the client's responsibility to inform others if they choose to do so.

    🔑 CN: Management of care; CL: Analyze

2. **2.** Under the policy for valuables, the nurse documents the description on an envelope with the client, the client and nurse sign the envelope, and the valuables envelope is locked in the safe. The other options increase the risk for loss or damage to the client's valuables.

    🔑 CN: Management of care; CL: Analyze

3. **3.** Sexually transmitted infections are communicable diseases that must be reported. The nurse is responsible for reporting these diseases to the appropriate public health agency and otherwise maintaining the client's confidentiality. The client's family cannot request the release of medical information without the client's consent. An HCP's prescription is not a substitute for a client's consent to release medical information in the absence of a communicable disease.

    🔑 CN: Management of care; CL: Analyze

4. **4.** In a life-threatening emergency where time is of the essence in saving life or limb, consent is not required. This client has a Glasgow Coma Scale score of 7, which indicates a comatose state. The client cannot be aroused, withdraws in a purposeless manner from painful stimuli, exhibits decorticate posturing, and may or may not have brain stem reflexes intact. The placement of the ICP monitor is crucial to determine cerebral blood flow and prevent herniation. The HCP should insert the catheter in this emergency. The client's fiancée cannot sign the consent because until the couple is married or the fiancée has designated power of attorney, the fiancée is not considered the client's next of kin. The HCP does not need to get a consultation from another HCP. When consent is needed for a situation that is not a true emergency, two nurses can receive verbal consent by telephone from the client's next of kin.

    🔑 CN: Management of care; CL: Apply

5. **4.** The nurse ensures client safety during transport and therefore requests another cart for transport. The method of transportation and the person transporting the client are documented by the nurse responsible for the transfer. The other options do not ensure client safety. Although the clasp needs to be repaired, the nurse's first action should be to request another cart with a functional clasp. Using a draw sheet to secure the client during transfer would not be a safe method of transporting the client. Contacting the security department is not appropriate.

    🔑 CN: Safety and infection control; CL: Analyze

6. **3.** One of the best strategies to help empower clients to manage their health is to ask them their view of situations and respond to what they say. This technique acknowledges that clients' opinions have value and relevance to the interview. It also promotes an active role for clients in the process. The use of a questionnaire or written instructions is a means of obtaining information but promotes a passive client role. Asking whether clients have questions encourages participation but, alone, does not acknowledge their views.

    🔑 CN: Management of care; CL: Analyze

7. **2, 3, 4, 5.** Socialization and communication, in addition to increased activity, are all means to aid in the prevention of self-injury. Education of family members may foster the development of strategies to prevent self-injury; hence, mitten restraints could be avoided. Applying lotion after bathing may not be appropriate when the skin is broken and not intact.

    🔑 CN: Management of care; CL: Analyze

8. **1.** When the client verbalizes that life is not worth living anymore, the nurse needs to ask the client directly about suicide by asking, "Are you thinking about killing yourself?" Asking this question does not provoke suicide but conveys concern, understanding, and the worth of the client. Commonly, the client experiences a sense of relief that someone finally hears them. It also helps the nurse plan responsible care by identifying the client who is at risk for suicide. The nurse should then evaluate the seriousness of the suicidal ideation

by inquiring about the intent and plan. Stating "Things will get better" offers hope too soon without first evaluating the intent of the suicidal ideation. Asking "Why do you think that way?" implies a lack of understanding and knowledge on the part of the nurse. Major depression usually is endogenous and biochemically based. Therefore, the client may not know why they do not want to live. Saying "You should not feel that way" admonishes the client, decreases self-worth, and conveys a lack of understanding.

CN: Psychosocial integrity; CL: Analyze

9. **1, 4, 5.** Lamotrigine, an antiepileptic, is used as a mood stabilizer for clients with bipolar disorder and has been found to be effective for the depressive phase of bipolar disorder. Common adverse effects are dizziness, headache, sedation, tremors, nausea, vomiting, and ataxia. The development of a rash needs to be reported and evaluated by the health care provider because it could indicate the start of a severe systemic rash such as Stevens-Johnson syndrome or a toxic epidermal necrolysis, which would necessitate the discontinuation of lamotrigine. Hyperthermia in conjunction with muscle rigidity suggests the development of neuroleptic malignant syndrome, a life-threatening complication associated with olanzapine.

CN: Pharmacological and parenteral therapies; CL: Analyze

10. **3, 4, 5.** The client has a stage II pressure ulcer. The nurse should take measures to relieve the pressure, treat the local infection, and protect the wound. The nurse should keep the ulcer covered with a protective dressing. The client should be turned every 2 hours, and an alternating pressure mattress should be used to relieve pressure on the buttocks. The head of the bed should be elevated no more than 30 degrees. All wounds have bacteria, and obtaining frequent cultures (unless prescribed otherwise) is not necessary.

CN: Safety and infection control; CL: Analyze

11. **2, 5, 6.** HCTZ is a thiazide diuretic used in the management of mild-to-moderate hypertension and in the treatment of edema associated with heart failure, renal dysfunction, cirrhosis, corticosteroid therapy, and estrogen therapy. It increases the excretion of sodium and water by inhibiting sodium reabsorption in the distal tubule of the kidneys. It promotes the excretion of chloride, potassium, magnesium, and bicarbonate. Side effects include drowsiness, lethargy, and muscle weakness but not muscle twitching. Although there may be abdominal cramping, there is no diarrhea. The client does not become confused as a result of taking this drug.

CN: Pharmacological and parenteral therapies; CL: Analyze

12.

STEP 1

1, 2, 3. An oral temperature above 99.5°F (37.5°C) is considered a fever. A normal heart rate for a 4-year-old runs between 80 and 120 bpm, with an average of 110 bpm. Rates above 120 bpm are considered elevated. Normal respirations are 20 to 30 breaths/min. Rates above 30 breaths/min are abnormal. Blood pressures of 99+/−20 over 65+/−20 mm Hg are considered normal. Oxygen saturations above 95% are normal.

CJ: Case study; Step 1: Recognize cues; CL: Analyze

13.

STEP 2

2, 3, 4, 6, 7, 8. The client is presenting with lethargy, weight loss, low urine output, changes in temperature, heart rate, and respiration. Additional information is needed to determine if the client is experiencing dehydration and if the dehydration is mild, moderate, or severe. In pediatric clients, assessments include determining if the capillary refill is delayed, how sunken the eyes appear, how dry the mucous membranes are, if tears are absent when crying, if the skin is warm or cool to touch, and how decreased the skin turgor is. Bowel sounds indicate intestinal activity but are not a measure of hydration. Assessing posturing is done as part of a Glasgow Coma Scale score to assess neurologic function.

CJ: Case study; Step 2: Analyze cues; CL: Analyze

14.

STEP 3

The top priorities for this client are treating the **fluid volume deficit** *and the* **vomiting**.

The client has a fluid volume deficit causing severe dehydration and requires immediate treatment to prevent shock. Oral rehydration therapy is a key element in the treatment plan for pediatric dehydration. Treating the vomiting and any associated nausea will increase the likelihood of success using oral rehydration therapy. Short-term diarrhea is the intestine's way of ridding of an irritant or infection. It may become necessary to treat the underlying cause when diarrhea persists or is severe. Low-grade fevers play a part in fighting infections and typically respond to rest and fluids. Correcting the fluid volume deficit will most likely improve the fever.

CJ: Case study; Step 3: Prioritize hypothesis; CL: Analyze

15.

STEP 4		
−/+	Nursing	☐ Vital signs every 30 minutes ☒ Clear liquids and advance diet as tolerated ☐ Weights every shift
	Medications	☒ Ondansetron IV now ☐ Acetaminophen with codeine orally every 4 hours as needed (PRN) for fever. ☒ 250 mL lactated Ringer's IV fluid bolus now
	Laboratory	☒ Urine culture ☒ Stool culture ☒ Electrolytes

The nurse would expect orders to begin oral rehydration therapy with clear liquid and to advance the diet as tolerated. Treating the nausea with ondansetron would make attempts with oral rehydration more successful. A 10- to 20-mL/kg fluid bolus would be anticipated to correct the severe dehydration and may help with the nausea. Urine cultures are needed to rule out urinary tract infections, which can also cause nausea, vomiting, and fever. Stool cultures are indicated to determine if antimicrobial therapy is needed to treat the diarrhea. Electrolytes are needed to determine if there has been potassium or sodium loss as a result of the vomiting and diarrhea. There is no need to assess vital signs every 30 minutes. Daily weights are all that is indicated. Acetaminophen has been prescribed for the fever, but there is no indication for adding codeine, which may increase nausea.

🗝 CJ: Case study; Step 4: Generate solutions; CL: Create

16.

STEP 5
0/1 **1.** The nurse should request a prescription to continue the home cetirizine taken for allergies. Loperamide is an antidiarrheal medication that is not recommended for children under the age of 6 years.

🗝 CJ: Case study; Step 5: Take action; CL: Apply

17.

STEP 6			
0/1	Assessment Findings	Effective	Ineffective	Unrelated
	Respiratory rate		X	
	Heart rate	X		
	Temperature	X		
	Urine output	X		
	Stool culture			X
	Oral intake	X		
	Capillary refill		X	

Signs that fluid volume deficit is improving include decreases in the elevated heart rate and temperature. The expected urine output is 1 mL/kg per hour, and voiding immediately after treatment is a sign of improved hydration. The ability to take oral fluids indicates that hydration and the antiemetic have improved the nausea. A normal respiratory rate is 20 to 30 breaths/min in a 4-year-old child. A respiratory rate of 14 breaths/min is low and could indicate progressing shock. A finding that the capillary refill is now 3 seconds is a sign that perfusion is worsening. A finding of a negative stool culture is unrelated to treatment with a fluid bolus and antiemetic.

🗝 CJ: Case study; Step 6: Evaluate outcomes; CL: Evaluate

18. 3. The nurse needs to inform the client's sibling that it takes 2 to 4 weeks before a full clinical effect occurs with the drug. The nurse should let the sibling know that the client will gradually get better and symptoms of depression will improve. Telling the sibling that the client is experiencing very serious depression does not give them important information about the medication. Additionally, this statement may cause alarm and anxiety. Conveying the sibling's concern to the HCP does not provide the sibling with the necessary information about the client's medication. Telling the sibling that the client's medication may need to be changed is inappropriate because a full clinical effect occurs after 2 to 4 weeks.

🗝 CN: Pharmacological and parenteral therapies; CL: Analyze

19. 2. Chest pain and dyspnea are signs of pneumothorax and should be treated immediately. Delayed puberty is common in adolescents with CF and is caused by poor nutrition. Poor weight gain is common in children with CF because so little is absorbed in the small intestine. Large, foul-smelling stools indicate noncompliance with taking enzymes and should be addressed, but respiratory complications are the greatest concern.

🗝 CN: Physiological adaptation; CL: Analyze

20. 3. The client is exhibiting temporary side effects associated with beginning lithium therapy. Therefore, the nurse should continue the lithium and explain to the client that the temporary side effects of lithium will subside. Common side effects of lithium are nausea, dry mouth, diarrhea, thirst, mild hand tremor, weight gain, bloating, insomnia, and light-headedness. Immediately notifying the HCP about these common side effects and obtaining a stat lithium level are not necessary actions at this point. Hyponatremia is known to contribute to lithium toxicity, not hypernatremia. Notifying the HCP, assessing sodium intake, and obtaining lithium levels should be considered if symptoms worsen or persist.

🔑 CN: Pharmacological and parenteral therapies; CL: Analyze

21. **1.** Thyroid replacement is a lifelong maintenance therapy. The medication is usually given as one dose in the morning. It cannot be tapered or discontinued because the client needs thyroid supplementation to maintain health. The medication cannot be discontinued after the TSH level is normal; the dose will be maintained at the level that normalizes the TSH concentration.

🔑 CN: Pharmacological and parenteral therapies; CL: Apply

22. **4.** The client's statement, "I know I'm getting sick when I don't need much sleep and start buying things," indicates insight into their illness because the client recognizes symptoms that can lead to relapse. The statement "I enjoy feeling high; I don't need much sleep then and get really creative" gives no indication that the client recognizes the detrimental effects of bipolar disorder. The statements about not needing medicine in another week and being cured indicate the client's lack of understanding about the chronic nature of the disorder. The client is not cured of bipolar disorder, but symptoms of the disorder are usually managed when the client is stabilized on medication. Medication may be needed by the client for many years or throughout the client's life.

🔑 CN: Psychosocial integrity; CL: Evaluate

23. **3.** The most appropriate response is to continue all treatments and attempt to stabilize the client using fluid replacement without administering blood or blood products. It is imperative that the health care team respects the client's religious beliefs and wishes, even if they are not those of the health care team. Discontinuing all measures is not an option. The health care team should continue to provide the best care possible and does not need to notify the attorney.

🔑 CN: Management of care; CL: Analyze

24.

0/1

Action to Take	Potential Conditions	Parameters to Monitor
Notify the health care provider	Premature ventricular contractions	Need for defibrillation
Administer 5 mg metoprolol IV push as prescribed		Cardiac rhythm

The client is having premature ventricular contractions (PVCs). Frequent PVCs can lead to ventricular tachycardia, ventricular fibrillation, and cardiac arrest. The nurse should administer metoprolol, a beta-blocker, intravenously to slow the heart rate and establish a regular rate and rhythm. The nurse should monitor the client's rhythm, which is expected to revert to a normal sinus rhythm after metoprolol is administered. The nurse should also notify the health care provider of the changes in cardiac rhythm and anticipate that the client might need additional intervention such as defibrillation. The nurse should continue to monitor the client's heart rate and rhythm and prepare to defibrillate the client per agency protocol if necessary. The client is in an ICU, which is staffed with a team of health care professionals with expertise in managing cardiac events, so it would not be necessary to call the rapid response team. When the client has a regular cardiac rhythm, the nurse can monitor the oxygen level and apply oxygen as needed, assess the client for chest pain, and monitor all vital signs.

🔑 CJ: Standalone bowtie; CL: Elevate

25. **4.** NSAIDs irritate the gastric mucosa and should be taken with food. NSAIDs should be taken on a regular basis to maintain blood levels of the drug, not just when the client is experiencing pain. If the client's care plan involves doing joint exercises, the client should do them after taking the NSAID when the drug level has peaked. Antacids may interfere with the absorption of NSAIDs.

🔑 CN: Pharmacological and parenteral therapies; CL: Analyze

26. **1.** When administering an injection using the Z-track method, the nurse should hold the gauze pledget against the site while removing the needle from the muscle to help seal off the track left by the needle in the tissue. The Z-track technique does not speed the spread of the medication or lessen the discomfort of an injection. Wiping the skin with alcohol prior to administering the injection prevents the likelihood of microorganisms from entering the body.

🔑 CN: Pharmacological and parenteral therapies; CL: Apply

27. **3.** When a client talks about not having a problem with alcohol, the nurse needs to point out how alcohol has gotten the client into trouble. Concrete facts are helpful in decreasing the client's denial that alcohol is a problem. Approaches such as questioning the client about how much alcohol the client consumes each day, confronting the client about being intoxicated 2 days ago, or asking the client about their reasons for not staying sober allow the client to use defense mechanisms, such as rationalization, projection, and minimization, to explain their actions. Therefore, these approaches are not helpful.

🔑 CN: Psychosocial integrity; CL: Analyze

28. **1, 3, 2, 4.** There are two acceptable ways of removing PPE. The nurse should remove the dirtiest items first. Typically, these items are the gloves followed by the gown. In the alternative method, the gloves and gown may be removed at the same time. It is then recommended that the nurse perform hand hygiene and remove the goggles, which may fit over the mask. Finally, the mask is removed from behind. The nurse should then perform hand hygiene again when all PPE has been removed.

CN: Safety and infection control; CL: Apply

29. **4.** The nurse should first obtain a serum glucose level for more accurate information about the client's glucose level. The nurse should not wait for 30 minutes to obtain another finger stick when more accurate information can be obtained with a serum glucose level. The nurse should have more information about the glucose level before contacting the HCP. It is not necessary to start an intravenous infusion at this point.

CN: Management of care; CL: Analyze

30. **1.** A client who has not been deemed a danger to self or others or who has not been declared incompetent retains the right to refuse treatment. Legal protocols need to be followed to initiate treatment against an adult client's wishes, even if the family wishes treatment to occur. Punitive threats of retaliation or loss of privileges are ethically unacceptable in administering treatment.

CN: Management of care; CL: Analyze

31. **3.** The most appropriate intervention is to offer the client frequent oral hygiene care to moisten the dry oral mucosa. Reexplaining why the client cannot drink may be helpful but will not relieve the thirst. Ice chips cannot be given to a client who is on NPO status. Diverting the client's attention does not help manage the thirst.

CN: Basic care and comfort; CL: Analyze

32. **2, 3, 4.** This client is at risk for pressure ulcers because of age, being on bed rest, and being incontinent. The nurse assesses all pressure points and the groin area, assures that the client changes positions every 2 hours, and has the client wear incontinence pads containing absorbent material (specially designed to absorb many times its weight in water) or disposable incontinence briefs. Sanitary napkins are not designed to contain or absorb urine. Anchoring a Foley catheter increases the risk for infection.

CN: Reduction of risk potential; CL: Analyze

33. **3.** Infant formula should never be heated in the microwave; the microwave can cause the formula to warm unevenly, leading to burns in the infant's mouth. Plastic bottle liners may also burst when heated in the microwave. Keeping water heaters at 120°F (49°C) is recommended to prevent tap water scalding injuries in small children. Setting the hot water heater a couple of degrees cooler will help keep hot water in the house cooler (recommended since 1974 by the Consumer Product Safety Commission). Small children are at risk for scald injury from hot tap water because of their decreased reaction time, their curiosity, and the thermal sensitivity of their skin. Avoiding holding infants while drinking coffee can prevent possible spills onto them. Keeping cords tied up on the counter prevents children from pulling on dangling cords and spilling hot liquids over themselves.

CN: Safety and infection control; CL: Evaluate

34. **1.** The client understands the instructions when they say they should avoid contact sports because they may result in injury to the client and the fetus. Learning to ski while pregnant is not recommended because injury may occur. Scuba diving should be avoided because depth pressures could cause fetal damage. Hot tubs should be avoided during the first trimester because sitting in them can result in fetal hyperthermia and fetal hypoxia. Mild exercises, such as walking, can help strengthen the muscles and prevent some discomforts such as backache.

CN: Health promotion and maintenance; CL: Evaluate

35. **1.** An appropriate outcome for the client with rheumatoid arthritis is that the client will adopt self-care behaviors to manage joint pain, stiffness, and fatigue and be able to perform activities of daily living. Range-of-motion (ROM) exercises can help maintain mobility, but it may not be realistic to expect the client to maintain full ROM. Depending on the disease progression, there may be further development of pain and joint deformity, even with appropriate therapy. It is important for the client to understand the importance of taking the prescribed drug therapy even if symptoms have abated.

CN: Reduction of risk potential; CL: Analyze

36. **1, 5.** The postexposure management plan after a needlestick injury when the client has hepatitis B must be instituted immediately. The nurse should wash the site of the needlestick with soap and water. The nurse should also notify the supervisor, who will then report the incident to the appropriate risk management department. It is not necessary to use an antiseptic agent. Because the nurse has had the hepatitis B vaccine, it is not necessary to have a booster dose or a blood test.

🔑 CN: Pharmacological and parenteral therapies; CL: Apply

37. 2. Many falls occur when older clients attempt to get to the bathroom at night. The risk is even greater in an unfamiliar environment. The use of a nightlight in the bathroom enables the older adult client to see the way to the bathroom. Keeping the lights on in the room at all times may contribute to sensory overload and prevent adequate rest. Raised side rails paradoxically contribute to falls when the older client tries to climb over them to get to the bathroom. The upper side rails may be raised, but it is not recommended that all four side rails be elevated. Medical alert systems are seldom indicated for clients without cognitive impairments.

🔑 CN: Safety and infection control; CL: Analyze

38.

STEP 1

−/+ **3, 5, 6.** The client reports feeling that their heart is racing and skipping indicating a need to check heart rhythm, pulse, and blood pressure for any changes. Because the client is feeling slightly short of breath, the nurse should also check oxygen saturation using a pulse oximeter on room air.

🔑 CJ: Case study; Step 1: Recognize cues; CL: Understand

39.

STEP 2

Client Finding	Dehydration	Atrial Fibrillation
1. Increased pulse	X	X
2. Increased respiration	X	X
3. Decreased skin turgor	X	
4. Decreased oxygen saturation		X
5. Decreased urine output	X	
6. Decreased blood pressure	X	X

Note: Each column must have at least one response option selected.

Dehydration causes a decrease in circulating blood volume and a decrease in blood pressure. The body will try to compensate for the decrease in blood pressure by increasing the heart rate and respirations. A decrease in urine output and skin turgor are also caused by dehydration. The oxygen saturation will not decrease because the hemoglobin in the blood retains the normal ability to carry oxygen.

Atrial fibrillation results in an increased, irregular heart rate. Often, the client with atrial fibrillation will have a lowered blood pressure, and because the heart is not able to perfuse the body as well, they will also have increased respirations with decreased oxygen saturation.

🔑 CJ: Case study; Step 2: Analyze cues; CL: Analyze

40.

STEP 3

R *The client's* **cardiac assessment** *is highly suggestive of the priority problem of* **atrial fibrillation**.

The client's cardiac assessment, including symptoms of feeling like the heart was racing and skipping, vital signs, and the ECG strip, are highly suggestive of atrial fibrillation. The respiratory assessment did reveal changes because of the client's atrial fibrillation; however, these symptoms could also have been from dehydration. The client's fluid assessment did not reveal changes.

🔑 CJ: Case study; Step 3: Prioritize hypothesis; CL: Create

41.

STEP 4

Potential Intervention	Indicated	Nonessential	Contraindicated
Request an order for adenosine			X
Request an order to decrease the IV fluid to 50 mL/h		X	
Request an order for a prophylactic anticoagulant	X		
Prepare the client for defibrillation			X
Request an order for a calcium channel blocker	X		
Request an order to initiate oxygen	X		

The nurse should anticipate that the health care provider will prescribe the following medications that are indicated for the treatment of atrial fibrillation. A calcium channel blocker such as diltiazem is used to control arrhythmias and slow the heart rate. The client is in atrial fibrillation and is at risk for blood clots, and the nurse should anticipate that the health care provider will order an anticoagulant. Because the client is feeling slightly short of breath and the oxygen saturation is 92%, the nurse should prepare to place the client on oxygen. It is not necessary to change the infusion rate of the IV fluid at this time. It would be contraindicated to administer adenosine because this drug slows or blocks conduction through the atrioventricular node to administer adenosine. If medication is not able to convert the client's atrial fibrillation to a normal rhythm, the next option is to attempt synchronized cardioversion; however, defibrillation is not recommended.

🔑 CJ: Case study; Step 4: Generate solutions; CL: Analyze

42.

STEP 5

Orders	
Today 1945	<u>Obtain a 12-lead electrocardiogram</u>
	<u>Obtain daily</u> international normalized ratio <u>levels</u>
	<u>Give diltiazem 20 mg IV bolus</u>; then start a drip at 5 mg/h
	Draw a basic metabolic panel and complete blood count
	Start warfarin 5 mg orally daily
	<u>Place on oxygen at 2 L via nasal cannula</u>; increase to keep oxygen saturation greater than 96%
	Start a second peripheral IV

It is important to obtain a 12-lead electrocardiogram to verify the client's heart rhythm. Once the rhythm is confirmed as atrial fibrillation, the nurse should administer the diltiazem IV bolus to try to convert the client out of atrial fibrillation. The nurse should place the client on oxygen immediately because the client is short of breath and the oxygen saturation is 92%. After the nurse completes these priorities, the nurse can request the laboratory studies, administer the warfarin, and establish the second peripheral intravenous line.

🔑 CJ: Case study; Step 5: Take action; CL: Apply

43.

STEP 6

Assessment Finding	Improved	No Change	Declined
Normal sinus rhythm per ECG	X		
Blood pressure 102/60 mm Hg		X	
Heart rate 78 bpm	X		
Oxygen saturation 92% with 2 L oxygen per nasal cannula			X
Conversing with nurse		X	

The client is now in normal sinus rhythm with a heart rate within normal range, and their condition has improved. The client's blood pressure has not significantly improved, and the client was able to converse with the nurse the entire time. The client's oxygen saturation was 92% on room air earlier, and it has not increased with the addition of 2 L of nasal oxygen, which shows a decline and may require further action.

🔑 CJ: Case study; Step 6: Evaluate outcomes; CL: Evaluate

44. 2. Hydrochlorothiazide is a thiazide diuretic. Muscle weakness can be an indication of hypokalemia. Polyuria is associated with this diuretic, not urinary retention. Confusion and diaphoresis are not side effects of hydrochlorothiazide.

🔑 CN: Pharmacological and parenteral therapies; CL: Analyze

45. 1. The ability to remember an old song is related to long-term memory, which persists after short-term memory is lost. Therefore, the nurse should respond by providing the son with this information. Stating that the nurse is happy to hear about the change and that the client is getting better is inappropriate and inaccurate because it ignores the issue of long-term versus short-term memory. Telling the client not to get their hopes up because the improvement is only temporary is inappropriate. The information provided does not indicate that the client has expressive aphasia, which would be suggested by the statement that the client cannot talk to their child.

🔑 CN: Psychosocial integrity; CL: Analyze

46. 4. Tingling and numbness of the toes would be the earliest indication of circulatory impairment. Inability to move the toes and cyanosis are later indicators. Cast tightness should be investigated because it can lead to circulatory impairment; it is not, however, an indicator of impairment.

🔑 CN: Reduction of risk potential; CL: Analyze

47. 1. The nurse should initiate fetal and contraction monitoring for this client upon arrival at the unit. This gives the nurse data regarding changes in fetal and maternal contraction status before completing the other prescriptions. Next, betamethasone would be given to begin the maturation process of the fetal lungs. The nurse should then start an intravenous infusion to provide a line for immediate intravenous access, if needed, and provide hydration for the client. The nurse should obtain the urine specimen before administering any antibiotic therapy if prescribed.

🔑 CN: Management of care; CL: Analyze

48. 3, 4, 1, 2. Because external stimuli can greatly contribute to agitation, the nurse should teach the client that the first step is to go to a quiet area, then enlist the help of others, and finally take medication. Taking the lorazepam first would help decrease anxiety quickly, thus diminishing agitation. If the lorazepam is not successful, the client could take the oral haloperidol to help clear the client's thoughts and decrease agitation.

🔑 CN: Management of care; CL: Analyze

49. 1. Cancer pain is best managed with a combination of medications, and the nurse should plan with each client individually to find the treatment regimen that works best. Cancer pain is commonly undertreated because of fear of addiction. The client who is in pain needs the appropriate level of analgesic and needs to be reassured that addiction is unlikely. Cancer pain is best treated with regularly scheduled doses of medication, rather than only when the pain becomes acute. As drug tolerance develops, the dosage of the medication can be increased without changing the medication.

🔑 CN: Basic care and comfort; CL: Analyze

50. -/+ **4, 5.** The client needs further instructions when they say, "I can continue to work at my job at the automobile factory until labor starts" and "I will need weekly frequent stress tests until birth." The goal is to avoid preterm labor. Because the client is experiencing severe hydramnios, the client will most likely be maintained on bed rest to increase uteroplacental circulation and reduce pressure on the cervix. Stress tests, which assess the fetus's responses to contractions, carry the risk for causing preterm labor, especially in clients with known risks. If a stress test is indicated, it is usually done very near term and is seldom repeated. The nurse should expect that the client may need frequent nonstress tests to monitor fetal well-being. Hydramnios has been associated with increased weight gain caused by increased amniotic fluid volume. Hydramnios has been associated with gastrointestinal disorders in the fetus, such as tracheoesophageal fistula with stenosis or intestinal obstruction. The client should continue to eat high-fiber foods and should avoid straining, which could lead to ruptured membranes. Stool softeners may also be prescribed. The client should report any symptoms of fluid rupture or labor.

🔑 CN: Reduction of risk potential; CL: Evaluate

51. 2. Irradiated skin can become dry and irritated, resulting in itching and discomfort. The client should be instructed to clean the skin gently and apply nonperfumed, nonirritating lotions to help relieve dryness. Taking an antihistamine does not relieve the skin dryness that is causing the itching. Heat should not be applied to the area because it can cause further irritation. Medicated ointments should not be applied to the skin without the prescription of the radiation therapist.

🔑 CN: Reduction of risk potential; CL: Evaluate

52. 3. The nurse is required to check the name and a second identifier. This varies by institution but typically includes the client's birth date or account number. The health care provider's name and room number may change during a health care encounter. Although the nurse should note if the client is allergic to the medication, verifying allergies is not a client identifier.

🔑 CN: Pharmacological and parenteral therapies; CL: Apply

53. 1. The nurse's first action after the removal of an NG tube is to provide the client with oral hygiene. Then it is appropriate to give the client liquids to drink if the client is no longer on nothing-by-mouth status. There is no association between the removal of an NG tube and having the client cough and deep breathe. Auscultating the client's bowel sounds should be done before the removal of the NG tube.

🔑 CN: Reduction of risk potential; CL: Analyze

54. -/+ **1, 3, 4, 6.** The nurse can administer first aid by rinsing the area with cool water and removing clothing in the area. Because the burns are near the neck, the nurse should then call for transport to a hospital. The client's age and the extent of the burns require care by a health care team. Additionally, the nurse should consider that the client may be experiencing older adult abuse and investigate further as needed. The nurse should refrain from applying antibiotic cream or covering the area with a sterile dressing.

🔑 CN: Safety and infection control; CL: Analyze

55. 2. At this time, the infant can be given the DTaP and IPV vaccines. The fact that the child's sibling is immunosuppressed because of chemotherapy is not a reason to withhold the vaccines. The fact that the child has a cold is not grounds for delaying the immunizations. However, if the child had a high fever, the immunizations would be delayed.

🔑 CN: Health promotion and maintenance; CL: Analyze

56. 2. Major car crashes can induce feelings similar to those of people who experience other kinds of disasters and crime. Therefore, the nurse should also be prepared to assist the passengers with their feelings of victimization. Passengers may mourn the loss of a vacation, but with no fatalities, major grief reactions are not expected. Other personnel can take calls from relatives while the nurse helps the passengers. Psychiatric hospitalization is a premature assumption.

🔑 CN: Psychosocial integrity; CL: Analyze

57. 1. When placed on the abdomen, a neonate pulls the legs up under the body, which puts tension on the perineum. Therefore, after surgery, the neonate should be positioned either supine with the legs suspended at a 90-degree angle or on either side with the hips elevated.

🗝 CN: Reduction of risk potential; CL: Evaluate

58. 1. Teenagers usually enjoy activities with peers rather than socializing with their parents, siblings, or younger children. Peer relationships help the adolescent develop self-identity.

🗝 CN: Health promotion and maintenance; CL: Analyze

59. 2. The urinary appliance should be emptied before the pouch is one-third to one-half full to prevent urinary reflux. The appliance should be attached to a leg bag at night to allow for adequate drainage; it should not be clamped. The urinary appliance is not changed daily. If no leakage occurs and the client's skin remains free from irritation, the appliance can be left in place for 1 week or more. The client can ambulate as tolerated.

🗝 CN: Reduction of risk potential; CL: Analyze

60. 1. Preoxygenating the client before suctioning helps prevent the development of hypoxia during the procedure. The suction catheter is inserted about 12.7 to 15 cm (5 to 6 inches) into the cannula. A bolus of 3 to 5 mL of sterile normal saline solution may be inserted into the cannula before suctioning to stimulate coughing and loosen secretions. The nurse uses sterile technique when suctioning a client, not clean technique.

🗝 CN: Physiological adaptation; CL: Apply

61. 3. Because the toddler has a severe diaper rash, it may be best to change all that the parents are doing. The buttocks need to be washed thoroughly with mild soap and dried well. In fact, it is helpful to leave the diaper off and expose the buttocks to the air. Baby wipes commonly contain additives and perfumes that may be irritating to the baby's sensitive skin. The diaper needs to be changed more often than every 4 to 6 hours. Otherwise, the moist diaper environment will continue to irritate the skin, causing the rash to worsen. Powder has limited absorbing ability and will most likely irritate the area more. In addition, some powders contain perfumes or are scented and can irritate the skin.

🗝 CN: Basic care and comfort; CL: Analyze

62. -/+ 1, 2, 5. The common presenting symptoms of infectious mononucleosis vary greatly but commonly include fever, malaise, sore throat, and swollen lymph glands (lymphadenopathy). Skin rash, cold symptoms, abdominal pain, and weight loss are rarely presenting symptoms.

🗝 CN: Reduction of risk potential; CL: Analyze

63. 1. The nurse should place the nondominant hand above the symphysis pubis and the dominant hand at the umbilicus to palpate the fundus. This prevents uterine inversion and trauma, which can be very painful to the client. The nurse should ask the client to assume a supine, not side-lying, position with the knees flexed. The fundus can be palpated in this position, and the perineal pads can be evaluated for lochia amounts. The fundus should be massaged gently if the fundus feels boggy. Vigorous massaging may fatigue the uterus and cause it to become firm and then boggy again. The nurse should ask the client to void before the fundal evaluation. A full bladder can cause discomfort to the client, the uterus to deviate to one side, and postpartum hemorrhage.

🗝 CN: Health promotion and maintenance; CL: Apply

64. 2. Administration of an epidural anesthetic can result in a hypotensive effect on maternal blood pressure. Therefore, the priority assessment is the client's blood pressure. Ephedrine or wedging the client to a position to keep pressure off the vena cava, such as on the left side, can be used to elevate maternal blood pressure should it drop too low. Epidural anesthesia has no effect on the level of consciousness or the client's cognitive function. Although the client's contraction pattern may decrease in frequency after administration of the anesthesia, the priority assessment is the client's blood pressure. After blood pressure is maintained, contractions can be assessed.

🗝 CN: Pharmacological and parenteral therapies; CL: Analyze

65. 4. Hypokalemia is one of the most common causes of digoxin toxicity. It is essential that the nurse carefully monitor the potassium levels of clients taking digoxin to avoid toxicity. Low serum potassium levels can cause cardiac dysrhythmias. Sodium, magnesium, and calcium levels are not significantly affected by the use of digoxin.

🗝 CN: Pharmacological and parenteral therapies; CL: Apply

66. 2. Evidence indicates that acetaminophen with codeine provides pain relief for most clients with moderate pain. Because the progress notes indicate that the client is obtaining relief from the morphine for more than 4 hours and has moderate pain, the nurse can suggest that the client try taking the acetaminophen with codeine every 3 hours. The goal for this client is to gradually use less pain medication. The client can be encouraged to ambulate, but that will not be sufficient to manage the postoperative pain at this point.

🗝️ CN: Pharmacological and parenteral therapies; CL: Analyze

67.

STEP 1

-/+ Nurse's Notes

A 43-year-old female presents to the clinic reporting **frequent urination, blurred vision**, and an **open sore on the ankle that is slowly healing**.
  The client states the symptoms have been ongoing for the past few weeks. The client denies any medical history and reports they do not take any medications at this time besides ibuprofen for the occasional headache.
  The client weighs 250 lb (113.4 kg) and has a blood pressure of 132/87 mm Hg and a heart rate of 78 bpm. The respiration rate is 12 breaths/min, and the lungs are clear and equal bilaterally. The skin is appropriate for ethnicity, warm, and dry. A small sore on the ankle was noted with minimal, nonodorous drainage. The client reports having a constantly dry mouth and needs to urinate almost every hour. The client also reports having blurred vision that comes and goes but has noticed it more over the past few months.

The symptoms that require further follow-up include frequent urination, blurred vision, and an open sore. The nurse should be concerned that these symptoms could indicate the client has a chronically elevated blood glucose level. Other symptoms that the nurse may assess for include increased hunger and frequent infections. Chronically high blood glucose levels can, over time, lead to poor blood circulation, weaken the immune response, and lead to poor and delayed skin repair. The client's blood pressure, heart rate, and respirations are within normal ranges. The client is overweight, but this is not of immediate concern at this time. The client takes ibuprofen occasionally, but taking this medication is not contraindicated for this client.

🗝️ CJ: Case study; Step 1: Recognize cues; CL: Understand

68.

STEP 2

-/+ **1, 4, 6.** The client's blood glucose level, hemoglobin A1C of 8.8, and urinalysis are consistent with type 2 diabetes. The client's white blood cells, hemoglobin, and sodium levels are all within normal limits and are not associated with type 2 diabetes.

🗝️ CJ: Case study; Step 2: Analyze cues; CL: Analyze

69.

STEP 3

R The client is at risk for chronic complications associated with type 2 diabetes such as **peripheral neuropathy** as evidenced by the client's **sore on the ankle**.

The client is at risk for chronic complications associated with type 2 diabetes such as peripheral neuropathy, a microvascular complication that can cause poor circulation to the extremities and is evidenced by poor healing and open sores. The client can reduce potential risks through appropriate diet and exercise. Diabetic ketoacidosis is not a chronic complication of diabetes, but it is a serious complication that is most often seen in people with type 1 diabetes. It occurs when the body does not produce enough insulin and produces high levels of blood acids called *ketones*. Oliguria occurs when an adult urinates less than 400 mL daily. Bladder training is not required for this client as they can control their bladder. Hypoglycemia would be an acute side effect for the client, not a chronic complication.

🗝️ CJ: Case study; Step 3: Prioritize hypothesis; CL: Apply

70.

STEP 4

0/1

Include in the Discharge Plan	Include in the Discharge Plan	Not Essential to Include in Discharge Plan
1. Assess that the client is ready for the learning experience.	X	
2. Assess the client's preferred learning style.	X	
3. Schedule the client to be seen by an outpatient dietician for diet planning.	X	
4. Schedule the client to be seen by an outpatient neurologist for blurred vision.		X
5. Ask the client to watch a video about type 2 diabetes before being discharged.		X
6. Teach the client how to check blood glucose at home.		X
7. Provide the client with sufficient time to ask questions during the education.	X	

The nurse should determine if the client is ready to learn about the care plan. The client may be overwhelmed receiving the news of the diagnosis and may need time to process the information, and the nurse can recommend a follow-up appointment if needed. The nurse should also determine the learning style preference of the client so the nurse can provide the appropriate forms of educational materials, such as written materials, videos, or links to appropriate information on the internet. The client would benefit from a scheduled appointment with a dietician to plan a diet appropriate for the client's needs and the addition of the metformin. The nurse should also provide the client with enough time to process the new information and ask questions. A neurologist is not necessary at this time because the blurred vision is associated with hyperglycemia and may resolve once the client's insulin level is regulated. The client should focus on improving the diet and increasing exercise. The client will not need to check blood glucose levels throughout the day and will need to only schedule regular follow-ups with the health care provider to have it monitored. The client will need time to process the diagnosis and care management plan; the client likely will not learn much from viewing a video at this time.

🔑 CJ: Case study; Step 4: Generate solutions; CL: Create

71.

STEP 5

–/+ 2, 3, 4, 6. The nurse should emphasize that it is important for the client to withhold the medication for 48 hours after any imaging procedure that uses contrast dye due to the increased risk for renal failure. The nurse should inform the client that metformin reduces intestinal absorption of glucose and increases insulin sensitivity and commonly causes gastrointestinal upset. The drug can also cause an increase in lactic acidosis, especially when taken with alcohol, but it does not cause a disulfiram-like effect. Metformin does not facilitate the pancreas to produce more insulin, which also significantly reduces the potential for hypoglycemia unless the client has a poor diet or engages in strenuous exercise.

🔑 CJ: Case study; Step 5: Take action; CL: Apply

72.

STEP 6

–/+ 1, 2, 3, 5, 6. The client should follow a healthy diet that is lower in calories and fats along with taking prescribed medication to prevent further complications. The client should schedule an appointment with a dietician or nutritionist to facilitate a meal plan. Many smartphone applications have been developed to encourage food and portion tracking and should be encouraged. The client should call the health care provider if they begin to show signs of irregular heartbeat, dizziness, light-headedness, muscle aches, or abdominal pain as this may be a sign of accumulating lactic acid. The client should begin to schedule annual ophthalmology and podiatry appointments. The nurse should instruct the client to have regular exercise such as walking or an exercise class to decrease insulin resistance and allow the body to utilize the natural insulin more efficiently. The nurse should remind the client that they only need to have their hemoglobin A1C checked two times a year if they are not receiving insulin.

🔑 CJ: Case study; Step 6: Evaluate outcomes; CL: Evaluate

73. 1. Infants at age 7 months are not capable of drinking from a cup without spilling. At age 6 months, infants can partially lift their weight on their hands, enjoy imitating sounds, and are developing separation anxiety.

🔑 CN: Health promotion and maintenance; CL: Analyze

74. 3. According to Erikson, a child of 13 years is normally seeking to meet the need to develop a personal identity. Personal values are a component of this identity. Developing a conscience is a component of achieving initiative during the preschool years. Developing a sense of competence is a component of achieving industry in the school-age years. Developing a lifetime vocation is a component of achieving generativity in adulthood.

🔑 CN: Psychosocial integrity; CL: Analyze

75. 3. The third maneuver is used to identify the presenting part. This maneuver is used to identify the part of the fetus that lies over the inlet to the pelvis. While facing the client, the nurse places the tips of the first three fingers on the side of the woman's abdomen above the symphysis pubis and palpates deeply around the presenting part to identify its contour and size. The first maneuver involves using the tips of the fingers of both hands to palpate the uterine fundus. The second maneuver identifies the back of the fetus, and the fourth maneuver identifies the cephalic prominence.

🔑 CN: Reduction of risk potential; CL: Apply

76. 4. Having the client deep breathe hourly is the most appropriate action for the **UAP** to take to help prevent pulmonary complications. The client should be turned at least every 2 hours or as needed, but this will not prevent pulmonary complications as effectively as deep breathing. Keeping the client's head elevated will not prevent pulmonary complications. Suctioning the client is not a UAP's responsibility, nor does it prevent pulmonary complications.

🔑 CN: Management of care; CL: Evaluate

77. 4. By asking the client to tell more about how the client is feeling, the nurse is not making any assumptions about what is troubling the client. The nurse should acknowledge the client's feelings and encourage the client to discuss them. Saying that this situation must be frustrating involves assumptions by the nurse about why the client is crying and is not a therapeutic response. Asking how long the client has been unable to comb their hair takes the focus off the client's feelings and inhibits therapeutic communication. Inquiring why the client's spouse has not helped insinuates that the spouse is not helping enough, which is inappropriate, takes the focus off the client's feelings, and inhibits therapeutic communication.

CN: Psychosocial integrity; CL: Analyze

78. 3, 4, 5. The goal is to promote health in this client who has stress incontinence. Participating in a weight-loss program or support group may decrease the intra-abdominal pressure that is contributing to the incontinence. Participating in swimming, bicycling, or low-impact exercise is beneficial to weight loss. Kegel exercises are helpful in developing muscle control. Wearing adult diapers will absorb leaked urine and prevent excoriation. Clients with urinary stress incontinence are encouraged to avoid drinks with caffeine and alcohol. Perineal care is essential to prevent skin breakdown, but the client does not require a Foley or straight catheter at this time.

CN: Health promotion and maintenance; CL: Analyze

79. 2. The parent's expressions of stress and grief and the adolescent's behavior and drug use could be preludes to suicide, especially because another member of the family succeeded in suicide. Suicide attempts are more likely in families in which there has been a previous suicide attempt or suicide death, especially for young people. Although the family's emotional states are important, one is not more important than the other. Obviously, the parent's ability to emotionally support the adolescent in this crisis has been compromised, but the safety of both family members supersedes this concern.

CN: Safety and infection control; CL: Analyze

80. 1. The nurse must first use at least two ways to identify clients. This is done to make sure that each client gets the correct medication and treatment. Although positioning the client in the bed, explaining the sequential compression therapy to the client, and determining the size of sleeve that is needed are actions the nurse should perform, none of these would be the first action.

CN: Physiological adaptation; CL: Apply

81. 20, Low Risk. This client's only risk factor is IV access, which places this client at low risk for a fall. The nurse must remember to reevaluate a client's risk for falls after any change in condition, upon transfer to another unit within the hospital, or after a fall. In most acute care facilities, a fall risk assessment is completed at least every 24 hours, if not every shift.

CN: Safety and infection control; CL: Evaluate

82. 1, 2, 5. The first trimester is when the couple works through the psychological task of accepting the pregnancy. These statements describe the client and their partner coping with the pregnancy, how it feels, and how it will impact their lives. The feelings include pleasure, excitement, and ambivalence. Wondering what the baby will look like and planning for the baby's room occur later in the pregnancy.

CN: Health promotion and maintenance; CL: Analyze

83. 1, 2, 4, 5. There are many reasons why clients may not be taking prescribed medications. The nurse should identify possible reasons and refer the client to the appropriate resources. The cost of medications is a common reason for not following health management plans. The nurse can refer the client to a case manager who can determine if the client has insurance that can cover the cost. The nurse can also determine if the client is taking the least expensive form of the drug and, if not, contact the health care provider to inquire about a change in prescription. Insufficient knowledge regarding how to take the medication can also prevent proper self-administration. The nurse should determine if the client is using the medication appropriately and if additional or alternative pain management strategies would help. Clients may stop taking medication when symptoms are gone or take more on days when they are not feeling well. It is important for the nurse to take the time to educate the client on the importance of taking the medication on a consistent basis.

CN: Management of care; CL: Analyze

84. 3. Accumulation of air in the pleural cavity after a crushing chest injury may be assessed by unilateral diminished or absent breath sounds and is indicative of a pneumothorax. The nurse should notify the health care provider. An oxygen saturation of 70% is expected when a client has a crushing chest injury. Fremitus is a sign of increased lung consolidation. Moderate-to-severe pain is an expected finding following a crushing chest injury.

CN: Physiological adaptation; CL: Analyze

85. 1. The biophysical profile typically measures five parameters to assess the fetus: fetal breathing, movement, and tone; amniotic fluid volume; and fetal heart reactivity. It does not measure placenta placement, amniotic fluid color, or gestational age.

CN: Physiological adaptation; CL: Evaluate

Comprehensive Test

This test has 120 questions. Time yourself as you take the test so you can determine the approximate amount of time it takes to complete this many questions. This test represents an exam length halfway between the 85-question minimum and 150-question maximum exam length.

1. The unit secretary who transcribes the health care provider's (HCP's) prescriptions asks the nurse to interpret an illegible prescription. The nurse should:
   ☐ 1. ask the client if they take this medication.
   ☐ 2. call the pharmacist to see if this is a drug the client takes.
   ☐ 3. contact the HCP to clarify the prescription.
   ☐ 4. tell the unit secretary what the prescription is and to rewrite it clearly.

2. A client with cholecystitis is taking propantheline bromide. What should the nurse tell the client to expect as a result of taking this drug?
   ☐ 1. increased bile production
   ☐ 2. decreased biliary spasm
   ☐ 3. absence of infection
   ☐ 4. relief from nausea

3. The nurse refers the parents of a child with cystic fibrosis to an organization that helps families with children who have this disease. What does the nurse determine is the desired outcome from this referral?
   ☐ 1. assistance finding tutors to educate the child at home
   ☐ 2. obtaining genetic counseling to determine the likelihood of having another child with cystic fibrosis
   ☐ 3. meeting with other parents of children with cystic fibrosis for mutual support
   ☐ 4. securing financial assistance to purchase medications for their child

4. A client tells the nurse that "the hospital food is horrible." What should the nurse tell the client?
   ☐ 1. "The staff is doing the best it can to cook in such large quantities."
   ☐ 2. "I'll report this to the health care provider."
   ☐ 3. "Would you like to speak with the dietitian about the food and meal selection?"
   ☐ 4. "I don't like the hospital cafeteria food either."

5. A client had a thrombotic cerebrovascular accident and now has flaccid hemiplegia on the right side. The nurse notes the client is confused. The client is receiving anticoagulant therapy and an antihypertensive drug. When can the health care team begin rehabilitation for this hospitalized client?
   ☐ 1. after beginning anticoagulant therapy
   ☐ 2. on admission to the hospital
   ☐ 3. when the client can understand the directions of the health care team
   ☐ 4. as directed by the physical therapist

6. A client has been involuntarily committed to a hospital after being assessed as being dangerous to self or others. The client has lost which right?
   ☐ 1. the right to refuse medications and treatments
   ☐ 2. the right to send and receive uncensored mail
   ☐ 3. freedom from seclusion and restraints
   ☐ 4. the right to leave the hospital against medical advice

7. The nurse cares for a client taking valproic acid for bipolar disorder. Which client statement indicates that further teaching about this medication is necessary?
   ☐ 1. "I need to take the pills at the same time each day."
   ☐ 2. "I can chew the pills if necessary."
   ☐ 3. "I can take the pills with food."
   ☐ 4. "I need to call my health care provider if I start bruising easily."

8. The nurse is making rounds and observes a client who is resting in bed (see figure). The unlicensed assistive personnel (UAP) has just turned the client from their back to the side-lying position. What should the nurse do **next**?

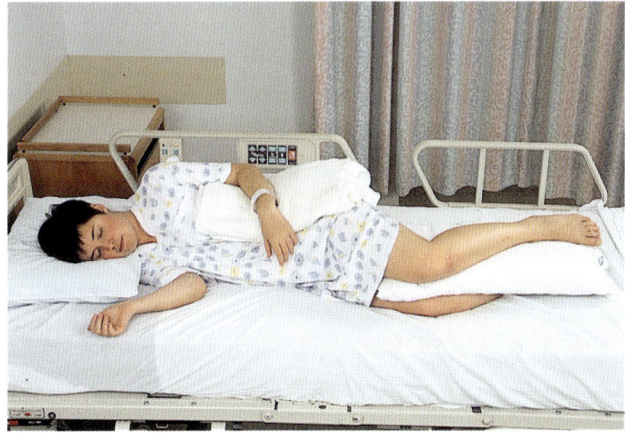

☐ 1. Elevate the head of the bed to 30 degrees.
☐ 2. Ask the UAP to add a pillow under the right arm.
☐ 3. Inspect the skin at pressure points from the back-lying position.
☐ 4. Assist the UAP in moving the client closer to the head of the bed.

9. A client is having elective surgery under general anesthesia. Who is responsible for obtaining the informed consent?
☐ 1. the nurse
☐ 2. the surgeon
☐ 3. the anesthesiologist
☐ 4. the social worker

10. The family of an older adult with terminal cancer asks about having hospice services. What should the nurse teach the family about hospice?
☐ 1. Hospice care focuses only on the needs of the client.
☐ 2. Only inpatient settings are used to provide hospice care.
☐ 3. Professional health care workers are used exclusively to staff hospice units.
☐ 4. Hospice services provide supportive care for the client and family.

11. The nurse cares for a child who has been receiving long-term steroid therapy. The nurse should assess the child for which complication?
☐ 1. usual behavior and temperament
☐ 2. loss of weight from baseline
☐ 3. development of truncal obesity
☐ 4. demonstration of a growth spurt

12. STEP 1

The nurse receives a report on a 12-hour-old neonatal client.

Nurse's Notes

0700:
Born by spontaneous vaginal birth to a primigravida client 12 hours ago, the term newborn is breastfeeding and rooming in. The birth parent had a temperature at birth of 102°F (38.8°C). Apgar scores were 7 and 8. The newborn's birth weight was 3200 g. The newborn's vital signs are temperature (T) 97.4°F (36.3°C); heart rate (HR) 140 bpm; and respiration rate (RR) 66 breaths/min. The newborn has acrocyanosis and audible grunting and has not voided or passed meconium.

➢ Which assessment(s) require **immediate** follow-up? Select all that apply.

☐ 1. Temperature
☐ 2. Heart rate
☐ 3. Respiratory rate
☐ 4. Color
☐ 5. Breath sounds
☐ 6. Urine output
☐ 7. Meconium

13. STEP 2

The nurse receives a report on a 12-hour-old neonatal client.

Nurse's Notes

0700:
Born by spontaneous vaginal birth to a primigravida client 12 hours ago, the term newborn is breastfeeding and rooming in. The birth parent had a temperature at birth of 102°F (38.8°C). Apgar scores were 7 and 8. The newborn's birth weight was 3200 g. The newborn's vital signs are temperature (T) 97.4°F (36.3°C); heart rate (HR) 140 bpm; and respiration rate (RR) 66 breaths/min. The newborn has acrocyanosis and audible grunting and has not voided or passed meconium.

▶ For each additional assessment the nurse can make, specify if the information is helpful or not helpful in determining the infant's risk for an acquired infection.

Assessment	Helpful	Not Helpful
Activity levels	○	○
Blood pressure	○	○
Feeding behaviors	○	○
Known maternal infections	○	○
Occipital frontal circumference	○	○
Pulse oximetry	○	○

14. STEP 3

The nurse receives a report on a 12-hour-old neonatal client.

Nurse's Notes

0700:
Born by spontaneous vaginal birth to a primigravida client 12 hours ago, the term newborn is breastfeeding and rooming in. The birth parent had a temperature at birth of 102°F (38.8°C). Apgar scores were 7 and 8. The newborn's birth weight was 3200 g. The newborn's vital signs are temperature (T) 97.4°F (36.3°C); heart rate (HR) 140 bpm; and respiration rate (RR) 66 breaths/min. The newborn has acrocyanosis and audible grunting and has not voided or passed meconium.

0715:
Pulse oximetry shows an oxygen saturation of 94% in room air. The client's BP is 72/44 mm Hg in the right arm.

The nurse obtains oxygen saturation and blood pressure readings.

▶ Complete the sentence from the list of drop-down options.

The nurse determines the client **most** likely has [moderate dehydration / early-onset sepsis / congenital heart disease]

evidenced by the [respiratory status / urine output / blood pressure]

and [temperature. / heart rate. / color.]

15. STEP 4

The nurse receives a report on a 12-hour-old neonatal client.

Nurse's Notes

0700:
Born by spontaneous vaginal birth to a primigravida client 12 hours ago, the term newborn is breastfeeding and rooming in. The birth parent had a temperature at birth of 102°F (38.8°C). Apgar scores were 7 and 8. The newborn's birth weight was 3200 g. The newborn's vital signs are temperature (T) 97.4°F (36.3°C); heart rate (HR) 140 bpm; and respiration rate (RR) 66 breaths/min. The newborn has acrocyanosis and audible grunting and has not voided or passed meconium.

0715:
Pulse oximetry shows an oxygen saturation of 94% in room air. The client's BP is 72/44 mm Hg in the right arm.

▶ Which diagnostic test(s) does the nurse anticipate will be included in the plan of care? Select all that apply.

- ☐ 1. Complete blood count
- ☐ 2. Blood culture
- ☐ 3. Stat bilirubin level
- ☐ 4. Chest x-ray
- ☐ 5. C-reactive protein
- ☐ 6. Urine drug screen
- ☐ 7. Stool culture

16. STEP 5

The nurse receives a report on a 12-hour-old neonatal client.

Nurse's Notes

0700:
Born by spontaneous vaginal birth to a primigravida client 12 hours ago, the term newborn is breastfeeding and rooming in. The birth parent had a temperature at birth of 102°F (38.8°C). Apgar scores were 7 and 8. The newborn's birth weight was 3200 g. The newborn's vital signs are temperature (T) 97.4°F (36.3°C); heart rate (HR) 140 bpm; and respiration rate (RR) 66 breaths/min. The newborn has acrocyanosis and audible grunting and has not voided or passed meconium.

0715:
Pulse oximetry shows an oxygen saturation of 94% in room air. The client's BP is 72/44 mm Hg in the right arm.

Orders

- Start intravenous (IV) dextrose in water (D10W) at 13 mL per hour.
- Give ampicillin 300 mg IV every 12 hours.
- Give gentamicin 7.5 mg IV every 24 hours.
- Obtain a trough level of gentamicin before the second dose.

➤ The nurse receives orders to begin antibiotics on the newborn. Which nursing action(s) are indicated? Select all that apply.

☐ 1. Administer the medications on a syringe pump.
☐ 2. Infuse ampicillin and genatamycin simultaneously.
☐ 3. Administer gentamycin slowly over 30 minutes.
☐ 4. Obtain the trough level 1 hour after the gentamicin infusion.
☐ 5. Monitor for signs and symptoms of renal toxicity.
☐ 6. Hold the second dose of gentamicin pending trough level results.
☐ 7. Report the trough level to the health care provider.
☐ 8. Check for birth parent drug allergies before administering antibiotics.

17. STEP 6

The nurse receives a report on a 12-hour-old neonatal client.

Nurse's Notes

0700:
Born by spontaneous vaginal birth to a primigravida client 12 hours ago, the term newborn is breastfeeding and rooming in. The birth parent had a temperature at birth of 102°F (38.8°C). Apgar scores were 7 and 8. The newborn's birth weight was 3200 g. The newborn's vital signs are temperature (T) 97.4°F (36.3°C); heart rate (HR) 140 bpm; and respiration rate (RR) 66 breaths/min. The newborn has acrocyanosis and audible grunting and has not voided or passed meconium.

0715:
Pulse oximetry shows an oxygen saturation of 94% in room air. The client's BP is 72/44 mm Hg in the right arm.

0800:
The client was placed on 2 L of oxygen per nasal cannula. Lab tests were drawn. A chest x-ray was done. An IV was started in the left hand. Antibiotics were started.

1000:
The neonate has decreased tone with periodic apnea. The blood glucose level is 60 mg/dL (3.3 mmol/L). Vital signs are T 100.4°F (38°C); HR 146 bpm; RR 40 breaths/min; and BP 70/42 mm Hg. The pulse oximetry reading is 97% on 2 L of oxygen.

Orders

- Start intravenous (IV) dextrose in water (D10W) at 13 mL per hour
- Ampicillin 300 mg IV every 12 hours
- Gentamicin 7.5 mg IV every 24 hours
- Obtain a trough level of gentamicin before the second dose

The nurse reviews the client's status 2 hours later.

➤ Highlight the findings that suggest the infant's sepsis may be worsening. Answer choices have been underlined.

Nurse's Notes

1000:
The neonate has decreased tone with periodic apnea. The blood glucose level is 60 mg/dL (3.3 mmol/L). Vital signs are T 100.4°F (38°C); HR 146 bpm; RR 40 breaths/min; and BP 70/42 mm Hg. The pulse oximetry reading is 97% on 2 L of oxygen.

18. The nurse manager has assigned a nurse as the circulating nurse for a surgical abortion. The nurse has a religious objection and wishes to refuse to participate in the abortion. What should the nurse manager of the operating room do?
☐ 1. Require the nurse to do this assignment.
☐ 2. Change the assignment, and record the behavior on the nurse's evaluation.
☐ 3. Change the assignment without comment.
☐ 4. Change the assignment to circulate, but have the nurse prepare the equipment.

19. A client is taking phenytoin as an antiepileptic medication. What should the nurse instruct the client to do?
☐ 1. Obtain increased iron from a pill.
☐ 2. Increased the calcium in the diet.
☐ 3. Schedule twice-yearly dental examinations.
☐ 4. Have yearly eye examinations.

20. A hospitalized 5-year-old is pulseless, and after verifying the child is not breathing, the nurse begins chest compressions. Where should the nurse apply pressure?
- ☐ 1. on the lower sternum with the heel of one hand
- ☐ 2. midway on the sternum with the tips of two fingers
- ☐ 3. over the apex of the heart with the heel of one hand
- ☐ 4. on the upper sternum with the heels of both hands

21. The nurse instructs a client with coronary artery disease on the proper use of nitroglycerin. The client has had two previous episodes of coronary artery disease. At the onset of chest pain, what should the client do?
- ☐ 1. Call 911 when 3 nitroglycerin tablets taken every 5 minutes are not effective.
- ☐ 2. Call 911 when 5 nitroglycerin tablets taken every 5 minutes are not effective.
- ☐ 3. Take 1 tablet and then immediately call 911.
- ☐ 4. Go to the emergency department if 2 nitroglycerin tablets taken 5 minutes apart are not effective.

22. The nurse is coaching an older adult who has been diagnosed with high serum lipids and leads a sedentary lifestyle. The goal is to increase the amount of exercise this client currently performs. After assessing the client's interests and setting an acceptable goal with the client, the nurse understands that which exercise will offer the client the **most** health benefits while being practical to implement?
- ☐ 1. jogging three to five times per week for 30 to 60 minutes
- ☐ 2. playing golf three times per week for 60 minutes
- ☐ 3. walking three to five times per week for 30 to 60 minutes
- ☐ 4. swimming once a week for 60 minutes

23. A client is to take methotrexate orally for severe rheumatoid arthritis. What should the nurse tell the client about taking this drug? Select all that apply.
- ☐ 1. "This drug will slow the progression of joint damage."
- ☐ 2. "You should avoid the chance of becoming bruised."
- ☐ 3. "Plan to increase the protein in your diet."
- ☐ 4. "Your health care provider will monitor your blood work to determine liver disease and blood count."
- ☐ 5. "Limit or avoid the use of alcoholic drinks."
- ☐ 6. "Increase your fluid intake to 3500 mL per day."

24. An older adult is constipated and tells the nurse that this has not happened before. What should the nurse tell the client?
- ☐ 1. "Constipation is an expected problem at your age. Wait to see if this continues."
- ☐ 2. "You need to eat more fiber. I'll tell the dietician."
- ☐ 3. "You need to drink more water. I'll start a record so you can keep track."
- ☐ 4. "This may be a sign of a more serious problem; I'll report this to your health care provider (HCP)."

25. A client is receiving gentamicin sulfate intravenously. Before administering the next dose, the nurse reviews the peak and trough serum levels. The nurse uses this information to do what?
- ☐ 1. Adjust the dosage to the therapeutic range.
- ☐ 2. Avoid inducing an allergic reaction.
- ☐ 3. Minimize side effects.
- ☐ 4. Reach therapeutic levels more quickly.

26. The nurse is teaching a client with type 1 diabetes how to determine how effectively they are managing the balance of diet, exercise, and insulin. Which method of documenting this balance would be **most** appropriate?
- ☐ 1. fasting serum glucose level
- ☐ 2. 1-week dietary recall
- ☐ 3. home log of blood glucose levels
- ☐ 4. glycosylated hemoglobin level

27. The nurses have instituted a falls prevention program. Which strategy will have the **highest** likelihood of preventing falls?
- ☐ 1. putting a falls risk sign on the clients' doors
- ☐ 2. having the client wear a color-coded armband
- ☐ 3. making rounds of the unit and clients' rooms
- ☐ 4. keeping all beds in a low position

28. A client is receiving a unit of packed red blood cells. Before the transfusion started, the client's blood pressure was 90/50 mm Hg, pulse rate was 100 bpm, respirations were 20 breaths/min, and temperature was 98°F (36.7°C). Fifteen minutes after the transfusion starts, the client's blood pressure is 92/54 mm Hg, pulse is 100 bpm, respirations are 18 breaths/min, and temperature is 101.4°F (38.6°C). What should the nurse do **first**?
- ☐ 1. Stop the transfusion.
- ☐ 2. Raise the head of the bed.
- ☐ 3. Administer acetaminophen.
- ☐ 4. Offer the client a cool washcloth.

29. A client is receiving opioid epidural analgesia. The nurse should notify the health care provider (HCP) if the client has which finding(s)? Select all that apply.
  ☐ 1. blood pressure of 80/40 mm Hg and baseline blood pressure of 110/60 mm Hg
  ☐ 2. respiratory rate of 14 breaths/min and baseline respiratory rate of 18 breaths/min
  ☐ 3. report of crushing headache
  ☐ 4. minimal clear drainage on the dressing
  ☐ 5. pain rating of 3 on a scale of 0 to 10

30. Which dietary strategy **best** meets the needs of a client with acquired immunodeficiency syndrome (AIDS)?
  ☐ 1. Tell the client to eat large meals frequently.
  ☐ 2. Encourage mega doses of nutritional supplements.
  ☐ 3. Instruct the client to cook foods thoroughly and adhere to safe food-handling practices.
  ☐ 4. Tell the client to prepare food in advance and leave it out to eat small amounts throughout the day.

31. The nurse examines a 6-week-old dark-skinned infant. There are large spots of deep blue pigmentation across the infant's buttocks. The nurse should identify this sign as characteristic of which finding?
  ☐ 1. nevus flammeus
  ☐ 2. telangiectatic nevi
  ☐ 3. infant milia
  ☐ 4. Mongolian spots

32. A nulliparous client has been given a prescription for oral contraceptives. The nurse should instruct the client to report which sign to the health care provider (HCP) immediately?
  ☐ 1. blurred vision
  ☐ 2. nausea
  ☐ 3. weight gain
  ☐ 4. mild headache

33. An older adult is admitted to the hospital with nausea and vomiting. The client has a history of heart failure and is being treated with digoxin. The client has been nauseated for a week and began vomiting 2 days ago. Laboratory values indicate hypokalemia. Because of these clinical findings, the nurse should assess the client carefully for:
  ☐ 1. chronic renal failure.
  ☐ 2. exacerbation of heart failure.
  ☐ 3. digoxin toxicity.
  ☐ 4. metabolic acidosis.

34. A woman is using progestin injections for contraception. When does the nurse instruct the client to return for the next injection?
  ☐ 1. 1 month
  ☐ 2. 3 months
  ☐ 3. 4 months
  ☐ 4. 6 months

35. STEP 1

The nurse cares for a 15-year-old male client with sickle cell anemia in the emergency department.

Admission Note

The client presented with a 3-day history of diarrhea and generalized body pain rated as an 8 on a scale of 0 to 10. The client also reports chest pain. Vital signs are temperature 102°F (38.9°C); heart rate 122 bpm; respiration rate 40 breaths/min; and blood pressure 132/84 mm Hg. The pulse oximetry reading is 95% in room air. The client's current weight is 110 lb (50 kg). The client is currently on 3 L of oxygen via nasal cannula. The client cannot provide a urine sample at this time. A complete blood count and an electrolyte panel are pending.

➤ What assessment(s) require **immediate** follow-up? Select all that apply.

☐ 1. Urine output
☐ 2. Oxygen saturation
☐ 3. Pain
☐ 4. Vital signs
☐ 5. Diarrhea

36. STEP 2

The nurse cares for a 15-year-old male client with sickle cell anemia in the emergency department.

Admission Note

The client presented with a 3-day history of diarrhea and generalized body pain rated as an 8 on a scale of 0 to 10. The client also reports chest pain. Vital signs are temperature 102°F (38.9°C); heart rate 122 bpm; respiration rate 40 breaths/min; and blood pressure 132/84 mm Hg. The pulse oximetry reading is 95% in room air. The client's current weight is 110 lb (50 kg). The client is currently on 3 L of oxygen via nasal cannula. The client cannot provide a urine sample at this time. A complete blood count and an electrolyte panel are pending.

➤ For each additional assessment the nurse can make, indicate if the information is helpful or not helpful in determining the client's risk for sickle cell anemia crisis.

Assessment	Helpful	Not Helpful
Acetaminophen use	○	○
Abdominal palpation	○	○
Breath sounds	○	○
Conjunctival color	○	○
Exposure to extreme temperatures	○	○
Recent dental procedures	○	○
Vaccination status	○	○

37. STEP 3

The nurse cares for a 15-year-old male client with sickle cell anemia in the emergency department.

Admission Note

The client presented with a 3-day history of diarrhea and generalized body pain rated as an 8 on a scale of 0 to 10. The client also reports chest pain. Vital signs are temperature 102°F (38.9°C); heart rate 122 bpm; respiration rate 40 breaths/min; and blood pressure 132/84 mm Hg. The pulse oximetry reading is 95% in room air. The client's current weight is 110 lb (50 kg). The client is currently on 3 L of oxygen via nasal cannula. The client cannot provide a urine sample at this time. A complete blood count and an electrolyte panel are pending.

Laboratory Results

Lab	Results	Reference Range
White blood cells	1.4×10^3 cells/mm³ (14×10^9/L)	$4.5–10.5 \times 10^3$ cells/mm³ ($4.5–10.5 \times 10^9$/L)
Hemoglobin	10 g/dL (100 g/L)	Ages 6–16 years: 10.3–14.9 g/dL (103–149 g/L)
Hematocrit	31% (.31 proportion of 1.0)	Ages 6–16 years: 32%–42% (0.32–0.42 proportion of 1.0)
Sodium	140 mEq/L (140 mmol/L)	135–145 mEq/L (135–145 mmol/L)
Potassium	3.2 mEq/L (3.2 mmol/L)	3.5–5.2 mEq/L (3.5–5.2 mmol/L)

The nurse reviews the client's lab test results.

➤ What are the top two priorities the nurse should **immediately** address for this client?

- ☐ 1. anemia
- ☐ 2. infection
- ☐ 3. hydration
- ☐ 4. pain
- ☐ 5. oxygenation

38. STEP 4

The nurse cares for a 15-year-old male client with sickle cell anemia in the emergency department.

Admission Note

The client presented with a 3-day history of diarrhea and generalized body pain rated as an 8 on a scale of 0 to 10. The client also reports chest pain. Vital signs are temperature 102°F (38.9°C); heart rate 122 bpm; respiration rate 40 breaths/min; and blood pressure 132/84 mm Hg. The pulse oximetry reading is 95% in room air. The client's current weight is 110 lb (50 kg). The client is currently on 3 L of oxygen via nasal cannula. The client cannot provide a urine sample at this time. A complete blood count and an electrolyte panel are pending.

Laboratory Results

Lab	Results	Reference Range
White blood cells	1.4×10^3 cells/mm^3 (14×10^9/L)	$4.5–10.5 \times 10^3$ cells/mm^3 ($4.5–10.5 \times 10^9$/L)
Hemoglobin	10 g/dL (100 g/L)	Ages 6–16 years: 10.3–14.9 g/dL (103–149 g/L)
Hematocrit	31% (.31 proportion of 1.0)	Ages 6–16 years: 32%–42% (0.32–0.42 proportion of 1.0)
Sodium	140 mEq/L (140 mmol/L)	135–145 mEq/L (135–145 mmol/L
Potassium	3.2 mEq/L (3.2 mmol/L)	3.5–5.2 mEq/L (3.5–5.2 mmol/L)

The health care provider (HCP) diagnoses the client with sickle cell crisis and writes orders to admit the client to the pediatric unit.

➤ For each possible order, specify if it is anticipated or not anticipated to include in the plan of care.

Possible Order	Anticipated Order	Not Anticipated
Activity ad lib	☐	☐
Broad-spectrum antibiotics	☐	☐
Chest x-ray	☐	☐
Intravenous (IV) fluid at 1.5 times the maintenance rate	☐	☐
Parenteral opioid analgesic agents	☐	☐
Pulmonary function tests	☐	☐
Supplemental oxygen to maintain saturation at 100%	☐	☐

39. STEP 5

The nurse cares for a 15-year-old male client with sickle cell anemia in the emergency department.

Admission Note

The client presented with a 3-day history of diarrhea and generalized body pain rated as an 8 on a scale of 0 to 10. The client also reports chest pain. Vital signs are temperature 102°F (38.9°C); heart rate 122 bpm; respiration rate 40 breaths/min; and blood pressure 132/84 mm Hg. The pulse oximetry reading is 95% in room air. The client's current weight is 110 lb (50 kg). The client is currently on 3 L of oxygen via nasal cannula. The client cannot provide a urine sample at this time. A complete blood count and an electrolyte panel are pending.

Laboratory Results

Lab	Results	Reference Range
White blood cells	1.4×10^3 cells/mm³ (14×10^9/L)	$4.5–10.5 \times 10^3$ cells/mm³ ($4.5–10.5 \times 10^9$/L)
Hemoglobin	10 g/dL (100 g/L)	Age 6–16 years: 10.3–14.9 g/dL (103–149 g/L)
Hematocrit	31% (.31 proportion of 1.0)	Age 6–16 years: 32%–42% (0.32–0.42 proportion of 1.0)
Sodium	140 mEq/L (140 mmol/L)	135–145 mEq/L (135–145 mmol/L
Potassium	3.2 mEq/L (3.2 mmol/L)	3.5–5.2 mEq/L (3.5–5.2 mmol/L)

Orders

Day 1
- Bed rest
- Titrate oxygen to maintain saturation above 95%
- IV of dextrose 5% in 0.9% normal saline (D5/0.9 NS) at 150 mL per hour
- Ceftriaxone 2 g IV every 24 hours
- Morphine sulfate 5 mg IV every 3 hours
- Obtain chest x-ray
- Obtain blood cultures
- Collect sputum specimen
- Call HCP if the pain rating is higher than 8 on a scale of 0 to 10

The nurse on the pediatric unit reviews the client orders. The nurse is working with unlicensed assistant personnel (UAP).

➤ Which task(s) can be delegated to an unlicensed assistant personnel (UAP)? Select all that apply.

- ☐ 1. Assessing pain levels
- ☐ 2. Assisting with a bed bath
- ☐ 3. Transporting the client to the radiology department for a chest x-ray
- ☐ 4. Recording intake and output
- ☐ 5. Increasing oxygen support if saturation falls below 90%
- ☐ 6. Collecting a sputum specimen

40. STEP 6

The nurse cares for a 15-year-old male client with sickle cell anemia in the emergency department.

Admission Note

The client presented with a 3-day history of diarrhea and generalized body pain rated as an 8 on a scale of 0 to 10. The client also reports chest pain. Vital signs are temperature 102°F (38.9°C); heart rate 122 bpm; respiration rate 40 breaths/min; and blood pressure 132/84 mm Hg. The pulse oximetry reading is 95% in room air. The client's current weight is 110 lb (50 kg). The client is currently on 3 L of oxygen via nasal cannula. The client cannot provide a urine sample at this time. A complete blood count and an electrolyte panel are pending.

Laboratory Results

Lab	Results	Reference Range
White blood cells	1.4×10^3 cells/mm^3 (14×10^9/L)	$4.5–10.5 \times 10^3$ cells/mm^3 ($4.5–10.5 \times 10^9$/L)
Hemoglobin	10 g/dL (100 g/L)	Age 6–16 years: 10.3–14.9 g/dL (103–149 g/L)
Hematocrit	31% (.31 proportion of 1.0)	Age 6–16 years: 32%–42% (0.32–0.42 proportion of 1.0)
Sodium	140 mEq/L (140 mmol/L)	135–145 mEq/L (135–145 mmol/L)
Potassium	3.2 mEq/L (3.2 mmol/L)	3.5–5.2 mEq/L (3.5–5.2 mmol/L)

Orders

Day 1
- Place the client on bed rest.
- Titrate oxygen to maintain saturation above 95%.
- Give IV of dextrose 5% in 0.9% normal saline (D5/0.9 NS) at 150 mL per hour.
- Administer ceftriaxone 2 g IV every 24 hours.
- Administer morphine sulfate 5 mg IV every 3 hours.
- Obtain a chest x-ray.
- Obtain blood cultures.
- Collect a sputum specimen.
- Call the HCP if the client's pain rating is higher than 8 on a scale of 0 to 10.

Day 4
- Discharge the client.
- Complete sickle cell management education.
- Schedule a follow-up appointment in 1 week.

The nurse has implemented the plan of care and is now preparing to discharge the client 4 days after an admission for sickle cell crisis.

➤ The nurse is evaluating the parent's understanding of education. For each parent statement, indicate if the statement by the parent is effective or ineffective.

Parent Statement	Effective	Ineffective
"My teen can participate in all school activities except contact sports like football."	○	○
"I will restrict fluids on my child."	○	○
"If my child has a fever, I can manage it at home with acetaminophen every 4 hours for the first 48 hours."	○	○
"My child is at risk for a stroke."	○	○
"I will tell the school nurse about my 15-year-old's diagnosis so the nurse can contact me with any signs of infection."	○	○
"My child will require penicillin prophylaxis."	○	○
"My teen may require long-acting pain medication."	○	○
"My teen would benefit from a diet high in folic acid such as vegetables and fruits."	○	○

41. While the nurse is caring for a multigravid client at 39 weeks' gestation in active labor whose cervix is dilated to 7 cm and completely effaced at +1 station, the client says, "I need to push!" What should the nurse do **next**?
☐ 1. Turn the client to the left side.
☐ 2. Tell the client to push when they have the urge.
☐ 3. Have the client pant quickly during the contraction.
☐ 4. Tell the client to focus on an object in the room to relax.

42. The nurse is teaching a client with chronic renal failure who is taking antibiotics about which signs and symptoms of potential nephrotoxicity to report. The nurse should tell the client to report which change(s) in the color of the urine? Select all that apply.
☐ 1. straw-colored
☐ 2. cloudy
☐ 3. smoky
☐ 4. pink
☐ 5. pale yellow

43. The nurse is teaching a client with heart failure about reducing fluid retention. Which strategy will be **most** effective in reducing a client's fluid retention?
☐ 1. low-sodium diet
☐ 2. walking for 20 minutes three times a week
☐ 3. restricting fluid intake
☐ 4. elevating the feet

44. During a physical examination, the nurse observes a copper bracelet on a client's wrist. The client states that they are wearing it to treat their arthritis. What should the nurse do?
☐ 1. Recognize that the client is wearing a protective object they believe prevents illness.
☐ 2. Inform the client that this is not a helpful practice, and ask the client to remove the bracelet.
☐ 3. Tell the client that wearing the bracelet is a form of quackery and not to use the bracelet as a treatment.
☐ 4. Encourage the client to continue wearing the copper bracelet because this is a medically supported treatment for arthritis.

45. The heart rate of a newly born term neonate is regular at 142 bpm. What should the nurse do **next**?
☐ 1. Notify the neonate's health care provider (HCP).
☐ 2. Check for the presence of cyanosis.
☐ 3. Assess the heart rate again in 3 hours.
☐ 4. Document this as a normal neonatal finding.

46. The nurse is teaching a client with diabetes insipidus about using desmopressin nasal spray. The therapeutic effects of desmopressin nasal spray are obtained when the client no longer has which symptom?
☐ 1. polydipsia
☐ 2. nasal congestion
☐ 3. headache
☐ 4. blurred vision

47. A client is recovering from an infected abdominal wound. Which foods should the nurse encourage the client to eat to support wound healing and recovery from the infection?
☐ 1. chicken and orange slices
☐ 2. cheeseburger and French fries
☐ 3. cheese omelet and bacon
☐ 4. gelatin salad and tea

48. The nurse is preparing a client for surgery. Although the client can speak English, English is the client's second language. When the nurse asks the client to explain the surgery that is scheduled, the client is unable to provide an accurate answer. What should the nurse do **next**?
☐ 1. Explain the procedure in detail to the client, and assess the client's understanding.
☐ 2. Contact the client's family to explain the surgery.
☐ 3. Notify the health care provider that the client cannot explain the scheduled surgery.
☐ 4. Document the client's response in the electronic medical record.

49. A toddler admitted in respiratory distress keeps pulling at the oxygen mask, trying to remove it. Which intervention(s) are initially indicated? Select all that apply.
☐ 1. Apply wrist restraints.
☐ 2. Have the parent read to the child.
☐ 3. Administer a sedative.
☐ 4. Encourage the parent to hold the child.
☐ 5. Tell the child the mask will help them breathe better.
☐ 6. Ask the parent to leave the child's bedside.

50. The nurse is developing a plan of care for a client who has joint stiffness because of rheumatoid arthritis. Which measure will be the **most** effective in relieving stiffness?
☐ 1. a warm shower before performing activities of daily living
☐ 2. aspirin after activity to decrease inflammation
☐ 3. a 4.5-kg (10-lb) weight loss to limit stress on joints
☐ 4. cold compresses to joints for 30 minutes to relieve stiffness

51. A client is taking large doses of aspirin daily to treat rheumatoid arthritis. The nurse should instruct the client to tell the health care provider (HCP) when having:
- ☐ 1. abdominal cramps.
- ☐ 2. tinnitus.
- ☐ 3. rash.
- ☐ 4. low blood pressure.

52. A multigravid client at 26 weeks' gestation with a history of pregnancy-induced hypertension (PIH) asks the nurse about traveling by air internationally to visit their parent, who wishes to see the client before they give birth. Which response by the nurse is **most** appropriate?
- ☐ 1. "Air travel at this point in your pregnancy can lead to preterm labor."
- ☐ 2. "You can travel by airplane as long as you take frequent walks during the trip."
- ☐ 3. "You need to avoid traveling because of your history of PIH."
- ☐ 4. "You would be placing yourself and your fetus at risk for regional communicable diseases."

53. A pregnant client does not have funds to purchase adequate, nutritious food. The client works part-time at a low-wage job and has two other children. The nurse can refer the client to which type of assistance?
- ☐ 1. home-delivered meals
- ☐ 2. neighbors who can provide food
- ☐ 3. the client's employer
- ☐ 4. food bank

54. The client has various sensory impairments associated with type 1 diabetes. The nurse determines that the client needs further instruction when the client makes which statement? I will:
- ☐ 1. carefully test the temperature of my bathwater.
- ☐ 2. avoid kitchen activities.
- ☐ 3. avoid hot water bottles or heating pads.
- ☐ 4. inspect my skin daily for pressure points and injury.

55. The nurse is providing discharge instructions to a client with peripheral venous disease. The nurse should include which information in the discussion with this client? Select all that apply.
- ☐ 1. Avoid prolonged standing and sitting.
- ☐ 2. Limit walking so as not to activate the "muscle pump."
- ☐ 3. Keep extremities elevated on pillows.
- ☐ 4. Keep the legs in a dependent position.
- ☐ 5. Use a heating pad to promote vasodilation.

56. A distraught parent tells the telehealth nurse that their child spends lots of time in their room, the child's grades are falling, and the child has given away a few of their favorite video games. What is the **most** appropriate action for the nurse?
- ☐ 1. Give the parent the telephone number for the local crisis hotline.
- ☐ 2. Have the parent take the adolescent to the nearest mental health outpatient facility now.
- ☐ 3. Make a same-day appointment for the adolescent with their usual health care provider.
- ☐ 4. Obtain more history information from the parent before making a decision.

57. A school-age child is admitted to the hospital with acute rheumatic fever with chorea-like movements. Which eating utensil should the nurse remove from the meal tray?
- ☐ 1. fork
- ☐ 2. spoon
- ☐ 3. plastic cup
- ☐ 4. drinking straw

58. A client's catheter is removed 4 days after transurethral resection of the prostate (TURP). The client is experiencing urinary dribbling. What should the nurse do?
- ☐ 1. Teach the client Kegel exercises.
- ☐ 2. Obtain a urine culture and sensitivity analysis to screen for a urinary infection.
- ☐ 3. Encourage voiding every hour to prevent dribbling.
- ☐ 4. Inform the client that the dribbling will stop after a few days.

59. The parent of a 2-month-old infant with colic states, "I don't know what to do anymore. My baby is up in the middle of the night crying all the time." What should the nurse tell the parent to do? Select all that apply.
- ☐ 1. Walk the floor holding the baby at night.
- ☐ 2. Take the infant for a short drive in the car.
- ☐ 3. Allow the infant to cry it out in the crib.
- ☐ 4. Offer cereal to fill the baby's stomach.
- ☐ 5. Try combining multiple interventions.

60. After the application of an arm cast, the client has pain on passive stretching of the fingers, finger swelling and tightness, and loss of function. Based on these data, the nurse anticipates that the client may be developing:
- ☐ 1. delayed bone union.
- ☐ 2. compartment syndrome.
- ☐ 3. fat embolism.
- ☐ 4. osteomyelitis.

61. The nurse is preparing a client who has just had a myocardial infarction for following an exercise program at home. Which type of exercise is **most** appropriate?
- ☐ 1. weight lifting with increasing weight two times a week
- ☐ 2. walking for 20 to 30 minutes most days of the week
- ☐ 3. strength training using elastic exercise bands
- ☐ 4. jogging for 1 mile three times a week

62. While assessing a 4-day-old neonate born at 28 weeks' gestation, the nurse cannot elicit the neonate's Moro reflex, which was present 1 hour after birth. The nurse notifies the health care provider (HCP) because this may indicate which complication?
- ☐ 1. postnatal asphyxia
- ☐ 2. skull fracture
- ☐ 3. intracranial hemorrhage
- ☐ 4. facial nerve paralysis

63. The nurse teaches the client with anxiety about the appropriate use of lorazepam. Which statement indicates that the client understands the nurse's teaching?
- ☐ 1. "I can take my medicine whenever I feel anxious."
- ☐ 2. "It's okay to double my dose if I need to."
- ☐ 3. "My medicine isn't for the everyday stress of life."
- ☐ 4. "It's safe to have a glass of wine while taking this medicine."

64. The health care provider prescribes a maternal blood test for alpha-fetoprotein for a nulligravid client at 16 weeks' gestation. When developing the teaching plan, the nurse bases the explanations on the understanding that this test is used to detect which condition?
- ☐ 1. neural tube defects
- ☐ 2. Rh incompatibilities
- ☐ 3. inborn errors of metabolism
- ☐ 4. lecithin-sphingomyelin ratio

65. An unlicensed assistive personnel (UAP) recorded a client's 0600 blood glucose level as 126 mg/dL (7 mmol/L) instead of 216 mg/dL (12 mmol/L). The UAP did not recognize the error until 0900 but reported it to the nurse right away. What should the nurse do **first**?
- ☐ 1. Complete an incident report.
- ☐ 2. Wait and observe the client for symptoms of hyperglycemia.
- ☐ 3. Reprimand the UAP for the error.
- ☐ 4. Call the health care provider (HCP).

66. A client recovering from an abdominal hysterectomy has pain in the right calf. What should the nurse do **next**?
- ☐ 1. Palpate the calf to note pain.
- ☐ 2. Measure the circumference of both calves, and note the difference.
- ☐ 3. Have the client flex and extend the leg and note the presence of pain.
- ☐ 4. Raise the right leg and lower it to detect changes in skin color.

67. STEP 1

The nurse is caring for a 48-year-old female client admitted to the medical-surgical unit with heart failure.

▷ Highlight the findings that require follow-up. Answer choices have been underlined.

Nurse's Notes

Today: 0700
A 48-year-old female client was admitted last night at 2130 for heart failure recurrence. The client has a history of congestive heart failure, hypertension, and chronic renal disease and is allergic to beta-blockers. The client is alert and oriented and denies pain or shortness of breath. A few crackles are heard in the bases of the lungs. There is 1+ pitting edema in the lower legs and feet, and pedal pulses are palpable. Vital signs are temperature (T) 98.9°F (37.2°C); pulse (P) 96 bpm; respiration rate (RR) 14 breaths/min; blood pressure (BP) 118/70 mm Hg; and pulse oximetry reading 97% on 2 L of oxygen via nasal cannula.

Nurse's Notes

Today: 0700
A 48-year-old female client was admitted last night at 2130 for heart failure recurrence. The client has a history of congestive heart failure, hypertension, and chronic renal disease and is allergic to beta-blockers. The client is alert and oriented and denies pain or shortness of breath. <u>A few crackles are heard in the bases of the lungs. There is 1+ pitting edema in the lower legs and feet</u>, and <u>pedal pulses are palpable</u>. Vital signs are <u>temperature (T) 98.9°F (37.2°C)</u>; <u>pulse (P) 96 bpm</u>; <u>respiration rate (RR) 14 breaths/min</u>; <u>blood pressure (BP) 118/70 mm Hg</u>; and <u>pulse oximetry reading 97% on 2 L of oxygen via nasal cannula</u>.

68. STEP 2

The nurse is caring for a 48-year-old female client admitted to the medical-surgical unit with heart failure.

Nurse's Notes

Today: 0700
A 48-year-old female client was admitted last night at 2130 for heart failure recurrence. The client has a history of congestive heart failure, hypertension, and chronic renal disease and is allergic to beta-blockers. The client is alert and oriented and denies pain or shortness of breath. A few crackles are heard in the bases of the lungs. There is 1+ pitting edema in the lower legs and feet, and pedal pulses are palpable. Vital signs are temperature (T) 98.9°F (37.2°C); pulse (P) 96 bpm; respiration rate (RR) 14 breaths/min; blood pressure (BP) 118/70 mm Hg; and pulse oximetry reading 97% on 2 L of oxygen via nasal cannula.

Today: 0800
The client is alert and oriented. The client denies pain but continues to have shortness of breath. Crackles are heard in the lower half of the lungs. There is 2+ pitting edema in the lower legs and feet, and pedal pulses are palpable. Vital signs are T 98.9°F (37.2°C); P 108 bpm; BP 160/90 mm Hg; and oxygen saturation 92% on 2 L of oxygen via nasal cannula.

Laboratory Results

Labs	Value	Date	Time
Sodium	140 mEq/L (140 mmol/L)	Adults: 135–145 mEq/L (135–145 mmol/L)	Yesterday 2200
Potassium	5 mEq/L (5 mmol/L)	Adults: 3.5–5.2 mEq/L (3.5–5.2 mmol/L)	Yesterday 2200
Blood urea nitrogen (BUN)	28 mg/dL (10 mmol/L)	8–20 mg/dL (2.9–7.5 mmol/L)	Yesterday 2200
Creatinine	1.7 mg/dL (129.6 mol/L)	Women: 0.6–1.1 mg/dL (53–97 mol/L)	Yesterday 2200
Glucose	80 mg/dL (4.4 mmol/L)	Adults: less than or equal to 110 mg/dL (less than or equal to 5.6 mmol/L)	Yesterday 2200
White blood cell (WBC) count	6.8×10^3 cells/mm^3 (6.8×10^9/L)	$4.5–10.5 \times 10^3$ cells/mm^3 ($4.5–10.5 \times 10^9$/L)	Yesterday 2200
Hemoglobin	11.2 g/dL (112 g/L)	Women: 12–16 g/dL (120–160 g/L)	Yesterday 2200
Hematocrit	30% (0.30 proportion of 1.0)	Women: 36%–48% (0.36–0.48 proportion of 1.0)	Yesterday 2200
Brain natriuretic peptide (BNP)	506 pg/mL (506 ng/dL)	Less than 100 pg/mL to 400 pg/mL	Yesterday 2200

The nurse reviews the Nurse's Notes and the laboratory results.

➤ Complete the following sentence by choosing from the list of options.

The client's morning assessment and lab results indicate a(n) [improvement / no change / worsening]

of the client's [hypertension. / heart failure. / renal disease. / allergies]

69. STEP 3

The nurse is caring for a 48-year-old female client admitted to the medical-surgical unit with heart failure.

Nurse's Notes

Today: 0700
A 48-year-old female client was admitted last night at 2130 for heart failure recurrence. The client has a history of congestive heart failure, hypertension, and chronic renal disease and is allergic to beta-blockers. The client is alert and oriented and denies pain or shortness of breath. A few crackles are heard in the bases of the lungs. There is 1+ pitting edema in the lower legs and feet, and pedal pulses are palpable. Vital signs are temperature (T) 98.9°F (37.2°C); pulse (P) 96 bpm; respiration rate (RR) 14 breaths/min; blood pressure (BP) 118/70 mm Hg; and pulse oximetry reading 97% on 2 L of oxygen via nasal cannula.

Today: 0800
The client is alert and oriented. The client denies pain but continues to have shortness of breath. Crackles are heard in the lower half of the lungs. There is 2+ pitting edema in the lower legs and feet, and pedal pulses are palpable. Vital signs are T 98.9°F (37.2°C); P 108 bpm; BP 160/90 mm Hg; and oxygen saturation 92% on 2 L of oxygen via nasal cannula.

➤ Which finding(s) are indicative of heart failure? Select all that apply.

- ☐ 1. Pitting edema
- ☐ 2. Crackles in lungs
- ☐ 3. Fatigue
- ☐ 4. Slow heart rate
- ☐ 5. Cough
- ☐ 6. Shortness of breath upon lying down
- ☐ 7. Increased appetite
- ☐ 8. Weight gain

Laboratory Results

Labs	Value	Normal Range	Date
Sodium	140 mEq/L (140 mmol/L)	Adults: 135–145 mEq/L (135–145 mmol/L)	Yesterday 2200
Potassium	5 mEq/L (5 mmol/L)	Adults: 3.5–5.2 mEq/L (3.5–5.2 mmol/L)	Yesterday 2200
Blood urea nitrogen (BUN)	28 mg/dL (10 mmol/L)	8–20 mg/dL (2.9–7.5 mmol/L)	Yesterday 2200
Creatinine	1.7 mg/dL (129.6 mol/L)	Women: 0.6–1.1 mg/dL (53–97 mol/L)	Yesterday 2200
Glucose	80 mg/dL (4.4 mmol/L)	Adults: less than or equal to 110 mg/dL (less than or equal to 5.6 mmol/L)	Yesterday 2200
White blood cell (WBC) count	6.8×10^3 cells/mm³ (6.8×10^9/L)	$4.5–10.5 \times 10^3$ cells/mm³ ($4.5–10.5 \times 10^9$/L)	Yesterday 2200
Hemoglobin	11.2 g/dL (112 g/L)	Women: 12–16 g/dL (120–160 g/L)	Yesterday 2200
Hematocrit	30% (0.30 proportion of 1.0)	Women: 36%–48% (0.36–0.48 proportion of 1.0)	Yesterday 2200
Brain natriuretic peptide (BNP)	506 pg/mL (506 ng/dL)	Less than 100 pg/mL to 400 pg/mL	Yesterday 2200
Sodium	145 mEq/L (145 mmol/L)	Adults: 135–145 mEq/L (135–145 mmol/L)	Today 0600
Potassium	5.5 mEq/L (5.5 mmol/L)	Adults: 3.5–5.2 mEq/L (3.5–5.2 mmol/L)	Today 0600
BUN	30 mEq/L (10.7 mmol/L)	8–20 mg/dL (2.9–7.5 mmol/L)	Today 0600
Creatinine	2.0 mg/dL (152.5 mol/L)	Women: 0.6–1.1 mg/dL (53–97 mol/L)	Today 0600
Glucose	82 mg/dL (4.6 mmol/L)	Adults: less than or equal to 110 mg/dL (less than or equal to 5.6 mmol/L)	Today 0600
WBC count	6.5×10^3 cells/mm³ (6.5×10^9/L)	$4.5–10.5 \times 10^3$ cells/mm³ ($4.5–10.5 \times 10^9$/L)	Today 0600
Hemoglobin	12.2 g/dL (122 g/L)	Women: 12–16 g/dL (120–160 g/L)	Today 0600
Hematocrit	35% (0.35 proportion of 1.0)	Women: 36%–48% (0.36–0.48 proportion of 1.0)	Today 0600
BNP	700 pg/mL (700 ng/dL)	100–400 pg/mL (100–400 ng/dL)	Today 0600

70. STEP 4

The nurse is caring for a 48-year-old female client admitted to the medical-surgical unit with heart failure.

Nurse's Notes

Today: 0700
A 48-year-old female client was admitted last night at 2130 for heart failure recurrence. The client has a history of congestive heart failure, hypertension, and chronic renal disease and is allergic to beta-blockers. The client is alert and oriented and denies pain or shortness of breath. A few crackles are heard in the bases of the lungs. There is 1+ pitting edema in the lower legs and feet, and pedal pulses are palpable. Vital signs are temperature (T) 98.9°F (37.2°C); pulse (P) 96 bpm; respiration rate (RR) 14 breaths/min; blood pressure (BP) 118/70 mm Hg; and pulse oximetry reading 97% on 2 L of oxygen via nasal cannula.

Today: 0800
The client is alert and oriented. The client denies pain but continues to have shortness of breath. Crackles are heard in the lower half of the lungs. There is 2+ pitting edema in the lower legs and feet, and pedal pulses are palpable. Vital signs are T 98.9°F (37.2°C); P 108 bpm; BP 160/90 mm Hg; and oxygen saturation 92% on 2 L of oxygen via nasal cannula.

The nurse receives the report on the client, reviews the morning lab test results, and completes the morning assessment. The nurse is planning care for the client.

➤ Indicate if the anticipated health care provider's (HCP's) orders would be indicated, nonessential, or contraindicated for the care of the client.

Potential Intervention	Indicated	Nonessential	Contraindicated
1. Request an order for spironolactone.	○	○	○
2. Request an order to increase the oxygen flow rate to keep oxygen saturation greater than 96%.	○	○	○
3. Request an order for furosemide.	○	○	○
4. Request an order for physical therapy.	○	○	○
5. Request an order to change the peripheral IV to a saline lock.	○	○	○
6. Request an order for a low-sodium diet.	○	○	○

Laboratory Results

Labs	Value	Normal Range	Date
Sodium	140 mEq/L (140 mmol/L)	Adults: 135–145 mEq/L (135–145 mmol/L)	Yesterday 2200
Potassium	5 mEq/L (5 mmol/L)	Adults: 3.5–5.2 mEq/L (3.5–5.2 mmol/L)	Yesterday 2200
Blood urea nitrogen (BUN)	28 mg/dL (10 mmol/L)	8–20 mg/dL (2.9–7.5 mmol/L)	Yesterday 2200
Creatinine	1.7 mg/dL (129.6 mol/L)	Women: 0.6–1.1 mg/dL (53–97 mol/L)	Yesterday 2200
Glucose	80 mg/dL (4.4 mmol/L)	Adults: less than or equal to 110 mg/dL (less than or equal to 5.6 mmol/L)	Yesterday 2200
White blood cell (WBC) count	6.8×10^3 cells/mm³ (6.8×10^9/L)	4.5–10.5×10^3 cells/mm³ (4.5–10.5×10^9/L)	Yesterday 2200
Hemoglobin	11.2 g/dL (112 g/L)	Women: 12–16 g/dL (120–160 g/L)	Yesterday 2200
Hematocrit	30% (0.30 proportion of 1.0)	Women: 36%–48% (0.36–0.48 proportion of 1.0)	Yesterday 2200
Brain natriuretic peptide (BNP)	506 pg/mL (506 ng/dL)	Less than 100 pg/mL to 400 pg/mL	Yesterday 2200
Sodium	145 mEq/L (145 mmol/L)	Adults: 135–145 mEq/L (135–145 mmol/L)	Today 0600
Potassium	5.5 mEq/L (5.5 mmol/L)	Adults: 3.5–5.2 mEq/L (3.5–5.2 mmol/L)	Today 0600
BUN	30 mEq/L (10.7 mmol/L)	8–20 mg/dL (2.9–7.5 mmol/L)	Today 0600
Creatinine	2.0 mg/dL (152.5 mol/L)	Women: 0.6–1.1 mg/dL (53–97 mol/L)	Today 0600
Glucose	82 mg/dL (4.6 mmol/L)	Adults: less than or equal to 110 mg/dL (less than or equal to 5.6 mmol/L)	Today 0600
WBC count	6.5×10^3 cells/mm³ (6.5×10^9/L)	4.5–10.5×10^3 cells/mm³ (4.5–10.5×10^9/L)	Today 0600
Hemoglobin	12.2 g/dL (122 g/L)	Women: 12–16 g/dL (120–160 g/L)	Today 0600
Hematocrit	35% (0.35 proportion of 1.0)	Women: 36%–48% (0.36–0.48 proportion of 1.0)	Today 0600
BNP	700 pg/mL (700 ng/dL)	100–400 pg/mL (100–400 ng/dL)	Today 0600

71. STEP 5

The nurse is caring for a 48-year-old female client admitted to the medical-surgical unit with heart failure.

Nurse's Notes

Today: 0700
A 48-year-old female client was admitted last night at 2130 for heart failure recurrence. The client has a history of congestive heart failure, hypertension, and chronic renal disease and is allergic to beta-blockers. The client is alert and oriented and denies pain or shortness of breath. A few crackles are heard in the bases of the lungs. There is 1+ pitting edema in the lower legs and feet, and pedal pulses are palpable. Vital signs are temperature (T) 98.9°F (37.2°C); pulse (P) 96 bpm; respiration rate (RR) 14 breaths/min; blood pressure (BP) 118/70 mm Hg; and pulse oximetry reading 97% on 2 L of oxygen via nasal cannula.

Today: 0800
The client is alert and oriented. The client denies pain but continues to have shortness of breath. Crackles are heard in the lower half of the lungs. There is 2+ pitting edema in the lower legs and feet, and pedal pulses are palpable. Vital signs are T 98.9°F (37.2°C); P 108 bpm; BP 160/90 mm Hg; and oxygen saturation 92% on 2 L of oxygen via nasal cannula.

Orders

Scheduled Medications

Drug Name	Scheduled Time	Dose	Route	Scanned Medication	Scanned Client
Furosemide	0600, 1400	40 mg	IV		
Metoprolol	2000	100 mg	Oral		
Hydrochlorothiazide	0800	12.5 mg	Oral		
Digoxin	0800	0.125 mg	Oral		
Hydralazine	0600, 1400, 2200	225 mg	Oral		
Bupropion	0800	150 mg	Oral		

The nurse is preparing to administer the client's 0800 medications and reviews the medication administration record.

➤ Which action(s) should the nurse take? Select all that apply.

☐ 1. Check the blood pressure before giving the medications.
☐ 2. Give the furosemide and hydralazine because they were not charted as being administered at 0600.
☐ 3. Check the radial pulse for 60 seconds before giving the digoxin.
☐ 4. Call the night shift nurse to ask if the furosemide and hydralazine were administered.
☐ 5. Withhold the metoprolol, and check with the HCP.
☐ 6. Change the second dose of the furosemide to 1800 so the doses are 12 hours apart.
☐ 7. Inject each 20 mg of furosemide over 1 to 2 minutes.

Laboratory Results

Labs	Value	Normal Range	Date
Sodium	140 mEq/L (140 mmol/L)	Adults: 135–145 mEq/L (135–145 mmol/L)	Yesterday 2200
Potassium	5 mEq/L (5 mmol/L)	Adults: 3.5–5.2 mEq/L (3.5–5.2 mmol/L)	Yesterday 2200
Blood urea nitrogen (BUN)	28 mg/dL (10 mmol/L)	8–20 mg/dL (2.9–7.5 mmol/L)	Yesterday 2200
Creatinine	1.7 mg/dL (129.6 mol/L)	Women: 0.6–1.1 mg/dL (53–97 mol/L)	Yesterday 2200
Glucose	80 mg/dL (4.4 mmol/L)	Adults: less than or equal to 110 mg/dL (less than or equal to 5.6 mmol/L)	Yesterday 2200
White blood cell (WBC) count	6.8×10^3 cells/mm³ (6.8×10^9/L)	$4.5–10.5 \times 10^3$ cells/mm³ ($4.5–10.5 \times 10^9$/L)	Yesterday 2200
Hemoglobin	11.2 g/dL (112 g/L)	Women: 12–16 g/dL (120–160 g/L)	Yesterday 2200
Hematocrit	30% (0.30 proportion of 1.0)	Women: 36%–48% (0.36–0.48 proportion of 1.0)	Yesterday 2200
Brain natriuretic peptide (BNP)	506 pg/mL (506 ng/dL)	Less than 100 pg/mL to 400 pg/mL	Yesterday 2200
Sodium	145 mEq/L (145 mmol/L)	Adults: 135–145 mEq/L (135–145 mmol/L)	Today 0600
Potassium	5.5 mEq/L (5.5 mmol/L)	Adults: 3.5–5.2 mEq/L (3.5–5.2 mmol/L)	Today 0600
BUN	30 mEq/L (10.7 mmol/L)	8–20 mg/dL (2.9–7.5 mmol/L)	Today 0600
Creatinine	2.0 mg/dL (152.5 mol/L)	Women: 0.6–1.1 mg/dL (53–97 mol/L)	Today 0600
Glucose	82 mg/dL (4.6 mmol/L)	Adults: less than or equal to 110 mg/dL (less than or equal to 5.6 mmol/L)	Today 0600
WBC count	6.5×10^3 cells/mm³ (6.5×10^9/L)	$4.5–10.5 \times 10^3$ cells/mm³ ($4.5–10.5 \times 10^9$/L)	Today 0600
Hemoglobin	12.2 g/dL (122 g/L)	Women: 12–16 g/dL (120–160 g/L)	Today 0600
Hematocrit	35% (0.35 proportion of 1.0)	Women: 36%–48% (0.36–0.48 proportion of 1.0)	Today 0600
BNP	700 pg/mL (700 ng/dL)	100–400 pg/mL (100–400 ng/mL)	Today 0600

72. STEP 6

The nurse is caring for a 48-year-old female client admitted to the medical-surgical unit with heart failure.

Nurse's Notes

Today: 0700
A 48-year-old female client was admitted last night at 2130 for heart failure recurrence. The client has a history of congestive heart failure, hypertension, and chronic renal disease and is allergic to beta-blockers. The client is alert and oriented and denies pain or shortness of breath. A few crackles are heard in the bases of the lungs. There is 1+ pitting edema in the lower legs and feet, and pedal pulses are palpable. Vital signs are temperature (T) 98.9°F (37.2°C); pulse (P) 96 bpm; respiration rate (RR) 14 breaths/min; blood pressure (BP) 118/70 mm Hg; and pulse oximetry reading 97% on 2 L of oxygen via nasal cannula.

Today: 0800
The client is alert and oriented. The client denies pain but continues to have shortness of breath. Crackles are heard in the lower half of the lungs. There is 2+ pitting edema in the lower legs and feet, and pedal pulses are palpable. Vital signs are T 98.9°F (37.2°C); P 108 bpm; BP 160/90 mm Hg; and oxygen saturation 92% on 2 L of oxygen via nasal cannula.

Orders

Scheduled Medications

Drug Name	Scheduled Time	Dose	Route	Scanned Med	Scanned Client
Furosemide	0600, 1400	40 mg	IV		
Metoprolol	2000	100 mg	Oral		
Hydrochlorothiazide	0800	12.5 mg	Oral		
Digoxin	0800	0.125 mg	Oral		
Hydralazine	0600, 1400, 2200	225 mg	Oral		
Bupropion	0800	150 mg	Oral		

The nurse has administered the morning medications to the client and is evaluating the outcomes of administering the medication.

➤ For each finding, specify if the finding indicates that the client's condition has improved, has not changed, or has declined.

Finding	Improved	Not Changed	Declined
1. Urine output of 1000 mL	○	○	○
2. Blood pressure of 86/60 mm Hg	○	○	○
3. 1+ pitting edema of the legs and feet	○	○	○
4. Oxygen saturation of 96% with 2 L oxygen	○	○	○
5. Heart rate of 102 bpm	○	○	○

Laboratory Chart

Labs	Value	Date	Time
Sodium	140 mEq/L (140 mmol/L)	Adults: 135–145 mEq/L (135–145 mmol/L)	Yesterday 2200
Potassium	5 mEq/L (5 mmol/L)	Adults: 3.5–5.2 mEq/L (3.5–5.2 mmol/L)	Yesterday 2200
Blood urea nitrogen (BUN)	28 mg/dL (10 mmol/L)	8–20 mg/dL (2.9–7.5 mmol/L)	Yesterday 2200
Creatinine	1.7 mg/dL (129.6 mol/L)	Women: 0.6–1.1 mg/dL (53–97 mol/L)	Yesterday 2200
Glucose	80 mg/dL (4.4 mmol/L)	Adults: less than or equal to 110 mg/dL (less than or equal to 5.6 mmol/L)	Yesterday 2200
White blood cell (WBC) count	6.8×10^3 cells/mm³ (6.8×10^9/L)	$4.5–10.5 \times 10^3$ cells/mm³ ($4.5–10.5 \times 10^9$/L)	Yesterday 2200
Hemoglobin	11.2 g/dL (112 g/L)	Women: 12–16 g/dL (120–160 g/L)	Yesterday 2200
Hematocrit	30% (0.30 proportion of 1.0)	Women: 36%–48% (0.36–0.48 proportion of 1.0)	Yesterday 2200
Brain natriuretic peptide (BNP)	506 pg/mL (506 ng/dL)	Less than 100 pg/mL to 400 pg/mL	Yesterday 2200
Sodium	145 mEq/L (145 mmol/L)	Adults: 135–145 mEq/L (135–145 mmol/L)	Today 0600
Potassium	5.5 mEq/L (5.5 mmol/L)	Adults: 3.5–5.2 mEq/L (3.5–5.2 mmol/L)	Today 0600
BUN	30 mEq/L (10.7 mmol/L)	8–20 mg/dL (2.9–7.5 mmol/L)	Today 0600
Creatinine	2.0 mg/dL (152.5 mol/L)	Women: 0.6–1.1 mg/dL (53–97 mol/L)	Today 0600
Glucose	82 mg/dL (4.6 mmol/L)	Adults: less than or equal to 110 mg/dL (less than or equal to 5.6 mmol/L)	Today 0600
WBC count	6.5×10^3 cells/mm³ (6.5×10^9/L)	$4.5–10.5 \times 10^3$ cells/mm³ ($4.5–10.5 \times 10^9$/L)	Today 0600
Hemoglobin	12.2 g/dL (122 g/L)	Women: 12–16 g/dL (120–160 g/L)	Today 0600
Hematocrit	35% (0.35 proportion of 1.0)	Women: 36%–48% (0.36–0.48 proportion of 1.0)	Today 0600
BNP	700 pg/mL (700 ng/dL)	100–400 pg/mL (100–400 ng/dL)	Today 0600

73. A 12-year-old has a fractured femur and is immobilized in traction as shown in the figure. What should the nurse do?

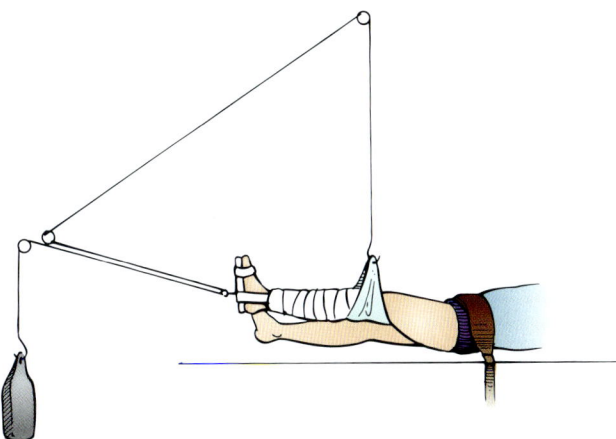

- ☐ 1. Add additional weight until the foot is only 5 cm (2 inches) from the bed.
- ☐ 2. Only offer foods that are easy to eat.
- ☐ 3. Place a pillow under the fractured leg to provide support.
- ☐ 4. Provide opportunities for age-appropriate activities.

74. A client's spouse arrives on the nursing unit 6 hours after the client's car collision, explaining that they have been out of town. The client's spouse is distraught because they were not at the hospital when the client was admitted. What should the nurse do **first**?
- ☐ 1. Allow the spouse to verbalize feelings and concerns.
- ☐ 2. Describe the client's medical treatment since admission.
- ☐ 3. Explain the nature of the injury, and reassure the spouse that the client's condition is stable.
- ☐ 4. Reassure the spouse that the important fact is that they are here now.

75. A client is scheduled to have a graded exercise test. What should the nurse explain to the client about the purpose of this test?

The test will determine how:
- ☐ 1. to set the incline gradient on a treadmill.
- ☐ 2. well the body reacts to controlled exercise stress.
- ☐ 3. far the client can walk.
- ☐ 4. long the client can walk.

76. The parent of an infant with hemophilia tells the nurse that they are planning to do homeschooling when the child reaches school age. The parent does not want their child in school because the teacher will not watch the child as well as the parent would. The parent's comments represent what common parental reaction to a child's chronic illness?
- ☐ 1. overprotection
- ☐ 2. devotion
- ☐ 3. mistrust
- ☐ 4. insecurity

77. A client with acute psychosis has been taking haloperidol for 3 days. When evaluating the client's response to the medication, the nurse understands that which comment reflects the **greatest** improvement?
- ☐ 1. "I know these voices aren't real, but I'm still scared of them."
- ☐ 2. "I'm feeling so restless, and I can't sit still."
- ☐ 3. "Boy, do I need a shower. I think it's been days since I've had one."
- ☐ 4. "I'm ready to talk about my discharge medications."

78. The nurse is administering an intravenous (IV) potassium chloride supplement to a client who has heart failure. Which information should the nurse consider when developing a plan of care for this client?
- ☐ 1. Hyperkalemia will intensify the action of the client's digoxin preparation.
- ☐ 2. The client's potassium levels will be unaffected by a potassium-sparing diuretic.
- ☐ 3. The administration of IV potassium chloride should not exceed 10 mEq per hour (10 mmol per hour) or a concentration of 40 mEq/L (40 mmol/L).
- ☐ 4. Metabolic alkalosis will increase the client's serum potassium levels.

79. The nurse is assessing a client who is incontinent for their risk for developing a pressure ulcer. The client is an 80-year-old woman who also has hypertension. Which factor contributes **most** to the client's risk for a pressure ulcer?
- ☐ 1. gender
- ☐ 2. incontinence
- ☐ 3. hypertension
- ☐ 4. age

80. A nurse is teaching a parenting class about how to prevent thrush (oral candidiasis). Which statement by a parent indicates more teaching is required?
☐ 1. "I will sterilize pacifiers."
☐ 2. "I should rinse my child's mouth after using a corticosteroid."
☐ 3. "If my child uses a spacer with asthma medications, I need to rinse it after each use."
☐ 4. "I should rinse my child's glass after each use."

81. A 10-year-old with a history of recent respiratory infection has swelling around the eyes in the morning and dark urine. What question should the nurse ask **first**?
☐ 1. "Has the child had a rash and fever?"
☐ 2. "Has the child had a sore throat?"
☐ 3. "Does the child have any allergies?"
☐ 4. "Does the child drink lots of liquids?"

82. The nurse is planning care for a client who had a total laryngectomy 24 hours ago. Which nursing action is the **priority** for this client?
☐ 1. Provide adequate nourishment.
☐ 2. Prevent skin breakdown around the stoma.
☐ 3. Maintain proper bowel elimination.
☐ 4. Keep the airway open.

83. A client is hearing voices that are telling the client to commit suicide. The client demands a knife to use on their wrists. The nurse calls for another team member to come to the room and provide assistance. Which is the **most** appropriate intervention for the nurse to implement?
☐ 1. Put the client in restraints after giving an intramuscular dose of medication.
☐ 2. Ask the client to talk about their anger and what is causing it.
☐ 3. Give oral doses of haloperidol and lorazepam as needed and prescribed.
☐ 4. Search the client's room for potential weapons while the client goes to the group meeting.

84. The nurse cares for a child with leukemia. Which measure is contraindicated when the nurse assists the child with oral hygiene?
☐ 1. applying petroleum jelly to the lips
☐ 2. cleaning the teeth with a toothbrush
☐ 3. swabbing the mouth with moistened cotton swabs
☐ 4. rinsing the mouth with a nonirritating mouthwash

85. The nurse gave the client the wrong medication. It is 2 hours later when the nurse realizes the error. What should the nurse do **first**?
☐ 1. Assess the client's condition.
☐ 2. Notify the health care provider (HCP) of the error.
☐ 3. Complete an incident report.
☐ 4. Report the error to the unit manager.

86. The nurse assesses a toddler in the emergency department for burns on both feet, both lower legs, and the buttocks. The only area not burned from the waist down is the inside of the back of the knee. The parents inform the nurse that the child stepped into the bathtub and then sat down in the water when the water was too hot. What should the nurse do in order of priority from first to last? All options must be used.

1. Provide fluid resuscitation and pain medications.
2. Assess burn depth in the different areas.
3. Document parent-child interactions.
4. Report the incident to the authorities.

87. The nurse is planning a health promotion class with a group of middle-age women. What information should the nurse include in the lesson plan about reducing the risk for developing osteoarthritis?
☐ 1. Follow a high-protein diet.
☐ 2. Exercise for 20 minutes at least twice a week.
☐ 3. Maintain a normal weight.
☐ 4. Take a multivitamin supplement daily.

88. A neonate circumcised with a Plastibell 1 hour ago is brought to their parent for feeding. What should the nurse instruct the parent to do?
☐ 1. Read a pamphlet about circumcision care.
☐ 2. Remove the petroleum jelly gauze in 24 hours.
☐ 3. Tell the nurse when the neonate voids.
☐ 4. Place petroleum jelly over the site every 2 hours.

89. The nurse cares for a term neonate diagnosed with transient tachypnea 2 hours after birth. Which intervention should the nurse anticipate using?
☐ 1. Monitor the neonate's color and cry every 4 hours.
☐ 2. Feed the neonate with a bottle every 3 hours.
☐ 3. Obtain extracorporeal membrane oxygenation equipment.
☐ 4. Provide warm, humidified oxygen in a warm environment.

90. A 25-year-old, 1-week postpartum, female client was brought to the clinic by their partner for concerns about their mental health.

> **Nurse's Note**
>
> A 24-year-old gravida 2 client delivered a healthy term neonate through a planned cesarean birth 7 days ago. Recovery progressed as expected, breastfeeding was going well, and the client and the baby were discharged on the third day. The partner reported that the client initially seemed okay but has since become progressively more tearful and disorganized. The partner is uncertain if the client has slept in the last 48 hours. This morning the partner became very concerned when they heard the client telling the infant that they knew the baby was really an alien. When confronted, the client stated, "God has told me what I need to do," but would not explain what that meant. The client has no mental health history but reports having a sibling with bipolar disorder.

The nurse reviews the client's admission data to begin the plan of care.

➤ Complete the diagram by circling the choices below to specify what condition the client is **most** likely experiencing, two actions the nurse should take to address that condition, and two parameters the nurse should monitor to assess the client's progress.

Actions to Take — Condition Most Likely Experiencing — Parameters to Monitor
Actions to Take — Parameters to Monitor

Risks for Condition	Potential Conditions	Parameters to Monitor
Arrange for immediate inpatient treatment	Baby blues	Sleep
Screen with a postpartum depression scale	Postpartum depression	Thought process
Refer to a postpartum depression support group	Postpartum psychosis	Breastfeeding
Ensure the client is not left alone with the infant	Schizophrenia	Infant care abilities
Schedule outpatient care with a mental health provider		Mood

91. The client is having peritoneal dialysis. During the exchange, the nurse observes that the flow of dialysate stops before all the solution has drained out. What should the nurse do **next**?
☐ 1. Have the client sit in a chair.
☐ 2. Turn the client from side to side.
☐ 3. Reposition the peritoneal catheter.
☐ 4. Have the client walk.

92. The nurse cares for several preterm infants in the special care nursery. Which action is **most** important for preventing nosocomial infections in these neonates?
☐ 1. using sterile supplies for all treatments
☐ 2. performing thorough handwashing before giving infant care
☐ 3. donning cover gowns for nurses and visitors to the unit
☐ 4. wearing a mask and changing it frequently when giving care

93. The nurse cares for a child in the immediate postoperative period after cleft palate repair. Which type of restraints is **best** for the nurse to use?
☐ 1. safety jacket
☐ 2. elbow restraints
☐ 3. wrist restraints
☐ 4. body restraints

94. A nulliparous client tells the nurse that during their last pelvic examination, the health care provider said that their uterus was in a severely retroverted position. The nurse determines that the client may experience which complication?
☐ 1. frequent vaginal infections
☐ 2. pain from endometriosis
☐ 3. severe menstrual cramping
☐ 4. difficulty conceiving a child

95. A client in severe respiratory distress is admitted to the hospital. When the nurse is assessing the client, what should the nurse do?
☐ 1. Obtain a brief health history.
☐ 2. Conduct a comprehensive physical examination.
☐ 3. Delay assessment until the client's respiratory distress is resolved.
☐ 4. Complete a focused assessment of the respiratory system.

96. A client has had a total hip replacement. When assessing the client, the nurse understands that which sign **most** likely indicates that the hip has dislocated?
☐ 1. abduction of the affected leg
☐ 2. loosening of the prosthesis
☐ 3. external rotation of the affected leg
☐ 4. shortening of the affected leg

97. A client with schizophrenia is withdrawn and suspicious of others and projects blame. The client's behavior reflects problems in which stage of development as identified by Erikson?
☐ 1. trust versus mistrust
☐ 2. autonomy versus shame and doubt
☐ 3. initiative versus guilt
☐ 4. intimacy versus isolation

98. The nurse is assessing a client who has just experienced a crisis. The nurse should **first** assess the client for which behavior?
☐ 1. capability of effective problem solving
☐ 2. increased level of anxiety
☐ 3. shortened attention span
☐ 4. seeks help from others

99. The nurse cares for a 55-year-old female client admitted to the mental health unit with alcohol withdrawal.

Flow Sheet

Vital Signs	10/24 2100	10/25 0100	10/25 0500	10/25 0900
	Temperature (T) 99°F (37.2°C) Pulse (P) 110 bpm Respiration rate (RR) 18 breaths/min Blood pressure (BP) 140/90 mm Hg Pulse oximeter 97% on room air (RA)	T 99.2°F (37.3°C) P 90 bpm RR 14 breaths/min BP 130/80 mm Hg Pulse oximeter 98% on RA	T 99°F (37.2°C) P 70 bpm RR 14 breaths/min BP 126/80 mm Hg Pulse oximeter 97% on RA	T 99°F (37.2°C) P 50 bpm RR 10 breaths/min BP 100/60 mm Hg Pulse oximeter 95% on RA
Nurse's Notes 10/24 2100	Intravenous (IV) dextrose 5% in water (D5W) at 60 mL/h was started in the left hand. Diazepam was administered. The client is oriented to person, place, and time.			
10/25 0100	The client is resting quietly.			
10/25 0500	The client is oriented to person, place, and time.			
10/25 0900	The client is confused.			

The nurse reviews the trends in the client's status.

➤ Complete the following sentence by using the list of drop-down options.

The **first** action the nurse should take is to [contact the health care provider (HCP). / increase the rate of the IV infusion. / attempt to arouse the client. / administer magnesium sulfate.]

100. A client with a new ileal conduit asks the nurse when to wear the appliance. What should the nurse tell the client?
☐ 1. "You need to wear your appliance all the time."
☐ 2. "You should wear your appliance after you irrigate."
☐ 3. "It's only necessary to wear your appliance at night."
☐ 4. "The appliance must be worn after your meals."

101. A child has been exposed to varicella. Which precaution should the nurse institute for infection control?
☐ 1. airborne precautions
☐ 2. droplet precautions
☐ 3. contact precautions
☐ 4. indirect contact precautions

102. Which nursing goal is appropriate for the nurse to make with a client who has multiple myeloma?
☐ 1. Achieve effective management of bone pain.
☐ 2. Recover from the disease with minimal disabilities.
☐ 3. Decrease episodes of nausea and vomiting.
☐ 4. Avoid hyperkalemia.

103. After an episode of severe pain, a client says to the nurse, "The pain really frightened me. I thought I was going to die." Which statement is the **most** appropriate response from the nurse?
☐ 1. "I understand that pain can be a frightening experience."
☐ 2. "Why were you frightened? You've had pain before."
☐ 3. "There's no need to be frightened of pain."
☐ 4. "Pain can't cause you to die. Try to relax."

104. A child returns to the pediatric unit after a bowel resection. Which action has the **highest** priority?
☐ 1. Administer intravenous (IV) fluids.
☐ 2. Keep the child on nothing-by-mouth status.
☐ 3. Monitor vital signs frequently.
☐ 4. Assess the child's pain level.

105. The nurse is obtaining a health history from a client who has recently been diagnosed with type 1 diabetes. Which statement indicates that the nurse should do further follow-up?
☐ 1. "I have some shortness of breath when I exercise."
☐ 2. "No matter how much I drink, I'm still thirsty all the time."
☐ 3. "I wake up early in the morning and can't go back to sleep."
☐ 4. "In the past couple of weeks, I've been having a lot of trouble urinating."

106. The nurse cares for a female client at 32-weeks' gestation admitted to the antenatal unit with severe preeclampsia.

Laboratory Values

Lab	Value	Reference Range
Serum magnesium	2 mg/dL (0.82 mmol/L)	Adults: 1.8–2.6 mg/dL (0.74–1.07 mmol/L).
Blood urea nitrogen (BUN)	30 mg/dL (10.71 mmol/L)	8–20 mg/dL (2.9–7.5 mmol/L)
Total bilirubin	1.5 mg/dL (25.66 µmol/L)	0.1–1.0 mg/dL (1.71–17.1 µmol/L)
Platelets	90,000 mm³ (90 × 10⁹/L)	Adults: 140,000–400,000/L (140–400 × 10⁹/L)
Hemoglobin	9.7 g/dL (97 g/L)	Women: 12–16 g/dL (120–160 g/L)
Hematocrit	29% (0.29 proportion of 1.0)	Women: 36%–48% (0.36–0.48 proportion of 1.0).

After reviewing admission lab test results, the nurse updates the client's care.

➢ Complete the diagram by circling the choices below to specify the condition the client is **most** likely experiencing, two actions to take, and two parameters the nurse should monitor to assess the effectiveness of the interventions.

Action to Take — Condition Most Likely Experiencing — Parameter to Monitor
Action to Take — — Parameter to Monitor

Action to Take	Potential Conditions	Parameters to Monitor
Administer corticosteroids	Disseminated intravascular coagulation (DIC)	Neurologic status
Transfuse platelets	HELLP syndrome	Bleeding
Administer magnesium sulfate	Idiopathic thrombocytopenia	Lecithin-sphingomyelin ratio
Transfuse whole blood	Liver failure	Urine output
Transfuse fresh frozen plasma		Jaundice

107. A young adult has been diagnosed with hypertrophic cardiomyopathy. The nurse should further assess the client for which complication?
 ☐ 1. angina
 ☐ 2. fatigue and shortness of breath
 ☐ 3. abdominal pain
 ☐ 4. hypertension

108. A parent suspects their toddler may have pinworms. The nurse should advise the parent to do the cellophane tape test at which time?
 ☐ 1. before an evening bath
 ☐ 2. after a bowel movement
 ☐ 3. first thing in the morning
 ☐ 4. after eating a meal

109. The nurse suspects a pregnant client has a fetus with a congenital anomaly and reviews the client's assessment data. Which finding provides the **most** evidence that the fetus might have a gastrointestinal tract anomaly?
 ☐ 1. meconium in the amniotic fluid
 ☐ 2. low implantation of the placenta
 ☐ 3. increased amount of amniotic fluid
 ☐ 4. preeclampsia in the last trimester

110. Using the Morse Fall Risk Scale (see exhibit), the nurse should initiate the **highest** fall risk precautions for which client?

Morse Fall Risk/Scale		
Item	Scale	Scoring
1. History of falling, immediate or within 3 months	No 0 Yes 25	
2. Secondary diagnosis	No 0 Yes 15	

3. Ambulatory aid
   Bed rest/nurse assist
   Crutches/cane/walker
   Furniture
	
	0
	15
	30	

4. IV/heparin lock	No 0 Yes 20	

5. Gait/transferring
   Normal/bed rest/immobile
   Weak
   Impaired
	
	0
	10
	20	

6. Mental status
   Oriented to own ability
   Forgets limitations
	
	0
	15	

☐ 1. Older adult client with diabetes admitted with new-onset confusion who reportedly fell at home last week, is currently on bed rest, and has normal saline infusing per saline lock

☐ 2. Alert and oriented client with quadriplegia admitted for wound care of a stage IV pressure ulcer, receiving intravenous (IV) antibiotics per a peripherally inserted central catheter

☐ 3. Client with a history of Parkinson's disease, admitted for pneumonia and receiving IV antibiotics, who has fallen at home but is able to ambulate with a cane and who during hospitalization has gotten out of bed without calling for assistance

☐ 4. Client with acute pancreatitis receiving morphine sulfate IV every 2 hours as needed for pain and no significant medical history, who smokes two packs of cigarettes per day, can be up independently, and has a steady gait

111. A 17-year-old gang member who is living on the streets is hospitalized after an overdose. When medically stable, the teen is admitted to the adolescent psychiatric unit of the same hospital. In what order of priority from first to last should the nurse explore the issues? All options must be used.

1. the reason the teen is not living with parents

2. the desire to leave or remain in the gang

3. the current level of suicidal risk

4. the desire to return home or go elsewhere after discharge

112. The nurse reviews the unit protocols. Which practice(s) can help assure client safety? Select all that apply.
☐ 1. reconciliation of medication prescriptions
☐ 2. communication among staff
☐ 3. placing culturally similar clients together
☐ 4. use of two unique identifiers
☐ 5. staff training

113. A nurse is planning care with a family of a 4-year-old in preschool who is often disruptive in class, is difficult to engage, and rarely speaks. The child flaps their arms and screeches when they are upset. What would be the **most** appropriate responses for the nurse to make to the parents? Select all that apply.
☐ 1. "Has your child received all their childhood immunizations? You know there is evidence that childhood immunizations play a role in the development of autism."
☐ 2. "Has your child been evaluated by a pediatrician? Your child seems to have some behaviors that are abnormal for a child of his age."
☐ 3. "How does your child behave at home? If you do not see acting out behavior at home, part of your child's problem may be dealing with new situations such as school."
☐ 4. "How do you respond if your child disobeys or acts out at home? If your techniques help, stop, or prevent negative behavior, perhaps the teachers can try similar measures at school."
☐ 5. "Have you considered private school? This environment does not seem right for your child."

114. A client asks to read their medical record. What should the nurse do?
☐ 1. Call the health care provider (HCP) to obtain permission.
☐ 2. Give the client information about how to request a copy of the medical record.
☐ 3. Tell the client to read the medical record when the HCP makes rounds.
☐ 4. Inform the client that an attorney needs to request access to the medical record.

115. A nurse is relieving the triage nurse in the labor and birth unit who is going to lunch. The report indicates that there are three clients having their vital signs assessed and a fourth client is on their way to the unit from the emergency department. In which order of priority from first to last should the nurse manage these clients? All options must be used.

1. the client with clear vesicles and brown vaginal discharge at 16 weeks' gestation
2. the client with right lower quadrant pain at 10 weeks' gestation
3. the client who is at term and has had no fetal movement for 2 days
4. the client from the emergency department at term who is screaming loudly because of labor contractions

116. The nurse is beginning the shift and is planning care for six clients on the postpartum unit. Three of the clients have immediate needs, and three of the clients are listed as "stable." For the **best** utilization of time and client safety, the nurse should make rounds on which client **first**?
☐ 1. the three clients who are reported to be stable
☐ 2. the birth parent with a 4-hour-old infant with an initial blood glucose of 33 mg/dL (1.8 mmol/L) and now at 45 mg/dL (2.5 mmol/L) who is breastfeeding their infant
☐ 3. a birth parent who had a spontaneous vaginal birth and received carboprost 1 hour ago for increased bleeding
☐ 4. a birth parent with a 3-day-old who had a bilirubin level of 13 mg/dL (220 µmol/L) 30 minutes ago and is now in a biliblanket at the parent's bedside

117. The nurse on the postpartum unit is caring for four couplets. There will be a new admission in 30 minutes. The new client is gravida 4 para 4 (G4 P4), speaks only Spanish, and has an infant who is in the special care nursery (SCN) for respiratory distress. The nurse should place the new client in a room with which client?
☐ 1. G4 P4 who is 2 days postpartum with an infant and who speaks Spanish only
☐ 2. G1 P1 who is 1 day postpartum with an infant in the SCN
☐ 3. G6 P6 who gave birth 4 hours ago by cesarean birth for fetal distress; infant at the bedside
☐ 4. G1 P1 who is a non–English-speaking client with an infant in the SCN for fetal distress

118. The nurse is developing a community health education program about sexually transmitted infections. Which information about women who acquire gonorrhea should be included?
☐ 1. Women are more reluctant than men to seek medical treatment.
☐ 2. Gonorrhea is not easily transmitted to women who are menopausal.
☐ 3. Women with gonorrhea usually have no symptoms.
☐ 4. Gonorrhea is usually a mild disease for women.

119. The nurse is planning care for a group of hospitalized clients. Which client is at **greatest** risk for falling? The client with:
☐ 1. three fractured ribs and a fractured left arm
☐ 2. episodes of syncope
☐ 3. angina
☐ 4. a fractured ankle

120. A child with meningococcal meningitis is being admitted to the pediatric unit. In preparation for the child's arrival, the nurse should perform which action **first**?
☐ 1. Institute droplet precautions.
☐ 2. Obtain the child's vital signs.
☐ 3. Ask the parent about medication allergies.
☐ 4. Inquire about the health of siblings at home.

Answers, Rationales, and Test-Taking Strategies

*The answers and rationales for each question follow below, along with keys (🔑) to the client need (CN) and cognitive level (CL) for each question. In addition, questions that measure clinical judgment will be coded (CJ). As you check your answers, use the **Content Mastery and Test-Taking Skill Self-Analysis** worksheet (tear-out worksheet in the back of the book) to identify the reason(s) for not answering the questions correctly. For additional information about test-taking skills and strategies for answering questions, refer to pages 12–51 in Part 1 of this book.*

1. **3.** Illegible writing is one of the most common reasons for medication errors. The nurse should contact the HCP to clarify the prescription. Neither the pharmacist, the nurse, nor the unit secretary can interpret or rewrite a prescription written by an HCP.

    🔑 CN: Management of care; CL: Analyze

2. **2.** Propantheline bromide is an anticholinergic used to decrease biliary spasm. Decreasing biliary spasm helps reduce pain in cholecystitis. Propantheline does not increase bile production or have an antiemetic effect, and it is not effective in treating infection.

    🔑 CN: Pharmacological and parenteral therapies; CL: Apply

3. **3.** An important function of support organizations for any health problem is to put parents of children with the condition in touch with each other. Other parents can commonly offer support and help. In some instances, organizations can offer assistance, such as providing equipment required for home care of their child with cystic fibrosis. These organizations do not obtain tutors for children, nor do they provide medications, financial assistance, or genetic counseling for parents.

    🔑 CN: Management of care; CL: Apply

4. **3.** Strategies for meeting client satisfaction include involving hospital department personnel to improve service. Saying, "The staff is doing the best it can," or, "I'll report this to the health care provider," does not offer a practical resolution to the client's problem. Expressing a personal dislike for the food negates the client's problem and does not offer a solution.

    🔑 CN: Management of care; CL: Analyze

5. **2.** Rehabilitation for a client who has sustained a cerebrovascular accident begins at the time the client is admitted to the hospital. The first goal of rehabilitation should be to help prevent deformities. This goal is achieved through such techniques as positioning the client properly in bed, changing the client's position frequently, and supporting all parts of the body in proper alignment. Passive range-of-motion exercises may also be started unless contraindicated. The fact that the client is receiving anticoagulant therapy or is confused does not prevent the health care team from starting rehabilitation. Although the physical therapist is an integral part of the health care team, all members can make sure the client is positioned correctly.

    🔑 CN: Management of care; CL: Analyze

6. **4.** An involuntarily admitted client loses the right to leave the hospital until the condition is stable enough that the client no longer poses a danger to self or others. While hospitalized, the client retains all civil rights such as receiving mail, making phone calls, refusing treatment, and also receiving the least restrictive treatment. If the involuntarily admitted client refuses treatment once admitted, the client will be evaluated for the need to receive treatment against their wishes to decrease the risk for self-harm or harm to others.

    🔑 CN: Management of care; CL: Analyze

7. **2.** Chewing the pill or capsule form of valproic acid can cause mouth and throat irritation and is contraindicated. Taking the pills at the same time each day is important to maintain the therapeutic effectiveness of the drug. Taking the pills with food is appropriate if the client is experiencing gastrointestinal upset. Valproic acid may cause clotting problems; therefore, bruising should be reported.

    🔑 CN: Pharmacological and parenteral therapies; CL: Evaluate

8. **3.** The client is positioned correctly in the side-lying position. While standing next to the client, the nurse should assess the client's skin for signs of breakdown, particularly at the elbows, back, hips, and heels where there were pressure points from the position in which the client was previously lying. It is not necessary to add another pillow under the arm, elevate the head of the bed, or move the client closer to the head of the bed.

    🔑 CN: Reduction of risk potential; CL: Evaluate

9. **2.** It is the role of the surgeon or the person performing the procedure to obtain informed consent. This consists of informing the client about the procedure, the risks of treatment, the side effects, other types of treatments available, and the effects without the procedure. Nurses, anesthesiologists, and social workers do not obtain informed consent.

CN: Management of care; CL: Apply

10. **4.** Hospice care focuses on supportive care for the client and family. Care for the family may continue throughout the bereavement period. Hospice care involves care of the client at home as well as in an inpatient setting. Although professional care is provided in hospice, family members, volunteers, and unlicensed assistive personnel (UAP) also participate in the care of the client.

CN: Basic care and comfort; CL: Apply

11. **3.** One of the side effects of steroid therapy is fat deposition on the trunk and face, producing classic Cushingoid signs. Therefore, the nurse should expect to find truncal obesity. Steroids also can cause altered moods or mood swings, so the child displaying their usual behavior would not be considered a complication. Typically, long-term steroid use results in weight gain, not weight loss. Steroids may inhibit the action of growth hormone; therefore, a growth spurt is not likely.

CN: Pharmacological and parenteral therapies; CL: Analyze

12.
STEP 1

1, 3, 5. The birth parent's fever suggests the infant could have been exposed to an infection during the birthing process. Temperature instability (less than 97.9°F [36.6°C] or greater than 99.7°F [37.6°C]), respiratory distress (seen here as a respiratory rate greater than 60 breaths/min), and grunting are signs of sepsis. A normal newborn heart rate ranges from 110 to 160 bpm. Acrocyanosis, or blue hands and feet, is a normal finding in the first 48 hours of life. Failure to void or pass meconium is not considered abnormal until an infant is 24 hours old.

CJ: Case study; Step 1: Recognize cues; CL: Analyze

13.
STEP 2

Assessment	Helpful	Not Helpful
Activity levels	X	
Blood pressure	X	
Feeding behaviors	X	
Known maternal infections	X	
Occipital frontal circumference		X
Pulse oximetry	X	

Acquired infections are those contracted during or after birth. Diagnosing infection in infants is challenging because symptoms are often nonspecific. Often the symptoms are that the infant does not look right. Behavior changes, such as lethargy, irritability, or poor feedings, are common signs of infection. Cardiovascular compromise can manifest as hypotension, tachycardia, bradycardia, or color changes. Respiratory compromise can manifest as tachypnea (respiration rate greater than 60 breaths/min), apnea, grunting, retractions, and low oxygen saturation. An abnormal occipital frontal circumference measurement can be associated with a congenital infection, but not an acquired infection.

CJ: Case study; Step 2: Analyze cues; CL: Analyze

14.
STEP 3

Potential answer: The nurse determines the client most likely has early-onset sepsis evidenced by the **respiratory status** *and* **temperature**.

The newborn is displaying signs and symptoms of early-onset neonatal sepsis, which is caused by an infection acquired in the birthing process. Increased metabolic needs to fight infection and address the low temperature (less than 97.9°F [36.6°C]) can lead to respiratory distress, seen here as a respiratory rate greater than 60 breaths/min, grunting, and a pulse oximetry reading of less than 95%. If the infant does not receive immediate treatment, the infection can cause multisystem organ failure or even death. There is no indication the infant is dehydrated because it is common for infants to only void one time within the first 24 hours of life, and the blood pressure and heart rate are normal. Congenital heart disease would be more suspected if central cyanosis or a murmur were present.

CJ: Case study; Step 3: Prioritize hypothesis; CL: Create

15.
STEP 4

1, 2, 4, 5. Signs and symptoms of infection are nonspecific and mimic other newborn problems. Additional testing is needed to confirm the presence and locations of infection. An elevated C-reactive protein can indicate inflammation. Both low and high white blood cell counts may indicate an infectious process. A chest x-ray can help determine the presence of pneumonia. Blood cultures are necessary to determine if there is a blood infection. Depending on the findings, urine and cerebral spinal fluid cultures may also be ordered. Although a bilirubin level may elevate with infection, the test does little to help determine the presence and nature of the infection. A urine drug screen does not help establish the presence of infection. Stool cultures are indicated when infants have diarrhea.

CJ: Case study; Step 4: Generate solutions; CL: Analyze

16.

STEP 5

1, 3, 5, 6, 7. Newborn antibiotics are most safely administered on a syringe pump that provides a precise rate of infusion. Gentamicin is ototoxic and nephrotoxic. These risks increase with higher serum drug levels. Slowly infusing gentamicin over 30 minutes helps control drug level spikes. Trough drug levels are drawn immediately before a second prescribed medication dose. The medication should be held until level results are obtained so adjustments in dosing can be made. The health care provider should be notified of the trough levels because the timing between gentamycin doses may need to be increased if levels are high. Antibiotics should not be infused simultaneously because medications may react with each other and if reactions recurred, it would not be possible to determine which medication caused the problem. It is not necessary to determine the birth parent's allergies because the IGE immunoglobins responsible for allergic reactions do not cross the placenta.

🔑 CJ: Case study; Step 5: Take action; CL: Apply

17.

STEP 6

Nurse's Notes

1000:
The neonate has decreased tone with periodic apnea. The blood glucose level is 60 mg/dL (3.3 mmol/L). Vital signs are T 100.4°F (38°C); HR 146 bpm; RR 40 breaths/min; and BP 70/42 mm Hg. The pulse oximetry reading is 97% on 2 L of oxygen.

Both high and low temperatures are concerning with neonatal sepsis. A fever of 100.4°F (38.0°C) in a child under 2 months of age requires investigation. Periods of apnea (pauses in respiration for more than 20 seconds or cessation of respiration of any duration accompanied by bradycardia [heart rate less than 100 bpm] or cyanosis) are symptoms of sepsis. Hypotonia is a worrisome sign of systemic illness with central nervous system involvement. A heart rate of 110 to 160 bpm, a respiratory rate of 30 to 60 breaths/min, and blood pressure between 50/30 mm Hg and 75/45 mm Hg are normal findings. Blood glucose levels of 40 to 60 mg/dL (2.2 to 3.3 mmol/L) are normal for a term neonate. The pulse oximetry reading improved with oxygen.

🔑 CJ: Case study; Step 6: Evaluate outcomes; CL: Evaluate

18. 3. The nurse should not be required to participate in an abortion if it contradicts the nurse's religious beliefs. The behavior should not be reflected negatively on the nurse's evaluation. Preparing equipment and supplies for the case may be viewed as the same as circulating for the case. The nurse has a right not to participate in an abortion unless it is an absolute emergency and no one else is available to care for the client.

🔑 CN: Management of care; CL: Analyze

19. 3. Phenytoin causes hyperplasia of the gums, and the client needs dental examinations twice a year and meticulous oral hygiene. Phenytoin therapy may contribute to a folic acid deficiency, but it is not related to iron or calcium metabolism. A need for frequent eye examinations is not related to the side effects of phenytoin, but the client should have regular eye exams as appropriate.

🔑 CN: Pharmacological and parenteral therapies; CL: Analyze

20. 1. The chest is compressed with the heel of one hand positioned on the lower sternum, two fingerbreadths above the sternal notch (at the nipple line). Fingertips are used to compress the sternum in infants, and the heels of both hands are used in adult cardiopulmonary resuscitation.

🔑 CN: Safety and infection control; CL: Apply

21. 1. Nitroglycerin tablets should be taken 5 minutes apart for 3 doses; if this is ineffective, 911 should be called to obtain an ambulance to take the client to the emergency department. The client should not drive or have a family member drive the client to the hospital.

🔑 CN: Pharmacological and parenteral therapies; CL: Analyze

22. 3. The client will obtain the most health benefits from aerobic exercises such as walking, biking, jogging, or swimming. Because the client has been sedentary, the nurse instructs the client to start the exercise program by walking slowly for 10 minutes four times a day and increasing to 30 to 60 minutes three to five times per week. Jogging is not a realistic exercise at this time. Playing golf is not considered an aerobic activity; therefore, it is not beneficial in lowering serum lipids. To promote cardiovascular changes, the client would need to swim more than once a week.

🔑 CN: Health promotion and maintenance; CL: Analyze

23. 1, 2, 4, 5. Methotrexate is used for clients with rheumatoid arthritis to decrease the progression of the disease and relieve pain. Side effects of methotrexate include decreased white blood cells and platelets and the potential for liver disease. The nurse should instruct the client to avoid infection and report signs such as fever, chills, or cough. The client should avoid contact sports that could cause bruising. The client should also limit the amount of alcohol use to avoid liver damage.

The client will have frequent blood tests to monitor liver enzymes and complete blood count. It is not necessary for the client to increase the protein in the diet or increase fluid intake to 3500 mL per day.

🗝️ CN: Pharmacological and parenteral therapies; CL: Apply

24. 4. The new onset of constipation may be a sign of a tumor or other health problems. Constipation is not an expected change of aging. Increasing fiber and fluid intake is helpful with constipation, but in this case, the client needs to be seen by an HCP to rule out a health problem.

🗝️ CN: Reduction of risk potential; CL: Analyze

25. 1. Peak and trough serum levels are used to adjust the dosage within a therapeutic range. Monitoring drug levels does not prevent allergic reactions. Preventing toxicity helps decrease the risk for some side effects but will not totally prevent them. Peaks and trough levels do not help achieve therapeutic levels more quickly because they are monitored only after a drug has been given long enough to achieve therapeutic levels.

🗝️ CN: Pharmacological and parenteral therapies; CL: Apply

26. 4. A glycosylated hemoglobin level gives the nurse data about the average blood glucose concentration over 2 to 3 months, providing a picture of the client's overall glucose control. A fasting serum glucose level gives a picture of the client's recent glucose level, not the overall effectiveness of the therapeutic regimen. A 1-week diet recall is not always accurate. Although a home log would provide some information about overall control and compliance, the log may not have all of the glucose levels recorded.

🗝️ CN: Reduction of risk potential; CL: Evaluate

27. 3. When making rounds, nurses can note a variety of risks in the clients' rooms, in the hallways, and in other areas where clients might be at risk. Using signs and color-coded armbands and keeping the bed in a low position are also useful measures, but making rounds offers the opportunity for nurses to intervene immediately and teach the client, family, and staff when risks are noted.

🗝️ CN: Safety and infection control; CL: Analyze

28. 1. The nurse's first action should be to stop the transfusion because the client is having a transfusion reaction. It is most important that the client not receive any more blood. Other measures may be appropriate after the transfusion has been stopped. The nurse should raise the head of the bed if the client becomes short of breath, but the client's respiration rate is currently still within the normal range. There is no need to administer acetaminophen to treat the client's temperature spike. The nurse can provide a cool washcloth for a headache or fever; however, this is not a priority.

🗝️ CN: Pharmacological and parenteral therapies; CL: Analyze

29. −/+ **1, 3, 4.** A drop in blood pressure to 80/40 mm Hg is significant and should be reported to the HCP. Hypotension and vasodilation may occur as a result of sympathetic nerve blockage along with pain nerve blockage. A report of a crushing headache suggests that the epidural catheter may be dislodged in the subarachnoid space rather than the epidural space. Epidural dressings should remain dry and intact. The presence of clear fluid on the dressing could indicate a cerebral spinal fluid leak or the leakage of medication. A respiratory rate of 14 breaths/min, although somewhat decreased from baseline, is within acceptable parameters. However, if the rate drops to 10 breaths/min or less, the HCP should be notified. A pain rating of 3 out of 10 suggests that pain is being relieved with the epidural analgesia.

🗝️ CN: Pharmacological and parenteral therapies; CL: Analyze

30. 3. A client with AIDS is immunocompromised, and food safety is an important concern. Food-borne illnesses and infections can be devastating to the client with AIDS, so the client should be encouraged to cook foods thoroughly and adhere to safe food-handling practices. Large, frequent meals are not necessary. Megadoses of vitamins can result in toxicities that may aggravate the client's clinical condition. Leaving food out encourages the growth of microorganisms.

🗝️ CN: Safety and infection control; CL: Analyze

31. 4. This finding describes Mongolian spots, or slate grey nevi, which are common in newborns of African, Asian, or Latin descent. Nevus flammeus, also known as "port-wine stain," is a permanent purple-red skin lesion made up of congested, dilated capillaries. Although they are typically found on the face, they may be found on other parts of the body. Telangiectatic nevi, or "stork bites," are pink lesions commonly found on the back of the neck. Milia are small white papules over the nose and cheek that indicate blocked sebaceous glands.

🗝️ CN: Health promotion and maintenance; CL: Analyze

32. 1. Blurred vision is a serious adverse effect of oral contraceptives, possibly because of severe hypertension as a result of the medication. If the client experiences blurred vision, they need to contact the HCP immediately. Nausea, weight gain, and mild headache are common and possibly bothersome side effects and should be noted. However, they do not need to be reported immediately unless they are severe, prolonged, or accompanied by other symptoms.

🗝 CN: Pharmacological and parenteral therapies; CL: Analyze

33. 3. Nausea and vomiting, along with hypokalemia, are likely indicators of digoxin toxicity. Hypokalemia is a common cause of digoxin toxicity; therefore, serum potassium levels should be carefully monitored if the client is taking digoxin. The earliest clinical signs of digoxin toxicity are anorexia, nausea, and vomiting. Bradycardia, other dysrhythmias, and visual disturbances are also common signs. Chronic renal failure usually causes hyperkalemia. With persistent vomiting, the client is more likely to develop metabolic alkalosis than metabolic acidosis. Exacerbations of heart failure would most likely manifest as signs and symptoms of fluid retention.

🗝 CN: Pharmacological and parenteral therapies; CL: Analyze

34. 2. At the time a client receives a progestin injection, a follow-up appointment should be made for 3 months later, not 1, 4, or 6 months later. The nurse should emphasize the need to adhere to the medication schedule to prevent an unplanned pregnancy. One of the most common reasons for failure of this contraceptive is lack of compliance to the appointment schedule for injections every 3 months.

🗝 CN: Pharmacological and parenteral therapies; CL: Apply

35.

STEP 1

-/+ **1, 3, 4, 5.** With sickle cell anemia, cells become elongated and crescent shaped and cannot freely move through blood vessels, so stasis, or sickling, occurs. During sickle cell crisis, a sudden severe onset of sickling occurs, and blood flow halts to the affected area, resulting in acute pain. Sickling of cells in the pulmonary vasculature can lead to chest pain or acute chest syndrome. A common prodrome for sickle cell crisis is fever and tachypnea, as seen here, that leads to pneumonia. This client's 3-day history of diarrhea and their inability to void suggest the client may be dehydrated, further complicating the sickle cell crisis. An oxygen saturation of 95% is within normal limits, even supplemental oxygen is being given, and does not warrant further intervention.

🗝 CJ: Case study; Step 1: Recognize cues; CL: Understand

36.

STEP 2		
Assessment	Helpful	Not Helpful
Acetaminophen use		X
Abdominal palpation	X	
Breath sounds	X	
Conjunctival color	X	
Exposure to extreme temperatures	X	
Recent dental procedures	X	
Vaccination status	X	

Gentle abdominal palpation can help determine if the client has an enlarged spleen or liver. An assessment of breath sounds can help identify if there are areas of the lungs filled with blood or if pneumonia is present. The eye sclera may become icteric (yellowed) from the release of bilirubin from the destruction of sickled cells during a crisis. Exposure to extreme temperatures can precipitate a crisis. Dental procedures can be a source of infection. Lacking age-appropriate immunizations increases the risk for infection. Acetaminophen is routinely used for pain management and does not present a special risk.

🗝 CJ: Case study; Step 2: Analyze cues; CL: Analyze

37.

STEP 3

3, 4. The child in a sickle cell crisis has three primary needs: pain relief, adequate hydration, and oxygenation to prevent further sickling and to halt the crisis. Since the client has adequate oxygenation and is on supplemental oxygen, the priorities to address are the pain and hydration. Sources of infection should be addressed but only after steps have been taken to treat the immediate pain crisis. The hemoglobin and hematocrit levels are within normal limits for a child with sickle cell anemia but should be monitored closely while the child is acutely ill.

🗝 CJ: Case study; Step 3: Prioritize hypothesis; CL: Create

38.

STEP 4

0/1

Possible Order	Anticipated Order	Not Anticipated
Activity ad lib		X
Broad-spectrum antibiotics	X	
Chest x-ray	X	
Intravenous (IV) fluid at 1.5 times the maintenance rate	X	
Parenteral opioid analgesic agents	X	
Pulmonary function tests		X
Supplemental oxygen to maintain saturation at 100%		X

Bed rest, not ambulation, should be encouraged to minimize oxygen demand and consumption. A broad-spectrum antibiotic that can act against a wide range of infections is indicated until the source of infection is identified. A chest x-ray is needed because of the chest pain and elevated respiratory rate to rule out pneumonia. Aggressive IV hydration is indicated including the option of running the IV at a higher rate. Relief of acute severe chest pain begins with opioid therapy, often parenteral morphine, which may be delivered via patient-controlled analgesia (PCA). Supplemental oxygen should be given to hypoxic clients and those who hypoventilate because of chest pain, but keeping the oxygen saturation at 100% is not needed. Pulmonary function tests would be indicated for those with underlying lung disease such as asthma or cystic fibrosis, not sickle cell anemia.

CJ: Case study; Step 4: Generate solutions; CL: Analyze

39.

STEP 5

–/+ 2, 4, 6. Tasks that can be delegated to UAP on the pediatric floor include assistance with bed baths, recording intake and output, and collecting nonsterile specimens. The client should be considered too unstable to be transported by a UAP without a registered nurse (RN). The pain assessment titration of oxygen are actions that must be initiated by an RN.

CJ: Case study; Step 5: Take action; CL: Apply

40.

STEP 6

0/1

Parent Statement	Effective	Ineffective
"My teen can participate in all school activities except contact sports like football."	X	
"I will restrict fluids on my child."		X
"If my child has a fever, I can manage it at home with acetaminophen every 4 hours for the first 48 hours."		X
"My child is at risk for a stroke."	X	
"I will tell the school nurse about my 15-year-old's diagnosis so my child can contact me with any signs of infection."	X	
"My child will require penicillin prophylaxis."	X	
"My teen may require long-acting pain medication."	X	
"My teen would benefit from a diet high in folic acid such as vegetables and fruits."	X	

Teens who have been admitted with sickle cell disease and crisis should regularly attend school and be allowed to play in all school activities except contact sports like football as this could result in a rupture of the enlarged spleen or liver. A cerebrovascular accident or stroke is an acute infarction in the brain and is a known complication of sickle cell disease. Due to a spleen that functions abnormally, the teen will always require prophylactic antibiotics prior to invasive procedures. The school nurse should be made aware of the teen's diagnosis and promptly notify parents of any infectious outbreaks. If the teen has more than one sickle cell crisis, they may develop chronic pain requiring long half-life opioid medication. Because of high cell turnover, folate stores are often depleted. Supplements or a diet high in folic acid replenishes the depleted folate stores needed for erythropoiesis.

During the summer, parents need to offer the teen frequent drinks to prevent dehydration and should not restrict fluids. Parents should be cautioned to bring their child to an HCP at the first indication of infection, especially a fever, and not wait 48 hours even if administering acetaminophen around the clock.

CJ: Case study; Step 6: Evaluate outcomes; CL: Evaluate

41. **3.** Panting will alleviate the client's urge to push. The client risks edema or tearing of the cervix if pushing begins before complete cervical dilation (10 cm) is achieved. Although turning the client to the left side improves uteroplacental blood flow, it will have no effect on diminishing the client's urge to push. Although focusing on an object in the room may help the client to relax, it will have no effect on diminishing the client's urge to push because of the pressure of a fetus at +1 station.

CN: Health promotion and maintenance; CL: Analyze

42. -/+ **2, 3, 4.** The client who is taking potentially nephrotoxic antibiotics should notify the health care provider (HCP) if the urine is cloudy, smoky, or pink; early signs of nephrotoxicity are manifested by changes in urine color. Straw-colored and pale-yellow-colored urine is normal.

🔑 CN: Pharmacological and parenteral therapies; CL: Analyze

43. **1.** In clients with fluid retention, sodium restriction may be necessary to promote fluid loss. Increasing exercise will not reduce fluid retention. Exercise will promote circulation, but it will not manage fluid retention. Restricting fluid intake will not reduce retained fluids; increased fluids will increase urine output and promote improved fluid balance. Elevating the client's feet helps promote venous return and fluid reabsorption but in itself will not reduce the volume of excess fluid.

🔑 CN: Reduction of risk potential; CL: Analyze

44. **1.** The client might wear objects as protection against specific medical disorders. Typically, these practices bring no harm to the client and should not be discouraged. The client should continue to be encouraged to follow the medical guidance of the health care provider. If the practice is not harming the client, it is inappropriate to label it quackery and demand that the client discontinue it. There is no medical evidence to support the wearing of a copper bracelet.

🔑 CN: Health promotion and maintenance; CL: Analyze

45. **4.** Normally, a neonate's heart rate should be between 120 and 160 bpm shortly after birth. The nurse should document this as a normal neonatal finding. The HCP does not need to be notified. Assessing for cyanosis is a routine assessment at birth, but with the neonate's heart rate at 142 bpm, cyanosis should be minimal and typically located in the hands and feet. Heart rate assessments are performed routinely according to facility protocol. For example, the heart rate is assessed soon after birth, every 15 minutes for 1 hour, every 30 minutes for 1 hour, and then every 4 hours.

🔑 CN: Health promotion and maintenance; CL: Analyze

46. **1.** The therapeutic effects of desmopressin nasal spray are relief from polydipsia and control of polyuria and nocturia in the client with diabetes insipidus. Side effects include nasal congestion and headache. Blurred vision is not related to desmopressin.

🔑 CN: Pharmacological and parenteral therapies; CL: Evaluate

47. **1.** Protein and vitamin C are particularly important in promoting wound healing and recovery from infection. A diet high in carbohydrates is also essential. Because the client with an infection commonly does not feel like eating, it is important that what the client eats be nutritious. Chicken and orange slices would help meet the client's protein and vitamin needs. A meal of a cheeseburger and fries or a cheese omelet and bacon are high in fat and do not contain as much vitamin C as the chicken and orange slices. Gelatin salad and tea contain minimal nutrients.

🔑 CN: Basic care and comfort; CL: Apply

48. **3.** The nurse should ask the health care provider to explain the surgery to the client again and ensure the client understands the procedure and the risks. If necessary, the nurse can call an interpreter. It is the role of the health care provider to explain the surgical procedure, not the nurse or the client's family. The nurse cannot continue to prepare the client until the health care provider has explained the surgery and the client agrees to proceed. The nurse should then document the client's response and the nurse's action after notifying the health care provider of the need to reexplain the procedure to the client.

🔑 CN: Reduction of risk; CL: Synthesis

49. -/+ **2, 4.** Children in respiratory distress need to be kept as quiet as possible to decrease respiratory and heart rates. Toddlers need a parent with them for security. The best way to quiet toddlers is to read to them or hold them. Restraints increase heart and respiratory rates. A sedative will mask the signs of further respiratory distress. Although toddlers can be told that a mask will help with breathing, they cannot understand the rationale and thus fully comprehend its importance. Asking the parents to leave the bedside will most likely result in the child becoming more upset, further contributing to respiratory distress.

🔑 CN: Basic care and comfort; CL: Analyze

50. **1.** Warm showers, baths, or hand soaks can help relieve joint stiffness and allow the client to more comfortably perform activities of daily living. Aspirin or other anti-inflammatory drugs should be taken before activity, not after, to help decrease inflammation and reduce joint pain and inflammation. Although weight loss may decrease stress on joints, pain and stiffness will continue to be a problem. Cold compresses are most effective for relieving joint pain, whereas moist heat is useful for decreasing pain and stiffness. When cold compresses are applied, their use should be limited to 10 to 15 minutes at a time to decrease the risk for tissue damage.

🔑 CN: Basic care and comfort; CL: Analyze

51. **2.** Tinnitus or ringing in the ears is a sign of aspirin toxicity and should be reported. Clients should be instructed to take aspirin as prescribed and avoid overdosage. Gastrointestinal symptoms associated with aspirin include nausea, heartburn, and epigastric discomfort caused by gastric irritation. Abdominal cramps, rash, and hypotension (low blood pressure) are not related to aspirin therapy.

🔑 CN: Pharmacological and parenteral therapies; CL: Analyze

52. **3.** Traveling is not advised because of the client's history of PIH. The client may be in jeopardy if complications occur and medical care is not available. In some cases, insurance companies will not cover the cost of medical care in foreign countries. Air travel is not associated with preterm labor, though some airlines advise clients who are at 28 weeks' gestation or beyond not to travel by air. Any travel that causes fatigue should be avoided. Any pregnant client should get frequent exercise while traveling to avoid venous stasis from prolonged sitting, but the priority is the client's history of PIH, which, if it occurs, could lead to complications. The client is not at greater risk for communicable diseases.

🔑 CN: Reduction of risk potential; CL: Analyze

53. **4.** The best option is a food bank; the nurse can guide the client to choose optimally nutritious foods. Home-delivered meals are expensive. Neighbors are unlikely to consistently provide sufficient food. The employer is not responsible for providing food.

🔑 CN: Management of care; CL: Apply

54. **2.** Safety concerns are essential for a client with sensory impairment. Water temperature should be tested carefully, hot water bottles should be avoided, and the skin should be inspected regularly. Independence and self-care are also important; the client should not be instructed to avoid kitchen activities out of fear of injury.

🔑 CN: Safety and infection control; CL: Evaluate

55. −/+ **1, 3.** Elevating the extremities counteracts the forces of gravity, promotes venous return, and reduces venous stasis, so the client would not be encouraged to keep the legs in a dependent position. Walking is encouraged to activate the muscle pump and promote collateral circulation. Prolonged sitting and standing lead to venous stasis and should be avoided. Although heat promotes vasodilation, the use of a heating pad is to be avoided to reduce the risk for thermal injury secondary to diminished sensation.

🔑 CN: Reduction of risk potential; CL: Create

56. **3.** These behaviors suggest that the adolescent is thinking of suicide. Because of these behaviors, it is imperative for the adolescent to see their health care professional as soon as possible to determine whether they are having suicidal thoughts. After the nurse makes the appointment, it would be appropriate to obtain more information. Giving the parent the telephone number for the local crisis hotline is appropriate after the appointment is made to ensure that the parent has additional support if the adolescent's behavior escalates and an emergency arises. Taking the adolescent to the nearest mental health outpatient facility now is not warranted unless the adolescent's behavior escalates.

🔑 CN: Psychosocial integrity; CL: Analyze

57. **1.** For a child with chorea-like movements, safety is of prime importance. Feeding the child may be difficult. Forks should be avoided because of the danger of injury to the mouth and face with the tines. Spoons, straws, and plastic cups pose little risk.

🔑 CN: Safety and infection control; CL: Analyze

58. **1.** After TURP, sphincter tone is poor, resulting in dribbling or incontinence. Kegel exercises can increase sphincter tone and decrease dribbling. Voiding every hour will not prevent dribbling or improve sphincter tone. It may take up to 12 months for urinary continence to be regained. Dribbling is not a sign of a urinary tract infection.

🔑 CN: Reduction of risk potential; CL: Analyze

59. −/+ **1, 2.** The nurse can encourage parents to implement soothing strategies one at a time to help reduce the infant's crying. These strategies can include reducing stimulation, carrying the infant, or trying the motion of a car ride. The more the infant cries, the more air is swallowed, adding to the colic pain. Cereal should not be offered until the infant is age 4 to 6 months because of the increased risk for food allergies. Additionally, cereal has not been found to help with colic. The nurse should recommend implementing one strategy at a time rather than multiple strategies to prevent overstimulation.

🔑 CN: Health promotion and maintenance; CL: Analyze

60. **2.** Compartment syndrome, caused by compression of blood vessels and nerves, can lead to irreversible muscle and nerve damage if not detected early. Common signs of compartment syndrome in the arm include pain unrelieved by analgesics, pain on passive extension of fingers, loss of function, numbness and tingling, pallor, coolness of the extremity, and decreased or absent peripheral pulse. Delayed bone union does not cause symptoms of neurovascular impairment. Fat embolism is characterized primarily by confusion and respiratory symptoms. Osteomyelitis is a bone infection and is manifested by signs and symptoms of inflammation and infection.

🗝️ CN: Reduction of risk potential; CL: Analyze

61. 2. The goal of exercise after a myocardial infarction is to increase cardiac strength and cardiac output. Cardiac rehabilitation programs include exercise that is individualized to the client and starts slowly. Walking is an exercise that most clients can tolerate; the goal is to be able to walk 30 minutes on most days. Weight lifting and other strength training programs do not provide sustained exercise. The client may be able to increase tolerance for exercise and begin jogging and alternating it with walking, but not until the client has increased tolerance for walking and is able to exercise on most days.

🗝️ CN: Health promotion and maintenance; CL: Analyze

62. 3. When the nurse cannot elicit the Moro reflex of a 4-day-old preterm infant and the Moro reflex was present at birth, intracranial hemorrhage or cerebral edema should be suspected. Other symptoms include lethargy, bulging fontanels, and seizure activity. Confirmation can be made by ultrasound. Postnatal asphyxia is suggested by respiratory distress, grunting, nasal flaring, and cyanosis. A skull fracture can be confirmed by radiography; however, it is unlikely to occur in a preterm neonate. Rather, it is more common in the large-for-gestational-age neonate. Facial nerve paralysis is indicated when there is no movement on one side of the face. This condition is more common in the large-for-gestational-age neonate.

🗝️ CN: Reduction of risk potential; CL: Analyze

63. 3. The statement, "My medicine isn't for the everyday stress of life," indicates an accurate understanding of the nurse's teaching about the use of lorazepam. Antianxiety agents like benzodiazepines are used to treat anxiety that is unmanageable by other means and beyond the client's ability to cope. For the drug to be effective, it must be taken as prescribed. Lorazepam can cause physical and psychological dependence. Tolerance can occur, and doubling the dose of lorazepam may increase the risk for tolerance. Lorazepam is a central nervous system depressant. When it is taken in combination with alcohol, the depressant effect increases, posing a danger to the client.

🗝️ CN: Pharmacological and parenteral therapies; CL: Evaluate

64. 1. A blood test for alpha-fetoprotein is recommended at 15 to 20 weeks' gestation to screen for certain chromosomal abnormalities and neural tube defects such as spina bifida. Chorionic villi sampling is used to detect chromosomal anomalies. Amniotic fluid amino acid determination is used to detect inborn errors of metabolism such as phenylketonuria. Amniocentesis is used to determine the lecithin-sphingomyelin ratio for fetal lung maturity, indicated by a ratio of 2:1, or chromosomal abnormalities. Rh incompatibilities are predicted with blood type testing measured with antigen tests.

🗝️ CN: Reduction of risk potential; CL: Apply

65. 4. The error should be reported to the HCP promptly; the HCP may write additional prescriptions. The nurse should complete an incident report because a potentially dangerous event happened during the client's care, but the first action is to call the HCP. The nurse should observe the client for symptoms of hyperglycemia but first must call the HCP and then complete an incident report. The UAP does not need to be reassigned for this error. The nurse does not need to reprimand the UAP for the error because the UAP already knows an error was made and has reported it to the nurse.

🗝️ CN: Management of care; CL: Analyze

66. 2. After abdominal pelvic surgery, the client is especially prone to thrombophlebitis. Measuring calf circumference can help detect edema in the affected leg. The calf should not be rubbed or palpated because a clot could be loosened and travel to the lungs as a pulmonary embolism. The Homan's sign, which is calf pain on dorsiflexion of the foot when the leg is raised, is sometimes associated with thrombophlebitis, but having the client flex and extend the leg does not provide useful assessment data. The leg will not change color when raised and lowered.

🗝️ CN: Reduction of risk potential; CL: Analyze

67.

STEP 1

Nurse's Notes

Today: 0700

A 48-year-old female client was admitted last night at 2130 for heart failure recurrence. The client has a history of congestive heart failure, hypertension, and chronic renal disease and is allergic to beta-blockers. The client is alert and oriented and denies pain or shortness of breath. <mark>A few crackles are heard in the bases of the lungs. There is 1+ pitting edema in the lower legs and feet</mark>, and pedal pulses are palpable. Vital signs are <mark>temperature (T) 98.9°F (37.2°C)</mark>; pulse (P) 96 bpm; respiration rate (RR) 14 breaths/min; <mark>blood pressure (BP) 118/70 mm Hg</mark>; and pulse oximetry reading 97% on 2 L of oxygen via nasal cannula.

The crackles in the bases of the lungs and 1+ pitting edema in the lower legs and feet indicate an accumulation of extra fluid resulting from heart failure and will require follow-up. The client's temperature is slightly elevated, and the nurse should monitor it frequently for further increase. The vital signs and pulse oximetry reading of 97% are within normal limits. The pedal pulses are palpable, indicating adequate blood flow and that they are not obstructed by the edema in the legs and feet.

CJ: Case study; Step 1: Recognize cues; CL: Analyze

68.
STEP 2

0/1 The client's morning assessment and lab results indicate a(n) **worsening** of the client's **heart failure**.

The client's continued shortness of breath despite oxygen, increase in crackles, increase in edema, and increased heart rate and blood pressure all are signs of heart failure. The abnormal laboratory findings of sodium, potassium, BUN, creatinine, hemoglobin, hematocrit, and BNP also indicate a decline in the client's status. While some of the assessment data and lab test results can indicate a worsening of the client's renal disease, they are all caused by the congestive heart failure. The client's blood pressure is elevated; however, this is also caused by the heart failure. The client is allergic to beta blockers, and should not receive a beta-blocker drug.

CJ: Case study; Step 2: Analyze cues; CL: Analyze

69.
STEP 3

−/+ 1, 2, 3, 5, 6, 8. Classic signs of heart failure are pitting edema, fluid in the lungs that presents as crackles and often a cough, fatigue, shortness of breath upon lying down, and weight gain. Clients with heart failure often will have an increase in heart rate and a decreased appetite. The heart rate for clients with heart failure increases, rather than decreases as the heart works harder to circulate accumulating fluid, rather than decreases. The client's appetite decreases.

CJ: Case study; Step 3: Prioritize hypothesis; CL: Create

70.
STEP 4

0/1

Potential Intervention	Indicated	Nonessential	Contraindicated
1. Request an order for spironolactone.			X
2. Request an order to increase the oxygen flow rate to keep oxygen saturation greater than 96%.	X		
3. Request an order for furosemide.	X		
4. Request an order for physical therapy.		X	
5. Request an order to saline lock the peripheral IV.	X		
6. Request an order for a low-sodium diet.	X		

The nurse should anticipate that the HCP will write orders to increase the oxygen flow rate due to oxygen saturation of 92%. To eliminate the extra fluid, the client needs a diuretic that will not retain potassium such as furosemide. The client should not be receiving IV fluids because the client is already in a hypervolemic state, and the nurse should establish a saline lock. The client's sodium levels are high, which helps retain fluid, and decreasing the amount of sodium intake will help reduce the hypervolemia. It is not essential to have physical therapy at this time; there are no indications of the need for physical therapy. Spironolactone is a potassium-sparing diuretic; thus, it would be contraindicated to administer it.

CJ: Case study; Step 4: Generate solutions; CL: Create

71.
STEP 5

−/+ 1, 4, 5, 7. The client is on several medications that will affect blood pressure, and the nurse should check the blood pressure before giving these medications to determine that the blood pressure is not dangerously low. The nurse must call the night shift nurse and ask if the furosemide and hydralazine were administered or administered and not charted. Furosemide IV is given slowly, with each 20 mg given over 1 to 2 minutes. The nurse should check the *apical* pulse for 60 seconds before giving digoxin. The client is allergic to beta-blocker drugs; metoprolol is a cardioselective beta-blocker, and the nurse should hold the medication and check with the HCP. The second dose of furosemide should remain at 1400 to help decrease the chance of nocturia.

CJ: Case study; Step 5: Take action; CL: Analyze

72.

STEP 6

0/1	Finding	Improved	No Change	Declined
	Urine output of 1000 mL	X		
	Blood pressure of 86/60 mm Hg			X
	1+ pitting edema of the legs and feet	X		
	Oxygen saturation of 96% with 2 L oxygen	X		
	Heart rate of 102 bpm		X	

The client has had a large urine output, their pitting edema has decreased to 1+ from 2+, and oxygen saturation is 96% on 2 L oxygen, indicating that the furosemide and hydrochlorothiazide have produced diuresis to decrease excess fluids. The client's pulse has not significantly improved; it could be remaining elevated because of the low blood pressure. The client's blood pressure has dropped below the normal level of adults possibly because of the furosemide, hydrochlorothiazide, and hydralazine.

🗝️ CJ: Case study; Step 6: Evaluate outcomes; CL: Evaluate

73. 4. Because the adolescent is positioned this way for an extended period, the nurse can help by finding age-appropriate activities that interest the client. The traction is set up correctly. Additional weights are not needed. A well-balanced diet with fiber should be offered; there is no indication that the client needs to have only easy-to-eat foods. A pillow under the leg would negate the effects of the traction.

🗝️ CN: Basic care and comfort; CL: Analyze

74. 1. Verbalizing feelings and concerns helps decrease anxiety and allows the family member to move on to understanding the current situation. Describing events or explaining equipment is appropriate when the person is not distraught and is ready to learn. Reassuring the family member does not allow verbalization of feelings and discounts the person's feelings.

🗝️ CN: Psychosocial integrity; CL: Analyze

75. 2. Graded exercise testing is a diagnostic and prognostic tool used to determine the physiologic responses to controlled exercise stress. The information gained from a graded exercise test can achieve diagnostic, functional, and therapeutic objectives for the client. Graded exercise tests involve the use of a treadmill, stationary bicycle, or arm ergometry. The information obtained from this test is not used to set the incline on the treadmill, and measuring the distance walked and the duration of the walk is not the purpose of a graded exercise test.

🗝️ CN: Reduction of risk potential; CL: Apply

76. 1. Overprotection is a typical parental reaction to chronic illness in a child. Characteristics include sacrifice of self and family for the child, failure to recognize the child's capabilities and sense of responsibility, placement of overly stringent restrictions on play and peer friendship, and a lack of confidence in other peoples' capabilities. Overprotection stems from an obsession with safety versus excessive devotion, mistrust, or insecurity.

🗝️ CN: Psychosocial integrity; CL: Analyze

77. 1. Knowing that the voices are not real is a reflection that haloperidol is effective in decreasing psychosis. Restlessness may be a side effect of haloperidol, but it is not an indication of improvement. Awareness of the need for an activity of daily living like showering is an indicator of improvement; however, recognizing that the voices are not real demonstrates a greater awareness of the client's disorder than the need for hygiene does. Wanting to prepare for discharge before stabilization reflects a denial of illness.

🗝️ CN: Pharmacological and parenteral therapies; CL: Evaluate

78. 3. Administration of IV potassium chloride should not exceed 10 mEq per hour (10 mmol per hour) or a concentration of 40 mEq/L (40 mmol/L) via a peripheral line. These limits are extremely important to prevent the development of hyperkalemia and the possibility of cardiac dysrhythmias. In a client with a dangerously low serum potassium level, cardiac monitoring and more than 10 mEq (10 mmol/L) of potassium per hour may be needed. Potassium-sparing diuretics may lead to hyperkalemia because they affect the kidney's ability to excrete excess potassium. Metabolic alkalosis can cause potassium to shift into the cells, thus decreasing the client's serum potassium levels. Hypokalemia can lead to digoxin toxicity.

🗝️ CN: Pharmacological and parenteral therapies; CL: Analyze

79. 2. Exposure to moisture can lead to maceration and the development of pressure ulcers. It is important for the client's skin to be kept clean and dry with prompt attention to cleanliness after incidents of incontinence. The client's gender and age and the presence of hypertension are not the most significant factors leading to pressure ulcers for this client.

🗝️ CN: Reduction of risk potential; CL: Apply

80. 4. A new glass should be used each time the child wants a drink; it is not enough to just rinse the glass. Thrush is a fungal infection. Children who regularly use a corticosteroid inhaler, use oral corticosteroids, or have received antibiotics disturbing normal flora are at risk. It can also occur chronically in children who have an immune disorder. To prevent reinfection, parents should sterilize bottle nipples and pacifiers. Children with asthma should rinse their mouth well with water after using a corticosteroid, and if a spacer (reduces the amount of medicine in the mouth and throat) is used, it also needs to be rinsed.

🗝️ CN: Health promotion and maintenance; CL: Evaluate

81. 2. In conjunction with the child's history of recent respiratory infection and report of dark urine, swelling around the eyes should lead the nurse to suspect acute glomerulonephritis. Therefore, the nurse should ask about a recent sore throat because a child with glomerulonephritis typically would have had a sore throat in the past 10 days. Asking about rash and fever are not as specific as asking about sore throats when assessing a child for glomerulonephritis. Allergies are unrelated to ark urine. Drinking lots of liquids is unrelated to periorbital edema.

🗝️ CN: Physiological adaptation; CL: Analyze

82. 4. During the first 24 hours after a total laryngectomy, maintaining a patent airway is a priority goal. After a total laryngectomy, the client will have a tracheostomy with increased secretions and will require suctioning and tracheostomy care. Providing adequate nutrition, preventing skin breakdown, and maintaining proper bowel elimination will be appropriate as the client recovers, but maintaining a patent airway is the initial priority goal.

🗝️ CN: Reduction of risk potential; CL: Analyze

83. 3. Haloperidol and lorazepam together decrease hallucinations and agitation, thus decreasing the risk for self-harm, so this is the most appropriate intervention. Putting the client in restraints is premature because danger is not imminent. Asking the client to talk about their anger is inappropriate because the client is beyond rational conversation. The nurse should not send the client to the group meeting without addressing the hallucinations. A room search is appropriate only after the crisis with the client is handled and ethically should be done with the client present.

🗝️ CN: Pharmacological and parenteral therapies; CL: Analyze

84. 2. The oral mucous membranes are easily damaged and are commonly ulcerated in the client with leukemia. It is better to provide oral hygiene without using a toothbrush, which can easily damage sensitive oral mucosa. Applying petroleum jelly to the lips, swabbing the mouth with moistened cotton swabs, and rinsing the mouth with a nonirritating mouthwash are appropriate oral care measures for a child with leukemia.

🗝️ CN: Basic care and comfort; CL: Analyze

85. 1. The nurse's first response to the error is to assess the client for any untoward reactions as a result of the error. Notifying the HCP and unit manager of the error as well as completing an incident report are all appropriate later actions, but the first action is to assess the client.

🗝️ CN: Management of care; CL: Analyze

86. 2, 1, 3, 4. When a child steps into hot water, they do not sit down in it. This child was held in the scalding water, and when they were held in the water, they abducted their knees (hence the areas not burned behind the knees). The nurse first assesses the extent of the burn and then assures fluid resuscitation and pain relief as needed. The nurse then documents what the parents report as well as the parent-child interaction. The burns appear to be from child abuse and must be reported to the authorities, which the nurse can do when the child is stable.

🗝️ CN: Management of care; CL: Create

87. 3. Obesity is a risk factor for osteoarthritis because it places increased stress on the joints. A high-protein diet, regular exercise, and vitamin supplements do not reduce a client's risk for developing osteoarthritis.

🗝️ CN: Health promotion and maintenance; CL: Create

88. 3. The nurse should instruct the parent to report the first voiding after the circumcision because edema could cause urinary obstruction. Although reading a pamphlet about circumcision care may be helpful, it may not be appropriate for all parents. Some parents could have difficulty reading or understanding the information. Petroleum jelly gauze is used with Gomco clamp circumcisions, not Plastibell. Petroleum jelly should not be used with Plastibell circumcision methods because the bell prevents further bleeding.

🗝️ CN: Health promotion and maintenance; CL: Analyze

89. 4. Symptoms of transient tachypnea include respirations as high as 150 breaths/min, retractions, flaring, and cyanosis. Treatment is supportive and includes the provision of warm, humidified oxygen in a warm environment. The nurse should continuously monitor the neonate's respirations, color, and behaviors to allow for early detection and prompt intervention should problems arise. Feedings are given by gavage rather than bottle to decrease respiratory stress. Obtaining extracorporeal membrane oxygenation equipment is not necessary but may be used for the neonate diagnosed with meconium aspiration syndrome.

🔑 CN: Physiological adaptation; CL: Analyze

90. 0/1

Risks for Condition	Potential Conditions	Parameters to Monitor
Arrange for immediate inpatient treatment	Postpartum psychosis	Sleep
Ensure the client is not left alone with the infant		Thought process

The client is displaying symptoms of postpartum psychosis, a rare mood disorder that manifests as severe mood lability, disorganized thinking, delusional beliefs, or hallucinations after giving birth. The loss of touch with reality makes this mood disorder more severe than baby blues or postpartum depression. While it is possible that the client has schizophrenia, the onset of that disorder tends to be more gradual. The client requires hospitalization and should not be left alone with the infant until they have been stabilized. Outpatient treatment and referrals to support groups are not appropriate because the client is at high risk for suicide or committing infanticide. A postpartum depression scale is not created to screen for psychosis. The two most important parameters to monitor are sleep and thought process. The nurse would expect the delusions or hallucinations to improve and the client to begin sleeping if treatment was effective. Mood decreases may persist long term after the resolution of the psychosis. Breastfeeding and infant care abilities are not good indicators of the client's progress because in the acute phase, the client will not be left alone with the newborn.

🔑 CJ: Standalone bowtie; CL: Create

91. 2. Fluid return with peritoneal dialysis is accomplished by gravity flow. Actions that enhance gravity flow include turning the client from side to side, raising the head of the bed, and gently massaging the abdomen. The client is usually confined to a recumbent position during the dialysis, so having the client sit in a chair or walk would not be the nurse's next action. The nurse should not attempt to reposition the catheter.

🔑 CN: Reduction of risk potential; CL: Analyze

92. 2. The number one cause of nosocomial infections in hospital units is not washing the hands. Nosocomial infections can be significantly reduced by thorough handwashing before caring for each infant. Sterile supplies are not necessary for all treatments. Cover gowns and masks, though helpful in reducing the risk for exposure to blood and body fluids, do not decrease the risk for nosocomial infection.

🔑 CN: Safety and infection control; CL: Analyze

93. 2. Recommended restraints for a child who has had palate surgery are elbow restraints. They minimize the limitation placed on the child but still prevent the child from injuring the repair with fingers and hands. A safety jacket or wrist or body restraints restrict the child unnecessarily.

🔑 CN: Safety and infection control; CL: Analyze

94. 4. Severe retroversion or anteversion may lead to infertility or difficulty conceiving a child because these positions can block the deposition or migration of sperm. The normal position of the uterus is tipped slightly forward. Frequent vaginal infections are commonly associated with diabetes or human immunodeficiency virus infection, not abnormal uterine positions. Pain from endometriosis (abnormal myometrial growth outside the uterus) is not associated with abnormal uterine positions. Severe menstrual cramping or dysmenorrhea (primary) is caused by increased prostaglandin production, not abnormal uterine positions. Secondary dysmenorrhea is associated with pelvic inflammatory disease or endometriosis.

🔑 CN: Health promotion and maintenance; CL: Analyze

95. 4. During an episode of acute respiratory distress, it is important that the nurse focus the assessment on the client's respiratory system and distress to quickly address the client's problem. Conducting a complete health history and a comprehensive physical examination can be deferred until the client's condition is stabilized. It is not appropriate to delay all assessments until the respiratory distress is resolved because the nurse must have data to guide treatment.

🔑 CN: Physiological adaptation; CL: Analyze

96. 4. The most likely indication of a dislocated hip is a shortening of the affected leg. Other indications of dislocation include increasing pain, loss of function to the extremity, and deformity. Abduction of the leg after total hip replacement is a desirable position to prevent dislocation. Loosening of the prosthesis does not necessarily indicate that the hip has dislocated. External rotation of the hip can occur without the hip being dislocated. However, a neutral position of rotation is the desired position.

🔑 CN: Physiological adaptation; CL: Analyze

97. 1. The client who is withdrawn and suspicious and projects blame is exhibiting problems in trust versus mistrust. Shame and doubt would be reflected as low self-esteem and suspiciousness. Guilt would be reflected in self-blame for all problems. Isolation would be reflected in a lack of long-term relationships.

🔑 CN: Psychosocial integrity; CL: Analyze

98. 2. During the first phase of a crisis, the client exhibits elevated levels of anxiety. If the client is able to use problem-solving capabilities, there is no crisis. A shortened attention span is a characteristic of the fourth phase of the crisis. Reaching out to others for help is indicative of the third phase of a crisis.

🔑 CN: Psychosocial integrity; CL: Apply

99. 0/1 The first action the nurse should take is to **contact the health care provider**.

The nurse should first contact the HCP. The client's vital signs and level of consciousness are deteriorating, indicating complications of withdrawal, which can be life-threatening. Increasing the rate of the infusion may cause fluid overload and has not been prescribed by the HCP. Arousing the client will not address the underlying problems. Magnesium sulfate is used to treat seizures precipitated by alcohol withdrawal, but the client is not demonstrating signs of actual or impending seizures.

🔑 CJ: Standalone trend; CL: Create

100. 1. An ileal conduit is a urinary diversion that requires the client to wear an appliance, or pouch, at all times, not just at night, because urine drains continuously. Ileal conduits are not irrigated. The urinary drainage is affected by fluid intake, not meals.

🔑 CN: Physiological adaptation; CL: Apply

101. 1. Children with varicella or suspected varicella should be treated under airborne precautions in addition to standard precautions. Varicella is transmitted by airborne nuclei. Droplet precautions are indicated for conditions such as pertussis, meningococcal pneumonia, and rubella. Contact precautions are indicated for conditions such as draining major abscesses, acute viral conjunctivitis, and *Clostridium difficile* gastroenteritis. Indirect contact is not a method of controlling infection. Rather, it is a mode of transmission involving contamination via some intermediate object, such as an instrument, needle, or dressing, or by hands that are not washed or gloves that are not changed between clients.

🔑 CN: Safety and infection control; CL: Analyze

102. 1. In multiple myeloma, neoplastic plasma cells invade the bone marrow and begin to destroy the bone. As a result of this skeletal destruction, pain can be significant. There is no cure for multiple myeloma. Nausea and vomiting are not characteristics of the disease, though the client may experience anorexia. The client should be monitored for signs of hypercalcemia resulting from bone destruction, not for hyperkalemia.

🔑 CN: Physiological adaptation; CL: Analyze

103. 1. The nurse's most appropriate response is to acknowledge and validate the client's concerns. Questioning the client's fears is not a therapeutic response and can make the client feel defensive. False reassurance that the client should not be afraid disregards the client's fears and does not promote further communication between the client and nurse. Dismissing the client's feelings and telling the client to relax do not encourage sharing of feelings.

🔑 CN: Psychosocial integrity; CL: Analyze

104. 3. In a child with abdominal surgery, it is important to check vital signs frequently to assess for internal bleeding. Administering IV fluids, assessing pain, and keeping the child on nothing-by-mouth status are all important, but monitoring vital signs frequently is the priority.

🔑 CN: Reduction of risk potential; CL: Analyze

105. 2. Polydipsia, or increased thirst, is a classic clinical manifestation of diabetes. The excessive loss of fluids is the result of the osmotic diuresis that occurs with glycosuria. It is unlikely that shortness of breath, early awakening, or trouble urinating are related to diabetes.

🔑 CN: Physiological adaptation; CL: Analyze

106.

0/1

Action to Take	Potential Conditions	Parameters to Monitor
Administer corticosteroids	HELLP syndrome	Neurologic status
Administer magnesium sulfate		Lecithin-sphingomyelin ratio

The anemia, increased bilirubin, and low platelets suggest that the client has HELLP syndrome (*h*emolysis, *e*levated *l*iver enzymes, *l*ow *p*latelet count). Additional liver function tests would help confirm the diagnosis. A diagnosis of DIC would be made based on visible bleeding and clotting studies. The client's thrombocytopenia is a result of the preeclampsia and is not idiopathic in nature. The bilirubin is not elevated enough to say the client is in liver failure. The client needs magnesium sulfate to prevent seizures and corticosteroids for fetal lung maturity. This client's hemoglobin, hematocrit, and platelets are not at critical levels to indicate these measures need interventions before the administration of magnesium sulfate and corticosteroids. The best indicator of the effectiveness of magnesium sulfate is improved neurologic status and prevention of seizures. A lecithin-sphingomyelin ratio of 2:1 predicts fetal lung maturity and would indicate the corticosteroids have been effective. While improved urine output is a positive outcome, it is secondary to preventing seizures. Magnesium sulfate and corticosteroids will have minimal effects on liver dysfunction, including bleeding and jaundice.

🗝 CJ: Standalone bowtie; CL: Create

107. 2. *Cardiomyopathy* is a broad term that includes three major forms: dilated, hypertrophic, and restrictive cardiomyopathies. The underlying etiology of hypertrophic cardiomyopathy is unknown; it is typically observed in young men but is not limited to them. Common symptoms are fatigue, low tolerance to activity related to the low ejection fraction, and shortness of breath. Angina may be observed if coronary artery disease is present. Abdominal pain and hypertension are not common.

🗝 CN: Physiological adaptation; CL: Analyze

108. 3. Pinworms come out of the rectum during the nighttime and early morning hours to lay eggs. Therefore, the best time to apply the tape to get results is in the early morning. The test should be done before a morning bath (if the child bathes in the morning), but doing the test before an evening bath, after a bowel movement, or after a meal may give false-negative results.

🗝 CN: Physiological adaptation; CL: Apply

109. 3. Increased amniotic fluid, known as hydramnios, occurs when the fetus has a congenital obstruction of the gastrointestinal tract, such as in the presence of a tracheoesophageal fistula. The fetus normally swallows amniotic fluid and absorbs the fluid from the gastrointestinal tract. Excretion then occurs through the kidneys and placenta. Most fluid absorption occurs in the colon. Absorption cannot occur when the fetus has a gastrointestinal obstruction. Meconium in the amniotic fluid, low implantation of the placenta, and preeclampsia could occur but are more specifically associated with fetal hypoxia.

🗝 CN: Health promotion and maintenance; CL: Analyze

110. 3. Using the Morse Fall Scale, risk factors for the client with a history of Parkinson's disease include a history of falling, secondary diagnosis, ambulatory aid, IV/heparin lock, weak gait/transfer, and forgetting limitations (100 points). The older adult client with diabetes is also high risk with a secondary diagnosis, history of falling, IV access, and confusion, but is on bed rest (75 points). Risks for the client with quadriplegia include IV access and secondary diagnosis (35 points). The client with acute pancreatitis is at risk because of their IV access only (20 points).

🗝 CN: Safety and infection control; CL: Analyze

111. 3, 2, 4, 1. Safety is the first priority, followed by the client's feelings about leaving the gang. If the client chooses to remain in the gang, the other issues are moot. If the client wishes to leave the gang, the issue of living arrangements becomes significant. If the client's wish is to return home, it would be important to discover the reasons why the teen left the home and explore if relationships can be repaired. If the client desires to live elsewhere, it would need to be a place safe from the gang. Foster or adoptive care is unlikely because the client is near 18 years of age.

🗝 CN: Safety and infection control; CL: Create

112. 1, 2, 4, 5. Client care safety is enhanced by the process of reconciling all medication prescriptions at least one time every 24 hours of hospitalization. This can rule out duplication of prescriptions, missing medication prescriptions, or alerting the staff to medications that should have been terminated. Communication among all staff members enhances client safety and prevents errors in written or in verbal format. The use of two identifiers should be consistently used to prevent wrong client and procedure errors. Staff training is an extremely valuable tool to educate and increase communication among staff members concerning existing or potential safety situations. Culturally similar clients are appreciative of being with someone who can speak their language or share thoughts and ideas, but this does not increase the safety of the clients.

🗝 CN: Safety and infection control; CL: Create

113. 2, 3, 4. The child's behavior appears to fit the criteria for autism, but suggesting the child's immunizations are causative is inaccurate according to recent research and dangerous regarding possibly convincing the parent to forego future immunizations. A better approach would be to suggest a full evaluation by a primary care provider, especially since symptoms could result from other illnesses or conditions. Inquiring about the child's behavior at home and the parent's discipline techniques would give the nurse a better idea of the home environment and could help determine whether this is a problem confined to the school setting or one that also occurs at home. Asking for the parent's input regarding discipline demonstrates a desire to involve them in problem solving. Suggesting a different school without a full evaluation does not address the problem.

🗝 CN: Psychosocial integrity; CL: Apply

114. 2. The nurse should tell the client how to request a copy of the medical record. In the meantime, the nurse should, within the nurse's scope of practice, answer any questions the client has. The client does not need the permission of the HCP and does not need to wait until the HCP is present to see the medical record. The client does not need an attorney to request a copy of the medical record.

🗝 CN: Management of care; CL: Apply

115. 4, 2, 1, 3. First, the nurse should assess the client from the emergency department who is screaming because they may be anywhere along the labor continuum and their status will be unknown until they have a vaginal examination to determine cervical effacement and dilation. The nurse should next assess the client with right lower quadrant pain because they may be experiencing an ectopic pregnancy or appendicitis and may need further evaluation by the health care provider (HCP). The client with clear vesicles and brown vaginal discharge is experiencing a molar pregnancy and will need to have a dilation and curettage (D&C) procedure to evacuate the vesicles; this condition will not jeopardize the life of the client if no intervention occurs within an hour. The client who is at term without fetal movement is a priority from an emotional standpoint if there is no heartbeat when they are evaluated, but the physical status of the fetus with no fetal movement for 2 days will not change if not seen within the next ½ hour, and the nurse can see this client last. The emotional care for this client will be extensive if there is a diagnosis of fetal demise, and the nurse should plan the time to be available to support this client as needed.

🗝 CN: Management of care; CL: Create

116. 3. The client most in need of validating safety is the client who has received carboprost 1 hour ago for increased bleeding. That client's bleeding level needs to be documented as having been evaluated at the beginning of the shift to determine if it has decreased to within normal limits (i.e., saturating less than one pad per hour). The three stable clients will need to have an initial assessment by the oncoming nurse but can wait until the nurse can first assess the client who is receiving carboprost. The client with the 4-hour-old infant is able to breastfeed to maintain the blood glucose level, and the client with the 3-day-old infant in the biliblanket is stable at this point.

🗝 CN: Management of care; CL: Analyze

117. 1. The ability to communicate with a person of the same language would be an advantage because it is an opportunity for socialization and support for the new birth parent who speaks Spanish. If a Spanish-speaking birth parent were placed with the client who also had a baby in the SCN, they would have no communication opportunity, and the same would apply to rooming with the client who has had a cesarean birth. The language of the client who is non–English speaking has not been identified, and the nurse cannot assume that it is Spanish.

🗝 CN: Management of care; CL: Analyze

118. 3. Many women who acquire gonorrhea have no symptoms or experience mild symptoms that are easily ignored. They are not necessarily more reluctant than men to seek medical treatment, but they are more likely not to realize they have been affected. Gonorrhea is easily transmitted to all women and can result in serious consequences, such as pelvic inflammatory disease and infertility.

🗝 CN: Management of care; CL: Create

119. 2. The client with syncopal episodes is at the greatest risk for falling. The nurse should assess the client's gait and balance and the syncopal episodes. The client with upper-body fractures and the client with angina are not at risk for falling. The client with a fractured ankle could be at risk for falling but is at less risk than the client with syncope.

🗝 CN: Management of care; CL: Analyze

120. 1. The child with meningococcal meningitis requires droplet precautions for at least the first 24 hours after effective therapy is initiated to reduce the risk for transmission to others on the unit. After the child has been placed on droplet precautions, other actions, such as taking the child's vital signs, asking about medication allergies, and inquiring about the health of siblings at home, can be performed.

🗝 CN: Management of care; CL: Analyze

3

Comprehensive Test

This test has 150 questions. Time yourself as you take the test so you can determine the approximate amount of time it takes to complete this many questions. This test reflects the maximum number of questions you might receive on the actual licensing exam.

1. The parent of a 2-week-old infant brings the child to the clinic for a checkup. The parent expresses concern about the baby's breathing because the infant breathes quickly for a while and then breathes slowly. The nurse interprets this finding as an indication of what factor?
   ☐ 1. a normal pattern in infants of this age
   ☐ 2. the need for an apnea monitor
   ☐ 3. a need for close monitoring by the parent
   ☐ 4. the need for a chest radiograph

2. When conducting preoperative preparations, the nurse determines that the client speaks only Spanish, a language the nurse does not understand. The surgeon needs to obtain the client's informed consent. What is the **best** way for the nurse to facilitate having the client sign an informed consent?
   ☐ 1. Have the client call a family member to act as an interpreter.
   ☐ 2. Have the client sign the Spanish language surgical consent form.
   ☐ 3. Call the Spanish language interpreter to translate the surgeon's explanation of the procedure, risks, and alternatives to obtain the client's consent and answer the client's questions.
   ☐ 4. Notify the surgical charge nurse of the situation.

3. The nurse is assessing a client with chronic obstructive pulmonary disease. The client weighs 200 lb (90.7 kg) and is 6 feet (183 cm) tall. Using the diagram shown here, how should the nurse describe the client's chest in the record in the health history?

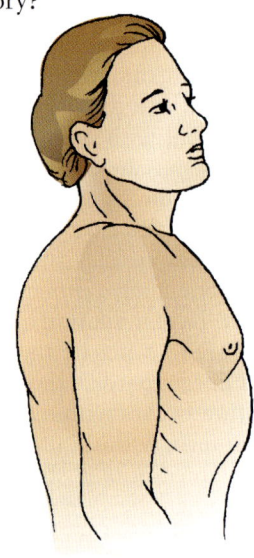

   ☐ 1. barrel shaped
   ☐ 2. indicative of lifting weights
   ☐ 3. normal for an adult's age, height, and weight
   ☐ 4. showing the effects of long-term use of bronchodilators

4. The parents of a child with cystic fibrosis express concern about how the disease was transmitted to their child. What information should the nurse give the clients?
   ☐ 1. A disease carrier also has the disease.
   ☐ 2. Two parents who are carriers may produce a child who has the disease.
   ☐ 3. A disease carrier and an affected person will never have children with the disease.
   ☐ 4. A disease carrier and an affected person will have a child with the disease.

5. The nurse cares for a client with grandiose delusions. Which intervention(s) should the nurse incorporate into the plan of care? Select all that apply.
☐ 1. Accept the client while not arguing with the delusion.
☐ 2. Focus on the feeling or meaning of the delusion.
☐ 3. Focus on events and topics based in reality.
☐ 4. Confront the client's beliefs.
☐ 5. Interact with the client only when the client is based in reality.

6. A parent reports they cannot afford the antibiotic azithromycin, which was prescribed by the health care provider (HCP) for a toddler's otitis media. What is the nurse's **best** response?
☐ 1. Instruct the parent on the importance of the medication.
☐ 2. Ask the parent if they have considered using any medical assistance programs in the community.
☐ 3. Confer with the HCP about whether a less expensive drug could be prescribed.
☐ 4. Consult with the social worker.

7. The nurse cares for a client who is euphoric and intrusive and interrupts other clients engaged in conversations to the point where they get up and leave or walk away. Which response is **most** helpful?
☐ 1. "When you interrupt others, they leave the area."
☐ 2. "You're being rude and uncaring."
☐ 3. "You should remember to use your manners."
☐ 4. "You know better than to interrupt someone."

8. The nurse transfers a multigravid client who is at 25 weeks' gestation with preeclampsia from the obstetrical intensive care unit to the antenatal unit. What information is essential to include in the transfer report to safely manage this client? Select all that apply.
☐ 1. record of blood pressure trends
☐ 2. record of urine protein
☐ 3. edema characteristics
☐ 4. client use of dietary sodium
☐ 5. fetal position
☐ 6. fetal heart rate pattern

9. The nurse is assessing fetal presentation in a multiparous client. The figure here indicates which presentation?

☐ 1. frank breech
☐ 2. complete breech
☐ 3. footling breech
☐ 4. vertex

10. A client believes they are experiencing premenstrual syndrome (PMS). The nurse should **next** ask the client about what symptom?
☐ 1. menstrual cycle irregularity with increased menstrual flow
☐ 2. mood swings immediately after menses
☐ 3. tension and fatigue before menses and through the second day of the menstrual cycle
☐ 4. midcycle spotting and abdominal pain at the time of ovulation

11. A hospitalized adolescent with type 1 diabetes mellitus is weak and nauseated with poor skin turgor. The nurse notes a fruity odor to the client's breath. The client uses lispro insulin. The last meal was lunch, 2 hours ago. Place the nursing actions in the order in which the nurse should perform them. All options must be used.

| 1. Obtain a fingerstick test for blood glucose. |
| 2. Start an intravenous (IV) infusion with normal saline solution. |
| 3. Administer insulin lispro. |
| 4. Notify the health care provider (HCP). |

12. A nurse is planning care for a hospitalized school-age child and is delegating care to a pediatric care assistant. When a nurse delegates a task to an unlicensed assistive personnel (UAP), which factor is **most** important?
☐ 1. The nurse has observed the UAP perform the task.
☐ 2. The child and UAP have established a positive relationship.
☐ 3. The task is appropriate for that individual's preparation.
☐ 4. The UAP has previously performed the task.

13. While assessing a neonate at age 24 hours, the nurse observes several irregularly shaped, red, flat patches on the back of the neonate's neck. The nurse interprets this as which finding?
☐ 1. stork bite
☐ 2. port-wine stain
☐ 3. newborn rash
☐ 4. café au lait spot

14. A client with Alzheimer's disease is started on a low dose of lorazepam because of agitation and a sleep disturbance. The nurse should assess the client for which complication?
☐ 1. nighttime agitation
☐ 2. extrapyramidal side effects
☐ 3. vomiting
☐ 4. anticholinergic side effects

15. The nurse is conducting a counseling session with a client experiencing posttraumatic stress disorder (PSTD) using a two-way video telehealth system from the hospital to the client's home, which is 2 hours away from the nearest mental health facility. What outcome(s) of using telehealth as a venue to provide health care to this client are expected? Select all that apply. The client will:
☐ 1. save travel time from the house to the health care facility.
☐ 2. avoid reliving a traumatic event that might be precipitated by visiting a health care facility.
☐ 3. experience a shorter recovery time than being treated on-site at a health care facility.
☐ 4. receive health care for this mental health problem.
☐ 5. obtain group support from others with a similar health problem.

16. A nurse who is not assigned to care for a client plans to access the client's electronic health record. In which circumstance does this planned action follow Health Insurance Portability and Accountability Act (HIPPA) guidelines?
☐ 1. The client is the nurse's child in the emergency department and has pending lab results.
☐ 2. The nurse had previously provided care to the client during past hospitalization.
☐ 3. The nurse is reporting lab results to the Code Blue team during resuscitation.
☐ 4. The client is the nurse's neighbor who asks the nurse to review the chart.

17. An older adult has few health problems, performs self-care, plays cards, and talks about "the good old days." The client wants to make "final" arrangements, such as completing an advance directive and planning and paying for a funeral and burial. What interpretation does the nurse make about the client?
☐ 1. The client is depressed and should be watched for further signs of depression.
☐ 2. The request is age-appropriate and should be honored.
☐ 3. The client should be placed on suicide precautions and seen by a psychiatrist.
☐ 4. The request suggests that the client has a premonition about dying soon and needs to talk about it.

18. A client with hydrocephalus reports having had a headache in the morning on arising for the last 3 days, but it disappears later in the day. What should the nurse do **next**?
☐ 1. Notify the health care provider (HCP).
☐ 2. Tell the client that this is normal because intracranial pressure (ICP) fluctuates throughout the day.
☐ 3. Instruct the client to increase fluid intake before going to bed to prevent a headache in the morning.
☐ 4. Advise the client to request pain medication from the HCP.

19. A primigravid client visits the clinic for a routine examination at 35 weeks' gestation. The client's blood pressure is near the baseline of 120/74 mm Hg with no proteinuria or evidence of facial edema. The client asks the nurse, "What should I take if I get an occasional headache after looking at my computer at work all day?" Which over-the-counter medicine does the nurse consider to be safest for occasional use by a pregnant client with no known risks?
☐ 1. acetaminophen
☐ 2. aspirin
☐ 3. ibuprofen
☐ 4. naproxen

20. An adolescent client has undergone an examination and had evidence collected after being sexually assaulted. The parent is overheard yelling to the child, "You're going to tell me who did this to you. What's their name?" Which is the nurse's **best** response?
- ☐ 1. "Please come with me. I need some important information."
- ☐ 2. "Stop yelling. You're being inappropriate."
- ☐ 3. "Please be quiet. You're not helping your child this way."
- ☐ 4. "If you don't stop yelling, I'll have to call Security."

21. A nurse is establishing priorities for home visits to a group of clients. Which client can be seen later on in the week?
- ☐ 1. a client recently diagnosed with terminal cancer with metastasis to the brain
- ☐ 2. a female client recently diagnosed with human immunodeficiency virus (HIV)
- ☐ 3. a client who is to demonstrate the ability to perform an insulin injection
- ☐ 4. a client with acquired immune deficiency syndrome (AIDS) with a CD4 count of fewer than 200 cells/mm^3

22. A 7-year-old child is admitted to the hospital with acute rheumatic fever. During the acute phase of the illness, which diversional activity would the nurse **most** discourage?
- ☐ 1. reading a book with the parent
- ☐ 2. playing with a doll with the nurse
- ☐ 3. watching the television with a sibling
- ☐ 4. playing video games with a roommate

23. The nurse is planning care for a client 1 day after having surgery to create a tracheostomy. Which nursing action is the **priority** goal for the client at this time?
- ☐ 1. Keep the secretions moist with saline.
- ☐ 2. Teach the client about tracheostomy care.
- ☐ 3. Relieve anxiety about breathing.
- ☐ 4. Maintain a patent airway.

24. **STEP 1**

The nurse cares for a 47-year-old male client who was involuntarily admitted for a psychiatric evaluation.

Admission Note

The client is a married adult. Today, the client got into a physical altercation with a customer at the auto dealership where they work. Police questioned the client's mental status and brought the client to the emergency department for evaluation. While at the emergency department, the client threatened to punch a hole in the wall after being told they could not take a walk. The client refused lunch, stating that they did not need to eat because they are "superior to all humans." The client requested to call their spouse and had a brief conversation. The client was angry after the phone call ended. The client refused vital signs and lab work. The client does not consent to have their spouse contacted for further information.

▸ Highlight the top two findings that require immediate follow-up. Answer choices have been underlined.

Admission Note

The client is a married adult. Today, the client <u>got into a physical altercation with a customer at the auto dealership where they work</u>. Police questioned the client's mental status and brought the client to the emergency department for evaluation. While at the emergency department, the client <u>threatened to punch a hole in the wall after being told they could not take a walk</u>. The client refused lunch, stating that they <u>did not need to eat because they are "superior to all humans."</u> The client <u>requested to call their spouse and had a brief conversation. The client was angry after the phone call ended</u>. The client <u>refused vital signs and lab work</u>. The client <u>does not consent to have their spouse contacted for further information</u>.

25. STEP 2

The nurse cares for a 47-year-old male client who was involuntarily admitted for a psychiatric evaluation.

Admission Note

The client is a married adult. Today, the client got into a physical altercation with a customer at the auto dealership where they work. Police questioned the client's mental status and brought the client to the emergency department for evaluation. While at the emergency department, the client threatened to punch a hole in the wall after being told they could not take a walk. The client refused lunch, stating that they did not need to eat because they are "superior to all humans." The client requested to call their spouse and had a brief conversation. The client was angry after the phone call ended. The client refused vital signs and lab work. The client does not consent to have their spouse contacted for further information.

➤ What assessment(s) are important for the nurse to make **next**? Select all that apply.

- [ ] 1. How long behavior changes have been present
- [ ] 2. Recent sleep patterns
- [ ] 3. Medication use
- [ ] 4. Location of spouse
- [ ] 5. Difficulty keeping track of thoughts
- [ ] 6. Increases in new activities
- [ ] 7. Perceptions of special powers
- [ ] 8. Recent reckless behaviors

26. STEP 3

The nurse cares for a 47-year-old male client who was involuntarily admitted for a psychiatric evaluation.

Admission Note

The client is a married adult. Today, the client got into a physical altercation with a customer at the auto dealership where they work. Police questioned the client's mental status and brought the client to the emergency department for evaluation. While at the emergency department, the client threatened to punch a hole in the wall after being told they could not take a walk. The client refused lunch, stating that they did not need to eat because they are "superior to all humans." The client requested to call their spouse and had a brief conversation. The client was angry after the phone call ended. The client refused vital signs and lab work. The client does not consent to have their spouse contacted for further information.

➤ Identify words from the choices below to fill in each blank found in the following sentence.

The finding of [_____] **most** suggests that the client is experiencing a(n) [_____] episode.

Word Choices
anger
depressive
dissociative
grandiosity
manic
violence

27. STEP 4

The nurse cares for a 47-year-old male client who was involuntarily admitted for a psychiatric evaluation.

Admission Note

The client is a married adult. Today, the client got into a physical altercation with a customer at the auto dealership where they work. Police questioned the client's mental status and brought the client to the emergency department for evaluation. While at the emergency department, the client threatened to punch a hole in the wall after being told they could not take a walk. The client refused lunch, stating that they did not need to eat because they are "superior to all humans." The client requested to call their spouse and had a brief conversation. The client was angry after the phone call ended. The client refused vital signs and lab work. The client does not consent to have their spouse contacted for further information.

➤ The health care team determines that the client needs to be transferred to the psychiatric unit with a diagnosis of bipolar disorder. For each possible order, specify if it is anticipated or not anticipated to include in the immediate plan of care.

Possible Order	Anticipated	Not Anticipated
As needed (PRN) medication for agitation	○	○
Close monitoring	○	○
Calorie count	○	○
Family meeting	○	○
Routine vital signs	○	○
Stat electrocardiogram	○	○
Routine lab tests	○	○

28. STEP 5

The nurse cares for a 47-year-old male client who was involuntarily admitted for a psychiatric evaluation.

Admission Note

The client is a married adult. Today, the client got into a physical altercation with a customer at the auto dealership where they work. Police questioned the client's mental status and brought the client to the emergency department for evaluation. While at the emergency department, the client threatened to punch a hole in the wall after being told they could not take a walk. The client refused lunch, stating that they did not need to eat because they are "superior to all humans." The client requested to call their spouse and had a brief conversation. The client was angry after the phone call ended. The client refused vital signs and lab work. The client does not consent to have their spouse contacted for further information.

Prescriptions

- Lithium carbonate 900 mg orally (PO) twice daily
- Haloperidol 5 mg intramuscularly (IM) now
- Lorazepam 2 mg IM now
- Diphenhydramine 50 mg IM now

➤ The health care provider prescribes medications to manage initial symptoms and prescribes lithium carbonate. What medication teaching(s) should the nurse provide about lithium carbonate? Select all that apply.

- ☐ 1. The side effects of lithium carbonate include weight gain.
- ☐ 2. It is important to monitor salt intake.
- ☐ 3. Take lithium carbonate at the same time each day.
- ☐ 4. Urinary retention is a common side effect.
- ☐ 5. Notify the health care provider immediately if severe diarrhea occurs.
- ☐ 6. Avoid caffeinated beverages.
- ☐ 7. Take lithium carbonate with meals.

29. STEP 6

The nurse cares for a 47-year-old male client who was involuntarily admitted for a psychiatric evaluation.

Admission Note

The client is a married adult. Today, the client got into a physical altercation with a customer at the auto dealership where they work. Police questioned the client's mental status and brought the client to the emergency department for evaluation. While at the emergency department, the client threatened to punch a hole in the wall after being told they could not take a walk. The client refused lunch, stating that they did not need to eat because they are "superior to all humans." The client requested to call their spouse and had a brief conversation. The client was angry after the phone call ended. The client refused vital signs and lab work. The client does not consent to have their spouse contacted for further information.

Prescriptions

- Lithium carbonate 900 mg orally (PO) twice daily
- Haloperidol 5 mg intramuscularly (IM) now
- Lorazepam 2 mg IM now
- Diphenhydramine 50 mg IM now

Nurse's Notes

Day 2

1730:
The client is accepting lithium. The client is participating in group unit activities but is easily distracted. The spouse visited briefly. The client reported that the visit went well, and the client was very optimistic about the future. The client was very talkative after the visit and appeared much happier. The client is eating small amounts of meals and slept 4 hours last night. Vital signs are temperature 99.2°F (37.3°C); pulse 82 bpm; respiration rate 16 breaths/min; and blood pressure 132/84 mm Hg.

➤ The nurse reviews the client's status at the end of the shift. Which finding(s) suggest the client's mania is not yet controlled? Select all that apply.

- ☐ 1. Distractibility
- ☐ 2. Elevated mood
- ☐ 3. Group participation
- ☐ 4. Sleep
- ☐ 6. Talkativeness
- ☐ 7. Vital signs

30. The nurse walks into the room of a client who has a "do-not-resuscitate" prescription and finds the client without a pulse, respirations, or blood pressure. What should the nurse do **first**?
- ☐ 1. Stay in the room, and call the nursing team for assistance.
- ☐ 2. Push the emergency alarm to call a code.
- ☐ 3. Page the client's health care provider (HCP).
- ☐ 4. Pull the curtain and leave the room.

31. The nurse has just received report on four clients. Which client should be seen **first**?
- ☐ 1. a client who had a cardiac catheterization 8 hours ago whose vital signs have been stable for the last 2 hours
- ☐ 2. a client diagnosed with asthma who just received respiratory therapy treatment
- ☐ 3. a client feeling sweaty and requesting antacid for stomach upset
- ☐ 4. a client with diabetes whose fingerstick blood glucose was 90 mg/dL 1 hour ago

32. The nurse is caring for a client who had an open cholecystectomy 24 hours ago. The client's vital signs have been stable for the last 24 hours, but the client now has a temperature of 101.1°F (38.4°C), a heart rate of 116 bpm, and a respiratory rate of 26 breaths/min. The client has an intravenous (IV) infusion running at a keep-open rate. The nurse contacts the health care provider (HCP) and receives several prescriptions (see chart). Which prescription should the nurse implement **first**?

Prescriptions

1. Continue to check vital signs every 2 hours.
2. Draw stat blood cultures × 2.
3. CT of abdomen.
4. Start broad-spectrum IV antibiotic 4 hours after blood cultures are drawn.
5. Draw CVC, CRP, ESR, and UA with culture and sensitivity if indicated.
6. Ensure client IV access for fluid bolus.

- ☐ 1. Obtain blood cultures.
- ☐ 2. Increase the rate of the IV infusion.
- ☐ 3. Obtain a computed tomography scan of the abdomen.
- ☐ 4. Chart vital signs.

33. The nurse is caring for a multigravid client in active labor when the nurse detects variable fetal heart rate decelerations on the electronic monitor. The nurse interprets this as the compression of which structure?
- ☐ 1. head
- ☐ 2. chest
- ☐ 3. umbilical cord
- ☐ 4. placenta

34. A neonate is experiencing respiratory distress and is using a neonatal oxygen mask. An unlicensed assistive personnel (UAP) has positioned the oxygen mask as shown. The nurse is assessing the neonate and determines that the mask:

- ☐ 1. is appropriate.
- ☐ 2. is too large.
- ☐ 3. is too small.
- ☐ 4. is positioned too low.

35. The nurse cares for a client who had a cesarean birth 8 hours earlier. Which finding(s) suggest that the client is developing disseminated intravascular coagulation (DIC)? Select all that apply.
- ☐ 1. petechiae on the arm where the blood pressure was taken
- ☐ 2. heart rate of 126 bpm
- ☐ 3. abdominal incision dressing with bright red drainage
- ☐ 4. platelet count of 80,000/mm³ (80 × 10⁹/L)
- ☐ 5. urine output of 350 mL in the past 8 hours
- ☐ 6. temperature of 98.4°F (36.9°C)

36. Three individuals with gunshot wounds are brought to the emergency department. The nurse should take which action to preserve forensic evidence on the clients' clothing?
- ☐ 1. Cut around bloodstains to remove clothing.
- ☐ 2. Place each item of clothing in a separate paper bag.
- ☐ 3. Place all wet clothing in a plastic bag.
- ☐ 4. Request that a police officer observe the removal of clothing.

37. The nurse is receiving a change of shift report on a group of clients. Which client should the nurse see **first**?
a client with:
- ☐ 1. wheezing and who has a PaO_2 of 79 and an oxygen saturation of 90% on room air
- ☐ 2. heart failure who has a PaO_2 of 75 and an oxygen saturation of 90% on a nonrebreather mask
- ☐ 3. chronic obstructive pulmonary disease (COPD) who has a PaO_2 of 65 and an oxygen saturation of 91% on 2 L via nasal cannula
- ☐ 4. a PaO_2 of 80 and an oxygen saturation of 93% on room air after being transferred from the operating room 30 minutes ago after having cardiac surgery

38. The nurse is caring for a client who does not speak the same language as the nurse. Which culturally appropriate action(s) are appropriate when the nurse is caring for this client? Select all that apply.
- ☐ 1. Look the client directly in the eye when asking questions.
- ☐ 2. Ask the client specific and direct questions.
- ☐ 3. Ask the client who they would identify to be the appropriate decision maker.
- ☐ 4. Arrange for an interpreter who speaks the client's dialect.
- ☐ 5. Point at the client using an index finger to show the client where to sit.

39. The nurse administers a tap water enema to a client. While the solution is being infused, the client has abdominal cramping. What should the nurse do **first**?
- ☐ 1. Clamp the tubing, and carefully withdraw the tube.
- ☐ 2. Temporarily stop the infusion, and have the client take deep breaths.
- ☐ 3. Raise the height of the enema container.
- ☐ 4. Rub the client's abdomen gently until the cramps subside.

40. The nurse teaches the parents of a school-age child with hemophilia about injury management. Which intervention(s) should the nurse teach the parents to use when the child develops bleeding into a joint? Select all that apply.
- ☐ 1. Have the child rest.
- ☐ 2. Apply heat to the joint area.
- ☐ 3. Begin factor VIII therapy.
- ☐ 4. Start physical therapy.
- ☐ 5. Apply a topical antifibrinolytic.

41. The nurse is teaching a client about using topical gentamicin sulfate. Which comment by the client indicates the need for additional teaching?
- ☐ 1. "I will avoid being out in the sun for long periods."
- ☐ 2. "I should stop applying when the redness is gone."
- ☐ 3. "I will call the health care provider (HCP) if the condition worsens."
- ☐ 4. "I should apply it to large open areas."

42. STEP 1

The nurse is caring for a 62-year-old male client with essential hypertension who has been admitted to an outpatient cardiac rehabilitation unit.

Nurse's Notes

The client states, "I've been feeling really dizzy when I stand up. I ran out of that blood pressure pill lisinopril 4 days ago, so I have been taking two of those water pills to make up for it. I did my rehab walking outside yesterday, but it was so hot and humid, and I ended up dripping with sweat. My mouth is dry, and my legs feel a little weak. I have a mild headache and my allergies have caused a stuffy nose. I had to start taking an over-the-counter decongestant. I did have some blood drawn yesterday."

Vital signs were taken supine, sitting, and standing. The pulse is slightly irregular. The cardiac monitor shows normal sinus rhythm with occasional premature ventricular contractions. Lung sounds are clear.

▸ Which finding(s) from the nurse's notes are the **most** concerning? Select all that apply.

- ☐ 1. mild headache
- ☐ 2. dizziness
- ☐ 3. dry mouth
- ☐ 3. normal sinus rhythm
- ☐ 4. stuffy nose
- ☐ 5. premature ventricular contractions
- ☐ 6. muscle weakness

43. STEP 2

The nurse is caring for a 62-year-old male client with essential hypertension who has been admitted to an outpatient cardiac rehabilitation unit.

Nurse's Notes

The client states, "I've been feeling really dizzy when I stand up. I ran out of that blood pressure pill lisinopril 4 days ago, so I have been taking two of those water pills to make up for it. I did my rehab walking outside yesterday, but it was so hot and humid, and I ended up dripping with sweat. My mouth is dry, and my legs feel a little weak. I have a mild headache and my allergies have caused a stuffy nose. I had to start taking an over-the-counter decongestant. I did have some blood drawn yesterday."

Vital signs were taken supine, sitting, and standing. The pulse is slightly irregular. The cardiac monitor shows normal sinus rhythm with occasional premature ventricular contractions. Lung sounds are clear.

Laboratory Results

Labs	Value	Norm	Date	Time
Sodium (serum)	152 mEq/L (152 mmol/L)	Adults: 135–145 mEq/L (135–145 mmol/L)	July 14	0700
Potassium (serum)	3.0 mEq/L (3.0 mmol/L)	Adults: 3.5–5.2 mEq/L (3.5–5.2 mmol/L)	July 14	0700
Chloride (serum)	100 mEq/L (100 mmol/L)	Adults: 96–106 mEq/L (96–106 mmol/L)	July 14	0700
Creatinine (serum)	1.0 mg/dL (88.4 µmol/L)	Men: 0.9–1.3 mg/dL (80–115 µmol/L)	July 14	0700
Blood urea nitrogen (BUN)	21 mg/dL (7.5 mmol/L)	8–20 mg/dL (2.9–7.5 mmol/L)	July 14	0700
Glucose	92 mg/dL (5.1 mmol/L)	Adults: less than or equal to 110 mg/dL (less than or equal to 5.6 mmol/L)	July 14	0700
White blood cell (WBC) count	6500/µL (6.5 × 10^9/L)	4.5–10.5 × 10^3 cells/mm^3 (4.5–10.5 × 10^9/L)	July 14	0700
Hemoglobin	15.4 g/dL (154 g/L)	Adult males: 14–17.4 g/dL (140–174 g/L)	July 14	0700
Hematocrit	50% (0.50)	In adult men, the value is 42%–52% (0.42–0.52)	July 14	0700
Platelet count	250,000/µL (250–400 × 10^9/L)	Adults, 140,000–400,000/µL (140–400 × 10^9/L)	July 14	0700

▸ The nurse reviews the client's lab results. Complete the following sentence using the list of options.

The client's laboratory results are consistent with
| anemia |
| fluid volume overload |
| hypokalemia |
| hyperglycemia |

which increases the client's risk for
| dysrhythmias |
| hypoxemia |
| tetany |
| stroke |

and is likely related to taking
| lisinopril. |
| hydrochlorothiazide. |

44. STEP 3

The nurse is caring for a 62-year-old male client with essential hypertension who has been admitted to an outpatient cardiac rehabilitation unit.

Nurse's Notes

The client states, "I've been feeling really dizzy when I stand up. I ran out of that blood pressure pill lisinopril 4 days ago, so I have been taking two of those water pills to make up for it. I did my rehab walking outside yesterday, but it was so hot and humid, and I ended up dripping with sweat. My mouth is dry, and my legs feel a little weak. I have a mild headache and my allergies have caused a stuffy nose. I had to start taking an over-the-counter decongestant. I did have some blood drawn yesterday."

Vital signs were taken supine, sitting, and standing. The pulse is slightly irregular. The cardiac monitor shows normal sinus rhythm with occasional premature ventricular contractions. Lung sounds are clear.

Laboratory Results

Labs	Value	Norm	Date	Time
Sodium (serum)	152 mEq/L (152 mmol/L)	Adults: 135–145 mEq/L (135–145 mmol/L)	July 14	0700
Potassium (serum)	3.0 mEq/L (3.0 mmol/L)	Adults: 3.5–5.2 mEq/L (3.5–5.2 mmol/L)	July 14	0700
Chloride (serum)	100 mEq/L (100 mmol/L)	Adults: 96–106 mEq/L (96–106 mmol/L)	July 14	0700
Creatinine (serum)	1.0 mg/dL (88.4 µmol/L)	Men: 0.9–1.3 mg/dL (80–115 µmol/L)	July 14	0700
Blood urea nitrogen (BUN)	21 mg/dL (7.5 mmol/L)	8–20 mg/dL (2.9–7.5 mmol/L)	July 14	0700
Glucose	92 mg/dL (5.1 mmol/L)	Adults: less than or equal to 110 mg/dL (less than or equal to 5.6 mmol/L)	July 14	0700
White blood cell (WBC) count	6500/µL (6.5 × 10^9/L)	4.5–10.5 × 10^3 cells/mm^3 (4.5–10.5 × 10^9/L)	July 14	0700
Hemoglobin	15.4 g/dL (154 g/L)	Adult males: 14–17.4 g/dL (140–174 g/L)	July 14	0700
Hematocrit	50% (0.50 proportion of 1.0)	In adult men, the value is 42%–52% (0.42 to 0.52 proportion of 1.0)	July 14	0700
Platelet count	250,000/µL (250–400 × 10^9/L)	Adults, 140,000–400,000/µL (140–400 × 10^9/L)	July 14	0700

Vital Signs

	July 15	July 15	July 15
Time	1400	1406	1410
Position	Supine	Sitting	Standing
Heart rate (HR)	88 bpm	94 bpm	114 bpm
Blood pressure (BP) systolic	134 mm Hg	132 mm Hg	110 mm Hg
Blood pressure (BP) diastolic	84 mm Hg	78 mm Hg	72 mm Hg
Respiratory rate	20 breaths/min		
Oxygen (O$_2$) saturation	95%		
Temperature	98.4°F (36.9°C)		
Pain on 0–10 scale	0	0	0

➤ The nurse analyzes the vital signs trends in supine, sitting, and standing positions. For each assessment finding, specify if the finding is expected or unexpected.

Finding	Expected	Unexpected
Systolic BP 132 mm Hg sitting	○	○
Diastolic BP 78 mm Hg sitting	○	○
HR 94 bpm sitting	○	○
Systolic BP 110 mm Hg standing	○	○
Diastolic BP 72 mm Hg standing	○	○
HR 114 bpm standing	○	○

45. STEP 4

The nurse is caring for a 62-year-old male client with essential hypertension who has been admitted to an outpatient cardiac rehabilitation unit.

Nurse's Notes

The client states, "I've been feeling really dizzy when I stand up. I ran out of that blood pressure pill lisinopril 4 days ago, so I have been taking two of those water pills to make up for it. I did my rehab walking outside yesterday, but it was so hot and humid, and I ended up dripping with sweat. My mouth is dry, and my legs feel a little weak. I have a mild headache and my allergies have caused a stuffy nose. I had to start taking an over-the-counter decongestant. I did have some blood drawn yesterday."

Vital signs were taken supine, sitting, and standing. The pulse is slightly irregular. The cardiac monitor shows normal sinus rhythm with occasional premature ventricular contractions. Lung sounds are clear.

Vital Signs

	July 15	July 15	July 15
Time	1400	1406	1410
Position	Supine	Sitting	Standing
Heart rate (HR)	88 bpm	94 bpm	114 bpm
Blood pressure (BP) systolic	134 mm Hg	132 mm Hg	110 mm Hg
Blood pressure (BP) diastolic	84 mm Hg	78 mm Hg	72 mm Hg
Respiratory rate	20 breaths/min		
Oxygen (O_2) saturation	95%		
Temperature	98.4°F (36.9°C)		
Pain on 0–10 scale	0	0	0

Laboratory Results

Labs	Value	Norm	Date	Time
Sodium (serum)	152 mEq/L (152 mmol/L)	Adults: 135–145 mEq/L (135–145 mmol/L)	July 14	0700
Potassium (serum)	3.0 mEq/L (3.0 mmol/L)	Adults: 3.5–5.2 mEq/L (3.5–5.2 mmol/L)	July 14	0700
Chloride (serum)	100 mEq/L (100 mmol/L)	Adults: 96–106 mEq/L (96–106 mmol/L)	July 14	0700
Creatinine (serum)	1.0 mg/dL (88.4 μmol/L)	Men: 0.9–1.3 mg/dL (80–115 μmol/L)	July 14	0700
Blood urea nitrogen (BUN)	21 mg/dL (7.5 mmol/L)	8–20 mg/dL (2.9–7.5 mmol/L)	July 14	0700
Glucose	92 mg/dL (5.1 mmol/L)	Adults: less than or equal to 110 mg/dL (SI, less than or equal to 5.6 mmol/L)	July 14	0700
White blood cell (WBC) count	6500/μL (6.5 × 10^9/L)	4.5–10.5 × 10^3 cells/mm^3 (4.5–10.5 × 10^9/L)	July 14	0700
Hemoglobin	15.4 g/dL (154 g/L)	Adult males: 14–17.4 g/dL (140–174 g/L)	July 14	0700
Hematocrit	50% (0.50 proportion of 1.0)	In adult men, the value is 42%–52% (0.42–0.52 proportion of 1.0)	July 14	0700
Platelet count	250,000/μL (250–400 × 10^9/L)	Adults, 140,000–400,000/μL (140–400 × 10^9/L)	July 14	0700

➤ The nurse is teaching the client about managing their care at home. For each potential instruction, indicate if the action is essential, nonessential, or inappropriate.

Potential Intervention	Essential	Nonessential	Inappropriate
1. Communicate the need to obtain timely medication refills	○	○	○
2. Obtain a list of the allergens that cause nasal congestion			
3. Inquire whether the client keeps medications in a pill case	○	○	○
4. Instruct to avoid outdoor exercise in extreme temperatures	○	○	○
5. Teach to change positions very slowly	○	○	○
6. Suggest using nonsteroidal antiinflammatory drugs (NSAIDs) to treat headaches	○	○	○
7. Explain that weakness is to be expected when taking antihypertensive medications	○	○	○

46. STEP 5

The nurse is caring for a 62-year-old male client with essential hypertension who has been admitted to an outpatient cardiac rehabilitation unit.

Nurse's Notes

The client states, "I've been feeling really dizzy when I stand up. I ran out of that blood pressure pill lisinopril 4 days ago, so I have been taking two of those water pills to make up for it. I did my rehab walking outside yesterday, but it was so hot and humid, and I ended up dripping with sweat. My mouth is dry, and my legs feel a little weak. I have a mild headache and my allergies have caused a stuffy nose. I had to start taking an over-the-counter decongestant. I did have some blood drawn yesterday."

Vital signs were taken supine, sitting, and standing. The pulse is slightly irregular. The cardiac monitor shows normal sinus rhythm with occasional premature ventricular contractions. Lung sounds are clear.

Vital Signs

	July 15	July 15	July 15
Time	1400	1406	1410
Position	Supine	Sitting	Standing
Heart rate (HR)	88 bpm	94 bpm	114 bpm
Blood pressure (BP) systolic	134 mm Hg	132 mm Hg	110 mm Hg
Blood pressure (BP) diastolic	84 mm Hg	78 mm Hg	72 mm Hg
Respiratory rate	20 breaths/min		
Oxygen (O_2) saturation	95%		
Temperature	98.4°F (36.9°C)		
Pain on 0–10 scale	0	0	0

Laboratory Results

Labs	Value	Norm	Date	Time
Sodium (serum)	152 mEq/L (152 mmol/L)	Adults: 135–145 mEq/L (135–145 mmol/L)	July 14	0700
Potassium (serum)	3.0 mEq/L (3.0 mmol/L)	Adults: 3.5–5.2 mEq/L (3.5–5.2 mmol/L)	July 14	0700
Chloride (serum)	100 mEq/L (100 mmol/L)	Adults: 96–106 mEq/L (96–106 mmol/L)	July 14	0700
Creatinine (serum)	1.0 mg/dL (88.4 μmol/L)	Men: 0.9–1.3 mg/dL (80–115 μmol/L)	July 14	0700
Blood urea nitrogen (BUN)	21 mg/dL (7.5 mmol/L)	8–20 mg/dL (2.9–7.5 mmol/L)	July 14	0700
Glucose	92 mg/dL (5.1 mmol/L)	Adults: less than or equal to 110 mg/dL (less than or equal to 5.6 mmol/L)	July 14	0700
White blood cell (WBC) count	6500/μL (6.5 × 10^9/L)	4.5–10.5 × 10^3 cells/mm^3 (4.5–10.5 × 10^9/L)	July 14	0700
Hemoglobin	15.4 g/dL (154 g/L)	Adult males: 14–17.4 g/dL (140–174 g/L)	July 14	0700
Hematocrit	50% (0.50 proportion of 1.0)	In adult men, the value is 42%–52% (0.42–0.52 proportion of 1.0)	July 14	0700
Platelet count	250,000 μL (250,400 × 10^9/L)	Adults, 140,000–400,000/μL (140–400 × 10^9/L)	July 14	0700

The nurse is preparing the client for discharge from the rehabilitation unit.

➤ Which plan(s) should the nurse include in the discharge teaching? Select all that apply.

☐ 1. Begin an exercise program as tolerated.
☐ 2. Avoid over-the-counter medications that are contraindicated for clients with essential hypertension.
☐ 3. Hold hydrochlorothiazide until the follow-up visit.
☐ 4. Learn how to monitor BP.
☐ 5. Limit sodium to 1500 mg a day (1 teaspoon).
☐ 6. Recheck serum potassium in 3 days.
☐ 7. Follow a DASH (Dietary Approaches to Stop Hypertension) diet.

47. STEP 6

The nurse is caring for a 62-year-old male client with essential hypertension who has been admitted to an outpatient cardiac rehabilitation unit.

Nurse's Notes

The client states, "I've been feeling really dizzy when I stand up. I ran out of that blood pressure pill lisinopril 4 days ago, so I have been taking two of those water pills to make up for it. I did my rehab walking outside yesterday, but it was so hot and humid, and I ended up dripping with sweat. My mouth is dry, and my legs feel a little weak. I have a mild headache and my allergies have caused a stuffy nose. I had to start taking an over-the-counter decongestant. I did have some blood drawn yesterday."

Vital signs were taken supine, sitting, and standing. The pulse is slightly irregular. The cardiac monitor shows normal sinus rhythm with occasional premature ventricular contractions. Lung sounds are clear.

Vital Signs

	July 15	July 15	July 15
Time	1400	1406	1410
Position	Supine	Sitting	Standing
Heart rate (HR)	88 bpm	94 bpm	114 bpm
Blood pressure (BP) systolic	134 mm Hg	132 mm Hg	110 mm Hg
Blood pressure (BP) diastolic	84 mm Hg	78 mm Hg	72 mm Hg
Respiratory rate	20 breaths/min		
Oxygen (O_2) saturation	95%		
Temperature	98.4°F (36.9°C)		
Pain on 0–10 scale	0	0	0

Laboratory Results

Labs	Value	Norm	Date	Time
Sodium (serum)	152 mEq/L (152 mmol/L)	Adults: 135–145 mEq/L (135–145 mmol/L)	July 14	0700
Potassium (serum)	3.0 mEq/L (3.0 mmol/L)	Adults: 3.5–5.2 mEq/L (3.5–5.2 mmol/L)	July 14	0700
Chloride (serum)	100 mEq/L (100 mmol/L)	Adults: 96–106 mEq/L (96–106 mmol/L)	July 14	0700
Creatinine (serum)	1.0 mg/dL (88.4 µmol/L)	Men: 0.9–1.3 mg/dL (80–115 µmol/L)	July 14	0700
Blood urea nitrogen (BUN)	21 mg/dL (7.5 mmol/L)	8–20 mg/dL (2.9–7.5 mmol/L)	July 14	0700
Glucose	92 mg/dL (5.1 mmol/L)	Adults: less than or equal to 110 mg/dL (less than or equal to 5.6 mmol/L)	July 14	0700
White blood cell (WBC) count	6500/µL (6.5 × 10^9/L)	4.5–10.5 × 10^3 cells/mm³ (4.5–10.5 × 10^9/L)	July 14	0700
Hemoglobin	15.4 g/dL (154 g/L)	Adult males: 14–17.4 g/dL (140–174 g/L)	July 14	0700
Hematocrit	50% (0.50 proportion of 1.0)	In adult men, the value is 42%–52% (0.42 to 0.52 proportion of 1.0)	July 14	0700
Platelet count	250,000/µL (250–400 × 10^9/L)	Adults, 140,000–400,000/µL (140–400 × 10^9/L)	July 14	0700

The nurse is evaluating whether the client understands when to contact the health care provider.

➤ The client understands the instructions when they note that which finding(s) require **immediate** follow-up? Select all that apply.

- ☐ 1. Thirst
- ☐ 2. Palpitations
- ☐ 3. Dizziness
- ☐ 4. Fatigue
- ☐ 5. Blurred vision
- ☐ 6. Swelling of the lips or tongue
- ☐ 7. Nasal congestion
- ☐ 8. Fainting
- ☐ 9. Dry cough

48. A client with angina shows the nurse the nitroglycerin tablets that the client carries in a plastic bag in a pocket. Where should the nurse teach the client to keep the nitroglycerin tablets?
☐ 1. in the refrigerator
☐ 2. in a cool, moist place
☐ 3. in a dark container to shield from light
☐ 4. in a plastic pill container where it is readily available

49. A client with a chronic mental illness who does not always take their medications is separated from their spouse and receives public assistance funds. The client lives with their parent and older sibling and manages their own medication. The client's parent is in poor health and also receives public assistance benefits. The client's sibling works outside the home, and the client's other parent is dead. Which issue should the nurse address **first**?
☐ 1. family support
☐ 2. marital communication
☐ 3. financial concerns
☐ 4. medication compliance

50. A client is receiving total parenteral nutrition (TPN). The nurse notices that the bag of TPN solution has been infusing for 24 hours but has 300 mL of solution left. What should the nurse do?
☐ 1. Continue the infusion until the remaining 300 mL is infused.
☐ 2. Change the filter on the tubing, and continue with the infusion.
☐ 3. Notify the health care provider (HCP), and obtain prescriptions to alter the flow rate of the solution.
☐ 4. Discontinue the current solution, change the tubing, and hang a new bag of TPN solution.

51. A client is being treated for acute low back pain. The nurse should report which of these clinical manifestations to the health care provider (HCP) **immediately**?
☐ 1. diffuse, aching sensation in the L4 to L5 area
☐ 2. new onset of footdrop
☐ 3. pain in the lower back when the leg is lifted
☐ 4. pain in the lower back that radiates to the hip

52. A client has had a central venous pressure line inserted. The nurse should **immediately** report which sign to the health care provider?
☐ 1. sharp pain on the affected side
☐ 2. urinary output of 50 mL per hour
☐ 3. heart rate of 88 bpm
☐ 4. discomfort at the insertion site

53. The nurse assesses a teenage girl's musculoskeletal system (see figure). What finding should the nurse document?

☐ 1. normal posture
☐ 2. kyphosis
☐ 3. scoliosis
☐ 4. lordosis

54. A client with a broken ulna reports having pain in the casted arm that is unrelieved by pain medication. The nurse assesses the arm and notes that the fingers are swollen and difficult to separate. After reviewing the health care provider's prescriptions, what should the nurse do **first**?
☐ 1. Administer morphine 2 mg intravenously.
☐ 2. Apply an ice bag to the fingers to relieve pain.
☐ 3. Elevate the arm on two pillows, and reassess in 30 minutes.
☐ 4. Notify the health care provider (HCP) about the swelling and pain.

55. While caring for a client and their 1-day-old neonate born vaginally at 30 weeks' gestation, the nurse explains the neonate's need for gavage feeding at this time instead of the client's plan for bottle-feeding. What should the nurse include as the rationale for this feeding plan?
- ☐ 1. The neonate has difficulty coordinating sucking, swallowing, and breathing.
- ☐ 2. A high-calorie formula, presently needed at this time, is more easily delivered via gavage.
- ☐ 3. Gavage feedings can minimize the neonate's increased risk for developing hypoglycemia.
- ☐ 4. This type of feeding, easily given in the isolette, decreases the neonate's risk for cold stress.

56. The nurse is giving preoperative instructions to a client who will have a reversal of a colostomy. What should the nurse prepare the client to expect during the immediate postoperative period? Select all that apply.
- ☐ 1. nasogastric (NG) tube attached to low intermittent suction
- ☐ 2. administration of intravenous (IV) fluids
- ☐ 3. daily measurement of abdominal girth
- ☐ 4. calculation of intake and output every 8 hours
- ☐ 5. assessment of vital signs every 6 hours

57. The nurse is assessing a client for signs of a blood transfusion reaction. Which finding indicates the client is having a transfusion reaction?
- ☐ 1. hypertension
- ☐ 2. diaphoresis
- ☐ 3. polyuria
- ☐ 4. warm skin

58. A client has been receiving total parenteral nutrition (TPN) for the last 5 days. Before the nurse discontinues the infusion, the infusion rate is slowed. What complication of TPN infusion should the nurse assess the client for as the infusion is discontinued?
- ☐ 1. essential fatty acid deficiency
- ☐ 2. dehydration
- ☐ 3. rebound hypoglycemia
- ☐ 4. malnutrition

59. A client with diabetes has been diagnosed with hypertension, and the health care provider has prescribed atenolol, a beta-blocker. When the nurse is teaching the client about the drug, what should they tell the client about how it may interact with the client's diabetes?

Atenolol may cause:
- ☐ 1. a decrease in the hypoglycemic effects of insulin.
- ☐ 2. an increase in the hypoglycemic effects of insulin.
- ☐ 3. an increase in the incidence of ketoacidosis.
- ☐ 4. a decrease in the incidence of ketoacidosis.

60. The nurse is caring for an older adult client who has experienced sensorineural hearing loss. The nurse anticipates that the client will exhibit which symptom?
- ☐ 1. difficulty hearing high-pitched sounds
- ☐ 2. problems with speaking clearly
- ☐ 3. inability to assign meaning to sound
- ☐ 4. vertigo when changing positions

61. **STEP 1**

The nurse is caring for a 25-year-old female primigravid client at 36 weeks' gestation in the prenatal clinic.

History and Physical

System	Findings
Cardiorespiratory	Pulse (P) 86 bpm; respiration rate (RR)18 breaths/min; blood pressure (BP) 156/100 mm Hg; and 1+ ankle edema
Neurologic-musculoskeletal	The client reports a headache starting this morning. The headache did not respond to acetaminophen. The client reports seeing flashing lights with headache.
Fluid and nutrition	Weight gain is 3.3 lb (1.5 kg) since the 34-week visit. Urine dipstick is +3 for protein.
Obstetric	Reports experiencing one or two contractions an hour. Fundal height is 35 cm, and the fetal heart rate (FHR) is 170 bpm. A cervical exam revealed that the client is dilated 1 cm.

➤ Which finding(s) require **immediate** follow-up? Select all that apply.

- ☐ 1. Contractions
- ☐ 2. Headache
- ☐ 3. Visual disturbances
- ☐ 4. Blood pressure
- ☐ 5. Weight gain
- ☐ 6. Urine dipstick
- ☐ 7. Fundal height
- ☐ 8. Fetal heart rate
- ☐ 9. Cervical dilation

62. STEP 2

The nurse is caring for a 25-year-old female primigravid client at 36 weeks' gestation in the prenatal clinic.

History and Physical

System	Findings
Cardiorespiratory	Pulse (P) 86 bpm; respiration rate (RR) 18 breaths/min; blood pressure (BP) 156/100 mm Hg; and 1+ ankle edema
Neurologic-musculoskeletal	The client reports a headache starting this morning. The headache did not respond to acetaminophen. The client reports seeing flashing lights with headache.
Fluid and nutrition	Weight gain is 3.3 lb (1.5 kg) since the 34-week visit. Urine dipstick is +3 for protein.
Obstetric	Reports experiencing one or two contractions an hour. Fundal height is 35 cm, and the fetal heart rate (FHR) is 170 bpm. A cervical exam revealed that the client is dilated 1 cm.

➤ For each client finding below, specify if it is **most** consistent with the diagnosis of mild preeclampsia or severe preeclampsia.

Finding	Mild Preeclampsia	Severe Preeclampsia
BP	○	○
Headache	○	○
Urine dipstick	○	○
Visual changes	○	○
Fetal tachycardia	○	○

63. STEP 3

The nurse is caring for a 25-year-old female primigravid client at 36 weeks' gestation in the prenatal clinic.

History and Physical

System	Findings
Cardiorespiratory	Pulse (P) 86 bpm; respiration rate (RR) 18 breaths/min; blood pressure (BP) 156/100 mm Hg; and 1+ ankle edema
Neurologic-musculoskeletal	The client reports a headache starting this morning. The headache did not respond to acetaminophen. The client reports seeing flashing lights with headache.
Fluid and nutrition	Weight gain is 3.3 lb (1.5 kg) since the 34-week visit. Urine dipstick is +3 for protein.
Obstetric	Reports experiencing one or two contractions an hour. Fundal height is 35 cm, and the fetal heart rate (FHR) is 170 bpm. A cervical exam revealed that the client is dilated 1 cm.

➤ Complete the following sentences by circling the correct answers from the list of options.

The client is at greatest risk for [pulmonary edema. / seizure. / stroke.]

To prevent complications, the client **most** likely requires immediate hospitalization and treatment with [antihypertensives. / anticonvulsants. / uterotonics.]

64. STEP 4

The 25-year-old female primigravid client at 36 weeks' gestation is transferred to the labor and delivery unit with a diagnosis of severe preeclampsia.

History and Physical

System	Findings
Cardiorespiratory	Pulse (P) 86 bpm; respiration rate (RR) 18 breaths/min; blood pressure (BP) 156/100 mm Hg; and 1+ ankle edema.
Neurologic-musculoskeletal	The client reports a headache starting this morning. The headache did not respond to acetaminophen. The client reports seeing flashing lights with headache.
Fluid and nutrition	Weight gain is 3.3 lb (1.5 kg) since the 34-week visit. Urine dipstick is +3 for protein.
Obstetric	Reports experiencing one or two contractions an hour. Fundal height is 35 cm, and the fetal heart rate (FHR) is 170 bpm. A cervical exam revealed that the client is dilated 1 cm.

Nurse's Notes

1100:
A 36-week-gestation client is admitted to the maternity unit for preeclampsia. The client reports a headache accompanied by seeing flashing lights. Clonus is present. Membranes remain intact. Vital signs are 97.9°F (36.6°C); P 88 bpm; RR 20 breaths/min; and BP 160/105 mm Hg. The pulse oximeter reading is 97% on room air. FHR is 165 bpm.

➤ Select the anticipated provider orders from each of the following categories. Each category must have at least one response option selected.

Category	Anticipated Order
Activity	☐ Bathroom privileges
	☐ Quiet environment
	☐ Seizure precautions
Medications	☐ Magnesium sulfate infusion
	☐ Magnesium sulfate bolus
	☐ Intrapartum antibiotics
Monitoring	☐ Intermittent fetal monitoring
	☐ Complete blood count (CBC) and clotting studies daily
	☐ Complete metabolic panel and magnesium levels

65. STEP 5

The nurse cares for a 25-year-old female primigravid client at 36-weeks' gestation who was transferred to the labor and delivery unit with a diagnosis of severe preeclampsia.

History and Physical

System	Findings
Cardiorespiratory	Pulse (P) 86 bpm; respiration rate (RR) 18 breaths/min; blood pressure (BP) 156/100 mm Hg; and 1+ ankle edema.
Neurologic-musculoskeletal	The client reports a headache starting this morning. The headache did not respond to acetaminophen. The client reports seeing flashing lights with headache.
Fluid and nutrition	Weight gain is 3.3 lb (1.5 kg) since the 34-week visit. Urine dipstick is +3 for protein.
Obstetric	Reports experiencing one or two contractions an hour. Fundal height is 35 cm, and the fetal heart rate (FHR) is 170 bpm. A cervical exam revealed that the client is dilated 1 cm.

Nurse's Notes

1100:
A 36-week-gestation client is admitted to the maternity unit for preeclampsia. The client reports a headache accompanied by seeing flashing lights. Clonus is present. Membranes remain intact. Vital signs are 97.9°F (36.6°C); P 88 bpm; RR 20 breaths/min; and BP 160/105 mm Hg. The pulse oximeter reading is 97% on room air. FHR is 165 bpm.

Prescriptions

Give magnesium sulfate intravenously (IV) 4 g in 100 mL lactated Ringer's solution over 15 minutes.
Then begin magnesium sulfate IV 10 g in 500 mL lactated Ringers at 100 mL per hour.

➤ The nurse receives prescriptions to administer magnesium sulfate. Which action(s) should the nurse take when administering magnesium sulfate? Select all that apply.

☐ 1. Have two clinicians double-check the medication.
☐ 2. Infuse on an IV pump.
☐ 3. Provide one-on-one care during the initial administration.
☐ 4. Have naloxone antidote available.
☐ 5. Monitor urine magnesium levels.
☐ 6. Monitor deep tendon reflexes.

66. STEP 6

The 25-year-old female primigravid client at 37 weeks' gestation is admitted to the labor and delivery unit with preeclampsia.

History and Physical

System	Findings
Cardiorespiratory	Pulse (P) 86 bpm; respiration rate (RR) 18 breaths/min; blood pressure (BP) 156/100 mm Hg; and 1+ ankle edema.
Neurologic-musculoskeletal	The client reports a headache starting this morning. The headache did not respond to acetaminophen. The client reports seeing flashing lights with headache.
Fluid and nutrition	Weight gain is 3.3 lb (1.5 kg) since the 34-week visit. Urine dipstick is +3 for protein.
Obstetric	Reports experiencing one or two contractions an hour. Fundal height is 35 cm, and the fetal heart rate (FHR) is 170 bpm. A cervical exam revealed that the client is dilated 1 cm.

Nurse's Notes

1200:
A 36-week-gestation client is admitted to the maternity unit for preeclampsia. The client reports a headache accompanied by seeing flashing lights. Clonus is present. Membranes remain intact. Vital signs are 97.9°F (36.6°C); P 88 bpm; RR 20 breaths/min; and BP 160/105 mm Hg. The pulse oximeter reading is 97% on room air. FHR is 165 bpm.

1200:
The magnesium sulfate bolus is complete, and a maintenance dose started. The client reports nausea but no headache. FHR is 120 bpm with acceleration. No contractions. Urine output is 50 mL per hour. Deep tendon reflexes are +1. Mild wheezing is present bilaterally. Vital signs are T 97.9°F (36.6°C); P 86 bpm; RR 20 breaths/min; and BP 150/100 mm Hg. Pulse oximetry shows an oxygen saturation of 97% on room air.

Prescriptions

Give magnesium sulfate intravenously (IV) 4 g in 100 mL lactated Ringer's solution over 15 minutes.
 Then begin magnesium sulfate IV 10 g in 500 mL lactated Ringers at 100 mL per hour.

➤ The nurse has implemented the treatment plan. For each assessment, specify if the finding indicates that interventions for preeclampsia plan been effective, ineffective, or not related.

Assessment Finding	Effective	Ineffective	Not Related
Urine output	○	○	○
FHR	○	○	○
Contractions	○	○	○
Deep tendon reflexes	○	○	○
Nausea	○	○	○
Wheezing	○	○	○

---

67. The nurse is evaluating the effectiveness of fluid resuscitation during the emergency period of burn management. Which finding indicates that adequate fluid replacement has been achieved?
☐ 1. The body weight has increased.
☐ 2. The fluid intake is less than urinary output.
☐ 3. The urine output is more than 35 mL per hour.
☐ 4. The blood pressure is 90/60 mm Hg.

68. The parent of a child who is taking an antibiotic for bilateral otitis media tells the nurse that they have stopped the medicine since the child is better and they are saving the rest of the medication to use the next time the child gets sick. What should the nurse tell the parent?
☐ 1. "It's important to give the medicine as prescribed."
☐ 2. "How do you know your child's ears are cured?"
☐ 3. "Your child needs all of the medicine so the infection clears."
☐ 4. "Stopping the medicine will make the next ear infection harder to treat."

69. A client who comes to the emergency department with multiple bruises on the face and arms, a black eye, and a broken nose says that these injuries occurred when they fell down the stairs. The nurse suspects that the client may have been physically assaulted. What should the nurse do **next**?
☐ 1. Ask the client directly about the possibility of physical abuse.
☐ 2. Tell the client that it is difficult to believe that such injuries resulted from a fall.
☐ 3. Ask the client what they did to make someone beat them so badly.
☐ 4. Discuss with the client what they can do to deescalate the situation next time.

70. A client has blood loss following an automobile accident. The blood pressure on admission to the emergency department is 80/40 mm Hg. What is the **primary** goal for the care of the client at this time?
☐ 1. Achieve adequate tissue perfusion.
☐ 2. Preserve renal function.
☐ 3. Prevent hypostatic pneumonia.
☐ 4. Maintain adequate vascular tone.

71. A client with emphysema has been admitted to the hospital. The nurse should assess the client further for which symptom?
☐ 1. frequent coughing
☐ 2. bronchospasms
☐ 3. underweight appearance
☐ 4. copious sputum

72. A nurse has made a medication error. Which information is appropriate to include in the incident report?
☐ 1. an interpretation of the likely cause of the incident
☐ 2. what the nurse saw and did
☐ 3. the client's statement about the incident that occurred
☐ 4. the extenuating circumstances involved in the situation

73. The nurse is preparing a teaching plan for a client who is being discharged after being admitted for chest pain. The client had one previous myocardial infarction 2 years ago and has been taking simvastatin 40 mg for the last 2 years. After the nurse reviews the lab results for the client's cholesterol levels (see chart), what should the nurse do?

Laboratory Results		
Test	Result	Reference Range
Cholesterol total	195 mg/dL (5.05 mmol/L)	<200 mg/dL (<5.18 mmol/L)
Triglycerides	106 mg/dL (1.20 mmol/L)	<150 mg/dL (<1.69 mmol/L)
HDL-cholesterol	69 mg/dL (1.79 mmol/L))	>39 mg/dL (<1.03 mmol/L)

☐ 1. Ask if the client is taking the simvastatin regularly.
☐ 2. Tell the client that the cholesterol levels are within normal limits.
☐ 3. Instruct the client to lower the saturated fat in the diet.
☐ 4. Review the chart for lab reports of hemoglobin and hematocrit.

74. The nurse is reconciling medications with a client who is being discharged. Which information indicates there is a discrepancy?
☐ 1. There is agreement between the client's home medication list and current medication prescriptions.
☐ 2. There is justification for a difference in the medication prescriptions.
☐ 3. There is a lack of congruence between a client's home medication list and current medication prescriptions.
☐ 4. Sample medications have been included in the medication list.

75. An older adult's child is asking if their parent will need to have follow-up x-ray exams after a pneumonectomy for primary lung cancer. What should the nurse tell the adult child?
☐ 1. "The usual follow-up is chest x-ray and liver function tests every 3 months."
☐ 2. "The follow-up for your parent will be a chest x-ray and a computed tomography scan of the abdomen every year."
☐ 3. "No follow-up is needed at this time."
☐ 4. "The follow-up for your parent will be a chest x-ray every 6 months."

76. A 17-year-old client visits the clinic at 36 weeks' gestation. The client's blood pressure is 130/90 mm Hg. On previous visits, the blood pressure ranged from 100 to 110 mm Hg systolic and 70 to 80 mm Hg diastolic. Further assessment reveals slight edema of the hands and 1+ proteinuria. The nurse anticipates that the health care provider will **most** likely prescribe which treatment?
☐ 1. intravenous (IV) magnesium sulfate
☐ 2. oral labetalol
☐ 3. bed rest with bathroom privileges
☐ 4. hourly blood pressure checks

77. A female client who is 32 years of age has been diagnosed with stage 1 hypertension. The client's height is 5 feet 5 inches (165 cm), and her weight is recorded as 125 lb (56.6 kg). She reports that she frequently eats at "fast-food" restaurants and enjoys a glass of wine to relax on weekends. In developing a teaching plan for this client, the nurse should address which topic?
☐ 1. potential use of nitroprusside
☐ 2. adverse effects of alcohol
☐ 3. decreasing dietary caloric intake
☐ 4. low-sodium food choices

78. A client with a fractured leg has been instructed to ambulate without weight bearing on the affected leg. The nurse evaluates that the client is ambulating correctly if the client uses which crutch-walking gait?
☐ 1. two-point gait
☐ 2. four-point gait
☐ 3. three-point gait
☐ 4. swing-to gait

79. The nurse is assessing a young adult male client who has pain when urinating. The client states they think they have a sexually transmitted infection. When obtaining a health history, the nurse should ask the client if they are experiencing which symptom?
☐ 1. impotence
☐ 2. scrotal pain
☐ 3. penile lesion
☐ 4. urethral discharge

80. A client's blood pressure is 160/90 mm Hg. The health care provider prescribed "clonidine 1 mg by mouth now." The nurse sent the prescription to the pharmacy at 0710, but the medication still has not arrived at 0800. What should the nurse do **next**? Select all that apply.
☐ 1. Check all appropriate places on the unit to which the drug could have been delivered.
☐ 2. Check the client's blood pressure.
☐ 3. Call the pharmacy.
☐ 4. Go to the pharmacy to obtain the drug.
☐ 5. Use a pill from another client who is taking the same medication.

81. A 4-year-old who weighs 40 lb (18 kg) is brought to the emergency department with the sudden onset of a temperature of 103°F (39.4°C), a sore throat, and refusal to drink. The child will not lie down and prefers to lean forward while sitting up. What should the nurse do **next**?
☐ 1. Give 600 mg of acetaminophen rectally, as prescribed.
☐ 2. Inspect the child's throat for redness and swelling.
☐ 3. Have equipment to secure the airway available.
☐ 4. Obtain a specimen for a throat culture.

82. The nurse is assessing a group of clients with pain. Which client would benefit from the application of warm moist heat? A client with:
☐ 1. appendicitis
☐ 2. a recently sprained joint
☐ 3. a suspected malignancy
☐ 4. low back pain

83. A client is newly diagnosed with pernicious anemia. The nurse is teaching the client to increase vitamin B_{12} intake. Which is the **most** effective way for this client to increase vitamin B_{12} intake?
☐ 1. increasing dietary intake of vitamin B_{12}
☐ 2. taking an oral vitamin B_{12} replacement
☐ 3. taking vitamin B_{12} injections or nasal spray replacement
☐ 4. using chelation therapy

84. The nurse has received a prescription to add 20 mEq of potassium chloride to a 1000-mL bottle of IV fluid. The nurse has a 30-mL, multiple-dose vial of potassium chloride. The label reads 2 mEq/mL. How many milliliters should the nurse add to the IV fluid? Record your answer using a whole number.

_____ mL.

85. A client with major depression and suicidal ideation is suddenly calmer and more energetic. Which conclusion should the nurse reach?
☐ 1. The client is improving.
☐ 2. The client's medication dosage is too high.
☐ 3. The client is overstimulated.
☐ 4. The client is suicidal.

86. A multigravid client at 38 weeks' gestation is scheduled to undergo a contraction stress test. What should the nurse include in the explanation as the purpose of this test?
☐ 1. evaluation of fetal lung maturity
☐ 2. determination of the fetal biophysical profile
☐ 3. assessment of fetal ability to tolerate labor
☐ 4. determination of fetal response during movements

87. The nurse is teaching a client with emphysema how to do pursed-lip breathing. What is the expected outcome of using pursed-lip breathing?
☐ 1. increased oxygenation
☐ 2. prolonged exhalation
☐ 3. increase exercise tolerance
☐ 4. relief from shortness of breath

88. A nursing unit is using an automated medication dispensing system to track dispensing narcotics. What is the advantage of using an automated medication dispensing system?
☐ 1. It facilitates the change-of-shift count of narcotics.
☐ 2. It keeps a record of narcotic usage.
☐ 3. It allows nurses unmonitored access to narcotics.
☐ 4. It cancels the charges for narcotics.

89. The nurse cares for a 21-year-old pregnant client with vaginal bleeding in the emergency department.

Nurse's Notes

1100:
A 21-year-old client presented to the emergency department with pain in the right lower abdomen accompanied by small amounts of vaginal bleeding. The pain is constant and radiates to the shoulder. The client rates pain as a 7 on a scale of 0 to 10. The client had a positive pregnancy test and thinks they are 12-weeks pregnant. They have not yet started prenatal care. The client reports feeling dizzy and nauseated. Vital signs are temperature 97.2°F (36.2°C); pulse 110 bpm; respiration rate 30 breaths/min; and blood pressure 85/50 mm Hg. Pulse oximetry shows an oxygen saturation of 95% on room air.

The nurse is reviewing the client's assessment data to prepare the client's plan of care.

➤ Complete the diagram by circling the choices to specify the condition the client is most likely experiencing, two actions to take to address that condition, and two parameters the nurse should monitor to assess the client's progress.

Action to Take → Condition Most Likely Experiencing ← Parameter to Monitor
Action to Take → ← Parameters to Monitor

Actions to Take	Potential Conditions	Parameters to Monitor
Begin intravenous fluids	Abruptio placentae	Abdominal edema
Administer antibiotics	Inevitable abortion	Fetal heart rate
Request a stat ultrasound	Ectopic pregnancy	Mental status
Prepare for dilation and curettage (D&C)	Molar pregnancy	Increasing pain
Administer misoprostol		Urine output

90. Immediately following an automobile accident, a 21-year-old client has severe pain in the right chest from hitting the steering wheel, a compound fracture of the right tibia and fibula, and multiple lacerations and contusions. What is the **priority** nursing goal for this client?
☐ 1. Reduce the client's anxiety.
☐ 2. Maintain adequate oxygenation.
☐ 3. Decrease chest pain.
☐ 4. Maintain adequate circulating volume.

91. While assessing a primiparous client 8 hours after birth, the nurse inspects the episiotomy site, finding it edematous and slightly reddened. Which interpretation by the nurse is **most** appropriate?
☐ 1. The client needs application of an ice pack.
☐ 2. The episiotomy site is infected.
☐ 3. A hematoma will likely develop.
☐ 4. The client has had a repair of a vaginal laceration.

92. The nurse prepares a toddler for removal of a foreign body in the nasal passage by the health care provider. Which method of restraint should the nurse use?
☐ 1. jacket restraint
☐ 2. elbow restraint
☐ 3. parental holding restraint
☐ 4. mummy restraint

93. The nurse auscultates the lungs of a client who has been diagnosed with a tumor in the lung and notes wheezing over one lung. What additional assessment should the nurse make?
☐ 1. the presence of exudate in the airways
☐ 2. the client's history of smoking
☐ 3. an indication of pleural effusion
☐ 4. obstruction of the airway

94. A client is to have an insertion of a peripheral venous access device (VAD). After explaining the procedure to the client, the nurse will perform the steps from first to last in which order?
☐ 1. Apply the tourniquet, and select a vein for inserting the VAD.
☐ 2. Apply clean gloves, and cleanse the insertion site with an antiseptic swab.
☐ 3. Insert the VAD with the bevel up at a 10- to 30-degree angle.
☐ 4. Observe for blood return in the flashback chamber.

95. A nurse receives a report of a subtherapeutic lithium level on a client who has previously had normal drug levels. What hypothesis does the nurse make about the lithium level?
☐ 1. Lithium levels are often low in clients with recent gastrointestinal illnesses.
☐ 2. Doses may need to be increased as clients develop tolerance to lithium.
☐ 3. Nonadherence to lithium therapy is a major problem when treating bipolar disorder.
☐ 4. The client's disease has significantly worsened, requiring higher lithium doses.

96. A child with 20% second- and third-degree burns is admitted to the burn center. The child weighs 44 lb (20 kg). The nurse has started an intravenous (IV) infusion of lactated Ringer's solution and inserted an indwelling catheter. Which finding(s) indicate that the child is going into shock? Select all that apply.
☐ 1. Urinary output is 25 mL per hour.
☐ 2. Specific gravity is within normal limits.
☐ 3. Pain is 7 on a pain scale of 1 to 10.
☐ 4. Heart rate is elevated.
☐ 5. Blood pressure is dropping.

97. A client has been receiving radiation therapy for 3 weeks to treat cancer and has fatigue. The nurse should consider which factor when planning to help the client cope with the fatigue?
☐ 1. Fatigue is a temporary problem that requires no active intervention.
☐ 2. The cause of the fatigue should be determined.
☐ 3. Fatigue indicates that the client's cancer is not under control.
☐ 4. A balance of activity and rest will help manage the fatigue.

98. The nurse is teaching the client how to use crutches. The nurse should instruct the client to bear weight primarily on which part of the body?
☐ 1. axillae
☐ 2. elbows
☐ 3. upper arms
☐ 4. hands

99. The nurse admits a toddler with croup to the unit. What should the nurse do **first**?
☐ 1. Monitor vital signs.
☐ 2. Assess respiratory status.
☐ 3. Ensure adequate fluid intake.
☐ 4. Place a tracheostomy set at the bedside.

100. The nurse is caring for a 72-year-old male client who had a stent inserted via the right femoral artery to repair an abdominal aneurysm 6 hours ago.

Nurse's Notes

1000:
Vital signs are temperature (T) 99°F (37.2°C); heart rate (HR) 88 bpm; respiration rate (RR) 28 breaths/min; and blood pressure (BP) 150/82 mm Hg. The client has normal sinus rhythm and a urine output of 50 mL per hour. The client rates the pain as a 2 on a 10-point scale after receiving 3 mg morphine at 0930. An intravenous (IV) line is infusing 5% dextrose in water (D5W) at 125 mL per hour. Pedal pulses are present on palpation, and the dressing in the right groin is dry.

1100:
Vital signs are T 99°F (37.2°C); HR 90 bpm; RR 28 breaths/min; and BP 150/82 mm Hg. The client has normal sinus rhythm and a urine output of 55 mL per hour. The IV is infusing at 125 mL per hour. The right dorsalis pedis and posterior tibial pulses are strong on palpation, and the dressing at the incision site in the right groin is dry.

1130:
Unable to palpate the right dorsalis pedis or posterior tibial pulses.

➤ Complete the diagram by circling the choices below to specify what condition the client is **most** likely experiencing at 1100, two actions the nurse should take to address that condition, and two parameters the nurse should monitor to assess the client's progress.

Action to Take — Condition Most Likely Experiencing — Parameters to Monitor

Action to Take — Parameters to Monitor

Action to Take	Potential Conditions	Parameters to Monitor
Check urine output	Dehydration	IV infusion rate
Use Doppler to auscultate the presence of pedal pulses	Bleeding from incision	Urine output
Increase the drip rate of the IV infusion to 150 mL per hour	Diminished blood flow to renal artery	Bleeding at the incision site
Assess the incision site for bleeding	Obstruction of stent	Assess pedal pulses using Doppler
Notify the surgeon		Vital signs

101. The nurse is administering an intravenous (IV) replacement of 5% dextrose in water with potassium chloride. What should the nurse do **first**?
☐ 1. Add potassium chloride to the bag at the bedside.
☐ 2. Evaluate laboratory results for electrolytes.
☐ 3. Prime tubing using sterile technique.
☐ 4. Check the rate for IV push administration.

102. A 45-year-old client diagnosed with colon cancer states, "I don't want any treatment. I haven't seen any family members in 25 years. I'm a loner. Besides, I'll decide when and how I want to die." In which order of priority from first to last should the nurse perform the actions? All options must be used.

| 1. Ask the client what methods for suicide are available. |
| 2. Tell the client that the primary care provider will ask for a psychiatric consult. |
| 3. Ask the client about thoughts of suicide. |
| 4. Express concern for the client's feelings and safety. |

| |
| |
| |
| |

103. The nurse is auscultating the lung sounds of a client with long-standing emphysema. Which lung sounds are expected for this client?
☐ 1. fine crackles
☐ 2. diminished breath sounds
☐ 3. stridor
☐ 4. pleural friction rub

104. The nurse is planning a presentation on the topic of osteoporosis to a group of middle-age women. Which information should the nurse include in the presentation?
☐ 1. An early symptom of osteoporosis is the dowager's hump.
☐ 2. Women of African and Latinx origin are at greater risk.
☐ 3. Loss of height is an early symptom of the disease.
☐ 4. Conventional radiographs are usually used to confirm the disease.

105. The nurse is to administer an enteral feeding to an adult client. Before initiating the feeding, the nurse evaluates the gastric residual. What should the nurse determine from evaluating the gastric residual?
☐ 1. how well nutrients are being absorbed
☐ 2. if the client is receiving enough feeding
☐ 3. the extent of overdistention of the stomach
☐ 4. the presence of undigested formula

106. The nurse is teaching an older adult about taking medication for a urinary tract infection. Which nonverbal or verbal response(s) by the client indicate a need for further clarification and education? Select all that apply. The client:
☐ 1. says they will stop taking prescribed medications when the symptoms are relieved.
☐ 2. takes a long time to respond to the nurses' questions.
☐ 3. nods the head in agreement with what the nurse is saying.
☐ 4. wants to use traditional practices to relieve symptoms.
☐ 5. tells the nurse they prefer taking nonprescribed medications purchased from a neighborhood grocery store.

107. When planning the care for a client diagnosed with hepatitis A, the nurse should include which intervention(s)? Select all that apply.
☐ 1. Implement an exercise program.
☐ 2. Provide relief from nausea and vomiting.
☐ 3. Administer pain medication.
☐ 4. Encourage multiple small meals daily.
☐ 5. Plan frequent rest periods.

108. The nurse is assessing a client who has had a myocardial infarction. The nurse notes the cardiac rhythm shown. The nurse identifies that this rhythm is:

☐ 1. atrial fibrillation.
☐ 2. ventricular tachycardia.
☐ 3. premature ventricular contractions.
☐ 4. third-degree heart block.

109. The health care provider has ordered soft wrist restraints to prevent a client from pulling out a nasogastric tube. What action(s) should be included in the care plan when the client is restrained? Select all that apply.
☐ 1. Instruct the client not to move while the restraints are in place.
☐ 2. Observe the client in person or by video through a window or door for the first 15 minutes of restraint.
☐ 3. Secure the restraints to the side rails of the bed.
☐ 4. Check on the client every 30 minutes while the restraints are on.
☐ 5. Check on the client every 15 to 30 minutes per agency policy while the restraints are in place.

110. A client has been diagnosed with atrial fibrillation. The health care provider prescribed warfarin to be taken on a daily basis. The nurse instructs the client to avoid using which over-the-counter medication while taking warfarin?
☐ 1. aspirin
☐ 2. diphenhydramine
☐ 3. digoxin
☐ 4. pseudoephedrine

111. The nurse is teaching a client about taking carbamazepine. The nurse informs the client that this medication can affect other medications in which way?
☐ 1. It decreases the effects of oral anticoagulants.
☐ 2. It decreases the serum concentration of verapamil.
☐ 3. It increases the serum concentration of other anticonvulsants.
☐ 4. It increases the effects of oral contraceptives.

112. A client has been diagnosed with hepatitis A. Which nursing goal is **most** appropriate for the client?
☐ 1. Achieve control of abdominal pains.
☐ 2. Increase activity levels gradually.
☐ 3. Be able to breathe without difficulty.
☐ 4. Experience relief from edema.

113. The nurse teaches a parent how to care for their child during the first few days after surgery to repair a cleft lip. Which parental activity offers the **most** support to the child?
☐ 1. holding and cuddling the child
☐ 2. helping the child play with some toys
☐ 3. reading some of the child's favorite stories
☐ 4. staying at the bedside and holding the child's hand

114. The nurse works to reduce the number of children involved in automobile crashes who were not wearing seat belts. Which strategy is the **most** effective?
☐ 1. Contact the local government representative to discuss new legislation about child seat belts.
☐ 2. Attend a school board meeting to advocate for classes teaching children seat belt safety.
☐ 3. Call the town mayor's office with this information so that the mayor can discuss it with the media.
☐ 4. Start a letter-writing campaign to the school superintendent about seat belt importance.

115. The nurse is preparing to administer intramuscular (IM) morphine sulfate to a client who is in pain. On checking the health care provider's (HCP's) prescription, the nurse notes that the prescription states "morphine sulfate 60 mg IM every 4 hours as needed for pain." The usual dose of morphine is 10 to 15 mg. What is the **most** appropriate action for the nurse to take?
☐ 1. Administer the medication as prescribed.
☐ 2. Administer 15 mg of the drug.
☐ 3. Contact the HCP to verify the prescription.
☐ 4. Ask another nurse to review the prescription.

116. Following surgery for removal of a brain tumor, a client is coughing and short of breath and has a "bad" feeling. The nurse obtains the following vital signs: blood pressure of 80/60 mm Hg, pulse rate of 120 bpm, and respiratory rate of 30 shallow breaths/min. What should the nurse do **first**?
☐ 1. Call the neurosurgeon.
☐ 2. Place the client in the Trendelenburg position.
☐ 3. Consult the neurologic clinical nurse specialist (CNS).
☐ 4. Activate the rapid response team (RRT).

117. The nurse is giving discharge instructions to a client who has had a laparoscopic cholecystectomy. Which statement indicates that the client has understood the instructions?
☐ 1. "I need to maintain a low-fat diet for the next 6 months."
☐ 2. "I can remove the dressing from my incision tomorrow and take a shower."
☐ 3. "I can anticipate some nausea for several days after surgery."
☐ 4. "I can return to work in 4 to 6 weeks."

118. The nurse is planning staffing assignments for a group of clients. Which client is **most** appropriate for the nurse to assign to a nurse who normally works on the maternity unit?
☐ 1. a client in a halo traction brace following surgery for a cervical spine injury
☐ 2. a client who had an open appendectomy yesterday
☐ 3. a client with cancer who requires ventilator support
☐ 4. a client with amyotrophic lateral sclerosis showing signs of progression

119. The nurse in the clinic reviews the record of an 8-year-old male client with attention deficit hyperactivity disorder (ADHD).

Flow Sheet			
Weights	October 10 56.9 lb (25.8 kg)	November 10 55.1 lb (25 kg)	December 10 51.8 lb (23.5 kg)
Nurse's Notes	10/10. Methylphenidate extended release is prescribed for ADHD. 11/10. Parents state school performance has improved, but it is difficult to get the client up and ready for school in the morning unless the client is given the medication as soon as they wake up. 12/12. The client continues to do well at school, but the parents report the child does not eat breakfast or very much of their lunch at school. The client eats dinner, but only an average amount of food.		

➤ What intervention(s) should the nurse recommend initially to manage the client's weight loss? Select all that apply.

☐ 1. Eat a breakfast bar with a glass of milk with medication every morning.
☐ 2. Weigh the child daily each morning before breakfast.
☐ 3. Encourage three small meals with three snacks per day.
☐ 4. Request a prescription change to a nonstimulant drug to treat the ADHD.
☐ 5. Suggest supplementing the child's dinner with a high-protein drink.

120. A client who had transurethral resection of the prostate has dribbling urine after the Foley catheter is removed on the second postoperative day. The nurse notes that the client had 200 mL of urine output in the last 8 hours with a 1000-mL intake. What should the nurse do **first**?
☐ 1. Apply a condom catheter.
☐ 2. Assess for bladder distention.
☐ 3. Obtain a urine specimen for culture.
☐ 4. Teach the client Kegel exercises.

121. A child diagnosed with tinea is being treated with griseofulvin. What instructions should the nurse give the parents?
☐ 1. Give the medication before a meal.
☐ 2. Have the child avoid intense sunlight.
☐ 3. Give the medication for 10 days.
☐ 4. Encourage increased fluid intake.

122. A client undergoes cystoscopy with bladder biopsy. After the procedure, which action should the nurse take **first**?
☐ 1. Assess the patency of the Foley catheter.
☐ 2. Assess urine for excessive bleeding.
☐ 3. Percuss the bladder for distention.
☐ 4. Obtain a urine specimen for culture.

123. The nurse is assessing an infant who is 6 months of age and has a black eye; the infant is brought by the parent to the quick-care clinic. The parent reports that the daycare provider told them that the child "fell down the steps with a walker." What should the nurse do in order of priority from first to last? All options must be used.

1. Report the incident to the social services department.

2. Document findings accurately.

3. Ask the parent for details about the incident and the daycare center.

4. Place an ice bag on the infant's eye.

124. The nurse is talking with a client who was diagnosed with bulimia 3 months ago. The client needs more education about the illness if the client makes which comment(s)? Select all that apply.
☐ 1. "I know that this illness is chronic and intermittent. I'll always have to control it."
☐ 2. "If I start severely restricting my eating, I may be building up to a bingeing episode."
☐ 3. "When I'm not bingeing and purging, I can skip that eating disorder support group."
☐ 4. "I've made a real effort to be more social and involved in activities."
☐ 5. "My depression is gone, so I don't need my antidepressant any longer."

125. The nurse suspects that a newborn has an imperforate anus. Which assessment finding(s) support the nurse's hypothesis? Select all that apply.
☐ 1. failure to pass a first stool within 48 hours after birth
☐ 2. curdled vomitus
☐ 3. missing or moved opening to the anus
☐ 4. stool passes out of the vagina, base of penis, scrotum, or urethra
☐ 5. distended abdomen

126. When an infant resumes taking oral feedings after surgery to correct intussusception, the parents comment that the child seems to suck on the pacifier more since the surgery. The nurse explains that sucking on a pacifier:
☐ 1. provides an outlet for emotional tension.
☐ 2. indicates readiness to take solid foods.
☐ 3. indicates intestinal motility.
☐ 4. is an attempt to get attention from the parents.

127. Parents of a neonate who is 32 weeks of age ask the nurse, "Why does he have a feeding tube in his nose?" What is the nurse's **best** response?
☐ 1. The sucking, swallowing, and breathing are not coordinated.
☐ 2. There is no sucking reflex at this gestational age.
☐ 3. The stomach cannot digest formula or breast milk at this time.
☐ 4. The infant needs extra fluids to prevent dehydration.

128. The nurse is teaching a client how to prevent shoulder ankyloses following chest surgery. What should the nurse teach the client to do?
☐ 1. Turn from side to side.
☐ 2. Raise and lower the head.
☐ 3. Raise the arm on the affected side over the head.
☐ 4. Flex and extend the elbow on the affected side.

129. A client with a tracheostomy tube coughs and dislodges the tracheostomy tube. What should the nurse do **first**?
☐ 1. Call for emergency assistance.
☐ 2. Attempt reinsertion of tracheostomy tube.
☐ 3. Position the client in the semi-Fowler position with the neck hyperextended.
☐ 4. Insert the obturator into the stoma to reestablish the airway.

130. The experienced licensed practical/vocational nurse (LPN/VN) under the supervision of the registered nurse (RN) team leader is providing nursing care for an infant with respiratory syncytial virus. Which task(s) are appropriate for the RN to delegate to the LPN/VN? Select all that apply.
☐ 1. Auscultate breath sounds.
☐ 2. Administer prescribed aerosolized medications.
☐ 3. Initiate the nursing care plan.
☐ 4. Check oxygen saturation using pulse oximetry.
☐ 5. Complete an in-depth admission assessment.
☐ 6. Evaluate the parent's ability to administer aerosolized medications.

131. The nurse is assessing a client who reports having a back injury. What should the nurse ask the client about **first**?
☐ 1. family history of back problems
☐ 2. previous hospitalizations
☐ 3. personal history of illness
☐ 4. mechanism of injury

132. A client is taking metoprolol and hydrochlorothiazide. Which finding indicates the medications are having the desired effect? The client:
☐ 1. has lower blood pressure.
☐ 2. has an increased heart rate.
☐ 3. has improved circulation in the extremities.
☐ 4. has decreased dyspnea.

133. The nurse is examining an older adult client with possible rheumatoid arthritis. The nurse should ask the client if they having which symptom?
☐ 1. nausea
☐ 2. dizziness
☐ 3. fatigue
☐ 4. limitation of movement

134. The nurse conducts a telehealth visit with a breastfeeding 30-year-old female client.

> **Nurse's Notes**
>
> The client is a 30-year-old gravida 2 para 2 who had a cesarean birth 10 days ago because of breech presentation. The client reports the lochia alba is scant and the abdominal incision is healing. The newborn has been breastfeeding every 2.5 hours with each session lasting 20 to 40 minutes. This morning, the client developed a warm, red, painful right breast. The client has a temperature of 101°F (38.3°C) and flulike symptoms of head and body aches. The client states, "I have a burning sensation when I try to nurse with my right breast."

▶ The nurse is reviewing the Nurse's Notes to prepare the client's plan of care. Complete the diagram by circling the choices below to specify what condition the client is **most** likely experiencing, two actions the nurse should take to address that condition, and two parameters the nurse should monitor to assess the client's progress.

Action to Take → Condition Most Likely Experiencing ← Parameter to Monitor
Action to Take ↗   ↘ Parameter to Monitor

Action to Take	Potential Conditions	Parameters to Monitor
Apply antifungals	Engorgement	Infant weights
Administer antibiotics	Mastitis	Abscess development
Use nipple shields	Blocked milk duct	Bleeding nipples
Apply ice packs	Thrush	Infant's oral cavity
Encourage frequent emptying		Infant latch

135. The nurse instructs the client in mixing and administering regular and NPH insulin. Which statement indicates that the client needs additional instruction?
☐ 1. "I draw up the regular insulin first."
☐ 2. "I shake the bottle of NPH insulin before drawing it up."
☐ 3. "I store the insulin in a cool place."
☐ 4. "I insert the needle at a 90-degree angle."

136. A client is trying to lose weight at a moderate pace. If the client eliminates 1000 calories a day from the usual food intake, how many pounds/kilograms would the client lose in 1 week?
_____ lb/kg.

137. A client is prescribed buspirone 5 mg two times a day. Which statement(s) indicate that the client has understood the nurse's teaching about this drug? Select all that apply.
☐ 1. "This medicine will make me sleepy."
☐ 2. "Buspirone will relax my muscles."
☐ 3. "My anxiety will be gone in about 2 weeks."
☐ 4. "Buspirone will help me not to worry so much."
☐ 5. "I'll be able to focus better."

138. The nurse has delegated providing postmortem care of an adult to an unlicensed assistive personnel (UAP). The family does not wish to have an autopsy but is considering organ donation. After obtaining additional information from the family, the nurse should give the UAP which instruction(s)? Select all that apply.
☐ 1. Let the family stay as long as they like.
☐ 2. The family does not have any special requests about preparing the body.
☐ 3. Elevate the head of the bed.
☐ 4. Check two identifiers before starting postmortem care.
☐ 5. The family wishes to have the client's beard shaved.
☐ 6. Remove all indwelling lines and catheters.

139. A client with schizophrenia is responding well to risperidone and is no longer psychotic. After the nurse teaches the client about managing the illness, which statement by the client reflects a need for further intervention?
☐ 1. "I just don't know if I can remember to keep taking medicines every day."
☐ 2. "When my thoughts start racing, I know I need to relax more."
☐ 3. "I can name the side effects of risperidone, but I'm not having any."
☐ 4. "I don't listen to my parent's religious beliefs about not using medicines."

140. A client had a cast applied to the left femur to stabilize a fracture. To promote early rehabilitation, what should the nurse do?
☐ 1. Call the physical therapy team to provide passive exercise of the affected limb.
☐ 2. Teach the client how to do isometric exercises of the quadriceps.
☐ 3. Show the family how to do active range-of-motion exercises of the unaffected limb.
☐ 4. Obtain weights so the client can exercise the upper extremities.

141. The nurse has just received a change-of-shift report for four clients. Based on this report, the nurse should assess which client **first**?
☐ 1. a 38-year-old who underwent a mastectomy 2 days ago because of breast cancer and is having difficulty coping with the diagnosis
☐ 2. a 52-year-old with pneumonia and chronic back pain who is requesting pain medication
☐ 3. a 35-year-old admitted after a motor vehicle collision whose urine output has totaled 30 mL over the last 2 hours
☐ 4. an 84-year-old with resolving left-sided weakness who is slightly confused and has been awake most of the night

142. The nurse cares for a 14-year-old male client hospitalized with cystic fibrosis.

Nurse's Notes

An adolescent with a history of cystic fibrosis was admitted to the pediatric unit for increasing respiratory distress and possible pneumonia. The client states feeling fatigued, getting short of breath walking, and having chest pain on the right side that is rated at a 3 on a scale of 0 to 10. Rhonchi are heard on auscultation, with diminished breath sounds in the lower lobes. A weak nonproductive cough is noted. Chest x-ray results and sputum cultures are pending.

Vital signs are temperature 100.7°F (38.2°C); pulse 100 bpm; respiration rate 40 breaths/min; and blood pressure 132/88 mm Hg. Pulse oximetry shows an oxygen saturation of 95% on room air.

▸ Complete the diagram by circling the choices below to specify the condition the client is **most** likely experiencing, two actions to take to address that condition, and two parameters the nurse should monitor to assess the client's progress.

Action to Take — Condition Most Likely Experiencing — Parameters to Monitor
Action to Take — Parameters to Monitor

Action to Take	Potential Conditions	Parameters to Monitor
Administer nebulizer treatment	Airway obstruction	Blood gases
Assist with intubation	Pneumothorax	Chest x-rays
Assist with chest tube insertion	Pulmonary edema	Breath sounds
Perform chest physiotherapy	Reactive airway	Cough
Administer a diuretic		Pulse oximetry

143. A client who has obesity and diabetes and who has bilateral leg aching is to start cardiac rehabilitation with an exercise program. Using which exercise equipment will be **most** helpful to the client?
☐ 1. stationary bicycle
☐ 2. treadmill
☐ 3. elliptical trainer
☐ 4. stair climber

144. The nurse has received a change-of-shift report. The nurse should assess which client **first**?
☐ 1. a 72-year-old admitted 2 days ago with a blood alcohol level of 0.08
☐ 2. a 36-year-old with a chest tube due to spontaneous pneumothorax with a current respiratory rate of 18 breaths/min and oxygen saturation of 95% on oxygen at 2 L per nasal cannula
☐ 3. a 28-year-old who is 2 days post appendectomy with discharge prescriptions written and whose spouse is waiting to take them home
☐ 4. a 62-year-old admitted with a recent gastrointestinal (GI) bleeding whose hemoglobin is 13.8 g/dL (138 g/L)

145. A small-for-gestational-age infant is born with facial abnormalities and vision abnormalities. These abnormalities are likely caused by which maternal factor?
☐ 1. alcohol consumption
☐ 2. rubella exposure
☐ 3. tetracycline use
☐ 4. folic acid deficiency

146. An adolescent with cystic fibrosis has been placed on ciprofloxacin for a lung infection. Which statement from the client indicates the need for more teaching?
☐ 1. "I won't take this drug with any dairy products."
☐ 2. "I'll need to have drug levels drawn while I'm on this medication."
☐ 3. "I should immediately report any muscle or joint pain."
☐ 4. "If I miss a dose, I should take it as soon as I remember."

147. A client whose condition remains stable after a myocardial infarction is to gradually increase activity. Which sign **best** indicates that the activity is appropriate for the client?
☐ 1. edema
☐ 2. skin color
☐ 3. respiratory rate
☐ 4. weight

148. The parents of a 7-year-old child with glomerulonephritis ask what they can do to ensure that their other children do not develop the disease. The nurse should respond with which statement?
☐ 1. "If you suspect your child has a urinary tract infection (UTI), see your primary health care provider (HCP) right away."
☐ 2. "I'm afraid there's nothing you can do; glomerulonephritis is a genetic disorder."
☐ 3. "Glomerulonephritis isn't contagious, so your other children won't get the disease."
☐ 4. "If any of them develop a streptococcal infection, complete the course of prescribed antibiotics."

149. A client admitted for alcohol detoxification is taking disulfiram. The nurse should instruct the client to avoid ingestion of which food(s) or liquid(s)? Select all that apply.
☐ 1. aged cheeses
☐ 2. beer
☐ 3. communal wine at church
☐ 4. chocolates
☐ 5. cough syrup

150. A client has been admitted to the emergency department (ED) with bleeding from a gunshot wound to the abdomen. During transport, medics applied a pressure dressing to the wound, started an intravenous infusion of normal saline at a keep-open rate, applied nasal oxygen at 2 L per minute, and inserted a Foley catheter.

Vital Signs			
	0900	0930	1000
Heart rate	86 bpm	88 bpm	90 bpm
Blood pressure systolic	98 mm Hg	90 mm Hg	136 mm Hg
Blood pressure diastolic	65 mm Hg	60 mm Hg	60 mm Hg
Respiratory rate	26 breaths/min	28 breaths/min	18 breaths/min
Oxygen saturation	96%	93%	93%
Temperature	101.8°F (38.7°C)		101.8°F (38.7°C)
Urinary output	40		30

➤ The nurse reviews the record of vital signs. What should the nurse anticipate the primary care provider will order **next**? Select all that apply.

☐ 1. Administer epinephrine.
☐ 2. Inspect the abdominal dressing for bleeding.
☐ 3. Perform neurologic checks.
☐ 4. Increase the rate of infusion of fluids.
☐ 5. Add an infusion of lactated Ringer's solution.
☐ 6. Administer packed red blood cells.

Answers, Rationales, and Test-Taking Strategies

*The answers and rationales for each question follow below, along with keys (🗝) to the client need (CN) and cognitive level (CL) for each question. In addition, questions that measure clinical judgment will be coded (CJ). As you check your answers, use the **Content Mastery and Test-Taking Skill Self-Analysis** worksheet (tear-out worksheet in the back of the book) to identify the reason(s) for not answering the questions correctly. For additional information about test-taking skills and strategies for answering questions, refer to pages 12–51 in Part 1 of this book.*

1. **1.** The infant is exhibiting periodic breathing, which is normal in infants of this age. The infant typically alternates short periods of rapid, louder respirations with periods of slower, quieter respirations. Since the finding is normal there is no need for a monitor, close parental monitoring, or a chest x-ray.

   🗝 CN: Health promotion and maintenance; CL: Analyze

2. **3.** The surgeon is required to give the client explanations and have questions answered. The nurse has no way of assessing the client's understanding without the interpreter. The client should sign the Spanish consent form only after receiving an explanation of the procedure, its risks, and alternatives. A family member cannot be relied on to translate the surgeon's instructions. The nurse is commonly asked to witness the explanation and obtain the client's signature on the informed consent form. Informed consent is the provision of information concerning the procedure and its risks, not obtaining the client's signature on the form. The surgical charge nurse does not need to be notified.

   🗝 CN: Management of care; CL: Analyze

3. **1.** This client has a barrel chest. The anterior-posterior diameter of the chest is larger than the transverse diameter, as is characteristic of the client with chronic obstructive pulmonary disease. Although the client may be muscular from lifting weights, the barrel chest is not associated with the client's age, height, or weight. The use of bronchodilators will not change the shape of the client's chest.

   🗝 CN: Physiological adaptation; CL: Analyze

4. **2.** Cystic fibrosis is the most common inherited disease in children. It is inherited as an autosomal recessive trait, meaning that the child inherits the defective gene from both parents. The chances are one in four for each of this couple's pregnancies.

   🗝 CN: Reduction of risk potential; CL: Apply

5. **−/+ 1, 2, 3.** For the client with grandiose delusions, the nurse should accept the client but not argue with the delusion to build trust and the client's self-esteem. Focusing on the underlying feeling or meaning of the delusion helps meet the client's needs. Focusing on events and topics based in reality distracts the client from delusional thinking. Confronting the client's delusions or beliefs can lead to agitation in the client and the need to cling to the grandiose delusion to preserve self-esteem. Interacting with the client only when based in reality ignores the client's needs and therapeutic nursing intervention.

   🗝 CN: Psychosocial integrity; CL: Analyze

6. **3.** The nurse must act as an advocate for the client when the client cannot afford treatment. It may be possible to substitute a less expensive antibiotic. The correct procedure includes contacting the HCP to explain the parent's economic situation and request a substitution. For example, amoxicillin is more economical than azithromycin. If it is not possible to use another antibiotic, the nurse can explore other avenues with the parent, social worker, or both.

   🗝 CN: Management of care; CL: Analyze

7. **1.** Saying "When you interrupt others, they leave the area" is most helpful because it serves to increase the client's awareness of others' perceptions of the behavior by giving specific feedback about the behavior. The other statements are punitive and authoritative, possibly threatening to the client, and likely to increase defensiveness, decrease self-worth, and increase feelings of guilt.

   🗝 CN: Psychosocial integrity; CL: Analyze

8. **−/+ 1, 2, 3, 6.** The important information to be given to a client with preeclampsia includes blood pressure trends while being monitored and the protein that is and has been present in the urine because these are indicators of increasing eclampsia. Edema of the face, a history of headache, blurred vision, and epigastric pain are important as these also indicate worsening preeclampsia. The fetal position at 25 weeks is of minor importance as the fetus is constantly changing positions at this point in the pregnancy. The use of dietary sodium does not have an impact on preeclampsia. Glycosuria is an important consideration if this client has gestational diabetes but is not significant for the client with preeclampsia.

   🗝 CN: Safety and infection control; CL: Analyze

9. 3. Although breech presentations are rare, footling breech occurs when there is an extension of the fetal knees and one or both feet protrude through the pelvis. In frank breech, there is flexion of the fetal thighs and extension of the knees. The feet rest at the sides of the fetal head. In complete breech, there is flexion of the fetal thighs and knees; the fetus appears to be squatting. Vertex position occurs in 95% of births; in such cases, the head is engaged in the pelvis.

CN: Health promotion and maintenance; CL: Apply

10. 3. The timing of symptoms is important to the diagnosis of PMS. The client should keep a 3-month log of symptoms and menses. With PMS, the symptoms begin 3 to 7 days before menses and resolve 1 to 2 days after the menstrual cycle has started. Menstrual cycle irregularity and mood swings after menses are not related to PMS, and other causes should be investigated. Midcycle spotting and pain are related to ovulation.

CN: Health promotion and maintenance; CL: Analyze

11. 1, 4, 2, 3. The client is experiencing ketoacidosis. The nurse should first obtain the blood glucose level and then notify the HCP who will then prescribe the appropriate dose of insulin. Prior to administering the insulin, the nurse will start the IV infusion.

CN: Physiological adaptation; CL: Create

12. 3. Tasks that the UAP can undertake vary greatly. The nurse must be aware of the scope of the UAP's preparation and the policies of the health care agency. The important consideration is that the task is appropriate for that individual and is within the guidelines for practice at the health care agency. The UAP can perform complicated tasks within the scope of the preparation. Although the nurse observes the UAP and evaluates the UAP on their ability to perform the task, the most important aspect of delegation is to delegate within the UAP's educational preparation. A positive relationship with clients, while desirable, is not essential to delegation. Delegation involves giving clear directions and following up after the task has been delegated.

CN: Management of care; CL: Analyze

13. 1. Several irregularly shaped red patches, common skin variations in neonates, are termed *stork bites*. They eventually fade away as the neonate grows older. Port-wine stains are disfiguring darkish red or purplish skin discolorations on the scalp and face that may need laser therapy for removal. Newborn rash is typically generalized over the body, not localized to one body area, and is commonly raised. Café au lait spots are brown and typically found anywhere on the body. More than six spots or spots larger than 1.5 cm are associated with neurofibromatosis, a genetic condition of neural tissue.

CN: Health promotion and maintenance; CL: Analyze

14. 1. In the cognitively impaired client, benzodiazepines, such as lorazepam, can increase confusion and nighttime agitation. Extrapyramidal side effects are more common with antipsychotics. Vomiting and sweating are signs of benzodiazepine withdrawal. Anticholinergic side effects are more likely with antipsychotics and tricyclic antidepressants.

CN: Pharmacological and parenteral therapies; CL: Analyze

15. 1, 2, 4. Telehealth is becoming an increasingly available way for nurses to conduct counseling sessions with clients who are at a distance from a health care provider (HCP) or health care facility. The client saves travel time and can avoid precipitating symptoms associated with the stress disorder that might occur as a result of a visit to a health care facility. The client also can access care that might not otherwise be easily available. Treatment for PSTD is long term, and there is no evidence to suggest that telehealth versus face-to-face counseling shortens recovery time. Counseling sessions using telehealth technology are conducted on an individual basis between one client and an HCP, but group support may be available if required as a part of a treatment plan.

CN: Management of care; CL: Evaluate

16. 3. Although not directly assigned to the client's care, the nurse is participating on the team providing emergency resuscitative care when relaying information from the client's health record. To gain access to the client's health information, regardless of employment at the hospital where the client was receiving care, the nurse would need to sign the HIPPA releases, just as any parent would need to do. While the nurse may have provided care to a client in the past, the nurse does not have permission to access the client's records on the current admission if not assigned to provide care. Although the neighbor gave verbal permission to access the records, the permission is not in writing and therefore would be unauthorized access by the nurse.

CN: Management of care; CL: Analysis

17. **2.** Given the client's age, making final plans is age appropriate. The absence of any signs of ill health, depression, or suicidal ideation makes the other options inappropriate.

🔑 CN: Psychosocial integrity; CL: Analyze

18. **1.** ICP is highest in the early morning, and the client with hydrocephalus may be experiencing signs of increased ICP that need to be treated. The increased ICP is not related to fluid levels, and the nurse should not advise the client to increase fluid intake. While ICP does fluctuate during the day, it is highest in the morning, and the nurse should notify the HCP. Pain medication will not treat the potentially increasing ICP and may mask important signs of increasing ICP.

🔑 CN: Physiological adaptation; CL: Analyze

19. **1.** The nurse should instruct the client that symptoms from an occasional headache due to eye strain or continuous work at a computer can be relieved by acetaminophen. Although this drug causes prostaglandin inhibition, this effect is rapidly reversed and cleared with no apparent harmful effects in pregnancy. If the headaches become more frequent or severe, the client should be instructed to contact the health care provider (HCP) immediately. Aspirin should be avoided during pregnancy because it inhibits prostaglandin synthesis. It also decreases uterine contractility and may delay the onset of labor or prolong pregnancy and labor. Aspirin decreases platelet aggregation, possibly increasing the risk for bleeding. Ibuprofen and naproxen can lead to premature closure of the fetal ductus arteriosus and decreased amniotic fluid with prolonged use. They may also prolong pregnancy or labor because of their antiprostaglandin effects.

🔑 CN: Pharmacological and parenteral therapies; CL: Analyze

20. **1.** With this level of anger in a crisis, the parent needs simple but firm directions to leave the room, calm down, and then talk. Doing so relieves the adolescent of any pressure from the parent. Telling the parent to stop yelling or be quiet provides no concrete directions to the parent and may embarrass them in front of their child. Telling the parent that if they do not stop yelling, the nurse will call Security is a threat, possibly leading to an escalation of the situation.

🔑 CN: Psychosocial integrity; CL: Analyze

21. **2.** Female clients with HIV are at risk for acquiring the papillomavirus, which predisposes them to cancer. This client needs to have regular Papanicolaou (Pap) tests. Visiting this client could be delayed. Because of the safety risks and the need for pain management, the nurse visits the client with brain metastasis as soon as possible. A client with diabetes who may not inject insulin properly will be at great risk, and the nurse should plan to visit this client early as well. Because the client with a CD4 count of fewer than 200 cells/mm³ is at great risk for a fulminating infection, the nurse does not postpone the appointment.

🔑 CN: Management of care; CL: Analyze

22. **4.** School-age children video games and are commonly intense about following rules. Their play can become emotional. Adequate rest is of utmost importance during the acute stage of rheumatic fever. Therefore, playing a game with another child probably would be too strenuous. Such diversional activities as reading a book, playing with a doll, and watching television would be more satisfactory.

🔑 CN: Health promotion and maintenance; CL: Analyze

23. **4.** The priority for a client with a new tracheostomy is to maintain a patent airway. A new tracheostomy commonly causes bleeding and excess secretions, and the client may require frequent suctioning to maintain a patent airway. The nurse can keep the secretions moist as a part of the suctioning procedure. The nurse can help the client manage anxiety while maintaining the priority of a patent airway. While the nurse will begin teaching the client about self-care, this is not the priority at this time.

🔑 CN: Reduction of risk potential; CL: Analyze

24.

STEP 1

−/+ Admission Note

The client is a married adult. Today, the client got into a physical altercation with a customer at the auto dealership where they work. Police questioned the client's mental status and brought the client to the emergency department for evaluation. While at the emergency department, the client threatened to punch a hole in the wall after being told they could not take a walk. The client refused lunch, stating that they did not need to eat because they are "superior to all humans." The client requested to call their spouse and had a brief conversation. The client was angry after the phone call ended. The client refused vital signs and lab work. The client does not consent to have their spouse contacted for further information.

The nurse's immediate concerns are for the safety of the client and the health care workers caring for them. By threatening to punch a wall, the client demonstrates an immediate potential for violent behavior. Stating that they are superior to all humans is indicative of delusional thinking, and an inaccurate interpretation of an external reality places the client at risk for self-harm. The nurse should immediately follow up on these two findings and evaluate the client for suicidal or homicidal ideations. Follow-up with the client about the conversation with their spouse and follow up on what led to the altercation earlier in the day should happen later. After deescalating tensions, the nurse should encourage the client to cooperate with vital signs and allow their spouse to be contacted.

🗝️ CJ: Case study; Step 1: Recognize cues; CL: Analyze

25.

STEP 2

−/+ **1, 2, 3, 5, 6, 7, 8.** The nurse should assess the client for the severity and nature of the presenting mood disorder. Information about the length of time the symptoms have been present, the decreased need for sleep, and compliance with any prescribed medication regimen is important. The nurse should also assess if the client is having difficulty keeping track of thoughts, which may emerge from an interview. Assessing for increases in new activities will help determine if the client is experiencing increased goal directedness. The client has stated they believe they are superior. The nurse needs to determine what that means to the client to help determine safety needs. The client has already displayed reckless behavior by getting into an alteration. Knowing about other behaviors helps support the creation of a treatment plan. Determining the spouse's location is not a priority because consent has not been given to contact them.

🗝️ CJ: Case study; Step 2: Analyze cues; CL: Analyze

26.

STEP 3

0/1 The finding of **grandiosity** most suggests that the client is experiencing a(n) **manic** episode.

A statement of superiority to all indicates the client is experiencing grandiosity, which is part of the diagnostic criteria for manic episodes of bipolar depression. The client's reckless behavior is also suggestive of manic episodes. Although the client is displaying anger, that is not a defining behavior for depressive, dissociative, or manic episodes. The client is not displaying dissociative symptoms, which manifest as amnesia, alter personalities, or feelings that one is detached from one own's life. The client is also not displaying signs of sadness to suggest a depressive episode.

🗝️ CJ: Case study; Step 3: Prioritize hypothesis; CL: Analyze

27.

STEP 4

0/1

Possible Order	Anticipated	Not Anticipated
As needed (PRN) medication for agitation	X	
Close monitoring	X	
Calorie count		X
Family meeting		X
Routine vital signs	X	
Stat electrocardiogram		X
Routine labs	X	

The client has demonstrated a high risk for violence. PRN medication for agitation will decrease the chance of a violent outburst and possible injury. The client has a history of aggressive behavior and requires close monitoring for agitation and aggression. Routine vital signs and routine lab tests are typical at admission. There are no data to support requiring a calorie count at this time; however, the client's appetite should be monitored. The client does not consent to having their spouse contacted, and arranging a family meeting would violate the client's confidentiality. Baseline lab tests may be needed before beginning some medications. An ECG is a routine admitting order, but there are no data that support the client requiring a stat ECG, and pursuing this intervention may increase agitation.

🗝️ CJ: Case study; Step 4: Generate solutions; CL: Create

28.

STEP 5

−/+ **1, 2, 3, 5, 6, 7.** Weight gain is a common side effect of lithium carbonate. To be efficacious, lithium has to achieve a therapeutic blood level. The client should be taught to maintain a therapeutic level by taking lithium at the same time each day and by monitoring salt intake and avoiding caffeine. (High salt intake and caffeine consumption can reduce the serum level, the latter by increasing the rate of lithium excretion.) The client should be taught to take lithium with meals to decrease the occurrence of nausea, a common side effect. Urinary retention is not a known side effect of lithium.

🗝️ CJ: Case study; Step 5: Take action; CL: Apply

29.

STEP 6

−/+ **1, 2, 4, 5.** Classic signs of mania include elevated or irritable mood, sleeping little, talking rapidly, distractibility, racing thoughts, increased goal-related activities, and delusions. The client is still very distractible and showed elevated mood and increased talkativeness following a visit.

Sleeping 4 hours a night shows that sleep patterns are not yet normal. Participating in group activities is desirable behavior. The vital signs are unrelated to the mania.

🔑 CJ: Case study; Step 6: Evaluate outcomes; CL: Evaluate

30. 1. The nurse should call the nursing station to ask the nursing team for assistance. It is not necessary to page the HCP because this is not an emergency, but the nurse will need to notify the provider of the client's death and then also notify the family. A "code" should not be called because the client and family have designated a "do-not-resuscitate" status. Nursing personnel should begin postmortem care so that the family does not walk in unannounced to find their loved one deceased and looking disarrayed.

🔑 CN: Management of care; CL: Analyze

31. 3. Signs of indigestion and sweating can be signs of impending myocardial infarction that should be carefully assessed by the nurse. The client who had the cardiac catheterization has stable vital signs and should be reassessed after assessing the client with a potential impending myocardial infarction. The client who had respiratory therapy does not require immediate attention. The client with diabetes has a normal finger stick glucose level and does not require immediate attention.

🔑 CN: Management of care; CL: Analysis

32. 1. The nurse should first obtain blood cultures because subsequent treatment will be dependent on the results. The client has an IV infusion; the HCP did not write a prescription to increase the infusion rate. Unless indicated otherwise, the nurse can take the client's vital signs after scheduling the computed tomography scan and other laboratory work.

🔑 CN: Reduction of risk potential; CL: Analyze

33. 3. Variable decelerations are associated with compression of the umbilical cord. The nurse should alter the client's position and increase the intravenous fluid rate. Fetal head compression is associated with early decelerations. Severe compression of the fetal chest, such as during the process of vaginal birth, may result in transient bradycardia. Compression or damage to the placenta, typically from abruptio placentae, results in severe, late decelerations.

🔑 CN: Reduction of risk potential; CL: Analyze

34. 1. The mask is appropriate because it covers the nose and mouth and fits snugly against the cheeks and chin. The mask is not too low. Masks that are too large may cover the eyes. Masks that are too small obstruct the nose.

🔑 CN: Management of care; CL: Evaluate

35. -/+ 1, 2, 3, 4. DIC is diagnosed based on clinical symptoms and laboratory findings. Findings such as excessive and unusual bruising or bleeding over areas of tissue trauma, such as intravenous insertion or incision sites, or application of a blood pressure cuff should be reported to the health care provider. Tachycardia and diaphoresis also may be noted. Laboratory results reveal low platelet, fibrinogen, proaccelerin, antihemophilic factor, and prothrombin levels. Bleeding time is normal, and partial thromboplastin time is increased. A urine output of 350 mL in 8 hours indicates adequate renal function. Temperature is not an indication of DIC.

🔑 CN: Physiological adaptation; CL: Analyze

36. 2. Preserving forensic evidence is essential for investigative purposes following injuries that may be suspected as having criminal intent. The nurse places each item of clothing in a separate paper bag and labels it; wet clothing is hung to dry. The nurse does not cut or otherwise unnecessarily handle clothing, particularly clothing with evidence such as blood or body fluids. It is not necessary to have police present at this time, but the nurse should document all nursing care and use quotes around the clients' exact words where possible; documentation will become a part of the clients' medical records and can be subpoenaed for subsequent investigation.

🔑 CN: Management of care; CL: Analyze

37. 2. The nurse should first see the client with heart failure who is on a nonrebreather mask and only has an oxygen saturation of 90% and a PaO_2 of 75. This client is not responding appropriately to oxygen therapy and warrants further assessment. This client is most likely experiencing an exacerbation of heart failure, and gas exchange is not occurring at the capillary-membrane level in the lungs. The client with wheezing has an oxygen saturation of 90% on room air with a PaO_2 of 79, indicating that gas exchange is impaired but not severely. The client with COPD can have PaO_2 of 65 if damage to the lungs is underway. A client with COPD can be considered adequately oxygenated with oxygen saturation of 91% on 2 L via nasal cannula. The client who underwent cardiac surgery 30 minutes ago and has a PaO_2 of 80, which is within the normal range, and an oxygen saturation of 93% is considered normal. This client is not experiencing poor oxygenation because of the surgery.

🔑 CN: Management of care; CL: Analysis

38. -/+ **2, 3, 4.** Miscommunication is a common cause of error and a risk to safety. The use of interpreters is the most important first step to ensure client understanding and support self-determination related to decision-making. Asking specific and direct questions and directing the questions to the culturally appropriate decision maker are culturally congruent behaviors. Direct eye contact is disrespectful in some cultures. Calling or directing someone with an index finger is considered disrespectful in some cultures.

🗝️ CN: Psychosocial integrity; CL: Synthesis

39. 2. If the client begins to experience abdominal cramping during administration of the enema fluid, the nurse's first action is to temporarily stop the infusion and have the client take a few deep breaths. After the cramping subsides, the nurse can continue with the enema solution. If the cramping does not subside, the nurse should clamp the tubing and remove it. Raising the height of the container will increase the flow of fluid and cause the cramping to increase. Rubbing the abdomen while infusing the enema fluid will not stop the cramping.

🗝️ CN: Basic care and comfort; CL: Analyze

40. -/+ **1, 3.** When a child with hemophilia develops bleeding in a joint, the parents should have the child rest and begin factor VIII therapy. If therapy is started immediately, usually other interventions such as ice are not necessary. Heat causes vasodilation and promotes bleeding. Starting factor VIII immediately helps prevent chronic joint disease. Starting physical therapy further traumatizes the joint, possibly increasing the bleeding. Applying a topical agent does not control internal bleeding.

🗝️ CN: Reduction of risk potential; CL: Create

41. 4. The aminoglycoside antibiotic gentamicin sulfate should not be applied to large, denuded areas because toxicity and systemic absorption are possible. The nurse should instruct the client to avoid excessive sun exposure because gentamicin sulfate can cause photosensitivity. The client should be instructed to apply the cream or ointment for only the length of time prescribed because a superinfection can occur from overuse. The client should contact the HCP if the condition worsens after use.

🗝️ CN: Pharmacological and parenteral therapies; CL: Evaluate

42.

STEP 1

-/+ **2, 6, 7.** The nurse should recognize that dizziness, premature ventricular contractions, and muscle weakness are findings that are of most concern for the client who is taking medications for hypertension and who has a history of coronary artery disease. The dry mouth and stuffy nose are not of concern at this time. The nurse should continue to monitor the client's headache to determine if it is increasing. Normal sinus rhythm is an expected underlying rhythm. The nurse should monitor the client's vital signs, and electrolytes should be monitored.

🗝️ CJ: Case study; Step 1: Recognize cues; CL: Analyze

43.

STEP 2

0/1 The client's laboratory results are consistent with **hypokalemia**, which increases the client's risk for **dysrhythmias** and is likely related to taking **hydrochlorothiazide**.

A review of the lab results reveals hypokalemia, which increases the risk for cardiac dysrhythmias including premature ventricular contractions. Although the angiotensin-converting enzyme (ACE) inhibitor lisinopril is potassium sparing, the client has not taken it for 4 days and made the decision to double the dose of the hydrochlorothiazide. Hydrochlorothiazide is potassium wasting and likely a cause of the hypokalemia.

🗝️ CJ: Case study; Step 2: Analyze cues; CL: Analyze

44.

STEP 3

Finding	Expected	Unexpected
Systolic BP 132 mm Hg sitting	X	
Diastolic BP 78 mm Hg sitting	X	
HR 94 bpm sitting	X	
Systolic BP 110 mm Hg standing		X
Diastolic BP 72 mm Hg standing		X
HR 114 bpm standing		X

The systolic and diastolic blood pressure and heart rate taken in the sitting position are expected. The systolic blood pressure and pulse in the standing position are unexpected and are priority findings to report to the health care provider. The systolic BP decreased by 22 mm Hg, the diastolic BP decreased by 6 mm Hg, and the pulse increased by 20 bpm. A positional drop in the systolic blood pressure of 20 mm Hg or more, a drop in the diastolic blood pressure of 10 mm Hg or more, or a pulse increase of 20 bpm or more is indicative of orthostatic hypotension.

🗝️ CJ: Case study; Step 3: Prioritize hypothesis; CL: Analyze

45.

STEP 4

0/1	Potential Intervention	Essential	Nonessential	Inappropriate
1.	Communicate the need to obtain timely medication refills	X		
2.	Obtain a list of the allergens that cause nasal congestion		X	
3.	Inquire whether the client keeps medications in a pill case		X	
4.	Instruct to avoid outdoor exercise in extreme temperatures	X		
5.	Teach to change positions very slowly	X		
6.	Suggest using nonsteroidal antiinflammatory drugs (NSAIDs) to treat headaches			X
7.	Explain that weakness is to be expected when taking antihypertensive medications			X

It is essential that the nurse tell the client about the importance of refilling prescriptions on time because disruptions in taking prescribed antihypertensives can lead to rebound hypertension. Exercising in the hot weather may have contributed to the client's electrolyte fluid losses. The nurse should advise the client to exercise in the morning, evening, or indoors in hot weather and to arise slowly to decrease the risk for falling and injury. The list of seasonal allergens or use of a pill case will not provide essential information relevant to the client's current problem. It is inappropriate for the nurse to suggest that the client take NSAIDs to treat headaches because these drugs may reduce the effectiveness of ACE inhibitors and thiazide diuretics. Muscle weakness can be a sign of hypokalemia and is an important symptom for the client to report because they will likely be restarting the hydrochlorothiazide.

🔑 CJ: Case study; Step 4: Generate solutions; CL: Create

46.

STEP 5

-/+ **1, 2, 4, 5. 7.** The nurse should plan to instruct the client about managing high blood pressure. The client should begin an exercise program that includes 40 minutes of aerobic exercise three to four times a week. The nurse should instruct the client to read the label of over-the-counter medications such as decongestants or stimulants because they can increase blood pressure. Home blood pressure monitoring will provide information about the effectiveness of antihypertensive medications for both the client and the health care provider, and the nurse should instruct the client to keep a daily record and report trends that indicate the blood pressure is not within the normal limits of 120/80 mm Hg at rest. The client should drink water to rehydrate instead of caffeinated beverages, which can have a diuretic effect. The client should limit the intake of sodium to about 1 teaspoon a day. The client should limit the intake of caffeine to two drinks per day and limit the use of alcohol to one drink per day for women and two drinks per day for men. The client should follow a diet that will help manage their blood pressure. The DASH diet focuses on foods that help the client lose weight, maintain a normal blood sugar level, reduce sodium intake, and prevent potassium loss.

🔑 CJ: Case study; Step 5: Take action; CL: Apply

47.

STEP 6

-/+ **2, 3, 5, 6, 8.** The client should be able to identify palpitations, dizziness, blurred vision, and fainting as signs of potentially life-threatening effects. Swelling of the lips or tongue can signify the development of angioedema, an allergic reaction that can occur with an ACE inhibitor such as lisinopril. The client can tell the health care provider about concerns regarding thirst, fatigue, nasal congestion, or dry cough, but these do not warrant immediate action.

🔑 CJ: Case study; Step 6: Evaluate outcomes; CL: Evaluate

48. 3. Nitroglycerin in all dosage forms (sublingual, transdermal, or intravenous) should be shielded from light to prevent deterioration. The client should be instructed to keep the nitroglycerin in the dark container that is supplied by the pharmacy, and it should not be removed or placed in another container. Nitroglycerine should be kept at room temperature in a dry place; it is not needed to refrigerate the drug.

🔑 CN: Pharmacological and parenteral therapies; CL: Apply

49. 4. Medication noncompliance is a primary cause of exacerbation in chronic mental illnesses. Of the issues listed, medications should be addressed first. Other issues, such as family, marriage, and finances, can be addressed as client stabilization is maintained.

🔑 CN: Psychosocial integrity; CL: Analyze

50. 4. IV fluids should not be infused for longer than 24 hours because of the risk for bacterial growth in the solution. The appropriate action for the nurse to take is to discontinue the current TPN solution, change the tubing, and hang a new bag of

51. **2.** Neurologic symptoms, such as footdrop or bowel or bladder changes, should be reported to the HCP immediately. When musculoskeletal strain causes back pain, these symptoms may take 4 to 6 weeks to resolve. As an accompanying symptom of acute low back pain, the client may have a diffuse, aching sensation in the L4 to L5 area, pain in the lower back when the leg is lifted, or pain that radiates to the hip.

CN: Reduction of risk potential; CL: Analyze

52. **1.** Sudden, sharp pain with breathing or coughing on the affected side, tachypnea, dyspnea, diminished or absent breath sounds on the affected side, tachycardia, anxiety, and restlessness indicate a pneumothorax, which can be a complication of inserting a central venous pressure line. The other findings are within normal limits.

CN: Physiological adaptation; CL: Analyze

53. **4.** This girl has an exaggeration of the lumbar spine, swayback, or lordosis which is not a normal posture. Kyphosis is an increased convexity or roundness of the curve of the thoracic spine. Scoliosis is a lateral curvature of the spine.

CN: Health promotion and maintenance; CL: Analyze

54. **4.** The most appropriate action is to report the swelling, loss of mobility, and unrelieved pain to the HCP. These symptoms are indicators of neurovascular impairment. Administering opioids will not eliminate the cause of the problem, which is unrelieved pressure on nerves and blood supply. If prompt action (cutting the cast) is not taken to relieve the pressure, permanent muscular and neurologic injury may result. Applying the ice bag would have been appropriate earlier to decrease or prevent swelling, but applying it at this time could actually lead to further decreased circulation. The arm should be elevated, but the nurse cannot wait 30 minutes to reassess the client without risking permanent damage.

CN: Reduction of risk potential; CL: Analyze

55. **1.** Before 32 weeks' gestation, most neonates have difficulty coordinating sucking and swallowing reflexes along with breathing. Increased respiratory distress may occur with bottle-feeding. Bottle-feedings can be given after the neonate shows sucking and swallowing behaviors. High-calorie formulas can be given by bottle or by gavage feeding. Although frequent feeding prevents hypoglycemia, the feeding does not have to be given via a gavage tube. Although these neonates can be stressed by cold, they can be kept warm with blankets while being bottle-fed or fed while in the warm isolette environment.

CN: Health promotion and maintenance; CL: Apply

56. **1, 2, 4.** After bowel surgery, an NG tube attached to low intermittent suction is used to remove gastric fluids. The amount of fluid from the NG tube suction is important because it contributes to the client's overall fluid and electrolyte balance. IV fluids are used to maintain hydration, and intake and output are measured to determine hydration status. Postoperative vital signs are assessed more frequently than every 6 hours. Bowel sounds will be auscultated to determine when they return. Measuring abdominal girth is not necessary following colostomy reversal.

CN: Physiological adaptation; CL: Analyze

57. **2.** The nurse should assess for signs of impending shock such as diaphoresis. The client would have hypotension, dysuria, and cool skin.

CN: Pharmacological and parenteral therapies; CL: Analyze

58. **3.** When dextrose is abruptly discontinued, rebound hypoglycemia can occur. The nurse should assess the client for symptoms of hypoglycemia. Essential fatty acid deficiency is very unlikely to occur because some of these fatty acids are stored. Preventing dehydration or malnutrition is not the reason for tapering the infusion rate; the client's hydration and nutritional status and ability to maintain adequate intake must be established before TPN is discontinued.

CN: Pharmacological and parenteral therapies; CL: Apply

59. **2.** There is a direct interaction between the effects of insulin and those of beta-blockers. The nurse must be aware that there is a potential for increased hypoglycemic effects of insulin when a beta-blocker is added to the client's medication regimen. The client's blood sugar should be monitored. Ketoacidosis occurs in hyperglycemia. Although a decrease in the incidence of ketoacidosis could occur when a beta-blocker is added, the direct result is an increase in the hypoglycemic effect of insulin.

CN: Pharmacological and parenteral therapies; CL: Apply

60. 1. The client with sensorineural hearing loss has difficulty hearing high-pitched sounds. Aging and ototoxicity are two causes of sensorineural hearing loss. The client's ability to speak is not affected. The client who cannot assign meaning to sound has central hearing loss. Vertigo is commonly an indication of an inner ear problem.

🗝 CN: Physiological adaptation; CL: Analyze

61.

STEP 1

−/+ **2, 3, 4, 6, 8.** A headache with visual disturbances and elevated blood pressure could be symptoms of preeclampsia. A urine dipstick finding of protein in the urine suggests kidney dysfunction, which may also be associated with preeclampsia. A typical FHR is 110 to 160 bpm. The FHR of 170 bpm indicates tachycardia that may be associated with placental perfusion. The client is most likely experiencing Braxton Hicks or prodromal contractions, which is a normal finding and does not indicate impending labor until contractions become more regular and frequent. Typical weight gain near the end of pregnancy is approximately 1 lb or a half a kilogram. Although a weight gain of 3.3 lb (1.5 kg) in 2 weeks is high, it is not alarming. A fundal height is best understood on a growth curve, but findings within 2 cm of the gestational age generally suggest typical growth. A cervical dilation of 1 cm is not an uncommon finding in the last month of pregnancy.

🗝 CJ: Case study; Step 1: Recognize cues; CL: Analyze

62.

STEP 2

0/1

Finding	Mild Preeclampsia	Severe Preeclampsia
BP	X	
Headache		X
Urine dipstick		X
Visual changes		X
Fetal tachycardia		X

Preeclampsia is a pregnancy complication characterized by the development of high blood pressure after 20 weeks' gestation. The pathophysiology is poorly understood, but vasospasm and activation of the coagulation system lead to damage to other organ systems. Mild preeclampsia is often managed at home. Severe preeclampsia requires hospitalization. Mild preeclampsia is associated with systolic blood pressures between 140 and 160 mm Hg and diastolic pressures between 90 and 110 mm Hg. Other organ system involvement is more characteristic of severe preeclampsia. Headache and visual disturbances indicate central nervous system irritation. Protein findings in the urine of +3 are consistent with severe preeclampsia. Higher levels are suggestive of increased kidney involvement and severe preeclampsia. Fetal tachycardia indicates the preeclampsia is severe enough to affect placental perfusion.

🗝 CJ: Case study; Step 2: Analyze cues; CL: Analyze

63.

STEP 3

0/1 *The client is at greatest risk for **seizure**. To prevent complications, the client **most** likely requires immediate hospitalization and treatment with **anticonvulsants**.*

The client is showing signs of multiorgan system involvement more consistent with severe preeclampsia. Severe preeclampsia is best managed in the hospital. The plan of care for preeclampsia is focused on decreasing risk to both the birth parent and the baby. Although stroke and pulmonary edema are possible, the greatest risk for the client is developing eclampsia, which causes seizures. Eclampsia occurs in approximately 1 in 200 women with preeclampsia. Treatment with the anticonvulsant magnesium sulfate is the primary need. If the blood pressure becomes higher, antihypertensive agents may be added. Uterotonic agents, such as oxytocin, are used to induce labor. While delivery is the best treatment for the birth parent, delivery before 37 weeks' gestation increases risks for the baby and is not indicated before magnesium sulfate has been initiated.

🗝 CJ: Case study; Step 3: Prioritize hypothesis; CL: Analyze

64.

STEP 4

−/+

Category	Anticipated Order
Activity	☐ Bathroom privileges
	☒ Quiet environment
	☒ Seizure precautions
Medications	☒ Magnesium sulfate infusion
	☒ Magnesium sulfate bolus
	☐ Intrapartum antibiotics
Monitoring	☐ Intermittent fetal heart rate monitoring
	☒ Complete blood count (CBC) and clotting studies daily
	☒ Complete metabolic panel and magnesium levels

Rationale: Clients hospitalized with preeclampsia most typically are put on strict bed rest to help increase placental perfusion. A quiet environment is needed to reduce stimulation that might invoke a seizure. Clients are at high risk for seizures, and thus using a padded rail and having oxygen and suction equipment available is indicated. Clients typically receive a loading dose of 4 to 6 g of the anticonvulsant magnesium sulfate over 15 to 20 minutes followed by an hourly maintenance dose of, typically, 2 g per hour. The client does not have signs of infection to warrant antibiotics.

The client is at high risk for uteroplacental insufficiency, and thus continuous fetal heart rate monitoring is indicated. Laboratory tests are needed to monitor the disease progress and determine if the client is progressing to HELLP syndrome (Hemolysis, Elevated Liver Enzymes, Low Platelets). A CBC and clotting studies are needed to monitor for hemolysis and low platelets. A complete metabolic panel monitors electrolytes, liver, and renal function. Magnesium levels need to be obtained to monitor for toxicity once magnesium sulfate is started.

🗝️ CJ: Case study; Step 4: Generate solutions; CL: Create

65.

STEP 5

1, 2, 3, 6. Magnesium sulfate is considered a high-alert medication because there is serious risk for causing significant client harm when it is used in error. Safety precautions for all high-alert medications include medication verification by two providers. Magnesium sulfate should only be infused in an IV pump to accurately control the rate of infusion. One-on-one care is needed during the loading dose administration and for at least the first hour after starting magnesium sulfate to monitor for toxicity, including respiratory depression. Calcium gluconate, not naloxone, is the antidote for magnesium sulfate. The nurse should monitor serum magnesium levels closely. Urine magnesium levels are more useful in diagnosing long-term magnesium deficit. Monitoring deep tendon reflexes helps the nurse identify toxicity. Therapeutic magnesium sulfate levels are 4 to 7 mEq/dL (1.6 to 2.9 mmol/L). At 10 mEq/dL (4.11 mmol/L), clients may lose deep tendon reflexes.

🗝️ CJ: Case study; Step 5: Take action; CL: Apply

66.

STEP 6

Assessment Finding	Effective	Ineffective	Not related
Urine output	X		
FHR	X		
Contractions			X
Deep tendon reflexes	X		
Nausea		X	
Wheezing		X	

Diuresis is a sign that a client has had a good response to magnesium. A fetal heart rate of 120 bpm with accelerations is a reassuring pattern, suggesting the placenta is well perfused. The 1+ deep tendon reflexes without clonus indicate the magnesium has reduced central nervous system irritability. Magnesium sulfate is sometimes used to prevent preterm labor, but here the treatment plan is geared at preventing complications of preeclampsia, not preventing contractions. Epigastric pain suggests that the preeclampsia may be affecting the liver. Wheezing may suggest the development of pulmonary edema.

🗝️ CJ: Case study; Step 6: Evaluate outcomes; CL: Evaluate

67. 3. A urine output of 30 to 50 mL per hour indicates adequate fluid replacement in the client with burns. An increase in body weight may indicate fluid retention. A urine output greater than fluid intake does not represent a fluid balance. Depending on the client, blood pressure of 90/60 mm Hg could indicate the presence of a hypovolemic state; by itself, it does not indicate adequate fluid replacement.

🗝️ CN: Physiological adaptation; CL: Evaluate

68. 3. Commonly, when a child appears better, the parents stop the medication. Unfortunately, the infection remains. Therefore, the nurse needs to explain that all of the medication must be administered to clear up the infection. Explaining why the medicine should be continued is more helpful to parents than saying it needs to be given. Telling the parent that stopping the medication will make the next ear infection harder to treat does not focus on the present issue.

🗝️ CN: Pharmacological and parenteral therapies; CL: Analyze

69. 1. Many clients who experience abuse are hesitant to talk about it and need help to do so. The nurse should ask the client directly about abuse when it is suspected, using a sensitive, empathetic, and compassionate approach. In this way, the client can feel comfortable revealing information about the abuse. Telling the client that it is difficult to believe the injuries resulted from a fall is not helpful because it is blameful and puts the client on the defensive. Asking the client what they did to make someone hit them or discussing what they can do the next time blames and alienates the client.

🗝️ CN: Psychosocial integrity; CL: Analyze

70. 1. A primary outcome for the care of the client in shock is to achieve adequate tissue perfusion, thus avoiding multiple organ dysfunction. While the lungs and kidneys are susceptible to injury, maintaining tissue perfusion will help avoid tissue damage. Vasoconstriction occurs as a compensatory mechanism to maintain perfusion until the client enters the irreversible stage of shock.

🗝️ CN: Reduction of risk potential; CL: Evaluate

71. 3. The client with emphysema is commonly underweight in appearance. The weight loss may be caused by the increased energy required to support the work of breathing. Frequent coughing, bronchospasms, and copious sputum are clinical manifestations of chronic bronchitis.

CN: Physiological adaptation; CL: Analyze

72. 2. The incident report includes only what the nurse saw and did—the objective data. The nurse does not try to interpret the likely cause of the incident, include statements from the client about the incident, or comment on extenuating circumstances.

CN: Management of care; CL: Apply

73. 2. The serum cholesterol is within the normal range for this client, indicating the medication is effective. Since the cholesterol levels are within normal limits, it is likely that the client is taking the medication. Asking may indicate the nurse has doubts or mistrusts that the client is taking the medication. The client does not need to change the diet at this point. Hemoglobin and hematocrit are not affected by simvastatin; since liver damage is a side effect of simvastatin, the nurse could review the liver function studies.

CN: Pharmacological and parenteral therapies; CL: Analyze

74. 3. The medications prescribed for, administered to, or dispensed to the client while under the care of a health care organization are compared with those on the list, and any discrepancies (e.g., omissions, duplications, potential interactions) are resolved. A complete list of the client's medications is communicated to the next provider of service when a client is referred or transferred to another setting, service, practitioner, or level of care within or outside the organization. The complete, accurate list of medications is also provided to the client on discharge from the organization. The next provider of service checks the Medication Reconciliation List again to make sure it is accurate and in concert with any new medications to be prescribed.

CN: Safety and infection control; CL: Analyze

75. 4. Follow-up after a pneumonectomy because of lung cancer generally involves semiannual chest x-rays. Recurrence usually occurs locally in the lungs and may be identified on chest x-rays. Follow-up after cancer treatment is an important component of the treatment plan. Unless there are indications of other problems, the health care provider will likely not order an abdominal computed tomography scan.

CN: Reduction of risk potential; CL: Analyze

76. 3. A client exhibiting mild preeclampsia is initially treated with activity restriction. Bed rest, or lying on the left side, decreases pressure on the vena cava and improves circulatory blood flow. Restriction of visitors and a quiet environment are also necessary. IV magnesium sulfate, a central nervous system depressant, is usually prescribed for the client with severe preeclampsia. Labetalol is used for the client with severe preeclampsia. Frequent monitoring of the client's blood pressure is important. However, hourly blood pressure checks are more routinely prescribed for the client with severe preeclampsia. Additionally, the client needs to rest, and checking the blood pressure hourly could interfere with their ability to rest.

CN: Reduction of risk potential; CL: Analyze

77. 4. Lifestyle modification to lower blood pressure includes weight reduction in clients who are overweight, reducing the intake of dietary sodium, and an increase in physical activity. Client teaching involves instruction on a low-sodium diet because of the propensity for high-sodium foods at fast-food restaurants. The client is of normal weight, and alcohol intake is in moderation. Nitroprusside is a treatment for hypertensive crisis.

CN: Physiological adaptation; CL: Analyze

78. 3. The three-point gait, in which the client advances the crutches and the affected leg at the same time while weight is supported on the unaffected extremity, is the appropriate gait of choice. This allows for non–weight bearing on the affected extremity. The two-point, four-point, and swing-to gaits require some weight bearing on both legs, which is contraindicated for this client.

CN: Reduction of risk potential; CL: Evaluate

79. 4. Urethritis is usually the initial clinical manifestation of gonorrhea in men. The symptoms include a profuse, purulent discharge and dysuria. Complications are uncommon, but they include prostatitis and sterility. Impotence, scrotal pain, and penile lesions are not associated with gonorrhea.

CN: Safety and infection control; CL: Analyze

80. 1, 2, 3. The nurse should first check to see if the medication has been misplaced, check the client's blood pressure to determine the immediacy of administering the drug, and then call the pharmacy to check that the medication was delivered. Although the nurse needs to obtain and administer the medication as soon as possible, it is inappropriate for the nurse to go to the pharmacy and request the drug without first calling the pharmacy. The nurse should not use another client's medication.

    CN: Safety and infection control; CL: Analyze

81. 3. The child is exhibiting signs and symptoms of possible epiglottitis. As a result, the child is at high risk for laryngospasm and airway occlusion. Therefore, the nurse should have intubation equipment and a tracheostomy tube and setup readily available should the child experience an airway occlusion. Although acetaminophen is an antipyretic, the dosage of 600 mg to be administered rectally is too high. A typical 4-year-old weighs approximately 40 lb (18 kg). The recommended dose is 12.5 mg. When any type of respiratory illness, and especially epiglottitis, is suspected, putting any object, including a tongue depressor for inspection or a cotton-tipped applicator to obtain a throat culture, in the back of the mouth or throat or having the child open the mouth is inappropriate because doing so may predispose the child to laryngospasm or occlusion of the airway by a swollen epiglottis.

    CN: Reduction of risk potential; CL: Analyze

82. 4. Direct application of warm moist heat would benefit a client with low back pain because the heat relaxes muscle spasms. Heat should not be applied to a client who has appendicitis because it can lead to rupture of the appendix and peritonitis. Ice is applied to recently sprained joints to help decrease edema. Applying heat to the area of a suspected malignancy can increase blood flow to the tumor and promote nourishment of the cancer cells.

    CN: Basic care and comfort; CL: Analyze

83. 3. The client with pernicious anemia will require lifelong supplementation of vitamin B_{12}, available through injection or nasal spray administration. It must be given in these forms to ensure absorption. Oral vitamin B_{12} would not be absorbed because the client lacks the intrinsic factor in the stomach necessary for absorption. Chelation therapy is used to extract metals at toxic levels such as in lead poisoning.

    CN: Pharmacological and parenteral therapies; CL: Apply

84. 10 mL. To administer 20 mEq of potassium chloride, the nurse needs to administer 10 mL. The following formula is used to calculate the correct dosage:

$$20\,mEq / X\,mL = 2\,mEq / 1\,mL$$
$$X = 10\,mL$$

    CN: Pharmacological and parenteral therapies; CL: Apply

85. 4. When a client with major depression and suicidal ideation displays a sudden elevation in mood, seems calmer, has more energy, and is more peaceful, the nurse should judge these behaviors as an indication that a suicide attempt is imminent. These symptoms may indicate relief from ambivalent thoughts about suicide and that the client has an immediate plan for suicide.

    CN: Psychosocial integrity; CL: Analyze

86. 3. The purpose of a contraction stress test is to determine fetal response during labor. If late decelerations are noted with the contractions, the test is considered positive or abnormal. Fetal lung maturity is evaluated through amniocentesis to obtain the lecithin-sphingomyelin ratio. The nonstress test is part of the biophysical profile. Determining fetal response during movements is evaluated as part of the nonstress test.

    CN: Reduction of risk potential; CL: Apply

87. 2. The primary reason for instructing the client with emphysema about how to pursed-lip breathe is to prolong exhalation. Prolonging exhalation helps prevent bronchiolar collapse and the trapping of air. It does not directly prevent respiratory infection. Because pursed-lip breathing affects the expiratory phase of the respiratory cycle, it does not affect oxygenation. It may decrease shortness of breath, but this is not the primary reason for the technique.

    CN: Reduction of risk potential; CL: Apply

88. 2. The primary purpose of the automated dispensing machine for nurses is to keep an up-to-date record of the narcotic usage and count. The automated dispensing machine has eliminated the need for change-of-shift counts for narcotics. It does not include unmonitored access by nurses to narcotics, which would not be considered an advantage. The pharmacy has direct information about the narcotics being used on the client at what intervals and by whom, and it automatically records the charges of narcotics used. Not recording the charges would not be an advantage.

    CN: Management of care; CL: Apply

89.

Actions to Take	Potential Conditions	Parameters to Monitor
Begin intravenous fluids	Ectopic pregnancy	Mental status
Request a stat ultrasound		Urine output

The one-sided radiating pain with light vaginal bleeding most suggests that the client has an ectopic pregnancy. The low blood pressure, tachycardia, and increased respiratory rate suggest that the fallopian tube has ruptured and there is internal bleeding. Intravenous fluids are needed immediately to treat shock. A stat ultrasound is indicated to confirm the diagnosis. An abruptio placenta is characterized by bleeding after 20 weeks' gestation. Bleeding from an inevitable abortion is typically heavy with cramping pains. Molar pregnancy bleeding is dark brown and may not be painful. Surgical treatment is needed for an ectopic pregnancy with a ruptured fallopian tube. A D&C, a procedure done to scrape the uterine lining, is a treatment option for an inevitable abortion or molar pregnancy. Misoprostol causes the cervix to dilate and can be used as an alternative treatment to a D&C for an inevitable abortion. There is no indication that the client's problems are related to infection to prioritize antibiotics. The client is at risk for shock. Mental status and urine output can indicate the adequacy of perfusion. Abdominal edema is a late sign of a tubal rupture in ectopic pregnancy. Pain is already severe, so increases are not likely to help the nurse understand if the client's condition is worsening. It is not necessary to monitor the fetal heart rate because the pregnancy is not viable.

CJ: Standalone bowtie; CL: Create

90. 2. Blunt chest trauma can lead to respiratory failure. Maintenance of adequate oxygenation is the priority for the client. Decreasing the client's anxiety is related to maintaining effective respirations and oxygenation. Although pain is distressing to the client and can increase anxiety and decrease respiratory effectiveness, pain control is secondary to maintaining oxygenation, as is maintaining adequate circulatory volume.

CN: Physiological adaptation; CL: Analyze

91. 1. An episiotomy that is edematous and slightly reddened 8 hours after birth is normal. Therefore, the nurse should offer the client an ice pack to provide some relief from the perineal pain for the first 24 hours. An infection is present if greenish, purulent drainage is observed from the site. The edema and discoloration of the episiotomy at this time after birth are normal and do not indicate that a hematoma is likely to develop. A laceration when repaired should appear intact with edges well approximated, clean, and dry.

CN: Health promotion and maintenance; CL: Analyze

92. 4. Because a toddler is strong and moves frequently, the child needs to be restrained during the removal procedure by a total body restraint. To protect the child, a mummy restraint is best because the arms, legs, chest, and head can be fully restrained. A jacket restraint would immobilize only the child's upper body. Elbow restraints would immobilize only the child's arms. The parent should be available to provide comfort before and after the procedure but not to hold the child down during the procedure.

CN: Safety and infection control; CL: Analyze

93. 4. Wheezing over one lung in the presence of a lung tumor is most likely caused by obstruction of the airway by a tumor. Exudate would be more likely to cause crackles. The client's history of smoking would not cause unilateral wheezing. Pleural effusion would produce diminished or absent breath sounds.

CN: Physiological adaptation; CL: Apply

94. 1, 2, 3, 4. The nurse should first apply the tourniquet and then select a vein for inserting the VAD. The tourniquet slows the venous return and allows the nurse to identify an appropriate vein. The nurse should then put on clean gloves and cleanse the insertion site with an antiseptic swab. The nurse may wear gloves while applying a tourniquet, but the insertion site must be cleansed immediately prior to the insertion of the VAD. Next, the nurse should insert the VAD with the bevel up at a 10- to 30-degree angle. These steps must be performed to ensure proper placement and prevent infection and are completed before observing for blood return or securing the device with a clear adhesive dressing.

CN: Reduction of risk potential; CL: Synthesis

95. 3. One of the most serious problems in mental health is nonadherence to medication therapy. In clients with a previous history of therapeutic lithium levels, the nurse should assess if the client is taking the medication as prescribed. Loss of sodium during gastrointestinal illnesses can lead to lithium toxicity. Tolerance is not a complication of lithium. Although a client would manifest increased bipolar symptoms with low lithium levels, worsening of the disease would not cause the levels to drop.

CN: Pharmacological and parenteral therapies; CL: Analyze

96. 4, 5. The child is observed for shock that can occur following a severe burn. Shock is noted by the increasing heart rate and dropping blood pressure. This child has an adequate urine output (more than 1 mL/kg body weight), and the specific gravity is within normal range. Pain is expected and is not an indicator of shock.

CN: Physiological adaptation; CL: Analyze

97. **4.** The plan of care to treat fatigue associated with radiation therapy should include encouraging the client to remain active and plan scheduled rest periods as necessary before activity. Engaging in activities, such as walking, has been shown to decrease the cycle of fatigue, anxiety, and depression that can occur during treatment. Fatigue is a very common side effect of radiation therapy that typically begins during the third or fourth week of treatment and persists until after treatment ends. The presence of fatigue does not mean that the cancer is not responding to treatment or that the client has developed another health problem.

CN: Reduction of risk potential; CL: Analyze

98. **4.** The proper use of crutches requires supporting the body weight primarily on the hands. Improper use of crutches can cause nerve damage from excess pressure on the axillary nerve, and undue weight bearing on the elbows and arms.

CN: Reduction of risk potential; CL: Apply

99. **2.** For the child with croup, assessing the child's respiratory status is the priority. It is especially important to assess airway patency because laryngeal spasms can occur suddenly. After the nurse has assessed the toddler's respiratory status, having a tracheostomy set at the bedside would be the next priority. Monitoring vital signs is important, as is ensuring adequate fluid intake to keep secretions loose, but assessing respiratory status is key.

CN: Physiological adaptation; CL: Analyze

100.

Actions to Take	Potential Conditions	Parameters to Monitor
Notify the surgeon	Possible obstruction of stent	Assess pedal pulses using Doppler
Use Doppler to auscultate the presence of pedal pulses		Urine output

Following surgery for placement of a stent to manage an aortic aneurysm, the nurse should assess the client for signs of obstruction to the stent as indicated by lack of blood flow distal to the site of stent insertion. The nurse should first palpate the dorsalis pedis and posterior tibial pulses, and if they are not able to identify their presence, they should next use a Doppler to auscultate the pulses. Because the nurse was able to palpate the dorsalis pedis and posterior tibial pulses at 1000 and 1100 and then not at 1130, the nurse now should attempt to use the Doppler to auscultate the pulses. The nurse should notify the surgeon of this change. Obstruction of the stent can also affect the renal artery, and the nurse should monitor the urine output. At 1000 the urine output was within normal limits (30 to 50 mL per hour), but the nurse should continue to monitor the client for any change in intake and output. The IV has been infusing at the prescribed rate, and there is no indication or order to increase the rate. The nurse should also continue to assess the dressing at the incision site.

CJ: Standalone bowtie; CL: Evaluate

101. **2.** IV solutions are prescribed based upon the fluid and electrolyte status of the client, so laboratory results should be monitored first. Safety recommendations are for standard premixed solutions. If solutions are not premixed, additives are completed by the pharmacy, not at the bedside. Potassium chloride is never given by IV push because this could be fatal. Administration guidelines require no more than 10 mEq (10 mmol/L) of potassium chloride be infused per hour on a general medical-surgical unit. An infusion device or pump is required for safe administration.

CN: Pharmacological and parenteral therapies; CL: Analyze

102. **3, 1, 4, 2.** Even with such a blatant suicide clue, it is still important to confirm that the client is truly suicidal. Then, it is crucial to know what methods of suicide are available to the client. Before the nurse asks for a psychiatric consult, the client needs to understand that the nurse cares, is empathetic, and will take actions to protect the client from harm.

CN: Safety and infection control; CL: Create

103. **2.** In emphysema, the anteroposterior diameter of the chest wall is increased. As a result, the client's breath sounds may be diminished. Fine crackles are present when there is fluid in the lungs. Stridor occurs as a result of a partially obstructed larynx or trachea; stridor can be heard without auscultation. A pleural friction rub is present when pleural surfaces are inflamed and rub together.

CN: Physiological adaptation; CL: Analyze

104. **3.** Loss of height and back pain are early indications of the disease that are caused by collapse of the vertebrae. Later signs include the dowager's hump and loss of the waistline. The dowager's hump is a later sign of osteoporosis that occurs when the vertebrae can no longer support the upper body in an upright position. Fair-skinned, small-boned, White, and Asian women are at greater risk for osteoporosis. Conventional radiographs are little help because more than 30%

of the bone mass must be lost before the disease is detected. High-density bone scans can detect the disease earlier.

🔑 CN: Health promotion and maintenance; CL: Analyze

105. 3. The primary reason for evaluating gastric residual is to determine whether gastric emptying has been delayed and the stomach is becoming overdistended from the feeding. With delayed gastric emptying, the possibility of aspiration of the feeding into the lungs is increased. It is not possible to determine how well the client's body is absorbing nutrients or whether the client is receiving enough feeding by checking the gastric residual. It is not necessary to keep partially digested formula separate from undigested formula.

🔑 CN: Reduction of risk potential; CL: Apply

106. -/+ 1, 5. When the nurse is teaching the client about taking medication, it is important to understand both verbal and nonverbal communication. Many factors, including the client's age, culture, economic situation, and health practices, influence what health information the client will receive from health professionals and be able to integrate into their own health maintenance plan. The nurse should recognize that the client will need additional information if the client states they will stop taking the medication before finishing the prescription or if the client indicates they will take over-the-counter medication that they purchase at a neighborhood grocery instead. The nurse should allow sufficient time for the client to respond, and rather than thinking a nod of the head indicates agreement, ask for a verbal response to be sure the client understands what the nurse is saying. If the client would like to incorporate traditional health care practices into the medication plan, the nurse can determine if those practices are compatible with taking the medication.

🔑 CN: Psychosocial integrity; CL: Synthesis

107. -/+ 2, 4, 5. Clients with hepatitis A commonly experience fatigue and altered nutrition due to anorexia and nausea. Because of the severe fatigue associated with hepatitis, clients are encouraged to rest and restrict activity during the active phase of the disease. It is important that frequent rest periods be planned throughout the day. Clients may experience nausea and vomiting; thus, providing relief is important. Small, frequent meals help clients manage the anorexia associated with hepatitis. An exercise program is not appropriate because the client needs to rest. Clients with hepatitis do not experience pain. All medications administered to clients with hepatitis need to be evaluated for their potential for hepatotoxicity.

🔑 CN: Physiological adaptation; CL: Analyze

108. 4. Third-degree heart block occurs when atrial stimuli are blocked at the atrioventricular junction. Impulses from the atria and ventricles are conducted independently of each other. The atrial rate is 60 to 100 bpm; the ventricular rate is usually 10 to 60 bpm.

🔑 CN: Reduction of risk potential; CL: Analyze

109. -/+ 2, 5. The application of restraints places the client in a vulnerable, confined position. When the restraints are first applied, the nurse should observe the client for the first 15 minutes either by staying in the room, using a video monitor, or observing the client through a window or door. Then, the nurse should check on the client every 15 to 30 minutes, according to agency policy, while restrained to make sure that the client is safe. The client should be able to move while the restraints are in place. Telling the client not to move is an unrealistic expectation, and the client should be able to move limbs and reposition within the limits of the restraints. The restraints should be removed every 2 hours to provide skin care and exercise the extremities. Restraints should not be secured to the side rails; they should be secured to the movable bed frame so that when the bed is adjusted, the restraints will not be pulled too tightly.

🔑 CN: Safety and infection control; CL: Analyze

110. 1. Aspirin is an antiplatelet medication. The use of aspirin is contraindicated while taking warfarin because it will potentiate the drug's effects. Diphenhydramine and pseudoephedrine do not affect blood coagulation. Digoxin is not an over-the-counter medication; it requires a prescription.

🔑 CN: Pharmacological and parenteral therapies; CL: Analyze

111. 1. The nurse should inform the client that carbamazepine can decrease the effects of oral anticoagulants. Carbamazepine can increase the serum concentration of verapamil and can decrease the serum concentration of other anticonvulsants and the effects of oral contraceptives.

🔑 CN: Pharmacological and parenteral therapies; CL: Apply

112. **2.** Viral hepatitis causes fatigue. It is important for the client to rest to allow the liver to recover. Activity levels are resumed gradually as the client begins to recover. Abdominal pain is not a common manifestation of hepatitis. The client typically does not have difficulty breathing or experience edema.

🗝 CN: Physiological adaptation; CL: Analyze

113. **1.** The parent should be encouraged to hold and cuddle the child to provide needed emotional support. Such activities as helping the child play with toys, reading stories, and staying with the child would not be contraindicated, but these activities do not offer as much emotional support as holding and cuddling.

🗝 CN: Psychosocial integrity; CL: Analyze

114. **2.** The best strategy to affect child seat belt safety is to attend the school board meeting and advocate for educational programming. The programming could be simple and done quickly. This action also targets the best audience.

🗝 CN: Health promotion and maintenance; CL: Analyze

115. **3.** The most appropriate action is to contact the HCP to verify that the prescription is correct. Although 60 mg of morphine is a significant dose, the amount of morphine administered to a client can vary widely, especially if a client has been taking morphine for an extended period and has developed a tolerance to the medication. The safest approach is for the nurse to verify prescriptions that do not appear to fall within the norm. Administering the medication without verification is unsafe. The nurse cannot decide to reduce the amount of a prescribed medication without a prescription. Asking another nurse to review the prescription is not inappropriate; however, checking with the HCP to verify the prescription should be done.

🗝 CN: Pharmacological and parenteral therapies; CL: Analyze

116. **4.** RRTs, or medical emergency teams, provide a team approach to evaluate and treat immediately clients with alterations in vital signs or neurologic deterioration. Calling the neurosurgeon or consulting the CNS may not result in a rapid response. The Trendelenburg position is usually used in treating shock, but because the client has had brain surgery, the head should not be lower than the trunk.

🗝 CN: Physiological adaptation; CL: Analyze

117. **2.** Postoperative care after a laparoscopic cholecystectomy includes removal of the dressing from the incisional site the day after surgery and allowing the client to bathe or shower. The client can resume a normal diet but may wish to follow a low-fat diet for a few weeks after surgery. Nausea is not expected to last for several days after surgery. The client usually can return to work within 1 week.

🗝 CN: Reduction of risk potential; CL: Evaluate

118. **2.** The nurse who usually works in a maternity unit has more experience with clients who have had abdominal surgery similar to a cesarean birth and should be assigned to a client who will closely match the nurse's experience level. The nurse should assign the client in halo traction to a nurse who has experience with the traction equipment. The client with cancer needing ventilation and the client with progressing amyotrophic lateral sclerosis require care from a nurse who has more experience with clients with these needs.

🗝 CN: Management of care; CL: Synthesis

119. **-/+ 1, 3.** Weight loss is a common side effect of methylphenidate. Because the child's symptoms are controlled with the stimulant, the first action should be to increase the child's oral intake before the medication's side effects begin. The child is less likely to experience medication-related anorexia if they eat a small meal before the medication peaks in the morning. Frequent small meals and snacks are more likely to be tolerated than large meals. Weight should be monitored, but daily weights can lead to obsessions with weight and are seldom recommended for children. A high-protein drink could work; however, the child would be taking in all their calories in the evening, which is not best nutritionally. A change of medication should be the last resort if other interventions do not work because methylphenidate is the most effective medication for ADHD and has been successful with this child.

🗝 CJ: Standalone trend; CL: Create

120. **2.** The imbalance between the client's intake and output indicates that the client may be retaining urine since the removal of the Foley catheter. The nurse's first action is to validate this assumption by assessing for bladder distention. Applying a condom catheter will not relieve urinary retention; condom catheters are meant to be used for incontinence. A urine specimen for a culture is obtained if a urinary infection is suspected, but this is not a priority at this point. Kegel exercises are helpful in controlling urinary dribbling but do not treat retention.

🗝 CN: Reduction of risk potential; CL: Analyze

121. **2.** Griseofulvin is associated with photosensitivity reactions. Therefore, the nurse should instruct the parents to have the child avoid intense sunlight. Griseofulvin is best absorbed when administered after a high-fat meal. Treatment with griseofulvin typically lasts for at least 1 month. There are no indications that increased fluid intake affects absorption.

CN: Pharmacological and parenteral therapies; CL: Analyze

122. **2.** After cystoscopy with biopsy, the nurse would assess for excessive hematuria, which might indicate hemorrhage caused by the biopsy. Catheters are not routinely inserted after cystoscopy. The nurse would not assess for bladder distention unless the client was having difficulty voiding. Urine cultures are not routinely prescribed after cystoscopy.

CN: Reduction of risk potential; CL: Analyze

123. **4, 3, 2, 1.** The nurse first assesses and manages the physical effects of the eye injury by placing an ice pack on the eye to reduce swelling. Next, the nurse obtains as much information about the situation and the daycare center as possible. The nurse documents all physical assessment findings and information provided by the parent. Because an infant who is 6 months of age should not be in a walker unattended and black eyes do not occur from falls with walkers, this is a potential child abuse incident; therefore, the nurse reports the incident as such using the agency's reporting structure (usually, social services department reports the incidents to the authorities).

CN: Management of care; CL: Create

124. **3, 5.** Not attending the support group consistently and not taking the antidepressant may lead to a relapse, and the client needs this information. Bulimia is chronic and intermittent and involves cycles of bingeing, purging, and restrictive eating. Increased socialization and activities promote healthy relationships.

CN: Psychosocial integrity; CL: Evaluate

125. **1, 3, 4, 5.** An imperforate anus is an anorectal anomaly involving the absence of an anus, or the opening in the wrong position. Classic symptoms include failure to pass meconium in the first 48 hours of life, abdominal distention, passing stool from an opening other than the anus, and a missing or moved anal opening. Curdled vomiting is associated with digestive rather than obstructive disorders.

CN: Physiological adaptation; CL: Analyze

126. **1.** Sucking provides the infant with a sense of security and comfort. It also is an outlet for releasing tension. The infant should not be discouraged from sucking on the pacifier. Fussiness after feeding may indicate that the infant's appetite is not satisfied. Sucking is not manipulative in the sense of seeking parental attention.

CN: Health promotion and maintenance; CL: Analyze

127. **1.** At 32 weeks' gestation, a neonate has limited ability to coordinate sucking, swallowing, and breathing. The sucking reflex is present at 32 weeks' gestation, but the neonate cannot coordinate the reflex with swallowing and breathing. The stomach has the capacity for digestion at this gestational age. There are no indications that this neonate is dehydrated.

CN: Basic care and comfort; CL: Analyze

128. **3.** The nurse should teach a client who has undergone chest surgery to raise the arm on the affected side over the head to help prevent shoulder ankylosis. This exercise helps restore normal shoulder movement, prevents stiffening of the shoulder joint, and improves muscle tone and power.

CN: Reduction of risk potential; CL: Analyze

129. **2.** The nurse's first action should be to attempt to replace the tracheostomy tube immediately so that the client's airway is reestablished. Although the nurse may also call for assistance, there should be no delay before attempting reinsertion of the tube. The client is placed in a supine position with the neck hyperextended to facilitate reentry of the tube. The obturator is inserted into the replacement tracheostomy tube to guide insertion and is then removed to allow passage of air through the tube.

CN: Management of care; CL: Analyze

130. **1, 2, 4.** LPN/VNs work collaboratively with colleagues in health care to assess, plan, and deliver quality nursing services. The experienced LPN/VN is capable of gathering data and observations, including breath sounds and pulse oximetry. Administering medications, such as aerosolized medications, is within the scope of practice for the LPN/LVN. The actions that are within the scope of practice for the professional RN include independently completing the admission assessment, initiating the nursing care plan, and evaluating a parent's abilities, as these activities require additional education and skills.

CN: Management of care; CL: Analyze

131. 4. The mechanism of injury is always the most critical information to obtain from a client with a musculoskeletal injury. In the event of a back injury, the mechanism of injury provides the greatest clue as to the extent of the injury and the proper treatment plan. The other questions are important but will not give the critical information needed related to this specific problem and injury.

🗝️ CN: Reduction of risk potential; CL: Analyze

132. 1. Antihypertensive medications such as metoprolol and hydrochlorothiazide work to lower the blood pressure by reducing peripheral resistance or decreasing cardiac output; the effectiveness of these drugs is noted by a lowering of the blood pressure. Vasodilators are used to improve peripheral circulation. Cardiac stimulants and antiarrhythmic drugs are used to increase heart rate. Although cardiac problems can cause dyspnea, the use of drugs to manage dyspnea depends on the underlying cause.

🗝️ CN: Pharmacological and parenteral therapies; CL: Evaluate

133. 3. Typical early signs of rheumatoid arthritis are nonspecific and not necessarily related to specific joint pain. Common early symptoms include fatigue, anorexia, weight loss, and generalized feelings of stiffness. Joint swelling and limitation of movement usually occur later as joint involvement becomes more specific. Dizziness is not a sign of rheumatoid arthritis. Nausea is not typically associated with the disease process but can be related to medications prescribed to treat rheumatoid arthritis.

🗝️ CN: Physiological adaptation; CL: Analyze

134.

0/1	Actions to Take	Potential Conditions	Parameters to Monitor
	Encourage frequent emptying	Mastitis	Infant latch
	Administer antibiotics		Abscess development

The client is exhibiting signs and symptoms of mastitis, a breast infection characterized by flulike symptoms. Engorgement is typically bilateral and occurs in the first few days after birth. Clients have pain but not fever. Breastfeeding thrush is most associated with cracked nipples or nipple pain. Blocked or plugged milk ducts are characterized by palatable lumps. The underlying infection indicated by the elevated temperature indicates that treatment with antibiotics will be needed. The nurse should contact the health care provider to obtain a prescription for antibiotics. The client should continue to breastfeed the infant from both breasts. Frequent breastfeeding, or breast pumping, is encouraged for anyone having a breast infection. Antifungals are indicated for breastfeeding thrush. The client does not report nipple pain to suggest that a nipple shield may be indicated. Icepacks are used to treat engorgement. The nurse should monitor the client for the development of localized infection in the form of a breast abscess. The nurse should monitor the latch because research suggests that most inflammatory breast problems will resolve with latching help to ensure complete milk removal. There is no need to monitor the infant's weight at this point, and there is no reason to suspect bleeding nipple will develop if cracked nipples are not present. The infant's oral cavity would need to be assessed if thrush was present.

🗝️ CJ: Standalone bowtie; CL: Create

135. 2. When instructing the client about mixing two types of insulin in the same syringe, the nurse should instruct the client about how to handle the insulin and which one to draw up first. NPH insulin should be rolled between the palms to mix it before drawing it up; shaking it will introduce air bubbles into the solution, which can cause inaccurate dosing. The nurse should also verify that the client understands they should draw up the most rapid-acting insulin first; the client states they are drawing up the regular insulin first. Additionally, the nurse can verify that the client understands to store the insulin in a cool place and inject the insulin at a 90-degree angle.

🗝️ CN: Pharmacological and parenteral therapies; CL: Evaluate

136. 2 lb or 0.9 kg. One lb or 0.45 kg of weight is approximately equivalent to 3500 calories. Removing 1000 calories a day results in a 2-lb (0.9-kg) weight loss per week (7000 calories divided by 7 days). A client who wanted to lose 1 lb (0.45 kg) in a 7-day period would need to cut out 500 calories a day (3500 calories divided by 7 days). It is unsafe to try to lose more than 2 lb (0.9 kg) a week.

🗝️ CN: Health promotion and maintenance; CL: Apply

137. 🔢 **4, 5.** Buspirone is not a benzodiazepine but acts as a serotonin agonist. Serotonin is the neurotransmitter implicated in depression. Buspirone reduces symptoms of worry, apprehension, difficulty with concentration, and irritability. Buspirone takes 1 to 6 weeks to be effective with full therapeutics benefits taking 3 to 6 weeks to occur. It does not cause muscle relaxation or produce dependence, withdrawal, or tolerance.

🗝️ CN: Pharmacological and parenteral therapies; CL: Evaluate

138. -/+ **1, 2, 3, 4, 5.** Before delegating postmortem care to the unlicensed assistive personnel (UAP) the nurse should speak with the family to identify their wishes about postmortem care and then share that information with the UAP. Some families would like to remain with the relative, and the nurse and UAP should respect cultural norms and family needs and allow as much time as they need to begin the grieving process. Before shaving a client's beard, the nurse should always check with the family or in the chart for the client and family's preference and verify the hospital's policy about shaving the head and communicate this information to the UAP. The nurse should consult with the family about any preparation requests such as wearing special clothing or jewelry and explain to the UAP if there are or are not any special requests. The nurse and UAP should always use two identifiers before providing care. It is important to elevate the head of the bed to prevent pooling of blood and discoloration from pooling blood. In the case of a potential organ donation, indwelling lines should not be removed.

🗝️ CN: Basic care and comfort; CL: Application

139. 1. The major cause of relapse is nonadherence to the medication treatment plan. If the client is worried about remembering to take the medicines on a regular basis, it is a warning sign to the nurse that the client may be at risk for noncompliance. The nurse needs to discuss strategies to help the client establish a new routine such as using digital reminders, integrating medications into a daily routine, and utilizing family support systems when available. Understanding when to relax and the side effects of medicines are positive findings. Choosing not to listen to a family member's negative beliefs about medication is also a positive finding.

🗝️ CN: Psychosocial integrity; CL: Evaluate

140. 2. The nurse should teach the client how to do isometric exercise, which is the contraction of the quadriceps muscle without movement of joint, to maintain muscle strength. The physical therapy team may assist the client later and will then teach the client how to do active exercises and crutch walking if prescribed. The client will be able to move the unaffected limb; the family will not need to assist. If the client will be using crutches, building upper extremity strength will be helpful, but the immediate need is to maintain and develop strength in the quadriceps.

🗝️ CN: Health promotion; CL: Analyze

141. 3. Urine output should be at least 500 mL in 24 hours (20 mL/h); this client's output has been just 15 mL/h for the past 2 hours requiring further assessment by the nurse. The nurse should first assess all clients and address physiological needs including pain control and safety measures; the nurse should then take time with the client having difficulty coping in order to listen and further determine the client's needs.

🗝️ CN: Management of care; CL: Analyze

142.

	Actions to Take	Potential Conditions	Parameters to Monitor
0/1	Administer nebulizer treatment	Airway obstruction	Cough
	Perform chest physiotherapy		Breath sounds

Clients with cystic fibrosis have tenacious mucus in the lungs that is difficult to expel, leading to lung infections. The history, elevated respiratory rate, rhonchi, diminished breath sounds, and nonproductive cough most indicate the client has obstructed airways. Absent breath sounds on one side are more consistent with a pneumothorax. Increased coughing is typically seen with reactive airways or pulmonary edema. The priority interventions are to perform chest physiotherapy and to give nebulizer treatments, which can help dilate bronchi and thin secretions. Diuretics, chest tubes, and intubation are not indicated. The nurse should monitor the cough and breath sounds to determine the effectiveness of the interventions. The child already has a normal oxygenation status, so pulse oximetry or blood gas is not the best indicator of treatment effectiveness. While chest x-rays can help confirm a diagnosis of pneumonia, they have limited use when trying to manage the ongoing problem of ineffective airway clearance in clients with cystic fibrosis

🗝️ CJ: Standalone bowtie; CL: Create

143. 1. The stationary bicycle is the most appropriate training modality because it is a non–weight-bearing exercise. The time that the individual exercises on the stationary bicycle is increased with improved functional capacity. The other exercise equipment requires exercising while standing.

🗝️ CN: Health promotion and maintenance; CL: Analyze

144. 1. The nurse should closely monitor the client admitted with an elevated blood alcohol level for several hours for signs and symptoms of withdrawal, administering sedation as needed; delirium tremens, the most severe form of withdrawal, usually peaks at 48 to 72 hours following the last drink. The client with the chest tube is not in any distress and has no pressing needs. For an older client who has had GI bleeding, a hemoglobin level of 13.8 g/dL (138 g/L) is within normal limits. After assessing all the clients' needs, the nurse will prepare the client who had an appendectomy for discharge as soon as possible.

🗝️ CN: Reduction of risk potential; CL: Analyze

145. 1. Fetal alcohol syndrome is characterized by central nervous system damage, poor growth, and specific facial stigmata. As many as 90% of children with fetal alcohol syndrome have eye abnormalities. Congenital syphilis is more frequently associated with preterm birth, and tetracycline use is associated with dental abnormalities. Folic acid deficiency contributes to neural tube defects.

🗝️ CN: Reduction of risk potential; CL: Analyze

146. 2. Therapeutic serum drug monitoring is not routinely done with ciprofloxacin. This medicine should not be taken with dairy products or other significant sources of calcium such as collard greens, calcium supplements, calcium carbonate antacids, or calcium-fortified juice. Clients may take a missed dose as soon as they remember. If it is very close to the time of the next dose, the missed dose should be omitted. The client should not take a double dose.

🗝️ CN: Pharmacological and parenteral therapies; CL: Evaluate

147. 3. Physical activity is gradually increased after a myocardial infarction while the client is still hospitalized and through a period of rehabilitation. The client is progressing too rapidly if activity significantly changes respirations, causing dyspnea, chest pain, a rapid heartbeat, or fatigue. When any of these symptoms appear, the client should reduce activity and progress more slowly. Edema suggests a circulatory problem that must be addressed but does not necessarily indicate overexertion. Cyanosis indicates a reduced oxygen-carrying capacity of red blood cells and indicates a severe pathology. It is not appropriate to use cyanosis as an indicator of overexertion. Weight loss indicates several factors but not overexertion.

🗝️ CN: Reduction of risk potential; CL: Analyze

148. 4. The most common noninfectious renal disease in children is acute poststreptococcal glomerulonephritis. Ensuring that children diagnosed with streptococcal infections complete a full course of antibiotics will decrease their risk for developing acute glomerulonephritis. Parents should contact the primary HCP if they suspect a UTI; however, glomerulonephritis is not caused by a UTI. Glomerulonephritis is not a genetic disease, and it is not contagious.

🗝️ CN: Reduction of risk potential; CL: Apply

149. -/+ **2, 3, 5.** The client who is taking disulfiram is advised to avoid all forms of alcohol, including beer, communal wine at church, and cough syrup; these can trigger a serious physical reaction. Aged cheeses and chocolate are to be avoided by the client taking monoamine oxidase inhibitors.

🗝️ CN: Pharmacological and parenteral therapies; CL: Apply

150. -/+ **1, 4, 5.** As noted on the progress record, the increasing heart rate, increasing systolic blood pressure, and decreasing diastolic blood pressure along with the decreased urine output indicate the client is going into hemorrhagic shock. The nurse should anticipate that the health care provider will order epinephrine to increase the client's blood pressure and will increase the rate of the intravenous infusion rate to manage hypovolemia. The health care provider will likely also order a second intravenous infusion line to administer lactated Ringer's solution to counteract the acidosis caused by fluid loss. Ultimately, the client may need packed red blood cells, but the health care provider will obtain the results of a complete blood count first.

🗝️ CJ: Standalone trend; CL: Analyze

Comprehensive Test

This test has 85 questions. Time yourself as you take the test so you can determine the approximate amount of time it takes to complete this many questions. This test reflects the minimum number of questions you might receive on the actual licensing exam.

1. A primigravid client at 26 weeks' gestation asks the nurse what causes heartburn during pregnancy. The nurse should explain to the client that heartburn during pregnancy is usually caused by which factor?
   - ☐ 1. increased peristaltic action during pregnancy
   - ☐ 2. displacement of the stomach by the diaphragm
   - ☐ 3. decreased secretion of hydrochloric acid
   - ☐ 4. backflow of stomach contents into the esophagus

2. A 4-year-old child is admitted for cardiac catheterization. Which is **most** important to include as the nurse teaches this child about cardiac catheterization?
   - ☐ 1. a plastic model of the heart
   - ☐ 2. a catheter that will be inserted into the artery
   - ☐ 3. the child's parents
   - ☐ 4. other children undergoing a catheterization

3. The nurse is caring for a newborn who is experiencing opioid withdrawal. To calm the infant, the nurse should include which interventions in the plan of care? Select all that apply.
   - ☐ 1. Swaddle the infant in a blanket.
   - ☐ 2. Use slow vertical rocking.
   - ☐ 3. Dim lighting around the crib.
   - ☐ 4. Provide fast-tempo music.
   - ☐ 5. Plan care around infant cues.

4. The nurse receives a report on four infants (see graphic). Which infant should the nurse see **first**?

Baby	Age	Gestational Age	Last Vital Signs/All Were Taken 15 Minutes Ago	Last Feeding	Additional Comments
A	30 minutes old	40 weeks	Temperature (T) = 97.3°F (36.3°C) Heart rate = 120 bpm Respiratory rate = 56 breaths/min	Not fed yet	No labs have been drawn
B	24 hours old	35 weeks	T = 97.7°F (36.5°C) Heart rate = 164 bpm Respiratory rate = 48 breaths/min	3 hours ago	Glucose 45 mg/dL (2.5 mmol/L) 30 minutes ago [Reference range, day 2: ≥45 mg/dL (2.5 mmol/L)]
C	48 hours old	36 weeks	T = 98.4°F (36.9°C) Heart rate = 146 bpm Respiratory rate = 38 breaths/min	4 hours ago	Bilirubin level of 5 mg/dL (85.5 µmol/L) 24 hours ago [Reference range, day 2: <10 mg/dL (171.0 mmol/L)]
D	72 hours old	37 weeks	T = 99.5°F (37.5°C) Heart rate = 110 Respiratory rate = 40 breaths/min	5 hours ago	Needs hearing screen before discharge in 1 hour

   - ☐ 1. A, 30 minutes 40 weeks
   - ☐ 2. B, 24 hours 35 weeks
   - ☐ 3. C, 48 hours 36 weeks
   - ☐ 4. D, 72 hours 37 weeks

5. The nurse is assessing the home care needs of a group of clients. Which client(s) qualify for home care services? Select all that apply.
The client:
- ☐ 1. requiring monitoring of prothrombin time due to (warfarin) therapy
- ☐ 2. needing additional instruction about preparing food in a low-sodium diet
- ☐ 3. who has episodes of vertigo that result in falls
- ☐ 4. who has multiple sclerosis with an open, draining lesion on the foot
- ☐ 5. who needs stronger lenses for glasses

6. The nursing staff has finished restraining a combative client. In addition to determining whether anyone was injured, the staff is mandated to evaluate the incident to obtain which outcome?
- ☐ 1. Coordinate documentation of the incident.
- ☐ 2. Resolve negative feelings and attitudes.
- ☐ 3. Improve the use of restraint procedures.
- ☐ 4. Calm down before returning to the other clients.

7. Two parents who are arguing in their infant's room, with voices raised and getting louder, start to hit each other. The infant is crying. Which action should the staff nurse take **next**?
- ☐ 1. Try to reason with both of the parents.
- ☐ 2. Ask one of the parents to leave the room.
- ☐ 3. Call security to come and break up the fight.
- ☐ 4. Remove the infant from the room.

8. A 2-month-old infant is at risk for an ileus after surgery to correct intussusception. What should be included in a focused assessment for this complication? Select all that apply.
- ☐ 1. measurement of urine specific gravity
- ☐ 2. assessment of bowel sounds
- ☐ 3. characteristics of the first stool
- ☐ 4. measurement of gastric output
- ☐ 5. bilirubin levels

9. A nurse is assessing a client with a history of myocardial infarction who is in the surgical unit following gastric resection. The client has chest pains. The nurse obtains the electrocardiogram (ECG) shown (see figure). What should the nurse do **first**?

- ☐ 1. Administer oxygen.
- ☐ 2. Inspect the client's incision.
- ☐ 3. Call the rapid response team.
- ☐ 4. Reposition the ECG electrodes.

10. | STEP 1

The nurse is caring for a 72-year-old male client in the emergency department (ED).

Nurse's Notes

Today: 1000
The client's spouse reports finding the client clutching their chest and short of breath while shoveling snow about 45 minutes ago. The client has a history of hypertension and hypercholesterolemia. The client has chest pain rated an 8 on a 0 to 10 scale. The pain radiates to the left shoulder and left jaw. Vital signs are temperature (T) 98.9°F (37.2°C); pulse (P) 120 bpm; respiration rate (RR) 24 breaths/min; and blood pressure (BP) 162/98 mm Hg. The pulse oximetry reading is 91% on room air. Upon assessment, the client is cool, diaphoretic, and short of breath. The lungs are clear, and capillary refill is 3 seconds. The client is alert and oriented to person, place, and time.

▶ Highlight the client findings that would require follow-up. Answer choices have been underlined.

Nurse's Notes

Today: 1000
The client's spouse reports finding the client clutching their chest and short of breath while shoveling snow about 45 minutes ago. The client has a history of hypertension and hypercholesterolemia. The client has <u>chest pain rated an 8 on a 0 to 10 scale</u>. The <u>pain radiates to the left shoulder and left jaw</u>. Vital signs are temperature (T) 98.9°F (37.2°C); <u>pulse (P) 120 bpm</u>; <u>respiration rate (RR) 24 breaths/min</u>; and <u>blood pressure (BP) 162/98 mm Hg</u>. <u>The pulse oximetry reading is 91% on room air</u>. Upon assessment, the <u>client is cool</u>, <u>diaphoretic</u>, and short of breath. The lungs are clear, and <u>capillary refill is 3 seconds</u>. The client is alert and oriented to person, place, and time.

11. STEP 2

The nurse is caring for a 72-year-old male client in the ED. The nurse obtains updated assessment data on the client.

Nurse's Notes

Today: 1000
The client's spouse reports finding the client clutching their chest and short of breath while shoveling snow about 45 minutes ago. The client has a history of hypertension and hypercholesterolemia. The client has chest pain rated an 8 on a 0 to 10 scale. The pain radiates to the left shoulder and left jaw. Vital signs are temperature (T) 98.9°F (37.2°C); pulse (P) 120 bpm; respiration rate (RR) 24 breaths/min; and blood pressure (BP) 162/98 mm Hg. The pulse oximetry reading is 91% on room air. Upon assessment, the client is cool, diaphoretic, and short of breath. The lungs are clear, and capillary refill is 3 seconds. The client is alert and oriented to person, place, and time.

Today: 1015
The client continues to have chest pain rated an 8 and radiating to the left shoulder and left jaw. Vital signs are T 98.9°F (37.2°C); P 126 bpm; RR 26 breaths/min; BP 174/98 mm Hg; and pulse oximetry reading of 90% on room air. Telemetry shows sinus tachycardia with ST elevation.

➢ For each finding below, specify if the finding is consistent with the disease process of myocardial infarction, pneumonia, or pulmonary embolism. Each finding may support more than one disease process.

Client Finding	Myocardial Infarction	Pneumonia	Pulmonary Embolism
1. Chest pain	☐	☐	☐
2. Tachycardia	☐	☐	☐
3. Shortness of breath	☐	☐	☐
4. Hypoxemia	☐	☐	☐
5. Hypertension	☐	☐	☐
6. Rhythm strip of sinus tachycardia with ST elevation	☐	☐	☐

Note: Each column must have at least one response option selected.

12. STEP 3

Nurse's Notes

Today: 1000
The client's spouse reports finding the client clutching their chest and short of breath while shoveling snow about 45 minutes ago. The client has a history of hypertension and hypercholesterolemia. The client has chest pain rated an 8 on a 0 to 10 scale. The pain radiates to the left shoulder and left jaw. Vital signs are temperature (T) 98.9°F (37.2°C); pulse (P) 120 bpm; respiration rate (RR) 24 breaths/min; and blood pressure (BP) 162/98 mm Hg. The pulse oximetry reading is 91% on room air. Upon assessment, the client is cool, diaphoretic, and short of breath. The lungs are clear, and capillary refill is 3 seconds. The client is alert and oriented to person, place, and time.

Today: 1015
The client continues to have chest pain rated an 8 and radiating to the left shoulder and left jaw. Vital signs are T 98.9°F (37.2°C); P 126 bpm; RR 26 breaths/min; BP 174/98 mm Hg; and pulse oximetry reading of 90% on room air. Telemetry shows sinus tachycardia with ST elevation.

➢ Identify the anticipated health care provider order(s). Select all that apply.

- ☐ 1. Obtain a 12-lead ECG.
- ☐ 2. Obtain a spiral computed tomography (CT) scan of the chest.
- ☐ 3. Obtain lab tests: cardiac enzymes.
- ☐ 4. Start intravenous (IV) dextrose 5% in water (D5W).
- ☐ 5. Start oxygen at 2 L per nasal cannula.
- ☐ 6. Give sublingual nitroglycerin every 5 minutes up to three times as needed (PRN).

13. STEP 4

The nurse is caring for a 72-year-old male client in the cardiac care unit (CCU).

Nurse's Notes

Today: 1000
The client's spouse reports finding the client clutching their chest and short of breath while shoveling snow about 45 minutes ago. The client has a history of hypertension and hypercholesterolemia. The client has chest pain rated an 8 on a 0 to 10 scale. The pain radiates to the left shoulder and left jaw. Vital signs are temperature (T) 98.9°F (37.2°C); pulse (P) 120 bpm; respiration rate (RR) 24 breaths/min; and blood pressure (BP) 162/98 mm Hg. The pulse oximetry reading is 91% on room air. Upon assessment, the client is cool, diaphoretic, and short of breath. The lungs are clear, and capillary refill is 3 seconds. The client is alert and oriented to person, place, and time.

Today: 1015
The client continues to have chest pain rated an 8 and radiating to the left shoulder and left jaw. Vital signs are T 98.9°F (37.2°C); P 126 bpm; RR 26 breaths/min; BP 174/98 mm Hg; and pulse oximetry reading of 90% on room air. Telemetry shows sinus tachycardia with ST elevation.

Today: 1500
The client has been admitted to the CCU after receiving a drug-eluting stent in the mid-anterior descending artery. Vital signs are T 97°F (36.1°C); P 110 bpm; RR 24 breaths/min; and BP 140/88 mm Hg. Pulse oximetry reading is 93% on room air. Telemetry shows normal sinus rhythm. A stent was inserted via the right groin; the dressing is dry and intact. Pedal pulses are present in both legs. An IV infusion of normal saline is infusing at 125 gtts per minute. The client reports they do not have chest pain. The client voided 200 mL of clear urine. The spouse is visiting.

The nurse has reviewed the Nurse's Notes from 1500 and is planning care for the client.

➤ Which action(s) should be included in the care plan? Select all that apply.

- ☐ 1. Inspect the stent insertion site for bleeding.
- ☐ 2. Increase the IV infusion to 150 gtts per minute.
- ☐ 3. Request an order for nasal oxygen.
- ☐ 4. Request a prescription for an antihypertensive drug.
- ☐ 5. Position the client in the semi-Fowler position.
- ☐ 6. Discuss plans for discharge with the client and spouse.
- ☐ 7. Catheterize the client for residual urine.

14. STEP 5

Nurse's Notes

Day 1: 1000
The client's spouse reports finding the client clutching their chest and short of breath while shoveling snow about 45 minutes ago. The client has a history of hypertension and hypercholesterolemia. The client has chest pain rated an 8 on a 0 to 10 scale. The pain radiates to the left shoulder and left jaw. Vital signs are temperature (T) 98.9°F (37.2°C); pulse (P) 120 bpm; respiration rate (RR) 24 breaths/min; and blood pressure (BP) 162/98 mm Hg. The pulse oximetry reading is 91% on room air. Upon assessment, the client is cool, diaphoretic, and short of breath. The lungs are clear, and capillary refill is 3 seconds. The client is alert and oriented to person, place, and time.

Day 1: 1015
The client continues to have chest pain rated an 8 and radiating to the left shoulder and left jaw. Vital signs are T 98.9°F (37.2°C); P 126 bpm; RR 26 breaths/min; BP 174/98 mm Hg; and pulse oximetry reading of 90% on room air. Telemetry shows sinus tachycardia with ST elevation.

Day 1: 1500
The client has been admitted to the CCU after receiving a drug-eluting stent in the mid-anterior descending artery. Vital signs are T 97°F (36.1°C); P 110 bpm; RR 24 breaths/min; and BP 140/88 mm Hg. Pulse oximetry reading is 93% on room air. Telemetry shows normal sinus rhythm. A stent was inserted via the right groin; the dressing is dry and intact. Pedal pulses are present in both legs. An IV infusion of normal saline is infusing at 125 gtts per minute. The client reports they do not have chest pain. The client voided 200 mL of clear urine. The spouse is visiting.

Day 2: 0800
The client slept most of the night. Vital signs are T 98.6°F (37°C); P 90 bpm; RR 22 breaths/min; and BP 140/86 mm Hg. The pulse oximetry reading is 94% on room air. Telemetry shows normal sinus rhythm. The stent site dressing is dry. Pedal pulses are present in both legs. The client denies having chest pain. The health care provider told the client they will be discharged today.

Orders

Today 0930	Discharge to home
	Metoprolol XL 100 mg daily
	Clopidogrel 75 mg daily
	One baby aspirin daily
	Nitroglycerin 0.6 mg tablet – 1 sublingual every 5 minutes up to three times PRN
	Lovastatin 20 mg daily
	Cimetidine 200 mg daily
	Start on a heart-healthy diet
	Schedule cardiac rehabilitation follow-up

The nurse receives the health care provider's discharge orders.

➤ When developing a discharge teaching plan, the nurse should include which instruction(s)? Select all that apply.

☐ 1. Tell the client to have 30 minutes of rigorous exercise 5 days each week.
☐ 2. Discuss differences between stable and unstable angina.
☐ 3. Instruct how to take nitroglycerin.
☐ 4. Explain the use and side effects of the calcium channel blocker.
☐ 5. Explain the beta-blocker medication.
☐ 6. Instruct how to take the anticoagulant.
☐ 7. Remind the client to take 324 mg of baby aspirin daily.
☐ 8. Tell the client how to take the proton pump inhibitor.
☐ 9. Ensure the client understands what is included in a heart-healthy diet.

15. STEP 6

Nurse's Notes

Day 1: 1000
The client's spouse reports finding the client clutching their chest and short of breath while shoveling snow about 45 minutes ago. The client has a history of hypertension and hypercholesterolemia. The client has chest pain rated an 8 on a 0 to 10 scale. The pain radiates to the left shoulder and left jaw. Vital signs are temperature (T) 98.9°F (37.2°C); pulse (P) 120 bpm; respiration rate (RR) 24 breaths/min; and blood pressure (BP) 162/98 mm Hg. The pulse oximetry reading is 91% on room air. Upon assessment, the client is cool, diaphoretic, and short of breath. The lungs are clear, and capillary refill is 3 seconds. The client is alert and oriented to person, place, and time.

Day 1: 1015
The client continues to have chest pain rated an 8 and radiating to the left shoulder and left jaw. Vital signs are T 98.9°F (37.2°C); P 126 bpm; RR 26 breaths/min; BP 174/98 mm Hg; and pulse oximetry reading of 90% on room air. Telemetry shows sinus tachycardia with ST elevation.

Day 1: 1500
The client has been admitted to the CCU after receiving a drug-eluting stent in the mid-anterior descending artery. Vital signs are T 97°F (36.1°C); P 110 bpm; RR 24 breaths/min; and BP 140/88 mm Hg. Pulse oximetry reading is 93% on room air. Telemetry shows normal sinus rhythm. A stent was inserted via the right groin; the dressing is dry and intact. Pedal pulses are present in both legs. An IV infusion of normal saline is infusing at 125 gtts per minute. The client reports they do not have chest pain. The client voided 200 mL of clear urine. The spouse is visiting.

Day 2: 0800
The client slept most of the night. Vital signs are T 98.6°F (37°C); P 90 bpm; RR 22 breaths/min; and BP 140/86 mm Hg. Pulse oximetry reading is 94% on room air. Telemetry shows normal sinus rhythm. The stent site dressing is dry. Pedal pulses are present in both legs. The client denies having chest pain. The health care provider told the client they will be discharged today.

Orders

Today 1130	Discharge to home
	Metoprolol XL 100 mg daily
	Clopidogrel 75 mg daily
	One baby aspirin daily
	Nitroglycerin 0.6 mg tablet – 1 sublingual every 5 minutes up to three times PRN
	Lovastatin 20 mg daily
	Cimetidine 200 mg daily
	Start on a heart-healthy diet
	Schedule cardiac rehabilitation follow-up

The nurse is caring for a client in the CCU. On the client's third day in the unit, the nurse is evaluating if the client understands how to take the nitroglycerine.

➤ Which statement(s) indicate the client knows how to use the nitroglycerine? Select all that apply.

The client will:

- ☐ 1. sit down before taking the nitroglycerin.
- ☐ 2. not take nitroglycerin if it tastes bitter.
- ☐ 3. take the nitroglycerin with a glass of water.
- ☐ 4. hold the nitroglycerine under the tongue until it is absorbed.
- ☐ 5. take a second nitroglycerine tablet if they do not obtain pain relief within 5 minutes.
- ☐ 6. call 911 if they continue to have chest pain after taking the second tablet.

16. Several clients have been admitted to the emergency department. The nurse should assess these clients in which order from first to last? All options must be used.
The client who is:

| 1. 12 years of age with a fractured tibia |
| 2. 8 years of age with small lacerations to legs and arms |
| 3. 16 years of age with a "sore throat" |
| 4. 6 months of age with diarrhea and dehydration |
| |
| |
| |
| |

17. Which urine output indicates that a 5-month-old weighing 15 lb (6.8 kg) and being treated for dehydration has a normal urine output?
☐ 1. 1 to 2 mL/kg per hour
☐ 2. 4 to 5 mL/kg per hour
☐ 3. 6 to 8 mL/kg per hour
☐ 4. 10 to 12 mL/kg per hour

18. A client has undergone a vasectomy. The nurse instructs the client that they can begin having unprotected intercourse at what time following the surgery?
☐ 1. when desired because sterilization is immediate
☐ 2. as soon as scrotal edema and tenderness resolve
☐ 3. when the sperm count reflects sterilization
☐ 4. after 6 to 10 ejaculations

19. A client is admitted to the hospital with a diagnosis of suspected pulmonary embolism. Prescriptions include oxygen 2 to 4 L per minute per nasal cannula, oximetry at all times, and intravenous (IV) administration of 5% dextrose in water at 100 mL per hour. The client has increasing dyspnea and has a respiratory rate of 32 breaths/min. The oxygen flow rate is set at 2 L per minute. What should the nurse do **first**?
☐ 1. Increase the oxygen flow rate from 2 to 4 L per minute.
☐ 2. Call the health care provider (HCP) immediately.
☐ 3. Provide reassurance to the client.
☐ 4. Obtain a sample for arterial blood gas analysis.

20. A 10-month-old child has cold symptoms. The birth parent asks how they can clear the infant's nose. What would be the nurse's **best** recommendation?
☐ 1. Use a cool air vaporizer with plain water.
☐ 2. Use saline nose drops and then a bulb syringe.
☐ 3. Blow into the child's mouth to clear the infant's nose.
☐ 4. Administer a nonprescription vasoconstrictive nose spray.

21. A health care provider (HCP) is calling the pediatric unit and asking the nurse to go into the medical record for the test results of a fellow pediatrician. How should the nurse respond to this request?
☐ 1. Verify that the caller is the HCP of record or has a need to know.
☐ 2. Access the medical record, and give the HCP the test results.
☐ 3. Decline to give the HCP the information requested.
☐ 4. Determine whether the nurse can access the medical record.

22. Which finding should **first** alert the nurse that a child is hemorrhaging after a tonsillectomy?
☐ 1. mouth breathing
☐ 2. frequent swallowing
☐ 3. requests for a drink
☐ 4. increased pulse rate

23. The nursing staff on the antepartum unit has leuprolide acetate and medroxyprogesterone acetate in the pharmacy for their clients. The nursing staff observed that the vials are similar in size and shape and could be confused. To promote client safety, the nursing staff should take which action(s)? Select all that apply.
☐ 1. Petition the pharmacy to relocate one drug away from the other product.
☐ 2. Move the drugs to a new position within the medication administration system during the night shift.
☐ 3. Communicate concerns, measures to remedy, and final decisions to all staff.
☐ 4. Leave repositioning of drugs to pharmacy staff to resolve.
☐ 5. Collaborate with pharmacy staff to develop a location that works well for both groups.

24. An adolescent client is hospitalized with bacterial meningitis. At 1730, the client's parent reports their child is "burning up." The nurse is reviewing the client's medication administration records in the medical record.

Medication	Time	Reason	Initial
Ibuprofen 200 mg orally (PO) as needed (PRN) every 3 to 4 hours for a temperature (T) higher than 99°F (37.2°C)	0910	T 100°F (37.8°C)	LM
	1315	T 100°F (37.8°C)	LM
	1615	T 101°F (38.3°C)	LM

The health care provider (HCP) has prescribed ibuprofen 325 mg every 3 to 4 hours for a temperature over 99°F (37.2°C). The child's temperature at 1730 is 102.5°F (39.1°C). What should the nurse do **first**?
☐ 1. Notify the HCP.
☐ 2. Initiate a tepid sponge bath.
☐ 3. Institute seizure precautions.
☐ 4. Administer another dose of ibuprofen.

25. The nurse from the postanesthesia care unit (PACU) is transferring a client to an orthopedic unit. Which is the **most** appropriate way for the nurse in the PACU to communicate the "hand-off-of-care" report with the nurse on the orthopedic unit?
☐ 1. Send an email to the receiving nurse on the orthopedic unit.
☐ 2. Give a written report to a transporter who is bringing the client to the receiving nurse.
☐ 3. Call the nurse on the orthopedic unit and give a verbal report.
☐ 4. Send the unit clerk from PACU to give the prescription list directly to the nurse on the orthopedic unit.

26. Which response would be **most** appropriate for the nurse when comforting a primiparous client whose critically ill neonate born at 25 weeks dies while the birth parent is present?
☐ 1. "This is probably for the best because the baby's organs were so immature."
☐ 2. "You should try to get pregnant again soon to get over this loss."
☐ 3. "You can stay with your baby as long as you want and say anything you want."
☐ 4. "If you want me to, I can call the chaplain to stay with you."

27. The nurse is developing a care plan for a female child who is 12 years of age and receiving surgery to correct idiopathic scoliosis. Which postoperative problem is a **priority**?
☐ 1. pain control
☐ 2. hypotension
☐ 3. prevention of pressure wounds
☐ 4. infection control

28. The nurse teaches a client taking desmopressin nasal spray about how to manage treatment. The nurse determines that the client needs additional instruction when the client makes which comment?
☐ 1. "I should check for sores in my nose while taking this medication."
☐ 2. "I should use the same nostril each time I take the medicine."
☐ 3. "I should report nasal congestion."
☐ 4. "I should report any signs of respiratory infection."

29. A nurse is assessing a client who is receiving clozapine. The nurse reviews the medical record. What should the nurse do **next**?

Vital Signs		
Date Time	06/12 0800	06/12 1200
Temperature	98°F (36.7°C)	98°F (36.7°C)
Pulse	140	148
Respirations	22	24
Blood pressure	120/80 mm Hg	122/84 mm Hg

☐ 1. Administer the clozapine, and tell the client to lie down.
☐ 2. Withhold the clozapine, and tell the client to go to an exercise group.
☐ 3. Administer the clozapine, and notify the health care provider (HCP).
☐ 4. Withhold the clozapine, and notify the HCP.

30. When fluids by mouth are appropriate for the infant after surgery to correct intussusception, the nurse **most** likely would initiate which type of feeding?
☐ 1. cereal-thickened formula
☐ 2. full-strength formula
☐ 3. half-strength formula
☐ 4. oral electrolyte solution

31. The rapid response team arrives in the room of a client who has had a cardiac arrest. The nurse on the team should **first** apply which piece of monitoring equipment?
☐ 1. electrocardiogram (ECG) electrodes
☐ 2. pulse oximeter
☐ 3. blood pressure cuff
☐ 4. Doppler pulse detection unit

32. The nurse is assessing a client for heroin addiction. Which finding indicates the client has used heroin?
- ☐ 1. sclera red and bloodshot
- ☐ 2. pupils small and constricted
- ☐ 3. pupils large and dilated
- ☐ 4. drooping eyelids

33. Which action is **most** important when the nurse is planning pain management for a client after a lobectomy for lung cancer?
- ☐ 1. repositioning the client immediately after administering pain medication
- ☐ 2. reassessing the client after administering pain medication
- ☐ 3. reassuring the client after administering pain medication
- ☐ 4. readjusting the pain medication dosage as needed

34. STEP 1

The nurse cares for a 4-year-old male client brought to the clinic with a rash.

History

The parent reports the client has not been feeling well for 2 days. This morning, the client developed itchy blisters over their trunk and in their mouth. The client now does not want to drink. The client has a history of a systolic murmur and atrial septal defect (ASD) repair with closure at 2 years of age. The client has done well since and is not on any routine medications. The other parent was deployed overseas 6 months ago, and the client goes to a babysitter full-time. There are three other children in the family, all under the age of 10. The parent is unsure of their immunization status.

Vital signs are temperature 103°F (39.5°C); heart rate 120 bpm; respiration rate 30 breaths/min; and blood pressure 100/50 mm Hg. The client weighs 36 lb (16.3 kg).

➢ What finding(s) are **most** important for the nurse to follow up on? Select all that apply.
- ☐ 1. Temperature
- ☐ 2. Heart rate
- ☐ 3. Respiratory rate
- ☐ 4. Blood pressure
- ☐ 5. Rash
- ☐ 6. Atrial septal defect
- ☐ 7. Fluid intake
- ☐ 8. Immunization status

35. STEP 2

The nurse cares for a 4-year-old male client brought to the clinic with a rash.

History

The parent reports the client has not been feeling well for 2 days. This morning, the client developed itchy blisters over their trunk and in their mouth. The client now does not want to drink. The client has a history of a systolic murmur and atrial septal defect (ASD) repair with closure at 2 years of age. The client has done well since and is not on any routine medications. The other parent was deployed overseas 6 months ago, and the client goes to a babysitter full-time. There are three other children in the family, all under the age of 10. The parent is unsure of their immunization status.

Vital signs are temperature 103°F (39.5°C); heart rate 120 bpm; respiration rate 30 breaths/min; and blood pressure 100/50 mm Hg. The client weighs 36 lb (16.3 kg).

Nurse's Notes

Multiple pruritic papular and vesicular lesions are noted over the body, centered at the trunk. Additional papular lesions are on the palate and oral mucosa. No lesions are present on the hands or face. The client is lethargic but cooperative. Mucous membranes are sticky. Skin is warm to touch, and capillary refill is less than 2 seconds. There is no tenting.

Immunization records indicate one varicella and one measles, mumps, and rubella vaccine. Other immunizations are up to date.

➢ Complete the following sentence from the list of drop-down options.

Pruritic, popular, and vesicular rashes are characteristic findings with [measles / rubella / varicella],

which is primarily spread by a/an [airborne / contact / droplet] mode of transmission.

36. STEP 3

The nurse cares for a 4-year-old male client brought to the clinic with a rash.

History

The parent reports the client has not been feeling well for 2 days. This morning, the client developed itchy blisters over their trunk and in their mouth. The client now does not want to drink. The client has a history of a systolic murmur and atrial septal defect (ASD) repair with closure at 2 years of age. The client has done well since and is not on any routine medications. The other parent was deployed overseas 6 months ago, and the client goes to a babysitter full-time. There are three other children in the family, all under the age of 10. The parent is unsure of their immunization status.

Vital signs are temperature 103°F (39.5°C); heart rate 120 bpm; respiration rate 30 breaths/min; and blood pressure 100/50 mm Hg. The client weighs 36 lb (16.3 kg).

Nurse's Notes

Multiple pruritic papular and vesicular lesions are noted over the body, centered at the trunk. Additional papular lesions are on the palate and oral mucosa. No lesions are present on the hands or face. The client is lethargic but cooperative. Mucous membranes are sticky. Skin is warm to touch, and capillary refill is less than 2 seconds. There is no tenting.

Immunization records indicate one varicella and one measles, mumps, and rubella vaccine. Other immunizations are up to date.

➤ The client receives a diagnosis of varicella. Which two complications are the child **most** at risk for developing?

- ☐ 1. dehydration
- ☐ 2. meningitis
- ☐ 3. pneumonia
- ☐ 4. skin infection
- ☐ 5. seizures

37. STEP 4

The nurse cares for a 4-year-old male client brought to the clinic with a rash.

History

The parent reports the client has not been feeling well for 2 days. This morning, the client developed itchy blisters over their trunk and in their mouth. The client now does not want to drink. The client has a history of a systolic murmur and atrial septal defect (ASD) repair with closure at 2 years of age. The client has done well since and is not on any routine medications. The other parent was deployed overseas 6 months ago, and the client goes to a babysitter full-time. There are three other children in the family, all under the age of 10. The parent is unsure of their immunization status.

Vital signs are temperature 103°F (39.5°C); heart rate 120 bpm; respiration rate 30 breaths/min; and blood pressure 100/50 mm Hg. The client weighs 36 lb (16.3 kg).

Nurse's Notes

Multiple pruritic papular and vesicular lesions are noted over the body, centered at the trunk. Additional papular lesions are on the palate and oral mucosa. No lesions are present on the hands or face. The client is lethargic but cooperative. Mucous membranes are sticky. Skin is warm to touch, and capillary refill is less than 2 seconds. There is no tenting.

Immunization records indicate one varicella and one measles, mumps, and rubella vaccine. Other immunizations are up to date.

➤ The nurse speaks with the health care provider about the treatment plan for a child with chickenpox. Which medication(s) should be included in the plan of care? Select all that apply.

- ☐ 1. nonsteroidal anti-inflammatory drugs
- ☐ 2. antihistamine medications
- ☐ 3. acetaminophen
- ☐ 4. antibiotics
- ☐ 5. calamine lotion
- ☐ 6. varicella vaccine

38. STEP 5

The nurse cares for a 4-year-old male client brought to the clinic with a rash.

History

The parent reports the client has not been feeling well for 2 days. This morning, the client developed itchy blisters over their trunk and in their mouth. The client now does not want to drink. The client has a history of a systolic murmur and atrial septal defect (ASD) repair with closure at 2 years of age. The client has done well since and is not on any routine medications. The other parent was deployed overseas 6 months ago, and the client goes to a babysitter full-time. There are three other children in the family, all under the age of 10. The parent is unsure of their immunization status.

Vital signs are temperature 103°F (39.5°C); heart rate 120 bpm; respiration rate 30 breaths/min; and blood pressure 100/50 mm Hg. The client weighs 36 lb (16.3 kg).

Nurse's Notes

Multiple pruritic papular and vesicular lesions are noted over the body, centered at the trunk. Additional papular lesions are on the palate and oral mucosa. No lesions are present on the hands or face. The client is lethargic but cooperative. Mucous membranes are sticky. Skin is warm to touch, and capillary refill is less than 2 seconds. There is no tenting.

Immunization records indicate one varicella and one measles, mumps, and rubella vaccine. Other immunizations are up to date.

Orders

1. Administer over-the-counter (OTC) acetaminophen as needed (PRN) for fever or pain.
2. Provide OTC diphenhydramine PRN for itching.
3. Give oatmeal baths PRN.
4. Apply calamine lotion two to three times a day until the lesions heal.
5. Encourage adequate oral intake.
6. Keep the child home until all the rash has crusted.
7. Contact the health care provider's office if the client's condition deteriorates.

➢ The health care provider has made a diagnosis of varicella for the 4-year-old client and written orders. What other action(s) should the nurse take before sending the client home from the clinic? Select all that apply.

☐ 1. Contact the daycare center about the exposure.
☐ 2. Determine the varicella risk for other family members.
☐ 3. Ensure the child will take fluids.
☐ 4. Teach parents about OTC medications to avoid.
☐ 5. Schedule a return appointment in 3 days.

39. **STEP 6**

The nurse cares for a 4-year-old male client brought to the clinic with a rash.

History

The parent reports the client has not been feeling well for 2 days. This morning, the client developed itchy blisters over their trunk and in their mouth. The client now does not want to drink. The client has a history of a systolic murmur and atrial septal defect (ASD) repair with closure at 2 years of age. The client has done well since and is not on any routine medications. The other parent was deployed overseas 6 months ago, and the client goes to a babysitter full-time. There are three other children in the family, all under the age of 10. The parent is unsure of their immunization status.

Vital signs are temperature 103°F (39.5°C); heart rate 120 bpm; respiration rate 30 breaths/min; and blood pressure 100/50 mm Hg. The client weighs 36 lb (16.3 kg).

Nurse's Notes

Multiple pruritic papular and vesicular lesions are noted over the body, centered at the trunk. Additional papular lesions are on the palate and oral mucosa. No lesions are present on the hands or face. The client is lethargic but cooperative. Mucous membranes are sticky. Skin is warm to touch, and capillary refill is less than 2 seconds. There is no tenting.

Immunization records indicate one varicella and one measles, mumps, and rubella vaccine. Other immunizations are up to date.

Orders

1. Administer over-the-counter (OTC) acetaminophen as needed (PRN) for fever or pain.
2. Provide OTC diphenhydramine PRN for itching.
3. Give oatmeal baths PRN.
4. Apply calamine lotion two to three times a day until the lesions heal.
5. Encourage adequate oral intake.
6. Keep the child home until all the rash has crusted.
7. Contact the health care provider's office if the client's condition deteriorates.

▶ The nurse is preparing to discharge the client and is evaluating the parent's understanding of the discharge education. For each parent statement, indicate if the statement by the parent indicates understanding or not understanding.

Parent Statement	Understanding	Not Understanding
"My child is contagious 1 day before the rash and 6 days after."	○	○
"My child can return to school once all lesions have crusted over."	○	○
"Since my child had an ASD repair, prophylactic antibiotics are needed."	○	○
"I will give my child aspirin for comfort."	○	○
"I will trim my child's fingernails regularly."	○	○
"I will give my child an oatmeal bath every night."	○	○
"My child can get shingles later in life."	○	○

40. A client with bipolar disorder, mania, has flight of ideas and grandiosity and becomes easily agitated. To prevent harmful behaviors, the nurse should take which action **initially**?
☐ 1. Encourage the client to stay in their room.
☐ 2. Seclude the client at the first sign of agitation.
☐ 3. Tell the client to seek out staff when feeling agitated.
☐ 4. Instruct the client to ask for medication when agitated.

41. The nurse should assess a child with newly diagnosed hyperthyroidism for which sign(s) or symptom(s)? Select all that apply.
☐ 1. weight gain
☐ 2. dry skin
☐ 3. constipation
☐ 4. rapid pulse
☐ 5. heat intolerance

42. The nurse plans care for four birth parents and their newborns. After reviewing the clients' medical records, the nurse should make rounds on which client **first**?
- ☐ 1. an 18-year-old with an uncomplicated spontaneous vaginal birth 12 hours ago who has abdominal cramps
- ☐ 2. a 35-year-old with an uncomplicated vaginal birth 4 hours ago; the nurse's notes indicated the client soaked two peripads over the last 2 hours; fundus is firm
- ☐ 3. a 16-year-old with a cesarean birth 4 hours ago, diagnosed with preeclampsia and receiving magnesium sulfate at 2 g per hour; reflexes are 2+, and the nurse's notes indicate the client has a headache; vital signs are temperature 99.4°F (37.4°C), pulse 88 bpm, respiration rate 20 breaths/min, and blood pressure 128/86 mm Hg
- ☐ 4. an 18-year-old who had a caesarian birth 2 days ago and now has severe breast pain; vital signs are temperature 99.8°F (37.7°C), pulse 96 bpm, and respiration rate 22 breaths/min

43. A nurse is evaluating the proper use of crutches by a client who has fractured the right leg. Which statement indicates the client is using the correct technique?
- ☐ 1. "I move my left leg forward first as I swing forward on my crutches."
- ☐ 2. "I need to increase my arm strength because my arms tingle after I use my crutches."
- ☐ 3. "I padded the tops of my crutches so that I can lean more comfortably on my crutches."
- ☐ 4. "I feel pressure on the palms of my hands when I am walking with my crutches."

44. The nurse cares for a child receiving a blood transfusion. The child becomes flushed and is wheezing. What should the nurse do **first**?
- ☐ 1. Notify the health care provider (HCP).
- ☐ 2. Administer oxygen.
- ☐ 3. Switch the transfusion to normal saline solution.
- ☐ 4. Take the child's vital signs.

45. A client who is allergic to penicillin has a prescription to receive cefazolin. What should the nurse do **first**?
- ☐ 1. Ask if the client has taken cefazolin before without an adverse response.
- ☐ 2. Verify the prescription with the health care provider (HCP).
- ☐ 3. Administer the cefazolin as prescribed.
- ☐ 4. Observe the client closely for urticaria.

46. The parent of a preschool-age child tells the nurse that the child is hyperactive and something needs to be done. Which response by the nurse would be **most** appropriate initially?
- ☐ 1. "What makes you think your child is hyperactive?"
- ☐ 2. "What do you think needs to be done?"
- ☐ 3. "How does your child behave normally?"
- ☐ 4. "Does the preschool teacher think your child is hyperactive?"

47. A client's 1200 blood glucose level was inaccurately documented as 310 mg/dL (17.2 mmol/L) instead of 130 mg/dL (7.2 mmol/L). This error was not noticed until 1300. The nurse administered the sliding scale insulin for a blood glucose level of 310 mg/dL (17.2 mmol/L). What should the nurse do **first**?
- ☐ 1. Notify the health care provider (HCP).
- ☐ 2. Assess the client for hypoglycemia.
- ☐ 3. Consult with the clinical pharmacist.
- ☐ 4. Call the charge nurse.

48. An older infant who has been injured in an automobile accident is to wear a splint on the injured leg. The parent reports that the infant has become mobile even while wearing the splint. What should the nurse advise the parent to do?
- ☐ 1. Notify the health care provider (HCP) immediately to adjust the treatment plan.
- ☐ 2. Confine the infant to one room in the apartment.
- ☐ 3. Keep the infant in the splint at night, removing it during the day.
- ☐ 4. Remove any unsafe items from the area in which the infant is mobile.

49. One hour before surgery, a client asks the nurse about the risks of the surgical procedure. Which statement by the nurse is **most** appropriate?
- ☐ 1. "What are your concerns? I can answer any questions that you have."
- ☐ 2. "There are several risks. Did the surgeon tell you about them?"
- ☐ 3. "It's important that your questions are answered and you understand the risks before you have surgery. I'll contact the surgeon."
- ☐ 4. "Actually, the risks associated with this procedure are minimal. The surgeon has performed this surgery many times."

50. The nurse is assessing fetal position in a 32-year-old female client in the eighth month of pregnancy. From the figure, how would the nurse document the fetal position?

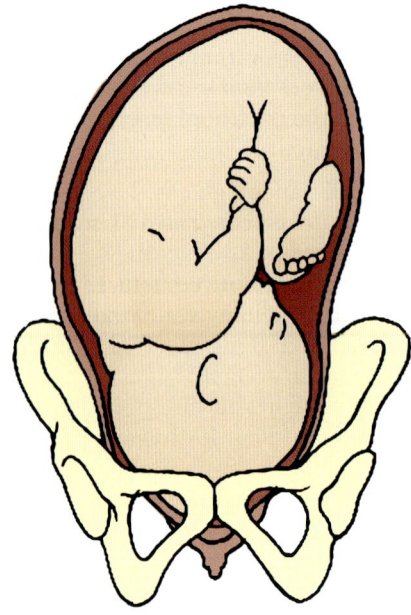

☐ 1. left occipital transverse
☐ 2. left occipital anterior
☐ 3. right occipital transverse
☐ 4. right occipital anterior

51. The nurse should instruct a client who is taking dexamethasone and furosemide to report which symptom?
☐ 1. excitability
☐ 2. muscle weakness
☐ 3. diarrhea
☐ 4. increased thirst

52. A client with a suspected diagnosis of lung cancer has a bronchoscopy with biopsy. Following the procedure, what should the nurse do?
☐ 1. Encourage the client to gargle with oral lidocaine to decrease throat irritation.
☐ 2. Monitor the client for signs of pneumothorax.
☐ 3. Administer pain medication as needed to relieve mediastinal discomfort.
☐ 4. Advise the client not to talk until the gag reflex returns.

53. A nurse is preparing to administer 500 mL of an intravenous solution to a child over 12 hours via tubing that delivers microdrips at 60 gtt/mL. At what rate should the nurse infuse the solution?
_____ gtt/min.

54. An older adult client hospitalized 4 days ago for treatment of acute respiratory distress has become confused and disoriented. The client has been picking invisible items off blankets and has been yelling at the client's child who is not in the room. The family tells the nurse that the client has been treated for anxiety with alprazolam for years, but alprazolam is not on the current medication list. Which safety measure(s) should be implemented? Select all that apply.
☐ 1. The client should be placed on withdrawal precautions and treatment started immediately.
☐ 2. The client should be placed in soft restraints.
☐ 3. A prescription should be obtained to help with the hallucinations.
☐ 4. The client's child should not visit until the client is better.
☐ 5. The client's medical and mental status should be evaluated frequently and treated as needed.

55. The parent of a toddler tells the nurse their child is "fussy" and not as "easygoing" as their other children. The parent is having difficulty feeding the child because the child fusses and cries when served a meal. What instructions should the nurse give the parent?
☐ 1. Allow the child to determine when feeding should occur.
☐ 2. Do not feed the child if they cry.
☐ 3. Provide structured feeding times and routines.
☐ 4. Give the child finger foods, and let them eat when they want.

56. Prior to a client's discharge from the hospital, the nurse is instructing the client about performing tracheostomy care at home. Which information should the nurse include in the instructions?
☐ 1. Remove the inner cannula every 2 hours for cleaning.
☐ 2. Secure the tracheostomy ties with a square knot.
☐ 3. Use cut gauze under the neck plate to protect the skin.
☐ 4. Suction the inner cannula on completion of the procedure.

57. The nurse finds an unopened bag of intravenous (IV) 50% dextrose in a sink in the nursing unit. What should the nurse do with the IV bag?
☐ 1. Leave it where it was found, and notify the charge nurse.
☐ 2. Send it to the pharmacy.
☐ 3. File an incident report.
☐ 4. Discard it in a sharps container.

58. The nurse is teaching an unlicensed assistive personnel (UAP) about the care of clients with self-mutilation. Which statement by the UAP would indicate teaching about self-mutilation has been effective?
  ☐ 1. "It's a means of getting what the person wants."
  ☐ 2. "It's a nonserious event that can be ignored."
  ☐ 3. "It's a way to express anger and rage."
  ☐ 4. "It's a form of manipulation."

59. A client is experiencing symptoms of early alcohol withdrawal. The client's blood pressure is 150/85 mm Hg, and the pulse is 98 bpm. What should the nurse do?
  ☐ 1. Administer lorazepam.
  ☐ 2. Administer an antihypertensive.
  ☐ 3. Assign an unlicensed assistive personnel to sit with the client.
  ☐ 4. Notify the health care provider.

60. Which diet instruction(s) are appropriate when teaching a client in the early stages of cirrhosis about nutritional needs? Select all that apply.
  ☐ 1. "Limit your caloric intake so that you don't become overweight."
  ☐ 2. "An adequate intake of protein is important to your health."
  ☐ 3. "I encourage you to eat small, frequent meals."
  ☐ 4. "Restrict your fluid intake to 1000 mL a day."
  ☐ 5. "Limit your alcohol intake to one glass of wine daily."

61. A client has received tissue plasminogen activator (t-PA) or alteplase recombinant therapy. What should the nurse do to protect the client?
  ☐ 1. Use the radial artery to obtain blood gas samples.
  ☐ 2. Maintain arterial pressure for 10 seconds.
  ☐ 3. Administer intramuscular (IM) injections.
  ☐ 4. Encourage physical activity.

62. On the first postpartum day, the nurse is caring for a primiparous client who speaks very little English. The nurse observes that the client has been bottle-feeding their neonate on occasion, but most of the neonatal care is being performed by the client's parent-in-law. Which action would be **most** appropriate?
  ☐ 1. Notify the social worker because bonding may be affected.
  ☐ 2. Document the unusual maternal behavior in the client's medical record.
  ☐ 3. Determine whether this is a cultural practice for the client and their family.
  ☐ 4. Obtain a prescription to make a home visit after the client's discharge.

63. A client whose job requires extensive use of a computer has developed carpal tunnel syndrome. The nurse should instruct the client to prevent which situation?
  ☐ 1. decreased circulation to the brachial nerve
  ☐ 2. muscle atrophy resulting from disuse
  ☐ 3. median nerve compression
  ☐ 4. progressive flexion contracture of the wrist

64. A client is admitted to the emergency department following an overdose of barbiturates. What should the nurse do **first**?
  ☐ 1. Assess ventilation and assist ventilation as needed.
  ☐ 2. Monitor the blood pressure.
  ☐ 3. Prepare to administer blood products.
  ☐ 4. Place the client in the Trendelenburg position.

65. A client who is recovering from transurethral resection of the prostate (TURP) experiences urinary incontinence and has decreased the fluid intake because of the incontinence. What is the nurse's **best** response to the client?
  ☐ 1. "Yes, limiting your fluids can decrease your incontinence."
  ☐ 2. "Limiting your fluids will cause kidney stones."
  ☐ 3. "Drink eight glasses of water a day, and urinate every 2 hours."
  ☐ 4. "If your incontinence continues, we will reinsert your catheter."

66. A female client is taking oral contraceptives. The nurse teaches the client that which medications may interfere with oral contraceptive efficacy?
  ☐ 1. antihypertensives
  ☐ 2. antibiotics
  ☐ 3. diuretics
  ☐ 4. antihistamines

67. A 28-year-old female client is prescribed danazol for endometriosis. The nurse should instruct the client to report which symptoms to the health care provider?
  ☐ 1. headaches
  ☐ 2. weight loss
  ☐ 3. increased libido
  ☐ 4. hair loss

68. To which unlicensed assistive personnel should the nurse assign a male orthodox Muslim client who needs complete morning care?
  ☐ 1. Judy, who has two other clients requiring complete morning care
  ☐ 2. Joe, who has one client requiring complete morning care
  ☐ 3. Jill, who has four clients requiring partial morning care
  ☐ 4. Jim, who has five clients requiring partial morning care

69. A client with chronic renal failure is experiencing central nervous system (CNS) changes caused by uremic toxins. Which nursing approach would be **most** appropriate for addressing these CNS changes?
☐ 1. Allow the client to grieve for body image changes.
☐ 2. Restrict foods that are high in potassium.
☐ 3. Restrict fluid intake to 1000 mL a day.
☐ 4. Assess the client's mental status regularly.

---

70. | STEP 1

The nurse cares for a 20-year-old male college student in the emergency department with suspected substance abuse.

Admission Note

1000:
The client was brought to the emergency department by a friend after the client became drowsy with slurred speech and vomited on the way to class. The friend reported that the client seemed okay when they were picked up to go to class. The friend reported that the client has a history of "partying hard" but did not know what they might have used this morning. Respirations are shallow, and the skin is pale and clammy. The client is sleepy but responds when shaken. Pupils are pinpoint. Vital signs are temperature (T) 99.5°F (37.5°C); pulse (P) 54 bpm; respiration rate (RR) 10 breaths/min; blood pressure (BP) 100/52 mm Hg; and pulse oximetry reading of 88% on room air (RA).

▶ Which three findings require **immediate** follow-up?

☐ 1. Blood pressure
☐ 2. Heart rate
☐ 3. Level of consciousness (LOC)
☐ 4. Respiratory rate
☐ 5. Oxygen saturation
☐ 6. Pupillary reactions
☐ 7. Vomiting

---

71. | STEP 2

The nurse cares for a 20-year-old male college student in the emergency department with suspected substance abuse.

Admission Note

1000:
The client was brought to the emergency department by a friend after the client became drowsy with slurred speech and vomited on the way to class. The friend reported that the client seemed okay when they were picked up to go to class. The friend reported that the client has a history of "partying hard" but did not know what they might have used this morning. Respirations are shallow, and the skin is pale and clammy. The client is sleepy but responds when shaken. Pupils are pinpoint. Vital signs are temperature (T) 99.5°F (37.5°C); pulse (P) 54 bpm; respiration rate (RR) 10 breaths/min; blood pressure (BP) 100/52 mm Hg; and pulse oximetry reading of 88% on room air (RA).

▶ For each of the client findings, indicate if the signs are consistent with alcohol, amphetamine, or opioid overdose. Each finding may support more than one type of overdose.

Findings	Alcohol	Amphetamines	Opioid
Respiratory depression	☐	☐	☐
Vomiting	☐	☐	☐
Decreased LOC	☐	☐	☐
Pinpoint pupils	☐	☐	☐

Note: Each column must have at least one response option selected.

72. STEP 3

The nurse cares for a 20-year-old male college student in the emergency department with suspected substance abuse.

Admission Note

1000:
The client was brought to the emergency department by a friend after the client became drowsy with slurred speech and vomited on the way to class. The friend reported that the client seemed okay when they were picked up to go to class. The friend reported that the client has a history of "partying hard" but did not know what they might have used this morning. Respirations are shallow, and the skin is pale and clammy. The client is sleepy but responds when shaken. Pupils are pinpoint. Vital signs are temperature (T) 99.5°F (37.5°C); pulse (P) 54 bpm; respiration rate (RR) 10 breaths/min; blood pressure (BP) 100/52 mm Hg; and pulse oximetry reading of 88% on room air (RA).

➤ Complete the following sentence from the list of drop-down options.

The client is at **highest** risk for developing [cardiogenic shock / respiratory arrest / generalized seizure]

as evidenced by the client's [neurologic assessment / respiratory assessment / cardiovascular assessment].

73. STEP 4

The nurse cares for a 20-year-old male college student in the emergency department with suspected substance abuse.

Admission Note

1000:
The client was brought to the emergency department by a friend after the client became drowsy with slurred speech and vomited on the way to class. The friend reported that the client seemed okay when they were picked up to go to class. The friend reported that the client has a history of "partying hard" but did not know what they might have used this morning. Respirations are shallow, and the skin is pale and clammy. The client is sleepy but responds when shaken. Pupils are pinpoint. Vital signs are temperature (T) 99.5°F (37.5°C); pulse (P) 54 bpm; respiration rate (RR) 10 breaths/min; blood pressure (BP) 100/52 mm Hg; and pulse oximetry reading of 88% on room air (RA).

➤ The client receives the diagnosis of opioid overdose. What intervention(s) does the nurse anticipate including in the plan of care? Select all that apply.

- ☐ 1. Administer naloxone.
- ☐ 2. Monitor respirations for 1 hour.
- ☐ 3. Obtain a urine drug screen.
- ☐ 4. Provide oxygen.
- ☐ 5. Secure the airway.

74. STEP 5

The nurse cares for a 20-year-old male college student in the emergency department with suspected substance abuse.

Admission Note

1000:
The client was brought to the emergency department by a friend after the client became drowsy with slurred speech and vomited on the way to class. The friend reported that the client seemed okay when they were picked up to go to class. The friend reported that the client has a history of "partying hard" but did not know what they might have used this morning. Respirations are shallow, and the skin is pale and clammy. The client is sleepy but responds when shaken. Pupils are pinpoint. Vital signs are temperature (T) 99.5°F (37.5°C); pulse (P) 54 bpm; respiration rate (RR) 10 breaths/min; blood pressure (BP) 100/52 mm Hg; and pulse oximetry reading of 88% on room air (RA).

Orders

Provide respiratory support if needed.
- Titrate oxygen to keep saturation greater than 94%.

Give naloxone nasal spray 4 mg/0.1 mL in one nostril as needed PRN for a RR less than 12 breaths/min.
- May repeat every 2 to 3 minutes PRN for up to four doses

Obtain a urine drug screen.

Monitor for at least 6 hours after discontinuing respiratory support and last naloxone dose.

Call if the client experiences signs or symptoms of opioid withdrawal.

On discharge:
- Give a take-home naloxone kit.
- Provide home harm-reduction teaching.
- Refer to the addiction clinic.

➤ The nurse receives a prescription to administer naloxone nasal spray. For each possible step, indicate if the step is appropriate or not appropriate when giving nasal naloxone.

Possible Steps	Appropriate	Not Appropriate
Only give naloxone if the client is having some respiratory effort.	○	○
Position the client with the head titled back before inserting the nozzle.	○	○
Begin rescue breathing at 10 breaths/min if respirations remain depressed after giving naloxone.	○	○
Give a second dose from the same vial if respirations remain depressed after 2 to 3 minutes.	○	○
Place the client on the side if breathing resumes.	○	○

75. STEP 6

The nurse cares for a 20-year-old male college student in the emergency department with suspected substance abuse.

Admission Note

1000. The client was brought to the emergency department by a friend after the client became drowsy with slurred speech and vomited on the way to class. The friend reported that the client seemed okay when they were picked up to go to class. The friend reported that the client has a history of "partying hard" but did not know what they might have used this morning. Respirations are shallow, and the skin is pale and clammy. The client is sleepy but responds when shaken. Pupils are pinpoint. Vital signs are temperature (T) 99.5°F (37.5°C); pulse (P) 54 bpm; respiration rate (RR) 10 breaths/min; blood pressure (BP) 100/52 mm Hg; and pulse oximetry reading of 88% on room air (RA).

Orders

Provide respiratory support if needed.
- Titrate oxygen to keep saturation greater than 94%.

Give naloxone nasal spray 4 mg/0.1 mL in one nostril as needed PRN for a RR less than 12 breaths/min.
- May repeat every 2 to 3 minutes PRN for up to four doses

Obtain a urine drug screen.

Monitor for at least 6 hours after discontinuing respiratory support and last naloxone dose.

Call if the client experiences signs or symptoms of opioid withdrawal.

On discharge:
- Give a take-home naloxone kit.
- Provide home harm-reduction teaching.
- Refer to the addiction clinic.

Flow Sheet

Time	1000	1015	1018	1035
T	99.5°F (37.5°C)			98.6°F (37°C)
P	54 bpm	56 bpm	66 bpm	105 bpm
RR	10 breaths/min	10 breaths/min	12 breaths/min	16 breaths/min
BP	100/52 mm Hg	96/54 mm Hg	100/60 mm Hg	116/70 mm Hg
Pulse oximetry	88% RA	90% RA	95% 2 L oxygen via nasal cannula	96% RA
Note	Drowsy, shallow respirations, pinpoint pupils	Naloxone nasal spray given in right nostril. Oxygen started at 2 L per nasal cannula.	Naloxone nasal spray given in left nostril. The client is more alert.	The client is alert and oriented but anxious and states feeling achy. Pupils are 3 mm. Slight tremors are noted. Skin is warm and dry. The client was weaned off oxygen.

➢ The nurse monitors the client after two doses of naloxone. Which finding(s) would indicate the client may be experiencing opiate withdrawal after receiving naloxone? Select all that apply.

☐ 1. anxiety
☐ 2. pain
☐ 3. pupils
☐ 4. tremors
☐ 5. heart rate
☐ 6. blood pressure
☐ 7. skin

76. A female client is treated for trichomoniasis with metronidazole. What should the nurse tell the client about this medication?
- ☐ 1. The medication should not alter the color of the urine.
- ☐ 2. The client should discontinue oral contraceptive use during this treatment.
- ☐ 3. The client should avoid alcohol during treatment and for 24 hours after completion of the drug.
- ☐ 4. The client's partner does not need treatment.

77. A client is in the advanced stages of osteoarthritis. Which statement **best** describes the pain that occurs in the advanced stage of the disease?
- ☐ 1. Pain occurs with minimal activity.
- ☐ 2. Crepitation develops and intensifies pain.
- ☐ 3. Joints are symmetrically affected by pain.
- ☐ 4. Fatigue accompanies pain.

78. Allopurinol is prescribed for a client who has chronic gout. Which comment indicates that the client understands how to take the allopurinol?
- ☐ 1. "I'll take the medication whenever my joints hurt."
- ☐ 2. "I must take this drug on an empty stomach."
- ☐ 3. "I should drink plenty of fluids when taking allopurinol."
- ☐ 4. "I shouldn't take aspirin when taking allopurinol."

79. A parent calls the nurse to report that their toddler has just been burned on the arm. What should the nurse advise the parent to do **first**?
- ☐ 1. Pack the arm in ice, and then take the child to the closest emergency department.
- ☐ 2. Rub the burned area with an antibacterial ointment, and then call the child's health care provider (HCP).
- ☐ 3. Run cool water over the burned area, and then wrap it in a clean cloth.
- ☐ 4. Call the child's HCP immediately, and then wrap the arm in a clean cloth.

80. The nurse is caring for a 75-year-old female client who had a right hip replacement 2 days ago.

Nurse's Notes

Today 0705:
The client has incisional pain and requires 4 mg of morphine every 3 to 4 hours since surgery. Morphine 4 mg via intravenous (IV) push was administered as per the health care provider's prescription of 4 mg every 3 to 4 hours for pain. The client voided 300 mL of urine. Vital signs are temperature (T) 99°F (37.2°C); heart rate (HR) 86 bpm; respiration rate (RR) 20 breaths/min; blood pressure (BP) 126/82 mm Hg; and 93% oxygen saturation on room air.

1000:
Vital signs are T 99°F (37.2°C); HR 86 bpm; RR 16 breaths/min; BP 126/82 mm Hg; and 93% oxygen saturation on room air. The client reports pain of 9 on a scale of 0 to 10 at the incision site on the right hip.

➤ Complete the diagram by circling the choices below to specify what condition the client is most likely experiencing at 1000, two actions the nurse should take to address that condition, and two parameters the nurse should monitor to assess the client's progress.

Action to Take — Condition Most Likely Experiencing — Parameter to Monitor
Action to Take — Parameter to Monitor

Action to Take	Potential Conditions	Parameters to Monitor
Administer 3 mg morphine	Narcotic dependence	Activity level
Ask the client to wait 30 minutes before the next dose	Narcotic tolerance	Respirations
Administer 4 mg of morphine	Postoperative pain	Pain level
Notify the physical therapy team to ambulate the client in 20 minutes	Depression of respirations	Urinary output
Ambulate the client before administering morphine		Oxygen saturation

81. A client with osteomyelitis of the left great toe has pain with partial weight bearing, unsteady gait, and general weakness. Based on these data, the nurse should institute which safety measures?
- ☐ 1. bed rest
- ☐ 2. airborne precautions
- ☐ 3. referral to physical therapy
- ☐ 4. falls precautions

82. A client receiving a blood transfusion begins to have chills and a headache within the first 15 minutes of the transfusion. What should the nurse do **first**?
- ☐ 1. Administer acetaminophen.
- ☐ 2. Take the client's blood pressure.
- ☐ 3. Discontinue the transfusion.
- ☐ 4. Check the infusion rate of the blood.

83. A client takes isosorbide dinitrate as an antianginal medication. Which statement indicates that the client understands the adverse effects of the drug?
- ☐ 1. "I should take my pulse before taking the medication."
- ☐ 2. "I should take isosorbide dinitrate with food."
- ☐ 3. "I'll need to change positions slowly so I won't get dizzy."
- ☐ 4. "It's important that I report any swelling in my ankles."

84. The nurse is performing the initial assessment on a middle-age female client recently diagnosed with Cushing's syndrome. The nurse reviews the history and physical (see chart). The nurse should develop a plan with the client to manage which effect(s)? Select all that apply.

History and Physical		
A recent ground-level fall resulting in multiple bruises on both arms and left shoulder		
A slow-healing laceration on the right hand from a fall 2 weeks prior		
Muscle weakness		
Unable to sleep more than 2 to 3 hours at a time		
Moon-faced appearance		
Oily skin		
Recent 20 lb (9.1 kg) weight gain		
Vital signs	BP:	148/94 mm Hg
	Heart rate:	96/strong/regular
	Respirations:	20/regular/unlabored
	Pain:	Denies

- ☐ 1. low blood volume
- ☐ 2. risk for injury
- ☐ 3. slow healing
- ☐ 4. changes in physical appearance
- ☐ 5. risk for infection

85. The nurse is instructing the spouse of a client who had an incision and drainage procedure for an abscess on how to care for the wound at home. What information should the nurse give the spouse about cleaning the wound?
- ☐ 1. Clean the incision and drainage sites simultaneously.
- ☐ 2. Clean from the incision site to the drainage site.
- ☐ 3. Clean from the drainage site to the incision site.
- ☐ 4. Clean each site independently.

Answers, Rationales, and Test-Taking Strategies

The answers and rationales for each question follow below, along with keys (🔑) to the client need (CN) and cognitive level (CL) for each question. In addition, questions that measure clinical judgment will be coded (CJ). As you check your answers, use the **Content Mastery and Test-Taking Skill Self-Analysis** *worksheet (tear-out worksheet in the back of the book) to identify the reason(s) for not answering the questions correctly. For additional information about test-taking skills and strategies for answering questions, refer to pages 12–51 in Part 1 of this book.*

1. **4.** Heartburn is caused when stomach contents enter the distal end of the esophagus, producing a burning sensation. To avoid heartburn during pregnancy, the client should avoid spicy foods, eat smaller, more frequent meals, and avoid lying down after eating. Peristalsis usually decreases during the latter half of pregnancy. Displacement of the stomach by the uterus, not the diaphragm, may contribute to heartburn. Increased, not decreased, secretion of hydrochloric acid also contributes to heartburn during pregnancy.

    🔑 CN: Basic care and comfort; CL: Apply

2. **3.** The most important aspect of teaching a preschooler is to have the family members there for support. Preschoolers are able to understand information that is individualized to their level. Including a plastic model of the heart and a catheter as part of the preoperative preparation may be helpful. The other family members will understand the heart model and catheter better than the preschooler will.

    🔑 CN: Reduction of risk potential; CL: Analyze

3. **-/+ 1, 2, 3, 5.** Swaddling, vertical rocking, reducing environmental stimuli like lighting, and planning care around infant cues help drug-exposed infants exhibit age-appropriate state modulation. Fast-tempo music will be too simulating to the infant.

    🔑 CN: Basic care and comfort; CL: Analyze

4. **1.** Of the infants the nurse received a report on, infant A is the most unstable and vulnerable. The infant is only 30 minutes old and is transitioning to extrauterine life. The other three infants will need assessments and care but are currently stable.

    🔑 CN: Management of care; CL: Analyze

5. -/+ **3, 4.** The National Association for Home Care (NAHC) defines "home care" as services for people who are recovering, disabled, or chronically ill and who need treatment or support to function effectively in the home environment. The client with multiple sclerosis and an open lesion is at risk for infection and will require assistance with managing the lesion. Prothrombin monitoring is usually done at the clinic or health care provider's (HCP's) office. Diet instruction can be accomplished at a health care facility or a dietitian's office. The client with vertigo should be monitored for safety in the home. Clients receiving home care services are usually under the care of an HCP with the focus of care being treatment or rehabilitation. Lenses for glasses can be evaluated at an eye clinic or an ophthalmologist's office; a prescription for stronger lenses could be written.

CN: Management of care; CL: Evaluate

6. 3. Although coordinating documentation, resolving negative feelings, and calming down are goals of debriefing after a restraint, the ultimate outcome is to improve restraint procedures.

CN: Safety and infection control; CL: Analyze

7. 4. The situation is escalating, and the nurse's priority is to protect the infant from harm. Therefore, the removal of the infant from this situation should be the first action by the nurse. At this point, trying to reason with the parents or asking one of the parents to leave the room would be ineffective and may serve to further escalate the situation. Calling security is necessary, but only after the nurse has removed the infant from the room.

CN: Safety and infection control; CL: Analyze

8. -/+ **2, 3, 4.** A postoperative ileus is a functional obstruction of the bowel. Assessment of bowel sounds, the first stool, and the amount of gastric output provide information about the return of gastric function. Measurement of urine specific gravity provides information about fluid and electrolyte status; bilirubin levels provide information about liver function, and neither of these tests needs to be included in a focused assessment for ileus.

CN: Reduction of risk potential; CL: Analyze

9. 3. The client has ventricular fibrillation, a dysrhythmia that can lead to cardiac arrest. Given the client's history, the nurse should call the rapid response team to initiate interventions to avoid cardiac arrest. After calling the team, the nurse can administer oxygen. Taking time to inspect the incision delays the necessary intervention. This ECG strip does not show loose electrodes.

CN: Management of care; CL: Analyze

10.

STEP 1

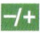

Nurse's Notes

Today: 1000
The client's spouse reports finding the client clutching their chest and short of breath while shoveling snow about 45 minutes ago. The client has a history of hypertension and hypercholesterolemia. <mark>The client has chest pain rated an 8 on a 0 to 10 scale.</mark> The <mark>pain radiates to the left shoulder and left jaw.</mark> Vital signs are temperature (T) 98.9°F (37.2°C); <mark>pulse (P) 120 bpm; respiration rate (RR) 24 breaths/min; and blood pressure (BP) 162/98 mm Hg.</mark> The <mark>pulse oximetry reading is 91% on room air</mark>. Upon assessment, the <mark>client is cool, diaphoretic,</mark> and short of breath. The lungs are clear, and <mark>capillary refill is 3 seconds</mark>. The client is alert and oriented to person, place, and time.

The nurse should plan to follow up on the client's chest pain that is radiating to the client's left shoulder and jaw, which is indicative of a myocardial infarction. The client's vital signs are of concern, particularly the elevated pulse, respirations, and blood pressure. The client is short of breath, and oxygen saturation is low on pulse oximetry. The client is also diaphoretic. These signs are also related to a diagnosis of myocardial infarction. The client's skin that is cool to touch and the capillary refill are not the most significant findings right now and will return to normal once the client's underlying problem is treated.

CJ: Case study; Step 1: Recognize cues; CL: Analyze

11.

STEP 2

Client Finding	Myocardial Infarction	Pneumonia	Pulmonary Embolism
1. Chest pain	X	X	X
2. Tachycardia	X	X	X
3. Shortness of breath	X	X	X
4. Hypoxemia	X	X	X
5. Hypertension	X		
6. Rhythm strip of sinus tachycardia with ST elevation	X		

Chest pain, shortness of breath, tachycardia, hypoxemia, and hypertension are classic signs of a myocardial infarction. The rhythm strip of sinus tachycardia with an ST elevation is also a clinical sign of a possible ST-elevation myocardial infarction

(STEMI). Chest pain, tachycardia, shortness of breath, and hypoxemia can also be findings associated with pneumonia and pulmonary embolism. However, these disease processes do not also cause elevated blood pressure or show a rhythm strip of sinus tachycardia with an ST elevation.

CJ: Case study; Step 2: Analyze cues; CL: Analyze

12.

STEP 3

1, 3, 5, 6. The nurse anticipates that the health care provider will order a 12-lead ECG and cardiac enzyme studies to confirm that the client had a myocardial infarction. The client would benefit from oxygen to help provide more oxygen to help the injured heart muscle. Nitroglycerin is a vasodilator that is used to help relieve chest pain, and this is the recommended protocol for providing nitroglycerin. A spiral CT scan of the chest would be ordered if the health care provider suspected a pulmonary embolism. A peripheral IV would be needed, but the preferred IV fluid would be an isotonic solution such as 0.9% sodium chloride (NaCl) rather than D5W, which is a hypotonic solution and draws fluid out of the intravascular compartment.

CJ: Case study; Step 3: Prioritize hypothesis; CL: Analyze

13.

STEP 4

1, 5, 6. The nurse should continue to inspect the stent for bleeding and infection. The client will be able to breathe better in a semi-Fowler position. The nurse should begin discharge planning as soon as possible, and because the spouse is present, the nurse can explain what to expect on discharge and answer any questions. The IV infusion is running at the prescribed rate, and there is no indication to increase it. The client's oxygen saturation, though changed from a previous reading, is within normal range. The blood pressure is in the normal range for this client at this point in the care plan, and the nurse can review the discharge orders to note if an antihypertensive medication has been written. The client has voided a sufficient amount of urine following the procedure; it is not necessary to catheterize the client to check for residual urine.

CJ: Case study; Step 4: Generate solutions; CL: Create

14.

STEP 5

2, 3, 5, 6, 7, 8, 9. The nurse should instruct the client about the difference between stable versus unstable angina to be sure they understand when there is an emergency. The client will need to follow a heart-healthy diet that includes reducing dietary cholesterol and sodium due to hypercholesterolemia and elevated blood pressure. The client is being referred to cardiac rehabilitation for exercise where they will be monitored during exercise, and the strenuousness will increase gradually. The client will also need instruction regarding medications: nitroglycerin, metoprolol (a beta-blocker), clopidogrel (an antiplatelet), lovastatin, cimetidine (an H2 receptor blocker), and baby aspirin. The nurse should not advise 30 minutes of rigorous exercise immediately; the client will increase exercise gradually and as tolerated. The health care provider has not prescribed a calcium channel blocker or a proton pump inhibitor. A baby aspirin is 81 mg (324 mg is four baby aspirin).

CJ: Case study; Step 5: Take action; CL: Apply

15.

STEP 6

1, 4, 5, 6. The client should sit down before taking nitroglycerin because it can cause the blood pressure to drop and the client can feel dizzy, thus presenting a risk for falls. The nitroglycerine tablet should taste bitter; it is taken sublingually, not with water. After taking nitroglycerin, the client should notice an improvement of symptoms, such as less chest pain and a decrease in sweating, shortness of breath, or both. If the client does not notice improvement, they can take another nitroglycerin in 5 minutes. If there is no improvement after the second dose, the client should call an ambulance.

CJ: Case study; Step 6: Evaluate outcomes; CL: Evaluate

16. 4, 1, 2, 3. The infant who is 6 months of age with diarrhea is seen first because of the risk for further dehydration, and the nurse immediately starts an intravenous (IV) infusion. The client who is 12 years of age is seen next; this child requires urgent care but can wait several hours. The client who is 8 years of age can be seen next; this client requires nonurgent care and will respond to assessment and first aid. The last client to receive care is the client who is 16 years of age; this client is considered nonurgent and likely will not require the services of the emergency department.

CN: Management of care; CL: Create

17. 1. Normal urine output for an infant is 1 to 2 mL/kg per hour.

CN: Physiological adaptation; CL: Evaluate

18. 3. After vasectomy, a sperm analysis will be performed every 4 to 6 weeks. A sperm-free analysis is necessary before the client can be considered sterile. Sperms gradually disappear from the ejaculate. Clients must be informed that conception is possible in the immediate postvasectomy period.

CN: Health promotion and maintenance; CL: Apply

19. **1.** The first action is to increase the oxygen flow rate from 2 to 4 L per minute to help ensure adequate oxygenation for the client. Although it is important to notify the HCP for additional prescriptions and to obtain further assessment data, such as arterial blood gas measurements, it is a priority to support the client's cardiopulmonary system. It would be appropriate to reassure the client while these other interventions are occurring.

CN: Management of care; CL: Analyze

20. **2.** Although a cool air vaporizer may be recommended to humidify the environment, using saline nose drops and then a bulb syringe before meals and at nap and bedtimes will allow the child to breathe more easily. Saline helps to loosen secretions and keep the mucous membranes moist. The bulb syringe then gently aids in removing the loosened secretions. Blowing into the child's mouth to clear the nose introduces more organisms to the child. A nonprescription vasoconstrictive nasal spray is not recommended for infants because if the spray is used for longer than 3 days, a rebound effect with increased inflammation occurs.

CN: Reduction of risk potential; CL: Analyze

21. **1.** The nurse should determine if the HCP is the HCP of record and should have access to the information in the medical record. The medical record is not for public access. The nurse would not give client information to any HCP or refuse to give information without first determining the HCP of record and if the HCP has a legitimate need to know. As an employee, the nurse should have access to medical records, but it is not acceptable to enter a medical record without justification.

CN: Management of care; CL: Analyze

22. **2.** An initial sign of hemorrhaging after a tonsillectomy is swallowing frequently as mucus and blood combine to increase secretions. Mouth breathing is expected after surgery because the child's mouth is very dry and the throat is sore. Because the child has been without fluids for some time, the child usually is thirsty and asks for a drink. Increased pulse rate is a later sign of hemorrhage.

CN: Reduction of risk potential; CL: Analyze

23. **1, 3, 5.** Notifying the pharmacy of the nursing concerns is an appropriate first action. The nursing staff should work cooperatively with the pharmacy to develop a system that works well for both the nursing staff and the pharmacy. Constant communication with all nursing staff during the quality improvement process is integral to the final approval process of both groups. Moving the drugs to a new position within the medication system during an off shift may create errors as medications are inserted into the system in a certain position. Leaving the decisions to the pharmacy staff eliminates the input provided by the nursing staff, which is a vital link between medication and the client.

CN: Management of care; CL: Analyze

24. **1.** Because the client's temperature continues to rise in spite of recently administering ibuprofen, the nurse notifies the HCP. After notifying the HCP, the nurse can bathe the client with tepid water. If the temperature cannot be lowered shortly, the client is also at risk for seizures; the nurse pads the side rails and observes for seizure activity. The nurse cannot administer another dose of ibuprofen without the HCP's prescription.

CN: Physiological adaptation; CL: Apply

25. **3.** The Joint Commission and the Health Council of Canada both mandate interactive handoff communication that allows the opportunity for questioning between the giver and receiver of client information, including up-to-date information regarding the client's care, treatment and services, current condition, and any recent or anticipated changes. Nurses have primary responsibility and accountability for the utilization of all nursing care provided to clients. The nurse retains the right and has the responsibility to refrain from delegating specific activities based on individual client care needs, caregiver expertise, and client care program requirements.

CN: Management of care; CL: Apply

26. **3.** When a neonate dies, the birth parent should be allowed to stay with the baby as long as they want and say anything they want. The parent is grieving and needs time with the neonate. A photograph should be taken in case the parent wants a photograph at a later time. Telling the parent that this is for the best is inappropriate because such a statement discounts the parent's feelings. Advising the parent to get pregnant again to get over the loss is not helpful because the parent needs time to grieve and be with the neonate. The nurse should remain near the parent and not delegate this responsibility to the hospital's chaplain. A chaplain or other religious member can be contacted if the parent desires.

CN: Psychosocial integrity; CL: Analyze

27. **1.** Clients typically have considerable pain for the first few days after surgery and require frequent administration of pain medication, preferably the use of opioids administered intravenously on a regular schedule or patient-controlled analgesia (PCA). The other problems are all possible complications following this type of surgery, but the priority, until noted otherwise, is to provide adequate pain control.

🗝️ CN: Physiological adaptation; CL: Apply

28. **2.** The client who is taking desmopressin nasal spray should not use the same naris for administration each time. The client should alternate nares every dose. The client should observe for and report promptly signs and symptoms of nasal ulceration, congestion, or respiratory infection.

🗝️ CN: Pharmacological and parenteral therapies; CL: Evaluate

29. **4.** Because clozapine can cause tachycardia, the nurse should withhold the medication if the pulse rate is higher than 140 bpm and notify the HCP. Giving the drug or telling the client to exercise could be detrimental to the client.

🗝️ CN: Pharmacological and parenteral therapies; CL: Analyze

30. **4.** When a child is ready to take fluids by mouth postoperatively, clear liquids are given initially. If clear liquids are tolerated, the concentration and amount of oral feedings are gradually increased. This means advancing to half-strength formula and then to full-strength formula while increasing the amount given with each feeding.

🗝️ CN: Basic care and comfort; CL: Analyze

31. **1.** The nurse should first apply the ECG electrodes to the client's chest. If the client is found to be in ventricular fibrillation, the immediate priority is to defibrillate the client. Pulse oximetry is not an immediate priority. The client's oxygenation is evaluated in a code situation using arterial blood gas analysis. The client's blood pressure is evaluated after the ECG rhythm has been established. A portable Doppler ultrasound unit may be needed to check for the presence of a pulse or to check the blood pressure in a code situation.

🗝️ CN: Safety and infection control; CL: Analyze

32. **2.** Heroin causes pinpoint pupils. Marijuana causes the eyes to appear red and bloodshot. Cocaine use causes pupils to dilate. Drooping of the eyelids is not typically associated with the use of any substance.

🗝️ CN: Pharmacological and parenteral therapies; CL: Analyze

33. **2.** It is essential for the nurse to evaluate the effects of pain medication after it has had time to act. Although other interventions may be appropriate, continual reassessment is most important to determine the effectiveness and need for additional intervention, if any. Repositioning could provide some comfort, but an assessment of the client's pain level is essential. Reassuring the client is important, but it will be of no value unless the nurse evaluates the client's pain level. To readjust the pain dosage is appropriate only if titration is prescribed by the health care provider.

🗝️ CN: Basic care of comfort; CL: Analyze

34.
STEP 1

−/+ **1, 5, 7, 8.** Assessment findings of a fever with a rash suggest an infectious process that needs investigation. Children who refuse to drink can quickly become dehydrated during periods of acute illness, especially when a fever is present. Some vaccine-preventable diseases present with a rash. Thus, the nurse needs to check the immunization record to see if there are risks.

An ASD is a congenital heart defect that occurs when there is a hole between the left and right atria chambers of the heart. Due to advances in evaluation and treatment, children who undergo successful closure of an ASD are expected to survive and thrive without long-term sequelae. It is good practice to notate this part of the client's history, but at present, it does not need further follow-up. The heart rate and respiratory rates are on the high end of the normal range for a 4-year-old, which can be expected with fever. The blood pressure of 100/50 mm Hg is normal for a child this age.

🗝️ CJ: Case study; Step 1: Recognize cues; CL: Analyze

35.
STEP 2

0/1 *Pruritic, popular, and vesicular rashes are characteristic findings with* **varicella**, *which is primarily spread by a/an* **airborne** *mode of transmission.*

The rash associated with the common childhood illness, varicella (chickenpox), is characterized by pink or red papules and small fluid-filled blisters that eventually break and crust over. The rash typically appears first on the trunk and then spreads to other areas of the body. Varicella is primarily spread by small airborne droplets. Clients often have fever, headaches, or malaise 24 to 48 hours before the rash appears and are contagious during this time. The disease may also be spread by contact with open lesions. Macular measles and rubella are both much rarer diseases and are characterized by red maculopapular rashes that typically begin on the face. Measles is spread by the airborne route, whereas rubella is spread through large droplets.

🗝️ CJ: Case study; Step 2: Analyze cues; CL: Analyze

36.

STEP 3

0/1 **1, 4.** The child has a fever and is not taking fluids. The sticky mucous membranes and lethargy indicate that the child is already experiencing mild to moderate dehydration. Scratching pruritic lesions commonly leads to secondary bacterial infections of the skin. Pneumonia and meningitis are possible, but they are much rarer compared with the risk for dehydration and skin infection. Seizures are also possible but uncommon. Seizures, when they do occur, may be febrile or associated with neurologic complications of varicella.

🗝️ CJ: Case study; Step 3: Prioritize hypothesis; CL: Analyze

37.

STEP 4

–/+ **2, 3, 5.** Antihistamine medications are often used to decrease itching. Common ones prescribed to reduce itching in varicella include diphenhydramine and loratadine. Topical treatment with calamine lotion two to three times daily also decreases itching. Acetaminophen is the drug of choice to treat fever and mild pain. Using nonsteroidal antiinflammatory medications with varicella has been associated with more severe secondary infections. Antibiotics are not used to treat viral infection and would only be needed if a secondary infection occurred. Giving a vaccine during moderate to severe illness is contraindicated. Once a child develops natural varicella, future vaccination is usually not indicated. A provider may check titers at some point to determine the adequacy of life-long immunity.

🗝️ CJ: Case study; Step 4: Generate solutions; CL: Create

38.

STEP 5

–/+ **2, 3, 5.** The nurse should determine the varicella risk for the three other children in the home by reviewing their vaccine status. Immediate vaccination is indicated for any family member who is behind on the varicella vaccine and not showing symptoms. The child needs to be able to take fluids to meet the criteria for home care. The parents should be taught to avoid giving the child nonsteroidal antiinflammatory drugs because of the association with Reye syndrome. The parent or health department would be expected to contact the daycare center. Bringing the child back to the clinic in 3 days could potentially expose other clients to varicella. The child does not need to return to the clinic unless they develop complications.

🗝️ CJ: Case study; Step 5: Take action; CL: Apply

39.

STEP 6

0/1

Parent Statement	Understanding	Not Understanding
"The child is contagious 1 day before the rash and 6 days after."	X	
"My child can return to school once all lesions have crusted over."	X	
"Since my child had an ASD repair, prophylactic antibiotics are needed."		X
"I will give my child aspirin for comfort."		X
"I will trim my child's fingernails regularly."	X	
"I will give my child an oatmeal bath every night."	X	
"My child can get shingles later in life."	X	

Varicella is very pruritic, and it is important to reduce opportunities for secondary infections from scratching. Keeping the child's fingernails clipped is essential. The parent's statements about communicability, oatmeal baths, and returning to school are accurate. Since the child has had chickenpox, they most likely have lasting immunity but may develop shingles later in life if the virus is reactivated. Administration of aspirin during varicella is contraindicated because of the possible development of Reye syndrome in children. Children who are well healed from cardiac surgery, such as an ASD repair, do not require antibiotic prophylaxis.

🗝️ CJ: Case study; Step 6: Evaluate outcomes; CL: Evaluate

40. **3.** Initially, the nurse would tell the client to seek out staff when feeling agitated or upset to prevent violent episodes. Doing so helps the client to redirect negative feelings in an appropriate manner, such as by talking. Encouraging the client to stay in their room is inappropriate because it does not help the client deal with their feelings. Secluding the client at the first sign of agitation is not indicated and may be perceived by the client as punishment. Instructing the client to ask for medication when agitated would not be the initial course of action. The nurse would interact with the client and direct the client to an activity to decrease their anxiety before intervening with any required medication.

🗝️ CN: Psychosocial integrity; CL: Analyze

41. **–/+** **4, 5.** Rapid pulse, heat intolerance, diarrhea, exophthalmos, and accelerated linear growth are more characteristic of hyperthyroidism, which is caused by an autoimmune response to thyroid-

stimulating hormone receptors. Weight gain, dry skin, and constipation are characteristic of hypothyroidism, which results from a deficiency in the secretion of thyroid hormone.

🔑 CN: Physiological adaptation; CL: Analyze

42. 2. The criterion for hemorrhage is saturating one pad per hour. The 35-year-old who delivered 4 hours ago had saturated a peripad per hour. Even though the client's fundus is firm, they may have experienced a cervical laceration, which would be the source of the bleeding. The client needs to be evaluated first, based on the bleeding. The 18-year-old who has abdominal cramps is within normal limits for a G2 P2 and is experiencing afterbirth pains normally seen in a multiparous client; they will need pain medication. The 16-year-old who had a cesarean birth and is taking magnesium sulfate is stable with adequate urinary output and normal reflexes. Their vital signs are within normal limits for a postpartum client. The headache is the one area of concern for this client. The 18-year-old who is 2 days postpartum with breast pain may be experiencing their milk coming in, though it does not indicate whether they are breast- or bottle-feeding; either situation may find a birth parent with milk developing within their system. The vital signs for this client are slightly elevated, but this may be from the milk coming in and would require nursing evaluation, but this is not an emergency.

🔑 CN: Management of care; CL: Analyze

43. 4. It is normal for the client to feel pressure on the palms of the hands when walking with crutches. The client should move their affected (right) leg forward first as they swing forward with the crutches. Leaning on the crutches can apply pressure to the axillae, leading to neurovascular impairment. If the client's arms are tingling after they use their crutches, the client is probably applying pressure on their axillae when walking.

🔑 CN: Reduction of risk potential; CL: Evaluate

44. 3. The child is having a reaction to the blood transfusion. The priority is to stop the blood transfusion but maintain an open venous access for medication or high fluid volume delivery. Thus, switching the transfusion to normal saline solution would be done first. Since the child is having difficulty breathing, applying oxygen would be the next action. Additionally, vital signs are taken to determine the extent of circulatory involvement. Then the HCP would be notified, and, if necessary, the crash cart would be obtained.

🔑 CN: Pharmacological and parenteral therapies; CL: Analyze

45. 1. A client who has an allergy to penicillin may have a cross-sensitivity to cefazolin, a first-generation cephalosporin, and the drug should be given with caution. The nurse should ask the client whether the client has taken cefazolin before. The nurse should inform the pharmacy of the client's allergy after asking the client about prior use of cefazolin. The medication should not be administered until the nurse first inquires about the client's exposure to cefazolin and then consults the pharmacist or HCP. Observing the client for urticaria is appropriate but is not an initial response.

🔑 CN: Safety and infection control; CL: Analyze

46. 1. The best approach by the nurse is to determine why the parent thinks the child is hyperactive. Some children are very active but do not have the necessary defining characteristics of hyperactivity. Asking what the parent thinks needs to be done, how the child behaves normally, and if the preschool teacher thinks the child is hyperactive would be an appropriate follow-up question once more information is gathered from the parent to determine whether the child indeed is hyperactive.

🔑 CN: Physiological adaptation; CL: Analyze

47. 2. The nurse should first assess the client because a hypoglycemic reaction is likely to occur. At this time, the nurse also should give the client a fast-acting simple carbohydrate. Then the nurse should notify the HCP for prescriptions to prevent or treat severe hypoglycemia. The nurse could consult the clinical pharmacist until able to contact the HCP, but the first action is to assess the client to have accurate information to report. When the situation has been resolved, the nurse should document the incident and report the incident to the charge nurse.

🔑 CN: Management of care; CL: Analyze

48. 4. Safety is the priority in caring for this infant. Infants adapt easily, increasing mobility even with a splint in place. Therefore, the birth parent needs to ensure that the area in which the infant is mobile is safe. There is no need to contact the HCP to alter the treatment plan. Confining the infant to one room may not allow the child to achieve normal development. The child needs different environments for maximum development. The infant needs to wear the splint as prescribed by the HCP to ensure optimal healing.

🔑 CN: Safety and infection control; CL: Analyze

49. **3.** The client must have adequate disclosure of the risks associated with the surgery before signing the consent form. It is the surgeon's responsibility to explain the risks of any procedures and to obtain the client's informed consent. If the nurse suspects that the client has not been truly informed, it is the responsibility of the nurse to act as a client advocate and contact the surgeon to provide additional information to the client. It is not appropriate to have the client go to surgery without understanding the risks. The nurse should not minimize the procedure or dismiss the client's concerns.

🔑 CN: Management of care; CL: Analyze

50. **4.** In a right occipital anterior lie, the occiput faces the right anterior segment of the birth parent's pelvis. In a left occipital transverse lie, the occiput faces the parent's left hip. In a left occipital anterior lie, the occiput faces the left anterior segment of the parent's pelvis. In a right occipital transverse lie, the occiput faces the parent's right hip.

🔑 CN: Physiological adaptation; CL: Analyze

51. **2.** The nurse should instruct the client who is taking dexamethasone and furosemide to observe for signs and symptoms of hypokalemia, such as malaise, muscle weakness, vomiting, and a paralytic ileus, because both dexamethasone and furosemide deplete serum potassium. This combination of drugs does not cause the client to become excitable or have diarrhea or thirst.

🔑 CN: Pharmacological and parenteral therapies; CL: Analyze

52. **2.** After a bronchoscopy with a biopsy, the nurse should monitor the client for signs of pneumothorax as well as hemorrhage. The client should not gargle with oral lidocaine; this will not allow the gag reflex to return. The client should not have any mediastinal discomfort after a bronchoscopy; if pain does occur, it should be reported promptly to the health care provider. It is not necessary to tell the client not to talk until the gag reflex returns.

🔑 CN: Reduction of risk potential; CL: Analyze

53. 42 gtt/min
The number of drops the client should receive each minute is determined as follows:

500 mL/12 hours = between 41 and 42 mL to be infused each hour

42 mL × 60 (drop factor) = 2520 drops to be infused each hour

2520 drops/60 minutes = 42 drops to be infused every minute

🔑 CN: Pharmacological and parenteral therapies; CL: Apply

54. ⊟ **1, 3, 5.** Especially in older adults, alprazolam withdrawal requires immediate and aggressive treatment. Hallucinations are frightening for the client and family. Changes in medical and mental status can occur quickly in older adults, and the client must be monitored closely. Restraints are not indicated for the client and would likely aggravate the confusion and agitation. There is no need to restrict the client's child from visiting at this point.

🔑 CN: Pharmacological and parenteral therapies; CL: Create

55. **3.** Each child has unique temperaments and energy levels, and parents must adapt parenting strategies for each child. Children who are easily upset do better in structured environments where they can learn what to expect. Easygoing children can manage flexible feeding times. Not feeding the child when they cry will not promote nutrition and does not provide the structure that will help the child learn appropriate eating behaviors. Children who are very active and always "on the go" respond well to eating food that can be carried in their hand and eating more frequently.

🔑 CN: Health promotion and maintenance; CL: Analyze

56. **2.** When a client is performing tracheostomy care, it is important that the tracheostomy ties be securely tied to prevent dislodgment of the tube. It is not necessary to remove the inner cannula every 2 hours for cleaning. Routine cleaning is usually performed every 8 hours. The nurse should tell the client to use precut tracheostomy dressings under the neck plate to protect the skin surrounding the stoma. Cutting and using a gauze dressing can cause loose gauze fibers to enter the airway. The inner cannula should be suctioned before cleaning, not afterward.

🔑 CN: Reduction of risk potential; CL: Apply

57. **2.** The nurse should send the unopened bag of IV 50% dextrose found in the sink to the pharmacy. A concentrated medication such as 50% dextrose could be lethal if inadvertently administered and should not be stored outside the pharmacy. An incident report is not necessary in this situation. The sharps container is not the appropriate method for the disposal of this medication.

🔑 CN: Safety and infection control; CL: Analyze

58. **3.** Self-mutilation is a way to express anger and rage and is commonly seen in clients with borderline personality disorder. It typically is a cry for help, an expression of intense anger, helplessness, or guilt. When a client is experiencing numbness or feelings of unreality, self-mutilation induces physical pain that validates the person's being alive because of the ability to feel the physical pain. Self-mutilation is not a means of getting what the person wants. It is not used as a form of manipulation, though it is often misinterpreted as such. Self-mutilation is a serious behavior that is harmful to the self and cannot be ignored.

CN: Management of care; CL: Evaluate

59. **1.** Lorazepam, a benzodiazepine, is commonly used to decrease the symptoms of central nervous system (CNS) irritability in a client who is experiencing early symptoms of alcohol withdrawal. An antihypertensive will not treat the underlying CNS irritability. If the lorazepam is effective, it will not be necessary to have someone sit with the client. At this point, it is not necessary to notify the health care provider.

CN: Management of care; CL: Analyze

60. **2, 3.** Appropriate diet instructions for the client in the early stages of cirrhosis include ensuring an adequate intake of protein and eating small, frequent meals. There is no need to limit protein intake unless the client has evidence of hepatic encephalopathy. Additionally, fluid intake is not restricted unless the client has significant ascites or edema (these typically occur later in the disease). Because of gastrointestinal dysfunction, small, frequent meals are frequently better tolerated than three regular meals. Clients with cirrhosis should be encouraged to increase their caloric intake instead of restricting it. Alcohol intake in any amount is discouraged.

CN: Physiological adaptation; CL: Analyze

61. **1.** The nurse should use the radial artery to obtain blood gas samples because it is easier to maintain firm pressure there than on the femoral artery. Nursing interventions to protect the client who has received t-PA or alteplase recombinant therapy include maintaining arterial pressure for 30 seconds because it takes longer for coagulation to occur with the thrombolytic agent on board. IM injections are contraindicated during thrombolytic therapy. The nurse should prevent physical manipulation of the client, which can cause bruising.

CN: Reduction of risk potential; CL: Analyze

62. **3.** In many cultures, the time after the birth of the neonate is a time for the parent to heal from the birth. The appropriate action by the nurse is to determine whether this is a cultural practice for this client and their family. If so, the client is behaving within their cultural practices. Teaching should be provided to both the parent and their parent-in-law. There is no indication that bonding is not taking place. Lack of bonding might be indicated if the client did not show any interest in the neonate. Documenting the client's maternal behavior in the medical record is a routine task. However, the nurse should not assume that this behavior is unusual because it may be reflective of the client's cultural framework. A home visit is not warranted unless there is evidence of infant neglect or the family needs additional follow-up or teaching.

CN: Health promotion and maintenance; CL: Analyze

63. **3.** Carpal tunnel syndrome is a condition in which the median nerve becomes compressed in the wrist. The brachial nerve is not affected. Carpal tunnel syndrome may be the result of a systemic disease, such as rheumatoid arthritis or diabetes mellitus, or it may be an occupational hazard for people whose jobs require repetitive hand movements such as someone who works long hours on a computer. It is not a condition resulting from disuse. The wrists do not develop flexion contractures with carpal tunnel syndrome.

CN: Physiological adaptation; CL: Analyze

64. **1.** Barbiturates can cause significant respiratory depression. The nurse's first action is to immediately assess the respiratory status and assist in bag-mask-valve ventilation as needed. Monitoring the vital signs is important, but respiratory care takes precedence over blood pressure. Without other injuries, blood products are not necessary. Placing the client in the Trendelenburg position will put pressure from the abdominal contents onto the diaphragm and further impair breathing.

CN: Pharmacological and parenteral therapies; CL: Analyze

65. **3.** Clients who have undergone TURP need to be instructed to maintain an adequate fluid intake despite urinary dribbling or incontinence. The client should be advised to drink at least eight glasses of water a day to dilute the urine and help prevent urinary tract infections. Maintaining a voiding schedule of every 2 hours can help decrease incidents of incontinence. Teaching the client Kegel exercises is also beneficial for strengthening sphincter tone. The nurse should not encourage the client to decrease fluids. It is not necessarily true that a decreased intake will cause renal calculi. Threatening the client with a catheter is not beneficial, and it is not the treatment of choice for a client who is experiencing incontinence from TURP.

🗝️ CN: Reduction of risk potential; CL: Analyze

66. 2. Broad-spectrum antibiotics can cause decreased efficacy of oral contraceptives, placing the client at risk for an unplanned pregnancy. When a client is prescribed a course of antibiotics, a backup method of contraception should be used. Antihypertensive agents, diuretics, and antihistamine medications do not interfere with oral contraceptive efficacy.

🗝️ CN: Pharmacological and parenteral therapies; CL: Apply

67. 1. Adverse effects of danazol include headaches, dizziness, irritability, and decreased libido. Masculinization effects, such as deepened voice, facial hair, and weight gain, also may occur.

🗝️ CN: Pharmacological and parenteral therapies; CL: Analyze

68. 2. The nurse should assign the Muslim male client who needs complete morning care to Joe. Muslim men cannot be cared for by female nurses. The nurse must also consider workload, and Joe has the lightest assignment.

🗝️ CN: Management of care; CL: Analyze

69. 4. CNS changes include such symptoms as apathy, lethargy, and decreased concentration. Seizures and coma can also occur. The nurse should assess the client's level of consciousness at regular intervals and maintain client safety. Allowing the client to express feelings related to body image changes and restricting foods high in potassium and fluid intake are all appropriate activities, but they are not related to the CNS changes.

🗝️ CN: Physiological adaptation; CL: Analyze

70.
STEP 1

0/1 3, 4, 5. The most urgent findings are decreased respirations, decreased LOC, and low oxygen saturation. The respiratory rate of fewer than 12 breaths/min and drowsiness are cause for concern because they indicate central nervous system depression. The low respiratory rate and shallow respirations are most likely causing the low oxygen saturation. Peripheral nervous system effects associated with opioid abuse include pinpoint pupils, constipation, and decreased gastric, biliary, and pancreatic secretions. The pulse and blood pressure are borderline. However, the respiratory depression is the immediate concern.

🗝️ CJ: Case study; Step 1: Recognize cues; CL: Analyze

71.
STEP 2

−/+

Findings	Alcohol	Amphetamines	Opioid
Respiratory depression	X		X
Vomiting	X	X	X
Decreased LOC	X		X
Pinpoint pupils			X

Vomiting can occur with overdoses of all three substances. Alcohol intoxication manifests as slurred speech and impaired coordination and judgment and progresses to decreased LOC and respiratory depression. Opioid overdoses are characterized by respiratory depression, decreased LOC, and pinpoint pupils. Amphetamine overdoses are characterized by dilated pupils, increased vital signs, and increased alertness that progresses to tremors, confusion, circulatory collapse, and seizures.

🗝️ CJ: Case study; Step 2: Analyze cues; CL: Analyze

72.
STEP 3

R The client is at **highest** risk for developing **respiratory arrest** as evidenced by the client's **respiratory assessment**.

Death from opioid overdose most often comes from the effects of the drug on the parts of the brain that regulate breathing. The shallow respirations and slow respirations indicate a respiratory arrest is likely to occur. The client has low blood pressure, changes in consciousness, and pallor, which are consistent with cardiogenic shock, but the heart rate and breathing are not rapid as would be expected. Also, the client does not have chest pain or shortness of breath. The nurse would look for signs of increased central nervous system irritation to support the hypothesis that the client was most at risk for a seizure. Pinpoint pupils and drowsiness are signs of central nervous system depression.

🗝️ CJ: Case study; Step 3: Prioritize hypothesis; CL: Analyze

73.
STEP 4

−/+ 1, 3, 4, 5. The nurse anticipates giving the antidote for an opioid overdose, which is naloxone either as an injectable or a nasal spray. Airway compromise is one of the greatest risks to clients with opioid overdose, making securing the airway important. Supplemental oxygen should be given until oxygen saturation can be maintained at least 95% in room air. The nurse anticipates obtaining a urine drug screen to help determine the type of opioid used and the possibility of polysubstance abuse. How long clients are monitored depends on the amount of naloxone needed to reverse the symptoms and the type of opioid overdose. The minimum monitoring time would be 2 hours after treatment for lower-risk clients and 6 to 12 hours for higher-risk clients.

🗝 CJ: Case study; Step 4: Generate solutions; CL: Create

74.

STEP 5

0/1

Possible Steps	Appropriate	Not Appropriate
Only give naloxone if the client is having some respiratory effort.		X
Position the client with the head tilted back before inserting the nozzle.	X	
Begin rescue breathing at 10 breaths/min if respirations remain depressed after giving naloxone.	X	
Give a second dose from the same vial if respirations remain depressed after 2 to 3 minutes.		X
Place the client on the side if breathing resumes.	X	

Naloxone should be given as soon as an opioid overdose is suspected. A client does not have to be breathing for the medication to work. To give the nasal spray, the nurse should tilt the client's head back, insert the plunger all the way, and administer the dose. If the client does not start breathing, or if the respiratory effort is depressed, the nurse should check for a pulse and begin rescue breathing at a rate of 1 breath every 6 seconds or 10 breaths per minute. If the client resumes breathing, they should be placed in the recovery position on their side. Naloxone spray comes as a single dose. If a second dose is needed, a new vial is used, and the dose is given in the alternate nostril.

🗝 CJ: Case study; Step 5: Take action; CL: Apply

75.

STEP 6

−/+ **1, 2, 4, 5.** Administration of naloxone can cause a precipitated withdrawal that gives symptoms that are the opposite of an opioid high or overdose. These symptoms can include sudden intense pain, anxiety, tachycardia, hypertension, tremors, sweating, nausea, and vomiting. Though the symptoms are uncomfortable, they are rarely life-threatening. Normal pupil size is 2 to 4 mm. The client's blood pressure and skin are within normal limits.

🗝 CJ: Case study; Step 6: Evaluate outcomes; CL: Evaluate

76. 3. Metronidazole can cause a disulfiram-like reaction if it is taken with alcohol. Tachycardia, nausea, vomiting, and other serious interaction effects can occur. Metronidazole will make the urine a darker color. Oral contraceptives should never be discontinued with trichomoniasis. The partner also requires treatment to prevent retransmission of infection.

🗝 CN: Pharmacological and parenteral therapies; CL: Analyze

77. 1. In the advanced stages of osteoarthritis, pain can occur with minimal activity or even when the client is at rest. Crepitation can be present at any stage of the disease and does not exacerbate pain. Joints are not symmetrically affected by the disease. Symmetric joint involvement and fatigue are characteristics of rheumatoid arthritis.

🗝 CN: Physiological adaptation; CL: Analyze

78. 3. It is important that the client force fluids to 3000 mL a day to avoid the development of renal calculi when taking allopurinol. Allopurinol must be taken consistently to be effective in the treatment of gout. The drug should be taken after meals to avoid gastrointestinal distress. Although the client can take aspirin when taking allopurinol, both drugs can cause gastrointestinal irritation, and the practice is not recommended if the client is sensitive to the medications.

🗝 CN: Pharmacological and parenteral therapies; CL: Evaluate

79. 3. The best advice for the nurse to give the child's birth parent is to run cool water over the burned area to stop the burning process. Then the area should be wrapped in a clean cloth. Once these initial actions are completed, the parent can call the child's HCP. Packing the arm in ice may cause more damage to the burned area because cold can cause burns just as heat can. For most burns, it is not advised to apply ointment until the area has been evaluated.

🗝 CN: Physiological adaptation; CL: Analyze

80.

0/1

Action to Take	Potential Conditions	Parameters to Monitor
Administer 4 mg of morphine	Postoperative pain	Pain level
Notify the physical therapy team to ambulate the client in 20 minutes		Respirations

Each client has a different reaction to pain, and on the third postoperative day, the client is still experiencing pain. The nurse can administer the 4-mg dose of morphine as prescribed. The client is not developing dependence (craving the drug to relieve symptoms of withdrawal) or tolerance (needing higher doses to achieve the same effect) to the morphine; the prescribed dose at the prescribed interval is helping the client manage the pain. The nurse, while helping the client manage the pain with the prescribed pain medication, can also assist the client in reducing the postoperative pain by encouraging the client to ambulate and use distraction, mindfulness, and other alternative pain management strategies. Following orthopedic surgery, physical therapists (PTs) or PT assistants are usually the ones to ambulate the client, and if they are not available, it is the nurse's responsibility. Narcotics can cause respiratory depression, but at this time the client's respirations are within normal limits, even though there is a change in the respiratory rate from 20 breaths/min to 16 breaths/min at 1000. The nurse should continue to monitor the client's oxygen saturation and encourage deep breathing. The client's urinary output is within normal limits, and the nurse will continue to record intake and output.

🔑 CJ: Standalone bowtie; CL: Analyze

81. **4.** The client is at risk for falling, and the nurse should initiate falls precaution. The client does not require airborne precautions. There is no indication the client needs a referral to physical therapy. The client should be encouraged to maintain mobility.

🔑 CN: Reduction of risk potential; CL: Analyze

82. **3.** Chills and a headache are signs of a febrile, nonhemolytic blood transfusion reaction, and the nurse's first action should be to discontinue the transfusion as soon as possible and then notify the health care provider (HCP). Antipyretics and antihistamines may be prescribed. The nurse would not administer acetaminophen without a prescription from the HCP. The client's blood pressure should be taken after the transfusion is stopped. Checking the infusion rate of the blood is not a pertinent action; the infusion needs to be stopped regardless of the rate.

🔑 CN: Pharmacological and parenteral therapies; CL: Analyze

83. **3.** Common adverse effects of isosorbide are lightheadedness, dizziness, and orthostatic hypotension. Clients should be instructed to change positions slowly to prevent these adverse effects and to avoid fainting. Ankle swelling is not related to isosorbide administration. The client does not need to take their pulse before taking the medication. The client does not need to take the medication with food.

🔑 CN: Pharmacological and parenteral therapies; CL: Evaluate

84. -/+ **2, 3, 4, 5.** Cushing's syndrome results from excessive levels of cortisol. Some effects of excessive adrenocortical activity include musculoskeletal changes, and the client may be at risk for injury and falls. There is excessive protein catabolism causing muscle wasting, decreased inflammatory response, and potential for delayed healing and infection. The increased cortisol levels cause a moon-faced appearance to which clients must adjust. The skin becomes thin and fragile, and the client is also at risk for infection. Increased cortisol levels do not cause deficient fluid volume.

🔑 CN: Management of care; CL: Analyze

85. **4.** The sites should be treated as separate sites to avoid cross-contamination. This adheres to the principle of cleaning from the least contaminated area to the most contaminated area. Each site is considered a separate area for wound care.

🔑 CN: Safety and infection control; CL: Apply

5

Comprehensive Test

This test has 120 questions. Time yourself as you take the test so you can determine the approximate amount of time it takes to complete this many questions.

1. The nurse has just received the change-of-shift report on clients in the labor, birth, recovery, and postpartum unit. Which of these clients should the nurse assess **first**?
   ☐ 1. an 18-year-old single primigravid client, in labor for 9 hours, with cervical dilation at 6 cm, 0 station, contractions occurring every 5 minutes, and receiving epidural anesthesia
   ☐ 2. a 24-year-old primiparous client who gave vaginal birth to a 7-lb, 3-oz (3260-g) neonate 1 hour ago, has a firm fundus and scant lochia rubra, and is attempting to breastfeed
   ☐ 3. a 26-year-old multigravid client, in labor for 8 hours, with cervical dilation at 8 cm, 1+ station, contractions every 3 to 4 minutes, and receiving no anesthesia
   ☐ 4. a 30-year-old multiparous client who gave birth to a 6-lb, 5-oz (2863-g) neonate by cesarean 3 hours ago, has a firm fundus and scant lochia rubra, and is receiving morphine by patient-controlled analgesia

2. The nurse is to administer ergonovine maleate 200 mcg intramuscularly. The ampule label reads 0.2 mg/mL. The nurse should administer how many milliliters? Record your answer using a whole number.

   _____ mL.

3. An infant is admitted to the hospital with dehydration secondary to viral gastroenteritis. Which room assignment is the **most** appropriate for this infant?
   ☐ 1. a semiprivate room with an 8-year-old child who has had an appendectomy
   ☐ 2. a semiprivate room with a 10-year-old child with a closed head injury
   ☐ 3. a private room
   ☐ 4. a semiprivate room with a 4-year-old child with leukemia

4. The nurse should be especially alert for what problem when caring for a term neonate, who weighed 10 lb (4500 g) at birth, 1 hour after a vaginal birth?
   ☐ 1. hypoglycemia
   ☐ 2. hypercalcemia
   ☐ 3. hypermagnesemia
   ☐ 4. hyperbilirubinemia

5. The nurse is giving care to an infant in an oxygen hood (see figure). Which intervention(s) are indicated? Select all that apply.

   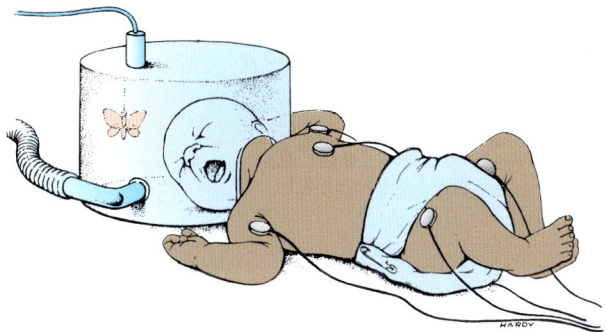

   ☐ 1. Assure that the oxygen is not blowing directly on the infant's face.
   ☐ 2. Place the butterfly mobile on the outside of the hood.
   ☐ 3. Immobilize the infant with restraints.
   ☐ 4. Remove the hood for 10 minutes every hour.
   ☐ 5. Encourage the parents to visit the child.

6. A nurse assesses an 82-year-old client for depression. Because of the client's age, the nurse's assessment should be guided by which factor?
   ☐ 1. Sadness of mood may be masked by other symptoms.
   ☐ 2. Impairment of cognition usually is not present.
   ☐ 3. Psychosomatic tendencies do not tend to dominate.
   ☐ 4. Antidepressant therapies are less effective in older adults.

7. The nurse teaches a pediatric client about an upcoming procedure. Which approach indicates that the nurse has selected the correct technique for the client's developmental level?
☐ 1. using dolls and stories to prepare school-age children
☐ 2. preparing an adolescent 1 day in advance of the procedure
☐ 3. using puppets and storytelling to prepare a preschooler
☐ 4. preparing a toddler 1 hour before the procedure

8. An abused child is admitted to the hospital, and the nurse is aware that a court appearance may be necessary. To plan for this eventuality, the nurse understands that what should be the **priority**?
☐ 1. Remember the parents' and child's behavior when the child was admitted.
☐ 2. Document physical findings and behaviors observed during the child's admission.
☐ 3. Formulate subjective opinions about the cause of any injuries.
☐ 4. Prepare answers to questions that may be asked by the attorneys.

9. When assessing a client withdrawing from alcohol, the nurse notes that the client is anxious, experiencing nausea, is restless, and has a tremor when both arms are extended. What should the nurse do **next**?
☐ 1. Continue to assess the client.
☐ 2. Move the client to a quieter room.
☐ 3. Administer a benzodiazepine as prescribed.
☐ 4. Transfer the client to an acute care psychiatric unit.

10.

STEP 1

The nurse is caring for a 20-year-old male college sophomore at the Campus Health Center.

Nurse's Notes

Today: 1100
A 20-year-old college sophomore with moderate persistent asthma states that at soccer practice today they got short of breath with little relief from a prescribed albuterol inhaler, and the coach asked the client to go to the student health center. The client is sneezing and has a runny nose. The client has been using the albuterol inhaler as needed, which, until today, has provided relief. The last use of the albuterol inhaler was 30 minutes ago.
  Vital signs are temperature (T) 99°F (37.2°C); pulse (P) 110 bpm; respiration rate (RR) 26 breaths/min; blood pressure (BP) 128/86 mm Hg; and oxygen saturation 92%. Lung sounds have bilateral expiratory wheezes with diminished sounds at bases, and the client reports shortness of breath. Nasal drainage is clear, and the nares are slightly red. Other physical assessments are within normal ranges.

➤ Which top four client findings require follow-up by the nurse?

☐ 1. Clear nasal drainage
☐ 2. Bilateral expiratory wheezes
☐ 3. Red nares
☐ 4. Oxygen saturation 92%
☐ 5. Short of breath
☐ 6. P 110 bpm
☐ 7. RR 26 breaths/min

11. STEP 2

The nurse is caring for a 20-year-old male college sophomore at the Campus Health Center.

Nurse's Notes

Today: 1100
A 20-year-old college sophomore with moderate persistent asthma states that at soccer practice today they got short of breath with little relief from a prescribed albuterol inhaler, and the coach asked the client to go to the student health center. The client is sneezing and has a runny nose. The client has been using the albuterol inhaler as needed, which, until today, has provided relief. The last use of the albuterol inhaler was 30 minutes ago.
    Vital signs are temperature (T) 99°F (37.2°C); pulse (P) 110 bpm; respiration rate (RR) 26 breaths/min; blood pressure (BP) 128/86 mm Hg; and oxygen saturation 92%. Lung sounds have bilateral expiratory wheezes with diminished sounds at bases, and the client reports shortness of breath. Nasal drainage is clear, and the nares are slightly red. Other physical assessments are within normal ranges.

Today: 1115
Vital signs are P 106 bpm; RR 24 breaths/min; BP 122/82 mm Hg; and oxygen saturation 92%. Lung sounds have bilateral expiratory wheezes throughout, and the client is using intercostal muscles while breathing.

➤ Highlight the findings that show a worsening of the client's condition at 1115. Answer choices have been underlined.

Nurse's Notes

Today: 1100
A 20-year-old college sophomore with moderate persistent asthma states that at soccer practice today they got short of breath with little relief from a prescribed albuterol inhaler, and the coach asked the client to go to the student health center. The client is sneezing and has a runny nose. The client has been using the albuterol inhaler as needed, which, until today, has provided relief. The last use of the albuterol inhaler was 30 minutes ago.
    Vital signs are temperature (T) 99°F (37.2°C); pulse (P) 110 bpm; respiration rate (RR) 26 breaths/min; blood pressure (BP) 128/86 mm Hg; and oxygen saturation 92%. Lung sounds have bilateral expiratory wheezes with diminished sounds at bases, and the client reports shortness of breath. Nasal drainage is clear, and the nares are slightly red. Other physical assessments are within normal ranges.

Today: 1115
Vital signs are P 106 bpm; <u>RR 24 breaths/min</u>; <u>BP 122/82 mm Hg</u>; and <u>oxygen saturation 92%</u>. Lung sounds have <u>bilateral expiratory wheezes throughout</u>, and the client is <u>using intercostal muscles</u> while breathing.

---

12. STEP 3

The nurse is analyzing cues and determining the client's priority health problem.

Nurse's Notes

Today: 1100
A 20-year-old college sophomore with moderate persistent asthma states that at soccer practice today they got short of breath with little relief from a prescribed albuterol inhaler, and the coach asked the client to go to the student health center. The client is sneezing and has a runny nose. The client has been using the albuterol inhaler as needed, which, until today, has provided relief. The last use of the albuterol inhaler was 30 minutes ago.
Vital signs are temperature (T) 99°F (37.2°C); pulse (P) 110 bpm; respiration rate (RR) 26 breaths/min; blood pressure (BP) 128/86 mm Hg; and oxygen saturation 92%. Lung sounds have bilateral expiratory wheezes with diminished sounds at bases, and the client reports shortness of breath. Nasal drainage is clear, and the nares are slightly red. Other physical assessments are within normal ranges.

Today: 1115
A: P 106 bpm; RR 24 breaths/min; BP 122/82 mm Hg; and oxygen saturation 92%. Lung sounds have bilateral expiratory wheezes throughout, and the client is using intercostal muscles while breathing.

➤ Complete the following sentence by choosing from the list of options.

The client is at risk for [cardiac failure / respiratory failure / anxiety.]

To prevent further complications, the nurse should immediately [start rescue breathing. / notify the health care provider. / have the client use an albuterol inhaler.]

13. STEP 4

The nurse has received these orders from the health care provider.

Nurse's Notes

Today: 1100
A 20-year-old college sophomore with moderate persistent asthma states that at soccer practice today they got short of breath with little relief from a prescribed albuterol inhaler, and the coach asked the client to go to the student health center. The client is sneezing and has a runny nose. The client has been using the albuterol inhaler as needed, which, until today, has provided relief. The last use of the albuterol inhaler was 30 minutes ago.

Vital signs are temperature (T) 99°F (37.2°C); pulse (P) 110 bpm; respiration rate (RR) 26 breaths/min; blood pressure (BP) 128/86 mm Hg; and oxygen saturation 92%. Lung sounds have bilateral expiratory wheezes with diminished sounds at bases, and the client reports shortness of breath. Nasal drainage is clear, and the nares are slightly red. Other physical assessments are within normal ranges.

Today: 1115
Vital signs are P 106 bpm; RR 24 breaths/min; BP 122/82 mm Hg; and oxygen saturation 92%. Lung sounds have bilateral expiratory wheezes throughout, and the client is using intercostal muscles while breathing.

Orders

Today: 1120	Medrol 20 mg daily for 7 days; start at home today
	Albuterol 2.5 mg per nebulizer four times per day and every 4 hours as needed. Give the first dose in Campus Health.

➤ Identify steps the nurse should take when administering the medication. Use actions from the box below to fill each box in the following sentence.

The nurse should first
[_____], then
[_____], then
[_____], then
[_____], and finally
[_____].

Nursing Actions

Verify allergies

Verify medication with orders

Verify the client's name and date of birth

Reassess the client for the effects of the medication

Administer medication

14. STEP 5

The nurse gives the client the albuterol inhaler and observes the client to be sure they use the inhaler correctly.

Nurse's Notes

Today: 1100
A 20-year-old college sophomore with moderate persistent asthma states that at soccer practice today they got short of breath with little relief from a prescribed albuterol inhaler, and the coach asked the client to go to the student health center. The client is sneezing and has a runny nose. The client has been using the albuterol inhaler as needed, which, until today, has provided relief. The last use of the albuterol inhaler was 30 minutes ago.

Vital signs are temperature (T) 99°F (37.2°C); pulse (P) 110 bpm; respiration rate (RR) 26 breaths/min; blood pressure (BP) 128/86 mm Hg; and oxygen saturation 92%. Lung sounds have bilateral expiratory wheezes with diminished sounds at bases, and the client reports shortness of breath. Nasal drainage is clear, and the nares are slightly red. Other physical assessments are within normal ranges.

Today: 1115
Vital signs are P 106 bpm; RR 24 breaths/min; BP 122/82 mm Hg; and oxygen saturation 92%. Lung sounds have bilateral expiratory wheezes throughout, and the client is using intercostal muscles while breathing.

Today: 1130
Vital signs are P 120 bpm; RR 18 breaths/min; BP 124/84 mm Hg; and oxygen saturation 96%. Lung sounds have bilateral expiratory wheezes throughout. The client has tremors and is "feeling anxious."

Orders

Today: 1120	Medrol 20 mg daily for 7 days; start at home today
	Albuterol 2.5 mg per nebulizer four times per day and every 4 hours as needed. Give the first dose in Campus Health.

➤ Identify the observation(s) the nurse should make as the client uses the inhaler to the box on the right. Select all that apply.

- ☐ 1. Sit up 90 degrees.
- ☐ 2. Shake the inhaler.
- ☐ 3. Blow out the air in the lungs.
- ☐ 4. Loosely seal the lips around the inhaler mouthpiece.
- ☐ 5. Quickly inhale at the same time as the inhaler is activated.
- ☐ 6. Hold the breath for 10 seconds.

15. STEP 6

After the client uses the albuterol nebulizer treatment, the nurse prepares the client for discharge. The nurse evaluates the outcomes of administering albuterol before discharging the client to home.

Nurse's Notes

Today: 1100
A 20-year-old college sophomore with moderate persistent asthma states that at soccer practice today they got short of breath with little relief from a prescribed albuterol inhaler, and the coach asked the client to go to the student health center. The client is sneezing and has a runny nose. The client has been using the albuterol inhaler as needed, which, until today, has provided relief. The last use of the albuterol inhaler was 30 minutes ago. Vital signs are temperature (T) 99°F (37.2°C); pulse (P) 110 bpm; respiration rate (RR) 26 breaths/min; blood pressure (BP) 128/86 mm Hg; and oxygen saturation 92%. Lung sounds have bilateral expiratory wheezes with diminished sounds at bases, and the client reports shortness of breath. Nasal drainage is clear, and the nares are slightly red. Other physical assessments are within normal ranges.

Today: 1115
Vital signs are P 106 bpm; RR 24 breaths/min; BP 122/82 mm Hg; and oxygen saturation 92%. Lung sounds have bilateral expiratory wheezes throughout, and the client is using intercostal muscles while breathing.

Today: 1130
Vital signs are P 120 bpm; RR 18 breaths/min; BP 124/84 mm Hg; and oxygen saturation 96%. Lung sounds have bilateral expiratory wheezes throughout. The client has tremors and is "feeling anxious."

Orders

Today: 1120	Medrol 20 mg daily for 7 days; start at home today
	Albuterol 2.5 mg per nebulizer four times per day and every 4 hours as needed. Give the first dose in Campus Health.

> For each finding below, specify if the finding indicates that the client's condition has improved, has not changed, or has declined.

Finding	Improved	Not Changed	Declined
RR 12 breaths/min	○	○	○
Oxygen saturation 96%	○	○	○
Expiratory and inspiratory wheezes	○	○	○
Use of accessory muscles	○	○	○
Slight shaking of hands	○	○	○

16. Which action should the nurse include in the plan of care for a child with leukemia who has an absolute neutrophil count of 400/mm³ (0.4×10^9/L)?
- ☐ 1. Restrict staff and visitors with active infections.
- ☐ 2. Place the child in strict isolation.
- ☐ 3. Consult with the primary care provider to administer an antiemetic.
- ☐ 4. Increase the child's oral fluid intake.

17. The nurse finds a client lying on the floor next to the bed. After returning the client to bed, assessing for injury, and notifying the health care provider (HCP), the nurse fills out an incident report. What should the nurse do **next**?
- ☐ 1. Give the incident report to the nurse-manager.
- ☐ 2. Place the incident report on the medical record.
- ☐ 3. Call the family to inform them.
- ☐ 4. Omit mentioning the fall in the medical record documentation.

18. The nurse is caring for four clients in labor. Which client is at **most** risk for a postpartum hemorrhage?
- ☐ 1. a client who is a gravida 4 para 3 with a history of polyhydramnios with this pregnancy
- ☐ 2. a client who is a gravida 1 para 0 at 34 weeks' gestation with mild pregnancy-induced hypertension
- ☐ 3. a client who is a gravida 4 para 0 with diet-controlled gestational diabetes being induced at term
- ☐ 4. a client who is a gravida 2 para 1 term pregnancy with a history of genital herpes

19. The parent of a 2-year-old child who has been bitten by the family dog asks the nurse what to do about the bite, which appears to be a minor injury. What should the nurse tell the parent?
- ☐ 1. "You need to take the child to the local urgent care center immediately."
- ☐ 2. "Wash the bite area with lots of running water, and then call your health care provider (HCP)."
- ☐ 3. "Determine when the child's latest tetanus vaccine was administered."
- ☐ 4. "Make an appointment to see the child's HCP now to start rabies shots."

20. The nurse is conducting a routine risk assessment at a prenatal visit. Which question would be the **best** to screen for intimate partner violence?
  ☐ 1. "Is your partner excited about your pregnancy?"
  ☐ 2. "How safe do you feel in your home?"
  ☐ 3. "Does your partner have an arrest record?"
  ☐ 4. "Does your partner own a gun?"

21. A nurse is obtaining the history of an infant with suspected acute otitis media. What should the nurse ask the parent about?
  ☐ 1. position of the infant when taking a bottle
  ☐ 2. covering the infant's ears when out in the cold
  ☐ 3. thoroughly drying the infant's ears after a bath
  ☐ 4. immunization status of the infant

22. A 7-year-old client has been diagnosed with bacterial meningitis. Who should receive chemoprophylaxis?
  ☐ 1. all children at the school
  ☐ 2. all household contacts and close contacts
  ☐ 3. the entire community
  ☐ 4. household contacts only

23. The nurse is preparing to suction a tracheostomy for a client with methicillin-resistant *Staphylococcus aureus* (MRSA) (see figure). What should the nurse do **next**?

  ☐ 1. Wear a powered air purifying respirator (PAPR) face shield.
  ☐ 2. Use goggles that include the hairline.
  ☐ 3. Change to a surgical mask.
  ☐ 4. Proceed to suction the client's tracheostomy.

24. The nurse discusses safety and accident prevention with the parent of a 9-month-old. The nurse understands that the teaching has been effective when the parent makes which statement?
  ☐ 1. "I make sure that I keep my cleaning supplies locked up."
  ☐ 2. "Sometimes my baby plays in the bathroom when I'm cleaning in there."
  ☐ 3. "I've enrolled my baby in an infant water safety classes."
  ☐ 4. "I've found that those child-protective cabinet locks don't work very well."

25. When the nurse is assessing a child receiving tobramycin sulfate, which finding(s) would indicate that the child is experiencing adverse effects? Select all that apply.
  ☐ 1. increased blood pressure
  ☐ 2. weight gain
  ☐ 3. rash
  ☐ 4. fever
  ☐ 5. ringing in the ears
  ☐ 6. decreased heart rate

26. A hospitalized client fell on the floor and sustained a small laceration on the hand that requires stitches. The intern will suture the client's hand at the client's bedside and asks for bupivacaine with epinephrine and a suture kit to suture the laceration. Which issue should be resolved before proceeding with suturing?
  ☐ 1. the intern's ability to suture
  ☐ 2. the client's room as an aseptic environment
  ☐ 3. bupivacaine with epinephrine used as the local anesthetic
  ☐ 4. the cosmetic effect from not having a plastic surgeon do the suturing

27. A 5-lb 8-oz (2.5-kg) baby was born 1 hour ago to a 19-year-old primigravida. What are the **priority** nursing assessments for the nurse to monitor?
  ☐ 1. jaundice and physical assessment
  ☐ 2. vital signs and gestational age assessments
  ☐ 3. feedings and vital signs
  ☐ 4. Apgar and gestational age assessments

28. A client at 37 weeks' gestation is scheduled for an ultrasound. What should the nurse instruct the client to do **before** the test?
  ☐ 1. Drink 1 to 2 L of fluid.
  ☐ 2. Take nothing by mouth after midnight before the test.
  ☐ 3. Plan to remain in the clinic for 4 hours after the test.
  ☐ 4. Eat a high-fiber meal after the test.

29. Which is true regarding delegation of client-care responsibilities? Select all that apply.
  ☐ 1. The nurse must know the nursing model that underlies care at the institution.
  ☐ 2. The nurse delegates in accordance with demands on their time.
  ☐ 3. The nurse confirms that the unlicensed assistive personnel has experience with the delegated activity.
  ☐ 4. The nurse retains the right to determine which tasks are delegated.
  ☐ 5. The nurse must document that the task has been delegated and to whom.

30. The nurse is evaluating the outcome of therapy for a client with osteoarthritis. Which finding indicates the goals of therapy have been met?
  ☐ 1. Joint degeneration has been arrested.
  ☐ 2. The client is able to self-administer gold compound safely.
  ☐ 3. The client feels better than on hospital admission.
  ☐ 4. Joint range of motion has improved.

31. A child with partial- and full-thickness burns is admitted to the pediatric unit. What should be the **priority** at this time?
  ☐ 1. preventing wound infections
  ☐ 2. evaluating vital signs frequently
  ☐ 3. maintaining fluid and electrolyte balance
  ☐ 4. managing the child's pain

32. A normal, healthy 2-month-old infant is brought to the clinic for the first diphtheria, tetanus, and acellular pertussis (DTaP) immunization. Which route is appropriate to administer this vaccine?
  ☐ 1. oral
  ☐ 2. intramuscular
  ☐ 3. subcutaneous
  ☐ 4. intradermal

33. Assessment of a client in active labor reveals the following: moderate discomfort; cervix dilated 3 cm, 0 station, and completely effaced; and fetal heart rate of 136 bpm. What should the nurse plan to do **next**?
  ☐ 1. Assist the client with comfort measures and breathing techniques.
  ☐ 2. Turn the client from the left side-lying position to the right side-lying position.
  ☐ 3. Prepare the client for epidural anesthesia to relieve pain.
  ☐ 4. Instruct the client that internal fetal monitoring is necessary.

34. STEP 1

The nurse cares for an 8-month-old female client admitted to the pediatric unit for vomiting.

Admission Note

The 8-month-old client with unresolved irritability, decreased oral (PO) intake, and vomiting for the past 2 days was admitted for observation and workup. The parents report the infant is otherwise healthy and happy with no significant medical history or allergies. Immunizations are up to date. The client's siblings, ages 5 and 7 years, are both recently recovering from norovirus. The client's diaper is dry. Vital signs are temperature (T) 97.7°F (36.5°C); heart rate (HR) 110 bpm; respiration rate (RR) 32 breaths/min; and pulse oximetry reading 97%. Weight is 22 lb (10 kg). A peripheral intravenous (IV) line of 5% dextrose in normal saline was started at 40 mL per hour in the left hand. Electrolytes, a stool culture, and a complete blood count are pending. The client is on contact precautions with strict intake and output (I&O). Other admission orders are routine.

➤ Which assessment(s) require follow-up? Select all that apply.
  ☐ 1. Irritability
  ☐ 2. PO intake
  ☐ 3. Vomiting
  ☐ 4. Exposure to norovirus
  ☐ 5. Pending lab test results
  ☐ 6. Urine output
  ☐ 7. Vital signs

35. STEP 2

The nurse cares for an 8-month-old female client admitted to the pediatric unit for vomiting.

Admission Note

The 8-month-old client with unresolved irritability, decreased oral intake, and vomiting for the past 2 days was admitted for observation and workup. The parents report the infant is otherwise healthy and happy with no significant medical history or allergies. Immunizations are up to date. The client's siblings, ages 5 and 7 years, are both recently recovering from norovirus. The client's diaper is dry. Vital signs are temperature (T) 97.7°F (36.5°C); heart rate (HR) 110 bpm; respiration rate (RR) 32 breaths/min; and pulse oximetry reading 97%. Weight is 22 lb (10 kg). A peripheral intravenous (IV) line of 5% dextrose in normal saline was started at 40 mL per hour in the left hand. Electrolytes, a stool culture, and a complete blood count are pending. The client is on contact precautions with strict intake and output (I&O). Other admission orders are routine.

➤ For each additional assessment the nurse can make, indicate if the information is helpful or not helpful in determining the infant's risk for dehydration.

Assessment	Helpful	Not Helpful
BP	○	○
Anterior fontanelle	○	○
Activity level	○	○
Breast and bottle feeds	○	○
Presence of Babinski reflex	○	○
Number of wet diapers in the past 24 hours	○	○
Previous weight	○	○
Urine specific gravity	○	○

36. STEP 3

The nurse cares for an 8-month-old female client admitted to the pediatric unit for vomiting.

Admission Note

The 8-month-old client with unresolved irritability, decreased oral intake, and vomiting for the past 2 days was admitted for observation and workup. The parents report the infant is otherwise healthy and happy with no significant medical history or allergies. Immunizations are up to date. The client's siblings, ages 5 and 7 years, are both recently recovering from norovirus. The client's diaper is dry. Vital signs are temperature (T) 97.7°F (36.5°C); heart rate (HR) 110 bpm; respiration rate (RR) 32 breaths/min; and pulse oximetry reading 97%. Weight is 22 lb (10 kg). A peripheral intravenous (IV) line of 5% dextrose in normal saline was started at 40 mL per hour in the left hand. Electrolytes, a stool culture, and a complete blood count are pending. The client is on contact precautions with strict intake and output (I&O). Other admission orders are routine.

Diagnostics Report

Labs	Result	Reference Range
Sodium	136 mEq/L (136 mmol/L)	135–145 mEq/L (135–145 mmol/L)
Potassium	3.0 mEq/L (3.0 mmol/L)	3.5–5.2 mEq/L (3.5–5.2 mmol/L)
White blood cells	5×10^3 cells/mm^3 (5×10^9/L)	$4.5–10.5 \times 10^3$ cells/mm^3 ($4.5–10.5 \times 10^9$/L)
Hemoglobin	13 g/dL (130 g/L)	Age 6 months to 1 year: 9.9–14.5 g/dL (99–145 g/L)
Hematocrit	39% (.39)	Age 6 months to 1 year: 29%–43% (0.29–0.43 proportion of 1.0)
Blood urea nitrogen	30 mg/dL (10.7 mmol/L)	8–20 mg/dL (2.9–7.5 mmol/L)

Radiology: Nine pea-sized metallic foreign bodies clustered together in the abdomen
Impression: Radiogram is consistent with ingestion of magnets

The nurse reviews the diagnostic reports.

➤ Complete the sentences by identifying the correct word(s) from the list of word choices.

The nurse must first address the client's _____.

Then the client will **most** likely need treatment for a(n) _____ that is causing the vomiting.

Word Choices

- Bleeding
- Dehydration
- Bowel obstruction
- Infection
- Intestinal perforation
- Poisoning

37. STEP 4

The nurse cares for an 8-month-old female client admitted to the pediatric unit for vomiting.

Admission Note

The 8-month-old client with unresolved irritability, decreased oral intake, and vomiting for the past 2 days was admitted for observation and workup. The parents report the infant is otherwise healthy and happy with no significant medical history or allergies. Immunizations are up to date. The client's siblings, ages 5 and 7 years, are both recently recovering from norovirus. The client's diaper is dry. Vital signs are temperature (T) 97.7°F (36.5°C); heart rate (HR) 110 bpm; respiration rate (RR) 32 breaths/min; and pulse oximetry reading 97%. Weight is 22 lb (10 kg). A peripheral intravenous (IV) line of 5% dextrose in normal saline was started at 40 mL per hour in the left hand. Electrolytes, a stool culture, and a complete blood count are pending. The client is on contact precautions with strict intake and output (I&O). Other admission orders are routine.

Diagnostics Report

Labs	Result	Reference Range
Sodium	136 mEq/L (136 mmol/L)	135–145 mEq/L (135–145 mmol/L)
Potassium	3.0 mEq/L (3.0 mmol/L)	3.5–5.2 mEq/L (3.5–5.2 mmol/L)
White blood cells	5 × 10^3 cells/mm^3 (5 × 10^9/L)	4.5–10.5 × 10^3 cells/mm^3 (4.5–10.5 × 10^9/L)
Hemoglobin	13 g/dL (130 g/L)	Age 6 months to 1 year: 9.9–14.5 g/dL (99–145 g/L)
Hematocrit	39% (.39)	Age 6 months to 1 year: 29%–43% (0.29–0.43 proportion of 1.0)
Blood urea nitrogen	30 mg/dL (10.7 mmol/L)	8–20 mg/dL (2.9–7.5 mmol/L)

Radiology: Nine pea-sized metallic foreign bodies clustered together in the abdomen
Impression: Radiogram is consistent with ingestion of magnets

Nurse's Notes

1300:
The client was transferred to the unit from the PACU following an exploratory laparoscopy for foreign body removal. The client has six small abdominal incisions that are clean, dry, and intact. The client has an IV of D5W/0.45 normal saline with 2 mEq potassium chloride (KCl)/100 mL at 40 mL/hour in the left hand. Vital signs are T 98.7°F (37°C); HR 110 bpm; RR 32 breaths/min, pulse oximetry reading 97%. Pain is rated as a 4 on the Faces, Legs, Activity, Cry, Consolability (FLACC) Pain scale.

➤ What orders should the nurse request to manage the infant's pain?

- ☐ 1. IV morphine patient-controlled analgesia (PCA)
- ☐ 2. acetaminophen per rectum
- ☐ 3. PO ibuprofen
- ☐ 4. heat therapy (hot packs)
- ☐ 5. cold therapy (cold packs)
- ☐ 6. activity orders: out of bed to parent's arms

38. STEP 5

The nurse cares for an 8-month-old female client admitted to the pediatric unit for vomiting.

Admission Note

The 8-month-old client with unresolved irritability, decreased oral intake, and vomiting for the past 2 days was admitted for observation and workup. The parents report the infant is otherwise healthy and happy with no significant medical history or allergies. Immunizations are up to date. The client's siblings, ages 5 and 7 years, are both recently recovering from norovirus. The client's diaper is dry. Vital signs are temperature (T) 97.7°F (36.5°C); heart rate (HR) 110 bpm; respiration rate (RR) 32 breaths/min; and pulse oximetry reading 97%. Weight is 22 lb (10 kg). A peripheral intravenous (IV) line of 5% dextrose in normal saline was started at 40 mL per hour in the left hand. Electrolytes, a stool culture, and a complete blood count are pending. The client is on contact precautions with strict intake and output (I&O). Other admission orders are routine.

Diagnostics Report

Labs	Result	Reference Range
Sodium	136 mEq/L (136 mmol/L)	135–145 mEq/L (135–145 mmol/L)
Potassium	3.0 mEq/L (3.0 mmol/L)	3.5–5.2 mEq/L (3.5–5.2 mmol/L)
White blood cells	5×10^3 cells/mm^3 (5×10^9/L)	$4.5–10.5 \times 10^3$ cells/mm^3 ($4.5–10.5 \times 10^9$/L)
Hemoglobin	13 g/dL (130 g/L)	Age 6 months to 1 year: 9.9–14.5 g/dL (99–145 g/L)
Hematocrit	39% (.39)	Age 6 months to 1 year: 29%–43% (0.29–0.43 proportion of 1.0)
Blood urea nitrogen	30 mg/dL (10.7 mmol/L)	8–20 mg/dL (2.9–7.5 mmol/L)

Radiology: Nine pea-sized metallic foreign bodies clustered together in the abdomen
Impression: Radiogram is consistent with ingestion of magnets

Nurse's Notes

1300:
The client was transferred to the unit from the PACU following an exploratory laparoscopy for foreign body removal. The client has six small abdominal incisions that are clean, dry, and intact. The client has an IV of D5W/0.45 normal saline with 2 mEq potassium chloride (KCl)/100 mL at 40 mL/hour in the left hand. Vital signs are T 98.7°F (37°C); HR 110 bpm; RR 32 breaths/min; and pulse oximetry reading 97%. Pain is rated as a 4 on the Faces, Legs, Activity, Cry, Consolability (FLACC) Pain scale.

Orders

Diagnosis: Status post exploratory laparoscopy; foreign body removal

- Diet of clear liquids; advance as tolerated
- Vital signs every 2 hours
- IV of D5W/0.45 normal saline with 2 mEq KCl/100 mL at 40 mL per hour. May discontinue when taking oral fluids well.
- Strict I&O
- Acetaminophen 120 mg suppository per rectum every 6 hours as needed for pain
- Call for an oxygen saturation less than 92%, a RR greater than 40 breaths/min, or changes in status

The child is progressing well and has started to exhibit signs of hunger 8 hours after surgery. The nurse reviews the client's orders and assigns tasks to the unlicensed assistive personnel (UAP).

➤ For each possible nursing action, indicate if it is appropriate or not appropriate to delegate to the UAP.

Possible Actions	Appropriate to Delegate to the UAP	Not Appropriate to Delegate to the UAP
Offer the first bottle of clear liquids	○	○
Change and weigh the infant's diaper	○	○
Comfort the infant with lullabies	○	○
Silence pump alarms while the infant is napping	○	○
Restock the client's rooms with additional diapers	○	○
Assist holding the client during dressing changes	○	○

39. STEP 6

The nurse cares for an 8-month-old female client admitted to the pediatric unit for vomiting.

Admission Note

The 8-month-old client with unresolved irritability, decreased oral intake, and vomiting for the past 2 days was admitted for observation and workup. The parents report the infant is otherwise healthy and happy with no significant medical history or allergies. Immunizations are up to date. The client's siblings, ages 5 and 7 years, are both recently recovering from norovirus. The client's diaper is dry. Vital signs are temperature (T) 97.7°F (36.5°C); heart rate (HR) 110 bpm; respiration rate (RR) 32 breaths/min; and pulse oximetry reading 97%. Weight is 22 lb (10 kg). A peripheral intravenous (IV) line of 5% dextrose in normal saline was started at 40 mL per hour in the left hand. Electrolytes, a stool culture, and a complete blood count are pending. The client is on contact precautions with strict intake and output (I&O). Other admission orders are routine.

Diagnostics Report

Labs	Result	Reference Range
Sodium	136 mEq/L (136 mmol/L)	135–145 mEq/L (135–145 mmol/L)
Potassium	3.0 mEq/L (3.0 mmol/L)	3.5–5.2 mEq/L (3.5–5.2 mmol/L)
White blood cells	5×10^3 cells/mm^3 (5×10^9/L)	$4.5–10.5 \times 10^3$ cells/mm^3 ($4.5–10.5 \times 10^9$/L)
Hemoglobin	13 g/dL (130 g/L)	Age 6 months to 1 year: 9.9–14.5 g/dL (99–145 g/L)
Hematocrit	39% (.39)	Age 6 months to 1 year: 29%–43% (0.29–0.43 proportion of 1.0)
Blood urea nitrogen	30 mg/dL (10.7 mmol/L)	8–20 mg/dL (2.9–7.5 mmol/L)

Radiology: Nine pea-sized metallic foreign bodies clustered together in the abdomen
Impression: Radiogram is consistent with ingestion of magnets

Nurse's Notes

1300:
The client was transferred to the unit from the PACU following an exploratory laparoscopy for foreign body removal. The client has six small abdominal incisions that are clean, dry, and intact. The client has an IV of D5W/0.45 normal saline with 2 mEq potassium chloride (KCl)/100 mL at 40 mL/hour in the left hand. Vital signs are T 98.7°F (37°C); HR 110 bpm; RR 32 breaths/min; and pulse oximetry reading 97%. Pain is rated as a 4 on the Faces, Legs, Activity, Cry, Consolability (FLACC) Pain scale.

Orders

Diagnosis: Status post exploratory laparoscopy; foreign body removal

- Diet of clear liquids; advance as tolerated
- Vital signs every 2 hours
- IV of D5W/0.45 normal saline with 2 mEq KCl/100 mL at 40 mL per hour. May discontinue when taking oral fluids well.
- Strict I&O
- Acetaminophen 120 mg suppository per rectum every 6 hours as needed for pain
- Call for an oxygen saturation less than 92%, a RR greater than 40 breaths/min, or changes in status

Day 2:
- Discontinue IV.
- Discharge the client to home.
- Provide home safety education.
- Make a follow-up appointment in 3 days.

The nurse receives orders to discharge the client and is evaluating the parent's understanding of home safety discharge education.

➢ For each finding, specify if the parent's statement indicates if the teaching is understood or not understood.

Parent Statement	Understood	Not Understood
"I will check the floors and area my baby can reach regularly for small objects."	○	○
"I need to check my baby's toys to make sure they don't have small pieces that could be swallowed."	○	○
"I will make sure that battery covers are secure on remote controls, key fobs, or musical books."	○	○
"I know how to use the Heimlich maneuver if my infant starts choking."	○	○
"I will begin teaching my child about what objects should not be put in the mouth."	○	○
"If I think my baby has swallowed a small object, I will try to get them to vomit the object as soon as possible."	○	○

40. The nurse observes that a client who has received midazolam for conscious sedation is having shallow respirations at a rate of 8 to 10 breaths/min. The heart rate is 75 bpm; blood pressure is 95/65 mm Hg. What should the nurse do? Select all that apply.
    ☐ 1. Encourage the client to deep-breathe.
    ☐ 2. Have respiratory resuscitation equipment nearby.
    ☐ 3. Administer oxygen as prescribed.
    ☐ 4. Contact the health care provider for a prescription for naloxone.
    ☐ 5. Notify the anesthesiologist.

41. A client newly diagnosed with deep vein thrombosis (DVT) of the left lower left extremity is on bed rest. What should the nurse instruct the unlicensed assistive personnel (UAP) providing routine morning care for the client to do?
    ☐ 1. Check that the legs are in a low, dependent position.
    ☐ 2. Ensure that the lower extremity is elevated.
    ☐ 3. Massage the leg and foot with lotion.
    ☐ 4. Place one or two pillows under the client's left knee.

42. The nurse is conducting a medication reconciliation for a client who is being admitted to the hospital. Which is true about the medication reconciliation process? Select all that apply.
    ☐ 1. Medication reconciliation is an important client safety goal.
    ☐ 2. Medication reconciliation is designed to obtain and communicate an accurate list of a client's home medications across the continuum of care.
    ☐ 3. Only nurses or health care providers (HCPs) can be involved in medication reconciliation.
    ☐ 4. Medications are considered reconciled if a medication prescription exists that is therapeutically equivalent to the one prior to admission.
    ☐ 5. A medication is considered to be any medication prescribed by an HCP.

43. A charge nurse asks a newly graduated registered nurse (RN) who normally works on a medical-surgical nursing unit to take care of two clients in the coronary care unit. The nurse has not had experience with taking care of clients on monitors or using the medications that these clients are taking. What should the new nurse do?
    ☐ 1. Accept the assignment, and then plan to ask the nurses in the coronary care unit to administer the medications for these clients.
    ☐ 2. Explain to the charge nurse about their level of experience and express concerns about this assignment.
    ☐ 3. Tell the charge nurse that the assignment was to the medical-surgical unit and refuse to go to the coronary care unit.
    ☐ 4. Ask the charge nurse if the assignment can be reduced to taking care of one client.

44. The nurse assesses a adolescent's musculoskeletal system. According to the figure, the nurse should note that the adolescent has which condition?

    ☐ 1. kyphosis
    ☐ 2. lordosis
    ☐ 3. spondylolisthesis
    ☐ 4. scoliosis

45. A child with type 1 diabetes is admitted to the emergency department with hot and dry skin, rapid and deep respirations, and a fruity odor to their breath. Which task, when performed by a new graduate registered nurse (RN), requires the RN preceptor to intervene?
    ☐ 1. assessment of the child's vital signs every 15 minutes
    ☐ 2. verification of the child's prescription for intravenous insulin infusion
    ☐ 3. providing encouragement to the child to drink some orange juice
    ☐ 4. verification of child's glucose by finger stick

46. A parent describes that they are trying to get their toddler to eat well but mealtimes have become increasingly frustrating. Which behavior would the nurse suggest that the parent modify to make meals a more pleasant experience?
    ☐ 1. keeping mealtimes to about 20 minutes
    ☐ 2. eating in an environment with few distractions
    ☐ 3. keeping food portions small
    ☐ 4. offering several healthy choices

47. A client is admitted to the emergency department with myasthenia crisis. What should the nurse do for this client? Place the nursing actions in order of highest priority to lowest priority. All options must be used.

1. Check if the client missed a dose of medication.

2. Assess the client for signs of infection.

3. Check the gag reflex.

4. Prepare for intubation.

48. The nurse is beginning the shift and is assessing the oxygen exchange on a neonate. The nurse reviews the medical record for a pulse oximetry reading for the last 8 hours.

Flow Sheet

Pulse Oximetry					
Time	0700	0900	1100	1300	1500
Reading	95%	90%	90%	90%	86%

The pulse oximetry reading at 1530 is 75% taken on the infant's right wrist. What should the nurse do **first**?

☐ 1. Administer oxygen via a mask.
☐ 2. Obtain a pulse oximeter reading in a lower extremity.
☐ 3. Reassess the oximetry reading in 30 minutes.
☐ 4. Draw blood gases for oxygen and carbon dioxide levels.

49. A client with a history of peptic ulcer disease is admitted to the hospital. Initial assessment reveals that the blood pressure is 96/60 mm Hg, with a heart rate of 120 bpm. The client just vomited coffee-ground–like material. Based on these data, what should the nurse do **first**?

☐ 1. Administer an antiemetic.
☐ 2. Prepare to insert a nasogastric (NG) tube.
☐ 3. Collect data regarding recent client stressors.
☐ 4. Place the client in a modified Trendelenburg position.

50. As a nurse begins the shift on the obstetrical unit, there are several new admissions. When anticipating priorities for the shift, the client with which condition would be a candidate for induction?

☐ 1. preeclampsia
☐ 2. active herpes
☐ 3. face presentation
☐ 4. complete placenta previa

51. In the early postoperative period following abdominal surgery, the nurse notes a bright red, 3″ × 5″ (7.6 × 12.7 cm) area of drainage on the client's dressing. What should be the nurse's **first** action in response to this observation?

☐ 1. Ignore it because drainage is normal.
☐ 2. Increase the intravenous (IV) flow rate.
☐ 3. Take the client's vital signs.
☐ 4. Change the dressing.

52. A 6-year-old client is diagnosed with attention deficit hyperactivity disorder (ADHD). When asking this client to complete a task, the nurse should use which techniques to communicate **most** effectively with the client?

☐ 1. Obtain eye contact before speaking, use simple language, and have them repeat what was said. Praise them if they complete the task.
☐ 2. Fully explain to the client the actions required of them and offer verbal praise and a food reward for task completion.
☐ 3. Explain to the client what they are to do and the consequences if they do not comply, and follow through with praise or consequences as appropriate.
☐ 4. Demonstrate to the client what they are to do, have them imitate the nurse's actions, and give a food reward if they complete the task.

53. Which instruction is **most** important for the nurse to include in the teaching plan for a client who is taking phenelzine?

☐ 1. Eat a normal amount of salt in the diet.
☐ 2. Drink 10 to 12 glasses of water each day.
☐ 3. Allow 10 days to achieve therapeutic effects.
☐ 4. Avoid foods high in tyramine.

54. Two days after being placed in a cast for a fractured femur, the client suddenly has chest pain and dyspnea. The client is confused and has an elevated temperature. The nurse should assess the client for which health problem?

☐ 1. osteomyelitis
☐ 2. compartment syndrome
☐ 3. venous thrombosis
☐ 4. fat embolism syndrome

55. An adolescent client on the psychiatric unit shows signs of mild intoxication. When questioned, the client states that another client gave them beer, and they refuse to name the client. What should the nurse do **next**?

☐ 1. Telephone the client's parents.
☐ 2. Call an interdisciplinary team meeting.
☐ 3. Urge the client to tell who gave them the beer.
☐ 4. Call the primary care provider.

56. A client with benign prostatic hypertrophy is being transferred from the emergency department to a surgery unit. Which information should be included in the report from the nurse in the emergency department to the nurse responsible for admitting the client?
☐ 1. "A urine specimen was obtained from the client and sent to the laboratory for analysis."
☐ 2. "The client was catheterized, and 1100 mL of urine was obtained. The urine appeared cloudy, and a specimen was sent to the laboratory."
☐ 3. "The client is very cooperative. The client is comfortable now that their bladder has been emptied. They have no ill effects from catheterization."
☐ 4. "The client was in the emergency department for 3 hours because of bladder distention. The client is fine now but is being admitted as a possible candidate for surgery."

57. A nurse administers indomethacin to a neonate. What should the nurse do to ensure that the nurse has identified the neonate correctly? Select all that apply.
☐ 1. Verify the infant's full name with the parent.
☐ 2. Ask another nurse to confirm that this is the neonate for whom the medication has been prescribed.
☐ 3. Check the neonate's identification band against the medical record number.
☐ 4. Verify the date of birth from the medical record with the date of birth on the neonate's identification band.
☐ 5. Compare the number on the crib with the number on the neonate's identification band.

58. Which statement indicates that the client with a peptic ulcer understands the dietary modifications to follow at home?
☐ 1. "I should eat a bland, soft diet."
☐ 2. "It's important to eat six small meals a day."
☐ 3. "I should drink several glasses of milk a day."
☐ 4. "I should avoid alcohol and caffeine."

59. The client with a nasogastric (NG) tube has abdominal distention. What should the nurse do **first**?
☐ 1. Call the health care provider (HCP).
☐ 2. Irrigate the NG tube.
☐ 3. Check the function of the suction equipment.
☐ 4. Reposition the NG tube.

60. The nurse instills 5 mL of normal saline before suctioning a client's tracheostomy tube. Which finding indicates the instillation is effective?
☐ 1. The secretions are thinned.
☐ 2. The client coughs.
☐ 3. There is minimal friction when the catheter is passed into the tracheostomy tube.
☐ 4. There is humidification for the respiratory tract.

61. A client with emphysema is receiving continuous oxygen therapy. Depressed ventilation is likely to occur unless the nurse ensures that the oxygen is administered in which way?
☐ 1. cooled
☐ 2. humidified
☐ 3. at a low flow rate
☐ 4. through a nasal cannula

62. Before cataract surgery, the nurse is to instill several types of eye drops. The surgeon writes prescriptions for 5 gtt of antibiotic in OD and 3 gtt of topical steroid drops in OD. What should the nurse do **next**?
☐ 1. Contact the surgeon to rewrite the prescription.
☐ 2. Administer the antibiotic in the left eye and the steroid in the right eye.
☐ 3. Administer both types of drops in the right eye.
☐ 4. Contact the pharmacist for clarification of the prescription.

63. A client with rheumatoid arthritis tells the nurse that they feel "quite alone" in adjusting to changes in their lifestyle. Which response by the nurse will be **most** effective?
☐ 1. referring the client and partner for counseling to decrease the sense of isolation
☐ 2. suggesting that the client develop a hobby to occupy their time
☐ 3. telling the client about a community arthritis support group
☐ 4. recommending that the client discuss their feelings with their religious advisor

64. Which laboratory test should the nurse monitor when the client is receiving warfarin sodium therapy?
☐ 1. partial thromboplastin time (PTT)
☐ 2. serum potassium
☐ 3. arterial blood gas (ABG) values
☐ 4. prothrombin time (PT)

65. A client who had transurethral resection of the prostate (TURP) 2 days earlier has lower abdominal pain. What should the nurse do **first**?
☐ 1. Auscultate the abdomen for bowel sounds.
☐ 2. Administer an oral analgesic.
☐ 3. Have the client use a sitz bath for 15 minutes.
☐ 4. Assess the patency of the urethral catheter.

66. The nurse is preparing to administer the IV dose of imipenem-cilastatin and finds the previous dose's minibag hanging without having been infused. What should the nurse do?
☐ 1. Discard the full partial fill of imipenem-cilastatin found hanging at the client's bedside.
☐ 2. Check the identifying information of the full partial fill of imipenem-cilastatin found hanging at the client's bedside.
☐ 3. Determine when the client received the last dose of the imipenem-cilastatin.
☐ 4. Administer the new partial fill of imipenem-cilastatin.

67. A client with a moderate level of anxiety is pacing quickly in the hall and tells the nurse, "Help me. I can't take it anymore." What would be the nurse's **best** initial response?
☐ 1. "It would be best if you would lie down until you are calmer."
☐ 2. "Let's go to a quieter area where we can talk if you want."
☐ 3. "Try doing your relaxation exercises to calm down."
☐ 4. "I'll get some medicine to help you relax."

68. A client is receiving a tube feeding and has developed diarrhea, cramps, and abdominal distention. What should the nurse do? Select all that apply.
☐ 1. Change the feeding apparatus every 24 hours.
☐ 2. Use a higher volume of formula because the formula may be too hypotonic.
☐ 3. Slow the administration rate.
☐ 4. Use a diluted formula, gradually increasing the volume and concentration.
☐ 5. Anticipate changing to a lactose-free formula.

69. A middle-age client who has smoked two packs of cigarettes for the last 10 years is admitted with a diagnosis of lung cancer. The client reports having "no appetite" and exhibits symptoms of anorexia. The client is 5 feet, 8 inches (173 cm) tall and weighs 112 lb (50.8 kg). The client is now scheduled for a left lung lobectomy. The nurse should include which factor when planning to prevent postoperative pulmonary complications?
☐ 1. The client tends to keep feelings to themselves.
☐ 2. The client ambulates and can climb one flight of stairs without dyspnea.
☐ 3. The client is middle age.
☐ 4. The client's weight relative to height is low.

70. STEP 1

The nurse is providing care to a 37-year-old female client in the fourth stage of labor following a spontaneous vaginal birth.

Nurse's Notes

1200:
The gravida 5, para 4, abortion 0 client delivered a 9-lb, 4-oz (4.2 kg) female neonate at 42 weeks' gestation. The client's membranes were ruptured for 20 hours, and the amniotic fluid was meconium stained. The client had an unmedicated birth with a 3-hour labor after contractions began. The client has a grade 3 perineal tear repair and does not have an intravenous (IV) line. The client is bottle-feeding.

1215:
The fundal height is one fingerbreadth below the umbilicus, and the fundus is firm. Lochia is moderate rubra. Vital signs are temperature (T) 99.7°F (37.6°C); pulse (P) 88 bpm; respiration rate (RR) 16 breaths/min; and blood pressure (BP) 120/70 mm Hg. The patient rates pain as a 4 on a scale of 0 to 10.

1230:
The fundal height is at the umbilicus, and the fundus is boggy. The peripad is saturated. Vital signs are T 99.7°F (37.6°C); P 98 bpm; RR 18 breaths/min; and BP 116/68 mm Hg. The pulse oximetry reading is 97% on room air. Pain is rated as a 6 on a scale of 0 to 10.

▸ Highlight the top three findings at the 30-minute check that require **immediate** follow-up. Answer choices have been underlined.

Nurse's Notes

1230:
The fundal height is at the umbilicus, and the fundus is boggy. The peripad is saturated. Vital signs are T 99.7°F (37.6°C); P 98 bpm; RR 18 breaths/min; BP 116/68 mm Hg; and pulse oximetry reading 97% on room air. Pain is rated as a 6 on a scale of 0 to 10.

71. STEP 2

The nurse is providing care to a 37-year-old female client in the fourth stage of labor following a spontaneous vaginal birth.

Nurse's Notes

1200:
The gravida 5, para 4, abortion 0 client delivered a 9-lb, 4-oz (4.2 kg) female neonate at 42 weeks' gestation. The client's membranes were ruptured for 20 hours, and the amniotic fluid was meconium stained. The client had an unmedicated birth with a 3-hour labor after contractions began. The client has a grade 3 perineal tear repair and does not have an intravenous (IV) line. The client is bottle-feeding.

1215:
The fundal height is one fingerbreadth below the umbilicus, and the fundus is firm. Lochia is moderate rubra. Vital signs are temperature (T) 99.7°F (37.6°C); pulse (P) 88 bpm; respiration rate (RR) 16 breaths/min; and blood pressure (BP) 120/70 mm Hg. The patient rates pain as a 4 on a scale of 0 to 10.

1230:
The fundal height is at the umbilicus, and the fundus is boggy. The peripad is saturated. Vital signs are T 99.7°F (37.6°C); P 98 bpm; RR 18 breaths/min; and BP 116/68 mm Hg. The pulse oximetry reading is 97% on room air. Pain is rated as a 6 on a scale of 0 to 10.

➤ For each client finding, indicate if it is a risk factor for bleeding-associated uterine atony, lacerations, or retained placental fragments. Each risk factor may be associated with more than one condition.

Risk Factor	Uterine Atony	Lacerations	Retained Fragments
High parity	☐	☐	☐
Maternal age	☐	☐	☐
Length membranes were ruptured	☐	☐	☐
Length of labor	☐	☐	☐
Fetal size	☐	☐	☐

Note: Each column must have at least one response option selected.

72. STEP 3

The nurse is providing care to a 37-year-old female client in the fourth stage of labor following a spontaneous vaginal birth.

Nurse's Notes

1200:
The gravida 5, para 4, abortion 0 client delivered a 9-lb, 4-oz (4.2 kg) female neonate at 42 weeks' gestation. The client's membranes were ruptured for 20 hours, and the amniotic fluid was meconium stained. The client had an unmedicated birth with a 3-hour labor after contractions began. The client has a grade 3 perineal tear repair and does not have an intravenous (IV) line. The client is bottle-feeding.

1215:
The fundal height is one fingerbreadth below the umbilicus, and the fundus is firm. Lochia is moderate rubra. Vital signs are temperature (T) 99.7°F (37.6°C); pulse (P) 88 bpm; respiration rate (RR) 16 breaths/min; and blood pressure (BP) 120/70 mm Hg. The patient rates pain as a 4 on a scale of 0 to 10.

1230:
The fundal height is at the umbilicus, and the fundus is boggy. The peripad is saturated. Vital signs are T 99.7°F (37.6°C); P 98 bpm; RR 18 breaths/min; and BP 116/68 mm Hg. The pulse oximetry reading is 97% on room air. Pain is rated as a 6 on a scale of 0 to 10.

➤ Complete the sentence from the list of drop-down options.

The client is **most** likely experiencing a postpartum hemorrhage due to [uterine atony. / perineal laceration. / retained fragments.]

Untreated, the client is greatest risk for developing [hypovolemic shock. / uterine prolapse. / uterine infection.]

73. STEP 4

The nurse is providing care to a 37-year-old female client in the fourth stage of labor following a spontaneous vaginal birth.

Nurse's Notes

1200:
The gravida 5, para 4, abortion 0 client delivered a 9-lb, 4-oz (4.2 kg) female neonate at 42 weeks' gestation. The client's membranes were ruptured for 20 hours, and the amniotic fluid was meconium stained. The client had an unmedicated birth with a 3-hour labor after contractions began. The client has a grade 3 perineal tear repair and does not have an intravenous (IV) line. The client is bottle-feeding.

1215:
The fundal height is one fingerbreath below the umbilicus, and the fundus is firm. Lochia is moderate rubra. Vital signs are temperature (T) 99.7°F (37.6°C); pulse (P) 88 bpm; respiration rate (RR) 16 breaths/min; and blood pressure (BP) 120/70 mm Hg. The patient rates pain as a 4 on a scale of 0 to 10.

1230:
The fundal height is at the umbilicus, and the fundus is boggy. The peripad is saturated. Vital signs are T 99.7°F (37.6°C); P 98 bpm; RR 18 breaths/min; and BP 116/68 mm Hg. The pulse oximetry reading is 97% on room air. Pain is rated as a 6 on a scale of 0 to 10.

Orders

1235:
Postpartum hemorrhage protocol:

- Establish IV access if not present.
- Begin 1000 mL of lactated Ringer's solution at 500 mL per hour.
- Administer 10 units of oxytocin intramuscularly (IM).
- Perform vigorous fundal massage for at least 15 seconds.
- Weigh blood-soaked materials.
- Take vital signs, including oxygen saturation and level of consciousness, every 5 minutes.
- Administer oxygen to maintain a pulse oximetry reading of greater than 95%.
- Type and crossmatch for 2 units of red blood cells stat.
- Empty the bladder with a straight catheter or place an indwelling catheter.

The nurse notifies the healthcare provider of the client's status and receives orders to activate the postpartum hemorrhage protocol.

➢ Highlight the three orders the nurse should implement first. Answer choices have been underlined.

Orders

1235:
Postpartum hemorrhage protocol:

- <u>Establish IV access if not present.</u>
- <u>Begin 1000 mL of lactated Ringer's solution at 500 mL per hour.</u>
- <u>Administer 10 units of oxytocin intramuscularly (IM).</u>
- <u>Perform vigorous fundal massage for at least 15 seconds.</u>
- <u>Weigh blood-soaked materials.</u>
- <u>Take vital signs, including oxygen saturation and level of consciousness, every 5 minutes.</u>
- <u>Administer oxygen to maintain a pulse oximetry reading of greater than 95%.</u>
- <u>Type and crossmatch for 2 units of red blood cells stat.</u>
- <u>Empty the bladder with a straight catheter or place an indwelling catheter.</u>

74. STEP 5

The nurse is providing care to a 37-year-old female client in the fourth stage of labor following a spontaneous vaginal birth.

Nurse's Notes

1200:
The gravida 5, para 4, abortion 0 client delivered a 9-lb, 4-oz (4.2 kg) female neonate at 42 weeks' gestation. The client's membranes were ruptured for 20 hours, and the amniotic fluid was meconium stained. The client had an unmedicated birth with a 3-hour labor after contractions began. The client has a grade 3 perineal tear repair and does not have an intravenous (IV) line. The client is bottle-feeding.

1215:
The fundal height is one fingerbreath below the umbilicus, and the fundus is firm. Lochia is moderate rubra. Vital signs are temperature (T) 99.7°F (37.6°C); pulse (P) 88 bpm; respiration rate (RR) 16 breaths/min; and blood pressure (BP) 120/70 mm Hg. The patient rates pain as a 4 on a scale of 0 to 10.

1230:
The fundal height is at the umbilicus, and the fundus is boggy. The peripad is saturated. Vital signs are T 99.7°F (37.6°C); P 98 bpm; RR 18 breaths/min; and BP 116/68 mm Hg. The pulse oximetry reading is 97% on room air. Pain is rated as a 6 on a scale of 0 to 10.

Orders

1235:
Postpartum hemorrhage protocol:

- Establish IV access if not present.
- Begin 1000 mL of lactated Ringer's solution at 500 mL per hour.
- Administer 10 units of oxytocin intramuscularly (IM).
- Perform vigorous fundal massage for at least 15 seconds.
- Weigh blood-soaked materials.
- Take vital signs, including oxygen saturation and level of consciousness, every 5 minutes.
- Administer oxygen to maintain a pulse oximetry reading of greater than 95%.
- Type and crossmatch for 2 units of red blood cells stat.
- Empty the bladder with a straight catheter or place an indwelling catheter.

1250:
- Give misoprostol 0.8 mg per rectum stat.

The uterus fails to firm after oxytocin IM and vigorous massage. IV access has been established. The nurse receives additional orders for misoprostol. The pharmacy sends four 200-mcg tablets of misoprostol to the unit.

➤ Complete the sentences by using the list of drop-down options.

The nurse determines that the misoprostol [dose is not clear. / order is appropriate. / route is an error.]

The nurse should [administer four tablets per rectum. / request an order for the oral route. / question the total dose to administer.]

75. STEP 6

The nurse is providing care to a 37-year-old female client in the fourth stage of labor following a spontaneous vaginal birth.

Nurse's Notes

1200:
The gravida 5, para 4, abortion 0 client delivered a 9-lb, 4-oz (4.2 kg) female neonate at 42 weeks' gestation. The client's membranes were ruptured for 20 hours, and the amniotic fluid was meconium stained. The client had an unmedicated birth with a 3-hour labor after contractions began. The client has a grade 3 perineal tear repair and does not have an intravenous (IV) line. The client is bottle-feeding.

1215:
The fundal height is one fingerbreath below the umbilicus, and the fundus is firm. Lochia is moderate rubra. Vital signs are temperature (T) 99.7°F (37.6°C); pulse (P) 88 bpm; respiration rate (RR) 16 breaths/min; and blood pressure (BP) 120/70 mm Hg. The patient rates pain as a 4 on a scale of 0 to 10.

1230:
The fundal height is at the umbilicus, and the fundus is boggy. The peripad is saturated. Vital signs are T 99.7°F (37.6°C); P 98 bpm; RR 18 breaths/min; and BP 116/68 mm Hg. The pulse oximetry reading is 97% on room air. Pain is rated as a 6 on a scale of 0 to 10.

1250:
Oxytocin was given. An IV was started in the left arm. Labs were sent. The uterus fails to firm after massage.

0100:
Misoprostol was given.

0130:
The fundus is firm. The client is saturating one peripad per hour and is diaphoretic. Vital signs are T 99.7°F (37.6°C); P 100 bpm; RR 18 breaths/min; BP 104/50 mm Hg; and pulse oximetry 97% on room air.

Orders

1235:
Postpartum hemorrhage protocol:
- Establish IV access if not present.
- Begin 1000 mL of lactated Ringer's solution at 500 mL per hour.
- Administer 10 units of oxytocin intramuscularly (IM).
- Perform vigorous fundal massage for at least 15 seconds.
- Weigh blood-soaked materials.
- Take vital signs, including oxygen saturation and level of consciousness, every 5 minutes.
- Administer oxygen to maintain a pulse oximetry reading of greater than 95%.
- Type and crossmatch for 2 units of red blood cells stat.
- Empty the bladder with a straight catheter or place an indwelling catheter.

1250:
- Give misoprostol 0.8 mg per rectum stat.

The nurse reassesses the client 30 minutes after implementing the treatment protocol.

➤ Which finding(s) suggest that the client's status is still declining and progressing toward shock? Select all that apply.

☐ 1. fundus
☐ 2. vaginal bleeding
☐ 3. diaphoresis
☐ 4. pulse
☐ 5. Respiratory rate
☐ 6. Blood pressure

76. When developing the plan of care for a 12-year-old child who is to receive chemotherapy that is associated with nausea and vomiting, the nurse should plan to administer an antiemetic at which time?
☐ 1. 30 minutes after the chemotherapy has started, then as needed
☐ 2. 30 minutes before the chemotherapy starts, then routinely
☐ 3. when the 12-year-old client requests medication for nausea, then as needed
☐ 4. on starting the chemotherapy infusion, then routinely

77. The membranes of a multigravid client in active labor rupture spontaneously, revealing greenish-colored amniotic fluid. How does the nurse interpret this finding?
☐ 1. passage of meconium by the fetus
☐ 2. maternal intrauterine infection
☐ 3. Rh incompatibility between the birth mother and the fetus
☐ 4. maternal sexually transmitted disease

78. A client is suspected of having a slow gastrointestinal bleed. The nurse should assess the client for which sign?
☐ 1. increased pulse
☐ 2. nausea
☐ 3. tarry stools
☐ 4. abdominal cramps

79. After a client undergoes a lobectomy for lung cancer, the nurse instructs the client to perform deep-breathing exercises. What is the expected outcome of these exercises?
☐ 1. Decrease blood flow to the lungs for rest and increased surface alveoli ventilation.
☐ 2. Elevate the diaphragm to enlarge the thorax so that the lung surface area available for gas exchange is increased.
☐ 3. Control the rate of airflow to the remaining lobe to decrease the risk for hyperinflation.
☐ 4. Expand the alveoli, and increase the lung surface available for ventilation.

80. A client with diabetes who takes insulin has a blood glucose level of 40 mg/dL (2.27 mmol/L). What should the nurse offer the client to begin to raise the blood glucose level? Select all that apply.
  ☐ 1. one-half cup (120 mL) of orange juice
  ☐ 2. one cup (240 mL) of milk
  ☐ 3. one-quarter cup (60 mL) of tuna
  ☐ 4. one tablespoon (15 mL) of peanut butter
  ☐ 5. one slice of bread
  ☐ 6. one-half cup (120 mL) of regular soda

81. When preparing to draw up 8 units of a short-acting insulin and 20 units of a long-acting insulin in the same syringe, the nurse should use which technique?
  ☐ 1. Inject air in the vial with the long-acting insulin first.
  ☐ 2. Draw up the long-acting insulin first.
  ☐ 3. Draw up either insulin first.
  ☐ 4. Use a high-dose insulin syringe.

82. The birth parent of an infant with iron deficiency anemia asks the nurse what they could have done to prevent the anemia. The nurse should teach the birth parent that it is helpful to introduce solid foods into the infant's diet at which age?
  ☐ 1. 3 months
  ☐ 2. 6 months
  ☐ 3. 8 months
  ☐ 4. 10 months

83. The nurse is caring for a client who is having an acute asthma attack. The nurse should notify the health care provider when the client has which symptom?
  ☐ 1. loud wheezing
  ☐ 2. tenacious, thick sputum
  ☐ 3. decreased breath sounds
  ☐ 4. persistent cough

84. A client has had a cardiac catheterization. The femoral dressing has a bright bloody drainage. What should the nurse do **first**?
  ☐ 1. Assess the airway.
  ☐ 2. Administer oxygen.
  ☐ 3. Apply pressure to the site.
  ☐ 4. Assess the pulse in the left extremity.

85. Bacterial conjunctivitis has affected several children at a local daycare center. A nurse should advise which measure to minimize the risk for infection?
  ☐ 1. Close the daycare center for 1 week to control the outbreak.
  ☐ 2. Restrict the infected children from returning for 48 hours after treatment.
  ☐ 3. Perform thorough handwashing before and after touching any child in the daycare center.
  ☐ 4. Set up a conference with the parents of each child to explain the situation carefully.

86. The nurse is evaluating the client's risk for having a pressure sore. Which is the **best** indicator of risk for the client's developing a pressure sore?
  ☐ 1. nutritional status
  ☐ 2. circulatory status
  ☐ 3. mobility status
  ☐ 4. orientation status

87. The nurse is planning care for a 65-year-old male client who had a lobectomy yesterday to remove a cancerous tumor in the right inferior lobe.

> **Nurse's Notes**
>
> **0800:**
> Vital signs are temperature (T) 99.8°F (37.7°C); heart rate (HR) 88 beats/min; respiration rate (RR) 22 breaths/min; blood pressure (BP) 120/86 mm Hg; and oxygen saturation per pulse oximeter 92%. Breath sounds in the left lung are normal; in the right lower lung they are diminished. The dressing is dry and intact; the chest tube is fluctuating. The client was administered 10 mg of morphine for incisional pain that is rated as an 8 on a scale of 0 to 10. The intravenous (IV) line is running at 30 mL per minute, with no signs of infiltration. The client was turned to the back, and the head of the bed was elevated to 30 degrees.
>
> **0900:**
> The client has been given reassurance. Vital signs are T 99.0°F (37.2°C); RR 24 breaths/min; BP 120/88 mm Hg; and oxygen saturation on pulse oximeter 90%. Breath sounds in the right lower lung are diminished; the left lung is clear. The client rates the incisional pain as 3 on a scale of 0 to 10.

➤ Complete the diagram by circling the choices below to specify the condition the client is most likely experiencing, the two most needed nursing actions to take, and two parameters the nurse should monitor to determine the effectiveness of the actions.

Action to Take	Condition Most Likely Experiencing	Parameters to Monitor
Action to Take		Parameters to Monitor

Possible Actions to Take	Potential Conditions	Parameters to Monitor
Administer oxygen at 6 L/min per face mask	Chest tube occlusion	Incisional pain
Administer morphine	Incisional pain	Oxygen saturation
Assist the client to use an incentive spirometer	Lung infection	Incision site
Turn the client to the left side	Decreased oxygenation, right lung	Chest tube drainage
Milk the chest tube		Breath sounds

88. While the nurse is assisting a client to ambulate as part of a cardiac rehabilitation program, the client has midsternal burning. What should the nurse do **next**?
☐ 1. Stop and assess the client further.
☐ 2. Obtain the client's blood pressure and heart rate.
☐ 3. Call for help, and place the client in a wheelchair.
☐ 4. Administer nitroglycerin.

89. A client has been taking dexamethasone for 2 weeks. Which statement by the client indicates they need follow-up teaching? The nurse evaluates a client's knowledge as deficient when the client makes which comment?
☐ 1. "I can't stop the medication all at one time."
☐ 2. "If I forget a dose, I'll take it when I remember it."
☐ 3. "When I get a cold, I need to let my health care provider (HCP) know."
☐ 4. "I need to watch for an allergic reaction when I first start taking this pill."

90. A 3-month-old has moderate dehydration. The nurse should assess the client for which sign of moderate dehydration?
☐ 1. oliguria
☐ 2. bulging eyes
☐ 3. sunken posterior fontanelle
☐ 4. pale skin color

91. The nurse is assessing a client who is suspected of being in the early symptomatic stages of human immunodeficiency virus (HIV) infection. Which indication of infection should the nurse detect during this stage?
☐ 1. whitish-yellow patches in the mouth
☐ 2. dyspnea
☐ 3. bloody diarrhea
☐ 4. raised, hyperpigmented lesions on the legs

92. A primiparous client who is breastfeeding develops endometritis on the third postpartum day. What instructions should the nurse give to the client?
☐ 1. The neonate will need to be bottle-fed for the next few days.
☐ 2. The condition typically is treated with intravenous (IV) antibiotic therapy.
☐ 3. The client may require oxytocin and frequent uterine massage.
☐ 4. The client needs to remain in bed in a side-lying position as much as possible.

93. After instructing a primiparous client who is breastfeeding on how to prevent nipple soreness during feedings, the nurse determines that the client needs further instruction when they make which statement?
☐ 1. "I should position the baby the same way for each feeding."
☐ 2. "I should make sure the baby grasps the entire areola and nipple."
☐ 3. "I should air-dry my breasts and nipples for 10 to 15 minutes after the feeding."
☐ 4. "I shouldn't use a hand breast pump if my nipples get sore."

94. A client who has Ménière's disease is experiencing an acute attack of vertigo. What should the nurse do to help the client manage the attack?
☐ 1. Darken the client's room and provide a quiet environment.
☐ 2. Give the client cheese and crackers.
☐ 3. Administer acetaminophen.
☐ 4. Offer carbonated fluids.

95. To reduce urethral irritation, where should the nurse tape the female client's Foley catheter?
☐ 1. inner thigh
☐ 2. groin area
☐ 3. lower abdomen
☐ 4. lower thigh

96.

The nurse cares for a 72-year-old female client with a history of alcohol use disorder on the medical-surgical unit the day after a left knee placement.

Nurse's Notes

Postoperative Day 2

0700:
The client was agitated, reported sleeping little last night, and refused breakfast. The client was given oral (PO) pain medication for left knee pain that was rated as a 6 on a scale of 0 to 10.

0800:
The nurse entered the room because the client was heard from the hall to be shouting "get the spiders out of here!" The client was found highly agitated, confused, and oriented to person only and had moderate hand and tongue tremors. Beads of sweat were visible on the client's forehead. A pool of vomit was found by the bed. The left knee dressing was also found on the floor. The incision remains intact. The client's spouse, returning from the cafeteria, verifies that the client's typical alcohol consumption included drinking a bottle of vodka a day. Vital signs are temperature 100°F (37.8°C); pulse 116 bpm; respiration rate 24 breaths/min; blood pressure 168/94 mm Hg; and pulse oximetry reading 96% in room air. The health care provider and the rapid response team were paged.

The nurse reviews the client's changes and updates the plan of care.

➤ Complete the diagram by circling the choices below to specify the condition the client is **most** likely experiencing, two actions to take immediately, and two parameters the nurse should monitor to assess the client's progress.

Action to Take — Potential Condition — Parameter to Monitor
Action to Take — Parameter to Monitor

Action to Take	Potential Conditions	Parameters to Monitor
Administer intramuscular (IM) haloperidol	Korsakoff psychosis	Blood alcohol levels
Perform gastric lavage	Delirium tremens	Alcohol withdrawal assessment scores
Administer intravenous (IV) diazepam	Wernicke encephalopathy	Vital signs
Initiate seizure precautions	Alcohol overdose	Memory changes
Administer PO thiamine		Glasgow Coma Scale score

97. The nurse assesses a client who is receiving a tube feeding. Which situation would require prompt intervention from the nurse?
☐ 1. The client is sitting upright in bed while the feeding is infusing.
☐ 2. The feeding that is infusing has been hanging for 8 hours.
☐ 3. The client has a gastric residual of 25 mL.
☐ 4. The feeding solution is at room temperature.

98. A client has been taking furosemide for 2 days. The nurse should review the laboratory record for changes in which blood level?
☐ 1. an elevated blood urea nitrogen (BUN)
☐ 2. an elevated potassium
☐ 3. a decreased potassium
☐ 4. an elevated sodium

99. Prior to administering plasminogen activator (t-PA) to a client admitted with a stroke, the nurse should verify which information about the client? Select all that apply.
☐ 1. is older than 65 years
☐ 2. has had symptoms of the stroke less than 3 hours
☐ 3. has a blood pressure within normal limits
☐ 4. does not have active internal bleeding
☐ 5. has not had an alcoholic beverage within the last 8 hours

100. How does the nurse identify the type of presentation shown in the figure?

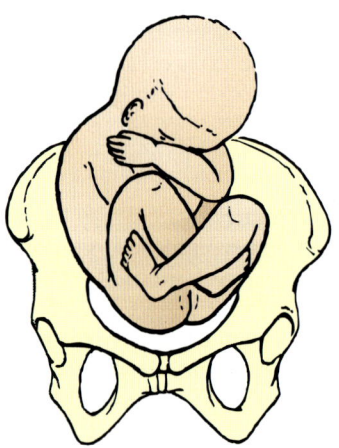

☐ 1. frank breech
☐ 2. compound breech
☐ 3. complete breech
☐ 4. incomplete breech

101. Following cardiac bypass surgery, the client has been referred to a cardiac rehabilitation exercise program. The client has type 1 diabetes and has bilateral leg discomfort with walking. The client is exercising using a stationary bicycle. The nurse should evaluate the client's response to exercise by assessing the presence of which condition?
☐ 1. diabetic neuropathy
☐ 2. muscle atrophy
☐ 3. Raynaud's disease
☐ 4. transient ischemic attacks

102. A client who has been taking diazepam for 3 months for skeletal muscle spasms and lower back pain has stopped taking the medication 2 days ago because it was no longer helping. Now the pain has increased. The nurse should assess the client for which sign(s) of withdrawal? Select all that apply.
☐ 1. insomnia
☐ 2. euphoria
☐ 3. bradycardia
☐ 4. diaphoresis
☐ 5. tremor
☐ 6. vomiting

103. An intravenous (IV) infusion is to be administered through a scalp vein on an infant's head. What should the nurse tell the parents to prepare them for the procedure?
☐ 1. It may be necessary to remove a small amount of hair from the infant's scalp.
☐ 2. A sedative will be given to help keep the infant quiet.
☐ 3. Visiting the infant will be delayed until the infusion has been completed.
☐ 4. Holding the infant will be contraindicated while the infusion is being administered.

104. A nurse is caring for a child with type 1 diabetes mellitus at camp. The child is irritable and has a headache. What should the nurse do **first**?
☐ 1. Administer 2 oz (60 mL) of orange juice.
☐ 2. Notify the health care provider (HCP) about the child's status.
☐ 3. Check the child's blood glucose level.
☐ 4. Send the child back to the planned activities.

105. A client is to learn to self-administer insulin. Which health professional should be involved in teaching the client?
☐ 1. nurse and client because both need to be responsible for teaching
☐ 2. health care provider (HCP) and client because the HCP is the manager of care and the client is the main participant
☐ 3. client because the client is best able to identify their needs and how to meet them
☐ 4. client, nurse, pharmacist, and HCP so the client can participate in planning care with the entire team

106. A multigravid client at 36 weeks' gestation who is visiting the clinic for a routine visit begins to sob and tells the nurse, "My partner has been beating me up once in a while since I became pregnant, but I can't bring myself to leave them because I don't have a job and I don't know how I would take care of my other children." What is the **priority** action by the nurse at this time?
☐ 1. Contact a social worker for assistance and family counseling.
☐ 2. Help the client make concrete plans for the safety of the client and their children.
☐ 3. Tell the client that they should not allow anyone to hit them or their children.
☐ 4. Provide the client with brochures on the statistics about domestic violence.

107. Several children were admitted yesterday. In which order of priority from first to last would the nurse assess these children? All options must be used.

1. a 3-month-old infant with respiratory syncytial virus and stable vital signs
2. a 10-month-old infant with pneumonia and a respiratory rate of 50 breaths/min
3. a 3-year-old child with acute pyelonephritis and a temperature of 104.5°F (40.3°C)
4. a 12-year-old child with a fractured femur and a lacerated liver

108. A client admitted with a diagnosis of dementia becomes agitated and violent. The nurse is reviewing the client's medication record. Which prescribed medication would be expected to reduce agitation?
☐ 1. tacrine
☐ 2. ergoloid
☐ 3. diazepam
☐ 4. risperidone

109. While performing cardiopulmonary resuscitation (CPR) on a 5-year-old child, the nurse palpates for a pulse. Which site is **best** for checking the pulse during CPR in a 5-year-old child?
☐ 1. femoral artery
☐ 2. carotid artery
☐ 3. radial artery
☐ 4. brachial artery

110. A child with tetralogy of Fallot and a history of severe hypoxic episodes is to be admitted to the pediatric unit. What would be **most** important for the nurse to have at the bedside?
☐ 1. morphine sulfate in a syringe ready to administer
☐ 2. oxygen tubing and flow meter plugged in
☐ 3. blood pressure cuff and stethoscope
☐ 4. suction tubing and equipment

111.
The nurse cares for a 2-year-old male client hospitalized with diarrhea and mild dehydration.

Laboratory Results

Stool Microscopy	Result	Reference Range
White blood cells	Many	Negative
Red blood cells	Few	Negative
Parasites	Negative	Negative
Stool culture	Results	Reference range
Pathogenic *Escherichia coli*	Positive	Negative
Salmonella	Negative	Negative

The nurse reviews the lab report from the client's stool specimen.

➢ Complete the sentence from the list of options.

The action the nurse should perform **first** is [cleanse and protect the child's anal area. / instruct the family to wash all home bed linens. / institute enteric precautions. / start an intravenous infusion.]

112. A client is voiding small amounts of urine every 30 to 60 minutes. What should the nurse do **first**?
☐ 1. Palpate for a distended bladder.
☐ 2. Catheterize the client for residual urine.
☐ 3. Obtain a urine specimen for culture.
☐ 4. Encourage an increased fluid intake.

113. When making rounds, the nurse should assess which client **first**?
☐ 1. a 16-month-old child with periorbital cellulitis who is to be discharged today
☐ 2. a 7-year-old child who had an appendectomy yesterday and developed peritonitis
☐ 3. a 10-year-old child in sickle cell crisis who has just been admitted
☐ 4. a 16-year-old adolescent receiving a third day of chemotherapy

114. Which intervention should the nurse suggest to a parent to relieve itching in a child with chickenpox?
☐ 1. generous amounts of fine baby powder
☐ 2. oatmeal preparation baths
☐ 3. soft towels moistened with hydrogen peroxide
☐ 4. cool compresses moistened with a weak salt solution

115. A woman who has preeclampsia is receiving magnesium sulfate 20 g per 500 mL of lactated Ringer's solution via an infusion pump. The prescribed rate of infusion is 2 g per hour. How many milliliters per hour should the nurse set the infusion pump for? Record your answer using a whole number.

_____ mL per hour.

116. A 16-year-old primigravida client at 36 weeks' gestation who has had no prenatal care experienced a seizure at work and is being transported to the hospital by ambulance. What should the nurse do upon the client's arrival?
☐ 1. Position the client in a supine position.
☐ 2. Auscultate breath sounds every 4 hours.
☐ 3. Monitor the vital signs every 4 hours.
☐ 4. Admit the client to a quiet, darkened room.

117. A client's chest tube is connected to a drainage system with a water seal. The nurse notes that the fluid in the water seal column is fluctuating with each breath that the client takes. How should the nurse interpret this finding?
☐ 1. There is an obstruction in the chest tube.
☐ 2. The client is developing subcutaneous emphysema.
☐ 3. The chest tube system is functioning properly.
☐ 4. There is a leak in the chest tube system.

118. The nurse discovers that a hospitalized client with stage 4 esophageal cancer and major depression has a gun in the home. What is the **best** nursing intervention to help the client remain safe after discharge?
    - ☐ 1. Give the client the number of a 24-hour crisis phone line for use, if needed.
    - ☐ 2. Tell the health care provider (HCP) that the client is too high risk for discharge at this time.
    - ☐ 3. Have the client promise to use the gun only for home protection.
    - ☐ 4. Talk with the HCP about requiring gun removal as a condition of discharge.

119. A client with severe osteoarthritis and decreased mobility is moved to an assisted living facility. The nurse notices that the client smells of alcohol, is slurring words, and has six wine bottles in the trash. The client tells the nurse, "Those are my other pain medicines." Which statement(s) by the nurse are appropriate? Select all that apply.
    - ☐ 1. "I didn't realize that your pain was not being managed with your current medication."
    - ☐ 2. "It's important for me to know how many bottles of wine you drank this week."
    - ☐ 3. "I'm worried about the amount of wine you are drinking and its effects on your balance."
    - ☐ 4. "How are you getting all this wine?"
    - ☐ 5. "I'm calling your health care provider (HCP) to have all of us talk about better pain control without the wine."

120. Which child **most** needs a referral for developmental language delay?
    - ☐ 1. the 1-year-old child who does not have three words
    - ☐ 2. the 18-month-old child who only points to one body part
    - ☐ 3. the 2-year-old child who only combines two words
    - ☐ 4. the 4-year-old child who is difficult to understand

Answers, Rationales, and Test-Taking Strategies

*The answers and rationales for each question follow below, along with keys (🔑) to the client need (CN) and cognitive level (CL) for each question. In addition, questions that measure clinical judgment will be coded (CJ). As you check your answers, use the **Content Mastery and Test-Taking Skill Self-Analysis** worksheet (tear-out worksheet in the back of the book) to identify the reason(s) for not answering the questions correctly. For additional information about test-taking skills and strategies for answering questions, refer to pages 12–51 in Part 1 of this book.*

1. **3.** The client who should be assessed first is the multigravid client who has been in labor for 8 hours and whose cervix is 8-cm dilated at 1+ station with contractions every 3 to 4 minutes. A multigravid client typically has a shorter labor and would be expected to deliver before a primigravid client whose cervix is dilated 6-cm. This client's station is 1+, which means that the birth of the fetus is imminent. The other two clients have given birth more than an hour ago and are stable with firm a fundus.

    🔑 CN: Management of care; CL: Analyze

2. **1 mL**

    First, convert micrograms to milligrams:
    $$200 \text{ mcg} = 0.2 \text{ mg}.$$
    Then:
    $$0.2 \text{ mg} / X \text{ mL} = 0.2 \text{ mg}/1 \text{ mL}$$
    $$X = 1 \text{ mL}.$$

    🔑 CN: Pharmacological and parenteral therapies; CL: Apply

3. **3.** Viral gastroenteritis may be communicable, and all the other children are already at risk for infection. The infant should be placed in a private room.

    🔑 CN: Safety and infection control; CL: Analyze

4. **1.** The neonate would be considered large for gestational age (LGA) because the neonate weighs more than 4000 g (90th percentile). Therefore, the nurse needs to assess for the possibility of complications. Hypoglycemia is a problem for the LGA neonate because glycogen stores are quickly used to maintain the weight. Other common complications for an LGA neonate include hyperbilirubinemia from the bruising and polycythemia, cephalhematoma,

caput succedaneum, molding, phrenic nerve paralysis, and a fractured clavicle. However, hyperbilirubinemia would not be evident 1 hour after birth. Hypercalcemia is not usually found in the LGA neonate. Hypocalcemia is common in infants of birth mothers with diabetes. Hypermagnesemia may occur in neonates whose birth mothers received large doses of magnesium sulfate to treat severe preeclampsia.

   CN: Reduction of risk potential; CL: Analyze

5. **1, 2, 5.** When an oxygen hood is used, the nurse should be sure the oxygen source is not directed at the infant's face to avoid skin irritation. Mobiles can be used to provide visual stimulation, but they should not be placed inside of the hood where they are a potential choking hazard. It is not necessary to restrain the infant unless there is an indication to do so, and the health care provider has written the prescription. There should be as little movement in and out of the hood as possible to maintain the warm and humid oxygen levels. The nurse should encourage the parents to visit the child and provide verbal and tactile stimulation.

   CN: Physiological adaptation; CL: Analyze

6. **1.** Older adult clients are a high-risk group for depression. The classic symptoms of depression frequently are masked, and depression presents differently in the aging population. Depression in late life is underdiagnosed because the symptoms are incorrectly attributed to aging or medical problems. Impairment of cognition in a previously healthy older adult client or psychosomatic problems may be the presenting symptom of depression. Antidepressant therapy is usually effective.

   CN: Psychosocial integrity; CL: Analyze

7. **3.** Preschool-age children are best prepared for procedures using play techniques such as puppets and storytelling. School-age children have a grasp of logic and respond well to diagrams, illustrations, videos, and books. Adolescents need to feel that they have had input into their care. They also need more time to build self-confidence. It is best to prepare adolescents a week in advance of a procedure. Toddlers should be prepared just before a procedure will occur.

   CN: Health promotion and maintenance; CL: Apply

8. **2.** When nurses deal with child abuse, the priority is the accurate and complete documentation of physical findings and observed behaviors on the child's record. Court proceedings usually occur sometime after the nurse's involvement with the child and family, and memories fade. Thus, careful documentation of the facts, not hearsay or subjective opinion, is essential. Objective data, not subjective opinions, are key. Preparing answers to questions that may be asked by the attorneys is not a priority for the nurse when the child is admitted. This may become appropriate later.

   CN: Management of care; CL: Analyze

9. **3.** The client is exhibiting signs and symptoms of withdrawal, and the nurse should administer the benzodiazepine to manage the anxiety, nausea, and restlessness and to prevent seizures. After administering the medication, the nurse will continue to assess the client and ensure the client is in a quiet environment. There is no need to transfer this client to the psychiatric unit based on the information provided.

   CN: Psychosocial adaptation; CL: Evaluation

10.

    STEP 1

    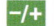 **2, 4, 5, 7.** Bilateral expiratory wheezes, shortness of breath, increased respirations, and lower than normal oxygen saturation are all findings of an acute asthma exacerbation and need immediate intervention. Clear nasal drainage is a normal finding indicating a lack of infection. The pulse is higher than normal, most likely due to the recent use of the albuterol. The red nares are likely caused by irritation.

       CJ: Case study; Step 1: Recognize cues; CL: Understand

11.

    STEP 2

    Nurse's Notes

    Today: 1100
    A 20-year-old college sophomore with moderate persistent asthma states that at soccer practice today they got short of breath with little relief from a prescribed albuterol inhaler, and the coach asked the client to go to the student health center. The client is sneezing and has a runny nose. The client has been using the albuterol inhaler as needed, which, until today, has provided relief. The last use of the albuterol inhaler was 30 minutes ago.
       Vital signs are temperature (T) 99°F (37.2°C); pulse (P) 110 bpm; respiration rate (RR) 26 breaths/min; blood pressure (BP) 128/86 mm Hg; and oxygen saturation 92%. Lung sounds have bilateral expiratory wheezes with diminished sounds at bases, and the client reports shortness of breath. Nasal drainage is clear, and the nares are slightly red. Other physical assessments are within normal ranges.

    Today: 1115
    Vital signs are P 106 bpm; RR 24 breaths/min; BP 122/82 mm Hg; and oxygen saturation 92%. Lung sounds have bilateral expiratory wheezes throughout, and the client is using intercostal muscles while breathing.

The oxygen saturation is lower, the nurse hears wheezes throughout the lungs, and the client is using accessory muscles when breathing now. These all indicate a worsening of the client's condition.

🔑 CJ: Case study; Step 2: Analyze cues;
CL: Understand

12.

STEP 3

0/1 The client is at risk for **respiratory failure**. To prevent further complications, the nurse should immediately **notify the health care provider**.

The client's respiratory status has declined, and the client is at risk for respiratory failure. The nurse needs to immediately notify the health care provider to request orders to continue care. The client is still able to breathe independently, so rescue breathing is not needed at this time. The client is not demonstrating signs of anxiety as would be noted in verbalization or changes in behavior. The nurse does not have a prescription to give the albuterol.

🔑 CJ: Case study; Step 3: Prioritize hypothesis;
CL: Analyze

13.

STEP 4

0/1 The nurse should first **verify the client's name and date of birth**, then **verify allergies**, then **verify medication with orders**, then **administer medication**, and finally **reassess the client for the effects of the medication**.

The nurse should first verify the client's name and date of birth, and then the nurse can assess the client's allergies before giving any medications. The medication must be verified with the health care provider's orders before being given. After administering the medication, the nurse should reassess the client for the effects of the medication.

🔑 CJ: Case study; Step 4: Generate solutions;
CL: Create

14.

STEP 5

−/+ 1, 2, 3, 6. The nurse should observe the client for the correct use of the albuterol inhaler. The client should sit up at 90 degrees to be able to expand the lungs fully. The client should shake the inhaler to mix the medication. The client should tightly seal their lips around the mouthpiece. The client should slowly and deeply inhale at the same time as the inhaler is activated. After inhaling the medication, the client should hold their breath for 10 seconds to help the medication go deeply into the lungs and then exhale to blow out the air in the lungs.

🔑 CJ: Case study; Step 5: Take action; CL: Apply

15.

STEP 6

0/1

Finding	Improved	Not Changed	Declined
RR 12 breaths/min	X		
Oxygen saturation 96%		X	
Expiratory and inspiratory wheezes			X
Use of accessory muscles			X
Slight shaking of hands		X	

The client's condition has improved. A RR of 12 breaths/min is within the normal range and would indicate that the client's respiratory status has improved. There has not been a change in the oxygen saturation level; the level of 95% is about the same as the earlier 96% level. Some continued shaking of hands would be normal from the albuterol. The client's condition has declined because the client still has wheezes progressing to wheezing both on expiration and inspiration and is using accessory muscles to breathe.

🔑 CJ: Case study; Step 6: Evaluate outcomes;
CL: Evaluate

16. **1.** The child's neutrophil count is low (the normal range is 3000 to 5000 cells/mm³ [3 to 5 × 10⁹/L]), predisposing the child to infection. If an infection occurs, the child will have difficulty combating it. Therefore, staff and visitors should be restricted to those without an active infection. Typically, neutropenic precautions, not strict isolation, would be used to protect the child from exposure to infection. The hospitalized child would be placed in a private room with visitors and staff screened for illnesses. The client's temperature would be monitored every 4 hours. Low neutrophil counts do not increase the likelihood of vomiting; therefore, an antiemetic is not needed. Increasing the child's oral fluid intake may be necessary; however, doing so is unrelated to the child's neutrophil count.

🔑 CN: Safety and infection control;
CL: Analyze

17. **1.** The incident report should be given to the nurse-manager. The incident report should not be placed on the medical record because it is considered a confidential communication and cannot be subpoenaed by a client or used as evidence in lawsuits. It is appropriate, ethical, and legally required that the fall be documented in the medical record. Unless there is a change in the client's condition reflecting an injury from the fall, there is no need to notify the family. If the family does need to be notified, the nurse-manager or the HCP should place the call.

🔑 CN: Management of care; CL: Analyze

18. **1.** The client who has had three prior births and has polyhydramnios has the potential for uterine atony and would be most at risk for a postpartum hemorrhage. The client at 34 weeks' gestation with mild pregnancy-induced hypertension would be at minimal risk because the uterus is not extraordinarily distended at this gestation. The gravida 4 para 0 client, who has diet-controlled gestational diabetes, has a risk for hemorrhage from being induced, but their uterus should be able to contract appropriately after the birth as long as there is no history of macrosomia. A history of genital herpes is not a risk factor for a postpartum hemorrhage.

🔑 CN: Reduction of risk potential; CL: Analyze

19. **2.** General wound care is appropriate initially. This includes washing the bite area with lots of water because infections occur frequently with animal bites, especially those on the arms or hands. Next, the parent should be advised to follow up with the child's HCP. A trip to the local care center would be warranted if the bite injury was extensive or there was severe bleeding. Although knowledge of when the child last had a tetanus vaccination is important, the child's wound takes priority. For rabies injections, there needs to be a history of rabies or unusual behavior in the pet.

🔑 CN: Physiological adaptation; CL: Analyze

20. **2.** The act of screening for intimate partner violence is a key intervention to help open doors for at-risk women to discuss ways to improve their safety and well-being. Asking clients how safe they feel in their home is an open-ended, nonjudgmental way to elicit perceptions of safety. Asking if a partner is excited about a pregnancy is not a good screening question because many couples are not excited to learn of an unplanned pregnancy. However, couples with healthy relationships eventually adjust. Having an arrest record and gun ownership do not automatically equate to having a history of violence.

🔑 CN: Safety and infection control; CL: Analyze

21. **1.** A significant association between feeding position and otitis media exists. Children fed in a supine position have a high incidence of otitis media because of the reflux of milk into the eustachian tubes during feedings. Keeping the infant's ears covered when out in the cold or thoroughly drying the ears after a bath has not been identified as a contributing factor to an infant's development of ear infections. Although the infant's immunization status is always important to ascertain, other factors, such as the position of the infant when taking a bottle, have more impact.

🔑 CN: Reduction of risk potential; CL: Analyze

22. **2.** Chemoprophylaxis should be given to household contacts and close contacts only. To prevent community outbreaks, chemoprophylaxis with rifampin 600 mg twice a day for 2 days or a single dose of ciprofloxacin 500 mg is indicated.

🔑 CN: Reduction of risk potential; CL: Analyze

23. **4.** The nurse is wearing protective personnel equipment appropriate for suctioning the client: goggles, gown, and respirator mask. It is not necessary to wear a PAPR face shield to suction a tracheostomy. A surgical mask does not provide maximum protection. The nurse must wear protective personnel equipment when caring for a client with a MRSA infection.

🔑 CN: Safety and infection control; CL: Apply

24. **1.** A major goal of safety and accident prevention focuses on having all cleaning supplies and medications locked up as infants become mobile. The child should not play in the bathroom even if the parent is present because the child will think that it is okay to play with these items when the parent is not present. Water safety classes are not recommended for children under the age of 1 year. The child-protective cabinet locks should work unless they were installed incorrectly or are defective.

🔑 CN: Safety and infection control; CL: Evaluate

25. 3, 4, 5. Common adverse effects of tobramycin include nephrotoxicity, ototoxicity, fever, and rash. Hypertension, weight gain, and decreased heart rate are not associated with this drug.

🔑 CN: Pharmacological and parenteral therapies; CL: Analyze

26. **3.** The nurse should question the use of a local anesthetic agent with epinephrine on the hands or feet because the epinephrine is a vasoconstrictor and can cause ischemia and gangrene of extremities. The nurse should suggest that the intern use bupivacaine without epinephrine as the local anesthetic agent. An intern should be trained in suturing small superficial incisions, and the cosmetic effect should be acceptable. The client's room should be a sufficiently aseptic environment because there is no other client in the room.

🔑 CN: Management of care; CL: Analyze

27. **3.** Infants should be monitored for hypoglycemia, temperature stability, and respiratory distress. The answer that best includes these components is monitoring the infant's feedings and vital signs. Apgar assessments are done at 1 and 5 minutes of age, not at 1 hour of age. The gestational age assessment is important for this infant but, after completion, does not require additional monitoring. The infant should be regularly assessed for jaundice as part of the physical assessment, but this is not the priority assessment at this time.

CN: Basic care and comfort; CL: Analyze

28. **1.** The client should plan to drink 1 to 2 L of fluid before an ultrasound to ensure a full bladder, which provides better visualization of the fetus. The client does not need to be on nothing-by-mouth status before the test. The client does not need to remain in the clinic for 4 hours after the test. However, if the client were scheduled for a contraction stress test, they would be observed as an outpatient for 1 to 4 hours after the test to make certain that the contractions had stopped. The client does not need to eat a high-fiber meal after the test. A high-fiber meal typically is indicated after certain radiographic procedures, such as an upper gastrointestinal series.

CN: Reduction of risk potential; CL: Apply

29. **-/+** **1, 3, 4.** Delegation involves the reassignment or transfer of selected aspects of a job to selected persons in selected situations. Although responsibility for the completion of a task or activity can be delegated, the accountability for that task remains with the registered nurse (RN). In delegating nursing acts, functions, or tasks, the RN must consider the nursing model to determine the appropriate delegation of assignment. Prior to delegation, the RN validates that the non-RN caregiver has orientation and experience in completion of the activity. The amount of time the nurse has does not direct the delegation procedure; the focus is on the task and capability of the staff to whom the task is delegated. It is not necessary to document that the task has been delegated and to whom; however, the outcome of the task should be documented by the nurse.

CN: Management of care; CL: Apply

30. **4.** One outcome criterion for the client with osteoarthritis is improved joint mobility. It is probably not possible to arrest the disease. Gold compound is administered to clients with rheumatoid arthritis, not osteoarthritis. Outcome criteria should be specific; feeling better is too general to be useful.

CN: Basic care and comfort; CL: Evaluate

31. **3.** Although monitoring vital signs frequently is important, for the first few days the primary concern in burn care is fluid and electrolyte balance, with the goal being to replace fluid and electrolytes lost. With burns, fluid and electrolytes move from the interstitial spaces to the burn injury and are lost. These must be replaced. Once the child's fluid and electrolyte status has been addressed and fluid resuscitation has begun, preventing wound infection is a priority, and efforts to control the child's pain can be initiated.

CN: Reduction of risk potential; CL: Analyze

32. **2.** The DTaP vaccine is given intramuscularly and often in combination with other vaccines. The inactivated polio vaccine may be given in either the intramuscular or subcutaneous route. The rotavirus vaccine is given orally. There are no approved intradermal vaccines for 2-month-old infants.

CN: Pharmacological and parenteral therapies; CL: Apply

33. **1.** The client's assessment findings indicate that the client is in the latent phase of the first stage of labor. Therefore, the nurse should plan to assist the client with comfort measures and breathing techniques to relieve discomfort. The client can move around, walk, or ambulate at this phase of labor. If the client chooses to remain in bed, a left side-lying position provides the greatest perfusion. It is too early for the client to have an epidural anesthetic. Epidural anesthesia is usually administered when the cervix is dilated 4 to 5 cm. The fetal heart rate is normal, so internal fetal monitoring is not warranted at this time.

CN: Health promotion and maintenance; CL: Analyze

34.

STEP 1

-/+ **1, 2, 3, 4, 5.** An infant with unresolved irritability, decreased PO intake, and vomiting for 2 days suggests that the child may be dehydrated. The nurse should try to determine when the client last had a wet diaper to determine how severe the dehydration may be. An infant with recent exposure to close ill contacts, such as siblings with a history of norovirus, should generate a high level of suspicion as a contagion. With norovirus, children develop "stomach flu" symptoms, such as vomiting and diarrhea 12 to 48 hours after exposure. The nurse needs to follow up on the pending lab test results, which can help determine if the child has norovirus or another gastrointestinal infection and help determine the severity of the dehydration. The posterior fontanelle typically closes by 8 weeks of age. All vital signs are normal for this age.

CJ: Case study; Step 1: Recognize cues; CL: Analyze

35.

STEP 2

0/1

Assessment	Helpful	Not Helpful
BP	X	
Anterior fontanelle	X	
Activity level	X	
Breast and bottle feeds		X
Presence of Babinski reflex		X
Number of wet diapers in the past 24 hours.	X	
Previous weight	X	
Urine specific gravity	X	

Common assessment findings for the infant with dehydration will include hypotension and a sunken fontanelle. With preverbal children, activity levels such as extreme irritability or listlessness should be closely assessed as infants do not have the ability to make their hydration needs known. The most precise method of assessing fluid deficit in children is a comparison to pre-illness weight. A weight loss of 5%, 10%, or 15% predicts the degree of dehydration as mild, moderate, or severe. An infant or toddler should generate 4 to 6 well-saturated diapers per day. If a parent reports less, there should be a heightened concern for dehydration. Urine specific gravity findings higher than 1.030 suggest dehydration. In a healthy newborn, the Babinski reflex is a positive normal sign. Breast- and bottle-feeding is typical at 8 months and does not help determine a child's risk for dehydration.

CJ: Case study; Step 2: Analyze cues; CL: Analyze

36.

STEP 3

0/1 The nurse must first address the client's **dehydration**. Then the client will most likely need treatment for a(n) **bowel obstruction** that is causing the vomiting.

The client's vomiting is caused by the ingestion of foreign bodies, which may be causing partial intestinal obstruction. Excessive vomiting can lead to fluid and electrolyte imbalances, which leads to hypokalemia and dehydration, as evidenced by the low potassium and high blood urea nitrogen. The laboratory results do not show current evidence of bleeding or infection; however, those risks would increase if perforation occurred. Ingestion of magnets places clients at risk for intestinal damage more so than poisoning.

CJ: Case study; Step 3: Prioritize hypothesis; CL: Analyze

37.

STEP 4

−/+ 2, 6. The goal of pain management in children is to optimize pain relief while minimizing adverse events. Nonopioids such as acetaminophen are useful for mild to moderate pain. The preferred route would be rectal for an infant who recently had both surgery and general anesthesia as the medicine will be most readily absorbed in the rectal vault. Nonpharmacologic methods such as holding a child may be comforting at all ages and may help the 8-month-old infant cope with pain. PO or gastric medication routes will not be well absorbed immediately following gastrointestinal surgery. Ibuprofen and other nonsteroidal antiinflammatory medications would be contraindicated due to increased bleeding risk. PCA has been used successfully for children older than 5 years but would not be indicated for a child who is unable to communicate their needs. A continuous infusion of morphine would not be the medication of choice for an infant because of the risk for respiratory depression. If the child developed greater levels of pain, interval dosing of opioids should be utilized. The direct application of heat or cold on a fresh surgical incision would be contraindicated as an infant's skin could quickly develop redness, burns, or blisters.

CJ: Case study; Step 4: Generate solutions; CL: Analyze

38.

STEP 5

0/1

Possible Actions	Appropriate to Delegate to the UAP	Not Appropriate to Delegate to UAP
Offer the first bottle of clear liquids		X
Change and weigh the infant's diaper	X	
Comfort the infant with lullabies	X	
Silence pump alarms while the infant is napping		X
Restock the client's rooms with additional diapers	X	
Assist holding the client during dressing changes	X	

In the pediatric setting, a UAP can provide a basic level of care such as changing an infant's diaper, recording I&O, singing lullabies, restocking client rooms, and assisting the nurse with various tasks such as dressing changes. The UAP should not offer the first bottle to an infant after gastrointestinal surgery. In a family-centered care environment, this task should be done by the nurse, or closely assessed by the nurse if the parent provides the first bottle, to assess for discomfort or aspiration. The UAP should not press any alarms on an IV pump as the nurse needs to know when IV fluids or medications are complete.

CJ: Case study; Step 5: Take action; CL: Apply

39.

STEP 6

Parent Statement	Understood	Not Understood
"I will regularly check the floors and areas my baby can reach for small objects."	X	
"I need to check my baby's toys to make sure they don't have small pieces that could be swallowed."	X	
"I will make sure that battery covers are secure on remote controls, key fobs, or musical books."	X	
"I know how to use the Heimlich maneuver if my infant starts choking."		X
"I will begin teaching my child about what objects should not be put in the mouth."	X	
"If I think my baby has swallowed a small object, I will try to get them to vomit the object as soon as possible."		X

Home safety should focus on teaching the parent to keep all small objects out of reach of the infant, including checking floors and toys for small pieces that can easily be swallowed. Items that have button-cell batteries can cause severe injury or death if ingested. Backs on such items should be secure. Infants as young as 8 to 12 months can learn simple requests such as "no" or "not for mouth" when they put nonfood items in their mouths. If an infant begins to choke, the preferred action is to do back blows and abdominal thrusts. The Heimlich maneuver is used on children older than 1 year. If a child swallows an object, the parents should call the health care provider or poison control. The parent should not induce vomiting because it may cause esophageal trauma.

CJ: Case study; Step 6: Evaluate outcomes; CL: Evaluate

40. **1, 2, 3.** The nurse should help the client take deep breaths. Resuscitation equipment should always be nearby when a client is recovering from anesthesia. The nurse can administer the oxygen as needed. The nurse does not need to contact the health care provider for a prescription for naloxone because naloxone is the antidote for morphine, not midazolam. It is not necessary to contact the anesthesiologist at this time.

CN: Reduction of risk; CL: Analyze

41. 2. DVT causes edema; therefore, the UAP should elevate the extremity to promote venous return. Dependent positioning is appropriate for a client with arterial insufficiency. Placing a pillow under the knee would position the foot in a low position, and pressure behind the knee may obstruct venous flow. Massaging the extremity could dislodge the thrombus.

CN: Management of care; CL: Analyze

42. **1, 2, 4.** A National Patient Safety Goal of the Joint Commission is to accurately and completely reconcile medications across the continuum of care. The requirement is that there is a process for comparing the client's current medications with those prescribed for the client while under the care of the health care organization. Clients are most at risk during transitions in care (hand-offs) across settings, services, providers, or levels of care. The development, reconciliation, and communication of an accurate medication list throughout the continuum of care are essential in the reduction of transition-related adverse drug events. The client or client's family is an integral component of medication reconciliation, particularly at the point of admission to, and discharge from, a health care facility. Any medications that the client uses, for example, over-the-counter medications, must be included in the reconciliation process.

CN: Pharmacologic and parenteral therapies; CL: Apply

43. 2. The nurse should not accept an assignment to "float" to another nursing unit for which the nurse does not have experience or adequate preparation. The first step is to discuss the situation with the person making the assignment; if the situation is not resolved, the newly graduated nurse should ask to speak with the supervisor.

CN: Management of care; CL: Analyze

44. 4. The teenage girl has scoliosis, the lateral deviation of the spine. Kyphosis is noted by a forward curvature of the shoulders. Lordosis is an inward curvature of the lower back. Spondylolisthesis is a slipping of the vertebrae out of position. Pain is the main finding with this condition, not curvature of the spine.

CN: Health promotion and maintenance; CL: Analyze

45. 3. The client is exhibiting symptoms that are consistent with hyperglycemia. The RN does not give any additional glucose. All of the other interventions are appropriate for this client. The new graduate RN notifies the health care provider about the assessment findings.

CN: Management of care; CL: Analyze

46. 4. It is best to keep choices simple for young children. Too many choices increase the likelihood of creating a picky eater. Mealtimes should be kept short to align with a toddler's attention span. Distraction, especially television, should be minimized so the child can focus on eating. Small portions are less overwhelming for small children.

CN: Health promotion and maintenance; CL: Apply

47. **4, 3, 2, 1.** Clients with myasthenia crisis have severe muscle weakness that may result in respiratory failure requiring mechanical ventilation. The nurse's first action is to focus on assuring an adequate airway by preparing for intubation. The nurse can then assess for a gag reflex for risk for aspiration. Once the airway and risk for aspiration are assured, the nurse can assess the client for infection and medication schedule.

🔑 CN: Physiological adaptation; CL: Create

48. **1.** The oxygen levels for this neonate have dropped during the last 8 hours; the nurse should administer oxygen as the neonate is not obtaining adequate oxygenation on room air. The recommended pulse oximetry reading in a term neonate is 95% to 100%. Obtaining a pulse oximeter reading in a lower extremity is done to screen for congenital heart defects. The priority is to correct the hypoxia first before gathering other assessments. Waiting to reassess the neonate could cause the neonate to have inadequate oxygen levels unnecessarily. Although blood gases may be drawn, the first action is to administer the oxygen.

🔑 CN: Management of care; CL: Analyze

49. **2.** The nurse should prepare to insert an NG tube. The data collected provide evidence that the client is experiencing an upper gastrointestinal bleed secondary to a peptic ulcer. The client will be placed on nothing-by-mouth status, and an NG tube will be inserted to provide gastric decompression and alleviate vomiting. Administering antiemetics is not a priority action for a client who is hypotensive and vomiting coffee-ground emesis. Assessment of client stressors is appropriate after emergency care has been provided and the client stabilized. A modified Trendelenburg position is inappropriate for clients who are vomiting.

🔑 CN: Reduction of risk potential; CL: Analyze

50. **1.** The client with preeclampsia would be a candidate for the induction process because ending the pregnancy is the only way to cure preeclampsia. A client with active herpes would be a candidate for a cesarean birth to prevent the fetus from contracting the virus while passing through the birth canal. The woman with a face presentation will not be able to give birth vaginally due to the extended position of the neck. The client with a complete placenta requires a cesarean birth.

🔑 CN: Management of care; CL: Analyze

51. **3.** The sudden onset of bright red drainage of this magnitude needs to be further assessed. Assessing vital signs is an important nursing action to determine whether there have been any changes in the client's status. Additional steps would include reinforcing the dressing and notifying the health care provider (HCP). Increasing the IV flow rate does not address the bleeding. Changing the dressing would be done only if the HCP prescribed it.

🔑 CN: Reduction of risk potential; CL: Analyze

52. **1.** Because the client with ADHD is easily distractible, it is important to obtain eye contact before explaining the task. Simple language and having them repeat what they are told is necessary because of the client's age. Praise encourages the client to repeat the task in the future as well as building the client's self-esteem. A full explanation with verbal praise and a food reward is inappropriate because a food reward increases the chance that the child will expect a physical reward for completing tasks. In addition, a full explanation might be too confusing for someone their age. Explaining consequences focuses on punishment, rather than praise. Although demonstration followed by imitation is an effective teaching method, rewarding with food fosters dependence on food reward for task completion.

🔑 CN: Psychosocial integrity; CL: Analyze

53. **4.** A client who is taking phenelzine, a monoamine oxidase inhibitor, needs to avoid foods that are rich in tyramine because this food-drug combination can cause hypertensive crisis. The client should be given a list of foods to avoid and should report headaches, palpitations, and a stiff neck to the health care provider (HCP) immediately. The client does not need to restrict or add salt to the diet. Drinking 10 to 12 glasses of water each day is important to teach the client who is receiving lithium therapy. Antidepressant drugs take 2 to 4 weeks to achieve therapeutic effects.

🔑 CN: Pharmacological and parenteral therapies; CL: Analyze

54. **4.** Clients with fractures of the long bones such as the femur are particularly susceptible to fat embolism syndrome (FES). Signs and symptoms include chest pain, dyspnea, tachycardia, and cyanosis. Changes in mental status are caused by hypoxemia and can be the first symptoms noted in FES. The client can also be restless and febrile and can develop petechiae. Osteomyelitis is an infection of the bone; signs and symptoms of osteomyelitis do not include respiratory symptoms. Compartment syndrome causes signs of localized neurovascular impairment, not systemic symptoms. Venous thrombosis occurs in the lower extremities and is caused by venous stasis.

🔑 CN: Reduction of risk potential; CL: Analyze

55. **2.** In this situation, the nurse should call a community meeting. The community meeting serves as a forum for clients to voice their opinions about the environment, receive feedback from staff and other clients, and discuss community concerns, including exploring the problems of daily living. The community meeting can be used to increase peer support and handle confrontation when necessary. For adolescents, peer pressure is generally more effective in changing behavior than the staff's influence. Telephoning the client's parents or urging the client to tell on their friends is authoritative and may lead to increased mistrust of the staff. Calling a primary care provider is not necessary at this time. Rather, a community meeting would be helpful to discuss the problem.

CN: Management of care; CL: Analyze

56. **2.** A report about the client's condition should be as clear, pertinent, and concise as possible. It should be free of subjective information that could be interpreted differently by different caregivers. The report mentioning that a specimen was sent to the laboratory does not indicate how much urine had been drained from the client's bladder and how the urine appeared. The report describing the client as cooperative is subjective and provides only limited client data. The report that mentions that the client was in the emergency department for 3 hours does not mention the treatment provided.

CN: Management of care; CL: Analyze

57. -/+ **1, 3, 4.** The nurse should use at least two sources of identification prior to administering medication to any client, such as the medical record number and the client's date of birth. Verifying the infant's full name with the parent provides an additional verification. It is not safe practice to ask another nurse to verify the correct neonate. It is also not safe to use the room number or crib number as a source of identification because neonates' locations in the hospital change frequently.

CN: Safety and infection control; CL: Apply

58. **4.** Caffeinated beverages and alcohol should be avoided because they stimulate gastric acid production and irritate the gastric mucosa. The client should avoid foods that cause discomfort; however, there is no need to follow a soft, bland diet. Eating six small meals daily is no longer a common treatment for peptic ulcer disease. Milk in large quantities is not recommended because it actually stimulates further production of gastric acid.

CN: Reduction of risk potential; CL: Evaluate

59. **3.** When a client with an NG tube exhibits abdominal distention, the nurse should first check the suction machine. If the suction equipment is functioning properly, the nurse should take other steps, such as repositioning the tube or checking tube patency by irrigating it. If these steps are not effective, the HCP should be called.

CN: Reduction of risk potential; CL: Analyze

60. **1.** The primary purpose of instilling 5 mL of normal saline solution before suctioning a tracheostomy tube is to thin the secretions to be suctioned. The saline may stimulate a cough; however, this is not the reason for using saline. The tracheostomy tube is larger than the suction catheter, so the catheter will easily pass into the tube without lubrication. Humidification is provided by a nebulizer if needed.

CN: Reduction of risk potential; CL: Evaluate

61. **3.** The client with emphysema has a chronically elevated carbon dioxide level. As a result, the normal stimulus for breathing in the medulla becomes ineffective. Instead, peripheral pressoreceptors in the aortic arch and carotid arteries, which are sensitive to oxygen blood levels, stimulate respirations. This is in response to low oxygen levels that have developed over time. If the client receives high concentrations of oxygen, the blood level of oxygen will rise excessively, the stimulus for respiration will decrease, and respiratory failure may result. Oxygen is not cooled. Humidification or administration of the oxygen through a nasal cannula will not prevent depressed ventilation if the flow rate of the oxygen is too high.

CN: Physiological adaptation; CL: Apply

62. **1.** The nurse should not administer drugs without a complete prescription. In this case, the prescription does not contain information about dosage and uses abbreviations that can cause confusion. The surgeon must write a prescription using complete dosages and without abbreviations before the nurse administers the drugs. Relying on the pharmacist for clarification is inappropriate.

CN: Management of care; CL: Analyze

63. **3.** The client should be encouraged to join the community arthritis support group so that they can share their feelings with others who are facing similar experiences with this chronic illness and can identify with their concerns. A hobby will not help the client resolve their feelings of being alone. Seeking counseling or discussing their feelings with a religious advisor may be helpful, but these activities will not necessarily help the client to understand that there are many individuals who must adjust their lifestyles because of arthritis and that they are not alone.

🗝️ CN: Health promotion and maintenance; CL: Analyze

64. 4. Warfarin sodium interferes with clotting. The nurse should monitor the PT and evaluate for the therapeutic effects of warfarin sodium. A therapeutic PT is between 1.5 and 2.5 times the control value; the PT should be established by the health care provider. It may also be reported as an international normalized ratio, a standardized system that provides a common basis for communicating and interpreting PT results. The PTT is monitored in clients who are receiving heparin therapy. Serum potassium levels and ABG values are not affected by warfarin.

🗝️ CN: Pharmacological and parenteral therapies; CL: Analyze

65. 4. The lower abdominal pain is most likely caused by bladder spasms. A common cause of bladder spasms after TURP is blood clots obstructing the catheter; therefore, the nurse's first action should be to assess the patency of the catheter. Auscultating the abdomen for bowel sounds would be appropriate after the patency of the catheter has been established. The nurse should assess for bladder spasms before administering an analgesic. A sitz bath would not relieve bladder spasms that are caused by an obstructed catheter.

🗝️ CN: Physiological adaptation; CL: Analyze

66. 3. The nurse should first determine whether the client received the last dose of imipenem-cilastatin. If the client did not receive the last dose, the nurse should notify the health care provider (HCP) that the client did not receive the dose, receive prescriptions, document, implement the prescriptions, and complete an incident report. The nurse should not automatically discard the partial fill of imipenem-cilastatin found at the client's bedside until further investigation is done. The nurse should recognize the cost of medications such as imipenem-cilastatin and consult the pharmacist after identifying information on the partial fill bag that was found. After verifying all information, the nurse can administer the new partial fill of imipenem-cilastatin so that the client can receive the antibiotic on time.

🗝️ CN: Safety and infection control; CL: Analyze

67. 2. For a client with moderate anxiety, the nurse should initially lead the client to a less stimulating environment and help them discuss their feelings. Doing so helps the client to gain control over anxiety that could be overwhelming. Telling the client that it would be best to lie down until they are calmer is not appropriate because the client is too anxious to benefit from this intervention. Suggesting that the client try relaxation exercises could be helpful after the nurse takes the client to a less stimulating environment and allows the client to vent and discuss their feelings. Getting some medication to help the client relax is an intervention that the nurse would carry out later after trying to help the client decrease anxiety through ventilation and relaxation exercises.

🗝️ CN: Psychosocial integrity; CL: Analyze

68. −/+ 1, 3, 4, 5. Although about 50% of diarrhea in clients receiving tube feedings is caused by sorbitol-containing medications, the nurse should assess for other possible causes. Diarrhea can occur as a result of bacterial contamination if fresh formula is not used or stored in a refrigerator or if the feeding apparatus is not changed at least every 24 hours. Lactose intolerance, rapid formula administration, low serum albumin level, and hypertonic solutions may also cause diarrhea. Hypotonic solutions would not be a likely cause of diarrhea, abdominal distention, or cramping.

🗝️ CN: Basic care and comfort; CL: Analyze

69. 4. Risk factors for postoperative pulmonary complications include malnourishment, which is indicated by the low weight relative to the client's height. Although keeping feelings inside can be problematic, it would not be considered a postoperative risk for pulmonary complications. The absence of dyspnea on exertion is not indicative of postoperative complications. The client's age does not necessarily place them at increased risk.

🗝️ CN: Reduction of risk potential; CL: Analyze

70.

STEP 1
−/+ **Nurse's Notes**
1230: The fundal height is at the umbilicus, and <mark>the fundus is boggy. The peripad is saturated</mark>. Vital signs are <mark>T 99.7°F (37.6°C)</mark>; <mark>P 98 bpm</mark>; RR 18 breaths/min; <mark>BP 116/68 mm Hg</mark>; and <mark>pulse oximetry reading 97% on room air</mark>. Pain is rated as a 6 on a scale of 0 to 10.

Following birth, the myometrium of the uterus needs to contract around the open blood vessels where the placenta implanted to control excessive bleeding. A contracted uterus feels firm. A boggy uterus is not contracted and thus allows bleeding. Soaking a peripad in a half hour is worrisome because soaking more than one peripad an hour is a sign of a postpartum hemorrhage. A pulse greater than 90 bpm may be a sign of hypovolemia related to blood loss. Approximately 1 hour after birth, the fundus rises to the level of the umbilicus, so the fundal height is an expected finding. Sustained temperature increases of 100.4°F (38°C) are signs of infection, but minor elevations may be related to inflammation from birth. The RR, BP, and oxygen saturation are all within normal limits. The pain level is most likely attributed to the diminishing effects of any anesthetic given during the perineal tear repair and can be treated with ice and an analgesic.

CJ: Case study; Step 1: Recognize cues; CL: Analyze

71.

STEP 2

Risk Factor	Uterine Atony	Lacerations	Retained Fragments
High parity	X		
Maternal age	X		X
Length of time membranes were ruptured	X		
Length of labor		X	
Fetal size	X	X	

Overdistention is a major factor that affects the uterus's ability to contract. Having more than four pregnancies and a large baby are major factors related to overdistention. Being over 35 years of age and the risk for infection from a 20-hour rupture of membranes are additional risk factors for uterine atony. Being over the age of 30 is a risk factor for retained placental fragments. The client had a rapid labor and a large baby. Both of these factors are risks for perineal lacerations. If the length of labor were long, it would have been a risk factor for uterine atony.

CJ: Case study; Step 2: Analyze cues; CL: Analyze

72.

STEP 3

0/1 *The client is most likely experiencing a postpartum hemorrhage due to* **uterine atony**. *Untreated, the client is at greatest risk for developing* **hypovolemic shock**.

A postpartum hemorrhage that occurs in the first 24 hours after birth is considered an early hemorrhage. Hemorrhages occurring after 24 hours are considered late. The finding of a boggy uterus most indicates uterine atony. Although the client has a perineal tear, uterine atony is the most common cause of an early hemorrhage. There is no evidence that the placenta was not fully expelled to suggest placental fragments are contributing to the bleeding. Untreated, the hemorrhage can lead to hypovolemic shock. The most common link between hemorrhage and infection is that infection is a risk factor for developing a hemorrhage. The causes of uterine prolapse are multifactorial and cannot be solely attributed to a hemorrhage.

CJ: Case study; Step 3: Prioritize hypothesis; CL: Analyze

73.

STEP 4

Orders

1235:
Postpartum hemorrhage protocol:
- Establish IV access if not present.
- Begin 1000 mL of lactated Ringer's solution at 500 mL per hour.
- Administer 10 units of oxytocin intramuscularly (IM).
- Perform vigorous fundal massage for at least 15 seconds.
- Weigh blood-soaked materials.
- Take vital signs, including oxygen saturation and level of consciousness, every 5 minutes.
- Administer oxygen to maintain a pulse oximetry reading of greater than 95%.
- Type and crossmatch for 2 units of red blood cells stat.
- Empty the bladder with a straight catheter, or place an indwelling catheter.

The first nursing priority is to stop the bleeding. This is done by administering IM oxytocin and massaging the fundus. The next priority is to establish venous access, which is needed to provide volume replacement and give additional medication. Drawing the type and crossmatch can occur after IV fluids have been started. Vital signs will be assessed after the priority interventions have been implemented. The need for oxygen will be established after the vital signs have been reassessed. Placing a catheter is one of the last interventions to implement.

CJ: Case study; Step 4: Generate solutions; CL: Analyze

74.

STEP 5

0/1 *The nurse determines that the misoprostol* **order is appropriate**. *The nurse should* **administer four tablets per rectum.**

Misoprostol is a prostaglandin that can be given to treat a postpartum hemorrhage. When given per rectum, tablets are rapidly absorbed from the rectal mucosa. The order is for 0.8 mg, which also equals 800 mcg. The drug on hand is 200 mcg tablets; thus, it is appropriate to give four tablets per rectum.

CJ: Case study; Step 5: Take action; CL: Apply

75.

STEP 6

−/+ 3, 4, 6. Diaphoresis is a symptom of shock. An increased heart rate and diastolic BP of less than 60 mm Hg are signs that the fluid volume deficit is increasing. A firm fundus is desirable. Saturating only one peripad an hour indicates the bleeding is returning to expected amounts. A RR of 18 breaths/min is normal.

🗝 CJ: Case study; Step 6: Evaluate outcomes; CL: Evaluate

76. 2. Administering an antiemetic before beginning chemotherapy and then routinely around the clock helps prevent nausea and vomiting. Waiting until the client requests it may be too late because nausea is already present.

🗝 CN: Pharmacological and parenteral therapies; CL: Analyze

77. 1. Greenish-colored amniotic fluid is caused by the passage of meconium, usually secondary to a fetal insult during labor. Meconium passage also may be related to an intact gastrointestinal system of the neonate, especially those neonates who are full term or of postdate gestational age. Amnioinfusion may be used to treat the condition and dilute the fluid. Cloudy amniotic fluid is associated with an infection caused by bacteria or a sexually transmitted disease. Severe yellow-colored fluid is associated with Rh incompatibility or erythroblastosis fetalis.

🗝 CN: Health promotion and maintenance; CL: Analyze

78. 3. Black, tarry stools indicate the presence of a slow upper gastrointestinal bleed. The longer the blood is in the system, the darker it becomes as the hemoglobin is broken down and iron is released. Vital sign changes, such as an increased pulse, are not evident with slow gastrointestinal bleeds. Nausea and abdominal cramps can occur but are not definitive signs of gastrointestinal bleeding.

🗝 CN: Physiological adaptation; CL: Analyze

79. 4. Deep breathing helps prevent microatelectasis and pneumonitis and also helps force air and fluid out of the pleural space into the chest tubes. It does not decrease blood flow to the lungs or control the rate of airflow. The diaphragm is the major muscle of respiration; deep breathing causes it to descend, thereby increasing the ventilating surface.

🗝 CN: Reduction of risk potential; CL: Apply

80. −/+ 1, 2, 5, 6. To treat a low blood glucose level, the nurse should provide the client with approximately 15 g of carbohydrate and monitor the blood glucose level within 15 minutes. The orange juice, milk, bread, or soda would provide approximately 15 g of carbohydrate. Meat or fish, such as tuna, does not contain carbohydrate. Processed peanut butter may contain small amounts of carbohydrate, but it is also high in fat and protein. Peanut butter is not a good option to raise a blood glucose level in a timely manner.

🗝 CN: Physiological adaptation CL: Analyze

81. 1. The air is injected into the long-acting insulin first. Air is then injected into the short-acting insulin, and the short-acting insulin is withdrawn. Then the long-acting insulin is withdrawn. It does matter which insulin is drawn up first because the nurse does not want to contaminate the short-acting insulin with the long-acting insulin. It is not necessary to use a high-dose insulin syringe to prepare 28 units of insulin.

🗝 CN: Pharmacological and parenteral therapies; CL: Apply

82. 2. Solids should be introduced at 6 months. Full-term infants use up their prenatal iron stores within 4 to 6 months after birth. Milk contains insufficient iron.

🗝 CN: Health promotion and maintenance; CL: Apply

83. 3. Diminished breath sounds during an acute asthma attack are a serious sign of airway obstruction, fatigue, and impending respiratory failure. Wheezing, coughing, and the production of sputum indicate the presence of airflow through the lungs and are less ominous symptoms.

🗝 CN: Physiological adaptation; CL: Analyze

84. 3. A moderate amount of bloody drainage could indicate active bleeding. The priority action is to apply pressure to the area and call for help. Assessing the airway or pulse or administering oxygen does not address the bleeding.

🗝 CN: Reduction of risk potential; CL: Analyze

85. 3. Bacterial conjunctivitis is very contagious. Attention should be paid to thorough handwashing, a major means of stopping the transmission of the disease. Closing the daycare center for 1 week is not necessary because thorough handwashing will stop the spread of the infection. Keeping the children out for 48 hours is not necessary. A child may return to daycare after being treated for 24 hours. Although the parents of each child should be told about the outbreak, doing so will not help to curtail or prevent the spread of the infection.

🗝️ CN: Safety and infection control; CL: Analyze

86. 3. The client's mobility status is the best indicator of risk for the development of a pressure sore. Nutritional and circulatory status are other factors that can contribute to pressure sore development, but immobility, even in the presence of adequate nutrition and circulation, is the leading cause of pressure sores. Disorientation can cause a client to neglect to make needed position changes, but the underlying factor will be immobility.

🗝️ CN: Reduction of risk potential; CL: Analyze

87.

Possible Actions to Take	Potential Conditions	Parameters to Monitor
Assist the client to use an incentive spirometer	Decreased oxygenation, right lung	Oxygen saturation
Turn the client to the left side		Breath sounds

Following a right lobectomy, the client has decreased oxygenation in the right lower lung as noted by diminished breath sounds and decreasing oxygen saturation. The chest tube is fluctuating, indicating it is not blocked; there is no need to milk the tube to facilitate drainage. The client has incisional pain relieved by morphine; the nurse should continue to monitor the effectiveness of the pain medication, but it is not yet time for the next dose. The client's temperature is within normal limits following surgery; there are no signs of infection. The oxygen saturation level decreased slightly, and the client's breath sounds in the affected lung are diminished; the most immediate intervention to improve oxygenation levels is to turn the client and assist the client to use the incentive spirometer. Supplementary oxygen will likely be provided, but the client's oxygen saturation is not sufficiently low that administration by face mask would be necessary. The nurse should continue to monitor the oxygenation saturation and the client's breath sounds.

🗝️ CJ: Standalone bowtie; CL: Create

88. 1. The nurse should stop and assess the client further. A chair should be available for the client to sit down. Obtaining the client's blood pressure and heart rate is important when the client is exercising. These values can be used to predict when the oxygen demand becomes greater than the oxygen supply. Calling for help is not necessary for the midsternal burning. If the health care provider has prescribed nitroglycerin, the nurse can administer it; however, stopping the activity may restore the oxygen balance.

🗝️ CN: Physiological adaptation; CL: Analyze

89. 2. The statement, "If I forget a dose, it's no big deal, I'll just take it when I remember it," indicates a knowledge deficit. The nurse should reinforce that the client should take dexamethasone as prescribed and at the same time each day. The drug has to be tapered off and cannot be stopped abruptly. The HCP should be notified when the client is under additional stress (e.g., infection, surgery, illness). The client can have an allergic reaction to inactive ingredients contained in dexamethasone.

🗝️ CN: Pharmacological and parenteral therapies; CL: Evaluate

90. 1. A child with moderate dehydration, described as a loss of 50 to 90 mL/kg of body fluid, would have oliguria, gray skin color, increased pulse rate, and poor skin elasticity. Sunken eyes, not bulging, are a sign of dehydration. The anterior fontanelle may be sunken, but the posterior fontanelle is normally closed by 6 to 8 weeks of age. A child with mild dehydration, described as a loss of less than 50 mL/kg of body fluid, would have pale skin color, decreased skin elasticity, decreased urine output, and normal or increased pulse rate.

🗝️ CN: Physiological adaptation; CL: Analyze

91. 1. Oropharyngeal candidiasis, or thrush, is the most common infection associated with the early symptomatic stages of HIV infection. Thrush is characterized by whitish-yellow patches in the mouth. Various other opportunistic diseases can occur in clients with HIV infection, but they tend to occur later, after the diagnosis of acquired immunodeficiency syndrome has been made. Dyspnea can be indicative of pneumonia, which is caused by a variety of infective organisms. Bloody diarrhea is indicative of cytomegalovirus infection. Hyperpigmented lesions are indicators of Kaposi sarcoma.

🗝️ CN: Physiological adaptation; CL: Analyze

92. 2. Postpartum infection is a leading cause of maternal mortality in the United States. Typical treatment for the condition is IV antibiotic therapy with drugs such as clindamycin, gentamicin, or both. Cultures of the lochia will also be obtained. The neonate can continue to breastfeed as long as the birth mother desires. A switch to bottle-feeding is not necessary. The uterus tends to be firm, with increased cramping to rid the uterus of the infection. The client should be encouraged to remain in the Fowler position when in bed to allow for drainage of the lochia.

🗝️ CN: Physiological adaptation; CL: Analyze

93. 1. The parent needs further instruction when they say, "I should position the baby the same way for each feeding." This can contribute to sore nipples. The position should vary for each feeding to prevent repeated pressure on the same area each time. Grasping the entire areola and nipple will help decrease nipple soreness. Air-drying the breasts and not using a hand pump will also help decrease nipple soreness.

🗝️ CN: Health promotion and maintenance; CL: Evaluate

94. 1. During an acute attack of vertigo, it is best for the client to lie down in a darkened, quiet room and avoid sudden position changes. Because vertigo is frequently accompanied by nausea and vomiting, the client will not want to eat or drink. Headaches are not a component of the vertigo attack. Fluids are usually administered parenterally to maintain hydration and administer medications.

🗝️ CN: Basic care and comfort; CL: Analyze

95. 1. To reduce urethral irritation and allow drainage, the nurse should tape the Foley catheter to a female client's inner thigh. Taping the catheter also prevents excessive traction against the bladder neck. Taping the catheter to the groin or lower abdomen would not allow for proper drainage and would cause urethral discomfort. Taping the catheter to the lower thigh would pull on the catheter and cause urethral irritation.

🗝️ CN: Reduction of risk potential; CL: Apply

96.

0/1

Action to Take	Potential Conditions	Parameters to Monitor
Initiate seizure precautions	Delirium tremens	Alcohol withdrawal assessment scores
Administer intravenous (IV) diazepam		Vital signs

The history of alcohol abuse, the sudden appearance of neurologic symptoms, and vomiting suggest that the client is experiencing delirium tremens (DT), a severe form of alcohol withdrawal. Wernicke encephalopathy is a degenerative brain disorder that primarily affects memory. Korsakoff psychosis is a complication of Wernicke encephalopathy that includes behavioral changes and confusion. An alcohol overdose would manifest as central nervous system depression. The client with DT is at high risk for seizures. Priority interventions include administering a benzodiazepine and implementing seizure precautions. Antipsychotics are sometimes needed, but IM medications are erratically absorbed, and haloperidol can decrease the seizure threshold. Clients should be kept on nothing-by-mouth (NPO) status to prevent the risk for aspiration until symptoms improve. If thiamine supplementation is needed it should be given IV. Gastric lavage is the treatment for alcohol overdose. The nurse should regularly monitor the client's status using a scale validated to assess alcohol withdrawal severity. The nurse should monitor vital signs to help prevent complications from life-threatening arrhythmias or respiratory failure. Blood alcohol levels do not help predict recovery from withdrawal. The Glasgow Coma scale best monitors clients with a traumatic brain injury. Memory changes are best used to assess long-term cognitive problems such as dementia.

🗝️ CJ: Standalone bowtie; CL: Create

97. 2. Feeding solutions that have not been infused after hanging for 8 hours should be discarded because of the increased risk for bacterial growth. Sitting the client upright during the feeding helps prevent aspiration of the feeding. A gastric residual of 25 mL is considered acceptable. A gastric residual of 100 to 150 mL, or a residual greater than 100% of the previous hour's intake, indicates delayed emptying. The feeding solution should be at room or body temperature.

🗝️ CN: Pharmacological and parenteral therapies; CL: Analyze

98. 3. Furosemide is a loop diuretic and inhibits the reabsorption of sodium and chloride from the proximal and distal renal tubules and the loop of Henle. Furosemide promotes sodium diuresis, resulting in a loss of potassium and serious electrolyte imbalances. Furosemide does not affect the BUN level.

🗝️ CN: Pharmacological and parenteral therapies; CL: Analyze

99. -/+ **2, 3, 4.** Contraindications for t-PA or alteplase recombinant therapy include current active internal bleeding, a duration of 3 hours or longer since the onset of symptoms of a stroke, and severe hypertension. Age older than 65 years and having had an alcoholic beverage are not contraindications for the therapy.

🗝️ CN: Pharmacological and parenteral therapies; CL: Analyze

100. 3. For a complete breech, the buttocks present, the feet and legs are flexed on the thighs, and the thighs are flexed on the abdomen. For a frank breech, the buttocks present with the hips flexed and the legs extended against the abdomen and chest. This is the most common type of breech presentation. For a compound breech, the buttocks present together with another part, such as a hand. This is a rare occurrence. For an incomplete breech, one or both feet or the knees extend below the buttocks. This can also be termed a single footling or double footling breech.

🔑 CN: Health promotion and maintenance; CL: Analyze

101. 1. A common complication of diabetes is diabetic neuropathy. Diabetic neuropathy results from the metabolic and vascular factors related to hyperglycemia. Damage leads to sensory deficits and peripheral pain. Muscle atrophy can result from disuse, but it is not a direct consequence of diabetes. Raynaud's disease is associated with vasospasms in the hands and feet. Transient ischemic attacks involve the cerebrum.

🔑 CN: Physiological adaptation; CL: Analyze

102. -/+ 1, 4, 5, 6. Diazepam is a benzodiazepine that causes symptoms of withdrawal when stopped abruptly. The nurse should assess the client for tremors, agitation, irritability, insomnia, vomiting, sweating, tachycardia, headache, anxiety, and confusion. Bradycardia and euphoria or elevated mood are not symptoms of benzodiazepine withdrawal.

🔑 CN: Pharmacological and parenteral therapies; CL: Analyze

103. 1. Parents are typically quick to notice changes in their infant's physical appearance. The removal of the infant's hair may be upsetting to them if they have not been told why it is being done. Hair may be removed on the scalp at the site of needle insertion for IV therapy to provide better visualization and a smooth surface on which to attach tape to secure the needle. Sedatives are not ordinarily prescribed before IV fluid administration. In most instances, it is acceptable for parents to visit their infant while the IV solution is infusing. Holding the infant is encouraged to provide comfort.

🔑 CN: Pharmacological and parenteral therapies; CL: Analyze

104. 3. The most appropriate initial response by the nurse would be to test the child's blood glucose level. The child's symptoms are consistent with hypoglycemia but could also be used by the child to avoid participation in planned activities. Administering milk or fruit juice during a mild reaction may also be appropriate if testing cannot be done. Notifying the HCP may be appropriate after the child's glucose level has been obtained and emergency treatment has been initiated if the child is experiencing hypoglycemia. Returning the child to previous activities is not appropriate until either testing or administering treatment has been done.

🔑 CN: Physiological adaptation; CL: Analyze

105. 4. Learning goals are most likely to be attained when they are established mutually by the client and members of the health care team, including the nurse, pharmacist, and the HCP. Learning is motivated by perceived problems or goals arising from unmet needs. The perception of the unmet needs must be the client's; however, the nurse, pharmacist, and HCP help the client arrive at their own perception of the need or reason to learn.

🔑 CN: Management of care; CL: Evaluate

106. 2. In this situation, the client has indicated that they are not willing to leave the abusive partner because of potential economic concerns and other children in the household. The nurse should explain the cycle of abuse (e.g., tension-building phase, battering incident, and honeymoon phase). The priority intervention is to assist the client to make concrete plans for the safety of the client and their children. The client should identify the safest, quickest routes out of the house and be able to identify where they will go once the cycle of violence escalates. Contacting a social worker at this time is not appropriate because the client is not ready to leave the abusive situation. The nurse can tell the client that these services are available, but it is up to the client to determine whether a referral is necessary. Telling the client that they should not allow anyone to hit them or their children does not assist the client to make plans for their safety and the children's safety should the violence escalate. The client may have a flat affect or feel extreme humiliation from the abuse. The client may also be feeling that the abuse is their fault. When the client is ready to leave the abusive situation and receive continuous counseling, efforts can be made to increase their self-esteem and prevent additional violence. The client should be made aware of the available services in the community for people who are involved in abusive relationships. The location and phone numbers for available shelters should be provided to the client. Giving a brochure related to the statistics about violence is not helpful and, if found by the abuser, may lead to further violence.

🔑 CN: Safety and infection control; CL: Analyze

107. 4, 3, 2, 1. The child whose condition could change most quickly should be assessed first, and the most stable child should be assessed last. The child with a lacerated liver is at the highest risk for a rapid change in condition. Therefore, this child should be assessed first because the child is at high risk for hemorrhage. The next child to be assessed is the 3-year-old child with pyelonephritis and fever. The fever needs to be acted upon, but this assessment is not as critical as that for the child with a lacerated liver. The normal respiratory rate for a 10-month-old infant is 30 breaths/min. Although the infant is tachypneic, this is expected with pneumonia. Additionally, the infant is not in acute respiratory distress. However, the increased respiratory rate needs evaluation, so the 10-month-old infant should be assessed before the 3-month-old infant with respiratory syncytial virus who has stable vital signs and is not in acute distress.

⚿ CN: Management of care; CL: Create

108. 4. Risperidone is prescribed for severe agitation and has a rapid response. Ergoloid and tacrine stabilize and may improve the cognitive functioning of clients with dementia. Diazepam is an antianxiety agent that would not have the desired effect on the client's severe agitation, violence, and bizarre thoughts.

⚿ CN: Pharmacologic and parenteral therapies; CL: Analyze

109. 2. Checking the carotid artery pulse in a child during CPR provides information about perfusion of the brain. The brachial pulse is checked in an infant because the infant's short and typically fat neck makes it difficult to palpate the carotid pulse. The femoral and radial arteries might indicate perfusion to the peripheral body sites, but the critical need is for adequate circulation to the brain.

⚿ CN: Physiological adaptation; CL: Apply

110. 2. Because the child has a history of severe hypoxic episodes, having oxygen readily available at the bedside is most important. Should the child experience another hypoxic episode, oxygen could be administered easily and quickly. Although morphine causes peripheral dilation, which causes the blood to remain in the periphery, decreasing system volume and oxygen administration is the priority. Also, morphine is a controlled substance and must be stored securely at all times. Typically, a child with tetralogy of Fallot with episodes of hypoxia does not require suctioning.

⚿ CN: Physiological adaptation; CL: Analyze

111. **0/1** *The action the nurse should perform first is to* **institute enteric precautions.**

The stool specimen indicates the client has *E. coli* in their stool. The nurse institutes enteric precautions and ensures that those who come in contact with the child perform good hand hygiene and wear a gown to prevent spread of infection.

Restoring fluid balance is a goal of therapy, but because the dehydration is mild, oral rehydration is the first choice for replacing fluids. The nurse also cleanses and protects the anal area from irritation from the diarrhea, but on an ongoing basis and not as the priority for care. It is not necessary for the family to wash all of their bed linens as only those in contact with the client are contaminated.

⚿ CJ: Standalone trend; CL: Analyze

112. 1. When a client voids frequent, small amounts, the nurse should suspect that the client is retaining urine. Palpating for a distended bladder is the first assessment that the nurse should perform to verify this suspicion. Obtaining a prescription to catheterize for residual urine may be appropriate as a follow-up activity. Obtaining a urine specimen for culture is not a first priority. The nurse would not encourage an increased fluid intake until further assessment of the situation is completed.

⚿ CN: Management of care; CL: Analyze

113. 3. Of the clients listed, the newly admitted client should be assessed first. This is the client who is likely to be unstable and in pain. The child to be discharged today would be considered the most stable and therefore would be assessed last.

⚿ CN: Management of care; CL: Analyze

114. 2. Because of their colloidal properties, oatmeal preparation baths typically help relieve the itching associated with chickenpox. Calamine lotion can also be used if there are no open lesions. Baby powder is unlikely to relieve itching because it acts primarily to absorb moisture. A soft towel moistened with hydrogen peroxide is unlikely to relieve itching. Rather, hydrogen peroxide is used to clean wounds. A cool compress moistened with a weak salt solution is unlikely to relieve itching because it does not have any antipruritic properties.

⚿ CN: Basic care and comfort; CL: Analyze

115. 50 mL per hour.

$$X = 500 \text{ mL}/20 \text{ g} \times 2 \text{ g/h}$$

$$X = 50 \text{ mL/h}$$

⚿ CN: Pharmacological and parenteral therapies; CL: Apply

116. 4. Because of the age and report of a seizure, the client is probably experiencing eclampsia, a condition in which convulsions occur in the absence of any underlying cause. Although the actual cause is unknown, adolescents and women older than 35 years are at higher risk. The client's environment should be kept as free of stimuli as possible. Thus, the nurse should admit the client to a quiet, darkened room. Clients experiencing eclampsia should be kept on the left side to promote placental perfusion. In some cases, edema of the lungs develops after seizures and is a sign of cardiovascular failure. Because the client is at risk for pulmonary edema, breath sounds should be monitored every 2 hours. Vital signs should be monitored frequently, at least every hour.

 CN: Management of care; CL: Analyze

117. **3.** Fluctuation of fluid with respirations in the water seal column indicates that the system is functioning properly. If an obstruction were present in the chest tube, fluid fluctuation would be absent. Subcutaneous emphysema occurs when air pockets can be palpated beneath the client's skin around the chest tube insertion site. A leak in the system is indicated when bubbling occurs in the water seal column.

 CN: Reduction of risk potential; CL: Apply

118. **4.** The only action that keeps the client safe is removal of the gun. If the HCP is considering discharge, the client is medically stable and will not be able to remain in the medical hospital any longer. The client's lack of current suicidal ideation means they cannot be hospitalized for psychiatric reasons. While helpful, the crisis phone line number and the client's promise do not ensure safety.

 CN: Safety and infection control; CL: Analyze

119. **1, 2, 3, 5.** Acknowledging the client's concern about pain and expressing the nurse's concern about the client's condition are important to help the client open up and gain further assessment of pain in this client. Awareness of the amount of wine consumption in a week will be helpful to guide which kind of detoxification will be needed. Expressing the nurse's concern about the client's safety is important. How the client is getting the wine is least important because there are so many possibilities, such a weekly shopping trips in the facility van or having friends or family bring it in. Notifying the primary care provider about the situation and arranging for a joint conference are important for the client's safety and recovery.

 CN: Safety and infection control; CL: Apply

120. **4.** More than 90% of children have speech that is totally intelligible at 4 years of age. Having one word at 1 year is the expectation. Having three words is a 15-month milestone. Pointing to one body part at 18 months and combining two words at 2 years would be a normal finding.

 CN: Health Promotion and maintenance; CL: Analyze

6

Comprehensive Test

This test has 150 questions. Time yourself as you take the test so you can determine the approximate amount of time it takes to complete this many questions. This test reflects the maximum number of questions you may receive on the actual licensing exam.

1. After a bronchoscopy with biopsy, the nurse assesses the client. The nurse should report which finding to the health care provider?
   - ☐ 1. green sputum
   - ☐ 2. dry cough
   - ☐ 3. hemoptysis
   - ☐ 4. laryngeal stridor

2. A nurse is caring for a client who has undergone a total laryngectomy for laryngeal cancer. The client has a history of smoking. What information is important to include in discharge teaching? Select all that apply.
   - ☐ 1. Provide humidity at home.
   - ☐ 2. Follow a bland diet.
   - ☐ 3. Learn how to suction.
   - ☐ 4. Have communication rehabilitation with a speech pathologist.
   - ☐ 5. Attend a smoking cessation program.

3. The client received electroconvulsive therapy (ECT) an hour ago and now has a headache. Which response by the nurse is **best**?
   - ☐ 1. "A headache is common after ECT."
   - ☐ 2. "I'll get some acetaminophen for you."
   - ☐ 3. "A nap will help you feel better."
   - ☐ 4. "Eat your breakfast, and then let me know how you feel."

4. The nurse interprets the rhythm strip (see figure) from a client's bedside monitor as which rhythm?

   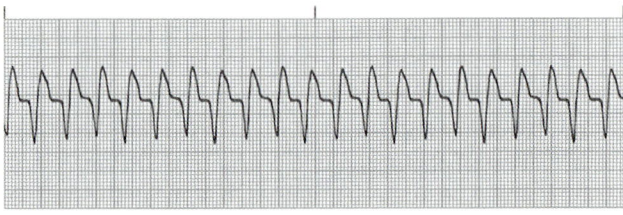

   - ☐ 1. normal sinus rhythm
   - ☐ 2. sinus tachycardia
   - ☐ 3. ventricular tachycardia
   - ☐ 4. ventricular fibrillation

5. The nurse cares for a client who is 12 weeks pregnant and speaks Spanish only. Which intervention(s) should the nurse include in the plan of care at the client's initial visit? Select all that apply.
   - ☐ 1. Provide brochures in the client's native language.
   - ☐ 2. Refer the client to a high-risk clinic.
   - ☐ 3. Discuss cultural differences, and emphasize the differences between cultures.
   - ☐ 4. Arrange for an interpreter for the client's appointments.
   - ☐ 5. Discuss contraception and options.
   - ☐ 6. Review dietary intake, and discuss nutrition.

6. When assessing speech development, the nurse should refer which child for further re-evaluation?
   - ☐ 1. a 4-month-old who laughs out loud
   - ☐ 2. a 10-month-old who says "dada" and "mama"
   - ☐ 3. a 1-year-old who says three to five words
   - ☐ 4. an 18-month-old who only says "no"

7. A client is admitted with numbness and tingling of the feet and toes after having an upper respiratory infection and flu for the past 5 days. Within 1 hour of admission, the client's legs are numb to the hips. What should the nurse do **next**? Select all that apply.
☐ 1. Notify the family of the change.
☐ 2. Notify the health care provider (HCP) of the change.
☐ 3. Place respiratory resuscitation equipment in the client's room.
☐ 4. Check for advancing levels of paresthesia.
☐ 5. Have the client perform ankle pumps.

8. When assessing a client with heart failure, the nurse should **immediately** report which finding(s) to the health care provider (HCP)? Select all that apply.
☐ 1. bibasilar crackles
☐ 2. blood pressure 108/62 mm Hg, heart rate 88 bpm
☐ 3. oxygen saturation 94% on room air
☐ 4. 2-lb (0.9-kg) weight gain in 5 days
☐ 5. urine output of 20 mL per hour
☐ 6. confusion

9. A client with paranoia is having a delusion. While the client is having the delusion, what nursing intervention is **most** indicated?
☐ 1. Assist the client to relieve anxiety.
☐ 2. Ask the client what is causing the feelings of anxiety.
☐ 3. Present reality when the client asks about the delusion.
☐ 4. Allow the client to express anger and intense emotions in appropriate ways.

10. STEP 1

The nurse is caring for a 33-year-old female client at a 6-week postpartum follow-up appointment following a term cesarean birth.

Nurse's Notes

The client is breastfeeding exclusively and taking prenatal vitamins. The client does not have lochia and notes not having a period since birth. The client reports not sleeping and crying constantly. The client is a single parent and states feeling isolated from family. The client has a 2-year-old child at home, but the other parent of the baby is not involved. The client needs a note to go back to work in the next week and is still trying to find daycare. They note feeling like a horrible parent. The client has lost half of the weight gained during pregnancy.

▶ Highlight the findings requiring **immediate** follow-up. Answer choices have been underlined.

Nurse's Notes

The client is breastfeeding exclusively and <u>taking prenatal vitamins</u>. The client does not have lochia and notes not <u>having a period since birth</u>. The client reports <u>not sleeping</u> and <u>crying constantly</u>. The client is a single parent and states <u>feeling isolated from family</u>. The client has a 2-year-old at home, but the <u>other parent of the baby is not involved</u>. The client <u>needs a note to go back to work in the next week</u> and is <u>still trying to find daycare</u>. They <u>note feeling like a horrible parent</u>. The client has <u>lost half of the weight gained during pregnancy</u>.

11. STEP 2

The nurse is caring for a 33-year-old female client at a 6-week postpartum follow-up appointment following a term cesarean birth.

Nurse's Notes

The client is breastfeeding exclusively and taking prenatal vitamins. The client does not have lochia and notes not having a period since birth. The client reports not sleeping and crying constantly. The client is a single parent and states feeling isolated from family. The client has a 2-year-old child at home, but the other parent of the baby is not involved. The client needs a note to go back to work in the next week and is still trying to find daycare. They note feeling like a horrible parent. The client has lost half of the weight gained during pregnancy.

▶ For each of the client findings, indicate if the finding is a risk factor for postpartum depression or not a risk factor for postpartum depression.

Possible Findings	Risk Factor	Not a Risk Factor
Age over 30	○	○
Breastfeeding	○	○
Being single	○	○
Stressful life events	○	○
Sleep deprivations	○	○
Second pregnancy	○	○

12. STEP 3

The nurse is caring for a 33-year-old female client at a 6-week postpartum follow-up appointment following a term cesarean birth.

Nurse's Notes

The client is breastfeeding exclusively and taking prenatal vitamins. The client does not have lochia and notes not having a period since birth. The client reports not sleeping and crying constantly. The client is a single parent and states feeling isolated from family. The client has a 2-year-old child at home, but the other parent of the baby is not involved. The client needs a note to go back to work in the next week and is still trying to find daycare. They note feeling like a horrible parent. The client has lost half of the weight gained during pregnancy.

Circle word(s) from the choices below to complete the following sentence.

➤ The top priority is for the nurse to address the client's _____.

Word Choices
imbalanced nutrition
ineffective coping
powerlessness
risk for suicide
social isolation
sleep disturbances

13. STEP 4

The nurse is caring for a 33-year-old female client at a 6-week postpartum follow-up appointment following a term cesarean birth.

Nurse's Notes

The client is breastfeeding exclusively and taking prenatal vitamins. The client does not have lochia and notes not having a period since birth. The client reports not sleeping and crying constantly. The client is a single parent and states feeling isolated from family. The client has a 2-year-old child at home, but the other parent of the baby is not involved. The client needs a note to go back to work in the next week and is still trying to find daycare. They note feeling like a horrible parent. The client has lost half of the weight gained during pregnancy.

The nurse begins to develop the client's plan of care.

➤ For each possible intervention, specify if the intervention is indicated or not indicated.

Possible Intervention	Indicated	Not Indicated
Postpartum depression screening	○	○
Thyroid screening	○	○
Mental health referral	○	○
Diazepam prescription	○	○
Self-care education	○	○

14. STEP 5

The nurse is caring for a 33-year-old female client at a 6-week postpartum follow-up appointment following a term cesarean birth.

Nurse's Notes

The client is breastfeeding exclusively and taking prenatal vitamins. The client does not have lochia and notes not having a period since birth. The client reports not sleeping and crying constantly. The client is a single parent and states feeling isolated from family. The client has a 2-year-old child at home, but the other parent of the baby is not involved. The client needs a note to go back to work in the next week and is still trying to find daycare. They note feeling like a horrible parent. The client has lost half of the weight gained during pregnancy.

Orders

1. Nursing:
   a. Screen for postpartum depression
   b. Postpartum depression education
2. Labs:
   a. Thyroid-stimulating hormone (TSH), T3, and T3 uptake
3. Referrals:
   a. Mental health referral

The nurse receives orders from the health care provider.

➢ When screening for postpartum depression, indicate if each action is essential or not essential.

Action	Essential	Not Essential
Screen for postpartum depression with a standardized screening tool	○	○
Have a second provider repeat the screen	○	○
Compare screening results with screenings done prior to hospital discharge	○	○
Refer clients with positive screens for a confirmatory diagnosis	○	○
Seek immediate care for clients who answer positively to self-harm questions	○	○

15. STEP 6

The nurse is caring for a 33-year-old female client at a 6-week postpartum follow-up appointment following a term cesarean birth.

Nurse's Notes

The client is breastfeeding exclusively and taking prenatal vitamins. The client does not have lochia and notes not having a period since birth. The client reports not sleeping and crying constantly. The client is a single parent and states feeling isolated from family. The client has a 2-year-old child at home, but the other parent of the baby is not involved. The client needs a note to go back to work in the next week and is still trying to find daycare. They note feeling like a horrible parent. The client has lost half of the weight gained during pregnancy.

Orders

1. Nursing:
   a. Screen for postpartum depression
   b. Postpartum depression education
2. Labs:
   a. Thyroid-stimulating hormone (TSH), T3, and T3 uptake
3. Referrals:
   a. Mental health referral

The nurse provides postpartum depression education.

➢ Which finding(s) would indicate the teaching has been effective? Select all that apply.

☐ 1. "If I need an antidepressant, I will need to stop breastfeeding."
☐ 2. "I should try to connect with friends or family several times a week."
☐ 3. "Keeping my home clean and free of clutter will reduce my anxiety."
☐ 4. "I will try to make time to do something I enjoy on most days."
☐ 5. "I should limit my alcohol intake to two drinks a day."
☐ 6. "It is critical that I get 8 hours of sleep a night."
☐ 7. "Connecting with other parents who feel this way can help."
☐ 8. "I know the phone number to call if I feel I can't cope."

16. The nurse teaches a pregnant client about the need to take supplemental vitamins with iron during pregnancy. The nurse should instruct the client to take the iron with which liquid to promote maximum absorption?
☐ 1. milk
☐ 2. tea
☐ 3. hot chocolate
☐ 4. orange juice

17. The nurse is reviewing the laboratory values of a client receiving clozapine. Which laboratory value should the nurse report to the health care provider (HCP)?
☐ 1. white blood cell (WBC) count of 3500/μL (3.5 × 10⁹/L)
☐ 2. hemoglobin level of 8.2 g/dL (82 g/L)
☐ 3. sodium level of 136 mEq/L (136 mmol/L)
☐ 4. hyaline casts in the urinalysis

18. Four hours after a cast has been applied for a fractured ulna, the nurse assesses that the client's fingers are pale and cool and capillary refill is delayed for 4 seconds. How should the nurse interpret these findings?
☐ 1. Nerve impairment is developing in the fingers.
☐ 2. Arterial blood supply to the fingers is decreased.
☐ 3. Venous stasis is occurring in the fingers.
☐ 4. The finding is normal for this recovery period.

19. Which nursing intervention(s) are appropriate when creating a plan of care to promote the development of a preschooler? Select all that apply.
☐ 1. Provide anticipatory guidance for parents.
☐ 2. Help the parents understand their child's behavior.
☐ 3. Identify deviations from normal growth and development patterns.
☐ 4. Determine the child's future development.
☐ 5. Send the child to a daycare center.

20. An adolescent client is hospitalized with acute glomerulonephritis. The nurse reviews the client's urine chemistry laboratory reports as noted below. Which finding does the nurse draw to the attention of the health care provider (HCP)?

Laboratory Results

Test	Results
Urine specific gravity	1.035 (1.035)
Protein	12 mg/24 h (120 mg/L)
Potassium	35 mEq/24 h (35 mmol/L)
Creatinine	2 mg/24 h (17.6 mmol/L)

☐ 1. urine specific gravity
☐ 2. protein
☐ 3. potassium
☐ 4. creatinine

21. A neonate receives an intravenous (IV) infusion of dextrose 10% administered by an infusion pump. The nurse should verify the alarm settings on the infusion pump at which times? Select all that apply.
☐ 1. when the infusion is started
☐ 2. at the beginning of each shift
☐ 3. when the neonate returns from x-ray
☐ 4. when the neonate moves in the crib
☐ 5. after the parents have visited

22. The nurse administers an intramuscular injection to an infant. Indicate the appropriate site for this injection.

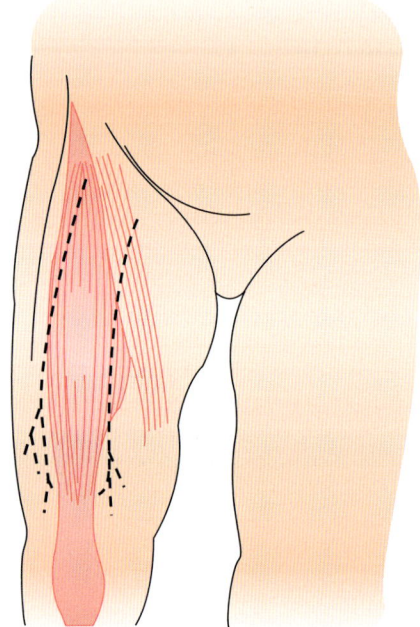

23. A client with diabetes is doing a "teach-back" by explaining to the nurse how to care for the feet at home. Which statement indicates that the client understands proper foot care?
☐ 1. "When I injure my toe, I'll plan to put iodine on it."
☐ 2. "I should inspect my feet at least once a week."
☐ 3. "It's okay to go barefoot in the house."
☐ 4. "It's important to dry my feet carefully after my bath."

24. The nurse observes a parent of a child with cystic fibrosis performing chest percussion. The nurse determines that the skill is being done correctly when the parent uses which technique?
☐ 1. firmly but gently striking the chest wall to make a popping sound
☐ 2. gently striking the chest wall to make a slapping sound
☐ 3. percussing over an area from the umbilicus to the clavicle
☐ 4. placing a blanket between the parent's hand and the child's chest

25. To prevent the development of peripheral neuropathies associated with isoniazid administration, what should the nurse teach the client to do?
  ☐ 1. Avoid excessive sun exposure.
  ☐ 2. Follow a low-cholesterol diet.
  ☐ 3. Obtain extra rest.
  ☐ 4. Supplement the diet with pyridoxine (vitamin B_6).

26. A nurse is planning care for a client who has heart failure. Which goal is appropriate for a client with excess fluid volume?
  ☐ 1. A weight reduction of 20% will occur.
  ☐ 2. Pain will be controlled effectively.
  ☐ 3. Arterial blood gas values will be within normal limits.
  ☐ 4. Serum osmolality will be within normal limits.

27. After the nurse teaches the parents of a 15-month-old child who has undergone cleft palate repair how to use elbow restraints, which statement by the parents indicates effective teaching?
  ☐ 1. "We'll keep the restraints in place continuously until our health care provider says it's okay to remove them."
  ☐ 2. "We can take off the restraints while our child is playing, but we'll make sure to put them back on at night."
  ☐ 3. "The restraints should be taped directly to our child's arms so that they'll stay in one place."
  ☐ 4. "We'll remove the restraints temporarily at least three times a day to check the skin and then put them right back on."

28. The nurse administers prednisone to a preschool child with nephrosis. What should the nurse do to ensure that the nurse has identified the child correctly? Select all that apply.
  ☐ 1. Ask another nurse to confirm that this is the correct dose and the correct client for whom the prednisone has been prescribed.
  ☐ 2. Check the child's identification band against the medical record number.
  ☐ 3. Verify the date of birth from the medical record with the date of birth on the client's identification band.
  ☐ 4. Compare the room number on the bed with the number on the client's identification band.
  ☐ 5. Ask the parent to state the client's full name.

29. A client is scheduled to have surgery to relieve an intestinal obstruction. Prior to surgery, the nurse should verify that the client has followed which preoperative instructions?
  ☐ 1. discontinued use of blood thinners
  ☐ 2. eaten a low-residue diet
  ☐ 3. practiced abdominal-strengthening exercises
  ☐ 4. signed a last will and testament

30. The nurse is preparing to administer propranolol to a client for control of migraine headaches. The client also has a prescription for sumatriptan as needed for a headache. The client's pulse rate is 56 bpm. What should the nurse do **next**?
  ☐ 1. Contact the health care provider (HCP).
  ☐ 2. Assess blood pressure.
  ☐ 3. Administer oxygen.
  ☐ 4. Administer sumatriptan.

31. A nurse is instructing a client about using nitroglycerin patches to prevent tolerance to the drug. What should the nurse instruct the client to do?
  ☐ 1. Remove the patch every night.
  ☐ 2. Use the patch only when chest pain occurs.
  ☐ 3. Change the site of the patch every day.
  ☐ 4. Apply the patch only on alternate days.

32. A client's abdominal incision eviscerates. What should the nurse do **first**?
  ☐ 1. Take the client's vital signs, and call the health care provider.
  ☐ 2. Lower the client's head and elevate the feet.
  ☐ 3. Cover the incision with a dressing moistened with sterile normal saline solution.
  ☐ 4. Start an emergency infusion of IV fluids.

33. The nurse is admitting a 4-year-old with a possible meningococcal infection. Which type of isolation is indicated?
  ☐ 1. airborne precautions
  ☐ 2. contact precautions
  ☐ 3. droplet precautions
  ☐ 4. standard precautions

34. STEP 1

The nurse is caring for a 32-year-old female client admitted for symptoms of schizophrenia.

Admission Note

1500:
The client, who has a history of schizophrenia, was brought to the emergency department (ED) this morning by their parents after the client stopped leaving their apartment 4 days ago. The client was found disheveled in bed with the shades pulled and the lights off. The client told their parents that aliens coming to Earth were stealing their thoughts. The parents report that a similar episode occurred 6 months ago. After that hospitalization, the client got a job, was taking an online class, and made a couple of friends.
In the ED, the client stayed in bed with the covers pulled over their head. The client refused food and fluid and stated, "the aliens want to sedate me." The client refused vital signs and refused to answer most of the admission questions; however, they did report not sleeping because they need to stay awake to watch for aliens. The client's affect is flat, and they appeared apathetic toward themselves and their parents.

▶ Which three findings need **immediate** follow-up?

☐ 1. Heightened mood
☐ 2. Nutritional status
☐ 3. Refusal of care
☐ 4. Thought patterns
☐ 5. Sleep patterns
☐ 6. Work status

35. STEP 2

The nurse is caring for a 32-year-old female client admitted for symptoms of schizophrenia.

Admission Note

1500:
The client, who has a history of schizophrenia, was brought to the emergency department (ED) this morning by their parents after the client stopped leaving their apartment 4 days ago. The client was found disheveled in bed with the shades pulled and the lights off. The client told their parents that aliens coming to Earth were stealing their thoughts. The parents report that a similar episode occurred 6 months ago. After that hospitalization, the client got a job, was taking an online class, and made a couple of friends.
In the ED, the client stayed in bed with the covers pulled over their head. The client refused food and fluid and stated, "the aliens want to sedate me." The client refused vital signs and refused to answer most of the admission questions; however, they did report not sleeping because they need to stay awake to watch for aliens. The client's affect is flat, and they appeared apathetic toward themselves and their parents.

▶ For each finding, specify if the finding represents positive symptoms of schizophrenia, negative symptoms of schizophrenia, or neither.

Findings	Positive Symptoms	Negative Symptoms	Neither Positive Nor Negative Symptoms
Not leaving apartment	○	○	○
Disheveled appearance	○	○	○
Believes in aliens	○	○	○
Refusal of care	○	○	○
Sleep disturbance	○	○	○
Marijuana use	○	○	○
Flat affect	○	○	○

36. STEP 3

The nurse is caring for a 32-year-old female client admitted for symptoms of schizophrenia.

Admission Note

1500:
The client, who has a history of schizophrenia, was brought to the emergency department (ED) this morning by their parents after the client stopped leaving their apartment 4 days ago. The client was found disheveled in bed with the shades pulled and the lights off. The client told their parents that aliens coming to Earth were stealing their thoughts. The parents report that a similar episode occurred 6 months ago. After that hospitalization, the client got a job, was taking an online class, and made a couple of friends.
In the ED, the client stayed in bed with the covers pulled over their head. The client refused food and fluid and stated, "the aliens want to sedate me." The client refused vital signs and refused to answer most of the admission questions; however, they did report not sleeping because they need to stay awake to watch for aliens. The client's affect is flat, and they appeared apathetic toward themselves and their parents.

➤ Complete the following sentence by choosing from the list of options.

The client is **most** likely experiencing [insomnia. / mood lability. / psychosis]

The priority intervention is to administer a(n) [antipsychotic. / sedative. / mood stabilizer]

37. STEP 4

The nurse is caring for a 32-year-old female client admitted for symptoms of schizophrenia.

Admission Note

1500:
The client, who has a history of schizophrenia, was brought to the emergency department (ED) this morning by their parents after the client stopped leaving their apartment 4 days ago. The client was found disheveled in bed with the shades pulled and the lights off. The client told their parents that aliens coming to Earth were stealing their thoughts. The parents report that a similar episode occurred 6 months ago. After that hospitalization, the client got a job, was taking an online class, and made a couple of friends.
In the ED, the client stayed in bed with the covers pulled over their head. The client refused food and fluid and stated, "the aliens want to sedate me." The client refused vital signs and refused to answer most of the admission questions; however, they did report not sleeping because they need to stay awake to watch for aliens. The client's affect is flat, and they appeared apathetic toward themselves and their parents.

Orders

- Admit to the psychiatric unit
- Routine orders
- Risperidone 2 mg orally (PO) stat
- Olanzapine 10 mg PO daily

The nurse receives orders to admit the client to the psychiatric unit.

➤ For each possible outcome, specify if the possible outcome is **most** appropriate for the acute psychotic phase of treatment or after stabilization.

Possible Outcome	Acute Psychotic Phase Outcomes	After Stabilization Outcomes
Not injure self or others	○	○
Maintain daily routines for eating and sleeping	○	○
Establish contact with reality	○	○
Interact with the nurse	○	○
Participate in therapeutic interventions	○	○
Express thoughts in an acceptable manner	○	○
Demonstrate independence in self-care	○	○

38. STEP 5

The nurse is caring for a 32-year-old female client admitted for symptoms of schizophrenia.

Admission Note

1500:
The client, who has a history of schizophrenia, was brought to the emergency department (ED) this morning by their parents after the client stopped leaving their apartment 4 days ago. The client was found disheveled in bed with the shades pulled and the lights off. The client told their parents that aliens coming to Earth were stealing their thoughts. The parents report that a similar episode occurred 6 months ago. After that hospitalization, the client got a job, was taking an online class, and made a couple of friends.
In the ED, the client stayed in bed with the covers pulled over their head. The client refused food and fluid and stated, "the aliens want to sedate me." The client refused vital signs and refused to answer most of the admission questions; however, they did report not sleeping because they need to stay awake to watch for aliens. The client's affect is flat, and they appeared apathetic toward themselves and their parents.

1900:
The client spent most of the day in their room in bed with the covers pulled over their head and refused vital signs and lab tests. They refused to participate in unit activities or come out for meals. The client ate crackers and drank approximately 500 mL of juice and 250 mL of decaffeinated tea. They stated that the aliens have poisoned the food and that some of the staff are aliens in disguise. The client refused to bathe and was observed walking in the hallway, holding a small stuffed bear given to them by their roommate. The client was also observed frequently stopping to look behind and around them and whispering to themselves and occasionally nodding their head. They requested paper and tape and made a "shield" to put on their door to keep the aliens away.

Orders

- Admit to the psychiatric unit
- Routine orders
- Risperidone 2 mg orally (PO) stat
- Olanzapine 10 mg PO daily

➤ When preparing the hand-off report, the nurse should recommend monitoring the client for the persistence of which symptom(s)? Select all that apply.

☐	1. grandiose delusions
☐	2. auditory hallucinations
☐	3. paranoia
☐	4. tangentiality
☐	5. catatonic excitement
☐	6. hypervigilance
☐	7. flight of ideas

39. STEP 6

The nurse is caring for a 32-year-old female client admitted for symptoms of schizophrenia.

Admission Note

1500:
The client, who has a history of schizophrenia, was brought to the emergency department (ED) this morning by their parents after the client stopped leaving their apartment 4 days ago. The client was found disheveled in bed with the shades pulled and the lights off. The client told their parents that aliens coming to Earth were stealing their thoughts. The parents report that a similar episode occurred 6 months ago. After that hospitalization, the client got a job, was taking an online class, and made a couple of friends.
In the ED, the client stayed in bed with the covers pulled over their head. The client refused food and fluid and stated, "the aliens want to sedate me." The client refused vital signs and refused to answer most of the admission questions; however, they did report not sleeping because they need to stay awake to watch for aliens. The client's affect is flat, and they appeared apathetic toward themselves and their parents.

1900:
The client spent most of the day in their room in bed with the covers pulled over their head and refused vital signs and lab tests. They refused to participate in unit activities or come out for meals. The client ate crackers and drank approximately 500 mL of juice and 250 mL of decaffeinated tea. They stated that the aliens have poisoned the food and that some of the staff are aliens in disguise. The client refused to bathe and was observed walking in the hallway, holding a small stuffed bear given to them by their roommate. The client was also observed frequently stopping to look behind and around them and whispering to themselves and occasionally nodding their head. They requested paper and tape and made a "shield" to put on their door to keep the aliens away.

2100:
The client received the first dose of olanzapine 10 mg PO.

2245:
The client was found sitting on the bed with their head pulled to one side. The client stated they could not move their head and felt like their throat was closing.

Orders

- Admit to the psychiatric unit
- Routine orders
- Risperidone 2 mg orally (PO) stat
- Olanzapine 10 mg PO daily

The nurse evaluates the client's status at the end of the shift.

➢ Complete the following sentence by using the list of drop-down options:

The nurse determines that the client's behavior indicates that they are experiencing [torticollis, catatonia, hallucinations,]

which is caused by [increased anxiety. the olanzapine. worsening psychosis.]

The nurse should call the health care provider to obtain a prescription for [lorazepam. diphenhydramine. haloperidol.]

40. While preparing to administer medications to a client, the nurse compares the medication in the medication box with the health care provider's (HCP) prescriptions and discovers that the HCP has prescribed oral prednisone 15 mg for a client with cirrhosis and the medication in the client's medication box is prednisolone 5 mg. What should the nurse do **next**?
    ☐ 1. Call the pharmacy for prednisone 15 mg.
    ☐ 2. Notify the charge nurse or supervisor.
    ☐ 3. Call the HCP for clarification.
    ☐ 4. Contact the pharmacy about the discrepancy.

41. A parent calls the clinic after their 4-year-old choked on a peanut. The parent reports performing abdominal thrusts and the child is breathing normally now. What should the nurse tell the parent to do?
    ☐ 1. Bring the child to the emergency department to check for airway obstruction.
    ☐ 2. Test the child's urine for blood from internal bleeding.
    ☐ 3. Call the health care provider if the child begins to sweat and feels dizzy.
    ☐ 4. Observe the child for difficulty breathing because the abdominal thrusts may have caused a pneumothorax.

42. The nurse is assessing Apgar scores for a neonate at birth and at 5 minutes after birth.

    Flow Sheets

	Apgar at Birth	Apgar 5 Minutes after Birth
Heart rate	120 bpm	100 bpm
Respirations	Slow	Irregular
Color	Blue extremities	Pink
Muscle tone	Flexion of extremities	Moving all four extremities
Reflexes	Grimace	Cough

    What should the nurse do **next**?
    ☐ 1. Notify the neonatologist on call.
    ☐ 2. Continue to assess the neonate.
    ☐ 3. Apply an oxygen mask.
    ☐ 4. Rub the neonate's extremities.

43. A nurse is concerned that a nurse colleague is diverting a narcotic medication. The nurse notes that the colleague administers pain medication in greater amounts than the nurse does when taking care of the same clients. These clients report unrelieved pain. What should the nurse do **next**? Select all that apply.
    ☐ 1. Remain focused on their own client assignment.
    ☐ 2. Continue to monitor the colleague's behavior.
    ☐ 3. Report concerns to the supervisor.
    ☐ 4. Ask the colleague about the clients' lack of pain relief.
    ☐ 5. Ignore the situation as this is a supervisory responsibility.

44. When developing a teaching plan for a client with an infected decubitus ulcer, the nurse should tell the client that which factor is **most** important for healing?
    ☐ 1. adequate circulatory status
    ☐ 2. scheduled periods of rest
    ☐ 3. balanced nutritional diet
    ☐ 4. fluid intake of 1500 mL a day

45. The nurse gives anticipatory guidance to the parents of a 5-month-old infant about toy safety. What toys should the nurse recommend?
    ☐ 1. plastic toy cars
    ☐ 2. wooden puzzles
    ☐ 3. stuffed animals
    ☐ 4. soft, washable toys

46. The nurse reviews the client's laboratory report to determine the client's blood level of valproic acid, which is 35 mcg/mL (243 µmol/L). Based on this report, what should the nurse do **first**?
    ☐ 1. Withhold the next dose of valproic acid.
    ☐ 2. Notify the health care provider (HCP).
    ☐ 3. Give the next dose as prescribed.
    ☐ 4. Take the client's vital signs.

47. A nurse cares for a client who gave birth to a term neonate at 0600. At 1600, the client has a distended bladder and is reporting pain of 5 on a scale of 0 to 10. The nurse reviews the client's output record. What should the nurse do **first**?

    Intake and Output

Output Record				
Time	0800	1000	1100	1600
	30 mL	50 mL	30 mL	60 mL

    ☐ 1. Apply a warm, moist towel over the bladder.
    ☐ 2. Ask the client to sit on the toilet while the nurse runs water from the faucet.
    ☐ 3. Administer acetaminophen with codeine.
    ☐ 4. Use an in-and-out catheter to empty the bladder.

48. The nurse observes that a client with a history of panic attacks is hyperventilating. What action should the nurse take?
☐ 1. Have the client breathe into a paper bag.
☐ 2. Instruct the client to put the head between the knees.
☐ 3. Give the client a low concentration of oxygen by nasal cannula.
☐ 4. Tell the client to take several deep, slow breaths and exhale normally.

49. The registered nurse (RN) is teamed with a licensed practical/vocational nurse (LPN/VN) in caring for a group of cardiac clients on a pediatric unit. Which action by the LPN/VN indicates the nurse should intervene **immediately**?
☐ 1. The LPN/VN assists a child to the bathroom 2 hours after a cardiac catheterization.
☐ 2. The LPN/VN places an infant having a cyanotic episode in a knee-chest position.
☐ 3. The LPN/VN checks a child's apical heart rate prior to administering digoxin.
☐ 4. The LPN/VN brings breakfast to a child who is scheduled for an electrocardiogram.

50. The nurse cares for an infant following the surgical repair of a cleft lip. What does the nurse determine is the **priority** goal for this client?
☐ 1. Manage pain.
☐ 2. Prevent infection.
☐ 3. Increase mobility.
☐ 4. Develop parenting skills.

51. When caring for a client with hepatitis B, which situation would expose the nurse to the virus?
☐ 1. contact with fecal material
☐ 2. a blood splash into the nurse's eyes
☐ 3. touching the client's arm with ungloved hands while taking a blood pressure
☐ 4. disposing of syringes and needles without recapping

52. The nurse observes a group of children in a daycare center. Which child warrants further assessment?
☐ 1. a child who is 12 months of age who has bruises on one side of the head
☐ 2. a child who is 3 years of age with a spiral fracture of the ulna whose mother does not know how the injury occurred
☐ 3. a child who is 4 years of age who wears the same clothes to the center every day
☐ 4. a child who is 2 years of age who has frequent episodes of untreated conjunctivitis

53. A client who had a hip replacement at 0900 is receiving an autologous blood transfusion that was started at 1100. At the change of shift (1500), the nurse working on the day shift reports that there is 50 mL of the unit of blood remaining to be infused. Which is a **priority** nursing action for the nurse working on the evening shift?
☐ 1. Keep the blood transfusing at the same rate.
☐ 2. Increase the rate so it will infuse by 1600.
☐ 3. Discontinue the blood transfusion at the beginning of the shift.
☐ 4. Maintain the current rate, and discontinue the blood transfusion at 1700.

54. A client undergoes a nephrectomy. In the immediate postoperative period, which nursing intervention has the **highest priority**?
☐ 1. Monitor blood pressure.
☐ 2. Encourage the use of the incentive spirometer.
☐ 3. Assess urine output hourly.
☐ 4. Check the flank dressing for urine drainage.

55. A client is receiving digoxin, and the pulse range is normally 70 to 76 bpm. After assessing the apical pulse for 1 minute and finding it to be 60 bpm, the nurse should do what **first**?
☐ 1. Notify the health care provider (HCP).
☐ 2. Withhold the digoxin.
☐ 3. Administer the digoxin.
☐ 4. Notify the charge nurse.

56. A client on a psychiatric care unit has muscle spasms in the neck and stiffness in other muscles, and the eyes are rolling upward. The client had two as-needed (PRN) doses of haloperidol in the last 6 hours. Of the drugs that have been prescribed for the client PRN (see chart), which drug should the nurse administer?

Prescriptions

- Lorazepam 1 mg IM
- Amantadine 100 mg PO
- Diphenhydramine 25 mg PO
- Benztropine 0.5 mg IM

☐ 1. lorazepam
☐ 2. amantadine
☐ 3. diphenhydramine
☐ 4. benztropine

57. After the birth of a neonate at 38 weeks' gestation, the nurse dries the neonate and places the neonate skin to skin on the birth parent's chest. The nurse performs this action based on the understanding that one neonatal response to cold stress involves which factor?
☐ 1. metabolism of brown adipose tissue
☐ 2. decreased utilization of glycogen stores
☐ 3. decreased utilization of calorie stores
☐ 4. increased shivering to keep warm

58. When developing the teaching plan for a primiparous client who is bottle-feeding their term neonate for the first feeding, what information should the nurse include?
☐ 1. Fill the entire nipple of the bottle with formula.
☐ 2. All term babies have well-developed sucking skills.
☐ 3. Bubble the baby after 2 oz (60 mL) of formula has been taken.
☐ 4. Propping of the bottle results in too much air being taken in by the baby.

59. A client has back pain 10 minutes after a unit of packed red blood cells (RBCs) was started. The client's pulse, blood pressure, and respirations are stable and similar to vital signs obtained before infusing the RBCs. What should the nurse do? Select all that apply.
☐ 1. Turn off the infusion of the packed RBCs.
☐ 2. Flush the Y-tubing with normal saline to clear the line.
☐ 3. Send the remaining blood to the lab.
☐ 4. Prepare for cardiopulmonary resuscitation.
☐ 5. Obtain a urine specimen to send to the laboratory.

60. A primiparous client 4 hours after a vaginal birth and manual removal of the placenta voids for the first time. The nurse palpates the fundus, noting it to be 1 cm above the umbilicus, slightly firm, and deviated to the left side, and notes painless dark red blood mixed with clots. The nurse notifies the health care provider based on the interpretation that the assessment indicates which problem?
☐ 1. perineal lacerations
☐ 2. retained placental fragments
☐ 3. cervical lacerations
☐ 4. urine retention

61. Two family members are visiting their parent who is experiencing acute delirium. They are upset that their parent is so disoriented. "They know who we are, but that's about it. We don't know what to say." What should the nurse tell the family? Select all that apply.
☐ 1. "Answer questions simply, honestly, slowly, and clearly."
☐ 2. "Correct your parent when they are hearing and seeing things that are not there."
☐ 3. "Occasionally remind them of the time, day, and place when they don't remember."
☐ 4. "Include your parent in your conversation, instead of talking about them while present."
☐ 5. "Raise your voice a bit so you're sure your parent hears you."

62. A 26-year-old is being treated for delirium due to acute alcohol intoxication. The client is restless, does not want to stay seated, and has a staggering gait. What should the nurse do **first**?
☐ 1. Place the client in a chair with a waist restraint.
☐ 2. Provide one-to-one supervision of the client until detoxification treatment can begin.
☐ 3. Ask the client to sit in a chair next to the Nurse's station.
☐ 4. Decrease stimuli by putting the client in bed with the room door closed.

63. A nurse is analyzing a client's intake and output. The client has a temperature of 102°F (38.9°C) and is receiving 2400 mL of intravenous (IV) fluids per 24 hours because the client is to have nothing by mouth. What information should the nurse obtain before taking action?
☐ 1. the client's body mass index
☐ 2. the amount of insensible fluid loss through the lungs and skin
☐ 3. when the client last ate
☐ 4. the IV fluid intake during the last 8 hours

64. A 5-month-old infant is brought to the emergency department with vomiting and diarrhea, which the parent states started 3 days ago. The nurse should conduct a focused assessment for which sign(s) or symptom(s)? Select all that apply.
☐ 1. decreased or absent tearing
☐ 2. dry mucous membranes
☐ 3. sunken fontanelle
☐ 4. clear, pale yellow urine
☐ 5. bounding pulse

65. A client gives birth to a neonate at 30 weeks' gestation. The neonate is stable on minimal ventilator settings. The client's previous infant, who was born at 24 weeks' gestation, did not survive. The family is Roman Catholic and requests that the neonate be baptized as soon as possible. What response by the nurse is **most** appropriate?
☐ 1. "What would you like me to do to help arrange the baptism?"
☐ 2. "Are you requesting the baptism because you are concerned that your infant might die?"
☐ 3. "We have a unit chaplain who rounds daily and can perform the baptism."
☐ 4. "Your baby is much older and much more stable than the baby you lost."

66. A client with bipolar disorder, manic phase, shows little interest in eating. What should the nurse do to help the client meet recommended daily allowances of nutrients?
☐ 1. Give the client half of a meat and cheese sandwich to carry with them.
☐ 2. Inform the client that snacks are available only if they eat properly at mealtime.
☐ 3. Tell the client to sit alone at mealtime so that they will not be distracted by others.
☐ 4. Teach the client about proper nutrition.

67. A client has bursitis in the subacromial bursa. A nurse determines that the client understands teaching when the client makes which statement?
☐ 1. "I'll apply moist heat to my shoulder for 20 minutes three times each day."
☐ 2. "I'll lift 30-lb (13.5-kg) weights at least three times each day."
☐ 3. "I'll place an ice pack on my shoulder for 20 minutes three times each day."
☐ 4. "I'll perform 360-degree circles with my arms extended at least three times daily."

68. A client has just undergone a lumbar puncture (LP). Which finding should the nurse **immediately** report to the health care provider (HCP)?
☐ 1. The client's oral intake was 1200 mL in the past 8 hours.
☐ 2. The client required analgesia for a headache.
☐ 3. A moderate amount of serous fluid was noted on the lumbar dressing.
☐ 4. The client is concerned about the test results.

69. The nurse is reviewing the lab report below for a client in hospice care with breast cancer and brain metastasis. According to the information in the chart, what should the nurse do **next**?

Laboratory Results		
Test	Result	Normal Range
Potassium	4.0 mEq/L (4.0 mmol/L)	3.5–5.2 mEq/L (3.5–5.2 mmol/L)
Sodium	142 mEq/L (142 mmol/L)	135–145 mEq/L (135–145 mmol/L)
Chloride	100 mEq/L (100 mmol/L)	96–106 mEq/L (96–106 mmol/L)
Calcium	12.4 mg/dL (3.1 mmol/L)	8.2 and 10.2 mg/dL (2.05–2.54 mmol/L)

☐ 1. Document these results on the medical record.
☐ 2. Report the elevated potassium level immediately.
☐ 3. Report the elevated calcium level immediately.
☐ 4. Refrain from reporting the results because the client is in hospice care.

70. **STEP 1**

The nurse is caring for a 75-year-old male client who has been brought to the emergency department by the client's spouse.

> Highlight the findings that require the nurse to follow up. Answer choices have been underlined.

Nurse's Notes

Today: 0900
A 75-year-old client was brought to the emergency department by their spouse who reports the client is experiencing sudden-onset drowsiness. The client has had a urinary tract infection treated with oral cephalexin for the past 5 days. The client's pupils are equal, round, and respond to light, and the client is oriented to time and place.
Admission vital signs are temperature (T) 101.8°F (38.8°C); pulse (P) 92 bpm; respiration rate (RR) 28 breaths/min; and blood pressure (BP) 88/40 mm Hg. Oxygen saturation per pulse oximeter is 95%.

Nurse's Notes

Today: 0900
A <u>75-year-old</u> client was brought to the emergency department by their spouse who reports the client is experiencing sudden-onset <u>drowsiness</u>. The client has had a <u>urinary tract infection</u> treated with oral cephalexin for the past 5 days. The client's pupils are equal, round, and respond to light, and the client is oriented to time and place.
Admission vital signs are <u>temperature (T) 101.8°F (38.8°C)</u>; <u>pulse (P) 92 bpm</u>; <u>respiration rate (RR) 28 breaths/min</u>; and <u>blood pressure (BP) 88/40 mm Hg</u>. <u>Oxygen saturation per pulse oximeter is 95%</u>.

71. STEP 2

The nurse is caring for a 75-year-old male client who has been brought to the emergency department by the client's spouse.

Nurse's Notes

Today: 0900
A 75-year-old client was brought to the emergency department by their spouse who reports the client is experiencing sudden-onset drowsiness. The client has had a urinary tract infection treated with oral cephalexin for the past 5 days. The client's pupils are equal, round, and respond to light, and the client is oriented to time and place.
Admission vital signs are temperature (T) 101.8°F (38.8°C); pulse (P) 92 bpm; respiration rate (RR) 28 breaths/min; and blood pressure (BP) 88/40 mm Hg. Oxygen saturation per pulse oximeter is 95%.

➢ For each assessment finding below, specify if the finding is consistent with urinary tract infection or septic shock. Each finding may support more than one disease process.

Client Findings	Urinary Tract Infection	Septic Shock
T 101.8°F (38.8°C)	☐	☐
RR 28 breaths/min	☐	☐
BP 98/40 mm Hg	☐	☐
P 94 bpm	☐	☐
Oxygen saturation 91%	☐	☐

Note: Each column must have at least one response option selected.

72. STEP 3

The nurse is caring for a 75-year-old male client who has been brought to the emergency department by the client's spouse.

Nurse's Notes

Today: 0900
A 75-year-old client was brought to the emergency department by their spouse who reports the client is experiencing sudden-onset drowsiness. The client has had a urinary tract infection treated with oral cephalexin for the past 5 days. The client's pupils are equal, round, and respond to light, and the client is oriented to time and place.
Admission vital signs are temperature (T) 101.8°F (38.8°C); pulse (P) 92 bpm; respiration rate (RR) 28 breaths/min; and blood pressure (BP) 88/40 mm Hg. Oxygen saturation per pulse oximeter is 95%.

0930:
Vital signs are T 101.8°F (38.8°C); P 96 bpm; RR 28 breaths/min; BP 84/38 mm Hg; and oxygen saturation 91%.

The client is becoming confused and unable to follow commands. The client voided 150 mL of cloudy urine.

➢ Complete the following sentence by choosing from the list of options.

The client is at risk for developing
| stroke |
| hypoxia |
| renal failure |
| septic shock |

as evidenced by the client's
| vital signs. |
| oxygen level. |
| neurologic assessment. |
| urinary output. |

73. STEP 4

The nurse is caring for a 75-year-old male client who has been brought to the emergency department by the client's spouse.

Nurse's Notes

Today: 0900
A 75-year-old client was brought to the emergency department by their spouse who reports the client is experiencing sudden-onset drowsiness. The client has had a urinary tract infection treated with oral cephalexin for the past 5 days. The client's pupils are equal, round, and respond to light, and the client is oriented to time and place.
Admission vital signs are temperature (T) 101.8°F (38.8°C); pulse (P) 92 bpm; respiration rate (RR) 28 breaths/min; and blood pressure (BP) 88/40 mm Hg. Oxygen saturation per pulse oximeter is 95%.

0930:
Vital signs are T 101.8°F (38.8°C); P 96 bpm; RR 28 breaths/min; BP 84/38 mm Hg; and oxygen saturation 91%.
The client is becoming confused and unable to follow commands. The client voided 150 mL of cloudy urine.

Orders

- Start oxygen at 2 L per minute per nasal cannula
- 5% dextrose in normal saline (D5NS) 1000 mL every 8 hours
- Vancomycin 500 mg intravenously (IV) every 6 hours
- Norepinephrine 0.01 to 3.3 mcg/kg per minute IV infusion
- Insert an indwelling urinary catheter
- Urine culture and sensitivity stat
- Arterial blood gas (ABG) stat
- Blood urea nitrogen (BUN) and creatinine

The nurse reviews the health care provider's orders and develops a care plan.

➢ Which nursing action(s) should the nurse include when developing a care plan and preparing to implement the health care provider's orders? Select all that apply.

☐	1. Start a peripheral IV.
☐	2. Start an arterial line.
☐	3. Question the order for oxygen at 2 L per minute.
☐	4. Place leads for continuous cardiac monitoring.
☐	5. Question the order for the indwelling catheter.
☐	6. Maintain accurate intake/output records.
☐	7. Explain the plan of care to the client and spouse.

74. STEP 5

The nurse is caring for a 75-year-old male client who has been brought to the emergency department by the client's spouse.

Nurse's Notes

Today: 0900
A 75-year-old client was brought to the emergency department by their spouse who reports the client is experiencing sudden-onset drowsiness. The client has had a urinary tract infection treated with oral cephalexin for the past 5 days. The client's pupils are equal, round, and respond to light, and the client is oriented to time and place.
Admission vital signs are temperature (T) 101.8°F (38.8°C); pulse (P) 92 bpm; respiration rate (RR) 28 breaths/min; and blood pressure (BP) 88/40 mm Hg. Oxygen saturation per pulse oximeter is 95%.

0930:
Vital signs are T 101.8°F (38.8°C); P 96 bpm; RR 28 breaths/min; BP 84/38 mm Hg; and oxygen saturation 91%.
The client is becoming confused and unable to follow commands. The client voided 150 mL of cloudy urine.

Orders

- Start oxygen at 2 L per minute per nasal cannula
- 5% dextrose in normal saline (D5NS) 1000 mL every 8 hours
- Vancomycin 500 mg intravenously (IV) every 6 hours
- Norepinephrine 0.01 to 3.3 mcg/kg per minute IV infusion
- Insert an indwelling urinary catheter
- Urine culture and sensitivity stat
- Arterial blood gas (ABG) stat
- Blood urea nitrogen (BUN) and creatinine

The nurse has established IV access and inserted the indwelling urinary catheter.

➤ Highlight the three orders the nurse should implement **right away**. Answer choices have been underlined.

Orders

- <u>Start oxygen at 2 L per minute per nasal cannula</u>
- 5% dextrose in normal saline (D5NS) 1000 mL every 8 hours
- <u>Vancomycin 500 mg intravenously (IV) every 6 hours</u>
- <u>Norepinephrine 0.01 to 3.3 mcg/kg per minute IV infusion</u>
- <u>Insert an indwelling urinary catheter</u>
- <u>Urine culture and sensitivity stat</u>
- Arterial blood gas (ABG) stat
- Blood urea nitrogen (BUN) and creatinine

75. STEP 6

The nurse is caring for a 75-year-old male client who has been brought to the emergency department by the client's spouse.

Nurse's Notes

Today: 0900
A 75-year-old client was brought to the emergency department by their spouse who reports the client is experiencing sudden-onset drowsiness. The client has had a urinary tract infection treated with oral cephalexin for the past 5 days. The client's pupils are equal, round, and respond to light, and the client is oriented to time and place.
Admission vital signs are temperature (T) 101.8°F (38.8°C); pulse (P) 92 bpm; respiration rate (RR) 28 breaths/min; and blood pressure (BP) 88/40 mm Hg. Oxygen saturation per pulse oximeter is 95%.

0930:
Vital signs are T 101.8°F (38.8°C); P 96 bpm; RR 28 breaths/min; BP 84/38 mm Hg; and oxygen saturation 91%.
The client is becoming confused and unable to follow commands. The client voided 150 mL of cloudy urine.

Orders

- Start oxygen at 2 L per minute per nasal cannula
- 5% dextrose in normal saline (D5NS) 1000 mL every 8 hours
- Vancomycin 500 mg intravenously (IV) every 6 hours
- Norepinephrine 0.01 to 3.3 mcg/kg per minute IV infusion
- Insert an indwelling urinary catheter
- Urine culture and sensitivity stat
- Arterial blood gas (ABG) stat
- Blood urea nitrogen (BUN) and creatinine

Vital Signs

Vital Signs	0900	0930	1000
HR	92 bpm	96 bpm	94 bpm
BP systolic	88 mm Hg	84 mm Hg	92 mm Hg
BP diastolic	40	38 mm Hg	50 mm Hg
RR	28 breaths/min	28 breaths/min	28 breaths/min
Oxygen saturation	95%	91%	94%
T	101.8°F (38.8°C)		101.8°F (38.8°C)
Urinary output	Voided 150 mL		Per catheter 40 mL

➤ The nurse administered norepinephrine at 0930 and reassesses the client's condition at 1000. Which vital sign(s) indicate the order for norepinephrine has been effective? Select all that apply.

- ☐ 1. Heart Rate
- ☐ 2. Systolic BP
- ☐ 3. Diastolic BP
- ☐ 4. Respiratory Rate
- ☐ 5. Oxygen saturation
- ☐ 6. Temperature
- ☐ 7. Urinary output

76. A nurse is caring for a primigravid client at 40 weeks' gestation in active labor. Assessments include: cervix 5 cm dilated; 90% effaced; station 0; cephalic presentation and fetal heart rate baseline 135 bpm, decreases to 125 bpm shortly after the onset of 5 uterine contractions and returns to baseline before the uterine contraction ends. Based on this assessment, what action should the nurse take **first**?
    ☐ 1. Position the client on the left side, and administer oxygen via face mask.
    ☐ 2. Document the findings on the client's medical record, and continue to monitor labor progress.
    ☐ 3. Perform a vaginal examination to rule out umbilical cord prolapse.
    ☐ 4. Notify the health care provider (HCP) immediately, and prepare for an emergency cesarean birth.

77. An adult with a peritonsillar abscess has been hospitalized. Upon assessment, the nurse determines the client has a temperature of 103°F (39.4°C), body chills, and leukocytosis. The client begins to have difficulty breathing. In what order from first to last should the nurse perform the actions? All options must be used.

    | 1. Call the health care provider (HCP). |
    | 2. Open the airway. |
    | 3. Start an IV access site. |
    | 4. Explain the situation to the family. |
    | |
    | |
    | |
    | |

78. A client who is receiving a blood transfusion suddenly experiences chills and a temperature of 101°F (38.3°C). The client also has a headache and appears flushed. In what order from first to last should the nurse perform the actions? All options must be used.

    | 1. Obtain a blood culture from the client. |
    | 2. Send the blood bag and administration set to the blood bank. |
    | 3. Stop the blood infusion. |
    | 4. Infuse normal saline to keep the vein open. |
    | |
    | |
    | |
    | |

79. A client in surgery has an endotracheal tube (ET) in place. The nurse should call a time-out if which requirement(s) are **not** in place? Select all that apply.
    ☐ 1. an identification band
    ☐ 2. postoperative pain medication
    ☐ 3. an intravenous (IV) line
    ☐ 4. oxygen administration
    ☐ 5. an anesthetist/anesthesiologist

80. A multiparous client at 16 weeks' gestation is diagnosed as having a fetus with probable anencephaly. The client has decided to continue the pregnancy based on religious beliefs and donate the neonatal organs after the death of the neonate. Which action by the nurse would be **most** appropriate?
    ☐ 1. Explore their own feelings about the issues of anencephaly and organ donation.
    ☐ 2. Contact the client's clergy to discuss the client's options related to the pregnancy.
    ☐ 3. Advise the client that the prolonged neonatal death will be very painful to watch.
    ☐ 4. Ask the client if they have discussed this with their family.

81. The nurse cares for a client who is breathing rapidly, is pacing back and forth across the room, and has their lips tightly closed and their arms crossed tightly across their chest. What should the nurse do **first**?
☐ 1. Assist the client to a safe, calm environment.
☐ 2. Place the client in an isolation room.
☐ 3. Ask the client why they are so anxious.
☐ 4. Administer buspirone as needed.

82. A nurse is planning care for a regressed, chronically ill client diagnosed with schizophrenia. What is the **most** appropriate milieu?
☐ 1. confrontation and peer pressure to break down the client's denial
☐ 2. reminder that all clients must participate fully in unit self-governance
☐ 3. required attendance at group activities with equal participation from all clients
☐ 4. nurturance and supportive interaction focusing on individual needs

83. The nurse is caring for a client who has been diagnosed with deep vein thrombosis. When assessing the client's vital signs, the nurse notes an apical pulse of 150 bpm, a respiratory rate of 46 breaths/min, and blood pressure of 100/60 mm Hg. The client appears anxious and restless. What should be the nurse's **first** course of action?
☐ 1. Call the rapid response team.
☐ 2. Administer a sedative.
☐ 3. Try to elicit a positive Homans sign.
☐ 4. Increase the flow rate of intravenous (IV) fluids.

84. Assessment of a primigravid client in active labor reveals cervical dilation at 9 cm with complete effacement and the fetus at +1 station. What is the **most** appropriate action for the nurse to take when the health care provider (HCP) prescribes morphine 2 mg intramuscularly (IM) for the client?
☐ 1. Administer the medication in the left ventrogluteal muscle.
☐ 2. Be certain that naloxone is at the client's bedside.
☐ 3. Ask the HCP to validate the dosage of the drug.
☐ 4. Refuse to administer the medication to the client.

85. A client has been hospitalized with a diagnosis of myasthenia gravis. The client has been talking on the phone. The nurse enters the room right after the client has recovered from choking on a sandwich. What should the nurse do **next**?
☐ 1. Instruct the client to sit at a 30-degree angle in bed when eating.
☐ 2. Tell the client to swallow when the chin is tipped down on the chest.
☐ 3. Remind the client to rest after eating.
☐ 4. Encourage the client not to talk while eating.

86. A client with a T2 to T3 spinal cord injury suddenly has a throbbing headache and blurred vision. The client is flushed and sweating on the upper trunk and face, and the hairs on the arms are raised. What should the nurse do **first**?
☐ 1. Raise the head of the bed.
☐ 2. Assess for hypotension.
☐ 3. Check the client for a distended bladder.
☐ 4. Logroll the client to see if the client is lying on a foreign object.

87. A 17-year-old unmarried primigravida client at 10 weeks' gestation tells the nurse that their family does not have much money and their dad just got laid off from work. What should the nurse do **first**?
☐ 1. Instruct the client on methods for low-cost, highly nutritious meal preparation.
☐ 2. Determine whether the client qualifies for local assistance programs.
☐ 3. Refer the client to a social worker for enrollment in a food assistance program.
☐ 4. Ask the client if they have a job and the amount of income earned.

88.

The nurse cares for an 8-year-old male child at a well-child visit.

Flowsheet

Age	Heart Rate	Respiration Rate	Blood Pressure (BP)	BP Percentiles	Height	Weight	Body Mass Index (BMI)	BMI for Age
8 years	88 bpm	22 breaths/min	112/72 mm Hg	82/84 mm Hg	55 inches (140 cm)	86 lb (39 kg)	20	95th

Labs	Results					Reference Range		
Total cholesterol	198 mg/dL (5.1 mmol/L)					<200 mg/dL (5.1 mmol/L)		
HbA1c	5.6% (0.06 proportion of total hemoglobin)					<5.7% (0.06 proportion of total hemoglobin)		

Nurse's Notes

The client likes school and uses a booster seat in the car. No one in the family smokes. The client likes video games but does not like sports. They sleep about 8 hours a day. They report having a good appetite but state they do not like vegetables. The family eats fast food most nights of the week and drinks soda with dinner.
The birth parent reports having gestational diabetes and borderline high cholesterol and is currently overweight. The family history is positive for type 2 diabetes and cardiovascular disease in the maternal grandmother. Immunizations are up to date.

➤ Complete the diagram by circling the choices below to specify the condition the client is **most** likely experiencing, two actions to take to address that condition, and two parameters the nurse should monitor to assess the client's progress.

Action to Take — Condition Most Likely Experiencing — Parameter to Monitor
Action to Take — — Parameter to Monitor

Action to Take	Potential Conditions	Parameters to Monitor
Establish structure for meals, activity, screen time, and sleep	Hypertension	Daily weights
Encourage 60 minutes of structured exercise per day	Prediabetes	Weekly blood pressures
Involve the entire family in the eating plan	Obesity	Calorie and carbohydrate counts
Teach daily calorie, carbohydrate, and sodium Limits	Metabolic syndrome	Physical activity patterns
Teach home blood pressure monitoring		Sugary beverage intake

---

89. A client has impairments in immediate recall and short-term memory. A nurse is planning for the client's daily activities. Which action by the nurse would be **most** effective?
   ☐ 1. Write out the client's schedule in large print, and show the client where the schedule is placed.
   ☐ 2. Describe each activity and the time of the events at the beginning of the day.
   ☐ 3. Take the client to each activity if the client does not attend on time.
   ☐ 4. Tell the client about each activity 10 minutes before it begins.

90. The nurse has been assigned to care for several postpartum clients and their neonates on a birthing unit. Which client should the nurse assess **first**?
   ☐ 1. a multiparous client at 48 hours postpartum who is being discharged
   ☐ 2. a primiparous client at 2 hours postpartum who gave vaginal birth to a term neonate
   ☐ 3. a multiparous client at 24 hours postpartum whose infant is in the special care nursery
   ☐ 4. a primiparous client at 48 hours postpartum after cesarean birth of a term neonate

91. A 4-year-old child who has been ill for 4 hours is admitted to the hospital with difficulty swallowing, a sore throat, and severe substernal retractions. The child's temperature is 104°F (40°C), and the apical pulse is 140 bpm. The white blood cell count is 16,000/mm³ (16 × 10⁹/L). What is the **priority** for nursing intervention?
☐ 1. infection
☐ 2. airway obstruction
☐ 3. difficulty breathing
☐ 4. potential for aspiration

92. Which baseline laboratory data should be established before a client is started on tissue plasminogen activator or alteplase recombinant?
☐ 1. potassium level
☐ 2. Lee-White clotting time
☐ 3. hemoglobin level, hematocrit, and platelet count
☐ 4. blood glucose level

93. A client is scheduled to undergo an upper gastrointestinal (GI) series. The nurse should give the client which instruction(s) in preparation for the test? Select all that apply.
☐ 1. "You will need to take a stool softener before the test to promote evacuation of the barium."
☐ 2. "Don't eat or drink for 8 hours before the test."
☐ 3. "You can expect white stools for about 48 hours after the test."
☐ 4. "You'll experience mild stomach pain during the test."
☐ 5. "It's okay for you to smoke before the test."

94. The nurse interprets the rhythm strip below from a client's bedside monitor as which rhythm?

☐ 1. normal sinus rhythm
☐ 2. sinus tachycardia
☐ 3. atrial fibrillation
☐ 4. ventricular tachycardia

95. The nurse is preparing to give an intramuscular (IM) injection to an underweight client. Which site is the safest?
☐ 1. deltoid
☐ 2. dorsogluteal
☐ 3. vastus lateralis
☐ 4. triceps

96. The nurse is planning to teach the client how to properly use a metered-dose inhaler to treat asthma. The nurse should tell the client to use which procedure?
☐ 1. Rinse the mouth after each use of a steroid inhaler.
☐ 2. Inhale quickly when administering the medication.
☐ 3. Inhale the medication, and then exhale through the nose.
☐ 4. Cough and deep-breathe before inhaling the medication.

97. A client who is receiving a blood transfusion begins to have difficulty breathing. The nurse notes an elevated blood pressure and a cough. Based on these signs, the nurse should prepare to manage which complication?
☐ 1. anaphylactic reaction
☐ 2. circulatory overload
☐ 3. sepsis
☐ 4. acute hemolytic reaction

98.

The nurse cares for a 17-year-old male client with abdominal pain in the emergency department.

Admission Note

1230:
The client has pain and tenderness of the abdomen, particularly on the left upper quadrant that radiates to the left shoulder. The client reports the pain began after a fall. The client took 200 mg of ibuprofen before coming to the emergency department, which helped the pain slightly. The client currently rates pain as a 6 on a scale of 0 to 10 and also reports feeling lightheaded and appears diaphoretic. The skin is cool to touch. The client's history is positive for Epstein-Barr virus diagnosed 7 days ago. Vital signs are temperature 100.2°F (37.9°C); pulse 94 bpm; respiration rate 26 breaths/min; blood pressure 78/40 mm Hg; and pulse oximetry reading 95% on room air. A bedside ultrasound is pending.

The nurse reviews the client's assessment data to prepare the plan of care.

➤ Complete the diagram by circling the choices below to specify the condition the client is **most** likely experiencing, two actions to treat that condition, and two parameters to monitor.

Action to Take — Condition Most Likely Experiencing — Parameter to Monitor
Action to Take — Parameter to Monitor

Action to Take	Potential Conditions	Parameters to Monitor
Give an intravenous fluid bolus	Reye syndrome	Urine output
Administer antibiotics	Ruptured spleen	Liver functions
Prepare for surgery	Liver inflammation	Levels of consciousness
Insert a gastric tube	Acute appendicitis	Gastric output
Administer corticosteroids		Intracranial pressure

99. The nurse is teaching a client with peptic ulcer disease how to take sucralfate. Which statement indicates that the client understands how to take the medication?
☐ 1. "I should take the sucralfate every evening at bedtime."
☐ 2. "It's important that I take this drug on an empty stomach."
☐ 3. "I should avoid milk products while taking this drug."
☐ 4. "I should have my hemoglobin checked monthly while taking sucralfate."

100. The nurse is conducting an admission interview with a client and is assessing for risk factors related to the client's safety. The nurse should include which targeted assessment(s)? Select all that apply.
☐ 1. suicide or self-harm ideation
☐ 2. incentives that motivate the client
☐ 3. recent use of substances of abuse
☐ 4. allergic reactions or adverse drug reactions
☐ 5. dietary preferences

101. An adult client has bacterial conjunctivitis. What should the nurse teach the client to do? Select all that apply.
☐ 1. Use warm saline soaks four times per day to remove crusting.
☐ 2. Apply topical antibiotic without touching the tip of the tube to the eye.
☐ 3. Wash the hands after touching the eyes.
☐ 4. Avoid touching the eyes.
☐ 5. Observe isolation procedures by staying in the bedroom until the redness in the eye disappears.

102. Which action(s) by the nurse will **most** likely ensure that the correct client receives a medication? Select all that apply.
☐ 1. Have the client state their name.
☐ 2. Check the name on the armband with the name on the medication.
☐ 3. Learn to recognize the client.
☐ 4. Check the client's room number.
☐ 5. Compare the date of birth on the client's medical record to the date of birth on the client's armband.

103. The nurse-manager is developing a "read-back" procedure to reduce medication administration errors. What is the purpose of the "read-back" requirement? Select all that apply.
  ☐ 1. to prohibit prescriptions and test results from being communicated verbally or by telephone
  ☐ 2. to make sure that prescriptions and test results that are communicated verbally or by telephone are clear to the receiver of the information
  ☐ 3. to make sure that prescriptions and test results that are communicated verbally or by telephone are confirmed by the individual giving the information
  ☐ 4. to minimize the risk for nonauthorized personnel from giving prescriptions that are communicated verbally or by telephone
  ☐ 5. to encourage the use of electronic medical records

104. A female client who is hospitalized for an eating disorder weighs 15 lb (6.8 kg) less than the ideal body weight. Which goal is a **priority** for this client?
  ☐ 1. attending all eating disorder support groups
  ☐ 2. eating bigger meals at breakfast
  ☐ 3. gaining 1 lb (0.5 kg) per week
  ☐ 4. reporting an improved self-image

105. A client with jaundice has had poor appetite, nausea, and two episodes of emesis in the past 2 hours. The client reports having spasms in the stomach area. The client does not have pruritus. The nurse should develop a care plan for which symptom **first**?
  ☐ 1. nausea
  ☐ 2. poor appetite
  ☐ 3. jaundice
  ☐ 4. abdominal spasms

106. The nurse is planning care for a group of clients who are at risk for the development of pressure ulcers. What should the nurse do **first**?
  ☐ 1. Identify at-risk clients on admission to the health care facility.
  ☐ 2. Place at-risk clients on an every-2-hour turning schedule.
  ☐ 3. Automatically place clients in specialty beds.
  ☐ 4. Provide at-risk clients with a high-protein, high-carbohydrate diet.

107. The nurse is teaching a young adult female who has a severe gonorrheal infection about the disease. The client understands the implications of the disease when they make which statement?
  ☐ 1. "Once I'm treated, I'll have immunity."
  ☐ 2. "My partner doesn't need treatment."
  ☐ 3. "I won't have any more problems once I learn to protect myself."
  ☐ 4. "I could have trouble getting pregnant."

108.

The nurse is admitting a 30-year-old male with a gunshot wound to the abdomen to the emergency department. The emergency medical technicians give a hand-off-of-care report to the nurse.

Admission Notes

The client has received a gunshot wound to the abdomen. Vital signs are temperature 97.0°F (36.1°C); heart rate 132 bpm; respiration rate 28 breaths/min; and blood pressure 84/60 mm Hg. Oxygen saturation by pulse oximeter is 89%.
The dressing on the wound is 90% saturated with frank blood. An intravenous (IV) line was established with 1000 mL normal saline infusing at a keep-open rate. The client is yelling "save me, save me" and crying out in pain.

➤ Complete the diagram by circling the choices below to specify the condition the client is **most** likely experiencing, the two most needed actions to take, and two parameters the nurse should monitor to determine the effectiveness of the interventions.

Action to Take — Condition Most Likely Experiencing — Parameter to Monitor
Action to Take — Parameter to Monitor

Possible Actions	Potential Conditions	Parameters to Monitor
Start oxygen per nasal catheter	Wound infection	Oxygenation levels
Type and crossmatch blood	Tachycardia	Dressing saturation
Insert an indwelling catheter	Hypovolemic shock	Pain level
Increase IV fluids	Pain	Urine output
Administer a narcotic for pain		Intake and output

109. After the nurse teaches the parent of a child with a spica cast about skincare, which parental action would indicate the need for additional teaching?
☐ 1. application of powder to the skin under the cast
☐ 2. inspection of the cast edges for smoothness
☐ 3. application of plastic film to cover the perineal cast area
☐ 4. inspection of areas inside the cast

110. The nurse-manager is teaching the staff about the medication reconciliation policy. The nurse teaches the staff that reconciliation is needed to ensure that clients are on the correct medications in which situation(s)? Select all that apply.
☐ 1. admission to the hospital
☐ 2. transfer to the nursing home
☐ 3. transfer of a client from surgery to the surgical unit
☐ 4. admission to a home health agency from the hospital
☐ 5. move from a double room to a single room on the same unit

111. A client is ready to be discharged following an inguinal hernia repair. Which criteria must the client meet before the nurse can discharge the client? Select all that apply.
☐ 1. has transportation home via a taxicab
☐ 2. is able to tolerate oral fluids
☐ 3. has pain rated as a 5 on a scale of 0 to 10
☐ 4. can walk to the bathroom unassisted
☐ 5. has voided

112. The nurse is administering eye drops to a client with glaucoma. Which technique is correct for instilling the eye drops?
☐ 1. in the lower conjunctival sac
☐ 2. near the opening of the lacrimal ducts
☐ 3. on the cornea
☐ 4. on the scleral surface

113. The nurse is teaching an older adult how to prevent falls. What should the nurse tell the client?
☐ 1. Turn on bright lights in the room so the client can see items in the room.
☐ 2. Instruct the client to rise slowly from a supine position.
☐ 3. Encourage the client not to use assistive devices as they reduce independence.
☐ 4. Instruct the client not to exercise painful joints.

114. A client scheduled for hip replacement surgery wishes to receive their own blood for the upcoming surgery. What should the nurse do?
☐ 1. Document the client's request on the medical record.
☐ 2. Notify the hematology laboratory.
☐ 3. Notify the surgeon's office.
☐ 4. Call the blood bank.

115. A client is using an over-the-counter nasal spray containing pseudoephedrine to treat allergic rhinitis. Which instruction about this medication would be **most** appropriate for the nurse to provide for the client?
☐ 1. Prolonged use of nasal spray can lead to nasal infections.
☐ 2. Pseudoephedrine is an addictive drug and must be used cautiously.
☐ 3. Overuse of pseudoephedrine can lead to increased nasal congestion.
☐ 4. A common side effect of pseudoephedrine nasal spray is thrush.

116. A 4-year-old child is admitted for an appendectomy. What is the **most** appropriate way for the nurse to prepare the child for surgery?
☐ 1. Explain how to use a patient-controlled analgesia (PCA) pump for pain control.
☐ 2. Permit the child to play with the blood pressure cuff, electrocardiogram (ECG) pads, and a face mask.
☐ 3. Show the child a video about the surgery.
☐ 4. Show the child a visual analog scale (VAS) based on a scale from 0 to 10.

117. The nurse is working on a hospital's birthing unit when a primigravid client in active labor is to receive morphine. As the nurse enters the medication room, the nurse observes a coworker slipping a vial of morphine into the side pocket of the uniform. Which action would be **most** appropriate?
☐ 1. Contact the hospital's security chief.
☐ 2. Notify the supervisor of the unit.
☐ 3. Tell the coworker of the incident.
☐ 4. Notify the federal drug agents about the incident.

118.

The nurse is caring for a 28-year-old female primigravid client at 8-weeks' gestation seen at the first prenatal visit.

Laboratory Results

Test	Result	Reference
ABO/Rh	O/Negative	O, A, B, or AB positive or negative
Antibody screen	Negative	Negative
Rubella AB immunoglobulin G (IgG)	Nonimmune	Immune
Hepatitis B surface antigen	Negative	Negative
White blood cells (WBCs)	5.23×10^3 cells/mm³ (5.23×10^9/L)	$4.5–10.5 \times 10^3$ cells/mm³ ($4.5–10.5 \times 10^9$/L)
Red blood cells (RBCs)	3.5×10^6/μL (3.5×10^{12}/L)	Women: 3.6–5 million/μL ($3.6–5 \times 10^{12}$/L)
Hemoglobin (HGB)	11.5 g/dL (115 g/L)	Women: 12–16 g/dL (120–160 g/L)
Hematocrit (HCT)	35% (0.35)	Women: 36%–48% (0.36–0.48 proportion of 1.0)
Mean corpuscular volume (MCV)	79 μm³ (79 fL)	80–100 μm³ (80–100 fL)

The nurse is reviewing the client's lab values to plan for the client's plan of care.

➤ Complete the diagram by circling the choices below to specify the condition the client is **most** likely experiencing, two actions to take to address that condition, and two parameters the nurse should monitor to assess the client's progress.

Action to Take — Condition Most Likely Experiencing — Parameters to Monitor

Action to Take — Parameters to Monitor

Action to Take	Potential Conditions	Parameters to Monitor
Provide nutrition counseling	Hepatitis B infection	Weight gain
Schedule catch-up vaccinations	Iron deficiency	Presence of fever
Begin iron supplementation	Rh incompatibility	Activity tolerance
Administer immunoglobulin	Rubella infection risk	Skin rashes
Provide disease prevention counseling		Evidence of jaundice

119. Which information should the nurse include when teaching the family and a client who was prescribed benztropine, 1 mg orally twice daily, about the drug therapy?
☐ 1. The drug can be used with over-the-counter cough and cold preparations.
☐ 2. The client should not discontinue taking the drug abruptly.
☐ 3. Antacids can be used freely when taking this drug.
☐ 4. Alcohol consumption with benztropine therapy need not be restricted.

120. A client has nephrotic syndrome. To aid in the resolution of the client's edema, the health care provider prescribes 25% albumin. In addition to an absence of edema, the nurse should evaluate the client for which expected outcome?
☐ 1. crackles in the lung bases
☐ 2. blood pressure elevation
☐ 3. cerebral edema
☐ 4. cool skin temperature in lower extremities

121. A client has polycystic kidney disease. The client asks the nurse, "How did I get these fluid-filled bubbles on my kidneys?" How should the nurse respond to help the client understand the risk factors for this disease?
☐ 1. "Secondhand smoke puts you at greater risk for developing cysts."
☐ 2. "Exposure to dyes used to color fruits and vegetables increases the risk for polycystic kidney disease."
☐ 3. "There is a higher incidence of polycystic kidney disease among blood relatives."
☐ 4. "Drinking alcohol daily allows the kidneys to develop cysts."

122. The nurse is working on a birthing unit with an unlicensed assistive personnel (UAP). The nurse determines that the UAP understands the type of information to report to the nurse when the UAP reports which information about one of the clients?
☐ 1. an episode of nausea after administration of an epidural anesthetic
☐ 2. contractions 3 minutes apart and lasting 40 seconds
☐ 3. evidence of spontaneous rupture of the membranes
☐ 4. sleeping after administration of intravenous (IV) nalbuphine

123. The nurse is to administer a bolus starting dose of heparin to a child who is taking penicillin. What should the nurse do? Select all that apply.
☐ 1. Check that the dose is appropriate for the child's weight.
☐ 2. Note that the onset of the medication will be immediate.
☐ 3. Follow the administration of the bolus of heparin with an intravenous (IV) infusion of heparin 10 units/kg per hour.
☐ 4. Monitor partial thromboplastin time (PTT).
☐ 5. Discontinue the penicillin until the PTT is at a therapeutic level.

124. A client is receiving epidural analgesia and has not voided for the last 5 hours. Which action should the nurse take **first**?
☐ 1. Encourage oral intake of fluids.
☐ 2. Palpate for bladder distention.
☐ 3. Review renal laboratory values.
☐ 4. Stop the infusion of medication.

125. The nurse is preparing to start an intravenous (IV) infusion. Before inserting the needle into a vein, the nurse applies a tourniquet to the client's arm. Which finding indicates the tourniquet has been applied correctly?
☐ 1. The veins are distended.
☐ 2. The veins do not "roll."
☐ 3. The arm is immobilized.
☐ 4. Arterial circulation is occluded.

126. A young adult has been admitted to the hospital for a biopsy to confirm the diagnosis of bone cancer. The nurse should assess the client for which condition(s)? Select all that apply.
☐ 1. cough
☐ 2. dyspnea
☐ 3. pain
☐ 4. swelling
☐ 5. fever
☐ 6. anorexia

127. A nurse on the labor and birth unit transfers a primiparous client and their term neonate to the mother-baby unit 2 hours after the client gave vaginal birth to the neonate. Which information is a **priority** for the nurse to report to the nurse receiving the client on the mother-baby unit?
☐ 1. firm fundus when gentle massage is used
☐ 2. evidence of bonding well with the neonate
☐ 3. labor that lasted 12 hours with a 1-hour second stage
☐ 4. temperature of 99°F (37.4°C) and pulse rate of 80 bpm

128.

The nurse assesses a neonate at 8 hours of age.

Flow Sheet

Time	0300	0700	1100
Color	acrocyanosis	acrocyanosis	central cyanosis
Respirations	50 breaths/min, breath sounds clear, no nasal flaring retractions, or grunting	60 breaths/min, breath sounds clear, no nasal flaring retractions, or grunting	90 breaths/min, breath sounds clear, no nasal flaring retractions, or grunting
Heart rate	120 bpm	128 bpm	142 bpm
Temperature	97.7°F (36.5°C)	98.9°F (37.2°C)	98°F (37°C)

➤ After reviewing the client's assessment data, what action(s) should the nurse take? Select all that apply.

☐ 1. Change the neonate's position.
☐ 2. Encourage the baby to cry.
☐ 3. Notify the health care provider (HCP).
☐ 4. Suction the nose and mouth.
☐ 5. Obtain a pulse oximeter reading.
☐ 6. Obtain blood pressures in all four extremities.
☐ 7. Place a nasogastric tube.

129. A nurse is admitting an older adult female client to the gynecology surgical unit. When the nurse asks the client what medication they are taking at home, the client responds that they are taking a little red pill in the morning and a white capsule at night for their blood pressure. What should the nurse do **next**?
☐ 1. Consult the pharmacist regarding identification of the medications.
☐ 2. Show pictures to the client from the *Physician's Desk Reference* to identify the medications.
☐ 3. Consult the previous medical record from 2 years ago, and notify the health care provider regarding medications that must be prescribed.
☐ 4. Ask a family member to bring the medications from home in the original vials for proper identification and administration times.

130. A client who had undergone an abdominal hysterectomy is in the recovery room. The surgeon has prescribed a 250-mL bolus of normal saline over 1 hour to replace blood loss. The intravenous (IV) solution infusing in the client was 1000 mL normal saline with 40 mEq of potassium chloride at 100 mL per hour. What should the nurse do? Select all that apply.
☐ 1. Increase the IV infusion rate to 250 mL per hour for 1 hour.
☐ 2. Add 250 mL of normal saline to the current infusion bag, and continue at 100 mL per hour.
☐ 3. Connect a 250-mL bag of normal saline to the Y-connector, and calculate to infuse over 1 hour.
☐ 4. Contact the health care provider regarding continuation of the primary IV infusion during the bolus infusion.
☐ 5. Administer the normal saline bolus via an IV infusion pump.

131. The nurse working on the mother-baby unit teaches the client about the facility's measures to prevent infant abduction. What precaution(s) does the nurse discuss? Select all that apply.
☐ 1. "Carry your baby in your arms back to the nursery if you plan to nap."
☐ 2. "Infant footprints and a color photograph are taken soon after birth."
☐ 3. "Only let staff wearing an appropriate identification (ID) badge transport your baby."
☐ 4. "Notify the staff about anyone who appears unusual."
☐ 5. "Make sure the staff compares your ID bracelets with your baby's daily."

132. The health care provider (HCP) is calling in a prescription for ampicillin for a neonate. What should the nurse do? Select all that apply.
☐ 1. Write down the prescription.
☐ 2. Ask the HCP to come to the hospital and write the prescription on the medical record.
☐ 3. Repeat the prescription to the HCP over the telephone.
☐ 4. Ask the HCP to confirm that the prescription is correct.
☐ 5. Ask the nursing supervisor to cosign the telephone prescription as transcribed by the nurse.

133. The nurse is planning care for a client who has been experiencing a manic episode for 6 days and is unable to sit still long enough to eat meals. Which choice will **best** meet the client's nutritional needs at this time?
☐ 1. a green salad topped with chicken pieces
☐ 2. a peanut butter sandwich
☐ 3. a bowl of vegetable soup
☐ 4. favorite foods from home

134. A female client who gave birth to a healthy baby 6 hours ago is having cramps in their legs. Upon further assessment, the nurse identifies leg pain on dorsiflexion. What action should the nurse take?
☐ 1. Tell the client to massage the area.
☐ 2. Apply warm compresses to the area.
☐ 3. Instruct the client on how to do ankle pumps.
☐ 4. Notify the health care provider (HCP).

135. After instructing a middle-age client about osteoporosis after menopause, the nurse determines that the client needs further instruction when the client makes which statement?
☐ 1. "A standard serving of yogurt is the equivalent of one glass of milk."
☐ 2. "Women who don't eat dairy products should consider calcium supplements."
☐ 3. "Women of African descent are at the greatest risk for osteoporosis."
☐ 4. "Estrogen therapy at menopause can reduce the risk for osteoporosis."

136. A young adult is hospitalized with a seizure disorder. The client, who is in a bed with padded side rails, has a tonic-clonic seizure. In what order from first to last should the nurse take the actions? All options must be used.

1. Loosen clothing around the client's neck.

2. Turn the client on their side.

3. Clear the area around the client.

4. Suction the airway.

---

137. A client with metastatic cancer of the liver tells the nurse about being concerned about the prognosis. How should the nurse respond to the client?
☐ 1. Provide information for the client to consider a liver transplantation.
☐ 2. Assure the client that the prescribed medications will shrink all tumor sites.
☐ 3. Explain the effects of chemotherapy.
☐ 4. Place emphasis on providing symptomatic and comfort measures.

---

138. The nurse is on a medical-surgical unit caring for a 72-year-old male client who had their gallbladder removed yesterday.

Output Record

Date and Time	T-Tube
4/7	
1200	50 mL
1600	60 mL
2000	60 mL
4/8	
0000	70 mL
0400	70 mL
0800	10 mL

➤ At 0800, the nurse reviews the input/output record to determine the amount of T-tube drainage. After reviewing the output record (see chart), what should the nurse do **next**? Select all that apply.

☐ 1. Report the 24-hour drainage amount at 1200.
☐ 2. Clamp the T-tube.
☐ 3. Evaluate the T-tube for patency.
☐ 4. Irrigate the T-tube.
☐ 5. Notify the surgeon.
☐ 6. Ask the unlicensed personnel (UAP) to empty the drainage apparatus.

---

139. A client with osteoarthritis purchased a copper bracelet to wear and tells the nurse that there is less pain now. Which response by the nurse is **most** appropriate?
☐ 1. Tell the client that copper is best applied as copper-lined gloves.
☐ 2. Warn the client not to spend any more money on quackery such as bracelets.
☐ 3. Instruct the client to remove the bracelet because the copper in it can interfere with salicylate metabolism.
☐ 4. Acknowledge that the client feels better, but encourage the client to continue with the prescribed therapy.

---

140. A client with a history of a left radical mastectomy is being admitted for abdominal surgery. The client has a swollen left arm. What should the nurse do to protect the client's swollen arm?
☐ 1. Take the blood pressure only in the unaffected arm.
☐ 2. Start an intravenous (IV) line in the affected arm.
☐ 3. Encourage a dependent position of the affected arm.
☐ 4. Allow blood draws in the affected arm.

141. After a nasogastric (NG) tube has been inserted, which finding helps the nurse determine that the tube is in the proper place?
☐ 1. The client is no longer gagging or coughing.
☐ 2. The pH of the aspirated fluid is measured.
☐ 3. Thirty milliliters of normal saline can be injected without difficulty.
☐ 4. A whooshing sound is auscultated when 10 mL of air is inserted.

142. A client has been diagnosed with early alcoholic cirrhosis. The client should be taught that which behavior could potentially reverse the pathologic changes occurring in the liver?
☐ 1. Do not become fatigued.
☐ 2. Avoid drinking alcohol.
☐ 3. Eliminate smoking.
☐ 4. Eat a high-carbohydrate, low-fat diet.

143. A client is admitted to the emergency department with sudden onset of chest pain. Which prescription(s) should the nurse implement **immediately**? Select all that apply.
☐ 1. Provide oxygen.
☐ 2. Administer nitroglycerin.
☐ 3. Administer aspirin.
☐ 4. Insert a Foley catheter.
☐ 5. Administer morphine.
☐ 6. Administer acetaminophen.

144. To reduce the possibility of catheter-related urinary tract infections (CAUTIs), the nurse should take which precaution?
☐ 1. Use sterile technique when providing catheter care.
☐ 2. Ensure that clients who are incontinent have indwelling urinary catheters.
☐ 3. Minimize urinary catheter use and duration of use in all clients.
☐ 4. Clean the periurethral area with antiseptics.

145. An older adult admitted with new-onset confusion, headache, poor skin turgor, bounding pulse, and urinary incontinence has been drinking copious amounts of water. Upon reviewing the lab results, the nurse discovers a sodium level of 122 mEq/L (122 mmol/L). What action(s) should the nurse take? Select all that apply.
☐ 1. Encourage fluids to 2000 mL in 24 hours.
☐ 2. Keep partial side rails up.
☐ 3. Restrict fluids to 800 mL in 24 hours.
☐ 4. Tell the family they may get the client up to walk in the halls.
☐ 5. Prepare to insert a Foley catheter.
☐ 6. Notify the health care provider (HCP).

146. Following the creation of an ileostomy, a client states, "I'm really worried about how I'm going to manage this thing." What should the nurse do **first**?
☐ 1. Remind the client to focus energy on getting healthy.
☐ 2. Determine the client's exact concerns about the ileostomy.
☐ 3. Arrange a meeting with the client's case manager.
☐ 4. Encourage the client's spouse to talk with the client.

147. A client who is being treated for nonhealing diabetic foot ulcers tells the nurse angrily, "I'm so frustrated with my doctors. The wound care doctor tells me this won't heal and I need to have my toes amputated, and another doctor tells me I need to keep going with the antibiotics and dressing changes so I can save my foot. I just want to go home!" After listening to the client's concerns, what should the nurse do?
☐ 1. Contact the client's case manager to set up a care conference.
☐ 2. Assure the client that the health care providers (HCPs) know what they are doing.
☐ 3. Remind the client of the responsibilities for health habits regarding diabetes.
☐ 4. Review the HCPs' progress notes with the client.

148. While making rounds, the nurse enters a client's room and finds the client on the floor between the bed and the bathroom. In which order of priority from first to last should the nurse take the actions? All options must be used.

1. If no acute injury, get help, and carefully assist the client back to bed.
2. Document as required by the facility.
3. Assess the client's current condition and vital signs.
4. Notify the client's health care provider (HCP) and family.

149. A neonate born at 30 weeks' gestation and weighing 2000 g is admitted to the neonatal intensive care unit. What nursing measure will decrease insensible water loss in a neonate?
☐ 1. bathing the baby as soon after birth as possible
☐ 2. use of eye patches with phototherapy
☐ 3. use of humidity in the incubator
☐ 4. use of a radiant warmer

150. A septic preterm neonate's intravenous (IV) line was removed due to infiltration. The nurse **prioritizes** restarting the IV to help which complication?
☐ 1. fever
☐ 2. hyperkalemia
☐ 3. hypoglycemia
☐ 4. tachycardia

Answers, Rationales, and Test-Taking Strategies

*The answers and rationales for each question follow below, along with keys (🔑) to the client need (CN) and cognitive level (CL) for each question. In addition, questions that measure clinical judgment will be coded (CJ). As you check your answers, use the **Content Mastery and Test-Taking Skill Self-Analysis** worksheet (tear-out worksheet in the back of the book) to identify the reason(s) for not answering the questions correctly. For additional information about test-taking skills and strategies for answering questions, refer to pages 12–51 in Part 1 of this book.*

1. 4. Laryngeal stridor is characteristic of respiratory distress from inflammation and swelling after bronchoscopy. It must be reported immediately. Green sputum indicates infection and would occur 3 to 5 days after bronchoscopy. A mild cough or hemoptysis is typical after bronchoscopy. If a tissue biopsy specimen was obtained, sputum may be blood streaked for several days.

🔑 CN: Reduction of risk potential; CL: Analyze

2. -/+ **1, 3, 4, 5.** Home care for a client with a total laryngectomy should include a high-humidity environment, laryngectomy tube care and suctioning, speech rehabilitation, and smoking cessation. The client is not restricted to a bland diet.

🔑 CN: Management of care; CL: Create

3. 2. Administering acetaminophen to the client with a post-ECT headache is the best action. Stating a headache is common after ECT and that napping will help the client feel better may be true, but it does not offer the client pain relief. Telling the client to eat breakfast and then to let the nurse know how the client feels conveys a lack of understanding to the client and dismisses the client's concern.

🔑 CN: Basic care and comfort; CL: Analyze

4. 3. This rhythm is ventricular tachycardia, which is characterized by an absent P wave and a heart rate of 140 to 220 bpm. Ventricular tachycardia requires immediate intervention, usually with lidocaine.

🔑 CN: Physiological adaptation; CL: Analyze

5. -/+ **1, 4, 6.** Providing culturally sensitive care includes providing printed material in the client's native language. There is nothing to indicate that this client is a high-risk pregnancy. Discussing cultural differences is not a priority or important at the first visit. Clients need to have an interpreter for each prenatal visit to translate and interpret questions. Contraceptive options are not a priority for the first prenatal visit. Reviewing dietary intake and discussing nutrition are important components of early prenatal care.

🔑 CN: Health promotion and maintenance; CL: Create

6. 4. An 18-month-old child should be able to say 10 or more words. Lack of speech development may indicate a lack of social stimulation, a hearing deficiency, or developmental delay. Referring the child for an evaluation may increase the child's chance of reaching the child's potential. A 4-month-old child with a healthy central nervous system and normal mental development should be able to laugh out loud if the child's environment has been caring and the child's needs are met safely and consistently. Children at age 10 months should be able to say the words "dada" and "mama" in response to the appropriate person. A 1-year-old child should have the ability to speak three to five words plus "mama" and "dada."

🔑 CN: Health promotion and maintenance; CL: Analyze

7. -/+ **2, 3, 4.** A client who has been admitted for numbness and tingling in the lower extremities that advances upward, especially after having a viral infection, has clinical manifestations characteristic of Guillain-Barré syndrome. The HCP must be notified of the change immediately because this disease is progressively paralytic and should be treated before paralysis of the respiratory muscles occurs. The nurse must assess the client continuously to determine how fast the paralysis is advancing. The family does not need to be called in to visit until the client is stabilized and emergency equipment is placed at the bedside. Performing ankle pumps will not relieve the numbness or change the course of the disease.

 CN: Management of care; CL: Analyze

8. 5, 6. The nurse reports signs of decreased tissue perfusion to the HCP; these include a decrease in urine output and confusion. Crackles, edema, and weight gain are monitored closely, but they are not as high a priority as decreasing tissue perfusion. Vital signs and oxygen saturation are within normal limits.

 CN: Physiological adaptation; CL: Analyze

9. 3. When a client is experiencing delusion, the nurse should present reality. The nurse should tell the client that they do not hear the voice, see the image, or experience whatever other manifestation of the delusion that the client is experiencing. The client with paranoia is delusional, related to anxiety states, but cannot manage the anxiety at this moment. Allowing expressions of anger or other intense emotions may be harmful to the client or others. Nurses should avoid "why" questions because such questions tend to make the client defensive.

 CN: Management of care; CL: Analyze

10.

STEP 1

Nurse's Notes
The client is breastfeeding exclusively and taking prenatal vitamins. The client does not have lochia and notes not having a period since birth. The client reports not sleeping and crying constantly. The client is a single parent and states feeling isolated from family. The client has a 2-year-old at home, but the other parent of the baby is not involved. The client needs a note to go back to work in the next week and is still trying to find daycare. They note feeling like a horrible parent. The client has lost half of the weight gained during pregnancy.

Normal baby blues typically last 2 weeks. Constant crying at 6 weeks indicates a more serious mood disorder. Not sleeping can increase the severity of depression symptoms and contributes to psychosis. Feeling isolated and that they are a horrible parent are symptoms of depression. While not having the other parent involved may indicate social isolation, it is most critical to understand why the client feels isolated. Having a second child that needs childcare in 1 week and the need to return to work in 1 week are important findings, but they are not as urgent as addressing the major depression symptoms. Continued breastfeeding, no lochia or period, and taking prenatal vitamins are typical findings. It is also normal to lose half of the weight gained in pregnancy by the 6-week recheck.

 CJ: Case study; Step 1: Recognize cues; CL: Understand

11.

STEP 2

Possible Findings	Risk Factor	Not a Risk Factor
Age over 30		X
Breastfeeding		X
Being single	X	
Stressful life events	X	
Sleep deprivations	X	
Second pregnancy		X

The cause of postpartum depression is thought to be a combination of hormonal, metabolic, and psychosocial components. Being single without a partner is a major risk for postpartum depression. Stressful events such as losing a job or domestic violence are major risk factors Sleep deprivation can contribute to hormonal imbalances, which affect the body's ability to regulate mood. Age less than 20, not older age, is a risk factor for postpartum depression. Breastfeeding is considered to decrease the risk for postpartum depression, though it may be associated with sleep deprivation. First pregnancies are considered a risk factor for postpartum depression because they are most associated with unrealistic expectations.

 CJ: Case study; Step 2: Analyze cues; CL: Analyze

12.

STEP 3

The top priority is for the nurse to address the client's **risk for suicide.**

Postpartum depression carries a high risk for suicide. The priority is for the nurse to assess the client's risk for self-harm or harm to the baby. The nurse should then address the social isolation and make appropriate referrals. Lack of sleep is very important to address because it increases the risk for developing psychosis. Sleep deprivation may be amenable to a short-term intervention. Low self-esteem, powerlessness, and ineffective coping are all problems that typically need cognitive behavioral therapy or group therapy to resolve. The nurse would monitor the client's weight loss to ensure it remains within normal limits, but at this time the client's nutritional status is not a top problem.

 CJ: Case study; Step 3: Prioritize hypothesis; CL: Analyze

13.

STEP 4		
0/1 Possible Intervention	Indicated	Not Indicated
Postpartum depression screening	✗	
Thyroid screening	✗	
Mental health referral	✗	
Diazepam prescription		✗
Self-care education	✗	

The nurse can anticipate conducting a focused screening for postpartum depression, which will help inform the plan of care. The nurse would anticipate an order to check the client's thyroid levels because symptoms of thyroid dysfunction can mimic depression or be another physiological factor contributing to sleep disturbances and a mood disorder. Referral to a mental health professional is needed to make a diagnosis and determine the best antidepressant or psychotherapy treatment options. The relationship between sleep and perinatal mood disorders is significant. The nurse may anticipate the need for a short-term sleep aid, but benzodiazepines, like diazepam, accumulate in the serum of breastfed infants with repeated doses and are generally not recommended. Teaching the client self-care care strategies such as asking for help, avoiding isolation, and taking breaks are important to help recovery.

CJ: Case study; Step 4: Generate solutions; CL: Analyze

14.

STEP 5		
0/1 Action	Essential	Not Essential
Screen for postpartum depression with a standardized screening tool	✗	
Have a second provider repeat the screen		✗
Compare screening results with screenings done prior to hospital discharge		✗
Refer clients with positive screens for a confirmatory diagnosis	✗	
Seek immediate care for clients who answer positively to self-harm questions	✗	

Screening for a postpartum or prenatal mood disorder should be done using a reliable and valid standardized tool such as the Edinburg Postnatal Depression Scale. A positive screening highly suggests the client has postpartum depression. However, the diagnosis must be confirmed by a health care provider qualified to make that medical diagnosis, and other medical problems or comorbidities must be ruled out. Any positive findings of suicide ideation should be seen immediately by a mental health professional for a lethality assessment and possible hospitalization. It is not necessary to have a second provider readminister the same screening test on the same day. Postpartum screening results are meant to assess a client's status. While results from previous screenings may be useful to understand client changes, they may not be readily available and are not necessary to assess a client's status.

CJ: Case study; Step 5: Take action; CL: Apply

15.

STEP 6

–/+ 2, 4, 7, 8. Connecting with friends and family helps break the cycle of isolation. Doing something the client enjoys such as a hobby, watching a movie, or exercising helps improve mood. Connecting with other mothers who have postpartum depression is a form of social support. Knowing where to call when a client is overwhelmed, whether it is a mental health hotline number or that of a trusted friend, is important to reduce the risk for self-harm or harm to the baby. Many antidepressants are considered safe to take during breastfeeding. Statements about needing to keep the house clean show that the client may be hanging on to unrealistic expectations. Alcohol is best avoided, and drinking two drinks a day is considered heavy drinking for a woman. If the client is exclusively breastfeeding, it is unrealistic to expect to get 8 hours of sleep a night. Rather, the nurse should help teach the client ways to get the most rest.

CJ: Case study; Step 6: Evaluate outcomes; CL: Evaluate

16. 4. Absorption of supplemental iron and nonmeat sources of iron is enhanced by combining them with meat or a good source of vitamin C. An acidic environment enhances iron absorption. Therefore, taking the iron on an empty stomach or with orange juice would be most effective. If gastrointestinal upset occurs, the client may take the drug with meals. However, doing so reduces iron absorption by 40% to 50%. Because milk interferes with the absorption of iron, the client should avoid taking the iron with milk. Tea has been shown to interfere with the absorption of iron. Therefore, the client should avoid taking the iron with tea. Hot chocolate, a milk product, interferes with iron absorption. Thus, the client should avoid taking the iron with hot chocolate.

CN: Basic care and comfort; CL: Analyze

17. 1. A low WBC count may indicate the development of agranulocytosis, a serious life-threatening side effect of clozapine, and should be reported immediately. While a hemoglobin level of 8.2 mg/dL (8.2 g/L) is low, it is not life-threatening. The sodium level of 136 mEq/L (136 mmol/L) is normal. Hyaline casts are usually caused by dehydration and indicate the need for more fluids.

CN: Management of care; CL: Analyze

18. 2. The pallor and cool temperature of the fingers and the decreased return time for capillary refill indicate decreased arterial blood supply to the fingers. These findings are not normal for any time in the recovery process. Nerve impairment includes numbness, tingling, and impaired movement of the fingers. Signs of venous stasis include edema and reddening of the fingers, not pallor and cool temperature.

🗝 CN: Physiological adaptation; CL: Analyze

19. -/+ 1, 2, 3. Goals for promoting healthy development in preschoolers include anticipatory guidance, helping parents understand their child's behavior, identifying deviations from the norm, and assessing parent-child interaction. No one can assess or determine the child's future development, and trying to do so can limit the potential the child may achieve. Although learning to interact with others is important, sending the child to a daycare center is not essential to promote healthy development. The nurse can encourage the parents to provide opportunities for the child to play with others.

🗝 CN: Psychosocial integrity; CL: Create

20. 1. The nurse verifies that the HCP has noted the elevated specific gravity. Clients with glomerulonephritis have concentrated urine from oliguria caused by the inflammation of the glomeruli. The other laboratory results are within normal range.

🗝 CN: Reduction of risk potential; CL: Analyze

21. -/+ 1, 2, 3. The alarm settings on infusion pumps should be verified at the time the infusion is started, at the beginning of each shift, and when the client is moved. The neonate can move in bed, but if the alarm is triggered, the nurse should verify the settings. Unless the neonate has moved or been taken out of the crib, it is not necessary to check alarm settings after the parents visit.

🗝 CN: Safety and infection control; CL: Apply

22. The vastus laleralis in the thickest part of the anterolateral thigh is a safe injection site for infants. The needle should be inserted at a 90-degree angle to the long axis of the femur.

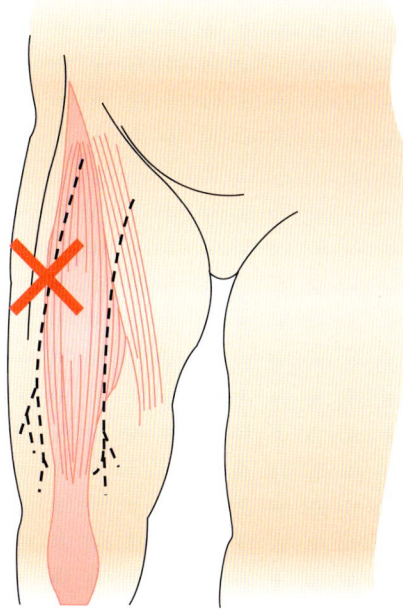

🗝 CN: Safety and infection control; CL: Apply

23. 4. It is important to dry the feet carefully after a bath to prevent a fungal infection. Clients with diabetes should seek medical attention when they injure their toes or feet to prevent complications. Iodine is highly toxic to the tissues. Clients with diabetes should inspect their feet daily and should wear shoes that support their feet while in the house.

🗝 CN: Reduction of risk potential; CL: Evaluate

24. 1. The parent should firmly yet gently strike the chest wall with the hand cupped to make a hollow popping sound. A slapping sound indicates that an incorrect technique is being used. The area over the rib cage is percussed to loosen mucus from the underlying lung passages. The child should wear a thin piece of clothing (T-shirt) over the chest area to protect the skin without diminishing the effect of the percussion.

🗝 CN: Reduction of risk potential; CL: Evaluate

25. 4. Isoniazid competes for the available vitamin B₆ in the body and leaves the client at risk for developing neuropathies related to vitamin deficiency. Supplemental vitamin B₆ is routinely prescribed to address this issue. Avoiding sun exposure is a preventive measure to lower the risk for skin cancer. Following a low-cholesterol diet lowers the individual's risk for developing atherosclerotic plaque. Rest is important in maintaining homeostasis but has no real impact on neuropathies.

🗝️ CN: Pharmacological and parenteral therapies; CL: Analyze

26. 4. Serum osmolality indicates the water balance of the body. A normal plasma osmolality between 275 and 295 mOsm/kg (mmol/kg) indicates that the fluid volume excess has been resolved. A weight reduction of 10% may not necessarily return the client to a state of normal serum osmolality. Clients with excess fluid volume do not necessarily have pain or abnormal arterial blood gas values.

🗝️ CN: Physiological adaptation; CL: Analyze

27. 4. Elbow restraints help keep the child from placing fingers or any other object in the mouth that would cause injury to the operative site. The restraints are worn at all times except when they are removed to check the skin. Because of the risk for skin breakdown, the restraints are removed periodically during the day to assess the child's underlying skin. It is advisable to remove only one restraint at a time while keeping hold of the child's hand on the unrestrained side. Toddlers are quick and usually want to explore the area in the mouth that the surgery has made feel different. The restraints should be in place at all times during sleep and play to prevent inadvertent injury to the operative site. Taping the restraints directly to the skin is not advised because skin breakdown can occur when tape is reapplied to the same area over several weeks. The restraints can be fastened to clothing to keep them from slipping.

🗝️ CN: Safety and infection control; CL: Evaluate

28. –/+ **2, 3, 5.** The nurse should use at least two sources of identification before administering medication to any client. The identification can include the medical record number and the client's date of birth. It is not necessary to check the client and dose for this drug with another nurse. It is also not safe to use the room number or bed number as a source of identification as clients' locations in the hospital are frequently changed. A parent may be used as an additional safety check with very young children because the nurse cannot assume that the child will give a correct first name.

🗝️ CN: Safety and infection control; CL: Apply

29. 1. Nurses should verify that clients having surgery discontinued the use of any blood thinners to prevent postoperative bleeding. Prior to bowel resection, the client should follow a high-residue diet with increased fluids. Abdominal-strengthening exercises are not necessary before this surgery. Clients may write a will before surgery, but the nurse does not have to inquire about it.

🗝️ CN: Reduction of risk potential; CL: Analyze

30. 2. One of the actions of propranolol, a drug used in the treatment of migraine headaches, is to inhibit arterial vasodilation. The nurse should assess the client's blood pressure to evaluate the overall circulatory response to the medication. Until the nurse determines the client's blood pressure, there is no immediate need to contact the HCP. There is no immediate need to administer oxygen. The client has not indicated pain; it is not necessary to administer the sumatriptan at this time.

🗝️ CN: Pharmacological and parenteral therapies; CL: Analyze

31. 1. The client may become tolerant of the antianginal effects of nitrates. Removing nitrates for 8 hours each day is usually effective in preventing tolerance. Nitrate patches should not be used on an as-needed basis. Sites should be rotated daily to prevent skin irritation, but this is not related to tolerance. Removing the patch for only 8 hours is sufficient to prevent tolerance, and skipping days could impact the drug's effectiveness.

🗝️ CN: Pharmacological and parenteral therapies; CL: Apply

32. 3. When an incision eviscerates, it is a medical emergency. The nurse's first response is to apply a sterile dressing that has been moistened with sterile normal saline solution. The client should also be placed in semi-Fowler position to release any tension on the abdominal area. Vital signs should be taken, and an IV line may be started for emergency treatment; however, the first action is to protect the wound and abdominal contents.

🗝️ CN: Reduction of risk potential; CL: Analyze

33. 3. Meningococcal infections are spread through close mucous membrane or respiratory contact with large respiratory droplets. Meningococcal infections are not spread by small airborne organisms or contact with a person's skin or contaminated items. Standard precautions, used when touching body fluids, are not sufficient to prevent the spread of meningitis.

🗝️ CN: Safety and infection control; CL: Apply

34.

STEP 1

0/1 **2, 4, 5.** The nurse most needs to follow up on the client's thought patterns, nutritional status, and sleep patterns. Belief in aliens indicates the client is experiencing delusions. Based on the client's history and refusal of food, it is unclear how long it has been since the client has eaten or drank. Sleep disturbances often precede psychosis. Apathy reflects a flattened versus heightened mood. The client has the right to refuse care. The client's work status is a low priority.

 CJ: Case study; Step 1: Recognize cues; CL: Analyze

35.

STEP 2

0/1

Findings	Positive Symptoms	Negative Symptoms	Neither Positive Nor Negative Symptoms
Not leaving apartment		X	
Disheveled appearance		X	
Believes in aliens	X		
Refusal of care		X	
Sleep disturbance			X
Marijuana use			X
Flat affect		X	

Delusions, such as believing in aliens, and hallucinations are classified as positive symptoms of schizophrenia. Medications can help control positive symptoms. Apathy, flat affect, social isolation, and loss of drive to perform self-care are negative symptoms of schizophrenia that may persist over time and present a major barrier to recovery. Although persons with schizophrenia have impaired sleep, this is not considered to be negative or positive symptoms. Rather it may be a factor that contributes to the development of psychosis.

 CJ: Case study; Step 2: Analyze cues; CL: Analyze

36.

STEP 3

0/1 The client is most likely experiencing **psychosis**. The priority intervention is to administer a(n) **antipsychotic**.

The client is demonstrating a disconnection from reality, which most suggests the diagnosis of psychosis. The primary treatment for psychosis is an antipsychotic medication. Although clients with schizophrenia may be prescribed benzodiazepines and mood stabilizers, these are not classified as antipsychotics. The client may at some point need a sedative prescription for sleep, but a sedative will not treat the underlying psychosis.

CJ: Case study; Step 3: Prioritize hypothesis; CL: Analyze

37.

STEP 4

0/1

Possible Outcome	Acute Psychotic Phase Outcomes	After Stabilization Outcomes
Not injure self or others	X	
Maintain daily routines for eating and sleeping		X
Establish contact with reality	X	
Interact with the nurse	X	
Participate in therapeutic interventions	X	
Express thoughts in an acceptable manner	X	
Demonstrate independence in self-care		X

Treatment during the acute psychotic phase is typically in an inpatient setting. Care focuses on stabilizing the client's thought process and maintaining safety. Appropriate outcomes include preventing injuries, establishing contact with reality, interacting with the nurse, expressing thoughts in an acceptable manner, and participating in the therapeutic regiment. Once the client has been stabilized, the focus of care shifts to helping the client learn to live independently. Maintaining daily routines and independence in self-care are appropriate outcomes after the client has been stabilized.

CJ: Case study; Step 4: Generate solutions; CL: Analyze

38.

STEP 5

−/+ **2, 3, 6.** Whispering to self, yelling out, and nodding the head suggest that client is responding to voices that they are hearing, or auditory hallucinations. Taping a shield to their door and believing the food is poisoned by aliens and that some staff are aliens indicate paranoia, or the feeling that one is being threatened. The client is also demonstrating hypervigilance by frequently stopping to look behind and around them.

Delusions of grandeur are false, fixed beliefs that are an inflated view of self. The client is delusional, but their delusions are persecutory, not grandiose. Tangentiality occurs when a topic of conversation is changed to an entirely different topic that detours from the original focus of the conversation. Catatonic excitement is hyperactivity characterized by purposeless and abnormal movements. Flight of ideas occurs when the topic of a conversation changes rapidly and repeatedly.

 CJ: Case study; Step 5: Take action; CL: Apply

39.

STEP 6

0/1 *The nurse determines that the client's behavior indicates that they are experiencing* **torticollis** *that was caused by* **the olanzapine**. *The nurse should call the health care provider to obtain an order for* **diphenhydramine**.

When a client experiences torticollis, the muscles of their neck pull their head to the side. The client is unable to move the neck. Catatonia is characterized by a trancelike state. The client's statements about not being able to move the head indicate the client is still communicating and not in a catatonic state. If the client were experiencing a tactile hallucination, they would still be able to move their head. Torticollis is a dystonic reaction that is caused by antipsychotic drugs such as olanzapine, not increased anxiety or psychosis. One treatment for torticollis is diphenhydramine 25 to 50 mg given intramuscularly or intravenously. Torticollis may also be treated with anticholinergic medications. Haloperidol is an antipsychotic, which could worsen symptoms. Lorazepam is a benzodiazepine used to treat seizures, anxiety, or sleep disorders.

 CJ: Case study; Step 6: Evaluate outcomes; CL: Evaluate

40. **4.** The nurse should contact the pharmacy and report the error and check the discrepancy with the actual prescription. The nurse must be vigilant when comparing medication in the medication box with the prescription; prednisolone, for example, is three to five times more potent than prednisone. The nurse cannot make a pharmacy substitution change without prescriptive authority. The prednisolone is not returned until a clarification prescription is obtained to determine the substitution drug and dosage are correct. It is not necessary to contact the charge nurse or supervisor as the nurse must first clarify the prescription with the HCP. The nurse reports the incident according to agency policy and notifies all involved of the change in the prescription.

 CN: Pharmacological and parenteral therapies; CL: Analyze

41. **1.** The nurse should instruct the mother to bring the child to the emergency department. If aspirated, nuts may swell, leading to an airway obstruction after the initial event; endoscopy may be required to remove remaining fragments. Bleeding from trauma to internal organs after abdominal thrusts is rare. There are no signs of shock to suggest anaphylaxis. There is no indication of the presence of a pneumothorax.

 CN: Physiological adaptation; CL: Analyze

42. **0/1** **2.** The neonate's Apgar score has been improving since birth. (The birth score is 6; the current score is 9.) The nurse should continue to assess the neonate. There is no indication that oxygen is needed since the color is improving, and stimulating the baby is not necessary as the baby is now flexing the extremities.

 CJ: Standalone trend; CL: Analyze

43. **–/+** **3, 4.** In accordance with ethical principles and the nurse's role to serve as an advocate for clients and protect their safety, the nurse must report the colleague's suspicious behaviors to the supervisor. It would also be appropriate to follow up with the colleague to address continued client reports of lack of pain relief. Deciding to avoid getting involved places the nurse's license at risk. Nurses are also responsible for reporting concerning behaviors of a nurse colleague.

 CN: Management of care; CL: Evaluate

44. **1.** Adequate circulatory status is the most important factor in the healing process of an infected decubitus ulcer. Blood flow to the area must be present to bring nutrients and prescribed antibiotics to the tissues. Rest and a balanced diet are essential to health maintenance but are not the priority for healing an infected decubitus ulcer. A fluid intake of 2000 to 3000 mL a day, if not contraindicated, is recommended to provide hydration to the client's tissues.

 CN: Reduction of risk potential; CL: Analyze

45. **4.** Soft, washable toys are appropriate for infants, who tend to place everything in their mouths. These toys are not harmful. Plastic toys cannot be manipulated by a child of this age, and the child would put the car in the mouth, which may not be safe due to small parts that may be swallowed or aspirated. Games and puzzles are too advanced for a 5-month-old, and the child could put the pieces in the mouth and swallow them. Some stuffed animals have eyes that can be swallowed or aspirated.

 CN: Reduction of risk potential; CL: Apply

46. **3.** The nurse should give the next dose as prescribed because the blood level is 35 mcg/mL, which is lower than the normal range of 50 to 100 mcg/mL. Withholding the next dose, notifying the HCP, and taking the client's vital signs are not indicated in this situation.

 CN: Pharmacological and parenteral therapies; CL: Analyze

47. 4. The client is not emptying their bladder after repeated attempts. The nurse should now use an in-and-out catheter to empty the bladder. While the other comfort measures may be helpful, this client has not completely emptied their bladder since birth and will be at risk for a urinary tract infection and postpartum hemorrhage.

CN: Management of care; CL: Analyze

48. 1. The best way to ease symptoms caused by hyperventilation is to have the client breathe into a paper bag. This helps raise the carbon dioxide level, which encourages deeper, slower breathing. The symptoms of hyperventilation will not be alleviated by having the client put the head between the knees, giving the client low concentrations of oxygen, or having the client take deep, slow breaths and exhaling normally.

CN: Basic care and comfort; CL: Analyze

49. 1. Because the femoral artery is usually used as the access site during cardiac catheterization, children are required to remain on bed rest (with the head only slightly elevated) for several hours after the procedure to avoid arterial bleeding at the site. A knee-chest position is the correct position for an infant during a cyanotic episode as it will create peripheral resistance to the extremities, shunting blood to the heart. The apical heart rate is assessed prior to administering this medication; administration can be performed by an experienced LPN/VN, although medication is checked with the RN prior to administration. Because echocardiography is noninvasive, there is no need to withhold meals before this procedure.

CN: Management of care; CL: Analyze

50. 2. After surgery, the most important nursing goal is to prevent infection. Surgery involves an incision, which places the infant at risk for infection. The infant with this type of procedure does have discomfort, which can be relieved with acetaminophen, and managing pain is important but not the priority. The infant may be in arm restraints or have the cuff of the sleeve pinned to the diaper or pants. It is important that the infant not touch the incision line or disrupt the sutures, but the infant is not at risk for problems related to immobility. There is no indication that the parents need to improve their skills, but the nurse can support the family as they would be reacting normally with a first reaction of shock.

CN: Reduction of risk potential; CL: Analyze

51. 2. Hepatitis B virus is spread through contact with blood, body fluids contaminated with blood, and such body fluids as cerebrospinal, pleural, peritoneal, and synovial fluids; semen; and vaginal secretions. The risk for transmission of hepatitis B through feces is low. Touching the client without gloves is acceptable when there is no danger of contact with blood or body fluids. Recapping a used needle is a common source of needlestick injuries; needles should be properly disposed of uncapped.

CN: Safety and infection control; CL: Apply

52. 2. Signs of child abuse include injury with a history that is inconsistent with the nature of the injury or unusual injuries for the age of the child. A spiral fracture of a child is always investigated as potential child abuse as this injury is often caused by twisting of an extremity. It is not unusual for a child who is learning to walk to have bruises. Wearing the same clothes is not an indication of abuse or neglect. The child with conjunctivitis requires health care, but having frequent episodes is not an indication of abuse or neglect.

CN: Reduction of risk potential; CL: Analyze

53. 3. In most agencies, it is a policy to discard the autologous blood after 4 hours of transfusing, due to an increased risk for infection. Increasing the infusion rate could cause fluid overload. Monitoring blood transfusions is a serious nursing responsibility, and because it is the change of shift, there is increased risk for error.

CN: Pharmacological and parenteral therapies; CL: Analyze

54. 3. After a nephrectomy, a specific aspect of immediate postoperative management includes monitoring urine output at least hourly. Monitoring blood pressure and encouraging the use of incentive spirometry are other important considerations, but because of the surgical disruption of the urinary system, urine output is a priority. Measurement of urine output should also include an estimation of the amount of urine drainage on the flank dressing.

CN: Physiological adaptation; CL: Analyze

55. 2. The nurse's initial response should be to withhold the digoxin. The nurse should then notify the HCP if the apical pulse is 60 bpm or lower because of the risk for digoxin toxicity. The charge nurse does not need to be notified, but the nurse needs to document the notification and follow-up in the medical record.

CN: Pharmacological and parenteral therapies; CL: Analyze

56. 4. Dystonic adverse effects of haloperidol, especially oculogyric crises, are painful and frightening. Intramuscular (IM) benztropine is the fastest and most effective drug for managing dystonia. Lorazepam is an antianxiety medication and is not effective for the treatment of dystonia. Although amantadine and diphenhydramine can be used for extrapyramidal symptoms, oral medications do not work as quickly, and amantadine may worsen psychotic symptoms.

CN: Pharmacological and parenteral therapies; CL: Analyze

57. 1. Neonates burn brown adipose tissue (fat) as a response to cold stress. In addition, there is increased utilization of glycogen and calorie stores. Hypoglycemia may result from becoming stressed by a cold environment. Neonates do not have the ability to shiver.

CN: Health promotion and maintenance; CL: Apply

58. 1. Formula should fill the entire nipple of the bottle while the baby is sucking. This decreases the amount of air taken in by the baby; taking in too much air can lead to regurgitation. Not all babies at term are born with well-developed sucking skills. Some neonates are sleepy and do not suck well. For the first feeding, the baby should be bubbled after taking one-fourth to one-half ounce of formula and then again when the infant has finished the feeding. Bottle propping can lead to aspiration, decreased infant bonding, and aspiration of formula. However, it is not associated with the intake of too much air.

CN: Health promotion and maintenance; CL: Analyze

59. -/+ 1, 3, 4, 5. When a client begins to have back pain with the administration of blood, the nurse should suspect a hemolytic reaction, and the blood transfusion should be stopped immediately. Any remaining blood and the tubing should be sent to the lab. The nurse should prepare for a reaction from mild to severe, including the need for cardiopulmonary resuscitation, because even a small amount of mismatched blood can lead to a major reaction. The nurse should obtain a urine specimen to send to the laboratory to check for hemoglobin because RBC hemolysis filters through the kidneys from the reaction. The nurse should stop the IV line with the Y-tubing for the blood and not flush the line with saline so that the client does not receive any more blood. The tubing should be changed so that a tube without blood can be used for infusions.

CN: Pharmacological and parenteral therapies; CL: Analyze

60. 2. At 4 hours postpartum, the fundus should be midline and at the level of the umbilicus. Whenever the placenta is manually removed after birth, there is a possibility that all of the placenta has not been removed. Sometimes, small pieces of the placenta are retained, a common cause of late postpartum hemorrhage. The client is exhibiting signs and symptoms associated with retained placental fragments. The client will continue to bleed until the fragments are expelled. Perineal and cervical lacerations are characterized by bright red bleeding and a firmly contracted fundus at the level that is expected. Urine retention is characterized by a full bladder, which can be observed by a bulge or fullness just above the symphysis pubis. Also, the client's fundus would be deviated to one side and boggy to the touch.

CN: Reduction of risk potential; CL: Analyze

61. -/+ 1, 3, 4. Clear communication is crucial for a client with delirium. The family must include the client in all conversations and keep them oriented to time and place. It is inappropriate to argue with a client's hallucinations because they are real to the client. Speaking more loudly will not help this client hear more distinctly and may increase the client's confusion.

CN: Management of care; CL: Analyze

62. 2. One-to-one supervision provides safety until appropriate detoxification can be given. Restraints are the last intervention after less restrictive alternatives have been tried. It is unlikely that the client can cooperate with staying in a chair. Putting the client in bed in their room puts the client at risk for falling, and a closed door prevents close observation.

CN: Safety and infection control; CL: Analyze

63. 2. Insensible fluid loss is invisible vaporization from the lungs and skin and assists in regulating body temperature. The amount of water loss is increased by accelerated body metabolism, which occurs with increased body temperature. The client's body mass index does not directly influence calculating fluid therapy.

CN: Pharmacological and parenteral therapies; CL: Analyze

64. -/+ 1, 2, 3. Clinical manifestations of dehydration include decreased tearing; dry mucous membranes; sunken fontanelles; weight loss; behavioral changes; scanty, concentrated urine; and a thready, fast pulse. Clear, pale yellow urine would indicate adequate hydration. A bounding pulse would indicate fluid volume excess.

CN: Physiological adaptation; CL: Analyze

65. 1. Patient-centered care involves honoring client preferences. It is common practice to baptize infants who are at risk for death in the Roman Catholic faith. While a 30-week gestation infant on minimal ventilator settings would be expected to survive, the family has had real experiences with neonatal death, and spiritual practices can provide comfort. The nurse should ask the family about their preferences and try to honor them. The family may indeed be requesting the baptism because they are fearful their infant might die. The nurse can reassure the family that the infant is doing well but must also respect the client's spiritual preferences. After the family shares their preferences, the nurse can offer the local chaplain as a resource.

🔑 CN: Psychosocial integrity; CL: Apply

66. 1. The best nursing intervention is giving the client finger foods high in protein and calories that they can eat while they pace or walk. Informing the client that snacks are available if they eat properly at mealtime is inappropriate because the client is too busy and distracted to sit and eat an entire meal. Telling the client to sit alone at mealtime to decrease distractions will not help because the client is in a manic state, is easily distracted, and needs to move. Teaching the client about proper nutrition ignores the need for adequate intake. The client would be unable to focus on the nurse's teaching.

🔑 CN: Basic care and comfort; CL: Analyze

67. 1. Moist heat is a nonpharmacologic pain management strategy that may alleviate pain and reduce the dose of analgesic medication, if required. Heat dilates blood vessels and decreases inflammation. Lifting and circular exercises will aggravate the already inflamed joint. Cold constricts blood vessels.

🔑 CN: Basic care and comfort; CL: Evaluate

68. 3. For an LP, a needle is inserted into the subarachnoid space to obtain a specimen of spinal fluid for diagnostic testing. Fluid on the lumbar dressing indicates cerebrospinal fluid (CSF) leakage and must be reported to the HCP immediately. The client should be encouraged to drink fluids after an LP to facilitate production of CSF. It is normal to have a mild headache because of the removal of CSF samples for laboratory analysis. Although the concerns of the client should be discussed with the HCP at some point, the CSF leakage is a priority and should be reported immediately.

🔑 CN: Reduction of risk potential; CL: Analyze

69. 3. The normal calcium level is 9.0 to 10.5 mg/dL (2.25 to 2.63 mmol/L). Hypercalcemia is commonly seen with malignant disease and metastases. The other laboratory values are normal. Hypercalcemia can be treated with fluids, furosemide, or the administration of calcitonin. Failure to treat hypercalcemia can cause muscle weakness, changes in level of consciousness, nausea, vomiting, abdominal pain, and dehydration. Although the client is on hospice care, they will still need palliative treatment. Comfort and risk reduction are components of hospice care.

🔑 CN: Reduction of risk potential; CL: Analyze

70.

STEP 1

> **Nurse's Notes**
>
> **Today: 0900**
> A 75-year-old client was brought to the emergency department by their spouse who reports the client is experiencing sudden-onset drowsiness. The client has had a urinary tract infection treated with oral cephalexin for the past 5 days. The client's pupils are equal, round, and respond to light, and the client is oriented to time and place.
> Admission vital signs are temperature (T) 101.8°F (38.8°C); pulse (P) 92 bpm; respiration rate (RR) 28 breaths/min; and blood pressure (BP) 88/40 mm Hg. Oxygen saturation per pulse oximeter is 95%.

The nurse should recognize that the client's age, present history of a urinary tract infection, and drowsiness are not normal. The client has a fever, an elevated heart rate, and an elevated respiratory rate, and the client's blood pressure indicates hypotension. The focused neurologic assessment is within normal limits. The oxygen saturation is within the normal range of 95% to 100%.

🔑 CJ: Case study; Step 1: Recognize cues; CL: Analyze

71.

STEP 2

Client Findings	Urinary Tract Infection	Septic Shock
T 101.8°F (38.8°C)	X	X
RR 28 breaths/min		X
BP 98/40 mm Hg		X
P 94 bpm		X
Oxygen saturation 91%		

Note: Each column must have at least one response option selected.

Clients with a urinary tract infection have an elevated temperature, but blood pressure, heart rate, respiration rate, and oxygen saturation remain in normal ranges. Older adults with an infection are at high risk for sepsis, which can progress quickly to septic shock. The nurse should analyze cues that indicate the client's condition is changing. Clients with septic shock have an elevated temperature due to infection, a respiratory rate above 22 breaths/min; a heart rate greater than 90 bpm, and a blood pressure less than 90/40 mm Hg.

  CJ: Case study; Step 2: Analyze cues; CL: Analyze

72.

STEP 3

R *The client is at risk for developing* **septic shock** *as evidenced by the client's* **vital signs**.

The client is at risk for developing septic shock as indicated by the change in vital signs from 0900 to 0930 (drop in blood pressure, increased heart rate, and increased respiratory rate). Although the oxygen saturation per pulse oximeter has dropped to 91%, hypoxemia is diagnosed at 90% and lower when using a pulse oximeter. The changes in neurologic status (confusion and ability to follow commands) are not indicative of stroke but are consistent with the other findings related to septic shock. The urinary output is within normal limits at this time and does not indicate renal failure.

  CJ: Case study; Step 3: Prioritize hypothesis; CL: Analyze

73.

STEP 4

−/+ **1, 2, 4, 6, 7**. The nurse should plan to implement the nursing care plan and health care provider's orders. The nurse should start a peripheral IV to administer fluids and medications and establish an arterial line to monitor blood pressure and obtain arterial blood gas samples. The nurse should also initiate continuous monitoring of cardiac rhythm. The nurse should insert an indwelling urinary catheter to monitor urinary output more accurately; a urinary output of 30 to 50 mL per hour is a sign of progressing shock and potential renal failure. The order for oxygen at 2 L per minute per nasal catheter is correct because the client's oxygen saturation on the pulse oximeter has dropped, and when the arterial line is established, the nurse can obtain a more accurate assessment of arterial oxygen levels. The nurse should also explain the plan of care to the client and spouse.

  CJ: Case study; Step 4: Generate solutions; CL: Analyze

74.

STEP 5

−/+

Orders

- Start oxygen at 2 L per minute per nasal cannula
- 5% dextrose in normal saline (D5NS) 1000 mL every 8 hours
- Vancomycin 500 mg intravenously (IV) every 6 hours
- Norepinephrine 0.01 to 3.3 mcg/kg per minute IV infusion
- Insert an indwelling urinary catheter
- Urine culture and sensitivity stat
- Arterial blood gas (ABG) stat
- Blood urea nitrogen (BUN) and creatinine

The nurse should first administer the norepinephrine because the client's blood pressure is dropping. Next, the nurse should administer the oxygen because the client's oxygen level has dropped. Then, the nurse should administer vancomycin, a broad-spectrum antibiotic, to manage the urinary tract infection. Managing the urinary tract infection is a priority, and the health care provider has ordered a high-dose, broad-spectrum antibiotic given intravenously to manage the infection until the results of the urine culture and sensitivity can be obtained.

  CJ: Case study; Step 5: Take action; CL: Analyze

75.

STEP 6

−/+ **1, 2, 3, 4, 5, 7**. Norepinephrine is a vasopressor and will cause the systolic and diastolic blood pressure to increase because of the constriction of blood vessels, and it will increase the heart rate and the respiration rate. The urinary output will increase as a result of improved renal perfusion. The client's urinary output is within normal range per output that has been measured by the urine from the indwelling catheter. The client's oxygen saturation has improved because of pulmonary vasoconstriction. The drug does not alter the client's temperature.

  CJ: Case study; Step 6: Evaluate outcomes; CL: Evaluate

76. 2. The nurse would document these findings as "early" decelerations. Early decelerations are thought to be the result of vagal nerve stimulation caused by compression of the fetal head during labor. They are considered normal physiologic responses to labor and do not require any intervention. Early decelerations do not require position change or oxygen as they are not a sign of fetal distress. Variable decelerations are thought to be due to umbilical cord compression. Early decelerations are not an emergency and do not require immediate reporting to the HCP or preparing for cesarean birth.

  CN: Management of care; CL: Analyze

77. 2, 3, 1, 4. An open airway is essential to survival. The nurse should first ensure an open airway. Next, the nurse should start an IV and then notify the HCP. Finally, the nurse should inform the family of the situation and, if appropriate, allow them to remain with the client.

  CN: Management of care; CL: Create

78. 3, 4, 1, 2. The client is experiencing a septic reaction to the blood transfusion. The nurse's first action is to stop the infusion and notify the health care provider and blood bank. The nurse then uses an infusion of normal saline to keep the vein open. Next, the nurse obtains a sample of the client's blood for a blood culture, and last, the nurse sends the blood bag and the administration set to the blood bank for culture.

🔑 CN: Pharmacological and parenteral therapies; CL: Create

79. −/+ **1, 3, 4, 5.** The nurse is responsible for the client's safety in the operating room. The nurse should call a time-out if the client is not properly identified with an identification band. In addition, an IV line and oxygen should always be established when an ET tube is placed. This practice applies whenever a client's airway is compromised enough for intubation to occur, not only in the operating room environment. An anesthetist or anesthesiologist should be present during surgery to manage the airway. Postoperative pain medication is administered in the recovery room.

🔑 CN: Safety and infection control; CL: Analyze

80. 1. Anencephaly is a neural tube defect that is not compatible with life, though some infants with anencephaly live for several days before death occurs. When the client has decided to continue the pregnancy and donate the neonatal organs after the death of the neonate, the nurse should remain nonjudgmental. The nurse should explore their feelings about the issue of anencephaly and organ donation. The nurse should not make judgments about the client's position, nor should the nurse try to persuade the client to terminate the pregnancy. Contacting the client's clergy to explore the client's options is not appropriate. The client may have already discussed the matter with their minister. Telling the client that the neonate's death will be prolonged and painful is not helpful. Death may occur very soon after birth. Contacting the client's family members is not appropriate. The client may wish not to discuss the matter with their family.

🔑 CN: Management of care; CL: Analyze

81. 1. The nurse should first ensure the safety of the severely anxious client in a safe, quiet, environment. The nurse should not leave the client alone. Asking the client "why" is not therapeutic. Buspirone is a maintenance medication that will not help relieve anxiety immediately.

🔑 CN: Management of care; CL: Analyze

82. 4. Due to the client's psychosis and difficulty coping, a positive, supportive environment is essential to limit further regression and help the client engage in their own treatment. Confrontation and peer pressure are the type of milieu more suited to a chemically dependent client. While involvement in self-governance can be therapeutic, forcing a psychotic client to participate in self-governance before they are ready could actually hinder treatment and recovery. Although group activities are commonly required in treatment programs, a client who is very disturbed or confused is not forced to attend. Also, the client must participate when and how the client feels comfortable, rather than mandating a specific amount of participation. Equal participation by clients does not ensure a therapeutic milieu or speed the client's recovery.

🔑 CN: Psychosocial integrity; CL: Analyze

83. 1. Pulmonary embolism is a potentially life-threatening complication of deep vein thrombosis. The client's change in mental status, tachypnea, and tachycardia indicate a possible pulmonary embolism. The nurse should promptly call the rapid response team. Administering a sedative without further evaluation of the client's condition is not appropriate. There is no need to elicit a positive Homans sign; the client is already diagnosed with deep vein thrombosis. Increasing the IV flow rate may be an appropriate action but not without first notifying the health care provider.

🔑 CN: Reduction of risk potential; CL: Analyze

84. 4. The nurse should refuse to administer the medication to the client because of the risk for respiratory depression in the neonate. Morphine, given IM, peaks in 30 to 60 minutes and lasts 4 hours. Based on the assessment findings, the client most likely will be giving birth within that time frame, increasing the risk for respiratory depression in the neonate, a serious consequence. Therefore, the nurse should not administer the drug. Naloxone should be readily available whenever opioids that can result in respiratory depression are used. Asking the HCP to validate the dosage is not necessary.

🔑 CN: Management of care; CL: Analyze

85. 2. Bending the chin down toward the chest decreases the risk for food entering the trachea and causing aspiration into the lungs. The client should sit up at a 90-degree angle when eating. Eating and talking increase the risk for aspiration as well as muscle fatigue; the nurse should encourage the client to avoid talking while chewing and swallowing. The client should rest before eating because muscle fatigue can contribute to choking.

🔑 CN: Reduction of risk potential; CL: Analyze

86. 1. The client with a spinal cord injury above T6 who suddenly experiences clinical manifestations of autonomic stimulation, such as flushing, sweating, and piloerection, is demonstrating life-threatening autonomic dysreflexia. The cluster of manifestation results from noxious stimuli, such as a full bladder, or lying on a foreign object, such as a plastic cap or crinkled paper, which the client cannot feel. As soon as the noxious stimulus is removed, the manifestations begin to subside. When the client demonstrates clinical manifestations of autonomic dysreflexia, the nurse should first elevate the head of the bed immediately to decrease the intracerebral pressure caused by the hypertension that developed from autonomic stimulation. The nurse can next check for a distended bladder or foreign object. The client's blood pressure will be elevated; the nurse should assess vital signs frequently.

🗝️ CN: Management of care; CL: Analyze

87. **3.** The nurse should refer the client to a social worker to help them enroll in a food assistance program, which provides foods such as milk, cereal, and infant formula. Instructing the client in low-cost, highly nutritious meal preparation will not meet the client's need for additional funds for food. Determining whether the client qualifies for state assistance is part of the role of the social worker, not the nurse. Asking the client if they have a job and the amount of income earned is not within the role of the nurse. The social worker can determine whether the family income guidelines are met for state and federal assistance.

🗝️ CN: Management of care; CL: Analyze

88.

Action to Take	Potential Conditions	Parameters to Monitor
Establish structure for meals, activity, screen time, and sleep	Obesity	Physical activity patterns
Involve the entire family in the eating plan		Sugary beverage intake

0/1

Children with a BMI for age at the 95th percentile and above are considered obese. Hypertension is not diagnosed until the BP reaches the 95th percentile compared with children who are the same sex, age, and height. The lab findings are within normal limits, suggesting the child does not have prediabetes and metabolic syndrome. The nurse should teach the parents to establish healthy structures related to family meals, physical activity, and sleep to help slow the child's weight gain as they grow. The nurse should also teach the parents to involve the entire family in the eating plan so that the child does not feel singled out. Children should be encouraged to be physically active for 60 minutes per day, but the nurse should focus on free play, helping the child find activities they enjoy versus promoting structured exercise. Dietary guidance should focus on healthy eating patterns versus calorie or macronutrient counts. The nurse should monitor the child's physical activity and sugary beverage intake. Once-weekly or even monthly weigh-ins are better measures for long-term weight control progress than daily weights as weight can fluctuate slightly from day to day. Blood pressure monitoring is not needed.

🗝️ CJ: Standalone bowtie; CL: Create

89. **4.** Telling the client about one activity at a time with 10 minutes' notice gives the client time to prepare for that activity. Writing out the schedule does not ensure that the client will remember to look at it. It is overwhelming to explain an entire day's schedule all at once to a client diagnosed with dementia. Leading a client to an activity after the fact does not allow the client to prepare.

🗝️ CN: Psychosocial integrity; CL: Analyze

90. **2.** The primiparous client at 2 hours postpartum who gave birth to a term neonate vaginally should be assessed first because this client is at risk for postpartum hemorrhage. Early postpartum hemorrhage typically occurs during the first 24 hours postpartum. Once the nurse has assessed the client's fundus, lochia, and vital signs, a determination about the stability of the client can be made. After this assessment, the nurse can provide care to the other clients, who are of lesser priority than the primiparous client who recently gave birth.

🗝️ CN: Management of care; CL: Analyze

91. **2.** The child's signs and symptoms in conjunction with the acute onset suggest possible croup or epiglottitis. The priority diagnosis at this time is airway obstruction. The airway may become completely occluded by the epiglottis at any time. Although the child has an infection and the client has respiratory distress, the immediate priority is to establish and maintain a patent airway. No evidence is provided to support the potential for aspiration.

🗝️ CN: Reduction of risk potential; CL: Analyze

92. **3.** The baseline laboratory data that are established before a client is started on tissue plasminogen activator or alteplase recombinant include hematocrit, hemoglobin level, and platelet count. The potassium level, Lee-White clotting time, and blood glucose levels do not affect the use of these drugs.

🗝️ CN: Reduction of risk potential; CL: Apply

93. -/+ **2, 3.** The client should be instructed not to eat or drink for 8 to 12 hours before the test. Stools will be white for up to 72 hours following the procedure as the barium is eliminated from the body. Laxatives and fluids will be encouraged after the procedure to help prevent barium impaction, but the client will not be given stool softeners or laxatives before the procedure. The client should not experience pain during the procedure. The nurse should also instruct the client to stop smoking at midnight the night before the test.

🗝️ CN: Reduction of risk potential; CL: Apply

94. 3. This rhythm is atrial fibrillation. It is characterized by an irregular QRS interval, no definite P waves before the QRS waves, and a ventricular rate greater than 100 bpm.

🗝️ CN: Reduction of risk potential; CL: Analyze

95. 3. The vastus lateralis site is the preferred IM site for all ages because it does not have any major nerves or blood vessels located near it. The deltoid and dorsogluteal muscles have major nerves and blood vessels located nearby. The triceps is not an acceptable muscle for IM injections because it is not well developed in most clients.

🗝️ CN: Pharmacological and parenteral therapies; CL: Apply

96. 1. Clients should be instructed to rinse their mouths after using a steroid inhaler to avoid developing thrush. Clients should also be instructed to inhale slowly through the mouth and then hold the breath as they count to 10 slowly. It is not necessary for the client to cough and deep-breathe before using the inhaler.

🗝️ CN: Pharmacological and parenteral therapies; CL: Analyze

97. 2. The symptoms of difficulty breathing, elevated blood pressure, and cough are indicative of circulatory overload. Circulatory overload occurs when blood is infused more rapidly than the circulatory system can accommodate. Anaphylactic reactions are manifested by urticaria, wheezing, and shock. Sepsis begins with a rapid onset of chills and fever. An acute hemolytic reaction is typically manifested by chills, fever, low back pain, and flushing.

🗝️ CN: Pharmacological and parenteral therapies; CL: Analyze

98.

0/1	Action to Take	Potential Conditions	Parameters to Monitor
	Give an intravenous fluid bolus	Ruptured spleen	Urine output
	Prep for surgery		Levels of onsciousness

Pain over the left upper abdomen, left-sided rib pain, and referred pain are signs of a ruptured spleen, a common complication associated with the Epstein-Barr virus. Liver inflammation and acute appendicitis are most often associated with right-sided abdominal pain. Reye syndrome, associated with aspirin use during viral infections, manifests as swelling of the liver and brain. The client is displaying signs and symptoms of shock, including low blood pressure, elevated heart rate, elevated respirations, diaphoresis, light-headedness, and cool skin. The care priorities are to restore fluid volume and stop the bleeding. This is accomplished through administering intravenous fluids and performing an emergency splenectomy. The need for antibiotics and gastric decompression can be determined during or after surgery. Corticosteroids would be indicated if the client had Reye syndrome. The nurse needs to closely monitor the client's perfusion to prevent complications of shock. Monitoring levels of consciousness helps determine the adequacy of cerebral perfusion. Monitoring urine output helps determine if there is adequate renal perfusion. Liver function tests would be needed if the client had liver inflammation or Reye syndrome. Monitoring gastric output may be necessary after surgery but is more likely to be needed in a client with appendicitis.

🗝️ CJ: Standalone bowtie; CL: Create

99. 2. Sucralfate should be taken on an empty stomach 1 hour before or 2 hours after meals and at bedtime. It is usually taken four times a day. There is no need to avoid milk products while taking the drug. Sucralfate does not affect hemoglobin levels.

🗝️ CN: Pharmacological and parenteral therapies; CL: Evaluate

100. -/+ **1, 3, 4.** When assessing client safety, the nurse assesses suicide thoughts or plans, recent use of illicit drugs (as they may cause impaired judgment or thought processes), and previously experienced allergic reactions and adverse reactions to medications. Note that safety involves many aspects of care. Incentives and diet preferences (allergies would be previously noted) are not directly related to safety, though they may be part of an overall assessment.

🗝️ CN: Reduction of risk potential; CL: Analyze

101. -/+ **1, 2, 3, 4.** The client with conjunctivitis can use warm soaks to remove crusting. The nurse should teach the client to dispose of the soaks by wrapping them in a separate bag to avoid spreading bacteria. Topical antibiotics are used to treat the infection. The client should avoid contaminating the tip of the medication dispenser. Bacterial conjunctivitis requires containing the spread of the infection. The client should avoid touching their eyes. If the client does touch their eyes, the client should wash their hands after touching their eyes. The client does not need to be isolated.

🔑 CN: Reduction of risk potential; CL: Create

102. 2, 5. Two sources of identification must be confirmed before administering medication to a client. A source of information can be the client's record number, name, or date of birth, as noted on the client's armband. A client may be confused or hard of hearing and may give a wrong name or answer to a wrong name; thus, having the client state their name or respond to their name is not safe practice. Client recognition is not sufficient identification for administering medication. Clients change rooms frequently, so a room number is not a source of identification for administering medication.

🔑 CN: Pharmacological and parenteral therapies; CL: Apply

103. 2, 3. A National Patient Safety Goal of the Joint Commission is to improve the effectiveness of communication among caregivers. The requirement for verbal or telephone prescriptions, or for telephonic reporting of critical test results, is to verify the complete prescription or test result by having the person receiving the information record and "read back" the complete prescription or test result. Effective communication that is timely, accurate, complete, unambiguous, and understood by the recipient reduces error and results in improved client safety. "Read-back" procedures are not intended to discourage or prohibit telephone communications among health care providers (HCPs) or to promote the use of electronic medical records. Safety procedures, such as provider identification codes, are in place for HCPs to give verbal or telephone prescriptions.

🔑 CN: Management of care; CL: Apply

104. 3. The actual desired weight gain of 1 lb (0.5 kg) per week is the most measurable goal for the client. Attending all eating disorder support groups is a goal, but it is not as important as actual weight gain. The client can eat a larger meal at breakfast and then not eat sufficient food and overexercise for the remainder of the day. The client's improved self-image is important, but actual weight gain is the priority.

🔑 CN: Physiological adaptation; CL: Analyze

105. 1. The nurse should first plan to relieve the nausea and vomiting; if these continue, the client is at risk for dehydration and electrolyte imbalance. The client's poor appetite is likely related to the underlying health problem and is not the priority; the nausea may adversely affect the appetite, and relieving the nausea may allow the client an opportunity to eat and drink. The client has jaundice but does not have uncomfortable symptoms such as pruritus. The abdominal spasms may be related to nausea and vomiting and can be assessed again when the nausea and vomiting have stopped.

🔑 CN: Reduction of risk potential; CL: Analyze

106. 1. All clients who are at risk for pressure ulcer development should be identified on admission to health care facilities so that preventive actions can be implemented by the nursing staff. These preventive actions need to be individualized to the client, so automatic placement of all at-risk clients on an every-2-hour turning schedule, a specialty bed, or a high-protein, high-carbohydrate diet is not appropriate.

🔑 CN: Reduction of risk potential; CL: Apply

107. 4. With a severe gonorrheal infection, scarring of the fallopian tubes may occur, and becoming pregnant may be difficult or impossible. If the client's partner is not treated, the client can be reinfected. There is no immunity against gonorrhea, and, if exposed again, the client can again become infected. Although a condom may provide some protection against contracting gonorrhea, it is not adequate protection against the condition and will not help clear up an existing infection. It is only with proper antibiotic administration that the condition can be eradicated.

🔑 CN: Safety and infection control; CL: Evaluate

108.

Possible Actions	Potential Conditions	Parameters to Monitor
Increase IV fluids	Hypovolemic shock	Intake and output
Start oxygen per nasal catheter		Oxygenation levels

The client is experiencing hypovolemic shock from loss of blood and entering the progressive stage of shock. The client's vital signs indicate a drop in blood pressure and increased heart rate, increased respiratory rate, and a drop in oxygen saturation on room air per pulse oximetry. Tachycardia is evident, but this is consistent with hypovolemic shock and is not the primary problem. The client is likely anxious and is in pain but these factors do not immediately threaten the client's safety; after the client is stabilized, the nurse can calm the client, sedate as necessary, and offer pain medication. The client is at risk for wound infection, and once the client is stabilized, the health care provider (HCP) may prescribe an antibiotic, but this potential problem is not acutely time-dependent. In collaboration with the HCP, the nurse should first increase the rate of IV fluids and, as ordered, infuse a crystalloid solution to offset hypovolemia and the associated lack of tissue perfusion. The nurse can next start oxygen per nasal catheter as ordered with the goal of promoting perfusion. The HCP may also prescribe a vasopressor to increase the blood pressure to improve tissue perfusion. It is important to closely monitor intake and output to gauge the progression of hypovolemic shock.

 CJ: Standalone bowtie; CL: Create

109. **1.** Powder should not be applied to the skin beneath the cast because powder can cause irritation and skin breakdown. The parent would need further teaching about avoiding this measure. Checking the smoothness of the cast edges, covering the cast around the perineum, and inspecting inside the cast are all appropriate actions for the child with a spica cast to help prevent skin breakdown.

 CN: Basic care and comfort; CL: Evaluate

110. **1, 2, 3, 4.** The goal of "medication reconciliation" is to ensure that clients are on the right medication after any transfer, admission, or discharge. It is not necessary to reconcile the medications if the client moves to a different room on the same floor. It is estimated that more than half of medication errors occur during these transitions, and medication reconciliation can reduce errors by 70% or more. The Joint Commission requirements mandate medication reconciliation programs.

 CN: Pharmacological and parenteral therapies; CL: Apply

111. **2, 4, 5.** To meet the criteria for discharge from same-day surgery, the postoperative client must be able to take fluids by mouth, walk without hypotension, void, and be escorted by a responsible adult who will drive the client home. Transportation home via a taxicab is not a sufficient escort to assist a client home after surgery. The client may be discharged with severe pain as long as the client can ambulate safely. The nurse should make sure the client has a prescription for pain medication.

 CN: Reduction of risk potential; CL: Evaluate

112. **1.** Eyedrops are correctly instilled by placing them in the lower conjunctival sac. Eyedrops should not be placed near the lacrimal ducts, to decrease the chance of the medication being systemically absorbed. Placing the drops on the cornea or sclera is uncomfortable for the client and may cause the medication to run out of the eye socket instead of being absorbed.

 CN: Pharmacological and parenteral therapies; CL: Evaluate

113. **2.** Normal age-related changes can predispose older adults to falling and include vision, hearing, cardiovascular, musculoskeletal, and neurologic changes. One of the most common problems facing older adults is the loss of tissue elasticity that affects the arteries. This loss of elasticity results in a decrease in tissue recoil and leads to changes in blood pressure with position changes. When they rise too quickly from a supine position, they feel light-headed and dizzy and can fall. The nurse should instruct clients to change positions slowly and to dangle the legs a few minutes when arising from a supine position. When aging, the lens of the eye becomes sensitive to very bright light that can cause a glare and visual disturbances that can lead to falls. Rooms should be well lit, but not with bright lights that cause a glare. Neurologic changes are seen in impaired reflexes and thus postural instability. This loss of postural stability leads to falls. Assistive devices (hand rails, cane, walkers) help reduce falls and promote independence. If joint pain develops and remains untreated, it can cause older adults to become sedentary or immobile. This disuse of muscles contributes to muscle weakness and falls. Nursing interventions should be directed at encouraging regular ambulation and joint movement (range of motion).

 CN: Reduction of risk potential; CL: Analyze

114. **3.** The nurse should call the surgeon's office so that arrangements can be made for the client to donate a unit of their blood for possible future autotransfusion. This must be done in sufficient time before surgery so that the client is not at risk for being anemic at the time of the scheduled procedure. The client's request must be scheduled through the surgeon's office because the surgeon has ultimate responsibility for the client. The nurse can document that the surgeon's office was notified of the client's request. Notifying the hematology laboratory or blood bank is not an appropriate response.

🔑 CN: Pharmacological and parenteral therapies; CL: Analyze

115. **3.** Overuse of nasal spray containing pseudoephedrine can lead to rhinitis medicamentosa, which is a rebound effect causing increased swelling and congestion. The use of pseudoephedrine nasal spray does not cause infections or thrush. Pseudoephedrine is not addictive.

🔑 CN: Pharmacological and parenteral therapies; CL: Analyze

116. **2.** The best way to teach a child about surgery is through play. The nurse can let the child handle the items that will be used for monitoring, such as the blood pressure cuff and the ECG pads. The child will become more familiar with the face masks they see the surgical team wearing in the operating room after playing with one and wearing it before surgery. A child of this age group does not understand detailed explanations of how to use equipment, such as a PCA, a VAS, or even a video. The pain scale that should be used for children is the FACES scale.

🔑 CN: Basic care and comfort; CL: Analyze

117. **2.** When a nurse observes the theft of an opioid, it is the responsibility of the nurse to report the incident to the supervisor of the unit. The supervisor of the unit can confront the coworker and notify the hospital's chief of security about the incident. In some situations, the drug-abusing coworker may be offered drug counseling. In situations in which the drugs are being sold, the police should be notified. The nurse should not confront the coworker because this may put the nurse in danger. It is not the responsibility of the nurse to notify federal drug agents about the incident.

🔑 CN: Management of care; CL: Analyze

118.

0/1

Action to Take	Potential Conditions	Parameters to Monitor
Provide nutrition counseling	Iron deficiency	Weight gain
Begin iron supplementation		Activity tolerance

The client's low RBCs, HGB, HCT, and MCV suggest that they are experiencing iron deficiency anemia. Untreated, the problem will worsen as the fetus grows and begins to store iron. Nutrition counseling and iron supplementation should begin. Clients with anemia are at risk for poor weight gain and low activity tolerance. The Rh-negative client can become sensitized if they are carrying an Rh-positive fetus. The sensitization most typically happens in the birth process and most induces risk in future pregnancies. Rh immune globulin will be given around the 28th week to manage the risk. If sensitization occurs, the nurse would monitor the newborn, not the birth parent, for jaundice. The client is not immune to rubella but cannot receive the live vaccine while pregnant. Rubella presents as low-grade fever, respiratory symptoms, headache, and rash. Herd immunity makes the risk for contracting rubella relatively low, and there are no special precautions the client needs to take. The client should be given the rubella vaccine after the baby is born. The client is hepatitis B surface antigen negative, meaning they do not have an active hepatitis B infection.

🔑 CJ: Standalone bowtie; CL: Create

119. **2.** The nurse should teach the client and family the importance of not discontinuing benztropine abruptly. Rather, the drug should be tapered slowly over a 1-week period. Benztropine should not be used with over-the-counter cough and cold preparations because of the risk for an additive anticholinergic effect. Antacids delay the absorption of benztropine, and alcohol in combination with benztropine causes an increase in central nervous system depression; concomitant use should be avoided.

🔑 CN: Pharmacological and parenteral therapies; CL: Analyze

120. **2.** Albumin is a colloid that remains in the intravascular space, pulling fluid out of the intracellular and interstitial space. The client with nephrotic syndrome loses excessive amounts of protein, mainly albumin, in the urine. Because fluid is drawn into the intravascular space, blood pressure will increase. Crackles in the lung bases and cerebral edema are signs of circulatory overload or fluid volume excess. When edema is present in the lower extremities, the skin feels cool to the touch unless an infection is present.

🔑 CN: Physiological adaptation; CL: Evaluate

121. **3.** Although it is not clearly understood why cysts form in polycystic kidney disease, the condition is known to be inherited. Environmental exposures such as smoking and breathing secondhand smoke promote the development of bladder cancer. Although drinking alcohol requires the kidneys to excrete the alcohol, it is not thought to cause the kidneys to develop cysts. Exposure to dyes used in foods does not increase the risk for polycystic disease.

CN: Physiological adaptation; CL: Analyze

122. 3. The nurse expects the UAP assigned to several clients in labor to notify the nurse if the UAP observes that one of the clients has evidence of spontaneous rupture of the membranes. When the membranes rupture spontaneously, there is danger of a prolapsed cord, a medical emergency requiring a cesarean birth. Nausea may occur after administration of an epidural anesthetic, but this is not a priority or emergency. Having contractions that are 3 minutes apart and last for 40 seconds is normal during active labor. Because nalbuphine is an analgesic, it is normal for a client to fall asleep after IV administration of this drug.

CN: Management of care; CL: Evaluate

123. 1, 2, 4. Heparin dosage in children is based on the child's weight. A bolus of heparin is administered by the IV route, and the onset of action is immediate. The PTT is an indicator of the effectiveness of heparin. Following the heparin with a continuous infusion of heparin would cause life-threatening anticoagulation in this child. Penicillin and cephalosporins potentiate the effects of heparin, so the heparin must be carefully titrated to obtain maximum effect without causing an overdose. However, the antibiotic should not be discontinued.

CN: Pharmacological and parenteral therapies; CL: Analyze

124. 2. Urinary retention is a common occurrence with epidural analgesia. The nurse should first assess for bladder fullness. There is no indication that the client has a low fluid intake; encouraging fluids is not warranted. A review of laboratory results, specifically blood urea nitrogen and creatinine, may be indicated if urinary retention is first excluded as the cause. The infusion should only be stopped in an emergent situation such as excessive sedation.

CN: Management of care; CL: Analyze

125. 1. Applying a tourniquet obstructs venous blood flow and, as a result, distends the veins. A tourniquet does not stabilize veins or immobilize the arm, nor is it applied to occlude arterial circulation.

CN: Pharmacological and parenteral therapies; CL: Apply

126. 1, 2, 3, 4. Cough and dyspnea can be present at the time of diagnosis of bone cancer, indicating that the cancer has metastasized to the lungs. About one-quarter of all adolescents with bone cancer have lung metastasis at the time of diagnosis. Pain and swelling result from the inflammation caused by the bone tumor and the increased vascularity of the tumor. At the time of diagnosis, fever, anorexia, and decreased range of motion have not occurred. The tumor involves the bone, so there is pain when pressure is exerted on the involved bone, but range of motion is not affected. Fever and anorexia can occur if extensive metastasis has occurred.

CN: Physiological adaptation; CL: Analyze

127. 1. The priority assessment is that the client has a firm fundus when gentle massage is used. This indicates that the client's fundus may be soft or "boggy" when it is not massaged. The receiving nurse should assess the client's fundus soon after admission and continue to monitor the client's fundus, lochia, and pulse rate. Postpartum hemorrhage is associated with uterine atony. Maternal-infant bonding is a process that usually starts on day 2 and ends at week 1. A 12-hour labor is normal. The temperature and pulse are within normal limits.

CN: Management of care; CL: Analyze

128. 3, 5, 6. The neonate is experiencing quiet tachypnea with central cyanosis, which is a sign of possible congenital heart disease. The nurse should obtain pulse oximeter readings and notify the HCP. Blood pressures in all four extremities should be obtained on any newborn with a suspected congenital heart defect. Differences of more than 20 mm Hg between the upper and lower extremities may indicate ductal-dependent defects. The baby is showing no signs of increased work of breathing, except an increased respiratory rate. Breath sounds are clear; therefore, suctioning is not necessary and may cause further distress because of trauma to the nasal passage. Changing the neonate's position would have no impact on the cyanosis. Encouraging the baby to cry would increase the distress by decreasing oxygen consumption. Newborns are obligate nose breathers, and placing a nasogastric tube could increase distress by causing a partial nasal obstruction.

CJ: Standalone trend; CL: Apply

129. 4. It is critical for medication safety to know the name, dosage, and times of administration of the medication taken at home. The family should bring the medication bottles to the hospital. The nurse should document the medication on the medical record from the bottles to ensure accuracy before the medication is prescribed and administered. The pharmacist is a helpful resource, but the safest way to identify the medication is in its original container. It is not safe to assume the client could correctly identify the medications from a drug book. The medication regimen may have changed since the record 2 years ago.

🗝️ CN: Pharmacological and parenteral therapies; CL: Analyze

130. −/+ **3, 4, 5.** The additional fluids should run through a separate line using a Y-connector. The nurse must contact the surgeon to clarify if the client should receive the additional 100 mL per hour of IV fluids containing potassium chloride during the bolus infusion. A rapid infusion of potassium chloride can cause hyperkalemia with adverse cardiac outcomes such as arrhythmias. Bolus infusions of IV fluids should be run via an infusion pump to avoid excess fluid administration. Increasing the current IV infusion rate or adding additional fluids to the existing infusion is not safe because the current infusion contains potassium.

🗝️ CN: Pharmacological and parenteral therapies; CL: Analyze

131. −/+ **2, 3, 4.** Infants should always be transported in a bassinette or crib in the hallways. A baby in arms outside of a parent room should trigger activation of infant abduction protocols. Footprints and a photograph taken by 2 hours after birth serve as ID should there be an unforeseen separation from the parent. Clients should only let staff wearing appropriate ID take their baby from their room. Clients should notify staff if they see anyone who looks suspicious on the unit. ID badges should be matched each and every time an infant is taken from or returned to the parent not just on a daily basis.

🗝️ CN: Safety and infection control; CL: Apply

132. −/+ **1, 3, 4.** The nurse should write down the prescription, read the prescription back to the HCP, and receive confirmation from the provider that the prescription is correct as understood by the nurse. It is not necessary for the HCP to come to the hospital to write the prescription on the medical record or to have the nursing supervisor cosign the telephone prescription.

🗝️ CN: Safety and infection control; CL: Apply

133. 2. Giving the client finger foods that have protein, carbohydrates, and calories supplies energy and allows the client to eat while on the move. A salad or soup is very difficult for the client to eat while moving and may not supply the nutrients needed. Favorite foods from home may or may not be appropriate to eat while walking.

🗝️ CN: Basic care and comfort; CL: Apply

134. 4. The client is experiencing signs of thrombophlebitis. The nurse should notify the HCP because emboli formation is a potential risk. Massaging the area may cause the thrombus to dislocate and become an embolus. Warm compresses will increase circulation to the area and may precipitate embolus formation. Ankle pump exercises are helpful in preventing thrombophlebitis but will not prevent further risk for embolus formation at this time.

🗝️ CN: Reduction of risk potential; CL: Analyze

135. 3. Small-boned, fair-skinned women of northern European descent are at the greatest risk for osteoporosis, not women of African descent. One standard serving of yogurt is the equivalent of one glass of milk. Women who do not eat dairy products, such as women who are lactose intolerant, should consider using calcium supplements. Inadequate lifetime intake of calcium is a major risk factor for osteoporosis. Estrogen therapy, or some of the newer medications that are not estrogen based, can greatly reduce the incidence of osteoporosis.

🗝️ CN: Reduction of risk potential; CL: Evaluate

136. 3, 1, 2, 4. The goal of care for a client who is having a seizure is to prevent respiratory arrest and aspiration. The nurse should first clear the area around the client. Next, the nurse should loosen clothing around the client's neck and turn the client on the side. As needed, the nurse can then suction the airway and administer oxygen.

🗝️ CN: Reduction of risk potential; CL: Create

137. 4. There is no cure for metastatic cancer of the liver; palliative nursing care is required. Liver transplants are not recommended for a client with widespread malignant disease. Prescribed medications will not make metastatic lesions shrink. There is nothing to indicate that the client is receiving chemotherapy; therefore, explaining its effects would not be helpful.

🗝️ CN: Physiological adaptation; CL: Analyze

138. -/+ **3.** The T-tube should drain approximately 300 to 500 mL in the first 24 hours, and after 3 to 4 days the amount should decrease to less than 200 mL in 24 hours. With the sudden decrease in drainage at 0800, the nurse should immediately assess the tube for obstruction of flow that can be caused by kinks in the tube or the client lying on the tube. The nurse should also assess the drainage color for signs of bleeding. The tube should not be irrigated or clamped without a prescription. It is not necessary to notify the surgeon unless the tubing remains obstructed. The UAP should not empty the drainage apparatus.

    CJ: Standalone trend; CL: Analyze

139. 4. The nurse should acknowledge that the client feels better but should also remind the client to continue the drug therapy and other self-care activities of rest, exercise, joint protection, and adequate nutrition. Wearing the copper-lined gloves is not harmful, and the nurse should not instruct the client to remove the gloves or label it quackery. Copper does not interfere with salicylate metabolism.

    CN: Psychosocial integrity; CL: Analyze

140. 1. Lymphedema occurs frequently after radical mastectomy when lymph nodes are removed. Aplasia, or the absence of lymph nodes, prevents proper lymph drainage. The tissue swelling is caused by obstructed lymph flow in the extremity. The blood pressure is taken in the unaffected arm to avoid further accumulation of lymphedema. An IV line should not be started in the affected arm. The nurse would encourage the client to elevate the extremity above the level of the heart. Blood draws in the affected arm should not be allowed.

    CN: Physiological adaptation; CL: Analyze

141. 2. Measuring the pH of the aspirated gastric fluid is the most accurate determination of the placement of the NG tube. A pH lower than 4 indicates that the tube is in the stomach. Whether or not the client is gagging or coughing is not an accurate way to determine if the tube is placed correctly. No fluids should be inserted into the tube until the placement has been determined. Inserting air into the tube and listening for the resulting whoosh can be used, but this is not as accurate as pH measurement.

    CN: Reduction of risk potential; CL: Evaluate

142. 2. Alcoholic cirrhosis is associated with excessive alcohol intake. In the early stages, the liver develops fatty changes. If alcohol intake stops, the fatty changes can be reversed. Avoiding overexertion is important in the client with cirrhosis, but it does not reverse the disease. Stopping smoking is a positive, healthy lifestyle change, but it does not have an impact on cirrhosis. A diet high in carbohydrates and low in fat is also recommended for the client with cirrhosis, but the diet does not reverse the pathologic changes that have occurred in the liver.

    CN: Reduction of risk potential; CL: Analyze

143. -/+ **1, 2, 3, 5.** When emergently managing chest pain, the nurse can use the memory mnemonic *MONA* to plan care: morphine, oxygen, nitroglycerin, and aspirin. A Foley catheter is not included in the emergent management of chest pain and can be inserted when the pain has been relieved and the client is stable. Acetaminophen is not used to manage chest pain.

    CN: Physiological adaptation; CL: Analyze

144. 3. Minimizing urinary catheter use and duration of use in all clients, particularly those at higher risk for CAUTI or mortality from catheterization such as women, older adults, and clients with impaired immunity, will reduce the opportunity for infection. The nurse should avoid the use of urinary catheters for clients who are incontinent; a bladder training program and frequent use of the toilet are preferred; external catheters may be used if necessary in incontinent clients. The nurse should not clean the periurethral area with antiseptics; cleansing the meatal surface during daily bathing or showering is appropriate. Using sterile technique to help reduce CAUTI is not necessary. Hand hygiene immediately before and after insertion or any manipulation of the catheter device or site is sufficient.

    CN: Reduction of risk potential; CL: Analyze

145. -/+ **2, 3, 5, 6.** The client is hyponatremic; the nurse should notify the HCP, restrict fluids, and prepare to insert a Foley catheter to ensure accurate intake and output. Side rails should be up to maintain client safety; it is not safe for the client to be ambulating in the hallway with family at this time. Encouraging fluids would not be beneficial and could be harmful.

    CN: Physiological adaptation; CL: Analyze

146. 2. While it is important to present options and help find solutions to the client's financial concerns, the nurse must first listen carefully to those concerns and allow the client to verbalize related emotions to identify the client's needs. Reminding the client to focus on getting well does not address the client's concerns or needs. Arranging a meeting with the case manager is premature as the nurse needs to first determine what the client's needs are. Until the nurse understands the client's needs, the nurse should not encourage the spouse to discuss the client's bill with the business office.

☞ CN: Management of care; CL: Analyze

147. 1. The nurse is ultimately responsible to coordinate the client's care while hospitalized; therefore, it is the nurse's responsibility to arrange a care conference to help get the client's questions, concerns, and frustrations addressed. Assuring the client that the HCPs know what they are doing does not address the client's concern or frustration with receiving conflicting information. While it is true that the client is ultimately responsible for health, asking the client to accept the consequences is a form of blaming the client. The HCPs' progress notes will not provide information that will address the client's concern or resolve the conflicting courses of action that the two HCPs are proposing.

☞ CN: Management of care; CL: Analyze

148. 3, 1, 4, 2. The nurse should first assess the client and then, if there is no acute injury, help the client get back into bed. The nurse must notify the HCP and the family of the client who fell and, finally, document the event on the client's health record.

☞ CN: Safety and infection control; CL: Create

149. 3. Adding humidity to the incubator adds moisture to the ambient air, which helps decrease the insensible water loss. Bathing and the use of eye patches have no impact on insensible water loss. The use of a radiant warmer will increase the insensible water loss by drawing moisture out of the skin.

☞ CN: Reduction of risk potential; CL: Analyze

150. 3. Neonates who are septic use glucose at an increased rate. During the time the IV is not infusing, the neonate is using the limited glucose stores available to a preterm neonate and may deplete them. Hypoglycemia is too little glucose in the blood; without the constant infusion of IV glucose, hypoglycemia will result. Fevers and hyperkalemia are not related to glucose levels. Tachycardia is the result of untreated hypoglycemia.

☞ CN: Reduction of risk potential; CL: Analyze

Appendices

State, Provincial, and Territorial Boards of Nursing   1219

Bibliography   1223

Credits   1224

State, Provincial, and Territorial Boards of Nursing

Alabama Board of Nursing
PO Box 303900
Montgomery, AL 36130-3900
Phone: 1-800-656-5318
Fax: (334) 293-5201
Website: http://www.abn.alabama.gov

Alaska Board of Nursing
550 W. Seventh Avenue, Suite 1500
Anchorage, AK 99501-3567
Phone: (907) 269-8160
Fax: (907) 269-8156
Website: https://www.commerce.alaska.gov/web/cbpl/ProfessionalLicensing/BoardofNursing.aspx

College of Registered Nurses of Alberta
11620 168 Street
Edmonton, AB T5M 4A6
Phone: 1 (800) 252-9392
Fax: (780) 452-3276
Website: https://www.nurses.ab.ca/

Arizona State Board of Nursing
1740 W Adams St. Suite 2000
Phoenix, AZ 85007
Phone: (602) 771-7800
Website: http://www.azbn.gov

Arkansas State Board of Nursing
University Tower Building
1123 S. University Avenue, Suite 800
Little Rock, AR 72204-1619
Phone: (501) 686-2700
Fax: (501) 686-2714
Website: https://www.arsbn.org

British Columbia College of Nurses and Midwives (BCCNM)
900 – 200 Granville St
Vancouver, BC V6C 1S4
Canada
Phone: (604) 742-6200
Website: https://www.bccnm.ca/Pages/Default.aspx

California State Board of Registered Nursing
1747 N. Market Boulevard, Suite 150
Sacramento, CA 95834
Phone: (916) 322-3350
Fax: (916) 574-8637
Website: http://www.rn.ca.gov

Colorado Board of Nursing
1560 Broadway Street, Suite 1370
Denver, Colorado 80202
Phone: (303) 894-2430
Fax: (303) 894-2821
Website: https://www.colorado.gov/pacific/dora/Nursing

Connecticut Board of Examiners for Nursing
Department of Public Health
410 Capitol Avenue, MS# 13PHO
PO Box 340308
Hartford, CT 06134-0308
Phone: (860) 509-7603
Fax: (860) 509-8457
Website: https://portal.ct.gov/DPH/Public-Health-Hearing-Office/Board-of-Examiners-for-Nursing/Board-of-Examiners-for-Nursing

Delaware Board of Nursing
861 Silver Lake Boulevard
Cannon Building, Suite 203
Dover, DE 19904
Phone: (302) 744-4500
Fax: (302) 739-2711
Website: https://dpr.delaware.gov/boards/nursing/

District of Columbia Board of Nursing
Department of Health
Health Professional Licensing Administration
899 N. Capitol Street, NE
Washington, DC 20002
Phone: (877) 672-2174
Fax: (202) 724-5145
Website: https://dchealth.dc.gov/node/149382

Florida Board of Nursing
4052 Bald Cypress Way, Bin C02
Tallahassee, FL 32399-3252
Phone: (850) 245-4125
Fax: (850) 245-4172
Website: http://floridasnursing.gov

Georgia Board of Nursing
237 Coliseum Drive
Macon, GA 31217-3858
Phone: (478) 207-2440
Fax: (877) 371-5712
Website: https://sos.ga.gov/georgia-board-nursing

Hawaii Board of Nursing
Professional and Vocational Licensing Division
PO Box 3469
Honolulu, HI 96801
Phone: (808) 586-2965
Website: https://cca.hawaii.gov/pvl/boards/nursing/

Idaho Board of Nursing
11341 W. Chinden Blvd.
Boise, ID 83714
Phone: 208-334-6620
Website: http://ibn.idaho.gov

Illinois Department of Professional Regulation
555 West Monroe Street, 5th Floor
Chicago, IL 60661
Phone: 1 (888) 473-4858
Website: https://www.idfpr.com/profs/Nursing.asp

Indiana State Board of Nursing
Professional Licensing Agency
402 W. Washington Street, Room W072
Indianapolis, IN 46204
Phone: (317) 234-2043
Fax: (317) 233-4236
Website: https://www.in.gov/pla/nursing.htm

Iowa Board of Nursing
River Point Business Park
400 S.W. 8th Street, Suite B
Des Moines, IA 50309-4685
Phone: (515) 281-3255
Fax: (515) 281-4825
Website: https://nursing.iowa.gov

Kansas State Board of Nursing
Landon State Office Building
900 S.W. Jackson Street, Suite 1051
Topeka, KS 66612
Phone: (785) 296-4929
Fax: (785) 296-3929
Website: http://www.ksbn.org

Kentucky Board of Nursing
312 Whittington Parkway, Suite 300
Louisville, KY 40222
Phone: (502) 429-3300
Fax: (502) 429-3311
Website: https://kbn.ky.gov/Pages/index.aspx

Louisiana State Board of Nursing
17373 Perkins Road
Baton Rouge, LA 70810
Phone: (225) 755-7500
Fax: (225) 755-7584
Website: http://www.lsbn.state.la.us

Maine State Board of Nursing
161 Capitol St
Augusta, ME 04333
Phone: (207) 287-1133
Fax: (207) 287-1149
Website: http://www.maine.gov/boardofnursing

College of Registered Nurses of Manitoba (CRNM)
890 Pembina Highway
Winnipeg, MB R3M 2M8
Phone: (204) 774-3477
Fax: (204) 775-6052
Website: http://www.crnm.mb.ca

Maryland Board of Nursing
4140 Patterson Avenue
Baltimore, MD 21215
Phone: (410) 585-1900
Fax: (410) 358-3530
Website: http://mbon.maryland.gov

Massachusetts Board of Registration in Nursing
Commonwealth of Massachusetts
250 Washington Street
Boston, MA 02108
Phone: (617) 973-0900
Fax: (617) 973-0984
Website: https://www.mass.gov/orgs/board-of-registration-in-nursing

Michigan Department of Licensing and Regulatory Affairs
Bureau of Health Professions
611 W. Ottawa Street
PO Box 30670
Lansing, MI 48909
Phone: (517) 241-0199
Fax: (517) 241-9416
Website: http://www.michigan.gov/lara

Minnesota Board of Nursing
1210 Northland Drive Suite 120
Mendota Heights, MN 55120
Phone: (612) 617-3000
Fax: 651-688-1841
Website: https://mn.gov/boards/nursing/

Mississippi Board of Nursing
713 Pear Orchard Road
Suite 300
Ridgeland, MS 39157
Phone: (601) 957-6300
Fax: (601) 957-6301
Website: https://www.msbn.ms.gov/Pages/Home.aspx

Missouri State Board of Nursing
3605 Missouri Boulevard
PO Box 656
Jefferson City, MO 65102-0656
Phone: (573) 751-0681
Fax: (573) 751-0075
Website: http://www.pr.mo.gov/nursing.asp

Montana State Board of Nursing
PO Box 200513
Helena, MT 59620-0513
Phone: (406) 444-6880
Website: http://boards.bsd.dli.mt.gov/nur

Nebraska Advanced Practice Registered Nurse Board
Office of Nursing and Nursing Support
DHHS, Division of Public Health, Licensure Unit 301 Centennial Mall South
Lincoln, NE 68509-4986
Phone: (402) 471-4376
Fax: (402) 742-1163
Website: https://dhhs.ne.gov/licensure/Pages/Nurse-Licensing.aspx

Nevada State Board of Nursing
5011 Meadowood Mall Way, Suite 300
Reno, NV 89502
Phone: (775) 687-7700
Fax: (775) 687-7707
Website: http://nevadanursingboard.org

Nurses Association of New Brunswick
165 Regent Street
Fredericton, NB E3B 7B4
Phone: (506) 458-8731
Fax: (506) 459-2838
Website: http://www.nanb.nb.ca

Nurses Association of Registered Nurses of Newfoundland and Labrador
55 Military Road
St. John's, NL A1C 2C5
Phone: (709) 753-6040
Fax: (709) 753-4940
Website: https://www.arnnl.ca

New Hampshire Board of Nursing
7 Eagle Square
Concord, NH 03301
Phone: (603) 271-2152
Website: https://www.oplc.nh.gov/new-hampshire-board-nursing

New Jersey Board of Nursing
PO Box 45010
124 Halsey Street, 6th Floor
Newark, NJ 07101
Phone: (973) 504-6430
Fax: (973) 648-3481
Website: https://www.njconsumeraffairs.gov/nur/Pages/default.aspx

New Mexico Board of Nursing
6301 Indian School Road, NE
Albuquerque, NM 87110
Phone: (505) 841-8340
Fax: (505) 841-8347
Website: http://nmbon.sks.com/

New York State Board of Nursing
Education Building
89 Washington Avenue
2nd Floor West Wing
Albany, NY 12234
Phone: (518) 474-3817 ext. 120
Fax: (518) 474-3706
Website: http://www.op.nysed.gov/prof/nurse

North Carolina Board of Nursing
4516 Lake Boone Trail
Raleigh, NC 27607
Phone: (919) 782-3211
Fax: (919) 781-9461
Website: http://www.ncbon.com

North Dakota Board of Nursing
919 S. 7th Street, Suite 504
Bismark, ND 58504
Phone: (701) 328-9777
Fax: (701) 328-9785
Website: http://www.ndbon.org

Registered Nurses Association of Northwest Territories and Nunavut
#3 483 Range Lake Road
Yellowknife, NT X1A 3R9
Phone: (867) 873-2745
Fax: (867) 873-2336
Website: http://www.rnantnu.ca

Nova Scotia College of Nursing
120 Western Parkway, Suite 300
Bedford, NS B4B 0V2, Canada
Phone: (902) 444-6726
Fax: (902) 377-5188
Website: http://www.crnns.ca

Ohio Board of Nursing
17 S. High Street, Suite 660
Columbus, OH 43215-3466
Phone: (614) 466-3947
Fax: (614) 466-0388
Website: http://www.nursing.ohio.gov

Oklahoma Board of Nursing
2501 N. Lincoln Blvd., Ste. 207
Oklahoma City, OK 73105
Phone: (405) 962-1800
Fax: (405) 962-1821
Website: http://nursing.ok.gov/

College of Nurses of Ontario
101 Davenport Road
Toronto, ON M5R 3P1
Phone: (416) 928-0900
Fax: (416) 928-6507
Website: http://www.cno.org

Oregon State Board of Nursing
17938 S.W. Upper Boones Ferry Road
Portland, OR 97224
Phone: (503) 673-0685
Fax: (503) 673-0684
Website: https://www.oregon.gov/OSBN/pages/index.aspx

Pennsylvania State Board of Nursing
2601 N. 3rd Street
Harrisburg, PA 17110
Phone: (717) 783-7142
Fax: (717) 783-0822
Website: https://www.dos.pa.gov/ProfessionalLicensing/BoardsCommissions/Nursing/Pages/default.aspx

College of Registered Nurses of Prince Edward Island
45 Paramount Drive
Charlottetown PE C1E 0C6, Canada
Phone: 1(844)843-3933
Fax: (902) 628-1430
Website: https://www.crnpei.ca/

Ordre des infirmières et infirmiers de Québec
4200 Molson Street
Montreal, Quebec H1Y 4V4, Canada
Téléphone: (514) 935-2501
Télécopieur: (514) 935-1799
Website: http://www.oiiq.org

Rhode Island Board of Nursing
Registration and Nursing Education
105 Cannon Building
Three Capitol Hill
Providence, RI 02908
Phone: (401) 222-5700
Fax: (401) 222-3352
Website: http://health.ri.gov/licenses/detail.php?id=231

Saskatchewan Registered Nurses' Association
1-3710 Eastgate Drive
Regina, SK S4Z 1A5
Phone: (306) 359-4200
Fax: (306) 359-0257
Website: http://www.srna.org

South Carolina State Board of Nursing
110 Centerview Drive, Suite 202
Columbia, SC 29210
Phone: (803) 896-4550
Fax: (803) 896-4515
Website: https://llr.sc.gov/nurse/

South Dakota Board of Nursing
4300 South Louise Avenue, Suite 201
Sioux Falls, SD 57106-3115
Phone: (605) 362-2760
Fax: (605) 362-2768
Website: http://doh.sd.gov/boards/nursing

Tennessee State Board of Nursing
665 Mainstream Drive
Nashville, TN 37243
Phone: (615) 532-5166
Fax: (615) 741-7899
Website: https://www.tn.gov/health/health-program-areas/health-professional-boards/nursing-board/nursing-board/about.html

Texas Board of Nursing
333 Guadalupe Street, Suite 3-460
Austin, TX 78701
Phone: (512) 305-7400
Fax: (512) 305-7401
Website: http://www.bon.state.tx.us

Utah State Board of Nursing
Heber M. Wells Building, 4th Floor
160 East 300 South
Salt Lake City, UT 84111
Phone: (801) 530-6628
Fax: (801) 530-6511
Website: https://dopl.utah.gov/nur/index.html

Vermont State Board of Nursing
Office of Professional Regulation
Board of Nursing
89 Main Street, Floor 3
Montpelier, VT 05620-3402
Phone: (802) 828-2396
Fax: (802) 828-2484
Website: https://sos.vermont.gov/nursing/

Virginia Board of Nursing
Department of Health Professions
Perimeter Center
9960 Mayland Drive, Suite 300
Henrico, VA 23233
Phone: (804) 367-4515
Fax: (804) 527-4455
Website: www.dhp.virginia.gov/nursing

Washington State Nursing Care Quality Assurance Commission
Department of Health
PO Box 47864
Olympia, WA 98504-7864
Phone: (360) 236-4703
Fax: (360) 236-4738
Website: http://www.doh.wa.gov/LicensesPermitsandCertificates/NursingCommission

West Virginia Board of Examiners for Registered Professional Nurses
5001 MacCorkle Avenue, SW
Suite 203
South Charleston, WV 25303
Phone: (304) 744-0900
Fax: (304) 744-0600
Website: http://wvrnboard.wv.gov/Pages/default.aspx

Wisconsin Department of Safety and Professional Services
P.O. Box 8935
Madison, WI 53708-8935
Phone: (608) 226-2112
Website: https://dsps.wi.gov/pages/BoardsCouncils/Nursing/Default.aspx

Wyoming State Board of Nursing
130 Hobbs Avenue, Suite B
Cheyenne, WY 82002
Phone: (307) 777-7601
Fax: (307) 777-3519
Website: http://nursing.state.wy.us

Yukon Registered Nurses Association
Suite 204
4133-4th Avenue
Whitehorse, YT Y1A 1H8
Phone: (867) 667-4062
Fax: (867) 668-5123
Website: https://www.yrna.ca/

Bibliography

1. The Nursing Care of the Childbearing Family

Lippincott Williams & Wilkins. (2022). *Lippincott nursing procedures* (9th ed.). Philadelphia, PA: Author.

Pillitteri, A. (2017). *Maternal & child health nursing: Care of the childbearing and childrearing family* (8th ed.). Philadelphia, PA: Lippincott Williams & Wilkins.

Ricci, S., & Kyle, T. (2020). *Maternity and pediatric nursing* (4th ed.). Philadelphia, PA: Lippincott Williams & Wilkins.

2. The Nursing Care of Children

Kyle, T., & Carman, S. (2020). *Essentials of pediatric nursing* (4th ed.). Philadelphia, PA: Lippincott Williams & Wilkins.

Lippincott Williams & Wilkins. (2022). *Lippincott nursing procedures* (9th ed.). Philadelphia, PA: Author.

Pillitteri, A. (2017). *Maternal & child health nursing: Care of the childbearing and childrearing family* (8th ed.). Philadelphia, PA: Lippincott Williams & Wilkins.

Ricci, S., & Kyle, T. (2020). *Maternity and pediatric nursing* (4th ed.). Philadelphia, PA: Lippincott Williams & Wilkins.

3. The Nursing Care of Adults with Medical and Surgical Health Problems

Ellis, J., & Hartley, C. (2011). *Managing and coordinating nursing care* (5th ed.). Philadelphia, PA: Lippincott Williams & Wilkins.

Karch, A. (2022). *Lippincott's nursing drug guide*. Philadelphia, PA: Lippincott Williams & Wilkins.

Lippincott Williams & Wilkins. (2022). *Lippincott nursing procedures* (9th ed.). Philadelphia, PA: Author.

Marquis, B., & Huston, C. (2020). *Leadership roles and management functions in nursing* (10th ed.). Philadelphia, PA: Lippincott Williams & Wilkins.

Smeltzer, B., et al. (2021). *Brunner and Suddarth's textbook of medical-surgical nursing* (15th ed.). Philadelphia, PA: Lippincott Williams & Wilkins.

Taylor, C., et al. (2020). *Fundamentals of nursing* (10th ed.). Philadelphia, PA: Lippincott Williams & Wilkins.

Weber, J. R., & Kelley, J. (2021). *Health assessment in nursing* (7th ed.). Philadelphia, PA: Lippincott Williams & Wilkins.

4. The Nursing Care of Clients with Psychiatric Disorders and Mental Health Problems

Andrews, M., & Boyle, J. (2019). *Transcultural concepts in nursing care* (8th ed.). Philadelphia, PA: Lippincott Williams & Wilkins.

Boyd, M. A. (2017). *Psychiatric nursing: Contemporary practice* (6th ed.). Philadelphia, PA: Lippincott Williams & Wilkins.

Karch, A. (2022). *Lippincott's nursing drug guide*. Philadelphia, PA: Lippincott Williams & Wilkins.

Videbeck, S. (2019). *Psychiatric mental health nursing* (8th ed.). Philadelphia, PA: Lippincott Williams & Wilkins.

Credits

Chapter 1

Figure 1.1: Distribution of Content Copyright by the National Council of State Boards of Nursing, Inc. All rights reserved.
Table 1.1: Copyright by the National Council of State Boards of Nursing, Inc. All rights reserved.
Table 1.2: Copyright by the National Council of State Boards of Nursing, Inc. All rights reserved.
Table 1.3: Copyright by the National Council of State Boards of Nursing, Inc. All rights reserved.

Chapter 2

Figure 2.23: Copyright by the National Council of State Boards of Nursing, Inc. All rights reserved.

The Nursing Care of the Childbearing Family

Test 1

Q 60: Modified from LifeART image copyright © [2019] Lippincott Williams & Wilkins. All rights reserved.

Test 3

Q 5 (all options); Modified from Kennedy, B., & Baird, S. (2017), *Intrapartum Management Modules*. (5th ed.). Philadelphia: Wolters Kluwer.
Q 37: Adapted from Layon, A. J., Gabrielli, A., Yu, M., et al. (2018). *Civetta, Taylor, & Kirby's critical care medicine* (5th ed.). Philadelphia, PA: Wolters Kluwer.
Q 17: (all options): From Nettina, S. M. (2014). *The Lippincott manual of nursing practice* (10th ed.). Philadelphia, PA: Lippincott Williams & Wilkins.

The Nursing Care of Children

Test 1

Q5: Modified from Kennedy, B., & Baird, S. (2016). *Intrapartum management modules* (5th ed.). Philadelphia, PA: Wolters Kluwer.
Q 43: (all options): Adapted from Pillitteri, A. (2003). *Maternal and child nursing* (4th ed.). Philadelphia, PA: Lippincott Williams & Wilkins.

Test 2

Q 1: From Nettina, S. M. (2014). *The Lippincott manual of nursing practice* (10th ed.). Philadelphia, PA: Lippincott Williams & Wilkins.
Q 44: From Nettina, S. M. (2014). *The Lippincott manual of nursing practice* (10th ed.). Philadelphia, PA: Lippincott Williams & Wilkins.
Q 54: From Hatfield, N. T. and Kincheloe, C. (2021). *Introductory Maternity and Pediatric Nursing* (5th ed.). Philadelphia, PA: Lippincott Williams & Wilkins

Test 4

Q 23: From Nettina, S. M. (2014). *The Lippincott manual of nursing practice* (10th ed.). Philadelphia, PA: Lippincott Williams & Wilkins.
Q 35: LifeART image copyright © (2022). Lippincott Williams & Wilkins. All rights reserved.
Q 68: Modified from Ricci, S. S., Kyle, T., Carman, S. (2021). *Maternity and pediatric nursing* (4th ed.). Philadelphia, PA: Wolters Kluwer.

Test 5

Q 33: From Nettina, S. M. (2014). *The Lippincott manual of nursing practice* (10th ed.). Philadelphia, PA: Lippincott Williams & Wilkins.

Test 6

Q 9: From Pillitteri, A. (2003). *Maternal and child nursing* (4th ed.). Philadelphia, PA: Lippincott Williams & Wilkins.
Q 61: From Nettina, S. M. (2014). *The Lippincott manual of nursing practice* (10th ed.). Philadelphia, PA: Lippincott Williams & Wilkins.

Test 8

Q 33 (all options): From Nettina, S. M. (2014). *The Lippincott manual of nursing practice* (10th ed.). Philadelphia, PA: Lippincott Williams & Wilkins.
Q 37: From Ellis, J. R., & Bentz, P. M. (2007). *Modules for basic nursing skills*. Lippincott Williams &; Wilkins., in Nettina, S. M. (2014). *The Lippincott manual of nursing practice* (10th ed.). Philadelphia, PA: Lippincott Williams & Wilkins.

Test 9

Q 19: From Nettina, S. M. (2014). *The Lippincott manual of nursing practice* (10th ed.). Philadelphia, PA: Lippincott Williams & Wilkins.

The Nursing Care of Adults with Medical and Surgical Health Problems

Test 1

Q 63: Adapted from Weber, J. R. (2017). *Nurses' handbook of health assessment* (9th ed.). Philadelphia, PA: Wolters Kluwer.

Test 2

Q. 11: From Billings, D. (2009). *Lippincott's content review for NCLEX-RN*. Philadelphia, PA: Wolters Kluwer Health.

Q. 12 (options 1, 2, 4): From Nettina, S. M. (2014). *The Lippincott manual of nursing practice* (10th ed.). Philadelphia, PA: Lippincott Williams & Wilkins.

Q. 12 (option 3): Modified from Taylor, C. R., Lillis, C., et al. (2008). *Fundamentals of nursing: The art and science of nursing care* (6th ed.). Philadelphia, PA: Lippincott Williams & Wilkins.

Test 4

Q 24: From Nettina, S. M. (2014). *The Lippincott manual of nursing practice* (10th ed.). Philadelphia, PA: Lippincott Williams & Wilkins.

Q 44: From Carter, Pamela & Goldschmidt, Wanda. (2010). *Lippincott's Textbook for Long-Term Care Nursing Assistants: A Humanistic Approach to Caregiving*.

Test 7

Q 37: From Billings, D. (2009). *Lippincott's content review for NCLEX-RN*. Philadelphia, PA: Wolters Kluwer Health.

Test 10

Q 22: Modified from Jensen, (2014). *Nursing health assessment: A best practice approach* (2nd ed.). Philadelphia, PA: Wolters Kluwer Health.

Test 14

Q 84: From Nettina, S. M. (2014). *The Lippincott manual of nursing practice* (10th ed.). Philadelphia, PA: Lippincott Williams & Wilkins.

Q 88: From Nettina, S. M. (2014). *The Lippincott manual of nursing practice* (10th ed.). Philadelphia, PA: Lippincott Williams & Wilkins.

100: From Nettina, S. M. (2014). *The Lippincott manual of nursing practice* (10th ed.). Philadelphia, PA: Lippincott Williams & Wilkins.

Test 15

Q 1: Modified from Springhouse. (2004). *Nursing procedures* (4th ed.). Ambler, PA: Lippincott Williams & Wilkins.

Test 16

Q 27: From Carter, P., & Goldschmidt, W. (2010). *Lippincott's textbook for long-term care nursing assistants: A humanistic approach to caregiving*. Philadelphia, PA: Wolters Kluwer Health.

Q 40: From Nettina, S. M. (2014). *The Lippincott manual of nursing practice* (10th ed.). Philadelphia, PA: Lippincott Williams & Wilkins.

Postreview Tests

Comprehensive Test 1

Q 10: From Nettina, S. M. (2014). *The Lippincott manual of nursing practice* (10th ed.). Philadelphia, PA: Lippincott Williams & Wilkins.

Comprehensive Test 2

Q 8: From Smeltzer, S. C., & Bare, B. G. (2000). *Brunner & Suddarth's textbook of medical-surgical nursing* (9th ed.). Philadelphia, PA: Lippincott Williams & Wilkins.

Comprehensive Test 3

Q 53: From Brody, L.T. & Hall, C. M. (2018). *Therapeutic exercise moving toward function*. Philadelphia Wolters Kluwer.

Comprehensive Test 5

Q 5: From Nettina, S. M. (2014). *The Lippincott manual of nursing practice* (10th ed.). Philadelphia, PA: Lippincott Williams & Wilkins.

Q 23: From Taylor, C., Lillis, C., et al. (2008). *Fundamentals of nursing: The art and science of nursing care* (6th ed.). Philadelphia, PA: Lippincott Williams & Wilkins.

Q 44: From Pillitteri, A. (2003). *Maternal and child nursing* (4th ed.). Philadelphia, PA: Lippincott Williams & Wilkins.

Comprehensive Test 6

Q 22: Adapted from (2004). *Nursing procedures* (4th ed.). Ambler, PA: Lippincott Williams & Wilkins.

Tear-Out Resources

CONTENT MASTERY AND TEST-TAKING SKILL SELF-ANALYSIS

Use the chart below to identify the subject matter and the reason you missed the question. Place a checkmark in the columns for questions you did not answer correctly and why, and then total each column. The key (🔑) to effective review is to understand your knowledge deficits and focus additional review on those subjects and reasons for not answering the question.

Review Strategies

Test Number	Subject (care of childbearing family, care of children, care of adults, care of clients with psychiatric disorders and mental health problems)	Score

Total number of questions missed:
_____
_____
_____

Use the chart below to identify the subject matter and the reason you missed the question. Use the following codes to note the client need area of the question you missed:
MC, management of care; SI, safety and infection control; HM, health promotion and maintenance; PA, physiological adaptation; PI, psychosocial integrity; PP, pharmacological and parenteral therapies; RR, reduction of risk potential; BC, basic care and comfort.

Question #	Client need	Misread/ misunderstood the question	Missed key word(s)	Did not read all options	Changed answer	Missed certain types of questions (often multiple-response questions)	Missed next generation (NGN) types of questions (case studies; bow ties; trends)	Did not understand the subject matter	Did not recognize the rationale for the correct answer	Made an incorrect guess	Did not understand the meaning of the term in question	Other
1												
2												
3												
4												
5												
5												
6												
7												

(continued)

Question #	Client need	Misread/ misunderstood the question	Missed key word(s)	Did not read all options	Changed answer	Missed certain types of questions (often multiple-response questions)	Missed next generation (NGN) types of questions (case studies; bow ties; trends)	Did not understand the subject matter	Did not recognize the rationale for the correct answer	Made an incorrect guess	Did not understand the meaning of the term in question	Other
8												
9												
10												
11												
12												
13												
14												
15												
16												
17												
18												
19												
20												
21												
22												
23												
24												
25												
26												
27												
28												
29												
30												
31												
32												
33												
34												
35												
36												
37												
38												
39												
40												
41												
42												
43												
44												

Question #	Client need	Misread/ misunderstood the question	Missed key word(s)	Did not read all options	Changed answer	Missed certain types of questions (often multiple-response questions)	Missed next generation (NGN) types of questions (case studies; bow ties; trends)	Did not understand the subject matter	Did not recognize the rationale for the correct answer	Made an incorrect guess	Did not understand the meaning of the term in question	Other
45												
46												
47												
48												
49												
50												
51												
52												
53												
54												
55												
56												
57												
58												
59												
60												
61												
62												
63												
64												
65												
66												
67												
68												
69												
70												
71												
72												
73												
74												
75												
76												
77												
78												
79												
80												
81												

(continued)

Question #	Client need	Misread/ misunderstood the question	Missed key word(s)	Did not read all options	Changed answer	Missed certain types of questions (often multiple-response questions)	Missed next generation (NGN) types of questions (case studies; bow ties; trends)	Did not understand the subject matter	Did not recognize the rationale for the correct answer	Made an incorrect guess	Did not understand the meaning of the term in question	Other
82												
83												
84												
85												
86												
87												
88												
89												
90												
91												
92												
93												
94												
95												
96												
97												
98												
99												
100												
101												
102												
103												
104												
105												
106												
107												
108												
109												
110												
111												
112												
113												
114												

Question #	Client need	Misread/ misunderstood the question	Missed key word(s)	Did not read all options	Changed answer	Missed certain types of questions (often multiple-response questions)	Missed next generation (NGN) types of questions (case studies; bow ties; trends)	Did not understand the subject matter	Did not recognize the rationale for the correct answer	Made an incorrect guess	Did not understand the meaning of the term in question	Other
115												
116												
117												
118												
119												
120												
121												
122												
123												
124												
125												
126												
127												
128												
129												
130												
131												
132												
133												
134												
135												
136												
137												
138												
139												
140												
141												
142												
143												
144												
145												
146												
147												

(continued)

Question #	Client need	Misread/ misunderstood the question	Missed key word(s)	Did not read all options	Changed answer	Missed certain types of questions (often multiple-response questions)	Missed next generation (NGN) types of questions (case studies; bow ties; trends)	Did not understand the subject matter	Did not recognize the rationale for the correct answer	Made an incorrect guess	Did not understand the meaning of the term in question	Other
148												
149												
150												

- How many questions in each area of client needs did you miss?
- How does this compare with other exam results from this review?

Lower _____ Same _____ Higher _____ NA _____

If you missed questions because you misread questions, missed key words, or changed answers, review Lippincott Q&A Review for NCLEX-RN Part I.

If you missed questions because you did not remember or understand the content, review that content in Lippincott Q&A Review for NCLEX-RN Part II and your other nursing references.

If you missed questions because you guessed, were you missing because of "rapid guessing" to complete the test on time, or because of "random guessing," making a reasoned attempt to answer the question? Consider how you will approach "guessing" when you do not know the answer.

If you missed questions because you did not pace yourself, practice taking timed test questions and pacing yourself to allow sufficient time for all questions.

What is the pattern of the types of questions you are missing?

_____
_____
_____

What is your action plan for further study?

_____
_____
_____

LABORATORY VALUES REFERENCE GUIDE

Laboratory Test	Reference Range in Metric and SI Units
ABG pH	7.35–7.45 (7.35–7.45)
ABG PO_2	75–100 mm Hg (10–13.3 kPa)
ABG PCO_2	35–45 mm Hg (10–13.3 kPa)
ABG $SaPO_2$	95%–100% (0.09–0.1)
ABG HCO_3	22–26 mEq/L (22–26 mmol/L)
Cholesterol (total)	<200 normal (<5.2 mmol/L) 200–239 borderline (5.2–6.2 mmol/L) ≥240 high (≥6.2 mmol/L)
Blood urea nitrogen (BUN)	10–20 mg/dL (3.6–7.1 mmol/L)
Creatinine (serum)	0.9–1.4 mg/dL (80–124 µmol/L)
Glucose (fasting)	Normal ≤99 mg/dL (<5.5 mmol/L) Prediabetes 100–125 mg/dL (5.6–6.9 mmol/L) Diabetes ≥126 mg/dL (≥7 mmol/L) Preterm infants 40–60 mg/dL (2.2–3.3 mmol/L)
$HgbA_1C$	Normal <5.7% (<0.06) Prediabetes 5.7–6.4% (0.06) Diabetes ≥6.5% (≥0.07)
Hematocrit	Males: 42%–52% (0.42–0.52); females: 35%–47% (0.35–0.47)
Hemoglobin	Males: 13–18 g/dL (130–180 g/L); females: 12–16 g/dL (120–160 g/L)
White blood cells (WBC)	$4.5–10.5 \times 10^3$ cells/mm^3 ($4.5–10.5 \times 10^9$/L)
Platelets	140,000–450,000/mm^3 ($140–450 \times 10^9$/L)
Prothrombin time (PT)	9.5–12 seconds (9.5–12 seconds)
Partial thromboplastin time (PTT) & activated partial thromboplastin time (APTT)	20–39 seconds (20–39 seconds)
International normalized ratio (INR)	Normal: 1.0 (1.0) On warfarin therapy: 2.0–3.5 (2.0–3.5)
Potassium (serum)	3.5–5 mEq/L (3.5–5 mmol/L)
Sodium (serum)	135–145 mEq/L (135–145 mEq/L)